UNIVERSITY OF ROCHESTER LIBRARIES
3 9087 01376139 2

D1552119

SPORTS INJURIES

Mechanisms • Prevention • Treatment

SPORTS INJURIES

Mechanisms • Prevention • Treatment

EDITED BY

FREDDIE H. FU, M.D.

Blue Cross of Western Pennsylvania Professor of Orthopaedic Surgery
Vice Chairman / Clinical
Department of Orthopaedic Surgery
Chief, Division of Sports Medicine Head Team Physician, Athletic Department
University of Pittsburgh
Pittsburgh, Pennsylvania

DAVID A. STONE, M.D.

Assistant Professor of Orthopaedic Surgery
Division of Sports Medicine and Rehabilitation Medicine
Department of Orthopaedic Surgery
University of Pittsburgh
Pittsburgh, Pennsylvania

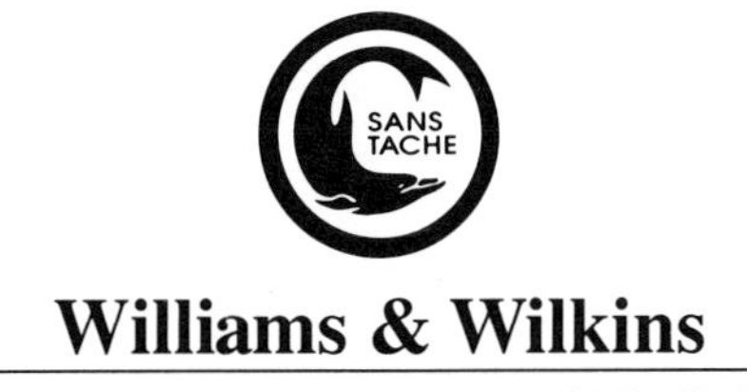

Williams & Wilkins

BALTIMORE • PHILADELPHIA • HONG KONG
LONDON • MUNICH • SYDNEY • TOKYO

A WAVERLY COMPANY

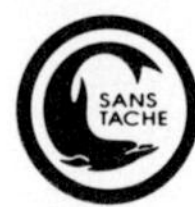

Editor: Timothy H. Grayson
Project Manager: Kathleen Courtney Millet
Copy Editors: Candace B. Levy, Harriet Felscher
Designer: Norman W. Och
Illustration Planner: Wayne Hubbel

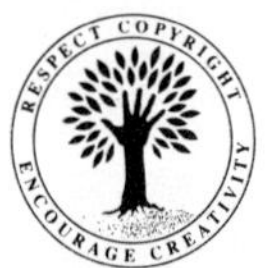

Accurate indications, adverse reactions, and dosage schedules for drugs are provided in this book, but it is possible that they may change. The reader is urged to review the package information data of the manufacturers of the medications mentioned.

Printed in the United States of America

Chapter reprints are available from the Publisher.

Library of Congress Cataloging in Publication Data

Sports injuries : mechanisms, prevention, and treatment / edited by Freddie H. Fu, David A. Stone.
p. cm.
Includes index.
ISBN 0-683-03388-3
1. Sports—Accidents and injuries. I. Fu, Freddie H. II. Stone, David A. (David Alan), 1952–
[DNLM: 1. Athletic Injuries—etiology. 2. Athletic Injuries—prevention & control. 3. Sports—physiology. 4. Sports Medicine. QT 260 S762945 1994]
RD97.S69 1994
617.1'027—dc20
DNLM/DLC
for Library of Congress

93-31440
CIP

94 95 96 97 98
1 2 3 4 5 6 7 8 9 10

DEDICATION

To my wife, Hilda; our son, Gordon; and our daughter Joyce.

FHF

To my parents, Joseph and Rosalind Stone; to my wife, Debra Bruckman, and our sons, Bradley and Todd; and to William F. Fishbaugh, M.D.

DAS

PREFACE

Sports Injuries was originally planned to be a second edition of the successful 1985 text edited by Schneider, Kennedy, and Plant, updated and modified to incorporate and order the proliferation of information concerning sports medicine over the past 8 years. But we also envisioned the book as a reference text for the "sports physician," someone interested in the spectrum of sports injuries. Thus, we added sections on conditioning, preseason evaluation, athletic training, and special interests, and we expanded the sections on treatment to provide a well-rounded, comprehensive approach to a variety of sports at all levels. In this way, the book could serve as an excellent starting point for those with a fledgling interest in sports medicine, but also become an enduring reference for the physician with a versatile sports-oriented practice. In addition, the book should be accessible to trainers and coaches whose concerns are the relatively common problems of their athletes. We wanted, however, to minimize the overlap that can result from overly ambitious efforts to be inclusive, a problem noted in the preface of the book by Schneider et al. Thus, we instructed the authors to select only the most common injuries in their particular field of expertise and to discuss them in a sports-specific manner. These chapters are supplemented by others emphasizing the treatment of specific joints and other aspects of sports medicine such as medical, dermatologic, and neurologic problems. In this way, we hope to provide a spectrum of opinions on treatment rather than a dogmatic approach.

The continued rapid expansion of sports medicine knowledge is being driven by basic science discoveries on wound healing and on tissue biomechanics. The increasing importance and sophistication of these topics makes inclusion of this information a necessity. The chapters written on soft tissue injury and biomechanics are among the new additions to the text that the reader will find helpful in approaching both the acute and chronic injury. Readers are sure to find them extremely well written and also enjoyable chapters to read.

Some physicians are more involved with the medical coverage of one-time sports events rather than with games. Road races, regattas, tennis and basketball tournaments are very popular everywhere, and the increasing need to provide coverage for these events requires an awareness of different medical issues and a different set of injuries than are normally confronted by a team physician. The sections on emergencies and on the administrative aspects of the marathon are designed to equip the sports physician for these situations.

The treatment of the injured athlete has become more complex in the last decade, so that creating a text with enduring appeal is a challenge. It is our hope that this new text is equal to that challenge and will serve as a solid foundation and an enduring reference in the years to come.

ACKNOWLEDGMENTS

Many people have contributed to the development of this project. We are above all indebted to our authors and their families and also to Ms. Dorothy Roman and Ms. Mary Yochum, who have handled the correspondence, coordinated the filing and transfer of documents, and provided perspective when necessary.

The members of the staff at Williams & Wilkins provided encouragement, expertise, and excellent technical support—our thanks go in particular to Katey Millet, Tim Grayson, and Margie Keating. This project would not have succeeded without them.

CONTRIBUTORS

Marlene Adrian, M.D.
Warrenton, Oregon

Steven L. Almany, M.D.
Staff Cardiologist,
William Beaumont Hospital,
Royal Oak, Michigan

Kenneth L. Anderson III, D.O.
Pacific Beach Urgent Care,
San Diego, California

Frank H. Bassett III, M.D.
Professor of Orthopaedic Surgery,
Duke University Medical Center,
Durham, North Carolina

Wilma Fowler Bergfeld, M.D.
Head, Section of Dermatopathology;
Consultant, Sports Medicine Department;
Cleveland Clinic Foundation,
Cleveland, Ohio

Robert O. Blanc, M.A., A.T.C.
Head Athletic Trainer/Clinical Instructor,
Sports Medicine Program,
University of Pittsburgh,
Pittsburgh, Pennsylvania

Paul A. Borsa, M.S., A.T.C.
Doctoral Candidate in Exercise Physiology/Athletic Training,
Clinical Instructor/Athletic Trainer,
University of Pittsburgh,
Pittsburgh, Pennsylvania

James P. Bradley, M.D.
Clinical Associate Professor,
Department of Orthopaedic Surgery,
University of Pittsburgh School of Medicine;
Director, Sports Medicine Center,
St. Margaret Memorial Hospital;
Team Physician, The Pittsburgh Steelers, National Football League,
Pittsburgh, Pennsylvania

Tony Brosky, P.T.
Coordinator of Physical Therapy,
University of Kentucky Sports Medicine Center,
Lexington, Kentucky

Neil A. Busis, M.D.
Clinical Assistant Professor of Neurology,
University of Pittsburgh School of Medicine,
Pittsburgh, Pennsylvania

David N.M. Caborn, M.D.
Director, Sports Medicine Center,
University of Kentucky,
Lexington, Kentucky

Peter J. Carek, M.D.
Postdoctoral Fellow, Sports and Occupational Medicine;
Clinical Instructor, Department of Family Practice;
University of Tennessee Medical Center,
Knoxville, Tennessee

Richard L. Carter, M.D.
Baptist Hospital of Miami Neuroscience Center;
Clinical Assistant Professor,
Department of Neurological Surgery,
University of Miami,
Miami, Florida

T. Jeff Chandler, ED.D., C.S.C.S., F.A.C.S.M.
Lexington Clinic Sports Medicine Center,
Lexington, Kentucky

Claire Chase, M.D.
Fellow in Traumatology,
Division of Thoracic Surgery,
Maryland Institute of Emergency Medical Service,
University of Maryland School of Medicine,
Baltimore, Maryland

Jerome V. Ciullo, M.D.
Clinical Assistant Professor,
Department of Orthopaedic Surgery,
Wayne State University and Michigan State University;
Hutzel Hospital/Detroit Medical Center,
Sports Medicine Center of Metro Detroit;
Troy, Michigan

Laura E. Clark, M.S., A.T.C.
Athletic Trainer/Clinical Instructor,
Sports Medicine Program,
University of Pittsburgh,
Pittsburgh, Pennsylvania

Thomas Crisp, M.B.B.S.
Clinical Academic Department of Sports Medicine,
The London Hospital Medical College;
Sports Injury Clinic,
The Royal London Hospital;
London, Great Britain

William M. Dillin, M.D.
The Kerlan Jobe Orthopaedic Clinic,
Inglewood, California

Lars-Gunnar Elmqvist, M.D., PH.D.
Department of Orthopaedics,
University Hospital,
Umea, Sweden

Dirk M. Elson, M.D.
Staff Dermatologist/Dermatopathologist,
Brooke Army Medical Center,
Fort Sam Houston, Texas

Richard D. Ferkel, M.D.
Clinical Instructor of Orthopaedic Surgery,
UCLA Center for Health Sciences,
Los Angeles, California;
Attending Surgeon,
Southern California Orthopedic Institute;
Van Nuys, California

Joseph F. Fetto, M.D.
Associate Professor,
Department of Orthopaedic Surgery,
New York University Medical Center,
New York, New York

John Lester Firth, M.B., F.R.C.S.(E)
Consultant Neurosurgeon,
Department of Neurosurgery,
University Hospital,
Queen's Medical Centre;
Clinical Teacher, Medical Schools,
University of Nottingham and University of Leichester;
Nottingham, United Kingdom

Peter J. Fowler, M.D., F.R.C.S.(C)
Professor of Orthopaedic Surgery,
Head, Section of Sports Medicine,
University of Western Ontario,
London, Ontario, Canada

Barry A. Franklin, PH.D.
Program Director,
Cardiac Rehabilitation and Exercise Laboratories,
William Beaumont Hospital,
Royal Oak, Michigan

Freddie H. Fu, M.D.
Blue Cross of Western Pennsylvania Professor of Orthopaedic Surgery;
Vice Chairman/Clinical
Department of Orthopaedic Surgery;
Chief, Division of Sports Medicine;
Head Team Physician, Athletic Department;
University of Pittsburgh,
Pittsburgh, Pennsylvania

William E. Garrett, Jr., M.D., PH.D.
Associate Professor of Orthopaedic Surgery and Cell Biology,
Duke University Medical Center,
Durham, North Carolina

Wayne K. Gersoff, M.D.
Assistant Professor Orthopaedic Surgery;
Director, Sports Medicine;
Department of Orthopaedics,
University of Colorado Health Sciences Center,
Denver, Colorado

Nöelle Grace, M.D., F.R.C.S.(C), F.A.C.S.
North York General Hospital,
Willowdale, Ontario, Canada

Larry J. Grollman, A.T.C.
Manager, Sports Medicine
Center for Sports Medicine and Rehabilitation,
Pittsburgh, Pennsylvania

Christopher D. Harner, M.D.
Assistant Professor of Orthopaedic Surgery;
Associate Medical Director;
Center for Sports Medicine and Rehabilitation,
University of Pittsburgh,
Pittsburgh, Pennsylvania

Jack Harvey, M.D.
Chief, Sports Medicine,
Orthopaedic Center of the Rockies,
Fort Collins, Colorado

Andrew M. Hauser, M.D.
Medical Director, Non-Invasive Laboratory,
William Beaumont Hospital,
Royal Oak, Michigan

Christine E. Haycock, M.D., F.A.C.S.
Professor Emeritus of Surgery,
University of Medicine and Dentistry of New Jersey,
Newark, New Jersey

James H. Herndon, M.D.
Professor and Chairman,
Department of Orthopaedic Surgery,
University of Pittsburgh,
Pittsburgh, Pennsylvania

Douglas H. Hildreth, M.D.
General and Vascular Surgery,
Medford Clinic,
Medford, Oregon

Linda L. Hildreth, R.N., B.S.N.
Nursing Administration,
Providence Hospital and Medical Center,
Medford, Oregon

Mary Lloyd Ireland, M.D.
Assistant Clinical Professor,
Division of Orthopaedics and Family Practice;
Team Orthopaedic Consultant,
University of Kentucky;
Team Physician,
Eastern Kentucky University,
Kentucky Sports Medicine,
Lexington, Kentucky

James J. Irrgang, P.T., A.T.C.
Director,
Center for Sports Medicine and Rehabilitation,
University of Pittsburgh,
Pittsburgh, Pennsylvania

Rebecca Jaffe, M.D., F.A.A.F.P., F.A.C.S.M.
Assistant Professor,
Thomas Jefferson University,
Philadelphia, Pennsylvania;
Associate Professor of Family Practice,
The Medical Center of Delaware;
Director, Pike Creek Sports Medicine Clinics,
Wilmington, Delaware;
Physician, United States Fencing Association Circuit Events

Jonathan S. Jaivin, M.D.
Attending Surgeon,
Southern California Orthopedic Institute,
Van Nuys, California

James P. Jamison, M.D.
Resident,
Department of Orthopaedic Surgery,
University of Pittsburgh,
Pittsburgh, Pennsylvania

Darren L. Johnson, M.D.
Assistant Professor of Orthopaedic Surgery,
Section of Sports Medicine,
University of Kentucky,
Lexington, Kentucky

Robert J. Johnson, M.D.
Professor,
Department of Orthopaedics and Rehabilitation,
University of Vermont College of Medicine,
Burlington, Vermont

Ruth Kamenski, M.S., P.T.
Sports Medicine Institute,
Pittsburgh, Pennsylvania

Michael J. Kaplan, M.D.
Resident,
Department of Orthopaedics and Rehabilitation,
University of Vermont College of Medicine,
Burlington, Vermont

W. Benjamin Kibler, M.D., F.A.C.S.M.
Lexington Clinic Sports Medicine Center,
Lexington, Kentucky

John B. King, M.B.B.S., F.R.C.S.
Director, Clinical Academic Department of Sports Medicine;
Senior Lecturer in Orthopaedic and Trauma Surgery,
The London Hospital Medical College;
Orthopaedic Surgeon,
Royal London Hospital;
London, Great Britain

Mininder S. Kocher, M.D.
Instructor of Orthopaedic Surgery,
Harvard Medical School,
Boston, Massachusetts

Wayne B. Leadbetter, M.D.
Clinical Assistant Professor of Orthopaedic Surgery,
Georgetown University School of Medicine;
Assistant Professor of Surgery,
Uniformed Services University of Health and Sciences;
Visiting Scientist, Wound Repair Enhancement Division,
Naval Medical Research Institute,
Bethesda, Maryland;
Medical Director,
Shady Grove Center for Sports Medicine and Rehabilitation,
Rockville, Maryland

Scott M. Lephart, PH.D., A.T.C.
Director, Sports Medicine/Athletic Training;
Assistant Professor, Education;
Assistant Professor of Orthopaedic Surgery;
University of Pittsburgh,
Pittsburgh, Pennsylvania

Jon A. Levy, M.D.
Clinical Instructor,
Department of Orthopaedic Surgery,
University of Pittsburgh;
Oakland Orthopaedic Associates,
Pittsburgh, Pennsylvania

John H. Lohnes, P.A.C.
Division of Orthopaedic Surgery,
Duke University Medical Center,
Durham, North Carolina

Michael G. Maday, M.D.
Orthopaedic Surgeon,
Midland Orthopaedic Associates,
Chicago, Illinois

Donald W. Marion, M.D.
Assistant Professor of Neurological Surgery;
Chief, Head Injury Service;
University of Pittsburgh School of Medicine,
Pittsburgh, Pennsylvania

Leslie S. Matthews, M.D.
Associate Professor,
Department of Orthopaedic Surgery,
The Johns Hopkins University School of Medicine;
Union Memorial Hospital,
Baltimore, Maryland

John R. McCarroll, M.D.
Methodist Sports Medicine Center,
Indianapolis, Indiana

Patrick J. McMahon, M.D.
Department of Orthopaedic Surgery,
University of Pittsburgh,
Pittsburgh, Pennsylvania

Roger H. Michael, M.D.
Associate Professor,
Department of Orthopaedic Surgery,
University of Maryland Medical Center;
Assistant Professor,
Department of Orthopaedic Surgery,
The Johns Hopkins University School of Medicine;
Union Memorial Hospital;
Baltimore, Maryland

Mark D. Miller, M.D.
Clinical Assistant Professor of Surgery,
Uniformed Services University of Health Sciences,
F. Edward Herbert School of Medicine,
Bethesda, Maryland

Jeffrey Minkoff, M.D.
Clinical Professor and Director of Sports Fellowships,
New York University Medical Center;
Attending Orthopaedic Surgeon,
Orthopaedic Institute; Hospital for Joint Disease; and
Lenox Hill Hospital;
Team Orthopedist, New York Islanders, National Hockey League;
New York, New York

Gabe Mirkin, M.D.
Associate Professor,
Department of Pediatrics,
Georgetown University School of Medicine,
Washington, DC

Raymond R. Monto, M.D.
Pennsylvania Orthopedic Associates,
Huntingdon Valley, Pennsylvania

Morey S. Moreland, M.D.
William F. and Jean W. Donaldson Professor;
Vice Chairman,
Department of Orthopaedic Surgery;
University of Pittsburgh School of Medicine;
Children's Hospital of Pittsburgh;
Pittsburgh, Pennsylvania

H. Andrew Motz, M.D.
Instructor,
Department of Orthopaedics,
University of Colorado Health Sciences Center,
Denver, Colorado

Julie A. Moyer, ED.D., A.T.C., P.T.
Pike Creek Sports Medicine Center,
Wilmington, Delaware

David L. Muller, M.D.
Resident,
Department of Orthopaedics and Rehabilitation,
University of Vermont College of Medicine,
Burlington, Vermont

Mark C. Mysnyk, M.D.
Assistant Clinical Professor,
Department of Orthopaedic Surgery,
University of Iowa School of Medicine;
Steindler Orthopaedic Clinic;
Iowa City, Iowa

Thomas C. Namey, M.D., F.A.C.P., F.A.A.S.P.
Chief, Section of Sports Medicine,
Associate Professor of Medicine, Human Performance,
and Sports Studies and Nutrition,
University of Tennessee Medical Center,
Knoxville, Tennessee

John A. Nyland, M.ED., P.T., A.T.C.
Doctoral Candidate,
Department of Kinesiology and Health Promotion,
University of Kentucky,
Lexington, Kentucky

Kevin O'Toole, M.D., F.A.C.E.P.
Assistant Professor of Medicine,
Division of Emergency Medicine,
University of Pittsburgh School of Medicine;
Director, Hyperbaric Medicine Program,
University of Pittsburgh Medical Center;
Pittsburgh, Pennsylvania

Mary L. O'Toole, PH.D.
Associate Professor,
University of Tennessee-Campbell Clinic;
Department of Orthopaedic Surgery,
University of Tennessee, Memphis;
Memphis, Tennessee

Ross Outerbridge, M.D.
National Team Physician, WSC;
Chief Resident,
Department of Orthopaedics,
University of British Columbia;
Vancouver, British Columbia, Canada

Robert C. Pashby, M.D., F.R.C.S.(C)
Assistant Professor of Ophthalmology,
University of Toronto Faculty of Medicine;
Active Staff, Department of Ophthalmology,
The Hospital for Sick Children and Mount Sinai Hospital;
Toronto, Ontario, Canada

Thomas J. Pashby, C.M., M.D., C.R.C.S.(C)
Emeritus Associate Professor of Ophthalmology,
University of Toronto Faculty of Medicine;
Honorary Consultant, Department of Ophthalmology,
The Hospital for Sick Children, Toronto Western Hospital,
and Centenary Hospital;
Toronto, Ontario, Canada

John F. Pepper, D.D.S., B.SC.D.
Willowdale, Ontario, Canada

John I.B. Pyne, M.D.
Resident,
Department of Orthopaedics and Rehabilitation,
University of Vermont College of Medicine,
Burlington, Vermont

Per A.F.H. Renstrom, M.D., P.H.D.
Professor,
Department of Orthopaedics and Rehabilitation,
University of Vermont College of Medicine,
Burlington, Vermont

E. Lee Rice, D.O., F.A.A.F.P.
San Diego Sports Medicine, Orthopedic and Family
Health Center,
San Diego, California

Karl A. Saleski, P.T., A.T.C.
Athletic Trainer/Clinical Instructor,
Sports Medicine Program,
University of Pittsburgh,
Pittsburgh, Pennsylvania

Jeffrey D. Shapiro, M.D.
Clinical Instructor,
Department of Orthopaedic Surgery,
Wayne State University;
Sports Medicine Center of Metro Detroit;
Troy, Michigan

Mark W. Shipman, M.D., F.A.C.E.P.
Wenatchee Emergency Physicians,
Wenatchee, Washington

Mark B. Silby, M.D.
Bradenton Orthopaedic Associates,
Bradenton, Florida

Barry G. Simonson, M.D.
Attending Orthopedic Surgeon,
North Shore University Hospital,
Cornell University Medical Center,
Manhassett, New York;
Associate Team Orthopedist, New York Islanders,
National Hockey League;
New York, New York

T. David Sisk, M.D.
Professor and Chairman,
University of Tennessee, Campbell Clinic;
Department of Orthopaedic Surgery,
University of Tennessee, Memphis;
Memphis, Tennessee

George A. Snook, M.D.
Consultant, University Health Services and Athletic
Teams,
University of Massachusetts,
Amherst, Massachusetts;
Lecturer in Orthopaedics,
University of Connecticut Medical School,
Farmington, Connecticut;
Hampshire Orthopaedics,
Northhamptom, Massachusetts

Richard A.Z. Sofranko, M.S.
Musculoskeletal Research Center,
Department of Orthopaedic Surgery,
University of Pittsburgh,
Pittsburgh, Pennsylvania

Wally Sokolowski, O.W.S.A.
Ontario Waterski Association,
Willowdale, Ontario, Canada

Dean G. Sotereanos, M.D.
Assistant Professor,
Department of Orthopaedic Surgery,
University of Pittsburgh,
Pittsburgh, Pennsylvania

David A. Stone, M.D.
Assistant Professor of Orthopaedic Surgery,
Division of Sports Medicine and Rehabilitation Medicine,
Department of Orthopaedic Surgery,
University of Pittsburgh,
Pittsburgh, Pennsylvania

Stephen Z. Turney, M.D., F.A.C.S.
Maryland Institute of Emergency Medical Service,
University of Maryland School of Medicine,
Baltimore, Maryland

Gerard P. Varlotta, D.O.
Clinical Instructor,
Department of Rehabilitation Medicine,
New York University;
Rusk Institute of Rehabilitation Medicine;
New York, New York

Vincent P. Verdile, M.D., F.A.C.E.P.
Associate Professor of Emergency Medicine,
Department of Emergency Medicine,
Albany Medical College,
Albany, New York

Kerry E. Waple, M.ED., A.T.C.
Athletic Trainer/Clinical Instructor,
Sports Medicine Program,
University of Pittsburgh,
Pittsburgh, Pennsylvania

W. Timothy Ward, M.D.
Associate Professor,
Department of Orthopaedic Surgery,
University of Pittsburgh,
Pittsburgh, Pennsylvania

Jon J.P. Warner, M.D.
Assistant Professor,
Department of Orthopaedic Surgery,
University of Pittsburgh,
Pittsburgh, Pennsylvania

Robert G. Watkins, M.D.
The Kerlan Jobe Orthopaedic Clinic,
Inglewood, California

Lawrence R. Wechsler, M.D.
Clinical Associate Professor of Neurology,
University of Pittsburgh School of Medicine,
Pittsburgh, Pennsylvania

Jeffery R. Weiss, M.S., P.T., A.T.C.
Physical Therapy Supervisor,
Allegheny Valley Hospital,
Center for Orthopaedics and Sports Medicine,
Natrona Heights, Pennsylvania

J.P.R. Williams, M.B.E., F.R.C.S.
Consultant Orthopaedic Surgeon,
Princess of Wales Hospital,
New South Wales, Australia

Robert P. Wills, M.D.
Clinical Instructor,
Department of Orthopaedics,
University of Washington;
Junior Partner, Orthopaedics International;
Seattle, Washington

Savio L-Y. Woo, P.H.D.
Professor and Vice Chairman for Research,
Department of Orthopaedic Surgery;
Professor, Department of Mechanical Engineering,
Director, Musculoskeletal Research Center,
University of Pittsburgh;
Pittsburgh, Pennsylvania

Shawn Wotowey, A.T.C.
Orthopaedic Center of the Rockies,
Fort Collins, Colorado

CONTENTS

SECTION ONE

Evaluation, Training and Special Concerns

SECTION TWO

Sports-Specific Injuries

SECTION THREE

Management and Treatment of Systemic and Regional Injuries

SECTION ONE

EVALUATION, TRAINING AND SPECIAL CONCERNS

1 / PRESEASON EVALUATION

David A. Stone and Robert O. Blanc

Introduction

The preparticipation evaluation is the team physician's initial opportunity to identify health problems of the team members. It is not a standardized exam, but one that is geared toward improving athletic performance, and, as such, should be sport- and position-specific. A great deal of controversy exists over what this evaluation should offer the athlete, how frequently it needs to be repeated, and what health problems it should seek to identify. Most authors agree that it should not be an alternative to the traditional health maintenance examination, although at the professional level, it often is. Ideally, the preparticipation evaluation is performed by a physician who understands the injury risk and the common injuries of the sport in question and appreciates the way injuries will affect the athlete's performance. The evaluation should also evaluate risk of sudden death, and it may evaluate fitness level.

The large majority of these evaluations are performed on adolescent athletes, and the bulk of the sports literature on the preseason evaluation concerns this group. However, recent trends toward organized sports participation by children, the increasing emphasis on early training to optimize performance in tennis and gymnastics as well as the prolonged success of older athletes in baseball and in track and field have made the literature on the preparticipation evaluation somewhat inadequate.

Common goals for the preparticipation evaluation are listed in Table 1.1. Although Smith et al. (1) have divided goals into primary and secondary categories, the authors believe that, in certain situations, those primary and secondary goals are interchangeable, especially at the professional level, where players are an investment to a team and where ensuring overall player health is a priority. At the college level, athletes often have no regular primary care physician and generally are healthy; therefore, the college athlete who develops medical problems is more likely to "slip through the cracks," and the initial preparticipation evaluation becomes an important tool in the overall assessment of the athlete's health. Because the National Collegiate Athletic Association (NCAA) mandates only one preparticipation evaluation during a college career, all goals should be met in the performance of this single exam.

Because athletes are generally perceived as "healthy," and athletics as "self selecting," general health screenings of athletes are viewed as largely unproductive. Risser et al. (2) performed a cost-benefit analysis of preparticipation examinations of 763 adolescents in two distinct geographically and socially different areas—one affluent and one indigent. Sixteen athletes (2.1%) were referred for further evaluation, but only two were disqualified, one for unilateral hydronephrosis, and one for subluxing patella, while another was treated (for a torn meniscus). The entire screening process was not considered cost effective, and the authors suggested using a history form to screen athletes or to widen the focus of the examination. Thompson et al. (3) performed a prospective study of 2670 high school athletes and noted that about 11% had some risk factors that could affect play and that required further evaluation. Only 1–2%, a figure comparable to that of Risser, had findings that contraindicated participation in certain sports. Musculoskeletal problems constituted about 67% of the risk factors; cardiovascular findings, 15%. Goldberg et al. (4) reviewed their results after screening 701 high school athletes and found that two (0.3%) required restriction for medical problems (one for multiple concussions and one for a ventricular arrhythmia) and seven (1%) restriction for orthopedic problems, predominantly for untreated knee ligament injuries or recent fractures.

Although these studies lend support to the concept of self-selection and the benign nature of the findings on these evaluations, other issues have become important in the overall screening process. As a consequence either of training, the use of ergogenic aids, or the exacerbation of underlying conditions, an athlete may develop various medical problems. Some of these, such as the athletic heart syndrome, are difficult diagnostic

Table 1.1.
Common Goals for Preparticipation Evaluation

Determine general health
Discover defects that limit participation
Uncover conditions predisposing to athletic injury
Bring athlete to optimal level of performance
Classify the athlete according to individual qualifications
Fulfill legal and insurance requirements for participation
Evaluate size and level of maturation in younger athletes
Improve fitness and performance
Counsel youths and answer personal health questions
Provide opportunities for disabled athletes to compete
Establish a physician-patient relationship

problems; others, such as exercise-induced bronchospasm, are more likely to be discovered in a preseason evaluation; and still others, such as systemic hypertension, could be the consequence of anabolic steroid use. There is, therefore, some controversy over whether a preseason physical should be viewed as a general health screen or solely as a tool to determine ability to play. As the team physician concept becomes more prevalent, the problem becomes more difficult, because the athlete's care will be split between the team physician and the primary care physician. The athlete may "see" the team physician yearly, but not undergo adequate health maintenance evaluation. We encourage all "team physicians" simply to make the "primary care" physician aware of any findings on the preparticipation evaluation—by use of a written form or by direct communication.

Components of the Examination

The factors that would enable a physician to predict injury in an athlete are still poorly defined. The sport, the level of competition, player experience, playing conditions, and coaching techniques all contribute to the risk of injury, but they are usually beyond the physician's control. Psychologic factors have been implicated (5) but are rarely evaluated. Strength imbalances have been shown to contribute to injury in some studies (6), but strength evaluations as part of the preseason physical are rarely performed. Flexibility imbalances around the hip and back also may contribute to injury risk (6) and can easily be detected, but these factors are also not a consistent predictor of injury in all studies. Strength and flexibility imbalances related to previous injuries may be a significant predisposing factor for injury. Thompson et al. (3) noted that almost 10% of the students in their study had conditions that were not serious but required attention before play. They singled out, in particular, patellofemoral syndrome and ligamentous instabilities at the ankle and knee. Risser et al. (2) found about 5% of their students had musculoskeletal problems that could be cleared for participation but still required treatment. Among 1268 preparticipation exams, Linder et al. (7) noted that the most frequently reported problems were previous injuries, previous hospitalizations, and joint problems. Shambaugh et al. (8) successfully used structural measures (Q-angle, bilateral weight, rear foot valgus, leg length inequality) to predict injury risk in basketball players. However, there was only one injury, and only 45 players were screened. These findings indicate that significant emphasis should be placed on musculoskeletal screening, as well as on a history of previous injuries and their treatment.

A variety of authors (1, 2, 7–17) have reviewed the patient history component of the preparticipation evaluation. Their recommendations range from as few as 6 questions to as many as 25 questions. These differences in detail from author to author reflect the lack of standardization in the entire process of screening athletes, as well as concern for overall health rather than simply sports participation. All authors agree that the evaluation must at least focus on a history of injury (causing residual impairment of performance), risk of sudden death (including murmurs, arrhythmias, hypertension, syncope, family history of sudden death), and history of concussion. Some authors (1, 10, 11,) correctly point out that screening for heat-related illness, exercise-induced bronchospasm, missing organs, and allergy history are a significant part of the athlete's history and should always be considered. Inquiring about the use of appliances (contact lenses, braces, dental bridges, glasses, etc.), last tetanus shot, and general medical condition are also recommended (1, 7, 9, 11). From sport to sport, emphasis on certain organ systems changes. Wrestlers, for example, can be disqualified from a match for impetigo or herpes simplex infection; thus, a history of skin infections is important for wrestlers. A history of amenorrhea in a distance runner would also be a significant finding. In a boxer, the discovery of significantly decreased visual acuity in one eye requires disqualification (17). The more familiar the examiner is with the sport, the more effective the history.

In his review of 2114 athletic screenings, Risser noted that 37% of athletes and their families failed to mention orthopedic problems even though they were aware of them (18). This observation makes a good orthopedic screening imperative. A simple demonstration of the authors' basic exam for the musculoskeletal screening is shown in Figures 1.1 to 1.9. Our rationale for these maneuvers is to demonstrate full painless range of motion in all joints. If this is not present, further evaluation of the joint becomes necessary. If the athlete's history indicates a previous injury, evidence of chronicity or failure of previous treatment should be sought. Because isolated muscle weakness or imbalances of frequently used muscles may predispose athletes to injury or poor performance, our evaluation includes a simple manual muscle test of any muscle "at risk." At the college level, the authors generally check knee and shoulder laxity for contact sports, but individual positions within a sport warrant different emphasis. For example, wide receivers in football should be checked for grip strength and hand function more closely than should linemen, but linemen should have a careful search for ankle anterior impingement symptoms, especially as their careers progress.

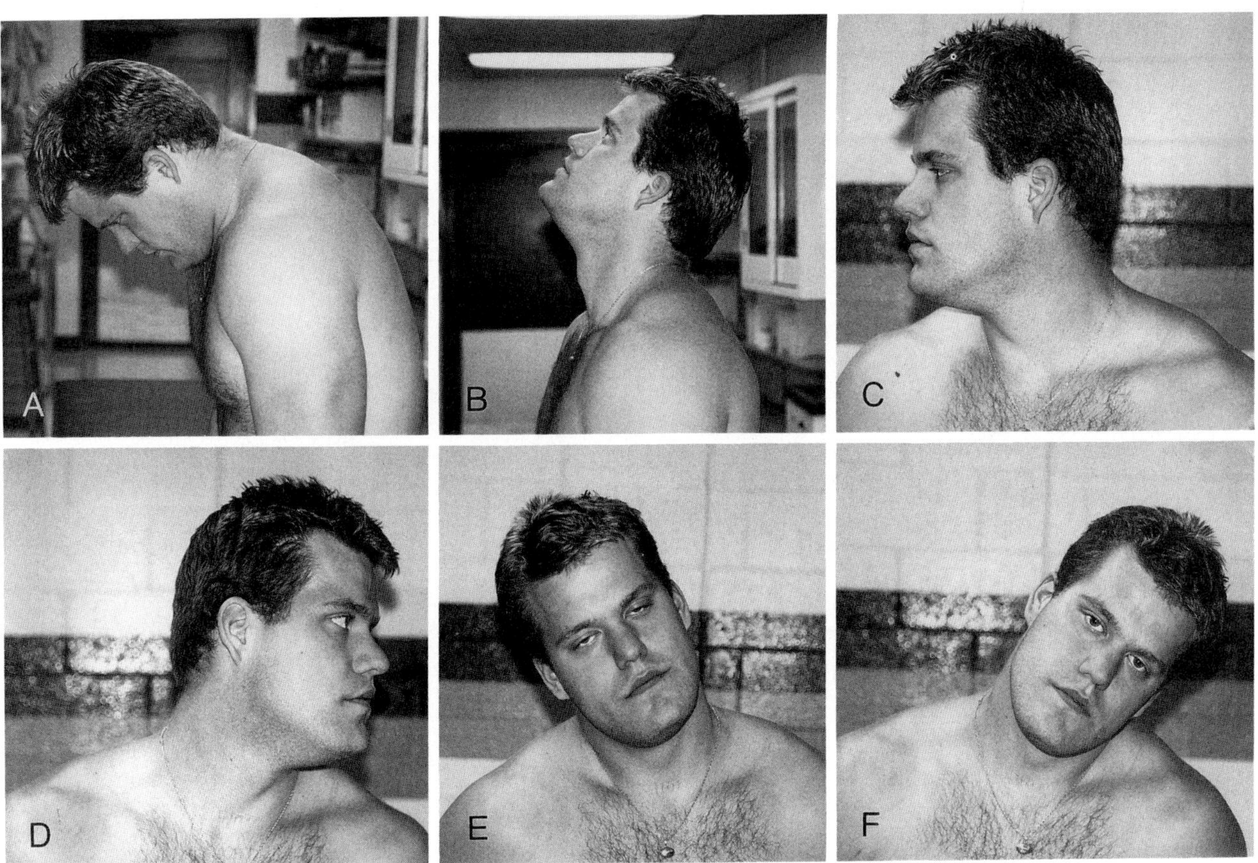

Figure 1.1. (A-F) Neck range of motion. All athletes should have full symmetric range of motion of the cervical spine. This is especially important in contact sports.

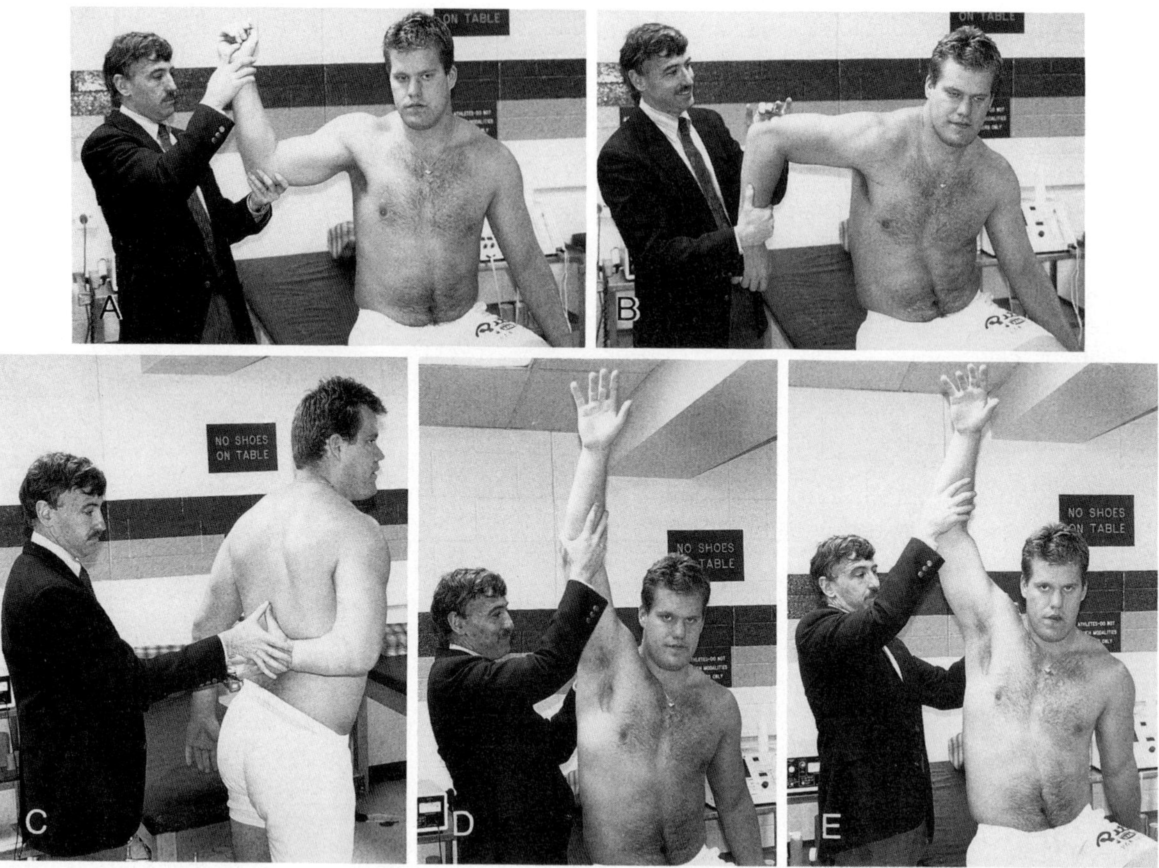

Figure 1.2. (A-E) Shoulder range of motion. Demonstrating full range of motion without pain is particularly important in throwing athletes who frequently lose internal range of motion.

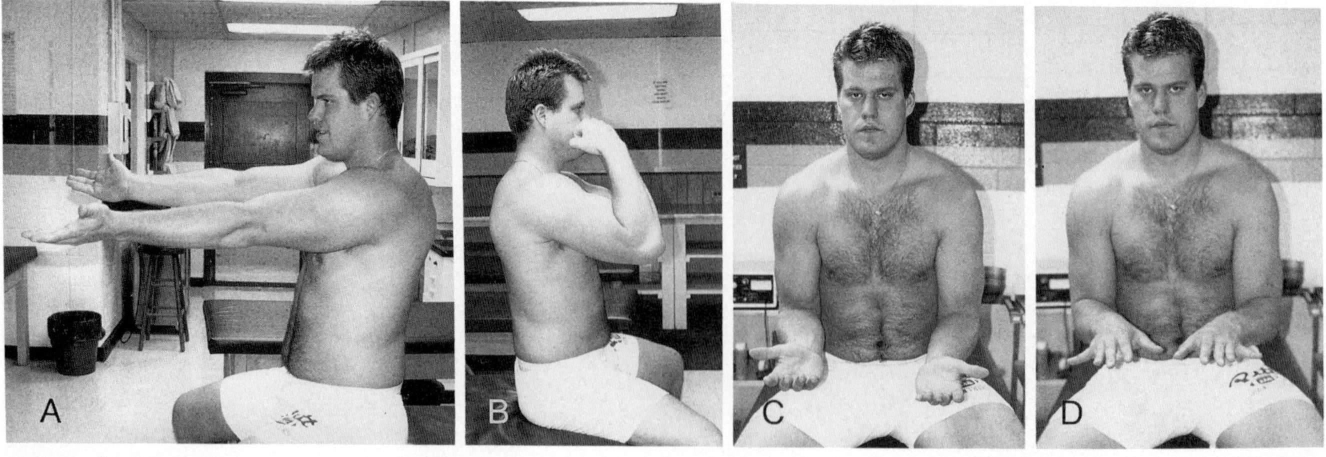

Figure 1.3. (A-D) Elbow range of motion. Full range of motion is often not present in throwing athletes. Flexion contractures should be noted.

In addition to the musculoskeletal screening, the adolescent athlete may benefit from an assessment of physical maturity. In 1975, Hafner (19) found that when boys aged 12–19 years were matched prior to competition according to sexual maturity, less than 2% of the athletes suffered injury. When they were matched by age, 50% suffered injuries that kept them from play for one week or more during the football season. Martens (20) noted that youngsters often dropped out of organized sports because of physical mismatching related to varied maturation. Kreipe (21) correlated self-assessed Tanner staging and grip strength, demonstrating significantly decreased grip strength in boys who were Tanner stage 3 or less. Self-assessment of Tanner staging can be used effectively in women who are difficult to stage. At present, no definition of maturity has been established. Tanner stage 3 boys are often considered at the greatest risk for epiphyseal damage because they are experiencing their most rapid growth, and Smith (22) considered this group inappropriate for contact sports. Since definitive epidemiologic evidence is still lacking, it is difficult to limit competition based solely on Tanner staging, but athletes and parents should be counseled when potential problems are obvious.

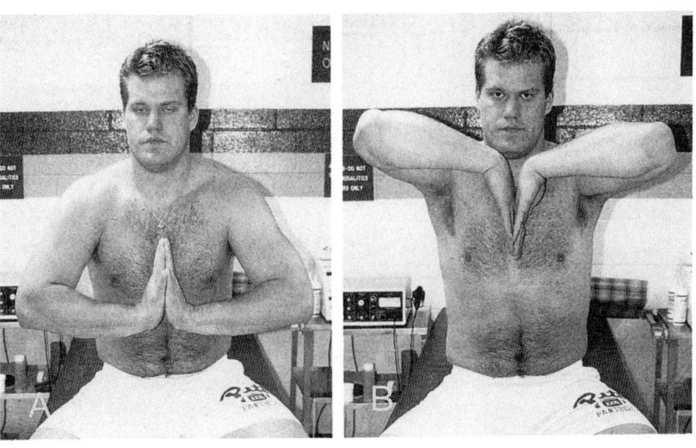

Figure 1.4. (A-B) Wrist range of motion. Full range of motion of the wrist is often absent in occult navicular fractures and carpal instabilities.

Cardiovascular screening is an important and occasionally confusing part of the preparticipation evaluation. Most young athletes who die suddenly do so without signs or symptoms of cardiac disease (23), but, in most cases, a structural lesion is present (23). Epstein and Maron (24) estimated that to identify a group of 1000 athletes with cardiovascular disease, one of whom will die, would require about 200,000 athletic screenings. The evaluation is complicated further by the training-induced changes frequently present on the athlete's cardiac exam and EKG (Fig.1.10). These changes are usually adaptations to training rather than evidence of pathology (25), but they can be difficult to interpret. In rare cases, an athlete will require catheterization (26). As a group, the changes are referred to as "the athletic heart syndrome" (27) and result from both endurance and strength training. The endurance athlete develops volume overload with an increase in left ventricular chamber size that rarely exceeds normal limits. Strength-trained athletes develop pressure overload from frequent isometric contractions and demonstrate left ventricular wall hypertrophy (27). Reduction or cessation of training can decrease the hypertrophy and has been used to distinguish between change caused by pathology versus training (28), although many athletes will not accept a reduction in training as part of their treatment.

The physical examination can demonstrate a variety of findings. Murmurs are present in 30–50% of endurance athletes, and third and fourth heart sounds are common (26). In strength-trained athletes, the left ventricular impulse is often displaced (29). Bradycardia is a common finding, with resting pulses as low as 25/min (30).

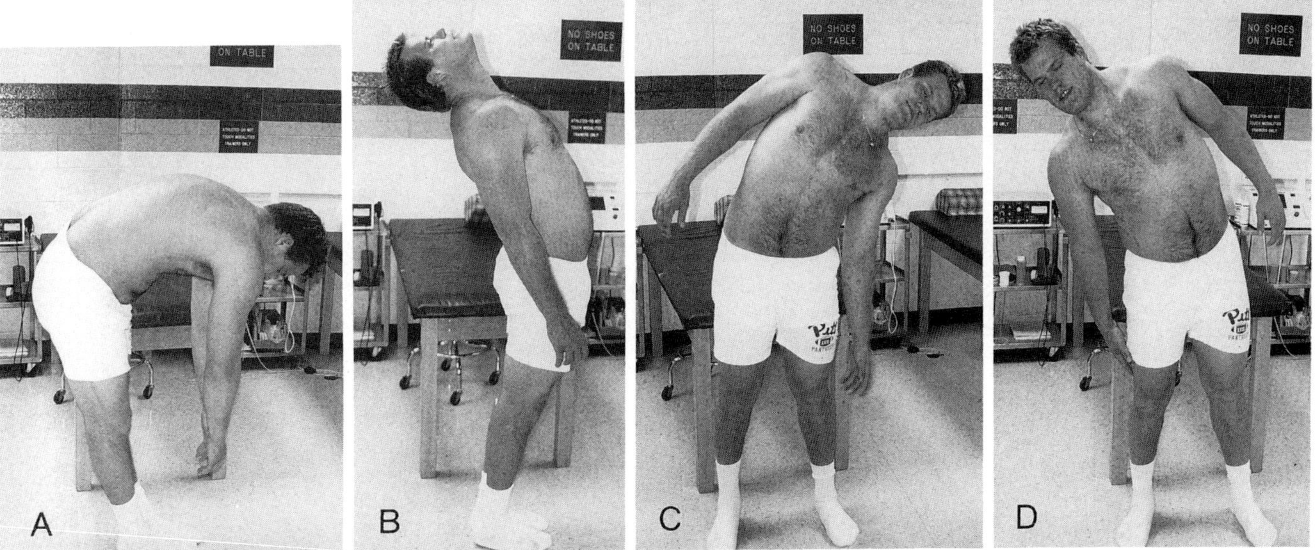

Figure 1.5. (A-D) Lumbar spine range of motion. Symptomatic spondylolisthesis often presents with limited range of motion. Limitations secondary to pain should be noted.

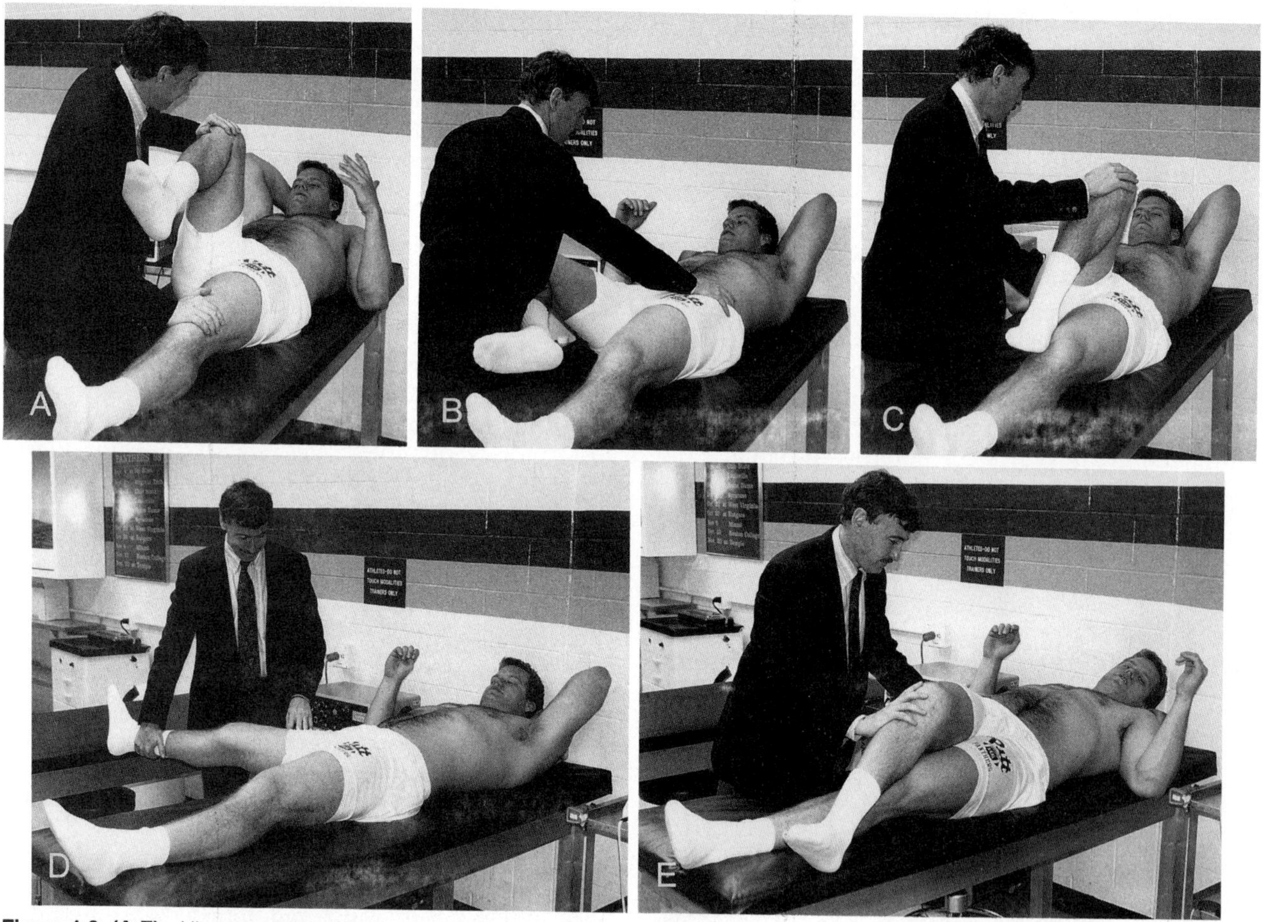

Figure 1.6. (A-E) Hip range of motion. Asymmetric range of motion of the hips is often seen in field goal kickers and soccer players.

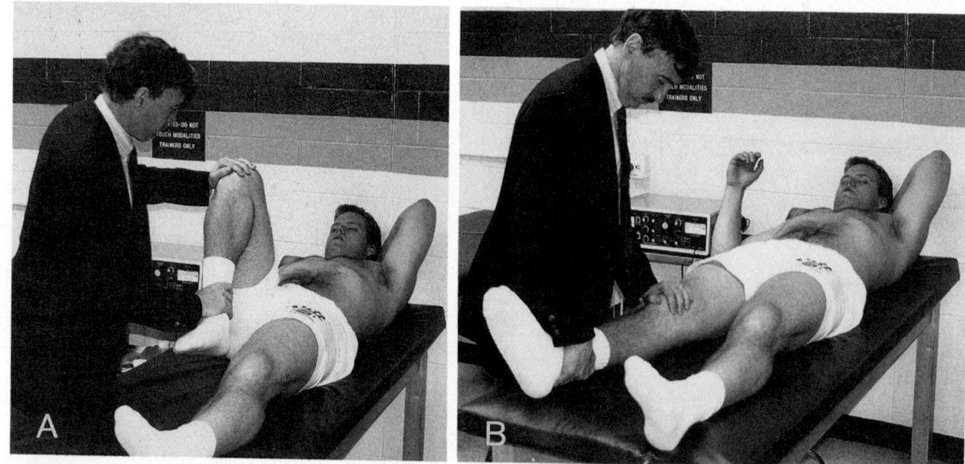

Figure 1.7. (A-B) Knee range of motion. The knee exam should include a check for full range of motion, a Lachman test, and a brief evaluation of the patellofemoral joint.

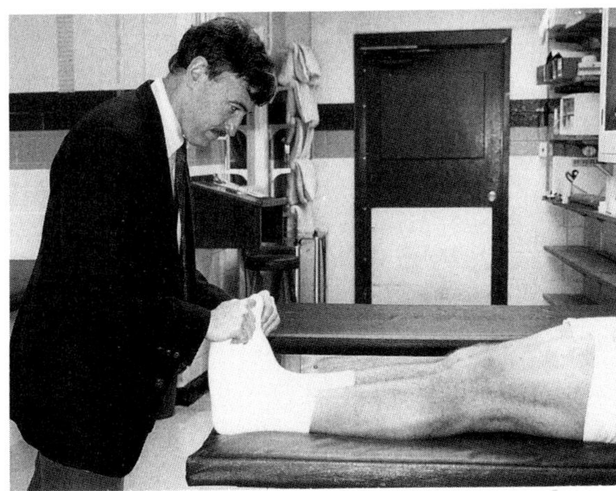

Figure 1.8. Ankle range of motion. Some authors simply check lower extremity motion by asking the athlete to squat.

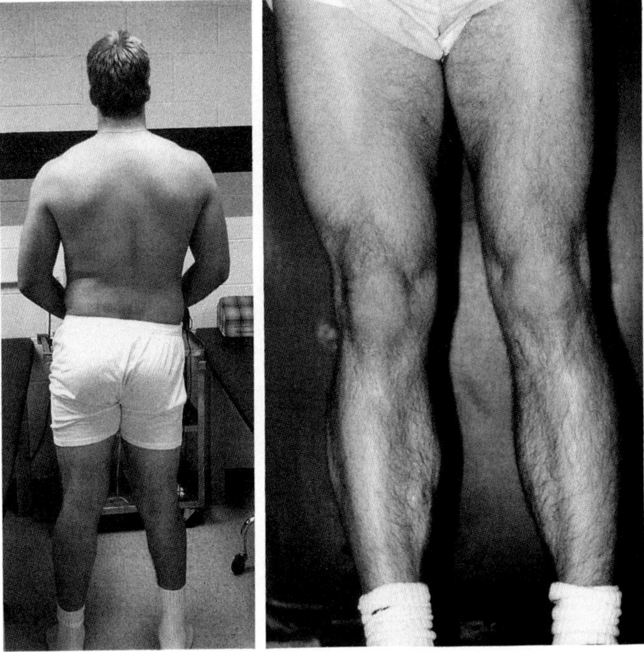

Figure 1.9. The preseason evaluation should always be performed in shorts for men and shorts and a halter top for women. **(A)** An athlete with a leg length discrepancy that is easily picked up in shorts. **(B)** An athlete with a history of partial meniscectomy who was noncompliant with rehabilitation.

EKG changes have been well described and include sinus bradycardia, atrioventricular conduction disturbances, first and second degree heart block, left and right ventricular hypertrophy, right axis deviation, prolonged Q-T interval, U waves, and tall T waves (31). Many of these changes disappear with exercise. The reader is referred to reviews for details (26, 32).

Young athletes who are victims of sudden death are usually males of junior high school age who participate most commonly in football and basketball (33). However, sudden death also occurs in college age athletes (34). Maron found that the most common lesion in this group was hypertrophic cardiomyopathy. The mechanism of death is unclear, although malignant ventricular arrhythmia is postulated. The characteristic systolic murmur is best heard along the left sternal border (35) and intensifies with the Valsalva maneuver, but it is not always heard (36), presenting an interesting diagnostic challenge. A rapid carotid upstroke can also be used to assist in making the diagnosis (35). Other frequently cited causes of sudden death include idiopathic concentric left ventricular hypertrophy, congenital anomalies of coronary arteries, aortic rupture, (usually secondary to Marfan's syndrome), and coronary artery disease (33). Less common conditions associated with sudden death include valvular heart disease; in particular, aortic stenosis; mitral stenosis; and mitral valve prolapse; myocarditis; conduction system abnormalities; and right ventricular dysplasia (27). The reader is referred the 16th Bethesda Conference on Cardiovascular Abnormalities in the Athlete for guidelines on these conditions (37).

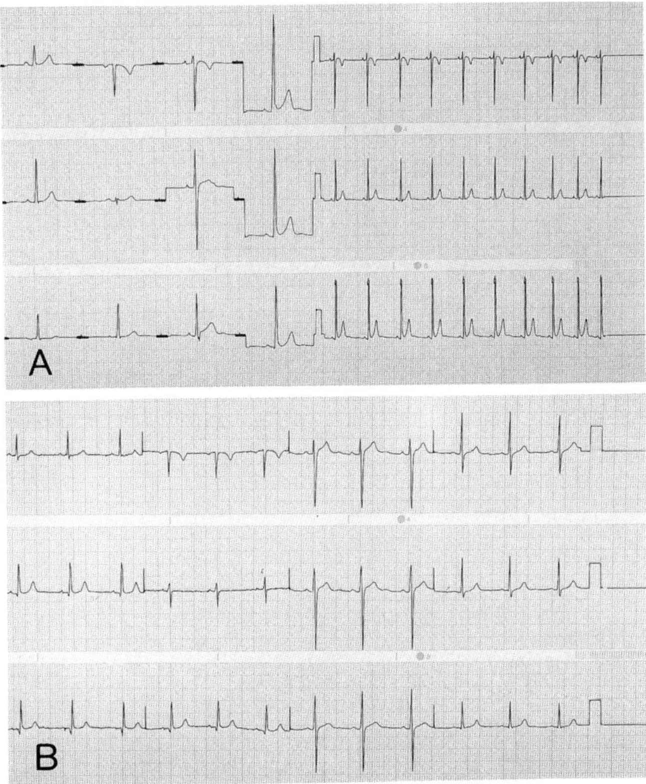

Figure 1.10. Cardiograms. **(A)** A 21-year-old cross-country runner demonstrating moderate voltage criteria for LVH. **(B)** An 18-year-old offensive tackle with essential hypertension and normal cardiogram. The athlete was cleared for participation.

The physical exam also should include an abdominal exam, especially if the athlete has recently had mononucleosis or abdominal trauma. Guidelines for returning the athlete to competition after these injuries are discussed in the section on abdominal injuries (Chapter 55). Risser (17) noted 4 abdominal problems in 2114 screenings, all involving the kidney. One case of asymptomatic hydronephrotic kidney was identified by physical examination.

An examination of the testes and a check for hernias should also be a part of the preparticipation evaluation.

An inguinal hernia is not a contraindication for participation but can be an occult source of abdominal pain or can become strangulated and require emergent treatment in the middle of a season. Testicular cancer is the most common cancer in the 20–40 year age group. Tanner staging can be performed with this part of the exam.

Visual exams are not considered a requirement in a preseason evaluation, although, as mentioned earlier, visual problems in boxers often contraindicate continued participation. Absence of one eye, field cuts, severe myopia, or strabismus are considered criteria for disqualification by some authors (11, 15). The presence of physiologic anisocoria is an important finding in the case of head injury (1).

Laboratory Evaluations

At the professional level, it is expected that athletes will undergo yearly blood tests, urine studies, chest radiographs, and cardiograms. These athletes are a substantial investment to their teams, and the cost of such an evaluation is minimal compared to the consequences of an important player being unavailable due

Table 1.2.
Recommendations for Participation in Competitive Sports[a]

Physical Condition	Contact/ Collision	Limited Contact/ Impact	Noncontact— Strenuous	Noncontact— Moderately Strenuous	Noncontact— Nonstrenuous
Atlantoaxial instability	No	No	Yes; In swimming, no butterfly, breast stroke or diving starts	Yes	Yes
Acute illness	Requires individual assessment (e.g., contagiousness, exacerbation of illness)				
Cardiovascular					
Carditis	No	No	No	No	No
Hypertension					
Mild	Yes	Yes	Yes	Yes	Yes
Moderate	Requires individual assessment				
Severe	Requires individual assessment				
Congenital heart disease	Patients with mild forms can be allowed a full range of physical activities; patients with moderate or severe forms or those who are postoperative should be evaluated by a cardiologist before athletic participation				
Absence or loss of function in one eye	Eye guards may allow the athlete to participate in most sports, but this must be judged on an individual basis				
Detached retina	Consult an ophthalmologist				
Inguinal hernia	Yes	Yes	Yes	Yes	Yes
Absence of one kidney	No	Yes	Yes	Yes	Yes
Enlarged liver	No	No	Yes	Yes	Yes
Musculoskeletal disorders	Requires individual assessment				
History of serious head or spine trauma, repeated concussions or craniotomy	Requires individual assessment		Yes	Yes	Yes
Convulsion disorder					
Poorly controlled	Yes	Yes	Yes	Yes	Yes
Well controlled	No	No	Yes; no swimming or weight lifting	Yes	Yes; no archery or riflery
Absence of one ovary	Yes	Yes	Yes	Yes	Yes
Pulmonary insufficiency	May be allowed to compete if oxygenation remains satisfactory during a graded stress test				Yes
Asthma	Yes	Yes	Yes	Yes	Yes
Sickle cell trait	Yes	Yes	Yes	Yes	Yes
Skin: boils, herpes, impetigo, scabies	While contagious, no contact sports or gymnastics using mats		Yes	Yes	Yes
Enlarged spleen	No	No	No	Yes	Yes
Absent or undescended testicle	Yes; certain sports may require a protective cup		Yes	Yes	Yes

[a]Adapted from American Academy of Pediatrics Committee on Sports Medicine. Recommendations for participating in competitive sports. Pediatrics 1988; 81:737–9.

to injury or illness. At the high school level, urinalysis and hemoglobin screening are often mandated, but neither test has been found to identify athletes who warrant disqualification (9). Kyle et al. (38) performed cholesterol level screening as part of the preparticipation evaluation and noted that 15% of their subjects had elevated cholesterol levels, using the 90th percentile for the students' age group as defined by the Lipid Research Clinic (39) data. The preparticipation evaluation is an excellent opportunity to look for exercise-induced bronchospasm, but routine exercise tests are considered unnecessary by most authors. In 1983, the American Academy of Pediatrics (AAP) Committee on Sports Medicine recommended against the use of routine laboratory evaluations in the preparticipation exam (40).

Disqualification

Disqualification of an athlete from participation is a decision that should be made with parents, coaches, and the athlete. A variety of guidelines have been created to assist the physician in this process, but these are only guidelines, and often break down in an individual situation. The initial guideline was created by the American Medical Association in 1976 (41), but it has become increasingly obsolete and has been replaced by the AAP recommendations from 1988 (Table 1.2) (42). It is recommended that the physician be familiar with them, but, as the guidelines themselves state, "Weigh whether the advantages gained by participating in athletics are worth whatever risks are involved." These risks can be classified by the amount of contact or by how strenuous they are (Table 1.3). More often than not, the athlete can be redirected to other sports or activities, and the physician should actively assist the athlete, coaches, and family in this process. The large majority of athletes will easily pass the evaluation, and almost all others will require some evaluation but ultimately also obtain clearance.

Table 1.3.
Classification of Sports by Contact and Strenuousness

		Noncontact		
Contact/Collision	Limited Contact/Impact	Strenuous	Moderately Strenuous	Non-strenuous
Boxing	Baseball	Aerobic dancing	Badminton	Archery
Field hockey	Basketball	Crew	Curling	Golf
Football	Bicycling	Fencing	Table tennis	Riflery
Ice hockey	Diving	Field		
Lacrosse	Field	Discus		
Martial arts	High jump	Javelin		
Rodeo	Pole vault	Shot put		
Soccer	Gymnastics	Running		
Wrestling	Horseback riding	Swimming		
	Skating	Tennis		
	Ice	Track		
	Roller	Weight lifting		
	Skiing			
	Cross-country			
	Downhill			
	Water			
	Softball			
	Squash, handball			
	Volleyball			

REFERENCES

1. Smith DM, Lombardo JA, Robinson JB. The preparticipation evaluation. Primary Care; Clinics in Office Practice 1991;18:777–807.
2. Risser WL, Hoffman HM, Bellah GG, et al. A cost benefit analysis of preparticipation sports examination of adolescent athletes. J of Sch Health 1985;55:270–273.
3. Thompson, TR, Andrish JT, Bergfeld JA. A prospective study of preparticipation sports examinations of 2670 young athletes: method and results. Cleve Clin Quart 1982;49:225–233.
4. Goldberg B, Saranti A, Witman BA, et al. Preparticipation sports assessment—An objective evaluation. Pediatrics 1980;66:736–745.
5. Jackson DW, Jarrett H, Bailey D, et al. Injury prediction in the young athlete: A preliminary report. Am J Sports Med 1978;6:6–14.
6. Knapik JJ, Jones BH, Bauman CL, et al. Strength, flexibility and athletic injuries. 1992; Sports Med 14:277–288.
7. Linder CW, DuRant RH, Seklecki RM, et al. Preparticipation health screening of young athletes. Results of 1268 examinations. Am J Sports Med 1981;9:187–193.
8. Shambaugh JP, Klein A, Herbert JH. Structural measures as predictors of injury in basketball players. Med Sci in Sports and Ex 1991;23:522–527.
9. Tanji JL. The preparticipation physical examination for sports. Am Fam Practitioner 1990;42:397–402.
10. Fields KB, Delaney M. Focusing the preparticipation sports examination. J of Fam Pract 1990;30:304–312.
11. Hulse E, Strong WB: Preparticipation evaluation for athletics. Ped in Rev 1987;9:173–182.
12. Jones R. The preparticipation, sport specific athletic profile examination. Semin in Adolesc Med 1987;3:169–175.
13. Dyment PG. Another look at the sports preparticipation examination of the adolescent athlete. J of Adolesc Health Care 1986;7:130S–132S.
14. Rowland TW. Preparticipation sports examination of the child and adolescent athlete: changing views of an old ritual. Pediatrician 1986;13:3–9.
15. Shaffer TE. The health examination for participation in sports. Pediatr Ann 1978;7:666–675.
16. Harvey J. The preparticipation examination of the child athlete. Clin Sports Med 1982;1:353–369.
17. O'Connor F, Tucker JB: Boxing. The preparticipation evaluation. Milit Med 1991;8:391–395.
18. Risser WL, Hoffman HM, Bellah GG. Frequency of preparticipation sports examinations in secondary school athletes: are the university interscholastic league guidelines appropriate? Tex Med 1985;81:35–39.
19. Hafner J. Problems in matching athletes: baby fat, peach fuzz, muscle and moustache. Sports Med 1975;3:96–98.
20. Martens R. The uniqueness of the young athlete: psychologic considerations. Am J Sports Med 1980;8:382–385.
21. Kreipe RE, Gewanter HL. Physical maturity screening for participation in sports. Pediatrics 1985;75:1076–1080.
22. Smith NJ: Medical issues in sports medicine. Pediatr Rev 1981;2;229–237.
22. Hergenroeder AC, Bricker JT. Preseason cardiovascular examination: A review. J Adolesc Health Care 1990;11:379–386.
23. Epstein SE, Maron BJ. Sudden death and the competitive athlete: perspectives on preparticipation screening studies. J Am Coll Cardiol 1986;7:220–230.
24. Maron BJ, Bodison SA, Wesley YE, et al. Results of screening a large group of intercollegiate competitive athletes for cardiovascular disease. J Am Coll Cardiol 1987;10:1212–1223.
25. Oakley DG, Oakley CM. Significance of abnormal electrocardiograms in highly trained athletes. Am J Cardiol 1982;50:985–989.
26. Huston TP, Puffer JC, Rodney WM. The athlete heart syndrome. New Engl J Med 1985;313:24–32.
27. Farenbach MC, Thompson PD: The preparticipation sports examination. Cardiovascular considerations for screening. Cardiol Clin 1992;10:319–328.

28. Lewis JF, Maron BJ, Diggs JA et al. Preparticipation echocardiographic screening for cardiovascular disease in a large predominantly black population of college athletes. Am J Cardiol 1989;64:1029–1033.
29. Ikaheimo MJ, Palatsi IJ, Takkunen JT. Noninvasive evaluation of the athletic heart: Sprinters versus endurance runners. Am J Cardiol 1979;44:24–30.
30. Chapman JH. Profound Sinus Bradycardia in the Athletic Heart Syndrome J Sports Med Phys Fitness 1982;22:45–58.
31. Hanne-Paparo N, Drory Y, Schoenfeld Y, et al. Common ECG changes in athletes. Cardiol 1976;61:267–278.
32. George KP, Wolfe LA, Burggraf GW. The "athletic heart syndrome." Sports Med 1990;11:300–323.
33. Maron BJ, Epstein SE, Roberts WC. Causes of sudden death in competitive athletes. J Am Coll Cardiol 1986;17:204–214.
34. Craven CM: Sudden death in a young athlete. A case report. Am J Sports Med 1992;20:621–623.
35. Powell MJ. Hypertrophic nondilated cardiomyopathy: Idiopathic hypertrophic subaortic stenosis and its variants. In: Johnson RA, Haber E, Austen WG eds. The practice of cardiology. Boston: Little Brown and Co., 1980:647–664.
36. Simons SM, Moriarity J. Hypertrophic cardiomyopathy in a college athlete. Med Sci Sports Exerc 1992;24:1321–1324.
37. Mitchell JH, Maron BJ, Epstein SE. 16th Bethesda Conference: Cardiovascular abnormalities in the athlete: Recommendations regarding eligibility for competition. J Am Coll Cardiol 1986;6:1186–1232.
38. Kyle JM, Walker RB, Jiales RR, et al. Student athlete cholesterol screening during routine precompetition examination. J Fam Pract 1991;33:172–176.
39. Lipid research clinics. Population studies databook. NIH Publication no 80-1527. NIH 1980;1:28–29.
40. American Academy of Pediatrics Committee on Sports Medicine. Sports medicine: Health care for young athletes. Evanston, IL; American Academy of Pediatrics, 1983.
41. American Medical Association, Committee on the Medical Aspects of Sports: Medical evaluation of the athlete: A guide. Chicago: American Medical Association, 1976.
42. Committee of sports medicine of the American academy of pediatrics. Recommendations for participation in competitive sports Pediatrics 1988;81;737–739.

2 / CONDITIONING AND TRAINING

Paul A. Borsa and Scott M. Lephart

Introduction

Exercise training and conditioning have become integral components of competitive athletic participation. Athletes, coaches, and athletic trainers concerned with enhancing athletic performance and minimizing the risk of athletic-related injury have developed the various elements of conditioning into scientifically based principles that focus on physiologic and metabolic adaptations that enhance efficiency and function of the human organism. Many sciences within the sports medicine discipline have contributed to the methodologic development of athletic conditioning in an effort to enable optimal physiologic function, resulting in peak performance characteristics for the athlete.

Training and conditioning involve a systematic modeling of the physiologic elements of the human organism that result from induced stress and use of the respective metabolic systems. The adaptations that occur following systematic conditioning include somatomorphic alterations, muscular strength and endurance, soft tissue proliferation and enhanced plasticity, central and peripheral cardiorespiratory efficiency, and the ability of all metabolic systems to withstand greater amounts of stress without fatigue or failure (1).

This chapter focuses on the elements of athletic performance that adapt to training and conditioning to enhance athletic performance. These elements include identifying those desirable characteristics for optimal athletic performance, means in which these characteristics can be quantified, modes that induce physiologic and metabolic adaptations, and methodologic approaches to implement efficiently and effectively training and conditioning of the athlete.

Conditioning the Athlete

Performance Characteristics

Although the specific requirements of each sport vary relative to specific skills necessary to perform the activity, there are general underlying functional components that are common to all performance. Strength, endurance, speed, and coordination are elements that lay the foundation of all sports activity (1). Regardless of the activity, whether it be cyclic or acyclic, these four characteristics are the limiting factors in the ultimate performance. Although the relevant importance of those components is a function of the particular sport, conditioning programs must ultimately address them all in an effort to enhance the athlete's performance and decrease the risk of injury.

Seldom does a sport demand any of these four functional components exclusively, and often the demand requires combinations of the components (1). For instance, many sports require both strength and speed, which is characterized as power. Other sports require strength to be exerted over extended periods of time, which is characterized as muscular endurance. Other activities demand the combination of speed and coordination that is characterized as agility. Finally, all performance characteristics necessitate mobility and muscular flexibility for ambulation. The ultimate success in optimizing a particular athlete's conditioning for a particular sport depends on implementing the appropriate exercises to enhance the aforementioned components needed for his or her sport.

Strength

Muscular strength is the tension generated within a muscle group(s) against a fixed resistance and angular velocity in one maximal effort (2, 3). Athletes require muscular strength to compete at high levels of exercise intensity. Strength is the combination of the structure of the muscle and neurologic stimulation that enables the muscle's functional unit to contract (1). Maximal strength development is, therefore, a combination of morphologic alteration, known as hypertrophy, and neurological adaptations, resulting in enhancing neural stimulation.

When a combination of force and speed of muscle contraction are necessary for performance, ultimate muscular power is desirable. Muscular power enhancement depends on the force and acceleration of contraction. Therefore, power training necessitates neuromuscular adaptations that increase the speed and force at which the muscular contraction takes place.

Endurance

For athletes whose performance demands sustained levels of strength, a key element of their conditioning is the enhancement of muscular endurance. Muscular endurance involves both strength and the ability to delay the onset of fatigue. Endurance in the general sense refers to an athlete's capacity to perform work over an extended period of time. The endurance capacity of an athlete is a function of the oxidative pathways, which are both centrally and peripherally mediated. Many factors affect aerobic endurance, including cardiorespiratory capacity and efficiency (transport), metabolic substrate availability, and cellular metabolic activity (use) (1). Also important is the power output (work load) in terms of skeletal muscle function. Therefore, conditioning responses for endurance athletes involves both mechanical (power output) and metabolic (substrate transport and utilization) adaptations. Because endurance activities usually induce fatigue, physical conditioning goals are to delay the onset of fatigue and to allow the athlete to work at high-intensity levels before fatigue is reached. These adaptations can only be achieved if the training sessions are intense enough to produce fatigue.

Speed

One of the most important characteristics for successful athletic performance is speed. Speed is defined as the capacity to move quickly and refers to locomotion (1). An athlete's speed is mediated predominantly by neuromuscular factors that include contractile capacities (power) and mechanical characteristics (gait and technique). Physiologically, speed adaptations are induced when selective neuromuscular units are enhanced through increased metabolic substrate availability and speed of muscular contractions (i.e., increasing the frequency and force of muscular contractions).

Coordination

Coordination is generally defined as harmonious action, as seen in muscles. This particular component of performance requires input from the other three components (strength, speed, and endurance) to allow the athlete to function at peak performance levels. The central nervous system (CNS) is the most rudimentary ordinate that mediates coordinated motion. The peripheral afferent and efferent branches of the CNS regulate coordinated motion by inhibiting and/or activating specific muscle groups, which produce movement patterns. Through repetition from physical training, the neuromuscular system is conditioned to provide the requisite movement patterns, or engrams, for developing the strength, speed, endurance, and agility that are necessary for athletic performance.

The general and specific movement patterns acquired with training are programmed centrally in the brain. The motor cortex and cerebellum play important roles in the acquisition of sophisticated movement patterns. The motor cortex is the learning center that programs the specific pattern, and the cerebellum is responsible for the precision and accuracy of that particular movement (1).

Coordination has been classified by Bompa (1) as general or specific, depending on the degree of complexity. General coordination encompasses normal body movement such as walking and climbing stairs. Specific coordination is the technical movements required for a specific sport. For instance, the tennis serve and basketball jump shot require specific movement patterns developed and fine-tuned through repetition. Sport-specific coordination may not carry over to general coordination as seen by the wrestler who is adept at his or her sport, yet grossly uncoordinated at basketball. On the other hand, general coordination has been attributed to athletes who are very skilled at their sport, e.g., Michael Jordan possesses both general and specific coordination.

Typed Activity

Athletic performance and exercise training is made up of various types of activities. These activities may be systematically broken down and categorized as cyclic, acyclic, or cyclic/acyclic combined (semicyclic). Cyclic movements are continuous activities that require identical movement patterns done repetitively. Distance running and cycling are sports that require cyclic movements. These particular athletes may show a coordinated gait pattern yet are not necessarily agile. Sprinters and jumping athletes are acyclic or cyclic/acyclic combined, and their sports may or may not require agility. Sports that require agility are acyclic or semicyclic in nature, mainly because these particular activities use common movement patterns done in repetition or in discontinuous cycles. Agility movements include activities that require constant directional changes such as forward/backward running, lateral movement, acceleration and deceleration, and diagonal cutting (Fig. 2.1) (1). Basketball, wrestling, gymnastics, and soccer are cyclic/acyclic combined sports that require high levels of agility. Because it is difficult to classify a sport as strictly acyclic, both acyclic and combined sports are referred to as semicyclic. Both cyclic and semicyclic activities require strength, speed, and endurance, but in varying degrees. The distance runner typically uses cy-

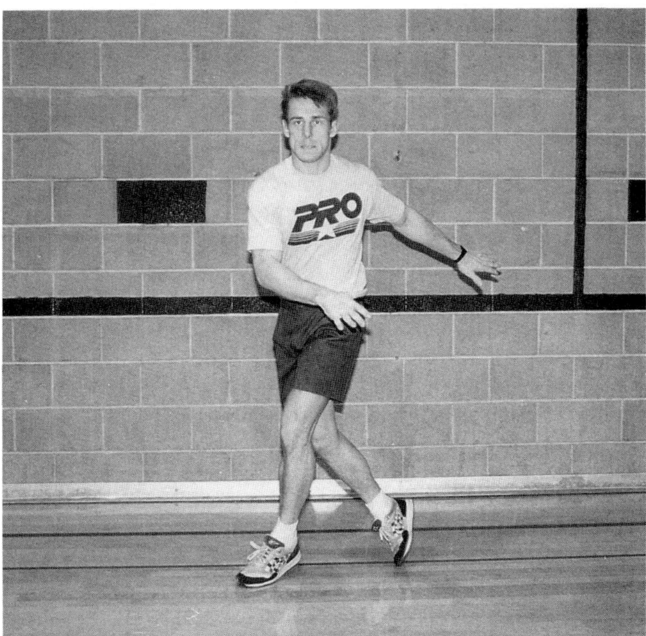

Figure 2.1. Agility is a performance characteristic important for activities requiring lateral mobility, acceleration and deceleration, and diagonal cutting.

clical movement coordinated over long durations, whereas the acyclical athlete requires greater levels of strength and speed to perform his or her sport at near maximal intensities.

The five characteristics of athlete performance are interrelated by the regulatory effects of the CNS. Coordinated movement, whether simple or complex, cyclic or semicyclic, requires varying amounts of strength, speed, and endurance. These three components of performance will be discussed throughout the chapter in regard to measurements, training, adaptation, and injury.

Body Composition

Morphometric structure and body composition are closely related to athletic performance (4–8) and susceptibility to injury during physical activity (9). As the athlete strives to maximize performance, he or she also must consider the ratio of lean body tissue to fat tissue.

The assessment of body composition involves the measurement and evaluation of the rudimentary structural components of the human body. Body composition is subdivided into body fat content (percent body fat) and lean body mass (LBM). Body fat is the adipose tissue deposited throughout the whole body and is classified as essential and nonessential. Essential fat is necessary for normal physiologic functioning. Essential fat is found in nerve myelination, blood lipids, and glandular hormones. Nonessential fat is the excess deposition of adipose tissue around the viscera, skeletal muscles, and subcutaneous fat layer. Lean body mass is the nonessential fat-free tissue that constitutes the remaining tissue of the body. This includes skeletal and smooth muscle (protein), bone (mineral), essential fat, and the volume of water within the various compartments of the body. The normal subdivision of lean tissues is total body water 73%, protein 19%, mineral 3%, and essential fat 5% (10).

Assessment techniques have been developed for estimating percent body fat (% BF) and LBM. Direct measurement of body composition was initially performed through chemical analysis of dissected human cadavers; the tissue was differentiated into fat and fat-free proportions for comparison (11). As a result of these direct methods, and more recent indirect methods such as the classic hydrostatic weighing studies done by Behnke at the naval academy, body density (BD) estimates for the "reference man and woman" were established (11, 12). Other examples of indirect methods to predict %BF and LBM include skinfold thickness and circumferential measurements.

Measurement of Body Composition

Hydrostatic Weighing. Hydrostatic weighing (underwater densiometry) is a method of estimating body composition by volumetrically measuring BD (Fig. 2.2) (13, 14). Volumetric measurements of a body submerged in water can be calculated through the application of Archimedes' principle, which states that the mass of an object is equal to its displacement volume when submerged in water (15). Specific gravity (SG) is a variable related to and often mentioned along with density. Specific gravity can be calculated by dividing the dry mass (M_d) of an individual by the loss of mass in water (M_w).

$$SG = \frac{M_d}{(M_d - M_w)}$$

The effect of water temperature on the bouyancy of the body when submerged is what separates specific gravity from BD. As a result, correction factors were incorporated into the prediction equations.

$$BD = \frac{\text{Mass}}{\text{Volume}} = \frac{M_d}{(M_d - M_w/D_w) - RLV}$$

or

$$BD = \frac{SG}{D_w} - RLV$$

where M_d is the dry mass or body weight in air; M_w, wet mass or body weight in water; RLV, residual lung volume; and D_w, density of water (correction factor). The ideal temperature for hydrostatic weighing is approximately 39.2°F (4°C), which is relatively uncomfortable for humans to withstand. Therefore, a correction factor (D_w) is incorporated in the BD equation as a means of statistically controlling for water temperature variation.

Residual lung volume (RLV) is the amount of air trapped in the lungs after a maximal exhalation and can be measured directly or indirectly by less reliable alternative methods. Because RLV is least affected by water

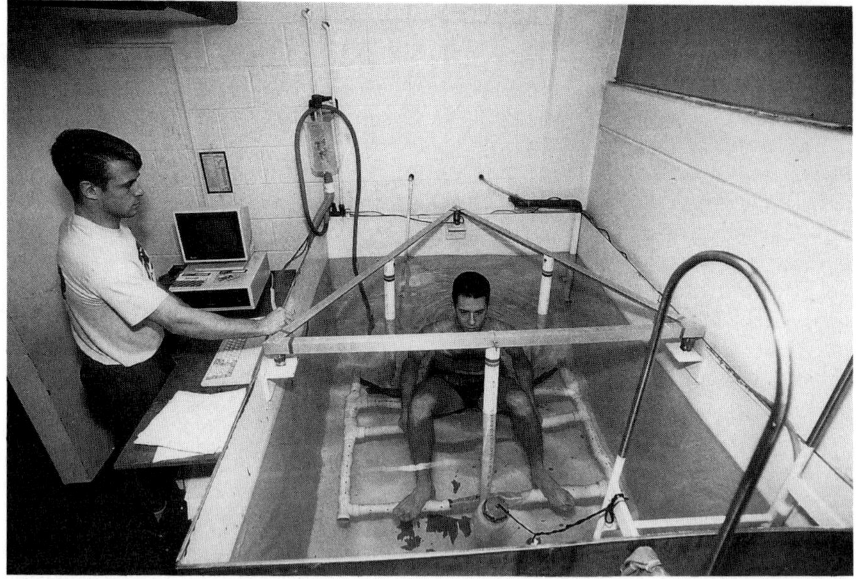

Figure 2.2. Hydrostatic weighing (underwater densitometry) measures body density by employing Archimedes' principle.

temperature, it is used most often with hydrostatic weighing and also is accountable as a potential source of error. Unaccountable sources of error are trapped air within the intestinal tract, hair, and excess clothing worn during assessment (10, 16).

Once BD is calculated, %BF and LBM are estimated through the use of a prediction equation. Siri (17) and Brozek et al. (18) have developed standard equations for calculating %BF by incorporating the BD value into an equation that uses constants derived from body density estimates of fat and fat-free tissue:

$$\text{Siri equation } \%BF = 495/BD - 450$$
$$\text{Brozek equation } \%BF = 4.570/BD - 4.215$$

Once %BF is determined, LBM can be calculated:

$$\text{Mass of fat } (M_f) = \%BF \times \text{total body mass (TBM)}$$
$$LBM = TBM - M_f$$

Recent investigations have identified other random sources of measurement error. For example, cadaveric analysis has shown LBM to be inconsistent compared with the reference man and woman as earlier described by Behnke (12). Other sources of random variation are age, gender, bone mineral content, and total body water (TBW). Although these sources of error exist, hydrostatic weighing is still considered to be the most reliable estimate of body composition (10, 20).

Skinfold Thickness. Percent body fat may be predicted from the measurement of the subcutaneous layer of adipose tissue at various anatomic sites on the body. The rationale for this method is based on the relationship between subcutaneous fat and whole body fat. Skinfold thicknesses are measured using calipers that measure the thickness of skin and subcutaneous fat (Fig. 2.3). The technique used for skinfold measurement permits the separation of skin and subcutaneous fat from the underlying muscle tissue.

Skinfolds provide reliable data concerning body fat distribution (21–24). Various sites throughout the body, believed to provide the most accurate predictions for overall body fat content, have been selected experimentally for caliper readings (21). The seven most popular sites are the subscapular, triceps, axilla, chest, abdomen, suprailium, and midthigh (21).

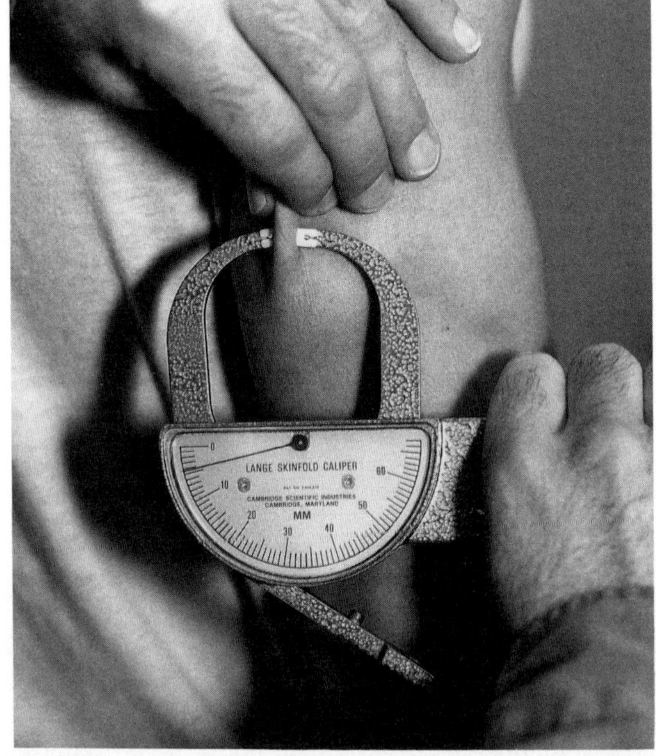

Figure 2.3. Skinfolds, indicators of subcutaneous fat, are measured with calipers.

All measurements are taken on the right side of the body while the subject is standing. The mean of two or three trials is recorded for each site. The measurement should be performed by an experienced technician who is capable of duplicating measures on a consistent basis. Several gender-specific regression equations for the prediction of %BF have been developed (12, 21–25). Once BD is estimated, the score is entered into the Brozek's or Siri's equation to compute %BF (17, 18).

Circumferential Measurements. Another method of estimating body fat is by measuring girth at specific an-anatomic sites on the body known to be target areas of fat deposition (Fig. 2.4) (26). It is a relatively quick, accurate, and inexpensive method to assess %BF and LBM. Often circumferential measurements are used to estimate %BF in obese individuals, because it is difficult to perform accurate skinfolds and underwater assessments. This method also can be used to identify quickly patterns of fat distribution on the body for comparison after weight loss. Body fat conversion tables estimate the %BF from the sum of the girth measures. Popular sites of measurement include the abdomen, buttocks, right thigh, right upper arm, right forearm, and right calf. The equations and tables are age and gender specific (15, 27).

Some methods combine skinfold and girth measurements to estimate body composition (10, 12, 21). Potential sources of error are inherent with the skinfold and girth methods. The intramuscular hydration level can obscure measures, and the texture and pliability of the skin and underlying fat layer also can cause erroneous measurements. To ensure valid measurements, the measurement instrument should be routinely calibrated.

Alternative Methods of Assessing Body Composition. The various methods of assessing body composition discussed thus far are all calculated through external or surface anthropometric measures. These measures are relatively simple, inexpensive, and reliable. Some alternative methods exist that are not generally used because of added expense and inconvenience to the patient. These methods are generally more accurate, as they use internal images for estimating body composition. Magnetic resonance imaging (MRI), computerized tomography, radiography, and ultrasound assessments of body composition use pictorial imaging techniques that delineate the tissues to measure the percent of bone, muscle, and fat (10, 15). Bioelectrical impedance and K^+ emission methods require electrochemical means of assessing BD. Body density may then be converted to %BF and LBM through the use of Siri's or Brozek's equation (10).

Strength Training

Physiology of Strength Training

As early as the ancient Olympic games, muscular strength has been acknowledged as an integral component to most athletic events. In general terms, strength is simply the force that can be generated when a muscle is contracting. Today's athlete is constantly striving to enhance muscular strength ultimately to enhance sport performance. Strength development is a function of muscle growth, which has been shown to occur 8 to 12 times greater in the athlete who engages in strength training than in the athlete who conditions by practicing only sport-specific activities (1). Thus strength training has become a specialized element in most competitive athletes.

The maximum force a muscle can generate is determined by the cross-sectional area of the muscle as well as the complex integration of the biochemical composition and neural input to that muscle. In addition, most strength characteristics are required for activities that involve limb motion, thus the limb biomechanics affect muscular contraction.

Muscular power is a component of strength and has become an important goal of strength-training programs. The strength of a muscle depends on the joint range of motion (ROM) in which the muscle acts. The rotary action of a muscle about a joint axis that produces force is referred to as torque. Muscular power is created by the torque generated and the speed of a muscular contraction. This dynamic action is essential to sports that require accelerated rates of force genera-

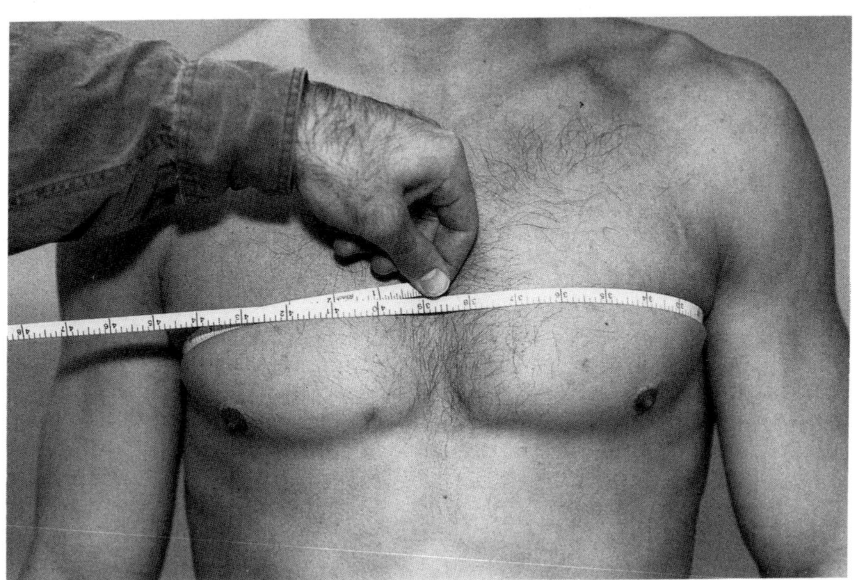

Figure 2.4. Circumferential (girth) measurements are also used to estimate body fat.

tion. This concept of strength-speed or power has become an important issue in strength training programs. Substantial attention is being directed toward the acquisition of strength-speed or "explosive" power. Research has shown a strong relationship between the generation of peak power and intramuscular concentrations of fast-twitch fibers (28). This implies that an athlete possessing inherent strength is more able to develop muscular power if he or she is endowed with a high concentration of fast-twitch (type II) muscle fibers.

Another component of strength-training is the acquisition of muscular endurance, which is defined as the capacity of a muscle group(s) to perform repeated contractions against a resistance. Depending on their sport, athletes need varying degrees of endurance training for those muscles that require force generation over protracted periods. Muscle fiber type has been found to play an important role in activities that require muscular endurance (29, 30). For instance, athletes who perform cyclic activities over prolonged periods, such as distance runners and swimmers, use mainly the type I and IIa fibers. Athletes who perform acyclic activities at high intensities for short bursts, such as baseball pitchers and tennis and volleyball players, use type IIa and IIb fibers.

Athletes train for muscular endurance in various ways. Some athletes use circuit resistance training (CRT), whereas other athletes use high-repetition progressive resistance exercise (PRE) or speed-specific isokinetic exercise to reduce the fatiguability of muscles. By reducing fatiguability, the muscles increase their capacity to metabolize lactic acid (30). Muscular endurance exercise induces aerobic and anaerobic metabolic system adaptations within the muscle, with the ultimate goal of maintaining forceful contractions (anaerobic power) over prolonged periods of time (aerobic power). Training also is sport specific, and some athletes require endurance-type activities. For instance, a baseball pitcher or swimmer may train the shoulder girdle muscles for endurance. Unfortunately, little research has been done to substantiate the most efficient means of acquiring muscular endurance, although many strength and conditioning experts use their own programs with varying degrees of success.

Adaptations to Strength Training

As the result of a strength-training program, certain morphologic and neural adaptations occur. Morphologically, the primary alteration that occurs is muscle hypertrophy or enlargement. For years there was considerable debate about whether hypertrophy (enlargement of muscle fibers) or hyperplasia (increased number of muscle fibers) was responsible for the increase in muscle size. Contemporary research has concluded that hyperplasia only occurs during the developmental stages of growth and maturation, and thus beyond adolescence most muscle growth is a function of hypertrophy (28). Hypertrophic changes occur from a number of mechanisms, primarily related to increasing muscle protein synthesis, which results in the anabolic process of muscle growth.

From a practical perspective, strength development needs to occur functionally, thus enhancing selected performance characteristics. It is, therefore, necessary to discuss functional strength that creates movement. The extent to which force is generated by a muscle through a range of motion is closely linked with neurally mediated activities. The neural components include intramuscular innervation and intermuscular coordination of the movement. Maximal muscular contraction is limited by the number of motor units that are activated. In addition to the hypertrophic changes that occur within the muscle fiber that enable greater force-generating capacity, an increase in motor unit activation occurs as a function of strength training. The combination of morphologic and neurologic adaptations results in a greater force-generating capacity per area of the muscle unit.

For strength gains to be functional, there needs to be enhanced capacity for movement through a range of motion. These adaptations are closely linked to the coordinated activity of the agonist, antagonist, and synergistic muscle groups that are neurally mediated. The activity of all of these muscle groups results in a coordinated movement which, as a result of intramuscular adaptations, results in greater potential for force to be generated through the desired motion.

For strength adaptations to occur within muscle tissue, the *overload principle* must be applied to the specific strength-training program. The overload principle is defined as the process of overloading a muscle or muscle group(s) with a resistance that exceeds a threshold, or level of intensity, by which adaptive changes occur within the muscle fiber. The mechanical and metabolic changes enable the muscle fiber to increase its force-generating capability (15, 28). The specific adaptations to imposed demands principle *(SAID principle)* is often equated with the overload principle, because both require training above threshold levels to prompt systematically the neuromuscular system to function more efficiently. The SAID principle applies to any training program and is specific to the demands of an athlete's sport. Strength developed functionally through sport-specific training involves activity that produces greater force with more precision. This involves neural intramuscular and intermuscular mediation. The overload principle is more general to the muscular system, and through the application of the SAID principle more functional strength is developed for sport-specific purposes. For example, a baseball pitcher requires overall upper- and lower-body strength; but specific to his or her position, the player requires sport-specific strength training of the shoulder girdle, hip, and thigh to maintain the muscular power and endurance needed for pitching.

Along with overload, any training and/or conditioning program must follow an agenda for incorporating intensity and volume (frequency and duration) and mode of exercise. These factors are the stimuli that dictate the systematic progress in functional performance and are manipulated according to the seasonal phase of training (see below).

Muscular strength, power, and endurance are developed through various modes of training. The training modes are specific to the type of force-generating capabilities within the exercising muscle. The four major modes of training discussed here are isometric, isotonic, isokinetic, and plyometric.

Modes of Strength Training

Isometric. Isometric contraction is classified as static, because the length of the muscle does not change in response to the generation of force within the muscle against an externally applied resistive force. Isometric training gained popularity in the late 1960s as a means of supplementation to other forms of resistance training. Early experimentation indicated muscular strength increases following isometric training programs (31, 32), although these adaptations were limited to the joint angle exercised. Strength and conditioning experts have used isometrics in an attempt to release "sticking points" that develop at specific angles within the range of motion (15). These adaptations have limitations relative to athletic performance; therefore, isometric exercise is most often limited to the early states of orthopedic rehabilitation when angular motion of anatomical joints is contraindicated (2). As a therapeutic modality, isometric exercise permits maximum tension generation within the muscle. This may retard disuse atrophy while also maintaining the normal neuromuscular firing patterns of the muscle groups. Functionally, isometric exercise rehabilitation and training is usually performed at various angles throughout the ROM of a particular joint, if not contraindicated. The static contraction is held for 5 to 10 sec with a specified protocol of sets and repetitions. This permits the muscle to generate force at various lengths and has been found to result in strength gains throughout the range exercised (33).

Isotonic. Isotonic training involves exercise at a fixed resistance with variable angular velocity occurring throughout the ROM. This type of exercise is different from isometric exercise in that the force generated within the muscle overcomes the external counterresistance, thus causing the muscle fibers to change their length. As a result, angular motion occurs in a specified range against a fixed resistance. Progressive resistance exercise (PRE) training is a popular mode of isotonic resistance training. In orthopedic rehabilitation, low to moderate PRE's are performed using rubberized tubing (Theraband or Sport Cord), free weights, or modified equipment machines such as the Nautilus or Universal systems (Fig. 2.5).

When exercising isotonically, the muscle changes length as a result of cross-bridge formation along the sarcomere. Muscular contractions occur concentrically (shorten) or eccentrically (lengthen). Both concentric and eccentric contractions have been shown to result in the development of muscular strength (34). Eccentric, or negative contractions, occur while the muscle is lengthening. Eccentric contractions generate greater tension within the muscle at higher angular velocities than concentric contractions (33). Concentric, or positive contractions, occur while the muscle shortens and has been shown to increase tension at slower angular velocities (33). Concentric contractions are equated with acceleration-type movements, such as the wind-up in baseball, while eccentrics are equated with deceleration-type movements such as the follow through in the baseball throw. Dudley et al. (34a) reported that a combination of concentric and eccentric contractions in resistance exercises produces the greatest gains in strength (34). Also, hypertrophy has been shown to occur in both type I and II muscle fibers (34).

From a training perspective, concentric exercise expends more muscle energy, while eccentrics impart greater damage to the muscle fiber. Therefore, eccentrics appear to be more economical, but concentrics appear to be safer. Thus, to minimize muscle damage and maximize energy, a slow progression in intensity and volume with a combination of both types of contrac-

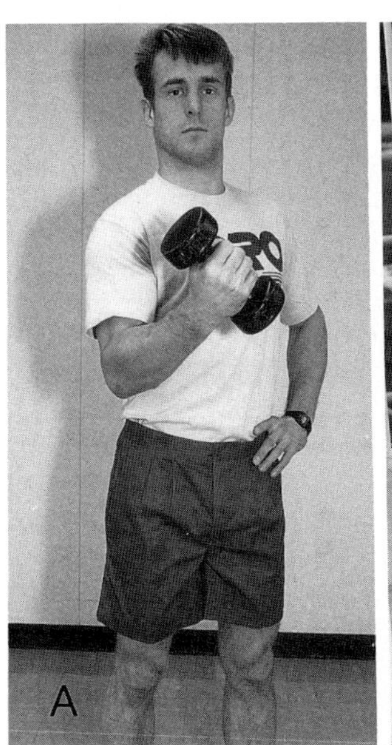

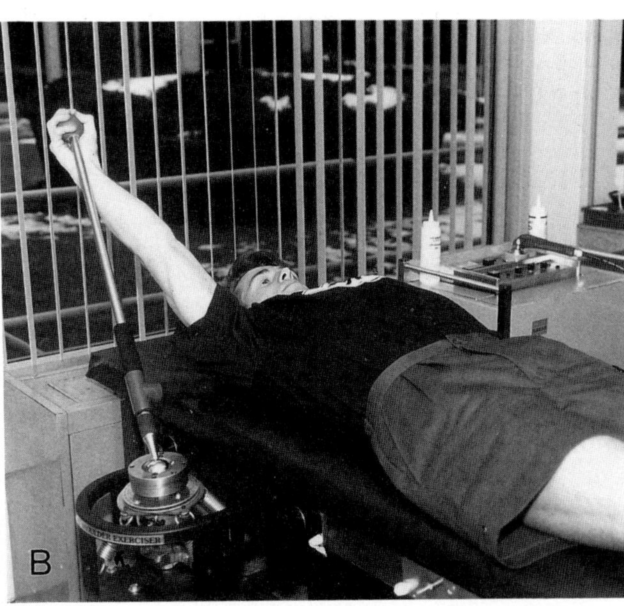

Figure 2.5. Strength training via the PRE method has various modes. **A,** Isotonic (dumbbells). **B,** multiaxial cable resistance.

tions should be prescribed to achieve safe and effective gains in muscular strength

Isokinetic. Isokinetic training is speed-specified exercise with accommodating resistance throughout the ROM. Isokinetic exercise permits the athlete to train at fast, intermediate, or slow angular velocities, with a counterresistive force matching the force exerted by the athlete. Isokinetic testing devices have the advantage of quantifying muscular force generated at preset speeds. In addition, isokinetics permit the measurement of muscular power and resistance to fatigue (endurance). Contemporary isokinetic devices are equipped with training programs for both concentric and eccentric exercise. Most commercially available isokinetic devices are interfaced with a computer that is able to store large quantities of information. Available devices are equipped for multijoint testing and exercise protocols. Much research has been devoted to isokinetic exercise, but little conclusive evidence has been forthcoming in regard to the proposed benefits as a testing and/or training device (33). Presently, isokinetic exercise has been used as a measurement tool to compare muscular strength and power; it also has been used as a strength-training modality. Furthermore, isokinetics have been recommended for use during the late stages of orthopedic rehabilitation owing to its proposed functional benefits, although researchers have shown that isokinetic scores do not correlate well with functional performance (35). The implementation of isokinetic devices for functional training has been recently questioned. Researchers now suggest that differences in the "kinetic chain" of force distribution is a major failure of isokinetic training, particularly in the lower extremities. Isokinetics are classified as "open kinetic chain," and most functional skills are performed under the "closed kinetic chain," thus accounting for the weak relationship between isokinetic parameters and functional performance (35).

Strength-Training Programs

In recent years the athlete's focus on strength development has escalated. Today's athletes devote extensive time to weight-training programs designed to develop functional strength specific to their sport. The basis for these programs evolved from DeLorme's progressive resistance exercise experiments (36). PRE programs follow the overload principle, which requires a systematic progression of resistance. This principle combined with a set training protocol of intensity, duration, and frequency will induce the specific muscle fiber adaptations discussed above (30). The following are some of the popular PRE programs used for strength development.

Progressive Resistance Exercise. DeLorme's PRE program is based on exercise that is performed at a percentage of the maximal amount of resistance (weight), in sets of 10 repetitions (2, 36). The progression occurs both within each session and between successive sessions as the athlete develops greater strength over the course of the program (Table 2.1). This form of strength training focuses mainly on isotonics. The training apparatus for PRE includes free weights, resistive tubing, circuit devices, and cable/pulley systems.

Recently, DeLorme's method of resistance training has been modified for purposes of orthopedic rehabilitation. Sanders's PRE program uses a formula based on percent of the individual's body weight to predict starting weight (Table 2.2) (2). Knight developed the daily adjusted progressive resistance exercise (DAPRE) programs, which allow for individual variations in progression (Table 2.3) (2). Berger further modified the DAPRE method by altering the number of repetitions from 10 to 6–8 for each of the three sets (Table 2.4) (2, 31).

Most clinicians and strength-training experts advise alternating PRE programs with moderate- to high-intensity resistance training to permit at least 48 hr recovery between PRE workouts. The recovery intervals permit muscle fiber repair and regeneration that not only acts as a prophylaxis against injury but also facilitates the necessary metabolic pathway adaptations that increase muscular strength.

Circuit Resistance Training. Circuit resistance training (CRT) is used mainly by endurance athletes who are interested in gaining muscular strength and endurance. CRT involves protracted periods of repeated muscle contractions followed by short periods of recovery between resistance machines.

Athletes begin training at a resistance level that is estimated to be 40% to 50% of their one-repetition maximum (1 RM). The 1 RM is a method of measuring absolute strength, using a one-repetition lift at maximum intensity. The process can be applied to all exercises (e.g., the squat or military press).

The circuits are arranged before the actual training sessions, and consist of 10 to 14 machines that exercise the major muscle groups of the body. The athlete begins the circuit by repeatedly lifting the set resistance for a specified period of time (30 sec) or number of repetitions (20 to 30), followed by a brief recovery period

Table 2.1.
DeLorme's Program

Set	Resistance	Repetitions
1	50% of 10 RM	10
2	75% of 10 RM	10
3	100% of 10 RM	10

Table 2.2.
Sander's Modified Program

Set	Resistance	Repetitions
4 sets (3 times per week)	100% of 5 RM	5
Day 1: 4 sets	100% of 5 RM	5
Day 2: 4 sets	100% of 3 RM	5
Day 3: 1 set	100% of 5 RM	5
2 sets	100% of 3 RM	5
2 sets	100% of 2 RM	5

Table 2.3.
Knight's DAPRE Program

Set	Resistance	Repetitions
1	50% of RM	10
2	75% of RM	6
3	100% of RM	Maximum
4	Adjusted working weight*	Maximum

**Adjusted Working Weight*

Number of Repetitions Performed during 3rd Set	Adjusted Working Weight during 4th Set	Next Exercise Session
0–2	Subtract 5–10 pounds	Subtract 5–10 pounds
3–4	Subtract 0–5 pounds	Same weight
5–6	Same weight	Add 5–10 pounds
7–10	Add 5–10 pounds	Add 5–15 pounds
11+	Add 10–15 pounds	Add 10–20 pounds

Table 2.4.
Berger's Program

Set	Resistance	Repetitions
3	100% of RM	6–8

(10 to 30 sec). The athlete moves to the next resistance machine in the circuit and continues the procedure until the entire circuit is completed. Theoretically, exercising the muscle at high repetitions with moderate resistance with limited recovery enables the athlete to maintain a heart rate (HR) that is sufficient for endurance adaptations to occur. CRT is a contemporary idea that has not been extensively studied scientifically, although initial findings are encouraging (15).

Plyometric Training. Plyometrics is a relatively new method of training that is gaining popularity among athletes that require explosive muscular power for performance. Plyometrics use the athlete's body mass as well as the force of gravity for resistance. The plyometric technique is performed by having the athlete repeatedly jump from and land on surfaces of different heights. Plyometric training employs the ballistic properties of skeletal muscle, resulting in the development of muscular strength for explosive power. The underlying premise of plyometrics is to train the muscle fibers to maximize their inherent elastic properties via the stretch/recoil response modulated by the myotactic reflex. (37). The myotactic reflex, or the muscle stretch reflex, occurs whenever a muscle is placed on stretch. The sudden implosive elongation of the muscle stimulates the muscle spindle, which in turn acts as a sensory relay to the CNS. Once the CNS has identified the intensity of the signal, a neural response indicated by the efferent pathways stimulates the muscle fibers to contract explosively. This activity is called a reflex because of the instantaneous response of the muscle. With training, adaptations occur within fast-twitch fibers that maximize not only the sensitivity of the stretch but, more important, the speed and number of motor units recruited for the resultant muscle contraction. The rapid change from stretch to recoil involves two types of muscle contractions. First, the muscle is elongated and loaded eccentrically. This decelerates the muscle in preparation for the recoil. The recoil involves the concentric contraction, which accelerates the explosive movement. This process also is known as the amortization phase. This coupling action has been found to take place within hundredths of a second, thus classifying the plyometric mechanism as a reflex.

A plyometric training program consists of explosive jumps and bounds on one or both legs in a vertical or horizontal direction. Various heights of jumping and landing are used in progression. Athletes should begin plyometric training at low intensity, working up to more intensive levels. Plyometrics may begin as general training and progress to a more functional and/or sport-specific activity. The progression from straight ahead to lateral and diagonal patterns of jumping is an example of a functional program for the athlete who requires high levels of agility. More vertical training will apply to those athletes seeking vertical displacement such as long jumpers, ice skaters, and volleyball and basketball players. Plyometrics also are performed for upper-body activities that require explosive muscle action. Shot-putters, gymnasts, and wrestlers may benefit from plyometric training as a means of gaining explosive power from the shoulder girdle (Fig. 2.6).

In summary, plyometric training uses the athlete's body mass and the force of gravity for resistance as the athlete repeatedly performs bounding (jumping) maneuvers. The major muscle groups that are usually exercised are the musculature surrounding the knee and hip joints. More recent techniques have been developed for the shoulder girdle, using external resistance such as medicine balls rather than body mass and gravity. The risk of orthopedic injury is high due to repetitive eccentric loading of the musculotendinous units, and therefore, proper warm-up techniques are indicated to increase the flexibility of muscle and connective tissue surrounding the involved joints.

Isokinetic Training. Isokinetic training is useful for speed-specific strength training. Fast and slow speed training have been studied with respect to gains in absolute strength as well as other parameters of muscle performance. Perrin et al. (38) revealed the benefits of isokinetic training on muscular strength and power, demonstrating that 7 weeks of fast speed training (270°/sec) is adequate for increases in peak torque (PT), torque acceleration energy (TAE), and average power at variable speeds (60°, 180°, and 270°/sec). Pipes and Wilmore (33) and Thomee et al. (39) in related studies also revealed strength gains from fast speed isokinetic training. It is suggested that the gains result from the adaptations within the fast-twitch (type II) fibers caused by increases in the fiber's cross-sectional area, metabolic function, and recruitment patterns. These reported strength gains also were found to carry over to slower speeds (33, 38, 39). In conclusion, fast speed

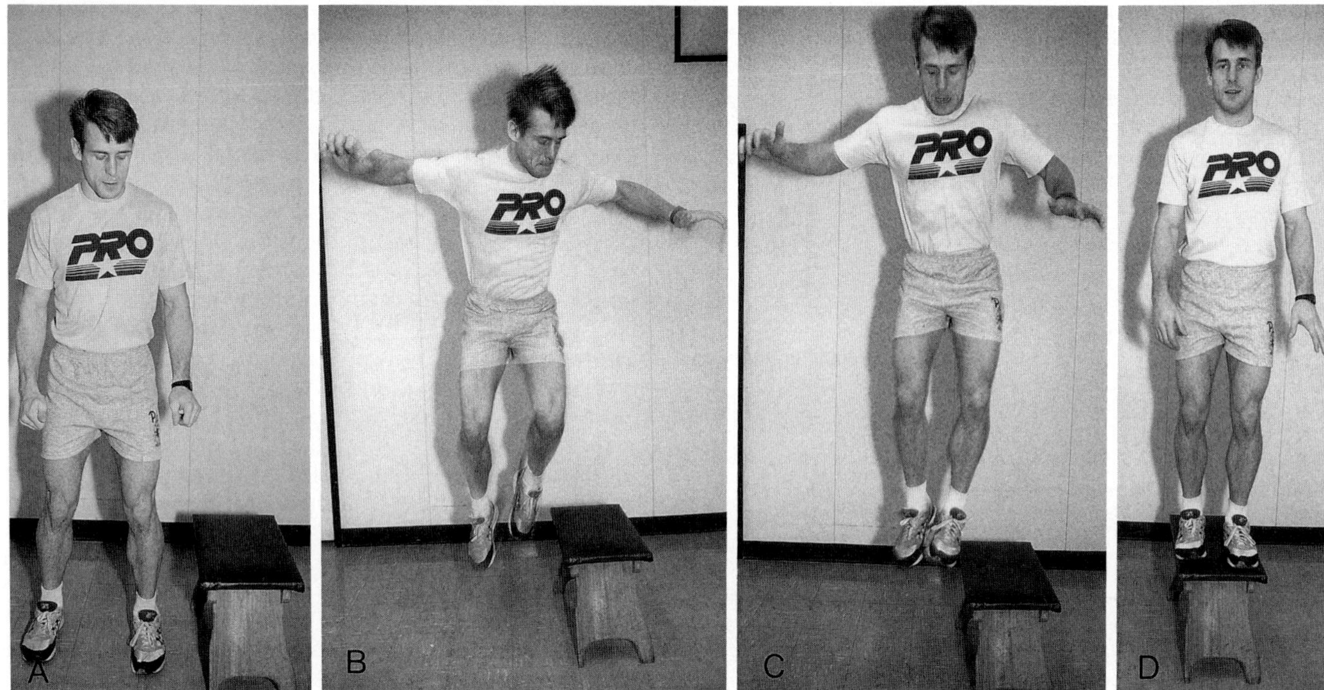

Figure 2.6. Plyometric training involves repetitious jumping from and landing on surfaces of various heights.

isokinetic exercise has been reported to increase muscular strength as well as power. Therefore, athletes who require muscular power may benefit from isokinetic resistance training at high angular velocities.

Increases in muscular strength and power are not beneficial unless they carry over to functional performance, and therefore, one must question the value of isokinetic strength gains for the purpose of performance enhancement. Recent investigations have revealed low correlations between isokinetic strength/power and functional performance (35). The lack of kinetic chain specificity is speculated to be responsible for the weak relationship.

Measurement of Muscular Strength, Power, and Endurance

Assessment of an athlete's strength using quantitative measurements is essential for determining baseline levels and progress during training. Objective strength data can be used to compare various individuals, identify strength gains during training, or provide evidence that one protocol is more effective than another. Because little is known about the etiology of strength gains, more research is necessary to identify which strength programs currently in use are the most beneficial (33, 40). Muscular strength may be measured in three different modes: isometrically, isotonically, and isokinetically.

Isometric. Isometric (static) strength assessments measure the maximal tension produced by a muscle or muscle group(s) independent of changes in muscle length (2, 15). Static measures can be obtained using cable tensiometry and/or dynamometry. Cable tensiometry has the potential to measure the static strength of specific muscles or groups of muscles at various joint angles. The cable is attached to a dynamometer that records the tension or force produced during an isometric contraction (Fig. 2.7). This method is effective for making strength measurements when joint motion is contraindicated. Furthermore, static measures are easily obtained clinically and are easily reproducible for bilateral or reciprocal muscle group comparisons. The dynamometer alone also can measure static strength. The dynamometer differs from the cable technique in that compressive forces are measured rather than tensile forces. Typically, grip strength is measured using a dynamometer (Fig. 2.8).

Isotonic. Isotonic (dynamic) strength measurements are assessed using a constant weight at variable angular velocities through a full range of joint motion. Isotonic assessments include the measurement of maximum weight moved through 1 RM (31, 41). This classic procedure is usually performed using barbell or dumbbell devices to provide a reference weight before planning a strength-training program. The most common 1 RM test is the bench press. This method effectively establishes a submaximal starting weight as a percentage of the 1 RM. The 1 RM isotonic strength assessment also is an efficient means of evaluating the strength of large groups of athletes (12, 41).

Isokinetic. Isokinetic assessment has recently become the standard for all muscle strength evaluation. With the innovation of computer technology, the assessment of muscular strength, power, and endurance can be quantified by interfacing dynamometers with digital microprocessor computers. Isokinetic assessments measure strength at preset angular velocities. Strength is measured as torque, a component of force and velocity. Isokinetic devices are speed controlled with accommodating resistance to maintain preset angular velocities. The velocity spectrum typically ranges from 0°/sec (isometric) to 300°/sec with contemporary isokinetic devices. The isokinetic devices provide rapid and accurate data relative to muscular strength, power, and endurance. These data permit the clinician to make rapid bilateral and reciprocal muscle group comparisons across a spectrum of test velocities (Figs. 2.9 and 2.10).

Isokinetic testing devices also can measure power and endurance at various angular velocities (low-high) and at accommodating resistances. Most joints of the body can be isolated for testing. The Cybex II Dynamometer (Lumex Inc., Ronkonkoma, NY) is a popular device used currently at many sports medicine clinics and universities. The main isokinetic parameters for measuring strength, power, and endurance are PT, TAE, average power, total work, and endurance. Isokinetic testing is an easy and reliable method to establish preseason strength measures, or strength progressions with rehabilitation programs.

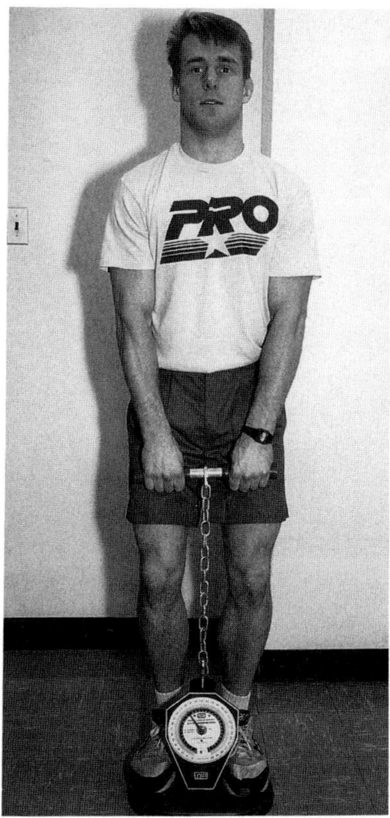

Figure 2.7. Cable tensiometry measures static strength of muscle group(s) through distaction forces. A cable is attached to a dynamometer.

Anaerobic Conditioning

Anaerobic conditioning is important for athletes who require near maximal, quick bursts of muscular power such as sprinters, rowers, and soccer and lacrosse players. Anaerobic conditioning results in the enhanced efficiency of anaerobic energy during exercise. This type of conditioning uses high-energy anaerobic pathways (ATP-CP) and glycolysis for generating the energy necessary to power skeletal muscle contractions.

Exercise that requires near maximal effort up to 2 to 3 min in duration is generated mainly by the anaerobic pathways adenosine triphosphate-creatine phosphate (ATP-CP) and glycolytic energy systems. The two energy systems are anaerobic in nature, because molecular oxygen is not assisting in the formation of the high-energy phosphates (ATP-CP). The ATP-CP system supplies the immediate source of fuel for approximately the first 10 sec of exercise or until the intracellular supply of ATP-CP is exhausted. After depletion of ATP-CP from the exercising cells, a quick shift to glycolysis occurs to continue the yield of ATP-CP. The glycolytic or short-term energy system uses the breakdown of glycogen to resynthesize the high-energy phosphates.

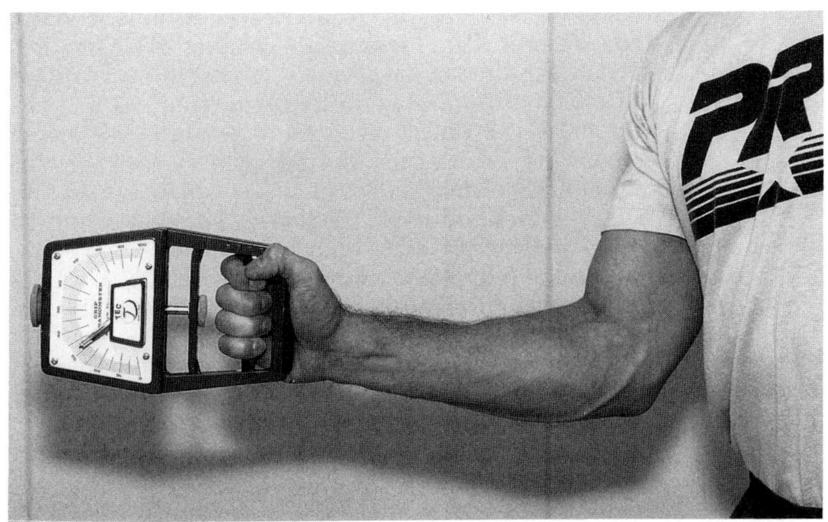

Figure 2.8. Static strength also can be measured with compressive forces on a hand-held dynamometer.

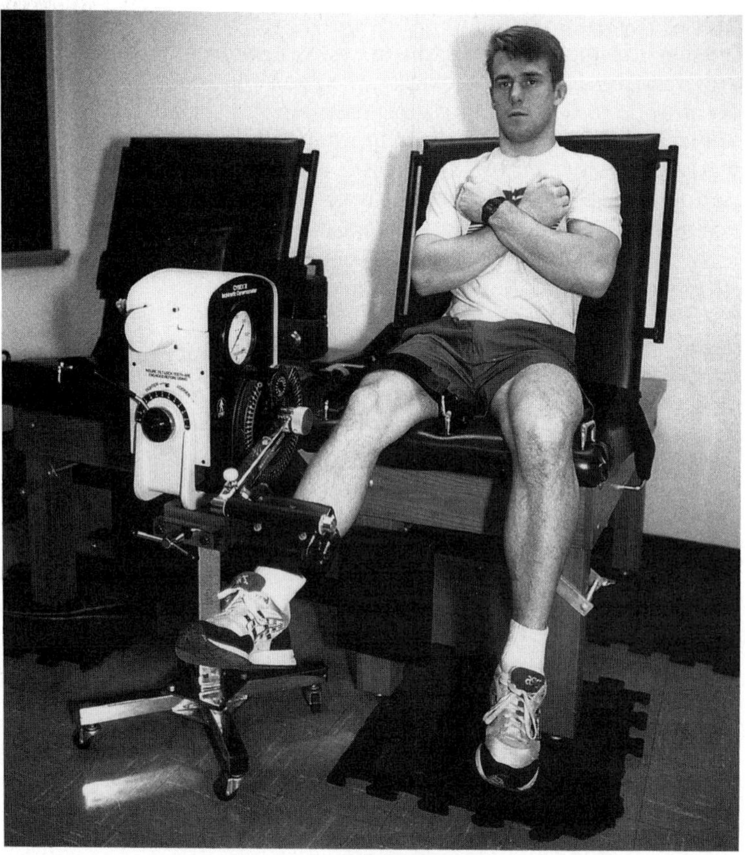

Figure 2.9. Isokinetic strength is quantitatively measured by a dynamometer interfaced with a computer.

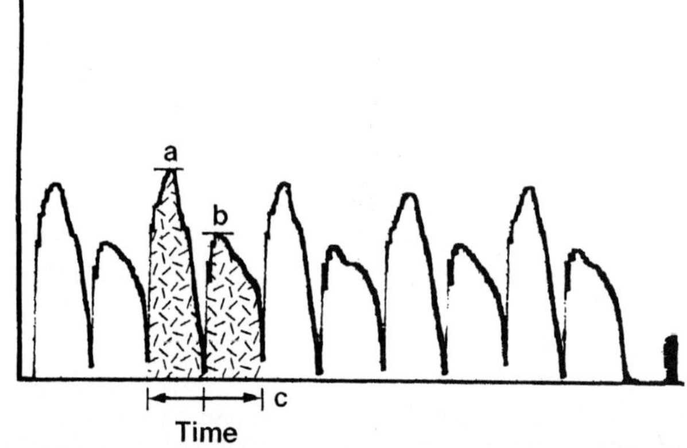

Figure 2.10. The computer printout from a Cybex II isokinetic testing device indicates strength and power output variables associated with knee extension (quadriceps, *a*) and knee flexion (hamstrings, *b*). The vertical axis, or amplitude, represents PT and the horizontal axis represents the total time *(c)* of the muscle contractions. The *shaded area* represents the total work output (torque times time of muscle contraction), and average power is computed by dividing the total work output by the time of contraction.

Immediate and Short-Term Exercise

Immediate (0 to 10 sec). High-intensity–short-duration activity is performed using predominantly fast-twitch, glycolytic muscle fibers (type IIb). These fibers are densely concentrated and consist of high-energy phosphate molecules, which generate most of the muscle contractions associated with activities that are explosive in nature.

Examples of activities that should be incorporated into a program that trains the immediate energy pathways include sport-specific and general-conditioning drills to enhance agility, sprint training (50, 100, 200, and 400 m), and plyometrics. Interval training also will induce metabolic adaptations within the type II fibers, resulting in increased use of ATP-CP for energy.

Short-Term (10 to 180 sec). Activities using the short-term energy pathway generally last from 10 to 180 sec and are powered by fast-twitch, glycolytic (FG) and intermediate fast oxidative glycolytic (FOG) muscle fibers (type IIa and IIb). Training to enhance glycolysis results in production of ATP-CP. Once the immediate ATP-CP sources are exhausted, the short-term pathway will break down glycogen to produce fresh supplies of ATP-CP. Exercise of high intensity (>60% max), and medium duration (30 to 120 sec) will condition this system to function more efficiently. The power output of this short-term, high-intensity system (75% to 90% of $\dot{V}_{O_2max}$ is referred to as an athlete's anaerobic capacity, because of the reliance on anaerobic metabolism for this type of activity (42).

Examples of short-term energy system training include interval training of distances ranging from 100 to 800 m; with short periods of recovery (30 to 60 sec). Resistance training, using high repetitions and low to moderate weight requires anaerobic pathways to provide muscular endurance and fatigue resistance during exercise. Isokinetic training also uses this energy system for muscular contractions at a variety of speeds.

Anaerobic Conditioning Programs

Sprint Training. Athletes that compete in sports that are acyclic and use the immediate energy pathway will benefit from exercises that require explosive power or sprinting. A variety of exercises have been found to be effective for enhancing the reaction time, speed of contractility, and explosive power. Speed athletes run interval sprints or, more recently, sprint against resistance. Many professional and intercollegiate football programs now have their speed athletes sprint with parachute like devices for increased resistance. Other methods of resistance sprinting include having the athlete run against resistive tubing or run in water. These methods follow the overload principle for specific adaptation enhancing the force and speed (acceleration) of contraction.

Athletes such as jumpers (high, long, and triple) and throwers (shot put, discus, hammer, and javelin) typically use plyometrics as a means to increase contractile strength or power. Isokinetic training at fast speeds also may enhance contractility, but the carryover to functional activities has not been proven scientifically.

Interval Training. Interval training is cyclic, incorporating high-intensity exercise for short (50 to 800 m) or moderate (1 mile repeats) distances or durations (10 sec to 6 min). This form of training is more beneficial during the preseason. The frequency of interval training is usually two to four times per week, with active recovery in between sessions. Modes of interval training may vary according to the sport and the specific demands of the sport. Some examples are running on a track, pedaling a stationary or nonstationary bicycle ergometer, and swimming. The anaerobic pathways are trained in combination with the aerobic pathway, although the anaerobic system receives the greatest benefits. Interval training is an efficient means of conditioning the body to function anaerobically. Athletes receive mechanical benefits from interval training; movements become more efficient, or economical. This energy-sparing benefit is significant for athletes who compete for time.

Isokinetic Training. New isokinetic equipment has been developed by Cybex (Lumex Inc., Ronkonkoma, NY) that provides isokinetic resistance during exercise. Cybex has designed a stationary bike and an upper body ergometer (UBE) that provide accommodating resistance at various work loads. Athletes use these devices to enhance their anaerobic power output.

Measurement of Anaerobic Power

Most of the immediate and short-term power output tests assess the athlete's ability to perform a maximal intensity activity, using either time or distance as the indicator of power output. Each measurement must be specific to the energy system that is being tested. For example, tests using immediate power will last approximately 1 to 10 sec, while tests for short-term power will last from approximately 30 sec to 3 min. When these systems are measured in human performance laboratories, they are recorded as units of power output or work. Power is generally expressed in standard units (as ft·lbs) or in metric units (as kg·m/min or sec), horsepower (HP), Newton meters (NM), or watts (W).

Immediate Tests

The most popular modes of measuring immediate power output use high-intensity explosive tests such as jumping, sprinting, stationary bicycling, and isokinetics.

Vertical Jump. The vertical jump assesses athletes' explosive power. The test is designed to isolate the musculature about the hip and thigh. The goal is to measure the displacement of the body vertically against the force of gravity. It is an easy test to conduct and can be used for large groups of athletes. The test is most applicable to volleyball, basketball, track and field, and other sports that rely heavily on the immediate energy system. The test is normalized to individual body weight by using the Lewis Nomogram (3).

The 40- or 50-Yard Dash. The 40- or 50-yard dash is a popular test for horizontal sprint speed. It is a test of acceleration more than of speed, with typical times ranging from 4 to 6 sec. Many sports such as football, use the 40-yard dash as a criterion measure for assessing speed. Sprint speed is highly related to tests of anaerobic power (43), and therefore, it may be used as a test of explosive power because of the short duration of the test.

Torque Acceleration Energy. Isokinetic testing devices have the capability of measuring specific parameters of power output. The Cybex II (Lumex Inc., Ronkonkoma, NY) measures TAE, which is a measure of the explosiveness of a muscle contraction, thus a work per unit time assessment, which defines power. TAE is defined as the total work produced in the first 1/8th of a muscular contraction. TAE has been found to correlate strongly with other tests of anaerobic power (44).

Margaria-Kalamen Step Test. The Margaria-Kalamen (M-K) step test was originally designed by Margaria et al. (45) and later modified by Kalamen (43). The test requires stair climbing at maximal speed and combines horizontal and vertical components, or vectorial displacements, against time. The subject starts 6 m from the stairs, and timing plates are situated on the third (start's timer) and ninth (stop's timer) step. The subject climbs the stairs at maximal speed making contact with the timing plates which record time in milliseconds. The time measure is incorporated into an equation used to calculate power output. The test has been proven valid and is readily used as a test of power (43–45).

Interrelationships of Tests

Lephart et al. (44) found strong relationships between TAE, the vertical jump, and the M-K step test. Furthermore, Kalamen (43) found strong relationships between the M-K step test and sprint speed. This suggests that these tests for immediate power may be used as valid indicators of anaerobic power under explosive conditions.

Short-Term Tests

100-, 200-, 400-, and 800-m Runs. These runs range in time from 10 sec to 2 to 3 min. The tests are valuable for assessing the anaerobic capacity of athletes who participate in sports that require extended periods of anaerobic power output such as middle-distance track, soccer, and basketball.

Bicycle Ergometer. The bicycle ergometer measures anaerobic power and/or capacity indirectly by measuring specific variables associated with power. The test protocols consist of pedaling a stationary bicycle ergometer at a preset resistance with near maximal levels of intensity for a specified period of time (Fig. 2.11). The wheel circumference, athlete's body weight, and number of repetitions are recorded and incorporated into an equation to calculate power output:

$$\text{Power (kg·m/min)} = \frac{\text{(No. of Reps) (Wheel Circumference [m]) (resistance [hg])}}{\text{Time (sec or min)}}$$

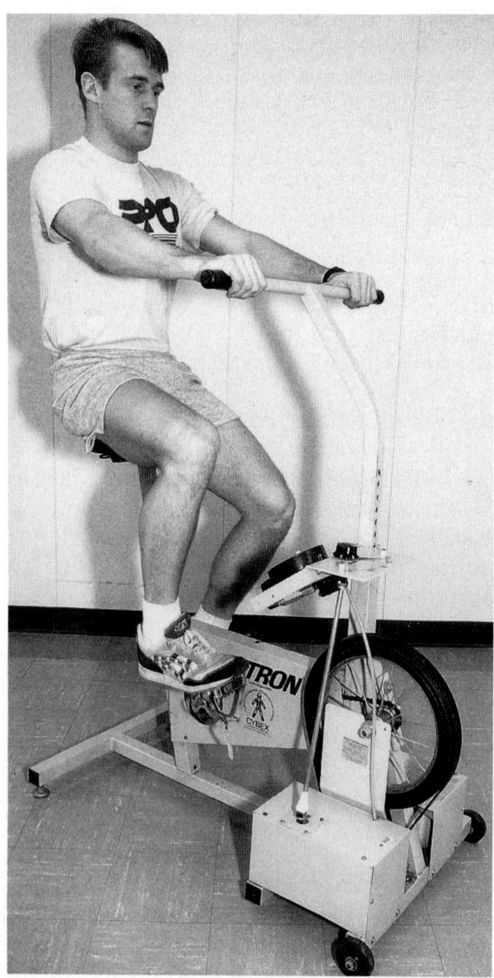

Figure 2.11. A stationary bicycle ergometer is a popular mode for measuring power output.

The most popular bicycle ergometer tests are the Gillum-Katch, Margaria-Kalamen, and Wingate tests for anaerobic power output (42–47).

Average Power, Total Work, and Endurance Ratio. Isokinetic testing devices also have the capability to measure anaerobic capacity by measuring torque production over the time it takes to perform muscle contractions at a constant angular velocity. Total work measures the sum total of power produced over time of contractions. Average power measures the total work produced divided by the time it takes for the entire set of contractions. Clinicians may assess muscular endurance through the 50% decrement test. This index of muscular endurance is assessed simply by recording the number of repetitions at a preset speed (i.e., 180° or 240°/sec) performed by the athlete before failing to produce 50% PT of the 100% PT (48). Another method used for assessing muscular endurance is the endurance ratio, which is calculated by dividing the work performed during the first five contractions by the work performed during the last five contractions when a preset number of repetitions (i.e., 25) are performed at a preset speed (i.e., 240°/sec).

Individual Differences

Several parameters may significantly effect individual scores of performance testing. Factors such as age, sex, motivational level, body weight and composition, and levels of skill and training create differences in scores, resulting in potential errors when compared with the normative data.

Aerobic Conditioning

Long-Term Exercise

Acquiring an aerobic base has often been suggested as a prerequisite to training. The term *aerobic* implies that oxygen is used to generate power for endurance exercise, whereas *base* describes a subthreshold level of aerobic power. Oxygen consumption, $\dot{V}_{O_2}$, is the volume of oxygen used in the process of cellular respiration. Aerobic conditioning involves submaximal endurance training for mainly cyclical activities with durations exceeding 3 min. Although an aerobic base is beneficial, it is important not to ignore the other metabolic systems associated with athletic performance. Dynamic exercise does not use one system exclusively but draws from both aerobic and anaerobic systems when necessary. For example, marathon runners principally use molecular oxygen (aerobic pathways) as their means of regenerating ATP-CP. But because marathoners run at high intensities ($\geq$ 75% to 80% $\dot{V}_{O_2max}$), they also use anaerobic pathways for the generation of muscular power. In addition, runners apply strategies that require short bursts of energy at particular points during the race to overtake an opponent. These bursts require energy supplied from the anaerobic (immediate and short-term) systems.

Unlike anaerobic conditioning, aerobic conditioning uses molecular oxygen to synthesize ATP-CP for energy. Aerobic metabolism oxidizes available substrates (glucose, free fatty acids, and amino acids) to form ATP. This consistent supply of ATP is sufficient to maintain low to moderate submaximal endurance exercise for prolonged periods of time. Therefore, to train this system, athletes must exercise for long durations (3 min to ≥ 1 hr) at low to moderate intensities (≤ 60% max). This training predominantly uses slow-twitch, oxidative (type I) fibers, which have high concentrations of oxidative enzymes and organelles. The fast-twitch, oxidative glycolytic, or intermediate, muscle fibers (type IIa) also are used, in smaller supply, to maintain aerobic power. Through training, the metabolic demands on these fibers increase, producing adaptations in the athlete's oxidative capability.

Examples of aerobic or endurance-type activities include distance training for running, cycling, rowing, stair climbing, cross-country skiing, and aerobics.

Aerobic Conditioning Program

Over-Distance Training. Over-distance training is performed purely for endurance benefits. Athletes who require an aerobic base or need endurance adaptations for long-distance events use over-distance, or long-slow distance (LSD), training. The athlete runs for protracted distances (> 5 miles) for long durations (> 30 min), at low to moderate intensity (40% to 70% $\dot{V}_{O_2max}$). This submaximal exercise produces peripheral adaptations commensurate with this type of activity. For example, the slow-twitch muscle fibers will increase oxygen consumption capacity by increasing mitochondrial and enzymatic efficiency. Lactic acid turnover also will be enhanced. This form of training is beneficial during the preseason for athletes who need to acquire an aerobic base or endurance for their sport.

Steady-Rate or Tempo Training. Steady-rate training has become popular among endurance athletes and is used as an adjunct to LSD and interval training. *Steady rate* implies that oxygen consumption is constant and proportional to the submaximal work load. The volume (frequency and duration) and intensity varies according to personal preferences and period of training. Tempo training may be implemented for sports that require aerobic power over an extended time period. Sports that may benefit include track (distance events), basketball, soccer, wrestling, lacrosse, and swimming.

Combined Program

Fartlek Training. *Fartlek* is a Swedish term meaning "speed play." This type of training is continuous aerobic exercise with interval periods of anaerobic bursts. Distance runners use this type of training to simulate competitive running. LSD running is combined with short periods of speed running. The intensities and durations are flexible with each athlete, thus protocols vary according to personal preference. Overall, this form of training lacks sophistication and is not scientifically recommended; but if done properly, all three systems may be trained simultaneously.

Hill Training. Hill training produces metabolic adaptations for power. The format consists of high-intensity running for specified distances. The hills may vary in grade and length; therefore, the athlete must titrate parameters such as repetition of climbs and recovery between climbs.

These types of training styles are not sport specific and may be formatted to apply to any sport. The training format should match the demands of the sport and also should be incorporated during the proper phase of training.

Measurement of Aerobic Power

$\dot{V}_{O_2max}$/Peak Testing. The most popular mode of directly measuring aerobic power is the $\dot{V}_{O_2max}$/peak test. The $\dot{V}_{O_2max}$/peak test is a volumetric measure of oxygen consumption taken when the muscles are at near maximal effort. The $\dot{V}_{O_2max}$ value is the highest volume of oxygen consumption, whereas $\dot{V}_{O_2peak}$ is the peak level relative to the mode of testing. The subject is tested on a motor-driven treadmill or stationary bicycle ergometer with a gas analyzer attached to his or her mouth, which analyzes the gas exchange ratio (CO_2:O_2). The exercise apparatus is interfaced with a computer, which calculates and prints the variables associated with this form of exercise. A graded, continuous-exercise test protocol is used to reach maximum intensity levels by increasing intensity in increments of time. Intensity is increased by increasing speed and grade of the treadmill and/or the resistance and RPMs of the bicycle ergometer, until the subject reaches the point of exhaustion, at which time the test is terminated. $\dot{V}_{O_2max}$ values are recorded by volume (ml), mass (kg), and time (min) (Fig. 2.12).

John Smith
Body weight = 65 kg
Humidity = 47%

Reports every 30 sec
Sample temperature = 22°C
Barometric pressure = 723 mm Hg

Time	Volume	$\dot{V}_{O_2}$	ml/kg	CO_2	RER	HR	RR
0:30	21.3	− 0.02	− 0.3	− 0.01	0.50	0	14
1:00	25.2	0.50	7.7	0.49	0.98	12	17

Figure 2.12. A computer printout from a graded exercise treadmill test quantifies variables associated with oxygen consumption during maximal or peak exercise. Volume is in liters per minute. *$\dot{V}_{O_2}$*, oxygen consumption (ml/kg/min); *CO_2*, ventilation; *RER*, respiratory exchange ratio; *HR*, heart rate; *RR*, respiratory rate. The variables are measured as a function of time.

Other Predictors of $\dot{V}_{O_2max}$. Several other tests may be used to predict or estimate $\dot{V}_{O_2max}$ through the use of a normative or predictor scale (49, 50). The mode of testing may vary, but all tests require submaximal efforts for a specified time. The tests are easily administered, but not always valid. These tests include endurance runs, step tests, and bicycle ergometer tests.

Endurance Runs. The Cooper 12-min run/walk measures the distance the athlete covers during 12 min. The distance is the criterion measurement, which is used to estimate $\dot{V}_{O_2max}$.

Maximal Heart Rate. Maximal heart rate (HR_{max}) tests require running or pedaling at a specified distance or time, while HR is assessed as the criterion measurement. HR_{max} values are then compared with prediction tables to estimate $\dot{V}_{O_2max}$.

Step Tests. The Howard and Queens step tests use cadence stepping of a known height and time. The recovery HR is measured, recorded, and then incorporated into a prediction equation to estimate $\dot{V}_{O_2max}$.

Bicycle Ergometer Tests. The YMCA test requires pedaling at a preset RPM level and time period. Interval HR measures are taken and compared with a normative data table for estimate of $\dot{V}_{O_2max}$.

Isokinetic Tests. The muscular endurance index (described above) may be used as a test of local muscular endurance.

Interrelationships of $\dot{V}_{O_2max}$ Tests. Relationships between $\dot{V}_{O_2max}$ and submaximal tests to estimate $\dot{V}_{O_2max}$ have been established with measurement errors varying between 10% and 20%. Cooper found a strong correlation between $\dot{V}_{O_2max}$ of air force personnel and the distance they could run/walk in 12 min ($r = .90$) (51). Some investigators have been unsuccessful in reproducing strong relationships among the tests, while other investigators have found a linear relationship between HR and oxygen consumption at submaximal exercise (51).

The limitations of estimates made from submaximal tests are implicit to the design of the particular test. Furthermore, $\dot{V}_{O_2max}$ has not been found to predict athletic performance strongly, although these tests do provide an avenue for the purpose of screening and classifying a large number of athletes in terms of aerobic fitness.

Year-Round Strength and Conditioning Program

The ever-increasing demand for excellence in athletic performance has prompted sports scientists and coaches to develop comprehensive 12-month strength and conditioning programs for their athletes. The premise for a year-round program is to develop and maintain various general and sport-specific performance parameters throughout the year. Most advocates of year-round programs will break down or cycle their program to attain peak performance levels at a preplanned time during the competitive season. This is known as periodization. For example, Olympic athletes train year round with the ultimate goal of peaking exactly when the Olympics begin. For the program to be successful, the athlete must abide by the principles of overload, specificity, and recovery. The variations of volume, intensity, and mode must be varied systematically and in a sophisticated manner to obtain maximal benefits. This section outlines a 12-month strength and conditioning program to demonstrate the benefit of a systematic format of training to achieve peak performance.

Periodization

The design and implementation of a periodized training program was introduced in the 1950s by Russian sports scientists (15). Their objective was to break down athletes' training into component parts that incorporated both short- and long-range goals. For most athletes, especially at the amateur, professional, and intercollegiate levels, the year is broken down into a preseason, precompetition, in-season competition, and postseason recovery.

The preseason objective is to attain a foundation or base level of fitness, whereas the precompetition phase is to work on technical skills in preparation for competition. The in-season phase of the program is dedicated to improving skills and technique while obtaining peak performance. Obtaining peak performance, or "peaking," is manifested from the combined increases of technique, strength, and conditioning. The postseason phase of the program is dedicated to recovery followed by the beginning of light training in preparation of the impending preseason training.

When designing the year-round program one must abide by certain parameters to achieve outcome goals. These parameters include volume (frequency times duration), intensity, and mode of training. If these parameters are not strictly monitored, unwanted setbacks such as overtraining, premature performance peaking, or chronic fatigue may result. The year-round program incorporates a strength and a conditioning phase, as both are integral to the athlete's overall performance.

Strength Program

Each sport has its specific requisites for muscular strength, although common objectives for strength acquisition apply to all sports. The outcome of strength training results in enhanced generation of muscular force by increasing morphologic and neurologic components of muscle contraction. Strength training uses resistance exercise and produces gains by employing the overload principle for specific muscles or muscle groups. The measurable gains in strength are a direct result of the overload principle in action. When the muscle is overloaded, the external force of resistance is significantly greater than the internal force of the muscle contraction(s); the result is hypertrophic changes that occur within the muscle fiber and that adapt to the external resistive forces. The overload force also results in enhanced recruitment of available motor units within the surrounding muscle tissue (15, 28). The combination of increased recruitment and hypertrophy permits greater force generation during muscle contraction(s). The strength phase has three important components that must be addressed to have a progressive and injury-free program: flexibility, sport-specific strength, and muscular endurance. The strength-training programs discussed earlier may be used by the athlete according to phase of training, personal preference, sport specificity, or accessibility for the athlete.

In addition to the development of muscle strength for the whole body, athletes must streamline their training to match their respective sport. This includes training the specific muscle groups that generate force for the techniques that are required for the athlete's performance. The SAID principle works in conjunction with the overload principle and involves sport-specific training, which will induce adaptations that improve athletic performance (15, 28). This component is generally addressed during the preseason and in-season training.

Flexibility training has been shown to improve joint ROM and prevent exercise-induced muscle injury (2, 3). Therefore, flexibility training is used as an adjunct to other types of training and conditioning. Flexibility exercises are classified as active, passive, or active assistive and are performed through "static" or ballistic stretching methods. Active stretching is performed solely by the athlete, whereas passive and active assistive require a partner. Static stretching is preferred before warmup. The slow progressive process of static stretching permits the muscle to lengthen efficiently without the risk of injury. Ballistic stretching uses fast, bouncing-type movements that require the muscle to respond quickly to the imposed changes in length. Ballistic stretching is performed after warmup and requires care because of the high risk of muscle injury (2, 3). Flexibility training will be addressed later in this chapter.

Conditioning Program

The way an athlete uses the three energy systems depends on his or her specific sport. Most sports combine speed with endurance for optimal levels of athletic performance. Soccer players need explosive power and speed for breakaway moves but also require an aerobic base to have enough energy to last through the match. When a conditioning protocol is developed, both the anaerobic and aerobic aspects of the sport must be addressed. For instance, to train effectively the immediate and short-term energy systems, an athlete must train at near maximal intensities for periods of 1 to 10 sec for explosive power and for 30 to 180 sec to increase anaerobic capacity. The transition from predominantly anaerobic to aerobic exercise requires a shift from glycolytic to oxidative pathways. This shift in metabolism requires protracted exercise at moderate to high intensity (70% to 85% $\dot{V}_{O_2max}$) for 2 to 3 minutes. The frequency of training intensity varies according to the season, but high-intensity training is normally alternated with low- to moderate-intensity training.

Concomitant with conditioning the metabolic pathways, the agility requisites also must be addressed. Agility drills for sports that demand balance, coordination, and lateral mobility condition the neuromuscular system for those types of activities.

Phases

As noted above, the 12-month program is divided into a preseason training, precompetition, in-season competition, and postseason recovery phase. The overall objectives of this program are to develop during the preseason, streamline during precompetition, maintain and peak during the in-season, and recover during the postseason. The principal components of athletic performance are strength development, anaerobic/aerobic conditioning, and skill acquisition. Each component is trained and used differently during each phase, according to the specific demands of the athlete's sport.

Preseason Training

Preseason training usually takes place in the 3 months before precompetitive training. It is the foundation from which the athlete develops his or her fitness base. Strength and conditioning are combined within this phase to prepare the athlete for precompetition, when training volume tapers and skill refinement takes precedent. Preseason training also may include active rehabilitation of acute and chronic injuries as well as the identification and correction of any preexisting weaknesses in technique and/or any musculoskeletal imbalances. The training consists of high-volume, moderate- to high-intensity exercise with gradual, progressive increases. Strength training involves low-repetition, high-resistance work, and conditioning consists of anaerobic and aerobic endurance activities.

Precompetition Phase

Precompetition usually begins 1 month before the in-season competition phase. The objectives here are to prepare the athlete for competition. During this phase, the athletes taper off from their high-volume preseason training and concentrate on sport-specific skills. For example, wrestlers use this period to refine their moves both on their feet (take downs) and on the mat (top and bottom). Precompetition workouts are shorter and at moderate- to high-intensity levels. The emphasis is on competition simulation. Strength and conditioning work continues, but their volume and intensity are not as great.

In-Season Competition Phase

The in-season competition phase includes peaking in terms of strength, power, conditioning, and technique. During the in-season phase of the program, general preseason strength and conditioning is streamlined and fine-tuned for sport-specific activities that relate to technique, speed of movement, and timing. The volume of practice time is often reduced to levels that will sustain the strength and conditioning that were established during the preseason. The intensity of the practice sessions are usually increased dramatically to mimic competition. By reducing the volume, the athlete maintains his or her conditioning and strength to meet the demands of the particular sport. The in-season phase lasts 3 to 4 months.

Postseason Recovery Phase

Immediately following the competitive season, most athletes rest 2 to 3 weeks to recover mentally, physically, and emotionally from the stress of competition. The athlete may wish to concentrate on other aspects of his or her life (e.g., coursework, family, friends, or hobbies). The following 3 to 4 months are used for active rest and recovery; the athlete engages in activities other than his or her sport. This practice is known as cross-training and can be an effective means for the athlete to stay active, fit, and injury-free without feeling burned out. This period also may be used for rehabilitation of any injuries incurred during the competitive season. Postseason recovery is important for long-term progress.

In summary, each program must follow the principles associated with exercise training. Overload, specificity, and timing are the crucial ingredients for the progressive increase in skill acquisition, strength, power, endurance, and recovery. Each program must take advantage of the overload and SAID principles to develop the requisite balance of strength and condition for a particular sport. In addition, the proper prescription of volume, intensity, and mode must be applied during the annual phases of training. This will produce a systematic progression in the performance parameters necessary to carry the athlete to proper peaks in training. The postseason recovery phase is a necessary component that permits mental, physical, and emotional rest to prepare the athlete for the next season.

Physiologic Effects of Training

Exercise training produces many biophysical adaptations that enable the athlete to meet the increased physiologic demands of strenuous exercise. Cardiovascular (CV), respiratory, and neuroendocrine adaptations occur as a result of endurance training and are centrally and peripherally manifested. These adaptations, identified below, provide the smooth transition from rest to exercise during endurance training.

Endurance training has shown to increase $\dot{V}_{O_2max}$ (29). Much debate has centered around the relative contributions of the central versus the peripheral system concerning the increase in oxygen consumption. Holloszy and Coyle (29) state that the great capacity of the CV system to deliver oxygen to the exercising muscles is the primary factor responsible for increases in oxygen consumption. Other researchers suggest that oxidative respiration (A-$\dot{V}_{O_2diff}$) is the primary rate-limiting factor during strenuous exercise (30). The oxygen consumption equation is

$$\dot{V}_{O_2} = Q(HR \times SV) \times A\text{-}V_{O_2diff}\ (Ca_{O_2} - Cv_{O_2})$$

Central Adaptations

As a result of exercise training, the CV system becomes more efficient in (1) transporting nutrients (oxygen, glucose, and hormones) to the exercising muscles, (2) extracting the nutrients from the blood, (3) removing metabolic wastes from the muscles, and (4) maintaining thermoregulation. With the onset of exercise, the CV system responds by increasing the cardiac output (Q), which is the volume of blood pumped from the heart per beat. This increase is the result of the increases in both the heart rate (HR) and stroke volume (SV).

Cardiac Output

Cardiac output has been shown to increase 6 liters/min for every 1 liter/min increase in $\dot{V}_{O_2}$ during strenuous exercise involving large muscle masses (52). The relationship between Q and $\dot{V}_{O_2}$ has been found to be consistent with all types of exercise (28, 53) and is regulated by the CNS. $\dot{V}_{O_2}$ is suggested to be the best noninvasive measurement of overall CV function (28, 52, 53).

Stroke Volume and Heart Rate

Stroke volume has been found to increase in proportion to the intensity of exercise until approximately 25% to 50% of $\dot{V}_{O_2max}$, when plateau effect occurs (28, 52). Further increases in Q are a result of increased HR, which also has been found to increase in direct proportion to exercise intensity. From a research standpoint, HR is the most consistent factor involved with increases in Q and $\dot{V}_{O_2}$ during exercise, and SV is considered the rate-limiting factor for determining individual differences in $\dot{V}_{O_2max}$ (28).

$\dot{V}_{O_2}$ and CV function depend on the relative amount of muscle mass used during exercise. For instance, exercises that use large muscle masses (e.g., cross-country skiing, cycling, and running) induce greater CV and $\dot{V}_{O_2}$ adaptations than exercises that use small or localized muscle masses (e.g., weight listing). Also, the volume (frequency and duration) of training will determine CV and $\dot{V}_{O_2}$ function.

Blood Pressure and Flow

As Q increases steadily, blood pressure rises to maintain adequate blood flow to the active tissues. Blood pressure (BP) is the product of cardiac output times the total peripheral resistance (TPR). During exercise, Q increases the volume of blood pumped from the heart, while TPR decreases blood flow (BF) to the inactive tissues and increases BF to the exercising muscles. The CNS regulates BP and BF at levels appropriate for the amount of muscle mass used or oxygen consumed during exercise (53). Increased areas of BF include the brain, heart (coronary), lungs (pulmonary), and skeletal muscles. Resting levels of BF (5 liters/min) have shown fivefold increases (up to 25 liters/min) with exercise at near maximal work loads (28). This adaptation maximizes BF to the exercising muscles and minimizes BF to inactive tissue (54). The ultimate adaptation is greater use of oxygen for peak levels of performance.

Ventilation

An often overlooked yet critical central adaptation to exercise is ventilation. Once venous blood returns to the heart, it is pumped into pulmonary circulation for gas exchange. During exercise, minute ventilation ($\dot{V}_E$) is increased linearly with Q, and this response is commonly known as the ventilatory perfusion ratio ($\dot{V}/\dot{Q}$). Chemoreceptors located in peripheral blood vessels returning deoxygenated blood to the heart are stimulated by high concentrations of carbon dioxide (CO_2). This stimulation causes the lungs to hyperventilate to expel the CO_2 in exchange for O_2. This adaptation is known as the perfusion percentage of blood gases (28). After oxygenation, the blood returns to the heart for transport and use at the periphery. Incidently, the energy cost of hyperventilation on the intercostal muscles is compensated through the increase in BF, as discussed previously.

Peripheral Adaptations

During exercise, BF to the peripheral vessels (arteries, capillaries, and veins) and active muscles increases. As a result of training, the working muscles become more efficient in extracting oxygen and returning carbon dioxide to the blood to meet the elevated metabolic demands of exercise. This process subserves oxidative respiration and is known physiologically as the atrio-venous oxygen difference ($A = \dot{V}_{O_2 diff}$).

Atriovenous Oxygen Difference and Oxygen Consumption

A linear increase in $A = \dot{V}_{O_2 diff}$ has been shown to occur with increases in exercise intensity (30, 55). Oxygen consumption by the active tissues increases until near maximal levels of exercise intensity, at which time a much-debated plateau in $\dot{V}_{O_2}$ has been shown to occur, indicating an oxidative peak. Any further increases in power output after the plateau is suggested to be from anaerobic mechanisms (30). The muscle tissue uses oxygen for oxidative metabolism, and as a result of this increase in oxygen consumption, the metabolic demand of exercise is met, allowing the athlete to train at higher levels of intensity.

Hematologic Adaptations

Hematologic adaptations to aerobic exercise training result in an increase in plasma volume (PV). This adaptation allows for facilitated nutrient and oxygen transportation and also compensates for the loss of TBW as a result of sweat loss (thermoregulation). The hemoconcentration of hemoglobin (Hb) does not change, although it may become diluted as a result of the increase in plasma volume. When the intensity of exercise increases, a shift in the O_2 dissociation curve (Bohr effect) occurs to facilitate gas exchange at the tissue level. This effect works in conjunction with $A = \dot{V}_{O_2 diff}$. When exercising at intensities near $\dot{V}_{O_2 max}$, the CNS will mediate hematologic responses through vasodilatory and/or constrictive mechanisms to satisfy the metabolic needs of the exercising muscles. At the cellular level, the muscle tissue is able to metabolize lactic acid more efficiently, which will enhance the efficiency of the exercising muscles.

Thermoregulation

The mechanisms involved with evaporative cooling have been found to increase in efficiency as a result of training (56). During exercise, the temperature of venous blood becomes elevated through conduction of heat produced from exercise. The blood is then shunted to the subcutaneous tissue layers where it is expelled to the environment. When sweat glands (apocrine and eccrine) are activated, the epidermal surface pores open, allowing heat to escape as a result of the evaporation of sweat. The cooled venous blood is then recirculated to the heart.

Fiber Type

Skeletal muscle contractions are generated by the muscle fibers concentrated within the tissue. Metabolic adaptations occur with exercise training and are specific to fiber type and format of training (endurance versus speed). Each athlete's fiber type ratio is genetically determined and does not change as a function of training. Research has indicated that metabolic capacity will, in some instances, adapt to the specific type of training (SAID principle), but the adaptations are fiber specific (15, 28). Furthermore, some exercise scientists suggest that an athlete's performance capacity may be predicted by the use of biomechanical profiles done from muscle biopsies (28). It has been observed that speed athletes are genetically endowed with a higher percentage of fast glycolytic (white) fibers, whereas predominantly endurance athletes have been found to possess a higher percentage of slow oxidative (red) fibers. Studies have found that speed athletes who combine speed and endurance training will develop the intermediate fast oxidative glycolytic fibers (15, 28, 57). This adaptation has been seen with elite track athletes who initially compete at middle distances (800 and 1500 m) and later become competitive marathoners as a result of combining speed and endurance training.

Neuroendocrine Adaptations

Neural

The role of the CNS during exercise is important in regard to regulating metabolic function. Sympathetic and parasympathetic stimulation of the central nervous system elicits specific CV changes in response to exercise. The adrenal glands release epinephrine and norepinephrine, and along with acetylcholine these hormones regulate the rate, force, and contraction speed of the heart (58). Peripherally, during exercise these hormones induce vasoconstriction of the vessels that supply inactive tissue and vasodilation of the vessels that supply active tissue, thus increasing transport of oxygenated blood for use as well as transporting heated venous blood to the cutaneous regions for evaporative cooling.

Endocrine

The effects of exercise on muscle tissue also result in a need for increased transport of fuel substrates into the muscle cell. Insulin, secreted by specialized cells located in the pancreas, facilitates substrate transport across cell membranes, and if the level of substrates in the blood drop below a certain threshold, the pancreas will release glucagon to maintain blood glucose levels. Thyroid and growth hormones are secondary hormones that also help to regulate fuel substrates at the cellular level as well as growth and repair of muscle tissue.

The hormones renin and angiotensin are released by the kidney as a defense mechanism against rapid fluctuations of plasma volume and blood pressure. These adapted responses maintain and/or increase PV and indirectly mediate BP and BF. This mechanism is primarily accomplished through vasoconstriction of renal arteries that redirects the blood back into general circulation. A secondary response of angiotensin is stimulation of the adrenal glands to release aldosterone, which increases salt and water retention at the kidney and cutaneous regions during evaporative cooling. This also indirectly maintains PV.

Implications for Exercise Training

As noted earlier, athletic performance and exercise training involve activities that are cyclic, acyclic, or cyclic/acyclic combined (semicyclic). Appropriate exercise training results in refined athletic performance that is sport specific. Sports that are cyclic involve technical skills or movement patterns that are repeated continuously for extended durations. Cycling, crew, gymnastics, swimming, and track and field are sports that may be classified as cyclic. Sports that are acyclic in nature involve nonrepetitive activities or spontaneous movement. Soccer, basketball, lacrosse, tennis, baseball, volleyball, and wrestling are sports that may be categorized as acyclic, although not exclusively. Most sports involve combinations of both cyclic and acyclic activities. These semicyclic sports integrate both repetitious and spontaneous activities. The sports mentioned as acyclic are classified as such because athletes perform by responding to external stimuli thus demanding spontaneous movement. External stimuli may be defined as anything in the immediate environment that changes in response to the activity, such as an opponent, a moving ball, or the field of play.

To train athletes to compete at optimal performance levels, sport-specific methods of training should be used to match the requirements of the sport. For example, each sport requires some degree of muscular strength, power, and endurance to overcome some form of external resistance that is inherent to the sport. Wrestlers must overcome the resistance provided by their opponents, and athletes whose sports require jumping (high and long jump, basketball, volleyball, etc.) must overcome the weight of their bodies and the force of gravity to propel themselves horizontally and vertically. Sports that involve throwing activities (baseball, volleyball, tennis, soccer, and shot put) require the athlete to propel the object horizontally and vertically, taking into consideration the weight of the object and the force of gravity. Most athletes also require muscular endurance to resist fatigue and to maintain maximal strength and power levels over long durations.

Each sport uses specific metabolic pathways to provide the necessary central and peripheral adaptations for maximal and submaximal exercises. Athletic performance requires input from both anaerobic and aerobic pathways, and the relative contributions of each pathway depends on the type of activity performed, its intensity, and its volume as well as the overall level of fitness and motivation of the athlete. Strenuous or near maximal intensity exercise demands the recruitment of both type I and II muscle fibers. During immediate anaerobic exercise, a higher percentage of type IIb fibers are recruited, whereas short-term anaerobic and long-term aerobic exercise use type I and IIa fibers. Compositionally, the muscle fibers vary according to capillary, mitochondrial, and enzyme density as well as cross-sectional area. Through endurance training, the FOG (IIa) fibers become more oxidative (30). For example, a speed athlete who develops a high percentage of FOG fibers has the potential to become more efficient at longer distances (i.e., marathon) as a result of the aerobic adaptations within the muscle fiber. Biomechanically, the speed of contraction does not change significantly, but the oxidative capacity of the muscle fiber has the ability to adapt. These adaptations also have been shown to be sport specific for the muscle groups trained for a particular sport. For example, runners and cyclists have demonstrated increases in type IIa fibers in the lower body, whereas swimmers, for example, have demonstrated the same adaptation in the upper body (29, 30). Interval training has been suggested by exercise scientists to be the best method for training both metabolic systems (aerobic and anaerobic) to adapt to strenuous exercise.

These adaptations will benefit athletes that compete in both cyclic and semicyclic sports, but semicyclic training will not produce the same adaptations as cyclic training. Semicyclic sports are usually discontinuous and do not function under the same metabolic conditions as cyclical sports. Furthermore, sports are aerobic. Sprinting is classified as a cyclic sport, yet functions under strictly anaerobic conditions.

Several acyclic or semicyclic sports require agility as well as other sport-specific technical skills. This component of athletic performance must be developed as part of the overall strength and conditioning program. General and sport-specific drills have been designed to enhance and/or refine agility and technique. Agility drills are general movement patterns that carry over to the demands of acyclic and semicyclic sports. These drills involve the combination of lateral, diagonal, and backward movements and include changing direction, stopping and starting, practicing carioca, and doing cutting maneuvers. Technique drills are more sport specific. The serve in tennis is an example of a technical skill that must be developed to optimal performance. In addition, athletic trainers recommend agility and sport-specific technical drills during the late stages of many rehabilitation programs.

In sum, each sport is classified according to the specific types of activity (cyclic, acyclic, semicyclic) used during performance. Furthermore, each sport has specific requirements for muscular strength, power, and endurance as well as for metabolic power and technical skills. To condition and train athletes effectively for a particular sport, sport-specific exercise training programs need to be designed to match the performance demands of that activity. Athletes who adhere to their training programs should benefit in terms of overall performance.

The Effects of Warming Up and Down

Any training and/or conditioning program is not complete without protection against injury. Proper warmup before exercise and a warmdown after exercise have been found to reduce the incidence and/or severity of overuse-type injuries and exercise-induced muscle damage (59–62).

Warming Up

The physiologic demands placed on the muscle fiber during strenuous exercise are often exceeded, causing injury to the musculotendinous unit (59–62). Therefore, an active warmup should include low-intensity exercise such as light jogging or pedaling on a stationary bike for short periods (5 min), followed by muscular stretching to increase tissue temperature and extensibility of the exercising muscles. The increase in tissue temperature results mainly from the heat produced during exercise, while the increase in tissue extensibility lubricates the exercising muscles and supplies them with oxygenated blood (63, 64). In addition, the warmup will initiate cardiorespiratory function.

Warming Down

After intense exercise it is beneficial to bring the muscle tissue temperature down gradually. This warmdown permits the exercising muscle(s) gradually to return to preexercise condition and also may help reduce the occurrence of exercise-induced muscle injury. Furthermore, stretching after warming down also is advocated to maintain flexibility levels and guard against postexercise muscle spasms (37).

Stretching as an Adjunct

A stretching program used as an adjunct to the warmup and warmdown increases the flexibility of the soft tissues about a joint (59–64). Flexibility has long been used as a component of rehabilitation and also has been found to enhance athletic performance and prevent the occurrence of musculotendinous injury (60, 63). Stretching should involve the major articulations and muscle groups for the upper and lower body. Repeated episodes of stretching the soft tissue structures about the major articulations will increase their range of motion. This is the result of mechanical adaptations within the musculotendinous unit that increase the soft tissue extensibility (59–64).

There are various stretching techniques for increasing and maintaining flexibility. The techniques most often used by athletes, coaches, and athletic trainers are presented below.

Techniques for Stretching

Static. Static stretching uses the progressive relaxation effects of soft tissue in response to a slow continuous stretch. This method involves stretching a muscle group(s) to a position of mild discomfort, then holding that position for a period of time (10 to 30 sec) (2, 62). This process should be repeated several times; the amount of stretch is increased in small increments with each repetition. Static stretching has been found to be an effective and safe means of increasing tissue extensibility (62). An advantage to this method of stretching is that it may be performed with or without a partner.

Ballistic. Ballistic stretching is the oldest and most often misused technique for stretching. These stretches use the stretch/relax reflex of muscle tissue (2) that occurs at very rapid speeds. The stretching technique involves repetitive bouncing motions, resulting in increased tissue extensibility. The bouncing motion causes the rapid, repetitive stretch of a muscle group. For example, if an athlete wishes to stretch the hamstrings, he or she would flex the trunk forward, which in turn would stretch the hamstrings. If the muscles are not properly warmed up or prestretched by other means, the sudden forces generated by the bouncing action of ballistic stretching may exceed the extensibility of the musculotendinous unit, inducing tissue damage (2).

Ballistic stretching does have applications to athletic performance when training for strength, speed, or power. Athletes that use plyometric training impose similar demands on the musculotendinous units, but at higher intensities. Therefore, ballistic stretching may be an effective precursor or warmup for plyometric training.

Proprioceptive Neuromuscular Facilitation. Proprioceptive neuromuscular facilitation (PNF) is a neurophysiologic phenomenon that was initially used as a rehabilitative modality; it is now used universally as a means of muscle stretching. PNF requires a partner to assist actively in the stretching process. The stretch/relax reflex is a neurophysiologic mechanism used to stretch specific muscle group(s). This reflex is inhibited by alternating the contract/relax phases of specific antagonist and agonist muscle groups. The contract/relax phases function to inhibit autogenically and reciprocally muscle resistance to stretch and allow for greater levels of tissue extensibility (2, 65, 66) (Fig. 2.13).

PNF methods are theoretically sound, yet their efficacy has not been proven scientifically. Personal testimonies and anecdotal evidence from trainers, coaches, and athletes provide support for this method of stretching.

All three stretching techniques have been found to increase flexibility, but their use requires some precaution. Most athletic trainers recommend warming up be-

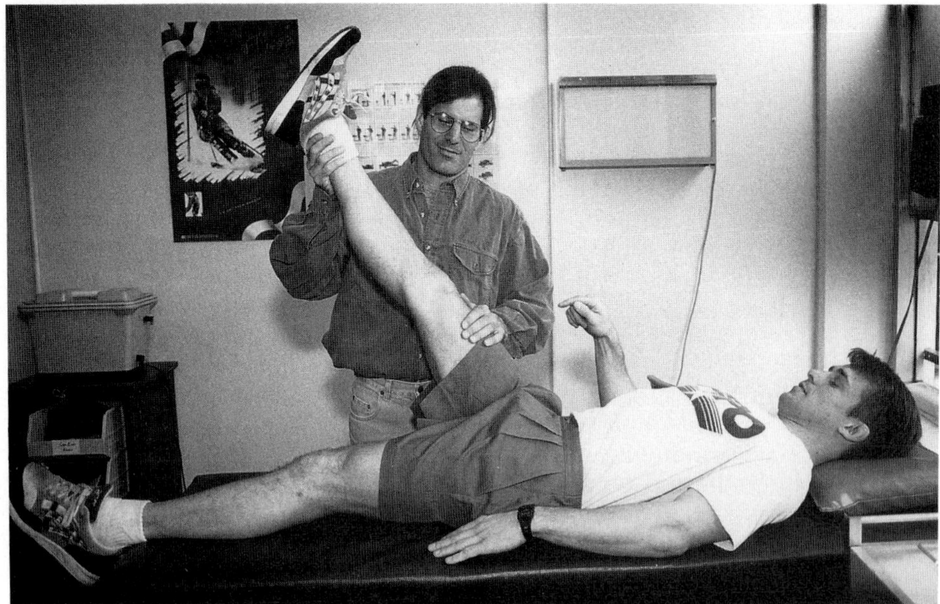

Figure 2.13. Proprioceptive neuromuscular facilitation (PNF) is a popular method of increasing muscle flexibility. A disadvantage to this method is that a partner is needed for active assistance.

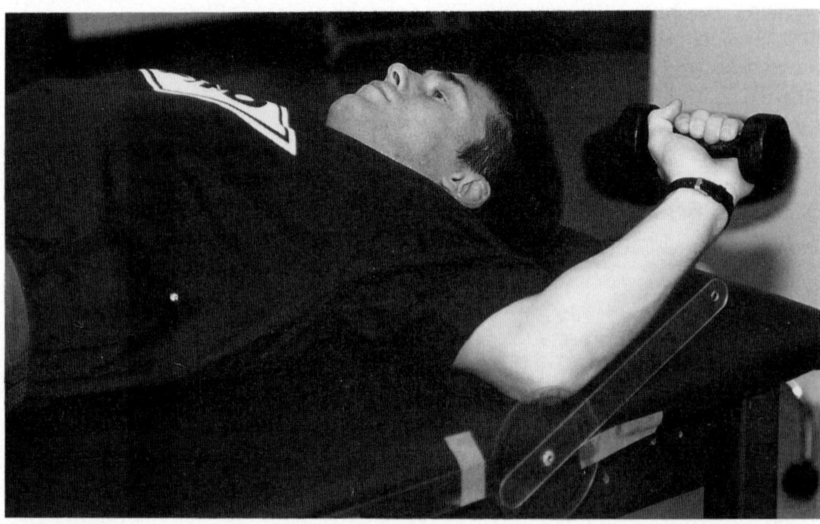

Figure 2.14. Any strength-training program should include flexibility training to increase strength throughout the entire ROM as well as to prevent injury.

fore stretching, especially for ballistic stretching. This technique should only be implemented when an athlete is thoroughly warmed up, because of the risk of injury. Static stretching is the most widely recommended method because it is safe, effective, and easy to perform. PNF, on the other hand, has been suggested to be the most effective in producing increases in flexibility (64, 67), but it requires a partner as well as some practical experience, because of its elaborate protocol.

In addition, significant relationships have been shown to occur between muscular strength and flexibility, and some experts suggest that strength training combined with a flexibility program may greatly enhance athletic performance (Fig. 2.14).

Pain Associated with Exercise

Pain associated with exercise is experienced by most athletes during their training. This pain may occur acutely during exercise or following exercise, depending on the physical condition of the athlete and the type and intensity of exercise. Exercise-induced pain is produced mechanically from damage to the contractile elements within the muscle fiber and/or metabolically from the accumulation of noxious chemicals within the muscle cell. This section discusses the major concepts, mechanisms, and management procedures involved with exercise-induced pain.

Acute Pain

Concept and Mechanisms

Functionally, the initial sign of acute pain during strenuous exercise is muscular fatigue (68) and is thought to be induced both mechanically and metabolically. The symptoms of acute pain are often described as the "burning" or unpleasant sensation felt within the muscle during strenuous exercise (69). The metabolic component associated with acute pain is thought to be caused by the accumulation of metabolites such as lactic acid and noxious chemicals at the cellular level (28, 70, 71). Some researchers suggest that mechanical damage or microtrauma to the contractile elements within the muscle fiber causes the initial sensations of acute pain (68, 70).

Management

The best treatment for pain associated with exercise is preparation. An athlete who is well-conditioned and physically trained will withstand the painful effects of strenuous exercise better than the untrained individual (72–74). A proper warmup and stretching program also may lessen the effects of acute pain during exercise (64). In addition, warming down followed by cryotherapy postexercise may decrease the associated effects of pain and muscle spasm commonly seen during the inflammatory response (37).

Exercise-Induced Muscle Damage

Concept and Mechanisms

Exercise-induced muscle damage occurs during strenuous and prolonged exercise and manifests long after exercise. The initial mechanism is thought to be mechanically induced through structural damage to the contractile elements of the muscle fiber (68, 75–78). High-intensity or prolonged exercise in which eccentric muscle contractions are used is thought to cause structural damage or microtrauma with metabolically induced secondary damage (75–79). The pain and stiffness of exercise-induced muscle damage is seen clinically as the loss of contractile force as well as pain with attempted movement. The symptoms experienced 24 to 72 hr (1 to 3 days) postexercise are clinically referred to as *delayed-onset muscle soreness* (DOMS). This form of retroactive pain may occur as a result of microtrauma to the fibers and the subsequent reparative phases of healing (75–79).

Management

Proper conditioning and training before strenuous exercise helps prevent the incidence and/or severity of exercise-induced muscle damage. A warmdown and stretching done postexercise have been suggested as effective safeguards against DOMS (37). Once DOMS is present, early treatment ($\leq$ 24 hr postexercise) of rest and cryotherapy often lessen the intensity of pain. Late treatment (24 to 72 hr postexercise) should focus on restoring the extensibility of muscle tissue. Warm whirlpools followed by low-intensity static stretching facilitate recovery from DOMS.

Summary

1. Although the specific requirements of each sport vary according to the skills necessary to perform the activity, there are general underlying functional characteristics that are common to all performance. Muscular strength, power, speed, endurance, and agility are elements that lay the foundation of all sports activity.
2. Sports are classified according to their degree of continuity. Cyclic sports are continuous and vary little in regard to technique. Acyclic and semicyclic sports are discontinuous and require a variety of movement patterns.
3. An athlete's body composition has been shown to be closely related to athletic performance and susceptibility to injury. Therefore, athletes should consider their ratio of lean body tissue to fat tissue.
4. The assessment of body composition involves the measurement of body density and the estimation of percent body fat and lean body mass. Hydrostatic weighing and skinfold thickness and circumferential measurements are methods used to estimate body composition.
5. Muscular strength is an integral component of athletic performance. Strength development is a function of muscular growth and adaptation. Muscular power is an extension of strength, combining strength and speed of muscular contraction. Muscular endurance is the ability of muscles to resist fatigue during work output.
6. Skeletal muscle is composed of fibers that are adaptable to exercise training. Hyperplasia and hypertrophy are specific adaptations that occur with strength training. Strength development needs to occur functionally, thus enhancing selected performance characteristics.
7. Muscular strength, power, and endurance are developed via various modes of training. The modes are specific to the type of force-generating capabilities within the exercising muscle. The four principal modes of strength training are isometric, isotonic, isokinetic, and plyometric. Using these modes, specific strength-training programs have been designed to develop functional strength specific to particular sports. Progressive resistance exercise, circuit resistance training, and plyometric training are some popular programs designed to develop functional strength.
8. Assessment of muscular strength, power, and endurance, using quantitative measurements, is essential for determining baseline data and progress of training. These factors can be objectively mea-

sured using isometric, isotonic, and isokinetic techniques.

9. Exercise that requires near-maximal effort up to 2 to 3 min is generated mainly by anaerobic pathways. Anaerobic power is divided into immediate and short-term power, depending on the duration of exercise. Immediate power uses high-energy phosphates, whereas short-term power uses glycogen to resynthesize the high-energy phosphates. The measurement of anaerobic power assesses the athlete's ability to perform maximal-intensity exercise, and each measurement must be specific to the energy system used.
10. Aerobic conditioning involves submaximal endurance exercise for activities exceeding 3 min. Aerobic conditioning enhances aerobic power, which uses oxygen to resynthesize the high-energy phosphates during exercise. The most popular method of assessing aerobic power is graded exercise tests, which measure oxygen consumption during intense exercise.
11. The ever-increasing demand for excellence in athletic performance has prompted sports scientists and coaches to develop comprehensive 12-month strength and conditioning programs for their athletes. Most advocates of the year-round program implement some form of periodization to attain peak performance levels at a preplanned time during the competitive season. The 12-month program is broken down into four phases: preseason, precompetition, in-season, and postseason.
12. For the year-round strength and conditioning program to be successful the athlete must abide by the principles of overload, SAID, timing, and recovery. The principles are applied progressively to develop the requisite balance of muscular strength, power, endurance, and skill needed for a particular sport. In addition, the prescription of volume, intensity, and mode of exercise must be applied during the annual phases of training. This prescription produces a systematic progression in the performance parameters necessary to carry the athlete to proper peaks in training. If these parameters are not strictly adhered to, unwanted setbacks such as overtraining, chronic fatigue, injury, and premature performance peaking may result.
13. Exercise training produces many biophysical adaptations that enable the athlete to meet the increased physiologic demands of strenuous exercise. These central and peripheral adaptations provide the smooth transition from rest to exercise during endurance training.
14. Proper warmup before exercise and a warmdown postexercise have been found to reduce the incidence and/or severity of overuse-type injuries and exercise-induced muscle damage. A stretching program used as an adjunct to the warmup and warmdown increases the flexibility of the soft tissues about a joint. Flexibility has long been used as a component of rehabilitation and also has been found to enhance athletic performance and prevent the occurrence of musculotendinous injury. Static, ballistic, and proprioceptive neuromuscular facilitation are the stretching techniques most often used by athletes, coaches, and trainers.
15. Pain associated with exercise is experienced by most athletes during training. This pain may occur acutely during exercise or following exercise, depending on the physical condition of the athlete and the type and intensity of exercise. Exercise-induced pain is produced mechanically from damage to the contractile elements within the muscle fiber and/or metabolically from the accumulation of noxious chemicals. The best treatment for exercise-induced pain is rest, warm whirlpools, light stretching, and cryotherapy.

REFERENCES

1. Bompa TO. Theory and methodology of training: the key to athletic performance. Dubuque, IA: Kendall/Hunt, 1983.
2. Prentice WE. Techniques of reconditioning. In: Prentice WE, ed. Rehabilitation techniques in sports medicine. St. Louis: CV Mosby, 1990:34–59.
3. Fox EL, Bowers RW, Foss ML. The physiological basis of physical education and athletics. 4th ed. Dubuque, IA: Brown, 1989.
4. Wilmore JH. Training for sport and activity: The physiological basis of the conditioning process. 2nd ed.: Boston: Allyn & Bacon, 1982.
5. Wilmore JH. Body composition in sport and exercise: directions for future research. Med Sci Sports Exerc 1983;15(1):21–31.
6. Keys A. The biology of human starvation. Minneapolis: University of Minnesota Press, 1950.
7. Cureton KJ, Sparling PB, Evans BW, Johnson SM, Kong JW, Purvis JW. Effect of experimental alterations in excess weight on aerobic capacity and distance running performance. Med Sci Sports 1978;10:194–199.
8. Montgomery DL. The effect of added weight on ice hockey performance. Phys Sportmed 1982;10(11):91–99.
9. Pollock ML, Gettman LR, Mileses CA, Bah MD, Durstine JL, Johnson, RB. Effects of frequency and duration of training on attrition and incidence of injury. Med Sci Sports 1977;4:31–36.
10. Lohman TG. Research progress in validation of laboratory methods of assessing body composition. Med Sci Sports Exerc 1984;16(6):596–603.
11. Clarys, JP. Gross tissue weights in the human body by cadaver dissection. Hum Biol 1984;56:459.
12. Behnke AR, Wilmore JH. Evaluation and regulation of body build and composition. Englewood Cliffs, NJ: Prentice-Hall, 1974;39–50.
13. Timson BF, Coffman JL. Body composition by hydrostatically weighing at total lung capacity and residual volume. Med Sci Sports Exerc 1984;16(4):411–414.
14. Katch FI. Practice curves and errors of measurement in estimating underwater weight by hydrostatic weighing. Med Sci Sports Exerc 1969;1(4):212–216.
15. McArdle WD, Katch FI, Katch VL. Exercise physiology: energy, nutrition, and human performance. 3rd ed. Philadelphia: Lea & Febiger, 1991.
16. Morrow JR, Jackson AS, Bradley PW, Hartung GH. Accuracy of measured and predicted residual lung volume on body density measurements. Med Sci Sports Exerc 1986;18(6):647–652.
17. Siri WE. Body composition from fluid spaces and density: analysis of methods. In: Techniques for measuring body composition. Washington, DC: National Academy of Sciences, 1961:223–244.
18. Brozek JF, Grande F, Anderson JT, Keys A. Densiometric analyses of body composition: revision of some quantitative assumptions. Ann N Y Acad Sci 1963;110:113–140.
19. Keys A, Brozek J. Body fat in adult man. Physiol Rev 1953;33:245–325.

20. Pollock ML, Jackson AS. Research progress in validation of clinical methods of assessing body composition. Med Sci Sports Exerc 1984;16(6):606–613.
21. Jackson AS, Pollock ML. Practical assessment of body composition. Phys Sportsmed 1985;13(5):76–90.
22. Sinning WE, Wilson JR. Validity of "generalized" equations for body composition analysis in women athletes. Res Q Exerc Sport 1983;55(2):153–160.
23. Sinning WE, Dolny DG, Little KD, et al. Validy of "generalized" equations for body composition analysis in male athletes. Med Sci Sports Exerc 1984;17(1):124–130.
24. Lohman TG. Skinfolds and body density and their relationship to body fatness: a review. Hum Biol 1981;53:181–225.
25. Katch FL, McArdle WD. Prediction of body density from simple anthropometric measurements in college age men and women. Hum Biol 1973;45:445–454.
26. Tran ZV, Weltman A. Generalized equations for predicting body composition from girth measurements [Abstract]. Med Sci Sports Exerc 1986;18(suppl):S32.
27. Oppliger RA, Tipton CM. Iowa wrestling study: cross-validation of the Tcheng-Tipton minimal weight prediction formulas for high school wrestlers. Med Sci Sports Exerc 1987;20(3):310–316.
28. Brooks, GA, Fahey TD. Exercise physiology: human bioenergetics and its applications. New York: Macmillan, 1985.
29. Holloszy JO, Coyle EF. Adaptations of skeletal muscle to endurance exercise and their metabolic consequences. J Appl Physiol Respir Environ Exerc Physiol 1984;56(4):831–838.
30. Noakes TD. Implications of exercise testing for prediction of athletic performance: a contemporary perspective. Med Sci Sports Exerc 1988;20:319–330.
31. Berger RA. Comparison of static and dynamic strength increases. Res Q 1962;33:329–333.
32. Gardner GW. Specificity of strength changes of the exercised and nonexercised limb following isometric training. Res Q 1963;34:98–101.
33. Pipes TV, Wilmore JH. Isokinetic vs isotonic strength training in adult men. Med Sci Sports Exerc 1975;7(4):262–274.
34. Kraemer WJ. Involvement of eccentric muscle action may optimize adaptations to resistance training. Sports Sci Exchange 1992;4(41).
34a. Dudley GA, Tesch PA, Miller BJ, Buchanan P. Importance of eccentric actions in performance adaptations to resistance training. Aviat Space Environ Med 1991;62:543–550.
35. Lephart SM, Perrin DH, Fu FH, Gieck JH, McCue FC, Irrgang JJ. Relationships between selected physical characteristics and functional capacity in the anterior cruciate ligament-insufficient athlete. J Orthop Sport Phys Ther 1992;16(4):174–181.
36. DeLorne TL, Watkins AL. Progressive resistance exercise. New York: Appleton Century Crofts, 1951.
37. Gamble JN. Strength and conditioning for the competitive athlete. In: Kulund DN. The injured athlete. 2nd ed. Philadelphia: JB Lippincott, 1988:111–150.
38. Perrin DH, Lephart SM, Weltman A. Specificity of training on computer obtained isokinetic measures. J Orthop Sports Phys Ther 1989;10(12):495–498.
39. Thomee R, Renstrom P, Grimby G, Peterson L. Slow or fast isokinetic training after knee ligament surgery. J Orthop Sports Phys Ther 1987;8(10):475–479.
40. Clarke DH. Adaptations in strength and muscular endurance resulting from exercise. In: Wilmore JH, ed. Exercise and sport science reviews. New York: Academic Press, 1973;1:73–102.
41. Mayhew JL, Ball TE, Bowen JL. Prediction of bench press lifting ability from submaximal repetitions before and after training. Sports Med Train Rehab 1992;3:195–201.
42. Katch VL, Weltman A. Interrelationship between anaerobic power output, anaerobic capacity and aerobic power. Ergonomics 1979;22(3):325–332.
43. Kalamen J. Measurement of maximum muscular power in man. Doctoral dissertation, Ohio State University, Columbus, 1968.
44. Lephart SM, Perrin DH, Manning JM, Gieck JH, McCue FC, Saliba EN. Torque acceleration as an alternative predictor of anaerobic power [Abstract]. Med Sci Sports Exerc 1987;19:59.
45. Margaria R, Aghemo P, Rovelli E. Measurement of muscular power (anaerobic) in man. J Appl Physiol 1966;21(5):1662–1664.
46. Patton JF, Duggan A. An evaluation of tests of anaerobic power. Aviat Space Environ Med 1987;58:237–242.
47. Komi PV, Rusko H, Vos J, Vihko V. Anaerobic performance capacity in athletes. Acta Physiol Scand 1977;100:107–114.
48. Pressley SC, Clark RD, Adams R, Lephart SM, Robertson RJ. A comparison of values obtained from the cybex II and kin-com II isokinetic dynamometers for peak torque and muscular endurance [Abstract]. Athletic Train 1991;26:150.
49. Fox E. A simple accurate technique for predicting maximal aerobic power. J Appl Physiol 1973;35(6):914–916.
50. Astrand P, Rhyming I. A nomogram for calculation of aerobic capacity (physical fitness) from pulse rate during submaximal work. J Appl Physiol 1954;7:218–221.
51. Baumgartner TA, Jackson AS. Measurement for evaluation in physical education. 2nd ed. Dubuque, IA: Brown, 1982.
52. Bevegard BS, Shepard JT. Regulation of the circulation during exercise in man. Physiol Rev 1967;47:178–213.
53. Rowell LB. Human circulation regulation during physical stress. New York: Oxford Press, 1986.
54. Lewis SF, Snell PG, Taylor WF, et al. Role of muscle mass and mode of contraction in circulatory responses to exercise. J Appl Physiol 1985;58:146–151.
55. Coyle EF. Cardiovascular function during exercise: neural control factors. Sport Sci Exchange 1991;4(34).
56. Saltin B, Hermansen L. Esophageal, rectal, and muscle temperature during exercise. J Appl Physiol 1966;21:1757–1762.
57. Skinner JS, McLellan TH. The transition from aerobic to anaerobic metabolism. Res Q Exerc Sport 1980;51(1):234–248.
58. Ekblom BA, Kilbom A, Soltysiak J. Physical training bradycardia and autonomic nervous system. Scand J Clin Lab Invest 1973;32:249–256.
59. Holt LE. Scientific stretching for sport (3-S). Halifax, N.S., Canada: Sports Research Ltd., 1976.
60. Anderson B, Beaulieu JE, Cornelius WL, Dominquez RH, Prentice WE, Wallace L. Roundtable: flexibility. Natl Strength Conditioning Assoc J 1984;6:10–22, 71–73.
61. Corbin CB, Noble L. Flexibility: a major component of physical fitness. J Phys Educ Rec 1980;51:23–60.
62. deVries HA. Evaluation of static stretching procedures for improvement of flexibility. Res Q 1962;33:222–229.
63. Sapega AA, Quendenfeld TC, Moyer RA, Butler RA. Biophysical factors in range of motion exercise. Phys Sportsmed 1981;9(12):57–65, 106.
64. Cornelius WL, Hands MR. The effects of a warm-up on acute hip joint flexibility using a modified PNF stretching technique. J Athletic Train 1992;27(2):112–114.
65. Osternig LR, Robertson RN, Troxel RK, Hansen P. Differential responses to proprioceptive neuromuscular facilitation (PNF) stretch techniques. Med Sci Sports Exerc 1989;22(1):106–111.
66. Prentice WE. A comparison of static stretching and PNF stretching for improving hip joint flexibility. Athletic Train JNATA 1983;18:56–59.
67. Wallin D, Ekblom B, Nordenborg T. Improvement of muscle flexibility: a comparison between two techniques. Am J Sports Med 1985;13:263–268.
68. Apple H-J, Soares J, Duarte JAR. Exercise, muscle damage and fatigue. Sports Med 1992;13(2):108–115.
69. Nolan MF. Pain: the experience and its expression. Clin Manage 1900;10(1):22–25.
70. Noakes TD. Effects of exercise on serum enzyme activities in humans. Sports Med 1987;4:2245–2267.
71. Beaver WL, Wasserman K. Muscle RQ and lactate accumulation from analysis of the $VCO_2 = VO_2$ relationship during exercise. Clin J Sports Med 1991;1:27–34.
72. Maxwell JH, Bloor CM. Effects of conditioning on exertional rhabdomyolysis and serum creatine kinase after severe exercise. Enzyme 1981;26:177–181.
73. Seaman R, Ianuzzo CD. Benefits of short-term muscular training in reducing the effects of muscular over-exertion. Eur J Appl Physiol 1988;58:257–261.
74. Schwane JA, Williams JS, Sloan JH. Effects of training on delayed muscle soreness and serum creatine kinase activity after running. Med Sci Sports Exerc 1989;19:584–589.
75. Clarkson PM, Nosaka K, Braun B. Muscle function after exercise-

induced muscle damage and rapid adaptation. Med Sci Sports Exerc 1991;24(5):512–520.
76. Byrd SK. Alterations in the sarcoplasmic reticulum: a possible link to exercise-induced muscle damage. Med Sci Sports Exerc 1991;24(5):531–536.
77. Armstrong RB, Warren GL, Warren JA. Mechanisms of exercise-induced muscle fibre injury. Sports Med 1991;12(3):184–207.
78. Friden J, Lieber RL. Structural and mechanical basis of exercise-induced muscle injury. Med Sci Sports Exerc 1991;24(5):521–530.
79. Potteiger JA, Blesing DL, Wilson GD. Effects of varying recovery periods on muscle enzymes, soreness, and performance in baseball pitchers. J Athletic Train 1992;27(1):27–31.

3 / THE ATHLETIC TRAINER

Robert O. Blanc, Laura E. Clark, Scott M. Lephart, Karl A. Salesi, and Kerry E. Waple

Athletic Training

Sports medicine is a multidisciplinary field that focuses on providing health care to athletes. The one profession that exclusively provides sports medicine services is athletic training. The athletic trainer is the primary health care provider for the athlete; he or she will use various other professionals to make up the sports medicine team when such professional expertise is required. The athletic trainer's role encompasses the athletic health care gamut from prevention of injuries to safely returning the athlete to activity following injury. For these reasons, it is the athletic trainer who is the focal professional of this multidisciplinary field.

The profession of athletic training has evolved from its early days of simply providing basic first aid and emergency management into its present-day sophistication, which has recently been acknowledged by the American Medical Association as an allied health profession. The National Athletic Trainer's Association (NATA) was formed in 1950 for the purpose of establishing and disseminating a knowledge base relative to injury prevention and management (1). Today the NATA has more than 9000 certified members practicing athletic training throughout the world.

Education Programs

Education programs were established in 1969 when the NATA approved its first program. The original athletic training education programs were designed to provide the student with a basic science foundation in human anatomy and physiology and an extensive clinical education in athletic training settings. In 1982, educational programs underwent significant changes following the landmark "Role Delineation Study" conducted by the NATA, which established the roles and responsibilities of the athletic trainer by surveying its members (2). As an result of this study, areas of emphasis were identified and academic programs restructured their curricula accordingly. Table 3.1 illustrates the subject matter requirements of current athletic training educational programs.

The academic curricula are structured to provide instruction in seven major task areas, which were established following the Role Delineation Study. Each of the task areas are weighed in terms of their relative importance to the practicing athletic trainer (Table 3.2). Within each task area, competencies have been established in the cognitive, psychomotor, and affective domains. These competencies provide the framework for the presentation of subject matter within the athletic training education programs.

The seven major task areas and their respective competencies are taught in both the classroom and clinical setting. Education programs can be either major academic degree programs (approved education programs) or interdisciplinary degree programs (internship programs) in which the student completes specific course requirements. The clinical component of the athletic training education program requires the student to accumulate 800 to 1500 hr of athletic training experience under the supervision of a certified athletic trainer. Those students enrolled in an NATA approved education program must accrue a minimum of 800 hr, whereas those students in an internship program must accrue a minimum of 1500 hr.

Certification

Upon completion of this designated education program, the prospective athletic trainer is eligible to take the certification examination administered by NATA. After the student passes the examination, he or she receives the credential of Athletic Trainer, Certified

Table 3.1.
Subject Matter Requirements of Approved Athletic Training Education Programs

Prevention of athletic injuries and illnesses
Evaluation of athletic injuries and illnesses
First aid and emergency care
Therapeutic modalities
Therapeutic exercise
Administration of athletic training programs
Human anatomy
Human physiology
Exercise physiology
Kinesiology and biomechanics
Nutrition
Psychology
Personal and community health
Instructional methods

Table 3.2.
Major Task Areas and Relative Importance in Athletic Training

Task Area	Importance
Prevention of athletic injuries	18
Evaluation and recognition of athletic injuries and medical referral	24
First aid and emergency care	22
Rehabilitation and reconditioning	20
Organization and administration of athletic training services	9
Counseling and guidance of athletes	3.5
Education of athletes, coaches, and student athletic trainers	3.5

(A.T.,C.). The certification examination reflects the responsibilities of an athletic trainer as identified by the Role Delineation Study and, therefore, reflects the education preparation. The examination evaluates the athletic trainer's proficiency in all three of the domains within each task area in both written and practical format.

Employment

Currently, the athletic trainer enjoys a wide array of employment opportunities. Entry-level athletic training positions exist in high schools, colleges and universities, professional sports organizations, and in private health care facilities. Today, many high school athletic training positions are available because of the recent exposure of the athletic training profession coupled with the institutions' awareness of liability relative to improper management of sport-related injuries. Athletic training positions vary within the high schools from exclusively providing athletic training services for the school district to a duel role of teacher/athletic trainer. In addition, some school districts contract athletic training services through local sports medicine clinics that employ athletic trainers.

College and university athletic training positions vary from providing athletic training services to an entire athletic department (usually in smaller colleges) to providing services to a select team or group of teams, along with the support of an athletic training staff. Athletic training staff at the larger universities may include 6 to 10 full-time certified athletic trainers and an array of both undergraduate and graduate student athletic trainers. Furthermore, some athletic training staff serve as academicians and scholars in those programs offering athletic training curricula at both the undergraduate and graduate level.

Athletic training positions in professional sports are limited and extremely competitive because there are relatively few teams at this elite level. Employment usually begins at the lower levels within organizations and promotion occurs internally. For example, Major League baseball trainers often spend a number of seasons working with the Minor League ball clubs and are only promoted to the Major League when head trainers retire or resign. Most professional football teams employ only two full-time trainers and initial employment is often a function of association with members of management.

The final primary area of employment for certified athletic trainers is in the private and corporate setting. Private sports medicine clinics have offered excellent opportunities for athletic trainers. The athletic trainer's responsibilities vary tremendously within the clinical setting, including assisting physicians and physical therapists who provide athletic-related health care to recreational athletes and providing high school athletic training services that are contracted by the clinic.

The remainder of this chapter focuses on the athletic trainer's role and responsibility in the health care of athletes. Specifically, the chapter focuses on the athletic trainer's contribution in the areas of prevention of athletic injuries, emergency management of athletic injuries, evaluation of athletic injuries, and rehabilitation of athletic injuries.

Prevention of Athletic Injuries

Prevention of athletic injurics and illnesses includes the following: reduction of risk factors; physical examination and screenings; conditioning programs; fitting, design, and maintenance of protective equipment; fitting and application of special pads and tapings; nutrition; and knowledge of environmental risks.

Reduction of Risk Factors

Injuries are inherent to sport. Athletic trainers have illustrated problematic areas through research, and changes have been initiated as the result of epidemiologic studies by sports medicine personnel (3–6). These efforts have focused on injury frequency, sport-specific injuries, and the mechanisms that results in these injuries. The primary focus of these studies has included head, neck, knee, and ankle injuries; heat illnesses; catastrophic injuries; and injury rates in contact sports.

A 3-year study by the NATA focused on high school football injuries (7). The study concluded that 60% of all football injuries occurred during practice, when most schools do not have a qualified on-site health care professional available. This study supported NATA's claim for the need of improved programs of injury management and the need for preventative care for high school athletes. NATA is promoting the need for athletic trainers to cover practices as well as games in high schools across the country. A certified athletic trainer who is present at practices can give prompt care to any injury and initiate rehabilitation programs as necessary. The athletic trainer also can inform the coaching staff of any unsafe drills or playing conditions that have resulted in injuries that could have been prevented.

As the rate of cervical spine fractures and paralytic spine injuries increased, research studies suggested that changes must occur to protect the players from injuries (8). Studies conducted on the injury rates associated with hockey and football have resulted in rule changes, equipment improvements, coaching technique changes, stricter penalties, and the improvement of officiating (4, 8, 9). Rule changes for the 1976 football season that eliminated the head as a primary and initial contact area for blocking and tackling was a significant act. These changes have resulted in a reduction of the number of fatalities since their inception (9). The emphasis on safer tackling techniques has contributed to the decline in direct fatalities. For the first time in nearly 60 years, no direct deaths were reported in high school football during the 1990 season (10).

Epidemiologic studies continue to provide valuable data on the number and mechanisms of injury and factors pertaining to the incidence of injury. Previous studies have lead to important rule changes and improvements in equipment that have significantly impacted the rate of injuries. As more athletic trainers conduct research on athletic injuries, there will be further reduction of injuries.

Preparticipation Examination

The preparticipation examination is a vital element of any sports medicine program. The athletic trainer and team physician should be involved in the planning, design, and implementation of the preparticipation examination for his or her athletes. This ensures that the physical is designed to evaluate the health status of the athlete and determine if the athlete can meet the demands of the sport safely. The physical examination is a tool used by the sports medicine staff to determine any weaknesses, problem areas, or preexisting injuries. Deficits in flexibility, strength, and range of motion also can be detected. Detection of problem areas and general health weaknesses before an injury or illness occurs gives the athletic trainer and athlete the opportunity to make corrections.

The physical examination is a screening designed to assess the overall health status of the athlete, primarily the musculoskeletal system and the cardiovascular system (11). Before the physical examination, the athletic trainer should have each prospective athlete complete a detailed medical history. The physical examination should include multiple stations that cover the following areas: height and weight; blood pressure and pulse; eye examination; urine analysis; ear, nose, and throat; heart, lungs and abdomen; cardiology; and an orthopedic examination. The height and weight, blood pressure and pulse, urinalysis, and eye examinations can be performed by student athletic trainers or certified athletic trainers. Internists, otolaryngologists, cardiologists, and orthopedists can staff the remaining stations with the team physicians.

In addition to the normal system and musculoskeletal assessment many preparticipation examinations include an electrocardiogram (ECG). The increase in ECG screening is the result of the increase in sudden death from unknown heart conditions in athletes. Many of these conditions may still go undetected, although the ECG along with a complete medical history and physical evaluation assist the sports medicine staff in detecting athletes who are susceptible to heart conditions before they occur.

Physical Conditioning and Training

Athletic trainers and coaches recognize that improper conditioning is one of the principal causes of sports injuries (12). Poor flexibility, muscular imbalance, and inadequate muscular and cardiovascular endurance are major causes of injuries to athletes. An athlete who has proper muscular balance and strength, cardiovascular conditioning, and flexibility is less likely to sustain an injury than an athlete who does not maintain good levels of conditioning year round. An appropriately organized training program works the soft and bony tissues of the body. Over time, stress and/or stretch positively affects these structures, increasing their blood supply, density, width, and strength (12).

It is important to design conditioning and training programs that adapt to the four phases of the sport: in-season; postseason; off-season; and preseason. Post-season programs must focus on physical restoration of the athlete's body, particularly if the athlete sustained any injury during the course of the season. This period should be used for any needed rehabilitation. If no rehabilitation is necessary, this phase should include low-intensity work and rest.

The off-season workout is a combination of cardiovascular, strength, and endurance exercises. The athlete may want to participate in an entirely different sport, yet one that requires physical exertion. The activity level should maintain the athlete's general muscular and cardiovascular fitness. The workouts, however, should be less strenuous than during the season, gradually increasing in intensity so that the athlete will be in good physical condition at the start of the preseason phase.

The need for maintaining general physical conditioning in the off-season cannot be overstressed by the athletic trainer. The athlete will find that by maintaining a high level of fitness in the off-season, the preseason will be much more productive and be less susceptible to injury (12). During the season, the competition schedule may not include enough strenuous activity to maintain preseason fitness levels. Athletes should undergo structured maintenance programs throughout the competitive season. This allows them to keep their level of cardiovasular fitness and maintain strength and flexibility throughout the entire season, reducing the risk of injury as the season progresses.

The athletic trainer must stress the importance of a well-rounded fitness program to both coaches and athletes. The program must include cardiovascular fitness, muscular strength and endurance, and flexibility for the program to benefit the athlete. The athlete who maintains preseason levels throughout the season and some semblance of conditioning during the off-season will be less prone to injury than those athletes that do not work out during the off-season.

Protective Equipment and Devices

The goal of protective sports equipment is to prevent injury to the athlete or to prevent further injury to an already injured part. Ideal protective equipment should cause minimal functional interference and should not be harmful to other participants. Practicality dictates that such equipment be simple to fit and maintain and be durable, reliable, and affordable (13).

Protective equipment designed to prevent injuries is used in contact sports and in sports for which participants are at risk from another player or object. Athletes in football, wrestling, field hockey, lacrosse, and ice hockey, for example, use various pieces of protective equipment. The National Operating Committee on Standards for Athletic Equipment (NOCSAE) is responsible for setting many of the standards for reconditioning equipment for these sports and for certifying new equipment (12, 14).

In determining which protective equipment to use, the athletic trainer must ask the following questions:

1. Is the particular protective device required by the rules of the sport?
2. Has research supported the use of the protective device in the prevention of injuries?
3. Is an exact fit of the protective item necessary to obtain adequate protection?
4. Is regularly scheduled maintenance and repair of each item of protective equipment necessary to preserve the protective qualities of that item?
5. Is the protective device to be worn during practice as well as competition?

Athletes, coaches and equipment personnel should inspect equipment on a regular basis. The athletic trainer should inform coaches and equipment personnel of any defective equipment.

Fabrication of Protective Devices

The athletic trainer is responsible for construction and design of protective devices. The limitations of a protective device are materials, budget, and the rules of the sport. Creativity and imagination are important assets for the athletic trainer. Protective devices will fall into one of the following four categories (12–14).

Taping. An athletic trainer's preparation includes acquisition of psychomotor competencies in the application of preventative and protective taping. The purpose of tape application is to provide functional support during a period of rehabilitation when the athlete is fit to participate but may require additional support. Taping should not be a replacement for proper rehabilitation of an injury, rather it should be used in conjunction with an extensive rehabilitation program.

Padding. Protective pads can be designed and constructed out of many different types of materials. Some of the materials commonly used by the athletic trainer include various types of felts and foams, cotton, gauze, tape, orthoplast, plaster, Fiberglas, hexalite and silicone (Fig. 3.1). There are a variety of materials that can be heated, molded into specific shapes, and fit individually to the athlete. Once cooled the material will return to its original density.

Pads are used to protect an area from further damage or to aid the athlete's recovery by adding support during rehabilitation. When creating a pad, the athletic trainer must follow the rules governing a specific sport. Each sport has specific rules concerning the type of materials that are allowed for practice and competition. These rules safeguard other athletes so that the protective pad does not become an offensive weapon.

Bracing. Most braces used by the athletic trainer are commercially produced. These braces include any type of neoprene sleeve, or prefabricated off-the-shelf brace (e.g., Anderson Knee Stabilizer, Omni Knee Brace, Aircast Ankle Brace, and Swedo Ankle Brace). These braces are worn during rehabilitation or during return to participation for protection. Custom-made braces are usually prescribed by physicians for injuries that require specific support following ligament-related injuries (Fig. 3.2).

Orthotics. The athletic trainer may design various types of foot orthotics to aid the athlete either as a preventative measure or to assist with injury management. Most of the orthotic devices constructed in the

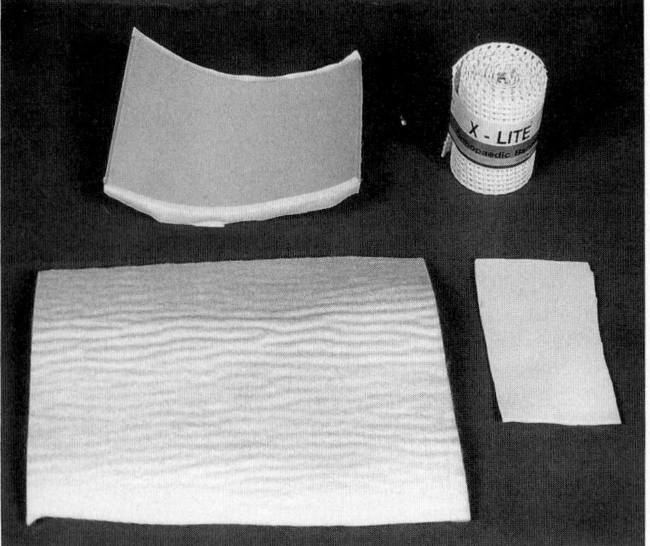

Figure 3.1. Materials for protective equipment. *Clockwise from upper left:* adhesive foam, hexalite, orthoplast, and Felt.

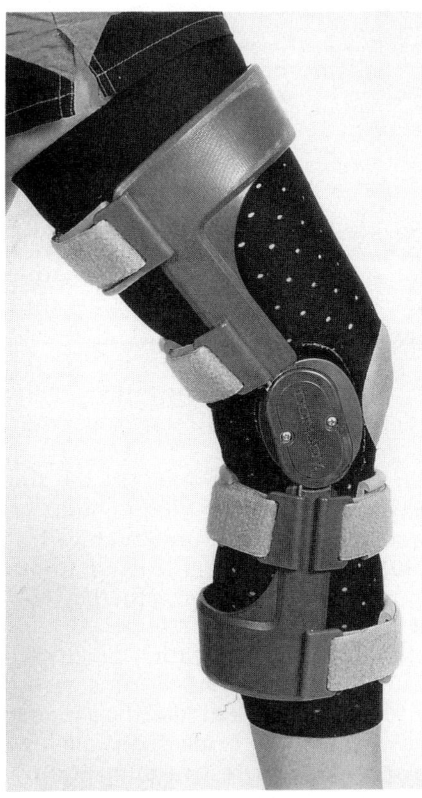

Figure 3.2. Postsurgical functional knee brace.

training room are made out of soft materials (foam or felt) and are temporary appliances. If an athlete has a structural problem, then he or she is referred to a podiatrist or someone specializing in prophylactic orthosis to obtain custom-made orthotics.

Nutrition

Athletes and coaches are easy targets for diet misinformation. In their desire to gain the edge over the competitor, they often lose sight of common sense. It is the role of the athletic trainer to educate and counsel the athletes, coaches, and administrators about all aspects of nutrition (12). This includes information concerning general nutrition, fluid replacement, pregame meals, and eating disorders.

The meals eaten the day before an event are more important than the preevent meal, but many coaches tend to overlook the meals 24 to 48 hr before an event. Athletes and coaches should be counseled on the importance of precompetition nutrition, because most budgets do not allow the team to eat at a training table together, except the meal just before a game. The athletic trainer should take an active role in planning the preevent meal, considering timing, location, size, composition, and availability. The meal should be eaten 3 to 4 hr before an event and should include predominantly carbohydrates and fluids that will be easily digested (3).

Eating Disorders

An eating disorder is a serious medical problem that may produce few obvious symptoms (15). Even though there is an increased awareness of eating disorders among the athletic population, they are difficult to diagnose because their complex and secretive nature. The key for the athletic trainer is to learn to distinguish between athletes with eating disorders and those whose behaviors only mimic such problems (3). Eating disorders occur most frequently in athletes who participate in sports with weight and/or body fat restrictions such as gymnastics, figure skating, wrestling, and ballet (10, 16). Two common eating disorders are bulimia and anorexia.

The athletic trainer must be able to disseminate information and dispel nutritional myths. They must train coaches, administrators, and others who work with the athletes to recognize the warning signs of eating disorders. Athletic trainers must help staff understand the physical and psychological effects of such disorders.

Once an athlete is suspected of having an eating disorder, an athletic trainer must have a referral plan for this individual. The athletic trainer may turn to a nutritionist, an eating disorders clinic, or a physician who specializes in such problems. Many athletes believe there is a stigma attached to professional counseling and will often avoid treatment. It is imperative that the athletic trainer insist that the athlete attend professional counseling sessions.

Environmental Risks

The athletic trainer must often respond to injuries produced by the environment in which the athlete participates (13). The areas of environmental concern to the athletic trainer are heat (hyperthermia) and cold (hypothermia).

Hyperthermia.

Heat illnesses are preventable, yet cases of heat exhaustion and death from heat stress continue to occur (14). Heat illnesses and injuries are a major concern to the athletic trainer who must inform the coaching staff about this environmental risk. Heat must be taken into account when planning practices and scheduling games. The sling psychrometer is used to determine the wet-bulb-globe temperature index. The athletic trainer and coach must clearly understand when environmental heat and humidity are at dangerous levels and restrict activity accordingly (12–14). Heat illnesses include heat cramps, heat exhaustion, and heat stroke (Table 3.3). The athletic trainer should be aware of the signs and symptoms of the heat illnesses and be able to make a differential diagnosis.

Fall sports, primarily football, cross-country, soccer, field hockey, and volleyball are the most susceptible to heat illness because practices and games are held late in the summer when the heat and humidity are high. Football is most often associated with heat illnesses. The protective equipment worn by football players decreases the athletes' ability to dissipate heat, and the added weight of the equipment increases heat production (14). Wrestlers also are extremely susceptible to heat illnesses as a result of self-imposed fluid and dietary restrictions.

Table 3.3.
Heat Illnesses

Illness	Symptoms	Skin Color	Sweating	Treatment
Heat cramps	Hot, fatigue	Flushed	Minimal to profuse	Fluids, cool down
Heat exhaustion	Headache, nausea, chills, dizziness, fatigue	Pale	Minimal to profuse	Cool down, ice towels, fluids, intravenous fluids
Heat stroke	Disorientation, confusion, unconsciousness	Flushed	Minimal to none	Cool down, reduce core temperature, transfer to emergency room

Normal body temperature is maintained through a balance of heat production versus heat loss (12, 13). If this system is not in balance, the athlete is susceptible to heat illness. Heat is eliminated from the body through convection, conduction, evaporation, and radiation. Most of these methods of heat loss rely on the environmental temperature being lower than body temperature. If the external temperature is higher than body temperature, the primary source of heat loss is evaporation of sweat, assuming that the ambient humidity is low enough to accept the moisture (13).

Since 1974 there has been a dramatic reduction in heat stroke deaths. Heat stroke and heat exhaustion are prevented by control of various factors in the conditioning program of the athlete (9). First, the athletes must slowly acclimatize to the new (warm) environment. The athletic trainer should monitor the athletes' workouts, especially those athletes who are obese, heavily muscled, or poorly conditioned. Initial practices for those sports that require protective equipment such as football, field hockey, and soccer should be conducted in T-shirts and shorts for several days to allow for acclimatization and conditioning.

Second, athletes who are susceptible to heat illnesses should be identified by the athletic trainer. As noted above, these are athletes who are obese, heavily muscled, or out of shape. One preventative measure is to weigh athletes before and after all practice sessions. Any athlete who has sustained a 3% to 5% weight loss per practice session that is not negated by the next session should be kept out of practice (12–14, 17).

Third, environmental conditions can be monitored using a sling psychrometer or the local weather service. Practice times must be adjusted according to the heat and humidity. Finally, an unlimited supply of fluids should be available to the athletes at practice. Frequent water breaks should be scheduled throughout practice. The athletes should be encouraged to drink plenty of fluids before, during, and after practice.

Hypothermia

The athletic trainer must take precautions in cold weather as well as hot. Decreasing temperature and wind can cause hypothermia, frostbite, or peripheral problems (14). The athletic trainer must help coaches and athletes recognize the signs and symptoms of cold disorders and inform them of the proper course of treatment. Common signs and symptoms of hypothermia include uncontrollable shivering, decreased coordination, decreased level of consciousness, sleeplessness, and apathy (12–14).

Sports susceptible to hypothermia are those that do not require heavy protective clothing and yet continue into the cooler seasons. Consequently, weather becomes a pertinent factor, particularly to athletes who are sweating and exhausted, thereby predisposing themselves to injury (12).

Prevention during cold weather practices and games should include the following: (*a*) instructing the athletes how to dress for cold weather practices; (*b*) instructing the athletes to bring spare gloves and socks; (*c*) making sure the athletes warm up properly; and (*d*) requiring proper fluid hydration.

Emergency Management of Athletic Injuries

Rarely is an injury sustained while participating in athletics considered to be an emergency. An emergency is defined as "an unforeseen combination of circumstances and the resulting state that calls for immediate action" (18). Because of the infrequency of such events, sports medicine personnel must be prepared for these situations. The athletic trainer is responsible for preparation and effective implementation of the emergency management of athletic injuries.

Emergency Plan

The most critical element in reacting to an emergency is time. A sport-specific management plan may eliminate costly mistakes or delays. A well-organized emergency plan may lessen the severity of injury and possibly save a life. Many variables must be addressed when developing an emergency plan, including the following:

1. Location of telephones (and accessibility during practice times), with numbers clearly listed
2. Proper communication of information
   a. Caller identifies self
   b. *Exact* location (special directions if needed)
   c. Exact nature of injury
   d. Call-back telephone number
3. Special entrances needed (including maps of all fields, buildings, and courses)
4. Define roles of personnel available
   a. Athletic trainer
   b. Coach and assistants

c. Student athletic trainers
d. Administrators
e. Local emergency medical service (EMS)
5. Medical helicopter landing zones.

Upon completion of this plan, the athletic trainers should review the procedures with coaches, administrators, team physicians, and the local EMS. A well-designed emergency plan involves cooperation of all personnel involved and the plan must be practical.

Patient Primary and Secondary Assessment

The priorities when assessing athletic injuries are similar to any injuries. The primary assessment includes evaluation of airway, breathing, and circulation (ABCs). If an injury to the spinal cord is suspected, stabilization of the head and neck must be obtained before proceeding with assessment. If the athlete is conscious a thorough history must be obtained before the physical assessment. The information from the history is especially important in emergencies.

Airway. Unless cervical spine injury is suspected, the airway should be opened with a head tilt–chin lift method.

Breathing. Breathing should be assessed by looking, listening, and feeling for air exchange from the mouth and nose. If breathing is not present, the attending personnel should begin mouth-to-mouth resuscitation, or mouth-to-mask if available.

Circulation. Assessment of circulation is performed by palpating the carotid artery in the neck. If no pulse is found, cardiopulmonary resuscitation (CPR) must be initiated. Massive bleeding also must be controlled if present.

If the findings of the primary survey are unimpressive, assessment should continue with a very thorough secondary survey. The secondary assessment includes a head-to-toe examination.

An integral portion of the secondary survey is monitoring vital signs. These include level of consciousness, pulse, blood pressure, skin temperature and color, respiration, and pupillary reaction. Level of consciousness (LOC), especially important for determining the effectiveness of brain tissue perfusion, is evaluated by conversing with the athlete and noting the appropriateness of the responses. The assessment must determine if the athlete is conscious; alert; and oriented to person, place, time, and purpose. While evaluating level of consciousness, it is important to note the injured athlete's behavior in general. Restlessness and anxiety are early signs of hypoxemia or internal bleeding (12). This sign can be easily overlooked.

Respiratory Injuries

The respiratory system is composed of the nasopharynx, oropharynx, laryngopharynx, trachea, and lungs (18). If this system is disrupted at any level for a period of time the result can be catastrophic.

Disruption of the respiratory system is rare in athletics but does occur. Problems most often observed at sporting events include obstruction by foreign object, trauma to the neck and larynx, closed head injuries accompanied by diminished levels of consciousness, and angioedema and anaphylaxis (18). Any irregularities in breathing patterns or cessation of respiration must be identified and corrected immediately. Cardinal signs of respiratory difficulty include nasal flaring, tracheal tugging, intercostal muscle retraction, use of diaphragm and neck muscles, and especially cyanosis (18).

Once the mechanism of the distress is identified, a decision can be made about the proper steps to correct the difficulty. Adjunctive equipment should be available and should be divided into basic and advanced life support.

Basic equipment for management of respiratory injuries includes a pocket mask, oropharyngeal airways, nasopharyngeal airways, a bag-valve-mask system (Fig. 3.3), and a suction unit. This equipment is easy to use; however, frequent practice with each piece is important to ensure familiarity in an emergency.

If advanced airway skill technicians are available, the following equipment should be included: laryngoscope with blades, a variety of endotracheal tube sizes, stylets, and Magill forceps. In addition, a prepackaged crycothyrotomy kit should be available in case a surgical airway is needed.

In the event of airway obstruction, the athletic trainer should follow the guidelines of the American Heart Association or the American Red Cross for management of foreign body obstruction. If acceptable results are not obtained, extraction by direct laryngoscopy should be attempted.

Airway obstruction from a head injury is usually caused by blockage of the airway by the athlete's tongue. This can be corrected by using basic airway control techniques such as the head tilt–chin lift maneuver.

As with any outdoor activity, an athlete may be a victim of an insect bite, and anaphylaxis is a distinct possibility. Epinephrine 1:1000 should be readily avail-

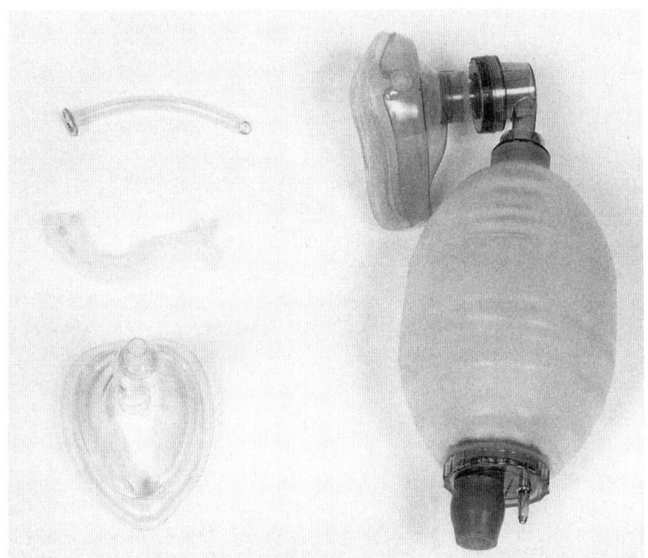

Figure 3.3. Airway equipment: bivalve mask, pocket mask, nasopharyngeal airway, and oral airway.

able. A dose of 0.3 to 0.5 ml for adults and 0.01 ml/kg for children should be administered by subcutaneous injection by the team physician (12).

Internal Injuries

Internal injuries are most often the result of blunt trauma. In the athletic setting, the forces needed to produce internal injury are most often inflicted by a projectile (hockey puck, baseball, etc.). Any injury to the abdomen should raise the suspicions of the athletic trainer. Blunt trauma to the abdomen is especially deceptive, because it may cause devastating injury with few external signs (19).

Athletes sustaining abdominal trauma should be closely monitored for 24 to 48 hr. If the athlete presents with abdominal pain, nausea, vomiting, rigidity, or discolorization around the umbilicus a further examination should be performed. An athlete with complaints of pain radiating into the left shoulder (Kehr's sign) may have sustained a ruptured spleen, which necessitates immediate medical attention.

Any athlete suspected of an internal injury should be treated for shock. Shock treatment includes ensuing an adequate airway, administering supplemental oxygen when warranted, placing the patient in a supine position and transporting him or her to the appropriate medical facility (18).

Musculoskeletal Injuries

Musculoskeletal injuries are by far the most common injuries seen by sports medicine specialists. Although these injuries are rarely life threatening, improper management may exacerbate the initial injury.

The most common signs of a musculoskeletal injury include swelling, ecchymosis, deformity, point tenderness, crepitus, guarding, and an open wound with bone ends exposed. If a fracture or dislocation is suspected, the injured region should be immobilized. Before immobilizing, the examiner should perform a neurovascular assessment, including distal pulses, sensation, and movement. If distal pulses are not present, immediate reduction or transport is required.

Splinting may be accomplished with any commercially available device. Rigid splints are usually made up of a padded board covered in vinyl and are held in place with cravats or an elastic bandage. Pneumatic splints are most often used for wrist, forearm, ankle, and lower leg fractures. These splints are inflated, compressing and stabilizing the fracture site. Traction splints are commonly used for femur fractures, whereas in-line traction is used to override muscular contraction.

A spine board is used to splint athletes with suspected spinal cord injuries. If the athlete is prone, he or she should be rolled as a unit to a supine position. The log roll method is most effective; four or five people are needed to assist (Fig. 3.4). One person should immobilize the head and control the immobilization process. A rigid cervical collar should be applied before spine boarding. The long board should be placed next to the athlete; the assistants roll the athlete while maintaining in-line axial alignments. The spine board should next be slid under the athlete as far as possible, followed by placing the athlete in a supine position on the board. The head must be immobilized by either a commercially available device or sand bags. Immobilization of the body is accomplished by placing straps over the thorax, hips, and legs.

Some variations are necessary when spine boarding a football player. Before moving the athlete, the face mask should be removed by cutting the plastic clips that attach the mask to the helmet (Fig. 3.5). If the player is wearing his shoulder pads and helmet, he should be immobilized with them in place. If just the helmet is worn, it must be removed to prevent flexion of the neck when lying supine. Removal of a football helmet should only be performed by persons who are familiar with this technique; two people should perform the re-

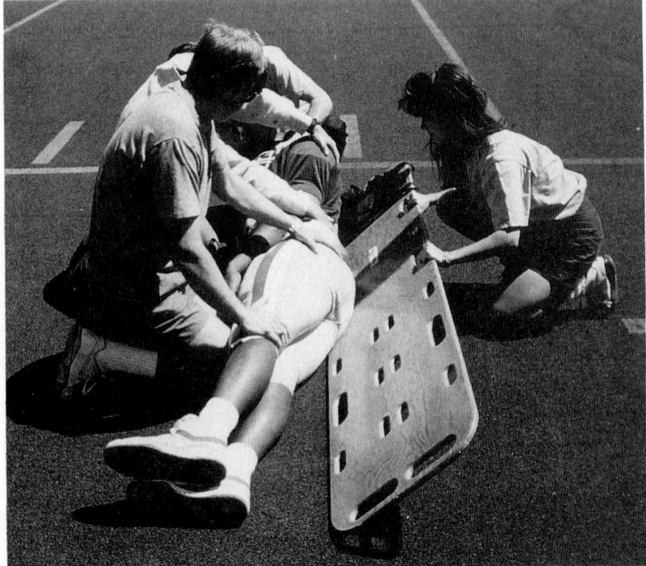

Figure 3.4. Using a spine board. The athlete is rolled to a supine position onto the spine board with axial alignment maintained.

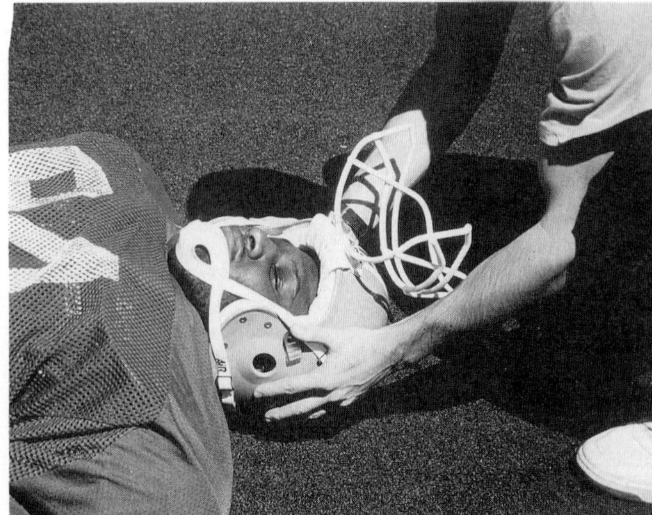

Figure 3.5. Face mask removal. The face mask can be cut away while maintaining stabilization of the head and neck.

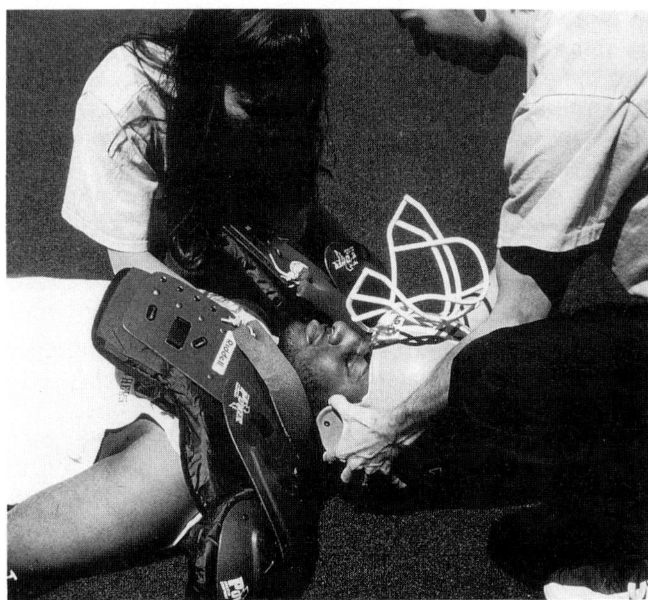

Figure 3.6. Helmet removal. The helmet may be removed by tilting it slightly forward.

moval. One person stabilizes the athlete's head by holding the helmet in axial alignment throughout the removal process. The second person should cut the clips to remove the face mask, cut the chin strap, and very carefully remove the two jaw pads by using a tongue depressor or similar object to pry open the snaps. The second person should next place one hand on the occiput, reaching as far into the helmet as possible; his or her other hand is on the mandible. On the second person's command, the first person should tilt the helmet slightly forward and slide it off the player's head (Fig. 3.6). The first person should then retake control of the athlete's head and place him in a neutral position. A rigid cervical collar can then be applied, and the athlete can be immobilized as described above.

Evaluation of Athletic Injury and Illness

Clinical Evaluation Process

The order in which the clinical examination components are assessed may vary slightly between clinicians; however, a basic systematic scheme should always be followed so that nothing is overlooked or forgotten (20, 21). As a result of the nature of the injury and amount of pain the athlete is experiencing, it is permissible to alter the procedure to avoid unnecessary movement of the injured area and eliminate the risk of further trauma. The athletic trainer is involved with a variety of situations and pathologies, ranging from acute and chronic injuries to various medical conditions and illnesses; thus only basic guidelines to the evaluation process will be presented here.

History

A comprehensive and detailed account of the injury is critical in the evaluation process to ensure accurate findings. A thorough history will alert the examiner to the type and extent of injury (21). The following information must be obtained subjectively from the athlete to help determine the etiology and provide the foundation for the subsequent evaluation.

1. Subjective complaint of the problem.
2. Mechanism of injury and the events that led to the onset of symptoms.
3. Feeling at time of injury (pop, snap, etc.).
4. Location and type of pain (ache, burning, etc.).
5. Duration and behavior of signs and symptoms.
6. Prior injury or surgery to either the involved or the noninvolved side.
7. Other present medical problems (allergies, medications, etc.).
8. Effectiveness of previous treatment (if any).

The exact location of pain may not be the most reliable indicator of the actual side or nature of the pathology. Nerve root syndromes, muscle spasms, inflammation, and other illness may refer pain to other areas, disguising the true origin of injury (22, 23). Therefore, it is important to view the history as only part of the whole evaluation process. More information is needed to assess objectively the type and extent of injury. It is important to note that the remainder of the evaluation serves to substantiate what was initially found in the history.

Observation

The purpose of observation is to identify any signs that could indicate the nature of the pathology. The examiner looks for any abnormalities and makes a bilateral comparison. As the athlete initially enters the training room an assessment should be made of his or her gait, identifying any noticeable lurches or obvious antalgic or compensatory gait changes. The examiner also should note the athlete's willingness to move as well as any changes in the carrying angles of different joints. Often overlooked but of great importance is the postural assessment. Correct posture is the position in which the minimum amount of stress will be applied to each joint (22). Care should be taken to observe the athlete from head to toe, looking for such things as head tilt, spinal alignment, articular alignment and foot abnormalities. Areas identified as abnormal must be noted and further assessed as the evaluation progresses. These areas may reveal conditions of hypomobility or hypermobility. Postural dysfunctions can be either primary or contributing causes of pain, or they may appear as resulting signs or symptoms.

The final stage of the observation should include identification of any obvious deformity or changes, including abnormal bony contours or deviations; asymmetric soft tissue size and shape; areas of muscle atrophy or hypertrophy; signs of swelling, ecchymosis, or infection; abnormal skin markings, hair patches, or scars; and skin color, texture, and general appearance. The examiner must be aware that the body is not normally perfectly symmetrical. Dominance of one side might produce changes in posture, especially in athletics. For example, a right-handed tennis player's shoulder may appear lower than the left. This is a normal compensatory change the body makes; however, it should be noted during observation because of any possible link to the pathology (23).

Upper/Lower Quarter Screening

In some cases extremity pain and dysfunction may be the result of either a cervical or lumbar spinal pathology. Therefore, before the clinician attempts an evaluation of an extremity, an upper or lower quarter screening examination may be appropriate to rule out a spinal disorder (Tables 3.4 and 3.5) (20, 21). Screening exams consist of a series of mobility, strength, and neurological tests designed to identify the exact location of the pathology. They are not specifically designed to identify the nature of the pathology (21). The upper quarter screen addresses the cervical spine, shoulder, elbow, wrist, and hand; whereas the lower quarter screen addresses the lumbar spine, sacroiliac area, hip, knee, ankle, and foot (24). These exams are basically quick overviews of both sections of the body to alert the examiner to areas that need to be examined in more detail. This component of the evaluation may be done following an initial history and observation, and the examiner should note any pain or limits in motion present. Once completed, the examination may continue to focus on the primary area of complaint. It is important to note, however, that if there is a clear history of trauma to a specific joint with no other unrelated signs or symptoms, this screening process may not be needed.

Table 3.4.
Summary of the Upper Quarter Screen

Postural assessment
Active range of motion of the cervical spine
Passive over pressures, if symptom free
Resisted cervical rotation (C1)
Resisted shoulder elevation (C2, C3, C4)
Resisted shoulder abduction (C5)
Active shoulder flexion and rotation
Resisted elbow flexion (C6)
Resisted elbow extension (C7)
Active range of motion of elbow
Resisted wrist extension (C6)
Resisted wrist flexion (C7)
Resisted thumb extension (C8)
Resisted finger abduction/adduction (T1)
Babinski's reflex test (upper motor neuron)

Adapted from Cyriax J. Textbook of orthopaedic medicine: diagnosis of soft tissue lesions. Vol. 1. 7th ed. London: Bailliere-Tindall, 1978.

Table 3.5.
Summary of the Lower Quarter Screen

Postural assessment
Active range of motion of the lumbar spine (FB, BB, RSB, LSB)
Toe raises (S1)
Heel walking (L4, L5)
Active rotation of the lumbar spine
Passive over pressures, if symptom free
Straight leg raise (L4, L5, S1)
Sacroiliac compression/distraction tests
Resisted hip flexion (L1, L2)
Passive range of motion of the hip
Resisted knee extension (L3, L4)
Active knee flexion and extension
Femoral nerve stretch
Babinski's reflex test (upper motor neuron)

Adopted from Cyriax J. Textbook of orthopaedic medicine: diagnosis of soft tissue lesions. Vol. 1. 7th ed. London: Bailliere-Tindall, 1978.

Palpation

Palpation is a method by which the examiner applies gentle, yet firm pressure over an area to identify skin texture, underlying defects, the type and extent of pain, and any abnormal sensations. The clinician should make sure the area to be palpated is relaxed and the region is well-supported. To ease the athlete's apprehension palpation should start on the noninvolved extremity so the athlete can become familiar with the process. The clinician progresses to the periphery of the injury and then to the actual site of pain.

Because referred tenderness can be so misleading, palpation should be done when the actual tissue at fault has been identified through previous range of motion assessments (22). In cases of clear trauma to an area, palpation may occur after the history and observation to rule out a fracture or dislocation before moving an athlete through a range of motion assessment. This will reduce the risk of further trauma, pain, and complications.

Active Range of Motion

Active movements are defined as the athlete's own ability to move a joint through an available range of motion (ROM). This allows for a general assessment of the athlete's willingness to move, irregular movement patterns, painful arcs of motion, the quality of the movement, and any other obvious restrictions or limitations. Specific joint isolation and stabilization is important to allow for pure movements.

Both contractile and inert tissues are stressed during active movements. Contractile tissue—muscle and tendons and their tenoperiosteal junctions—is stressed by both active contraction in one direction and passive stretch by movement in the opposite direction (20, 22). Inert tissue—joint capsules, ligaments, bursae, cartilage, and nerves—may be pinched or stretched during active movements, because of its orientation to the moving structures. Therefore, passive and resistive movements are needed to delineate further between contractile and inert tissue pathology. All range of motion assessments should be repeated several times to identify changes in the signs or symptoms, movement patterns, and strength.

Passive Range of Motion

Passive motion is accomplished by the clinician, who moves the joint through the available range of motion while the athlete is relaxed. No muscle contraction should be present. This technique assesses primarily inert tissue and may reveal any apparent hypomobility or hypermobility. As the terminal end of a range is approached, the examiner feels the sensation of the end point resistance, or end feel. The type and quality of the end feel should be noted and a bilateral comparison is made to reference normal. The most commonly identified normal end feels include bone to bone, soft tissue approximation, and tissue stretch. Abnormal end feels include muscle spasm, springy block (mechanical blocking), empty (no movement due to pain), and capsular (20, 22).

Appropriate knowledge of the normal end feels for each joint is imperative for valid assessment. It also is important to note whether pain and restriction appear together or separately. For example, in a typical sequence of pain, if pain is felt before the end point resistance is reached, one should be careful not to work through the pain or begin stretching. However, if the resistance of the end range is encountered before pain, aggressive stretching may be necessary and well-tolerated (22).

Resistive Range of Motion

Resistive movements assess the integrity of contractile tissue (Fig. 3.7). An isometric contraction is performed against the manual resistance applied by the examiner to identify any pain or weakness that is present. The joint should be placed in the midrange of motion, because it is the position in which minimal stress is placed on inert tissue and it allows for maximal recruitment of muscle fibers by mechanical advantage (20, 22). As resistance is applied, the examiner must isolate and stabilize the joint segment and muscle to be evaluated to eliminate any accessory joint motion. This excess motion will place stress on other tissues and may cause inappropriate and inaccurate feedback.

Different combinations of pain and weakness can be categorized to identify the severity and nature of the lesion. Resistive assessments can range from strong and pain free, indicating no contractile tissue lesion, to weak and painless, indicating neurologic dysfunction or muscle/tendon rupture (20, 22). Furthermore, resistive movements in the form of manual muscle tests may be employed to help the clinician subjectively quantify strength (Table 3.6) (13, 25).

Special Tests

During the final phase of the evaluation process, further and more specific testing help identify the particular site and/or extent of the pathology. Such testing may include ligamentous and capsular stress testing to quantify joint laxity and instability. In traumatic injuries involving moderate to severe tissue damage, initial pain and instability may cause the surrounding sup-

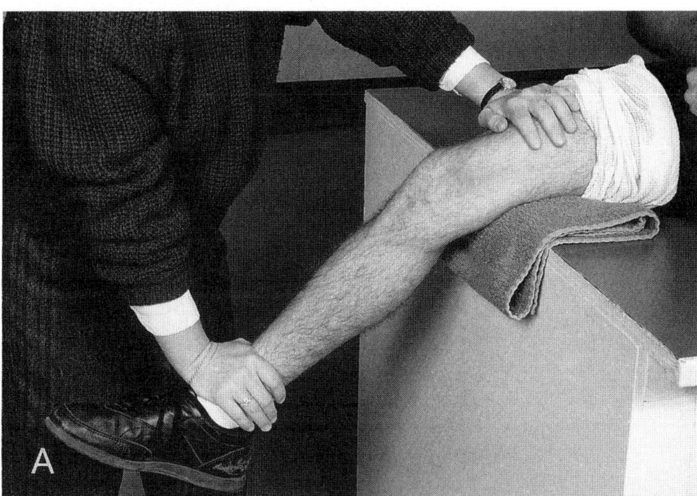

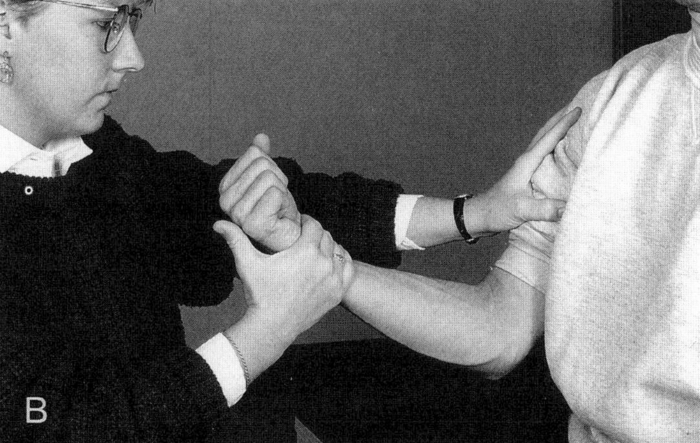

Figure 3.7. Manual muscle testing. **A,** Knee extension, **B,** Elbow flexion.

Table 3.6.
Resistive Range of Motion and Manual Muscle Tests—Grading Scale

Muscle Strength	Percent	Concentration	Grade
Complete ROM against gravity with *full* resistance	100	Normal	5
Complete ROM against gravity with *some* resistance	75	Good	4
Complete ROM against gravity with *no* resistance	50	Fair	3
Complete ROM with gravity eliminated	25	Poor	2
Evidence of a slight muscle contraction with no change in ROM	10	Trace	1
No evidence of muscle contraction	0	Zero	0

Adopted from Hunter-Griffin et al. Athletic training and sports medicine. 2nd ed. Park Ridge, IL: AAOS, 1991 and Kendall FP, McCreary EK. Muscle testing and function. 3rd ed. Baltimore: Williams & Wilkins, 1983.

portive muscles to spasm. This protective spasm or muscle-guarding response often masks the extent of injury by preventing true joint laxity to be reproduced and accurately assessed. In these situations, it is critical to perform the tests and assess joint instability at the beginning of the evaluation in a timely fashion to ensure an accurate impression.

A complete neurologic exam is often indicated to assess the integrity of the central and peripheral nervous systems. Motor and sensory functions of both nerve roots and peripheral nerves are evaluated to identify the exact site and/or level of the lesion. Myotomes, dermatomes, and corresponding reflexes (Fig. 3.8) should be compared bilaterally for any asymmetry or deficits, which would suggest possible spinal cord or nerve root pathology. Examples of specific neurologic tests may include Tinel's sign, which is elicited by tapping over a superficial peripheral nerve, creating an abnormally increased sensation or tingling along its corresponding distribution (20). This may indicate a peripheral nerve irritation, entrapment, or dysfunction. The Babinski reflex also may be tested by running a semisharp object along the plantar aspect of the foot. If the great toe

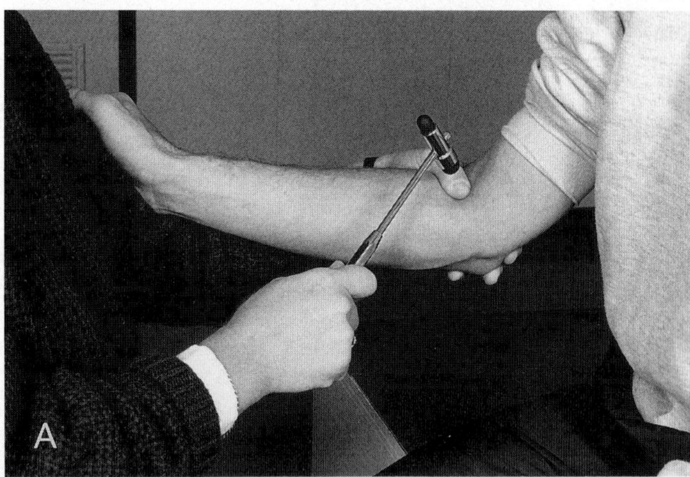

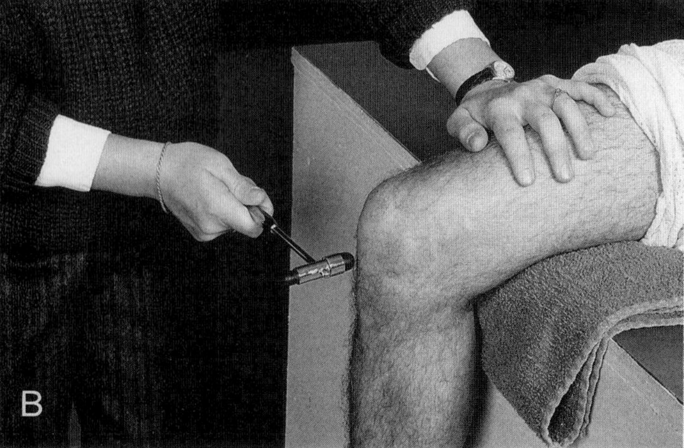

Figure 3.8. Reflex testing. **A,** Biceps/tendon reflex. **B,** patellar tendon reflex.

splays out into abduction, a positive test is noted, indicating an upper motor neuron lesion (20, 24).

Further diagnostic tests may be necessary to confirm suspicions produced in the evaluation. The use of roentograms, magnetic resonance imaging (MRI), bone scans, CT scans, blood tests, etc. can be useful to clarify subjective findings and document the extent of the injury (23).

Upon completion of all parts of the clinical evaluation, the examiner studies the relationship between the history and the objective and subjective signs and symptoms to determine the etiology and pathology. Once an impression is formed, medical referral and/or subsequent management and treatment may be determined.

Rehabilitation of Athletic Injuries

Before discussing athletic rehabilitation, it is important to distinguish between athletic rehabilitation and clinical or orthopedic rehabilitation. The intricacies of athletic rehabilitation are often overlooked by practitioners of orthopedic rehabilitation, who believe there is no difference between the two. The distinguishing elements include the following: (*a*) immediate acute care; (*b*) treatment on a more frequent basis; (*c*) psychological preparedness; and (*d*) functional return of the individual to high-level athletic activity.

When a weekend warrior sustains an ankle sprain, he or she applies heat or ice at home or goes to the hospital for an x-ray. This negligence of appropriate care can result in painful inflammation. An athlete under the care of a certified athletic trainer, on the other hand, will be immediately examined and treated with modalities designed to limit the effect of pain in inflammation. The athlete may eventually require an x-ray, but only after following thorough instructions regarding the use of ice or heat; ambulation with crutches, and use of compression bandages, braces, and splints. This immediate care rendered by the athletic trainer minimizes early stages of injury and enables the athlete to progress more rapidly through all aspects of rehabilitation.

The athletic trainer's relationship with an athlete can greatly enhance the rehabilitation of injuries. Once injured, the athlete typically progresses through four psychological phases: denial, anger, depression, and acceptance (13). These phases differ in intensity and sequence, and depending on the athlete and severity of the injury, some phases may be omitted. Athletic trainers and athletes often have a mutual respect and trust, which is essential in developing a positive goal and plan for the athlete's well-being and eventual return to competition. The trainer's sensitivity to the psychological aspects of an athlete's injury often accelerates the process of rehabilitation because of the positive focus the athlete will employ.

The rehabilitation program of an injured athlete can be divided into three basic stages: (*a*) acute care, or control of the inflammatory response; (*b*) subacute care, or physical reconditioning; and (*c*) chronic care, or return to activity. Each stage within the rehabilitation process should be clearly defined for the athlete, keeping in mind the athlete's design to return to full competitive participation. If the injury process requires a long rehabilitation time, several sets of goals may be needed within each stage of the process to motivate the athlete to return to full competitive activity.

Stage One: Acute Care

Acute care is a particular area of expertise of the athletic trainer. Appropriate acute care can prevent or minimize the effects of initial trauma, including hemorrhage and edema. Athletic trainers provide on-sight care of injuries, using typical acute care measures—such as protection, rest, ice, compression, and elevation (PRICE)—that minimize the effects of the initial inflammatory response.

Following an injury, protective devices can be used effectively and efficiently to assist in the healing process. These devices enable the athlete to rest the injured area adequately, and coupled with the use of modalities, pain and swelling of an injured area also are decreased (Fig. 3.9). The acute stage of rehabilitation focuses on minimizing initial hemorrhage and edema and slowing down the tissue metabolic rate through PRICE, which diminishes histamine release, thereby decreasing the inflammatory response. The athletic trainer is skilled in controlling and assessing the inflammatory phase of the injury. The use of PRICE and other modalities are determined by the inflammatory response to injury and treatment. Athletic trainers are well-versed in recognizing the signs of the inflammatory processes and in determining the appropriate modalities to allow rapid progression through the rehabilitation plan.

When treating the athlete during the acute stage of the rehabilitation program, the athletic trainer must be aware of healing process. This process is a series of phases that overlap one another; the phases are inflammatory, fibroplastic, and maturation. The goal of the trainer in this process is to avoid problems that may exacerbate the inflammatory process, which would delay healing. The ultimate product of proper acute care

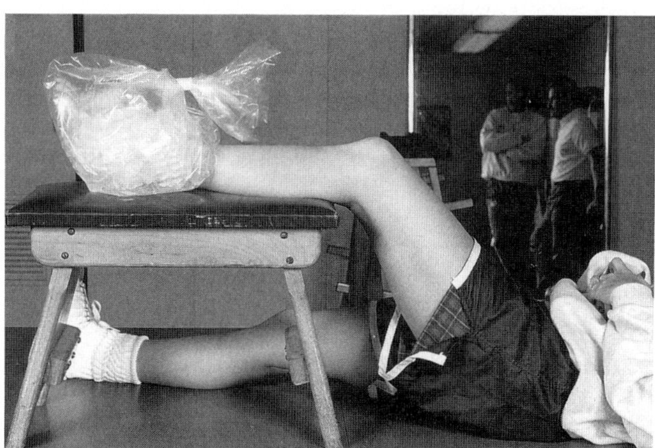

Figure 3.9. Ice and elevation are used to minimize swelling.

management is a strong functional scar that will permit full return to competitive activity.

The early stage of rehabilitation involves minimizing the effects of inflammation and enhancing repair of the pathologic tissue while also maintaining the athlete's overall conditioning wish. Deconditioning can result in exacerbation of the athlete's current injury. The athletic trainer's background in exercise physiology will help him or her design an activity program that will not exacerbate the symptoms of the injury, thus preventing the athlete's deconditioning. Such activities include alternate conditioning modes like cycling and pool therapy to prevent deconditioning and weight training to prevent general musculature atrophy of the noninvolved and noninjured sites. These alternate modes enable the athlete to maintain aerobic capacity and overall strength, resulting in the efficient return to activity upon healing of the injury.

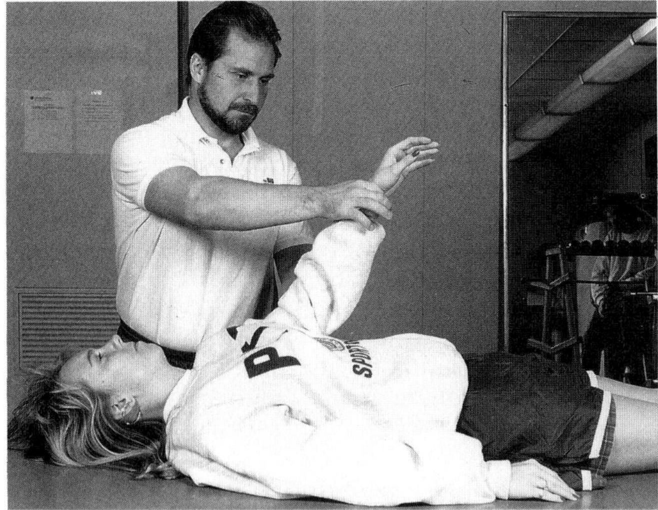

Figure 3.10. Active assistive range of motion. Assistance is provided by the clinician to increase range of motion during the subacute healing phase.

Stage Two: Subacute Care (Physical Conditioning)

Stage two rehabilitation begins when pain and swelling are controlled and the athlete does not require continued immobilization. The athlete may be placed in a removal splint or required to use an assistive device (see Fig. 3.2). The primary goals of the athletic trainer in stage two of the rehabilitation program is to restore range of motion, strength, and endurance to the effected site. The progression will be based on the physician's prescribed therapy as well as the athletic trainer's assessment of the status of the injury and will include subjective and objective variables such as the athlete's pain and limitation in range of motion, observable swelling, and strength deficits. In stage two of the rehabilitation program, the athletic trainer develops an individualized therapy plan for each athlete.

Restoring full ROM to an injured limb is of paramount importance to the rehabilitation process. ROM is typically measured against and compared with the normal contralateral limb. Occasionally, athletes such as javelin throwers and pitchers will not have normal symmetrical motion, although most athletes have equal range of motion bilaterally. Range of motion can easily be assessed using a goniometer, which identifies any deficits in range of motion and provides information about attainable ROM goals. Functional range of motion can be reestablished using a combination of passive, active assistive, and active exercises that facilitate normal motion and enhance strength to the injured limb.

Passive range of motion exercises are those exercises that are performed by the athletic trainer manually moving the athlete's limb. Active assistive range of motion exercises are performed by the athlete with the assistance of the athletic trainer, the goal is to reach the terminal limits of the motion (Fig. 3.10). Active range of motion exercises allow the athlete to perform within his or her full pain-free range of motion. Passive, active assistive, and active exercises are used to regain the full range of motion. When prescribing these exercises, the clinician must keep in mind the athlete's pain and any changes in inflammation that may be caused by any of these activities.

Modalities should be continued during stage two rehabilitation, because they play an important role in facilitating progression. Modalities of choice include moist heat packs and warm whirlpools, which increase blood flow to the effected area and help facilitate range of motion. In addition, once the tissues have been warmed, therapeutic massage can be used to release scar tissue and adhesions that can prevent normal range of motion. Occasionally, cold modalities can be used before activity in an attempt to minimize pain and enable the athlete to exercise within his or her range of motion comfortably. Following the therapeutic exercise, cold whirlpools and ice packs help minimize or prevent secondary swelling or effusion as a result of the activities.

There is a variety of equipment devices available to assist the athletic trainer with increasing the athlete's range of motion. These devices include the continuous passive motion machine that is used postoperatively and splints that can be used to provide a static stretch to areas where range of motion has been diminished because of adhesions. Isokinetic machines also are capable of providing static stretch to an extremity by isometrically setting the joint at various points throughout the range of motion.

As the athlete progresses through stage two and regains range of motion, the strengthening process should be initiated. In the early portion of the rehabilitation program strengthening can be performed daily, but as strength increases to approximately 25% of the noninjured muscle group the frequency should be decreased to alternate days to facilitate cellular adjustments in the muscle tissue (13). This allows for superior strength gains while minimizing the effects of inflammation caused by excessive frequency and intensity of exercise. Strength gains can be achieved through modes of strengthening, including isometrics, isotonics, and isokinetics. Isometric exercise are employed during the early stages of strengthening and can be used when range of motion needs to be limited. Isometrics help prevent significant disuse atrophy in an immobilized athlete. Isotonic exercises are performed through a range of motion with a fixed resistance. Isotonic exercise can be incorporated to an athlete's rehabilitation program when resistive exercise will not exacerbate the healing process.

There are many available programs that help an athlete increase strength. Examples of these progressive resistive strengthening programs are the DeLorme program (26), the Oxford technique (27), and Knight's Dapper program (28). Progressive resistive exercises are initiated once the athlete has completed a program of active exercise without signs of increased inflammation secondary to the exercise. If inflammation does appear, the exercise program should be curtailed until the inflammatory process is controlled.

The use of isokinetic devices in the rehabilitative process provides an advantage by allowing resistance to accommodate to pain and fatigue as the athlete exercises through the full range of motion. Recently, closed kinetic chain exercises are being advocated by many orthopedic surgeons, resulting in less reliance on isokinetic devices with lower extremity injuries. Certainly, isokinetics will continue to have a role in the rehabilitative process, but their continued use as the sole criterion for return to play has been eliminated from the athletic trainer's program (29).

Proprioceptive and coordination exercises in stage two of rehabilitation are extremely important. Following a non–weight-bearing period, coordination and balance will be compromised as a result of decreases in neurophysiologic stimuli (Fig. 3.11). Promoting balance and coordination during the early stages of rehabilitation are

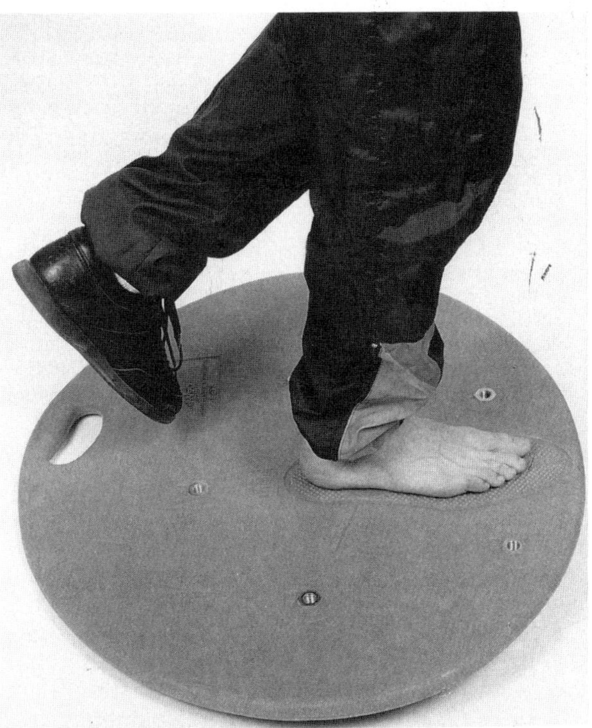

Figure 3.11. Proprioception training using a BAPS board.

important for the athlete in regaining not only the use of his or her limbs but also the self-confidence to perform.

Furthermore, it is important that the athlete appreciates the link between rehabilitation and participation. Thus functional activities that are sport specific should be implemented to ensure that the athlete remains motivated. Examples include pool exercises and the use of rubber tubing resistance activities that mimic or reproduce the motions involved in the desired sport (30). These sport-specific activities enhance the athlete's motivation while inducing adaptations specific to his or her functional requirements.

The goals that an individual makes in stage two of the rehabilitation program can easily be documented to provide a motivational tool for the athlete. Achievement of full range of motion, near-normal strength levels, and near-normal levels of power and endurance as well as increases in balance and coordination and maintenance of cardiovascular endurance provide the athlete with increased motivation.

Stage Three: Chronic Care (Return to Competition)

Return to competition is often the most difficult decision for both the athletic trainer and athlete. The decision must be based on a thorough assessment of the athlete's physical status to ensure that the risk of reinjury has been minimized.

Often the decision to return an athlete to competition is based on the athletic trainer's understanding of the mechanical demands of the sport and the athlete's ability to perform without the risk of injury. Obviously, if the athlete is unable to perform the basic mechanical movements of his or her sport, the likelihood of reinjury or injury to another area increases. It is the trainer's responsibility to ensure that the athlete's physical abilities are appropriate for the activity and that they are consistent with repeated use, thus lowering the likelihood of reinjury and preventing any injuries to other joints or musculoskeletal soft tissue caused by compensation for the injured region.

Another important, yet often neglected, component of returning the athlete to competition is the proprioceptive mechanisms, training of kinestatic awareness, and balance. The rehabilitation program at this point can thus be isolated to ensure that the athlete is able to perform certain activities that are functional within his or her sport without causing any abnormal mechanics at competitive speed. Activities such as jogging straight ahead, doing carioca, running figure eight's and zigzags, running and cutting at 45° cuts, and performing specific agility drills should be employed to ensure that the athlete is able to engage in all activities at full speed and without pain.

Upon returning the athlete to competition any splint, brace, or protective strapping should be considered to assist maintenance and provide additional stability. It is important for the athlete to understand that braces, taping, and splints do not replace the rehabilitation program but help the performance of his or her sport.

The return of normal strength, power, and endurance during the final phase of rehabilitation provide the athlete not only with the aforementioned functional requirements but also assist the athlete with the psychological component of rehabilitation and provide him or her with the confidence to return to competition without fear of reinjury. Information about preinjury strength, aerobic fitness, and power provides objective goals for the athlete.

Return to activity should be gradual and needs to be considered by the athletic trainer, athlete, and coach. This gradual return can be obtained in small-group activities such as one-on-one in basketball and performing full-court drills. Such practice enhances the athlete's confidence in his or her ability to perform. Once the athlete meets the requirements for his or her sport, the length of practice sessions can increase. Practice duration can vary from 25% to full practice, depending on the nature of the injury and any residual effects that may occur, such as swelling and pain, postactivity.

Before any athlete returns to competition, he or she must have regained full mechanical ability, balance, coordination, and general fitness. The athletic trainer must decide along with the physician whether taping or bracing will facilitate the athlete's activity without compromising his or her performance. The decision to return to play is made by the physician, athletic trainer, athlete, and coach based on the athlete's ability to fulfill all requirements demanded of his or her sport.

Athletic rehabilitation is made up of three stages. These stages often overlap, and each can last from 3 days to 6 months. Because of this variation in recovery time, the athletic trainer's role is critical with respect to return to play. Often the motivated athlete wants to return prematurely; however, the athletic trainer must make that decision, taking into consideration the initial care and the progress of the rehabilitation. Thus the athletic trainer plays an important role in deciding when to return the athlete to his or her sport at competitive level.

REFERENCES

1. O'Shea M. History of the NATA. Greenville, NC: National Athletic Trainers Association, 1980.
2. Grace P, Ledderman L. Role delineation study for the certification examination for entry-level athletic trainers. Athletic train 1985;17;264.
3. Peterson M, Peterson K. Eat to compete: a guide to sports nutrition. Chicago: Yearbook Medical Publishers, 1988.
4. Powell J. Pattern of knee injuries associated with college football 1975–1982. Athletic Train 1985;20(2):104–109.
5. Romstar J. No direct deaths in high school football. Phys Sportsmed 1991;19(9):48–49.
6. Scriber K, Matheny M. Knee injuries in college football: an 18 year report. Athletic Train 1990;25(2):127.
7. Duda M. Injury study supports need for more trainers. Phys Sportsmed 1989;17(4):30–31.
8. Brenda C. Catastrophic head and neck injuries in amateur hockey. Phys Sportsmed 1189;97(12):115–122.
9. Mueller F, Schindler R. Annual survey of football injury research 1931–1984. Athletic Train 1985;20(3):213–218.
10. Rosen LW, Hough DO. Pathogenic weight control behaviors of female college gymnasts. Phys Sportsmed 1988;16(9):141–144.
11. Herbert D. What standards exist for conducting and evaluating preparticipation examinations? Reporter 1991;(1):13–15.
12. Arnheim D, Prentice WE. Modern principles of athletic training. 8th ed. St. Louis: CV Mosby, 1993.
13. Hunter-Griffin LY et al. Athletic training and sports medicine. 2nd ed. Park Ridge, IL: AAOS, 1991.
14. Roy S, Irving R. Sports medicine: prevention, evaluation, management and rehabilitation. Englewood Cliffs, NJ: Prentice-Hall, 1983.
15. Dick RW. Eating disorders in NCAA athletic programs. Athletic Train 1991;26(2):137–140.
16. Grandjean A. Eating disorders—the role of the athletic trainer. Athletic Train 1991;26(2):105–112.
17. Francis K, Feinstein R, Brasher J. Optimal practice times for the reduction of risk of heat illnesses during fall football practice in the Southeastern United States. Athletic Train 1991;26(1):76–79.
18. Caroline NL. Emergency care in the street. 3rd ed. Boston: Little, Brown, 1987.
19. Feld F, Blanc R. Immobilizing the spine-injured football player. J Emerg Med Serv 1987;12:38–40.
20. Magee DJ. Orthopaedic physical assessment. Philadelphia: WB Saunders, 1987.
21. Saunders HD. Evaluation, treatment and prevention of musculoskeletal disorders. Minneapolis: Viking Press, 1985.
22. Cyriax J. Textbook of orthopaedic medicine: diagnosis of soft tissue lesions. Vol. 1. 7th ed. London: Bailliere-Tindall, 1978.
23. Kuland DN. The injured athlete. 2nd ed. Philadelphia: JB Lippincott, 1982.
24. Saunders HD. Evaluation of a musculoskeletal disorder. In: Gould JA, Davies GJ, eds. Orthopedic and sports physical therapy. St. Louis: CV Mosby, 1985:169–180.
25. Kendall FP, McCreary EK. Muscle testing and function. 3rd ed. Baltimore: Williams & Wilkins, 1983.
26. DeLorme T, Watkins A. Techniques of progressive resistance exercise. Arch Phy Med Rehab 1948;29:263.
27. Zinowieff AN. Heavy resistance exercise: the oxford technique. Br J Phys Med 1951;14:129.
28. Knight KL. Knee rehabilitation by the daily adjustable progressive exercise technique. Am J Sports Med 1979;7:336.
29. Lephart SM, Perrin DH, Minger K, Fu F. Functional performance tests for the anterior cruciate ligament insufficient athlete. Athletic Train 1991;26(2):44–50.
30. Rarick GL, Sufeldt V. Characteristics of young athletes. In: Thomas JR, ed. Youth sports guide for coaches and parents. Washington, DC: AAPHER, 1973.

4 / ENVIRONMENTAL FACTORS IN ATHLETIC PERFORMANCE

Wayne K. Gersoff and H. Andrew Motz

The environment in which we live contributes greatly to our lifestyles. The role of the environment is even more pronounced when its impact on exercise and athletic participation are considered. Although there are many components of the environment that can potentially impact our ability to exercise, only three will be considered in this chapter: cold, heat, and altitude. Each of these environmental factors will be reviewed in terms of their effects on athletic performance.

Effects of Heat on the Athlete

Thermoregulation

Hyperthermia

The main center for thermoregulation in the human body is the hypothalamus. This structure is a group of specialized nerve cells that serves to protect the body from the buildup or loss of heat. These cells are stimulated in two ways: (*a*) directly, by sensing change in the temperature of the blood perfusing them, and (*b*) indirectly, through special thermoreceptors in the skin. Once these cells are stimulated, there are five mechanisms to facilitate the loss of heat: radiation, conduction, convection, evaporation, and respiration.

Radiation

Heat is exchanged between all objects through electromagnetic waves. Through these waves, heat is transferred from warm objects to cooler objects. When the ambient temperature is lower than body temperature, heat is released from the body to objects in the environment. This exchange does not require molecular contact. However, if the objects in the environment are warmer than body temperature no net heat loss from the body occurs. This explains why thermoregulation is more efficient in the shade than in direct sunlight. The sun warms objects through radiation, and the objects in the environment are cooler when shaded. If they are cooler than body temperature, heat can be released. Generally, 50% of body heat is released through radiation. This avenue is lost when the ambient temperature exceeds body temperature.

Conduction

Conduction involves the direct transfer of heat from one object to another and requires molecular interaction. One of the first responses to increases in body temperature is vasodilation. This enables the body to transfer most of the core heat to the surface rapidly. The heat can be transferred from the surface molecules on the skin directly to clothing or air molecules. Again, this transfer depends on the environmental objects being cooler than body temperature. This phenomenon explains the cooling benefit of a wet shirt or wet towel.

Convection

Convection refers to the motion of fluids (gases or liquids) and their ability to carry molecules of higher temperature away from the body and replace them with cooler molecules. It is codependent on conduction for actual heat loss. The air or water molecules immediately adjacent to the skin are warmed by conduction. The convective currents then move these molecules away and replace them with other molecules that can be heated. If these convective currents are not present, the warmed molecules of air or water remain adjacent to the warm body and actually provide a layer of insulation that impedes further heat loss. Together, conduction and convection account for 15% of heat loss.

Evaporation

Although heat loss through evaporation accounts for only 30% of heat loss in normal situations, it is the principal physiologic defense mechanism against hyperthermia, because it does not depend on the ambient temperature to have an effect. As body temperature increases, the hypothalamus stimulates the cholinergic sympathetic fibers, which in turn stimulate the 3 million sweat glands in the human body. This stimulus causes the release of a hypotonic saline solution, which is then vaporized on the skin surface. For 1 g of saline solution vaporized, approximately 0.6 kcals of heat are removed. Because this occurs on the skin surface, it is the skin that is cooled. This in turn cools the blood, by convection and conduction, that supplies it. At high ambient temperatures, radiation, conduction, and convection all serve to increase body temperature because the objects around the body are equally as hot or hotter. In this situation, only evaporation will cool the body.

Studies have shown that the rate of sweating is directly proportional to the ambient temperature. The major limitation to this method of heat loss is humidity. Humidity refers to the amount of moisture in the air. For a given temperature, the air can only hold so much water. As this limit is reached, the relative humidity increases. As the vapor pressure in the air begins to approach that on the skin, less and less sweat will evaporate. Sweating, by itself, is not enough to release heat, and in fact, if sweat rolls off or is wiped off, its ability to release heat is lost.

Respiration

Respiration is not truly a different avenue of heat loss. It is actually a composite of the other four methods discussed above, although the heat loss does not occur on the skin surface. As cool air is inspired, heat is exchanged through radiation, conduction, and convection. In addition, vaporization occurs from the mucous membranes of lungs, and they are thus cooled. This accounts for less than 5% of normal heat loss.

Heat Injury

Although the body has developed means to lose heat, it is still overcome at times and heat injury can occur. There are three heat exposure syndromes that represent different levels of injury.

Heat Cramps

To ensure proper functioning of all muscles, a delicate balance of electrolytes and water must be maintained. During exercise in the heat, this balance can be altered through the loss of both electrolytes and water through perspiration. When this occurs, the involved muscles may spasm. Although any muscle can be affected, the most common is the calf muscle. These spasms are unrelated to the fibrillations of overexerted muscles or the spasms of injured (pulled) muscles.

As in all heat injuries, the best treatment is prevention. Proper ingestion of fluids—both in the days and hours preceding exercise and in the normal diet—is necessary to avoid cramps. Once cramps have occurred, the proper treatment is rest, passive stretching, and rehydration.

Heat Exhaustion

Heat exhaustion (also known as heat prostration or heat syncope) is a manifestation of an inadequate cardiovascular response to heat stress. During heat stress, blood is directed to the skin so that heat can be released. During exercise in the heat, the muscles also require more blood flow. These increased demands on blood volume require that blood be shunted from other bodily systems. In physically fit, well-acclimatized individuals, this dual stress can be compensated for by the cardiovascular system. However, in unfit or unacclimatized individuals, the stress is too much and central blood volume is insufficient to maintain cardiac output. The symptoms are, therefore, primarily those of shock: weak, rapid pulse; low blood pressure; dizziness or postural syncope; headache; pallor; nausea and/or vomiting; loss of appetite; urge to defecate; and general weakness. Body temperature is generally not elevated.

Treatment consists of lying down in a cool environment and hypotonic fluid replacement; in some cases, the fluids should be replaced intravenously. Athletes with heart disease or those who have recently had bouts of vomiting or diarrhea are most susceptible than other athletes.

Heat Stroke

Heat stroke represents a true medical emergency. The mortality rate is 20% to 75% if cooling is not effective. The cause of death is from damage to the cells of the central nervous system, and survivors may have persistent symptoms of nerve damage. Heat stroke may develop as a sequela to heat exhaustion or suddenly, without warning. Heat stroke represents a failure in the temperature-regulating system. It occurs most commonly in conditions of high ambient temperature and high humidity, but can occur in the absence of both. Under conditions of heat stress, the body cannot respond indefinitely. When dehydration occurs, sweat production stops. In high ambient temperatures, this is usually the last of the defense mechanisms and so the body temperature begins to climb. This is further aggravated by the increase in metabolic rate that accompanies increases in core temperature. The increased metabolic demands especially affect the central nervous system, and cell damage occurs when the demands are not met. Symptoms of heat stroke include mental status changes, emotional lability, and unsteady gait. The pulse is generally strong initially, respiration is rapid, and temperature is high. The skin is warm and *dry*. The athlete lapses into unconsciousness, and as further cell damage occurs, the pulse weakens and blood pressure drops.

Immediate treatment involves taking any steps available to lower body temperature; alcohol rubs, ice packs, and wet sheets with fans are acceptable temporary measures, but whole body immersion in a tub with iced water is best. Although cooling should be the priority, treatment for shock also may be necessary. Acetaminophen and aspirin are not helpful, because their antipyretic effects depend on intact heat-regulating mechanisms. *An important reminder:* Oral temperature is not an accurate indication of core temperature in athletes following exercise. Rectal temperatures are much more accurate and should be used for both diagnosis and subsequent monitoring of treatment.

Predisposing Factors

Although all athletes are susceptible to any of the heat illness syndromes, there are several factors that may place certain athletes at risk. In addition to discussing these factors, other popular misconceptions about heat illness also will be addressed.

Drugs

The most important class of drugs in heat illness are the diuretics. In cases of prescription use (hypertension, edema, etc.), the body usually makes adjustments over time in the cardiovascular system to decrease this risk. However, diuretics are abused by athletes required to make weight, especially wrestlers. The short-term use just before events does not allow compensation and puts the athletes at risk for thermal and cardiovascular breakdown. In addition, diuretics are known to interfere with neuromuscular function through an unknown mechanism that seems to be independent of fluid and electrolyte concentrations. Cathartics and laxatives also are abused by these athletes. In addition to dehydration, they are associated with potassium loss, which causes muscle weakness.

Although not technically a drug, salt tablets are often abused by athletes. Most Americans get adequate salt intake from their diets. Although athletes may lose salt through sweating, only small increases in dietary salt are usually needed to replace this loss. Salt tablets are known to cause abdominal cramping and the gastric electrolyte load. If not accompanied by adequate fluid intake, the excess salt will draw fluid out of the cells and exacerbate dehydration.

Acclimatization

Acclimatization involves neural, hormonal, and cardiovascular changes in response to repeated heat stress. Heat illness frequently occurs at the start of athletic training, before the body has had a chance to adapt to heat stress. This is independent of general conditioning as it is known to occur in individuals who are not changing their workouts, just their environment. The bulk of this process is complete within the first week of exposure and results in increased exercise capacity and decreased discomfort. The body adapts by becoming better able to shunt blood to the periphery with less cardiovascular compromise. There also is a lower threshold for sweating so that the heat-regulating system is turned on sooner, preventing increases in core temperature. Thus sweating soon after initiation of exercise is not an indication of being out of shape but of being acclimatized.

Obesity

Fatal heat stroke is known to occur more than three times more often in obese individuals than thinner individuals. The increase in metabolic requirements simply to move the heavier load stresses the heat-regulatory system. In addition, the fat serves as insulation that prevents conduction of heat to the skin surface.

Gender

Although men do sweat more and at lower core temperature, they do not possess better heat-regulating capabilities than women. If controlled for level of conditioning and acclimatization, women are able to tolerate heat as well as men. This indicates that women probably have better adapted circulatory responses for the release of heat.

Age

Although there is a delayed onset of sweating associated with advancing age, there is controversy as to whether this affects heat-regulating capabilities. Studies comparing young and middle-aged marathon runners showed no difference in ability to regulate temperature. The increased incidence of cardiac disease with age is probably the most likely explanation for any difference in heat tolerance.

Clothing

The choice of clothing may have the most pronounced effect on the body's ability to regulate heat for a variety of reasons. As discussed earlier, sweating only works to control heat if evaporation occurs. Dry clothing of any type absorbs the sweat from the skin before it has a chance to evaporate. Evaporation will only occur when the clothing is soaked. Many athletes like to change their shirts when they become soaked with sweat but this only inhibits the body's ability to regulate heat. The best choice is clothes that are made of a light-colored (to reflect radiant energy from the sun), loosely fitting (to enhance convection), highly absorbent material; the clothing should be left in place throughout the exercise. The use of sweat suits, especially in warm climates, is dangerous and of no benefit. They are usually made of synthetic, nonabsorbent material. Thus the relative humidity between the suit and the skin rises quickly, regardless of the humidity of the environment, because the moisture is not allowed to escape. Evaporation is retarded, convection and conduction are prevented, and the body increased temperature becomes difficult to regulate. As there is no documented advantage to the use of sweat suits in conditioning, athletes should be discouraged from wearing them. Football uniforms interfere with heat regulation in a similar way as well as increasing the metabolic load because of the increased weight the athlete must carry.

Heat injury syndromes are common and potentially life threatening. They also are totally preventable. Athletes should be made aware of these entities and instructed in simple methods of prevention: Avoid dehydration before exercise, properly rehydrate during and after exercise, condition, acclimatice, and wear proper clothing. Through these simple measures, heat injuries can be avoided.

Effects of Cold on the Athlete

Cold-related problems for the athlete represent one of the most common athletic environmental hazards.

Indeed, the cold can play an important role in any outdoor sport. Although cold-related problems are usually associated with winter sports such as skiing, skating, mountaineering, and snowshoeing, other sports also introduce risk, including running, cycling, swimming, and hiking.

Cold Weather Physiology

The human body represents a remarkable temperature-controlled machine. It has the ability to maintain a relatively constant body temperature in varying types of environments. Unfortunately, the human body has evolved in such a way that makes efficient acclimatization to cold very difficult. However, the human body has developed several mechanisms that not only generate body heat but also conserve body heat. The generation of body heat can be divided into four categories of mechanisms: basal heat production, muscular thermoregulatory heat, high-intensity exercise–induced heat, and mild- to moderate-intensity exercise–induced heat.

Basal heat production is associated with the heat that is produced by the normal metabolic processes of the body. Although this is sufficient to maintain the body under various resting conditions, it is relatively ineffective in generating body heat during the exposure to relatively colder environments.

Muscular thermoregulatory heat refers to the heat that is produced by the mechanisms of shivering. Along with the commencement of shivering, there also is an alteration in the circulatory flow to provide more heat to the internal organs. Therefore, the blood circulation from the toes, fingers, and facial structures will be affected first. In the event that cooling further progresses, the core body temperature will be lowered. Although shivering may increase heat production three to five times the basal level, it also has the negative effect of using large amounts of energy, which is reserved in the body. The actual act of shivering also can reduce coordination and useful movements that may be needed to perform tasks that will help conserve body heat.

High-intensity exercise–induced heat simply refers to the heat that is produced by the body during various activities, such as walking or running, in which there is increased muscular activity. Although this type of heat production can generate up to 10 times the basal heat generation, it can only be maintained for several minutes. This is because it rapidly exhausts the energy stored within the body.

Mild- to moderate-intensity exercise–induced heat is provided by the same mechanisms as other exercise-induced heat. However, because of the lower rate and intensity of exercise, this form of heat production is only approximately five times greater than the basal level. Because it uses less of the body's stored energy, it can be maintained for longer periods of time than high-intensity exercise–induced heat.

In addition to mechanisms for generating body heat, the body also has developed mechanisms for conserving body heat. These include superficial forms of constriction, body insulation, and external heat sources. In the event that the body is exposed to a cold environment, blood flow will be shunted away from the surface area of the body to the core. Blood is moved away from areas where it can easily lose heat to the cooler environment and brought to areas that greatly depend on optimal temperatures for their function. The body also insulates itself to conserve heat. The most common manner in which this is done is by layering subcutaneous fat in the body. Although not totally developed by the body itself, the application of external heat sources such as proper clothing or exposure to external sources of heat such as fire, sun, and hot food also provide insulation against heat loss. As mentioned earlier, the body also has several mechanisms of transferring heat. These are important in the processes involved in maintaining the steady state not only against hot environments but also against cold environments.

When discussing the various physiologic factors in cold weather and cold environments, consider the body to consist of a core and a shell. The core refers to internal structures such as the brain, heart, lungs, and abdominal organs. The shell refers to the skin, muscles, and extremities. When the shell temperature decreases and the core temperature is maintained, the result is local injuries to the shell. However, if the shell temperature decreases and the core temperature also decreases, then it is possible that systemic problems will develop.

Cold environments also will have an effect on the potential performance capabilities of the individual. Cold environments reduce the exercise efficiency of an individual. This is probably related to the fact that in the cold environment muscle function is decreased and nerve conduction can be slowed. In addition, if it gets cold enough for the body's mechanisms to be activated, the first mechanism to be implemented is shivering, which also will inhibit the performance of the individual.

Furthermore, it has also been shown that there are various predisposing factors for individuals to develop problems in a cold environment. These include inadequate insulation of the body, restricted peripheral circulation (Raynaud's disease or diabetes), fatigue, poor nutrition, the use of alcohol, the use of tobacco, age, and the body's ability to shunt the blood.

Specific Cold Injuries

Cold injuries can be classified as being either local or systemic. Local cold injuries result when the shell temperature, that of the skin and the peripheral tissues, is exposed to freezing temperatures but the core body temperature is maintained. If however, the cold induces a drop not only in the peripheral temperature but also in the core temperature, then more systemic manifestations such as hypothermia can be produced. In this section the local cold injuries—frostnip, chilblains, and frostbite foot—will be discussed along with the systemic injury of hypothermia.

Frostnip

Frostnip is a slow-developing condition that results in blanching or whiteness of the skin. This is usually associated with reversible ice crystal formation on the skin's surface. Frostnip usually will develop slowly and painlessly and usually affects the tips of the ears, nose, cheeks, chin, fingertips, and toes. Unfortunately, this condition is not first recognized by the victim but rather by a companion. Frostnip often is confused with frostbite. It is frequently seen in conditions of high wind, extreme cold, or both.

Most commonly no permanent tissue damage will be obtained from frostnip. It is important to treat this condition in an appropriate fashion to prevent tissue damage. The treatment that is recommended for frostnip is to provide warming of the effected tissue by the firm steady contact of a warm hand, by blowing hot breath on the effected tissue, or by holding the injured body part in either the axilla or the groin area. It is extremely important not to rub the skin with snow. This old folklore treatment can actually result in more damage to the tissue. As the tissue gradually warms and thaws out, the color returns and the victim may experience tingling in that body part. Indeed, several days after the tissue has warmed, the skin may continue to be red, and there may even be some flaking of the skin. As in all types of cold injuries, it is best to try to prevent their onset. There is no guaranteed prevention for frostnip, except to allow for adequate protection of exposed body parts and to recognize the environmental risk conditions.

Chilblains

Chilblains are commonly grouped with trench foot or immersion foot. The underlying etiology of this condition results from repeated exposure of bare skin to cold water or from wet cooling of an extremity for prolonged periods of time, usually at a temperature around freezing. Trench foot usually affects the lower extremity, and chilblains are found on the hands and feet. Initially, this condition damages the capillaries of the skin. With further progression of the injury, one can see necrosis or gangrene of the skin, underlying muscles, nerves, and other associated soft tissue. This injury initially results in red, swollen, hot, and tender skin. It can then progress to mottled skin with a pale or grayish blue tint. The usual initial symptoms are that of tingling, and/or burning. The extremity also may feel cold and numb.

Upon rewarming of the effected body part, there is a typical sequence of events. The skin may again become red, swollen, and hot. Areas of increased itchy sensations may develop. These areas may blister and/or develop localized gangrene. Interestingly enough, recurrence of this injury tends to happen in the same area of the body. This is probably related to some degree of permanent injury to the peripheral vascular system in that body part. The treatment of this particular entity depends on the cause. If the injury has developed secondary to exposure to a wet, cold environment, then the limb must be cleaned, dried, and carefully rewarmed. The rewarming of the limb should take place in an appropriate environment. If this environment is not available, then the limb is at risk for reexposure to increased cold. Unfortunately, there is no treatment for this entity once skin injury has been established. Therefore, all treatment should be geared to prevent recurrence and to protect the area that is injured from further exposure to cold.

Frostbite

Frostbite represents one of the worst local cold-related injuries. It is caused by the actual freezing of the soft tissue. The danger of frostbite must be considered very strongly whenever there is exposure to extreme cold. It is important to be aware of the effects of windchill, direct contact with frozen objects, and hypoxia from high altitudes as well. It also is believed that the abuse of internasal cocaine can increase the risk of nasal frostbite. The areas of the body that are commonly involved in frostbite injury are the fingertips, earlobes, tip of the nose, toes, and any exposed areas of skin. Frostbite can be classified into various stages based on the degree of injury. First-degree frostbite is usually associated with local pain or discomfort. There also is usually a numbness, redness, or swelling of the affected area. Second-degree frostbite displays all of the previously mentioned symptoms along with the development of a serous superficial blistering. Third-degree frostbite brings on the development of deep blistering, which is of a hemoserous nature. Fourth-degree frostbite involves the deep soft tissues. This includes bone and could result in possible mummification of the tissues, leading to the need for amputation.

Initially, the victim experiencing frostbite will develop swelling and redness of the effected body part. This is often preceded by itching or prickling sensations. After this initial appearance, the skin on the frostbitten area may appear white, often with a yellowish to bluish tint that gives it the appearance of wax.

The treatment of frostbite should be directed toward the prevention of any further injury to the tissue and to being able to prevent the necrosis of any damaged tissue. While it may appear to be a justifiable treatment, rubbing or massaging frostbitten tissues is strongly contraindicated. The accepted therapy for frostbite is rapid rewarming. In this regard, a whirlpool type of device is ideal. It is recommended that the water temperature be 40° to 42°C (104° to 108°F). The use of dry heat such as from a camp fire, car exhaust, or radiator is contraindicated. This type of rewarming is slow and the heat is often not equally distributed. In addition, because of numbness, there is a chance for the skin to become burned from this type of heat. If out in the field with a victim who is experiencing frostbite, it is strongly recommended not to thaw out the frostbitten part unless there is a mechanism available to keep it thawed. If the frostbitten part is thawed and then allowed to refreeze, there is a greater risk of more extensive damage. Depending on the extent of the frostbite and the penetration into the deeper tissues, the time of thawing can take from 30 to 45 min. It is important to note that upon rewarming of the frostbitten body part, the victim will experience pain. The degree of pain will be related to the degree of frostbite injury. The victim may need an analgesic to help him or her deal with the pain. It is extremely important to warn the victim that this pain on rewarming is not a dangerous sign, but rather part of the natural process of rewarming.

After the body part has been rewarmed and blood flow returns to the area, the injured tissue may appear mottled, blue, or purple. There also may be swelling, resulting in large blisters or gangrenous areas several days after treatment. These blisters may eventually form blackened necrotic areas of tissue. The area of necrotic tissue can easily be separated from the normal skin. The new skin is usually of a poorer quality than the original and appears to be very sensitive to cold.

The initial management of the frostbite injury after thawing should be of a protective nature. It should include the use of an antibiotic type of ointment to the skin. The skin also should be protected with soft sterile bandages. Whenever possible, blisters should be left intact, but they may require further debridement after arrival at a health-care facility. The involved skin should be protected from extreme contact. This can be done by either elevating the limb or designing a protective cradle around the limb to prevent any pressure. Anyone who has experienced a frostbite injury should be examined in a medical facility. It is generally recommended that all frostbite injuries greater than first-degree be observed in a hospital. It is often difficult to access viability accurately from the gross appearance of the damaged part. Therefore, it is necessary to observe such injuries over time. This is especially important when considering the possibility of amputation. Amputation should be delayed as long as possible to allow the tissues truly to demonstrated what is necrotic and what is salvageable.

Ultimately, the best way to treat frostbite is to prevent frostbite. There are many ways to prevent frostbite, and most important is to prepare for the environment. This requires the individual to be aware of not only the actual temperature but the temperature as affected by windchill factors. Prevention includes adequate and properly fitted clothing as well as protection of exposed body parts, e.g., hands, feet, nose, and ears. It also is extremely important to keep clothing dry and prevent subsequent chilling from the moist clothing next to the body. If a body part feels as though it were getting cold, the individual should move it continually and be careful not to keep it in one position for a long time. This is especially true with the toes and the hands. However, if the face is beginning to feel cold, it is important to use the facial muscles to help generate some heat in that area. Remember that when out in a harsh environment, it is imperative to observe the other people's faces and any other exposed skin for possible signs of frostbite injury.

Hypothermia

Unlike the previously discussed injuries, hypothermia is a systemic injury. Hypothermia will occur when the body's core temperature drops to less than 95°F (35°C). Hypothermia causes 500 to 700 deaths per year in the United States. It can occur at almost any altitude and in any temperature that is lower than body core temperature. Several types of individuals have been identified with an increased risk for hypothermia, including accident and trauma victims, the very young and very old, people with chronic metabolic disease, people with acute or chronic alcoholism and/or acute intoxication or drug overdose, and those that are mentally impaired.

Hypothermia has been classified as mild, moderate, or severe and within these classes as either being acute, subacute, or chronic. Mild hypothermia is diagnosed when the rectal core temperature (RCT) is greater than 95°F but less than 98.6°F. Moderate hypothermia is when the RCT is greater than 90°F but less than 95°F. Severe hypothermia occurs when the RCT drops to below 90°F.

Hypothermia represents a true medical emergency. It is important to recognize the condition as soon as possible. Once recognized, action should be taken to prevent the further loss of body heat and to rewarm the individual safely and quickly. While it might be difficult in the field, it certainly must be recognized that the development of cardiac ventricular fibrillation is a distinct possibility in these individuals. It is, therefore, imperative that care be taken in treating these individuals in the field, in transporting them, and also in rewarming them. Hypothermia must be suspected whenever an individual is found in a cold environment with an altered mental status. In addition, it also must be strongly considered if there is a history of trauma or cold water immersion. Any individual with hypothermia and altered mental status should not be given the opportunity to make important decisions because his or her judgment will certainly be impaired. To assess the degree of hypothermia in these individuals, a low temperature thermometer—one that is calibrated below 94°F—is needed. Both oral and axillary temperatures are relatively unreliable in this regard, and rectal temperatures must be taken.

Victims of hypothermia are very sensitive metabolically, especially in their cardiovascular system. Therefore, they must be handled very carefully and any unnecessary agitation must be avoided. As in any emergency, it is important to maintain an airway for respiration. The rewarming of an individual who has experienced hypothermia should be carefully done. The possible sources of heat for rewarming must be considered; however, the victim should not engage in vigorous exercise and should not be rubbed or massaged. The victim should not be immersed. If the individual experiences cardiopulmonary arrest, CPR should be initiated and continued until the victim is revived or death is pronounced. CPR should never be stopped because the patient appears to be clinically dead. This is common in people who are hypothermic, and often the patient will recover. It is imperative that an individual who has experienced cardiopulmonary arrest be transported to a medical facility as quickly as possible.

Specific Levels of Hypothermia. Mild hypothermia is characterized by a rectal core temperature of less than 98.6°F but greater than 95°F. The individual experiencing mild hypothermia will usually have a sensation of cold fingers and toes. They also may develop chills and shivering. On a physiological level, the victim will have an increased pulse rate and an increased respiratory rate. These individuals also may experience slight incoordination and a urinary urgency. Mild hypothermia is the most common of all stages of hypothermia and needs to be recognized, because of the possibility of an increase in severity. The individual experiencing mild hypothermia should be placed in a shelter that will protect him or her from the environmental factors. Any wet clothing needs to be replaced with dry clothing. Some type of external heat source should be developed, such as a fire. Efforts should be made to avoid heat loss from the individual as well. It is important when traveling in groups or competing in groups, that the earliest signs of hypothermia be recognized and all teammates participate in the treatment of the victim.

Moderate hypothermia involves increased fatigue and the loss of the shivering mechanism. There also is an increase in muscular uncoordination. These individuals have the potential to develop an altered mental state and also will not be good historians or reporters of their state. In addition, they will experience the numbing of the fingers and toes with actual functional loss. Moderate hypothermia needs to be treated immediately. It is important to recognize its development. Any individual demonstrating decreased signs of shivering, slow reactions, or any other altered state of mental capacity must be suspected of having developed moderate hypothermia and should be treated appropriately. The victim should be warmed and protected from the environment. If there is alteration of the mental state, the victim should not be given fluids or foods by mouth. If they are given by mouth and the patient is not fully awake, there is a risk of aspiration. Attention should be directed toward rewarming of the body core before the extremities.

Severe hypothermia results in a complete loss of shivering, marked confusion, inappropriate behavior, and visual disturbances. There also may be changing levels of consciousness. As the core body temperature continues to drop, especially if the RCT goes below 85°F, muscle rigor may develop. At the physiologic level, the victim's blood pressure, pulse, and respiratory rate are depressed. Pulmonary edema may develop as well. Such an individual is in severe danger of developing cardiac arrhythmias. If this victim develops any sign of cardiorespiratory compromise, he or she needs to be very closely monitored. Because the body core temperature is lowered, the hypothermia can be somewhat protective, and the victim may not require a high pulse or respiratory rate to support life. Indeed, if CPR is initiated before it is needed, an arrhythmia may develop because of the fragile state of the cardiac muscle. The severe hypothermia victim must be monitored very closely and transported safely to a medical facility as quickly as possible.

Prevention. The prevention of hypothermia is of the utmost importance. Hypothermia can effect any individual who is exposed to a cold environment, including competitive outdoor athletes, spectators, and recreational athletes. The human body cannot acclimatize well to the cold environment. There is some degree of adjustment, but it varies greatly with physical condition, overall health, nutrition, and age. Hypothermia can represent a life-threatening situation, and therefore, appropriate measures should be undertaken to prevent its development. Some ways to prepare for outdoor exposure and prevent hypothermia include the following: appropriate preparation for the worse conditions, appropriate food supplements for the duration of the outdoor exposure, appropriate fluid intake to avoid dehydration, appropriate clothing that may be placed in layers, clothing that is windproof and well-insulated and allows for water to evaporate, avoidance of becoming wet, avoidance of alcoholic beverages, recognition of high-risk situations and individuals at risk, and common sense.

Nature provides a wonderful arena for athletic activities at all levels. Unfortunately, the outdoors can be dangerous. It is important to be prepared to recognize any of the dangers that will cause injury to individuals in the outdoors. Those people who choose to recreate or compete in potentially dangerously cold environments also need to know how to prepare themselves for this participation and how to prevent both local and systemic injuries.

Effects of Altitude on the Athlete

Athletic performance at increased altitudes first became important during the 1968 Olympic Games in Mexico City. At that time, exercise physiologists and athletes were concerned about the effect that an altitude of 2237 m would have on their performance capabilities. Before this time, altitude was only the concern of mountaineers and other individuals who were doing labor at altitude. From the experience of mountaineers, it was known that certain types of tasks were difficult to perform at higher altitudes. The principal question, therefore, was which events would be affected by altitude. Since the 1968 Olympic Games in Mexico City, there has been a continuing growth of research into the effects of increased altitude on athletic performance. However, there are still many unanswered questions and there are many theories that are yet to be supported by well-organized research. This section delves into the areas of physiologic considerations, acclimatization, the general altitude disorders, and the effects of training and performance at altitude.

Physiologic Considerations

As altitude increases, there is a reduced availability of oxygen present for the body to use. For example, at sea level, the partial pressure of oxygen is 159 mm Hg; however, at 2438 m the partial pressure of oxygen is only 118 mm Hg. Thus at high altitude the body experiences a restriction of the oxygen delivery system, which is believed to show direct relationship with the decrease in total oxygen pressure and an inverse relationship to altitude.

The alteration in availability of oxygen has a direct effect on the pulmonary system as well. The effects on the pulmonary system also lead to various changes in the acid-base balance in the body. At altitude there is an increase in the rate of pulmonary ventilation when the individual is at rest and exercising. The increased ventilatory rate is actually a compensatory mechanism. To obtain the necessary amount of oxygen in the lung, the individual must breathe more rapidly because there is less oxygen available with each breath. This results in hyperventilation, which is similar to that seen at sea level. The result of hyperventilation is that carbon dioxide is forced out of the alveoli and its concentration rises in the blood. The increased carbon dioxide delivery to the blood raises the pH of the blood, which is called respiratory alkalosis. The kidneys immediately compensate for the respiratory alkalosis by removing excess bicarbonate in an effort to normalize the pH of the blood. Therefore, there is excretion of base and a decrease in the alkaline reserve.

The effects of altitude on the cardiovascular system can be divided into immediate effects and long-term effects. The immediate effects are the increase in submaximal heart rate and cardiac output. At altitude, the stroke volume remains the same or slightly decreases along with the maximal heart rate and cardiac output.

The long-term effects of altitude on the cardiovascular system include an increase in the submaximal heart rate and a decrease in the stroke volume, maximal heart rate, and maximal cardiac output. The submaximal cardiac output also will fall to rates below those seen at sea level.

The hematopoietic system also is effected by exposure to altitude. There is a loss in plasma volume that occurs upon arrival at a high altitude; however, this is believed to be a transient response. In addition, there is an increase in the number of red blood cells circulating throughout the body. This is demonstrated by not only the increase in hematocrit but also increases in hemoglobin and the total red blood cell count. The changes in the red blood cell count and hemoglobin allow the body to increase its oxygen-carrying capacity within a fixed volume of blood.

At the local cellular level, research has indicated that there is an increase in the capillarization of the skeletal muscle. Associated with this is an increase in the red blood cell organic phosphate 2,3-diphosphoglycerate (2,3-DPG), an increase in the number of mitochondria within the cell, and an increase in the number of aerobic enzymes.

Acclimatization

Acclimatization can be defined as the adaptive responses that the body undertakes to improve its tolerance to altitude hypoxia. For the individual involved in athletic competition at altitude, acclimatization requires not only physiologic but psychological components. At a physiologic level, the athlete's body needs to respond with an increase in red blood cell production and concentration and eventually an increase in the total blood volume. The monitoring of red blood cell concentration can be misleading, however, because immediate responses to altitude are hydration and loss of plasma volume. The athlete's body also must adjust acutely by increasing pulmonary ventilation, which will help regain a normal alveolar and arterial P_{O_2}.

On a psychological level, the athlete must adjust to what has been termed competitive acclimatization. This simply refers to the athlete learning to be able to compete at high altitude. While this does encompass the physiologic adaptations associated with training at altitude, it also must include the idea of actually being able to compete at altitude. This involves experience, which will allow the athlete to determine the best strategies for his or her own training and competition within his or her sport.

There is a great deal of variation among authorities regarding how long it takes to become totally acclimatized to altitude. It is generally agreed that for long-term acclimatization and total physiologic adaptation, the body requires between 6 and 8 weeks. A lot of the short-term adaptations that can take place greatly depend on the specific altitude. For example, it is generally accepted that for exposure of altitudes up to 2300 it may require up to 2 weeks for the body to become fairly acclimatized. It is estimated that it would then require 1 week more for each 610 m increase in altitude up to an altitude of 4572 m. Again, these are general guidelines and do not refer to fully acclimatized physiologic adaptations.

For the athlete that will be soon competing at altitude, it is recommended that intense training start as soon as possible after exposure to altitude and the period of acclimatization. Once the athlete is acclimatized, it is predicted that these effects will last from 2 to 3 weeks after returning to sea level. The aspects of training at altitude for performance at sea level will be discussed later.

Altitude Disorders

No one, not even the highly trained athlete, is immune from illnesses that can develop secondary to rapid exposure to high altitudes. The actual severity and onset of symptoms vary between individuals and the specific altitude. The symptoms that develop from altitude exposure are believed to be directly proportional to not only the repeated descent but the duration and degree of exertion. Symptoms also are inversely proportional to the amount of acclimatization and physical conditioning. In general, the initial signs and symptoms that are felt by the individual who is exposed to increased elevations are the result of hypoxia. This is a direct result of the physiologic response described above. It should be noted that the symptoms of altitude exposure can be present even at elevations as low as 1615 m. The disorders that are most commonly associated with acute altitude exposure are acute mountain sickness (AMS), high-altitude pulmonary edema (HAPE), and high-altitude cerebral edema (HACE).

Acute Mountain Sickness

Acute mountain sickness represents the mildest form of altitude disorder and can actually occur at almost any increased altitude. Most people that go to a high altitude from sea level will probably experience this type of disorder. Most commonly, the individual will notice a time lag of from 6 to 96 hr between the arrival at altitude and the onset of symptoms. The more common symptoms associated with acute mountain sickness are headaches, difficulty sleeping, dyspnea on exertion, loss of appetite, fatigue, light-headedness, weakness, and sometimes confusion and edema. If these symptoms associated with acute mountain sickness are recognized and care is taken to keep the body well hydrated and not overexerted, the individual can experience resolution after 72 hr. Many people experience AMS when going, for example, from Texas to the mountains of Colorado to go skiing.

High-Altitude Pulmonary Edema

A more severe disorder that can occur with exposure to higher altitudes is high-altitude pulmonary edema. High-altitude pulmonary edema represents a noncardiac form of pulmonary edema. Although symptoms may vary in severity, it certainly represents a dramatic form of altitude illness. The more common symptoms associated with HAPE are shortness of breath, increased respiratory rate, irritating cough, and sometimes hemoptysis. In addition to these symptoms, the diagnosis is strongly suspected when rales can be heard on auscultation of the chest.

Any athlete or individual who is suspected of having high-altitude pulmonary edema must be returned to a lower altitude as quickly and as safely as possible and must be given oxygen when possible. Because HAPE is often seen in the reascent of individuals to a higher altitude, any individual who experiences high-altitude pulmonary edema must be thoroughly reevaluated before being allowed to return to an increased altitude.

High-Altitude Cerebral Edema

Although uncommon, high-altitude cerebral edema represents the most dangerous and serious form of altitude sickness. HACE has been reported at altitudes as low as 2438 m, but it is usually considered rare below an altitude of 3658 m. The actual relationship between the development of high-altitude pulmonary edema and high-altitude cerebral edema remains uncertain. Individuals that are developing HACE will, like all altitude disorders, initially present with the signs and symptoms of acute mountain sickness. However, the individual with HACE will then experience increasing severity of headaches, which can often be followed by confusion, forgetfulness, emotional instability, hallucinations, motor weakness, and reflex changes. This entity may progress to not only coma but death. Increased cerebral pressure and swelling of the brain results in bradycardia upon initial evaluation of these people. The increased brain swelling also leads to impairment of judgment and coordination. As further swelling of the brain—especially the cerebellum—occurs, various ocular signs such as blurring of vision, papilledema, and retinal and vitreous hemorrhage may develop. As with high-altitude pulmonary edema, HACE victims must be moved to a lower altitude as quickly and as safely as possible.

Other Concerns

Although not directly considered to be altitude disorders, it is important to remember that at higher altitudes the ambient temperature is low and exposure ultraviolet light is high. The individual who will be competing or training under these conditions must remember not only to protect his or her skin with appropriate sun block but also to protect his or her eyes, so as not to damage the cornea and retina.

Preparation and Prevention of Illness

Although there are no specific guarantees for the prevention of any type of altitude disorder, several guidelines have been suggested for individuals who will be either competing or recreating at increased altitudes. One of the keys to minimizing the chances of developing acute mountain sickness for the athlete or the athletic team is to compete within 24 hr of arriving at the altitude destination. The authors have noted that if a team arrives in, e.g., Boulder or Denver the night before the competition, few athletes have difficulty with the altitude. Individuals who do not have the luxury of arriving at altitude 24 hr before their competition should try to allow at least 2 weeks for training at altitude. This will allow the fundamental physiologic adaptation to occur so that the individual is able to compete effectively. An individual who knows that he or she will be involved in athletics at a high altitude should begin preparation months before exposure, including the development of a high level of cardiovascular fitness. While this may not be of concern to the highly trained athlete, it will be to the recreational athlete.

Because of the acute loss of plasma volume and insensible water loss at altitude, it is strongly recommended and very necessary to drink lots of water or a fluid-replacement drink. Studies have shown that high-carbohydrate meals should be eaten at high altitudes, because they are easily digested, providing a high-energy source. Alcoholic beverages should be avoided because they contribute to dehydration of the body.

Mountaineers have recognized that the use of Diamox, a carbonic anhydrase inhibitor, lessens the effects of altitude. Unfortunately, Diamox has several side effects, including tingling of the ears and mouth, and should not be taken if there is any history of cardiac illness in the athlete. It also is considered a diuretic, and as such, Diamox is banned from use by competitors in the Olympics and many other international events.

Training and Performance

When training for events at altitude, the athlete must consider several important factors. It is important, of course, that the athlete understand the physiologic effects of altitude; however, he or she also must be aware of the effects that altitude will have on performance. In general, events or competitions that require strength and flexibility are not affected by altitude. Events that involve skill can be either negatively or positively affected by altitude exposure, depending on whether the activity involves a high-endurance or a high-speed component. Many athletes whose events involve speed through the air, for example, sprinting and cycling, usually achieved better results at altitude, because they are now moving through a less dense atmosphere. Swimmers, however, do not experience this phenomenon, because water at altitude is the same density as it is at sea level. Athletic events that require endurance are adversely affected by altitude, because of the lower blood oxygen concentration and the reduced atmosphere oxygen. Therefore, altitude does not adversely affect anaerobic events, but the decreased oxygen pressure does have a negative effect on aerobic activities. An interesting contradiction to this concept is seen with endurance events that do not involve running, for example, bicycling, speed skating, and nordic skiing. In these events, performance at altitude may be improved, because the positive aspects of decreased air resistance become more important than the negative effects of decreased oxygen availability.

When training for events at altitude, appropriate measures to prevent altitude sickness must be taken. In addition, it is important that the training program be designed to counterbalance the negative effects altitude has on endurance events. A prime consideration is the amount of time that is available for training. If the athlete has less than 1 week available for acclimatization, it is probably best for him or her to arrive at the event site just before competition. The ideal situation is to give the athlete several weeks at altitude before the competition, which would allow him or her to acclimatize.

There has been much discussion and research concerning the benefits of training at altitude for an athletic event that will occur at sea level. Unfortunately, much of the information about the effects of altitude training seem to be rather anecdotal. Research, however, does suggest that altitude-trained athletes have the capability to perform better at sea level than do equally trained athletes who train only at sea level. An important consideration in doing altitude training for sea-level events is the amount of time that is needed for training before returning to sea level. The athlete should probably train at least 2 weeks at altitude to prepare for the sea-level event. It is important also to consider the effects of going from a cooler and dryer atmosphere at altitude to a warmer and possibly humid environment at sea level. Upon returning to sea level, the effects of training at altitude are usually lost after 2 or 3 weeks. In all cases, it should be remembered that training at altitude alone is not a substitute for hard work and appropriate levels of training.

SUGGESTED READINGS

Adams WC, Fox RH, Fay AJ, MacDonald IC. Thermoregulation during marathon running in cool, moderate, and hot environments. J Appl Physiol 1975;38:1030–1037.

Avellini BA, Kamon E, Krajewski JT. Physiological responses of physically fit men and women to acclimation to humid heat. J Appl Physiol 1980;49:254–261.

Bass DE. Mechanisms of acclimatization to heat in man. Medicine 1955;34:323–332.

Boname JR, Wilhite WC. The acute treatment of heat stroke. South Med J 1967;60:885–887.

Boswick JA, Thompson JD, Jonas RA. The epidemiology of cold injuries. Surg Gynecol Obstet 1979;149:326–332.

Caldwell JE. Diuretic therapy, physical performance, and neuromuscular function. Phys Sportsmed 1984;12(6):73–78.

Casey MJ, Foster C, Hixson EG, Ryan AJ. Winter sports medicine. Contemporary exercise and sports medicine series. Philadelphia: FA Davis, 1990.

Claremont AD, Costill DL, Fink W, Van Handei P. Heat tolerance following diuretic induced dehydration. Med Sci Sports 1976;8:239–243.

Costill DL, Cote R, Fink W. Muscle water and electrolytes following varied levels of dehydration in man. J Appl Physiol 1976;40:6–11.

Davies CT. Effect of acclimatization to heat on the regulation of sweating during moderate and severe exercise. J Appl Physiol 1981;50:741–746.

Fox EL, Mathews DK, Kaufman WS, Bowers RL. Effects of football equipment on thermal balance and energy cost during exercise. Res Q 1966;37:332–339.

Fritz RL, Perrin DH. Cold exposure injuries: prevention and treatment. Clin Sports Med 1989;8(1):111–128.

Gledhill N. Blood doping and related issues: a brief review. Med Sci Sports Exerc 1982;14:183–189.

Golden FS. Recognition and treatment of immersion hypothermia. Proc Soc Med 1973;66:1058–1061.

Hackett PH. Acute mountain sickness. Semin Resp Med 1983;5:132–140.

Hackett PH, Rennie D. Rales, peripheral edema, retinal hemorrhage and acute mountain sickness. Am J Med 1979;67:214–218.

Horstman DH, Christensen E. Acclimatization to dry heat: active men vs. active women. J Appl Physiol 1982;52:825–831.

Houston CS. Altitude illness. Emerg Med Clin North Am 1984;2:503–512.

Houston CS. Going higher: the story of man at altitude. 3rd ed. Boston: Little, Brown, 1987.

Hultgren HN, Markovena EA. High altitude pulmonary edema epidemiologic observations in Peru. Chest 1978;74:372–376.

Jarrett F. Frostbite: current concepts of pathogenesis and treatment. Rev Surg 1974;31:71–74.

Larson EB, Roach RC, Schoene RB, Hornbein TF. Acute mountain sickness and acetozolamide: clinical efficacy and effect on ventilation. JAMA 1982;248:328–332.

Mangi R, Jokl P, Dayton OW. Sports fitness and training. New York: Pantheon Books, 1987.

Mathews DK. Physiological responses during exercise and recovery in a football uniform. J Appl Physiol 1969;26:611–615.

McArdle WD, Majel JR, Lesmes GR, Pechur GS. Metabolic and cardiovascular adjustment to work in air and water at 18, 25, 33 degrees Celsius. J Appl Physiol 1976;40:85–90.

McArdle WD, Majel JR, Spira RJ, Gergley TS, Toner MM. Thermal adjustment to cold-water exposure in resting men and women. J Appl Physiol 1984;56:1572–1577.

McFadden DM, Houston CS, Sutton JD, Powles ACP, Gray G, Roberts RS. High altitude retinopathy. JAMA 1981;245:581–586.

Nadel ER, Holmer I, Bergh U, Astrand PO, Stolwijk JA. Thermoregulatory shivering during exercise. Life Sci 1973;13:983–989.

Oelez O, Howald H, dePrampero PE. Physiological profile of world-class high altitude climbers. J Appl Physiol 1986;60:1734–1742.

Rennie D, Wilson R. Who should not go high. In: Sutton JR, Jones

NL, Houston CS, eds. Hypoxia: man at altitude. New York: Thieme-Stratton, 1982:186–190.
Robinson S. Training, acclimatization and heat tolerance. Can Med Assoc J 1967;96:795–800.
Rozycki TJ. Oral and rectal temperatures in runners. Phys Sportsmed 1984;12(8):105–108.
Schoene RB. Relationship of hypoxic ventilatory response to exercise performance on Mount Everest. J Appl Physiol 1984;56:1478–1484.
Schoene RB. Pulmonary edema at high altitude: review, pathophysiology, and update. Clin Chest Med 1985;6:507–517.
Smith MH, Sharkey BS. Altitude training: who benefits? Phys Sportsmed 1984;12(4):48–51.
Wells CS. Sexual differences in heat stress response. Phys Sportsmed 1977;5:79–84.
Wells CL, Horvath SM. Responses to exercise in a hot environment as related to the menstrual cycle. J Appl Physiol 1974;36:299–302.

5 / BIOMECHANICS OF KNEE LIGAMENTS RELATING TO SPORTS MEDICINE

Savio L-Y. Woo, Richard A. Z. Sofranko, and James P. Jamison

Introduction

Musculoskeletal soft tissues such as tendons and ligaments, are subjected to loads of widely varying intensities during sports activities. As a result, these structures are frequently the focus of injury. However, such injuries currently lack absolute, definitive treatments because of limited quantitative research. Consequently, their repair and subsequent rehabilitation frequently is based on the past experience of the physician. Given these circumstances, the importance of insight into the basic mechanical behavior of the tendons and ligaments becomes clear. Knowledge of the properties of these tissues and their responses to various physiologic conditions can provide a broader perspective on the processes of growth and development, tissue homeostasis, and healing. Armed with this information, more effective treatment modalities for injuries to these structures, both relatively minor and severely debilitating, may be developed.

This chapter concentrates primarily on biomechanics of knee ligaments, because an understanding of these principles is one of the keys to developing new methods of injury management. This discussion begins with a review of the basic biomechanical concepts, including engineering terminology, and experimental methodologies used to describe ligament behavior. This fundamental knowledge forms the framework for the discussion of the effects of strain rate, age, and skeletal maturation on the properties of knee ligaments as well as the effects of immobilization and exercise. Finally, recent experimental data on the healing and repair of knee ligaments will be summarized, including the use of substitute tissues such as autografts and allografts to restore ligament function.

Basic Biomechanics

Structural Properties

Tendons and ligaments consist of densely packed collagen fiber bundles that are oriented along the length of the tissue. They have nonlinear and time-dependent responses when subjected to tensile load (force, recorded in Newtons). The nonlinear response is thought to be caused by the progressive recruitment of collagen fibrils, as these fibrils lie in a "crimped" pattern when subjected to no external load. As a tensile load is applied and the tissue is stretched, more fibers gradually are straightened and begin to resist the tension (1). The time-dependent behavior of ligaments is thought to reflect the interactions of the viscoelastic collagen with the surrounding elastin and other ground substances.

Because the primary function of tendons and ligaments is to resist tensile loads, it is common practice to measure their biomechanical properties in tension. In the case of ligaments, tests are usually performed using a bone-ligament-bone complex, because it is difficult to clamp an isolated ligament (which is usually short and wide). The complex also provides a representation of the tissue's functional properties. Typically, a nonlinear and upwardly concave load-elongation curve that represents the structural properties of the bone-ligament-bone complex is obtained (Fig. 5.1). The shape and size of the whole curve as well as its individual sections reveal important characteristics. The first part is a nonlinear "toe" region, thought to result from the recruitment of collagen fibrils. Next is a linear region that ends just before the ligament fails. This curve characterizes the load, ultimate elongation, linear stiffness, ultimate load, and energy absorbed at failure (rupture), which are defined as follows.

Stiffness (measured in Newtons. [N]/mm). The relationship between load and elongation, measured as the slope of the linear portion of the load-elongation curve.

Ultimate Load (N). The highest load observed just before failure of the tissue during a tensile test. This parameter is often erroneously referred to as "tensile strength."

Ultimate Elongation (mm). The maximum distance a tissue can be stretched from its initial unloaded length to its length at failure.

Energy Absorbed at Failure (N-mm). The area under the

load-elongation curve between zero load and the ultimate load.

Mechanical Properties

To differentiate between the behavior of the bone-ligament interface and the midsubstance of the ligament, researchers also obtain a stress-strain curve that represents the mechanical properties of the ligament substance (Fig. 5.2). The stress of a ligament is defined as load per cross-sectional area (N/mm²). Measurements of the cross-sectional area of the ligament permit the tensile load to be converted to tensile stress. The strain is defined from the elongation of the tissue only and should exclude the length changes at the bone-ligament interface. Parameters obtained from the stress-strain curve include the modulus, tensile strength, ultimate strain, and strain energy density (see Fig. 5.2), which are defined as follows.

Modulus (N/mm²). The relationship between stress and strain, measured as the slope of the linear portion of the stress-strain curve.
Tensile strength (N/mm²). The maximum stress observed on the stress-strain curve before failure of the tissue.
Ultimate Strain (mm/mm). The strain at the point of failure, defined as length at failure minus the original length, which is then divided by the original length.
Strain Energy Density (N-mm). The area under the stress-strain curve, representing the amount of energy a specimen can absorb before failure.

For these measurements to be valid, the sample must have an adequate size, a relatively uniform cross-section along its length, and a large length:width ratio. These features are necessary because changes in cross-sectional area along the ligament would change the stress values, and the strain characteristics at the insertion sites (caused by stress concentration) would not be the same as those in the ligament substance. As a result, the stress at the insertion site is not equal to the stress in the midsubstance.

Viscoelastic Properties

Ligaments exhibit a time- and history-dependent (viscoelastic) response to load and elongation. Experimentally, this response appears as a time-dependent decrease in stress when the ligament is subjected to constant elongation (stress relaxation) or as an increase in length when the ligament is subjected to constant load (creep). In a stress-relaxation test, an instantaneous elongation is imposed on the ligament. As this elongation is held constant, the change in load, or stress, over time is recorded until equilibrium is reached (Fig. 5.3*A*). A creep test is performed by applying a constant load instantaneously to the ligament and measuring the elongation to the point of equilibrium (see Fig. 5.3*B*). Both the creep and stress-relaxation tests are more complicated than the more commonly used tensile test, in which a load is applied to the specimen to the point of rupture.

Another method employed to measure the viscoelastic behavior of ligaments is a cyclic loading and unloading test. During exercise, human ligaments experience repeated stretching and relaxation, which can result in a gradual reduction of stress in the tissue. For example, when the canine medial collateral ligament (MCL) was subjected to cyclic loading between prescribed strains of 1.6% and 2.4%, a time-dependent relaxation in the peak and valley stresses was observed (Fig. 5.4) (2). This phenomenon indicates that the tissue is becoming softened (relaxed) while undergoing a cyclic pattern of stress.

Experimental Methodology

Cross-Sectional Area Measurements

Various methods of measuring the cross-sectional area of ligaments and tendons have been devised. As mentioned earlier, these data are needed for calculation of the stress in the ligament. Methods of measurement fall into two general categories: contact and noncontact.

One contact method consists of measuring the width

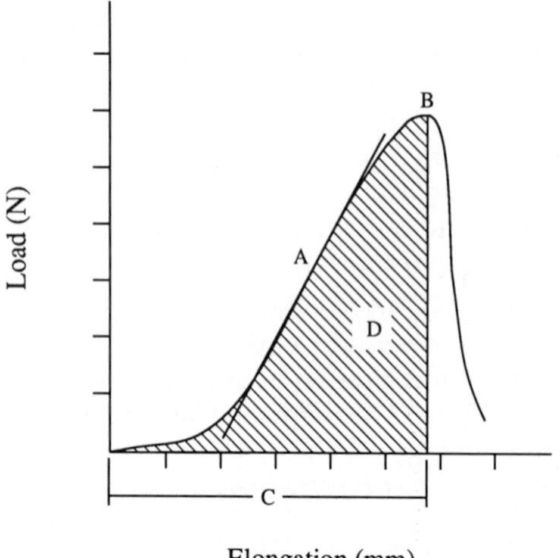

Figure 5.1. Load-elongation curve representing the structural properties of a bone-ligament-bone complex. *A*, stiffness; *B*, ultimate load; *C*, ultimate elongation; *D*, energy absorbed to failure.

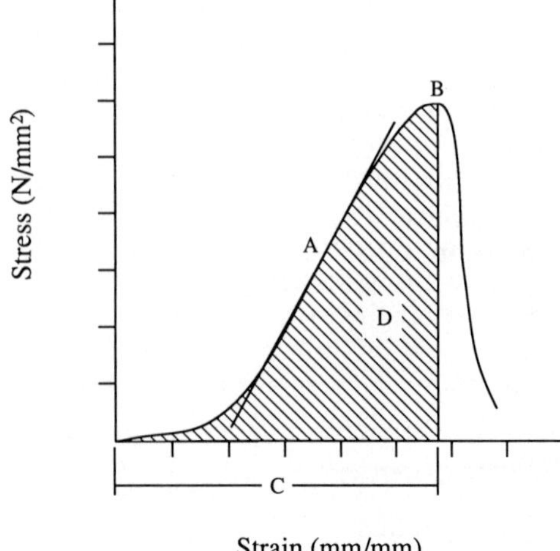

Figure 5.2. Stress-strain curve, representing the material properties of the tissue. *A*, modulus; *B*, tensile strength; *C*, ultimate strain; *D*, strain energy density.

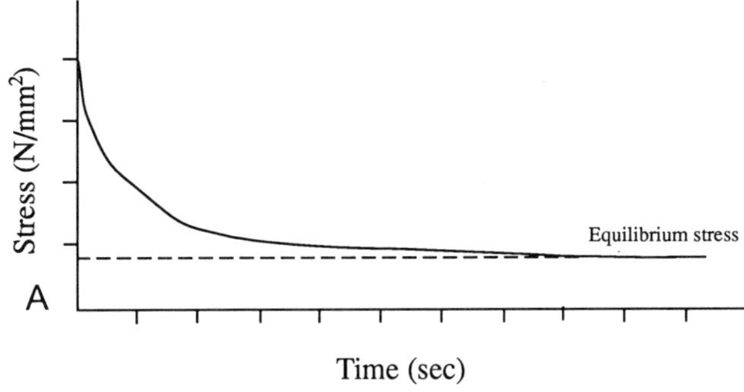

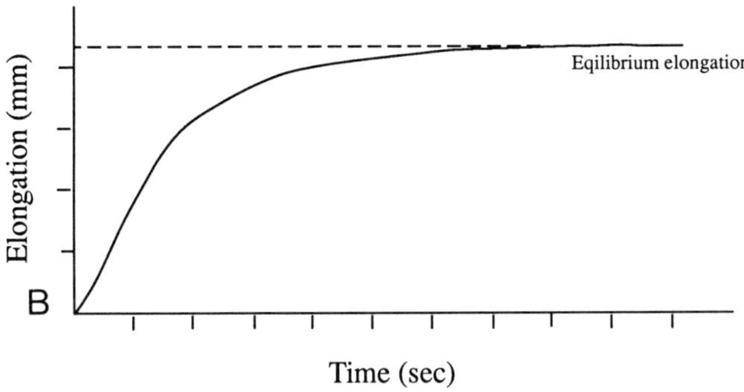

Figure 5.3. **A,** Relaxation test. **B,** Creep test.

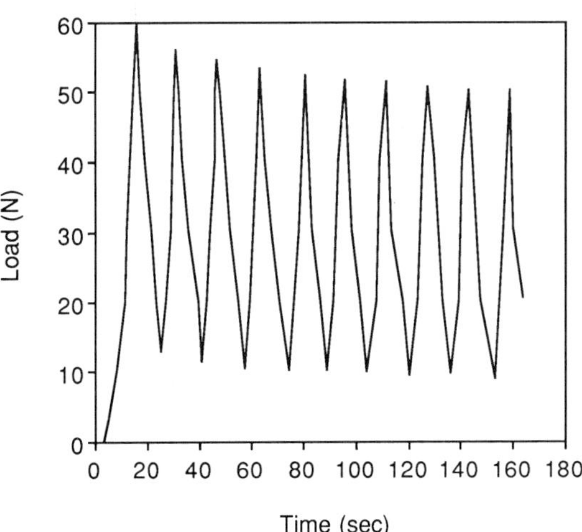

Figure 5.4. Cyclic loading and unloading of the canine medial collateral ligament. Reprinted by permission from Woo SLY, Gomez MA, Akeson WH. The time and history-dependent viscoelastic properties of the canine medial collateral ligament. J Biomech Eng 1981;103:293–298. © American Society of Mechanical Engineers.

and thickness of the ligament with a Vernier calipers to calculate area, assuming either a rectangular or an elliptical cross-section. However, this method can lead to large errors in ligaments that have an irregularly shaped cross-section, such as the anterior cruciate ligament (ACL) (3). By comparison, the area micrometer contact method measures the thickness of tissue compressed into a slot of known width. As a result, the tissue is deformed, and the area measured depends greatly on the pressure applied to the tissue (4, 5). Thus contact methods have the potential of producing measurements with relatively high degrees of inaccuracy.

The noncontact methods generally couple some types of optical system with image reconstruction, by avoiding contact, they do not distort the specimen. Noncontact methods include the shadow amplitude method (6), the profile method (7, 8), and the laser micrometer method (3, 9). For the laser micrometer technique, the specimen is placed perpendicular to a collimated laser beam. Profile widths of the specimen are obtained as the specimen is rotated 180° in small increments of rotation. The profile widths are then reconstructed by a computer to reproduce the cross-sectional shape and area of the specimen. For ligaments the accuracy is within ± 0.1 mm^2 (3).

Strain Measurements

The strain in a specimen generally is calculated using the formula $(l - l_0)/l_0$, where l is the specimen length during a test and l_0, a reference length (the original length at rest). Often, ligament strain is incorrectly determined by measuring the distance between the clamps, known as the clamp-to-clamp distance, used to secure the specimen to the testing apparatus. Because that distance includes the elongation at the insertion sites, which is quite different from that of the ligament alone, the measurement thus obtained cannot represent the tissue strain.

As in measurements of cross-sectional area, contact methods are one modality used to determine ligament strain. One such method employs mercury-filled silastic tubes that are sutured onto the fibers of the ligament and undergo a measurable change in resistance corresponding to a change in the length of the ligament fibers (10–13). This measurement then is converted to strain. Hall-effect strain transducers also have been used to measure ligament strain. These instruments are attached to ligaments via sharp barbs that penetrate the ligament substance (14). The change in distance between the barbs alters the strength of the magnetic field, which is converted to a proportional output of strain. A disadvantage of both methods is that the fixation of a device onto the ligament may alter the behavior of that ligament.

To avoid direct contact between the device and the ligament substance, noncontact methods such as the video dimension analyzer (VDA) system have been used to measure longitudinal ligament strain (Fig. 5.5) (15). Within this system, two or more reference lines are painted on the specimen perpendicular to the direction of strain. The VDA system superimposes two electronic "windows" over these reference lines and tracks the separation of the lines throughout the period of tissue elongation. The distances measured are reported as output voltages in terms of strain. The VDA system has now been improved so that transverse ligament strain can be measured as well, allowing the determination of a two-dimensional strain field (16).

Force Measurements

Many investigators have developed methods to measure ligament forces in intact joints. Lewis et al. (17) used buckle-type transducers for this purpose. With

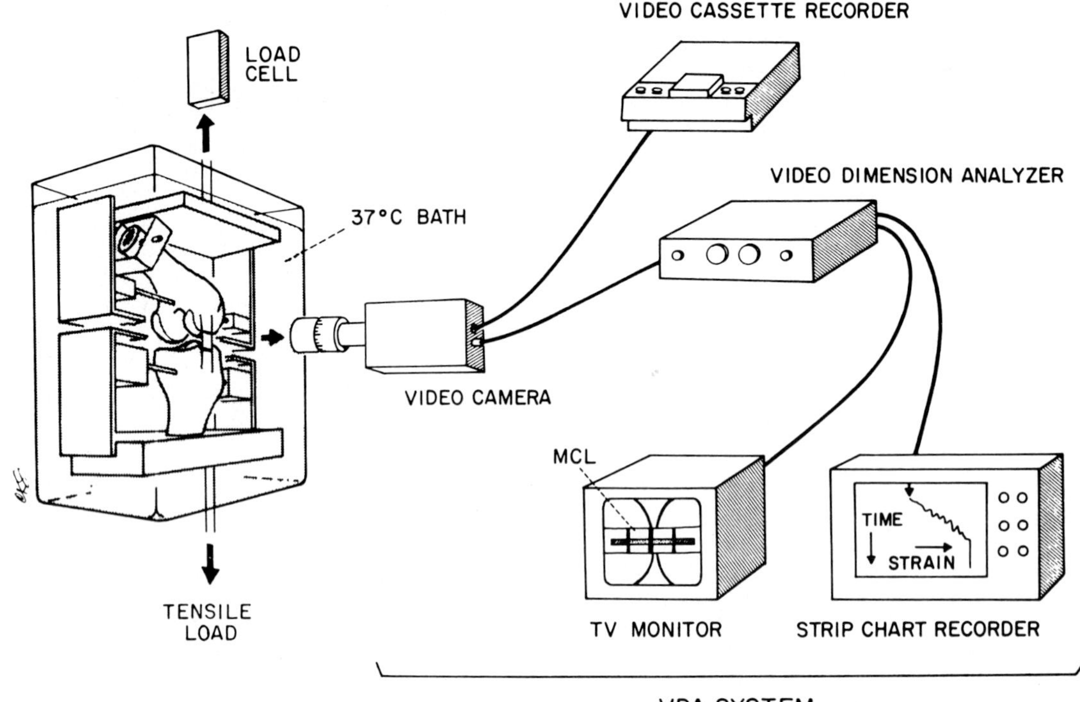

Figure 5.5 Video dimension analyzer system configured to measure the tensile strain in the medial collateral ligament (MCL) of the knee. Reprinted by permission from Woo SLY, Ohland KJ, Weiss JA. Aging and sex related changes in the biomechanical properties of the rabbit medial collateral ligament. Mech Ageing Devel 1990;56:129–142.

this technique, a ligament is passed through the transducer the same way a belt goes through a buckle. Lengthening of the ligament with the application of load then varies the output voltage of the transducer. A variation of this type of transducer was developed for use with tendons by An et al. (18). The tendon is passed through an S-shaped frame, and any lengthening of the tissue creates a proportional change in the output of the transducer.

Markolf et al. (19) directly measured the forces in the ACL by drilling a hole through the proximal tibia in line with the ligament. A load-cell, a device to measure force, was attached to the bone plug, and the force in the ACL was measured as the knee was subjected to various loads. In the authors' laboratory, loads in the human ACL were estimated via knee kinematics and a load-elongation curve of the ACL (20). To accomplish this, the motion of the knee during passive flexion under an anterior tibial load of 100 N was measured. The lengths of different portions of the ACL then were calculated from the recorded motion. All the soft tissue except the ACL was then removed from the joint, and load-elongation curves were obtained at different flexion angles for the entire ACL and for the anterior portion alone. Using the load-elongation curves and the length data, in situ loads on the intact ACL and on the ligament's anterior portion were determined.

Effects of Strain Rate

The majority of severe ligament injuries in athletes occur when the ligaments are subjected to high strain rates (percent per unit time). This terminology represents the instantaneous application of strain many times greater than that seen at normal physiologic conditions, an effect difficult to simulate experimentally. The authors have investigated the effects of a wide range of strain rates on ligament properties. Tensile tests were performed on skeletally immature (3.5 months old) and skeletally mature (8.5 months old) rabbits to assess the effects of strain rate and age. The structural properties of the femur-MCL-tibia complex (FMTC) were measured at rates of elongation (longitudinal extension or distraction) from 0.008 to 113 mm/sec, a range of more than 4 orders of magnitude. The structural properties at the lowest and highest extension rates differed only slightly, as the load-elongation curves were similar (Fig. 5.6). In the skeletally immature group, the ultimate load for the highest extension rate was 2.33 times greater than that for the lowest rate. Differences in these measurements also were evident in the skeletally mature specimens but were lower in magnitude. Failure, or rupture, of the FMTC was independent of the extension rate, as the skeletally mature specimens failed exclusively in the ligament substance while the skeletally immature specimens experienced failures at the insertion sites. Similar trends were noted for the mechanical properties of the MCL substance. The corresponding strain rates of the MCL substance were found in the range of 0.011% to 155%/sec. Again, the effects of strain rate for the two groups were not significant (Fig. 5.7). Changes in modulus were small at the different strain rates, while a 60% increase over 4 orders of magnitude was observed with respect to tensile strength (21).

The effects of slow, medium, and fast strain rates on

the properties of the rabbit anterior cruciate ligament (ACL) also have been studied (22). Only a small difference in modulus (the slope of the stress-strain curve), was observed between the slow (0.016%/sec) and medium (1.68%/sec) strain rates. However, the modulus at the fast strain rate (381%/sec) was 31% higher than those at the slower strain rates. In addition, the slow strain rate group absorbed 30% less energy. These findings show that the ACL is relatively insensitive to strain rate compared with bone (23).

Based on these studies, strain rate appears to have minimal impact on the mechanical properties of knee ligaments. On the other hand, the state of skeletal maturity does have a significant effect on the tensile properties of bone-ligament-bone complexes.

Effects of Maturation and Aging

The effects of skeletal maturation and aging on the MCL have been evaluated in female New Zealand white rabbits (24). Tests of the FMTCs from female rabbits aged 3.5 months, 6 months, 12 months, and 3 years showed that the structural properties of the FMTC dramatically increased from 6 to 12 months of age, after which differences between the age groups diminished (Fig. 5.8*A*). The mechanical properties of the ligament substance showed a similar trend (see Fig. 5.8*B*). This finding is of importance in that the age of skeletal maturity in the rabbit is 7 to 8 months. A significant finding of this study was that skeletally immature and mature specimens fail differently. All of the FMTCs from

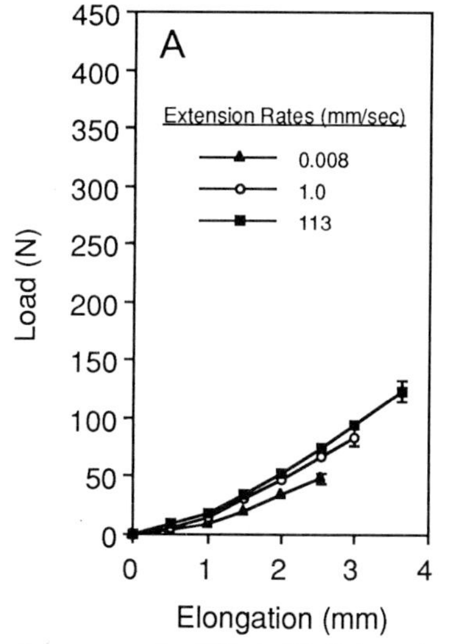

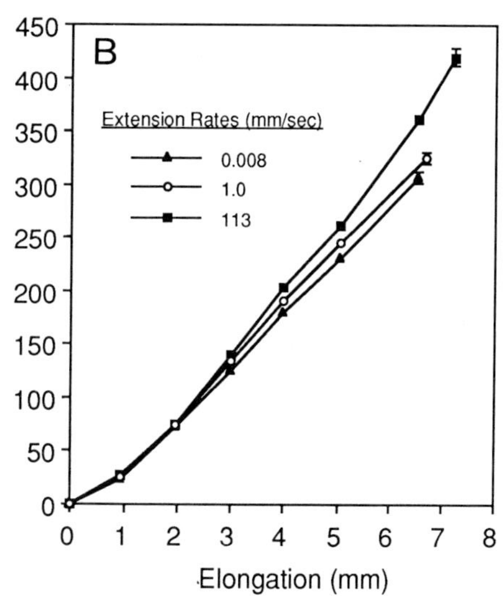

Figure 5.6. Load-elongation curves for (*A*) skeletally immature and (*B*) skeletally mature rabbit femur-medial collateral ligament-tibia complex at different extension rates. Reprinted by permission from Woo SLY, Peterson RH, Ohland KJ, Sites TJ, Danto MI. The effects of strain rate on the properties of the medial collateral ligament in skeletally immature and skeletally mature rabbits: a biomechanical and histological study. J Orthop Res 1990;8:712–721.

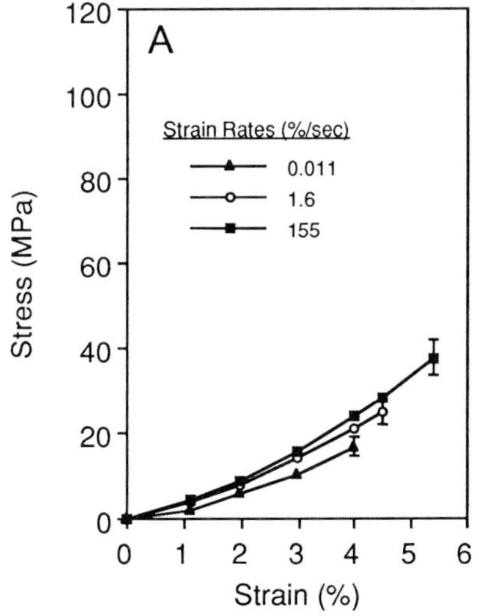

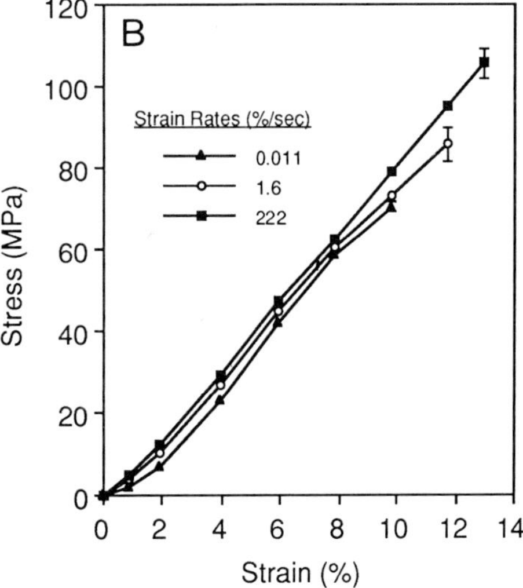

Figure 5.7. Stress-strain curves for (*A*) skeletally immature and (*B*) skeletally mature rabbit medial collateral ligament at different strain rates. Reprinted by permission from Woo SLY, Peterson RH, Ohland KJ, Sites TJ, Danto MI. The effects of strain rate on the properties of the medial collateral ligament in skeletally immature and skeletally mature rabbits: a biomechanical and histological study. J Orthop Res 1990;8:712–721.

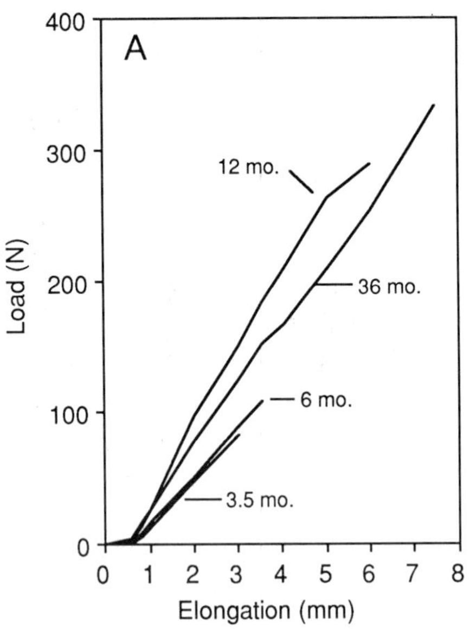

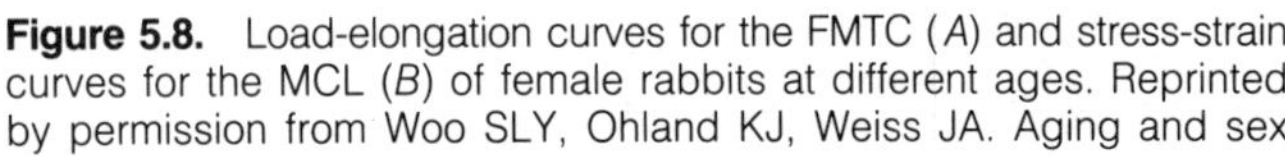
Figure 5.8. Load-elongation curves for the FMTC (*A*) and stress-strain curves for the MCL (*B*) of female rabbits at different ages. Reprinted by permission from Woo SLY, Ohland KJ, Weiss JA. Aging and sex related changes in the biomechanical properties of the rabbit medial collateral ligament. Mech Ageing Devel 1990;56:129–142.

rabbits with an open epiphysis failed by avulsion at the tibial insertion site, whereas after closure of the epiphysis, all failures occurred in the ligament substance. These results indicate that before skeletal maturation, the tibial insertion site is the weakest link in the complex. After skeletal maturation, the strength of the insertion site surpasses that of the ligament substance, and the ligament itself becomes the weakest link.

Most tensile studies of the ACL have been performed in animal models (2, 6, 23, 25–29) rather than humans, because young healthy donor tissue has been scarce (28). Recently though, the ultimate load and energy absorbed at failure were reported to be approximately 3 times greater for young donors (22 to 35 years old) than for older specimens (30). The linear stiffness and ultimate elongation also decreased with age. These values were found to be 34% and 45% greater, respectively, for the young donors than for the old group (aged 60 to 97 years). Based on these studies, it appears that maturation has a dramatic influence on the strength of the insertion sites, whereas aging has a strong effect on the strength of the ligament substance.

Tissue Homeostasis

In vivo studies of tissue homeostasis in response to increases and decreases in stress and motion can help to determine the effects of immobilization and remobilization (exercise) on injured ligaments. These data, in turn, can aid the physician in choosing the most appropriate repair and rehabilitative options.

Effects of Exercise

Studies have shown that exercise affects the various biomechanical properties of the ligament substance and the insertion sites. Using bush babies (*Galago senegalensis*), Tipton et al. (31) showed that a 20-week treadmill exercise program led to a significantly stronger patellar tendon than in a nonexercised control group, without changing the strength of the MCL-tibia junction. Viidik (25) demonstrated that the structural properties of the rabbit ACL greatly increased after 40 weeks of daily training. In addition, the exercised group exhibited faster relaxation and a greater amount of stress relaxation. Zuckerman and Stull (32) found a 35% increase in the ultimate load of the rat MCL and lateral collateral ligament (LCL) after the animals were exercised for 9-week periods of swimming or running (15 min/day, 5 days/week). In another study, Tipton et al. (33) demonstrated a 10% increase in both the FMTC ultimate load and the ultimate load:body weight ratio and a 20% increase in the energy absorbed at failure in rats that had undergone 10 weeks of treadmill endurance training. These results indicate that exercise increases the tensile properties of the ligament substance.

The effect of exercise on properties of knee ligaments from different age and gender groups has been studied by Tipton et al. (34). Exercise was found to significantly increase the tensile strength of the isolated LCL for 6- to 12-month-old rats, but not for 18- and 24-month-old rats. They also found that male rats experienced a significant increase in the ultimate load:body weight ratio of the FMTC in response to 10 to 15 weeks of exercise, but female rats did not (35).

In examining the effects of different types of endurance exercises, Tipton et al. (36) showed that running on a graded surface increased the ultimate load of the FMTC by 12%, whereas level running had no effect. Cabaud et al. (37) studied the influence of exercise frequency and duration on knee ligaments in rats. Treadmill exercising for 6 days/week over 8 weeks proved to be more effective than 3 days/week at increasing the structural properties of the femur-ACL-tibia complex (FATC). However, exercise periods of 30 min/day were more effective than periods of 60 min/day. Thus the higher-frequency, shorter-duration exercise regimen yielded the greatest increases in linear stiffness (7%), ultimate load (17%), and energy absorbed at failure (31%) compared with nonexercised controls. This same regimen also yielded a 20% increase in tensile strength and ultimate strain of the ACL.

The authors (38) have studied the effects of prolonged exercise on the biomechanical properties of the swine FMTC. After 12 months of scheduled exercise (8 months on an oval dirt track followed by 4 months on a treadmill), the structural properties of the FMTC increased. Specifically, a 14% increase in the linear stiffness, a 38% increase in the ultimate load when normalized to body weight, a 20% increase in the tensile strength, and a 10% increase in the ultimate strain were found. These results correlate well with the other studies mentioned.

The impact of lifelong exercise on the biomechanical properties of the FMTC has been investigated using beagles (39). The exercise program involved trotting on a treadmill at a speed of 3 km/hr for 75 min/day, 5 days/week, for a total period of 420 to 557 weeks (approximately 8 to 10 years). During the actual training sessions, the animals were fitted with an 11-kg backpack. Age-matched control animals were given ad lib cage activity for the same duration. Skeletally mature dogs approximately 10 months old also were tested to evaluate the effects of aging on the experimental subjects. The results indicate that lifelong exercise training had little or no effect on the structural properties of the FMTC. Neither linear stiffness, ultimate load, ultimate deformation, nor energy absorbed at failure were statistically different between the exercised and control animals. Nor were the mechanical properties of the MCL substance statistically different in the control and exercised groups. Age, however, had a marked effect on the mechanical properties of the MCL substance. The tensile strength of FMTC in 10-month-old beagles was 45% and 40% higher, and failure of the FMTC occurred at 41% and 36% higher strains than in those of the 8- to 10-year-old exercised and control groups, respectively. Therefore, the aging process may have negated the potential for positive effects of exercise.

Effects of Immobilization

Immobilization is frequently used in the treatment of musculoskeletal injuries. Such treatment is thought to protect the injured tissue from disruptive forces during the early healing period. However, joint immobility has profound negative effects on the soft connective tissues because it significantly compromises the biomechanical properties of the ligaments and ligament insertion sites.

Laros et al. (40) found that immobilization of the canine FMTC for 6, 9, or 12 weeks reduced the ultimate load:body weight ratio by approximately 27% compared with caged dogs. Immobilization also led to bone resorption and disruption of ligament fibers at the ligament tibial insertion site. Although complete reossification at the bone resorption sites occurred within 24 weeks after cast removal and the return to normal activity, the ultimate load:body weight ratio at the insertion site had not normalized by that time. There were no findings of ultrastructural alterations within the ligaments themselves in this study.

Noyes et al. (41) analyzed the effects of activity levels on the ACL of nonhuman primates. In the experimental group, the right lower limb was exercised daily, while the remainder of the body was immobilized in a cast. Such exercise was determined to be ineffective in preventing the detrimental effects of immobilization. Load-elongation curves of the exercised FATCs were similar to those of the immobilized limbs, and bone resorption was evident at the insertion sites of both the exercised and the immobilized specimens.

Lam et al. (42) and Walsh et al. (43) found that the viscoelastic behavior of the New Zealand white rabbit MCL was influenced by immobilization and skeletal maturation. During a cyclic stress-relaxation test, the amount of relaxation that occurred between the 1st and 10th cycles was significantly higher for the 3-month-old rabbits than for those that were 6, 9, and 12 months old. Furthermore, the normal maturation of the MCL was affected by immobilization. After 3 months of immobilization, the structural properties of the MCL in 6-month-old rabbits were found to be equivalent to those in 3-month-old rabbits. Similar results were found after as little as 1 month of immobilization. Because the structural properties of ligaments normally improve with skeletal maturity, these results indicate that immobilization can interfere significantly with the development of the FMTC.

The findings of several investigators have helped to explain how immobilization affects the soft tissues of the joint. Evans et al. (44) evaluated histologically rat knees that had been immobilized for 15 to 90 days and observed a proliferation of fatty connective tissue within the joint. By 30 days of immobilization, the adhesions formed by this tissue were well-established and were thought to contribute to joint stiffness. Langenskiöld et al. (45) noted periarticular soft tissue thickening after immobilizing rabbit knees in extension for only 2 weeks. After 12 more weeks of immobilization, they found that joint stiffness restricted knee motion to only 20° to 40°. In addition, Enneking and Horowitz (46) observed that prolonged immobilization can obliterate the joint space in humans.

Joint stiffness secondary to immobilization is a major clinical problem. To address this problem, immobilized joints have been evaluated quantitatively with the use of an arthrograph (47). This device measures the amount of torque and energy required to cycle a knee joint through a set range of motion. The magnitude of torque required to extend the knee to a predetermined angle of flexion represents the joint stiffness, and the area within the hysteresis loop represents the energy required for the joint motion. Joint stiffness in knees immobilized for 9 weeks was 10 times that of controls and required as much as 23 times more energy for the first cycle of motion. A similar study showed that compared with a control joint the extension of a joint that was immobilized for 9 weeks required an increased magnitude of torque and energy (48). This phenomenon is thought to be a result of the new collagen fibrils forming interfibrillar contacts, restricting the sliding of fibers in the joint capsule (47, 49).

The biomechanical change in the rabbit FMTC after immobilization and remobilization has been studied (50). The structural integrity of the bone-ligament-bone complex was found to be largely altered following 9 weeks of immobilization, with the ultimate load measuring 31% of control values (Fig. 5.9). Stress-strain curves revealed that immobilization was associated with a significant decrease in MCL modulus and that there was a time-dependent inverse relationship between immobilization and mechanical properties (Fig. 5.10). In addition, the cross-sectional area of the MCL was 78% and 79% of control values at 9 and 12 weeks of immobilization, respectively. After remobilization for 9 weeks, load-elongation data revealed similar structural properties in both the experimental and control specimens at lower loads. However, failure-inducing loads of the bone-ligament-bone complex in the remobilized specimens were 80% and 63% of control values, respectively, for those that had been immobilized for 9 and 12 weeks. Failure occurred by tibial avulsion in all of the animals that underwent immobilization without subsequent remobilization. After remobilization, the tibial avulsion rate was 60% and 80% in those immobilized for 9 weeks and 12 weeks, respectively, signifying a relative improvement in strength at the site of tibial insertion.

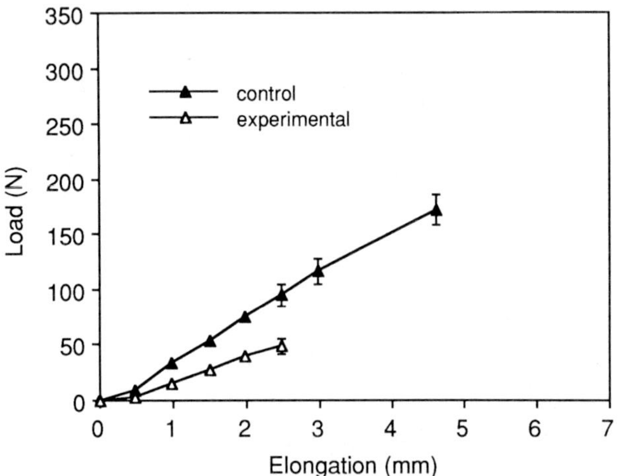

Figure 5.9. Load-deformation curves, representing the structural properties of the bone-ligament-bone complexes after 9 weeks of immobilization. Modified from Woo SLY, Gomez MA, Sites TJ, Newton PO, Orlando CA, Akeson WH. The biomechanical and morphological changes in the medial collateral ligament of the rabbit after immobilization and remobilization. J Bone Joint Surg 1987;69A:1200–1211.

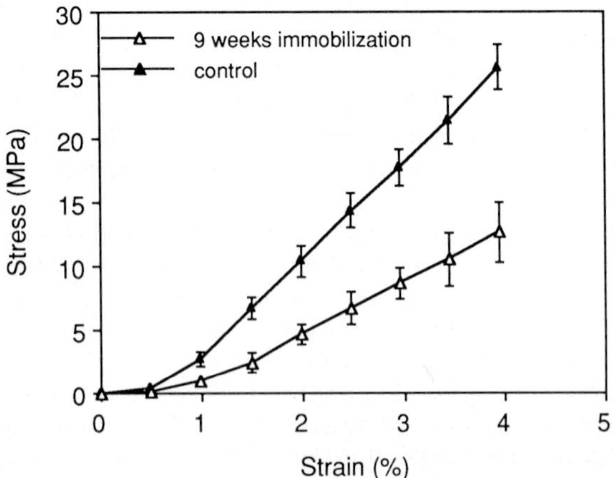

Figure 5.10. Stress-strain curves, representing the mechanical properties for control and experimental medial collateral ligaments after 9 weeks of immobilization. Modified from Woo SLY, Gomez MA, Sites TJ, Newton PO, Orlando CA, Akeson WH. The biomechanical and morphological changes in the medial collateral ligament of the rabbit after immobilization and remobilization. J Bone Joint Surg 1987;69A:1200–1211.

These findings correlate with histologic evaluations of the same specimens, which showed increased osteoclastic activity and bone resorption at the insertion sites after immobilization and partial recovery with remobilization. Overall, 1 year of remobilization was needed for normalization of the ligament-tibia complex. In contrast, the mechanical properties of the ligament substance quickly returned to normal following remobilization (Fig. 5.11). This study illustrated that remobilization will improve the structural properties of ligaments following immobilization but will not restore the original biomechanical state of the entire complex because the insertion site has residual weakness.

Metabolically, collagen turnover increased with immobility in similar groups of rabbits (51, 52). The rate of degradation was matched by the rate of synthesis during the first 9 weeks, but with longer periods of immobilization, the degradation outpaced synthesis, causing ligament atrophy. The authors suggest that this was because the new collagen synthesized during the immobility was not required to resist tensile loads. Therefore, its structure may have developed in a manner that restricts joint motion.

Healing and Repair

There are various approaches to the healing and repair of knee ligament tears, the options include immobilization versus no immobilization, conservative versus surgical treatment, and the choice of soft tissue autografts versus allografts for reconstruction. Midsubstance tears of the ACL are known to have limited healing capacity, whereas the MCL has a much greater propensity to heal. As a result, the MCL has been the focus of most studies on ligament healing and reconstruction has been targeted at the torn ACL.

Immobilization

In surgical treatment, immobilization to protect the newly formed repair tissue has been a commonly accepted practice (53, 54). However, this modality can result in a proliferation of fibro-fatty connective tissue and synovial adhesions that can lead to increased joint stiffness, all of which compromise ligament properties, as discussed previously (47, 50). Using the canine knee as a model, the authors compared the effects of no repair and no immobilization (group I) versus repair and im-

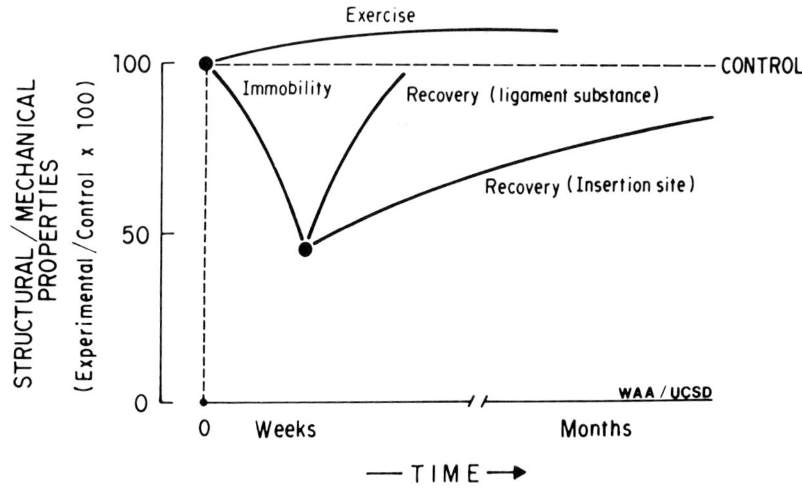

Figure 5.11. Plot of the physiologic response of bone-ligament-bone complex subjected to varying levels of activity. Reprinted by permission from Woo SLY, Gomez MA, Sites TJ, Newton PO, Orlando CA, Akeson WH. The biomechanical and morphological changes in the medial collateral ligament of the rabbit after immobilization and remobilization. J Bone Joint Surg 1987;69A:1200–1211.

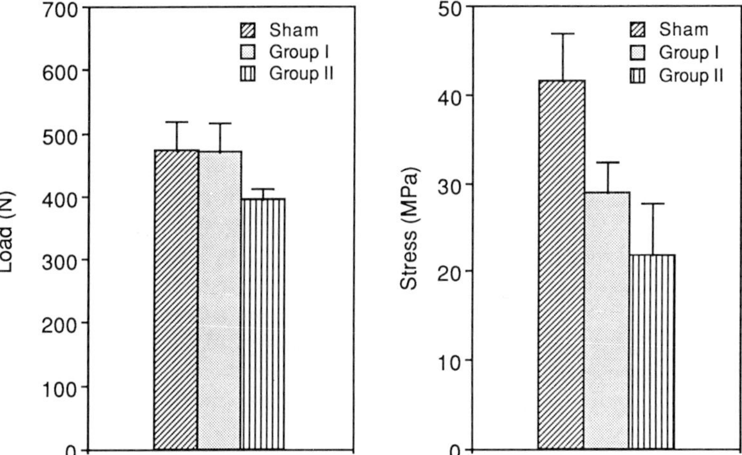

Figure 5.12. Ultimate load and tensile strength values for the sham group, group I (no repair or immobilization), and group II (repair followed by 6 weeks of immobilization). Modified from Inoue M, Woo SLY, gomez MA, Amiel D, Ohland KJ, Kitabayashi LR. Effects of surgical treatment and immobilization on the healing of the medial collateral ligament: a long-term multidisciplinary study. Connect Tissue Res 1990;25:13–26.

mobilization (group II) of the injured MCL (55). Histologic evaluation of the injury site 6 weeks after either approach showed some longitudinal alignment of fibroblasts. After 12 weeks, group II showed a more pronounced longitudinal alignment of fibers. These results are in agreement with previous studies (56, 57). At 48 weeks, the histologic findings in the healed MCL from both groups were similar to each other and to the normal MCL. However, the MCL collagen fiber orientation in the experimental groups remained irregular under polarized light microscopy.

Biomechanical testing revealed that varus-valgus knee instability was less at 48 weeks in group I, which was indistinguishable from controls. Tensile property evaluation of the FMTC showed that surgical treatment appeared to hinder linear stiffness in group II, but by 48 weeks it was equivalent to that of both the group I and the control knees. However, the ultimate load of the FMTCs from group II reached only 78% of control levels, compared with near-normal values for the group I specimens. The modulus of the MCL substance also did not differ between group I and control specimens at 48 weeks, whereas that of group II was only 41% of the control value (Fig. 5.12). The tensile strength of both experimental groups remained low at all times and, at 48 weeks, measured 58% of and 45% of controls for groups I and II, respectively.

As these findings demonstrate, the healed MCL is not the same as normal tissue, both histologically and biomechanically, suggesting the need to investigate methods of improving the quality of the healing tissue. In addition, these data illustrate that surgical repair and immobilization of isolated MCL injuries may not be an advantageous form of treatment. Immobilization has been shown to have adverse effects on the amount of collagen fiber oriented along the direction of the load (15, 50). Furthermore, it leads to greater osteoclastic activity in the tibial insertion site, resulting in a dramatic reduction in the strength of the bone-ligament-bone complex and in failures of the FMTC by tibial avulsion (50). However, these findings were observed in isolated MCL injuries. In the case of more severe and extensive knee injuries, controversy persists regarding the most desirable modality of treatment (58, 59).

Reconstruction

In contrast to MCL injuries, midsubstance ACL injuries often are treated by surgical reconstruction with an autograft or an allograft, especially in young, active patients who wish to return to athletic activities. Such surgical treatment is chosen based on convincing evidence that mid-substance ACL tears do not heal (60–62). In one study, 94% of patients with an acutely torn ACL still demonstrated instability 5 years after primary repair. Nevertheless, controversy exists as to the most optimal techniques and tissues to use for reconstructions. Ideally, tissue for ACL replacement should be readily available and should closely resemble the structural and mechanical properties of the native ligament before and after implantation (63–66). Currently, the search for tissue with these qualities is ongoing. The following sections describe the development and characteristics of ACL autografts and allografts.

Autografts

Many autologous tissues have been used for ACL replacement, including the central and medial thirds of the bone-patellar tendon (PT)-bone complex (67–73), the iliotibial tract (ITT) (29, 74, 75), the semitendinosus tendon (76–78), and the gracilis tendon (79). The use of bone-PT-bone grafts originally was described by Jones (67). This tissue has become the most popular graft material because it withstands the highest ultimate load and has bone blocks at each end of the graft for secure initial fixation at the femur and tibia.

Extensive investigation has been conducted into both the biologic and mechanical characteristics of autograft tissue used for ACL reconstruction. Histologically, the tissue has been found to progress from its initial avascular state at implantation to complete revascularization within 1 year. The autograft tissue also has some resemblance to a normal ACL (70).

ACL reconstructions with autograft tissue have been evaluated biomechanically in various animal models. In the rabbit model, autografts from the medial one-third of the PT have been tested at various time periods up to 1 year postoperatively. The structural properties of the autografts appeared to reach peak values at 30 weeks, when the ultimate load and stiffness were 15% and 24%, respectively, of the levels in control FATCs (73). In dogs, linear stiffness and ultimate load of implanted medial one-third PT grafts were 9% and 10% of isolated medial one-third PT control values, respectively, in the immediate postoperative period. By 3 months, the linear stiffness and ultimate load of the autografts were only 20% and 27% of control values, respectively (71). The data for autografts in goats (69) and monkeys (65) are slightly better, showing a general trend toward improvement of biomechanical properties with time. However, follow-up of most long-term animal studies (except those from monkeys) has revealed ultimate loads in autografts to be only 30% to 40% those of control groups.

Despite these experimental results, ACL reconstruction using autografts in humans has achieved success based on clinical examination. Nonetheless, the use of autologous tissue is not without drawbacks. Increased operative time is required for tissue harvesting, posing greater risk of neurologic sequelae from the tourniquet and greater risks from prolonged anesthesia. In addition, size constraints limit the available tissue, and the potential exists for postoperative complications such as infection or patellar tendon rupture at the donor site (80, 81). Consequently, alternatives to autograft reconstruction have been sought, leading to the consideration of the use of allografts.

Allografts

Allogenic ACL grafts eliminate many of the disadvantages of autologous grafts. With no need to harvest autologous tissue, operative time is decreased. Because normal tissue is not disrupted, there is no risk of infection or PT rupture at the donor site. In addition, tissue banks can provide a wide variety of graft types and sizes to fit the patient's needs. Postoperatively, patients regain function and the ability to resume normal activities, and the transplanted tissue remodels in the same manner as autografts (82–84). At 1 year after surgery, allografts have been found to be completely revascularized and histologically similar to autografts (83, 85).

The central one-third of the bone-PT-bone complex is the most popular allograft tissue, although the Achilles tendon and ACL also have been transplanted (83, 86, 87). Compared with autografts, allografts generally must be more carefully prepared for transplantation to maintain sterility and to reduce the possibility of disease transmission. Donors are screened thoroughly and the tissue is harvested using sterile technique. Tissue banks preserve allografts either by deep freezing or freeze drying. Cryopreservation by these methods may compromise the biomechanical properties of the allografts, although these deficiencies have not proven to be of clinical significance (63, 88–92). The ultimate load of flexor tendons has been shown to decrease after freeze drying, although results with other tissues contradict this finding (93–95). Deep freezing without subsequent drying of the ligament or tendon has been shown to have little or no effect on the mechanical properties of these tissues (28, 96, 97).

Efforts to eliminate transmittable disease pathogens from allograft tissue led initially to the development of sterilization with ethylene oxide. However, Roberts et al. (98) found that a high rate of failure, and a significant rate of graft dissolution occurred up to 2 years postoperatively in patients who received grafts treated in this manner. Radiographic examination of the operated knee showed joint space narrowing and the presence of osteophytes. Histologic evaluation of failed grafts detected an inflammatory response, tissue necrosis, and a lack of cellularity and collagen organization. Such failures may be caused by the presence of ethylene glycol and ethylene chlorhydrin, by-products of ethylene oxide that can cause graft dissolution. In addition, freeze-dried ethylene oxide debris has been shown to increase synoviocyte production of interleukin-1, a potent mediator of connective tissue inflammation and destruction (99).

Allografts are now sterilized using cobalt irradiation.

Gibbons et al. (84) and Butler et al. (100) have shown that doses of 2 Mrads of irradiation can eliminate most pathogens while producing no deleterious effects on the structural and mechanical properties of the frozen tissue. However, the effectiveness of irradiation in killing HIV and the hepatitis virus, both of great concern, remains in question. Butler et al. (101) found low-dose irradiation (2 Mrads) to cause minimal changes in the mechanical properties of allografts, whereas Paulos et al. (102) showed high doses (3 Mrads) to create significant changes. However, Haut and Powlison (103) demonstrated a 25% decrease in ultimate strength of a fresh-frozen specimen following irradiation at 2 Mrads and a 75% decrease if the specimen was first freeze-dried. In a different study, although the dimensions of the bone-PT-bone complex did not change from control values after 2 or 3 Mrads of cobalt irradiation, decreases in the mechanical properties of the grafts were noted after treatment with 3 Mrads (84).

At this time, however, the long-term effects of currently used preservation and sterilization techniques remain unknown. The actual antigenicity of fresh-frozen (deep-frozen) allografts is now being investigated in the authors' laboratory as well as by others. Before these techniques can be accepted definitively, their effects on the behavior of allograft tissue must be completely understood.

Summary

This chapter has provided some insight into the biomechanics of parallel-fiber connective tissue using knee ligaments as a model. Integral to understanding the behavior of these tissues is an appreciation of the differences in their structural and mechanical properties as determined from the load-elongation and stress-strain curves as well as viscoelastic properties. These basic principles form the foundation for studying the effects on the tissues that result from strain rate, maturation and aging, exercise and immobilization, and healing and repair.

Increased strain rate has been found to change the structural and mechanical properties of the skeletally immature rabbit FMTC and MCL; its effect on mature specimens was much less pronounced (21). In addition, the ACL was found to be relatively insensitive to strain rate (22). During skeletal maturation, the knee ligament of a rabbit demonstrated a considerable change in biomechanical properties, with minimal change thereafter. Failure occurred by avulsion at the tibial insertion site in the immature animals and at the MCL midsubstance in mature animals (24). Overall, the principal effect of maturation appears to be an increase in the structural properties of the insertion site. In the ACL of humans, structural properties and age show an inverse relationship; aging rapidly deteriorates the properties of the ligament (30).

Exercise has been found to be beneficial to properties of normal ligaments in general. Steady running regimens appear to have greater impact than does sprinting (33), and exercise on a grade is better than on a flat surface (36). Animals undergoing exercise periods of shorter duration but greater frequency seem to fare better (37). Concerning gender and age, the properties of ligaments in males improved more with exercise than in females, while those of younger animals improved more than in older subjects (34, 35). However, increasing age can erase the benefits of exercise (38).

Immobilization results in decreased strength of the ligament insertion site and increased bone resorption (40). It can delay the beneficial effects of skeletal maturation on the FMTC (42, 43) and lead to increased joint stiffness caused by adhesion formation, thickening, and increased interfibrillar contacts between collagen fibrils (48, 49). However, remobilization improves the impairments in structural properties of the FMTC and mechanical properties of the MCL substance that follow immobilization. The recovery of the mechanical properties of the MCL is quick and complete. However, although they improve, the structural properties of the FMTC never reach baseline levels because of insertion site weakness (50).

Isolated MCL tears have demonstrated no benefit from surgical repair and immobilization. In fact, injured MCLs subjected to neither repair nor immobilization appear histologically superior to those repaired surgically and immobilized. They also demonstrate improved biomechanical properties and less instability of the knee joint. On the other hand, ACL midsubstance tears heal poorly, often requiring reconstruction. Autograft tissue has proven to be successful clinically in the repair of ruptured ACLs, although its use is not free of complications. As a result, allograft reconstruction has been introduced, and it, too, has been clinically successful. However, questions remain regarding adequate measures for tissue sterilization and preservation and the effects of such processes on the mechanical properties of the tissue. Clearly, much work remains in the quest to understand the biomechanics of knee ligaments.

REFERENCES

1. Woo SLY, Young EP, Kwan MK. Fundamental studies in knee ligament mechanics. In: Daniel D, Akeson W, O'Connor J, eds. Knee ligament: structure, function, injury, and repair. New York: Raven, 1990:115–134.
2. Woo SLY, Gomez MA, Akeson WH. The time and history-dependent viscoelastic properties of the canine medial collateral ligament. J Biomech Eng 1981;103:293–298.
3. Woo SLY, Danto MI, Ohland KJ, Lee TQ, Newton PO. The use of a laser micrometer system to determine the cross-sectional shape and area of ligaments. A comparative study with two existing methods. J Biomech Eng 1990;112:426–431.
4. Walker LB, Harris EH, Benedict JV. Stress-strain relationship in human cadaveric plantaris tendon—a preliminary study. Med Elect Biol Eng 1964;2:31–38.
5. Ellis DG. Cross-sectional area measurements for tendon specimens: a comparison of several methods. J Biomech 1969;2:175–186.
6. Ellis DG. A shadow amplitude method for measuring cross-sectional areas of biological specimens. Paper presented at the Twenty-first Annual Conference on Engineering in Medicine and Biology, 1968.
7. Gupta BN, Subramanian KN, Brinker WO, Gupta AN. Tensile

strength of canine cranial cruciate ligaments. Am J Vet Res 1971;32:183–190.

8. Njus GO, Njus NM. A non-contact method for determining cross-sectional area of soft tissues. Trans Orthop Res Soc 1986;32:126.
9. Lee TQ, Woo SLY. A new method for determining cross-sectional shape and area of soft tissues. J Biomech Eng 1988;110:110–114.
10. Kennedy JC, Hawkins RJ, Willis RB. Strain gauge analysis of knee ligaments. Clin Orthop 1977;129:225–229.
11. Monahan JJ, Grigg P, Pappas AM, et al. In vivo strain patterns in the four major canine knee ligaments. J Orthop Res 1984;2:408–418.
12. Henning CE, Lynch MA, Glick KR. An in vivo strain gauge study of elongation of the anterior cruciate ligament. Am J Sports Med 1985;13:22–26.
13. Meglan D, Berme N, Zuelzer W. On the construction, circuitry and properties of liquid metal strain gauges. J Biomech 1988;21:681–685.
14. Arms SW, Pope MH, Boyle JB, Davigon PJ, Johnson RJ. Knee medial collateral ligament strain. Trans Orthop Res Soc 1982;7:47.
15. Woo SLY, Gomez MA, Woo YK, Akeson WH. Mechanical properties of tendons and ligaments. I. Quasi-static and nonlinear viscoelastic properties. Biorheology 1982;19:385–396.
16. Weiss JA, France EP, Bagley AM, Blomstrom GL. Measurement of 2-D strains in ligaments under uniaxial tension. Trans Orthop Res Soc 1991;17:662.
17. Lewis JL, Lew WD, Hill JA, et al. Knee joint motion and ligament forces before and after ACL reconstruction. J Biomech Eng 1989;111:97–106.
18. An KN, Berglund L, Cooney WP, Chao EYS, Kovacevic N. Direct in vivo tendon force measurement system [technical note]. J Biomech 1990;23:1269–1271.
19. Markolf KL, Gorek JF, Kabo JM, Shapiro MS. Direct measurement of resultant forces in the anterior cruciate ligament. An in vitro study performed with a new experimental technique. J Bone Joint Surg 1990;72A:557–567.
20. Takai S, Adams DJ, Livesay GA, Woo SLY. Determination of loads in the human anterior cruciate ligament. Trans Orthop Res Soc 1991;16:235.
21. Woo SLY, Peterson RH, Ohland KJ, Sites TJ, Danto MI. The effects of strain rate on the properties of the medial collateral ligament in skeletally immature and mature rabbits: a biomechanical and histological study. J Orthop Res 1990;8:712–721.
22. Danto MI, Woo SLY. The mechanical properties of skeletally mature rabbit anterior cruciate ligament and patellar tendon over a range of strain rates. J Orthop Res 1993:58–67.
23. Wright TM, Hayes WC. Tensile testing of bone over a wide range of strain rates: effects of strain rate, microstructure, and density. Med Biol Eng 1976;14:671–679.
24. Woo SLY, Ohland KJ, Weiss JA. Aging and sex related changes in the biomechanical properties of the rabbit medial collateral ligament. Mech Ageing Devel 1990;56:129–142.
25. Viidik A. Elasticity and tensile strength of the anterior cruciate ligament in rabbits as influenced by training. Acta Physiol Scand 1968;74:372–380.
26. Yoshiya S, Andrish JT, Manley MT, Bauer TW. Graft tension in anterior cruciate ligament reconstruction. An in vivo study in dogs. Am J Sports Med 1987;15:464–470.
27. Goldberg VM, Burstein A, Dawson M. The influence of an experimental immune synovitis on the failure mode and strength of the rabbit anterior cruciate ligament. J Bone Joint Surg 1982;64A:900–906.
28. Noyes FR, Grood ES. The strength of the anterior cruciate ligament in humans and rhesus monkeys. Age-related and species-related changes. J Bone Joint Surg 1976;58A:1074–1082.
29. O'Donoghue DH, Frank GR, Jeter GL, Johnson W, Zeiders JW, Kenyon R. Repair and reconstruction of the anterior cruciate ligament in dogs. Factors influencing long-term results. J Bone Joint Surg 1971;53A:710–718.
30. Woo SLY, Hollis JM, Adams DJ, Lyon RM, Takai S. Tensile properties of the human femur-anterior cruciate ligament-tibia complex: the effects of specimen age and orientation. Am J Sports Med 1991;19:217–225.
31. Tipton CM, Matthes RD, Vailas AC, Schnoebelen CL. The response of the *Galago senegalensis* to physical training. Comp Biochem Physiol 1979;63A:29–36.
32. Zuckerman J, Stull GA. Effects of exercise on knee ligament separation force in rats. J Appl Physiol 1969;26:716–719.
33. Tipton CM, Matthes RD, Maynard JA, Carey RA. The influence of physical activity on ligaments and tendons. Med Sci Sports 1975;7:165–175.
34. Tipton CM, Vailas AC, Matthes RD. Experimental studies on the influences of physical activity on ligaments, tendons and joints: a brief review. Acta Med Scand 1986;711(Suppl):157–168.
35. Tipton CM, Martin RK, Matthes RD, Carey RA. Hydroxyproline concentrations in ligaments from trained and nontrained rats. In: Howald H, Poortmans JR, eds. Metabolic adaption to prolonged physical exercise. Basel: Birkhauser Verlag, 1975:262–267.
36. Tipton CM, Matthes RD, Vailas AC. Influences de l'exercise sur les structures ligamentaires. In: Lacour J, ed. Facteurs limitant l'endurance humaine. Saint-Etienne, 1977:103–114.
37. Cabaud HE, Chatty A, Gildengorin V, Feltman RJ. Exercise effects on the strength of rat anterior cruciate ligament. Am J Sports Med 1980;8:79–86.
38. Woo SLY, Kuei SC, Gomez MA, Winters JM, Amiel D, Akeson WH. The effect of immobilization and exercise on the strength characteristics of bone-medial collateral ligament-bone complex. 1979 ASME Biomech Symp Appl Med Div 1979;32:67–70.
39. Wang CW, Weiss JA, Albright JP, Buckwalter JA, Woo SLY. The effects of long term exercise on the structural and mechanical properties of the canine medial collateral ligament. 1989 ASME Biomech Symp AMD 1989;98:69–72.
40. Laros GS, Tipton CM, Cooper RR. Influence of physical activity on ligament insertions in the knees of dogs. J Bone Joint Surg 1971;53A:275–286.
41. Noyes FR, Torvik PJ, Hyde WB, DeLucas JL. Biomechanics of ligament failure. II. An analysis of immobilization, exercise, and reconditioning effects in primates. J Bone Joint Surg 1974;56A:1406–1418.
42. Lam T, Frank C, Shrive N. Ligament viscoelastic behaviour changes with maturation. Trans Orthop Res Soc 1989;14:187.
43. Walsh S, Frank S, Chimich D, Lam T, Hart D. Immobilization inhibits biomechanical maturation of growing ligaments. Trans Orthop Res Soc 1989;14:253.
44. Evans EB, Eggers GWN, Butler JK, Blumel J. Experimental immobilization and remobilization of rat knee joints. J Bone Joint Surg 1960;42A:737–758.
45. Langenskiöld A, Michelsson JE, Videman T. Osteoarthritis of the knee in the rabbit produced by immobilization. Acta Orthop Scand 1979;50:1–14.
46. Enneking WF, Horowitz M. The intra-articular effects of immobilization on the human knee. J Bone Joint Surg 1972;54A:973–985.
47. Woo SLY, Matthews JV, Akeson WH, Amiel D, Convery FR. Connective tissue response to immobility: correlative study of biomechanical and biochemical measurements of normal and immobilized rabbit knees. Arthritis Rheum 1975;18:257–264.
48. Akeson WH, Amiel D, Woo SLY. Immobility effects on synovial joints: the pathomechanics of joint contracture. Biorheology 1980;17:95–110.
49. Akeson WH, Woo SLY, Amiel D, Matthews JV. Biomechanical and biochemical changes in the periarticular connective tissue during contracture development in the immobilized rabbit knee. Connect Tissue Res 1974;2:315–323.
50. Woo SLY, Gomez MA, Sites TJ, Newton PO, Orlando CA, Akeson WH. The biomechanical and morphological changes in the medial collateral ligament of the rabbit after immobilization and remobilization. J Bone Joint Surg 1987;69A:1200–1211.
51. Amiel D, Akeson WH, Harwood FL, Frank CB. Stress deprivation effect on metabolic turnover of the medial collateral ligament collagen. A comparison between nine- and 12-week immobilization. Clin Orthop 1983;172:265–270.
52. Amiel D, Woo SLY, Harwood FL, Akeson WH. The effect of immobilization on collagen turnover in connective tissue: a biochemical-biomechanical correlation. Acta Orthop Scand 1982;53:325–332.
53. O'Donoghue DH. Surgical treatment of fresh injuries to the major ligaments of the knee. J Bone Joint Surg 1950;32A:721–737.

54. Starke W. Fibular ligament rupture during growth. Unfallchirurg 1989;92:6–10.
55. Inoue M, Woo SLY, Gomez MA, Amiel D, Ohland KJ, Kitabayashi LR. Effects of surgical treatment and immobilization on the healing of the medial collateral ligament: a long-term multidisciplinary study. Connect Tissue Res 1990;25:13–26.
56. Korkala O, Rusanen M, Gronblad M. Healing of experimental ligament rupture: findings by scanning electron microscopy. Arch Orthop Trauma Surg 1982;102:179–182.
57. O'Donoghue DH, Rockwood CA Jr, Zaricznyj B, Kenyon R. Repair of knee ligaments in dogs. I. The lateral collateral ligament. J Bone Joint Surg 1961;43A:1167–1178.
58. Ellsasser JC, Reynolds FC, Omohundro JR. The non-operative treatment of collateral ligament injuries of the knee in professional football players. An analysis of seventy-four injuries treated non-operatively and twenty-four injuries treated surgically. J Bone Joint Surg 1974;56A:1185–1190.
59. Kannus P. Long-term results of conservatively treated medial collateral ligament injuries of the knee joint. Clin Orthop 1988;226:103–112.
60. Balkfors B. The course of knee-ligament injuries. Acta Orthop Scand Suppl 1982;198:1–99.
61. Odensten M, Lysholm J, Gillquist J. Suture of fresh ruptures of the anterior cruciate ligament. A 5-year follow-up. Acta Orthop Scand 1984;55:270–272.
62. Feagin JA Jr, Curl WW. Isolated tear of the anterior cruciate ligament: 5-year follow-up study. Am J Sports Med 1976;4:95–100.
63. Nikolaou PK, Seaber AV, Glisson RR, Ribbeck BM, Bassett FH. Anterior cruciate ligament allograft transplantation. Long-term function, histology, revascularization, and operative technique. Am J Sports Med 1986;14:348–360.
64. Clancy WG. Advances in biologic substitution for cruciate deficiency. In: Finerman G, ed. AAOS symposium on sports medicine: the knee. St. Louis: CV Mosby, 1985:222–229.
65. Clancy WG Jr, Narechania RG, Rosenberg TD, Gmeiner JG, Wisnefske DD, Lange TA. Anterior and posterior cruciate ligament reconstruction in rhesus monkeys: a histological, microangiographic, and biomechanical analysis. J Bone Joint Surg 1981;63A:1270–1284.
66. Grood ES, Butler DL, Noyes FR. Models of ligament repairs and grafts. In: Finerman G, ed. AAOS symposium on sports medicine: the knee. St. Louis: CV Mosby, 1985:169–181.
67. Jones KG. Reconstruction of the anterior cruciate ligament. A technique using the central one-third of the patellar ligament. J Bone Joint Surg 1963;45A:925–932.
68. Ryan JR, Droupp BW. Evaluation of tensile strength of reconstructions of the anterior cruciate ligament using the patellar tendon in dogs. South Med J 1966;59:129–134.
69. McPherson GK, Mendenhall HV, Gibbons DF, et al. Experimental, mechanical and histologic evaluation of the Kennedy ligament augmentation device. Clin Orthop 1985;196:186–195.
70. Arnoczky SP, Tarvin GB, Marshall JL. Anterior cruciate ligament replacement using patellar tendon. An evaluation of graft revascularization in the dog. J Bone Joint Surg 1982;64A:217–224.
71. Yoshiya S, Andrish JT, Manley MT, Kurosaka M. Augmentation of anterior cruciate ligament reconstruction in dogs with protheses of different stiffnesses. J Orthop Res 1986;4:475–485.
72. Hurley PB, Andrish JT, Yoshiya S, Manley M, Kurosaka M. Tensile strength of the reconstructed canine anterior cruciate ligament: a long-term evaluation of the modified Jones technique. Am J Sports Med 1987;15:393.
73. Ballock RT, Woo SLY, Lyon RM, Hollis JM, Akeson WH. Use of patellar tendon autograft for anterior cruciate ligament reconstruction in the rabbit: a long-term histologic and biomechanical study. J Orthop Res 1989;7:474–485.
74. Thorson EP, Rodrigo JJ, Vasseur PB, Sharkey NA, Heitter DO. Comparison of frozen allograft versus fresh autogenous anterior cruciate ligament replacement in the dog. Trans Orthop Res Soc 1987;12:65.
75. Holden JP, Grood ES, Butler DL, et al. Biomechanics of fascia lata ligament replacements: early postoperative changes in the goat. J Orthop Res 1988;6:639–647.
76. Cho KO. Reconstruction of the anterior cruciate ligament by semitendinosus tenodesis. J Bone Joint Surg 1975;57A:608–612.
77. Lipscomb AB, Johnston RK, Snyder RB, Brothers JC. Secondary reconstruction of anterior cruciate ligament in athletes by using the semitendinosus tendon. Preliminary report of 78 cases. Am J Sports Med 1979;7:81–84.
78. Mott HW. Semitendinosus anatomic reconstruction for cruciate ligament insufficiency. Clin Orthop 1983;172:90–92.
79. Noyes FR, Butler DL, Grood ES, Zernicke RF, Hefzy MS. Biomechanical analysis of human ligament grafts used in knee-ligament repairs and reconstructions. J Bone Joint Surg 1984;6A:344–352.
80. Roberts TS, Drez DJ Jr, Banta CJ III: Complications of anterior cruciate ligament reconstruction. In: Sprague NF III, ed. Complications in arthroscopy. New York: Raven, 1989;169–177.
81. Webster DA, Werner FW. Freeze-dried flexor tendons in anterior cruciate ligament reconstruction. Clin Orthop 1983;181:238–243.
82. Shino K, Inoue M, Horibe S, Hamada M, Ono K. Reconstruction of the anterior cruciate ligament using allogenic tendon: long-term follow-up. Am J Sports Med 1990;18:457–465.
83. Shino K, Kawasaki T, Hirose H, Gotoh I, Inoue M, Ono K. Replacement of the anterior cruciate ligament by an allogenic tendon graft. An experimental study in the dog. J Bone Joint Surg 1984;66B:672–681.
84. Gibbons MJ, Butler DL, Grood ES, Bylski-Austrow DI, Levy MS, Noyes FR. Effects of gamma irradiation on the initial mechanical and material properties of goat bone-patellar tendon-bone allografts. J Orthop Res 1991;9:209–218.
85. Shino K, Inoue M, Horibe S, Nagano J, Ono K. Maturation of allograft tendons transplanted into the knee. An arthroscopic and histological study. J Bone Joint Surg 1988;70B:556–560.
86. Jackson DW, Grood ES, Arnoczky SP, Butler DL, Simon TM. Freeze dried anterior cruciate ligament allografts. Preliminary studies in a goat model. Am J Sports Med 1987;15:295–303.
87. Vasseur PB, Rodrigo JJ, Stevenson S, Clark G, Sharkey N. Replacement of the anterior cruciate ligament with a bone-ligament-bone anterior cruciate ligament allograft in dogs. Clin Orthop 1987;219:268–277.
88. Arnoczky SP, Warren RF, Ashlock MA. Replacement of the anterior cruciate ligament using a patellar tendon allograft. An experimental study. J Bone Joint Surg 1986;68A:376–385.
89. Sullivan R, Fassolitis AC, Larkin EP, Read RB Jr, Peeler JT. Inactivation of thirty viruses by gamma irradiation. Appl Microbiol 1971;22:61–65.
90. Wright KA, Trump JG. Cooperative studies in the use of ionizing radiation for sterilization and preservation of biologic tissue: twenty years experience. In: International Atomic Energy Agency, ed. Sterilization and preservation of biologic tissues by ionizing radiation. Vienna: Editor, 1969:107–118.
91. Van Winkle W, Borich AM, Fogarty M. Destruction of radiation resistant microorganisms on surgical structures by ^{60}Co-irradiation under manufacturing conditions. In: International Atomic Energy Agency, ed. Radiosterilization of Medical Products. Vienna: Editor, 1967:169–180.
92. Cameron RR, Conrad RN, Sell KW, Latham WD. Freeze-dried composite tendon allografts: an experimental study. Plast Reconstr Surg 1971;47:39–47.
93. Thomas ED, Gresham RB. Comparative tensile strength study of fresh-frozen and freeze-dried human fascia lata. Surg Forum 1963;14:442–443.
94. Barad S, Cabaud HE, Rodrigo JJ. Effects of storage at −80°C as compared to 4°C on the strength of rhesus monkey anterior cruciate ligaments. Trans Orthop Res Soc 1982;7:378.
95. Webster DA, Werner FW. Mechanical and functional properties of implanted freeze-dried flexor tendons. Clin Orthop 1983;180:301–309.
96. Viidik A, Sanquist L, Magi M. Influence of postmortem storage on tensile strength characteristics and histology of rabbit ligaments. Acta Orthop Scand Suppl 1965;79:1–38.
97. Woo SLY, Orland CA, Camp JF, Akeson WH. Effects of postmortem storage by freezing on ligament tensile behavior. J Biomech 1986;19:399–404.
98. Roberts TS, Drez D Jr, McCarthy W, Paine R. Anterior cruciate ligament reconstruction using freeze-dried, ethylene oxide-sterilized, bone-patellar tendon-bone allografts. Two year results in thirty-six patients. Am J Sports Med 1991;19:35–41.

99. Silvaggio VJ, Fu FH, Georgescu HI, Evans CH: The induction of IL-1 by freeze dried ethylene oxide treated bone-patellar tendon-bone allograft wear particles. An in vitro study. Trans Orthop Res Soc 1991;16:207.
100. Butler DL, Oster DM, Feder SM, Grood ES, Noyes FR. Effects of gamma irradiation on the biomechanics of patellar tendon allografts of the ACL in the goat. Trans Orthop Res Soc 1991;16:205.
101. Butler DL, Noyes FR, Walz KA, Gibbons MJ. Biomechanics of human knee ligament allograft treatment. Trans Orthop Res Soc 1987;12:128.
102. Paulos LE, France EP, Rosenberg TD, et al. Comparative material properties of allograft tissues for ligament replacement: effects of type, age, sterilization, and preservation. Trans Orthop Res Soc 1987;33:129.
103. Haut RC, Powlison AC. Order of irradiation and lyophilization on the strength of patellar tendon allografts. Trans Orthop Res Soc 1989;14:514.

6 / REHABILITATION

James J. Irrgang

Introduction

Rehabilitation involves any procedure designed to maximize function after injury or illness. In sports medicine it includes procedures designed to restore athletes to their prior level of function within the shortest period of time. Rehabilitation begins immediately after the injury and progresses through the acute and subacute phases of injury or surgery, culminating in return to sport. For an athlete, it must also include a period of reconditioning to ensure optimal levels of fitness, including flexibility, strength, and endurance, which are necessary to achieve optimum performance and to minimize the risk of reinjury. Rehabilitation includes the application of therapeutic exercise and physical agents. Physical agents include various forms of heat, cold, electricity, and massage that are used to relieve pain and swelling and to aid in the healing process. Therapeutic exercise includes a variety of movements designed to restore function to the greatest possible degree in the shortest period of time and to attain high levels of physical conditioning.

Rehabilitation requires that athletic trainers and physical therapists have basic knowledge of the effects of exercise and physical agents. The purpose, indications, contraindications, and precautions of these procedures must be known. Athletic trainers and physical therapists must be able to relate the effects of the physical agents and therapeutic exercise to the rehabilitation goals for the athlete. Establishment of appropriate goals during rehabilitation is dependent upon the ability to assess the extent of injury and functional status of the injured athlete. An understanding of pathology and the healing process is also necessary to ensure appropriate rehabilitation. Anatomy, kinesiology, and biomechanics must also be considered when developing the rehabilitation program.

The ultimate goal of rehabilitation following athletic injury is to restore symptom-free movement and function, allowing individuals to return to their prior level of activity in the shortest time possible. Specific goals in the rehabilitation program are dependent on the phase of rehabilitation. They include limiting inflammation, decreasing pain and swelling, improving mobility and flexibility, improving muscle strength and endurance, improving cardiovascular endurance, and promoting coordination. Rehabilitation procedures must be designed to meet these goals. The injured athlete's must progress through the rehabilitation program as successive goals are accomplished.

Immobility and decreased activity adversely affect many tissues. Decreased stresses on bone due to prolonged immobilization, relief of weightbearing, or decreased muscle activity, result in decreased deposition of bone, while resorption remains unchanged, resulting in an overall decrease in bone mass.

Articular cartilage is dependent on synovial fluid for maintenance of its nutrition. Intermittent compression of joint surfaces enhances the exchange of synovial fluid within the articular cartilage. Prolonged immobilization adversely affects nutrition of articular cartilage and may result in adherence of the synovial membrane to the margins of the articular cartilage, preventing movement of synovial fluid into the underlying articular cartilage. The result of this synovial fluid deprivation is known as obliterative degeneration of articular cartilage (1). Continuous pressure of joint surfaces for a period as short as 8 days will deprive the articular cartilage of nutrition by movement of synovial fluid and can result in the development of a compression sore, also termed compression necrosis of the articular cartilage (1).

Prolonged immobilization of a joint also results in synovial adhesions that can limit motion. It can also decrease stiffness and strength of ligaments and joint capsules. Immobilization of the knee in rhesus monkeys resulted in a significant decrease in maximum load to failure, even after 12 months of reconditioning (2).

The response of muscle to decreased use is atrophy. Type I fibers atrophy faster than type IIa or IIb fibers (3). Immobilization also results in decreased oxidative capacity of the muscle fiber.

In the growing child, intermittent compression of the epiphyseal plate is necessary for growth of long bones. Immobilization and/or inactivity decrease normal intermittent pressures on the growth plate with a potential effect on growth.

Living tissues respond and adapt to the stresses placed upon them. The effects of increased stress upon the body result in changes that are essentially opposite to those imposed by the decreased use described above. Wolff's law states that bone adapts to the stresses placed upon it. Stresses from weightbearing and muscular contraction result in increased bone mass. Soft tissue structures respond in a similar manner. The SAID principle is an acronym coined by Wallis and Logan (4) from the phrase "specific adaptations to imposed demands." It implies that tissues adapt to altered patterns of use. Increased use results in specific adaptations of structure and/or function that enable those tissues to withstand the stresses imposed upon them. This is an important concept in rehabilitation. It implies that the degree of functional capacity achieved is dependent upon the intensity, duration, and frequency of exercise. In order to achieve the highest levels of structure and function, it is necessary to progressively increase the load applied to the tissues. During rehabilitation, tissues within the body must be stressed in a positive, progressive, and appropriately planned manner with the ultimate goal of improvement of overall function of the individual to meet the demands of his or her sport.

Rehabilitation of the injured athlete is a problem-solving process that can be depicted as a feedback loop. It includes assessment of the athlete and leads to development of needs, goals, and a plan of care. As the athlete progresses, the plan of care needs to be modified to allow for continued progress. Frequent reassessment of the athlete is required in order to do this. The ability to accurately evaluate and identify rehabilitation goals is critical to this process. The reader is referred to individual chapters for reviews of the physical examination of specific joints.

Forms of Therapeutic Exercise

Therapeutic exercise is defined as those movements designed to restore the greatest possible degree of function in the shortest period of time and to attain high levels of physical fitness. A therapeutic exercise program must consider the nature and severity of the illness or injury, the purpose of the exercise, sequencing, and progression of the exercise, as well as contraindications and precautions. In addition, the intensity, frequency, and duration of the exercise must be appropriate for the stage of inflammation, healing, and conditioning.

Therapeutic exercise can be categorized into static or dynamic exercise (Fig. 6.1). Static exercise includes isometric exercises in which no observable movement occurs. The length of the muscle appears constant; however, there is shortening at the sarcomere level. Isometric contractions occur when torque produced by muscle tension is equal to external resistance.

Dynamic exercise may be either active or passive. Active dynamic exercise results from voluntary contraction of muscles. Free active exercise occurs when muscles produce movement without application of additional external resistance. Free active exercise includes range of motion and stretching. Active range of motion exercise includes those movements within the unrestricted available range of motion that are produced by voluntary contraction of the individual's muscles. Active stretching exercises are those in which the athlete utilizes voluntary effort to move beyond the restricted range of motion. Range of motion exercises are performed to maintain motion, while stretching exercises are designed to increase motion.

Active resistive exercises are those exercises in which the individual utilizes voluntary muscle contraction to

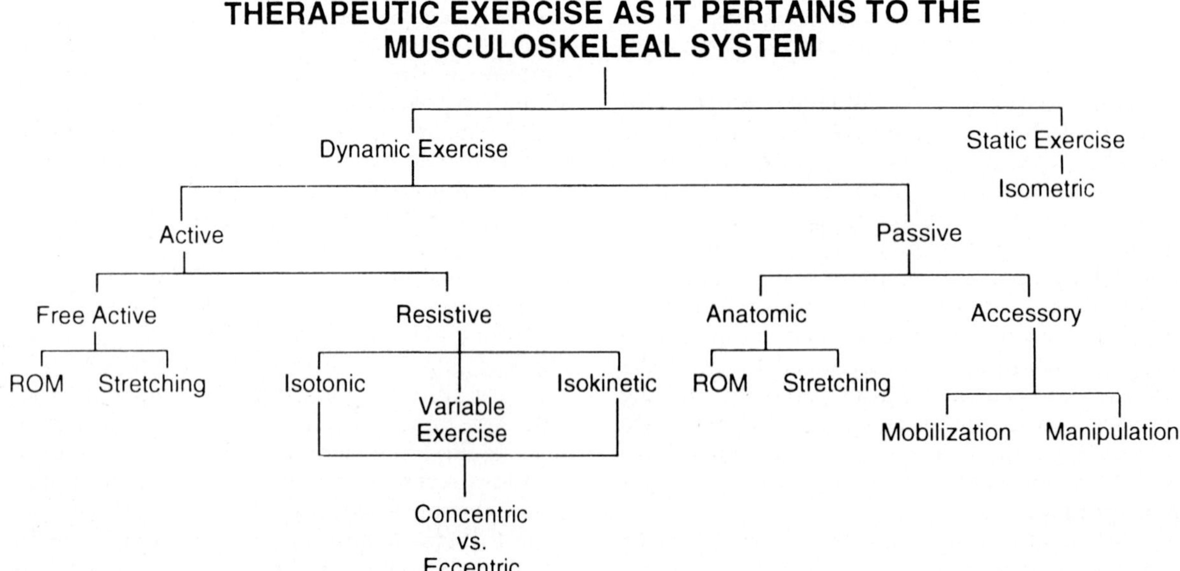

Figure 6.1. Scheme describing the categorization of therapeutic exercise as it pertains to treatment of the musculoskeletal system.

move against an applied resistance. The exercises include isotonic and isokinetic exercises.

Isotonic exercises, by definition, should result in constant tension within the muscle through the range of shortening (5). However, this condition rarely occurs and the term isotonic exercise has come to imply movement against a fixed external resistance. Motion against a fixed external resistance results in variable muscle tension due to the length-tension relationship of the muscle fiber itself and the changing mechanical advantage that the line of muscle action has on the skeletal system. Speed is not controlled during isotonic exercise.

Isokinetic exercise involves movement at a constant speed. External resistance is variable and accommodating. Resistance during isokinetic exercise is proportional to the effort put forth by the athlete.

Recently, variable resistance machines have been developed in an attempt to provide variable resistance that matches the torque curves produced by a particular muscle or muscle group. In variable resistance exercises, the resistance is not accommodating and the speed is not controlled.

Isotonic, isokinetic, and variable resistance exercises can be performed concentrically or eccentrically. Concentric contraction implies that the muscle shortens as it contracts, while an eccentric contraction implies lengthening as the muscle contracts. Concentric contractions are necessary to accelerate the body and eccentric contractions are necessary for deceleration. The force velocity relationship is different for each type of contraction. During a concentric contraction, the force created by the muscle decreases as the speed of contraction increases. During an eccentric contraction, however, the force created by the muscle increases as the speed of lengthening increases. This is believed to result from facilitation of the stretch reflex and stretching of the connective tissue component within the musculotendinous unit, both of which give rise to increased muscle tension with increased speed of lengthening. Concentric contractions occur when the internal force created by the muscle is greater than external resistance. Conversely, eccentric contractions occur when external resistance overcomes internal resistance created by the muscle. Eccentric exercise is associated with increased muscle soreness and increased injury.

Passive exercise occurs without voluntary muscular effort on the part of the athlete. Passive movement is the result of forces external to the body. Passive exercise can be either physiologic or accessory. Physiologic passive exercise implies angular displacement of the bone. These are movements that the patient could perform under voluntary muscular control. Passive physiologic motion can be performed either as range of motion or as stretching exercises. Passive physiologic range of motion is motion that occurs within the unrestricted range of motion. Passive stretching movements are those movements beyond the restricted range and are performed in an attempt to increase motion.

Accessory motions are those that the individual is not capable of producing by voluntary muscle action. Accessory motion includes motions of the joint surfaces that are necessary for normal physiologic movement of the joint and include distraction, compression, rolling, gliding, and spins of the joint surfaces. Passive accessory motion is performed to increase joint play, which is necessary for normal physiologic motion. Joint mobilization is passive accessory motion that is performed at slow speeds. Mobilization can be performed using oscillatory or sustained movements both to decrease pain, and to increase joint mobility. Manipulations are passive movements performed with a quick low-amplitude thrust at the end of the available range of motion. Manipulation is used to regain the final degrees of motion.

Both physiologic and accessory passive exercise can be graded in terms of the total amount of motion available at the joint (15). The normal range of motion for a joint is the amount of motion that is normal or expected for a particular joint. However, the available range of motion may be less than the normal range of motion for a particular joint. The total available range of motion is equal to motion in the unrestricted range and motion beyond the motion barrier that is achieved with overpressure. Grade I motion is a small amplitude movement at the beginning of the range of motion. Grade II motion is a large amplitude movement performed within the available range of motion, but not up to the motion barrier. Grade III passive motion is a large amplitude movement performed up to and beyond the motion barrier. Grade IV passive motion is a small amplitude movement performed at and beyond the motion barrier. Grade V movements are those high velocity, small amplitude movements performed beyond the motion barrier (Fig. 6.2).

Grade I and II movements constitute range of motion exercises and are used to maintain motion during the acute and early subacute phases when excessive motion may be detrimental to healing. Grade III and IV movements are stretching exercises used during the subacute and chronic stage of recovery to increase motion. Grade V motions include manipulations and are designed to increase motion and are discussed below.

Principles for Improvement of Range of Motion

Range of motion available at a particular joint is determined by the configuration of the joint surfaces as well as surrounding soft tissue structures such as the capsule, ligament, muscle, tendon, fascia and skin. The range of motion available at a particular joint is termed "joint range" (6). Joint range is measured in degrees with a goniometer. Muscle range is related to the functional excursion produced by muscles that cross the joint (6). The functional excursion of a muscle is the distance that it is capable of lengthening and shortening. For a one-joint muscle, the functional excursion is directly influenced by the joint that the muscle crosses. A one-joint muscle is expected to shorten and lengthen sufficiently to permit full active range of motion at the joint that it crosses. The functional excursion of multijoint

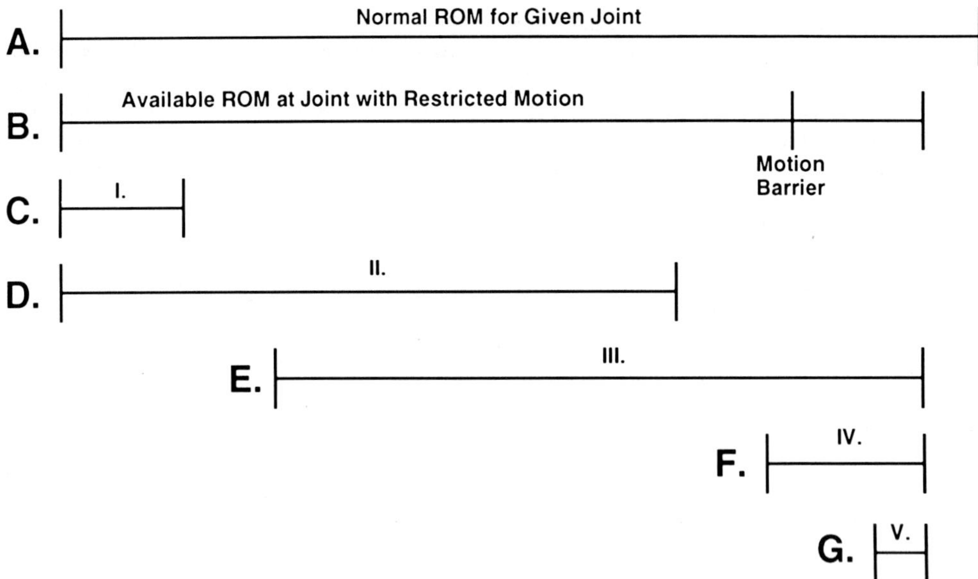

Figure 6.2. Grading system for passive motion. **A.** Normal range of motion (ROM) available for a given joint. **B.** Range of motion available for a joint with restricted motion. The motion barrier represents resistance to motion engaged near the end of the motion. Motion beyond the motion barrier is achieved with overpressure. **C.** Grade I motion—small amplitude movement at the beginning of the range. **D.** Grade II motion—large amplitude motion within the available range but not up to the motion barrier. **E.** Grade III motion—large amplitude movement up to and beyond the motion barrier. **F.** Grade IV motion—small amplitude motion at and beyond the motion barrier. **G.** Grade V motion—high velocity, small amplitude motion performed beyond the motion barrier.

muscles exceeds the joint range of any one of the joints that it crosses. Multijoint muscles, however, cannot lengthen or shorten sufficiently to simultaneously permit the extreme range of motion at all the joints that it crosses. For example, the hamstrings cannot lengthen sufficiently to permit simultaneous full hip flexion and full knee extension. In this position, the hamstrings are said to be passively insufficient. In the passive, insufficient position, further motion is limited by tension in the musculotendinous unit. Similarly, the hamstrings cannot shorten sufficiently to permit simultaneous full active knee flexion and hip extension. In this position, the hamstrings are said to be actively insufficient. In the active insufficient position, the muscle fibers cannot shorten any further and are ineffective in generating additional tension.

In order to increase motion, the properties of the tissue that limit the motion must be considered. Traditionally, these tissues are divided into noncontractile and contractile tissues. Noncontractile tissues include ligaments, tendons, capsule, fascia, connective tissue components of muscle and skin. The material strength of tissue is its ability to resist load or stress. Stress is defined as force per unit of cross-sectional area and can be tensile, compressive, or shearing. Strain is defined as the deformation that occurs in response to stress. It is typically expressed as a percentage of elongation (i.e., change in length divided by original length). The mechanical properties of tissue are often plotted in a stress/strain curve (Fig. 6.3) that relates strain as a function of stress for a given tissue. The toe region occurs at the beginning of the stress/strain curve. This is the region where little force is required to elongate the tissue. This probably represents straightening of the wavy pattern of connective tissue fibers. The elastic range consists of that area of the stress/strain curve in which the tissue returns to its original size and shape when the stress is removed. The upper end of the elastic range is termed the elastic limit. This is the point beyond which the tissue will not return to its original size or shape when the stress is removed. The plastic range of the stress/strain curve represents the range beyond the elastic limit that results in permanent elongation when the stress is removed. The upper end of the plastic range is associated with failure of the tissue. Sequential failure of col-

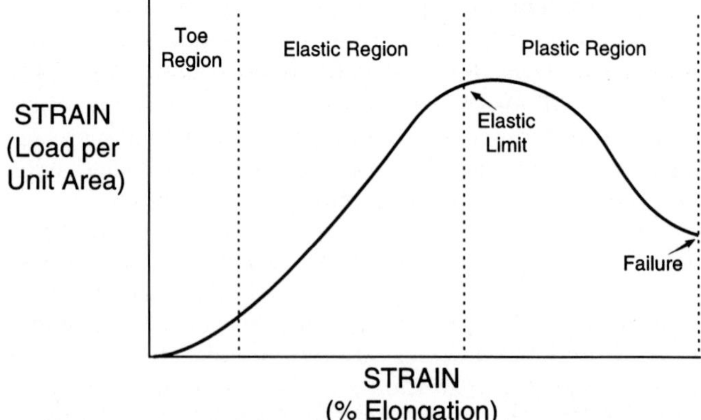

Figure 6.3. Typical stress/strain curve for connective tissue. Toe region represents the region where little stress is required to lengthen the tissue; it probably represents straightening of wavy pattern of collagen fibers. Elastic region is that portion of the curve in which tissue returns to its original length when the stress is removed. Plastic region is that portion of the curve that results in permanent elongation when the stress is removed. Modified from Kisner C, Colby LA. Therapeutic exercise: Foundations and Techniques. 2nd ed. Philadelphia: F.A. Davis, 1990.

lagen fibers in tendon occurs between 4–8% strain. Failure of the tissue occurs beyond 8–10% strain of the collagen fibers (7). This corresponds to 20–40% strain of the entire tendon (8).

Connective tissues is viscoelastic, that is, it exhibits properties of viscosity and elasticity. Elasticity refers to the tissue's ability to return to its original length when stress is removed. Viscosity refers to a tissue's ability to resist elongation. Due to the viscoelastic nature of connective tissue, it exhibits properties of creep, relaxation, and stiffness. Creep is the elongation of tissue that results from constant loading (Fig. 6.4). Creep can be increased by increasing tissue temperature (9). Relaxation is the progressive decrease in internal stress over time as a result of lengthening to a constant strain. Stiffness is the ability of the tissue to resist elongation and is indicated by the slope of the stress/strain curve shown in Figure 6.3. Since connective tissue is viscoelastic, stiffness is dependent on the rate of loading. Increased rate of loading is associated with greater stiffness.

The mechanical characteristics of connective tissue should be considered when attempting to increase range of motion. Lengthening of connective tissue requires plastic deformation that results in gradual rearrangement of the connective tissue. Adequate time must be provided for remodeling to prevent fatigue or rupture of the tissue, or both. Plastic deformation of connective tissue can be maximized by utilizing the principles of creep, relaxation, and stiffness. To maximize permanent lengthening, low magnitude forces should be applied for prolonged periods of time. This process can be facilitated by the use of heating modalities and by maintaining the lengthened position during the period of cooling (9).

The mechanical characteristics of contractile tissue must also be considered when attempting to increase range of motion. It should be remembered that muscle consists of both contractile and noncontractile components (10). The noncontractile components include the series elastic and parallel elastic components. The series elastic component includes the connective tissue that connects the muscle fiber to bone, while the parallel elastic component consists of the connective tissue that surrounds each muscle fiber. Lengthening the musculotendinous unit lengthens both the series and the parallel elastic component, producing a sharp rise in tension. As lengthening of the musculotendinous unit continues, mechanical disruption of the cross bridges begins, as the actin and myosin filaments slide apart and an abrupt lengthening of sarcomere occurs. This is termed "sarcomere give" (11). Sarcomeres are elastic and, when short-term stretch is removed, they return to their original length. This implies that short-term stretching is not effective in increasing the length of the contractile components of a muscle.

Plastic deformation of contractile tissue can be achieved with prolonged immobilization. Prolonged immobilization in the lengthened position results in the addition of sarcomeres and permanent lengthening of the contractile tissues. This occurs to maintain the greatest functional overlap of the actin and myosin filaments. Prolonged immobilization in the shortened position results in a decreased number of sarcomeres (12, 13).

The neurophysiologic properties of contractile tissue must also be considered when attempting to increase range of motion limited by musculotendinous structures. The muscle spindle is a sensory organ sensitive to muscle lengthening. Sudden stretching of the muscle results in lengthening of the muscle spindle and initiation of the monosynaptic stretch reflex. Consequently, sudden or ballistic stretching of musculotendinous units may cause the muscle to contract while it is being lengthened, thus resulting in increased soreness following ballistic stretching.

Another sensory organ, the Golgi tendon organ (GTO) is found in the musculotendinous junction and is sensitive to tension caused by passive stretching or active contraction of the musculotendinous unit. Excessive musculotendinous tension causes the GTO to discharge, inhibiting contraction. Stretching techniques such as contract/relax utilize the GTO to inhibit the muscle, contraction allowing it to lengthen.

Reciprocal inhibition occurs when the antagonist muscle is inhibited as an agonist muscle contracts. This

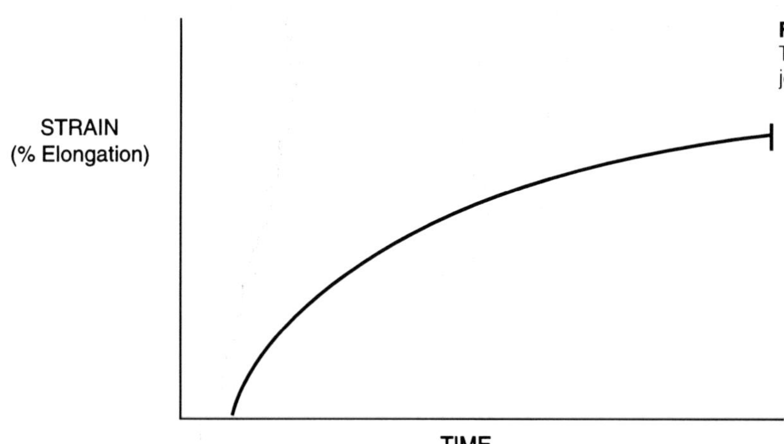

Figure 6.4. Graphic representation of phenomena of creep. Tissue undergoes gradual elongation over time when subjected to constant stress.

principle can also be incorporated into stretching techniques, such as contract/relax/contract and agonist contraction.

Range of motion exercises are exercises that are performed within the unrestricted range of motion in order to maintain joint mobility. They can be passive, active assistive, or active. Passive range of motion exercises are movements that are produced by an external force without voluntary muscular effort on the part of the athlete. The external force may be applied by an athletic trainer or therapist, another part of the athlete's own body, a machine, or gravity. Passive range of motion is indicated when the athlete is not able to move the body segment voluntarily or when voluntary muscle activity would be detrimental to the healing process. This technique can be used to limit the adverse effects of immobility and to demonstrate motion when teaching other forms of exercise. In addition, passive range of motion techniques may be applied prior to stretching. Passive range of motion will not prevent muscle atrophy or affect muscle strength or endurance. Nor will it improve circulation to the same extent as voluntary, active use of the muscles. True passive movement may be difficult to obtain when muscles are innervated.

Active range of motion exercises are exercises within the unrestricted range of motion that are produced by active voluntary muscle contraction. Active assistive exercises combine active voluntary contraction with an outside force to complete motion within the unrestricted range. Both active and active assistive range of motion exercises are used when the athlete is able to actively contract the muscles to move the segment and when there are no contraindications for active voluntary muscle contraction. Active and active assistive range of motion exercises can be used to:

1. Limit the adverse effects of immobility and maintain contractility of muscles;
2. Provide sensory feedback;
3. Provide a stimulus for maintaining integrity of bone;
4. Increase circulation;
5. Improve coordination and motor skills necessary for functional activities;
6. Improve strength of very weak muscles.

Sustained exercises involving large muscle groups can be used to improve cardiorespiratory function. It should be noted, however, that active assistive and active exercises cannot be used to strengthen or maintain strength of muscles that are already strong. It should also be noted that active exercises will only develop skill and coordination in the movement patterns utilized.

Range of motion exercises are contraindicated when motion is disruptive to the healing process. It is important to recognize signs of excessive exercise if range of motion exercises are performed acutely after injury. These signs include increased pain, swelling, warmth, redness, and loss of motion that persists for more than 1–2 hr after the exercise is completed. Range of motion exercises should not replace stretching exercises when the treatment goal is to increase range of motion.

Range of motion exercises may be performed in anatomic planes or in combined patterns incorporating movement in several planes simultaneously. Range of motion exercises also can be performed using sport-specific functional patterns. They should be performed within the pain-free range of motion. Motion beyond the available range of motion should not be forced. Generally 5–10 repetitions several times per day is adequate to limit the adverse effects of immobility. The athlete's response to range of motion exercises should be closely monitored and documented. Treatment must be modified as the athlete progresses.

Stretching exercises are designed to increase range of motion and lengthen pathologically shortened soft tissue structures. Stretching may be performed actively or passively. During passive stretching, the stretch is produced by external forces applied to the body. In active stretching, the stretching force is created by active voluntary contraction of the athlete's muscles. Active stretching allows for incorporation of the neurophysiological principles of stretching.

Flexibility is defined as the ability of the muscle to relax and yield to a stretching force (6). Flexibility exercises are used to increase length of the musculotendinous unit. The term flexibility exercise is often used synonymously with stretching exercise.

A contracture is a shortening of a muscle or other tissues that cross a joint that results in loss of motion. Contractures are defined by identifying the muscle group that limits the range of motion. For example, a lack of full knee extension would be termed a knee flexion contracture while a lack of full knee flexion would be termed a knee extension contracture. A myostatic contracture refers to an adaptive shortening of the musculotendinous unit that results in loss of motion. Tightness is a nonspecific term used to describe mild shortness of the musculotendinous unit that does not result in loss of joint motion. Tightness is common in multijoint muscles such as the hamstrings, rectus femoris and gastrocnemius. Tightness can be improved by self-stretching or flexibility exercises.

During passive stretching exercises, the stretching force is produced externally to the body. The external force can be applied manually or mechanically. Manual passive stretching exercises are generally of short duration lasting 15–30 sec per repetition. The stretch can be applied statically or ballistically. A slow static stretch is less likely to elicit a stretch reflex response. Ballistic stretching refers to a high-intensity, short-duration stretch that results in rapid lengthening of the muscle, which, in turn, stimulates the muscle spindle and facilitates a stretch reflex. The musculotendinous unit is susceptible to microtrauma with ballistic stretching. Ballistic stretching may be beneficial immediately before engaging in exercise, but should be performed only after a warm-up that includes slow static stretching.

Passive mechanical stretching is performed by applying a low (5–10 1b) external load to the shortened tissues for a prolonged period of time (15–30 minutes). Passive mechanical stretching may be performed with the use of ankle weights (Fig. 6.5) or other mechanical

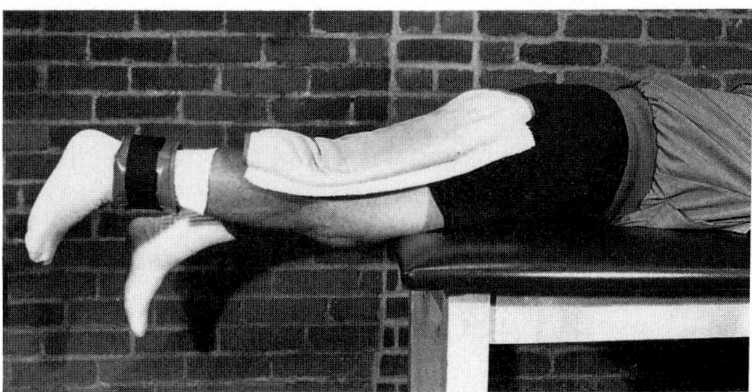

Figure 6.5. Passive mechanical stretching can be performed with the use of ankle weights or other similar equipment. In the prone position, an ankle weight applied to the distal leg can be used to increase knee extension. Low load is applied for prolonged period of time. Heat may be applied simultaneously to maximize plastic deformation.

equipment. Prolonged mechanical stretch may result in greater permanent lengthening of contractile and noncontractile tissues.

Neurophysiologic principles can be incorporated to relax muscles prior to elongation. This allows the contractile component to be lengthened more easily. These techniques can be used to stretch tight contractile structures such as that associated with muscle spasm more comfortably; however, they do not generally result in a permanent increase in length. Examples of neurophysiologic stretching techniques include contract/relax and contract/relax/contract. Contract/relax stretching techniques involve isometric contraction of the tight muscle followed by lengthening of the muscle. The prestretch contraction of the short muscle results in autogenic inhibition stimulation of the Golgi tendon organ. An example of contract/relax stretching technique to stretch the hamstrings would incorporate contraction of the hamstring by simultaneous hip extension and knee flexion, followed by passive lengthening of the hamstrings after the contraction has been completed.

Contract/relax/contract stretching techniques incorporate an isometric contraction of the tight muscle, followed by relaxation and contraction of the antagonistic muscle while the tight muscle is lengthened. Contract/relax/contract stretching techniques combine autogenic inhibition with the principle of reciprocal inhibition. A contract/relax/contract technique to lengthen the hamstrings would incorporate contraction of the hamstring by simultaneous hip extension and knee flexion, followed by relaxation of the muscle and contraction of the quadriceps and hip flexors while the hamstring is lengthened.

The athlete should be taught self-stretching techniques that incorporate use of the athlete's body weight with active inhibition to stretch the tight muscle. These should be performed following the passive stretching and active inhibition techniques described above. The athlete also should be instructed to perform self-stretching exercises several times daily to make continued gains in motion.

Stretching exercises are indicated when the athlete demonstrates limited range of motion in the subacute or chronic phases of healing. It is necessary to regain full motion necessary for athletic activity to avoid interference with sports-related skills. Stretching exercises also can be used to correct muscle imbalances that result when a muscle group is tight, and its opposing muscle group is weak. Generally, the tight muscle group should be stretched before strengthening exercises are performed to improve strength of the opposite muscle group. Stretching exercises may also be indicated before activity as a warm up and after activity as a cool down. Proper warm-up and cool down minimize the risk of musculotendinous injuries associated with physical activity and sports. Stretching exercises should avoid forcing the joint beyond the normal range of motion required for athletic activity. In carrying out these exercises, care should be taken to avoid creating a hypermobile joint. Stretching exercises should not be performed in the acute stages of healing. Stretching during this period may jeopardize the healing tissue and aggravate inflammation. During this time, range of motion exercise rather than stretching exercises should be used. Stretching exercises should not cause a persistent increase in pain that lasts longer than 1–2 hr. Caution must be used when stretching across the fracture site of a newly united fracture. Stretching exercises should not be used in an attempt to increase motion that is limited by a bony block.

Prior to stretching, a local application of heat or engagement in active exercise to elevate body temperature may be beneficial because it increases soft tissue extensibility. Massage and biofeedback may be employed to promote relaxation and decrease muscle spasm making it easier to stretch tight muscles. If mobility of a joint surface is limited, mobilization techniques should be utilized prior to stretching exercises.

In order to understand the principles of joint mobilization, which is used to restore normal movement of the joint surfaces, it is necessary to understand arthrokinematics and osteokinematics. Arthrokinematics refers to movement of the joint surfaces which are necessary for normal physiologic movement of the joint through a full range of motion. Movement of the joint surfaces include distraction, compression, rolling, gliding, and spinning. Osteokinematics refers to the angular displacement of the bone during physiologic motion (14).

The shape of the joint surfaces determines the amount and type of motion available at a joint. An ovoid joint is one in which one joint surface is convex and the other is concave. A sellar-shaped joint is one in which one surface is convex in one direction and concave in the opposite direction. The other joint surface is reciprocally shaped. (Fig. 6.6). The mechanical axis of the joint is a line perpendicular to the center of the joint surface (Fig. 6.7).

Angular movement of a bone about its axis of rotation is termed a swing. Rolling occurs when new points on one joint surface meet new points on an opposing joint surfaces much like a tire rolling along a road (Fig. 6.8*A*). Rolling of the joint surface always occurs in the

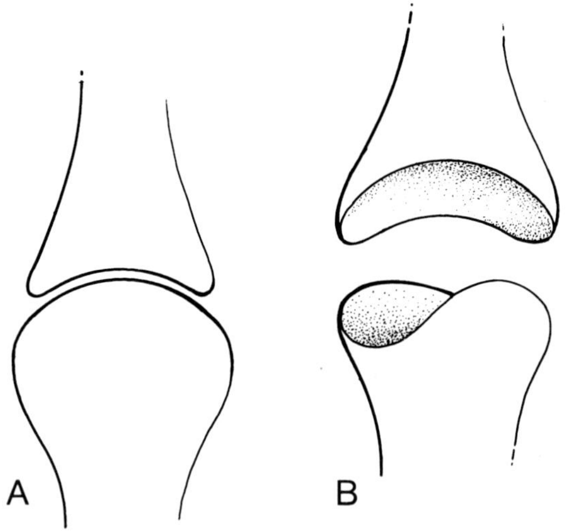

Figure 6.6. **A.** Ovoid joint—one surface is convex and the other surface is concave. **B.** Sellar joint—one surface is convex in one direction and concave in the opposite direction. Other joint surface is reciprocally shaped. Modified from Kisner C, Colby LA. Therapeutic exercise: Foundations and Techniques. 2nd ed. Philadelphia: F.A. Davis, 1990.

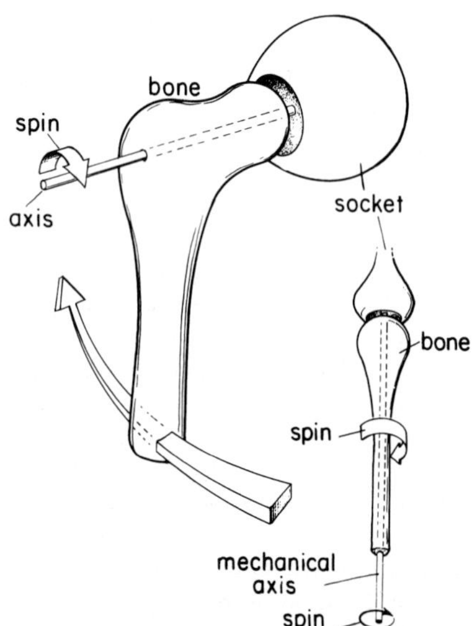

Figure 6.7. Mechanical axis is a line perpendicular to the center of the joint surface.

same direction as the swing of the bone. The joint surfaces are compressed on the side to which the bone is rolling and separated on the opposite side. This may traumatize articular surfaces when gliding of joint surfaces is limited.

Rolling does not occur in isolation during the normal movement of a joint. Rolling is accompanied by sliding of the joint surfaces to prevent the convex joint surface from the rolling off the concave surface. Sliding of joint surfaces involves the same point on one surface contacting new points on the opposing surface much like a locked tire sliding over a road (Fig. 6.8*B*). The direction of the gliding is dependent upon the shape of the articular surface. Convex joint surfaces glide in the direction opposite the swing of the bone while concave joint surfaces glide in the same direction as the swing of the bone. Normal joint motion combines both rolling and gliding of the joint surfaces. Joint mobilization techniques are designed to restore the normal gliding of joint surfaces that is necessary for physiologic motion.

Joint mobilization techniques can be used to increase joint play of hypomobile joints. Restoring normal joint play is necessary to restore full physiologic motion. Joint mobilization increases the extensibility of tight capsules and ligaments that limit mobility of the joint surfaces.

Joint mobilization can also be used to reduce pain and spasm. Small-amplitude, oscillatory joint mobilization stimulates joint mechanoreceptors and can inhibit the perception of pain. Joint mobilization techniques may also reduce pain by stimulating movement of synovial fluid and preventing fluidostasis.

Joint mobilization is contraindicated with hypermobile joints. These same techniques are also contraindicated during the period of active inflammation. During this period, joint mobilization will aggravate inflammation. Joint mobilization is also contraindicated in the presence of a large joint effusion in which the capsule is already stretched because of distention of the joint. Use of mobilization techniques following fractures should be delayed until there is radiographic evidence of union.

Proper application of joint mobilization techniques requires grading of the forces that are utilized. The Maitland or Australian system uses oscillatory techniques (15). Techniques are graded I through IV. Grade I oscillations are small amplitude movements at the beginning of the available range of motion. Grade II oscillations are large amplitude motions performed within the available range but not up to the motion barrier. Grade III oscillations are large amplitude motions performed up to and beyond the motion barrier. Grade IV oscillatory movements are small movements performed at and beyond the motion barrier. In the Australian system, grade I and II oscillatory motions are used to stimulate mechanoreceptors to decrease pain. Grade III and IV oscillatory movements are used to stretch tight structures in order to increase joint mobility and range of motion.

The Kaltenborn, or Norwegian, system utilizes sustained mobilization techniques (16). This system has three grades of motion. Grade I, also called piccolo motion, separates the joint surfaces just enough to equalize intraarticular and atmospheric pressure and is typically utilized to decrease pain. A grade II, or slack technique, removes the slack from the capsule and surrounding ligaments and can be utilized as a trial treatment to increase range of motion. Grade III, or stretch techniques, utilize sufficient force to stretch joint structures to improve mobility.

In general, the oscillatory motions of the Australian system are utilized to decrease pain while the sustained movements in the Kaltenborn system are utilized to improve joint mobility and range of motion.

Proper application of joint mobilization techniques requires a thorough examination of the involved joint

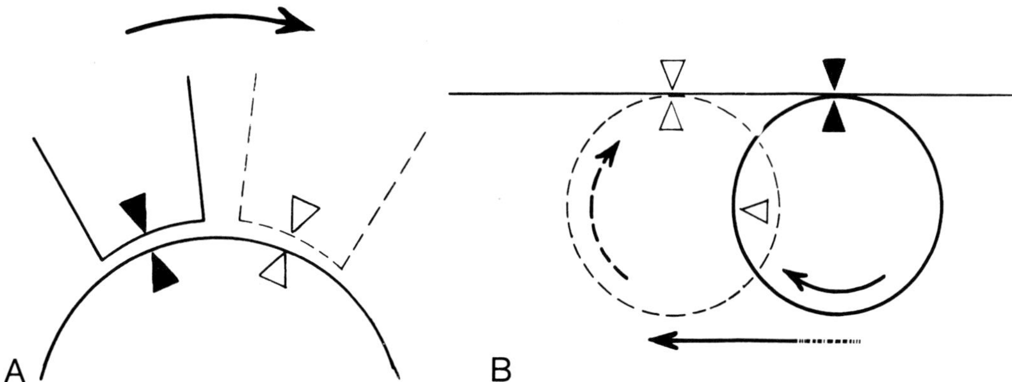

Figure 6.8. **A.** Representation of rolling. New points on one surface contact the new points on opposing surface. **B.** Representation of gliding. New points on one surface contact same point on opposing surface. Modified from Kisner C, Colby LA. Therapeutic exercise: Foundations and Techniques. 2nd ed. Philadelphia: F.A. Davis, 1990.

to determine the tissues limiting motion as well as the stage of pathology. The mobilizing force should be correlated with the sequence of pain to resistance of motion. Pain occurring before resistance to motion is reached indicates an acute condition. Mobilization for acute conditions should consist of grade I and II oscillating techniques to decrease pain and maintain joint play. Pain synchronous with resistance to motion indicates a subacute condition. A trial of gentle stretching should be utilized for subacute conditions. Grade III oscillatory or grade II (slack) mobilization techniques are appropriate for subacute conditions. Pain engaged after resistance to motion has been encountered is indicative of a chronic condition. Vigorous stretching is indicated for chronic conditions. Joint mobilization techniques for chronic conditions include grade III and IV oscillatory or grade III (stretch) sustained techniques.

Joint mobilization techniques should be utilized only when mobility testing reveals decreased joint play. Hypermobile joints should not be mobilized. Generally mobilization techniques are utilized when passive range of motion is limited in a capsular pattern with a capsular or firm end feel. Joint mobilization techniques may be utilized when passive range of motion is limited in a noncapsular pattern, if joint play is limited in the direction of the restricted motion.

When performing joint mobilization, the athlete should be positioned to promote relaxation and stabilization of the part to be mobilized. Initially mobilization should be performed with the joint in the position where the capsule has the greatest amount of laxity. This position generally occurs in the middle of the available range of motion. As range of motion improves, joint mobilization techniques can be performed in the restricted position. Forces should be applied as close to the opposing joint surfaces as possible. The area of contact with the hand should be as large as possible to improve patient comfort. The force of the mobilization technique should be graded according to the stage of the condition and the intended goals of treatment as described above.

The direction of movement is dictated by the direction of the restricted motion and the shape of the joint surface. The treatment plane is a plane perpendicular to a line from the axis of rotation to the center of the concave articulating surface (Fig. 6.9). When joint surfaces are distracted, the force should be applied perpendicular to the treatment plane. When gliding joint surfaces the forces should be applied parallel to the treatment plane, utilizing the following convex/concave rule: Concave joint surfaces should be glided in the direction of the limited swing of the bone, while convex surfaces should be glided in the direction opposite the limited swing of the bone. In performing joint mobilization techniques, angular motion of the bone should be minimized. Angular motion while gliding joint surfaces may result in compression of the joint surfaces which may damage the articular surface.

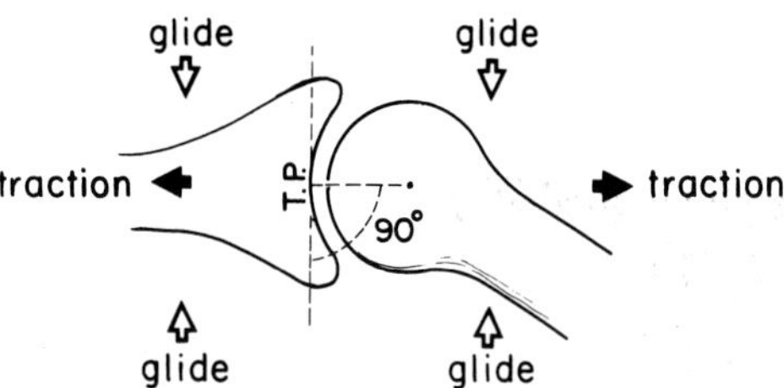

Figure 6.9. Treatment plane (T.P.) is a line perpendicular to the line drawn from axis of rotation for joint to center of concave joint surface. Force to distract the joint are applied perpendicular to the treatment plane. Forces to glide the joint are applied parallel to treatment plane. Modified from Kisner C, Colby LA. Therapeutic exercise: Foundations and Techniques. 2nd ed. Philadelphia: F.A. Davis, 1990.

When oscillatory joint mobilization techniques are performed, they should be performed at a rate of 1–2 cycles per sec for 1–2 min. When performing sustained joint mobilization techniques, they should be sustained for 5–15 sec and repeated 10 times. Joint mobility and range of motion should be assessed at the completion of joint mobilization. The athlete also should perform range of motion and stretching exercises as a follow-up treatment to joint mobilization. The athlete should be warned that it is common to experience some increase in soreness; however, this should subside within several hours.

Principles for Improvement of Muscle Performance

Rehabilitation of athletes must also address muscle performance that includes strength, power, and endurance. Strength is defined as the maximal force that a muscle can generate at a specified velocity. Force is a linear measure that changes the state of rest or motion of matter. When applied to the musculoskeletal system, muscle force causes rotation of a joint about its axis. Force is measured in newtons. Torque is the effectiveness of the force to produce rotation about an axis and is the product of force times the perpendicular distance from the line of action of the force to the axis of rotation. Torque is measured in newton meters. Work is force expressed through a distance with no limitation on time. Mathematically, work is force times distance. It is expressed in joules. Power is the rate of doing work per unit of time. It is expressed as force times distance over time, or as force times velocity. It is expressed as watts. Power is not force at high contractile velocities. Maximum power occurs at intermediate contractile velocities for concentric contractions. Endurance is the ability of the muscle or muscle group to perform work over time. It can be measured as the time a person is able to maintain a particular level of isometric force or power level involving a combination of concentric and eccentric contractions.

Strength of normal muscle is influenced by several factors. The amount of force that a muscle can generate is related to its cross-sectional size. Length of the muscle also influences force generation. According to the length-tension relationship, muscle can generate maximal force at its resting length. This is the position at which there is a maximum number of cross bridges between the actin and myosin filaments. As the muscle shortens, there is greater overlap of the actin-myosin filaments resulting in a decreased number of cross bridges. As a result of this, the force that a muscle can generate in a shortened position is decreased. The contractile force generated by a muscle also decreases as the muscle is lengthened beyond its resting position. However, there is increased force due to passive lengthening of the connective tissue. Therefore, the total force produced by the musculotendinous unit (including both contractile and noncontractile forces) increases as the muscle lengthens (Fig. 6.10).

The number of motor units recruited also influences the level of force generated. The level of force increases as the number of motor units recruited increases. According to Henneml's size principle, small motorneurons are recruited before large motorneurons. Small motorneurons innervate slow-twitch (type I) muscle fibers. These fibers produce low levels of force and are resistant to fatigue. Large motorneurons innervate fast-twitch (type II) muscle fibers. Fast-twitch muscle fibers produce high levels of force, but they fatigue rapidly. Since small motorneurons are recruited before large motorneurons, activities involving low levels of muscle tension are produced primarily by slow-twitch muscle fibers. As force requirements increase, progressively more fast-twitch fibers are recruited.

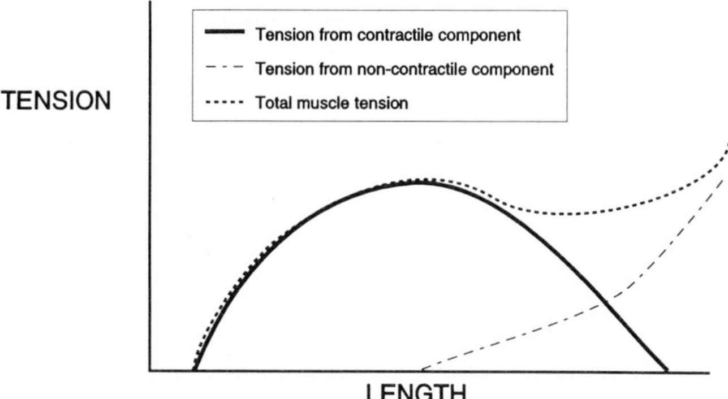

Figure 6.10. Relationship of contractile and noncontractile tension to total tension of a muscle. Contractile tension is greatest at the resting length for a muscle. As the muscle is shortened or lengthened, contractile tension decrease. Noncontractile tension increases as the muscle is lengthened. Total tension produced by a muscle is the sum of contractile and noncontractile tension.

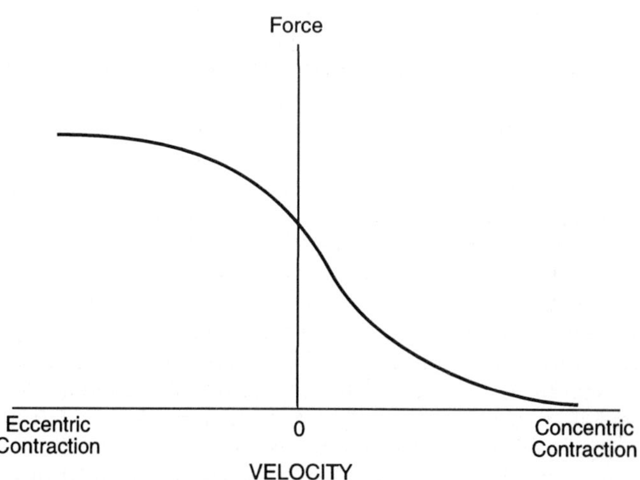

Figure 6.11. Force-velocity relationship for muscle. For concentric contraction, force decreases as the speed of shortening increases. For eccentric contraction, force increases up to some maximum value as the speed of lengthening increases. Modified from Curwin S, Stanish WD. Tendinitis: Its etiology and treatment. Lexington MA: DC Heath & Co, 1984.

The speed and type of muscle contraction also influence the amount of force that a muscle can generate. For concentric contractions, force decreases as speed increases, while, for eccentric contractions, force increases as speed increases up to some maximal value (Fig. 6.11). A maximal eccentric contraction produces greater force than a maximal isometric contraction and a maximal isometric contraction produces greater force than concentric contraction.

Motivation also influences the amount of force generated by a muscle. The individual must be willing and motivated to put forth maximum effort in order to generate maximum forces.

Strength training exercises are designed to increase the maximum force that a muscle can generate. Traditionally, strength training involves heavy-resistance, low-repetition exercise. The definition of heavy resistance varies for individuals and from muscle group to muscle group. Generally, heavy resistance is considered to mean the amount of weight that can be lifted for 6–12 repetitions before fatigue develops. Strength training exercises using heavy resistance are typically performed for 6–12 repetitions.

Response to strength training includes hypertrophy of muscle fibers. The increase in cross-sectional area of muscle fibers is related to increased contractile protein and the number of fibrils within the muscle fiber, as well as an increased density of the capillary bed surrounding individual muscle fibers. Hypertrophy also may be related to an increase in the connective tissue component of muscle. Heavy resistance training appears to selectively hypertrophy fast-twitch (type II) muscle fibers.

Hyperplasia is an increase in the number of muscle fibers that results from longitudinal splitting of muscle fibers. Hyperplasia has been observed in laboratory animals exposed to heavy resistance exercise (17, 18, 19); however, hyperplasia is controversial in humans. In response to strength training, individuals are able to recruit increased number of motor units. Improved recruitment and synchronization of motor units result in greater generation of muscle force. This may explain increases in strength early in the training program in the absence of hypertrophy. Biochemical changes associated with strengthening are small and inconsistent.

Endurance training makes use of low- to moderate-resistance high repetition exercises. Endurance training results in peripheral and central adaptations that improve an individual's ability to sustain work.

The peripheral adaptations are localized to the muscle or muscles involved in the endurance training exercises. The peripheral responses generally result in an improved oxidative capacity of the muscle fiber. This is a result of an increased concentration of myoglobin within the muscle fibers. Increased myoglobin concentration aids in the delivery of oxygen from the cell membrane to mitochondria. A muscle fiber's ability to oxidize carbohydrates and fats is improved. This is the result of an increase in the size, number and membrane surface area of mitochondria as well as an increase in the concentration and activity of oxidative enzymes. The intramuscular stores of adenosine triphosphate (ATP) and creatine phosphate (CP) are increased. There appears to be selective hypertrophy of slow-twitch (type I) muscle fibers; however, this may be modified by the intensity of the endurance exercise. High intensity endurance training (greater than 90%) results in improved endurance capabilities in type II fibers (20, 21). Anaerobic glycolysis is not appreciably affected by endurance training.

Cardiovascular responses to endurance training occur, if the training stimulus is sufficient. Generally, the cardiovascular responses to endurance training include increased cardiac output that is related to increased stroke volume. Resting heart rate and heart rate at a given work load decrease in response to endurance training.

Contraindications to resistive exercise include active inflammation and pain. Use of resistive exercise in the presence of active inflammation can lead to further tissue trauma and aggravate pain and swelling. Resistive exercises should be eliminated or reduced if they produce an increase in pain persisting more than several hours following exercise.

Several precautions should be observed when performing resistive exercises. These include avoidance of a Valsalva maneuver, which may cause a transient, but marked increase in blood pressure that places abnormal stress on the cardiovascular system. Athletes should be warned directly to avoid use of the Valsalva maneuver; they also should be instructed to exhale while performing resistance exercises—particularly during isometric and heavy resistance exercises.

Prolonged resistive exercises result in local muscular fatigue and total body fatigue. Local muscular fatigue is a diminished response of a muscle to sustain work. The fatigue may be due to disturbances in the contractile mechanism of the muscle, including decreased energy stores, insufficient oxygen, or lactic acid accumulation. Local muscular fatigue may also result from inhibitory influences from the central nervous system, pain, and discomfort. Total body fatigue occurs in response to prolonged resistance exercises and may result from decreased blood glucose or depletion of muscle and/or liver glycogen. No biologic marker of overtraining exists. Adequate time in the training program must be included for recovery from vigorous exercise in order to avoid fatigue. Recovery is associated with removal of lactic acid and with replenishment of energy and oxygen stores. Light exercise may facilitate recovery and recovery after each exercise session is required in order to improve performance. This requirement has implications for rehabilitation—particularly in the later stages, when the intensity of exercise is increased and more time for recovery is required from session to session.

The athlete must be observed carefully when performing resistance exercises to detect substitute motions in which alternate motions or muscles complete the motion when the prime movers are weak or fatigued. Use of substitute motion allows muscle weakness to persist. Substitute motions can be avoided by using appropriate amounts of resistance and instructing the athletes to perform the exercise precisely.

Resistance exercises may also result in the development of muscle soreness. Immediate muscle soreness develops during or directly after strenuous exercise. It may be related to muscle injury, ischemia, or the buildup of metabolites. Immediate onset of muscle soreness generally subsides quickly after exercise with rest.

By contrast, delayed onset muscle soreness develops 24–48 hr after vigorous exercise. Numerous causes have been postulated, none satisfactory. Accumulation of lactic acid in the muscle was one of the postulated causes; however, lactic acid is cleared approximately 1 hr after exercise. The reflex pain—spasm theory as proposed by Devries (22) held that ischemia produces pain that in turn produces a reflex muscle spasm. A positive feedback loop develops as spasm creates further pain and ischemia. The original evidence for this theory included increased EMG activity from muscles with delayed muscle soreness; however, this evidence has not been duplicated by others.

Currently, the most plausible explanation for delayed onset muscle soreness is microscopic tearing of muscle and/or connective tissue during vigorous exercise. Disruption of tissue results in inflammation and pain. This theory is supported by the observation that delayed onset muscle soreness is more common after eccentric exercise. Microtearing of muscle and connective tissue may be more pronounced as the muscle lengthens against resistance.

Prevention of delayed onset muscle soreness includes an appropriate period of warm up and cool down before and after the resistance exercise. In addition, delayed onset muscle soreness may be prevented by a gradual progression of the resisted exercise program and the avoidance of the eccentric component of exercise.

Isometric exercises are one form of resistive exercises in which the muscle contracts without an appreciable change in the length of the muscle or invisible joint motion. Since isometrics occur in the absence of joint motion, they can be used when motion is contraindicated. They are also easy to perform and require little equipment. However, isometric exercises develop strength only at the position at which the exercise is performed and they must be performed at 15–30° increments to develop strength throughout the full range of motion. Isometric exercises do not significantly improve endurance.

When performing isometric exercises, the athlete should be instructed to contract the muscle maximally, holding it for 5–10 sec to allow time for development of peak tension. The isometric exercises should be performed at multiple angles to improve strength throughout the range of motion. Submaximal isometrics can also be used to maintain mobility between muscle fibers during the healing phase.

Isotonic exercises make use of movement against a constant external resistance. They can be performed manually or mechanically to improve strength, power, and endurance. In order to improve muscle function, the overload principle must be applied, and the muscle must be progressively loaded by increasing resistance and/or repetitions in order to make continued improvements in function.

When designing an isotonic exercise program, specificity of the exercise must be considered. This means that the exercise program must be designed to strengthen the muscle or muscle groups and during specific functional activities. The speed of the exercise should match the speed of the functional movement. The resistive exercise program should also reproduce the type of contraction required during function. Isometric exercises should be utilized to develop muscles that stabilize the body or body segment. Concentric exercises should be utilized to develop muscles that are responsible for acceleration, while eccentric exercises should be used to develop muscles that are responsible for deceleration of the body. Specificity of the exercise program should also consider the intensity of force required by the muscles during activity. The exercises should be performed through the entire range of motion in which strength is required. When possible, functional exercise patterns should be utilized to develop strength. This implies the use of closed chain activities for the lower extremity and open chain activities for the upper extremity. During closed chain activities, the distal aspect of the extremity is fixed and motion occurs simultaneously at all joints that comprise the kinetic chain. During open chain activities, the distal extent of the extremity is free to move. In order for exercises to be specific, the variables must match the requirements and demands placed upon the athlete during functional activities.

When developing an isotonic exercise program, several variables—load, repetitions, sets and frequency—must be considered. Load is the amount of resistance used during the exercise. In order to improve strength, the load must be progressively increased. Repetitions are the number of times an exercise is performed in a given bout. The number of repetitions must be progressively increased in order to improve endurance. Sets are the number of bouts of repetitions that are performed. There are many combinations of sets and repetitions that can be used to improve strength and/or endurance. Frequency is the number of times the exercises are performed per day or week. Early in rehabilitation, isotonic exercises are usually submaximal and can be performed several times daily. As rehabilitation progresses to reconditioning, the isotonic exercising should become more vigorous, but should be performed less frequently in order to allow adequate time for recovery to prevent fatigue. Most heavy resistance exercise programs designed to improve strength are done every other day. Six weeks may be required in order to see increased strength.

The intensity of the exercise is dependent on the stage of inflammation and healing as well as the goals of the exercise program. Generally, submaximal exercises are utilized to increase muscle endurance. They are emphasized during the early stages of rehabilitation to protect healing tissues and avoid pain and further aggravation of the injury. Maximal exercises are used in the later stage of rehabilitation when the goal is to recondition the athlete to improve strength and power.

Several specific exercise regimes to improve strength have been proposed. DeLorme (23) proposed a technique of progressive resistive exercises (PRE's) that begins by establishing a 10 repetition maximum (RM) weight. This is defined as the amount of weight that can be lifted precisely 10 times, and is usually established by trial and error. In the scheme proposed by DeLorme, 3 sets of 10 repetitions are performed. The first set is against one-half 10 RM weight. The second set is against three-quarters 10 RM weight and the third set is against the full 10 RM weight. A new 10 RM weight is determined each week. The method proposed by DeLorme builds in a gradual warm-up.

The Oxford technique (24) is the opposite of the Delorme method. The first set is performed against the full 10 RM weight. The third set is performed against one-half of the 10 RM weight. This method attempts to accommodate for the effects of fatigue; however, warm-up is required before beginning.

Knight (25) proposed a program of daily adjustable progressive resistive exercises (DAPRE). The Dapre program attempts to objectively determine when and by how much to increase resistance. Knight originally proposed using a 6 RM weight, which is the amount of resistance that can be lifted precisely 6 times. Four sets of exercise are performed. The first set of 10 repetitions is performed with one-half 6 RM weight. The second set of 6 repetitions is performed with three-quarter 6 RM weight. The third set consists of as many repetitions as possible at the full 6 RM weight. The number of repetitions performed during the third set is used to determine the resistance for the fourth set. If more than 6 repetitions are performed during the third set, then the weight for the fourth set is increased. If less than six repetitions are performed for the third set, then the weight for the fourth set is decreased. The number of repetitions performed during the fourth set determines the amount of weight used for the next session.

The methods proposed by DeLorme, Oxford, and Knight make use of heavy resistance, low repetition exercise in an attempt to increase strength. It should be noted that heavy resistance exercise may be inappropriate for the early stages of healing. Heavy resistance may not be tolerated by the joint and the healing structures during this time. As a result of this consideration, exercises using submaximal resistance for greater repetitions may be performed during this period. The author commonly uses resistance that can be performed 30–50 repetitions. Use of heavy resistance exercises are delayed until the athlete enters the reconditioning phase of rehabilitation.

As noted above, isotonic exercises can be performed mechanically or manually. Mechanical resistance exercises have several advantages. The amount of resistance and the number of repetitions performed can quantify the patient's baseline level of muscle performance and progression. In addition, the athletes can see their progress when performing mechanical resistance exercise. This visible progress provides motivation. Resistance applied during mechanical resistance exercises is not limited by the strength of the athletic trainer or therapist. A variety of equipment can be used to provide mechanical resistance exercises.

During manual resistance exercises, resistance is applied by the therapist or athletic trainer. Manual resistance exercise can make use of dynamic or static muscular contractions and can be performed in the cardinal planes or more functional diagonal patterns. Proprioceptive neuromuscular facilitation (PNF) is a technique of manual resistance exercise that emphasizes movement in diagonal patterns.

The popularity of isokinetic exercise has increased over the last 20 years. During isokinetic exercise, the speed of exercise is controlled by a dynamometer. Most isokinetic dynamometers allow concentric and eccentric exercise from 0° to 450°/second. During isokinetic exercise, the resistance is accommodating and proportional to the effort put forth by the athlete. Research indicates there may be some carry-over of training from one speed to another. However, to ensure improvement in muscle performance across the spectrum of speeds, isokinetic training should be performed at a variety of contractile velocities (26). Ideally, the speed of exercise selected for isokinetic training should be comparable to the speed of movement required by function. However, it should be noted that angular velocity during function typically exceeds the speed of movement permitted by the isokinetic dynamometer. Caution must be used when performing isokinetic exercise to insure that further inflammation or injury does not occur. Inappropriate use of isokinetic exercise can be detrimental. During the earlier phases of rehabilitation, isokinetic exercise should be submaximal. Maximal isokinetic exercise should be reserved for the final stages of rehabilitation. Isokinetic testing has been utilized to measure muscle performance and to determine when an athlete is ready to return to full activity. However, there is little scientific validation for the use of isokinetic testing to predict athletic function.

Principles for Improvement of Proprioception

Recently there has been interest in the role that proprioception plays in the prevention and progression of injuries. Proprioception has been described as variation in the sense of touch that includes sensation of joint motion and joint position. Proprioception is mediated by sensory receptors that are located in the skin, in musculotendinous units, ligaments, and joint capsules. These sensory receptors transduce mechanical deformation to a neural signal that modulate conscious and unconscious responses. It has been hypothesized that proprioception is important for providing smooth, coordinated movement as well as protection and dynamic stabilization of joints.

Mechanoreceptors have been identified in the ankle (27), knee (28, 29, 30, 31, 32), and in the shoulder (33, 34). These receptors have been identified in the joint capsules, ligaments, menisci, labrum, and fat pads. Four types of joint mechanoreceptors have been described (27). Type I mechanoreceptors are Ruffini-like receptors that respond at rest and during movement to convey the direction, velocity, and amplitude of movement. They have a low threshold for excitation and they adapt slowly. Type II mechanoreceptors are pacinian-like receptors that have a low threshold for excitation and adapt rapidly. They are responsible for signaling acceleration and deceleration of the joint. Type III mechanoreceptors are similar to Golgi tendon organs that lie in the musculotendinous unit. They have a high threshold for excitation and are nonadapting. They respond at the extremes of motion and may be responsible for mediating protective reflex arcs. Type IV mechanoreceptors are free nerve endings that convey pain.

It has been proposed that joint mechanoreceptors mediate protective reflexes. Solomonow et al. (35) described an anterior cruciate ligament (ACL) hamstring arc in anesthetized cats. High-loading of the ACL resulted in increased electromyographic (EMG) activity in the hamstrings with electrical silence in the quadriceps. The increase in hamstring EMG activity was not evident when light to moderate loads were applied to the ACL. It was proposed that this ACL-hamstring reflex arc served to protect the ACL during high loading conditions. However, it is unknown if this reflex arc can protect the joint from injury if high loads are applied rapidly. Under rapid loading conditions, the ligament may be loaded and ruptured before sufficient muscle tension can be generated to protect the ligament. It is likely that similar reflex arcs exist in other joints.

Other proprioceptive reflexes originating from the joint capsule or musculotendinous unit probably exist. This was demonstrated by Solomonow et al., who reported increased hamstring EMG activity in a patient with an ACL-deficient knee during maximal slow-speed isokinetic testing of the quadriceps. The increased EMG activity occurred simultaneously with anterior subluxation of the tibia at approximately 40° of knee flexion and was associated with a sharp decrease in quadriceps torque and EMG activity. Since the ACL was ruptured, reflex contraction of the hamstrings could not have been mediated by receptors originating in the ACL. It was proposed that this reflex contraction was mediated by receptors in the joint capsule and/or hamstring muscles. It is likely that similar reflex arcs exist in other areas of the body.

Several clinical studies have evaluated proprioception in terms of the threshold to detection of passive motion and reproduction of joint position. Barrick et al. (36) demonstrated deficits in the threshold to detection of passive motion in subjects with a unilateral ACL deficient knee. Lephart et al. (37) studied threshold to detection of passive motion in patients who had undergone ACL reconstruction. Testing was performed at 15° and 45° of flexion. Three trials were performed moving into flexion/extension. The results indicated that threshold to detection of passive motion was less sensitive in the reconstructed knee compared to the noninvolved knee. In addition, threshold to detection of passive motion was more sensitive in the reconstructed and normal knee at 15° of flexion compared to 45° of flexion. The enhanced sensitivity to passive motion near full extension may be due to increased stress on the ligament, making it more sensitive to detection of motion. Kinesthetic deficits in the shoulder in patients after anterior glenohumeral dislocation were demonstrated by Smith and Brunolli (38). They found deficits in angular reproduction, threshold to detection of motion, and end range reproduction of joint angle in the shoulder that had been dislocated.

Injury to a joint may result in abnormal sensory feedback and altered neuromuscular control. Altered neuromuscular control may account for recurrent injury. Proprioceptive training following injury should attempt to maximize use of sensory information mediated by the joint structures and musculotendinous unit to dynamically protect the area. Proprioceptive training requires repetition to develop motor control of abnormal motion. Initially, control of abnormal motion requires conscious effort. Through repetition of training, motor control of abnormal motion may become automatic and occur subconsciously. This requires learning how to recruit muscles with the proper force, timing, and sequencing to protect the area. It should be noted, however, that the extent to which one can develop neuromuscular control of abnormal joint motion to dynamically stabilize a joint is currently unknown. Further research is required to determine the effectiveness of proprioceptive training to dynamically protect the injured area.

Initial proprioceptive activities are designed to enhance conscious awareness of joint position. This can be developed by asking the injured athlete to match and rematch the position of the joint with eyes closed. Proprioceptive neuromuscular facilitation techniques can also be used to enhance proprioception. Specifically, rhythmic stabilization can be used to enhance joint stability. This should initially be performed with the joint in the resting position. As the patient improves, dynamic stabilization can be performed at the extremes of motion. Likewise, the amplitude and velocity of the perturbances applied during the rhythmic stabilization can be increased.

For lower extremity injuries, proprioception can be developed by performing balance activities with the eyes open and closed. Initially, these are performed on a firm surface. With improvement in their sense of balance, athletes can be progressed to balancing on unstable surfaces such as a foam mat, miniramp or balance board.

Return to athletic activity must include a transference of proprioceptive training to athletic activity. This can be accomplished by slow, deliberate rehearsal of the particular activity to ensure that proper mechanics are being used. Visual feedback can be given with the use of mirrors or videotape. EMG biofeedback can be utilized to ensure that muscles are being recruited with the proper force, timing, and sequencing to protect the area.

A variety of sports-specific activities should be used to develop motor control of abnormal joint motion. To develop motor control, activities are generally progressed from slow speed to fast speed, from low force to high force, and from controlled to uncontrolled activities. Emphasis should be on establishing proper movement patterns to dynamically protect the area. General progression of activities to enhance proprioception and dynamic stability of the lower extremity progresses from walking to jogging, running, sprinting, acceleration and deceleration, jumping and cutting, pivoting, and twisting. The athlete's sport should determine specific activities for the upper extremity. The return to throwing for throwing athletes has been described by Papas et al. (39) and Blackburn et al. (40).

Return to throwing should progress from mirror throwing, followed by a short toss program, and finally, a long toss program. Velocity should be increased gradually as tolerated. The functional progression for return to activity must provide the athlete with adequate time to ensure a safe return to sport with minimal risk for reinjury.

Summary

The basic principles of rehabilitation for an injured athlete have been presented. These principles can be applied to rehabilitate the common musculoskeletal injuries that occur in athletics. Development of a rehabilitation program is a problem-solving process. It requires a thorough evaluation of the athlete in order to develop goals and a plan of care. The basic principles of rehabilitation reviewed in this chapter can be applied to accomplish specific rehabilitation goals. Finally, the athlete must be monitored continuously to ensure optimum progression through the rehabilitation program.

REFERENCES

1. Salter RB. Textbook of disorders and injuries of the musculoskeletal system. Baltimore: Williams and Wilkins, 1983.
2. Noyes FR, Torvik PJ, Hyde WB, et al. Biomechanics of ligament failure: II. An analysis of immobilization exercise and reconditioning effects in primates. J Bone Joint Surg 1974:1406–1418.
3. Appell HJ. Sports Med 1990;10:42–58.
4. Wallis EL, Logan GA. Figure improvement and body conditioning through exercise. Englewood Cliffs, NJ: Prentice-Hall, 1964.
5. Knuttgggen HG, Kraemer WJ. Terminology and measurement in exercise performance. J Appl Sport Sci Res 1987;1:1–10.
6. Kisner C, Colby LA. Therapeutic exercise: Foundations and techniques, 2ed. Philadelphia: F.A. Davis, 1990.
7. Curwin S, Stanish WD. Tendinitis: Its etiology and treatment. Lexington MA: DC Heath & Company, 1984.
8. Noyes FR, Keller CS, Grood ES, et al. Advances in the understanding of knee ligament injury repair and rehabilitation. Med Sci Sports Exerc 1984;16:427–443.
9. Lehmann JF, Masock AJ, Warren CG, Koblanski JN. Effect of therapeutic temperatures on tendon extensibility. Arch Phys Med Rehab 1970;51:481–487.
10. Soderberg GL. Kinesiology: Application to pathological motion. Baltimore: Williams and Wilkins, 1986.
11. Flitney FW, Hirst DG. Cross bridge detachment and sarcomere "give" during stretch of active frog's muscle. J Physiol 1978;276:449–465.
12. Tarbary JC, Tarbary C, Tardieu C, Tardieu G, Goldspink G. Physiological and structural changes in the cat's soleus muscle due to immobilization at different lengths in plaster casts. J Physiol 1972;224:231–244.
13. Williams PE, Goldspink G. The effect of immobilization on the longitudinal growth of striated muscle fibers. J Anat 1973;116:45–55.
14. Williams PL, Warwick R. Gray's anatomy. 36th ed. Philadelphia: W.B. Saunders Company, 1980.
15. Maitland GD. Peripheral manipulation, 3ed. London: Butterworth-Heinemann, 1991.
16. Kaltenborn F. Mobilization of the Extremity Joints: Examination and Basic Treatment Techniques. 3rd ed Oslo: Olaf Norlis Bokhandel, 1985.
17. Gonyea WJ, Erikson GC. Experimental model for study of exercise induced skeletal muscle hypertrophy. J Appl Physiol 1976;40:L630–633.
18. Gonyea WJ, Bonde-Petersen F. Alterations in muscle contractile properties and fiber composition after weight-lifting exercise in cats. Exp Neurol 1978;59:75–84.
19. Gonyea WJ, Bonde-Petersen F. Electromyographic analysis of two wrist flexor muscles studied during weight-lifting exercise in cats. Biomechanics 1978;6A:207–212.
20. Gollnick PD, Armstrong RB, Saltin B, et al. Effect of training on enzyme and fiber composition of human skeletal muscle. J Appl Physiol 1973;34:107–111.
21. Henriksson J, Reitman JS. Quantitative measures of enzyme activities in type I and type II muscle fibers in man after training. Acta Physiol Scand 1976;97:392–397.
22. DeVries H. Quantitative electromyographic investigation of the spasm theory of muscle pain. Am J Phys Med 1966;45:119–134.
23. DeLorme T, Watkins A. Technics of progressive resistance exercise. Arch Phys Med Rehabil 1948;29:263.
24. Zinowieff AN. Heavy resistance exercise: The Oxford technic. Br J Phys Med 1951;14:129.
25. Knight KL. Knee rehabilitation by the daily adjustable progressive resistive exercise technique. Am J Sports Med 1979;7:336–337.
26. Davies GJ. A compendium of isokinetics in clinical usage: Workshop and clinical notes. La Crosse, WI: S & S Publishers, 1984.
27. Wyke B. Articular neurology—a review. Physiother 1972;58:94–99.
28. DeAvila GA, O'Conner BL, Visco DM, et al. The mechanoreceptor innervation of the human fibular collateral ligament. J Anatomy 1989;162:1–7.
29. Katonis PG, Assimakopoulos AP, Agapitos MV, et al. Mechanoreceptors in the posterior cruciate ligament. Histological study on cadaveric knees. Acta Orthop Scand 1991;62:276–278.
30. Krenn V, Hofmann S, Engel A. First Description of mechanoreceptors in the corpus adiposum infrapatellar of man. Acta Anat 1990;137:187–188.
31. O'Conner BL, McConnaughey JS. The structure and innervation of cat knee menisci and their relation to a 'sensory hypothesis' of meniscal function. Am J. Anat 1978;1533:431–442.
32. Schultz RA, Miller DC, Kerr CS, et al. Mechanoreceptors in human cruciate ligaments: An historical study. J Bone Joint Surg 1984;66A:1972–1076.
33. Tomita Y, Ozaki J, Tamai S: Sensory nerve endings in the subacromial bursa. (Abstr) Acta Ortho Scand. 1992;63 (suppl 247):23.
34. Vangsess CT, Ennis M: Neural anatomy of the human glenoid labrum and shoulder ligaments. Presented at the 59th Annual Meeting of the American Academy of Orthopaedic Surgeons. Washington DC, Feb 24, 1992.
35. Solomonow M, Baraytta R, Zhou BH, Shoji H, Bose W, Beck C, D'Ambrosia R: The synergistic action of the anterior cruciate ligament and thigh muscles in maintaining joint stability. Am J Sports Med, 1987;15:207–213.
36. Barrack RL, Skinner HB, Buckley SL: Proprioception in the anterior cruciate ligament deficient knee. Am J Sports Med 1989;17:1–6.
37. Lephart SM, Kicher MS, Fu FH, Borsa PA, Harner CD: Proprioception following anterior cruciate ligament reconstruction. J Sports Rehab 1992;1:188–196.
38. Smith RL, Brunolli J: Shoulder kinesthesia after anterior glenohumeral joint dislocation. Phys Ther 1989;69(2):106–112.
39. Pappas AM, Zawachi RM, McCarthy CF: Rehabilitation of the pitching shoulder. Am J Sports Med 1985;13:223–235.
40. Blackburn TA, White B, McLeod WD, Wofford L: EMG analysis of posterior rotator cuff exercises. J Natl Ath Train Ass 1990;25–40–45.

7 / MEDICAL PROBLEMS OF THE ATHLETE

Gabe Mirkin

Physicians who treat athletes should know that exercise has profound effects on the body. Laboratory findings, such as hematuria, that are abnormal in sedentary people, may be normal in athletes. Drugs, such as β-blockers, that are regularly prescribed for sedentary people can markedly affect an athlete's ability to exercise. Some conditions, such as exercise-induced asthma, are associated with exercise. Certain diseases, such as diabetes, require special precautions during exercise. The most important aspect of treating athletes is to know how to evaluate and treat their signs and symptoms and advise them accordingly. This chapter walks through, step by step, the thought processes, procedures, laboratory tests, diagnoses, and treatments that are used when physicians treat medical problems in athletes.

Urinary Tract Effects

Exercise-Induced Pseudonephritis

Exercise-related proteinuria and microscopic hematuria that clear within 48 hr of stopping exercise are almost never signs of disease. The first step in evaluating these conditions is to check the urine 48 hr after all exercise is stopped. The vast majority of all cases of benign hematuria and/or proteinuria induced by exercise will clear by then, and virtually all will clear by 72 hr (1). Intravenous pyelography and cystoscopy may be indicated when *(a)* there is visible hematuria, *(b)* the urine is not free of blood or protein 48 hr after the athlete stops exercising, *(c)* an illness is associated with hematuria, and *(d)* the physician, athlete, or parent is concerned enough to want the evaluation.

Benign hematuria occurs in up to 60% of football players (2), 100% of hockey players (3), 73% of boxers (4), and 20% of marathon runners (1). Benign proteinuria has been reported to occur in 62% of adolescent sports physical examinations (5). Dehydration, prolonged exercise, hard body contact, hot weather, and hard pounding of the feet on the road increase an athlete's chances of developing hematuria.

Exercise-induced hematuria can come from the bladder or kidney. During exercise, renal plasma flow is diminished by almost 80%, which can lead to hypoxic damage to the glomeruli (6). Renal plasma flow is reduced even further by dehydration. Red blood cells that pass through glomeruli become dysmorphic, lose hemoglobin, and become misshapened. These changes appear to be caused by the trauma of passing through a glomerulus. Using these criteria, Reid et al. (7) have shown that most of the bleeding from running a marathon comes from the kidneys and most of the bleeding that comes from running shorter distances comes from the bladder. Localized contusions of the bladder are thought to be caused by repeated impacts of the posterior vesical wall against its base: in the interureteral bar extending laterally to each ureter, the posterior rim of the internal meatus, the lower posterior bladder wall, and the trigone (8).

Proteinuria

As mentioned earlier, exercise-induced proteinuria is usually a benign laboratory finding that clears within 48 hr of stopping exercise. It is caused by the following sequence: Exercise markedly reduces renal plasma flow, which markedly reduces glomerular filtration, causing increased glomerular permeability to serum protein.

Myoglobinuria

Conditioning helps protect muscles from releasing myoglobin (9). However, hard exercise, particularly in very hot weather, can cause rhabdomyolysis. The resultant release of small amounts of myoglobin is usually benign and is common in prolonged exercise, such as marathon running, and body-contact sports, such as playing football. No treatment is indicated. When myoglobinuria is associated with severe dehydration, it can cause renal damage (10). This usually occurs only in untrained individuals who undergo severe exertion in hot weather. Myoglobin, by itself, is not toxic. However, it is converted to hematin, which is toxic to renal tubules.

Simple urine tests can be used to differentiate between albuminuria, myoglobinuria, and hemoglobinuria. The dipstick method for protein will pick up only albumin, whereas the heat and sulfosalicylic acid precipitation test picks up all three. Therefore, a weakly positive dipstick for protein and strongly positive sulfosalicylic acid test implies that the urine contains either myoglobin or hemoglobin. A positive dipstick test for red blood cells (Hemastix) and absence of urinary red blood cells usually means that myoglobin is present (Table 7.1).

Hemoglobinuria

Hemoglobinuria is caused by repetitive trauma on the extremities, such as engaging in karate, playing the congo drums (11) and marching (12). The athlete complains of voiding very dark urine after significant hard exercise. The blood will show evidence of intravascular hemolysis with elevated serum hemoglobin and methemalbumin, and decreased serum haptoglobin (13). The urine shows granular casts suggestive of tubular injury. The condition is almost always benign, although acute renal failure has been reported (14).

Hematologic Effects

Blood Loss During Exercise

Athletes lose blood during exercise through intravascular hemolysis, gastrointestinal bleeding and hematuria. Intravascular hemolysis occurs with running and not with cycling, leading to the impression that it is caused by the force of the foot strike during running (15). A significant number of runners have been shown to have gastrointestinal bleeding (16) and hematuria (17). However, these blood losses rarely cause anemia and are usually of little clinical importance. Virtually all cases of guaiac positive stools and hematuria caused by heavy exercise will be clear of blood within 72 hr (1, 18).

Table 7.1.
Clinical States Associated with Myoglobinuria

Trauma with crush injuries
Heat stroke
Severe exercise
Seizures
Decreased muscle energy production (hypokalemia, hypophsphatemia, and genetic enzymatic deficiencies)
Muscle ischemia such as arterial insufficiency
Infections, such as Legionnaires disease
Toxins, such as alcohol and carbon monoxide
Polymyositis
Malignancy

Pseudoanemia

The vast majority of athletic-associated anemia is caused by a relative dilutional effect and is beneficial, because it allows the athlete to start competition with a larger blood volume and increased amounts of fluid. It is common for athletes to increase their blood volume by 10% within a few weeks of training (19), and one study demonstrated that trained athletes have a 20% higher plasma volume and hemoglobin (20). There are no known deleterious effects from this dilutional anemia as it is accompanied by an increase in red cell mass (21).

Blood Doping

Decreasing red blood cell concentration limits performance and increasing it improves performance. Exercise capacity is determined by oxygen uptake, which depends on the ability to move oxygen from the mouth (and nose) into the lungs (ventilation), from the lungs into the bloodstream (diffusion), from the blood in the lungs to the blood in the muscles (perfusion), and from blood into muscle cells. The limiting reaction, perfusion, depends on the strength of the heart to pump blood through the body and the ability of the blood to carry oxygen (22). Athletes can increase heart strength through intense training. The only way that they can increase the oxygen-carrying capacity of the blood is to increase the concentration of red blood cells. The gain of increased oxygen-carrying capacity is greater than the loss from the increased vascular resistance caused by increased viscosity (23). Blood doping appears to improve performance in athletic events requiring endurance (24). As far as the author knows, there are no reported deaths from autologous blood doping, although there are reports of U.S. Olympic team members getting hepatitis from heterologous transfusions. It was reported that 12 young, apparently healthy Dutch cyclists died, presumably because they had been given erythropoietin (EPO) to increase red blood cell cells (25). Administration of EPO can raise hematocrit to high levels and cause pulmonary embolism clots, myocardial infarction, and seizures with encephalopathy. The International Olympic Committee and the U.S. Olympic Committee have banned blood doping.

No Anemia, Decreased Ferritin

Athletes can be iron deficient, even though they are not anemic. More than 50% of the iron in the body is located in the iron reserves, such as the spleen, liver, bone marrow, lymph nodes, and other tissues. People do not become anemic from iron deficiency until the iron stores are depleted. Previous studies showed that iron deficiency, even without anemia, reduces endurance by lowering concentrations of muscle α-glycerol phosphate oxidase; this impairs glycolysis and leads to accumulation of lactic acid in muscles and blood (26). However, more recent studies show that iron deficiency does not impair endurance unless it also causes anemia.

True Anemias

True anemia can impair performance severely, so all cases of anemia must be evaluated, at the very least, with a complete blood count, reticulocyte count, and ferritin. Anemias can be caused by decreased output by the bone marrow, hemolysis, and blood loss.

A normal or elevated reticulocyte count means that the bone marrow is making red blood cells. As with nonathletes, anemias in athletes are classified into hypochromic and microcytic, normochromic and normocytic, and megaloblastic and normochromic.

Hypochromic, Microcytic Anemia

Almost all cases of hypochromic, microcytic anemia in athletes will be caused by iron deficiency or thalassemia. Less frequent causes include anemia of chronic inflammation and sideroblastic anemia.

A low serum ferritin level will almost always clinch a diagnosis of iron deficiency. The most dependable method to measure iron reserves is to examine stained bone-marrow sediment under a microscope. However, this procedure is painful and invasive, so serum ferritin levels are usually used to measure iron reserves. A low ferritin level is diagnostic of iron deficiency, but caution must be used in interpreting a normal or high level. In cases of extensive tissue damage, ferritin is released from the reticuloendothelial system into the bloodstream, raising blood levels. Thus regular intense exercise, acute infection, inflammation, liver disease, or malignancy can raise serum ferritin levels even though iron deficiency may be present. Therefore, ferritin levels may be elevated without iron overload, and normal in iron deficiency. If iron deficiency is suspected in the face of normal ferritin levels, repeat the test after athletes have not exercised for 3 days and after recovery, if they have an infection (27).

That diagnosis can be further confirmed if the serum iron is low and the iron binding capacity is elevated. A bone marrow aspirate lacking iron clinches the diagnosis of iron deficiency. In athletes, the most common causes of true anemia are iron deficiency from inadequate intake or excessive uterine or gastrointestinal bleeding.

Vegetarians are at increased risk for iron deficiency. Women who are iron deficient are likely to suffer from excessive menstrual bleeding. Men who are iron deficient are most likely to suffer from gastrointestinal bleeding.

Up to 25% of college women are iron deficient, even though fewer than 10% are anemic (28). Women who are anemic from iron deficiency and have a history of irregular periods or excessive menstrual bleeding should be referred to a gynecologist. Those with regular periods of normal flow need dietary instruction and iron supplementation. They should be encouraged to eat meat, fish, and chicken and be given 300 mg of ferrous sulfate once a day in a pill for at least 1 year. Iron deficiency is corrected slowly because high doses of iron can cause severe constipation or diarrhea.

Red blood cells from thalassemia patients usually demonstrate marked microcytosis and basophilic stippling and many are target cells. In contrast to iron deficiency, the hemoglobin A_2 is usually elevated in α-thalassemia, although it may be normal in β-thalassemia. Coexisting iron deficiency can mask the elevation of hemoglobin A_2 in β-thalassemia.

The anemia of chronic diseases, such as rheumatoid arthritis, is characterized by a low transferrin level, a low serum iron and total iron binding capacity, elevated ferritin and protoporphyrin, and normal hemoglobin A_2.

Sideroblastic anemia is diagnosed by the demonstration of ringed sideroblasts in the bone marrow. It can be genetic and can respond to pyridoxine, can be associated with drugs or tumors, or can be idiopathic (Table 7.2).

Normochromic, Normocytic Anemia

In athletes, the causes of normochromic, normocytic anemia are decreased production, hemolysis, and bleeding. Athletes with low reticulocyte counts and normal or high ferritin have bone marrows that are not producing red blood cells, even though they have adequate iron stores. They should be referred to a hematologist for evaluation. Those who have low reticulocyte counts and low ferritin should be treated with iron supplements. If their reticulocyte counts increase, they should be treated for iron deficiency as described above. If reticulocyte counts do not return to normal within 2 weeks, they should be referred to a hematologist.

Macrocytic, Normochromic Anemias

The megaloblastic anemias are caused by lack of vitamin B_{12} or folic acid, genetic disorders, and drug poisoning of DNA. Any neuropathy can be caused by lack of vitamin B_{12}. Blood tests for these vitamins should always be considered for the evaluation of unexplained pain, loss of sensation, or muscle disorder. If pernicious anemia is strongly suspected, a radioactive Schill-

Table 7.2.
Differential Diagnosis of Hypochromic, Microcytic Anemia

Test	Iron Deficiency	β-thalassemia	Chronic Disease	Sideroblastic Anemia
Serum iron	down	normal	down	up
Total iron binding capacity (TIBC)	up	normal	down	normal
Serum ferritin	down	normal	up	up
Red cell protoporphyrin	up	normal	up	up or normal
Hemoglobin A_2	down	up	normal	down

From Schafer AI, Bunn HF. Anemias of iron deficiency and iron overload. In: Braunwald E, Isselbacher KJ, Petersdorf RG, et al., eds. Harrison's principles of internal medicine. New York: McGraw-Hill, 1988:1420.

ing test should be given to prove decreased vitamin B_{12} absorption. Recent data show that pernicious anemia can be treated with daily 1000 mg vitamin B_{12} pills (29).

Sickle-Cell Disease

Sickle-cell disease limits exercise performance, primarily because of the anemia it causes. The degree of impairment is inversely proportional to the concentration of normal hemoglobin (30). Athletes who have sickle-cell trait appear to perform as well as people who have normal hemoglobin (31). Sickle-cell trait appears to restrict exercise only under conditions of infections, severe oxygen deprivation, and severe dehydration. Examples include exercising at high altitudes, swimming underwater, being in unpressurized airplanes, exercising for hours in hot weather, and exercising after drinking alcohol. People with sickle-cell trait may form clots when they suffer severe oxygen deprivation. Then, in these unusual situations, they can suffer splenic, renal, or heart muscle damage.

Liver Effects

Pseudohepatitis

Abnormal liver function tests are common in endurance athletes (32). During vigorous exercise, muscles are damaged and release intracellular enzymes into blood. Surprisingly, liver cells also release lesser amounts of their enzymes (33). The harder and more sustained the exercise, the greater the rise in serum enzymes (34). A marked elevation in serum enzymes indicates significant muscle damage from exercise and should serve as a warning signal for the athlete to rest, hydrate, and replace glycogen reserves.

Virtually all cases of exercise-elevated enzymes will return to normal within 3 days of cessation of exercise. If the athlete with elevated liver enzymes refuses or is unable to stop exercising, the physician can measure tissue-specific enzymes. Lactate dehydrogenase (LDH) and serum glutamic-oxaloacetic transaminase (SGOT) are found in both myocytes and hepatocytes. Serum glutamic-pyruvic transaminase (SGPT) and serum gamma glutamic transpeptidase (GGTP) are found only in hepatocytes. Creatine kinase (CK) is found in muscle and not in liver cells. For example, markedly elevated LDH, CK and SGOT associated with a normal or slightly elevated SGPT and GGTP should lead to a diagnosis of athletic pseudohepatitis. In that case, the only treatment is rest, hydration, and a carbohydrate-rich diet.

Jaundice with Normal Liver Enzymes

Screening physicals often detect athletes with elevated bilirubin levels and normal liver enzymes (27). These athletes often will give a history of left upper quadrant pain with extreme exertion. They should be checked for hemolytic anemia. If there is no evidence of hemolysis, they probably have Gilbert's syndrome, caused by a partial deficiency of glucuronyl transferase.

Starting in their third decade, 3% to 5% of healthy young adults develop elevated serum bilirubin levels with normal liver enzymes. Most of the bilirubin is unconjugated, with levels fluctuating between 1.2 and 3 mg/dl and rarely exceeding 5 mg/dl. Blood levels of bilirubin rise with fasting, surgery, fever, infections, alcohol ingestion, and exercise. When patients with this condition are placed on a diet containing 300 cals/day for 2 days, their bilirubin will increase by at least 1.5 mg/dl. Administration of 15 mg of phenobarbital three times a day will enhance glucuronyl transferase function and will usually return bilirubin levels temporarily to normal. No treatment is indicated for this condition, although a low-fat diet can reduce serum bilirubin levels.

Liver Disease

A diagnosis of hepatitis mandates a thorough search for the cause. In young, previously healthy athletes, ask about alcohol and drugs. Order blood tests for infectious diseases, such as mononucleosis, hepatitis A virus antigen, hepatitis B surface antigen, hepatitis C antibody, VDRL, HIV, cytomegalovirus IgM antibody, toxoplasmosis IgM antibody, and herpes antibody. Active hepatitis B and C can be treated with daily interferon injections.

The hepatitis-causing drugs that are used most frequently by athletes are anabolic steroids and cocaine. Other drugs that have been reported to cause hepatitis include blood pressure medicines (α-methyldopa), aspirin, acetaminophen, allopurinol, isoniazid, and antibiotics (sulfonamide and nitrofurantoin). Far less frequent causes include autoimmune diseases, Wilson's disease, and α-1-antitrypsin deficiency.

If no drug or infectious etiology is found, a CT scan is then ordered. If that is normal, it is up to the discretion of the physician whether a liver biopsy should be done. It is common for all of these tests to be normal and a diagnosis of "fatty liver" to be made.

Exercise for People with Liver Disease

Considerable disagreement exists whether people with hepatitis can exercise safely. Chalmers et al. (35) showed that patients with hepatitis improved as rapidly with ambulation as those who were put at strict bedrest. Exercise caused patients with bilirubin greater than 3 to have relapses, while it did not adversely affect those whose bilirubin was below 3 (36). Vigorous exercise after cessation of acute symptoms did not delay recovery in young, previously healthy army recruits (37). However, vigorous exercise during the preicteric state has led to fulminant disease and death (38).

Lorber (39) recommends that during hepatitis, there is no need for absolute bed rest, but vigorous exercise should be avoided, and that once the bilirubin is below 1.5, the athlete can resume light exercise. Patients with mononucleosis should not be allowed to participate in vigorous exercise until their spleen and liver have returned to normal size, usually in more than 4 weeks. Sometimes radiologic proof may be necessary to demonstrate this.

The Side Stitch During Exercise

Most previous explanations for the cause of pain behind the bottom right front ribs during hard exercise have been flawed. Lack of oxygen to the diaphragm is not plausible because the blood supply to the diaphragm is not shut off by running. Gas in the colon is not plausible because most people do not pass gas after the pain goes away.

The most reasonable explanation depends on the fact that the liver is held in place by ligaments that attach to the diaphragm. Humans have a fixed pattern of breathing during running. They breathe once for each two strides. They breathe out when one foot (80% of the time it's the right), strikes the ground. Breathing out causes the diaphragm to go up at the same time that the force of the footstrike causes the liver to drop down, stretching the hepatodiaphragmatic ligaments and causing pain.

The treatment for a side stitch is to stop running and use the hands to press the liver up against the diaphragm. Prevention involves doing situps to strengthen the abdominal muscles and running very fast in practice to strengthen the hepatodiaphragmatic ligaments.

Gastrointestinal Tract Effects

Runner's Diarrhea

One out of every four runners has suffered from cramps and diarrhea during competition, and one out of every three has had urgent bowel movements during a run (40). These symptoms are probably caused by exercise-induced giant contractions of the colon (41), rather than any effect it may have on the small intestine. Exercise does not accelerate food passage through the small intestine (42). Furthermore, exercise does not affect the absorption of food in the small intestine (44).

Most studies do not demonstrate that exercise accelerates transit time. For example, using first appearance of breath hydrogen, Keeling and Martin (45) showed that transit time to the colon is sped up by exercise: 44 min during fast walking, compared with 66 min during rest. Using ^{99m}Tc-labeled particles, Ollenshaw et al. (46) showed that transit time to the colon was not affected by exercise, 4.5, 5.4, and 4.1 hr for minimal, moderate and strenuous activity. Using breath hydrogen, Meshkinpour et al. (47) showed that exercise slows transit time, 55 min for resting and 89 min for exercise.

The key to treatment is to accelerate the transit of food through the small intestine by eating large amounts of food on the night before and morning of competition and to make sure that the colon is empty at the time of competition (Table 7.3). If this regimen does not alleviate symptoms, a 7-day trial of avoidance of all foods that contain dairy products may be attempted. Other foods for avoidance trials include those that contain caffeine (48) and those that contain gluten. If symptoms continue, 10 grains of aspirin before exercise should be tried. If that is ineffective, an evaluation by a gastroenterologist is indicated. The workup may include colonoscopy, stool cultures, breath hydrogen collection after food challenges, and a check for ova and parasites.

Table 7.3.
Strategy for Runners Who Develop Running-Associated Diarrhea

1. Eat a large meal that is rich in fiber on the night before competition (to speed up transit time).
2. Eat a large meal 5 hr before race time.
3. Continue to try to defecate up to immediately before race time.

Heart and Blood Pressure Effects

Pseudomyocarditis

In 1899, S.E. Henschen, professor of medicine at the University of Upsala, published the first report of the athletic heart in long-distance cross-country skiers. Carl von Rokitansky of Vienna had shown 50 years earlier that a large heart was a sign of disease (49). Its stretched ventricles had outgrown their meager blood supply. Even to this day, some people still think that exercise will harm the heart because they do not understand that there is a great difference between the strong heart of exercise and the weak one of heart failure. As an example of the dangers of exercise, they rarely cite Rokitansky, but they often cite the case of Phidippides, who, in 490 B.C., died in the Athens market after running through the plains of Marathon to bring news of the defeat of the Persians.

Endurance athletes often have chronic serum elevations in creatine kinase, and transient elevations in the muscle and brain isoenzymes of the heart-specific fraction of creatinine kinase (50). These findings could lead to a mistaken diagnosis of cardiomyopathy or coronary artery disease. In healthy endurance athletes who have no symptoms attributable to myocardial disease, these findings are probably caused by exercise-induced injury to skeletal muscle.

Exercise also can cause ECG changes that could be interpreted as abnormal in nonexercising individuals. This topic is covered in Chapter 8.

Blood Pressure

Athletes who have high blood pressure, but no target organ damage, should be allowed to compete in aerobic sports (51). However, there is inadequate information to show whether the extraordinary rise in blood pressure that accompanies strength training and strength competition can harm athletes. The blood pressure rise that is induced by lifting heavy weights is exaggerated in people who have hypertension (52). However, regular strength training can reduce the degree of rise in blood pressure (53).

Regular exercisers have lower systolic and diastolic blood pressures than sedentary people do (54). After starting an exercise program, normotensive people usually do not experience a reduction in blood pressure (55), but hypertensive individuals do (59). Therefore, the nonpharmacologic treatments for hypertension should include exercise in addition to weight reduction, low-fat diet, and the avoidance of stimulants.

Nonetheless, many people who exercise regularly still need to take medications to control their hypertension (Tables 7.4–7.7). The ideal medication should not limit their ability to exercise. Chick et al. (56) recommend that the ideal antihypertensive drug for exercisers should *not*

1. Depress myocardium during exercise.
2. Cause arrhythmias.
3. Decrease blood flow to exercising skeletal muscles.
4. Interfere with substrate use by muscle.

β-blockers and the calcium channel blocker verapamil impair left ventricular function during exercise. For example, the β-blocker propranolol at a dose of 240 mg/day limits the increase of $\dot{V}_{O_2max}$ normally associated with training (58). Nifedipine and diltiazem are far less likely to do this. Virtually all the other antihypertensives do not depress the myocardium. Neither β-blockers nor calcium channel blockers limit strength gains associated with weight training. β-blockers can help athletes in sports that require slow movements and great concentration, such as pistol shooting.

Diuretics decrease endurance by causing hypovolemia. They also can cause hypokalemia and hypomagnesemia, which increase susceptibility for arrhythmias.

There are little data to show whether antihypertensives reduce skeletal muscle perfusion or interfere with substrate usage by muscle, but all calcium channel blockers, all angiotensin-converting enzyme (ACE) inhibitors, clonidine, methyldopa, and prazosin have not been shown to restrict exercise performance (59). Furthermore, ACE inhibitors can reduce postexercise proteinuria, whereas β-blockers (acetobutolol), α-1-blockers (prazosin), and a nonsteroidal antiinflammatory (indomethacin) do not (60).

The following recommendations for the use of β-blockers are modified from those of Gordon and Duncan (61).

1. Because β-blockers can limit training and improvement in $\dot{V}_{O_2max}$, they should be prescribed with reservation to athletes who compete in sports that require endurance.
2. Because there are many drugs that will control hypertension and not cause fatigue and limitation in $\dot{V}_{O_2max}$, β-blockers should rarely be prescribed to treat hypertension in exercisers.
3. Because blockers offer some advantages over other drugs in the treatment of patients with coronary artery disease, they can be prescribed to these patients. However only β-1 selective blockers should be used.
4. Because exercise can offset the rise in low-density lipoprotein (LDL) cholesterol associated with taking β-blockers, most patients on β-blockers should be encouraged to exercise.
5. Because nonselective β-blockers increase susceptibility to hyperthermia, all patients on β-blockers should be cautioned about that complication during exercise, particularly in hot weather.
6. Because β-blockers slow heart rate and increase perceived exertion, most exercisers taking β-blockers should have special counseling regarding their exercise prescriptions based on exercise tests done while they are on medication.

Varicose Veins

The saphenous venous system delivers blood from the subcutaneous venous system to the deep veins under the muscles for transmission back to the vena cava.

Table 7.4.
Antihypertensive Drugs Not Recommended for Competitive Athletes in Endurance Sports

Verapamil
All β-blockers
All diuretics

Table 7.5.
Antihypertensives That Allow a Normal Cardiovascular Response

Captopril (and other ACE inhibitors)
Clonidine
Calcium channel blockers (except verapamil)
Guanabenz acetate
Methyldopa
Prazosin

Table 7.6.
Antihypertensives That May Interfere with Sexual Function

Prazosin	Rare cases of priapism
Phenoxybenzamine	Failure of ejaculation
Spironolactone	Gynecomastia in males, breast enlargement in females, occasional impotence
Methyldopa	Impotence, reduced libido, ejaculatory failure
Guanethidine	Ejaculatory failure, 50% impotence
Thiazide-type diuretics	Occasional impotence
Clonidine	Rare impotence, delayed ejaculation, gynecomastia
β-blockers	Occasional impotence
Captopril	Impotence
Guanethidine	Impotence
Guanabenz acetate	Impotence

Table 7.7.
Antihypertensive Medication and Lipids

Thiazide-type diuretics	Increases total cholesterol, LDL cholesterol, and triglycerides
β-blockers	Increases triglycerides and lowers HDL cholesterol
Spironolactone	Raises LDL cholesterol
α-blocker, prazosin	Lowers cholesterol
α-agonist, guanabenz acetate	Lowers cholesterol

Normally, bicuspid valves inside veins direct blood in one direction only from sistal to proximal and superficial to deep. When these valves become incompetent and allow blood to back up, the veins enlarge and become tortuous. Varicose veins are subcutaneous veins that have enlarged enough to be visible or symptomatic (62).

A sustained increase in intraabdominal pressure, retrograde blood flow or hydrostatic pressure will cause genetically susceptible people to develop varicose veins. So can direct trauma to a valve. Pregnancy, coughing, and standing enlarge varicose veins, while running and walking tend to be part of the treatment. Pregnancy and coughing increase intraabdominal pressure; standing increases hydrostatic pressure. Secondary varicosities can be caused by thromboses or or other obstructions in the veins underneath muscles.

Varicosities of the superficial veins rarely increase a person's chances of developing deep-vein thromboses (63) and are usually more a cosmetic and comfort problem than a danger to life. However, people who have superficial vein incompetence may be more likely to have valvular incompetence in the deep veins. When thrombophlebitis occurs, it is usually caused by trauma.

Usually varicosities do not cause symptoms. However, with prolonged standing, people who have varicosities complain of a feeling of heaviness and aching in their legs.

The treatment is aimed at reducing hydrostatic pressure. Support hose with ankle compression up to 30 mm Hg are helpful (64). Elevating the legs is beneficial. Running and walking decrease hydrostatic pressure because the pressure of pumping leg muscles is far greater than the increased resistance of intraabdominal pressure. So exercise can be part of treatment provided that it does not involve standing around for a long periods of time. Surgery is indicated only when symptoms become unbearable to the patient. Injections can help to eradicate varicosities in small superficial veins, but are of little value in larger ones. Excision of larger veins is not an indication to restrict vigorous exercise afterward.

Lung Effects

Respiratory Infections and the Common Cold

How Exercise Affects Immunity

There is no evidence that a regular exercise program helps prevent upper respiratory infections, although there are studies that show that hard exercise can both depress and increase some humoral factors of immunity (65–67). Other studies show no effect whatever on immune parameters (68). There is weak evidence that a single intense competition increases susceptibility to infection and that it may depress some parameters of immunity. There is some evidence that overtraining can increase a person's chances for infection.

Seriously training children had the same incidence of upper respiratory infections as their sedentary classmates (69). Athletic training does not affect the number of days absent from school (70). The incidence of tuberculosis was the same in trained and sedentary individuals (71). Furthermore, exposure to cold weather does not increase a person's susceptibility to colds on exposure to rhinovirus (72).

Runners who trained by running more than 15 miles/week suffered more frequent respiratory infections than those training fewer than 15 miles (73). Ultramarathon runners have increased incidence of upper respiratory infections in the 2-week period after competition (74). No data are available to show why this happens.

Okay to Exercise?

It is probably all right for athletes to continue training when they have upper respiratory infections, provided that their muscles do not hurt, they do not have a fever, and they do not feel very sick. However, each case should be decided on its own merits.

Forced swimming markedly increased myocardial damage in mice infected with coxsackievirus B3. Both fever and exercise markedly increase cardiac output. The combination of increased workload and viral myocarditis can cause a fatal arrhythmia (75). Exercising with painful muscles markedly increases susceptibility to injury. Infected muscles have reduced strength (76) and endurance (77), and glycolytic enzyme levels (78).

Prevention and Treatment

The cold virus is spread through the air and by the hands (79). One study showed that medical students increased their susceptibility to colds through rubbing their eyes (80). Therefore, virucidal hand washes and attempts to avoid nose picking and eye wiping can help to prevent colds.

The most effective treatment for the common cold is to warm and liquefy mucus. Indeed, warm chicken soup was found to increase the rate of mucus clearing and decrease nasal obstruction more effectively than warm or cold water (81). This led Rosner to respond that Maimonides was the first author to recommend what is now known as *bohbymycetin*, a term based on the Yiddish word for grandmother (82). Humidifiers and increased ingestion of fluids are also effective liquefiers. When the mucus turns thick and discolored, antibiotics may be of some benefit. Viruses depress granulocyte counts and increase susceptibility to secondary bacterial infections. Large doses of vitamin C, antihistamines, and decongestants have not been shown to prevent or reduce duration of the common cold (Table 7.8).

Exercise-Induced Asthma

The triad of exercise-induced coughing, shortness of breath, and wheezing does not comprise a specific dis-

Table 7.8.
Treatment of the Common Cold

1. Wash hands frequently (to prevent spread to others).
2. Drink fluids frequently.
3. Use humidification during the winter.
4. Take antibiotics when mucus is thick and discolored.

ease, any more than dust-induced asthma does. The asthmatic response caused by exercise is exactly the same as that caused by exposure to allergens, but no allergen is involved. All people who wheeze with exercise will wheeze with other stimuli, even though some think that exercise is the sole cause. When asthmatics exercise, the vast majority (even those who do not recognize symptoms) will have pulmonary functions demonstrating increased residual volume and many will have a decreased 1-sec forced-expiratory volume (83).

Exercise-induced asthma (EIA) affects 15% of the general population, 40% of people who have allergic rhinitis, and 80% of asthmatics (84). It is not caused just by exercise (85). Breathing hard and fast dries and cools the bronchial mucosa, which causes a rapid expansion of blood in the vascular plexi. This causes reactive hyperemia and edema within the airway wall (86). It can be caused by voluntary hyperventilation when the patient sits in one place, by rapid intravenous infusion of saline and by rapid exercise of the leg muscles pumping increased amounts of blood to the lungs. The most potent stimulus comes when the inspired air is cold and dry. That is why running is a much greater stimulus for EIA than cycling, which is a stronger stimulus than swimming, and exercising in a heated indoor facility in the winter often causes EIA.

When an asthmatic starts to breathe deeply and rapidly, there is progressive cooling of the bronchial mucosa. This gradually increases bronchospasm. The patient often does not notice the onset of symptoms until the bronchospasm reaches a peak at 6 to 12 min. If the athlete can persevere and is in good enough shape to continue exercising, the bronchospasm will gradually disappear during exercise. On the other hand, if the athlete stops when he or she first starts to wheeze, the coughing will often go on for hours.

Exercise can precipitate severe attacks in all people who have asthma, but there is no evidence that exercise per se is harmful. Asthmatics should be encouraged to exercise and compete in sports, provided that they are taught how to prevent and treat symptoms when they arise (Table 7.9).

However, asthmatics should not dive in deep water. Asthma attacks can and do occur under water. In the event of an attack while deep diving, failure to reach the surface quickly enough can cause severe hypoxia; coming up too rapidly can cause the bends.

A single attack of exercise-induced asthma can desensitize bronchial hyperactivity for up to 90 min (87). Therefore, 15 to 45 min before a competition, asthmatic athletes should gradually warm up to the point at which they are moving almost at race pace and are breathing hard and fast. Because EIA is caused by breathing dry and cold air, athletes can warm the air they breathe by inhaling air through a tube wrapped around and heated by their bodies. Such tubes are available, but are impractical for competition.

Exercise-induced asthma is just another form of asthma. Asthma is defined as inflammation of the mucosa causing obstruction of the bronchial tubes. Corticosteroids and cromolyn are the only asthma drugs that reduce inflammation, and "corticosteroids are the most effective anti-inflammatory drugs for the treatment of reversible-airflow obstruction" (88). Therefore, asthmatic athletes who have significant symptoms in the weeks before major competitions can be placed on systemic glucocorticoids until they clear and then be maintained on inhaled steroids until after competition. Isolated inhalations of glucocorticoids just before competition are ineffective in preventing EIA (Table 7.10).

All infections can precipitate and exacerbate asthmatic symptoms. It is extremely important to treat infections that occur 1 or 2 weeks before competition in asthmatic athletes. When asthmatic athletes present at that time with discolored respiratory mucus, sore throat, or fever, the author often takes nasal or throat cultures and prescribes an antibiotic.

Several medications can be taken before competition. Inhalation of a beta-2-adrenergic bronchodilator, such as terbutaline, salbutamol, or albuterol, immediately before competition can prevent EIA. These drugs do not improve performance in nonasthmatics, so they offer no ergogenic boost and should continue to be permitted in international competition (Table 7.11). Inhal-

Table 7.9.
Recommendations for Athletes with Asthma

1. Chose sports with short bursts (tennis and football), rather than continuous movement (cross-country skiing and long-distance running).
2. Chose sports that allow you to breathe moist warm air (swimming).
3. Try to compete in situations in which you can breathe warm moist air.
4. Warm up intensely before competition (a significant refractory period lasts up to 90 min).
5. Use medication as directed by your physician.

Table 7.10.
Drugs to Prevent Exercise Induced Asthma

Before Competition
- Albuterol, salbutamol, or terbutaline inhaler (2 sprays immediately before competition)
- Cromolyn inhaler 30 min before competition

If the Athlete Has Had Significant Asthma for the Weeks Leading Up to Competition
- Prednisone, 15 mg morning and 10 mg afternoon for 7 days or until clear, whichever comes first
- Athlete should then use a steroid inhaler (2 sprays, 4 times a day)
- If that does not control asthma, the athlete can take up to 4 sprays, 4 times a day

Table 7.11.
Antiasthmatic Medications Approved by the International Olympic Committee

Oral theophylline
Inhaled cromolyn
Inhaled and oral albuterol
Inhaled and oral terbutaline
Inhaled and oral corticosteroids

ing sodium cromolyn 30 min before competition will also prevent EIA but is less effective than inhaling β-2-adrenergics (90). Oral theophylline is far less effective than either β-2-adrenergics or cromolyn. Furthermore, therapeutic doses cause gastrointestinal upset, nausea, and headache.

Exercise for People Who Have Chronic Pulmonary Diseases

The degree of obstruction of oxygen transport into the bloodstream usually reflects the amount of disease and limitation of exercise. A regular, controlled program of supervised exercise can help to improve the quality of life for people with chronic pulmonary disease (COPD) (91). Exercise tolerance can be increased by exercise with medication and supplemental oxygen for those who become hypoxemic while breathing room air. Exercising on consecutive days increases muscle injury significantly, so people with COPD should not try to exercise more often than every other day. They should stop exercising when they experience increasing dyspnea.

Skin and Soft Tissue Effects

Exercise-Induced Anaphylaxis

Pruritus, urticaria, and angioedema that occur during and after exercising can be caused by an increase in body temperature (cholinergic urticaria); ingestion, inhalation, or contact with food, pollen, or other antigens (allergy), an irritant touching the skin (contact dermatitis); or no known cause (exercise-associated anaphylaxis) (92). Urticaria associated with exercise appears to be no different from urticaria caused by other factors. It occurs frequently in people who have a personal or family history of atopic dermatitis, rhinitis, asthma, and sinusitis (93) and is associated with a rise in whole blood histamine levels and an increase in circulating basophils (94, 95). One attack can lead to a relative refractory period for 24 hr.

Some authors have suggested that food eaten within 24 hr of exercise can trigger urticaria (96). However, the author has never seen a case of food-associated urticaria in which the patient did not also have urticaria or pruritus after eating the food at least once when he or she did not exercise. Pruritus can be induced by exercise when sweat activates an irritating chemical on the skin. Aspirin is the most common drug to cause this condition.

A workup can include evaluating patients for hidden infection, tumor, or collagen disease; exposing them to a warm bath or shower; asking them to exercise after fasting for 6 hr and testing them for allergies. If itching occurs without urticaria, ask the patient to change his or her body and laundry soaps. If that does not help, patch test the patient to a small piece of the clothes that touch his or her skin when the reaction occurs.

Usually, the medical evaluation is normal. Those who develop urticaria after a warm shower or bath have cholinergic urticaria (93). Those who do not develop urticaria after 6 hr of fasting usually do not have food allergy. Wheat is the most common reported food allergen (97, 96). Skin tests for food are of limited value because they are often negative, even when a food is the cause (98). Skin tests for pollens may be of value if the symptoms occur when specific pollens are in the air.

Table 7.12.
Medication Used to Treat Exercise-Induced Anaphylaxis

To Prevent an Attack
Benadryl, 50 mg
Hydroxazine, 50 mg
Cyproheptadine, 4 mg (do not use in hypertension or cardiovascular disease)
To Treat an Attack
Benadryl, 50 mg
To Treat Hypotension, Massive Facial Edema, and Shortness of Breath
Dexamethasone, 8 mg i.m. or i.v.
Aqueous adrenalin, 1/1000 dilution 0.3 ml i.m.
If shock, dopamine, 400 mg in 500 ml of W5W i.v. fluids

Symptoms can be reduced by taking antihistamines before exercise (99) of which ketotitin may be the most effective (100), exercising intensely repeatedly (101), avoiding exercise during pollen season when indicated; avoiding aspirin and certain foods when indicated (102), and taking cromoglycate by inhalation, which is more effective than by mouth (103).

An acute attack in which there is significant swelling of the respiratory tract or face, or hypotension, should be treated with an intramuscular injection of 8 mg (22 ml) dexamethasone. If indicated, 0.3 ml of 1/1000 dilution of aqueous adrenalin may be given. However, giving adrenalin without also giving a corticosteroid often does not stop the reaction. Hypotension can be treated with intravenous dopamine diluted in 500 ml of D5W (5% glucose solution) fluids (Table 7.12).

Neurologic Effects

Exercise-Induced Headaches

Exercise-associated headaches are common, although the exact incidence is unknown. They can be caused by great effort or trauma. A detailed discussion will be found in Chapter 45.

Diabetes Effects

Diabetics cannot be given a blank prescription for exercise, because intense muscular activity can either raise or lower blood sugar levels (Table 7.13). Exercise can be harmful when blood glucose levels are uncontrolled. When glucose exceeds 300 mg/dl and plasma ketones exceed 2 mmoles/liter, exercise raises blood sugar levels further. The resultant rise in catecholamines and growth hormone (104) increases glucogenesis and ketogenesis (105).

Exercise is healthful when blood sugar levels are controlled. Exercise usually markedly increases glucose use by muscles and blood sugar levels are lowered (105). Hypoglycemia is the main concern during exercise in diabetics who have received a subcutaneous injection

Table 7.13.
Cautions for Insulin-Dependent Diabetics

1. Commit to a regular exercise program. Irregular exercise can cause either high or low blood sugar levels.
2. Do not exercise when your blood sugar is above 300 mg/dl or when ketones are present in your blood or urine. You must correct these abnormalities first.
3. Always eat within 2 hr of exercising. Failure to do so can cause low blood sugar levels.
4. Always have food available during exercise. You can suffer from low blood sugar levels at any time.
5. If you have had a previous episode of low blood sugar, eat just before you exercise.
6. On days when you exercise, do not inject insulin into an area over a muscle that will be exercised heavily. This can cause low blood sugar levels.

Table 7.14.
Nonsteroidal Antiinflammatory Drugs

Salicylates
- Aspirin, 325–975 mg q. 4h. p.r.n. up to 4 mg per day
- Magnesium trisalicylate, 750–1000 mg q. 12h. p.r.n.
- Diflunisal, 500 mg q. 12h. p.r.n.
- Salsalate, 1000–1500 mg q. 12h. p.r.n.

Acetic Acids
- Diclofenac, 75–150 mg q. 8h. p.r.n.
- Flenac, 200–600 mg q. 8h. p.r.n.
- Tolmetin, 400–1200 mg q. 8h. p.r.n.

Anthranilic Acids (Fenemates)
- Meclofenamate, 50–100 mg q. 8h. p.r.n.
- Mefenamic acid, 250–q. 6h. p.r.n.

Indole/Indene Acetic Acids
- Sulindac 150–300 mg q. 12h. p.r.n.
- Indomethacin, 25 mg t.i.d. p.r.n. up to 150 mg per day

Propionic Acids
- Carpofen, 100–150 mg q. 12h. p.r.n.
- Fenoprofen, 200–600 mg q. 6h. p.r.n.
- Flurbiprofen, 150–300 mg q. 12h. p.r.n.
- Ibuprofen, 200–800 mg q. 6h. p.r.n. up to 3.2 mg per day.
- Ketoprofen, 50–100 mg q. 8h. p.r.n.
- Naproxen, 250–375 q. 12h. p.r.n.

Oxicams
- Piroxicam, 20 mg per day (caution: photosensitivity)

Pyrazolidinediones
- Phenylbutazone, 50–100 mg q. 8h. p.r.n.

Quinazolinones
- Proquazone, 200–300 mg q. 8h. p.r.n.

Pyranocarboxylic Acids
- Etodolac, 200–400 mg q. 8h. p.r.n.

From Knoben JE, Anderson PO, eds. Handbook of clinical drug data. Hamilton, IL: Drug Intelligence, 1988.

of insulin. Exercising the area that contains the injected insulin can cause high blood insulin levels, which prevent gluconeogenesis and increase glucose use. Diabetics who are treated with continuous infusions of insulin do not suffer from hypoglycemia (106). Hypoglycemia can occur up to 48 hr after exercise and is caused by increased muscle sensitivity to insulin. All exercising insulin-dependent diabetics require tight dietary and insulin control because exercise alone will not control their diabetes. Exercise increases muscle sensitivity, but not liver sensitivity, to insulin.

Muscles

Chronic Aches and Pains

Training for competitive sports requires repeated stresses and recoveries. Optimum training programs include training at the maximum stress that can be applied without causing injury, then applying a stress of that magnitude again only after the athlete has recovered. Delayed muscle soreness serves as the best available guide to maximize training and avoid injury. Athletes may be tempted to treat such soreness with nonsteroidal antiinflammatory drugs. However, there is no evidence that they hasten healing and they may mask symptoms and increase susceptibility to injury. Delayed muscle soreness starts 8 to 24 hr after exercise, reaches a maximal intensity at 1 to 3 days and then gradually subsides. The affected muscles are firm and tender and cannot contract with their maximum force (107). Exercise and pressure increase soreness. The muscle volume is increased by edema (108). Inflammation is not the cause, as evidenced by lack of granulocytosis (108). The soreness is felt to be caused by damage to the muscle fibers with disruption of Z lines (109) and release of enzymes into blood (110). Elevated environmental temperature and eccentric contractions increase soreness (111).

Nonsteroidal Antiinflammatory Drugs

NSAIDs and aspirin are widely used in the treatment of both acute and chronic sports injuries (Table 7.14). For the purpose of this discussion, aspirin will be lumped together with NSAIDs. The vast majority of studies show that when used with rest, ice, compression, and elevation, NSAIDs hasten return to competition (112). However, NSAIDs do not appear to shorten recovery periods for athletes with chronic overuse injuries (113). They can block pain and inflammation, but they also can delay healing. In lower doses, NSAIDs can decrease the amount of heat at the site of injury (114) and, by relieving pain, can decrease muscle spasm. In higher doses, they may reduce inflammation. NSAIDS block bradykinin and prostaglandin synthesis. E series prostaglandins sensitize nerve endings to the pain-producing effects of bradykinin and increase vascular permeability (115).

On the other hand, F series prostaglandins initiate wound healing (116), and NSAIDs have been shown to delay bone fracture healing (117).

Side Effects

Athletes with gastritis or stomach ulcers should try to avoid NSAIDs. If such athletes need to take these drugs, they should also take antiulcer medications, such as ranitidine and cimetidine.

Virtually all people who take NSAIDs regularly will have evidence of gastrointestinal bleeding, although many will have no symptoms whatever. NSAIDs also increase bleeding by inhibiting platelet aggregation, so they should not be used when there is a great chance for bleeding from trauma. This effect can last up to 10 days after a single dose. The NSAID choline magnesium trisalicylate is less likely than other NSAIDs to cause bleeding. Small doses of NSAIDs decrease renal excretion of uric acid, whereas high doses are uricosuric. Therefore, they should be given with caution to people who have gout. NSAIDs can cause renal damage, so they should not be given regularly to people who have kidney diseases.

NSAIDs should be used with caution during exercise in hot weather. They lower fever by causing vasodilation of the blood vessels in the skin and increasing sweating; therefore, in theory, they may increase fluid loss. During dehydration, prostaglandins are necessary to maintain renal plasma flow and glomerular filtration rate. In that case, prostaglandin inhibition may cause azotemia (118). On exposure to NSAIDs, a significant percentage of asthmatics suffer urticaria, angioedema, asthma, or anaphylactic shock.

Aspirin and NSAIDs

When NSAIDs are used together with aspirin, lower-than-expected blood levels of NSAIDs and an increased incidence of bleeding result. The combination appears to be less effective than when either drug is used alone. While NSAIDs and aspirin have equal antiinflammatory effects, higher doses of aspirin are required with an increased incidence of side effects. For significant antiinflammatory effect, at least 10 five-grain aspirin tablets per day are required. Almost all people on this dose of aspirin will suffer from gastrointestinal bleeding.

Chronic Fatigue in Athletes

Chronic fatigue is the seventh most common symptom in primary care (119). At some time in their lives, most athletes complain of a drop in performance, of not being able to finish their workouts, and that their muscles hurt and feel weak. Muscle glycogen depletion and chronic dehydration are the most likely causes. The recommended treatment is usually to ask the patient to stop training for a few days, or, at the very least, to stop intensive training and drink extra fluids and eat a little extra carbohydrates.

On the other hand, some athletes do not recover for months or even years (120). Other complaints often include muscle ache and headaches, amenorrhea, depression, inability to concentrate or stay awake, loss of libido, insomnia, constipation or diarrhea, enlarged lymph nodes, and frequent colds and injuries.

An evaluation should include a thorough search for a cause. More than 60% of chronic fatigue cases have no known cause (121). Depression and infections are the most common known causes. Fatigue is usually a presenting symptom of depression. Depression affects up to 25% of people who complain of chronic fatigue (122). Depression can be situational or chemical. Situational depression may not require medication and often can be treated with environmental changes and psychotherapy. Chemical depression is usually treated with medication.

Infection

Any infection can induce fatigue. Young, healthy athletes can have chronic sexually transmitted diseases. If indicated, order bacterial cultures of urine, nose, throat, vagina or semen, and chlamydia, gonorrhea, and herpes cultures of the cervix or urethra. There appears to be a specific chronic fatigue syndrome that has been shown to be associated with immune activation, although the specific infectious cause remains elusive (123). Epstein-Barr virus has not been shown to be the cause (124), but human T-cell lymphocytotrophic virus 1 (HTLV-1) and a spumavirus are suspect. Occasional cases may be caused by cytomegalovirus; hepatitis A, B, and C; toxoplasmosis; and other agents that cause mononucleosis-like syndromes.

Drugs

Frequent ingestion of alcohol can impair glycolysis and cause early muscle fatigue (125). All potassium-losing diuretics can cause hypokalemia and hypomagnesemia. The lipid-lowering drugs—lovostatin, gemfibrozil, niacin, and the clofibrates—can cause muscle fatigue and pain (126). The asthma drug salbutamol can cause muscle pain. Other causes include glucocorticoids, large doses of vitamin E, and cytotoxic drugs.

Potassium

Abnormalities in mineral metabolism are rare causes of chronic fatigue in athletes. Healthy athletes do not develop potassium deficiency. Because potassium is found in all foods, the only way to create a low-potassium diet with adequate caloric intake is to deprive the athlete of food and feed him or her hard candies all day long (127). Low blood levels of potassium are caused by vomiting, diarrhea, licorice, glucocorticoids, and diuretics. If bulimia is suspect, order a 24-hr urine for potassium. Vomiting causes a metabolic alkalosis, which forces the kidneys to conserve hydrogen ions and lose potassium.

Sodium

Sodium abnormalities are unusual causes of fatigue in healthy athletes. The average American takes in more than 4000 mg of sodium each day, although an individual needs only about 200 mg at rest and a maximum of 3000 mg when exercising extensively in hot weather. If the athlete is heat acclimatized, does not add salt to food or cooking, and does not use especially salty-tasting food, he or she will still take in around 300 mg sodium each day (128). Severe salt restriction is not recommended for the treatment of hypertension because it can raise blood pressure and LDL cholesterol (129).

High blood sodium levels are caused by dehydration, exogenous glucocorticoids, renal disease, and adrenal hyperfunction. Low blood levels are usually caused by dehydration, polydipsia, gastrointestinal disturbances such as vomiting and diarrhea, diuretics, renal disease, glucocorticoid deficiency, hypothyroidism, and severe salt restriction, usually in vegetarians.

Calcium

An elevated calcium level calls for a search for parathyroid or kidney disease, other hormonal disorders, tumors, and sarcoidosis. It also can be caused by drugs such as massive doses of vitamin A and D, thiazides, lithium, estrogens, and antiestrogens. Low calcium levels are caused by parathyroid and kidney disorders, a deficiency of vitamin D, pancreatitis, hypophosphatemia or hypomagnesemia, and administration of calcitonin or toxic doses of fluoride.

Magnesium

The author could find no reports of magnesium deficiency causing chronic fatigue syndrome in nonathletes, and magnesium supplements have been reported to improve clinical symptoms (130). Magnesium is the only mineral with a blood concentration that drops during exercise, but this drop is caused by magnesium moving from serum into red blood cells, fat, and muscle rather than acute loss through sweat (131).

More than 50% of American adults do not ingest their recommended dietary allowance for magnesium (132), and a deficiency of that mineral can cause early fatigue during exercise (133). It is prudent to measure blood magnesium levels in athletes who have chronic fatigue. However, because magnesium is primarily intracellular, blood values may not always be dependable. Low blood levels can be caused by diuretics. Magnesium supplements should not be given unless the athlete has low blood levels. Excess magnesium is a cathartic and can cause phosphate loss (134).

Other Causes

If indicated, tests can be ordered for hormonal abnormalities, tumors, primary muscle or neurological diseases, or immune diseases. The evaluation of most cases of chronic fatigue in athletes does not lead to a known cause.

REFERENCES

1. Siegel AJ, Hennekens CH, Solomon HS, et al. Exercise-associated hematuria findings in a group of marathon runners. JAMA 1979;241:391–397.
2. Boone AW, Haltiwanger E, Chambers RL. Football hematuria. JAMA 1955;158:1516–1520.
3. Fletcher DJ. Athletic pseudonephritis. Lancet 1977;1:910–914.
4. Amelar RD, Solomon C. Acute renal trauma in boxers. J Urology 1954;72:145–149.
5. Peggs JM, Reinhardt RW, O'Brien JM. Proteinuria in adolescent sports physical examinations. J Fam Pract 1986;22(1):80–81.
6. Castenfors J, Mossfeldt F, Piscator M. Effect of prolonged heavy exercise on renal function and urinary protein excretion. Acta Physiol Scand 1967;70:194–203.
7. Reid RI, Hosking DH, Ramsey EW. Haematuria following a marathon run: source and significance. Br J Urology 1987;59:133–136.
8. Blacklock NJ: Bladder trauma in the long-distance runner. Br Med J 1977;49:129–134.
9. Ritter WS, Stone MJ, et al. Reduction in exertional myoglobulinemia after physical conditioning. Arch Intern Med 1979;139:644–652.
10. Poortmans JR. Exercise and renal function. Sports Med 1984;1:25–28.
11. Caro XJ, Sathetlar PW, Mitchel DB, et al. Traumatic hemoglobinuria associated with congo drums. West J Med 1975;123:141–165.
12. Fleischer R: Ueber eine nene form von hemoglobinuria bein menschen. Klin Wochenschr 1881;47:691–702.
13. DuFaux B, Hoederath A, Streitberger I, et al. Serum ferritin, haptoglobin, and iron in middle and long-distance runners, elite rowers, and professional racing cyclists. Int J Sports Med 1981;2:43–46.
14. Pollard TD, Weiss IW. Acute tubular necrosis in a patient with march hemoglobinuria. N Eng J Med 1970;283:803–812.
15. Eichner ER. Runner's macrocytosis: a clue to footstrike hemolysis. Am J Med 1985;78:321–325.
16. Stewart JG, Ahlquist DA, et al. Gastrointestinal blood loss and anemia in runners. Ann Intern Med 1984;100:843–845.
17. Fletcher DJ. Athletic pseudonephritis. Lancet 1977;1:910.
18. McMahon LF, Ryan MJ, Larson D, et al. Occult gastrointestinal blood loss in marathon runners. Ann Int Med 1984;100:846.
19. Oscai LB, Williams BT, Hertig BA. Effect of exercise on blood volume. J Appl Physiol 1968;24:622–624.
20. Brotherhood J, Brozovic B, Pugh LDC. Haemotological status of middle and long distance runners. Br J Mol Med 1975;48:139–145.
21. Adner MM. Hematology. In: Strauss, RH ed. Sports medicine. Philadelphia: WB Saunders, 1984.
22. Davison AJ, Banister E, Taunton J. Rate limiting processes in energy metabolism. In: Taylor AW, ed. Applications of science and medicine to sport. Springfield, IL: Charles C Thomas, 1975:105–119.
23. Ekblom B, Goldbarg AN. Response to exercise after blood loss and reinfusion. J Appl Physiol 1972;33:175–180.
24. Brien AJ, Simon TL. The effects of red blood cell transfusion on 10-km race time. JAMA 1987;257:2761–2765.
25. Ramotar JE: Cyclists deaths linked to erythropoietin? Phy Sportsmed 1990;18(8):48–49.
26. Finch CA, Miller LR, Inamader AR, et al. Iron deficiency in the rat, physiological and biochemical studies on muscle dysfunction. J Clin Invest 1976;58:447.
27. Siegel AJ. Medical conditions arising during sports. In: Mirkin G, Shangold M, eds. Women and exercise: physiology and sports medicine. Philadelphia: FA Davis, 1993:227.
28. Scott DE, Pritchard JA. Iron deficiency in healthy young college women. JAMA 1967;199(12):147.
29. Lederle F. Oral cobalamin for pernicious anemia. JAMA 1991;265(1):94–95.
30. Miller DM, Winslow RM, et al. Improved exercise performance after exchange transfusion in subjects with sickle cell anemia. Blood 1980;56:1127–1131.
31. Murphy JR. Sickle cell hemoglobin (HbAS) in black football players. JAMA 1973;225:981–982.
32. Bunch TW. Blood test abnormalities in runners. Mayo Clinic Proc 1980;55:113–117.
33. Apple FS, Rogers MA. Serum and muscle alanine aminotransferase activities in marathon runners. JAMA 1984;252:626.
34. Siegel AJ, Silverman LM, Lopez RE: Creatine kinase elevations in marathon runners, relationship to training and competition. Yale J Biol Med 1980;53:275.
35. Chalmers TC, Eckardt RK, Reynolds WE, et al. The treatment of acute infectious hepatitis. Controlled studies of the effects of diet, exercise and reconditioning on the acute course of the disease and on the incidence of relapses and residual abnormalities. J Clin Invest 1955;34:1163–1235.
36. Swift WE Jr, Gardner HT, Moore DJ, Streitfield FH, Havens WD Jr. Clinical course in viral hepatitis and the effect of exercise on convalescence. Am J Med 1950;8:614.
37. Repsher LH, Frehern RK. Effects of early and vigorous exercise on recovery from infectious hepatitis. N Engl J Med 1969;281:1393–1396.
38. Krikler DM, Zilberg B: Hepatitis and activity. Lancet 1971;2:1046–1047.
39. Lorber SH: Gastrointestinal disorders. In: Bove AA, Lowenthal DT, eds. Exercise medicine, physiological principles and clinical applications. New York: Academic, 1983:279–290.
40. Sullivan, SN. The effect of running on the gastrointestinal tract. J Clin Gastroenterol 1984;6:461–465.

41. Dapoigny M, Sarna SK. Effects of physical exercise on colonic motor activity. Am J Physiol 1991;23:G646–G652.
42. Cammack J, Read NW, Cann PA, Greenwood B, Holgate AM. Effect of prolonged exercise on the passage of a solid meal through the stomach and small intestine. Gut 1982;23:957–961.
43. Harris A, Lindeman AK, Martin BJ. Rapid orocecal transit in chronically active persons with high-energy intake. J Appl Physiol 1991;70(4):1550–1553.
44. Harris A, Lindeman AK, Martin BJ. Rapid orocecal transit in chronically active persons with high-energy intake. J Appl Physiol 1991;70(4):1550–1553.
45. Keeling WF, Martin BJ. Gastrointestinal transit during mild exercise. J Appl Physiol 1987;63(3):978–981.
46. Ollerenshaw KJ, Norman S, Wilson C, Hardy JG. Exercise and small intestine transit. Nucl Med Commun 1987;8:105–110.
47. Meshkinpour H, Kemp C, Fairshter R. Effect of aerobic exercise on mouth-to-cecum transit time. Gastroenterology 1989;96:938–941.
48. Wald A, Back C, Bayless TM. Effect of caffeine on the human small intestine. Gastroenterology 1976;71:738–742.
49. Jokl E, Jokl P. Heart and sport. In: Brunner D, Jokl E, eds. The role of exercise in internal medicine. Basel: S. Karger, 1977:36–67.
50. Siegel AJ, Silverman LM, Holman BL. Elevated creatine kinase MB isoenzyme levels in marathon runners. JAMA 1981;246:1049.
51. Walther RJ, Tifft CP. High blood pressure in the competitive athlete: guidelines and recommendations. Phys Sportsmed 1985;13(5):93–114.
52. Fixler D, Laird P, Brown R, et al. Response of hypertensive adolescents to dynamic and isometric exercise stress. Pediatrics 1979;64:579–583.
53. Hoel BL, Lorentsen E, Lund-larsen PC. Hemodynamic responses to sustained hand grip in patients with hypertension. Acta Med Scand 1970;188:491–495.
54. Cooper B, Pollock M, Martin RP, et al. Physical fitness levels vs. selected coronary risk factors. JAMA 1976;236:166–169.
55. Ekblom B, Astrand PO, Saltin B, et al. Effect of training on circulatory responses to exercise. J Appl Physiol 1969;24:518–528.
56. Boyer JL, Kasch FW. Exercise therapy in hypertensive men. JAMA 1970;211:1668–1671.
57. Chick TW, Halperin AK, Gacek EM. The effect of antihypertensive medications on exercise performance: a review. Med Sci Sports Exerc 1988;20(5):447–454.
58. Stewart KJ, Effron MB, Valenti SA, Kelemen MH. Effects of diltiazem or propranolol during exercise training of hypertensive men. Med Sci Sports Exerc 1990;22(2):171–177.
59. Lowenthal DT, Broderman SJ. Exercise in renal and hypertensive disease. In: Bove AA, Lowenthal DT, eds. Exercise medicine physiological principles and clinical applications. New York: Academic, 1983.
60. Esnault, VKM, Potiron-Josse M, Testa A, Ginet JD, Le Carrer D, Guenel J. Captopril but not acebutolol, prazosin or indomethicin decreases post exercise proteinuria. Nephron 1991;58:437–442.
61. Gordon NF, Duncan JJ. Effect of beta blockers on exercise physiology: implications for exercise training. Med Sci Sports Exerc 1991;23(66):668–676.
62. Donaldson MC. Varicose veins in active people. Phys Sportsmed 1990;18(7):47–52.
63. Larson RH, Lofgren EP, Myers TT, et al. Long-term results after vein surgery. Study of 1,000 cases after 10 years. Mayo Clin Proc 1974;49(2):114–117.
64. Noyes LD, Rice JC, Kerstein MD. Hemodynamic assessment of high-compression hosiery in chronic venous disease. Surgery 1987;102(5):813–814.
65. Lewicki R, Tchorzewski H, Denys A, Kowalska M, Gokinska A. Effect of exercise on some parameters of immunity in conditioned sportsmen. Int J Sports Med 1987;8:309–314.
66. Edwards AJ, Bacon TH, Elms CA, Verardi R, Felder M, Knight SC. Changes in the populations of lymphoid cells in human peripheral blood following physical exercise. Clin Exp Immunol 1984;58:420–427.
67. Simon HB. The immunology of exercise. JAMA 1984;252(19):2735–2738.
68. Green RL, Kaplan SS, Rabin BS, Stantitski CL, Zdziarski U. Immune function in marathon runners. Ann Allergy 1981;47(2):73–75.
69. Osterback L, Qvarnberg Y. A prospective study of respiratory infections in 12-year old children actively engaged in sports. Acta Paediatr Scand 1987;76:944–949.
70. Shephard RJ, Corey P, Renzland P, Cox M. The influence of employee fitness and lifestyle modification program upon medical care costs. Can J Public Health 1982;73:259–263.
71. Dormer BA, Friedlander J, Jokl E. Physical efficiency and pulmonary tuberculosis. S Afr J Med Sci 1942;38:424–434.
72. Douglas RG, Lindgren KM, Couch RB. Exposure to cold environment and rhinovirus common cold. N Engl J Med 1968;279:742–747.
73. Nieman DC, Johanssen LM, Lee JW. Infectious episodes in runners before and after a roadrace. J Sports Med 1989;29:286–296.
74. Peters EM, Bateman ED: Ultramarathon running and upper respiratory tract infections. S Afr Med J 1983;64:582–584.
75. Roberts JA. Viral illnesses and sports performance. Sports Med 1986;3:296–303.
76. Friman G. Effect of acute infectious disease on isolated muscle strength. Scand J Clin Lab Invest 1977;37:303–308.
77. Arnold DL. Excessive intracellular acidosis of skeletal muscle on exercise in a patient with post-viral exhaustion syndrome. Lancet 1984;1:1367–1369.
78. Astrom E. Effect of viral and mycoplasma infections on ultrastructure and enzyme activities in human skeletal muscle. Acta Pathol Micr Immunol Scand 1976;84:113–122.
79. Gwaltney JM Jr, Moskalski PB, Hendley JO. Hand-to-hand transmission of rhinovirus colds. Ann Intern Med 1978;88:463–467.
80. Hendley JO, Wnetzel RP, Gwaltney, JR Jr. Transmission of rhinovirus colds by self inoculation. N Engl J Med 1973;288:1361.
81. Saketkhoo K, Adolph-Januszkiewicz BS, Sackner MA. Effects of drinking hot water, cold water and chicken soup on nasal mucous velocity and nasal airflow resistance. Chest 1978;74:4.
82. Rosner F. Hot chicken soup for asthma. Lancet 1979;2:1079.
83. Haynes RL, Ingram RH Jr, McFadden ER Jr. An assessment of the pulmonary response to exercise in asthma and an analysis of the factors influencing it. Am Rev Respir Dis 1976;114:739.
84. McCarthy P. Wheezing and breezing through exercise-induced ashtma. Phys Sportsmed 1989;17(7):125–130.
85. McFadden ER, Ingram RH. Exercise-induced asthma, observations on the initiating stimulus. N Engl J Med 1979;301:763–769.
86. McFadden ER. Exercise-induced asthma. J Allergy Clin Immunol 1991;88(3):318.
87. Edmunds AY, Tooley M, Godfrey S. The refractory period after exercise-induced asthma: its duration and relation to severity of exercise. Am Rev Respir Dis 1978;117(2):247–254.
88. National Heart, Lung, and Blood Institute, National Asthma Education Program Expert Panel Report (Albert Sheffer, chairman). Guidelines for the diagnosis and management of asthma. J Allergy Clin Immun 1991;88(3):452.
89. Meeuwisse WH, Hopkins SR, McKenzie DC, McGavin A. The effect of salbutamol on performance in elite non-asthmatic athletes. Med Sci Sports Exerc 1991;23(4):S134.
90. Rohr AS, Siegel SC, Katz RM, et al. A comparison of inhaled albuterol and cromolyn in the prophylaxis of exercise-induced bronchospasm. Ann Allergy 1987;59(2):107–109.
91. Hodgkin JE, Balcham OJ, Kass I, et al. Chronic obstructive airway disease, current concepts in diagnosis and comprehensive care. JAMA 1975;232:1243–1260.
92. Mirkin GB: Exercise-associated anaphylaxis. JAMA 1991;265(5):65.
93. Sheffer AL, Austen KF. Exercise-induced anaphylaxis. J Allergy Clin Immunol 1980;66(2):106–111.
94. Harries MG, Burge PS, O'Brien I, Cromwell O, Pepys J. Blood histamine levels after exercise testing. Clin Allergy 1979;9(5):437–441.
95. Casale TB, Keahy TM, Kaliner M. Exercise-induced anaphylactic syndrome. Insights into diagnostic and pathophysiologic features. JAMA 1986;255(15):2049–2052.
96. Kivity S, Sneh E, Greif J, Mekori YA. The effect of food and exercise on the skin response to compound 48/80 in patients with food-associated exercise-induced urticaria-angioedema. J Allergy Clin Immunol 1988;81(6):1155–1158.

97. Kushimoto H, Masked type I wheat allergy. Relation to exercise-induced anaphylaxis. Arch Dermatol 1985;121(3):355–360.
98. Sheffer AL, Austen KF. Exercise-induced anaphylaxis. J Allergy Clin Immunol 1980;66(2):106–111.
99. Kobza C, Black A, Abookaker J, Gibson JR, Harvey SG, Marks P. Acrivistine versus hydroxyzine in the treatment of cholinergic urticaria. A placebo-controlled study. Acta Derm Venereol (Stockh) 1988;68(6):541–544.
100. McClean SP, Arreaza EE, Lett-Brown MA, Grant JA. Refractory cholinergic urticaria successfully treated with ketotifen. 1989;83(4):738–741.
101. Kaplan AP, Natbony SF, Tawil AP, Fruchter L, Foster M. Exercise-induced anaphylaxis as a manifestation of cholinergic urticaria. J Allergy Clin Immunol 1981;68(4):319–324.
102. Sheffer AL. Exercise-induced anaphylaxis. N Engl Regl Allergy Proc 1988;9(3):215–217.
103. Hatty S, Mufti GJ, Hamblin TJ. Exercise-induced urticaria and angioedema with relief from cromoglycate insufflation. Postgrad Med J 1983;59(695):586–587.
104. Tamborlane WV, Sherwin RS, Koivisto V, Hendler R, Genel M, Felig P. Normalization of the growth hormone and catecholamine response to exercise in juvenile-onset diabetics treated with a portable insulin infusion pump. Diabetes 1979;28:785.
105. Wahren J, Hagenfeldt L, Felig P. Splanchnic and leg exchange of glucose, amino acids and free fatty acids during exercise in diabetes mellitus. J Clin Invest 1975;55:130.
106. Koivisto VA, Felig P. Effects of leg exercise on insulin absorption in diabetic patients. N Engl J Med 1978;298:7.
107. Komi PV, Rusko H. Quantitative evaluation of mechanical and electrical changes during fatigue loading of eccentric and concentric work. Scan J Rehab Med (Suppl) 1974;3:121–126.
108. Bobbert MF, Hollander AP, Huijing PA. Factors in delayed onset muscular soreness of man. Med Sci Sports Exerc 1986;18(1):75–81.
109. Friden J, Sjostrom M, Ekbloom B. Myofibrillar damage following intense eccentric exercise in man. Int J Sports Med 1983;4:170–176.
110. Triffletti P, Litchfield PE, Clarckson PM, Byrnes WC. Creatine kinase and muscle soreness after repeated isometric exercise. Med Sci Sports Exerc 1988;20(3):242–248.
111. Asmussen E. Observations on experimental soreness. Acta Rheum Scand 1956;2:109–116.
112. Santelli G, Tuccemei V, Cannestra FM. Comparative study with piroxicam and ibuprofen verses placebo in the supportive treatment of minor sports injuries. J Infect Med Res 1980;8:265–269.
113. Rhind V, Downiew WW, Bird HA, et al. Naproxen and indomethicin in periarthritis of the shoulder. Rheum Rehab 1982;21:51–53.
114. Giani E, Rocchi L, Tavoni A, Montanari M, Garagiola U. Telethermic evaluation of NSAIDs in the treatment of sports injuries. Med Sci Sports Exerc 1989;21(1):1–6.
115. Krane SM. Action of salicylates. N Engl J Med 1972;286:317.
116. Lord JT, Zibok VA, Cagle WD, et al. Prostaglandins in wound healing; possible regulation of granulation. In: Samuelson B, Ramwell PW, Paoletti R, eds. Advances in prostaglandin research. Vol. 2. New York: Raven, 1980.
117. Elves MW, Bayley I, Roylance PJ. The effect of indomethicin upon experimental fractures in the rat. Acta Orthop Scand 1982;53:35–41.
118. Calabrese LH, Rooney TW. The use of nonsteroidal anti-inflammatory drugs in sports. Phys Sportsmed 1986;14(2):89–87.
119. Kroenke K, Wood DR, Mangelsdorf AD, et al. Chronic fatigue in primary care. Prevalence, patient characteristics, and outcome. JAMA 1988;260(7):929–934.
120. Eichner ER. Chronic fatigue syndrome: searching for the cause and treatment. Phys Sportsmed 1989;17(6):142–152.
121. Jerret WA. Lethargy in general practice. Practitioner 1981;225(1355):731–737.
122. Manu P, Mathews DA, Lane TJ. The mental health of patients with a chief complaint of chronic fatigue. A prospective evaluation and follow-up. Arch Intern Med 1988;148(10):2213–2217.
123. Linday AL, Jessop C, Lenette ET, Levy JA. Chronic fatigue syndrome: clinical condition associated with immune activation. Lancet 1991;338:707–712.
124. Holmes GP, Kaplan JE, Stewart JA, et al. A cluster of patients with a chronic mononucleosis-like syndrome. Is Epstein-Barr virus the cause? JAMA 1987;257(17):2297–2302.
125. Rubin E. Alcoholic myopathy in heart and skeletal muscle. N Engl J Med 1979;301:28–35.
126. London SF, Gross KF, Ringel SP. Cholesterol-lowering agent myopathy (CLAM). Neurology 1991;41:1159–1160.
127. Costill D. Muscle water and electrolytes during acute and repeated bouts of dehydration. In: Parizkova J, Rogozkin VA, eds. Nutrition, physical fitness and health. Baltimore: University Park Press, 1978;1066–1115.
128. Mirkin GB. Nutrition for sports. In: Shangold MM, Mirkin GB eds. Women and exercise, physiology and sports medicine. Philadelphia: FA Davis, 1988:101.
129. Ruppert M, Diehl J, Kolloch A, et al. Short-term dietary sodium restriction increases serum lipids and insulin in salt-sensitive and salt-resistant normotensive adults. Klin Wochenschr 1991;69(Suppl 25):51–57.
130. Cox IM, Campbell MJ, Dowson D. Red blood cell magnesium and chronic fatigue syndrome. Lancet 1991;(337):1094–1095.
131. Wolfswinkel JM, Van Der Walt WH, Van Der Linde A. Intravascular shift in magnesium during prolonged exercise. South Afr J Sci 1983;79:37.
132. Morgan KJ, Stampley, GL, Zabin ME, Fischer DR. Magnesium and calcium dietary intakes of the United States population. J Am Coll Nutr 1985;4:195–206.
133. Keen CL, Gershwin ME, Lowney P, Hurley P, Stern JS. The influence of dietary magnesium intake on exercise capacity and hematological parameters in rats. Metabolism 1987;36:788–793.
134. Spencer H. Minerals and mineral interactions in human beings. J Am Diet Assoc 1986;86:864–867.

SUGGESTED READINGS

Appenzeller A. Sports medicine: fitness, training, injuries. Baltimore: Urban & Schwarzenberg, 1988.

Bove A, Lowenthal D. Exercise medicine physiologic principles and clinical applications. New York: Academic, 1983.

Shangold M, Mirkin G. Women and exercise: physiology and sports medicine. Philadelphia: FA Davis, 1993.

8 / CARDIOVASCULAR EVALUATION OF THE ATHLETE

Barry A. Franklin, Steven L. Almany, and Andrew M. Hauser

Cardiovascular evaluation of the athlete can yield important information relative to performance potential and abnormalities that may cause exercise-related symptoms and, in rare instances, sudden cardiac death. The evaluation may include a careful and complete medical history, physical examination, 12-lead electrocardiogram (ECG), and if clinically warranted, exercise stress testing (1, 2). Unfortunately, athletes often minimize symptoms in an effort to avoid restrictions on participation. Moreover, several studies now suggest that routine, intensive screening of athletes for potentially lethal cardiovascular conditions is impractical because of the small diagnostic yield (3–5), extremely high cost (5), and low incidence of sudden death during competition (1).

The purpose of this chapter is to review the functional and diagnostic basis and rationale for cardiovascular screening in athletes, with specific reference to acute injury, ECG anomalies, sickle cell, sudden cardiac death, and pathologic versus physiologic adaptive cardiac responses to training.

Energy Systems for Exercise

The body's cells do not directly use the glucose and free fatty acids obtained from the breakdown of food for energy. Instead, food is converted through a series of chemical reactions to an energy-rich compound, adenosine 5′-triphosphate (ATP), which serves as the "fuel" for all the energy-requiring processes within the cell. Figure 8.1 illustrates a simplified structure of an ATP molecule.

Somatic energy needs of the athlete may increase more than 20-fold in the transition from rest to maximal physical exertion (6). Because the available stores of ATP are extremely limited and capable of providing energy to maintain moderate- to high-intensity exercise for several seconds only, ATP must be constantly resynthesized. The energy (ATP) required for muscle contraction, biologic work, and athletic competition is produced by anaerobic and aerobic energy pathways. However, far more ATP is formed if oxygen is readily available to exercising muscle tissue. This process, referred to as aerobic metabolism, relies heavily on the cardiorespiratory system for the delivery of oxygen and nutrients and for the removal of waste products to maintain the internal equilibrium of the cells.

Anaerobic Versus Aerobic Production of ATP

Anaerobic pathways supply a rapid source of ATP for brief physical exertion of near-maximal intensity, such as a 440-yard run, 100-yard swim, and other activities that produce exhaustion quickly. ATP may be synthesized anaerobically (in the absence of oxygen) via the splitting of a phosphate molecule from another stored energy-rich compound (creatine phosphate) or the breakdown of carbohydrate within the cell (glycolysis) or both. It should be emphasized, however, that these processes supply only limited amounts of ATP, enough to sustain vigorous exercise for only several seconds.

Glycolysis results in the production of two molecules of ATP. However, these two ATP molecules represent only about 5% of the potential ATP that can be produced when the glucose molecule is completely degraded to carbon dioxide and water during subsequent aerobic reactions. In addition to the low ATP yield, anaerobic glycolysis results in the formation of lactic acid with associated muscle soreness and fatigue. Aerobic energy sources predominate, however, when the duration of exercise exceeds 2 min (Fig. 8.2) (7).

Because the anaerobic reactions of glycolysis release only about 5% of the available ATP, aerobic metabo-

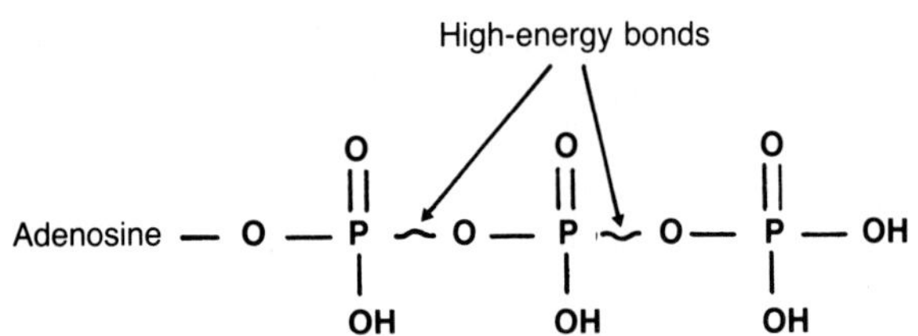

Figure 8.1. Simplified structure of an ATP molecule. ~, high-energy bonds.

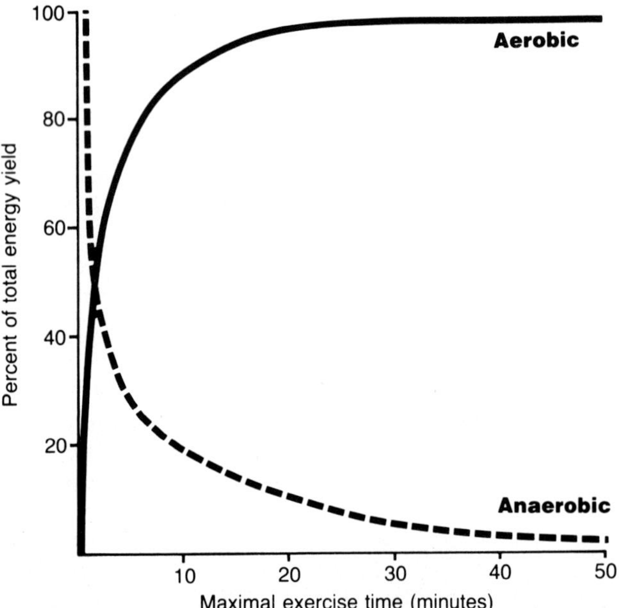

Figure 8.2. Relative contribution of aerobic and anaerobic metabolism during physical activity of increasing duration. As exercise time increases, the relative contribution of anaerobic energy sources decreases. Adapted from Åstrand PO, Rodahl K. Textbook of work physiology. New York: McGraw-Hill, 1970:304.

lism provides an additional means of extracting energy from the glucose molecule. Pyruvic acid molecules are ultimately converted to acetyl-CoA, which also can be formed by the degradation of fats and amino acids. This compound passes into the cell's mitochondria, where it is ultimately broken down in the presence of oxygen to carbon dioxide, water, and significant quantities of ATP. Indeed, more than 90% of the total ATP production occurs via the Krebs citric acid cycle.

Functional Exercise Testing

Maximal oxygen consumption ($\dot{V}_{O_2max}$) and anaerobic threshold largely determine the level of endurance activity that an athlete can sustain (6). Both of these variables can be measured during functional exercise testing.

Maximal Oxygen Consumption

The most widely recognized measure of cardiopulmonary fitness is the aerobic capacity or $\dot{V}_{O_2max}$ (8). This variable is defined physiologically as the highest rate of oxygen transport and use that can be achieved at maximal physical exertion.

Somatic oxygen consumption ($\dot{V}_{O_2}$) may be expressed mathematically by a rearrangement of the Fick equation:

$$\dot{V}_{O_2} = HR \times SV \times (Ca_{O_2} - Cv_{O_2})$$

where $\dot{V}_{O_2}$ is oxygen consumption in milliliters per minute, HR is heart rate in beats per minute, SV is stroke volume in milliliters per beat, and ($Ca_{O_2} - C_{O_2}$) is the arteriovenous oxygen difference in milliliters of oxygen per deciliter of blood. Thus it is apparent that both central and peripheral regulatory mechanisms affect the magnitude of body oxygen consumption.

Typical circulatory data at rest in a healthy, sedentary 30-year-old man are shown in Table 8.1. The absolute resting oxygen consumption (250 ml/min) divided by the man's body weight (70 kg) gives the energy requirement for basal homeostasis, termed 1 metabolic equivalent (MET), which is approximately 3.5 ml/kg/min. This expression of oxygen consumption is independent of body weight and thus relatively constant for all individuals (9). Furthermore, multiples of this value are often used to quantify respective levels of energy expenditure (10). Thus, if running at a 6-mph pace requires 10 times the resting energy expenditure, the aerobic cost is 10 MET, or 35.0 ml/kg/min.

Maximal oxygen consumption may be expressed on an absolute basis in liters per minute, reflecting total body energy output and caloric expenditure, where each liter of oxygen consumed is equivalent to 5 kilocalories (kcals). Because large people usually have a large absolute oxygen consumption simply by virtue of their large muscle mass, physiologists generally divide this value by body weight in kilograms to allow a more equitable comparison between individuals of different size. This variable, when expressed as milliliters of oxygen per kilogram of body weight per minute (ml/kg/min) or as METs, is considered the single best index of physical work capacity or cardiopulmonary fitness (11).

The typical 12-fold increase in oxygen transport and use achieved at maximal exercise is brought about by respective increases in the hemodynamic determinants of $\dot{V}_{O_2}$, e.g., a 4-fold increase in cardiac output and a 3-fold increase in arteriovenous oxygen difference ($4 \times 3 = 12$ MET). Table 8.2 provides representative maximal circulatory values for a sedentary 30-year-old man and a similarly aged world-class endurance athlete. The sedentary man can increase his oxygen uptake approximately 12 times from rest to maximal exercise (6). This is about half the $\dot{V}_{O_2max}$ of a world-class endurance athlete. The increased aerobic capacity in the athlete appears primarily the result of increased maximal cardiac output, secondary to an augmented stroke volume, rather than increased peripheral extraction of oxygen. With less than 10% variation in maximal heart rate and maximal systemic arteriovenous oxygen difference between athletes and nonathletes, $\dot{V}_{O_2max}$ may be used as an index of the inotropic capacity of the heart (12). Therefore, it is of major importance in the cardiovascular evaluation of the athlete.

Table 8.1.
Circulatory Data at Rest for a Healthy, Sedentary Man (70 kg)

	$\dot{V}o_2$ (ml/kg/min)	$\dot{V}o_2$ (liters/min)	MET	HR (beats/min)	SV (ml/beat)	$(Ca_{O_2} - Cv_{O_2})$ (ml/dl blood)
Rest	3.5[a]	0.25	1.0	70	70	5.1

[a] The average resting metabolic rate for all persons, regardless of body weight is 3.5 ml/kg/min, or 1 MET.

Table 8.2.
Typical Circulatory Data during Maximal Exercise for a Sedentary 30-year-old Man and a World-Class Endurance Athlete

	Maximal Oxygen Consumption (liters/min)	Maximal Oxygen Consumption (METs)	Maximal Cardiac Output (liters/min)	Maximal Heart Rate (beats/min)	Maximal Stroke Volume (ml/beat)	Maximal Arteriovenous Oxygen Difference (ml/dl blood)
Sedentary man	3.0	12.0	20.0	190	100	15.8
Endurance athlete	6.0	24.0	35.3	190	185	17.0

Determination of the $\dot{V}o_{2max}$

Maximal oxygen consumption is generally determined by measuring the volume and analyzing the oxygen content of expired air, corrected to standard temperature and pressure dry (STPD), using the following equation (13):

$$\dot{V}o_2 = \dot{V}E\ (FI_{O_2} - FE_{O_2})$$

where $\dot{V}E$ is the expired measured volume per minute, FE_{O_2} is the directly measured concentration of oxygen in expired air, and FI_{O_2} is the concentration of oxygen in the inspired air, normally 0.2093. Traditionally, this variable has been measured using an open circuit or Douglas bag technique. However, several automated systems are now available to measure $\dot{V}o_2$ and related respiratory variables during exercise testing.

It is inconvenient to measure $\dot{V}o_2$ directly because it requires sophisticated equipment, technical expertise, and frequent calibration; therefore, clinicians have increasingly sought to predict or estimate $\dot{V}o_{2max}$ from the treadmill speed and percent grade, or the cycle ergometer workload, expressed as kilogram meters per minute (14). The conventional Bruce (12) test is perhaps the most familiar and widely employed treadmill protocol that offers normative data on oxygen consumption so that aerobic capacity may be estimated from the workload attained (Fig. 8.3). Additional advantages include the rapid workload progression (which incorporates simultaneous increases in both speed and grade, limiting the duration of the test) and advanced stages to accommodate world-class endurance athletes.

Average $\dot{V}o_{2max}$ Values for Various Athletic Groups

$\dot{V}o_{2max}$ values (expressed relative to body weight) in national class and championship athletes vary from a high of 94 ml/kg/min, now reported in a cross-country skier, to values between 40 and 45 ml/kg/min for athletes participating in anaerobic-type sports (Fig. 8.4). Virtually all world-class endurance athletes, including cross-country skiers and elite distance runners and bicyclists, have a $\dot{V}o_{2max}$ between 70 and 80 ml/kg/min, whereas many other championship athletes have a $\dot{V}o_{2max}$ of 60 to 70 ml/kg/min (rope skippers, race walkers, swimmers, and rowers). In contrast, the reported $\dot{V}o_{2max}$ of professional football, tennis, and basketball players is between 40 and 50 ml/kg/min (15, 16). Although strenuous athletic training may produce a 25% or more increase in $\dot{V}o_{2max}$, it has become increasingly apparent that natural endowment, i.e., an exceptional genetic makeup, rather than training per se, plays the primary role in producing a gold-medal winner at an Olympic endurance event.

Anaerobic Threshold

Although the onset of metabolic acidosis during submaximal exercise has been traditionally determined by the measurement of blood lactate, an abrupt increase in arterial lactate may be noninvasively determined by assessment of expired gases during exercise testing, specifically minute ventilation ($\dot{V}E$) and carbon dioxide production ($\dot{V}co_2$) (17). The gas exchange anaerobic threshold (AT) signifies the peak workload or oxygen consumption at which energy demands exceed the circulation's ability to sustain aerobic metabolism. At this exercise intensity (the AT), energy release from anaerobic metabolism increases and a lactic acidemia results.

The physiology underlying the AT is attributed, at least in part, to the buffering of lactic acid, according to the following reaction:

$$\underset{\text{(lactic acid)}}{HLA} + \underset{\text{(sodium bicarbonate)}}{NaHCO_3} \rightarrow \underset{\text{(sodium lactate)}}{NaLa} + \underset{\text{(carbonic acid)}}{H_2CO_3} \rightarrow H_2O + CO_2$$

As lactic acid is produced and buffered by sodium bicarbonate in the blood, CO_2 is released in excess of that

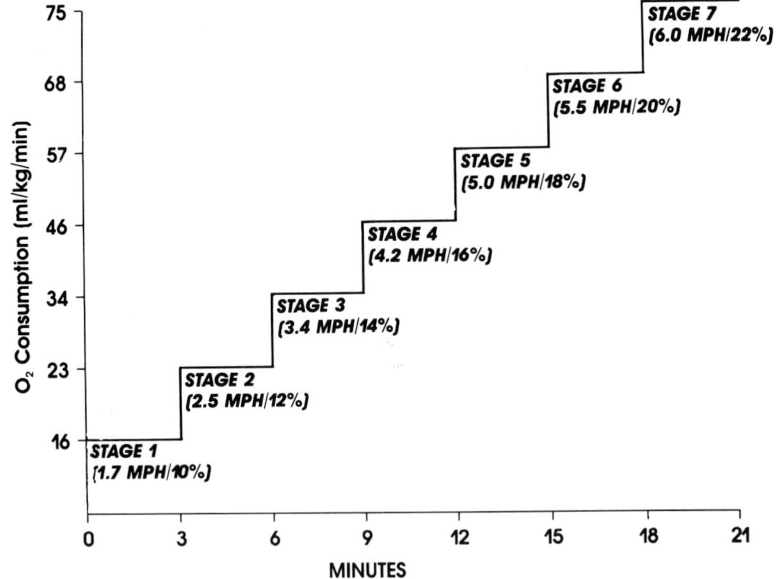

Figure 8.3. The standard Bruce treadmill protocol showing progressive stages (speed, percent grade) and the corresponding aerobic requirement, expressed in ml/kg/min.

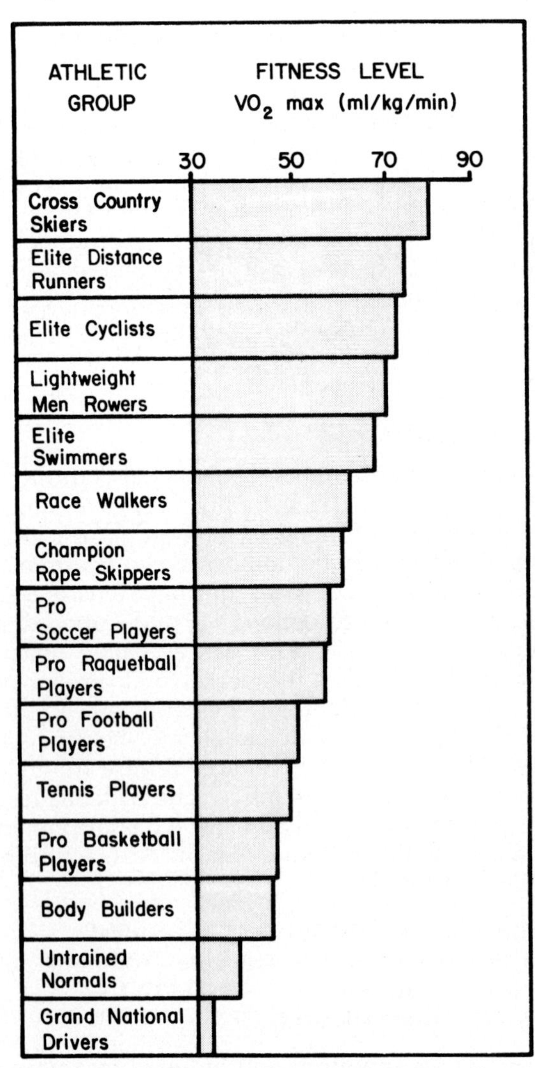

Figure 8.4. Average $\dot{V}_{O_2max}$ values (ml/kg/min) for various athletic groups.

produced by muscle metabolism. Because of the increased CO_2 production ($\dot{V}_{CO_2}$), the decreased pH of the blood, or both, minute ventilation exhibits a break point in linearity. At the AT, the values for $\dot{V}E$ and $\dot{V}_{CO_2}$ increase out of proportion to the intensity of exercise performed, i.e., they increase more abruptly than expected (Fig. 8.5) (18). This method correlates well with the lactate method and obviates the need to measure lactate in repeated blood samples.

The AT from respiratory gas measurements is often expressed as a percentage of the athlete's $\dot{V}_{O_2max}$. For example, an athlete with a $\dot{V}_{O_2max}$ of 4.25 liters/min whose break point in $\dot{V}E$ occurs at 3.20 liters/min would have an anaerobic threshold corresponding to 75% of his or her aerobic capacity (Fig. 8.6). It would be expected that this athlete would be able to maintain exercise intensities below 75% of his or her $\dot{V}_{O_2max}$ using a predominance of aerobic processes. Moreover, such exertion should be accomplished without inducing a significant increase in blood lactic acid and muscle fatigue. Although the AT typically corresponds to 4% to 64% of the $\dot{V}_{O_2max}$ in healthy, untrained persons (18), it generally occurs at a higher percentage of the $\dot{V}_{O_2max}$ (i.e., 70% to 90%) in endurance-trained athletes (19).

The $\dot{V}_{O_2max}$ has long been recognized as an important predictor of performance in endurance events. However, several studies (19–21) now suggest that the highest percentage of the $\dot{V}_{O_2max}$ that can be used over an extended duration, without incurring a significant increase in arterial lactate, may represent an even more important determinant of endurance performance. This suggests that the AT may be critical in determining optimal running speed during marathon races (22, 23).

Diagnostic Exercise Testing

Exercise stress testing is one of the most common evaluations performed in the assessment of sympto-

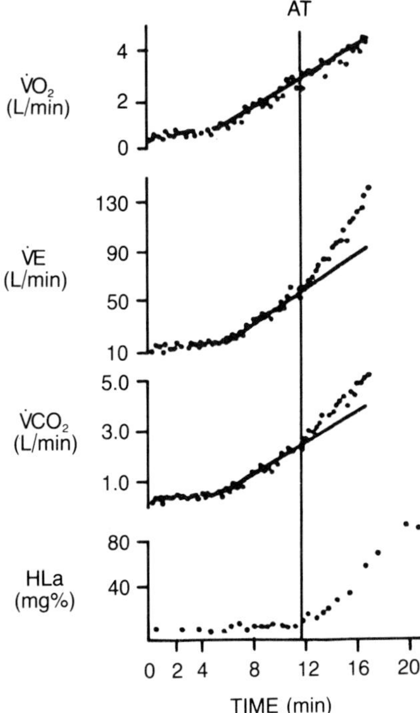

Figure 8.5. Relationship between intensity of exercise (oxygen consumption) and simultaneous, abrupt nonlinear increases in serum lactate (HLa), CO_2 production, and minute ventilation occurring at the anaerobic threshold (AT). Exercise was initiated at minute 4. Modified from Davis JA, Vodak P, Wilmore JH, et al. Anaerobic threshold and maximal aerobic power for three modes of exercise. J Appl Physiol 1976;41:544–550.

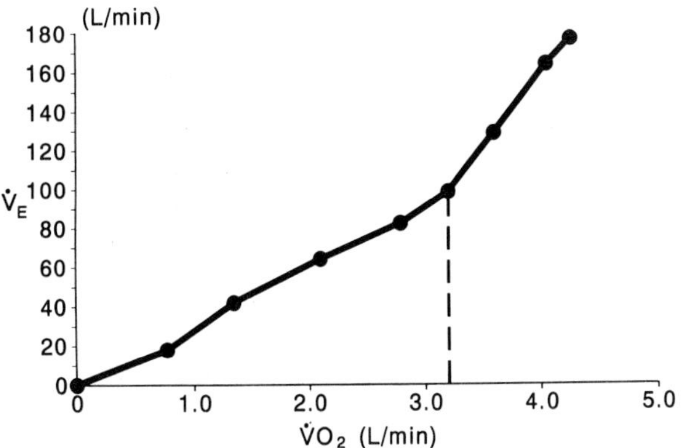

Figure 8.6. Relationship between intensity of exercise (oxygen consumption) and simultaneous, abrupt nonlinear increase in minute ventilation, signifying the anaerobic threshold. In this subject, the breakpoint occurred at 3.20 liters/min, corresponding to 75% of measured $\dot{V}_{O_2max}$ (4.25 liters/min).

matic athletes with suspected coronary artery disease (CAD) (2). The test is based primarily on the electrocardiographic response to exercise, with 1 mm or more of ST-segment depression used as an indicator of myocardial ischemia (Fig. 8.7). The conventional exercise ECG, however, has significant limitations in the diagnosis of occult CAD (24). In some instances, false-positive responses occur. In other words, exercise-induced ST-segment depression may be suggestive of underlying heart disease when, in fact, no disease is present. Conversely, when a patient is found to have significant cor-

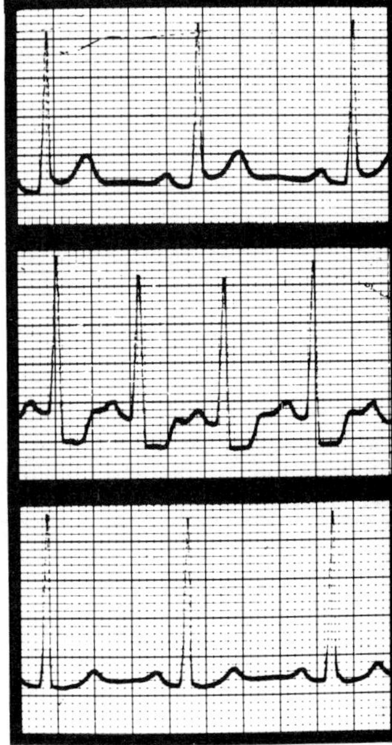

Figure 8.7. Top, resting electrocardiogram (V_5) before exercise testing. **Middle,** after several minutes of exercise, the subject demonstrated significant ST-segment depression and complained of mild substernal chest pain. **Bottom,** resting ECG 6 minutes after exercise is again representative of a normal ECG.

onary narrowing and fails to demonstrate exercise-induced ST-segment depression, his or her test is classified as false-negative.

Although the predictive accuracy of the exercise ECG seems reasonable, a 25% false-negative and a 15% false-positive rate highlight its limitations in detecting CAD. As a result, the need for exercise testing as a screening procedure in young, asymptomatic physically active adults has been questioned (25). Critics emphasize that the cost of mass screenings would be prohibitive and that the incidence of exercise-related cardiovascular complications in presumably healthy adults is extremely low (26). In addition, the significance of exercise-induced ST-segment depression is tenuous at best in persons with a low pretest likelihood of CAD.

Estimating Pretest Likelihood of Heart Disease

Clinicians now use three variables to estimate the risk of heart disease even before the exercise test is conducted. These variables, including age, gender, and symptoms, define a person's pretest risk or likelihood of disease (Table 8.3). The risk of disease may be even further defined by complementary information regarding blood pressure, smoking status, and lipid/lipoprotein profile. In general, the incidence of heart disease increases with advancing age. Moreover, at any given age, men are at a higher risk than women. Individuals who have anginal symptoms also have a greater pretest probability of disease than those who are free of symptoms. Accordingly, an asymptomatic 45-year-old woman has only a 1% chance of having significant CAD, whereas a 65-year-old man with typical angina has a high (94%) pretest risk of heart disease (27).

Table 8.3.
Pretest Likelihood of CAD (%) in Patients by Age, Gender, and Symptoms

	Asymptomatic		Nonanginal Chest Pain		Atypical Angina		Typical Angina	
Age	Men	Women	Men	Women	Men	Women	Men	Women
35	1.9	0.3	5.2	0.8	21.8	4.2	69.7	25.8
45	5.5	1.0	14.1	2.8	46.1	13.3	87.3	55.2
55	9.7	3.2	21.5	8.4	58.9	32.4	92.0	79.4
65	12.3	7.5	28.1	18.6	67.1	54.4	94.3	90.6

Adapted from Diamond GA, Forrester JS. Analysis of probability as an aid in the clinical diagnosis of coronary artery disease. N Engl J Med 1979;300:1350.

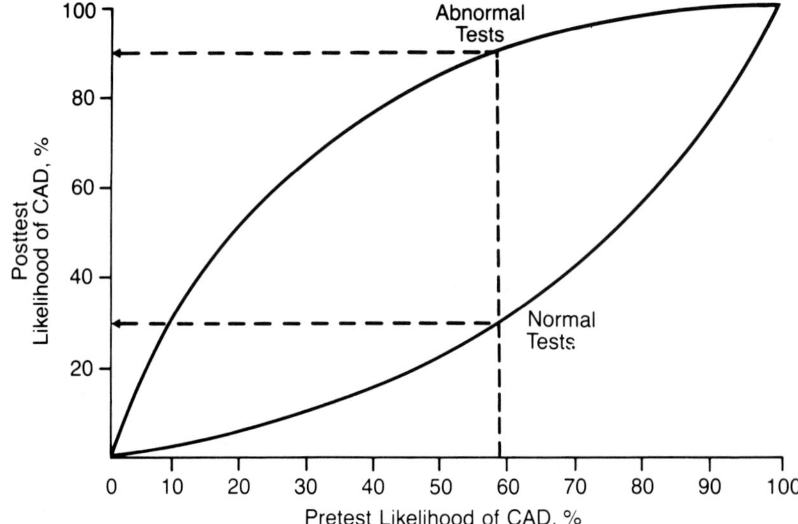

Figure 8.8. Impact of 59% pretest likelihood of CAD on posttest likelihood of disease when exercise ECG is normal (30%) and abnormal (90%). Sensitivity of exercise ECG is 75% and the specificity, 85%. Adapted from Epstein SE. Implications of probability analysis on the strategy used for non-invasive detection of coronary artery disease. Am J Cardiol 1980;46:491.

Determining Posttest Likelihood of Heart Disease

The results of the exercise test are considered along with the pretest risk to determine the posttest likelihood of disease. When the pretest risk of CAD is either very high or very low, a normal or abnormal ECG response has minimal influence on the posttest likelihood of disease. Thus, for the asymptomatic 45-year-old woman or 65-year-old man with angina, any findings from an exercise ECG would be of limited additional value in the diagnosis of CAD. Exercise stress tests have the greatest diagnostic impact in people with an intermediate pretest likelihood of disease, that is, in the 30% to 70% range of pretest probability (28). For example, a 55-year-old man with atypical angina has an approximate 59% likelihood of having significant CAD before any testing is done. After an exercise ECG, his likelihood of having significant CAD (posttest likelihood of disease) separates to about 90% if the test results are abnormal, demonstrating significant ST-segment depression, and about 30% if the test yields normal findings (Fig. 8.8). Thus, by applying Bayesian analyses, the need for additional diagnostic studies (e.g., myocardial perfusion imaging with thallium-201) or coronary arteriography can be defined more intelligently.

Acute Injury

Nonpenetrating (blunt) cardiac trauma is most commonly the result of high-speed deceleration accidents but can occur in contact sports. It should be suspected in cases of unexplained hypotension, dyspnea, chest pain, murmurs or rubs, or fractured ribs. It is the result of compression of cardiac structures between the spine and sternum, increases in intrathoracic pressure, deceleration injury (contrecoup), or combinations thereof.

Diagnosis depends on a high index of suspicion; complete physical examination; and when indicated, diagnostic studies such as chest radiographs, serial ECGs, and cardiac enzyme determinations. Only 50% of patients with significant chest trauma manifest ECG changes, with the most common finding being T-wave flattening or inversion. Elevation of the ST-segment in blunt trauma is unusual; however, it is not uncommon for ECG changes to be delayed for up to 48 hr. Abnormalities of conduction are common, and they are usually transient and rarely require permanent pacing. In cases for which the preliminary evaluation is highly suspicious, other evaluations should be considered such as echocardiograms, nuclear imaging, and occasionally angiography. Immediate complications can include myocardial necrosis ("cardiac contusion"), valvular injuries, and arrhythmias, whereas long-term complications include recurrent and constrictive pericarditis.

Electrocardiographic Changes and Arrhythmias

Resting sinus bradycardia (heart rate < 60 beats/min) is the most common ECG finding among endurance-trained athletes. Resistance-trained athletes less commonly display sinus bradycardia. Findings such as sinus arrhythmia, sinus pauses, first-degree atrioventricular (AV) block, second-degree AV block (Mobitz type I and II), complete heart block, wandering atrial pacemaker, and AV nodal rhythms also have been reported in highly trained athletes (229). These arrhythmias may be more common in older athletes and often occur at night and resolve with exercise (30).

Atrioventricular and intraventricular conduction delays are usually attributed to altered autonomic balance with enhanced parasympathetic tone. The duration and amplitude of the QRS complex can be at the upper limit of normal. Incomplete right bundle branch pattern is a common finding in endurance athletes (31). An early repolarization pattern, with its characteristic ST-segment and J-point elevation, also is a common finding, especially in young black males. Inversion of the T wave, a sign of potential ischemia in the nonathlete, is usually a benign finding, associated with other anomalies such as mitral valve prolapse and asymmetric septal hypertrophy.

Hypertrophic obstructive cardiomyopathy, the most common cardiovascular cause of sudden death in adolescents, is associated with an abnormal ECG in more than 90% of cases (1). Findings include deep and narrow Q waves in leads II, III, aVF, and V_2–V_6, without evidence of left ventricular hypertrophy. Because hypertrophic obstructive cardiomyopathy is an autosomal dominant disorder with variable penetrance, all first-degree relatives should be screened after the condition is diagnosed.

The treatment and prognosis of arrhythmias in athletes has received considerable attention, especially since the sudden death of college basketball star Hank Gathers. Most arrhythmias, including atrial and ventricular premature complexes and atrial tachycardias, are considered normal variants and are nonspecific for heart disease (32). Complex ventricular ectopy, including runs of ventricular tachycardia (such as the case of Hank Gathers), require extensive cardiologic evaluation before medical clearance for athletic participation. Symptoms such as syncope, presyncope, or dizziness (with or without accompanying arrhythmia); a family history of hypertrophic cardiomyopathy or sudden cardiac death; and/or complex ventricular ectopy mandate preparticipation screening (33, 34). All patients with evidence of preexcitation Wolff-Parkinson-White syndrome require evaluation by a cardiologist before participation in vigorous physical activity (2).

Sickle Cell

Sickle-cell trait has been associated with sudden cardiac death in blacks. Surprisingly, sickle-cell disease (the homozygous and more serious form with an occurrence of 0.15%) has been associated with only sporadic reports of sudden cardiac death, perhaps because of the more stringent restrictions that are often placed on these patients.

Sickle-cell trait occurs in approximately 8% of black Americans. In these patients, sickling of the abnormal hemoglobin can occur under conditions of low oxygen tension (altitude), dehydration, and acidosis. Cardiovascular manifestations can include anemia, vasoocclusive "crises," low arterial P_{O_2} and systolic ejection murmurs because of the hyperdynamic circulation. The trait as well as the disease are easily diagnosed with simple sickle preparations.

The etiology of sudden death in these patients is unclear. Several isolated reports have implicated heat stroke, leading to acute renal failure, as a causative factor, whereas others have described strenuous activity at elevations greater than 4000 feet (35). It is rare for sickle-cell patients to suffer acute myocardial infarction as a result of their disease. Correcting for extreme conditions of dehydration and low oxygen tension, there is no reason to preclude patients with sickle-cell trait or disease from participation in strenuous physical activity (36).

Sudden Cardiac Death

Sudden cardiac death is defined as death occurring within 1 hr of an unexpected cardiac event. Because of the high prevalence of cardiovascular disease in the United States and Americans' preoccupation with sports and exercise, there are numerous reports of exercise-related death. Although the exact etiology of sports-related sudden cardiac death is rarely known at the scene, autopsy series usually confirm some form of organic heart disease. Coronary artery disease appears to be the major killer of conditioned runners aged 40 years and older who die while running (37). Common findings, accounting for up to 85% of sports-related sudden cardiac death, include severe atherosclerosis, ruptured aorta, hypertrophic obstructive cardiomyopathy (CM), idiopathic left ventricular hypertrophy (LVH), myocardial bridging, and anomalous origin of the left coronary artery (2, 38–43). Less common findings include irregularities of the conduction system, myocarditis, right ventricular (RV) dysplasia, and mitral valve prolapse (1). Autopsy findings related to exercise-related sudden cardiac death seem to differ from those seen in non-sports-related sudden cardiac death (Table 8.4) (43). Thus the combination of exercise and a diseased or susceptible heart, rather than exercise itself, seems to be the principal acute cardiovascular risk of physical activity (44).

Siscovick et al. (45) reported that the relative risk of cardiac arrest during exercise compared with that at other times was 56 times greater among sedentary men and

Table 8.4.
Relative Frequencies of Sports- and Nonsports-Related Sudden Cardiac Death and Causes of Death

Characteristic	Sports Related	Nonsports Related
Age (mean)	26	32
Male	90%	75%
Female	10%	25%
Causes of death		
Severe CAD	Severe CAD	
Hypertrophic CM	Unknown	
Unknown	Idiopathic LVH	
Anomalous coronary	Marked hypertension/LVH	
Idiopathic LVH	Myocarditis	
Myocarditis	Hypertrophic CM	
RV dysplasia	Aortic dissection	

Adapted from Burke AP, Farb A, Virmani R, et al. Sports-related and non-sports related sudden cardiac death in young adults. Am Heart J 1991;121:568–575.

only 5 times greater among men with high levels of habitual activity. However, the total risk of cardiac arrest among habitually active men was only 40% of that for sedentary men. In other words, if an individual exercises vigorously for 1 hr/day, that person is more likely to experience a cardiac event during that period than during a comparable period of less vigorous activity, regardless of whether he or she is habitually active or sedentary. On the other hand, if he or she is physically active, compared with a sedentary person, he or she is at a lower overall risk for a cardiac event. These findings agree with the hypothesis that vigorous physical activity both protects against and provokes sudden cardiac death (46).

Implications for Athletes and Physicians

Although the salutary effects of regular physical activity are well-documented, there are limitations to the benefits that athletic training offers relative to the prevention of heart disease. Contrary to the speculation of a few overzealous enthusiasts (47), regular exercise, regardless of the intensity, duration, or both, does not confer immunity to CAD. Furthermore, neither superior athletic ability, habitual physical activity, nor the absence of cardiac risk factors guarantees protection against an exercise death (48).

Noakes et al. (49) reported clinical findings in 21 marathon runners who either died suddenly or developed anginal symptoms, demonstrating that CAD was the most common diagnosis. A total of 65% of all cardiovascular complications occurred during or within 24 hr of competitive events, and 86% of the runners had a very low high-density lipoprotein (HDL) to total cholesterol ratio (< 19%). Moreover, 81% developed premonitory symptoms, yet the majority continued to train or even race without seeking medical advice. These findings suggest that endurance athletes should not consider themselves immune to either sudden cardiac death or CAD and should seek medical advice immediately if they develop any symptoms suggestive of ischemic heart disease. Furthermore, physicians should not assume that highly trained athletes cannot have coronary or other life-threatening cardiac diseases such as hypertrophic CM. Rather, all symptomatic athletes should undergo exhaustive cardiovascular evaluation to exclude the possible presence of heart disease (2). However, the complete absence of ECG abnormalities and premorbid warning symptoms in some athletes indicates that not even these measures will prevent all cases of exercise-related cardiovascular complications.

Cardiac Adaptations in Endurance-Trained Athletes

Adaptive cardiac responses to isotonic training in endurance runners and swimmers are reflected by increased left ventricular (LV) volume and mass with insignificant alterations in resting ejection fraction (50). The resultant increased stroke volume is similar to alterations seen in chronic volume loading conditions and allows greater efficiency of pump function. Athletes participating in isometric exercise, such as shot-putters, power lifters, and wrestlers, tend to display relatively greater increases in LV wall thickness with unchanged chamber volumes, similar to the alterations that occur with chronic pressure loads such as hypertension and aortic stenosis (51, 52). Rowers who participate in combined heavy dynamic and isometric exercise develop measurable increases in both LV wall thickness and chamber dimension within months of training (52). Similar dimensional changes occur in trained cyclists (53). Most athletes display increased LV mass, even when normalized for body surface area (54). Enlargement of the right heart commonly occurs in long-distance runners but tends to remain proportionate in size to left-sided chambers (55).

Various conflicting studies have reported normal, augmented, and diminished ventricular performance in trained athletes. These observed differences may relate to altered loading conditions that diminish the ability of usual methods to evaluate accurately ventricular contractile performance (54). Because it is noninvasive, accurate, and repeatable over time, cardiac ultrasound provides an ideal imaging tool for the study of cardiac alterations that occur with exercise training. Accurate measurements of left ventricular wall thickness, volume, and mass as well as determination of other chamber sizes and cardiac contractility are all readily achieved using cardiac ultrasound. Currently, there is increasing interest in Doppler ultrasound measurement of blood flow velocity to evaluate the physiology of diastolic function. These ultrasound techniques far exceed the ability of the physical examination and radiographic methods to detect and discriminate between the pathologic and physiologic alterations that occur in patients and trained subjects.

Distinguishing Pathologic from Physiologic Changes in Athletes: The Cardiomyopathies

Because third and fourth heart sounds and ECG evidence for LVH frequently occur among trained individuals, and thus may suggest the presence of heart disease, it may be important to exclude pathologic changes in such subjects. The echocardiographic demonstration of symmetrical hypertrophy and normal contractility in the appropriate clinical setting may reveal the presence of physiologic hypertrophy (56). The hypertrophic cardiomyopathies are an important cause of sudden death in the young athlete. An autosomal dominant mode of inheritance is common; however, sporadic cases also occur. Murmurs detected during routine examination that suggest outflow obstruction or mitral insufficiency and abnormal ECG patterns, indicating hypertrophy or an infarction, may provide the first clue. A murmur that becomes softer when the athlete squats and louder when he or she stands up suggests hypertrophic cardiomyopathy (2). Young individuals with hypertrophic cardiomyopathy are especially prone to sudden death particularly when first-degree relatives have succumbed at an early age or when complex ventricular arrhythmias are observed during monitoring studies. A previous history of exertional syncope also portends a poor prognosis. Competitive exercise in such high-risk individuals should be prohibited. Among those with milder forms of hypertrophic cardiomyopathy, screening with 24-hr monitoring and exercise testing may allow participation in some competitive sports, although caution is advisable. Avoidance of dehydration is particularly important in these individuals.

Similarities in patterns of hypertrophy between individuals with hypertrophic cardiomyopathy and athletes who perform static exercise may, at times, be problematic (Table 8.5). In such cases it is helpful to examine first-degree relatives to see if they show the pattern of hypertrophy seen in hypertrophic cardiomyopathy. Evidence for ventricular outflow obstruction (presence of systolic anterior motion of the mitral valve leaflets and Doppler outflow tract gradients) and a pattern of septal "speckling" on echocardiography provide further support for pathologic hypertrophy. Patients with congestive (or "dilated") cardiomyopathy are generally easily distinguished by finding impaired LV contractility in association with enlarged LV chamber dimensions. Although a postviral or idiopathic etiology is most common in young individuals, other causes such as alcohol abuse and AIDS should also be considered.

Table 8.5.
Summary of Changes in LV Wall Thickness and Chamber Dimensions in Physiologic and Pathologic States

Sport	LV Thickness	LV Chamber Size
Physiologic states		
Long distance runners	↑[a]	↑↑
Power lifters, shot-putters, wrestlers	↑↑	↔
Cyclists, swimmers, rowers	↑	↑
Body builders	↑	↑
Sprinters	↔↑	↑
Pathologic states		
Hypertrophic cardiomyopathy	↑↑↑	↓
Congestive cardiomyopathy	↔↑	↑↑
Hypertension	↑↑	↔

[a] ↑, increased; ↓, decreased; ↔, unchanged.

Other Congenital Heart Diseases Presenting in Athletes

Although cardiomegaly, heart murmurs, and gallops are common among highly trained athletes (the so-called athlete's heart), pathologic causes should always be excluded by undertaking a careful history, physical examination, and cardiovascular testing, including electrocardiography and echocardiography. The more common causes of systolic heart murmurs found in association with congenital abnormalities include mitral regurgitation and midsystolic clicks caused by mitral valve prolapse, flow murmurs caused by atrial and ventricular septal defects, and ejection murmurs caused by aortic or pulmonic stenosis. A congenitally bicuspid aortic valve may present with an early systolic ejection sound at the base and systolic and diastolic murmurs related to valvular stenosis and insufficiency. The presence of significant aortic valvular stenosis may contraindicate competitive exercise; however, milder forms of stenosis and insufficiency may be well-tolerated. Static exercise, which markedly increases aortic pressure, should be especially avoided in those with significant aortic or mitral valvular insufficiency. A tall, thin body habitus with increased arm span, arched palate, arachnodactyly and lens abnormalities may suggest the presence of Marfan's syndrome. In this autosomal dominant inherited disorder, patients may present with a dilated ascending aorta, aortic insufficiency, and mitral prolapse. Aortic dissection is a feared and potentially fatal complication of this syndrome.

Acquired Valvular Heart Disease

Although the incidence of rheumatic heart disease has decreased markedly in the United States and other Western countries, it remains high in immigrants from underdeveloped or developing countries. Stenosis of the mitral valve may result in dyspnea during exercise, whereas the characteristic opening snap and soft apical diastolic rumble may be a subtle finding on cardiac examination. However, cardiac ultrasound is sensitive and specific to the identification and quantification of rheumatic lesions involving the mitral and aortic valves and should, therefore, be employed in the evaluation of all patients presenting with unexplained dyspnea. Endocarditis also may result in destruction of heart valves, and this diagnosis should be considered in the setting of new heart murmurs or dyspnea associated with fever.

Anabolic Steroids and the Heart

In addition to a variety of potentially serious adverse effects, the use of anabolic steroids results in disordered cholesterol metabolism. The resulting reduction in high-density lipoprotein (HDL) cholesterol is associated with an increased risk of developing premature CAD. All who provide health care to competitive ath-

Table 8.6.
Sample Questionnaire for Cardiovascular Screening of Athletes

1. Has it been more than 2 years since you had a physical exam that included a blood pressure reading and listening to the heart? ☐ Yes ☐ No
2. Have your parents or has a physician ever told you that you have a heart murmur? ☐ Yes ☐ No
3. Have you experienced resting or exertional chest pain, pressure, dizziness, or fainting within the past 2 years? ☐ Yes ☐ No
4. Has anyone in your family died suddenly at a young age (under age 45)? ☐ Yes ☐ No
5. Has a physician diagnosed anyone in your family with an abnormally thickened heart or Marfan's syndrome? ☐ Yes ☐ No
6. Do you use, or have you ever used, cocaine or anabolic steroids? ☐ Yes ☐ No
7. Has a physician ever suggested that you refrain from athletic competition? ☐ Yes ☐ No

Especially Important for Athletes Over Age 35:

8. Does your family (parents, grandparents, brothers, sisters) have a history of coronary artery disease, including heart attack, bypass surgery, balloon angioplasty, or angina, before age 65? ☐ Yes ☐ No
9. Do you smoke, have high blood pressure, high cholesterol, or diabetes? ☐ Yes ☐ No

If the answer to any of the above questions is yes, please give more details in the space below. A physician may need to review your medical status before you participate in sports.

____

____

____

____

WARNING: **Failure to answer these questions as honestly and accurately as possible may be hazardous to your health.**

Adapted from Ades PA. Preventing sudden death: cardiovascular screening of young athletes. Phys Sportsmed 1992;20(9):75–89.

letes should be aware of the current widespread use of anabolic steroids, even among high school students, and should be familiar with the hazards associated with their use (57).

Conclusion

The primary goal of cardiac preparticipation screening should be to determine whether the athlete has a history of syncope or chest pain, two of the most important symptoms for cardiovascular disease. Perhaps physicians can assess this information most economically with a questionnaire (Table 8.6), designed specifically to elicit a family history of sudden cardiac death or hypertrophic cardiomyopathy, Marfan's syndrome, or premature CAD (1). In such cases, additional studies such as echocardiography, treadmill testing, and lipid/lipoprotein profiling appear warranted. Sometimes the symptoms may reflect severe CAD or a potentially fatal arrhythmia. However, syncope or near syncope may also be the result of sympathetically mediated tachycardia, which may favorably respond to β-blocker therapy (2).

The Sixteenth Bethesda Conference (58) produced useful guidelines in screening for cardiovascular abnormalities in the athlete. The guidelines recommended that individuals with Marfan's syndrome or cystic medial necrosis avoid all sports involving body contact and high-intensity isotonic or isometric demands. It was suggested that low-risk patients with CAD could safely participate in nonvigorous competitive sports. On the other hand, high-risk patients with left ventricular dysfunction, exertional ischemia, or malignant ventricular arrhythmias should refrain from all competitive sports. Additional exercise recommendations for athletes with other cardiac conditions such as arrhythmias, hypertension, mitral valve prolapse, and valvular heart disease, were also listed.

The physician's role is to provide a clear recommendation of the advisability of sports participation based on the athlete's cardiovascular condition, the anticipated somatic and myocardial demands, and the associated risk. What an athlete does with a physician's recommendation to avoid sports participation is another matter. In some cases, he or she may seek a second opinion, hoping to avoid losing the opportunity to compete. If this reassurance fails to materialize, the athlete must ultimately ask this question: "Is my participation in competitive sports possibly worth dying for?"

REFERENCES

1. Ades PA. Preventing sudden death: cardiovascular screening of young athletes. Phys Sportsmed 1992;20(9):75–89.
2. Cheitlin MD. Evaluating athletes who have heart symptoms. Phys Sportsmed 1993;21(3):150–162.
3. Epstein SE, Maron BJ. Sudden death and the competitive athlete: perspectives on preparticipation screening studies. J Am Coll Cardiol 1986;7(1);220–230.
4. Lewis JF, Maron BJ, Diggs JA, et al. Preparticipation echocardiographic screening for cardiovascular disease in a large, predominantly black population of collegiate athletes. Am J Cardiol 1989;64:1029–1033.
5. Maron BJ, Bodison SA, Wesley YE, et al. Results of screening a large group of intercollegiate competitive athletes for cardiovascular disease. J Am Coll Cardiol 1987;10(6):1214–1221.
6. Franklin BA, Gordon S, Timmis GC. Fundamentals of exercise physiology: implications for exercise testing and prescription. In: Franklin BA, Gordon S, Timmis GC, eds. Exercise in modern medicine. Baltimore: Williams & Wilkins, 1989:1–21.

7. Åstrand PO, Rodahl K. Textbook of work physiology. New York: McGraw-Hill, 1970.
8. Taylor HL, Buskirk E, Henschel A. Maximal oxygen intake as an objective measure of cardiorespiratory performance. J Appl Physiol 1955;8:73–80.
9. Balke B. Experimental studies on the functional capacities of middle-aged and aging persons. J Okla State Med Assoc 1961;54:120–123.
10. Wilson PK, Bell CW, Norton AC. Rehabilitation of the heart and lungs. Fullerton, CA: Beckman Instruments, 1980.
11. Mitchell JH, Sproule BJ, Chapman CB. The physiological meaning of the maximal oxygen intake test. J Clin Invest 1958;37:538–547.
12. Bruce RA. Principles of exercise testing. In: Naughton JP, Hellerstein HK eds. Exercise testing and exercise training in coronary heart disease. New York: Academic Press, 1973:45–61.
13. Consolazio CF, Johnson RE, Pecora LJ. Physiological measurements of metabolic functions in man. New York: McGraw-Hill, 1963.
14. American College of Sports Medicine. Guidelines for graded exercise testing and exercise prescription. 4th ed. Philadelphia: Lea & Febiger, 1991.
15. Franklin BA, Kaimal KP, Moir TW, et al. Characteristics of national-class race walkers. Phys Sportsmed 1981;9:101–109.
16. Vander LB, Franklin BA, Wrisley D, et al. Physiological profile of national-class national collegiate athletic association fencers. JAMA 1984;252:500–503.
17. Wasserman K, Whipp BJ, Koyal SN, et al. Anaerobic threshold and respiratory gas exchange during exercise. J Appl Physiol 1973;35:236–243.
18. Davis JA, Vodak P, Wilmore JH, et al. Anaerobic threshold and maximal aerobic power for three modes of exercise. J Appl Physiol 1976;41:544–550.
19. Costill DL. Physiology of marathon running. JAMA 1972;221:1024–1029.
20. Costill DL, Fox EL. Energetics of marathon running. Med Sci Sports 1969;1:81–86.
21. Costill DL, Thomason H, Roberts E. Fractional utilization of the aerobic capacity during distance running. Med Sci Sports 1973;5:248–252.
22. Costill DL, Branam G, Eddy D, et al. Determinants of marathon running success. Int Z Angew Physiol 1971;29:249–254.
23. Rhodes EC, McKenzie DC. Predicting marathon time from anaerobic threshold measurements. Phys Sportsmed 1984;12:95–98.
24. Laslett LJ, Amsterdam EA. Management of the asymptomatic patient with an abnormal ECG. JAMA 1984;252:1744–1746.
25. Solomon H. Undue exertion: cardiac stress tests aren't worth the money—or the risk. The Sciences, 1986;(Jan–Feb):12–16.
26. Vander L, Franklin B, Rubenfire M. Cardiovascular complications of recreational physical activity. Phys Sportsmed 1982;10:89–98.
27. Diamond GA, Forrester JS. Analysis of probability as an aid in the clinical diagnosis of coronary-artery disease. N Engl J Med 1979;300:1350–1358.
28. Epstein SE. Implications of probability analysis on the strategy used for noninvasive detection of coronary artery disease. Am J Cardiol 1980;46:491–499.
29. Huston TP, Puffer JC, Rodney WM, et al. The athletic heart syndrome. N Engl J Med 1985;313:24–32.
30. Northcore RJ, McKillop G, Todd IC, et al. The effect of habitual sustained endurance exercise on cardiac structure and function. Eur Heart J 1990;11:17–22.
31. Lichtman J, O'Rourke RA, Klein A, et al. Electrocardiogram of the athlete. Arch Intern Med 1973;132:763–770.
32. Pantano JA, Oriel RJ. Prevalence of cardiac arrhythmias in apparently normal well trained runners. Am Heart J 1982;104:762–768.
33. Zehender M, Meinertz T, Keul J, et al. ECG variants and cardiac arrhythmias in athletes: clinical relevance and prognostic importance. Am Heart J 1990;113(6):1378–1391.
34. Furlanello F, Bettini R, Bertoldi A, et al. Arrhythmia patterns in athletes with arrhythmogenic right ventricular dysplasia. Eur Heart J 1989;10(suppl D):16–19.
35. Jones SR, Binder RA, Donowho EM, et al. Sudden death in the sickle cell trait. N Engl J Med 1970;282:323–325.
36. Diggs LW. The sickle cell trait in relation to the training and assignment of duties in the Armed Forces. III. Hyposthenuria, hematuria, sudden death, rehabdomyolysis, and acute tubular necrosis. Aviat Space Environ Med 1984;55:358–364.
37. Waller BF, Roberts WC. Sudden death while running in conditioned runners aged 40 years and over. Am J Cardiol 1980;45:1292–1300.
38. Maron BJ, Roberts WC, McAllister HA, et al. Sudden death in young athletes. Circulation 1980;62:218–229.
39. Morals AR, Romanelli R, Boucek RJ. The mural left anterior descending coronary artery, strenuous exercise and sudden death. Circulation 1980;62:230–237.
40. Thiene G, Nava A, Corrado D, et al. Right ventricular cardiomyopathy and sudden death in young people. N Engl J Med 1988;318:129–133.
41. Maron BJ, Epstein SE, Roberts WC. Causes of sudden death in competitive athletes. J Am Coll Cardiol 1986;7(1):204–214.
42. Corrado D, Thiene G, Nava A, et al. Sudden death in young competitive athletes: clinical pathologic correlations in 22 cases. Am J Med 1990;89(5):588–596.
43. Burke AP, Farb A, Virmani R, et al. Sports-related and non-sports related sudden cardiac death in young adults. Am Heart J 1991;121:568–575.
44. Franklin BA. Exertion-induced cardiovascular complications: is vigorous exercise worth the risk? Exerc Stand Malpractice Report 1988;2(3):33–41.
45. Siscovick DS, Weiss NS, Fletcher RH, et al. The incidence of primary cardiac arrest during vigorous exercise. N Engl J Med 1984;311:874–877.
46. Thompson PD, Mitchell JH. Exercise and sudden cardiac death: protection or provocation [editorial]. N Engl J Med 1984;311:914–915.
47. Bassler TJ. Marathon running and immunity to heart disease. Phys Sportsmed 1975;3:77–80.
48. Thompson PD, Stern MP, Williams P, et al. Death during jogging or running. A study of 18 cases. JAMA 1979;242:1265–1267.
49. Noakes TD, Opie LH, Rose AG, et al. Marathon running and immunity to coronary heart disease: fact versus fiction. In: Franklin BA, Rubenfire M, eds. Symposium on cardiac rehabilitation. Clinics in sports medicine. Vol. 3. Philadelphia: WB Saunders, 1984:527–543.
50. Gilbert CA, Nutter DO, Felner JM, et al. Echocardiographic study of cardiac dimensions and function in the endurance-trained athlete. Am J Cardiol 1977;40(4):528–533.
51. Morganroth J, Maron BJ, Henry WL, Epstein SE. Comparative left ventricular dimensions in trained athletes. Ann Intern Med 1975;82(4):521–524.
52. Raskoff WJ, Goldman S, Cohn K. The "athletic heart." Prevalence and physiological signficance of left ventricular enlargement in distance runners. JAMA 1976;236(2):158–162.
53. Bekaert I, Pannier JL, Van de Weghe C, et al. Non-invasive evaluation of cardiac function in professional cyclists. Br Heart J 1981;45(2):213–218.
54. Colan SD, Sanders SP, Borow KM. Physiologic hypertrophy: effects on left ventricular systolic mechanics in athletes. J Am Coll Cardiol 1987;9(4):776–783.
55. Hauser AM, Dressendorfer RH, Vos M, et al. Symmetric cardiac enlargement in highly trained endurance athletes: a two-dimensional echocardiographic study. Am Heart J 1985;109:1038–1044.
56. Roeske WR, O'Rourke, Klein A, et al. Noninvasive evaluation of ventricular hypertrophy in professional athletes. Circulation 1976;53(2):286–291.
57. Strauss RH, Wright JE, Finerman GAM, et al. Side effects of anabolic steroids in weight-trained men. Phys Sportsmed 1983;11(12):87–95.
58. Mitchell JM, Maron BJ, Epstein SE. Sixteenth Bethesda conference: cardiovascular abnormalities in the athlete. Recommendations regarding eligibility for competition. J Am Coll Cardiol 1985;6(6):1186–1232.

9 / DRUGS IN SPORTS

David A. Stone

Drugs in Sports

The use of drugs by athletes has become a highly charged, emotional issue. Coaches, athletes, physicians, teams, and regulatory bodies all choose sides and partners in an attempt to balance improved athletic performance and appropriate legal and ethical standards. Many athletes exist in an environment where athletic goals become the only priority and the normal checks and balances others often take for granted do not exist. An immature, impressionable, or superstitious athlete may be incapable of making the right decisions, let alone understanding the issues. The difficulty the average person would have in obtaining anabolic steroids or growth hormone does not exist in this environment, and the potential benefits to the athlete would far outweigh the side effects. Thus, lacking knowledge of scientific evidence of risk or benefit, and hoping to obtain an edge, or not to lose one, the athlete commits to a potentially dangerous course.

Drugs can be classified in a variety of ways.

1) By their legality,
2) By their help in training or performance,
3) By the condition that they treat, such as asthma medications, cold preparations, etc.,
4) By chemical action, such as diuretics, anabolic steroids, stimulants, etc.

None of these systems adequately describes their use, and many drugs fall into more than one category. For example nonsteroidal antiinflammatory drugs (NSAIDs) can control pain during training and also at the time of performance. Clenbuterol is a beta agonist, but also has some anabolic effects. In many respects, the best way to view a drug is by assessing why the athlete is taking it and what benefit they expect to derive from its use (Tables 9.1 and 9.2).

Ergogenic aids are usually defined as physical, mechanical, nutritional, psychological, or pharmacological substances or treatments that either directly improve physiological variables associated with exercise performance or remove subjective restraints which may limit physiological capacity (1). They include substances such as bee pollen, vitamins, vanadium, chromium, amino acids, boron, dietary manipulation, various herbs, as well as activities such as blood doping, soda loading, and phosphate loading. The use of many ergogenic aids is unsubstantiated by the medical and exercise physiology literature, but the risk of death or injury is also poorly defined in many cases.

Sodium Bicarbonate

Sodium bicarbonate ($NaHCO_3$) is presently considered an effective ergogenic aid for anaerobic events that are affected by the buildup of lactic acid in muscle, but are less than 4 minutes in duration. Traditionally, this includes the 400, 800, and 1500m races, but does not include longer runs, such as the marathon, which is more dependent on aerobic metabolism, or shorter springs, such as the 100m or 200m runs in which fatigue is unrelated to the buildup of lactic acid.

Following supramaximal contractions of muscle, intracellular pH decreases and lactate increases (2). The force of muscle contraction decreases as lactate and hydrogen ion accumulate (3). $NaHCO_3$ appears to enhance the buffering capacity of the extracellular environment, resulting in more efficient buffering of diffused H+ and lactate, and indirectly maintains intracellular pH. $NaHCO_3$ does not diffuse into muscle cells and cannot affect intracellular pH (3).

$NaHCO_3$ has long been considered an effective ergogenic aid. Dennig et al. (4) reported in the 1930s that $NaHCO_3$ could improve exercise performance in runners, but several other studies (5–7) performed later did not substantiate these results. In 1977, Jones et al. (8) were able to identify an ergogenic $NaHCO_3$ dosage and in 1983, Wilkes et al. (9) conducted a definitive study demonstrating the effectiveness of $NaHCO_3$, using a dose of 300 mg/kg body weight taken over a 2 hr period before practice in male varsity 800m and 1500m athletes. Calcium carbonate was used as a placebo. Five of the six subjects ran faster and the average improvement of 2.9 sec represented a distance estimated by the

Table 9.1.
NCAA Banned Drug Classes 1988 to 1989[a]

Psychomotor and central nervous system stimulants	
Amiphenazole	Meclofenoxate
Amphetamine	Methamphetamine
Bemigride	Methylphenidate
Benzphetamine	Nikethamide
Caffeine*	Norpseudoephedrine
Chlorphentermine	Pemoline
Cocaine	Pentetrazol
Cropropamide	Phendimetrazine
Crothetamide	Phenmetrazine
Diethylpropion	Phentermine
Dimethylamphetamine	Picrotoxine
Doxapram	Pipradol
Ethamivan	Prolintane
Ethylamphetamine	Strychnine
Fencamfamine	And related compounds
Sympathomimetic amines†	
Clorprenaline	Methoxyphenamine
Ephedrine	Methylephedrine
Etafedrine	Phenylpropanolamine
Isoetharine	Pseudoephedrine
Isoprenaline	And related compounds
Anabolic steroids	
Boldenone	Norethandrolone
Clostebol	Oxandrolone
Dehydrochlormethyl-testosterone	Oxymesterone
Fluoxymesterone	Oxymetholone
Mesterolone	Stanozolol
Methonolone	Testosterone‡
Methandienone	And related compounds
Nandrolone	
Substances banned for specific sports	
Rifle	Pindolol
Alcohol	Propranolol
Atenolol	Timolol
Metoprolol	And related compounds
Nadolol	
Diuretics	
Acetazolamide	Hydroflumethiazide
Bendroflumethiazide	Methyclothiazide
Benzthiazide	Metolazone
Bumetanide	Polythiazide
Chlorothiazide	Quinethazone
Chlorthalidone	Spironolactone
Ethacrynic acid	Triamterene
Flumethiazide	Trichlormethiazide
Furosemide	And related compounds
Hydrochlorothiazide	
Street drugs	
Heroin	THC (tetrahydrocannabinol)§
Marijuana§	

[a]Reprinted with permission from Haupt HA. Drugs in athletics. Clin Sports Med 1989; 8(3): 576 and from the 1988–1989 NCAA Drug Testing Program, p 8–9. Definition of positive depends on the following:

*For caffeine, if the concentration in urine exceeds 15 μg per mL.

†Refer to Section No. 3.5 of the drug-testing protocol or Executive Regulation 1-7-(c)-(5).

‡For testosterone, if the ratio of the total concentration of testosterone to that of epitestosterone in the urine exceeds 6.

§For marijuana and THC, if the concentration in the urine of THC metabolite exceeds 25 mg per mL.

authors of about 19m, often the difference between last and first in a college track meet. Subsequent studies have demonstrated an ergogenic "window" of 1 to 7 min of maximal exercise in which $NaHCO_3$ is effective (3). Nonetheless, it appears that novice runners,

Table 9.2.
Examples of the Doping Classes Banned by the USOC[a]

Generic Name	Example
Stimulants	
Amfepramone	Apisate, Tenuate, Tepanil
Amfetaminil	AM-1 (Germany)
Amiphenazole	Dapti, Daptizole, Amphisol
Amphetamine	Delcobese, Obetrol, Benzedrine, Dexedrine
Bemigride	Megimide
Benzphetamine	Didrex
Caffeine	12 μg/ml*
Cathine	(Norpseudoephedrine) Adiposetten N (Germany)
Chlorphentermine	Pre Sate, Lucofen
Clobenzorex	Dinintel (France)
Clorprenaline	Vortel, Asthone (Japan)
Cocaine	Surfacaine
Cropropamide	(component of "Micoren")
Crothetamide	(component of "Micoren")
Diethylpropion HCL	Tenuate, Tepanil
Dimetamfetamine	Amphetamine
Ephedrine	Tedral, Bronkotabs, Rynatuss, Primatene
Etafedrine	Mercodal, Decapryn, Nethaprin
Ethamivan	Emivan, Vandid
Etilamfetamine	Apetinil (Netherlands)
Fencamfamine	Envitrol, Altimine, Phencamine
Fenetylline	Captagon (Germany)
Fenproporex	Antiobes Retard (Spain), Appeitzugler (Germany)
Furfenorex	Frugal (Arg), Frugalan (Spain)
Isoetharine HCL	Bronkosol, Dronkometer, Numotac, Dilabron
Isoproterenol	Isuprel, Norisodrine, Metihaler-ISO
Meclofenoxate	Lucidril, Brenal
Mefenorex	Doracil (Arg), Pondinil (Switzerland), Rondimen (Germany)
Metaproterenol	Alupent, Metaprel (Oral Form-Tablets)
Methamphetamine*	Desoxyn, Met-Ampi
Methoxyphenamine	Ritalin, Orthoxicol Cough Syrup
Methylamphetamine	Desoxyn, Met-Ampi
Methylephedrine	Tzbraine, Methep (Germany, Great Britain)
Methylphenidate HCL	Ritalin
Morazone	Rosimon-Neu (Germany)
Nikethamide	Coramine
Pemoline	Cylert, Deltamin, Stimul
Pentetrazol	Leptazol
Phendimetrazine	Phenzine, Bontril, Plegine
Phenmetrazine	Preludin
Phentermine HCL	Adipex, Fastin, Ionamin
Phenylpropanolamine	Sinutab, Contac, Dexatrim
Picrotoxine	Cocculin
Pipradol	Meratran, Constituent of Alertonic
Prolintane	Villescon, Promotil, Katovit
Propylhexedrine	Benzedrex Inhaler
Pyrovalerone	Centroton, Thymergex
Strychnine	Movellan (Germany)
And related substances*	
Narcotic Analgesics	
Alphaprodine	Misentil
Anileridine	Leritine, Apodol
Buprenorphine	Buprenex
Codeine	Codicept (Germany), Codipertussin (Germany)
Dextromoramide	Palfium, Jetrium, D-Moramid, Dimorlin

Table 9.2. *continued*

Generic Name	Example
Dextropropoxyphen	Palfium, Jetrium, D-Moramid, Dimorlin
Diamorphine	Heroin
Dihydrocodeine	Synalogos DC, Paracodin
Dipipanone	Pipadone, Doconal, Wellconal
Ethoheptazine	Panalgin (Italy)
Ethylmorphine	Diosan Comp (Spain), Tracyl (France)
Levorphanol	Levo-Dromoran
Methadone HCL	Dolophine, Amidon
Morphine	Cyclimorph 10, Duramorph MST-Continus
Nalbuphine	Nubain
Pentazocine	Talwin
Pethidine (Europe)	Demerol, Centralgin, Dolantin, Dolosol, Pethold
Phenazocine	Narphen, Primadol
Trimeperdine	Demerol, Mepergan
And related compounds	
Hydrocodone	Hycodan, Tussionex
Oxocodone	Percodan, Vicodan
Oxomorphine	Narcan
Hydromorphone	Dilaudid
Tincture opium	Paregoric
Anabolic steroids	
Bolasterone	
Boldenone	Vebonol
Clostebol	Steranobol
Dehydrochlormethyl-Testosterone	Turnibol
Fluoxymesterone	Android F, Halotestin, Ora-testryl
Ultandren	
Mesterolone	Androviron, Proviron
Metandienone	Danabol, Dianabol
Metenolone	Primobolan, Primonabol-Depot
Methandrostenolone	Dianabol
Methyltestosterone	Android, Estratest, Methandren
Oreton, Testred	
Nandrobolic	Durabolin, Deca-Durabolin, Kabolin
Norethandrolone	Nilevar
Oxandrolone	Anavar
Oxymesterone	Oranabol, Theranabol
Oxymetholone	Anadrol, Nilevar, Anapolon 50, Adroyd
Stanozolol	Winstrol, Stroma
Testosterone*	Malogen, Malogex, Delatestryl, Oreton
And related compounds, ie, Danazol, Danocrine	
Testosterone†	
Beta Blockers	
Acebutolol	Sectral
Alprenolol	Aptine (France), Betacard (Austria), Sinalol (Japan)
Atenolol	Tenormin
Labetalol	Normodyne, Trandate
Metoprolol	Lopressor
Nadolol	Corgard
Oxprenolol	Apsolox, Oxanol (Spain), Trasacor (Japan)
Pindolol	Visken
Propanolol	Inderal
Sotalol	Betacardone (Arg), Sotalex (Germany)
Timolol	Blocadren
And related substances	
Diuretics	
Acetazolamide	Diamox, AK-ZOL, Dazamide
Amiloride	Midamor
Bendroflumethiazide	Naturetin
Benzthiazide	Aquatag, Exna, Hydrex, Mara-zide, Proaqua
Bumetanide	Bumex
Canrenone	Aldactone (Germany), Phanurane (France), Soldactone (Switzerland)
Chlormerodrin	Orimercur (Spain)
Chlortalidone	Hygroton, Hylidone, Thalitone
Diclofenamide	Daranide
Ethacrynic acid	Edecrin
Furosemide	Lasix
Hydrochlorothiazide	Esidrix, Hydro Diuril, Oretic, Thiuretic
Mersalyl	Mersalyl Injection
Spironolactone	Alatone, Aldactone
Triamterene	Dyrenium, Dyazide
And related substances	

[a]Reprinted with permission from Haupt HA. Drugs in athletics. Clin Sportsmed 1989; 8(3):577–579 and from Sports Mediscope. USOC Sports Medicine and Science Division Newsletter. 1988;7, (7):2–4.

*Vicks inhalers containing L-Desoxyephedrine (foreign produced inhalers do not contain this ingredient, but those sold in the USA do) used in excessive, non-recommended doses can produce the metabolite methamphetamine in the urine. Therefore, caution—Vicks Inhaler should not be used 48 hours before competition. Afrin Nasal Spray is an acceptable substitute if needed.

†The definition of a positive depends on the following: the administration of testosterone or the use of any other manipulation having the result of increasing the ratio in urine of testosterone/epitestosterone to above 6.

and even some marathon runners, appear to be using $NaHCO_3$ in longer events (Grollman L: Personal communication from manager of Pittsburgh Marathon, 1993).

Critical to the use of $NaHCO_3$ is the timing of the dosage. It would appear that the drug must be ingested less than 2 to 3 hours before competition (3). Side effects, in particular, abdominal pain and diarrhea, can be controlled by administering small frequent doses rather than a single large dose (10) and by consuming large amount of water to diminish the osmotic load on the stomach, but the runner who experiences running-induced gastrointestinal problems may find the drug intolerable. Half of the runners in the Wilkes et al. (9) study had urgent gastrointestinal distress within 1 hr of ingestion of $NaHCO_3$.

Growth Hormone

Human growth hormone (hGH) is a single chain polypeptide hormone composed of 191 amino acids with a molecular weight of about 22KDa (kilodaltons). Several "variants" of this molecule exist within the body. About 10% of hGH in the pituitary has a molecular weight of 20 KDa rather than the usual weight of 22KDa, and a large form of growth hormone, twice the size of hGH also exists, however it is probably a dimer rather than a precursor hormone (11). Growth hormone is produced by the somatotrophic cells in the anterior pituitary which contain a total of 5 to 10 mg of hGH (12). It is metabolized in the liver. The 24-hour secretion rate in young men is about 1 to 2 mg/day. Its plasma half-life is between 17 to 45 minutes (13), although some of its biologic effects are mediated by the somatomedins and last much longer.

Growth hormone is usually secreted in an intermittent, pulsatile fashion throughout the day. The largest peak occurs consistently 60 to 120 minutes after the onset of deep sleep (14). Athletes do not have a different pattern of hormone secretion than sedentary controls (15). Secretion is regulated by two hypothalamic peptides, growth hormone releasing hormone (GHR), and somatostatin. A variety of feedback mechanisms including drugs, nutritional status and diet, exercise, and levels of GHR and somatostatin control growth hormone release, all under the control of the 3′:5′-cyclic phosphate (cAMP) second messenger system (16). Athletes often use drugs, such as clonidine or levodopa, or nutritional supplements, such as arginine, to maximize secretion of growth hormone stimulation.

Growth hormone affects a variety of tissues in the body, including muscle, connective tissue, bone, and fat. Many of the physiologic effects are not completely understood and the ergogenic effects of growth hormone can be questioned. Nonetheless, its use by athletes is no longer anecdotal and with the increased emphasis on drug testing, substances like growth hormone that are not easily detectable with present methods are increasing in use although sparse epidemiologic data are available (17, 17a).

When hGH is given to GH deficient children, there is prompt stimulation of protein anabolism, increased intracellular transportation of amino acids, retention of nitrogen, and an increase in messenger RNA in muscle cells, enhanced synthesis of collagen in connective tissue, and increased intracellular catabolism of fat, resulting in increased circulation of free fatty acids, which can then be utilized as an energy source (12). Peripheral fat stores are reduced, and hepatic fat stores are increased (8). These anabolic actions are not sustained with repeated administration, and are often supplanted by insulin antagonism (12). Growth hormone inhibits the cellular uptake of glucose and decreases sensitivity to insulin. Total daily insulin production is increased. The retention of potassium, magnesium, and phosphate is also stimulated by hGH. Hypercalcuria occurs during the early weeks of hGH administration, and hGH has as a direct action on the proximal renal tubules, increasing reabsorption of phosphate (12).

Some of the effects of hGH are mediated by the somatomedins, which are peptides that resemble insulin in structure and in some actions. The somatomedins were originally given the names insulin-like growth factor I and II (IGF I and IGF II). The somatomedins can be synthesized by a number of cell types, but levels are growth hormone dependent. In growth hormone deficiency, levels of IGF I and IGF II are almost unmeasurable, while in acromegaly, levels are almost always elevated (19). In general, levels of IGF I are low in infancy, highest in adolescence, with a decline at the end of adolescence as adulthood is entered. They return to prepubertal levels after the age of fifty (16). The somatomedins have an anabolic and mitogenic effect on cartilage and fibroblasts, but the contributions of hGH and IGF I to growth have not been determined (20). In vitro, somatomedins have also been shown to have mitogenic effects on myocytes, osteocytes, adipocytes, and hepatocytes (11).

Among ergogenic aids hGH appears to be ideal. It is both anabolic and lipolytic, and it stimulates synthesis of collagen to strengthen connective tissue and to reduce risk of connective tissue injury from the forces generated by larger, more powerful muscles. Nonetheless, controversy over its effectiveness exists because animal studies on the effectiveness of growth hormone are not convincing. In 1952, Bigland and Jehring (21) treated fully grown normal rats with growth hormone for 21 days, and were matched with controls for activity and diet. At the end of the test period, growth-hormone-treated rats were 20% heavier and had quadriceps weights that were 26.6% greater. However, despite the increase in quadriceps size and muscle fiber cross sectional diameter of 6 to 12% the growth-hormone-treated quadriceps did not develop greater tension and did not perform as well as control animals on tests comparing tension per gram of muscle weight.

Apostolakis et al. (22) studied the effects of hGH on atrophied muscle in rats. He immobilized one leg and used the corresponding extremity for comparison. Growth hormone increased the weight of the atrophied muscles by 19% when compared to untreated controls, Twitch and tetanic contractions were increased by 58% and 65%, respectively, when compared with controls, but no increase in the tension produced was found in the normal, nonatrophied, contralateral controls. It is postulated that growth hormone increases collagen synthesis in muscle rather than muscle fiber synthesis (23).

The effects of obesity on growth hormone are clear. In obese patients, concentrations of hGH are normal or reduced (24); the typical increase in hGH levels in response to arginine infusion is blunted (25), although it is not in very muscular or overweight men (26); and the rise in hGH level that occurs with deep sleep is also reduced (27). Obese subjects treated with hGH show increases in oxygen consumption (28) and increased catabolism of fatty acids from adipose tissue.

The cost of a one-month supply of hGH is generally estimated at $350 (17). In the U.S., hGH is synthesized using recombinant DNA technology. Cadaveric hGH is associated with cases of Jacob-Creutzfeldt disease (29) and has not been available in the United States since 1986, but it is still available in foreign countries. Animal growth hormone preparations and foreign products are now considered to be the primary black market sources of growth hormone (30), but there is a significant difference in the structure of primate and human growth hormone from mammalian growth hormone, and human beings do not respond to growth hormone of nonprimate origin (31).

Blood Doping and Erythropoietin

Blood doping is a procedure in which normovolemic erythrocythemia is produced by transfusion of autologous or homologous red blood cells (RBCs). This technique was initially used to study hematologic control mechanisms for systemic transport of oxygen during acute hypoxic exposure (32) and demonstrated significant physiologic benefits not duplicated in subsequent studies that used refrigerated blood (33, 34), not freshly transfused blood. Gledhill (35) notes that 30 to 35% of the red cells are lost during the storage period due to aging and processing, and the reported increases in hemoglobin or hematocrit in all studies except the initial study were small. Because the ergogenic properties of normovolemic erythrocythemia are dependent on increasing hemoglobin concentration, studies that reinfused whole blood but did not increase hemoglobin concentration sufficiently would not be expected to demonstrate any benefit. In 1972, Ekblom et al. (36) demonstrated, in an uncontrolled study using refrigerated blood, an increase in maximal oxygen uptake and in all-out running time to exhaustion. Subsequently, studies using freeze-preserved RBCs also demonstrated ergogenic benefits (37, 38).

Blood doping results in augmented oxygen delivery to tissues, improved carbon dioxide transport, and acid-base balance. When transfusion takes place, a shift of protein-free plasma filtrate from the intravascular to interstitial compartment occurs, resolving the post-infusion hypervolemia. The resulting decrease in plasma volume produces a rapid restoration of normal blood volume in the presence of increased hemoglobin concentration. Following transfusion, both hemoglobin and hematocrit are elevated within 24 hours, and remain constant for the next 7 days. Over the next 15 weeks, values gradually return to control levels (39).

Erythropoietin acts in several ways to increase the number of circulating RBCs. Its primary action is to increase the number of erythroid precursors within the marrow, but it also acts on more mature erythroid progenitors and stimulates early release of immature RBCs (9). A normal person replaces about 1% of the circulating RBCs per day, but when stimulated by erythropoietin, the erythroid marrow can increase RBC production by 2 to 3 times, and with prolonged stimulation, by 10 times (40). Erythropoietin exists in two forms, an acidic glycoprotein with a molecular weight of 39,000, and a desialated form with a molecular weight of 34,000, which appears to be active in vitro but not in vivo (40).

Ekblom and Berglund (41) have demonstrated the ergogenic benefits of erythropoietin using time to exhaustion and $\dot{V}_{O_{2max}}$. Epidemiologic studies of its use by athletes have not been performed, and, as yet, assays for detection are still being developed. The recent deaths of Belgian and Dutch cyclists have led some authors to suspect erythropoietin use, but no definitive statements can be made (42).

Anabolic Steroids

Anabolic steroids are perhaps the most prevalent problem of the sports medicine community today. Patterns of use have been studied in a variety of populations, and all indications are that use is increasing in spite of drug testing, negative press, and concerns expressed by the medical community (43). Drugs that were once relegated only to weight lifters are now used throughout the spectrum of sport, including women's events and endurance events (44, 45). Much of the appeal of anabolic steroids is the perception that they are effective ergogenic aids and will work for anyone willing to use them in appropriate amounts and in conjunction with the proper training program—regardless of what exercise physiologists, physicians, or anyone else has to say (46). This is not an inappropriate point of view. While the medical and exercise physiology communities had difficulty proving the effectiveness of anabolic steroids (47, 48), athletes who knew they worked used them and did so effectively for many years before definitive evidence was available (49). There is still some question whether anabolic steroids are actually able to enhance athletic performance, because no study can ethically study the excessive doses used in a typical athlete's drug regimen (50), but it is generally accepted that they do enhance performance (45).

The initial demonstration of the anabolic effect of androgens is generally attributed to Kochakian and Murlin (51), who injected male hormone into castrated dogs, decreasing protein breakdown and achieving a positive nitrogen balance. In the late 1930s and early 1940s, testosterone was administered as an anabolic agent in patients with wasting and chronic disease (52). During World War II, it was used by the Germans to make soldiers more aggressive (53). In the early 1950s, the Soviets began experimenting with testosterone on their athletes, and at the 1956 Olympics, John B. Zeigler, an American medical officer witnessed their use and brought it to light. Following this discovery, the CIBA drug company and Dr. Ziegler collaborated on the development of methandrostenolone, a synthetic derivative of testosterone designed to enhance the anabolic effects of testosterone while minimizing the androgenic effects. Thus was the first of the anabolic-androgenic steroids born (45). Attempts to completely remove any androgenic side effects from these drugs have failed, leading some authors to call these drugs "anabolic-androgenic steroids" (49). Initially, these drugs had some medical indications in addition to their use by athletes, including the treatment of hypogonadal males, some anemias, angioneurotic edema, muscle injuries, endometriosis, osteoporosis, and impotence. However, indications have decreased over time, and, at present, tighter control over these drugs is becoming commonplace. Steroids approved for therapeutic uses include stanozolol (Winstrol), methandrostenolone (Dianabol), and nandrolone phenpropionate (Durabolin) (12).

Several different populations have been studied for steroid use (55–62); however, many of the recent studies have focused on adolescent use (58–61). In all studies, the primary reason participants used steroids, when stated, was to increase strength or athletic performance. Other reasons offered included improved physical appearance or social pressures, prevention and treatment of sports injuries, improved sexual performance, and increased sexual organ size. All studies indicated that medical knowledge of steroids and the side effects of their use were lacking. The study of Johnson et al. (60) demonstrated that information sources for anabolic steroid users were more likely to be peers or television than a physician or health professional. The percentage of subjects surveyed who used anabolic steroids ranged from 3 to 11.1%. Athletes tended to use steroids more than nonathletes, but almost 1/3 of all users in the Buckley et al (58) study were not athletes, and almost 2/3 of all users had started use before age 16. This trend towards early usage was highlighted by the survey of Radakovich et al. (19), who studied seventh-grade students' knowledge and use of anabolic steroids in an agricultural-industrial community and found a 3.8% overall use rate, (4.7% males, 3.2% females). Those students most interested in participating in football and wrestling used steroids significantly more often than those interested in other sports. Of the students who used steroids, 83% had tried other drugs, in particular, alcohol and marijuana.

When looking at older age groups, the use of steroids seems to increase in selected populations. The study by Pope et al. (53), demonstrated that 17% of college athletes were using anabolic steroids compared to 2% of all college males. Kersey (55) looked at the use of anabolic steroids in health club athletes with a mean age of 30 years and found that 15% were using or had used anabolic steroids. A study by Frankle et al. (63) found that more than 40% (110 of 250 interviewed) of all persons regularly training at gyms were using steroids.

Of as much interest as the populations using steroids is the way they are used. As described by Frankle et al. (63), use is cyclic, with athletes "cycling" on and off drugs for various periods of time. In Frankle's study, these cycles lasted from 4 to 18 weeks, with drug-free periods lasting from one month to one year. In the study by Strauss et al. (57), looking at women body builders, mean cycle length was 9.2+/−2.2 weeks, with an average of 3 cycles per year, although some body builders continued low-dose steroids between cycles. In the study by Perry et al, (43) cycle length was 7 to 14 weeks. Frankle also described "pyramiding"—the concept of starting with a low dose, increasing the dose over time, then tapering the dose gradually prior to stopping completely—and "stacking"—the use of multiple steroids at once, often a combination of oral and injectable agents. The female body builders of the Strauss et al. study used 3.1+/−1.7 anabolic agents, and, at peak usage, the combined dosage was nine times the manufacturers recommendation. Perry et al. (43) noted an average of 2 or 3 oral preparations and 2 long-acting injectable preparations, with dosages of the oral drugs close to manufacturers' recommendations, but dosages of the long-acting injectable preparations were 3 to 8 times those of controlled studies. Use in health clubs, according to Kersey (55), was less aggressive, with only 50% of users stacking and the majority of users employing 6 to 9 week cycles. Buckley et al. (58) found that 44% of the high school users in his study had "stacked," and 38% used injectable preparations.

Anabolic steroids have a wide variety of effects and side effects and these have been reviewed by a number of authors (45, 48, 49, 52, 57, 64–66). While most agree that the large majority of side effects resolve with cessation of the drug, it is clear from recent case reports that this is not always the situation; the consequences of steroid use can affect a variety of organ systems and even result in death (45, 67). Unfortunately, biologic variability makes predicting those at risk difficult, although prolonged useage would appear to be a risk factor. Alen et al. (68) studied endocrine responses in 7 male power lifters who self-medicated with black market steroids through their usual 12 week cycles. He found significant decreases in concentrations of thyroid stimulating hormone (TSH), thyroxine, free thyroxine, triiodothyronine (T_3), and thyroid hormone binding globulin (TBG). The value of T_3 uptake increased. Serum testosterone concentration increased, but so did serum estradiol levels. Luteinising hormone (LH) and follicle stimulating hormone (FSH) levels decreased substantially, resulting in decreased testicular testosterone production, characterized by low serum testosterone levels at 4 weeks and 9 weeks after the cycle was completed, an indication of prolonged suppression of the body's own testosterone production. In 5 of the 7 subjects, growth hormone levels increased 5- to 60-fold at some time during the study, which, the authors suggested, might strengthen the anabolic effects of the drugs.

Administration of anabolic steroids also reverses the LDL/HDL ratio, increasing levels of LDL, and decreasing levels of HDL (69–71). The effect may be less with testosterone as compared to its synthetic derivatives (70). There are several enzymes that affect lipid metabolism and that could be responsible for these changes. Lecithin cholesterol acyltransferase catalyzes the transfer of fatty acids from lecithin to cholesterol and assists in the conversion of HDL_3 to HDL_2. Apolipoprotein A-1, is an activator of LCAT and has been shown to be inhibited by stanozolol. Hepatic lipase is thought to hydrolyse phospholipids on the surface of HDL particles, irreversibly degrade apoproteins, and catalyze the hydrolysation of the fatty ester bond of triglycerides. In athletes using anabolic steroids, elevated hepatic lipase activity has been found. While the consequences of short term, intermittent use of anabolic steroids are not known, these data make continuous use appear quite dangerous (72).

The effects of anabolic-androgenic steroids on fibroblasts, in particular on tendons have been studied by a variety of authors (73). Initial results were equivocal, with some studies demonstrating depression of collagen synthesis and others enhancement. More recent work, however, has shown a more disconcerting bent. Michna (73) studied the effects of methandienone (Dianabol) on mice adapted to running on a treadmill and found considerable alterations in collagen fibril architecture between 1 week and 10 weeks. He felt that steroids produced time-dependent collagen abnormalities. Karpakka et al (73a) found a transitory effect on collagen biosynthesis in male rat tendon, using nandrolone decanoate (Deca-Durabolin) for up to 3 weeks. The changes were most marked in the first week, and by the third week had returned to baseline values. Wood et al. (74) studied the mechanical and morphologic changes of rat Achilles tendons after administration of nandrolone laurate (Laurabolin) for 6 weeks. Four groups were studied, 1) an exercise and anabolic steroid group, 2) an exercise-only group, 3) an anabolic steroid and rest group, and 4) a rest-only group. They found alterations in crimp length and angle most significant in the rats that were exercised on anabolic steroids. They concluded that anabolic steroids alter the mechanical properties of the tendon in a way that predisposes them to injury. Miles et al. (75) evaluated the effects of anabolic steroids and exercise on rats given both Winstrol (stanozolol) and Deca-Durabolin (nandrolone decanoate). He found that anabolic steroid use produced a stiffer tendon with increased cross-sectional area in the exercised group, but in the group that received anabolic steroids and was not exercised, no significant changes were noted. The reduced flexibility of the tendon reduced the energy the tendon could absorb before failure, making the tendon more susceptible to injury, despite the fact that the maximum force the tendon could absorb was not effected.

The effects of anabolic steroids on muscle are mediated in several different ways: 1) They improve utilization of ingested protein, increasing nitrogen retention (49). This effect is contingent upon adequate protein and calorie intake, and in the normal state of the body, is short lived. In castrated animals, the effect is prolonged, although steroids may depress appetite and actually may reduce body weight (64). 2) They promote the synthesis of protein in skeletal muscle and other tissues. This can result in an increase in lean body weight, as well as in muscular strength. In many of the studies on anabolic steroids, strength gains were unimpressive, especially for beginners. However, as noted by Lamb (64), those same gains at a championship level would be substantial, and experienced weight lifters tended to derive more benefit from the use of steroids than beginners did (64). Salmons (76) used nandrolone decanoate and electrical stimulation of different muscles in different species of animals (rabbit, mouse, rat, and guinea pig) to demonstrate that these drugs have a significant myotrophic effect. He noted that some muscles were more sensitive to the effects of the drug than others, and the differences were species-specific in some cases. 3) They can reverse the catabolic effects of glucocorticoids released during stress, in this case, intense training. This theory was first proposed by Mayer and Rosen (77), and many authors have embraced it (49). Salmons (76) looked at the benefits of nandrolone in adrenalectomized rats and did not find any difference in the effects of the drug on muscle size in the control group or in the adrenalectomized animals. More basic science research on this aspect of anabolic steroids needs to be performed. 4) There are substantial motivational effects. Athletes using anabolic steroids have described a variety of emotional states ranging from euphoria and diminished fatigue to increased aggressiveness (78), some of which appear to aid training.

In addition to the effects noted above, a variety of side effects have been noted. Strauss et al. (57) noted deepening of the voice, increased facial hair, clitoral enlargement, and menstrual irregularities in the female body builders he studied. Of the women in the study, 50% thought there was a decrease in breast size. It is important to note that these side effects, though undesirable, were tolerable to these women.

The cutaneous side effects of anabolic steroids have been reviewed by Scott (79), who noted cystic acne, androgenic alopecia, hirsutism, and jaundice as the most common manifestations, but he also described oily skin, seborrhea, and a variety of persistent bacterial and fungal skin infections. He noted that in the vast majority of cases, side effects were completely reversible with cessation of the drugs, although in some cases of androgenic alopecia, complete restoration of hair did not occur.

Nearly all of the oral anabolic steroids produce abnormal liver function (64). Most of the orally active steroids are produced by adding an alkyl group at C-17 of the D-ring in the testosterone nucleus to retard the degradation of the drug by the liver, and this is associated with hepatotoxic effects (80). Among the abnormalities described are abnormal liver function tests, (LFT's) most commonly alanine transferase (ALT), alkaline phosphatase, bilirubin, and aspartate transferase (AST), bromsulphalein retention, cholestatsis, and jaundice (49, 64). Liver tumors have also been associated with androgen useage in medical conditions and one death by hepatic carcinoma in a young body builder has been reported (67). Vesselinovitch et al. (81) noted that endogenous sex steroid hormones modify the development of tumors in both target organs (breast, gonads) and in the liver and kidney, possibly by influencing the enzymatic profile of the liver, potentially modifying clearance of environmental carcinogens or other mediators. Saborido et al. (80) were able to demonstrate that while using high doses of androgens in rats did not impair liver function, levels of cytochrome p-450 and cytochrome b5 were significantly reduced. Peliosis hepatitis, a condition characterized by cystic degeneration of the liver, has been associated with the use of androgens for medical conditions and with tuberculosis (66).

Although anabolic steroids have been associated with increased aggressiveness, increased or decreased sex drive, and mood swings (22), until the late 1980s, there were only 4 case reports of more significant psychiatric effects. Pope and Katz (82) solicited structured interviews using the DSM-III-R severe combined immunodeficiency disorders (SCID), comparing periods of steroid exposure with periods of no exposure on 41 athletes (39 men and 2 women) using anabolic steroids. They found that 9 patients (22%) displayed a full affective syndrome, and 5 (12%) displayed psychotic symptoms. Five (12.2%) subjects developed major depression while withdrawing from steroids, and recent concerns about potential addiction to these drugs have been voiced (66). Only a minority of the steroid users from whom they solicited interviews responded, and they felt that a significant underground subculture of users existed. Although the true incidence of severe psychologic and neurologic side effects of anabolic steroid use are still not clear, these may be among the most disabling side effects the steroid user experiences.

Anabolic steroid use has also been associated with several case reports of cardiomyopathy and myocardial infarction in apparently young, healthy males (83, 84). At present, no established cause and effect relationship between steroids and myocardial infarction or myocarditis exists. However, the timing of these events, and the lack of risk factors in these cases make this a source of concern for the potential user.

Case reports on prolonged hypogonadism following frequent "cycles" of anabolic steroids (85) and bilateral avascular necrosis of the femoral heads (86) have also been reported.

Stimulants

Stimulants are used by athletes to produce alertness, increase the ability to concentrate, and decrease sensitivity to pain. With the exception of caffeine, there is no hard scientific evidence that these drugs actually improve performance, although their ability to disguise the physiological symptoms of fatigue can seduce an athlete into believing they can (87).

Caffeine represents a legitimate ergogenic aid only for exercise performed for prolonged periods at 70 to 80% $\dot{V}_{O_2max}$ (88, 89). A variety of studies on human subjects have demonstrated its lack of effect on strength and power (90), although in vitro studies have established that large doses of caffeine can increase the force of muscle contraction (91).

Caffeine is a methylxanthine, one of a group of chemicals that includes theophylline and theobromine. They are found in more than 60 species of plants worldwide, including coffee beans, cocoa beans, cola nuts and tea leaves. The amount of caffeine in these sources varies considerably (Table 9.3), depending on the particular variety of bean or leaf, where it was grown, type of cut or grind, and length of brewing time. Cola nuts have very little caffeine and caffeine is usually added to soft drinks (Table 9.4). It is readily absorbed after ingestion and peak blood levels are attained within 30 minutes. Caffeine is also found in a variety of prescription and nonprescription medications, including cold remedies, pain relievers, weight control aids, and stimulants (92).

The ergogenic effect of caffeine is based on three possible mechanisms. 1) Increased affinity of myofilaments for calcium or increased release of calcium in the sarcoplasmic reticulum in skeletal muscle. 2) Accumulation of cyclic nucleotides by inhibition of phosphodiesterase. 3) Blockage of adenosine receptors (90, 93). Adenosine dilates blood vessels, slows the rate of cardiac pacemaker cells, and inhibits lipolysis (90, 93).

Of the three mechanisms, blockage of adenosine receptors may be the most important (90), and the effect on lipolysis would coincide with the traditional explanation for caffeine's effect on endurance exercise, namely, its effect on substrate utilization. Caffeine has been shown to promote lipolysis and fat metabolism, and to spare muscle glycogen utilization (89).

Other important physiologic effects of caffeine include its diuretic effect, which is mild compared to oral diuretics, but present even in mild doses, and its ability to increase basal metabolic rate by about 10% at doses of between 3 to 9 mg/kg. The half-life of caffeine is about 3.5 hours. The usual ergogenic dose is between 250 to 350 mg, or 5 mg/kg. Urine levels greater than 12 mcg/ml are considered doping in international competition (94). To attain these urine concentrations would require about 6 to 8 cups of coffee within 2 to 3 hours of test-

Table 9.3.
Caffeine Content of Various Soft Drinks[a]

Soft Drinks*	Caffeine (mg per 12-oz Serving)†
Sugar-Free Mr. PIBB	58
Mountain Dew	54
Mello Yello	52
TAB	46
Coca-Cola	46
Diet Coke	46
Shasta Cola	44
Shasta Diet Cola	44
Mr. PIBB	40
Dr Pepper	40
Sugar-Free Dr Pepper	40
Pepsi Cola	38.4
Diet Pepsi	36
Pepsi Light	36
RC Cola	36
Diet Rite	0
Canada Dry Diet Cola	0

[a]Reprinted with permission from Slavin JL, et al. Caffeine and sports performance. Phys Sportsmed 1985; 13(5):191.
*At least 70 types of soft drinks manufactured by the 12 leading bottlers contain no caffeine.
†Data obtained from the National Soft Drink Association.

Table 9.4.
Caffeine Content of Popular Beverages and Food[a]

Item	Caffeine (mg)*
Coffee (5-oz cup)	
Drip method	110–150
Percolated	64–124
Instant	40–108
Decaffeinated	2–5
Instant decaffeinated	2
Tea (loose or bags) (5-oz cup)	
One-minute brew	9–33
Three-minute brew	20–46
Five-minute brew	20–50
Tea products	
Instant tea (5-oz cup)	12–28
Iced tea (12-oz cup)	22–36
Cocoa	
Made from mix	6
Milk chocolate (1 oz)	6
Baking chocolate (1 oz)	35

[a]Reprinted with permission from Slavin JL, et al. Caffeine and sports performance. Phys Sportsmed 1985; 13(5):191.
*Data for caffeine content obtained from Consumers Union, Food and Drug Administration, National Coffee Association, and National Soft Drink Association.

ing. The accepted level for the NCAA is 15 mug/ml. Doses of 3 to 10 g are usually considered toxic. These doses produce plasma levels of about 500umol/L.

Amphetamines are sympathomimetic amines that function as central nervous system and adrenergic nervous system stimulants through both direct and indirect actions. Amphetamine, dextroamphetamine, and methamphetamine are so similar in their effects that they can only be differentiated from each other by laboratory analysis (95). While far more popular in the 1950s and late 1960s than at present, their use tends to be cyclic, and these drugs may once again become popular (96). There are studies demonstrating benefits in athletic performance from the use of amphetamines (97, 98), especially when speed endurance and power are essential; however, these studies have been criticized for not addressing factors such as coordination, judgment, and timing (99). Other studies (100) have not demonstrated these same benefits. While some authors (101) feel the amphetamine is being replaced by cocaine, others note that its place in sports is secure and still prevalent (102). Amphetamines are banned by both the National Collegiate Athletic Association (NCAA) and the United States Olympic Committee (USOC).

Amphetamines are excellent appetite suppressants, but significant tolerance to these drugs occurs, and they have numerous adverse reactions and side effects involving the cardiovascular and central nervous systems. Hypothermia is also a potential problem.

Cocaine use in sports appears to be still largely recreational, especially following its epidemic use in the 1980s (10) and the much publicized deaths of Len Bias and Don Rogers, although as with amphetamines, perceived benefits from use are mentioned by some authors (103).

While cocaine has no significant benefits, it has substantial side effects associated with its acute use, in addition to its risk of addiction. Lange et al. (104) studied the effects of intranasal cocaine on blood flow, dimensions of the coronary arteries, and on myocardial oxygen demand in patients undergoing cardiac catheterization. He noted increases in heart rate, arterial pressure, and myocardial oxygen demand as well as decreases in coronary sinus blood flow and the diameter of the left coronary artery. No patient had chest pain or electrocardiographic changes. Patients with coronary artery disease were no different from patients with normal arteries. The doses used were much smaller than those generally estimated in recreational use (2 mg/kg body weight versus 25 mg per "line" of cocaine, 4 to 20 times/day (105). The authors speculated that patients experiencing sudden death or myocardial infarction induced by cocaine had intense and sustained coronary vasoconstriction in response to high serum cocaine concentrations.

Isner et al. (106) reviewed the clinical and pathological findings in 26 patients in whom cocaine use was temporally related to acute myocardial infarction, myocarditis ventricular arrhythmias, sudden death, or a combination of these events. They found that the cardiac consequences of cocaine use are not limited to massive doses of cocaine and that seizure activity was not a prerequisite or complication of cardiac toxicity. All patients in their study used cocaine intranasally.

Roth et al. (107) reviewed their experience with acute rhabdomyolysis associated with cocaine use, identifying 39 patients. Mean serum creatine kinase level was 12,187 U/L with a range of 1756 to 39,000. There were 6 deaths, all of whom developed acute renal failure, liver dysfunction, and disseminated intravascular coagulation. The pathophysiology was unclear, with vasoconstriction and hyperthermia, both common responses to cocaine use, considered. Muscle injury this severe in an athlete could be a career threat.

Miscellaneous Drugs

Diuretics are used by athletes to mask substances in drug tests and to make weight in sports such as boxing, wrestling, and judo where weight classes define competition. Diuretics have been shown to decrease muscular work and exercise tolerance to the degree of the dehydration that is produced (108). Electrolyte imbalances must be looked for when use of diuretics is known.

Beta blockers are used in shooting events to steady the hand and decrease heart rates, avoiding the effect of cardioballistic vibrations. Because they decrease cardiac endurance in trained athletes, beta blockers are often not effective drugs for the treatment of hypertension in athletes (109).

Probenecid is used by anabolic steroid abusers to reduce urine concentration of anabolic steroids (109).

Drug Testing

Drug testing has become a part of life for many team physicians at the college and professional level. A working knowledge both of banned substances and testing methods is necessary when abuses occur. Initially, drug testing was performed to "create a level field" by banning substances that enhanced performance; however, the issues of "medical safety," (the need to control dangerous drugs) and "social acceptability," (i.e., recreational drugs) have also been incorporated into drug testing schemes (110).

The legal aspects of drug testing have been debated continuously since the deaths of Len Bias and Don Rogers in 1986. While support for drug testing programs remains strong, compulsory testing of urine may be considered a "search and seizure" and a violation of the Fourth Amendment (111). Methods of collecting urine and a coherent drug policy formulated through the athletic department of the university or team administration are absolute requirements for a good drug testing program. There is no substitute for making athletes aware of policy and banned substances. An emphasis on treatment rather than punishment must also be incorporated into the program.

A wide variety of screening techniques are available to detect the presence of drugs in the urine. Radioimmunoassays and enzyme multiplied immunoassay are considered questionable to poorly specific for detecting abuses. Gas, liquid, and thin layer chromatography are considered adequate. Gas chromatography combined with mass spectroscopy (GC/MS) is considered highly specific, and only GC/MS provides legally admissible data (112).

Analytical strategies to detect and confirm detection are based on available technology (Table 9.5). Preanalytical sample manipulations are difficult and require experience. Generally, trainers are the persons collecting samples of urine for transport to a laboratory facility, so that maintenance of the chain of custody becomes more important than specimen preparation. Decisions regarding whether or not to test for specific drugs as well as for potential masking agents are often based on cost. With the detection of anabolic steroids, preliminary GC/MS is performed and then confirmed with more specific techniques (112) (Fig. 9.1).

It is very clear that drug testing has not proven to be a good deterrent to drug use in sports. Understanding the drugs athletes use and why they are using drugs is only part of the solution. Education in training techniques that maximize performance without drug use should be our ultimate goal.

Table 9.5.
Approximate Drug Elimination Time[a]

Drug	Approximate Elimination Time
Stimulants, i.e. amphetamines and derivatives	1 to 7 days
Cocaine: occasional use	6 to 12 hours
Cocaine: repeated use within 48 hrs	3 to 5 days (CAUTION: possibly longer!)
Codeine and narcotics in cough medicines	24 to 48 hours
Tranquilizers	4 to 8 days
Marijuana (Tetrahydrocannabiol)	3 to 5 weeks
Anabolic Steroids:	
Fat-soluble injectable types	6 to 8 months
Oral or Water-soluble types	3 to 6 weeks
Over-the-counter cold medications containing ephedrine derivatives as decongestants	48 to 72 hours

[a]Reprinted with permission from Newsom MM, Waters D, Grice J. Colorado Springs, CO: USOC Drug Education Program, 1989:43.

REFERENCES

NaHCO3

1. Williams MH, Lindhejm M Schuster R. Effect of blood infusion upon endurance capacity and ratings of perceived exertion. Med Sci Sports 1978;10:113–118.
2. Mainwood GW, Worsley-Brown P. The effects of extracellular pH and buffer concentration of the efflux of lactate from frog sartorius muscle. J Physiol 1975; 250:1–22.
3. Linderman J. Fahey TD. Sodium bicarbonate ingestion and exercise performance; an update. Sports Med 1991;11:71–77.
4. Dennig H, Talbot JH, Edwards HT, et al. Effects of acidosis and alkalosis upon the capacity for work. J Clin Invest 1931;9:601–613.

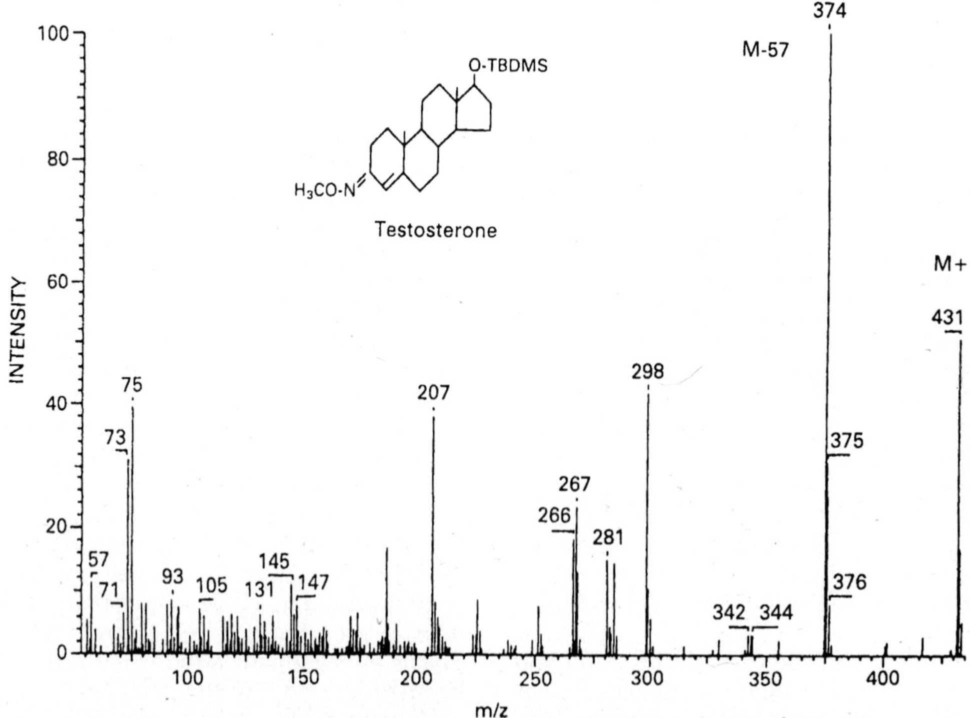

Figure 9.1. Electron impact spectrum of testosterone cypionate *(top)* after partial separation using direct exposure probe. The first peak in the reconstructed ion chromatogram *(bottom)* indicates where the selected scan was obtained. Reprinted with permission from Shipe JR. Mass spectrometry instrumentation in the 1990s. In: Shipe JR, Savory J, eds. Drugs in competitive athletics. Int. Union Pure and Applied Chemistry. Oxford: Blackwell, 1991:66.

5. Johnson WR, Black DH. Comparison of effects of certain blood alkalinizer and glucose upon competitive endurance. J Applied Physiol 1953;5:577–578.
6. Margaria RHT. Effect of alkalosis on performance and lactate formation in supramaximal exercise. Internationale Zeitschrift für Ängewandte Physiologie Einschliesslich Arbeitphysiologic 1971;29:215–223.
7. Poulus AJ, Docter HJ Wjestra HG. Acid-base balance and subjective feeling of fatigue during physical exercise. Eur J Appl Physiol 1974;33:207–213.
8. Jones NL, Sutton JR, Taylor R, et al. Effect of pH on cardiorespiratory and metabolic response to exercise. J App! Physiol 1977;43:959–964.
9. Wilkes D, Gledhill N Smyth R. Effect of acute induced metalbolic alkalosis on 800m racing time. Med Sci Sports Exerc 1983;15:277–280.
10. George KP, MacLaren DPM. The effect of induced alkalosis and acidosis on endurance running at an intensity corresponding to 4mM blood lactate. Ergonomics 1988;31:1639–1645.

Growth Hormone

11. Duagheday WH. Growth hormone: normal synthesis, secretion, control and mechanisms of action. In: LJ De Groot, ed. Endocrinology Philadelphia: WB Saunders, 1989:318–329.
12. Daugheday WH. The anterior pituitary. In: Wilson and Foster, eds. Williams Textbook of Endocrinology. Philadelphia: WB Saunders, 1985:577–611.
13. Shepard RJ, Sidney KH. Effects of physical exercise on plasma growth hormone and cortisol levels in human subjects. In: Wilmore and Keough, eds. Exercise and sports science reviews New York: Academic Press, 1975:1–30.
14. Mendelson WB. Studies of human growth hormone secretion in sleep and waking. Int Rev Neurobiol 1982;23:367.
15. Paxton SJ, Trinder J, Shapiro CM, et al. Effect of physical fitness and body composition on sleep and sleep-related hormone concentrations. Sleep 1984;7:339–346.
16. Rogol AD: Growth hormone: physiology, therapeutic use, and potential for abuse. In: Exercise and sport sciences reviews 1989:353–379.
17. Voy R: Drugs, Sport and Politics. Champaign, Ill: Leisure Press, 1991;57–66.
17a. Rickert VI, Pawlak-Morello C, Sheppard V, et al. Human growth hormone: A new substance of abuse among adolescents? Clin Pediatr 1992; Dec:723–726.
18. Bradley CA, Sodeman TM: Human growth hormone. Its use and abuse. Clinical Toxicology II. Clinics in Laboratory Medicine 1990;10:473–477.
19. Daughaday WH: Radioligand assays for insulin-like growth factor II. Methods Enzymol 1987;146A:248.
20. Schlechter NL, Russell SM, Spencer EM, et al.: Evidence suggesting that the direct growth-promoting effect of growth-hormone on cartilage in vivo is mediated by local production of somatomedin. Proc Natl Acad Sci USA 1986;83:7932.
21. Bigland B Jehring B. Muscle performance in rats, normal and treated with growth hormone. Physiol 1952;116:129–136.
22. Apostolakis M, Deligiannis A, Madena-Pyrgaki A. The effects of human growth hormone administration on the functional status of rat atrophied muscle following immobilization. Physiologist 1980;23(suppl):S111–112.
23. Macintyre JG. Growth hormone and athletes. Sports Med 1987;4:129–142.
24. Meistas MT, Foster GV, Margolis S, et al.: Integrated concentrations of growth hormone, insulin, C-peptide and prolactin in human obesity. Metabolism 1982;31:1224–1228.
25. Bray GA. The obese patient. Major problems in internal medicine Philadelphia: WB Saunders, 1976.
26. Kalkhoff R, Ferrou C. Metabolic differences between obese overweight and muscular overweight men. N Engl J Med 1971;284:1236–1239.
27. Bray GA: Obesity: An endocrine perspective. In: LJ Degroot, ed. Endocrinology. Philadelphia: WB Saunders, 1989:2303–2338.
28. Bray GA, Raben MS, Londono J, et al. Effects of triiodothronine, growth hormone, and anabolic steroids on nitrogen excretion and oxygen consumption of obese patients. J Clin Endocrinol Metab 1971;33:293–300.
29. Committee on Growth Hormone Use. Degenerative neurologic disease in patients formerly treated with growth hormone. J Pediatr 1985;107:10–12.
30. Council on Scientific Affairs. Drug abuse in athletes: Anabolic steroids and human growth hormone. JAMA. 1988;259:1703–1705.
31. Wallis M. The molecular evolution of pituitary growth hormone, prolactin and placental lactogen: A protein family showing variable rates of evolution. J Mol Evol 1981;17:10–18.

Blood Doping and Erythropoietin

32. Pace N, Lozner EL, Consolazio WV, et al. The increase in hypoxia tolerance of normal men accompanying the polycythemia induced by transfusion of erythrocytes. Am J Physiol 1947;148:152–163.
33. Gullbring B, Homgren A Sjostrand T, et al. The effect of blood volume variations on the pulse ratio in supine and upright positions and during exercise. Acta Physiol Scand 1960;50:62–71.
34. Robinson B, Epstein SE, Kahler RL, et al: Circulatory effects of acute expansion of blood volume: Studies during maximal exercise and at rest. Circ Res 1966;19:26–32.
35. Gledhill N: The ergogenic effect of blood doping. Phys SportsMed 1983;11(9):87–90.
36. Ekblom B, Goldbarg AN, Gullbring B: Response to exercise after blood loss and reinfusion. J Appl Physiol 1972;33:175–180.
37. Buick FJ, Gledhill N, Froese AB, et al. Effect of induced erythrocythemia on aerobic work capacity. J Appl Physiol 1980;48:636–642.
38. Williams MH, Wesseldine S, Somma T, et al. The effect of induced erythrocythemia upon 5-mile treadmill run time. Med Sci Sports Exerc 1981;13:169–175.
39. Anonymous. ACSM Position Stand on Blood Doping as an Ergogenic Aid [Editorial]. ACSM 1987;540–543.
40. Adamson JW, Kaushansky K, Powell JS, et al. Hormones and blood production. In: Degoot LJ ed. Endocrinology. Philadelphia: WB Saunders 1989:2612–2631.
41. Ekblom B, Berglund B. Effect of erythropoietin administration on maximal aerobic power. Scan J Med Sci Sports 1991;1:88–93.
42. Eichner ER. Sports anemia, iron supplements, and blood doping. Med Sci Sports Exerc 1992;24(suppl)S315–S318.

Anabolic Steroids

43. Perry PJ, Andersen KH, Yates WR: Illicit anabolic steroid use in athletes. A case series analysis. Am J Sports Med 1990;18:422–428.
44. Windsor R, Dumitru D: Prevalence of anabolic steroid use by male and female adolescents. Med Sci Sports Exerc 1989;21:494–497.
45. Voy R, Deeter KD: Drugs, sports and politics. West Point, NY: Leisure Press 1991.
46. Stamford BA, Moffatt R: Anabolic steroids: Effectiveness as an ergogenic aid to experienced weight trainers. J Sports Med Phys Fitness 1974;14:191–197.
47. Percy, EC. Ergogenic aids in athletics. Med Sci Sports Exerc 1978;10:298–303.
48. Ryan AJ. Anabolic steroids are fool's gold. Fed Proc 1981;40:2682–88.
49. Haupt HA, Rovere G. Anabolic steroids: A review of the literature. Am J Sports Med 1984;12:469–484.
50. Wilson JD. Androgen use by athletes. Endocr Rev 1988;9:181–199.
51. Kochakian CD, Murlin JR. The effect of male hormone on the protein and energy metabolism of castrate dogs. J Nutr 1935;10:437–459.
52. Mellion MB. Anabolic steroids in athletics. Am Fam Phys 1984;30:113–119.
53. Wade N. Anabolic steroids: Doctors denounce them but athletes aren't listening. Science 1972;176:1399–1403.
54. Hallagan JB, Hallagan LF, Snyder MB. Anabolic-Androgenic use by athletes sounding board. New Engl J Med 1989;321:1042–1045.
55. Kersey RD. Anabolic-Androgenic steroid use by private health club/gym athletes. J Strength Cond Res 1993;7:118–126.
56. Pope HG, Katz DL, Champoux R. Anabolic-androgenic steroid use among 1010 college men. Phys SportsMed 1988;16:75–81.
57. Strauss RH, Liggett MT, Lanese RR. Anabolic steroid use and perceived effects in ten weight-trained women athletes. JAMA 1985;253:2871–1873.

58. Buckley WE, Yesalis CE III, Friedl KE, et al. Estimated prevalence of anabolic steroid use among male high school seniors. JAMA 1988;260:3441–3445.
59. Windsor R, Dimitru D. Prevalence of anabolic steroid use by male and female adolescents. Med Sci Sports Exerc 1989;21:494–497.
60. Johnson MD, Jay MS, Shoup B. Anabolic steroid use by male adolescents. Pediatrics 1989;83:921–924.
61. Radakovich J, Broderick P, Pickell G. Rate of anabolic-androgenic steroid use among students in junior high school. JABFP 1993;6:341–345.
62. Dezelsky TL, Toohey JV, Shaw RS. Non-medical drug use behavior at five united states universities: A 15 year study. Bull Narc 1985;37:49–53.
63. Frankle M, Cicero J, Payne J. Use of anabolic androgenic steroids by athletes. JAMA 1984;252:482.
64. Lamb DR: Anabolic steroids in athletics: How well do they work and how dangerous are they? Am J Sports Med 1984;12:31–38.
65. Bomze JP, Cox MH: Anabolic steroids: A historical and clinical perspective. Nat Strength and Cond Assoc J 1991;13:42–46.
66. Haupt HA: Drugs in athletics. In office practice of sports medicine. Clinics in Sports Med 1989;561–583.
67. Overly WL, Dankkoff JA, Wang BK, et al. Androgens and hepatocellular carcinoma in an athlete. (Letter) Ann Int Med 1984;100:158–159.
68. Alen M, Rahkila P, Reinla M, et al. Androgenic-anabolic steroid effects on serum thyroid, pituitary and steroid hormones in athletes. Am J Sports Med 1987;15:357–361.
69. Alen M, Rahkila P, Marniemi J: Serum lipids in power athletes self administering testosterone and anabolic steroids. Int J Sports Med 1985;6:139–144.
70. Crist DM, Peake GT, Stackpole PJ: Alpha lipoproteinemic effects of androgenic anabolic steroids in athletes. Ann Sports Med 1985;2:125–128.
71. Cohen JC, Faber WM, Spinnler-Benade AJ et al. Altered serum lipoprotein profiles in male and female power lifters ingesting anabolic steroids. Phys Sports Med 1986;14:131–136.
72. Alen M, Rahkila P. Anabolic-androgenic steroid effects on endocrinology and lipid metabolism in athletes. Sports Med 1988;6:327–332.
73. Michna H. Organization of collagen fibrils in tendon: Changes induced by an anabolic steroid. Part I. Functional and ultrastructural studies. Virchow Arch (Cell Pathol) 1986;52:75–86.
73a. Karpakka JA, Pesola MK,Takala TES. The effects of anabolic steroids on collagen synthesis in rat skeletal muscle and tendon. Am J Sports Med 1992; 20:262–266.
74. Wood TO, Cooke PH, Goodship AE. The effect of exercise and anabolic steroids on the mechanical properties and crimp morphology of the rat tendon. Am J Sports Med 1988;16:153–158.
75. Miles JW, Grana WA, Egle D, et al. The effect of anabolic steroids on the biomechanical and histological properties of rat tendon. JBJS 1992;74-A 411–422.
76. Salmons S: Myotrophic effects of anabolic steroids. Vet Res Commun 1983;7:19–26.
77. Mayer M, Rosen F. Interaction of anabolic steroids with glucocorticoid receptor sites in rat muscle cytosol. Am J Physiol 1975;229:1381–1386.
78. Ariel G, Saville W. Anabolic steroids: The physiological effects of placebos. Med Sci Sports 1972;4:124–126.
79. Scott MJ. Cutaneous side-effects of anabolic-androgenic steroid use. Clin Sports Med 1989;1:5–16.
80. Saborido A. Vila J, Odriozola JM, et al. Effects of anabolizing androgens on hepatic monoxygenase activities. In: Shipe JR, Savory J, eds. drugs in competitive athletics. Blackwell Scientific Publications, 1991:121–127.
81. Vesselinovitch SD, Mihailovich N, Rao KVN. Potential role of synthetic sex steroids in hepatocarcinogenesis. In: Shipe JR, Savory J, eds. Drugs in competitive athletics. Blackwell Scientific Publications, 1991:97–106.
82. Pope HG, Datz DL. Affective and psychotic symptoms associated with anabolic steroid use. Am J Psychiatr 1988;145:487–490.
83. Menkis AH, Daniel JK, McKenzie N. et al. Cardiac transplantation after myocardial infarction in a 24-year-old bodybuilder using anabolic steroids. Clin J Sports Med 1991;1:138–140.
84. Mochizuki RM, Richter KJ. Cardiomyopathy and cerebrovascular accident associated with anabolic-androgenic steroid use. Phys Sports Med 1988;16:109–114.
85. Jarow JP, Lipshultz LI. Anabolic steroid induced hypogonadotropic hypogonadism. Am J Sports Med 1990;18:429–431.
86. Pettine KA. Association of anabolic steroids and avascular necrosis of femoral heads. Am J Sports Med 1991;19:96–98.

Stimulants

87. Percy EC. Ergogenic aids in athletics. Med Sci Sports 1978;10:298–303.
88. Costill DL, Dalsky GP, Fink WJ. Effects of caffeine ingestion on metabolism and exercise performance. Med Sci Sports 1978;10:155–158.
89. Essig D, Costill DL, Van Handel PJ: Effects of caffeine ingestion on utilization of muscle glycogen and lipid during leg ergometer cycling. Int J Sports Med 1980;1:86–90.
90. Dodd SL, Herb RA, Powers SK. Caffeine and exercise performance. An update. Sports Med 1993;15:14–23.
91. Fryer MW, Neering IR. Actions of caffeine on fast and slow twitch muscles of the rat. J of Phys 1989;416:435–454.
92. Slavin JL, Joensen DJ. Caffeine and sports performance. Phys Sports Med 1985;13:191–193.
93. DiPalma JR. Caffeine. AFP 1982;25:206–207.
94. U.S. Olympic Committee Drug Education Handbook 1989–1992:20.
95. Drugs of Abuse. U.S. Department of Justice, Drug Enforcement Agency 1988:36–44.
96. Gawin FH, Elinwood EH. Cocaine and other stimulants. actions, abuse, and treatment. N Eng J Med 1988;318:1173–1182.
97. Smith GM, Beecher HK. Amphetamine sulfate and athletic performance. JAMA 1959;170:542–557.
98. Chandler JV, Blair SN. The effect of amphetamines on selected physiological components related to athletic success. Med Sci Sports and Exerc 1980;12:65–69.
99. Wagner JC. Enhancement of athletic performance with drugs: An overview. Sports Med 1991;12:250–265.
100. Karpovich PV. Effect of amphetamine sulfate on athletic performance. JAMA 1959;170:558–561.
101. Haupt HA. Drugs in athletics. Office practice of sports medicine. Collins HR, ed. Clin Sports Med 1989;561–583.
102. Voy R, Deeter KD. Drugs, sport, and politics. Champaigne Ill: Leisure Press, 1991.
103. Puffer J. The use of drugs in swimming. Clinics Sports Med 1986;5:77–89.
104. Lange RA, Cigarroa RG, Yancy CW, et al. Cocaine-induced coronary-artery vasoconstriction. N Eng J Med 1989;321:1557–1606.
105. Tennant FS Jr: Dealing with cocaine use by athletes. Sports Med Dig 1984;6:1–3.
106. Isner JM, Kark Estes NA III, Thompson PD, et al. Acute cardiac events temporally related to cocaine abuse. N Eng J Med 1986;315:1438–1443.
107. Roth D, Alarcon FJ, Fernandez JA, et al. Acute rhabdomyolysis associated with cocaine intoxication. N Eng J Med 1988;319:673–677.

Miscellaneous Drugs

108. Caldwell JE. Diuretic therapy and exercise performance. Sports Med 1987;4:290–304.
109. Catlin DH, Hatton CK. Use and abuse of anabolic and other drugs for athletic enhancement Adv Intern Med, 1991;399–424.

Drug Testing

110. Catlin DH, Hatton CK: Use and abuse of anabolic and other drugs for athletic enhancement. Adv Intern Med 1991;399–424.
111. Curran WJ: Compulsory drug testing: The legal barriers. N Eng J Med 1987;316:318–321.
112. Dugal R, Masse R: Methodological imperatives and analytical requirements for the detection and identification of drugs misused in sport. In: Shipe JR, Savory J, eds. Drugs in competitive athletics. Blackwell Scientific Publications 1991;3–17.

10 / SPECIAL CONCERNS OF THE PEDIATRIC ATHLETE

Morey S. Moreland

"Adults are Obsolete Children"—*Dr. Seuss*

Introduction

The unique quality of growth potential imparts special characteristics to the musculoskeletal system of children and adolescents. Indeed, it is the special property of tissues in "transition" with the ability of creating newer and larger structures (bones, muscles, tendons, and ligaments) that require the clinician to understand the specific demands of sport on these tissue structures. The treating clinician as well must understand how these unique characteristics relate to the implicit healing capabilities in childhood injuries. Therefore, in diagnosing and treating injuries to children it is fundamental to understand that the child is not just a small adult, although, as noted by Dr. Seuss, the opposite may be true. This chapter will look at various common pediatric injuries and disorders and examine their relationship to sport activities in a manner that addresses the special concerns and difficulties in children as they relate to the potential mechanisms of injury and their diagnosis and management.

Special Considerations of Growth and Development

From birth to the completion of adolescence the child undergoes a remarkable change in size and body proportion. Height increases approximately 3.5 times, weight increases 20–25 times, and muscle mass increases about sevenfold (1). The attainment of these increases is not uniform throughout growth, but follows a generally declining growth velocity curve with the notable exception of the adolescent growth spurt. This period of rapid growth occurs during ages 10 to 14 years in females and 13 to 17 years in males (Fig. 10.1). In addition to size changes, body proportions related to the center of gravity (CG) change with respect to head size, truncal length and leg length (Fig. 10.2). In infants and young children, the CG is located in the midtrunk with a proportionally long trunk and short legs, while the adolescent attains a nearly adult form with a center of gravity centered at L4 and more equally proportioned leg length, truncal, and head length (2). With

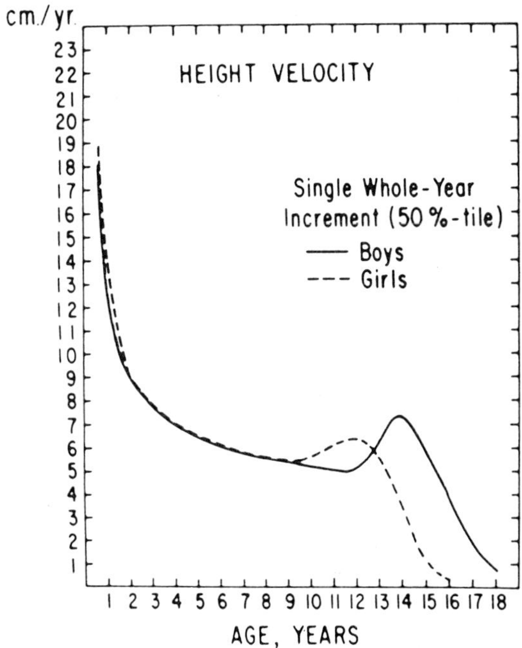

Figure 10.1. Height velocity: single whole-year increment (50th percentile for boys and girls). This chart compares only the boy and girl means from the Tanner study. The standard deviations have been removed. The relative velocity for boys (7.3 cm) is greater than that for girls (6.5cm) during the maximal year of growth. The data indicate a rapid deceleration following birth and a relatively short duration of acceleration during adolescence. Reprinted from Lowey GH. Growth and development of children. 7th ed. Chicago: Yearbook Medical Publishers, Inc., 1978.

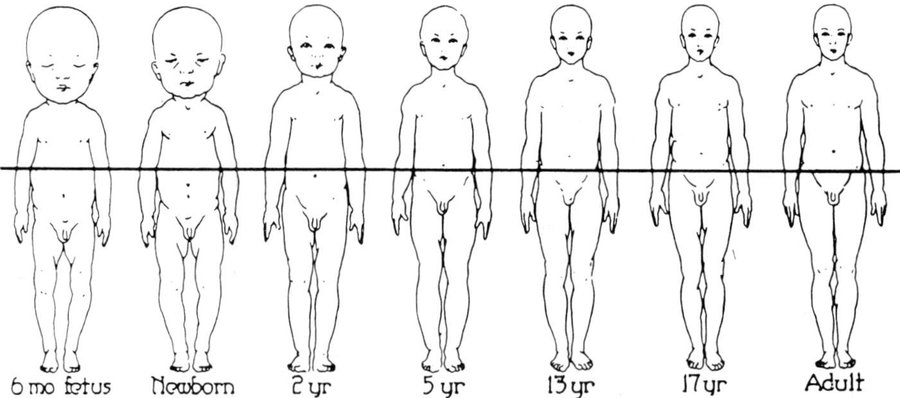

Figure 10.2. Height proportion. Ventral aspect of the body at intervals from the sixth fetal month to maturity. Body lengths are reduced to the same scale, and the transverse plane of gravity is represented by a transverse line. The relatively longer upper body height of earlier age may be seen. The distance of the center of gravity above the soles is expressed as an index or percent of statute and maintains a fairly constant ratio, ranging from 55.0 to 59.0 during the whole of the developmental period. Modified from Palmer CE. Studies of the center of gravity in the human body. Child Dev 1944;15:99–180.

increased interest in organized sports, the problems of differing body size among participating children has necessitated careful classification and monitoring to assure that the larger body mass and velocity attained, for example, in older children do not increase chances for injury or confer unfair competitive advantage. The lack of such monitoring remains a problem for unsupervised playground sport activities.

There also are physiologic differences in children throughout the span of their growth. Children require more O_2 for a given activity and rely on anaerobic metabolism less during periods of increased muscle activity. They have a less efficient thermoregulation system with fewer sweat glands (3) and they have higher heart rates and lower cardiac stroke volumes. Test of strength and endurance show progressive increases in the last half of childhood (4). Neuromuscular development is evident also in faster audio and visual reaction time (5), and in reaction and speed of movement (6).

Finally, and considering the uniqueness of the child's musculoskeletal system and possible response to injury, the specific specialized anatomic structures of growing bone must be considered.

While the bone substance of children is the same as adults, biomechanically, the bones of children have more flexible and elastic qualities, and especially in the younger child, they are less brittle in their behavior. In addition, in children the growth plate (physis) is most commonly considered the "weak link" in resisting forces, although tendon attachments into growing bones (apophysis), should also be considered vulnerable. These areas and their injury constitute a large percentage of what is commonly considered significant injury in children's sports. However, reporting variances make actual determination of the epidemiology of such injuries difficult to assess. As might be expected, reported injury rates vary depending on the sport. Garrick and Requa have reported injury rates for high school sports (Fig. 10.3), as reported by trainers over a two-year period with the total of 1197 injuries (17). As may be seen in this figure, the number of injuries requiring more than 5 days lost to a sport is only 31%. The sport's injury rates also rise with increasing age. In a study of POP Warner Football Players, injury rates rose from 2.8 per 100 players age 9 to 12 to 10.1 per 100 for age 11 to 14 (8). More organization, longer practice and playing times, and acquisition of advanced skill levels probably play a role in controlling this rate. These factors are especially important in view of the fact that at these ages the skeletal system is becoming mature, losing its cartilaginous weaker zones, and increasing muscle bulk, which on an anatomic basis should have a protective effect. Knowledge of the types of injury likely to cause symptomatic problems for the pediatric athlete, therefore, must include an understanding of the level of ma-

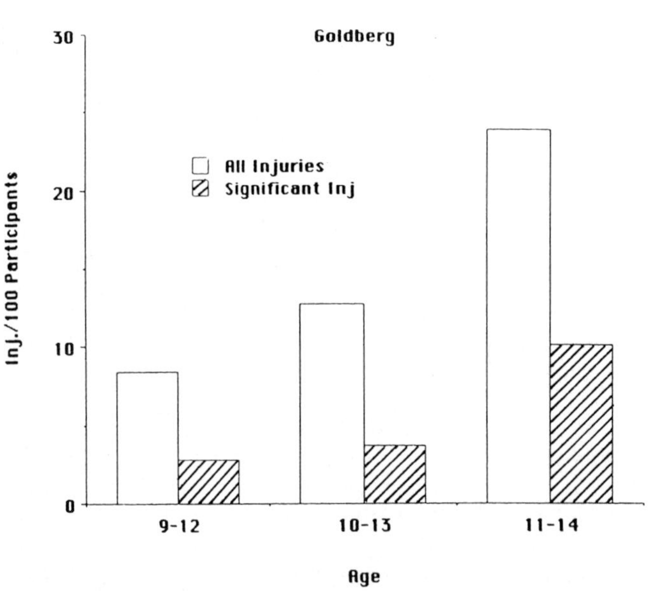

Figure 10.3. Injury rates in youth football. Reprinted from Goldberg B, Rosenthal PP, Nicholas JA. Injuries in youth football. Phys Sports Med 1984;12:122–132.

turity of the athlete and the level of demands placed on the participant by the sport.

Fractures in Children—Strains and Sprains

Skeletal trauma accounts for 10% to 15% of all childhood injuries and fractures of cartilaginous physis account for about 15% of all fractures in children (9, 10). In general, fracture rates for all locations in bones in children are slightly higher than in adults except for the elderly female. Overall, fractures in children account for 18% to 20% of all skeletal trauma, sprain and dislocations account for approximately 45% (11).

Mechanism

Fortunately, children's bones and, to some extent, soft tissues are more flexible than adults', allowing for greater energy absorption and deformation due to any external force. The periosteum surrounding the child's bone is thicker and retains a considerable capability for growth and remodeling. Fractures can occur because of twisting, bending, or direct blows, and fracture patterns are reflective of these forces. For example, twisting produces a torque often leading to a spiral fracture pattern, bending a short oblique pattern, and direct blows account for transverse pattern (12) (Fig. 10.4). Because of relative elasticity, greenstick or incomplete fractures are the fractures commonly seen, as are buckle fractures.

Disruptions of the physeal plate are usually classified by five types as initially described by Salter and Harris (13) (Fig. 10.5). In these injuries, the fracture line either goes through a portion of the growth plate, (type 1, 2, 3) or across it (type 4). In severe compression-type injuries, a crushing of the plate (type 5) may occur. In addition to serving a useful function for classification, the type of epiphyseal fracture implies various types of injury mechanism, e.g., shear or rotation for type 1, bending for type 2, 3, bending with compression for type 4, and compression alone for type 5. It is important to identify the pattern of the fracture because the potential for permanent damage of the growth mechanism increases with each type in the classification. In other words, less disruption usually occurs with type 1 versus the higher probability of disruption with type 5 (14).

Acute Trauma

Acute trauma, severe enough to produce a fracture, usually occurs as a result of a fall or a contact/collision between sport participants. In this instance, severe pain, inability to use the extremity, deformity and swelling, readily assist in making a diagnosis. The anatomic location of these findings whether it is at the end of a bone (epiphysis), the middle of the bone, (diaphysis), or in the junctional area in between (the metaphysis) may give the examiner further information on the likelihood of growth plate injury. Deformities about joints may represent either frank dislocation or complete separation of the epiphysis at the growth plate. Radio-

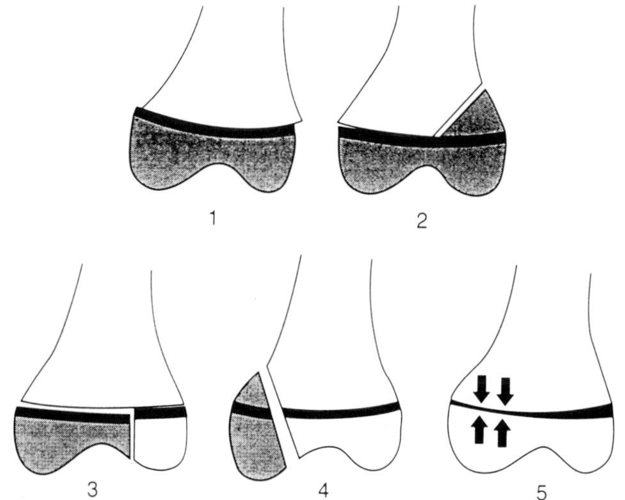

Figure 10.5. Salter-Harris classification of physeal injuries. The injuries are divided by the plane of the fracture line relative to the physis as growth plate. Reprinted from Staheli LT. Fundamentals of pediatric orthopaedics. New York; Raven Press, 1992.

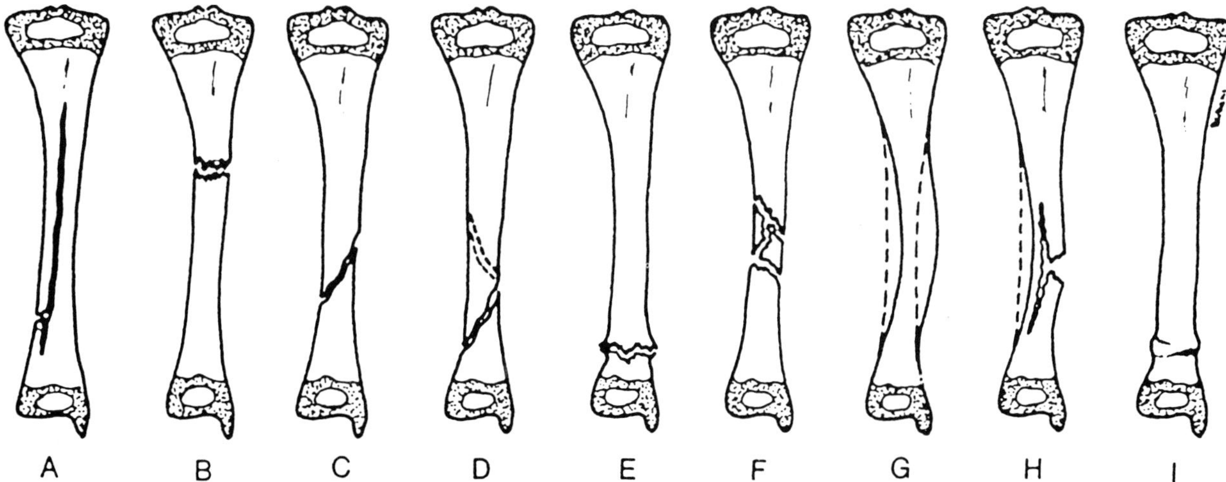

Figure 10.4. Schematic of tibia (3-year-old child) showing various types of fractures: **A,** longitudinal; **B,** transverse; **C,** oblique; **D,** spiral; **E,** impacted; **F,** comminuted; **G,** bowing (plastic deformation); **H,** greenstick; and **I,** torus. Reprinted from Ogden JA. Skeletal injury in the child. 2nd ed. Philadelphia: WB Saunders, 1990.

graphic examination is the single most helpful test for all musculoskeletal injury and should always include anterior/posterior and lateral views, or, at least, two views with 90° difference in orientation in order to adequately find and define the fracture. Occasionally, oblique views will be helpful, particularly for short oblique and nondisplaced fractures. Because the skeleton of each child is constantly changing with respect to maturation, it is helpful to obtain comparison x-rays of the opposite extremity in order to gain understanding of the normal skeletal pattern for that patient. This is particularly true since more or less of the cartilaginous anlage of the bone will be ossified and, therefore, appear on the x-ray. The appearance of secondary centers of ossification, while reasonably predictable by skeletal age, are somewhat variable with chronological age. Therefore, comparison x-rays may be helpful in determining what is normal for that child. In injuries without significant angulation and in injuries around joints, soft tissue swelling, clinically, and, as perhaps seen radiographically, may be helpful in assessing the location of the injury. For example, ligamentous injuries or injuries to a joint producing distention of the joint capsule suggest intraarticular hemorrhage and/or soft tissue hemorrhage and, thus, help determine the location and probability of either fracture or soft tissue disruption.

Acute trauma must be differentiated from chronic or repetitive trauma because the former is more likely to produce sudden onset of severe disruption occurring over a shorter period of time, whereas chronic injury often represents repetitive, less well-defined events or onset. Acute injuries in sports most commonly involve hand and wrist, ankle, knee, elbow, and shoulder and hip in that order. The relative frequency depends upon the nature of the sport. For example, hand and finger injuries are more common in baseball than in soccer. However, in soccer, ankle and knee injuries are much more frequent. An accurate physical exam that attempts to localize as closely as possible the anatomic area of maximum deformity, swelling, and pain will increase the likelihood of getting the appropriate x-ray. This will also increase the likelihood of initiating a proper focus of attention to adequately diagnose the problem and begin appropriate therapy.

Common pitfalls in diagnosing trauma problems in children include the failure to appreciate the cartilaginous injury, e.g., a Salter I fracture or a fracture through the cartilaginous portion of the epiphysis. Often, these injuries are mistakenly diagnosed as sprains because no frank fracture is seen radiographically. True sprains are less common in children than in adults, and injuries surrounding joints should be highly suspect as possible cartilaginous injuries rather than assumed to be "just a sprain." Conversely, since trauma seen both in organized activity and in free play activity is so common in children that symptoms of pain and swelling are often ascribed to an injury or a traumatic event, one should keep in mind that their symptoms could also represent an infection or a tumor. Careful history and follow-up is helpful to differentiate the nature of the symptoms.

Management

Careful assessment of the injured player is the first and foremost consideration of any acute injury. Surveying for other injuries and preventing further injury also has a high priority. With most injuries it is important to evaluate whether there is a fracture and/or instability, and indeed, if so, whether this is an open fracture or closed fracture. Open fractures involve any break in the skin in or around the fracture site and need application of a sterile dressing. Closed fractures are those in which the skin is intact. Initial field management involves immobilization with a splint and in those cases of extremity fracture or with a backboard for suspected spine trauma. Splinting should be done in a position satisfactory for transportation and in a position in which reasonable normal anatomic alignment can occur. Following radiographic confirmation of the diagnosis, the fracture or dislocation may need reduction, which is done under intravenous sedation, regional anesthesia, or, in some cases, general anesthesia. Compound open fractures usually need debridement and irrigation in addition to reduction.

Several unique features of children's fractures are helpful in the healing process. Because of the growth potential of the growth cartilage and periosteum, children's fractures tend to heal rapidly. In addition, because children are constantly making new and larger bones, they can correct angular deformities easily—a feature not present in most older adolescents and adults. Such remodelling may be seen in the distal forearm fractures as seen in Figure 10.6. The remodelling process in younger children may take up to 1 to 2 years but does not normally interfere with function. One disadvantage of managing children's fractures is the difficulty of monitoring activity levels during recovery. Cast immobilization is usually maintained from 6 to 10 weeks depending on the location and nature of the fracture. However, following cast removal, a period of rehabilitation of muscle strength and motion is necessary as is mechanical strengthening of the fracture site, which may take 6 months or longer. Obviously, return to sport activity requires this rehabilitative phase to be complete and often is frustrating for a young athlete, the coaches, and parents. Nonunion of fractures is rare in children and malunion with shortening or angulation can usually be avoided with careful follow-up. Healing periods become somewhat longer the closer the child is to adulthood, and, for that reason, there has been recent interest in internally fixing fractures in the adolescent which may lessen some of the time required for rehabilitation. This is probably true of femur fractures in the adolescent who is close to reaching skeletal maturity. Such a procedure may be seen in Figure 10.7. Additionally, fractures that occur around joints or through the epiphysis (types 3, 4) may need very accurate reduction in order to reconstruct the joint surface and accurately reapproximate the growth plate. In order to achieve this open reduction, internal fixation is frequently necessary. These fractures carry the biggest risk of potential long-term problems because of growth ar-

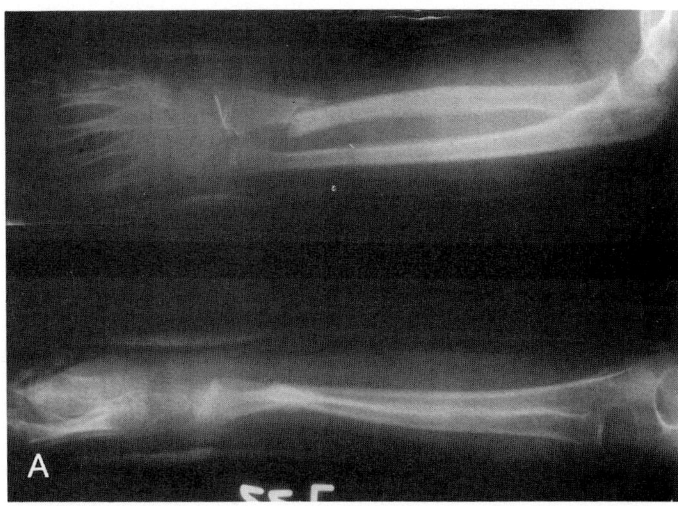

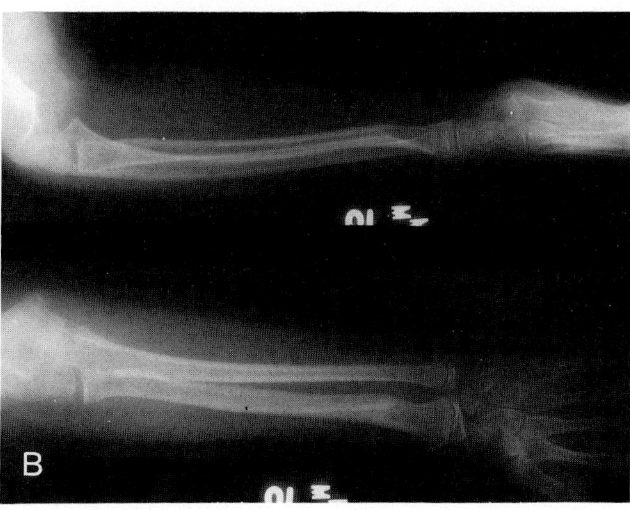

Figure 10.6. Nine-year-old female who sustained fractures of radius and ulna in a fall. **A.** Early radiographs at 1 month following fracture showing early bone remodelling of the fracture. **B.** Radiographs at 4 months showing further remodelling of the metaphysis and straightening of the bones.

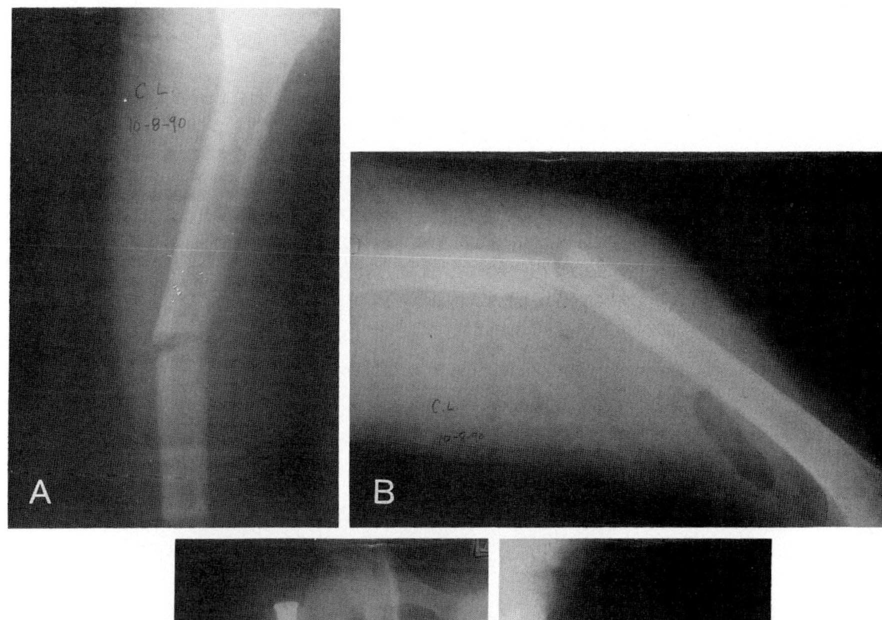

Figure 10.7. Radiographs of 15-year-old male, tackled while playing football sustaining a fractured right midshaft femur. (**A** and **B**). One week after placement of intermedulary rod for stabilization of fracture to allow crutch walking during healing (**C** and **D**).

rest, or because of an irregular joint surface leading to subsequent degenerative joint disease. This often needs to be brought to the attention of parents and coaches.

As indicated previously, not all injuries lead to significant acute symptoms, but may have longer term consequences. Figure 10.8 shows the result of an ankle injury sustained in a 13-year-old baseball player while sliding into second base. He had a moderate swelling over his left medial malleolus and could walk with pain. The initial radiograph showed little more than a slight irregularity at the distal tibial physis. He was casted for 4 weeks, had an uneventful recovery, and returned to sports in three months. However, a year and a half later, it was noted that the lower portion of his ankle was turning in; his x-rays showed a varus deformity of the distal tibia. The initial injury had been a type 5 epiphyseal injury with very little instability or deformity, but the proliferating cells of the epiphyseal plate had been damaged with subsequent failure to grow on the medial side while the lateral portion and the fibula continued to get longer. This required a surgical procedure both to arrest further fibular growth and lateral tibial growth as well as to realign the tibia. Fortunately, this event occurred near the end of growth and no significant leg length discrepancy occurred.

Sprains and Strains

While contusions are undoubtedly the most prevalent of all injuries in children competing in sports, just as they are in adults, true sprains of ligament and strains of muscle are uncommon. This is especially true for younger children, but not for the adolescent who begins to reflect injury patterns similar to adults. There are two anatomic reasons for this. First, children tend to have a much higher degree of ligamentous laxity, which allows accommodation of relatively greater excursions than are possible for adults. Secondly, there appears to be greater ability to sustain stretching of soft tissues. Descriptions of ligament injury (sprains) are commonly classified as mild, moderate and severe: mild are those in which only minor microscopic disruption occur with little clinical evidence of increased laxity; moderate, those in which microscopic injury is notable with swelling and increased excursion or laxity, but in which the fibers remain in continuity; and severe are those with gross injury and disruption of the ligament, severe swelling, and potential loss of joint stability revealed on clinical testing. Ligaments have a higher resistance to failure when rapid small loads are applied to them, and they have decreased resistance to failure with slow loading of large loads, for example, as those sustained with larger body mass. Similarly, strains that involve an injury to the muscle tendon complex are rarely seen in the younger athlete. When they do occur, they may appear as pain and swelling in the substance of the muscle, or at the muscle tendon junction. Short of violent injuries, tendon rupture is rare in the substance of the tendon, although occasionally avulsion of the tendon bone attachment may more commonly present as pain with point tenderness and loss of function. This is due to pain on use of the muscle tendon complex. These injuries usually involve a sudden deacceleration of a forcefully contracting muscle such as may occur while kicking a soccer ball or striking the

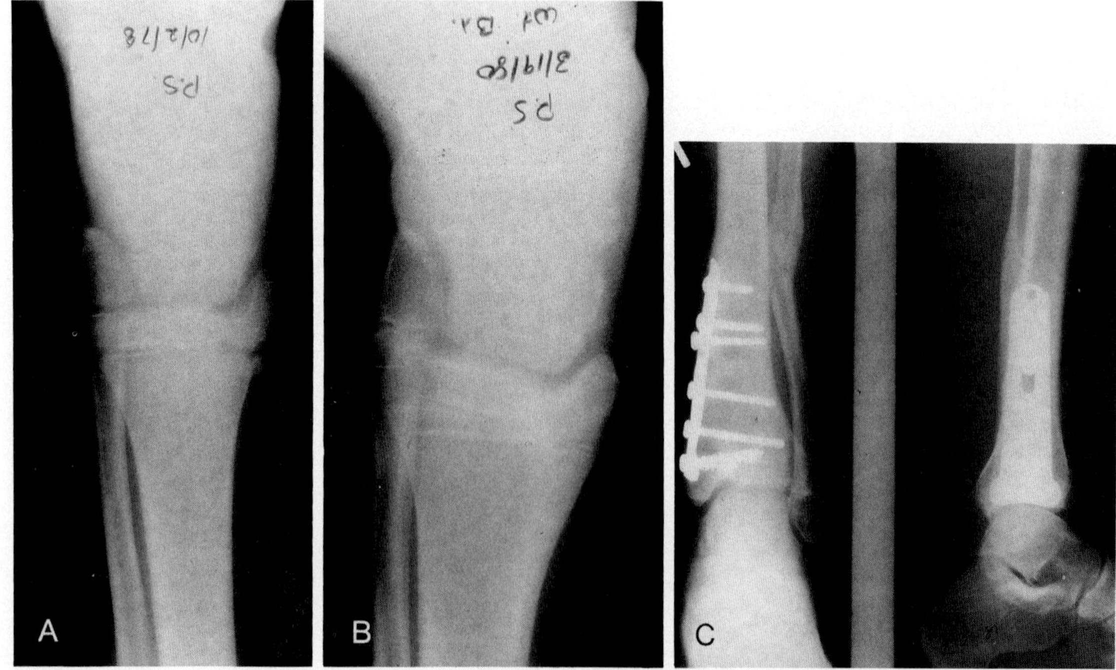

Figure 10.8. Radiographs of 13-year-old baseball player injured while sliding into second base. There was swelling and tenderness over the medial malleus. **A.** Epiphyseal plate disruption of the medial portion of the distal medial epiphysis. The leg was casted and no attempts at reduction were made. **B.** Radiographs 18 months later showing angular growth disturbance of distal tibia with fibula overgrowth. **C.** Two years after injury, radiographs showing operative correction with distal tibial osteotomy and completion of growth arrest of distal fibula and tibia.

ground with the foot. Such an injury may cause severe groin pain due to injury of the attachment of the rectus femora in front of the hip joint. Such injuries usually are associated with a specific forceful event and need to be distinguished from multiple small repetitive injuries that may lead to chronic changes at the tendon esthesis.

Treatment

Treatment for ligamentous injuries is tailored to the type of injury, but in all instances is designed to allow for the fibers of the ligament to heal as close as possible to their natural length to provide for subsequent stability. In mild injuries, rest until symptoms have abated with avoidance of subsequent stress to the ligament structures for 4–6 weeks until healing is complete is generally satisfactory. For injuries in which the ligament has been stretched, but is still in continuity (moderate injury), immobilization for several weeks followed by protective mobilization is generally sufficient. In most instances of complete disruption, similar treatment to those for moderate sprains will provide for adequate healing. The role of remodelling and subsequent growth of ligamentous structures in children is poorly defined at present.

Strains of the muscle/tendon complex can usually be managed by temporary immobilization for comfort, rest without stressing the complex for 2 to 3 weeks followed by rehabilitation and stretching. A program of increasing resistance exercises is exceptionally helpful for building up muscle strength. As in all sport activities, recovery from injury and return to previous competitive levels of activity require a graduated program of increasing participation.

Overuse Injuries

Once thought to be found only in elite and highly trained athletes, the effects of repetitive, subacute trauma to connective tissues producing symptoms are seen with increasing frequency in young adults. These same symptoms are also recognized in children who do not participate in organized sports, but participate vigorously in normal play activities. Symptoms of pain, particularly while performing an activity or immediately after an activity is often a reflection of microtrauma usually occurring in the muscle/tendon complex. The symptoms themselves most likely are the result of the inflammatory response to microdamage to the tissues, caused by repetitive stress. Primary anatomic sites where this may seen include tendon/bone junctions and muscle/tendon junctions in the growing portion of the bone to which the tendon attaches (apophysis or epiphysis).

Anatomy and Growth Considerations

As has already been mentioned, developing tissues of children present special consideration when analyzing the cause and location of injury to the musculoskeletal structures. The origin of muscles near the growth apophysis of the iliac crest, for example, or along the ischial tuberosity can be sites of irritation or frank inflammation. Since these sites are the anchor points for the contractile unit working distally, repetitive, forceful stresses are felt to be the initiating events of the inflammatory response, which, in fact, is the first phase of the repairing process. At the other end of the contractile apparatus, the distal anchor point is also commonly involved in much the same manner. The insertion site of the tendon and the bone represents a complex graded interdigitation of fibrous tissue into the cartilage of bone by histologically evident Sharpey's fibers. These attach to the periosteum, and a direct linkage of the collagen into the cortex through 4 distinct zones representing mineralization of the fibrocartilage occurs. This step-down attachment may serve a protective role in transmitting forces from the flexible tendon to the rigid bone structure (15). The blood vessels supplying the tendon and periosteum at the attachment appear to be completely separate from those supplying the chondro-osseous structures in the apophysis and epiphysis (16). Therefore, the exact mechanism which initiates inflammation as the result of microtears of the tendon near its insertion and which vessels might produce inflammatory response in the chondro-osseous structure is unknown. Complicating this issue in children is the fact that the "growth plate" for the tendon may be at the tendon/bone junction. Thus this active area of myelogenesis and fibrogenesis leading to modelling and remodelling may be the unique feature that lead to such notable anatomic changes as seen in Osgood-Schlatter disease of the tibial tubercle, and Sever's disease of the heel apophysis. These two processes are commonly classified as osteochondrosis, but are distinctly related to stress and inflammation. Along with Little Leaguer's elbow, an irregularity occurring along the common origin of flexors of the forearm and Sinding-Larson-Johannson syndrome with irritation at the inferior pole of the patella occasionally leading to ossification within the ligament, these situations represent a true apophysitis and are unique to children. In some manner yet to be determined, these processes represent the results of unique injury to growing tissues in children.

Medical Considerations

As with many other injuries to the musculoskeletal system in children, symptoms of overuse tend to be more common in the child as he reaches pre-adolescence. Whether this represents an anatomically unstable period for the skeleton or are related to growth or significant increase in structural demands or both is unclear.

Sever's Disease

Originally described as an injury (17) heel pain is the presenting symptom during or following activities and these symptoms may be bilateral. The clinical findings of point tenderness over the posterior aspect of the os calcis is common, rarely this tenderness may extend onto the plantar surface or dorsally along the tendo achilles. In a recent series, Micheli found that soccer was the sport most likely to present the problem. This was followed by basketball and gymnastics (18). The average age of diagnosis in this series was 11 years plus 10 months in boys and 8 years plus 8 months in girls.

Treatment follows the treatment plan for overuse syndromes in general. This includes rest until symptoms are relieved, then a gradual progressive rehabilitation program with return to activities. Many authors, including Micheli, feel that the rapid growth period and increased activities during the growth spurt lead to tight tendons. Therefore, stretching of the gastrocnemius/soleus complex and strengthening of the dorsiflexions of the ankle is recommended. It should be noted that the x-ray appearance of fragmentation of the apophysis as seen on the lateral x-ray probably represents normal variation in the pattern of calcification of the ossification center rather than abnormal calcification or abnormality. The addition of a quarter inch lift under the heel serves as a stress reducer and may help decrease the symptoms. Rarely are nonsteroidal antiinflamatory drugs (NSAIDs) necessary or helpful.

Osgood-Schlatter Disease

First reported in 1903 simultaneously by Osgood in Boston and Schlatter in Zurich, this common condition presents as pain and swelling over the proximal tibia at the sight of insertion of the intrapatellar tendon. Symptoms may begin from a direct blow or fall onto the region or may be present after sport activities. Most observers, including Osgood felt that this was representative of microevolutions from the insertion of the quadriceps mechanism (19). In a survey of 389 adolescent athletes Kujola have found Osgood-Schlatter symptoms in 21% versus only 4.5% in a nonathletic group (20).

The clinical symptoms are pain after activities, or a hypersensitivity and swelling anteriorly under the knee. Physical examination will confirm tenderness and variable increase in the prominence of the proximal tibial tubercle. Radiographs usually show no bony abnormalities though soft tissue swelling may be present (Fig. 10.9). In older adolescent or adult, a separate united fragment may occasionally be seen. The treatment is rest, usually begun by having a brief period of splinting. Graduated stepwise return to sports may be possible although a knee pad may be helpful for preventing accidental direct trauma. Modification of normal activities of knee bending, such as stair climbing and jumping, may be necessary in order for patients to remain asymptomatic. Contact sports may prove too difficult because of the chance of recurrent direct trauma. Hamstring stretching and isometric quadriceps strengthening may be helpful in rebalancing the muscle forces about the knee. The natural history of this disorder is for the symptoms to disappear with maturity, particularly with closure of the apophyseal plate anteriorly. This often alleviates the slight tibial prominence, which is usually asymptomatic. On rare occasions, there may be a small separate ossicle in the tibial tubercle that may remain painful as an adult and may require excision.

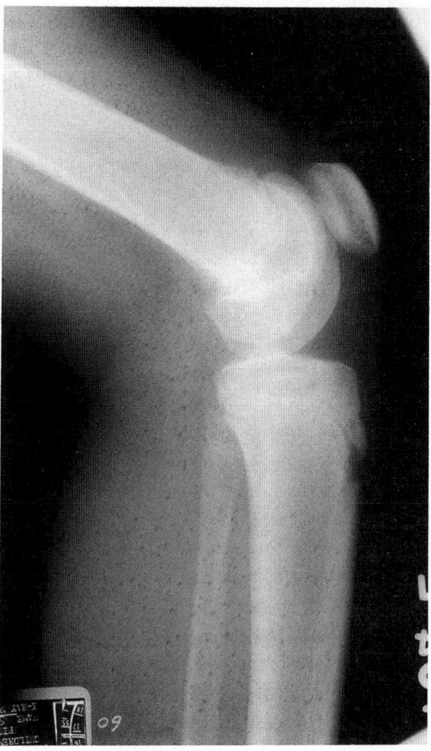

Figure 10.9. Lateral radiograph of a 12-year-old with complaints of anterior knee pain with jumping sports and with kneeling showing tibial apophysis that is slightly prominent but otherwise normal. Fragmentation of this apophysis is not always present in patients with Osgood-Schlatter disease.

Sinding/Larson, Johannson Disease

This is not a true disease process, but merely an expression of multiple microtraumas to the infrapatellar tendon at the knee. The pain and tenderness presents nearer the patella than that of Osgood-Schlatter, and x-rays in patients with long standing symptoms or frequent recurrent symptoms may show multiple calcifications of the inferior pole of the patella. Treatment is the same as for Osgood-Schlatter disease, and jumping activities and sports may have to be curtailed. Occasionally, excision of the bony ossicle is helpful in patients whose symptoms are recalcitrant to rest and gradual rehabilitation.

Little League Elbow/Epicondylar Apophysis

Frequent throwing activities may produce a valgus stress about the elbow that traumatizes the medial epicondylar attachments of the origin of the flexors of the wrist and fingers. Small fibrous disruptions of this tissue leads to inflammation and pain. This process seems to occur more commonly in the 10 to 14 year old male and usually involves the throwing arm only. Pain on palpation of the medial epicondyle coupled with the history will usually indicate the diagnosis. Radiographs may show some fragmentation and irregular ossification of the medial epicondyles. Rarely repeated trauma to the medial epicondyle region and associated swelling will produce compression of the ulna nerve. Treatment of Little League elbow involves rest and gradual supervised return to throwing activities. Changing the throwing style and limiting the number of innings pitched is usually effective. Little League elbow may be best equated with tennis elbow in its anatomic location and symptom complex. It should be distinguished from osteochondritis dessicans involving the medial condyle or the lateral capitellum region (Panner's disease) where irregular ossification of the joint surface occurs (Fig. 10.10). These conditions will be discussed separately later, but they are also found frequently in pitchers (20).

Stress Fractures

The common cause of the overuse symptom complex involving soft tissues is repetitive microstrains producing microscopic tissue damage. The subsequent reactive and reparative process produce the symptoms and what few findings will be present. The same process is present when microfractures occur due to repetitious stresses in bone. Stress fractures in children are less frequent than in adolescents or adults. Holkho and Orava surveyed 368 patients with stress fractures and found less than 10% in children less than 15-years-old, and 32% in the 16 to 19 years age group (21). In addition, the distribution of stress fractures is somewhat different in children. Stress fractures of the tibia represent about 50% of the total number of stress fractures whereas fractures, in the spine (pars interarticular) is more frequent in children particularly in gymnast and football players (23). Metatarsal stress fractures seem more common in adolescents than adults (22). The diagnosis requires a high degree of suspicion aided by a careful history of activities, including a history of change in training, training frequency and training techniques. Localized tenderness may be present, and plain radiographs may show periosteal new bone and thickening if the symptoms have been present for a sufficient period of time—usually longer than 1 month. A bone scan may be helpful, and those suspected patients should have normal plain radiographs.

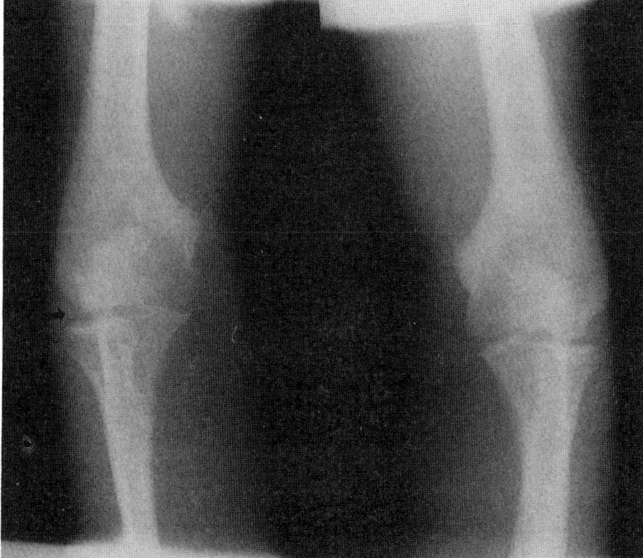

Figure 10.10. 14-year-old male with pain in elbow following prolonged throwing activities showing irregular ossification of the capitellum. (Panner's disease). Ossification of the lateral epicondyle may be delayed or form in an irregular fashion in Little League elbow.

Treatment consists of rest, avoidance of sport activities, and a carefully supervised return to activities in a stepwise manner. Occasionally in the very symptomatic, a brief period of casting may be necessary to begin the healing process. Tibial stress fractures may take greater than 6 months to heal completely and some pars interarticular fractures may never heal, though may become asymptomatic. Based on the presumption of too much activity too fast as a cause of this problem, careful training techniques may be important in both treatment and prevention. Ruben and Associates have shown that bone response to training loads will increase strength for two weeks and then in the third week may show decreased mineral content (24). Based on these same findings, it may be advisable to combine a two-week, intensive training period with at least one week of decreased training to allow bone strength to catch up and match muscle strength.

Osteochondrosis/Osteochondritis Dessicans

A variety of disorders occur in children in which pain is a primary symptom with radiographs showing an irregular ossification of the underlying epiphysis or secondary center of ossification. Since most of these disorders appear to involve the osseous and chondral portions of the bone at the articular ends, the general term osteochondrosis has been applied. Most of these disorders have been given an eponym associated with the individual who originally described the process. Most of these processes occur during periods of rapid growth of the skeletal system leading some authorities to feel that many of these processes may be related to hormonal dynamics. Disturbed circulation has been shown to lead to avascular necrosis in some portion of the epiphysis (25). Such an avascular process is clearly involved in those entities involving the proximal femoral epiphysis (Legg-Calvé-Perthes disease) and Kohler's disease of the tarsal navicula. As noted previously, irregular ossification of the calcaneal apophysis appears to show a fragmented calcification, but this does not appear to be related to true avascularity and usually goes on to a normal closure to the ossified portion of the apophysis. The role of trauma in the production of osteochondrosis is difficult to evaluate because of the frequency of its occurrence in children. In addition, histologic and pathologic confirmation have not shown specific fracture patterns. The role of direct trauma has been suggested as an inciting mechanism by Douglas and Rang (26). An inflammatory response once thought to be infection is most likely a reparative response. Bony repair of the process eventually occurs with healing, although not always with an epiphysis that is symmetrical with the normal site.

Legg-Calvé Perthes Disease

Originally described in 1913 after roentgenograms became available, this process appears to occur in chil-

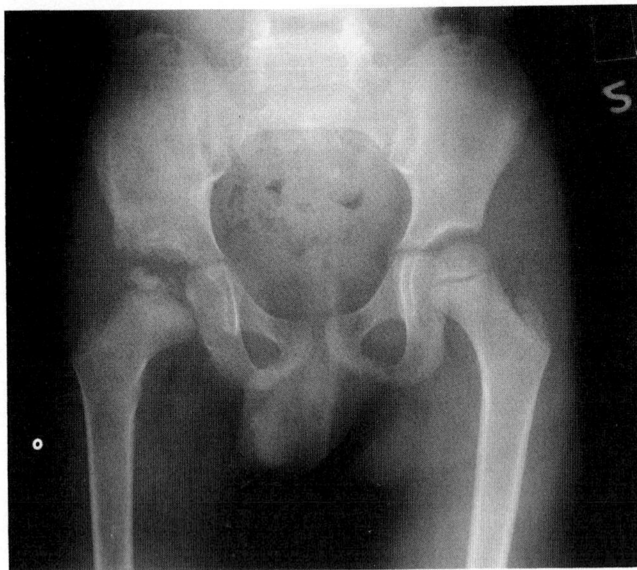

Figure 10.11. Nine-year-old male with Legg-Calvé-Perthes disease of right hip, showing shortening of the femoral neck and enlargement and fragmentation of the femoral head.

dren age 4 to 11. It usually presents as limping or as thigh or knee pain. More common in boys, it can be bilateral although it rarely has its onset in both hips simultaneously. Radiographs show variable irregularity of the capital femoral epiphysis, subchondral fractures as evidenced by radiolucency, and eventual fragmentation of the femoral head as seen on both the anterior/posterior and frog-leg lateral x-rays (Fig. 10.11).

The best method of treatment remains controversial, although some form of reduced activities, including walking and jumping, is common to all forms of treatment. Nonweight bearing with crutches during the acute phase may be helpful and an abduction cast or brace may be effective in keeping the femoral head located under the acetabulum—"containing" the femoral head—during the reparative process. Similarly, operative procedures designed to change the direction of the femoral head into the acetabulum or change the acetabulum over the femoral head to improve containments have been used. The goal of these therapies is to allow healing to occur, a process taking from 1 to 3 years depending on the age of the patient. The goal is to produce a femoral head that is as round as possible and contained within the acetabulum and to allow range of motion as normal as possible with fit of the femoral head in the acetabulum as good as possible. Often some flattening and enlargement of the femoral head occur during the healing process which may have implications for joint degeneration in the future. Because of the length of time necessary to heal this lesion, prolonged absence from running and jumping sports may be necessary. It should also be noted that while this process is not caused by sport participation per se, this diagnosis should be kept in mind when presented with a child with limping or with hip, thigh, or knee pain.

Kohler's Disease

This painful condition of childhood often presents with pain over the dorsal medial aspect of the foot after or during activity. Most common in the 3- to 10-year-old age group the characteristic finding on an AP and lateral radiograph is collapse and narrowing of the navicula with increased bone density. Over the course of 1 to 2 years, restoration of the navicular to near-normal size occurs in most (27). During that time, the use of orthotics to support the medial side of the foot with modification of sport and play activities facilitates resolution of this benign condition. Early use of cast immobilization may be helpful in accelerating the relief of symptoms (28).

Osteochondritis Dissecans

The term osteochondritis, once the term used for all osteochondrosis, has remained the current term of choice for those epiphyseal irregularities that involve the subchondral area immediately beneath the articular cartilage and most often involves the articular cartilage itself. Osteochondritis dissecans probably represents a specialized form of osteochondrosis whose underlying pathology represents an area of focal avascular necrosis of the subchondral region of the supporting articular surface with subsequent repair. An infectious etiology has not been supported in the literature, and the inflammatory response thought to be part of the process undoubtedly represents true tissue repair. Trauma has been suggested as a cause, but Mubarak and Carroll found no such specific association could be made (29). Genetic predisposition for a variation in the ossification patterns of normal development may play a role (30). There are three primary locations where these lesions are characteristically found; they are the medial femoral condyle of the knee, the posterior medial surface of the talus and the anterior/lateral portion of the humeral capitellum. These appear radiographically either as a radiolucent line or as an elliptical irregular area of ossification representing an isolated osteochondral unit usually 1 to 2 cm in size depending upon the joint involved (Fig. 10.12). The natural history of the healing of these lesions depends in part on the age of the patients, the symptoms at the time of presentation and the radiographic appearance. Pappas has classified this process into three categories based upon age (31). Category I involves young children up to the beginning of adolescence, defined as age 11 for girls and 13 for boys. The epiphyseal and articular regions have a considerable amount of growth remaining at this age, and lesions are sometimes not well developed. They occasionally are found as incidental findings on radiographs taken for other injuries. Category II includes the adolescent age group characterized by a period of rapid growth. Symptoms in this group are likely to occur especially with frequently repeated sport activity. They may involve not only pain in the knee joint, but swelling representing an effusion into the knee joint. Some of these patients have distinct symptoms of an osteo-

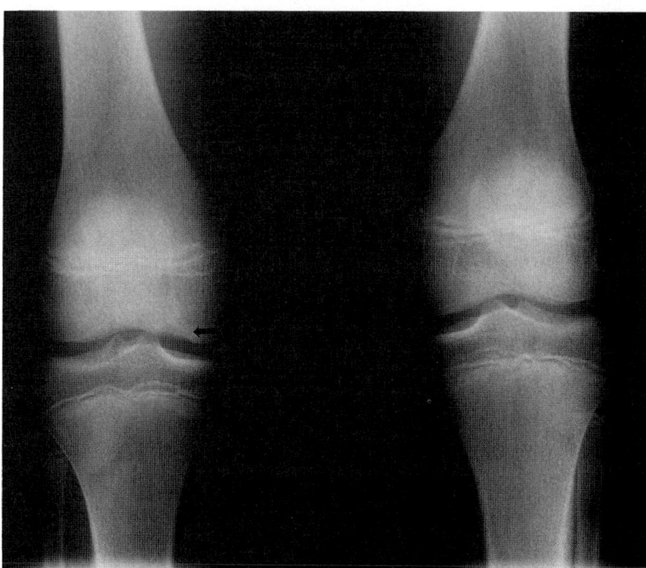

Figure 10.12. Osteochondritis dissecans of the knee in a 12-year-old with intermittent right knee symptoms of pain. Irregular ossification and radiolucency in the subchondral region of the medial condyle may be seen *(arrow)*.

chondral fragment, as evidenced by locking or catching. In addition to the radiolucent area seen on routine x-ray, improved visualization may be seen on other projections, particularly the intracondylar notch view of the knee. Tomograms of the joint may delineate the extent of the bony involvement. Magnetic resonance imaging (MRI) evaluation will often clarify the extent of the bone and cartilaginous involvement. Category III represents the post-adolescent period, or adult, who may also have a gradual onset of symptoms, but who is even more likely to have some degree of separation of the fragment and formation of loose bodies. In these individuals, the symptom complex will often include recurrent episodes of pain, swelling, and occasionally locking of the knee.

Knee Treatment

In younger children (category I), tenderness in the anterior joint line may be diagnostic of the problem of osteochondritis dissicans. In early involvement, frank radiographic changes may be less extensive and less apparent. If there is no history of locking and full range of motion of the joint exists, immobilization for a period of 3 to 6 weeks may make them asymptomatic. Following this, modification of sport activities may be necessary along with rehabilitation of the muscles. Most of these patients do well without further intervention. In those adolescent patients (category II), who have symptoms of long duration and well-established radiographic lesions, immobilization may be tried. If radiographic healing does not occur or if significant effusion or locking is present, then a more complete evaluation, including radiograph, MRI, and arthroscopy is important. Arthroscopic findings of a partially separated subosteochondral fragment may require drilling to reestablish circulation and/or pin fixation to reattach, if the fragment is large enough. A completely free fragment or loose bodies will need to be removed. It is much less likely for lesions in category III adult patients to heal and some form of fixation and/or excision will usually be necessary. Restriction of athletic activities to allow reconstruction of the bony integrity or fibrocartilaginous filling-in of the defect is an important part of the rehabilitative process as is the rehabilitation of the muscle/tendon complex.

Ankle Treatment

The ankle is less commonly affected by osteochondritis dessicans than is the knee, and the condition is usually somewhat more subtle in its production of symptoms. Diffuse ankle pain and swelling after physical activity may occur. Occasional locking or snapping of the ankle will be noted. Routine AP and lateral radiographs may show the lesion; however, often linear tomograms may be necessary to see the specific lesion well. Similar forms of therapy as described for the knee are applicable to this process as well.

Panner's Disease

Involvement of the anterior and lateral portions of the capitellum of the elbow may be the result of multiple, repeated loads associated with frequent throwing (31). It is postulated that repeated microfractures of the supporting subchondral region allow for collapse and subsequent separation of the cartilaginous surface. This commonly occurs in the younger ages (categories I, II) and is more common in boys (32). It is to be distinguished from medial epicondylitis, which is usually also due to throwing, but produces symptoms on the opposite side of the elbow. Radiographically, fragmentation is common. In addition to the subchondral radiolucency that occurs, and, particularly, in longstanding processes loose body formation is frequent, giving rise to locking and catching symptoms with elbow motion. In the milder forms, treatment consists of immobilization and a splint until symptoms have subsided, usually 3 to 6 weeks, followed by moderation of sport activities, especially throwing. This may require a change in sport emphasis, for example, giving up the position of pitcher at least until radiographic resolution occurs. For elbows with an effusion or a history of locking, an MRI or arthrogram may be helpful. Arthroscopic evaluation and debridement may be necessary both for diagnosis as well as removal of loose bodies.

Recent reports of upper extremity problems in young gymnasts with either Pannerlike lesions in the capitellum, or epiphyseal changes in the distal radius may demonstrate the need to be more aware of potential problems in a variety of sports that put increased repetitive stresses on the upper extremities.

Anterior Patella Pain Disorders

The patellofemoral articulation at the knee is an exceptionally important part of locomotion and thereby plays a role in almost all forms of sport activities. The extensor mechanism of the knee involves a complex relationship of the muscle/tendon complex where a sesamoid bone, the patella, facilitates the biomechanical function of active extension. It also plays an indirect role in controlled flexion of the knee. The patella generally is guided through flexion and extension by the articular congruity of its various facets and the femoral condyles while riding in the lateral condylar grove. Because of the attachment of the infrapatella tendon into the proximal tibial apophysis and the direction of pull of the quadriceps muscle mass, both of which are slightly lateral to the intercondylar groove, there tends to be an angular force created about the knee. This valgus force was described by Curveilhier as a Q angle (quadriceps angle) (34) (Fig. 10.13). The direction of the femoral groove helps determine the stability of the patella passively, but dynamic stability comes from both the medial and lateral retenacular fibers that attach the fibers to the patella, but also broadly into the deep fascia on the lateral and medial side of the proximal tibia. Any mechanical conditions that increase the Q angle will produce increased pressure during articulation, particularly over the lateral condyle and the lateral facet of the patella. In severe malalignment problems, especially those following traumatic disruptions of the medial retenacular structures, the patella may actually dislocate laterally.

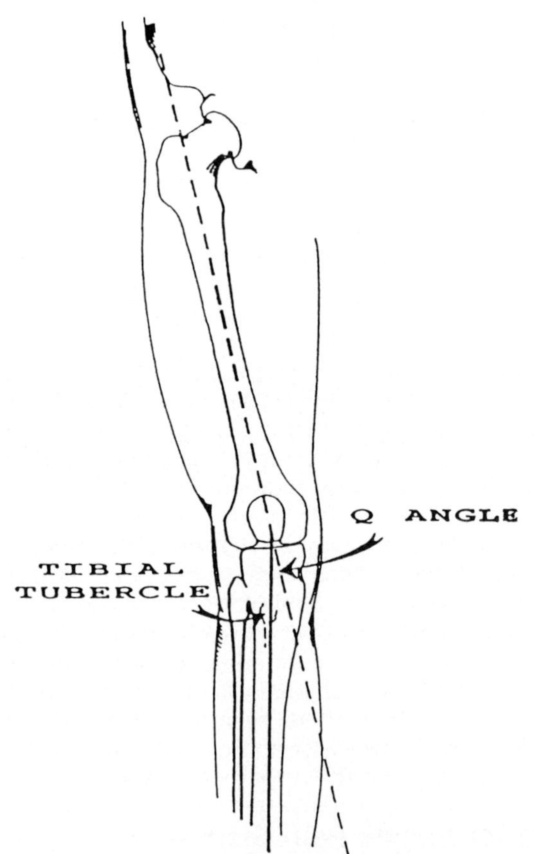

Figure 10.13. The Q-angle measurement of patella-femoral-tibial alignment as described by Cruveilhier (1791–1874). Reprinted from Talbott, JN A biographical history of medicine. Exerpts and essays on the men and their work. New York: Grune & Stratton, 1970.

In spite of the fact that younger children and preadolescents often have increased genu valgus as part of their normal developmental alignment pattern, anterior patellar pain and symptoms of instability are unusual. A prospective study of children and adolescents with patellofemoral pain has shown that less than 10% of these patients had symptoms below the age of 13 (35). Indeed, the patellofemoral pain in younger children may represent more of a soft tissue overuse problem, whereas in the older child or preadolescent, where patellar tracking problems may become more apparent, articular cartilage may occur.

Evaluation and Treatment

Children who have suffered a specific traumatic event involving the knee, especially if it involved frank dislocation of the patella, will usually have a dramatic history and clear findings indicating injured tissue with swelling, pain, and perhaps a laterally displaced patella. However, most often chronic patellofemoral problems present as diffuse anterior knee pain in the patella without a dramatic event. These symptoms are often made worse while participating in specific sport activities or other activities of daily living.

In younger patients, these symptoms may be difficult to elucidate, but by the time patellofemoral problems present as a common problem in the adolescent age group, these symptoms are better defined. Occasionally, there is a sense that the knee gives out or catches, but this represents pseudolocking and rarely are these true interarticular locking episodes. With most patellofemoral pain problems, an effusion in the joint is rare. Point tenderness at the edge of the patella, especially on the lateral side is common. Actively ranging the knee through an arc of motion from extension to flexion will give the examiner an idea of the direction of tracking of the knee cap in the groove. Evaluation of the Q angle may be helpful in determining abnormal tracking or positioning. A valgus knee deformity may contribute to the malalignment in the older adolescent. The side-to-side excursion of the patella when pushed in the extended knee may help to determine the glide of the patella in addition to determining increased laxity. If pushing the patella gives the patient the sense that there is instability or produces increase in pain, reproduce their symptoms and elicit an "apprehension sign." Subpatella crepitus, thought to indicate softening of the cartilage of the subchondral area of the patella, is a common finding event in the normal knee. Most patients with nontraumatic patellar pain syndrome have bilateral symptoms although one knee is commonly more involved than the other. Treatment is aimed at symptomatically managing this problem by modification of the demands upon the knee in the short-term and attempts at rehabilitation of the quadriceps mechanism in the long-term. Reducing the demands upon the knee often involves not only modifying sport activities and gym, but reducing other daily activities that produce significant knee use, for example, stair climbing, hill climbing, and frequently getting up and down out of chairs. Tight hamstrings must be stretched in order to reduce some of the forces across the patella. It may be advantageous to strengthen the vastus medialis specifically in order to help support the medial aspect of the patella and to prevent lateral tracking. Quadricep strengthening should be done through short arc-type exercises using no more than 25° to 30° of flexion to full extension in order to minimize compressive loads on the patella. The key to successful treatment of most adolescent patellofemoral problems depends upon a regular and consistent dedication to the above program. Elastic knee braces designed to support the patella from the sides may be helpful in some cases. Unless there is a significant tracking problem, most patellofemoral pain symptoms can be managed symptomatically. Patients can usually return to most sport activities in the long-term. The symptom complex may have a tendency to wax and wane over several years, but generally will respond to intermittent use of a program to reduce activities and to increased stretching and strengthening exercises of the thigh muscle. For those individuals with severe tracking problems, especially frank dislocation, or with such poor mechanics about the knee that abnormal forces are being brought to bear, a surgical realignment procedure done either from above or below the patella may be necessary to ensure normal knee function.

Spine and Sports

General

The spine represents a complex composite of supportive elements where the vertebral bodies, their facets, lamina, and spinous processes are supported by ligaments and an extensive paravertebral muscle system. The growing spine has some of the same risks for injury as has an adult spine—with the added caveat that secondary centers of ossification and growth plates exist in the vertebral bones just as they do in immature long bones and may be injured or affected by external or environmental forces. It is generally accepted that younger children have proportionally longer trunks and, therefore, a longer spine length than extremity length, although this proportionality changes with the attainment of adolescence and adulthood. Also, younger children generally have more flexible spines, in keeping with their generalized ligamentous flexibility as demonstrated in other joints throughout the body. The normal coronal plane alignment is straight (assuming equal leg length), while the sagittal plane alignment shows a normal cervical lordosis, a thoracic kyphosis, and a lumbar lordosis. Very young infants and toddlers generally have reduced lumbar lordosis, while juveniles in the 8 to 12 age group often exhibit increased functional lordosis in the lumbar spine. These are normal variations.

In contrast to adults, back pain in normal children is rare with the exception of Scheuerman's kyphosis and spondylolysis, as discussed below. More potentially serious problems such as fractures, infections, or tumors should be considered when examining the child who presents complaining primarily of back pain. Back pain with peripheral radiation symptoms into the lower extremities should also be taken as a potentially serious implication for neurologic abnormality. Otherwise, children and adolescents occasionally present with back fatigue, generalized muscle pain, and discomfort that may or may not be sport-related. This is more likely to be interscapular and paravertebral. It often is associated with excessive sport participation in much the same manner as other overuse problems. Occasionally, children and adolescents sitting for long periods of time while playing musical instruments, typing, or doing computer work present with interscapular pain that is usually related to fixation of the shoulder muscles in order to stabilize the arms, leading to fatigue symptoms.

Trauma to the Spine

Significant injury may occur to the spine in children participating in sports, and while rare, the outcomes can be disastrous. Fortunately, with closer supervision of the level of sport activities, avoidance of high risk behavior—for example, tackling with the head in football or spearing—the risk of significant problems has been reduced (36). The two highest risk areas are football and gymnastics or trampolinelike activity (37). Significant injuries include fracture or dislocation with or without neurologic injury. The cervical spine may be most liable to injury because of its relative lack of support. All complaints referable to the back or spine that appear related to a specific injury should be given serious consideration for a thorough evaluation.

One special circumstance related to the cervical spine and sport activities involves spinal instability at the C1, C2 level in patients with Down's syndrome (trisomy 21). Instability of this specific level has been estimated occur in 10% to 15% of children with this problem, although most of these patients are asymptomatic (38). Because of the asymptomatic nature of some of these children, questions have been raised about a particular need to assess children who are participating in sports. Recommendations of the American Academy of Pediatrics applicable to all children with Down's syndrome participating in sports include:

1. All children with Down's syndrome should be evaluated with lateral roentgenograms of the C1/C2 region in flexion, extension, and neutral position;
2. If signs of increased stability are present radiographically and neurologic symptoms are present, surgical stabilization should be entertained;
3. If radiographic instability exists and no symptoms are present, then follow-up examinations should be performed as often as yearly or sooner, and the children should not participate in contact sports, diving, or gymnastics;
4. Since the natural history is not known of the potential for developing radiographic signs if no instability exists and no radiologic abnormality is seen, these children should have an examination done at 2 to 3

year intervals. In light of the low frequency of occurrence and the very rare reported complications of these children participating in sports, these guidelines might seem restrictive, but until further natural history data and information are forthcoming, they should be followed.

Scoliosis

Classically, scoliosis is defined as lateral bending of the spine. Since, in the coronal plane, the spine is usually straight, theoretically any bending from the zero position would represent a "scoliosis," although we generally accept up to 10° of angulation as being within normal limits and not constituting a true scoliosis. While scoliosis may be caused by a wide variety of abnormalities, the most common type of scoliosis encountered in children who are participating in an otherwise normal sport activity is idiopathic scoliosis. This scoliosis has an unknown etiology and it occurs in otherwise healthy children. Often it appears for the first time during the adolescent growth spurt. Other causes of scoliosis, such as neurologic abnormalities as seen in children with cerebral palsy or congenital scoliosis as seen in children with an underlying osseous defect presenting from birth, occasionally are seen in children participating in sports. While muscular imbalance is thought to play a role in the development of scoliosis in patients with neuromuscular causes, the etiology of idiopathic scoliosis is not known. The vast majority of children with small curves do not progress during their adolescent growth spurt; however, some do with girls being somewhat more likely than boys. There are no clinical or radiographic indicators that can be used to predict progression, so that frequent repeated examination at 6 to 8 month intervals during the years of remaining growth are necessary to monitor the potential changes indicating a progressive deformity. In spite of the curvature of the spinal column that occurs with scoliosis, the spine retains its normal biomechanical integrity, and, therefore, most children with scoliosis may participate fully in all activities and are encouraged to do so to help maintain muscle strength in spinal flexibility. There are no known activities that either cause an increase or decrease in the progression of the curve. Anatomically, the curve can commonly be located in the thoracic region, the lumbar region, or both (Fig. 10.14). While the characteristic deformity is a lateral bending of the spinal column, scoliosis is anatomically a three-dimensional deformity with changes occurring in the sagittal plane as seen by flattening, usually in the thoracic spine, and also by a twisting or a rotation that occurs in the transverse plain of the body. It is the twisting that gives the apparent rib hump when bending forward.

The only two known effective therapeutic interventions are the use of a body brace called a thoracal–lumbo–sacral orthosis (TLSO) or surgery. The primary goal of brace therapy is to control the curve while it is still mild-to-moderate and prevent it from becoming severe. Children have to demonstrate a progression of

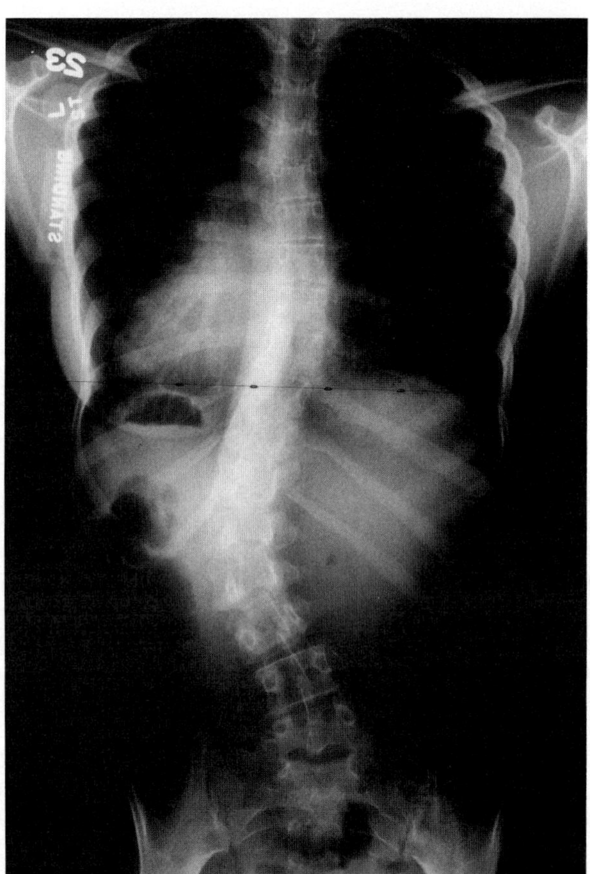

Figure 10.14. Adolescent idiopathic scoliosis in a 14-year-old female as seen from the back showing lateral bending and deviation of the spine and trunk giving an imbalance to the trunk. This curve is in the thoracolumbar region and is convex to the left.

the curve to a significant level before the brace will be effective, and they have to have growth remaining for it to be effective. Brace wearing is done most of the day and night during the remaining portion of the growth spurt, which may involve as much as 1 or 2 years. Full participation in sports may occur during brace treatment. In many instances, participation may occur with the brace on, but in instances when this interferes with the sport activity or is an endangerment to other participants, sport activities may take place without the brace. This is especially true for competitive sports in which the brace may be removed during practice and for competitions without any detrimental effects. In those children requiring surgery, there is usually a period of 8 months to 1 year following the surgery where sport participation is not allowed or is limited. After the spine fusion is complete, however, the patient may again return to most sport activities. While flexibility may be mildly disturbed in those individuals with surgery, most of these patients are returned to normal activities without limitations.

Kyphosis

The term kyphosis is often used in the pathologic sense and means an increased bending in the sagittal plane. While normal kyphosis exists in the thoracic spine, increase in this bending, hyperkyphosis, may produce a noticeable deformity. The presence of "poor posture" is often a concern of the parents of teenagers. This is usually due to hyperkyphosis that is flexible and often positionally related and fully correctable with an effort on the part of the patient to sit or stand in an erect manner. This is a common teenage habitus with no known consequences for permanent deformity in spite of parental concerns. This condition is also known as functional round back. It usually will respond to careful encouragement to the adolescent and improves with maturation. Occasionally, extension exercises of the paravertebral muscles may be helpful, particularly in nonathletic individuals, but sport participation should be encouraged.

Scheuermann's Kyphosis

This condition represents a hyperkyphosis or excessive kyphosis, usually in the thoracic region that involves actual structural changes in the endplates of the vertebral bodies. The cause is unknown, although its occurrence seems to be limited to the growing spine. There is usually an associated wedging of the vertebrae (Fig. 10.15). The deformity may be quite noticeable cosmetically. Most commonly it is associated with back pain, particularly during activities. If the symptom complex is mild and only occasional and the deformity is not terribly noticeable, a program of extension exercises and a moderation of activities may manage symptoms. At the completion of growth, the symptoms usually disappear spontaneously, probably associated with closure of the growth plate. In those patients who have a more significant deformity and whose symptoms are fairly constant during the day, the best management scheme may be with a specialized TLSO for a period of 1 to 2 years. Again, the symptoms usually disappear fairly rapidly with the use of bracing with the deformity at least partially corrected in many cases. In those individuals with severe deformities, frequently accompanied by marked symptoms, it may be necessary to perform surgical stabilization for improvement. Sport participation is encouraged in all of these patients except for those who have recently undergone surgical correction. Otherwise, the long-term outcome for patients with Scheuermann's kyphosis is satisfactory.

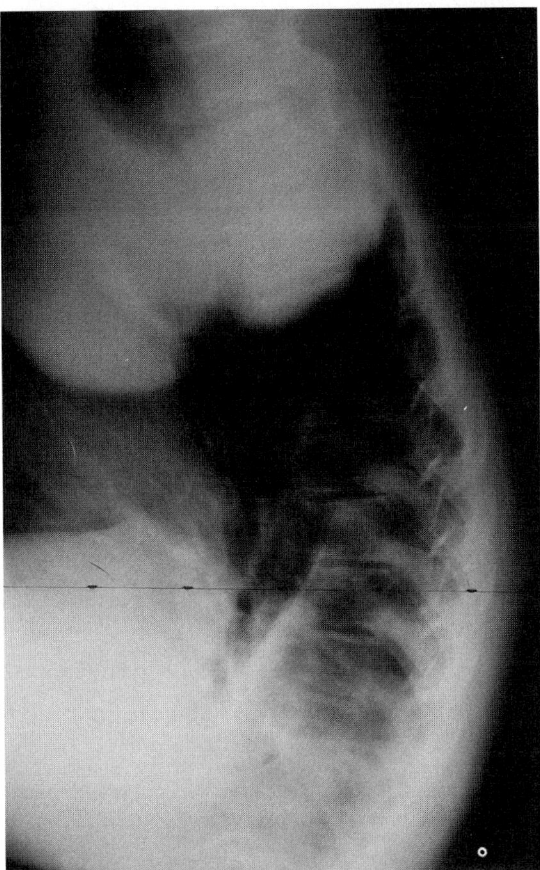

Figure 10.15. Scheuermann's kyphosis in an 11-year-old male with back pain and "poor posture." In addition to the kyphosis, end-plate irregularities (Smorals nodes) may be seen in the lower vertebral bodies and wedging may be seen in the vertebra of the upper thoracic vertebra.

Spondylolysis and Spondylolisthesis

Anatomical disturbance of the portion of the vertebral bodies posteriorly between the "superior" and "inferior" facets may produce structural and symptomatic problems in some patients. This area, known as the pars interarticulus, may show a defect on the anterior/posterior, lateral or oblique roentgenogram of the lumbar spine. This defect often is bilateral, although on occasion it may be seen on one side only. These findings are noted usually after the child or adolescent has presented with midline low back pain, although occasionally symptoms of posterior or lateral thigh pain may also accompany the back pain. This problem is not found in children less than 4 years of age. It has an incidence of 4% at age 6, and 6% in adults (39). Spondylolysis refers to the mere presence of the defect in the pars interarticulus area, while spondylolisthesis refers to a slippage or forward movement of one vertebral body onto another. The most common level of involvement is the L5 vertebrae with forward slipping of the body at L5 on S1 (Fig. 10.16). Occasionally, this may be seen also at the L4 or L3 level. The slipping process is gradual and may exist in a small portion of the adult population who are unaware that they have spondylolisthesis. Therefore, not all instances of pars interarticular defect are symptomatic. Trauma may play a role in the etiology of this problem, since there is an increased incidence of this problem among gymnasts and in interior linemen in professional football.

The clinical presentation, in addition to the presence of back pain, may show evidence of hamstring tightness or may show as limitation in motion in a straight leg raising test. Flattening of the lumbosacral region on standing may suggest displacement and the presence of spondylolisthesis. X-rays, as noted previously, often show a defect in the pars interarticulus and will clearly show the presence of slippage if it is occurring. Treatment is tailored to the specific problem at the time of presentation. If the onset is acute and symptoms seem related to a specific activity, x-rays may show a well-

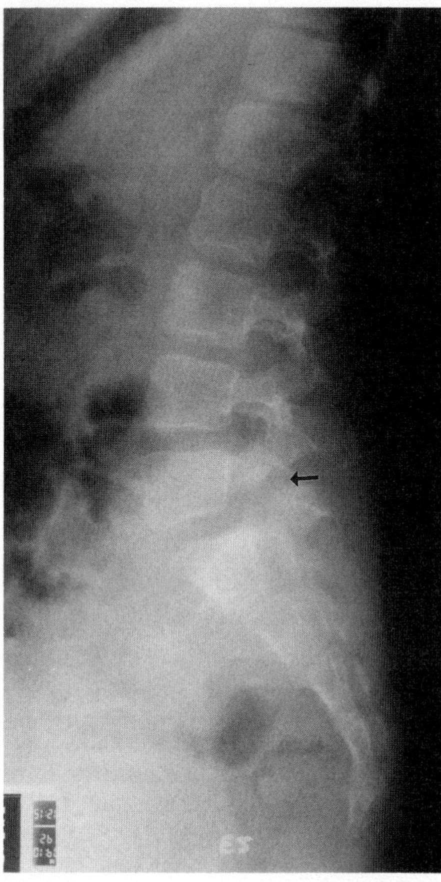

Figure 10.16. Spondylolisthesis of L5 on S1 (sacrum) in a 16-year-old with low back pain, initially only after sport activities, but becoming more constant with time. Lateral radiographs show forward slipping of the vertebrae body of L5 on S1 (sacrum) and the arrow marks the defect in the pars interarticularis.

defined defect in the pars and a bone scan may show evidence of increased activity in this region. In such a patient, an acute injury may be assumed that may respond to the application of a lumbar brace (modified anterior-opening TLSO). The healing of such defects has been described (40). Other children with a more long-standing symptom complex or a more notable defect appearing roentgenograms may respond symptomatically to the application of a brace for a 3 to 6 month period. If they remain asymptomatic, they may undergo a rehabilitation process that would include hamstring stretching and abdominal muscle strengthening. They may return on a gradual basis to their sport activities. They should be followed symptomatically, since very mild spondylolisthesis rarely progresses. In those with more severe slippage or documented radiographic progression, surgical stabilization and fusion may be necessary. Not unlike the rehabilitation from other spinal surgeries, there is an excellent chance to return to most sport activities and participate in fully and normal activities once satisfactory fusion has been obtained in about 8 months to 1 year.

REFERENCES

1. Tanner JM, Whitehouse RH, Takaishi M. Standards from birth to maturity for height, weight, height velocity, and weight velocity; british children, 1956, Part II. Arch Dis. Child 1966,41:613–35.
2. Palmer CE. Studies of the center of gravity in the human body, Child Dev 1944;15:99–180.
3. Bar-Or O. Importance of differences between children and adults for exercise testing and exercise prescription. In Skinner JS, ed. Exercise testing and exercise prescriptions for special cases: Theoretical bains and Clinical Application. Philadelphia: Lea & Febiger, 1987,59–65.
4. Ellis, JD, Carron AV, Bailey DA Physical performance in boys from 10 to 16 years. Hum Biol 1975:263–81.
5. Curetun TK, Barry AJ. Improving the physical fitness of youths: A report in the sports fitness school of the University of Illinois. Monogr Soc Res Child Dev 1964;29:Serial #95.
6. Carron AV, Bailey DA. A. Longitudinal examination of speed reaction and speed movement in young boys, ages 7–13 years. Hum Biol 1973,45:669.
7. Garrick JG, Requa RK. Injuries in high school sports. Pediatrics, 1978;61:465–469.
8. Goldberg B, Rosenthal PP, Nicholas JA. Injuries in youth football. Phys Sports Med 1984:12:122–132.
9. Hanlon, CR, Estes WC. Fractures in childhood, a statistical analysis. Am Surg 1954;87:312–323.
10. Ogden JA. Injury to the immature skeleton. In: Touloukian R. Pediatric trauma, 2nd ed. New York. John Wiley and Sons, 1990.
11. Hyattsville, MD: National Health Interview Survey, Data File. National Center for Health Statistics, 1990.
12. Ogden, John A. Skeletal injury in the child. 2nd ed. Philadelphia: W.B. Saunders Co, 1990.
13. Salter RB, Harris WR. Injuries involving the epiphyseal plate. Bone Joint Surg [AM], 1963;45A:587.
14. Staheli Lynn T. Fundamentals of pediatric orthopaedics. New York: Raven Press, 1992.
15. Woo, SL-Y Maynard J, et al. Ligament, Tendon, and Joint Capsule Insertions to Bone. In: Injury and repair of the musculoskeletal soft tissues, Woo, SL-Y, Buchwalter J, ed. Park Ridge, IL: American Academy of Orthopaedic Surgeons, 1987.
16. Dorfl, J. Vessels in the region of tenderness insertions, I. Chondro Physeal Insertion Folia Morphology, 1969;17:74–78.
17. Sever, JW. Apophysitis of the os calcis. N Y Med J May 1, 1912.
18. Micheli LJ, Ireland ML. Prevention and management of calcaneal apophysitis in children: An overuse syndrome., Pediatr Orthop 1987;7(1):34–38.
19. Ehrenborg G, Engfeldt B. Histologic changes in the Osgood-Schlatter lesions. Clin Scand 1962;124:89–105.
20. Kujala UM, Kuist M, Heinonen O. Osgood-Schlatter's disease in adolescent athletes. Retrospective study of incidence and duration. Am J Sports Med. 1985;13(4):236–41.
21. Hulkko A, Orava S. Stress fractures in athletes. Int J Sports Med 1987;8:221–226.
22. Devas MB. Stress fractures in children. Bone Joint Surg 1963;45B:520–541.
23. Walter NE, Wolf MD. Stress fractures in young athletes. Am J Sports Med 1977;5:165–170.
24. Rubin CT, Lonyon LE. Osteoregulatory mature of mechanical stimuli: Function is a determinant for adoptive remodeling in bone. J Orthop Res 1987;5:300–310.
25. Siffert RS. Classification of osteochondrosis. Clin Orthop 158:10–18, 1981.
26. Douglas G, Rang, Merca. The role of trauma in the pathogenesis of osteochondrosis. Clin Orthop 1981;158:28–32.
27. Ippolito E, Ricciari-Pollini PT, Falez F. Kohler's disease of the tarsal navicular. Long-term follow-up of 12 cases, J Pediatr Orthop 1984;4(4):416.
28. Williams GA, Cowell HR. Kohlers disease of the tarsal navicular. Clin Orthop 1981;158:53–58.
29. Mubarak SJ, Carroll NC. Familiar osteochondritis dissecans of the knee, Clin Orthop 1979;140:131–136.
30. Andrew, TA, Spivey J, Lindebaum RH. Familial osteochondritis dissecans and dwarfism. ACTA Orthop Scand 1981;52:579–523.

31. Pappas, AMJ. Osteochondrosis dissecans. Clin Orthop 1981;158:70–76.
32. Omer GE, Jr. Primary articular osteochondrosis. Clin Orthop 1981;158:70–76.
33. Maffulli H, Chan D, Aldridge MS. Derangement of the articular surfaces of the elbow in young gymnasts. J Ped Ortho 1992;12:344–350.
34. Wenger D, Rang M. The Art and Practice of Pediatric Orthopaedics. New York: Raven Press, 1993:242.
35. Gates C, Grana WA Patella femoral pain: A prospective study, Orthopedics, 1986;9:663–667.
36. Clark KS. A survey of sports-related spinal cord injuries in schools and colleges, J Safety Res 1977;9:140.
37. Toly JS, Vegco JJ, Seimett B. The national football head and neck injury registry: 14-year-report on cervical quadriplegia, 1971–1981. JAMA 1985;254:3439.
38. Pueschel SM, Scola FH. Atlontoxial instability in individuals with Downs syndrome: Epidemiologic, radiographic, and chemical studies, Pediatrics 1987;80.555.
39. Fredrickson BE, Baker D, McHolick WJ. The natural history of spondylolysis and spondylolisthesis. J Bone Joint Surg 1984;66A:699–707.
40. Rocke MD. Healing of the bilateral fracture of the pars interarticulus of the lumbar sacral arch. J Bone Joint Surg, 1950;32A:428.

11 / SPECIAL CONCERNS OF THE FEMALE ATHLETE

Mary Lloyd Ireland

Introduction

Physiologic, anatomic, and psychologic differences in females and males create certain unique patterns of illness and injury. Enhanced appreciation of these special situations will enable the practitioner to sharpen diagnostic skills and improve treatment of the female athlete. Unique illnesses are related to nutritional and hormonal balance. These illnesses include anorexia nervosa, bulimia, athletic amenorrhea, iron deficiency anemia, hormonal imbalance, pregnancy, and postmenopausal osteoporosis (1–4).

The majority of injuries are related to participation in the sport rather than the gender of the athlete (5–10). Anatomic differences in lower extremity alignment, less upper extremity strength, hormonal imbalance, and nutritional disorders increase chances for certain overuse injuries with intense training in females. Stress fractures in amenorrheic runners and upper extremity injuries in underdeveloped prepubertal gymnasts are common. There is an increased incidence of patellofemoral (PF) disorders and anterior cruciate ligament (ACL) injuries in females (11). Differences shown diagrammatically are the female's wider pelvis, increased flexibility, less developed musculature, less developed vastus medialis obliquus (VMO), narrower femoral notch and genu valgum, and external tibial torsion (Fig. 11.1). In the male, extremity alignment includes a narrower pelvis, more developed thigh musculature, VMO hypertrophy, less flexibility, wider femoral notch, genu varum, and internal or neutral tibia torsion (Fig. 11.2). Why do these overuse and ACL injuries occur? The reasons are multifactorial. In the past, studies were done on males only. More research is desperately needed in women's sports. Concerns over lasting injury and illness exist. Follow-up of a women's collegiate gymnastics team showed half of the athletes had less than fully recovered from their injuries three years after stopping competition (12).

With the increased awareness in the importance of fitness and the passage of Title IX ensuring equal rights for male and female athletes in federally supported institutions, the numbers of females participating in structured competitive and recreational athletics has skyrocketed during the past several decades. The history of competition of women at various levels—local, national, and international—is fascinating (13, 14). With this dramatic increase in participation, injury rates and patterns emerge. More research is needed in areas of female sport participation.

Sports of Participation

National Collegiate Athletic Association (NCAA) and United States Olympic Committee (USOC) recognize sports that are male and female combined, male only, and female only (Table 11.1). In NCAA competition, female-only sports are field hockey and softball. Male-only NCAA sports are water polo, baseball, football, ice hockey, and wrestling. Olympic sports that are female only are rhythmic gymnastics and synchronized swimming. Male-only Olympic sports are baseball, bobsled, boxing, ice hockey, modern pentathlon, ski jumping, nordic combined skiing, soccer, water polo, weight lifting, and wrestling. Sport biomechanics of the male- or female-only sports create uniquely different patterns and different incidence of injury.

Injury Rates

Since 1982, the NCAA Injury Surveillance System has been published with detailed injury information in 16 sports. The 4 comparable sports for men and women are gymnastics, basketball, soccer, and lacrosse. Female-only sports are softball and field hockey. Male-only sports are spring football, football, wrestling, ice hockey, and baseball.

For women, the highest overall injury rate in collegiate sports is gymnastics, followed by soccer, basket-

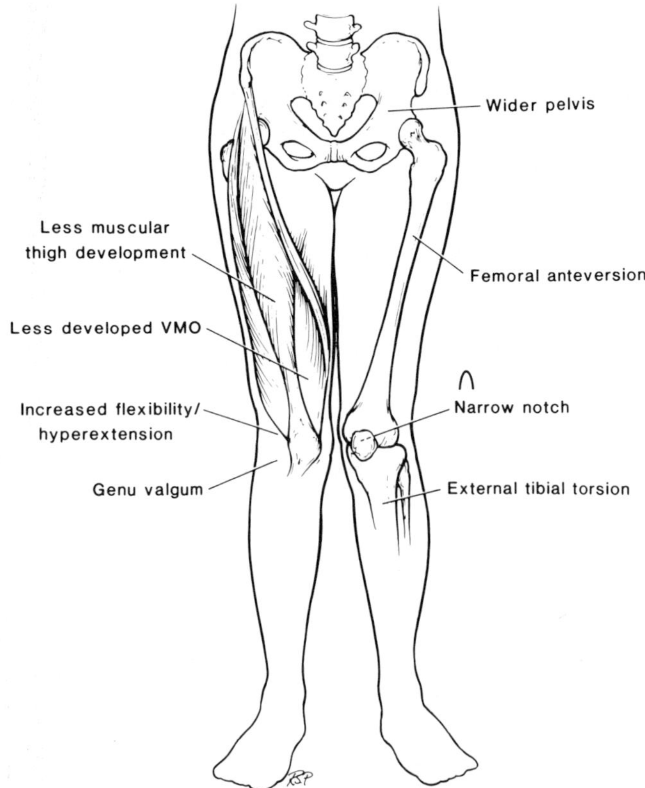

Figure 11.1 Diagram shows the lower extremity alignment that may predispose to certain overuse problems involving the hips and knees and especially ACL and patellofemoral injuries. Females have a wider pelvis, increased flexibility, less developed musculature, hypoplastic vastus medialis obliquus, narrow femoral notch, genu valgum, and external tibial torsion.

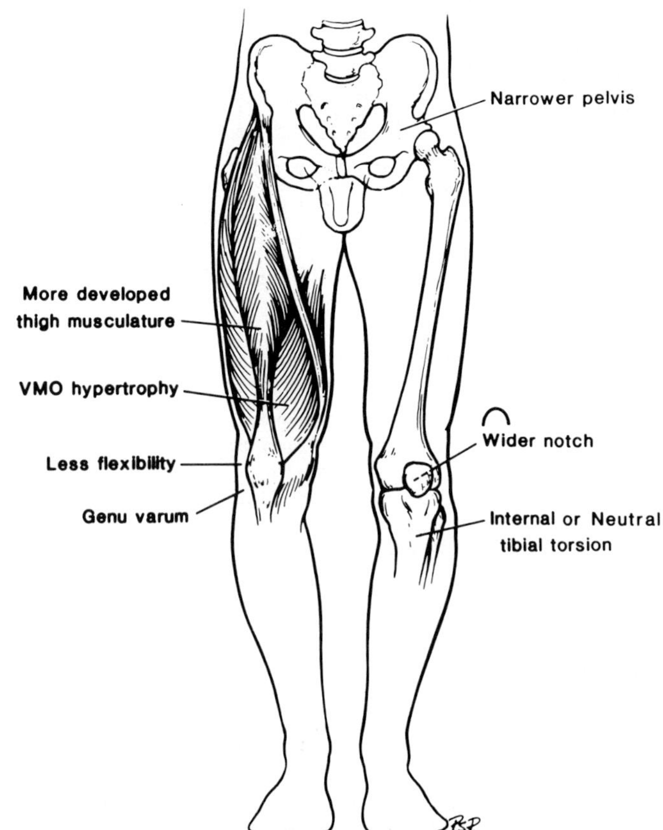

Figure 11.2 Males have a narrower pelvis, more developed thigh musculature, vastus medialis obliquus hypertrophy, less flexibility, wider femoral notch, more tendency toward a genu varum, and internal or neutral tibial torsion.

ball, field hockey, volleyball, lacrosse, and softball. The men's sports of spring football and wrestling had the highest injury rates (10) (Table 11.2). Equal occurrence of injury in practice and games were women's and men's soccer, lacrosse, field hockey, softball, and baseball. In gymnastics, about 80% of injuries occurred in practice (Table 11.2). Knowledge of injury rate and timing of occurrence allows the practitioner to plan coverage.

The type of injury for each of the 16 NCAA sports was analyzed (Table 11.3). The categories analyzed included contusion, tendinitis, incomplete ligament sprain, incomplete muscle tendon strain, complete muscle tendon strain, fracture and stress fracture, concussion, heat exhaustion, and inflammation. For completeness, the sixteen sports and all categories are included. The incidence of incomplete sprains was highest in spring football (Table 11.3) followed by women's gymnastics, wrestling, and men's soccer. Women's gymnastics lead the diagnoses of complete sprain, incomplete strain, and tendinitis. Concussion and heat exhaustion rarely occurred.

The rate at which a particular body part was injured was also analyzed (Table 11.4). The ankle was the most commonly injured joint. Women's gymnastics had the highest rates of lower back and foot injuries. The injured body parts for all sixteen sports are shown for comparison in this table.

There are many studies comparing male and female incidence of injury in similar sports (7, 8, 15). Using the National Athletic Injury Illness Reporting System, Whiteside (8) reported the order of highest to lowest incidence of injuries was basketball, gymnastics, softball in women (compared to basketball) gymnastics, and baseball in men. Men's and women's basketball had the highest relative injury frequency. Women had a relatively higher frequency rate of ankle injuries and fractures in basketball and gymnastics.

Injury type and rate were compared to six varsity sports at Indiana University during the 1977 to 1978 season (15). The highest injury rate was gymnastics (40%) with the most injuries occurring during practice, in tumbling, and in younger women. Most of the basketball injuries occurred on defense while guarding.

The ankle is the most commonly injured joint in many series (6, 8, 9, 15). In 19 female collegiate sports, injury rates were most common in basketball, followed by volleyball, field hockey, gymnastics, and track and field (16). In this survey of 361 colleges and universities, the injury-contributing factors in order were improper

Table 11.1.
Sports by Gender

Olympic Sports: Male / Female	Male Only	Female Only
Archery	Baseball	Rhythmic gymnastics
Athletics	Bobsled	Synchronized swimming
Basketball	Boxing	
Biathlon	Ice hockey	
Canoe / kayak	Modern pentathlon	
Cycling	Ski jumping	
Diving	Nordic combined skiing	
Equestrian	Soccer	
Fencing	Water polo	
Gymnastics, artistic	Weight lifting	
Field hockey	Wrestling	
Judo		
Luge		
Rowing		
Shooting		
Figure skating		
Speed skating		
Alpine skating		
Nordic skiing		
Swimming		
Team handball		
Tennis		
Table tennis		
Volleyball		
Yachting		

NCAA Sports: Combined	Male / Female	Male Only	Female Only
Fencing	Gymnastics	Water polo	Field hockey
Rifle	Volleyball	Baseball	Softball
Skiing	Basketball	Football	
	Cross country	Ice hockey	
	Lacrosse	Wrestling	
	Soccer		
	Swimming / diving		
	Tennis		
	Indoor / outdoor track		
	Golf		

training methods, inadequate facilities, and poor coaching techniques.

Sport Differences

Differences in sport biomechanics and training create certain specific injury patterns. The repetitive maneuvers of ballet, gymnastics, cheerleading, dance, and ice skating create circumstances for unique injuries. Gymnastic balance beam maneuvers may cause unusual injuries due to the apparatus (Fig. 11.3). In this collegiate gymnast, repetitive landings on the balance beam caused recurrent medial dislocations, one of which was open, of the left great toe from landing with the beam between the great and second toe causing the first metatarsophalangeal (MTP) dislocation. Medial stress views show severe instability of the left first MTP joint (Fig. 11.4*A*). Following a season of buddy taping of the toes, surgical reconstruction of the joint was performed. Intraoperative stress testing shows severe lateral instability of the left first metatarsophalangeal joint (Fig. 11.4*B*). There are reports of profiles and injuries in specific sports which include women rowers (17), professional ballerinas (18), and swimmers (19). Summarization of physiologic profiles provide excellent information (20–22).

Gender Differences

The diagnosis and treatment of the athletic female has been reviewed in detail. (4, 23). Excellent comparative studies of the genders have been done in the military setting (20, 24–26). Athletic women in the Navy were found to have more success than nonathletes in areas of stamina, strength, and self-discipline (26). Compared to males, women were found to be capable of equal efficiency and aerobic metabolism at the United States Military Academy (20). In a random review of 74 female and 74 male cadets, an increased incidence of stress fractures were found in females (24). Eleven fe-

Table 11.2.
Injury Rates per 1000 and Percentage in Practice and Games[a]

	Women				Men			
	Injury Rate per 1000	Total Injuries	Practice	Game	Injury Rate per 1000	Total Injuries	Practice	Game
Gymnastics	8.59	1634	78%	22%	5.06	415	81%	19%
Lacrosse	4.25	871	68%	32%	6.05	2554	54%	46%
Basketball	5.13	281	61%	39%	5.61	3386	65%	35%
Soccer	7.90	2540	51%	49%	7.87	5194	47%	53%
Volleyball	4.76	2823	65%	35%	x	x	x	x
Field Hockey	5.00	1526	59%	41%	x	x	x	x
Softball	3.90	1788	52%	48%	x	x	x	x
Spring Football	x	x	x	x	9.59	2129	94%	6%
Wrestling	x	x	x	x	9.41	4992	66%	34%
Football	x	x	x	x	6.57	29217	58%	42%
Baseball	x	x	x	x	3.37	3837	44%	56%
Ice Hockey	x	x	x	x	5.61	2908	32%	68%

[a]All data are shown as rate per 1000 athletic exposures for 1992–1993
Source: NCAA Injury Surveillance System, No. 9044–11/92

Table 11.3.
NCAA Injury Rate by Type of Injury[a]

	Contusion	Tendinitis	Ligament Sprain (incomplete tear)	Ligament Sprain (complete tear)	Muscle-tendon Strain (incomplete tear)	Muscle-tendon Strain (complete tear)	Fracture	Stress Fracture	Concussion	Heat Exhaustion	Inflammation
Gymnastics-W	0.98	0.30	2.73	0.46	2.43	0.03	0.30	0.30	0.19	0.00	0.25
Gymnastics-M	0.60	0.20	1.59	0.00	1.00	0.00	0.40	0.00	0.00	0.00	0.30
Basketball-W	0.50	0.21	1.79	0.21	0.78	0.03	0.28	0.20	0.17	0.00	0.18
Basketball-M	0.80	0.20	2.23	0.09	1.06	0.03	0.39	0.07	0.10	0.00	0.15
Soccer-W	0.92	0.33	2.12	0.23	2.20	0.07	0.44	0.25	0.23	0.04	0.32
Soccer-M	1.75	0.19	2.24	0.20	1.98	0.01	0.47	0.03	0.30	0.03	0.20
Lacrosse-W	0.18	0.18	1.08	0.12	1.83	0.00	0.09	0.33	0.09	0.00	0.33
Lacrosse-M	1.15	0.30	1.51	0.15	1.24	0.01	0.35	0.06	0.15	0.00	0.11
Field Hockey-W	0.84	0.33	0.88	0.12	1.10	0.02	0.33	0.10	0.08	0.08	0.18
Volleyball-W	0.23	0.23	1.51	0.05	1.02	0.02	0.13	0.04	0.05	0.02	0.15
Softball-W	0.51	0.30	0.55	0.11	0.86	0.03	0.34	0.01	0.10	0.00	0.06
Spring Football-M	1.25	0.18	3.23	0.25	1.98	0.03	0.55	0.03	0.20	0.00	0.13
Wrestling-M	0.69	0.06	2.46	0.14	1.63	0.04	0.27	0.03	0.31	0.03	0.08
Football-M	0.86	0.08	1.95	0.23	1.29	0.03	0.34	0.03	0.30	0.12	0.10
Ice Hockey-M	1.04	0.02	1.14	0.10	0.79	0.01	0.35	0.01	0.30	0.00	0.01
Baseball-M	0.44	0.28	0.59	0.06	1.15	0.01	0.25	0.02	0.05	0.00	0.05

[a]All data are shown as rate per 1000 athletic exposures in 1991–1992
Source: NCAA Injury Surveillance System, No. 9044–11/92

Table 11.4.
NCAA Injury Rate by Body Part[a]

	Neck	Shoulder	Wrist	Hand	Lower Back	Hips, Groin	Upper Leg	Knee	Patella	Lower Leg	Ankle	Foot
Gymnastics-W	0.22	0.41	0.30	0.05	0.96	0.25	0.46	1.48	0.03	0.49	1.91	0.71
Gymnastics-M	0.00	0.50	1.00	0.10	0.50	0.00	0.00	0.10	0.00	0.40	1.00	0.20
Basketball-W	0.02	0.21	0.05	0.09	0.33	0.21	0.25	0.92	0.10	0.24	1.38	0.27
Basketball-M	0.07	0.14	0.07	0.06	0.40	0.35	0.34	0.78	0.14	0.19	1.83	0.30
Soccer-W	0.32	0.25	0.07	0.01	0.27	0.37	1.45	1.27	0.08	0.71	1.76	0.41
Soccer-M	0.40	0.19	0.11	0.03	0.25	0.46	1.39	1.39	0.09	0.54	1.75	0.46
Lacrosse-W	0.00	0.03	0.03	0.03	0.21	0.45	0.69	0.63	0.06	0.66	0.84	0.27
Lacrosse-M	0.08	0.56	0.07	0.06	0.23	0.38	0.82	0.90	0.04	0.28	0.99	0.10
Field Hockey-W	0.02	0.12	0.04	0.10	0.16	0.14	0.73	0.47	0.22	0.35	0.69	0.24
Volleyball-W	0.02	0.40	0.01	0.07	0.38	0.12	0.27	0.52	0.15	0.15	1.17	0.11
Softball-W	0.03	0.63	0.08	0.15	0.24	0.08	0.22	0.45	0.06	0.13	0.39	0.08
Spring Football-M	0.53	1.33	0.08	0.05	0.35	0.28	1.28	1.80	0.20	0.30	1.70	0.18
Wrestling-M	0.60	1.18	0.09	0.10	0.38	0.14	0.22	1.66	0.11	0.17	0.75	0.06
Football-M	0.28	0.83	0.06	0.10	0.29	0.34	0.57	1.26	0.08	0.21	0.97	0.16
Ice Hockey-M	0.07	0.82	0.13	0.06	0.20	0.42	0.47	0.89	0.04	0.13	0.26	0.13
Baseball-M	0.02	0.80	0.09	0.08	0.07	0.10	0.33	0.29	0.04	0.11	0.32	0.05

[a]All data are shown as rate per 1000 athletic exposures for 1991–1992
Source: NCAA Injury Surveillance System, No. 9044–11/92

males and no males sustained stress fractures. Women had double the incidence of men's lower extremity injuries. However, men required an extra week to resolve their lower extremity injuries and required twice as much time to reach maximal improvement from back injuries as compared to women. Physiologic differences in men compared to women occur in aerobic fitness and resistive training. Compared to men, women midshipmen improved their fitness level more rapidly, and the disparities were often societal (27). Stress-related injuries were seen more often in women. As the women acclimated to the Naval Academy, similar numbers of serious injuries were seen. There is a comprehensive review of data comparing male and female athletes in areas of body composition and physique, muscle characteristics, strength, and cardiovascular endurance capacity (22). After age 10 to 12, there are significant differences in all aspects of physical performance. In the 18 to 22 year olds, body fat for females is 22% to 26% and males is 12% to 16%. In males, androgens create greater lean body weight. In females, estrogens contribute to the greater amount of fat weight. Detailed summaries of different sports comparing the genders include body composition, somatotype, muscle fiber, strength and cardiovascular endurance capacity, and O_2 max. Similarities in highly trained male and female athletes are lower-body strength (per unit of body weight), cardiovascular endurance capacity, body composition, and muscle fiber type. In females, a sedentary lifestyle after puberty may significantly contribute to the differences physiologically (22).

Gender differences in body composition and structural variables have been studied (21). Differences are similar in athletic females compared to males and nonathletic females compared to males. Total lean body mass is greater in males. Similar male and female ranking for fatness and leanness were reported with the lowest in runners and gymnasts and highest in basketball, volleyball and field events.

Work capacity studies show that, compared to men, women have more fat and less muscle, but only slight differences in the $\dot{V}_{O_{2max}}$ when expressed relative to body size and composition (28). Males have greater hemoglobin and higher red blood cell levels. In general, females are highly trainable and demonstrate the same physiologic training changes as males. The effects of aerobic exercises on training in symptomatic women with mitral valve prolapse were reviewed (29). Aerobic exercise was found to be a positive influence in the management of symptomatic women with mitral valve prolapse.

Women, like men, can experience significant increases in strength, power, and muscular endurance (30). Although upper body strength and development are less in females compared to males, sound strength training principles can decrease these differences as based on ratios to body weight. However, upper body strength in women, even with training, has, in some studies, remained only 30 to 50% of their male counterparts. Lower body strength comes much closer to parity.

The development of strength is usually the weakest link in the physiologic profile of the female athlete (22).

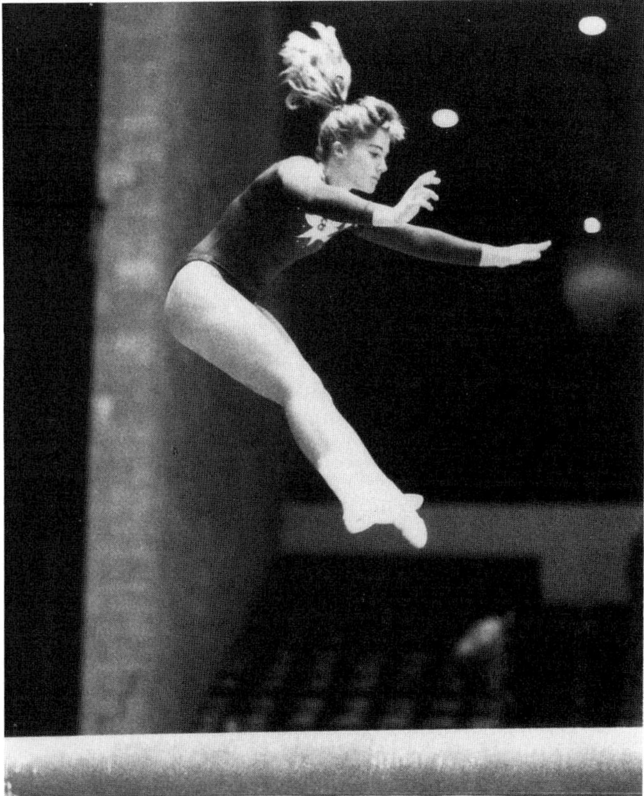

Figure 11.3 Gymnastic apparatus of the balance beam, which is unique in female sports, can result in certain unusual injuries.

Orthopaedic Considerations

Specific Joints

Knee

Injury Rates. Compared to males, PF disorders and ACL injuries are more common in females (9, 31–33). The knee is often injured in collegiate sports. The injuries can be matched to the sport (Table 11.5). The knee injury rates were categorized into the structures involved: ligaments (collateral, anterior cruciate, posterior cruciate), torn cartilage (meniscus), patella or patellar tendon. The collateral ligaments were most frequently injured in spring football, wrestling, football, and ice hockey. In comparable sports, the athletic exposure rate per 1000 ACL in the female involved more

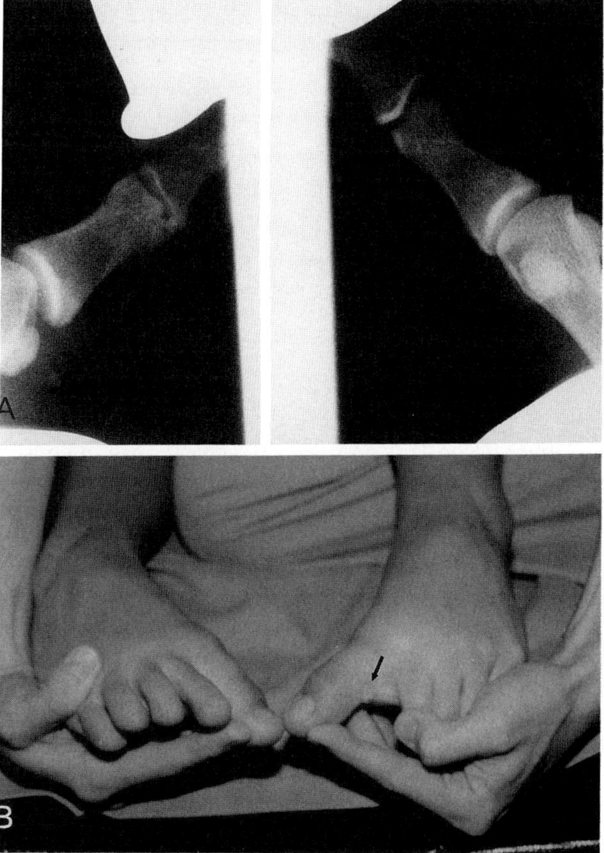

Figure 11.4 Collegiate gymnast sustained several injuries when landing on the beam. The force between her great toe and second toe on the left caused several medial dislocations, one of which was open. **(A)** Medial stress radiographs of both great toes medially show the severe medial instability without fracture. **(B)** Clinical stress test immediately prior to surgery. Note the previous scar from open dislocation *(arrow)*. She required reconstruction of the lateral structures of her left great toe.

Table 11.5.
NCAA Knee Injury Rate by Sport[a]

	Total # of Exposures	Collateral	Anterior Cruciate	Posterior Cruciate	Torn Cartillage (Meniscus)	Patella and/or Patella Tendon
Gymnastics-W	36,570	0.41	0.44	0.05	0.36	0.16
Gymnastics-M	10,048	0.10	0.00	0.00	0.00	0.00
Basketball-W	150,617	0.32	0.25	0.03	0.28	0.19
Basketball-M	175,023	0.21	0.07	0.01	0.14	0.24
Soccer-W	75,064	0.39	0.27	0.04	0.29	0.17
Soccer-M	148,959	0.53	0.13	0.08	0.19	0.23
Lacrosse-W	33,315	0.15	0.12	0.00	0.09	0.18
Lacrosse-M	71,032	0.32	0.21	0.00	0.13	0.11
Field Hockey-W	50,971	0.08	0.08	0.00	0.06	0.14
Volleyball-W	120,258	0.12	0.11	0.01	0.14	0.20
Softball-W	71,179	0.11	0.13	0.00	0.08	0.11
Spring Football-M	39,894	1.03	0.18	0.10	0.18	0.28
Wrestling-M	108,990	0.86	0.11	0.01	0.29	0.19
Football-M	744,698	0.69	0.21	0.03	0.25	0.14
Ice Hockey-M	99,863	0.69	0.08	0.01	0.03	0.06
Baseball-M	176,702	0.08	0.03	0.01	0.06	0.07

[a]All data are shown as rate per 1000 athletic exposures for 1991–1992
Source: NCAA Injury Surveillance System, No. 9044–11/92

Table 11.6.
Differential Diagnosis of Anterior Knee Pain

Inflammatory	Mechanical	Miscellaneous
Bursitis	Hypermobility	Reflex sympathetic
Prepatellar	Subluxation	dystrophy
Retropatellar	Dislocation	Ostechondritis dissecans
Pes anserinus	Patellofemoral stress	Fat pad syndrome
Tendinitis	syndrome	Systemic arthritides
Pes anserinus	Pathologic plica	Muscle Strain
Semimembranosus	syndrome	Stress fracture
Patellar	Osteochondral	Meniscal tear
Synovitis	arthrosis	Iliotibial band syndrome

often in gymnastics (0.44 to 0.00), basketball (0.25 to 0.07) and soccer (0.27 to 0.13). In lacrosse, the male more frequently injured the ACL (0.21 to 0.12). In sports, female gymnasts have the highest rate of knee injury. Women's gymnastics lead other women sports with involvement of the ACL, collateral ligament, and cartilage. The uniqueness of the sport and its apparatus, biomechanics, as well as the gymnast's body habitus, strength, ligamentous laxity and alignment are all factors which contribute to this increased injury rate.

Patellofemoral Stress Syndrome and Alignment. Anterior knee pain is common in females. The differential diagnosis is lengthy (Table 11.6). Categories include inflammatory (bursitis, tendinitis, synovitis), mechanical (subluxation, dislocation, patellofemoral stress syndrome, plica), and miscellaneous. The term chondromalacia, or softening of the articular cartilage, is a pathologic diagnosis; clinically, the use of PF (patellofemoral) stress syndrome is suggested. Excellent reviews of chondromalacia exist (34, 35).

PF stress syndrome is commonly seen in females who have microtraumatic forces, alignment abnormalities, forefoot pronation and tibial torsion. For comparison, normal alignment is shown (Fig. 11.5*A*). Abnormal alignment or miserable malalignment syndrome creates excessive lateral forces subluxing the patella. These include Q angle exceeding 15°, increased femoral anteversion, hypoplastic vastus medialis obliquus, external tibial torsion, forefoot pronation, and heel valgus (Fig. 11.5*B*). This malalignment is commonly seen in cheerleaders, gymnasts, dancers, and track athletes. A swimmer exhibits miserable malalignment syndrome as seen on front (Fig 11.5*C*) and side (Fig. 1.5*D*) clinical views. PF disorders are best treated with quadriceps strengthening, avoidance of knee extension machines and full squats, knee sleeves with pads, orthotics for weight bearing sports, and nonsteroidal anti-inflammatory medications. Surgical intervention should be a last consideration in PR stress syndrome and miserable malalignment syndrome.

Anatomically, the articular surface of the patella is the thickest of all and consists of medial, lateral, superior and inferior nonarticulating facet (Fig. 11.6). Great variability in the size and shape of patellar facets, the depth of the trochlear groove, and dynamic muscle forces result in clinical PF disorders. The contact areas and facets of the PF joint have been well identified. Aglietti (36) determined the contact areas based on the degree of flexion (Fig. 11.7). The greatest contact area and pressure occurs at 90° flexion. Patellar tracking is dependent on bony anatomy, alignment, muscular development, and on the type of loading with machines or sport.

Patellar Instability: Radiographic and Clinical Assessment. Because PF disorders and ACL injuries are more common in females, attention to specific radiographic views is key. Routine views are anterior posterior (AP), lateral, femoral notch, and bilateral patellar sunrise. Radiographic measurements and reviews of

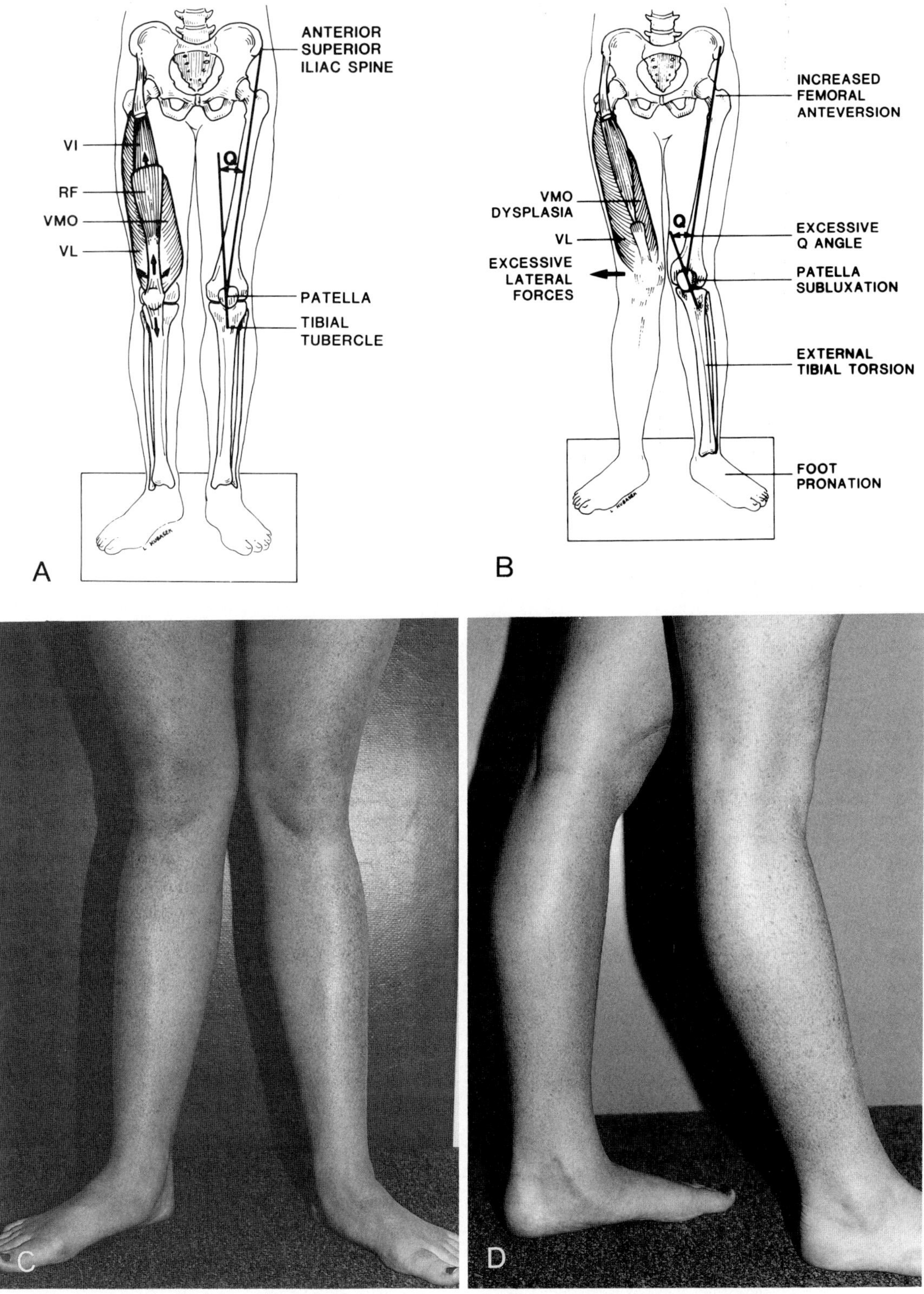

Figure 11.5 Patellofemoral disorders are common in females. **(A)** Normal alignment with normal Q angle measured from anterosuperior iliac spine central portion of the patella, patella to tibial tubercle of less than 15°, and normal musculature of developed vastus medialis obliquus, create forces that centralize the patella resulting in normal patellofemoral tracking. **(B)** Miserable malalignment syndrome consists of increased femoral anteversion, excessive Q angle, external tibial torsion, and foot pronation. All of these factors cause lateral patellar subluxation. This miserable malalignment syndrome is frequently seen in females. Clinical example of collegiate swimmer from the front **(C)** showing 20° genu valgum, external tibial torsion, hypoplastic vastus medialis obliquus, heel valgus, and pes planus with forefoot pronation. **(D)** Hyperflexibility of 20° hyperextension is seen from the side in a clinical view.

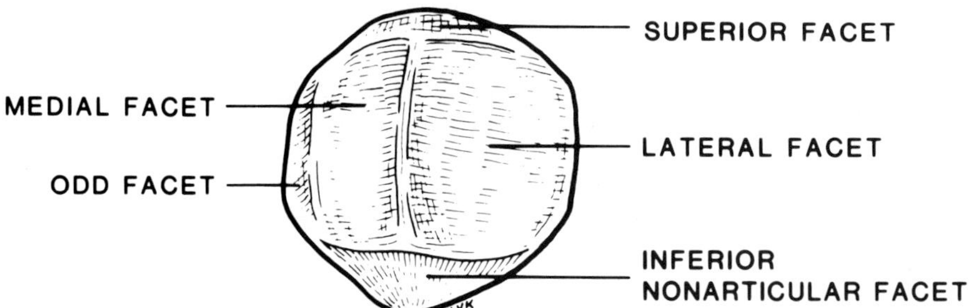

Figure 11.6 Articular surface of the patella demonstrates the anatomy of mediolateral odd patellar facets and the nonarticulating inferior and superior faces. Anatomy can be quite variable in size of the medial and lateral patellar facets.

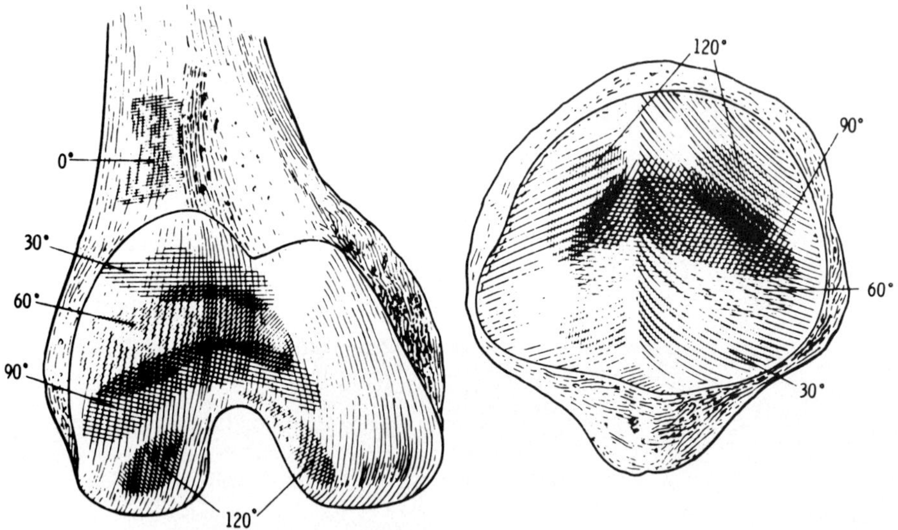

Figure 11.7 Patellofemoral contact areas are shaded at 0°, 30°, 60°, 90°, and 120° flexion in this right knee diagram. Femur *(lateral* to the *left* and *medial* to the *right)* and patella *(lateral* to the *right* and *medial* to the *left)* are shown. Reprinted with permission from Aglietti P, Insall JN, Walker PS, A New Patellar Prosthesis, Clin Ortho 1975;107:175.

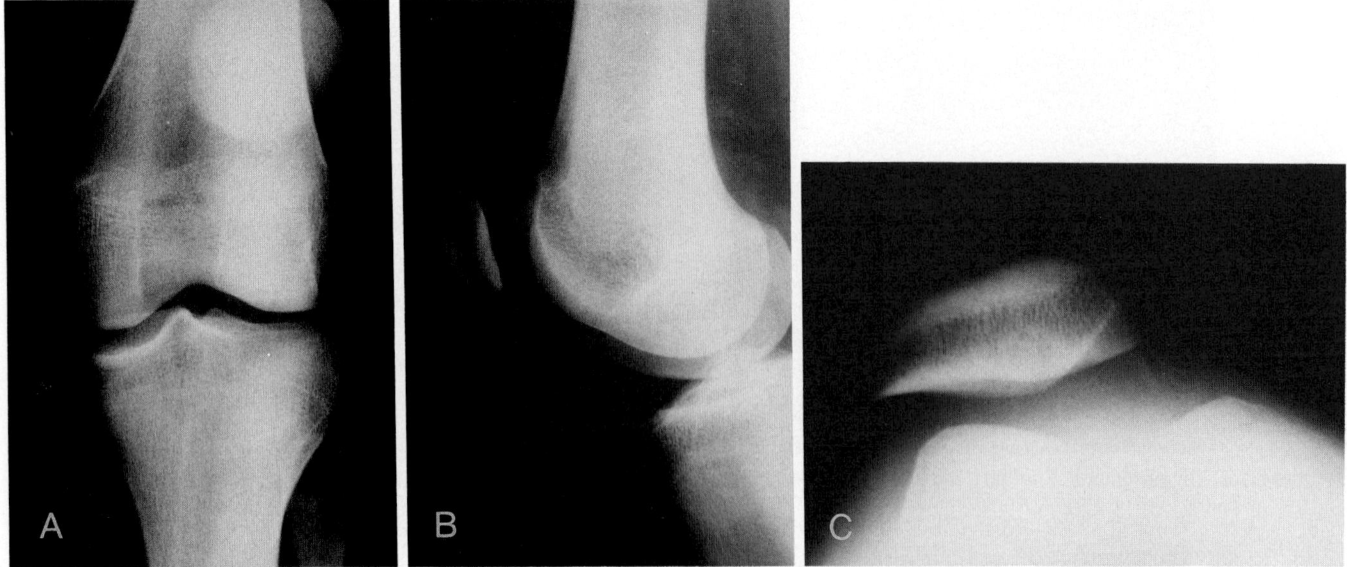

Figure 11.8 Routine plain radiographs include AP, lateral, and patellar view. Views of this left knee demonstrate patella alta. **(A)** On the AP view, the patella is significantly superolateral. **(B)** On lateral view, the measurement of the ratio of the patella to the patellar tendon is 0.5, confirming patella alta. Normal ratio is 0.8. **(C)** Hughston sunrise patellar view shows the lateral patellar subluxation, which is mildly symptomatic in this basketball athlete.

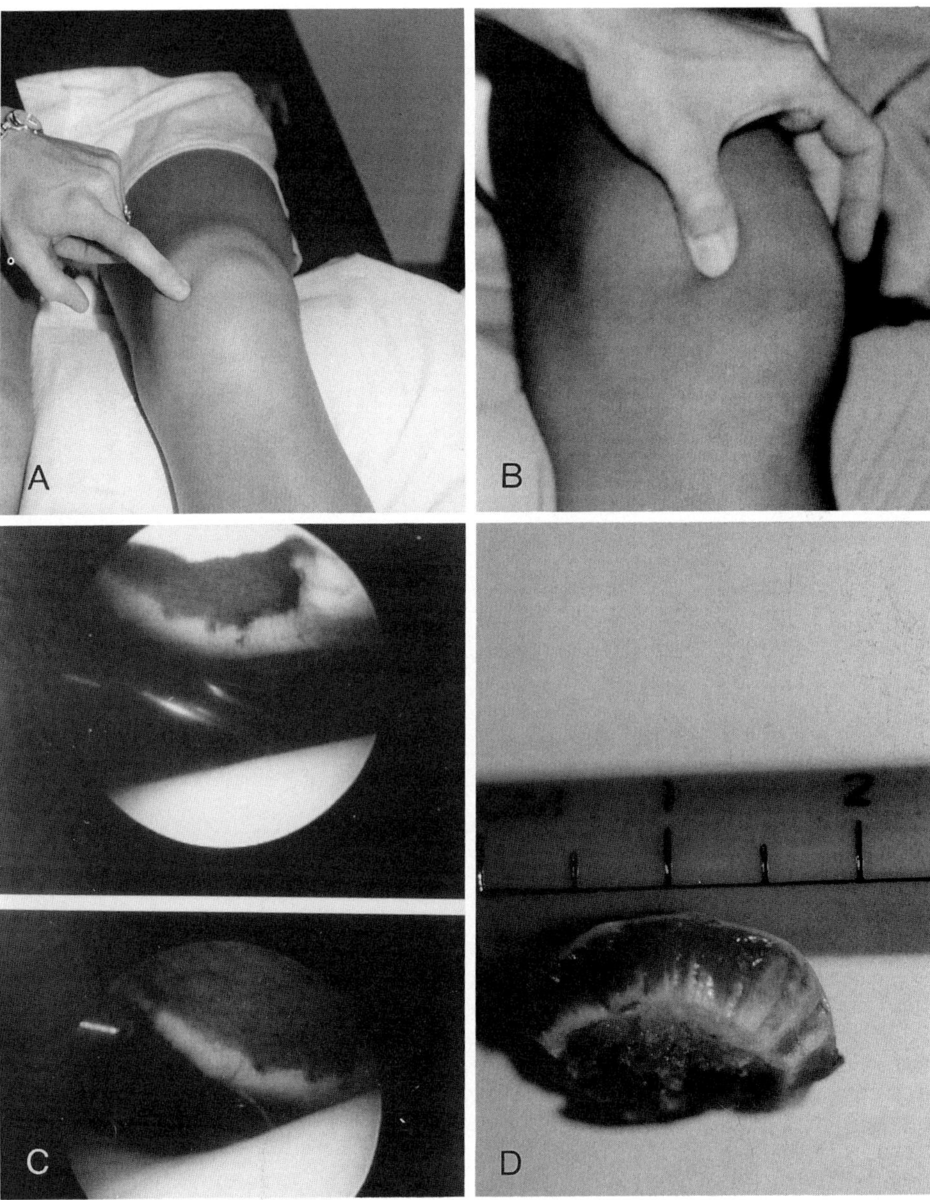

Figure 11.9 Clinical view of a swimmer who laterally dislocated her patella while walking down a stairwell. **(A)** Examiner points to the area of maximal tenderness. Note tense hemarthrosis. **(B)** Intraoperative exam documents lateral patellar instability. **(C)** Arthroscopic exam shows the debrided patellar above and normal trochlear groove below. **(D)** Excised loose patellar fragment is shown. Notice the very thick articular cartilage.

chondromalacia are important in the understanding of PF disorders (34). Measurement of length of a patella-to-patella tendon less than 0.8 is termed patella alta and greater than 0.8 is termed patella infera. This basketball athlete complained of anterior pain and swelling of her knee. Patella alta is demonstrated on AP and lateral views (Fig. 11.8*A*). Patella-to-patella tendon ratio is 0.5 and the Hughston patellar view shows lateral subluxation (Fig. 11.8*B*). The subject of these views returned successfully to competition with a quadriceps strengthening program and use of a neoprene sleeve with lateral pad.

An acute lateral patellar dislocation can be associated with an osteochondral fracture of the patella. This medial patellar facet fracture may not be seen on AP or lateral view. A Hughston patellar view including as much of the distal femur as possible is necessary. This patient with a severely swollen knee and pain over the medial retinaculum (Fig. 11.9*A*) sustained an acute lateral patella dislocation with medial osteochondral fracture. The intraoperative exam demonstrates lateral patellar instability (Fig. 11.9*B*). The arthroscopic view is of debrided patella and normal trochlear groove (Fig. 11.9*C*). The loose patellar fragment was removed arthroscopically. (Fig. 11.9*D*). The very thick articular cartilage and small amount of cancellous bone are well shown.

ACL Injury Rates. The four sports in which men and women compete are gymnastics, soccer, basketball, and lacrosse. The ACL was injured in females 3.5 times more often in basketball, 2.0 times more often in soccer as measured by rates per athletic exposure (9) (Table 11.7). In females, the highest rate of ACL injury was 0.44, whereas no male gymnast sustained an ACL injury. In lacrosse, males sustained ACL injuries 1.75 times more often than females.

Table 11.7.
NCAA ACL Injury Rate by Sport[a]

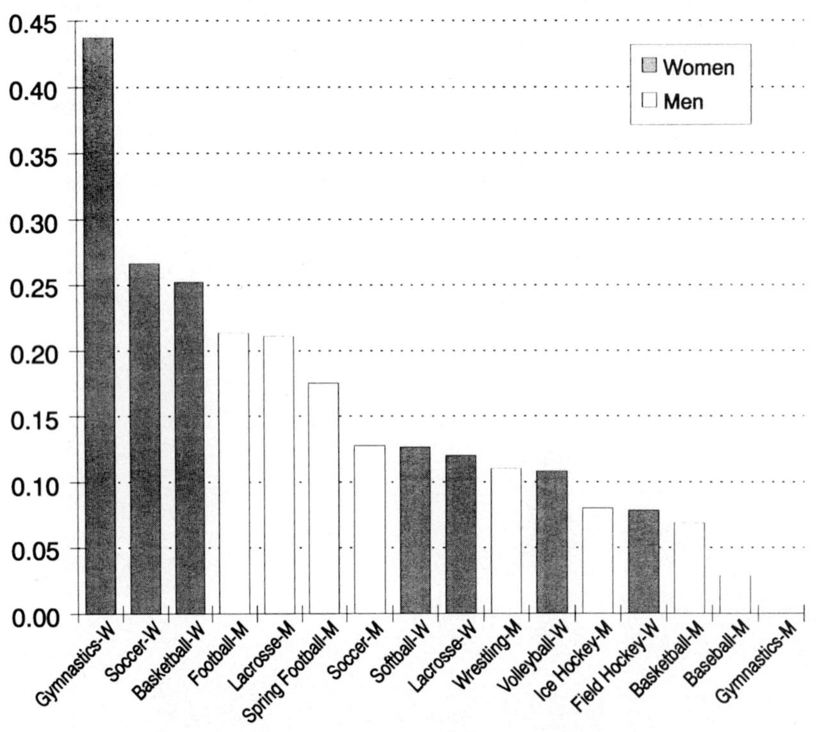

[a]All data is shown as rate per 1000 athletic exposures for 1991–1992
Source: NCAA Injury Surveillance System, No. 9044–11/92

Male and female basketball injuries at the professional level were compared (33). Compared to men, women were found to sustain more injuries, more sprains, and to have increased knee and thigh injuries. The most common injury involved the ankle. Women's injury frequency was 1.6 times greater than men.

An epidemiology survey of athletes invited to the U.S. Basketball Olympic Trials in 1988 showed that knee injuries ($P < .0001$) occurred more often in females compared to males and that females required surgery ($P < .0007$) more often than males (30). Of the 64 females, 17 required arthroscopy and 8 sustained an injury to the ACL. Of the 80 males, 3 sustained an injury to the ACL, while 3 required arthroscopy only. Factors contributing to this increased incidence of injury at the professional level (33) include differences in training, strengthening, weight lifting, shoes, floor, lower extremity alignment. Further investigation and prospective studies to determine why knee injuries involving the ACL are so common in females are needed.

ACL Research Projects. Some prospective studies have been done, but more research is needed. Studies analyzing differences in noninjured female volleyball and basketball athletes showed only one statistically significant difference in isokinetic strength testing and no differences in ligamentous laxity (37). This difference was with greater peak extension and higher hamstring-to-quadricep peak torque ratio in trail leg at 60° per sec in volleyball players. KT 1000 (Medmetric Company, San Diego, CA) testing showed no statistically significant anterior displacement comparing legs or sports. Further investigation with high speed video, taping, force plate analysis, and electromyography of lower extremity musculature is needed. Differences can be easily observed in volleyball and basketball. Cutting, one-footed positions, changing direction in basketball are shown in Figure 11.10. In volleyball, the position is more two-footed, straight ahead with less cutting and changing of direction (Fig. 11.11).

ACL Injuries: Radiographic and Clinical Assessment. Intraoperative view of a swollen right knee in a female basketball athlete undergoing ACL reconstruction is shown (Fig. 11.12). Notice the scar with severe keloid formation from her previous ACL reconstruction on the left. The elastin and collagen tissue in females may contribute to completeness of ACL tears and scar formation.

Femoral notch views are good for outlining the size, shape and contour of the notch and the articular surface. Narrow notch shape and size has been suggested as a contributing factor to ACL injuries. Letters can be used to classify notch shape (Fig. 11.13). The A-shaped notch on the right is commonly seen in ACL injuries. Other shapes are H, reverse U, or C shape (Fig. 11.13). Ratios of notch-to-femoral width can predict ACL injuries and incidence of bilaterality (38).

This high school basketball athlete was injured on offense while changing directions with the ball in a

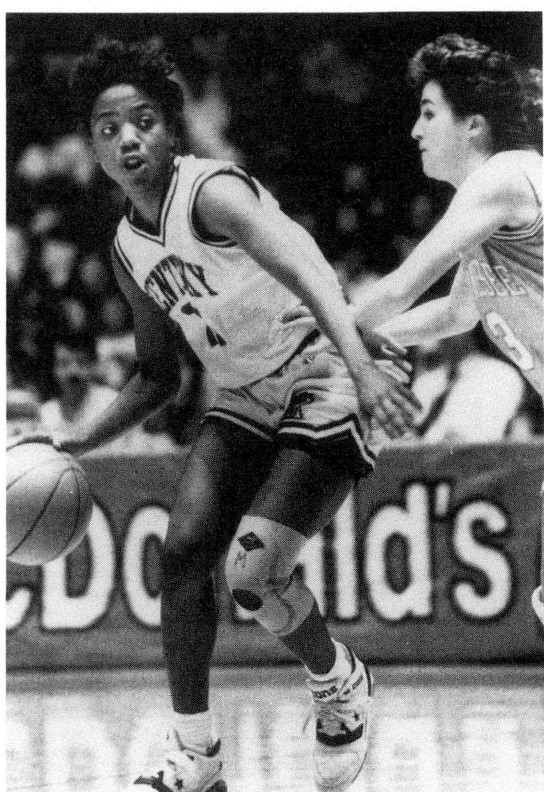

Figure 11.10 Although women's basketball is played similarly to men's, there are unique injury patterns most significantly involving the knee of increased incidence of knee injuries and anterior cruciate ligament tears. A collegiate basketball athlete is shown in one-footed position, eyes attempting to fake the opponent, and pivoting while making a drive for the basket.

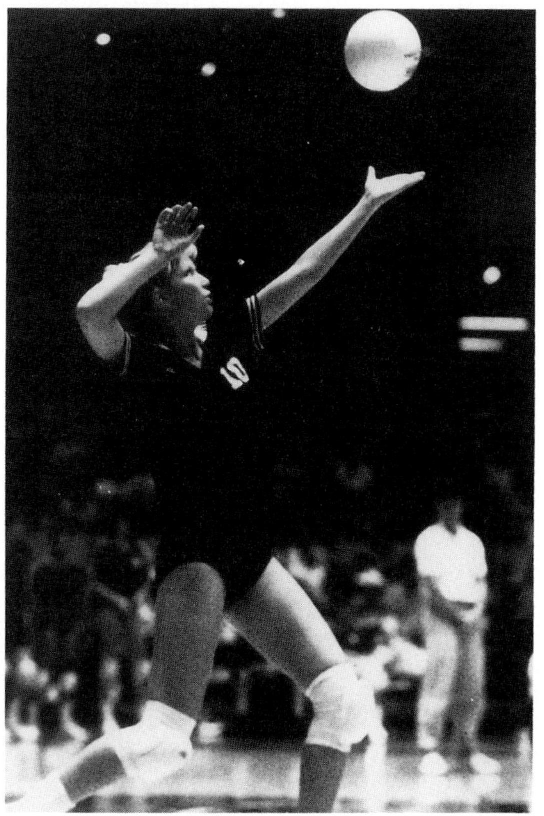

Figure 11.11 In volleyball, most injuries are from overuse and involve patellofemoral joint. A collegiate volleyball athlete is shown serving the ball with her eyes set straight forward and with positioning on both feet without rotation.

noncontact mechanism. She had a narrow A-shaped notch view (Fig. 11.14*A*). MRI scan shows abnormal ACL signal, narrow notch, and bone bruise of the lateral femoral condyle (Fig. 11.14*B*). Arthroscopy confirmed the MRI results of a mop-end ACL tear (Fig. 11.14*C top*) and osteochondral femoral condyle defect (Fig. 11.14*C bottom*). Due to their less muscular development and their lower extremity alignment differences, females rely more on the ACL and less on hamstring control. Ligamentous reconstruction should be considered in the ACL-dominant female who is at high risk for significant meniscal and articular surface injury.

Foot and Ankle

Tibiotalar impingement syndrome results from repetitive axial loading sports. Osteophyte formation of the distal tibia and dorsal talar neck causes loss of dorsiflexion range and anterior pain (Fig. 11.15*A*). Arthroscopic removal of osteophytes and partial synovectomy allow a return to sport with improved motion (Fig. 11.15*B*).

In ballet athletes, posterior impingement of the os trigonum can result in local pressure on the flexor hal-

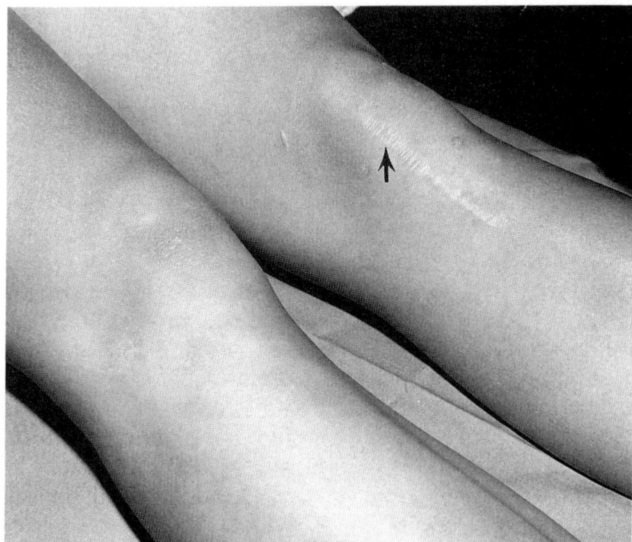

Figure 11.12 Photograph on the operating table of a collegiate female basketball athlete who will undergo right anterior cruciate ligament reconstruction. Note the right knee intra-articular swelling. Also note the keloid scar consistent with elastin stretching on her three-year-old left anterior cruciate ligament reconstruction *(arrow)*.

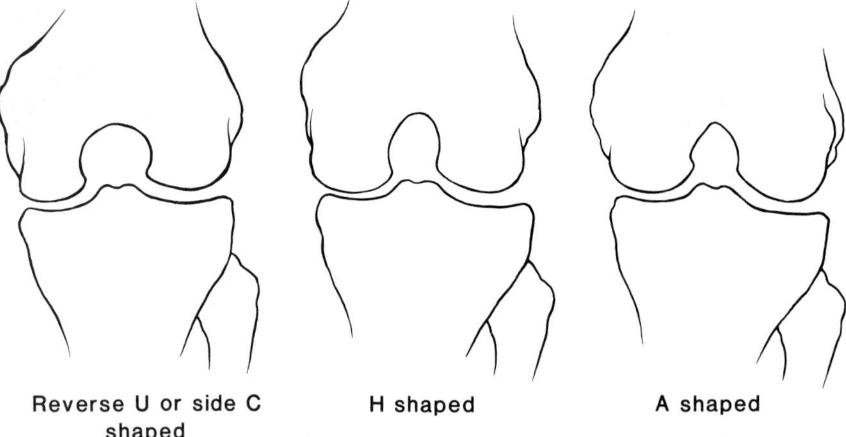

Figure 11.13 A proposed contributing factor to anterior cruciate ligament tears is the uniqueness of notch shapes. These have been seen as reverse C or U, H, and A in shape. The more narrow A shape and a low notch to femur ratio on notch views are common with ACL tears.

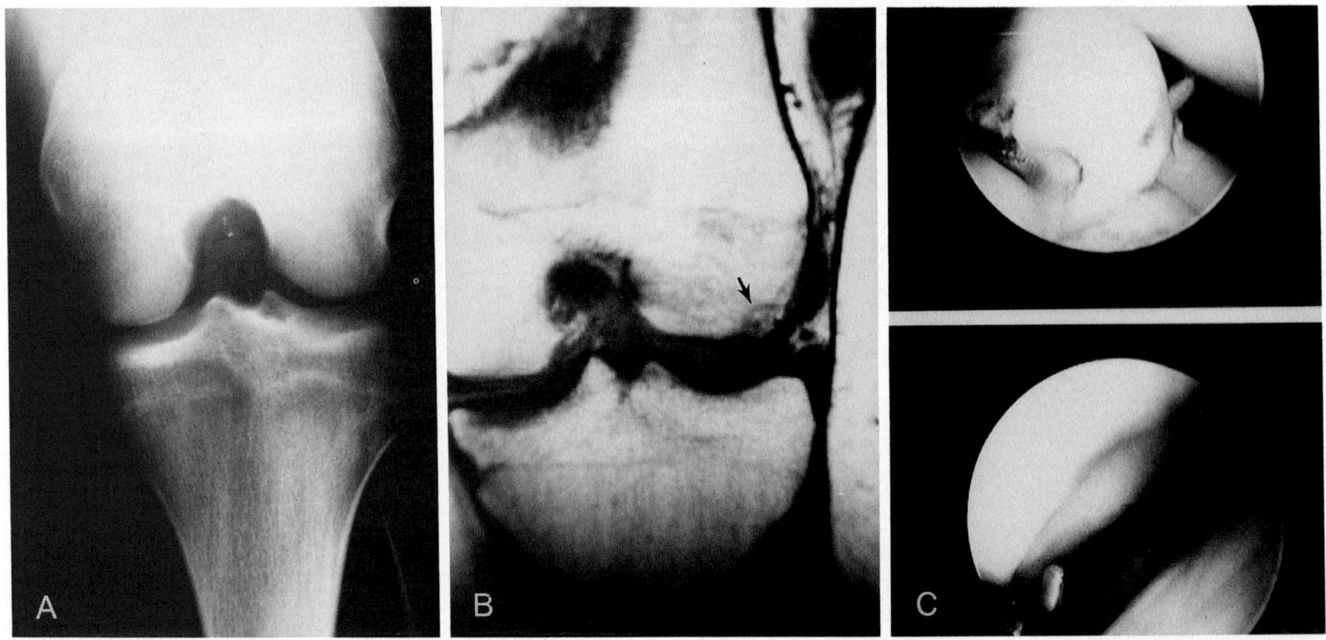

Figure 11.14 Female basketball athlete sustained an acute ACL tear. **(A)** The notch is A-shaped and narrow. **(B)** MRI scan shows on this AP view the narrowed notch and lack of signal in the notch consistent with an ACL tear. Osteochondral change in density of the lateral aspect of the femur is shown *(arrow)*. **(C)** Arthroscopic findings show mop end tear of the ACL *(top)* and probe pointing to osteochondral defect *(bottom)* seen on MRI view.

lucis longus. Pain in the posterior ankle is elicited by resistive testing of great toe plantar flexion. A cone lateral view before (Fig. 11.16*A*) and after (Fig. 11.16*B*) os trigonum excision is shown. Pain-free resumption of ballet activities was possible after surgery.

Tendon problems of the foot are common in females. Posterior tibial tendinitis is seen commonly in dance athletes with pes planus. Tendon problems are more common with the cavus foot. Accessory ossicles may be symptomatic at tendon insertions. This condition caused pain on eversion in this soccer athlete. A peroneus brevis accessory ossicle can be symptomatic. This os versalianum (Fig. 11.17), as shown preoperatively, required excision due to persistent pain.

Stress fractures should also be considered when evaluating soft tissue problems. In dance athletes, a second metatarsal stress fracture can occur at the Lisfranc joint (39).

A high ankle sprain was the working diagnosis in this basketball athlete who complained of continued pain. Radiographs revealed a fibula stress fracture, shown at diagnosis in Figure 11.18*A* and when healed four months later in Figure 11.18*B*.

Bunions (hallux valgus) are commonly encountered in the female athletes. Correction for cosmetic reasons should not be performed because a painful, although straight, great toe may result. Modification of the type of shoe worn is the mainstay of treatment (40). Severe clinical bunion abnormalities are commonly seen, but are usually asymptomatic. A Morton's foot with a short first metatarsal can result in a severe but painless hallux valgus, as in this dancer. (Fig. 11.19). Symptomatic stress fractures of the tibial (medial) sesamoid can mimic bunion pain. A work-up with plain films in this track athlete showed diffuse radiolucency on dorsiflexion sunrise sesamoid views (Fig. 11.20*A*). Increased activity on bone scan (Fig. 11.20*B*) confirmed the diagnosis.

Shoulder

With generalized laxity, sport dependent problems involving the shoulder occur. The vicious cycle of physiologic instability, rotator cuff weakness, pain, posterior tightness, and further imbalance results in persistent pain and dysfunction in overhead activities or in extremes of range of motion (Fig. 11.21). In younger females, joint laxity and decreased strength can cause shoulder problems. Restoration of normal range of motion and strength with proper sport biomechanics is the goal.

In swimmers, increasing joint distraction and repetitive microtrauma, "impingement syndrome," and pain are common (41). The exact diagnosis should be documented by noting the structure involved, severity, and acuteness. Treatment is strengthening, relative rest, and evaluation of biomechanics.

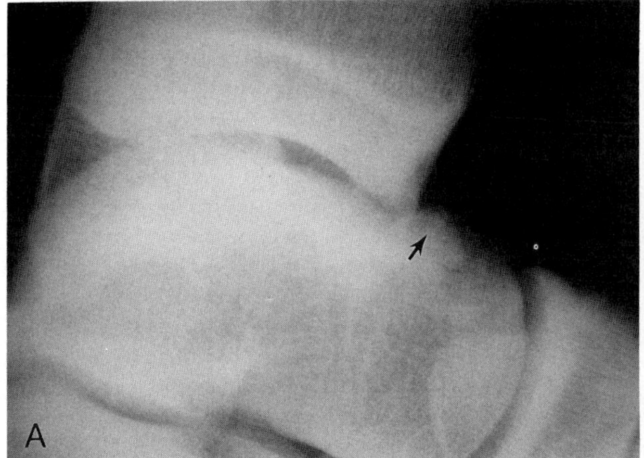

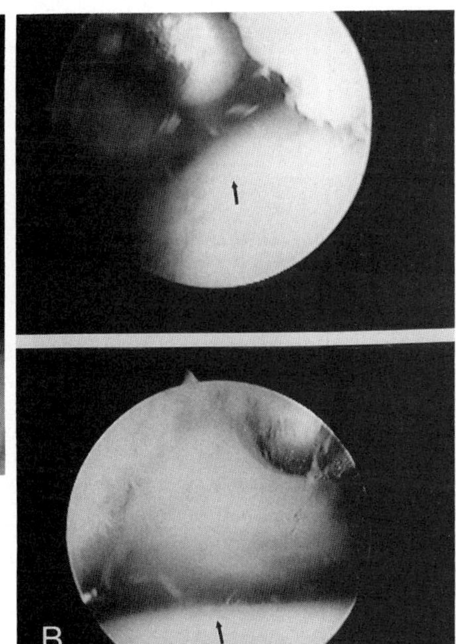

Figure 11.15 **(A)** Tibiotalar impingement syndrome is seen in a forced dorsiflexion lateral view with an osteophyte on the neck of the talus *(arrow)* with convexity instead of concavity. Impingement of the tibia and talus results in anterior compartment synovitis and limited dorsiflexion range. **(B)** Arthroscopic synovectomy and debridement of osteophytes has been successful. Resector and tibia are shown on upper side and talus *(arrow)* on the bottom.

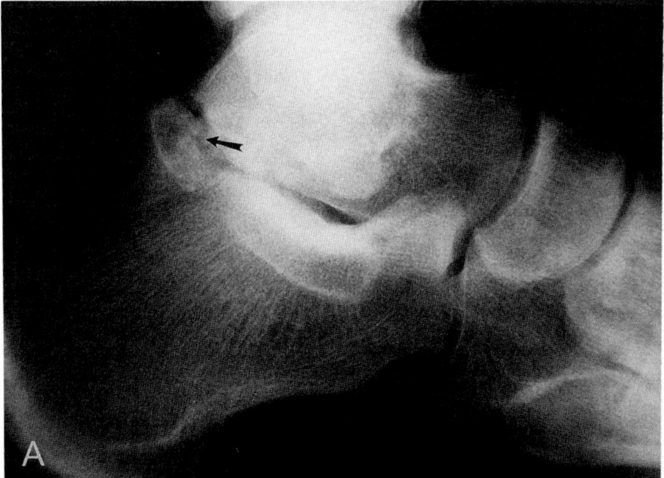

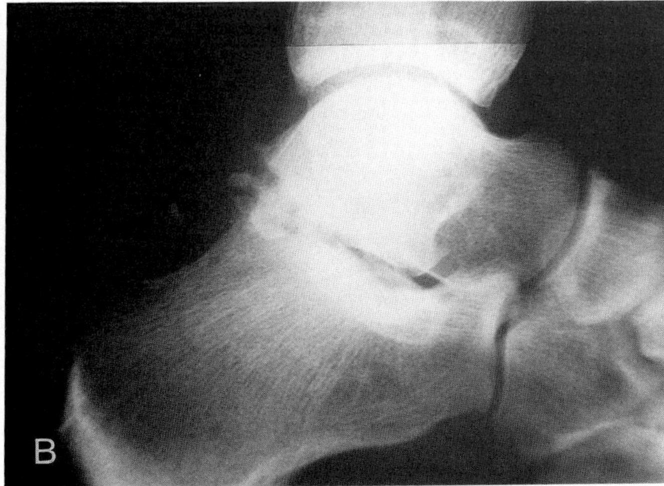

Figure 11.16 Ballet athletes who complain of posterior ankle and great toe pain can have a symptomatic os trigonum fracture. **(A)** A large os trigonum is seen in this ballet athlete who is having difficulty in doing repetitive en pointe maneuvers *(arrow)*. Nonunion and pressure on flexor hallucis longus result in posterior ankle pain and great toe flexion weakness. **(B)** Surgical excision of this lesion, as shown by postoperative lateral radiograph, resulted in a complete cure.

This synchronized swimmer with habitual posterior subluxation was able to compete at highly competitive levels. Note the prominent posterior contour with arm forward flexed and humeral head posteriorly subluxed (Fig. 11.22*A*). The patient smilingly feels the reduction as the examiner pushes forward (Fig. 11.22*B*). Associated generalized laxity and multidirectional instability are common. Operative results are inconsistent.

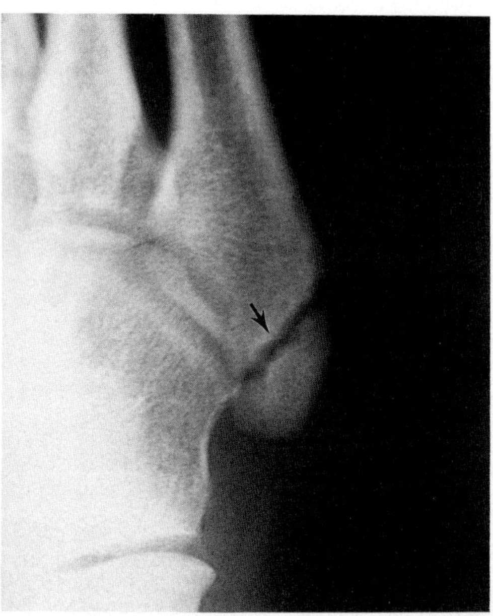

Figure 11.17 Symptomatic secondary ossification center at the base of the fifth metatarsal in this soccer athlete required excision. Os versalianum *(arrow)* was excised with uneventful return to full activities.

In competitive diving, the forces involving axial loading on water entry and extreme ranges of motion during the gymnastic portion of diving maneuvers result in combined rotator cuff and instability problems. Use of the shoulder as a weight bearing joint can lead to long-term dysfunction. In gymnastics, the shoulder is commonly injured (6, 9, 42). Sport specific strengthening program may prevent significant injuries.

Elbow

The female has an increased valgus carrying angle and ligamentous laxity compared to the male. Due to the increased lateral pressures and less upper extremity strength, repetitive axial loading activities are common.

Osteochondritis dissecans with resultant loose body formation should be considered in axial loading sports. This fourteen-year-old gymnast complained of locking of her elbow. Lateral plain radiograph (Fig. 11.23*A*) and CT scan (Fig. 39.23*B*) confirmed two osteocartilaginous loose bodies in the anterior compartment. Arthroscopic removal of loose bodies (Fig. 11.23*C*) fragments and debridement of the capitellum allowed return to her sport. The largest loose body is shown at time of arthroscopic removal (Fig. 11.23*D*). Posterior compartment loose bodies may also occur. Two large osteochondral fragments are well seen by plain radiographs (Fig. 11.24*A*) and CT scan (Fig. 11.24*B*). An elbow arthroscopy and loose body removal by small arthrotomy of the posterior compartment were done. Resolution of pain, return of full extension, and resumption of gymnastics were possible in this case.

Severe injuries can occur in cheerleading. This young female sustained an elbow dislocation when she landed

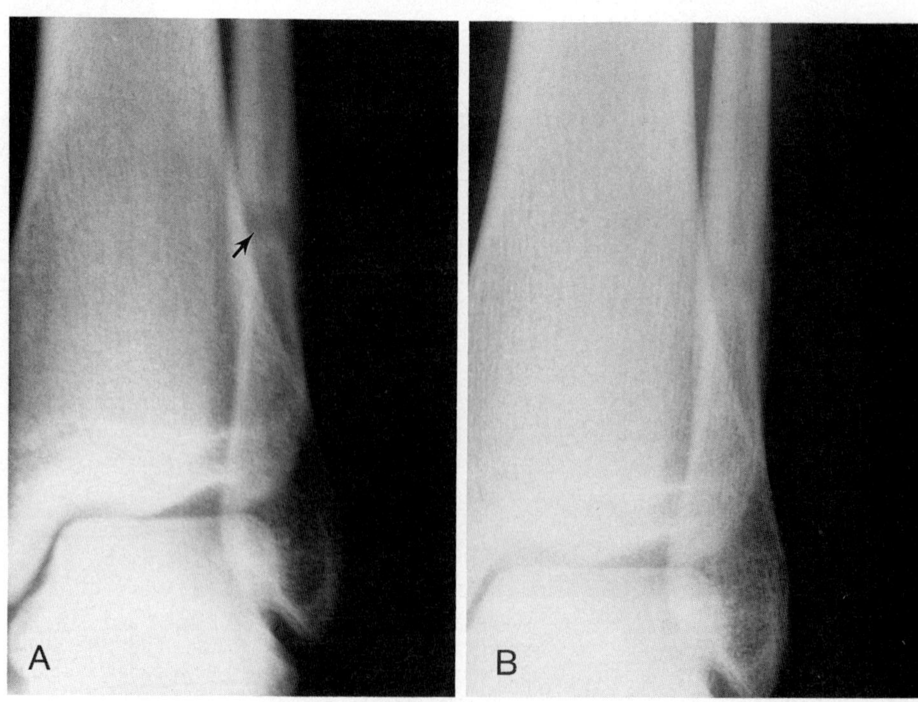

Figure 11.18 Fibula stress fractures can also cause problems with ankle pain as shown in this basketball athlete who had been having pain for several months. **(A)** A stress fracture of the fibula *(arrow)* is seen well above the ankle; this was confused for a high ankle sprain 4 months following a decrease in her activities. **(B)** Fibula fracture is asymptomatic clinically and healed radiographically.

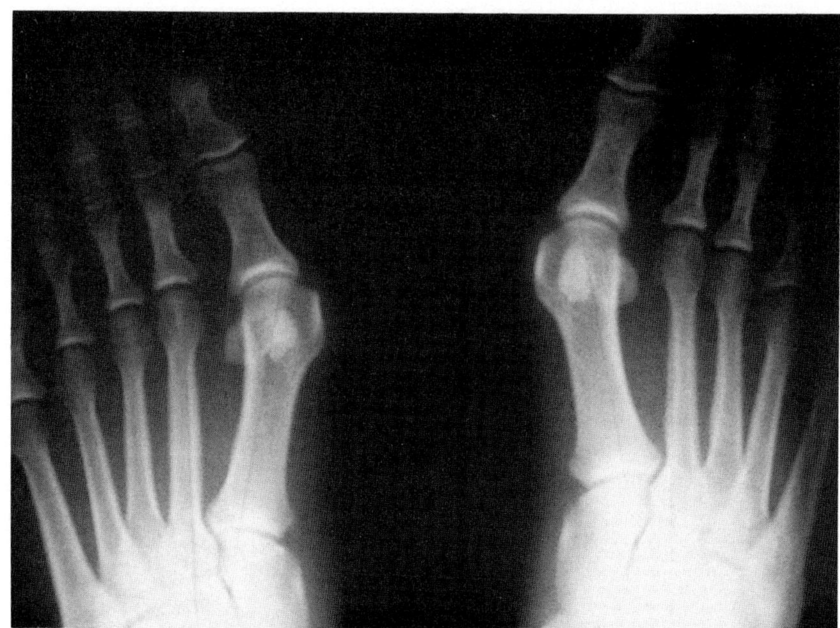

Figure 11.19 Bunions or hallux valgus are quite common in females, especially dance athletes. Standing AP views of both feet show hallux valgus, lateral subluxation of great toe and sesamoids, and short first metatarsal.

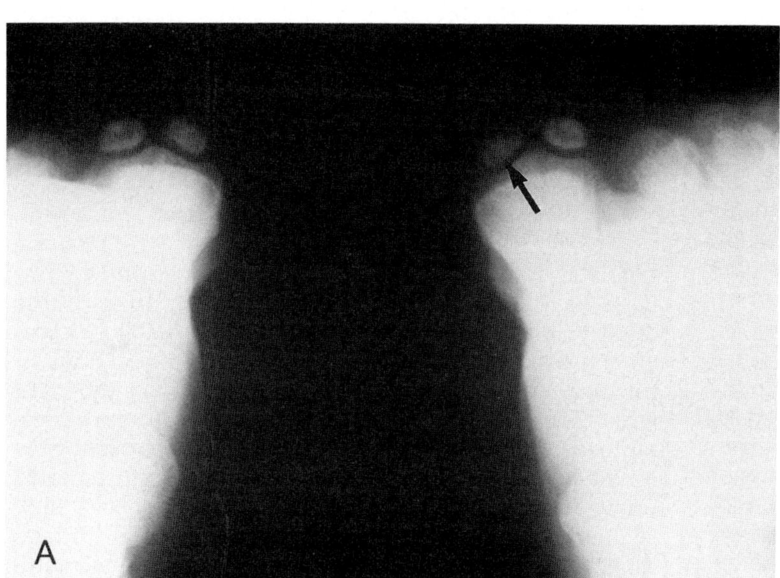

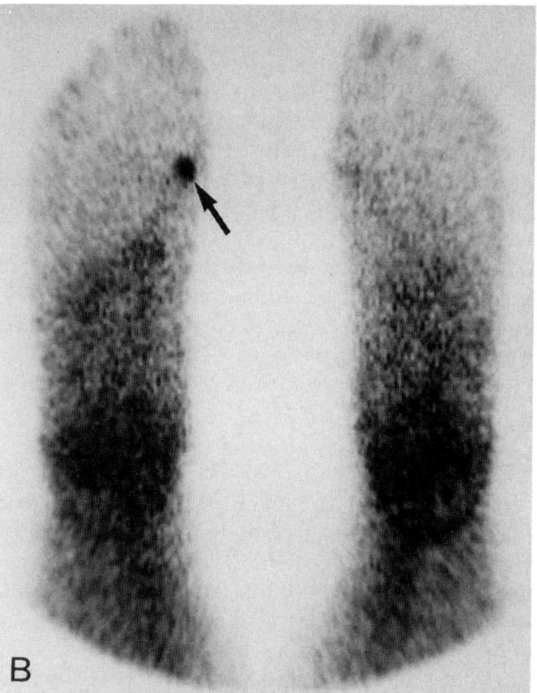

Figure 11.20 In runners, great toe pain, especially with pain on the plantar aspect, can be a sesamoid fracture. **(A)** Sunrise views show radiolucency of tibial *(medial)* sesamoid compared to fibular sesamoid *(lateral)* on right foot *(arrow)*. **(B)** Bone scan confirms a stress fracture of the sesamoid left foot. This was treated with padding, avoidance of running; healing occurred at 8 months clinically.

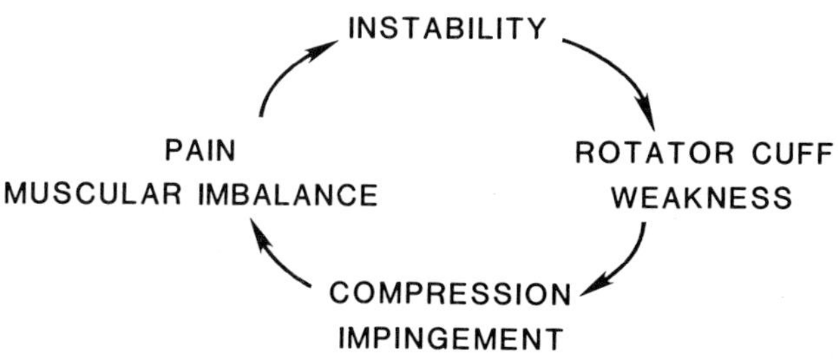

Figure 11.21 Vicious cycle of shoulder pain occurs especially in females when there is a physiologic instability that may be multi-directional, with rotator cuff weakness, subsequent pain, posterior tightness, and further weakness, and muscular imbalance.

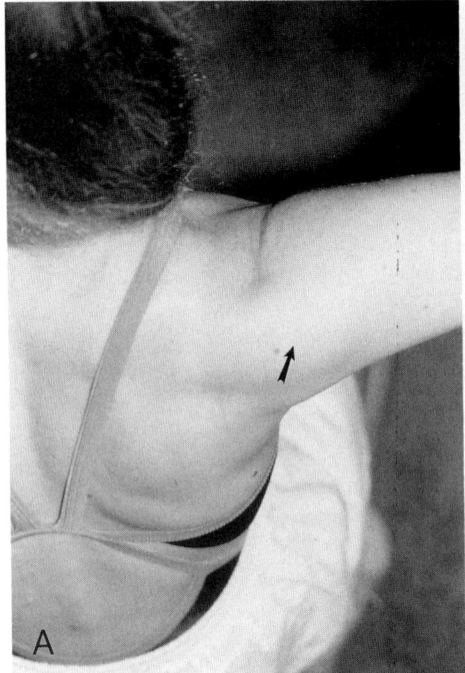

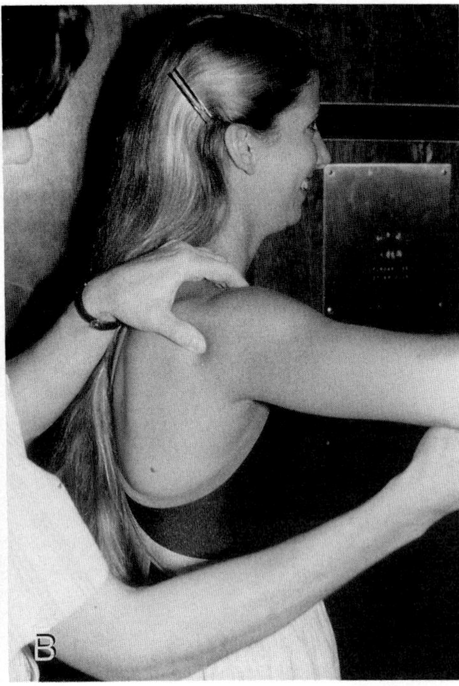

Figure 11.22 (A) This synchronized swimmer shows habitual posterior subluxation. She can voluntarily sublux posteriorly by moving arm anterior to axis of body and internally rotating. Notice the prominence of the subluxed posterior humeral head *(arrow)*. **(B)** Patient's dislocation is easily and painlessly reduced by posteriorly moving the arm and placing direct pressure by the examiner's thumb on the now reduced humeral head.

short from a double-back stunt. Attempted reduction by personnel at practice was not successful. AP and lateral elbow radiographs showed a posterolateral dislocation (Fig. 11.25*A*). A physical exam revealed absent radial pulse and pain, an ecchymotic area medially, and severe elbow swelling (Fig. 11.25*B*). Emergency arteriogram (Fig. 11.25*C*) showed absent filling of the brachial artery, although collateral filling was present. The hand was viable. Surgical exploration revealed an entrapped brachial artery. A cephalic vein patch to the brachial artery was required to restore normal vascularity.

Stress Fractures

In the military population, stress fractures were found to be more common in female cadets compared to males (25). The association of menstrual irregularity and stress fractures in collegiate female distance runners has been established (43). Several series report increased incidence of stress fractures in females (44–48). The association of stress fractures with low bone density, amenorrhea, and poor nutrition has been established (23, 33, 34). The association of nutritional habits and the incidence of stress fractures in ballet dancers was reviewed (49). Specific health concerns of female runners has been addressed (23, 50).

A detailed nutritional and gynecologic history must be obtained. Reviews of treatment by diet modification and hormonal replacement offer excellent guidelines (1, 3, 23, 51).

First Rib

First rib fractures are most commonly associated with major trauma. Stress fractures of the first rib have been reported in female rowers (52). In this ballet athlete, a delayed union (Fig. 11.26) occurred. The only mechanism of injury was repetitive lifting by her partner. Treatment was directed toward improvement of the dancer's nutrition and her hormonal status with avoidance of the specific lifting maneuvers that led to the injury. Resumption of full activities occurred at eight months following injury.

Wrist Injuries

Distal Radius Epiphyseal Fractures. Young gymnasts have been reported to have stress changes of the distal epiphysis (53). Repetitive axial compression forces on the distal radius can cause epiphyseal reactions or fracture. A Salter I distal radius occurred in the right wrist (Fig. 11.27*B*) in this gymnast. The normal distal radius epiphyseal plate is shown in comparison view on the left (Fig. 11.27*A*). This Salter type I fracture healed uneventfully. However, radial growth arrest with subsequent ulnar overgrowth can occur. Clinical and radiographic exams should be done until skeletal maturity is reached.

Even in the skeletally immature, navicular fractures occur. This gymnast complained of right wrist pain for three weeks. She had tenderness in the anatomic snuffbox, not distal radial. Radiographs showed a midwaist navicular fracture (Fig. 11.28).

This collegiate gymnast complained of wrist pain for three months. A work-up with normal plain views marked at the area of maximal tenderness (Fig. 11.29*A*), tomograms (Fig. 11.29*B*), and a bone scan (Fig. 11.29*C*) made the diagnosis of distal radius stress fracture with localized cyst. Successful treatment included dorsal taping blocking full dorsiflexion and relative rest.

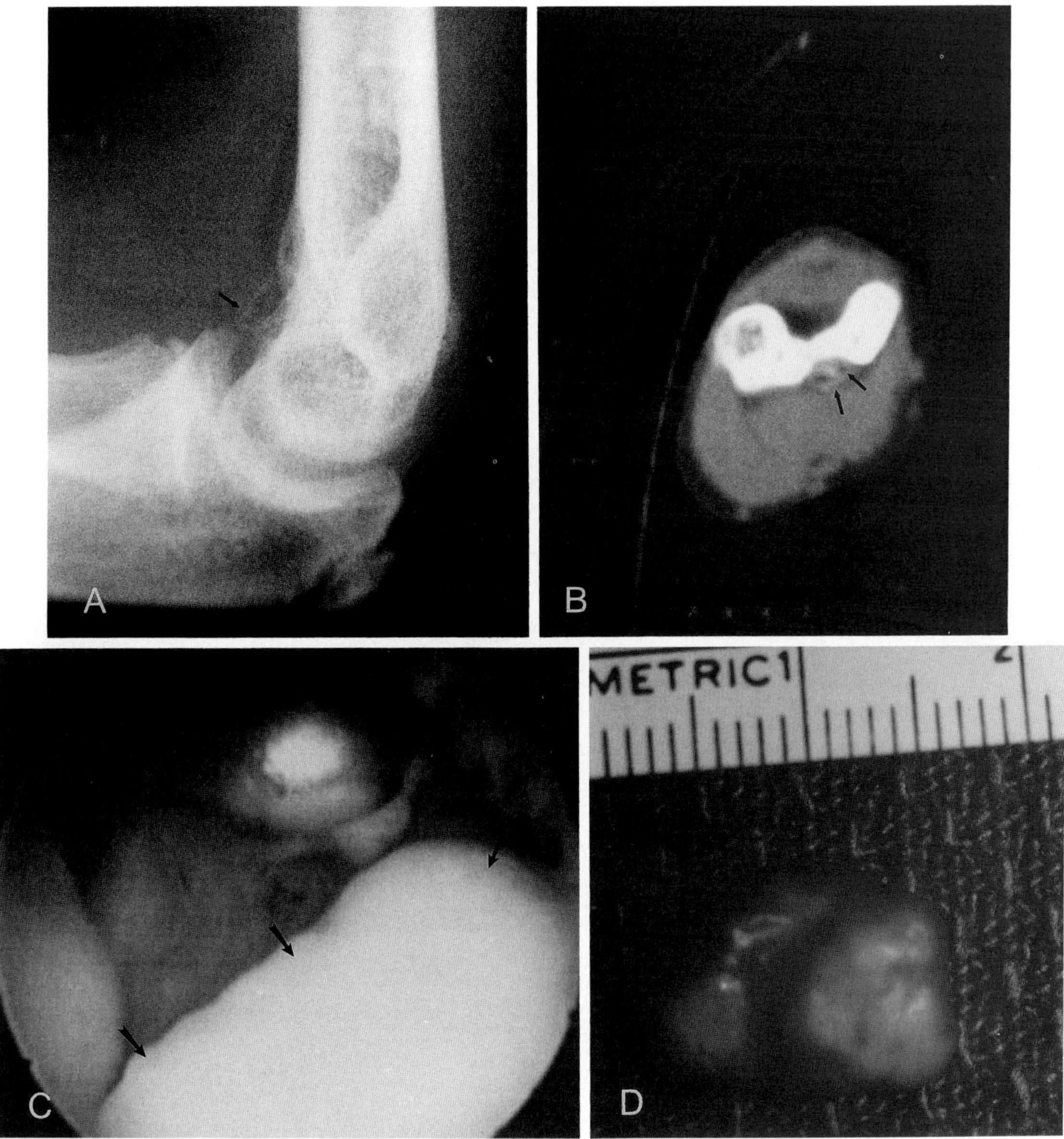

Figure 11.23 Fourteen-year-old gymnast complained of locking of her elbow. **(A)** Lateral plain radiographs show a large radiolucency in the anterior compartment. AP and oblique views did not show any significant area of osteochondral fracture. There was some flattening of the capitellum consistent with an osteochondritis dissecans. **(B)** A CT scan confirmed two osteocartilaginous loose bodies in the anterior compartment *(arrows)*. **(C)** Anterior loose body *(arrows)* is seen at time of arthroscopy. Anterior capsule and motorized resector are at the top. Arthroscopic removal of the loose bodies was successful. **(D)** Largest loose body is shown measuring 1.5 × 1.2 × 1.5 cm.

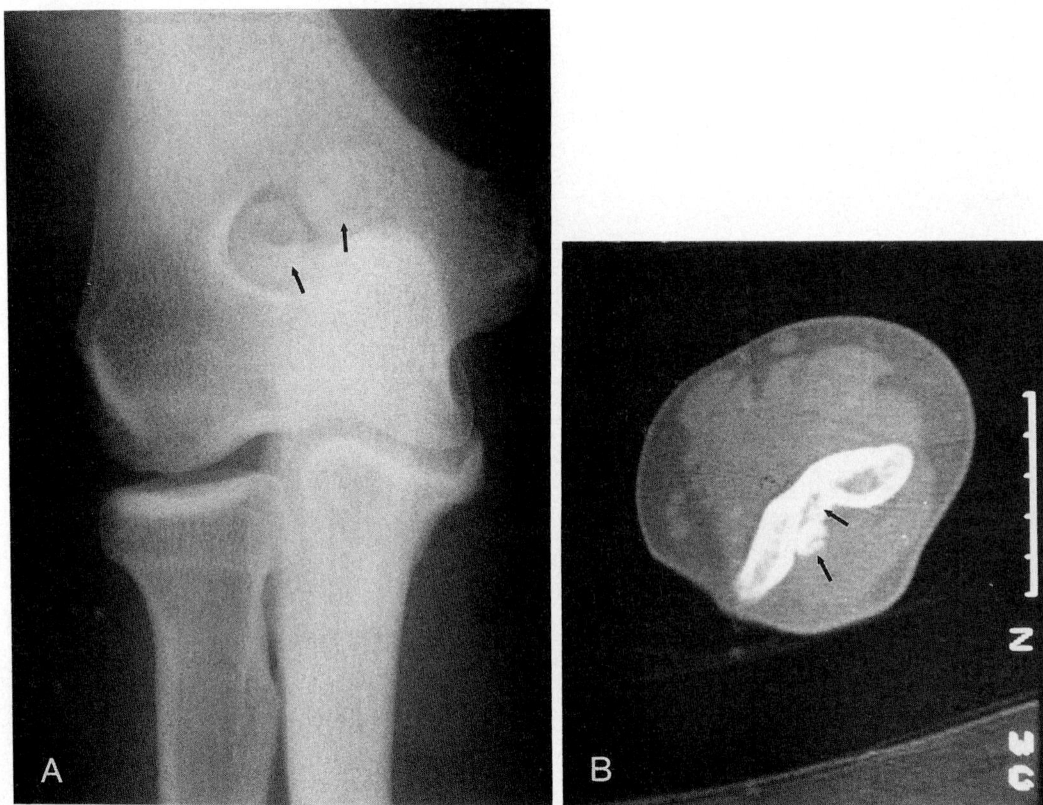

Figure 11.24 A collegiate gymnast complained of pain in her elbow posteriorly, when doing axial loading activities. She had a 10° flexion contracture and pain on bounce home passive extension testing. **(A)** AP radiographs of the elbow showed two large loose bodies in the posterior compartment *(arrows)*. **(B)** The location, size, and number of these were confirmed by CT scan showing the two large loose bodies in the posterior compartment of the olecranon fossa *(arrows)*. Arthroscopy and miniarthrotomy posteriorly resulted in full and painless range of motion.

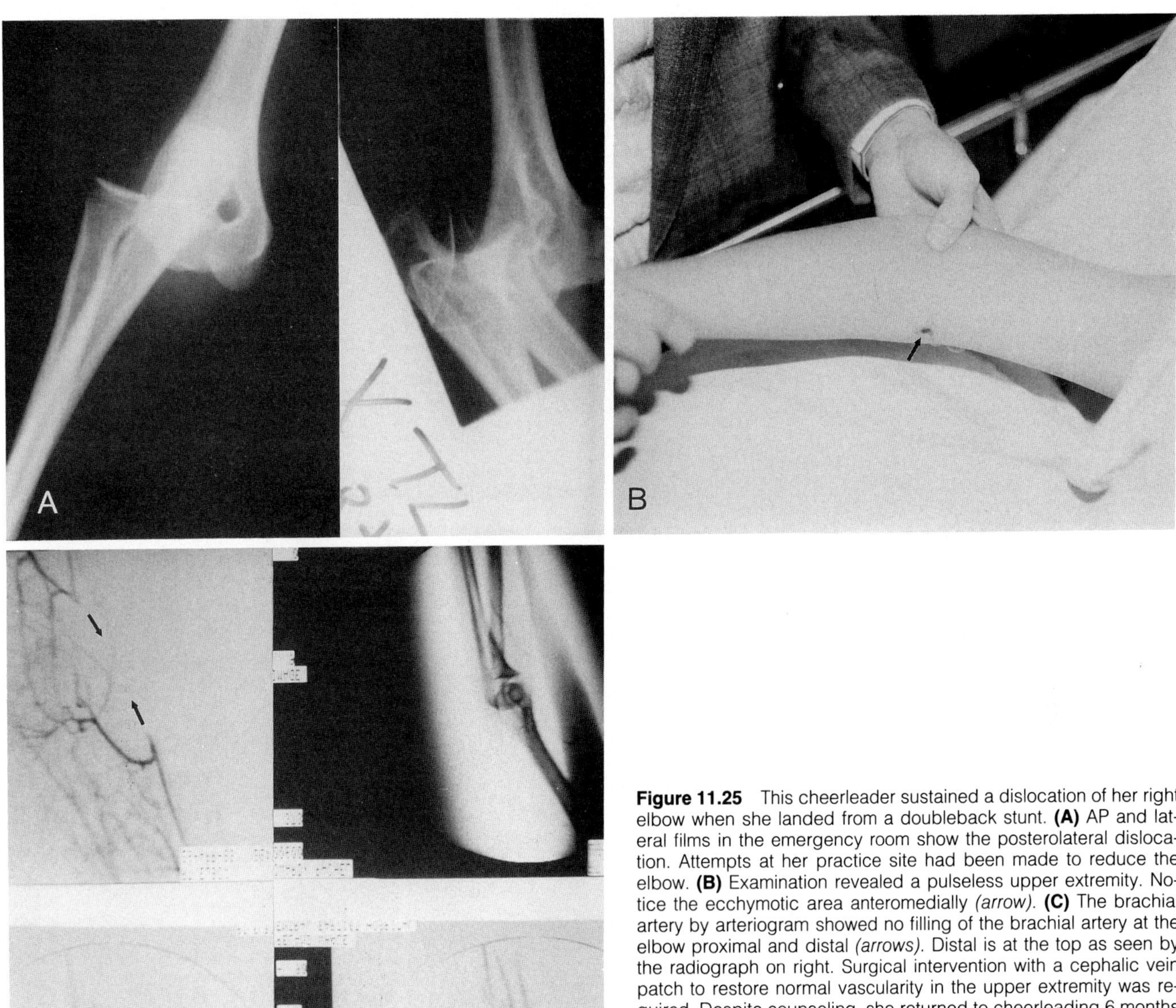

Figure 11.25 This cheerleader sustained a dislocation of her right elbow when she landed from a doubleback stunt. **(A)** AP and lateral films in the emergency room show the posterolateral dislocation. Attempts at her practice site had been made to reduce the elbow. **(B)** Examination revealed a pulseless upper extremity. Notice the ecchymotic area anteromedially *(arrow)*. **(C)** The brachial artery by arteriogram showed no filling of the brachial artery at the elbow proximal and distal *(arrows)*. Distal is at the top as seen by the radiograph on right. Surgical intervention with a cephalic vein patch to restore normal vascularity in the upper extremity was required. Despite counseling, she returned to cheerleading 6 months later with 10° to 140° range of motion in the elbow and full pronation and supination.

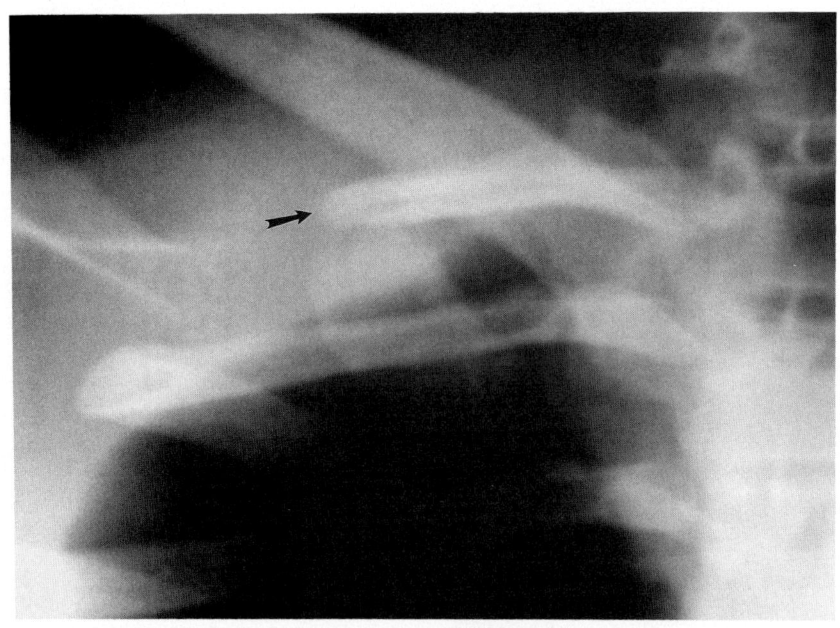

Figure 11.26 A ballet athlete sustained a left first rib fracture that went on to a delayed union. Notice the rounded edges of the proximal fragment *(arrow)*.

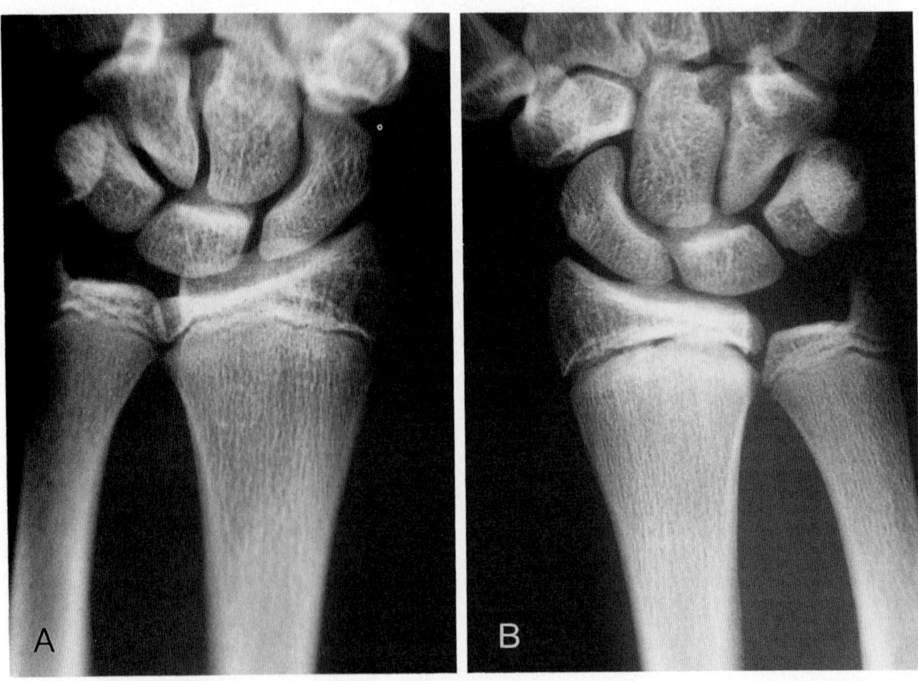

Figure 11.27 **(A)** A normal undulating epiphyseal plate on comparison view of the left wrist and **(B)** a widened epiphyseal plate on the right. This is a Salter I fracture of the distal radius in this gymnast.

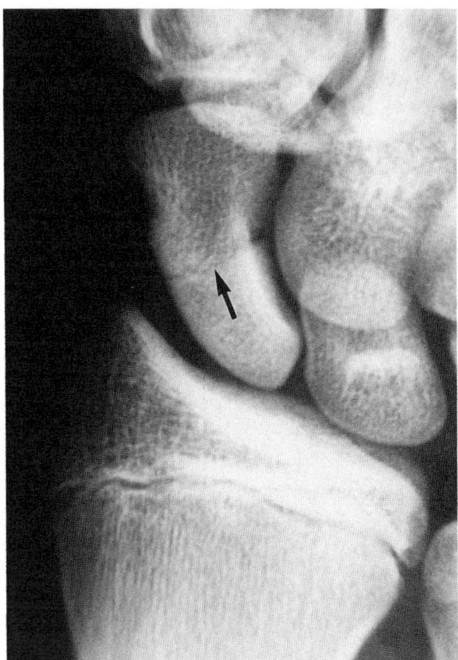

Figure 11.28 Acute midwaist navicular fracture is seen in this skeletally immature right wrist of a gymnast *(arrow)*.

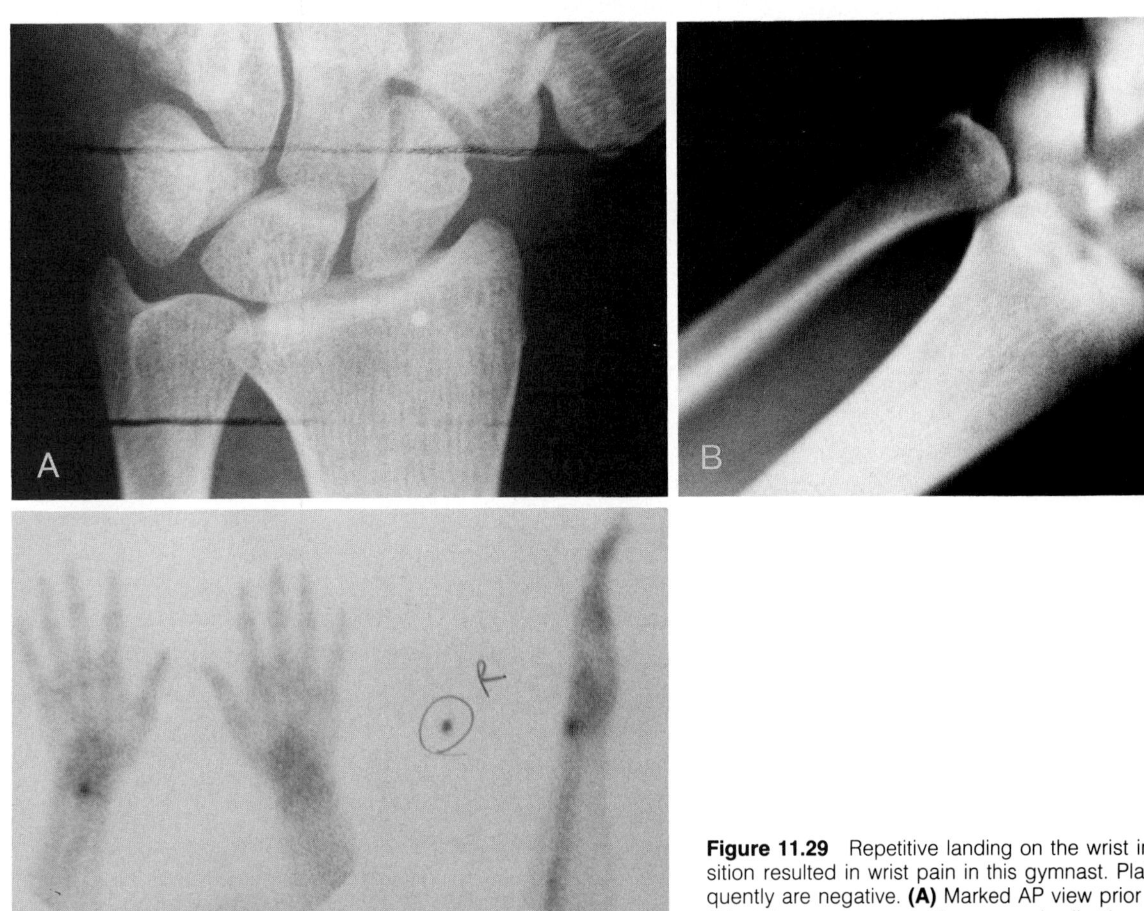

Figure 11.29 Repetitive landing on the wrist in a dorsiflexed position resulted in wrist pain in this gymnast. Plain radiographs frequently are negative. **(A)** Marked AP view prior to tomograms and **(B)** oblique tomograms show a cystic distal radius stress fracture confirmed by **(C)** bone scan. Increased activity in the dorsal central aspect of the right radius is shown.

Femoral Neck

There should be a high index of suspicion for fracture in track athletes with persistent groin pain. Iliopsoas or adductor strain could really be a femoral neck stress fracture. This middle distance and cross country track athlete complained of left hip pain for one month. She was amenorrheic and did not eat meat or drink milk. AP and lateral radiographs showed cortical reaction of the inferior (Fig. 11.30) and posterior (Fig. 11.30) femoral neck. An initial bone scan showed increased activity (Fig. 11.30). This compression side fracture was treated conservatively with nonweight bearing, swimming, nutritional counseling, and oral contraceptives. The fractures healed in six months clinically and radiographically as shown on AP view (Fig. 11.31). On the compression side, femoral neck stress fractures can be treated nonoperatively. If the fracture is on the superior or tensile side, percutaneous pinning before fracture displacement is recommended.

Tibial Fracture

The tibia is a common site for stress fractures. Use of marked views over the area of maximal tenderness to look for periosteal reactions is helpful. If plain films

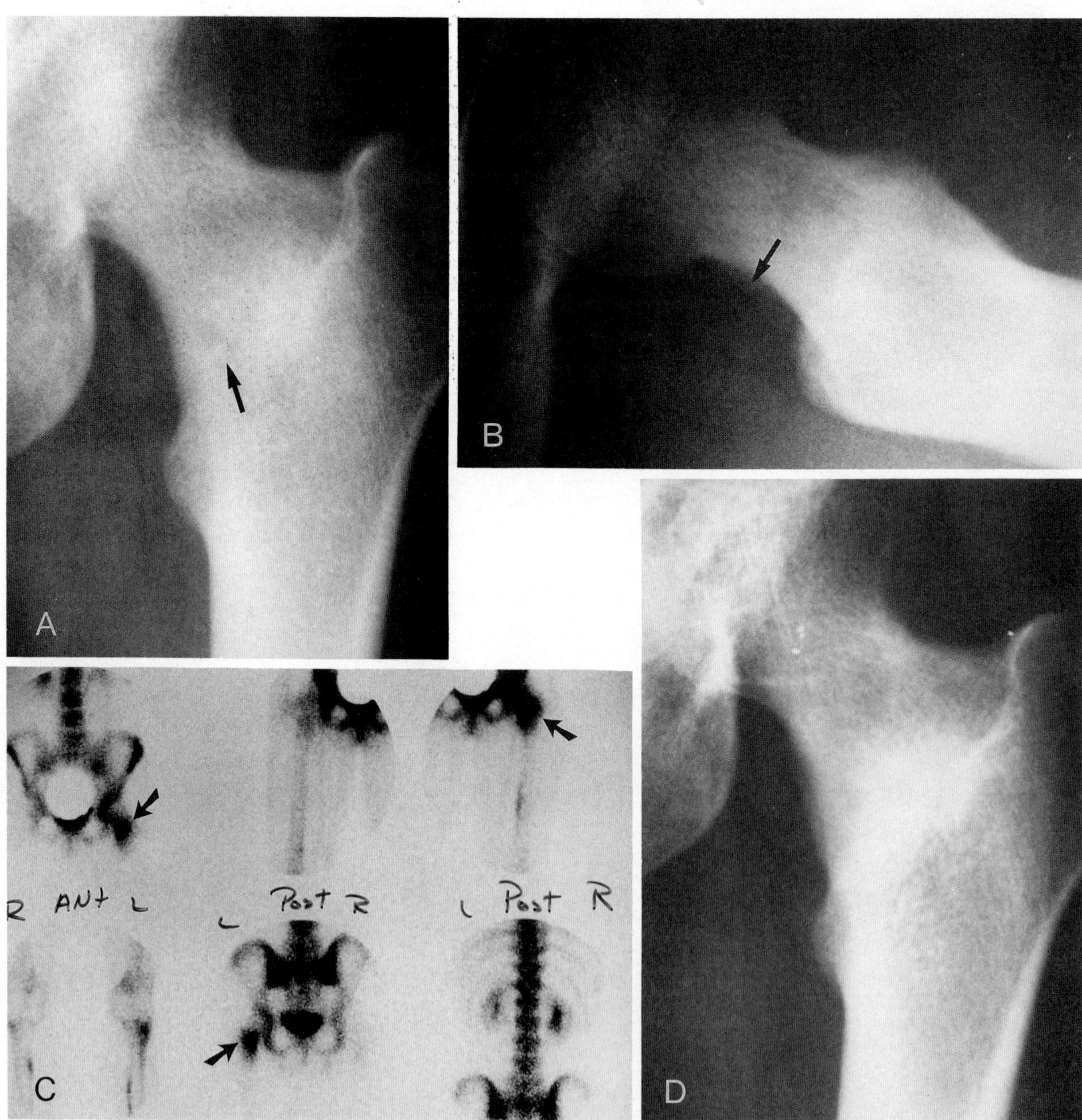

Figure 11.30 A collegiate middle distance and cross country track athlete had pain in her left hip for 1 month. Plain radiographs showed **(A)** an AP view with thickened medial cortex and radiolucency *(arrow)* and **(B)** a lateral view with periosteal reaction posteriorly *(arrow)*. The stress fracture on the compression side inferiorly can be treated nonoperatively. Tension or superior femoral neck fractures should be more aggressively treated with pinning prior to displacement. **(C)** A bone scan showed significant increase in activity in the inferior neck *(arrows)*. **(D)** Follow-up radiographs 6 months following documentation of the fracture showed femoral neck periosteal reaction.

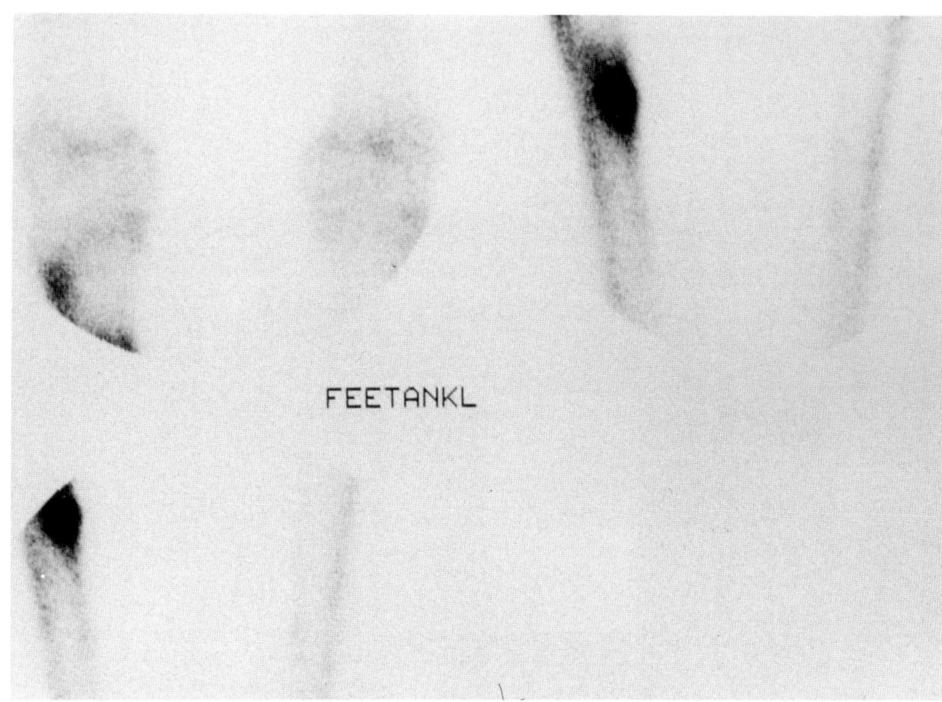

Figure 11.31 Tibial stress fractures are common at the proximal midthird junction and distal third junction. If plain radiographs are negative, a bone scan is helpful. Intensely increased activity of the medial proximal midthird junction is seen. Plain and marked views at area of maximal tenderness were negative in this soccer athlete.

are negative, a bone scan will confirm the diagnosis, as in this soccer athlete with midproximal third junction tibial stress fracture (Fig. 11.31) who had had normal radiographs.

The midthird anterior cortex stress fractures is important to recognize. Clinically, point tenderness and anterior tibial bow suggest this unique stress fracture. Plain radiographs of AP (Fig. 11.32*A*), lateral (Fig. 11.32*B*), and cone-marked lateral view at point of maximum tenderness (Fig. 11.32C) confirm the diagnosis. This is commonly seen in basketball athletes with varus and anterior bow of the tibia. Conservative management usually results in healing, as in this patient after six months. However, electrical stimulation or operative management has also been suggested (54).

Fibular Fractures

Repetitive loading such as tumbling, floor routines, cheerleading, and gymnastic maneuvers may result in fibular stress fractures. Pain localization to the lateral fibula and radiographs showing significant increased cortical thickness and a very small medullary cavity are the usual findings in athletes with fibular stress fractures. Tibiofibular views with the marker at the area of maximal tenderness suggest a fracture (Fig. 11.33*A*). Note the prior, now asymptomatic, healed fibular stress fracture just proximal to marked level in this collegiate cheerleader. A bone scan revealed intensely increased activity at the level of maximal tenderness (Fig. 11.33*B*). Successful treatment included compressive support and avoidance of tumbling activities for three months.

Metatarsal Fractures

The most common metatarsal stress fracture is the second, followed by the third. This track athlete was seen after callus formation was present on plain radiographs (Fig. 11.34). With localized swelling and tenderness over the diaphysis and callus on plain radiographs, the diagnosis was easily established.

Back Conditions and Fractures

Scoliosis

Scoliosis is more common in females than males. This skeletally immature eleven-year-old cheerleader has a 20° typical right thoracic curve with apex at thoracic level 8 shown on posteroanterior (PA) view (Fig. 11.35*A*). The lateral view (Fig. 11.35*B*) shows no thoracic kyphosis associated with flat back appearance. This cheerleader demonstrates a more acute 21° left upper lumbar curve on this PA view with apex at lumbar level 1 (Fig. 11.36).

Spondylolysis

Repetitive flexion extension activities result in stress fractures of the pars interarticularis or spondylolysis. The work-up of persistent back pain and a positive hyperextension test should include radiographs of AP, standing lateral, and obliques. The radiolucent defect in the pars interarticularis is best seen on oblique view (Fig. 11.37*A*). Increased activity on oblique view bone scan at the third lumbar level confirms the diagnosis of spondylolysis (Fig. 11.37*B*). Acquired spondylolysis will not progress to spondylolisthesis. In these athletes, spondylolysis and sciatica can occur simultaneously in a single patient. If there is nonunion of the pars interarticularis, posterior spinal fusion successfully eliminates pain. (Micheli LJ, personal communication 1984).

Spondylolisthesis

Standing lateral views are necessary to assess posterior spinal stability for spondylolisthesis. This colle-

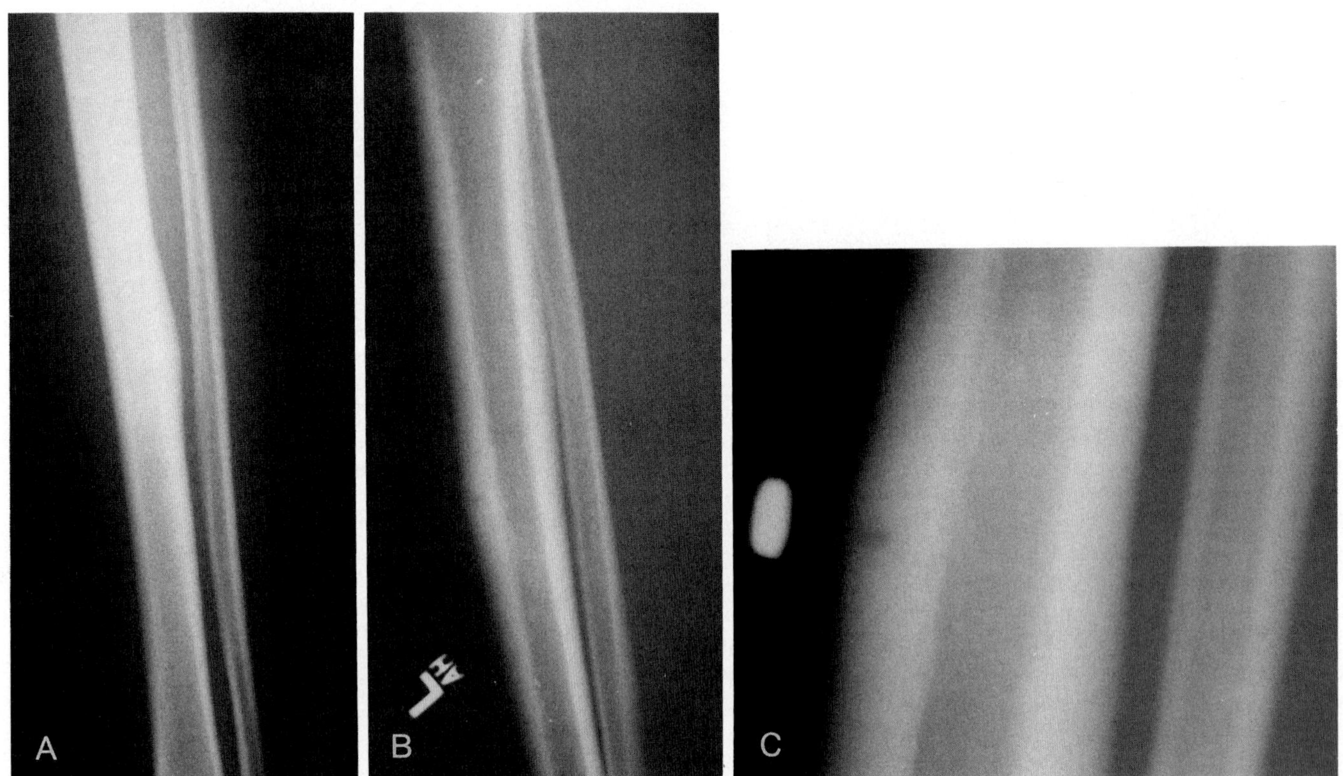

Figure 11.32 This female basketball athlete sustained a stress fracture in the midthird anterior cortex of the left tibia. **(A)** AP and **(B)** lateral view show the healing fracture now four months after onset of symptoms. **(C)** A metallic marker on lateral view at point of maximum tenderness helps confirm that the radiolucency seen is at the level of patient's pain. Conservative management in this patient resulted in complete healing.

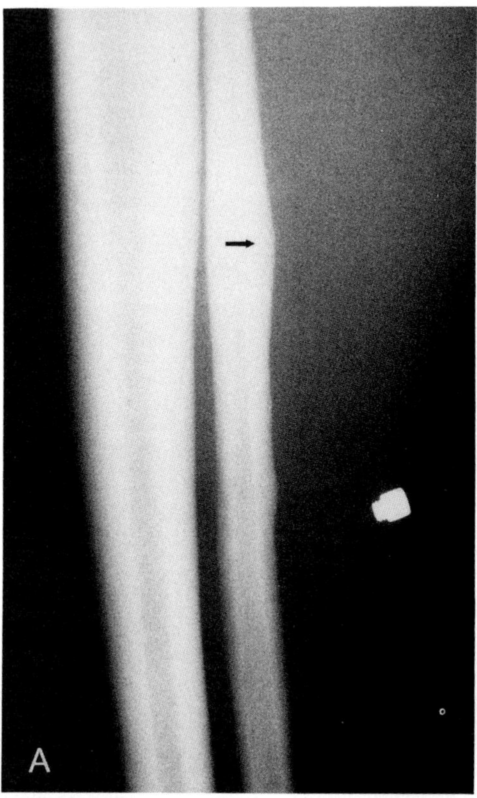

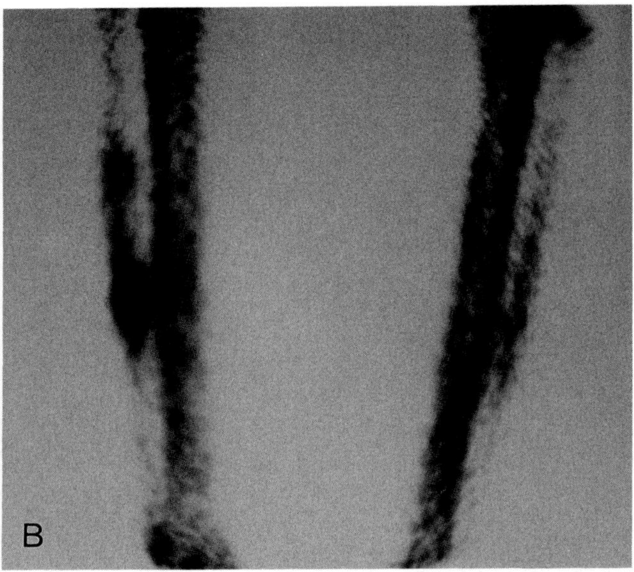

Figure 11.33 This collegiate cheerleader was evaluated for pain in the lateral calf. **(A)** A marked view revealed periosteal reaction at the midthird of the fibula. Notice the periosteal reaction just superior to level of symptoms *(arrow)*. The patient had a documented stress fracture of the fibula at this level 6 months prior to her new onset of symptoms. Notice the narrow intramedullary cavity. **(B)** A bone scan showed increased activity more intensely at the distal fracture level shown on the left as compared with the normal lower extremity on the right.

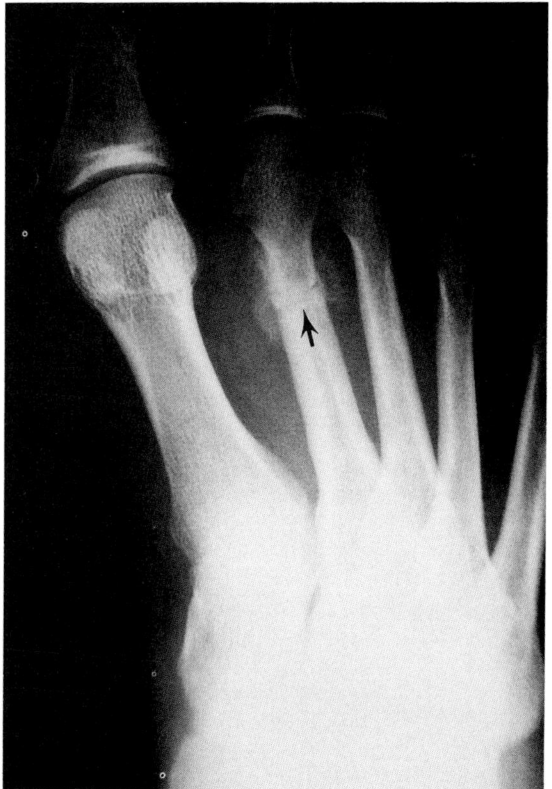

Figure 11.34 A callus is seen in this healing second metatarsal stress fracture in a female track athlete. On plain films, radiolucency of the fracture line *(arrow)* can be seen with abundant callus, which was palpable and painful over the second metatarsal diaphysis.

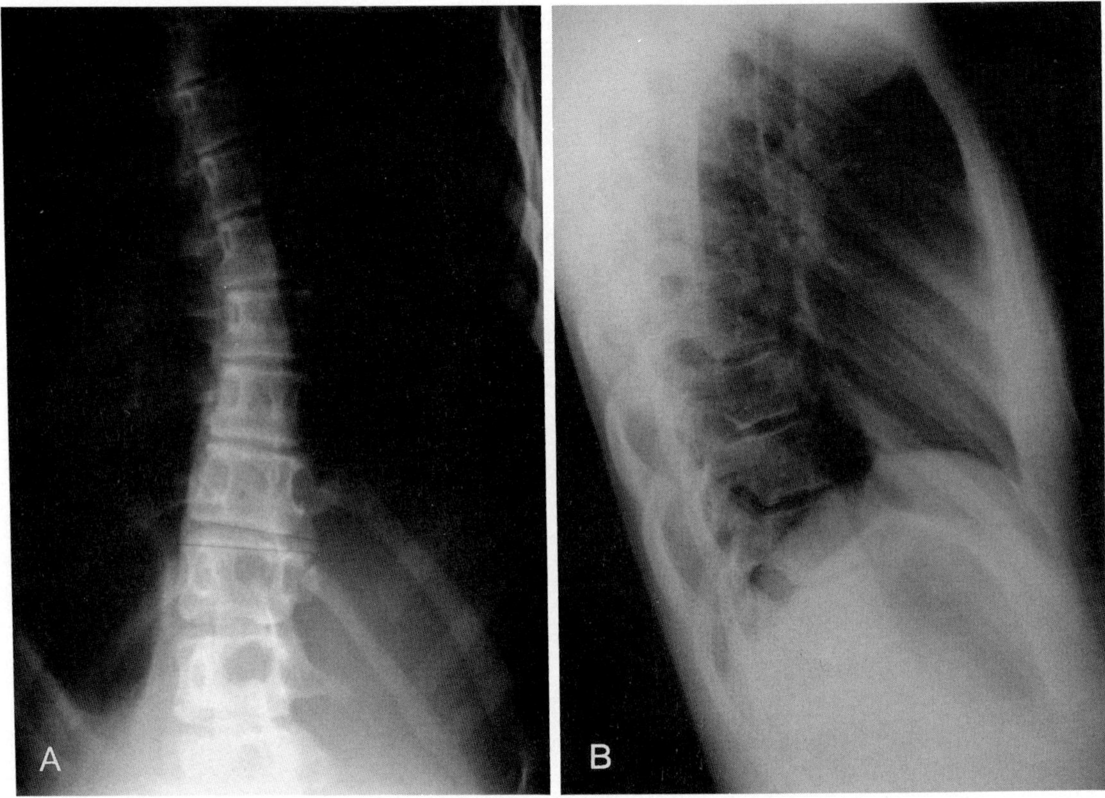

Figure 11.35 **(A)** Standing PA and **(B)** lateral views show a typical right 20° thoracic curve with apex at thoracic L-8 and no thoracic kyphosis in a skeletally immature 11-year-old basketball athlete.

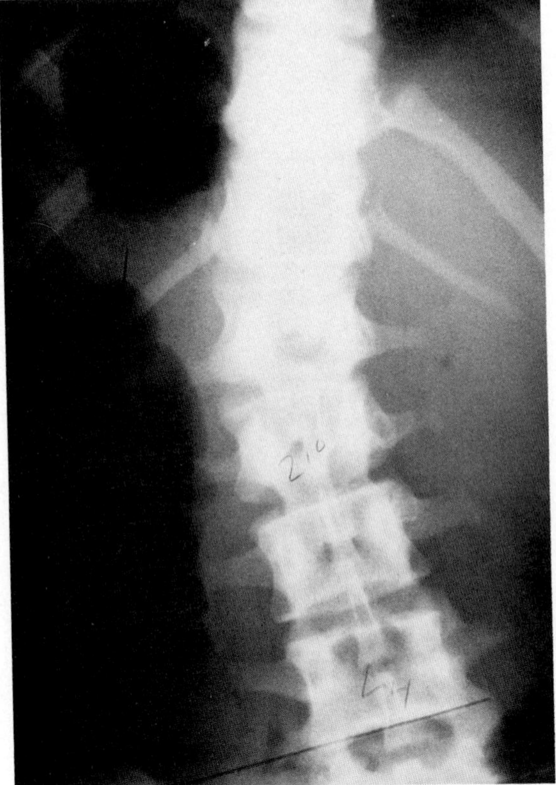

Figure 11.36 This cheerleader demonstrates a more unusual left upper lumbar curve measuring 21° with apex at L1.

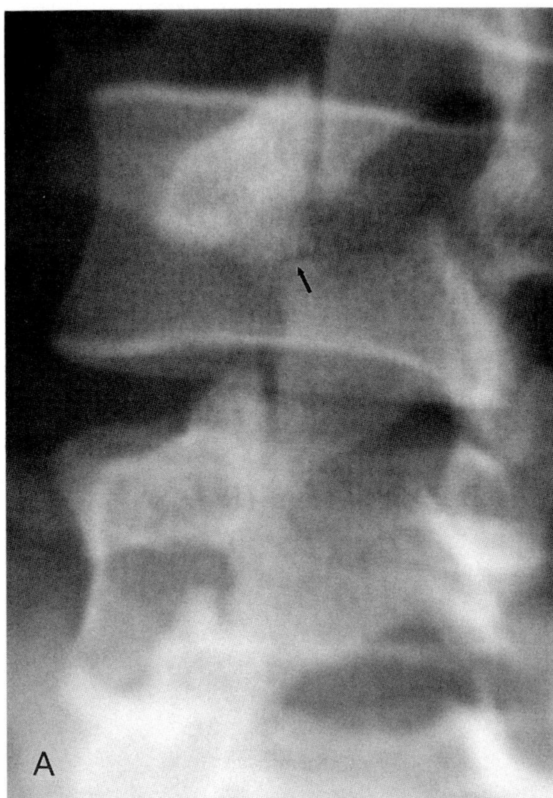

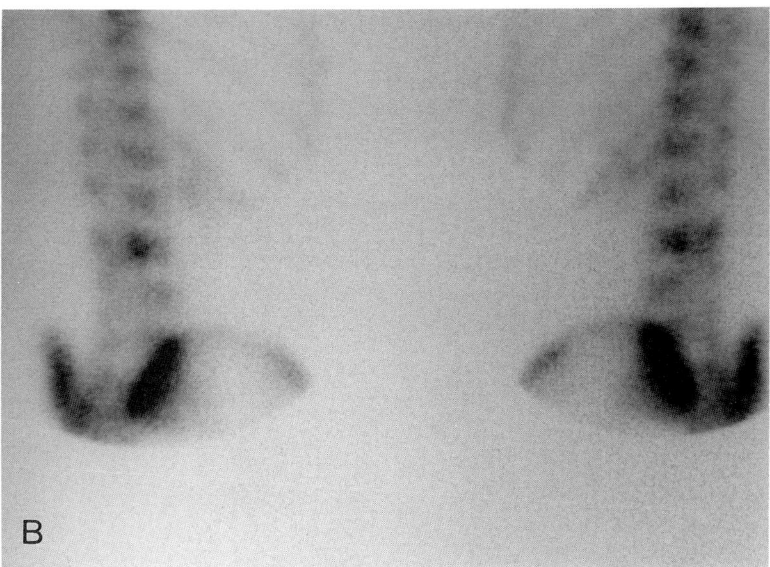

Figure 11.37 **(A)** An acute pars interarticularis defect in a cheerleader who had a positive hyperextension test is shown on an oblique marked radiograph *(arrow)*. **(B)** The acuteness of the spondylolysis is confirmed by increased activity on the bone scan at L4 level.

giate gymnast had a five-year history of occasional back pain. Standing lateral view showed L5-S1 grade IV spondylolisthesis, indicated by dotted lines (Fig. 11.38*A*). Oblique views showed two old radiolucencies in the pars interarticularis at L5 (Fig. 11.38*B*). This gymnast had previous back problems but none at the time of presentation. Her complaints were limited to lateral calf pain. A bone scan showed increased activity in fibula (Fig. 11.38*C*) but no increased activity in the lumbar spine (Fig. 11.38*D*).

Spondylolysis at different levels from a spondylolisthesis may also occur. In this cheerleader, an acute spondylolysis is shown in this oblique marked view (Fig. 11.39*A*). A bone scan showed increased activity at the marked level of pain but not at L5-S1 level. An old grade I spondylolisthesis is shown two levels lower than her level of pain (Fig. 11.39*B*).

Other Fractures

A vertebral body fracture at L5 occurred when this collegiate gymnast fell in a hyperflexed position from the top of the uneven parallel bars. A cone view better shows the fracture, which showed increased activity by bone scan (Fig. 11.40*A*). Anatomic variants or a limbus vertebra may look similar. Bone scan is helpful to establish the diagnosis and better counsel the athlete on the timing of a return to sport. A standing lateral view showed marked lordosis one month after injury (Fig. 11.40*B*).

Pedicle stress fracture has been reported in a ballet athlete (55) and documented by computed tomography (CT) scan (Fig. 11.41*A*). Lateral views showed radiolucency in posterior elements. The CT scan confirmed this diagnosis (Fig. 11.41*B*).

Psychologic

Young female participants in athletics improve self-confidence and overall performance, and enhancement of confidence with positive reinforcement is possible when females actively engage in sports (23, 56, 57). Young women who understand their motives for being involved in sports relate rewarding experiences. However, when maturity occurs, these goals may change and priorities are modified in some female athletes (56). Participating and excelling in athletics can be used as a springboard for dealing with stresses, competition, and challenges in both professional and personal spheres of life (32).

Nutrition

Adequate nutrition is of paramount importance for the athlete's health and successful performance. Reviews of nutritional concerns in the adolescent female (58) and older athlete (59) have been addressed. Particularly in the female athlete, diets are often imbalanced or contain inadequate nutritional components (23, 60–62). Studies comparing males and females in similar sports have emphasized major differences in caloric intake and diet type. Collegiate basketball players were compared, showing that males had twice the caloric intake. Nutritional supplements had a significant effect

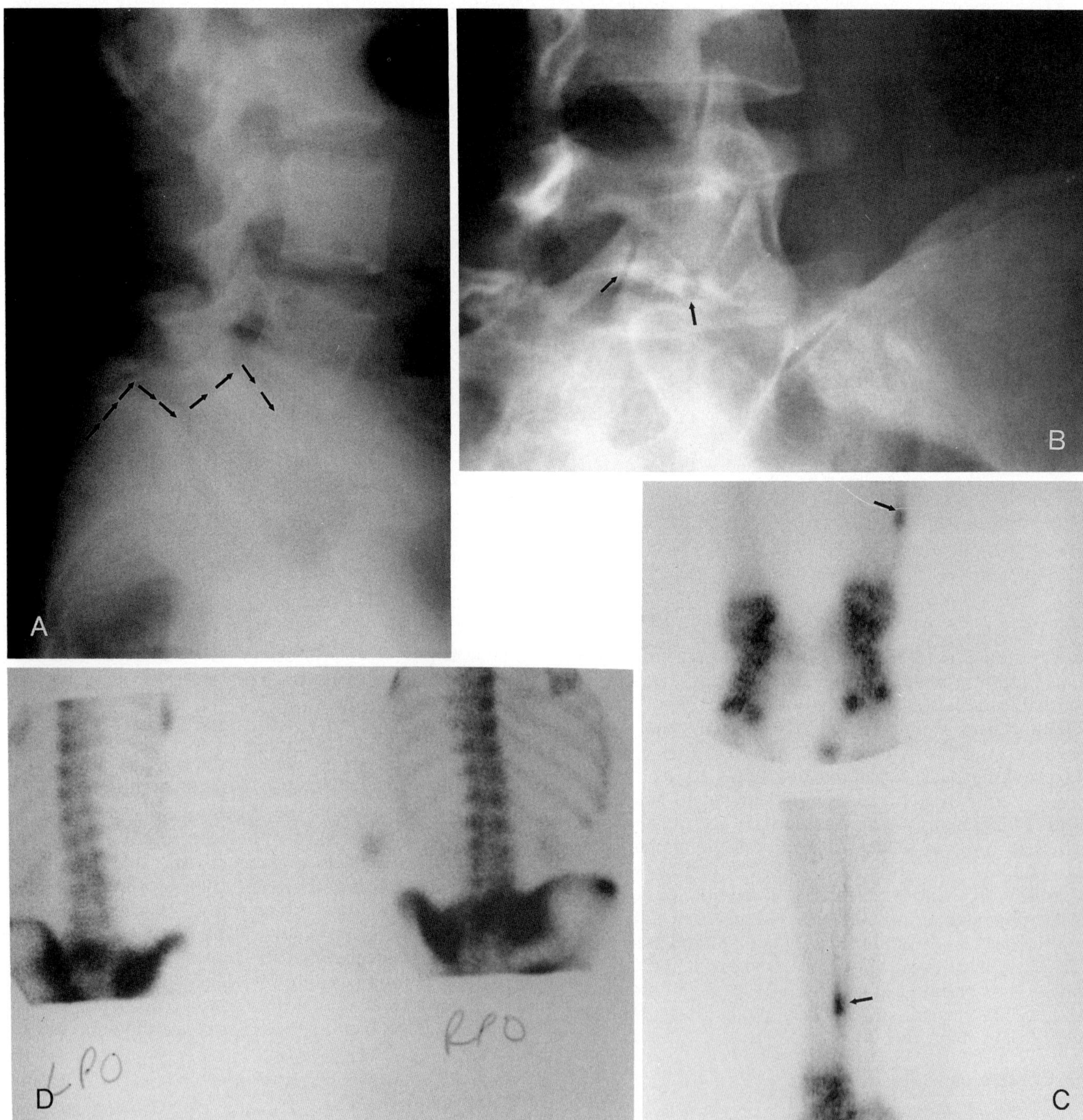

Figure 11.38 Standing lateral views are necessary to assess posterior spinal stability. **(A)** Standing lateral view of this collegiate level gymnast shows a grade IV spondylolysis L5-S1 level *(linear arrows)*. **(B)** Oblique view shows two levels of pars defect at the L5 level *(arrows)*. Patient was evaluated for pain in her fibula. She mentioned prior history of back problems and lateral radiograph was obtained. The patient was disqualified from continued collegiate competition due to subsequent low back pain and neurologic complaints. **(C)** The bone scan shows increased activity in the fibula consistent with a stress fracture *(arrows)* and **(D)** no increase in activity in the lumbar spine.

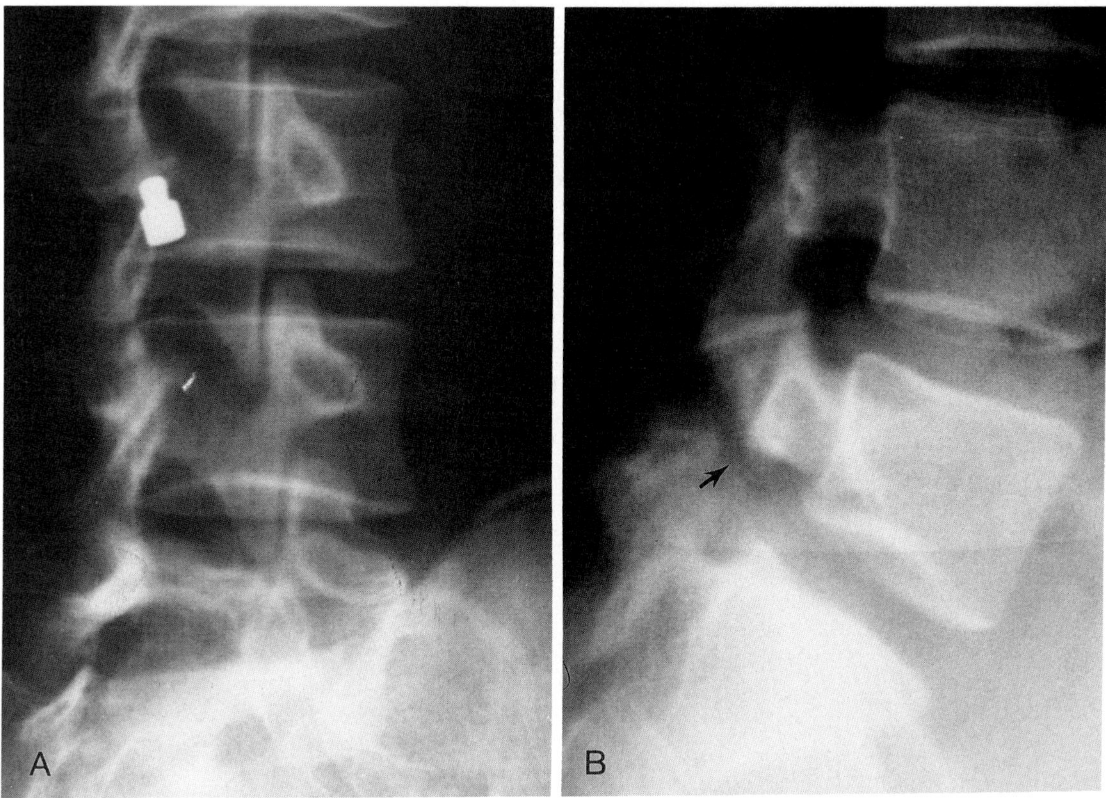

Figure 11.39 An old spondylolisthesis can be seen at a different level from an acute spondylolysis. **(A)** A marked oblique view at the level of pain is two levels above an old symptomatic grade I L5–S1 spondylolisthesis seen on **(B)** lateral view level. Note the radiolucency of posterior elements L5—S1 without significant slippage *(arrows)*.

on the total nutrient intake in the women (60). Compared to males, female skiers and marathoners consume fewer calories and have less intake of vitamins, proteins, and carbohydrates (63).

Poor diet can result in deficiency in the intake of carbohydrates, iron, calcium, zinc. Low calcium intake is associated with low bone density, stress fractures, and subsequent problems with osteoporosis (63, 64). Carbohydrate deficiency can result in glycogen depletion and increased onset of muscular fatigue. Zinc deficiency can result in increased injuries from microtrauma as well as changes in immune function. Iron deficiency can contribute to anemia and to poor thermal regulation, especially during exposure to cold.

Common nutritional problems contributing to poor performance are inadequate intake of fluids (65), carbohydrates (66), and excess fat intake (23, 65–68). Nutritional counseling for female athletes to stress the importance of proper ratios of food groups and other nutrients is needed. Nutritional educational programs are essential for improvement of the food choices and overall health in the female athlete (63, 65).

Fluid Intake

Fluid loss of only 1% of body weight during activity is a state of dehydration. Fluid depletion can occur in a very short period of time—in as little as 30 minutes (69). Simple weighing of athletes before and after activity to determine fluid loss is necessary. To maintain physiologic hydration, 16 ounces of fluid must be consumed for every pound lost in excess of body weight multiplied by .03 (69). Fluid intake schedules and discussions of the best hydration fluids have been published (63, 65, 66, 68, 69).

Diet Composition

Meals high in complex carbohydrates, such as starches of bread, whole grain cereals, pasta, legumes, and vegetables like potatoes are required to support all sports activity. The carbohydrate is a primary fuel for anaerobic work and the limiting fuel for aerobic endurance work (66). Many female athletes harbor the belief that starchy foods cause obesity (65). These athletes deprive themselves of starches, then suffer from increased injury and are prone to binge on high sugar, high fat snacks. High carbohydrate menu patterns of 60% carbohydrates are available for the athlete (63, 65, 66, 70).

Iron and calcium ingestion are of particular importance in female athletes. Calcium intake may need to be increased in athletes with amenorrhea. Iron deficiency anemia is very prevalent in females due to inadequate intake associated with normal menstruation (71, 72). Recognition of iron deficiency anemia and treatment with supplements and dietary counseling are necessary (73).

Screening for anemia in all athletes is recommended. In adolescent athletes with a serious commitment to exercise performance, screening of serum ferritin levels to

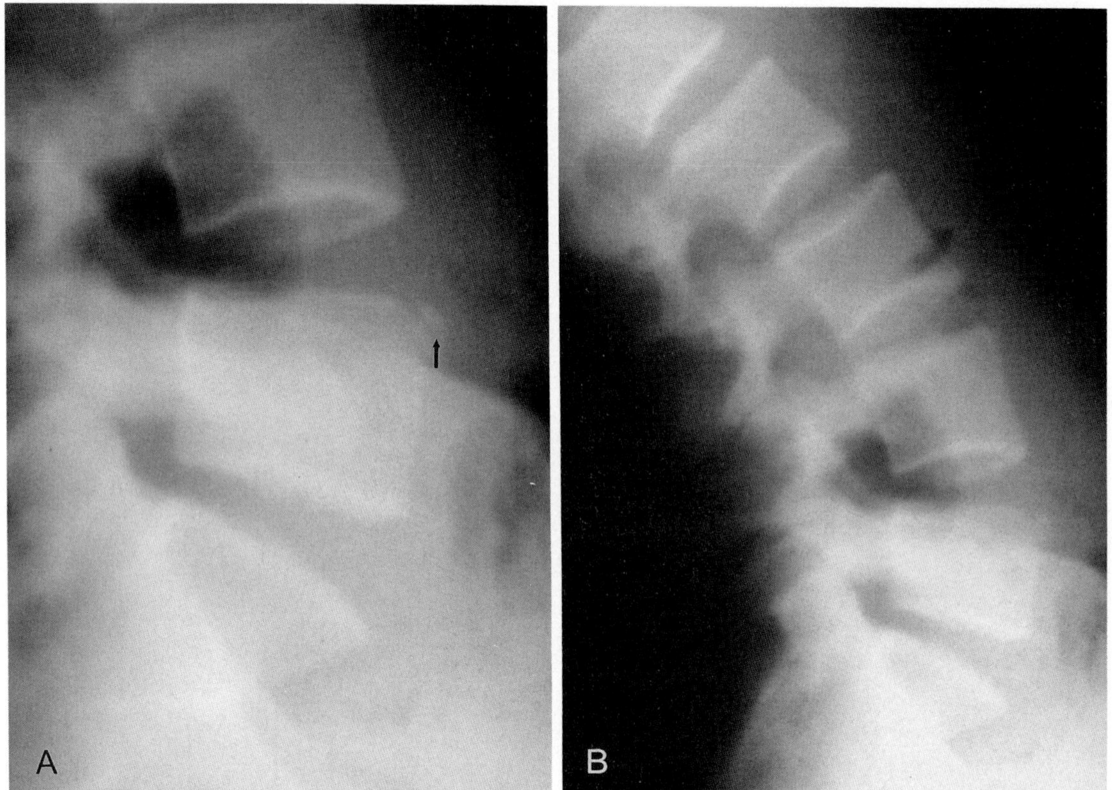

Figure 11.40 An acute avulsion at L5 occurred in this collegiate gymnast who fell from a top uneven parallel bar in a hyperflexion mechanism. **(A)** A cone view shows a superior vertebral body fracture *(arrow)*. **(B)** A standing lateral view 1 month following the injury shows excessive lordosis and healing of the L5 fracture.

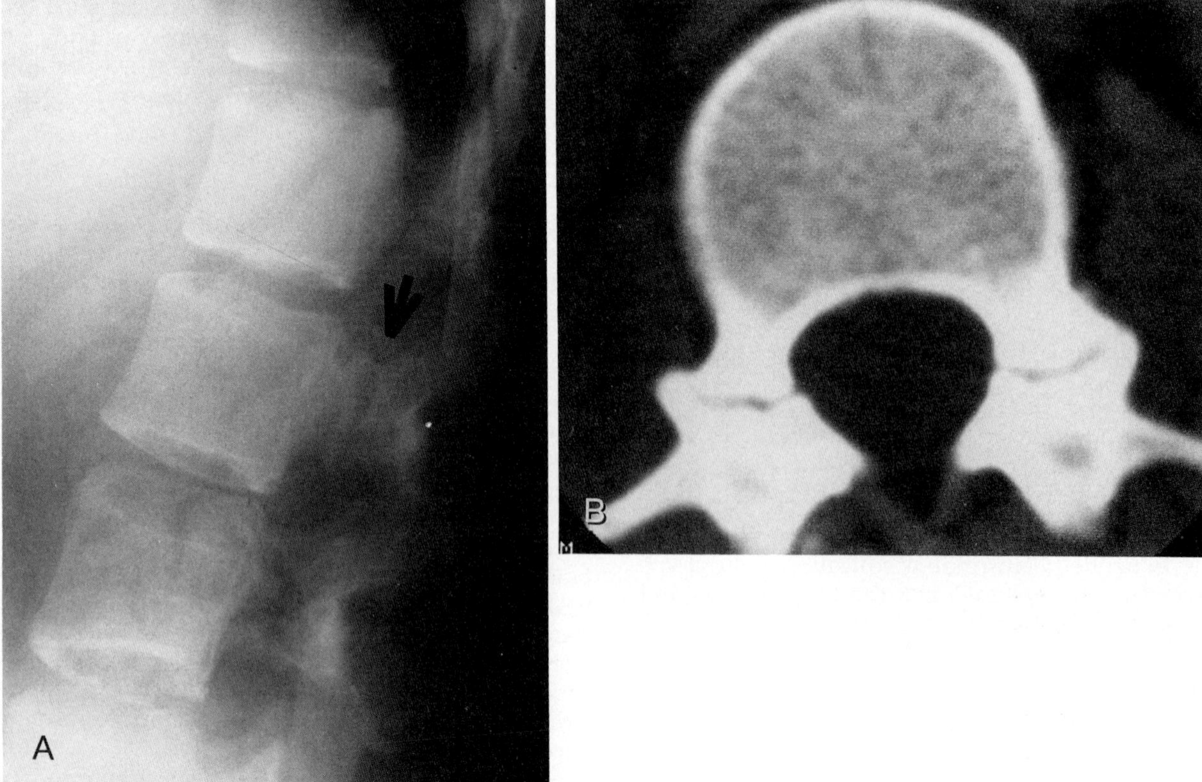

Figure 11.41 A pedicle stress fracture occurred in this ballet athlete. **(A)** A standing lateral view shows posterior element radiolucency *(arrow)*. **(B)** a CT scan confirmed the pedicle fracture.

determine a preanemic iron deficiency has been suggested (73).

Weight, body fat standards, height and weight standards are used as training goals for athletes. The coaching and medical staff must be aware of the proper methods to assess ideal body weight. It is best to employ standards that determine progress toward improved percentage of body fat. Methods for assessing body fat and guidelines for setting standards can be found in nutritional sports references (69, 74). (See Chapter 2.) Athletes carry more lean mass per height than the general population. Weight for height standards can be misleading (65). The athlete should be performing at ideal body weight. Contribution to compromised performance and behavior or to the eating disorders of anorexia nervosa and bulimia occurs when unrealistic body weights and body fat percentages are given by an uneducated member of the coaching or medical staff. Education of the athlete, the coaches, and the medical staff on athletic nutritional needs is mandatory. Consultation with dieticians familiar with needs of a particular sport can result in significant improvements in performance and decreases in injury and illness rates. We are what we eat!

Eating Disorders

Eating disorders are underdiagnosed and exist in epidemic proportions in female athletes. Estimates are that anorexia and bulimia affect as many as one-third of athletic females (75). The athlete, family, coaches, and medical staff should be aware of the very high incidence of eating disorders and nutritional misconceptions among young adolescent females. According to the American Psychiatric Association's definition, eating disorders are gross disturbances in eating behavior, typically beginning in adolescence or early adult life (76). Bulimia is fear of fatness but weight does not decrease below normal weight. Episodes of binge eating and vomiting are common in bulimia. Anorexia nervosa is a disorder with features of refusal to maintain body weight over minimal normal weight for age and height, intense fear of gaining weight or becoming fat, a distorted body image and amenorrhea. Anorexia is a misnomer since loss of appetite is rare. Bulimia and anorexia nervosa can both exist in a single patient.

In the athletic setting, frequent body weight measurements and teammate observation will help identify underlying problems. Denial of eating disorders is common. Cures are rare, so that early diagnosis of eating disorders is critical to hopes of reestablishing a nutritionally sound and normal patient.

Osteoporosis

Hormonal replacement and weight bearing exercise in the premenopausal stages reduces bone loss. Weight bearing activities in postmenopausal women appears to increase mineral content of bone (77). Weight bearing exercise will increase or maintain bone mass, but will not produce a large increase in bone mass (78). Regularly maintained athletic programs for adult women may reduce the rate of bone mass loss that occurs with age and especially postmenopausally (79–82). Patients with anorexia nervosa have reduced bone density that may be permanent. Bone density and mineral content in amenorrheic and eumenorrheic athletes and nonathletes have been quantitated. Further work on bone density is being done to develop normal values for single as well as dual photon densitometry normal values.

Gynecologic/Obstetric

Introduction

Hormonal balance, menarche, menstrual disorders, and menopause are unique considerations in the female athlete.

Normal Menarche

Puberty is the transition period between the juvenile state and adulthood, when the adolescent growth spurt occurs and when secondary sexual characteristics appear. Fertility is achieved and profound psychologic changes take place. It is also the time when many young athletes are initiating or finding their skills. In both males and females, there has been a trend toward early onset of puberty over the last 150 years. This is thought to result from improvement in socioeconomic conditions, nutrition, and general health. Although general trends vary, the average age of menarche in the United States is approximately 12.3 years. It appears that the more critical factor in the time of menarche is the percentage of total body fat, although critical height to weight ratios have been described also (83). Any factor affecting this critical percentage, the body fat ratio, can alter normal menarche. Due to multiple factors including variations in weight, accelerated activity level, and individual differences athletes are at great risk for delays in menarche or alteration in menstruation. Breast development also occurs when the estrogen production in the normal hypothalamic pituitary gonadal axis occurs. Poor nutrition and hormonal imbalance can alter normal development.

With the onset of puberty, the normal menstrual cycle occurs. Production of estrogen feeds back to the hypothalamic-pituitary axis to stimulate production of follicle stimulating hormone (FSH) and development of follicles within the ovary. The surge of a luteinizing hormone (LH) at midcycle results in ovulation, followed by an increase in progesterone production in the luteal phase of the cycle, and, subsequently, menses.

Delayed Menarche

Delayed age at menarche and increased incidence of oligomenorrhea and amenorrhea have been associated with training (84). Menarche in athletes appears to be delayed when compared to nonathlete sisters (85, 86). Premenarchal training does delay the onset of menses but not other pubertal changes (77).

Menstrual Abnormalities

Menstrual irregularities and nutritional abnormalities interrelate to increase the frequency and severity of injuries and illnesses. Differences in body composition between men and women may affect performance in environmental extremes (87). While the average women has a smaller surface area than her male counterpart, her ratio of body surface area (BSA) to weight is greater. In hot climates, women gain heat faster and have a smaller mass to store it in. In air temperature below skin temperature, women lose heat faster. In cold environments, increased subcutaneous fat enhances insulation in women, but the increased BSA/weight ratio in women allows greater heat loss, so that men and women with an equal percentage of body fat demonstrate no differences in metabolic rate, rectal temperature, or skin temperature.

Gynecologic concerns and menstrual dysfunction have been reviewed (51, 88). Decreased resting metabolic rates have been documented in amenorrheic runners (89). Unique gynecologic situations in the female dancer have been published (90). Women athletes with menstrual irregularity have an increased incidence of muscle injury (49). Premenopausal individuals with irregular menses are at increased risk for musculoskeletal injury (44).

Drinkwater (91) and Lutter (50) reviewed health concerns of women runners, including concerns about menstrual abnormalities and pregnancy. An association of athletic amenorrhea, major affective disorders, and eating disorders in runners has been suggested (92). The common occurrence of menstrual dysfunction in adolescents who are involved in intensive athletic activity or who limit their nutritional intake excessively has been established (93). Excessive exercise can alter body weight, decreasing the percentage of body fat, which in turn decreases estrogen production. In this situation, the hypothalamic pituitary ovarian axis is affected, and anovulation, abnormal bleeding, and amenorrhea occur. The association of menstrual dysfunction with low bone density has also been established (64, 91, 94). Lowered estrogen levels and decreased calcium binding in the bony matrix can cause osteoporosis (88). Oligomenorrheic runners have been noted to have decreased bone density compared with eumenorrheic runners (95).

Hypothalamic amenorrhea in dieters and athletic amenorrhea has been treated with estrogen replacement. Controversy exists over whether routine use of oral birth control pills should be implemented early in the treatment of athletic amenorrhea (32).

An excellent summary of indications, contraindications, benefits, and negative effects of oral contraceptives is presented by Kulpa (96). The athlete must understand the importance of taking her birth control pills regularly to prevent breakthrough bleeding and to report any side effects such as calf tenderness, chest pain, severe headaches, or visual symptoms. The basic problem of decrease in percentage body fat is not addressed.

Controversy exists about whether the use of oral birth control pills increases bone density. Use of birth control pills in the perimenopausal period may maximize genetic bone density (96). Runners who had never taken oral contraceptives were twice as likely to sustain stress fractures as runners taking birth control pills for more than one year (43). A definite decrease in the incidence of stress fractures in women athletes, particularly in gymnasts and cross country runners has occurred with the use of oral birth control pills at the University of Kentucky (Hager D, Caborn D, personal communication, 1992).

Athletic performance may be affected by the phases of the menstrual cycle. Exercise performance and muscle glycogen content are enhanced during the luteal phase (88, 96–98). Record breaking performances have occurred in all phases of the menstrual cycle.

Menstrual Abnormalities and Nutritional Disorders

The relationship between food intake, activity, leanness, and menstruation has been investigated. There are reviews of menstrual dysfunction of athletic women ranging from basic principles to evaluation and treatment literature (99–101). Other problems seen in athletic women are iron deficiency anemia and the association of affective disorders and eating disorders (71, 92). The causes of athletic amenorrhea continue to be debated and investigated. Low body fat and low weight have been shown to be a significant contributor to athletic amenorrhea (102–104). The association of the intensity of the athletic activity with changes in the menstrual cycle have also been explored (84, 105, 106). Stress and nutrition are critical factors in the development of menstrual abnormalities (107). Interaction between diet, particularly dietary fiber intake, decreased bone density, and menstrual dysfunction has been postulated (44). Reviews of athletic amenorrhea discuss its causes, complications, and management (108). Hormonal therapy and greater calcium intake have been suggested to treat the condition (108).

Interrelationships of diet and athletic activity, menstrual status and bone density in collegiate women have been reviewed (15, 75, 91, 109). Abnormality in one of these areas can result in increased illness and injury rates, with stress fractures as example.

Exercise and Pregnancy

Special consideration of exercise during pregnancy has been outlined in various articles (32, 110–117). When women who exercise routinely become pregnant, continuation of the same baseline program appears to be safe and should be encouraged. Women who have not exercised before pregnancy can cautiously begin an exercise program with the physician's permission. Guidelines for exercise in the pregnant and postpartum state have been set. Regular exercise is defined as a minimum of 3 periods of exercise per week. Strenuous exercises should be limited to 15 minutes. Exercise should not be done in a hot or humid environment or when mother is febrile. Maternal temperature should not exceed 38° centigrade. Conditioning during pregnancy is encouraged but it should be carried out in accordance with prior exercise patterns. Avoidance of jumping and loading activities lessens the risk of injury associated with presence of the hormone relaxin which stretches the ligaments. No supine exercises should be performed until after 4 months gestation. The maternal heart rate should not exceed 140 beats per minute. Appropriate warm-up and cool-down periods as well as the use of liquids is suggested. In the postpartum period of 4 to 6 weeks, women have been cautioned against exercise, although more research should be done in this area. In summary, for mental and physical health, during pregnancy, exercise according to above guidelines is suggested.

Breast Development

Hindle concisely reviewed the subject of the breast and its protective devices (118). The breast is composed of essential fat and sex-specific fat. There is no true change in breast size with exercise programs or with pectoralis-specific strengthening.

The breast is an endocrine end organ composed of fat, suspensory ligaments and ducts. The nipple is the end organ that receives the lactiferous, or mammary, ducts, and it is the most prominent part of the breast. Changes in weight and genetics influence breast size and shape. The development of this mammary gland occurs by hormonal influence, including estradiol growth hormone, hydrocortisone, insulin, oxytocin, progesterone, prolactin, and thyroxine. The glandular tissue responds to the menstrual cycle by changes in size and mitotic activity. Except for the period of pregnancy, the terminal duct units remain in a resting state.

Protective Devices

Sports Bras. Sports bras have design features of firm support of the breast, limitation of breast motion, and material which will not abrade the skin. The repetitive motion of exercise requires soft material to protect the nipple from abrasion or irritation. Small-breasted women attain comfort with a compression bra while large-breasted women require an encapsulation bra. Sports-type bras are recommended for women with larger breasts in order to limit motion to 2 cm in the vertical plane. The features important in a sports bra are the following: circumferential support, crisscross or Y construction, unstretchable straps, breathable material, no seams at the nipple area, no hooks or fasteners, and individualized fit. A sports bra should be comfortable during exercise and at rest.

Breast Problems

Breast Trauma. Breast discomfort related to sports activity is common. Use of sports bras and appropriate padding is beneficial. Nipple irritation caused by friction is more common in females and abrasions can result. Treatment is accomplished with local padding and lubricants. Breast trauma from contact is uncommon. When direct significant contact occurs, hematoma formation and prolonged pain can result. The recommended treatment is analgesics, support, and the avoidance of repetitive contact.

Fibrocystic Disease. The disorder is characterized by fibrous and cystic changes within the breast parenchyma. Since approximately 70% of women in the U.S. have this disorder, it is actually more unusual not to be affected by fibrocystic change. The precise cause of fibrocystic change remains unknown. Xanthines contained in caffeine and chocolate may accentuate the breast tenderness experienced by the individuals with fibrocystic change. Many women athletes are troubled with this disorder and experience cyclic breast discomfort. This can be relieved with the use of supportive bras and the restriction of caffeine in the diet.

Galactorrhea. Discharge from the nipples (galactorrhea) may be seen in normals. It also may be associated with irritation of the breast nipple or with the presence of a pituitary microadenoma. A pituitary microadenoma is a noninvasive lesion in the pituitary gland causing increase in the production of prolactin. Elevated prolactin levels inhibit normal menses and cause galactorrhea. Women athletes who present with a combination of amenorrhea and galactorrhea should be evaluated for a pituitary microadenoma.

Conclusion

Appreciation of the unique situations that exist for female athletes will improve their care and treatment. Medical personnel who have these added insights in their armamentarium can make diagnoses more efficiently and institute treatment earlier. The epidemic of knee injuries in females is of concern and requires further research. The high incidence of hormonal and nutritional imbalances increases the risk of stress fractures. These imbalances are common in the female athlete. Nutritional, gynecologic, and psychologic balance is vital to a healthy athlete. The eating disorders of anorexia nervosa and bulimia exist in epidemic proportions and treatment programs for these serious disorders must be instituted promptly. Certainly, encouragement of female participation in sports is beneficial to all, especially the athlete. The healthy female athlete can best be served by health professionals who appreciate these special and unique concerns.

ACKNOWLEDGMENTS

Special thanks to Carolyn Large, Transcriptionist; Pete Williams, PA-C, A.T.,C.; Lonnie Wright, B.A., Manager, Library Services, Central Baptist Hospital, Lexington, Kentucky; Sharon Wallace, R.D., D.Sc., Chief Clinical Dietician, Central Baptist Hospital, Nutrition Consultant for University of Kentucky Athletic Association; David Hager, M.D., Obstetrics and Gynecology.

REFERENCES

1. Agostini R. The athletic woman. In: Mellion MB, ed. Office management of sports injuries and athletic problems. Philadelphia: Hanley and Belfus 1988;76–88.
2. Hunter LY, Andrews JR, Clancy WG, Funk JR Jr. Common orthopaedic problems of female athletes. A.A.O.S: Instructional Course Lectures. 1982;31:126–151.
3. Roy S, Irvin R. The female athlete. In: Sports medicine: preven-

tion, evaluation, management, and rehabilitation. Englewood Cliffs, NJ: Prentice-Hall Inc. 1983:457–467.
4. Hale RW, ed. Caring for the exercising woman. New York: Elsevier, 1991.
5. Clarke KS, Buckley WE. Women's injuries in collegiate sports. Am J Sports Med 1980;8:187–191.
6. Garrick JG, Requa RK. Girls' sports injuries in high school athletics. JAMA 1978;239:2245–2248.
7. DeHaven KE, Linter DM. Athletic injuries: comparison by age, sport, and gender. Am J Sports Med 1986;14:218–224.
8. Whiteside PA. Men's and women's injuries in comparable sports. Phys Sportsmed 1980;8:130–136.
9. National Collegiate Athletic Association: NCAA injury surveillance system. Overland Park, Kansas: NCAA, 1991–1992.
10. National Collegiate Athletic Association: NCAA injury surveillance system. Overland Park, Kansas: NCAA, 1992–1993.
11. Ciullo, Jerome V. Lower extremity injuries. In: Pearl AJ, ed. The athletic female. Champaign, IL: Human Kinetics Pubs, 1993:267–305.
12. Wadley GH, Albright JP. Women's intercollegiate gymnastics: Injury patterns and "permanent" medical disability. Am J Sports Med 1993;21(2):314–320.
13. Lutter JM. A 20-year perspective: What has changed? In: Pearl AJ ed. The athletic female. Champaign, IL: Human Kinetics Pubs, 1993:1–10.
14. Hale RW. Historical perspective. In: Hale RW, ed. Caring for the exercising woman. New York, Elsevier 1991:1–3.
15. Ritter MA, Goie TJ, Albohn M. Sport-related injuries. Women's College Health 1980;28:267–268.
16. Gillete J. When and where women are injured in sports. Phys Sportsmed 1975;2:61–63.
17. Howell DW. Musculoskeletal profile and incidence of musculoskeletal injuries in lightweight women rowers. AM J Sports Med 1984;12:278–282.
18. Micheli LJ, Gillespie WJ, Walaszek A. Physiologic profiles of female professional ballerinas. Clin Sports Med 1984; Jan 3(1):199–209.
19. Marino M. Profiling swimmers. Clin Sports Med 1984:Jan 3(1):211–219.
20. Protzman RR. Physiologic performance of women compared to men. Am J Sports Med 1979;7:191–194.
21. Sady SP, Freedson PS. Body composition and structural comparisons of female and male athletes. Clin Sports Med 1984:3:755, 666.
22. Wilmore JH. The application of science to sport: Physiological profiles of male and female athlete. Canadian J Applied Sport Sciences. 1979;4(2):103–115.
23. Pearl AJ, ed. The athletic female. Champaign, IL: Human Kinetics Pubs, 1993.
24. Protzman RR, Bodnari LM. Women athletes. Am J Sports Med 1980;8:53–55.
25. Protzman R, Griffis C. Stress fractures in men and women undergoing military training. JBJS 1977;59A:825.
26. Good JE, Klein KM. Women in the military academies: US Navy (part 1 of 3). Phys Sportsmed 1989;17:99–106.
27. Cox JS, Lenz HW. Women midshipmen in sports. Am J Sports Med 1984 May–June;12(3):241–243.
28. Berg K. Aerobic function in female athletes. Clin Sports Med 1984;3:779–789.
29. Scordo KA. Effects of aerobic exercise training on symptomatic women with mitral valve prolapse. Am J Cardiol 1991; Apr 15;67(9):863–868.
30. Baechle TR. Women in resistance training. Clin Sports Med 1984;3:791–880.
31. Ireland ML, Wall C. Epidemiology and comparison of knee injuries in elite male and female United States basketball athletes. [Abstract] Med Sci Sports Exer 1990;22(2):582.
32. Ireland ML. Problems facing the athletic female. In: Pearl AJ ed. The athletic female. Champaign, IL: Human Kinetics Pubs 1993:11–18.
33. Zelisko JA, Noble HB, Porter M. A comparison of men's and women's professional basketball injuries. Am J Sports Med 1982;10:297–299.
34. Insall J. Disorders of the patella. In: Insall J, ed. Surgery of the knee. New York: Churchill Livingstone 1984:191–260.
35. Insall J, Falvo KA, Wise PW. Chondromalacia patella. JBJS 1976;58:1–8.
36. Aglietti P, et al. A new pattellar prosthesis. Clin Orthop 1975;179:175–187.
37. Colosimo AJ, Ireland ML: Isokinetic peak torque and knee joint laxity comparison in female basketball and volleyball college athletes. [Abstract] Med Sci Sports Exer 1991;23(suppl 4): S135.
38. Souryal TO, Moore HA, Evans JP: Bilaterality in anterior cruciate ligament injuries. Am J of Sports Med 1988;16(5):449–454.
39. Micheli LJ, Sohn RS, Solomon R: Stress fractures of the second metatarsal involving Lisfranc's joint in ballet dancers. JBJS 1985:67A:1372–1375.
40. Protera C. Women in sports: the price of participation. Phys Sportsmed 1986;14:149–153.
41. Richardson A, Jobe F, Collins SH. The shoulder in competitive swimming. Am J Sports Med 1980;8(3):159–163.
42. Snook G. Injuries in women's gymnastics: a five year study. Am J Sports Med 1979;7(4):242–244.
43. Barrow GW, Saha S. Menstrual irregularity and stress fractures in collegiate female runners. Am J Sports Med 1988;16(3):209–216.
44. Lloyd T, Buchanan JR, Bitzer S, Waldman CJ, Myers C, Ford BG. Interrelationships of diet, athletic activity, menstrual status, and bone density in collegiate women. Am J Clin Nutr 1987 Oct;46(4):681–684.
45. Sullivan D, Warren RF, Pavlov H, et al. Stress fractures in 51 runners. Clin Orthop 1984 Jul;187:188–192.
46. Hershman EB, Mailly T. Stress fractures. Clin in Sports Med 1990 Jan;9(1):183–214.
47. Matheson GO, Clement DB, McKenzie DC, et al. Stress fractures in athletes: a study of 320 cases. Am J Sports Med 1987 Jan–Feb;15(1):43–58.
48. Lloyd T. Diet and menstrual status as determinants of injury risk for the athletic female. In: Pearl AJ, ed. The athletic female. Champaign, IL: Human Kinetics Pubs, 1993: 61–80.
49. Frusztajer N, Dhuper S, Warren M, et al. Nutrition and the incidence of stress fractures in ballet dancers. Am J Clin Nutr 1990;51:779–783.
50. Lutter JM. Health concerns of women runners. Clin in Sports Med 1985;4:671–683.
51. Shangold MM. Gynecologic concerns in the woman athlete. Clin in Sports Med 1984;3(4):869–878.
52. Holden DL, Jackson DW. Stress fracture of the ribs in female rowers. Am J Sports Med 1985 Sep–Oct;13(5):342–348.
53. Roy S, Caine D, Singer KM. Stress changes of the distal epiphysis in young gymnasts. A report of twenty-one cases and a review of the literature. Am J Sports Med 1985 Sep–Oct;13(5):301–308.
54. Blank S. Transverse tibial stress fractures: a special problem. Am J Sports Med 1987 Nov–Dec;15(6):597–602.
55. Ireland ML, Micheli LJ. Bilateral stress fractures of the lumbar pedicles in a ballet dancer: a case report. J Bone Joint Surg 1987;69-A(1):140–142.
56. Stark JA, Toulouse A. The young female athlete: psychological considerations. Clin Sports Med 1984;3:909–921.
57. Corbin CB. Self-confidence of females in sports and physical activity. Clin Sports Med 1984:3:895–908.
58. Morgan BLO. Nutritional needs of the female adolescent. Healthcare of the Female Adolescent. New York: Haworth Press, 1984:15–28.
59. Grandjean RD. Nutritional concerns for the woman athlete. Clin Sports Med 1984;3(4)923–938.
60. Nowak RK, Knudsen KS, Schulz LO: body composition and nutrient intakes of college men and women basketball players. J Am Diet Assoc. 1988;88(5):575–578.
61. Kleiner SM, Bazzarre TL, Litchford MD. Metabolic profiles, diet, and health practices of championship male and female bodybuilders. J Am Diet Assoc 1990;(7):962–967.
62. Keith RE, Okeeffe KA, Alt LA, et al. Dietary status of trained female cyclists. J Am Diet Assoc 1989;(11):1620–1623.
63. Clark N. Nutritional problems and training intensity, activity level, and athletic performance. In: Pearl AJ, ed. The athletic female. Champaign, IL: Human Kinetics Pubs, 1993;165–168.
64. Myburgh KH, Hutchins J, Fataar AB, et al. Low bone density is

an etiologic factor for stress fractures in atheletes. Ann Intern Med 1990 Nov 15;113(10):754–759.
65. Clark N. Sports Nutrition Handbook. Champaign, IL: Leisure Press, 1990:135–148.
66. Berning Jr, Steen SN. Sports Nutrition for the 90's. Gaithersburg, MD: Aspen, 1991.
67. Faber M, Spinnler-Benade AJ, Daubitzer A. Dietary intake, anthropometric measurements and plasma lipid levels in throwing field athletes. Int J Sports Med 1990;11(2):140–145.
68. Smith NJ. Weight control in the athlete. Clin Sports Med 1984 Jul;3(3):693–704.
69. Bernadot D, ed. Sports Nutrition: A guide for the professional working with active people, 2nd ed. Chicago: Sports and Cardiovascular Nutrition Practice Group of the American Dietetic Association, 1993.
70. Hoffman CJ, Coleman E. An eating plan and update on recommended dietary practices for the endurance athlete. J Am Diet Assoc 1991;(3):325–330.
71. Risser WL, Lee EJ, Poindexter HB et al. Iron deficiency in females: its prevalence and impact on performance. Med Sci Sports Exerc 1988 Apr;20(2):116–121.
72. Rowland TW. Iron deficiency in young endurance athlete. In: Advances in Pediatric Sports Sciences. Champaign, IL: Human Kinetics Pubs, 1989:169–190.
73. Rowland TW. Iron deficiency in the athlete. Pediatr Clin North Am 1990;37(15):1153–1163.
74. Eisenman PA, Johnson SC, Benson JE. Coaches guide to nutrition and weight control. Champaign, IL: Leisure Press, 1990.
75. Clark N. Eating disorders among female athletes. In: Pearl AJ, ed. The athletic female; Champaign, IL: Human Kinetics Pubs, 1993:141–148.
76. American Psychiatric Association. Diagnostic and Statistical Manual of Mental Disorders. 3rd ed. Washington, D.C.: American Psychiatric Assoc., 1987.
77. Hale RW. Exercise, sports, and menstrual dysfunction. Clin Obstet Gynecol 1983 Sep;26(3):728–735.
78. Dalsky GP. The role of exercise in the prevention of osteoporosis. Compr Ther 1989;15(9):30–37.
79. Jacobson PC, Beaver W, Grubb SA, et al. Bone density in amenorrheic women: college athletes and older athletic women. J Orthop Res 1984;2(4):328–332.
80. Jones KP, Ravnikar VA, Tulchinsky D, et al. Comparison of bone density in amenorrheic women due to athletics, weight loss, and premature menopause. Obstet Gynecol 1985 Jul;66(1): 5–8.
81. Linnell SL, Stager JM, Blue PW, et al. Bone mineral content and menstrual regularity in female runners. Med Sci Sports Exerc 1984 Aug;16(4):343–348.
82. Rikli RE, McManis BG. Effects of exercise on bone mineral content in postmenopausal women. Res Q Exerc Sport 1990 Sep;61(3):243–249.
83. Frisch RE, McArthur JW. Menstrual cycles: fatness as a determinant of minimum weight for height necessary for their maintenance or onset. Science 1974;185:949–951.
84. Frisch RE, Gotz-Welbergen AV, McArthur JW et al. Delayed menarche and amenorrhea of college athletes in relation to age of onset of training. JAMA 1981 Oct 2;246(14):1559–63.
85. Stager JM, Wigglesworth JK, Hatler LK. Interpreting the relationship between age of menarche and prepubertal training. Med Sci Sports Exerc 1990 Feb;22(1):54–58.
86. Halfon ST, Bronner S. Determinants of physical ability in 7th grade school children. Eur J Epidemiol 1989 Mar;5(1):90–96.
87. Haymes EM. Environmental factors as they affect women. In: Hale RW, ed. Caring for the exercising woman. New York: Elsevier, 1991:37–45.
88. Noakes TD, Vanlend M. Menstrual dysfunction in female athletes. S Afr Med J 1988;73:350–355.
89. Myerson M, Gutin B, Warren MP, et al. Resting metabolic rate and energy balance in amenorrheic and eumenorrheic runners. Med Sci Sports Exerc 1991;23(1):15–22.
90. Shade AR. Gynecologic and obstetric problems of the female dancer. Clin Sports Med 1983;2(3):515–523.
91. Drinkwater BL, Bruemner B, Chesnut CH 3d. Menstrual history as a determinant of current bone density in young athletes. JAMA 1990 Jan 26;263(4):545–548.
92. Gadpaille WJ, Sanborn CF, Wagner WW Jr. Athletic amenorrhea, major affective disorders, and eating disorders. Am J Psychiatry 1987 Jul;144(7):939–942.
93. Mansfield MJ, Emans SJ. Anorexia nervosa, athletics, and amenorrhea. Pediatr Clin North Am 1989 Jun;36(3):533–549.
94. Baker E, Demers L. Menstrual status in female athletes: correlation with reproductive hormones and bone density. Obstet-Gynecol 1988 Nov;72(5):683–687.
95. Cook SD, Harding AF, Thomas KA et al. Trabecular bone density and menstrual function in women runners. Am J Sports Med 1987 Sep–Oct;15(5):503–507.
96. Kulpa PJ. Oral Contraceptives and the athletic female. In: Pearl AJ, ed. The athletic female. Champaign, IL: Human Kinetics Pubs, 1993:103–112.
97. Rebar RW. Exercise and the menstrual cycle. In: Pearl AJ, ed. The athletic female. Champaign, IL: Human Kinetics Pubs; 1993:59–75.
98. Nicklas BJ, Hackney AC, Sharp RL. The menstrual cycle and exercise: performance, muscle glycogen, and substrate responses.
99. Shangold M, Rebar RW, Wentz AC, et al. Evaluation and management of menstrual dysfunction in athletes. JAMA 1990 Mar 23–30;263(12):1665–1669.
100. Shangold MM. Menstrual irregularity in athletes: basic principles, evaluation, and treatment. Can J Appl Sport Sci 1982 June;7(2):68–73.
101. Baker ER. Menstrual dysfunction and hormonal status in athletic woman: a review. Fertil Steril 1981 Dec;36(6):691–696.
102. Sanborn CF, Albracht BH, Wagner WW Jr. Athletic amenorrhea: lack of association with body fat. Med Sci Sports Exerc 1987 Jun;19(3):207–212.
103. Sinning WE, Little KD. Body composition and menstrual function in athletes. Sports Med 1987 Jan–Feb;4(1):34–35.
104. Carlbert KA, Buckman MT, Peake GT, et al. Body composition of oligo/amenorrheic athletes. Med Sci Sports Exerc 1983;15(3):215–217.
105. Malina RM, Spirduso WW, Tate C, et al. Age at menarche and selected menstrual characteristics in athletes at different competitive levels and in different sports. Med Sci Sprts Exer 1978 Fall;10(3):218–222.
106. Eston RG. The regular menstrual cycle and athletic performance. Sports Med 1984 Nov–Dec;1(6):431–445.
107. Schweiger U, Laessle R, Schweiger M, et al. Caloric intake, stress, and menstrual function in athletes. Fertil Steril 1988;49(3):447–450.
108. Highet R. Athletic amenorrhea. An update on aetiology, complications and management. Sports Med 1989 Feb;7(2):82–108.
109. Arendt EA. Osteoporosis in the athletic female: amenorrhea and amenorrheic osteoporosis. In: Pearl AJ, ed. The athletic female. Champaign, IL: Human Kinetics Pubs, 1993:41–59.
110. Jarski RW, Trippett DL. The risks and benefits of exercises during pregnancy. J Fam Pract 1990 Feb;30(2):185–189.
111. Sady SP, Carpenter MW. Aerobic exercise during pregnancy. Special considerations. Sports Med 1989 Jun;7(6):357–375.
112. Hall DC, Kaufmann DA. Effects of aerobic and strength conditioning on pregnancy outcomes. Am J Obstet Gynecol 1987 Nov;157(5):1199–1203.
113. Mullinax KM, Dale E. Some considerations of exercise during pregnancy. Clin Sports Med 1986 Jul;5(3):559–570.
114. ACOG Home Exercise Programs: Exercise during pregnancy and the postnatal period. Washington DC, American College of Obstetricians and Gynecologists, 1985.
115. White J. Exercising for two: what's safe for the active pregnant woman. Phys Sportsmed 1992;20(5):179–186.
116. Wolfe LA, Hall P, Webb KA, et al. Prescription of aerobic exercise during pregnancy Sports Med 1989;8(5):273–301.
117. Artal R. Exercise and fetal responses during pregnancy. In: Pearl AJ, ed. The athletic female. Champaign, IL: Human Kinetics Pubs, 1993:103–117.
118. Hindle WH. The breast and exercise. In: Hale RW. Caring for the exercising woman. New York: Elsevier, 1991:83–92.

SECTION TWO

SPORTS-SPECIFIC INJURIES

12 / BASEBALL

Christopher D. Harner, James P. Bradley, Patrick J. McMahon, and Mininder S. Kocher

Introduction

Baseball is considered America's national pastime and has recently developed a large international following. In 1981, there were 4.5 million amateur baseball players in the United States (1), but baseball skills also are required in softball, which is the largest team sport in the country, with 40 million league players (2). Players of all ages enjoy the sport, and 52% of the participants are under 12 years of age (1). Many youngsters begin playing at age 6 or 7 and dream of playing professional baseball as adults.

Baseball is a noncontact sport with minimal protective gear. Therefore, it is commonly considered a safe sport. In fact, the relative incidence of injury in baseball is last among common competitive sports with 1.6 injuries per 1000 practices/games (3). Because of the large number of participants, however, baseball ranks second only to football in total number of injuries and fatalities (4). In 1981, the U.S. Consumer Product Safety Commission estimated that more than 900,000 injuries occur annually in baseball and that 35% of these injuries require emergency room visits (5). From 1973 to 1981, there were 183 baseball-related fatalities nationwide, with 40% of the fatalities in the 5- to 14-year-old age group (6).

This chapter addresses baseball injuries as they occur during different aspects of the game: throwing, hitting, sliding, catching, and fielding. Particular attention is focused on the mechanism, diagnosis, and prevention of injuries. Special mention also is made of vascular compromise and head/neck injuries.

Throwing

Biomechanics of Throwing

Overhead throwing is an elaborate, synchronous progression of body movements that starts in the legs and trunk, involves the upper extremities, and concludes in the rapid propulsion of the ball. It is essential to remember that the throwing mechanism is a total body activity. Parameters that determine the effectiveness of a thrower include (*a*) velocity; (*b*) accuracy, (*c*) spin production, and (*d*) endurance. A high level of neuromuscular control is required to ensure that the above parameters are achieved. Synchrony of muscular contractions and neurologic control throughout the body are essential to produce an effective throwing motion. Effectiveness also necessitates repetitive performance at a level that maximally stresses the physiologic limits of the upper extremities' anatomic components. A delicate balance exists between mobility and stability of the joints of the upper extremities while throwing, and maintenance of this fragile balance is paramount. The intricate interactions between static restraints (bone, capsule, and labrum) and the dynamic restraints (muscle) permit the versatile motion, precise positioning, and tremendous force that are imperative in efficient throwing. Small aberrations in the mechanisms that control stability have a significant and cumulative effect on upper extremity function and increase the risk of crossing the fine line between maximal throwing effectiveness and injury.

Multiple investigators have studied the complex biomechanics of throwing (7–14). Although the mechanics of throwing seem to differ slightly between player positions, in essence, the motions are quite similar. The majority of throwing studies have concentrated on the pitcher, because *(a)* the motion is more constant, *(b)* the collection of photographic and electromyographic (EMG) data is easier, and *(c)* pitchers frequently injure their arms.

The baseball pitch is divided into five stages: stage I is the stance phase, stage II is the windup or preparation phase, stage III is the cocking phase, stage IV is the short propulsive phase of acceleration, and stage V is the follow-through/deceleration phase (Fig. 12.1).

From a virtual standstill, a professional pitcher will accelerate a 142-g baseball to a release velocity of more than 90 mph in just 50 msec. Tremendous tensile, com-

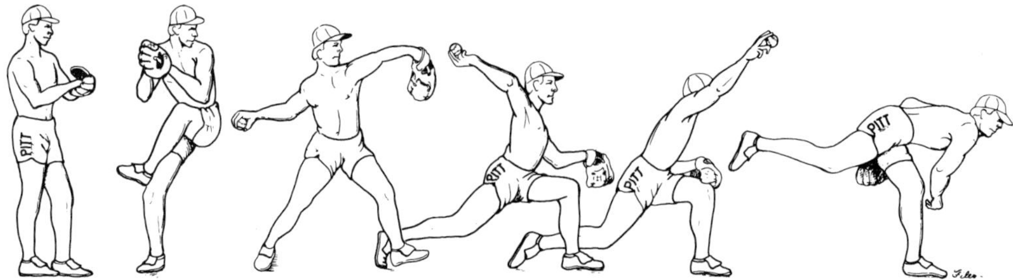

Figure 12.1. Phases of the baseball pitch. The baseball pitch is divided into five stages: stance, windup, cocking (early and late), acceleration, and follow-through.

pressive, and rotational forces must be created and dissipated in the upper extremities to achieve this action. Therefore, a detailed description of the throwing motion will help clarify how this force is generated, transmitted, and dissipated.

In the stance phase, the pitcher stands facing the batter with his or her shoulders parallel to the rubber. The pivot foot (right for right-handers) is positioned on the rubber.

In the windup phase, the body mechanics are quite individual. In general, windup begins with the stride foot (left for right-handers) coiling backward, away from home plate, and the arms swinging overhead. At this time, the position of the fingers on the ball is finalized while screened by the glove. The pivot foot rotates on the rubber as weight is transferred to it. This phase ends with the ball leaving the glove hand and the body balanced on the pivot foot. The EMG activity of the shoulder girdle and upper extremities is low during windup.

Cocking is divided into early and late stages. Early cocking starts with extension of the pivot leg, thus propelling the stride leg, nondominant upper extremity, and trunk forward. The gluteus maximus of the pivot leg is important in providing this propulsion. Temporarily, the dominant upper extremity lags behind the rest of the body. The upper trapezius upwardly rotates the scapula to place the glenoid in a stable position for the abducting humeral head. The deltoid and the supraspinatus concomitantly abduct the humeral head. The elbow is flexed by the brachioradialis. This phase is terminated as the stride foot contacts the ground. Early cocking pain is not typical in throwers, and aberrations in neuromuscular controls are seldom noted.

During late cocking, rapid forward motion of the trunk is noted (8). The dominant shoulder rotates forward. Inertia and gravity act on the arm in horizontal abduction, external rotation, and adduction; however, the arm does not move in the direction of these forces. Large torques are generated at the elbow and shoulder joints to overcome the inertial and gravitational forces. Static and dynamic restraints combine to stabilize both joints against these forces. In this position, the primary anterior stabilizer of the glenohumeral joint is the anterior inferior glenohumeral ligament (15). The pectoralis major and latissimus dorsi muscles appear to act as a dynamic sling to augment the inferior glenohumeral ligament (16). The scapulothoracic muscles protract and rotate the scapula upward to produce a stable platform for the humeral head, thus enhancing maximal humeral external rotation. During this phase, the elbow is experiencing considerable valgus stress that is localized to the medial stabilizers. Sometimes symptoms of anterior instability of the glenohumeral joint and medial instability of the elbow are demonstrated during this phase, secondary to an imbalance of the stabilizing mechanism (11).

The acceleration phase begins with maximal shoulder external rotation and terminates with ball release. The acceleration of the arm is coincident with the deceleration of the rest of the body, producing efficient transfer of energy to the arm and ball (8). A large glenohumeral joint compressive force (860 Nm), which has a stabilizing effect, is demonstrated during this phase. Synchronous muscular contraction about the glenohumeral joint balances the requirements of stabilization and rapid motion. The pectoralis major, latissimus dorsi, and subscapularis concentrically contract, propelling the humerus into rapid internal rotation. The humeral internal rotation torque is 14,000 inch-pounds with an angular velocity of 6100°/sec. (2, 8, 10). The pectoralis major and the latissimus dorsi are the primary propellers of the arm, whereas the subscapularis functions as a steering muscle to position the humeral head precisely in the glenoid. The internal rotation force is then transmitted to the forearm through the elbow. A large valgus stress is created at the elbow as the internal rotation force is transferred to the forearm and hand. Static stabilization at the elbow is absorbed by a tension force at the medial collateral ligament and a compressive force in the radiocapitellar joint. Dynamic stabilization is augmented by the wrist and finger flexors and pronator muscles that originate from the medial epicondyle. Elbow extension reaches a maximum angular velocity of 2200°/sec. (8, 10). Generally, athletes will note symptoms of elbow or shoulder dysfunction during this phase of throwing. Typical problems include *(a)* anterior subluxation of the shoulder, *(b)* medial ligamentous instability at the elbow, *(c)* ulnar neuritis pain, and *(d)* "catching" pain from posterior compartment pathology.

Follow-through is after ball release. The trunk and dominant lower extremity rotate forward. The shoulder continues to adduct and internally rotate to 30°, while the elbow terminates at about 50° of flexion and the forearm is pronated (8, 10). The remaining kinetic energy not transferred to the ball must be absorbed by the decelerating arm and body. Deceleration is estimated to be −500,000°/sec. at the elbow and shoulder, with an external rotation torque of approximately 15,000 inch-pounds at the humerus (8, 14). Deceleration of the arm is accomplished by simultaneous contraction of opposing muscles around the shoulder and elbow. Essential roles are played by the trapezius, serratus anterior, teres minor, latissimus dorsi, supinators, and extensors of the wrist and fingers. Posterior compartment elbow pathology and injury to the posterior glenohumeral joint stabilizers will commonly become apparent during this phase.

In summary, the throwing motion requires the rapid transmission of large amounts of kinetic energy through the upper extremities. The resultant kinetic energy in the throwing arm has been estimated to be 27,000 inch-pounds, which is four times the energy in the leg during a soccer kick (8). This produces huge torques in the musculoskeletal components involved, putting them at great risk for injury.

Proper Pitching Technique

The best way for a thrower to avoid injury is through conditioning techniques, proper body mechanics, and a vigorous warmup. McConnell (17) stressed the importance of proper pitching technique:

> It is possible to perfect baseball skills and at the same time avoid injury. . . . Very seldom do we hear of a player who executes a play properly, being injured. The man who knows how to throw, and uses this knowledge in throwing, doesn't pull a muscle in his arm.

The lessons learned from professional pitchers can be applied to all players on the team. John Sain, an ex-Major League pitcher and a pitching coach for the Atlanta Braves organization, believes that the most important lesson about proper body mechanics is throwing the ball in a natural way (18). This applies to all players, whether the ball is thrown from the outfield or the mound. When an outfielder throws the ball, he or she first takes a step backward and then lands on the opposite forefoot with the knee slightly flexed. A pitcher should do the same. When a pitcher overthrows to get more speed on the fastball, he or she tends to hyperextend the knee and land on the heel. This places sudden, large forces on the shoulder during the cocking phase of throwing. Also, all motions should be in the direction that the pitcher is throwing. This is most easily accomplished by planting the stride foot in the direction of the pitch.

When throwing in a natural fashion, the forearm is supinated during the cocking phase. With a smooth follow-through, the forearm moves from supination to pronation easily as the elbow extends. With deceleration of the upper extremity, the forearm should be in pronation.

The arm should be kept in shape throughout the year; however, many pitchers thrown their first ball of the year just before the season begins. Sain has an excellent year-round conditioning program. During each week of the off-season, professional pitchers throw for 5 days at half speed and then take 2 days of complete rest. The number of pitches should not exceed 120 per day. During the season, in a 4-day rotation, the workout as shown in Table 12.1 is recommended. These same principles apply to Little League throwers.

An off-season weight-training program should be built around light weights to build endurance, especially in the rotator cuff musculature. Both the anterior and posterior shoulder muscles should be included. Most people tend to forget the posterior shoulder muscles when weight training. Furthermore, strength in the legs and trunk are important for proper body mechanics. Emphasis also should be placed on flexibility.

Adequate warmup is essential to prevent injury. A total body warmup should be followed by general body stretching, including the legs, trunk, and upper extremities. Always warmup to pitch, do not pitch to warmup.

Finally, many people believe that side-arm pitchers place less stress on their shoulders. This is probably not true. Shoulder abduction is about the same for the over-the-top and the side-arm pitcher. Side-arm pitchers simply bend their trunks and extend their elbows more.

Shoulder Injuries

Injuries to the shoulder account for the majority of injuries to adult baseball players (19). Most of these injuries occur during the throwing motion. A professional baseball pitcher may play 30 to 40 games in a season. He or she may throw as many as 200 pitches in a game, many of these at high velocity (20). Although amateur pitchers may not play as many games in a season, they still try to throw the ball as fast as possible while maintaining accuracy. It is not surprising that shoulder pain is a frequent complaint among baseball pitchers.

Clinical assessment of shoulder injuries in athletes should not focus attention on the shoulder joint too quickly, because other disease processes may be overlooked. One must always be aware of other potential causes of shoulder pain when obtaining a history and physical exam from an injured player. Systemic phenomena, such as rheumatoid arthritis and calcium pyrophosphate crystalline disease, can result in shoulder pain. Pain also can be referred to the shoulder from the

Table 12.1.
Pitcher's In-Season Pitching Program

Day 1	Pitcher performs in the game
Day 2	Pitcher rests except for light exercises and gentle throwing
Day 3	Pitcher should toss the ball lightly 40 feet at half speed
Day 4	Pitcher throws from the mound to remove all stiffness and soreness; he or she should not throw for more than 15 min. The pitcher also exercises his or her entire body in anticipation of performing in the game the following day.

Modified from McConnell ME. How to play Little League baseball. New York, Ronald, 1960.

hand (e.g., carpal tunnel syndrome), neck (e.g., radicular symptoms), or chest (e.g., angina).

The history should be meticulous, including the patient's age, sex, and chief complaint. Loss of velocity, accuracy, and distance usually alert the thrower to injury more serious than usual aches and pains. The impact of the injury on the patient's activities of daily living may provide as many clues to the diagnosis as the impact of the injury on sports performance. A relevant review of systems and family history can aid in diagnosis of systemic diseases. Pain is a subjective symptom but careful assessment can provide insight into disease pathology. The duration, anatomic location, and character of the pain should be specifically assessed. In addition, the presence of night pain and analgesic requirements should be considered. The temporal relationship to sports activity and the postural relationship to arm motion should be obtained from the patient with shoulder pain. For example, a pitcher who complains of anterior shoulder pain during the cocking phase of the throwing motion usually has anterior shoulder instability and possibly impingement. The pitcher who has pain during the follow-through phase may have posterior shoulder instability. The onset of night pain, especially when lying on the affected side, may indicate a rotator cuff tear. Pain with overhead activities is indicative of impingement syndrome.

The physical exam of the shoulder consists of several phases: visual inspection; palpation; range-of-motion testing; neurologic appraisal; vascular assessment; and general physical evaluation. Visual inspection includes examining the skin and the contour of the entire shoulder girdle. Special attention should be given to areas of swelling or muscle atrophy. Side-to-side differences should be recorded with knowledge that there are some normal changes that occur in the throwing arm. For example, the musculature is usually hypertrophied and the scapula is often displaced slightly inferiorly in the throwing arm. Palpation should be performed from the neck to the fingers on all sides of the upper extremities. MRI, CT scans, and other diagnostic tests are used only to reinforce the physical findings. The differential diagnosis of shoulder pain in the throwing athlete is shown in Table 12.2.

Table 12.2.
Differential Diagnosis of Shoulder Pain in the Throwing Athlete

- I. Neck injury
- II. Acromioclavicular joint
- III. Glenohumeral joint
  - A. Instability
    - 1. Anterior
    - 2. Posterior
    - 3. Multidirectional
  - B. Degenerative joint disease
- IV. Rotator cuff
  - A. Edema and hemorrhage
  - B. Inflammation and fibrosis
  - C. Tears
- V. Biceps
  - A. Tendinitis
  - B. Subluxation
  - C. SLAP lesions
- VI. Humeral fracture
  - A. Microfracture (stress)
  - B. Macrofracture
- VII. Neurovascular entrapment
  - A. Suprascapular nerve
  - B. Thoracic outlet syndrome

Adult Shoulder Injuries

Neurologic Injury. Degenerative joint disease of the cervical spine can be confused with shoulder pathology. Many of these patients initially complain of shoulder pain, but neck pain is usually present on careful questioning. Physical exam supplemented with cervical spine x-rays enables one to localize the pathology correctly.

Thoracic outlet syndrome (TOS) refers to the compression of the nerves and vessels of the upper extremities as they pass under the clavicle and between the scalene muscles over the first rib (21–24). Symptoms are usually vague, making the diagnosis difficult. Typically, there is a long period of time from the onset of symptoms until the diagnosis is made. There is usually a history of paresthesia and pain that radiates down the lateral side of the neck, then moves into the shoulder and the medial side of the arm, and finally continues into the ring and little fingers. Physical findings are usually subtle. Although it is not specific for TOS, Adson's test is positive if there is a diminution of the radial pulse when the arm is abducted, the head is rotated toward the involved side, and a deep breath is held. TOS also is suggested if the patient experiences numbness and tingling when the hands are rapidly opened and closed with the upper extremities elevated. TOS is discussed in greater detail with other vascular injuries, later in this chapter.

Chronic neurologic injuries of the shoulder can present in baseball players of all ages. The neurologic exam should include complete sensory evaluation, testing of reflex arcs, observation for atrophy, and strength testing. The sympathetic system also should be tested for signs of reflex sympathetic dystrophy. Commonly, the throwing athlete has a long history of achy shoulder pain during the cocking phase. The suprascapular nerve originates from the superior trunk of the brachial plexus to innervate the supraspinatus and infraspinatus muscles. Along its path, there are two areas of the scapula where it can be tethered and compressed: the suprascapular notch and the neck of the spine (spinoglenoid notch) (25). Compression results in pain and weakness. Symptoms may preclude pitching more than one or two innings. In the chronic situation, the correct diagnosis can be elusive, because the disease has an insidious onset and vague symptoms. Muscle pain and diminished endurance are the important presenting symptoms. There is weakness of external rotation and sometimes of abduction, depending on the location of the compression. Ringel et al. (25) have shown that either the infraspinatus is involved alone or both muscles are involved. This depends on the location of the compression, which is demonstrated on physical exam by muscle atrophy in most cases. The trapezius overlies the supraspinatus muscle, but atrophy of this muscle can be appreciated as a depression over the supraspinatus fossa of the shoulder. Atrophy of the infraspinatus is easy to appreciate as a depression over the lower half of the scapula. Electromyography can be used to confirm the diagnosis. Suprascapular nerve palsy can be confused with rotator cuff tears, which present with pain in a similar area and weakness of the same musculature. Surgical exploration and decompression of the nerve generally gives good results when the nerve is compressed at the suprascapular notch. In this case the supraspinatus and infraspinatus muscles are both involved. However, if atrophy and EMG changes are confined to the infraspinatus muscle, the nerve is compressed at the spinoglenoid notch. In this situation, nonsurgical treatment is recommended, because surgical decompression is much more difficult and has not always been successful. The effects of chronic compression may not be reversible in either case. Thus this condition requires a meticulous history and physical exam for proper diagnosis early in the disease course.

Injury to the spinal accessory nerve results in trapezius muscle atrophy with symptoms of pain and weakness during shoulder abduction. Winging of the scapula, caused by long thoracic nerve palsy, is demonstrated by pushing against a wall with the arms outstretched. Range of motion and strength testing are important in making a correct diagnosis. A herniated nucleus pulposis (slipped disc) can cause nerve root compression in the neck with pain radiating down the arm in the distribution of the affected nerve. Strength and reflex testing are important to determine the severity of the functional impairment and the location of injury.

Persistent valgus stress to the medial side of the elbow, induced by throwing, may incite inflammation of the ulnar nerve in the cubital tunnel. During flexion, the ulnar nerve elongates an average of 4.7 mm and can translate over 7 mm medially because of the medial head of the triceps (26). The presenting clinical symptom is pain about the medial elbow, occasionally radiating distally along the ulnar aspect of the forearm into the hand. Numbness and tingling of the ring and little fingers is sometimes present. Additional symptoms include clumsiness, heaviness, and problems with grasp, especially after throwing. One must be aware of possible concomitant medial elbow instability when a throwing athlete complains of cubital tunnel symptoms.

Examination elicits tenderness over the cubital tunnel and the tunnel may feel thick and "doughy." Tinel's sign may be localized to the cubital tunnel. Neurologic abnormalities in the distribution of the ulnar nerve include hypoesthesia, interosseous wasting, and dry skin. Ulnar neuritis, in which the symptoms are mild and intrinsic atrophy is absent, usually responds well to conservative treatment. Rest and ice along with splint immobilization for 2 to 3 weeks have been helpful in reducing acute symptoms. Steroid injections into the cubital tunnel is not recommended, and surgical intervention is usually not required. Surgical decompression may be indicated in chronic relapsing cases or when intrinsic atrophy and weakness are present.

Acromioclavicular Joint. Acromioclavicular (AC) problems commonly begin with an acute injury, such as shoulder separation. In fact, follow-up of AC joint sprains reveals a significant number of residual symptoms with second-degree sprains probably resulting in the highest incidence (65%) (27). Regardless of the severity, most athletes with a shoulder separation can return to their sport in a few weeks. However, some athletes develop degenerative joint disease (DJD) of the AC joint. The diagnosis is made by careful palpation of the AC joint for tenderness and crepitus. The area of the AC joint will be painful with motion, especially horizontal adduction, which loads the clavicle. Acromioclavicular joint DJD can mimic other shoulder problems such as impingement syndrome. Initial treatment should include antiinflammatory medications and steroid injection. If this fails, distal resection of the clavicle yields good results. Arthroscopic resection also is a well-accepted approach, with results similar to the open procedure. Baseball players treated with distal clavicle resection have returned to competition with no loss of function, strength, or motion (28).

Impingement. The most common injuries that occur in the shoulder from throwing result from the constant irritation of anterior shoulder structures (1). Impingement is defined as compromise of the space between the coracoacromial arch and the proximal humerus. The coracoacromial arch includes the coracoid, the coracoacromial ligament, the acromioclavicular joint, the acromion, and the subacromial bursa. These structures make up the roof over the anterior glenohumeral joint. The supraspinatus tendon and the tendon of the long head of the biceps brachii are the most commonly compressed structures. When the humerus is flexed and internally rotated, the insertion of the supraspinatus tendon is brought under the coracoacromial arch and constant irritation can ensue. This is especially true when the space between the acromion and the humerus is further compromised by anterior acromial osteophytes. The athlete initially complains of pain in the anterior shoulder during the acceleration phase or sometimes during the follow-through phase. Initially, the pain resolves after a short period of rest. However, the condition relentlessly progresses if the offending activity is not stopped. With time, the pain becomes more intense, especially with forward flexion and internal rotation (impingement sign). Physical exam reveals tenderness with palpation of the anterior acromion and a positive impingement sign and test. Neer (29) divided impingement syndrome into three stages as described in Chapter 31. The symptoms are reversible during the early stages with rest, nonsteroidal antiinflammatory drugs (NSAIDs), and rotator cuff strengthening exercises done with the arm at the side. Because the insertion of the supraspinatus and biceps tendons lie anterior to the coracoacromial arch with the shoulder in a neutral position, any activities that require forward flexion should be restricted until symptoms resolve. In the majority of cases, stage I impingement resolves within 2 to 4 weeks. Stage II impingement persists longer and may take 3 months to improve. Often stage II and III impingement require surgical intervention. Classic teaching is that the patient needs to have 3 to 6 months of nonoperative treatment before any recommendation for surgery. This is not always realistic and must be modified based on the throwing athlete's skill level and demands in addition to the surgeon's comfort with impingement procedures. Current techniques of arthroscopic subacromial decompression and distal clavicle resection minimize the athlete's down time (4 to 6 weeks).

Rotator Cuff Disease. Rotator cuff disease has extrinsic and intrinsic etiologies (30). The extrinsic causes are forces acting outside the rotator cuff that cause injury to the tendons. Impingement syndrome, which Neer (31) implicated in 95% of rotator cuff tears, is an example of extrinsic rotator cuff disease. Extrinsic causes of rotator cuff disease also include instability of the glenohumeral joint. Jobe et al. (32) have shown that muscle activity becomes abnormal about the shoulder as it begins to sublux. In an attempt to stabilize the shoulder girdle, the scapula becomes fixed; the rotator cuff muscles attempt to substitute for the lost scapulothoracic motion; and muscle overuse and fatigue occur. If this condition persists, spasm and pain result. Muscle fatigue leads to abnormal shoulder kinematics and contributes to instability. A downward spiral then ensues. Eventually, instability results in the humeral head impinging on the coracoacromial arch. This situation is different from that of pure impingement, and a careful evaluation for shoulder instability is required. These patients occasionally report that the shoulder feels as though it were moving anteriorly. However, anterior shoulder pain is usually the only complaint. Careful physical examination reveals the subtle anterior instability. CT arthrogram may show an avulsion of the anterior-inferior labrum from the glenoid (Bankart lesion). Along with demonstrating the Bankart lesion, arthroscopy can show anterior labral fraying (the only lesion in some cases). Small posterior-lateral humeral head compression fracture (Hill-Sachs lesion) also may be present. Conservative treatment results in improvement of the symptoms in most cases. Because impingement is present, all exercises must be done with the affected upper extremity at the side as described below. Both the rotator cuff and the scapular rotator muscles are weak and must be strengthened. In this group of patients, an anterior acromioplasty only makes the instability worse. Surgery to reconstruct the anterior labrum and capsule may be required if physical therapy fails.

Intrinsic causes of rotator cuff disease include traction injuries and primary cuff degeneration not related to impingement syndrome. There is a critical zone of hypovascularity at the insertion of the supraspinatus tendon (33, 34). The majority of rotator cuff pathology occurs in this area. Uhthoff et al. (35) showed that most tears of the rotator cuff begin on the articular side of the tendon, which supports a role for intrinsic etiologies of rotator cuff disease. Nirschl (36) wrote of angiofibroblastic changes occurring in the tendon with secondary development of rotator cuff calcification, erosion, and impingement. Undoubtedly both extrinsic and intrinsic factors play a role in rotator cuff pathology.

Motion of all four joints (sternoclavicular, acromioclavicular, scapulothoracic, and glenohumeral) is essential to normal shoulder kinematics. This can be assessed both actively and passively. Differences between active and passive motion can be the result of neuromuscular deficiency such as a rotator cuff tear. Motion should always be compared with the contralateral shoulder. Brown et al. (37) found that Major League pitchers have different ranges of motion between the shoulders. In the pitching arm, with the shoulder in abduction, there is 11° less extension, 15° less internal rotation, and 9° more external rotation. Therefore, comparison with the contralateral arm should be done with this variance in mind.

Throwing a baseball subjects the rotator cuff to many insults (impingement, traction, and contusion), which can result in failure of the tendon fibers. Repeated, small episodes of partial rotator cuff tearing can occur. The incidence of partial rotator cuff tears rises with age. In a series of 233 patients with rotator cuff tears, Neer et al. (38) found 97% to occur in individuals over the age of 40 years. These patients commonly present with a long history of intermittent shoulder tendonitis that likely represents tendon fiber failure. Most full-thickness rotator cuff tears occur in a tendon that is already weakened by earlier pathology. Eventually, the patient experiences increasing shoulder pain that may wake him or her up at night, especially when sleeping on the affected shoulder. Elevation of the arm in the scapular plane against resistance becomes increasingly difficult, partly because of the tear and partly because of disuse atrophy. Samuilson and Binder (39) found the most common symptoms of complete rotator cuff tears to be pain, weakness in shoulder elevation, and subacromial crepitus. Partial rotator cuff tears are characterized by less severe symptoms. Nonoperative treatment of rotator cuff tears includes rotator cuff–strengthening exercises done with the arm at the side, NSAIDs, avoidance of precipitating activities, and steroid injections. Surgical repair in competitive athletes has had disappointing results. In a recent study, only 56% of patients were able to return to their former competitive level after surgical repair. Only 32% of the throwers were able to return to collegiate or professional sports at the same level (40).

Proper rehabilitation of the rotator cuff is essential for a full recovery from shoulder injury. All internal and external rotation exercises must be done with the arm at the side to eliminate pain from impingement. To strengthen the external rotators, the patient is instructed to lie on the side of the uninvolved shoulder with a small weight held in the hand as shown in Figure 12.2*A*. The shoulder is externally rotated, and the patient is then instructed to lie supine and a small weight is held in the hand as the patient internally rotates the shoulder (see Fig. 12.2*B*). These exercises also can be easily performed with elastic bands that have a progressive resistance to elongation. The scapular stabilizers can best be strengthened with a variation of the standard push-up. At the top of the exercise, the body is pushed as far from the floor as possible. This acts to protract the scapula, strengthening the stabilizers. Stretching exercises also should be done. These exercises should be supervised to ensure that the patient stretches only those muscle groups that are tight and does not place the shoulder in positions that may aggravate the pathology.

Anterior Instability. Dislocation of the shoulder joint usually occurs secondary to a single traumatic event. Subluxation is incomplete dislocation of the joint, in other words, contact between the joint surfaces remains. Subluxation is much more common in the throwing athlete secondary to chronic overuse. Anterior instability is discussed in more detail in Chapter 51.

Posterior Instability. Posterior shoulder instability is often unrecognized in throwing athletes. Pure dislocation of the joint is rare, but subluxation is not. There are two different mechanisms that can result in posterior instability. In the first situation, improper pitching technique causes repetitive microtrauma to the posterior capsule. The follow-through phase of the throwing motion is characterized by intense contraction of the shoulder muscles to decelerate the upper extremity. At this time, the shoulder is in the vulnerable position of flexion, adduction, and internal rotation. This creates high stresses in the posterior capsule. Repeated microtrauma, resulting from poor pitching technique, causes posterior capsule weakness and eventual humeral head subluxation. In the second situation, a single traumatic event initiates the instability. For example, a player falls on the outstretched throwing arm and has immediate posterior shoulder pain. After the pain subsides, throwing velocity and endurance decrease. This is accompanied by pain during the follow-through. Through either mechanism, the posterior capsule can become attenuated. Complete tears of the capsule from the glenoid, which commonly occur anteriorly, are less common posteriorly.

Patients with posterior shoulder instability complain of pain in the posterior shoulder, sometimes radiating along the scapula. However, anterior shoulder pain is not unheard of in these patients. A careful physical exam demonstrates the true pathology. Usually, the patient has pain with forward flexion, adduction, and internal rotation, and it may be possible to sublux the shoulder posteriorly in this position. The best way to feel the subluxation is to place the patient on the examination table in a supine position. The examiner puts his or her hand over the humeral head and positions the shoulder as described above. A posteriorly directed force applied to the humeral head, results in a palpable instability. During examination for glenohumeral instability, the examiner must always be aware of the patient's generalized ligamentous laxity. This is especially critical in the adolescent athlete (41). Radiographic examination may reveal a posterior glenoid spur (42). However, this lesion is extracapsular (19) and of questionable significance.

Some athletes can voluntarily sublux their shoulder. These patients have reached the last stage in the spectrum of instability patterns and do not have an associated psychological component. They should be treated like any other patient with posterior instability. This is in contrast to the patient with voluntary shoulder dislocation and drug-seeking behavior.

Rehabilitation results in symptomatic improvement in two-thirds of the cases (32). The external rotators as well as the posterior deltoid should be strengthened. This exercise program should be well-supervised and last for 6 months. Throwing technique also should be examined to eliminate any activity that may be placing additional stress on the posterior capsule.

Glenohumeral Degenerative Joint Disease. Osteoarthritis of the glenohumeral joint is rare in the

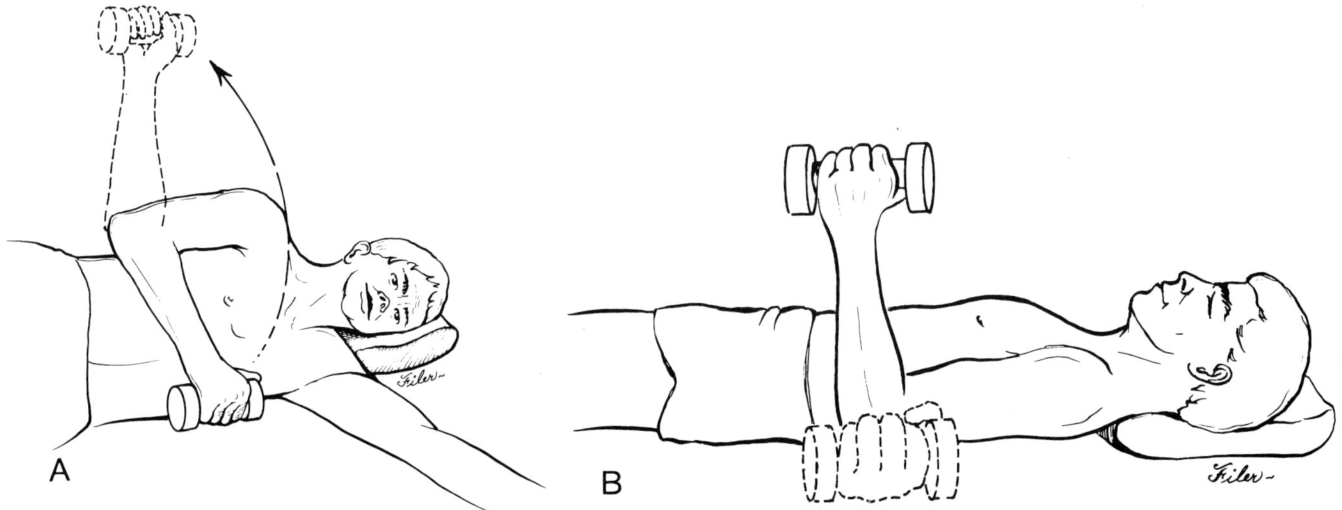

Figure 12.2. Rotator cuff strengthening exercises. **A,** External rotators. **B,** Internal rotators.

throwing athlete. Radiographic findings include joint space narrowing, subchondral sclerosis, peripheral osteophytes, and cystic changes. Inciting factors in young individuals include trauma and avascular necrosis of the humeral head.

Biceps Injury. The biceps tendon is difficult to palpate. Examination is performed by slowly internally and externally rotating the shoulder, feeling for the intertubercular groove of the humerus. Numerous stress tests have been described. All involve forced supination of the forearm trying to elicit pain in the bicipital groove.

Biceps tendon subluxation can be a source of anterior shoulder pain. O'Donoghue (44) described differences in the bicipital groove that can lead to subluxation. A shallow groove was more prone to subluxation with the internal and external rotation that occurs during the throwing mechanism. Tears of the superior glenoid labrum at the insertion of the biceps tendon are termed superior labral anterior to posterior (SLAP) lesions. First described in 1990 by Snyder et al. (45), SLAP lesions have recently received considerable attention. Snyder believed the lesion occurred after a fall on the outstretched arm when the shoulder was forward flexed and abducted. An injury also can occur from an eccentric muscle load on the biceps tendon during a single traumatic event or after repetitive microtrauma such as occurs during the follow-through phase of throwing.

In the authors' laboratory, it has been shown that the biceps tendon can stabilize the glenohumeral joint in a simulated dynamic shoulder model (46). When superior labral lesion was created, the stabilizing effect of the biceps tendon during the late cocking phase of throwing was eliminated in the model. EMG studies in pitchers with unstable shoulders show increased activity in the biceps muscle during this same phase of the throwing motion. This implies the biceps muscle plays a role in stabilizing the glenohumeral joint in the thrower with anterior instability.

Clinically, complaints include achy shoulder pain after a short period of throwing, and occasionally "popping" or "catching" in the shoulder joint. No imaging studies accurately define the SLAP lesion. Arthroscopic debridement has yielded encouraging results after short-term follow-up (45).

Microfracture/Macrofracture. The humerus is subject to enormous forces during the throwing mechanism. Several authors have found that the torques on the humerus during throwing are larger than the torque required to fracture the humerus (8, 47). Axial compressive forces on the humerus from muscular contraction are thought to be protective in preventing fracture. Although rare, these forces can result in stress fractures (47) or overt fractures (48). When an athlete complains of midupper arm pain, the physician is obligated to rule out a stress fracture. The authors have seen two cases of humeral fracture preceded by upper arm pain. These pitchers had minimally displaced spiral fractures that healed well with closed treatment. Rarely is open reduction and internal fixation indicated.

Pediatric Shoulder Injuries

Micheli (49) has noted several risk factors that predispose the pediatric athlete to injury. These include training errors, anatomic malalignment, repeated trauma to growing cartilage, and associated disease states.

Little League shoulder was first described by Dotter (50). This entity, further characterized by Adams (51), consists of pain in the shoulder occurring at the end of a hard throw. The onset can be insidious or acute and usually does not immediately stop the pitcher from throwing. Radiographs typically show uniform widening of the proximal humeral epiphysis compared with the contralateral shoulder. There is no evidence of displacement although Cahill et al. (52) feel that the repeated trauma of pitching results in disruption of the epiphyseal plate, thus causing fracture. They suggest that stress fractures result either from the large torque generated in the cocking and acceleration phases of throwing, or from the distraction force generated during acceleration. Other etiologies also have been proposed (51, 53). In all cases, the condition is self-limiting with the pain relieved by rest.

A young pitcher who complains of shoulder or upper-arm pain should be examined for other pathology as well. In this age group, musculoskeletal tumors are most commonly benign. A simple bone cyst is a solitary cystic defect of bone. The classic location of this lesion is in the proximal humerus of young children and the most common reason for clinical presentation is a fracture through the weakened bone. Radiographs reveal a well-defined lucent area in the bone with a thin sclerotic margin (Fig. 12.3). A pseudoloculated appearance can be present. When observed over time, the lesion appears to migrate away from the growing epiphysis. Treatment includes observation for small lesions and cast immobilization for lesions associated with fracture. Large lesions require steroid injection or bone grafting to ensure healing of the cyst.

Elbow Injuries

Baseball players can sustain a plethora of injuries to the elbow. The repetitious, high-velocity nature of the baseball throw induces chronic stresses at the elbow and particularly predisposes the elbow to overuse syndromes. Biomechanically, efficient throwing necessitates rapid forceful extension of the elbow, accompanied by significant valgus stress and finally pronation of the forearm. The angular velocity of the elbow while throwing can exceed 300°/sec. The normal valgus angle of the elbow in extension may specifically bias the medial aspect of the elbow to overuse injuries. The velocity and force required in repetitive throwing contributes to inflict microtrauma on the elbow and its stabilizers. Commonly, overuse injuries are encountered when the body's physiologic ability to heal lags behind incessant microtrauma. Each age group and proficiency level normally demonstrates specific injury patterns. Therefore, even though the throwing motion is similar in all ages, the typical sites of injury are much

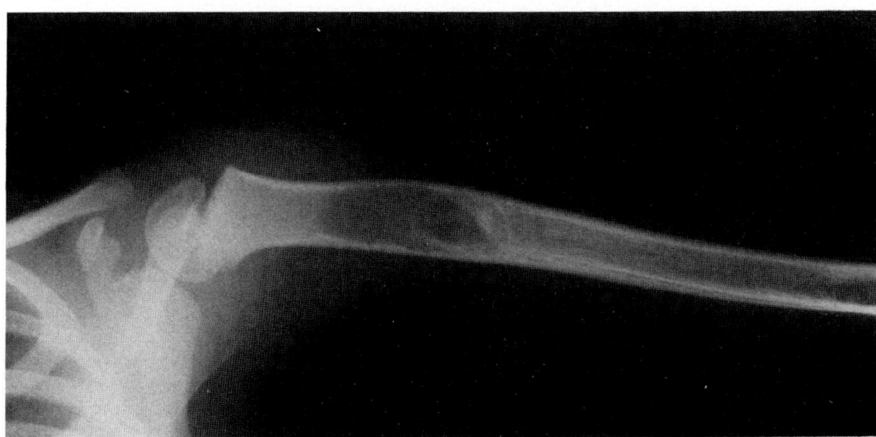

Figure 12.3. Simple bone cyst in the proximal humerus of an adolescent. AP radiograph reveals a well-defined radiolucent area in the humerus with a thin sclerotic margin.

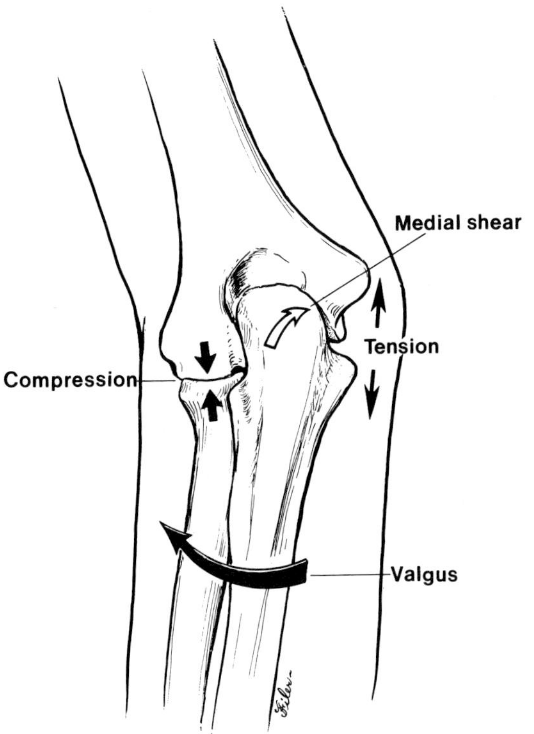

Figure 12.4. Forces at the elbow during throwing include medial tension, lateral compression, and posteromedial shear.

different when comparing immature and mature throwers. Four distinct areas are vulnerable to throwing stresses: *(a)* medial tension overload; *(b)* compression overload to the lateral surfaces; *(c)* posteromedial shear stresses; and *(d)* extension overload to the lateral restraints (54) (Fig. 12.4). In the mature thrower, the weakest link is the ligamentous and bony surface as opposed to the physis in immature throwers.

Adult Elbow Injuries

The differential diagnosis of adult elbow injuries is shown in Table 12.3.

Table 12.3.
Differential Diagnosis of Adult Elbow Injuries

Medial epicondylitis
Medial collateral ligament injury/neuritis
Ulnar neuritis
Lateral epicondylitis
Posterior compartment degenerative joint disease
Posterior compartment loose bodies

Medial Tension Overload. A significant tension force is absorbed by the medial elbow restraints during the late cocking and acceleration phases of the throwing cycle. The resultant force presents as tension on the medial epicondylar attachments of the flexor muscle origin and medial collateral ligaments. Chronic microtrauma to these structures can result in inflammation of the musculotendinous attachments on the medial epicondyle or scarring and attenuation of the medial collateral ligaments with possible rupture.

Inflammation of the medial epicondyle presents with pain and tenderness and positive provocative tests (pain with resisted wrist flexion and pronation). Initial treatment entails ice, rest from throwing, phonophoresis, and antiinflammatory agents. Recalcitrant cases will sometimes need local steroid injections at the site of maximal tenderness. Once symptoms have abated, a systematic regimen of strengthening exercises is helpful.

Inflammation and scarring of the medial collateral ligaments, secondary to insidious microtrauma, is much more demanding clinically. Diagnosis is difficult, with the athlete typically complaining of pain distal to the medial epicondyle during late cocking and acceleration. Associated ulnar neuritis symptoms may be present. Throwing velocity is decreased, and the athlete will have problems when accelerating the ball more than three-quarters normal velocity. Physical examination demonstrates deep tenderness at the site of the ligaments. Instability tests require sensitive fingers to detect subtle medial instability. Stress radiographs are technique dependent and are helpful only when positive.

Treatment of these injuries depends on the integrity of the medial ligament complex and the degree of joint instability. Most cases of medial ligament strain will resolve with conservative treatment, including ice, rest from pitching, phonophoresis, and antiinflammatory agents. Once acute symptoms subside, a strengthening protocol of the forearm flexors and pronators and a progressive throwing program is started as symptoms permit. Infrequently, chronic microtrauma of the ligament will cause a complete rupture with resultant medial instability. The history will include multiple bouts of medial elbow strain that have responded to conservative treatment. Suddenly, a single episode of "giving way" will occur, representing ligamentous rupture. Treatment depends on the goals of the athlete and the degree of instability. However, surgical reconstruction for acute ruptures of the medial collateral complex is usually necessary in high-level throwers.

Lateral Extension Overload. Lateral extension overload presents during the acceleration phase of throwing when rapid forearm pronation initiates a tension stress to the lateral musculotendinous origin. Repeated stress may induce lateral epicondylitis; however, the lateral ligamentous complex is rarely involved. Treatment is similar to that already described for medial epicondylitis.

Posteromedial Shear. Posteromedial shear with posterior compartment damage is common in adult throwers and develops in two phases of throwing. During late cocking and follow-through, the posterior compartment must absorb and dissipate the posteromedial shear force that develops. This force commonly induces three types of pathology: *(a)* posteromedial spurs; *(b)* pure posterior spurs; and *(c)* osteophytes on the floor of the olecranon fossa. All three of these sites may contribute to loose body formation. Treatment is initially conservative with attention to symptomatic control. Chronic posterior impingement and loose body symptoms usually necessitate arthroscopic removal of spurs and loose bodies.

Pediatric Elbow Injuries

Young throwers tend to have more elbow injuries than shoulder injuries (55). The term *Little League elbow* has been routinely used to describe a group of pathologic entities in and about the elbow joint in immature throwers. Each of these conditions, in fact, is a specific elbow injury with an individual personality as to prognosis and treatment. The typical problems in immature throwers include *(a)* medial epicondylar fragmentation and avulsion, *(b)* delayed or accelerated apophyseal growth of the medial epicondyle, *(c)* delayed closure of the medial epicondylar physis, *(d)* osteochondrosis and osteochondritis of the capitellum, *(e)* deformation and osteochondrosis of the radial head, *(f)* hypertrophy of the ulna, and *(g)* olecranon apophysitis with or without delayed closure of the olecranon apophysis (56–61). Many investigators have implicated these maladies to be secondary to the biomechanical throwing stresses placed on young, developing elbows (62–65). Exceptional forces are absorbed and transmitted by the elbow during throwing. These forces include traction, compression, and shear localized to the medial, lateral, and posterior elbow, respectively (55). Any or all of these forces may contribute to the alteration of normal osteochondral development of the elbow (66).

The cornerstone to successful treatment of Little League elbow is a timely, accurate diagnosis of the specific injury. A meticulous history and physical examination are the essential tools in achieving this goal, routine radiographs excluded. The use of special tests such as the arthrogram, CT scan, and MRI are often necessary in a confirmatory role rather than a diagnostic one.

Two of the most common abnormalities in the immature thrower are medial tension injuries and osteochondritis dissecans of the capitellum. Discussions of the remainder of the aberrances of Little League elbow can be found in Chapter 51. The differential diagnosis of pediatric elbow injuries is shown in Table 12.4.

Medial Tension Injuries. The most common complaints in immature throwers involve the medial aspect of the elbow. The athlete will complain of a triad of symptoms, including progressive medial pain, decreased effectiveness, and decreased throwing distance. The most common cause of the dysfunction is a subtle stress fracture involving the medial epicondylar physis. Radiographs will usually be negative, however, sometimes an irregular medial epicondylar epiphysis will be apparent. The salient physical finding is tenderness of the medial epicondyle. Generally, acute symptoms will subside with rest, ice, and nonsteroidal antiinflammatory agents. A flexibility, strengthening, and progressive throwing protocol is helpful after cessation of symptoms. Residual deformity and delayed fusion of the epicondyle is not common.

Conversely, if a more vigorous valgus stress is absorbed while throwing, an avulsion fracture through the medial epicondylar physis may occur. Sudden medial pain, point tenderness, and a flexion contracture are typical. Radiographs most often demonstrate a minimally displaced epicondylar fragment, although at times substantial displacement will be apparent (Fig. 12.5). Treatment depends on the amount of epicondylar displacement. Although controversy exists, the authors advocate an anatomic surgical reduction and do not accept any degree of medial epicondylar displacement.

Medial ligamentous ruptures in immature throwers seldom occur. These instabilities are much more prevalent in mature throwers, who have accumulated years of insidious microtrauma and scarring of the medial

Table 12.4.
Differential Diagnosis of Pediatric Elbow Injuries

Medial epicondyle injury
Osteochondrosis
Capitellum
Radial head
Osteochondritis dessicans of the capitellum
Hypertrophy of the ulna
Olecranon apophysitis

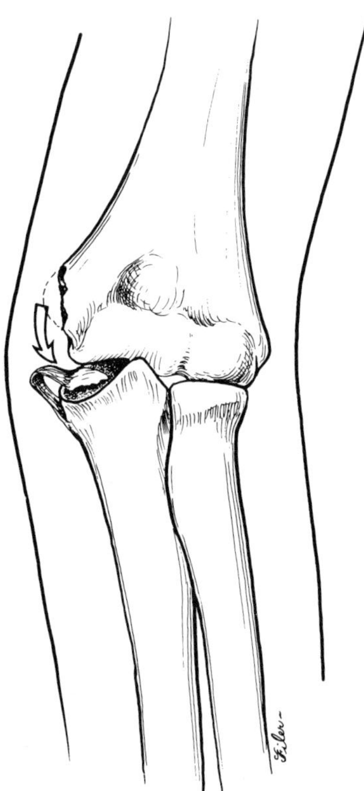

Figure 12.5. Displaced medial epicondylar fragment in the joint of immature thrower.

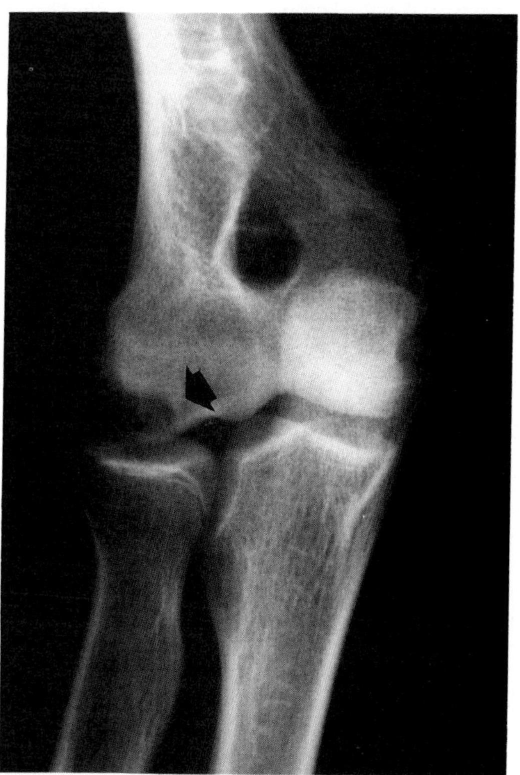

Figure 12.6. Osteochondritis dissecans of the capitellum in an immature thrower.

collateral complex. Treatment is usually conservative, involving initial immobilization followed by functional bracing and, finally, gradual rehabilitation. This rehabilitation protocol includes symptomatic control, range-of-motion exercises, and strength training. Surgical reconstruction of the medial collateral ligament complex is rarely indicated.

Lateral Compression Injuries. Osteochondritis dissecans (OCD) of the capitellum typically presents in young throwers between 13 and 16 years of age. They complain of dull lateral elbow pain associated with a flexion contracture and occasional locking. Radiographs demonstrate a focal island of subchondral bone demarcated by a rarefied zone, with or without loose bodies (Fig. 12.6). OCD can usually be delineated from Panner's disease (osteochondrosis) of the capitellum by age (younger than 7 to 12 years in Panner's) and x-ray presentation. Treatment of OCD is determined by lesion location, size, fixation, and condition of the articular cartilage. Type I lesions that are intact with no evidence of displacement or articular fracture require rest and splinting for 3 to 4 weeks followed by range-of-motion exercises. Protection of the elbow is continued until radiographic evidence of healing is apparent. Type II lesions present with fracture or fissuring of the articular surface and with partial displacement of the nonvascular fragment. Partially detached Type II lesions usually require elbow arthroscopy to evaluate the articular surface. Two modes of treatment are common: in situ pinning (large fragment) and removal and burring of the base of the lesion (small fragment). Type III lesions are completely detached, and loose body symptoms may be present. The avascular fragment is usually hypertrophied and rounded. The crater is obscured by fibrous tissue and is subsequently smaller than the fragment. Treatment requires arthroscopy, removal of the fragment, and burring of the crater. Late sequelae of OCD include loose bodies, residual deformity of the capitellum, and often residual elbow disability.

Vascular Compromise

Diagnosis of vascular compression injuries in the throwing athlete is difficult. The symptoms are usually vague and physical findings are often subtle. In addition, these injuries are relatively uncommon.

Vascular exam includes a number of tests for vascular compression in addition to skin exam and pulse palpation. Vascular injuries in athletes are related to chronic throwing effort. McCarthy et al. (67) evaluated 17 baseball players for vascular upper extremity conditions: 7 had thoracic outlet syndrome and the remaining 10 athletes had hand ischemia. The athletes with thoracic outlet syndrome had complaints of decreased endurance or severe finger ischemia from emboli (one athlete). All of the pitchers had a measurable loss of pitch velocity and were unable to pitch for more than three innings. Forearm pain, throwing arm heaviness, and hand coldness were present in some pitchers. Loss of pitching control was not a symptom. Physical diagnosis revealed a diminished pulse or a loud bruit in all but one athlete. Doppler ultrasonography and duplex scanning confirmed the presence of arterial compression in more than 90% of the athletes. Most of the athletes had compression of the subclavian artery behind the scalene musculature. Sometimes these injuries are the result of subclavian artery aneurysm with thrombosis. In this case, embolization can occur to the hand. Fortunately, these arterial injuries are rare. Compression of the subclavian artery can occur at the thoracic outlet by either a cervical rib or hypertrophied scalene musculature (23, 68). Treatment of TOS includes avoidance of all exacerbating activities and a carefully supervised program of muscle strengthening for the entire shoulder girdle. Postural training also may have a positive effect. Surgical decompression of the thoracic outlet can be approached in many ways (20–23). Compression of the posterior humeral circumflex artery (69), the suprascapular artery, or the subscapular artery (67) also can result in localized symptoms.

Rohrer et al. (70) examined 92 extremities in three groups: professional pitchers, nonpitching professional players, and nonathlete controls (70). They found 83% of the extremities had some compression of the axillary artery by the humeral head when the shoulder was in the position of abduction and external rotation. However, greater than 50% arterial compression was present in only 7.6% of the extremities, and a significant difference was not present among the three groups.

Itoh et al. (69) have documented circulatory disturbances in the throwing hand of baseball pitchers, resulting in finger pain, ulcers, and cyanosis. They proposed that the digital arteries sustain repeated compression and traction with ball release as they are entrapped between Cleland's ligament and a hyperextended proximal interphalangeal (PIP) joint. With surgical release of Cleland's ligament good recovery of circulation and return to throwing is possible. Pitchers who commonly throw the split-finger fastball may be particularly prone to developing circulatory disturbances in their throwing hands. This may be related to the extreme angular displacement between the index and long fingers required to perform this pitch.

Head and Neck Injuries

Baseball, although not considered a contact sport, results in surprisingly high numbers of head and neck injuries. Approximately half of baseball fatalities are the result of head and neck injuries (4). The U.S. Consumer Product Safety Commission estimates that 170,000 baseball-related injuries occur each year to the face, predominantly the mouth and the eyes (5). Head injuries are especially common in the 5- to 14-year-old age group, accounting for 40% of all baseball injuries (5). Numerous studies have found baseball to be the leading cause of youth, sports-related head injuries (6, 71).

The mechanisms of head and neck injury in baseball include ball impact, collision trauma, and sliding accidents. Between 40% and 70% of baseball-related youth eye injuries occur from being hit by a pitch while batting (71, 72). Bony trauma to the teeth, jaw, facial bones, nose, orbit, and skull also can result from being hit. Ocular injuries seen in baseball include lid lacerations, foreign bodies, hyphema (Fig. 12.7), vitreous hemorrhage, retinal detachment, optic nerve damage, and blindness (71, 72). Head-first sliding has been described as causing neck hyperflexion injuries that can result in quadriplegia (1). Neurologic sequelae, including subdural hematomas, also can result from head trauma during baseball.

Careful physical examination of a baseball player who has sustained a head or neck injury is essential. Clinical assessment must define the cause, type, location, and extent of injury. In every instance of significant head trauma, the neck should be stabilized in a cervical collar until the integrity of the spine is established. Types of traumatic head and neck injury include concussions, contusions, skull fracture, epidural hematomas, subdural hematomas, and spinal fractures. Any loss of consciousness, sensory change, motor deficit, neck stiffness, or altered mental status, other than a transient concussion with rapid recovery of all senses, should be aggressively pursued with a careful neurologic exam and further diagnostic tests to determine the extent of involvement. Significant facial soft tissue injury suggestive of bony involvement should be evaluated with appropriate diagnostic radiographs. When ocular involvement is suggested, a thorough eye exam, including evaluation of fundi, visual fields, acuity, and eye movements, is necessary to determine the extent of injury. Table 12.5 reviews important aspects concerning the exam of a patient with suspected head or neck injuries.

Baseball is being targeted as a sport that should require total head and face protection. Little League and professional baseball organizations require the use of batting helmets, base-running helmets, and catchers' helmets with face masks. Facial and ocular injuries resulting from baseball impact are largely preventable. The National Society to Prevent Blindness estimates 90% of ocular injuries resulting from sports are preventable and

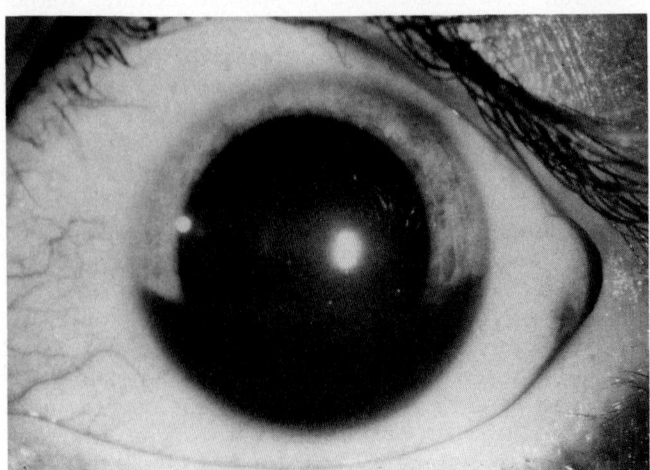

Figure 12.7. Hyphema. Blood in the anterior chamber of the eye in a batter hit by a pitch. Courtesy of JB Jeffers.

Table 12.5.
Head and Neck Injury Assessment

History	Loss of consciousness Temporal course of symptoms
General physical exam	Vital signs Neck stabilized (cervical collar) Other significant trauma Airway, breathing, circulation
Neurologic exam	Serial examinations Motor Sensory Reflexes Cranial nerves Mentation
Radiologic exam	Cervical spine (C1–C7) Skull
CT scans	Head Neck

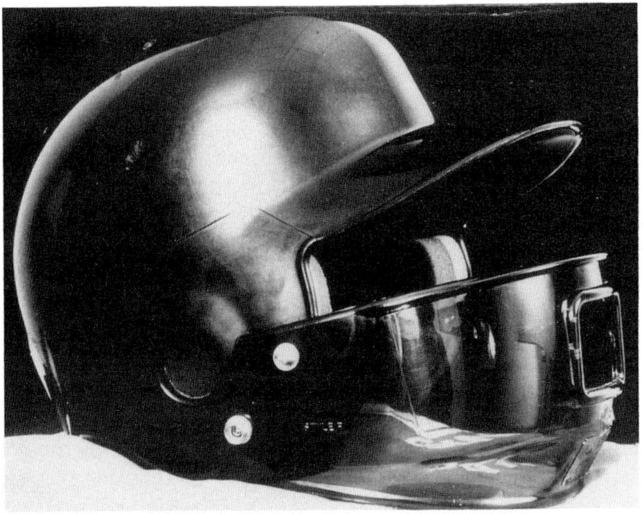

Figure 12.8. Commercially available polycarbonate face guard attached to a batting helmet to reduce head and face injuries. Courtesy of Home Safe Face Guards, Inc.

thus recommends that baseball batters and base runners be required to wear face guards (5). Much effort is being channeled into the research and development of protective equipment, including a presently available polycarbonate face guard (Home Safe-Face Guards Inc., Salem, Virginia) (Fig. 12.8) and improved energy-absorbing capabilities of baseball headgear (73).

Hitting

The ability to hit a baseball hurled 60 feet 6 inches at speeds greater than 90 mph is a skill that requires coordination, strength, quickness, and judgment. Most batting injuries result from being hit by a pitch. Soft tissue trauma and fractures can occur at the site of impact. Such injuries to the head and face were described above. In addition, batting injuries can occur during the swing itself as a result of either a full, uncontrolled swing (patellar dislocation) or direct impact with the bat handle (hook of the hamate fracture).

Gross (74) described a series of five softball players who dislocated the patella of their trailing legs while taking a full, uncontrolled swing. When the batter begins to swing, a valgus force is placed on the knee of the trailing leg with the foot fixed by cleats into the ground. As the quadriceps contracts with the trailing leg in flexion, the tibia rotates externally with respect to the femur. Thus the patella can be subluxed laterally out of the femoral sulcus with a resultant rupture of the medial capsular structures (75). Radiologic evaluation of the patellofemoral joint is made with standard knee views (AP, lateral) and with axial "sunrise" views of the knee in varying positions of flexion. The treatment of acute patellar dislocation is relocation, brief immobilization (less than 48 hr), and intensive quadriceps rehabilitation and subsequent conditioning. In the majority of cases, surgery can be avoided.

Isolated fractures of the hook of the hamate can occur while batting. In a series of 62 patients with hook of the hamate fractures described by Stark et al. (76), more than 80% of the fractures occurred while swinging a baseball bat, golf club, or tennis racquet. When a baseball bat is gripped, the butt of the bat is located over the distal and ulnar aspect of the hook. Thus if the centrifugal force of the swinging butt can overcome the grasping power of a right-handed batter, the end of the bat can fracture the hook of the left hamate. Patients with hook of the hamate fractures will usually complain of a dull, aching pain on the ulnar aspect of the wrist that worsens with passive or active extension. On physical exam, grip strength is usually decreased and palpation over the hook results in increased pain. Radiographically, most of the fractures can be diagnosed on a carpal tunnel view or a special oblique view of the supinated wrist. When the fracture is not apparent on either of these types of roentgenograms, a bone scan or a computerized tomography scan (Fig. 12.9) with the hands in the praying position should be made. There are many reports of acute hook of the hamate fractures that fail to heal after immobilization of the hand and wrist (77–80) or after open reduction and internal fixation (81). Because of the ligamentous and muscular attachments to the hamate, Stark et al. (76) suggest that

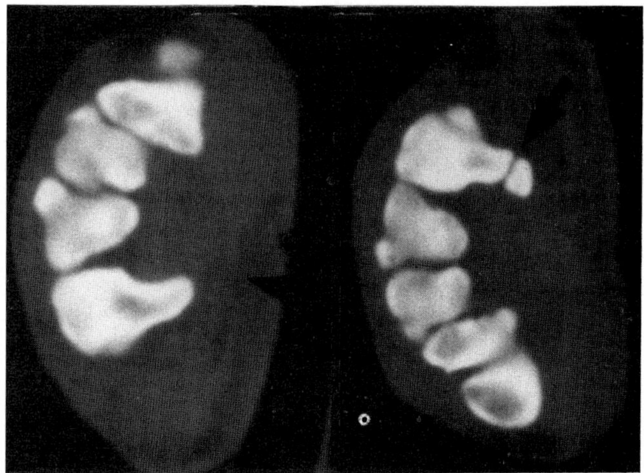

Figure 12.9. Hook of the hamate fracture. CT images of left (**left**) and right (**right**) carpal bones. Fracture of the hook of the hamate (*arrow*) is seen in the right wrist.

movement of the fingers and thumb tends to cause motion at the hamate fracture site and, therefore, prevents union even when the wrist and hand are immobilized. Thus hook resection is the treatment of choice and reliably eliminates symptoms, lessens the likelihood of subsequent sequelae, and returns most players to their previous level of activity in 8 weeks (76, 82, 83).

Sliding

Baseball sliding involves sprinting along a baseline and converting a vertical stance to a horizontal stance to arrive at a base while avoiding a fielder's tag. The two primary sliding techniques are head-first and feet-first.

Corzatt et al. (84) kinematically analyzed the head-first and feet-first sliding techniques of professional baseball players during game situations with high-speed cinematography. The act of sliding was divided into four distinct phases. In phase 1 of the feet-first slide (sprint phase), the base runner accelerates in the horizontal direction. Body lean is approximately 70° from horizontal, and the runner keeps the center of gravity ahead of the striding foot. In phase 2 (sliding position), the base runner leans back and the arms move behind the player in anticipation of the airborne and landing phases. In phase 3 (airborne phase), the position of the feet-first slide is characterized by extension of the lead leg with the trail leg flexed beneath and a semierect trunk posture. In phase 4 (landing phase), the runner hits the ground. In feet-first sliding, base contact is made with the extended leg, whereas body contact is made with the buttocks, lower back, and posterior thighs. In head-first sliding, forward lean is increased to approximately 30° from horizontal and the body position is lowered to assume a crouching position. The airborne phase of the head-first slide is much less distinct than in the feet-first slide and involves a prone position with arms forward and legs extended. Base contact is made with the forward arms while body contact is made with the chest and anterior thighs.

Sliding is responsible for a large proportion of injuries in baseball and softball. Investigators have estimated 41% to 71% of all softball injuries occur while sliding (85, 86). The mechanisms of sliding injuries include *(a)* shear force of the infield surface (abrasions and contusions), *(b)* rapid deceleration against a stationary base (ankle/hand fractures, ankle/hand ligamentous injuries, and knee ligamentous injuries), *(c)* collision injuries with a fielder (head injuries, fractures, and sprains), and *(d)* rapid acceleration from a standing position (hamstring pulls). Wheeler (85) investigated 55 sliding injuries during competitive softball games and found the following injury frequencies: ankle injuries, 46%; ankle fractures, 36%; knee injuries, 7%; and upper extremity injuries, 11%. Vertebral fractures can occur as a result of rapid deceleration against a stationary base or collision with a fielder. Most sliding injuries occur during the landing phase (phase 4) owing to the significant forces acting against the body during impact with the ground and the base. However, injuries can occur during the other phases of sliding as well (Table 12.6). Hamstring muscle strains during the sprint phase of base running are common baseball injuries and will be discussed in more detail later in this chapter. It is unclear whether feet-first sliding or head-first sliding results in a greater relative incidence of injuries, however, head-first sliding injuries tend to be more severe (1, 85).

Preventative measures to reduce the incidence of sliding injuries in baseball include the illegalization of sliding, the use of base-running helmets, instruction on proper sliding technique, improved musculoskeletal conditioning, and the use of recessed bases or break-away bases. Some Little League associations have disallowed head-first sliding or sliding altogether until a certain age is reached. However, the illegalization of sliding is impractical to the majority of participants and fans in a sport as steeped in tradition as baseball. Furthermore, the illegalization of sliding may result in increased numbers of collision and thrown ball injuries. Instruction and practice of proper sliding technique can be beneficial in organized settings such as Little League baseball (87). Aspects of proper sliding technique include keeping the lead foot (feet-first slide) or lead hand (head-first slide) elevated, starting the slide at the correct distance, maximizing body surface contact area, and avoiding last-minute hesitation (1, 87). At home plate, ankle injuries during sliding are less frequent because the base runner slides over, not into, the base (85). Hence, recessing second and third base as is home plate could reduce the number of sliding injuries; however, poor visualization of the bases by umpires is problematic. Janda et al. (2) demonstrated significant prevention of softball sliding injuries through the use of break-away bases by prospectively studying 633 games played on break-away base fields and 627 games played on stationary base fields (Fig. 12.10). A total of 45 sliding injuries occurred on the stationary base fields (1 injury for every 13.9 games), whereas two sliding injuries occurred on the break-away base fields (1 injury for every 316.5 games). In a 1035-game follow-up study on break-away base fields, only two sliding injuries occurred (1 injury for every 517.5 games) (88). Although break-away bases cost roughly twice as much as stationary bases, Janda et al. estimated that mandatory use of break-away

Table 12.6.
Sliding Injuries

Phase	Feet-First Sliding Injuries	Head-First Sliding Injuries
1: Sprint phase	Ankle sprains Hamstring strains	Ankle sprains Hamstring strain
2: Sliding position	Ankle sprains	Ankle sprains
3: Airborne phase		
4: Landing phase	Abrasions and contusions Lower extremity fractures Ankle/knee sprains	Abrasions and contusions Upper extremity fractures Wrist/elbow sprains Shoulder injuries Vertebral fractures

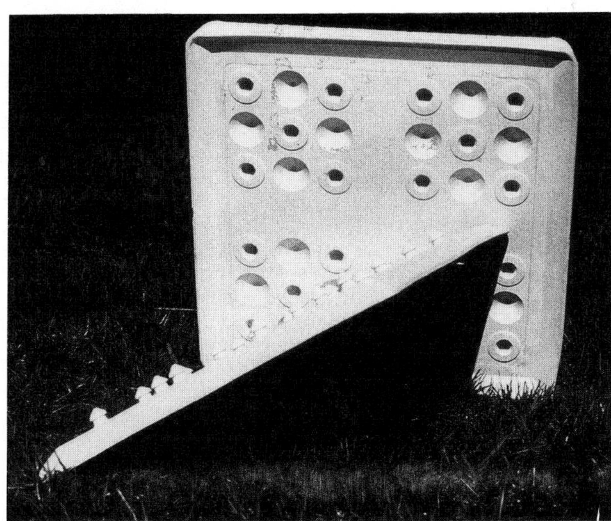

Figure 12.10. Break-away base. Anchored and detachable portions of a break-away base designed to reduce sliding injuries. Courtesy of DH Janda.

bases by recreational softball leagues could save $2.0 billion per year in acute care medical costs. It also was believed that break-away bases did not detract from the flow of the game or base visualization by umpires.

Catching

Catching of the thrown baseball is an exacting task that requires excellent hand-eye coordination. The catcher is considered to play the most physically demanding position in baseball as he or she is constantly getting up and down from a squatting position, receiving pitches, making throws, chasing foul balls, and avoiding collisions from the ball, bat, and base runner.

The mechanisms of catching injuries include chronic repetitive catching impact (digital ischemia); acute collisions with a base runner, ball, or bat (head injuries, fractures, and sprains); and meniscal lesions in the older catcher from constant squatting.

Catchers are predisposed to vascular injury in the gloved hand because of the sizable impact forces involved in catching 150 to 200 pitches per game, many of which exceed velocities of 90 mph (89). Sugawara et al. (90) demonstrated the presence of digital ischemia using angiograms and thermography in eight baseball players who presented with coolness and numbness in the index fingers of their catching hands. Physical exam of the involved hand demonstrated paleness, cyanosis, and a positive digital Allen's test. Thermograms and angiograms revealed an occluded index digital artery located at the distal interphalangeal joint more frequently than the proximal interphalangeal joint.

Lowry et al. (91) assessed 21 professional catchers and one collegiate catcher with Doppler flow studies and a modified digital Allen's test. These investigators found that only 41% of the catchers had normal left index finger circulation (catching hand), whereas 95% of the catchers had normal right-hand circulation (noncatching hand). Furthermore, the 9 catchers with normal left finger circulation reported the frequent use of a thick glove below their catcher's mitt. To assess the incidence of digital ischemia among baseball players, Sugawara et al. (90) surveyed 578 junior high school, high school, and college baseball players in Japan. The researchers found an increased frequency of digital ischemia among those positions involving the most repetitive catching: catchers and first base players. They also found an increased incidence of digital ischemia in players with more accumulated experience.

Preventative measures to reduce the incidence of catching injuries in baseball include hand padding, improved mitt design, protective equipment, and instruction on proper catching technique. Enhanced mitt padding or the use of a thick glove under the mitt may reduce the vascular changes in the catching hand that result from repetitive impact. Protective equipment is essential to avoid collision injury from a ball, bat, or base runner. Proper equipment for the catcher includes a padded mask, a helmet, a throat protector extending from the lower aspect of the mask to the clavicle, a chest protector, a protective groin cup, and well-fitting shin guards that include patellar shielding (92). Instruction for the catcher concerning proper tagging technique can reduce the number of base runner collision injuries and instruction concerning proper catching stance can reduce the number of bat and ball impact injuries. Protection of the noncatching hand, by placing it behind the back in one-handed catching or cupped behind the glove hand in two-handed catching, is also essential to avoid injuries from foul tips and wild pitches (Fig. 12.11).

Fielding

Fielding of fly balls and ground balls requires coordination, judgment, and sudden running. It is essential to the success of the team in the field.

The mechanisms of fielding injuries include *(a)* collision with players or the ballpark fence (head injuries,

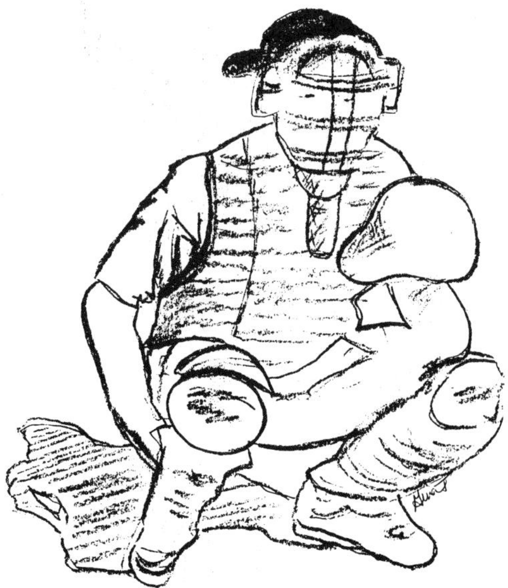

Figure 12.11. Catcher in protective gear, which includes padded glove, padded mask, helmet, throat protector, chest protector, groin cup, shin guards, and patellar shielding. Proper catching technique includes protection of the noncatching hand.

Table 12.7.
Grading of Hamstring Muscle Strains

Degree	Musculotendinous Unit	Pain	Swelling	Strength	Motion
First	No disruption	Mild	+	0	0
Second	Partial disruption	Moderate	+ +	–	–
Third	Complete disruption	Severe	+ + +	– –	– –

fractures, and sprains), *(b)* ball trauma from uncaught balls (head injuries and fractures), and *(c)* explosive bursts of muscle activity (muscle strains).

Strain of a muscle group from sudden activity after a period of inactivity is a common baseball injury. An acute strain is the result of a single violent force applied to the muscle and can be classified into three degrees, depending on the extent of injury (Table 12.7). Even a mild muscle strain can be distressing and debilitating to a competitive baseball player. However, it is essential that the muscle-tendon unit be given protected time to heal so that complete recovery and prevention of subsequent injury is ensured (93–95).

Preventative measures to reduce the incidence of fielding injuries in baseball include stretching exercises (95), good communication between players to avoid player collisions, and warning tracks around the outfield fence to avoid wall collisions.

Summary

Baseball is a fun and challenging sport enjoyed by players of all ages. Although not a particularly dangerous sport, baseball results in a substantial total number of injuries due to its large participation. Thus both the primary care physician and the orthopedic surgeon will see patients with baseball-related injuries and must be knowledgeable as to their diagnosis and treatment. A good history and thorough physical exam, augmented by selected diagnostic tests, will usually result in the appropriate diagnosis. Definitive, early treatment of injuries with close follow-up and the allowance of time for healing will result in good recovery and return to activity. An understanding of the mechanisms of injury associated with throwing, hitting, sliding, catching, and fielding is helpful in the prevention of injuries. Emphasis on good conditioning and proper technique will not only improve performance but also prevent injury. Through better understanding of the mechanism, diagnosis, treatment, and prevention of injury, it is possible to enhance the careers of players and make baseball an even safer sport.

REFERENCES

1. Collins HR, Lund D. Baseball injuries. In: Schneider RC, Kennedy JC, Plant MC, eds. Sports injuries: mechanisms, prevention, and treatment. Baltimore: Williams & Wilkins, 1986:64–77.
2. Janda DH, Wojtys EM, Hankin FM, Benedict MA. Softball sliding injuries: a prospective study comparing standard and modified bases. JAMA 1988;259:1848–1850.
3. Powell JW. Pros and cons of data-gathering mechanisms. In: Vinger PF, Hoerner EF, eds. Sports injuries: the unthwarted epidemic. Littleton: PSG, 1986:28–32.
4. Kraus JF, Conroy C. Mortality and morbidity from injuries in sports and recreation. Annu Rev Public Health 1984;5:163–192.
5. Caveness LS. Ocular and facial injuries in baseball. Int Ophthalmol Clin 1988;28:238–241.
6. Rutherford GW, et al. Overview of sports-related injuries to persons 5–14 years of age. Washington, DC: U.S. Consumer Product Safety Commission, 1981.
7. Bradley JP, Perry J, Jobe FW. The biomechanics of the throwing shoulder. Perspec Orthop Surg 1990;1:49–59.
8. Gainor BT, Piotrowski G, Puhl J, Allen WC, Hagen R. The throw: biomechanics and acute injury. Am J Sports Med 1980;8:114–119.
9. Glousman R, Jobe FW, Tibone JE, Moynes D, Antonelli D, Perry J. Dynamic EMG analysis of the throwing shoulder with glenohumeral instability. J Bone Joint Surg 1988;70A:220–226.
10. Gowan ID, Jobe FW, Tibone JE, Perry J, Moynes DR. A comparative EMG analysis of the shoulder during pitching: professional vs. amateur pitchers. Am J Sports Med 1987;15:586–590.
11. Jobe FW, Bradley JP. Rotator cuff injuries in baseball: prevention and rehabilitation. Sports Med 1988;6:377–387.
12. Jobe FW, Moynes DR, Tibone JE, Perry J. An EMG analysis of the shoulder in pitching: a second report. Am J Sports Med 1984;12:218–220.
13. Jobe FW, Tibone JE, Perry J, Moynes DR. An EMG analysis of the shoulder in throwing and pitching. A preliminary report. Am J Sports Med 1983;11:3–5.
14. Papas AM, Zawack RM, Sullivan TJ. Biomechanics of baseball pitching: a preliminary report. Am J Sports Med 1985;13:216–222.
15. Turkel SJ, Panio NW, Marshall JL, Girgis FG. Stabilizing mechanics preventing anterior dislocation of the glenohumeral joint. J Bone Joint Surg 1981;63A:1208–1217.
16. Digiovine N, Jobe F, Pink M, Perry M. An electromyographic analysis of the upper extremity in pitching. J Shoulder Elbow Surg 1992;1:15–25.
17. McConnell ME. How to play Little League baseball. New York: Ronald, 1960.
18. Sain J, Andrews JR. Proper pitching techniques. In: Zarins B, Andrews JR, Carson WG, eds. Injuries to the throwing arm. Philadelphia: WB Saunders, 1985:31–37.
19. Barnes DA, Tullus HS. An analysis of 100 symptomatic baseball players. Am J Sports Med 1978;6:63–67.
20. Pappas AM, Zawacki RM, McCarthy CF. Rehabilitation of the pitching shoulder. Am J Sports Med 1985;13:223–235.
21. Falconer MA, Li FWP. Resection of the first rib in costoclavicular compression of the brachial plexus. Lancet 1962;1:59.
22. Roos DB. Transaxillary approach to the first rib to relieve thoracic outlet syndrome. Ann Surg 1966;163:354–358.
23. Roos DB. Congenital anomalies associated with thoracic outlet syndrome. Anatomy, symptoms, diagnosis and treatment. Am J Surg 1976;132:771–778.
24. Adson AW, Caffey JF. Cervical rib: a method of anterior approach for relief of symptoms by resection of the scalenus anterior. Ann Surg 1927;85:839.
25. Ringel SP, Treihaft M, Carry M, Fischer R, Jacobs P. Suprascapular neuropathy in pitchers. Am J Sports Med 1990;18:80–86.
26. Jobe FW, Bradley JP. Ulnar neuritis and ulnar collateral ligament instabilities in overarm throwers. In: Torg JS, ed. Current therapy in sports medicine. Toronto: BC Decker, 1990:419–424.
27. Bergfeld JA, Andrish JT, Clancy WA. Evaluation of the acromioclavicular joint following first- and second-degree sprains. Am J Sports Med 1978;6:153–159.
28. Cook FF, Tibone JE. The Mumford procedure in athletes: an objective analysis of function. Am J Sports Med 1988;16:97–100.
29. Neer CS II. Anterior acromioplasty for the chronic impingement syndrome in the shoulder. A preliminary report. J Bone Joint Surg. 1972;54A:41–50.
30. Fu FH, Harner CD, Klein AH. Shoulder/impingement syndrome. A critical review. Clin Orthop 1991;269:162–173.
31. Neer CS II. Impingement lesions. Clin Orthop 1983;173:70–77.
32. Jobe FW, Tibone JE, Jobe CM, Kvitne RS. The shoulder in sports. In: Rockwood CA, Matsen FA, eds. The shoulder. Philadelphia: WB Saunders, 1990:961–990.
33. Codman EA. The shoulder: rupture of the supraspinatous tendon and other lesions in or about the subacromial bursa. Boston: Thomas Todd, 1934.

34. Rathbun JB, McNab I. The microvascular pattern of the rotator cuff. J Bone Joint Surg 1970;52B:540–553.
35. Uhtoff HK, Loehr J, Sarkar K. The pathogenesis of rotator cuff tears. In: Takagishi N, ed. The shoulder. Tokyo: Tokyo Professional Postgraduate Services, 1987:211.
36. Nirschi RP. Rotator cuff tendonitis: basic concepts of pathoetiology (American Academy of Orthopedic Surgeons Instructional Course Lecture No. 439). Las Vegas, NV: 4405, 1989.
37. Brown LP, Niehues SL, Harrah A, Yavorsky P, Hirshman HP. Upper extremity range of motion and isokinetic strength of the internal and external rotators in Major League baseball players. Am J Sports Med 1988;16:577–585.
38. Neer CS II, Flatow EL, Lech O. Tears of the rotator cuff: long term results of anterior acromioplasty and repair. Paper presented at the American Shoulder and Elbow Surgeons Fourth Meeting, Atlanta, February 1988.
39. Samilson RL, Binder WF. Symptomatic full thickness tears of the rotator cuff: an analysis of 292 shoulders in 276 patients. Orthop Clin North Am 1975;6:449–466.
40. Tibone JE, Elrod B, Jobe FW, et al. Surgical treatment of the rotator cuff in athletes. J Bone Joint Surg 1986;68A:887–891.
41. Grana WA, Moretz JA. Ligamentous laxity in secondary school athletes. JAMA 1978;240:1975–1976.
42. Bennett GE. Shoulder and elbow lesions of the professional baseball pitcher. JAMA 1941;117:510.
43. Neer CS II, Foster CR. Inferior capsular shift for involuntary and multidirectional instability of the shoulder. J Bone Joint Surg, 1980;62A:897–908.
44. O'Donoghue DH. Subluxing biceps tendon in the athlete. Am J Sports Med 1973;1:20.
45. Snyder SJ, Karzel RP, Del Pizzo W, Ferkel RP, Friedman MJ. SLAP lesions of the shoulder. Arthroscopy 1990;6:274–279.
46. Rodosky MW, Rudert MJ, Harner CD, Luo L, Fu FH. Significance of a superior labral lesion of the shoulder: a biomechanical study. Trans Orthop Res Soc 1990;15:276.
47. Sterling JC, Calvo RD, Holden SC. An unusual stress fracture in a multiple sport athlete. Med Sci Sports Exerc 1991;23:298–303.
48. Linn RM, Kreigshauser LA. Ball thrower's fracture of the humerus. A case report. Am J Sports Med 1991;19:194–197.
49. Micheli LJ. Overuse injuries in children's sports: the growth factor. Orthop Clin North Am 1983;14:337–360.
50. Dotter WE. Little Leaguer's shoulder: fracture of the proximal humeral epiphyseal cartilage due to baseball pitching. Guthrie Clin Bul 1953;23:68–72.
51. Adams JE. Bone injuries in very young athletes. Clin Orthop 1968;58:129–140.
52. Cahill BR, Tullos HS, Fain RH. Little League shoulder. J Sports Med Phys Fitness 1974;2:150–152.
53. Goff W. Legg-Perthes disease and related osteochondrosis of youth. Springfield, IL: Charles C Thomas, 1954.
54. Pappas AW. Elbow problems associated with baseball during childhood and adolescence. Clin Orthop 1986;701:84–90.
55. Inman VT, Saunders JB, Abbott LC. Observations on the function of the shoulder joint. J Bone Joint Surg 1944;26:1–30.
56. Trias A, Ray RO. Juvenile osteochondritis of the radial head: report of a bilateral case. J Bone Joint Surg 1963;45A:576–582.
57. Tullos HS, Ferwin WD, Woods GW. Unusual lesions of the pitching arm. Clin Orthop 1972;88:169–182.
58. Adams IE. Injury to the throwing arm: a study of traumatic changes in the elbow joints of boy baseball players. California Med 1965;102:127–132.
59. Gugenheim JJ, Stanley RF, Wood GW, et al. Little league survey: the Houston study. Am J Sports Med 1976;4:189–199.
60. Larson RL, Singer KM, Berstrom R, et al. Little League survey: the Eugene study. Am J Sports Med 1976;4:201–209.
61. Brogdon BG, Crow NC. Little Leaguer's elbow. Am J Roentgenol 1960;83:671–675.
62. Lipsomb AB. Baseball pitching injuries in growing athletes. Am J Sports Med 1975;3:25–34.
63. Brown R, Blazina ME, Kerlan RK. Osteochondritis of the capitellum. Am J Sports Med 1974;2:27–46.
64. Middleman ID. Shoulder and elbow lesions of baseball players. Am J Surg 1961;102:627–632.
65. Slager RF. From Little League to big league, the weak spot is the arm. Am J Sports Med 1977;5:37–48.
66. Bianco AJ. Osteochondritis dissecans. In: Morrey BF, ed. The elbow and its disorders. Philadelphia: WB Saunders, 1985:254–259.
67. McCarthy WJ, Yao JS, Schafer MF, et al. Upper extremity arterial injury in athletes. J Vasc Surg 1989;9:317–326.
68. Baumgartner F, Nelson RJ, Robertson JM. The rudimentary first rib: a cause for thoracic outlet syndrome with arterial compromise. Arch Surg 1989;124:1090–1092.
69. Itoh Y, Wakaro K, Takeda T, Murakami T. Circulatory disturbances in the throwing hand of baseball pitchers. Am J Sports Med 1987;15:264–269.
70. Rohrer MJ, Cardullo PA, Pappas AM, Phillips DA, Wheeler HB. Axillary artery compression and thrombosis in throwing athletes. J Vasc Surg 1990;11:761–768.
71. Nelson LB, Wilson TW, Jeffers JB. Eye injuries in childhood: demography, etiology, and prevention. Pediatrics 1989;84:438–441.
72. Grin TR, Nelson LB, Jeffers JB. Eye injuries in childhood. Pediatrics 1987;80:13–17.
73. Goldsmith W, Kabo JM. Performance of baseball headgear. Am J Sports Med 1982;10:31–37.
74. Gross RM. Acute dislocation of the patella: the mudville mystery. J Bone Joint Surg 1986;68A:780–781.
75. Hughston JC. Subluxation of the patella. J Bone Joint Surg 1968;50A:1003–1026.
76. Stark HH, Chao E, Zemel NP, Rickard TA, Ashworth CR. Fracture of the hook of the hamate. J Bone Joint Surg 1989;71A:1202–1207.
77. Andress MR, Peckar VG. Fracture of the hook of the hamate. Br J. Radiol 1970;43:141–143.
78. Bray TJ, Swafford AR, Brown RL. Bilateral fracture of the hook of the hamate. J Trauma 1985;25:174–175.
79. Carter PR, Eaton RG, Littler JW. Ununited fracture of the hook of the hamate. J Bone Joint Surg 1977;59A:583–588.
80. Egawa M, Asai T. Fracture of the hook of the hamate: report of six cases and the suitability of computerized tomography. J Hand Surg 1983;8:393–398.
81. Bryan RS, Dobyns JH. Fractures of the carpal bones other than lunate and navicular. Clin Orthop 1980;149:108–109.
82. Parker RD, Berkowitz MS, Brahms MA, Bohl WL. Hook of the hamate fractures in athletes. Am J Sports Med 1986;14:517–523.
83. Stark HH, Jobe FW, Boyes JH. Fracture of the hook of the hamate in athletes. J Bone Joint Surg 1977;59A:575–582.
84. Corzatt RD, Groppel JL, Pfautsch E, Boscardin J. The biomechanics of head-first versus feet-first sliding. Am J Sports Med 1984; 12:229–232.
85. Wheeler BR. Slow-pitch softball injuries. Am J Sports Med 1984;12:237–240.
86. Janda DH, Hankin FM, Wojtys EM. Softball injuries: cost, cause, prevention. Am Fam Physician 1986;33:143–144.
87. Little League Baseball, Inc. Play it safe. Williamsport, PA: LLB, 1989.
88. Janda DH, Wojtys EM, Hankin FM, Benedict ME, Hensinger RN. A three-phase analysis of the prevention of recreational softball injuries. Am J Sports Med 1990;18:632–635.
89. Rettig AC. Neurovascular injuries in the wrists and hands of athletes. Clin Sports Med 1990;9:389–417.
90. Sugawara M, Ogino T, Minami A, Seiichi I. Digital ischemia in baseball players. Am J Sports Med 1986;14:329–334.
91. Lowrey CW, Chadwick RO, Waltman EN. Digital vessel trauma from repetitive impact in baseball catchers. J Hand Surg 1976;1:236–238.
92. Christiansen T, Wilson K. Facial injuries in sports. Minnesota Med 1983;1:29–32.
93. O'Donoghue DH. Treatment of injuries to athletes. Philadelphia: WB Saunders, 1984:433–446.
94. Garrett WE Jr. Muscle strain injuries: clinical and basic aspects. Med Sci Sports Exerc 1990;22:436–443.
95. Glick JM. Muscle strains: prevention and treatment. Phys Sports Med 1980;8:73–77.

13 / BASKETBALL

Frank H. Bassett III

Basketball is a collision sport. In spite of rules and regulations aimed at minimizing body contact with other players, unplanned collisions do occur and injuries result. Injuries can also be the result of a player colliding with the backboard or the hard playing surface. Because basketball is a game that is played without protective equipment, such injuries can be serious. The majority of injuries, however, are minor and consist primarily of contusions and lacerations.

Foot

The most common problems of the foot in basketball players are those affecting the skin. Blisters, calluses, and corns are expected difficulties in the early part of the basketball season. These relate to the constant stopping and starting and pivoting that is required in this sport. Conditioning of the skin by skin toughening compounds help, but most skin problems can be prevented by proper fitting basketball shoes, wearing two pairs of socks that are cleaned daily and using moleskin or Band-Aids to minimize friction and pressure. The protection of such skin lesions by good foot care (lubricating ointments and sterile dressing) minimize discomfort and prevent infection of the skin, which can prolong recovery.

Injuries to the musculoskeletal anatomy of the foot are not rare. Sprains of the intertarsal or tarsometatarsal ligaments (Fig. 13.1) result from twisting injuries such as coming down with a rebound and landing on someone else's foot. If the arch of the foot is thereby bowed dorsally upward by the superimposed force of the elevated heel being driven toward a more cavus position, the dorsal tarsometatarsal ligaments are torn and a dislocation of one or all of the tarsometatarsal joints can result (1). Even if deformity is minimal, edema across the dorsum of the foot always provides a clue as to the seriousness of the injury. Radiographs are indicated to rule out a spread of the first and second cuneiform metatarsal joints and/or subluxation or dislocation of one or all of the tarsometatarsal joints. If a dislocation or a fracture-dislocation is present, then open reduction and internal fixation is mandatory.

Taping of the foot and ankle prophylactically often minimizes the seriousness of the sprain. Longitudinal arch supports and transverse metatarsal arch supports, while not routinely used to prevent sprains of the foot, are extremely helpful in basketball players with high-arched or flat feet.

Individuals with a particularly high arch are prone to microtears of the plantar fascia, and plantar fasciitis is commonly seen. A well-fitting longitudinal arch support relieves discomfort and prevents chronicity of the heel pain so often associated with plantar fasciitis. Nonsteroidal antiinflammatory drugs (NSAIDS) also are helpful on a long-term basis in limiting the duration and severity of the pain.

The complete tear of the plantar fascia, while not common, is a painfully disabling condition that prevents further practice or competition. The athlete usually feels something tear or pop and direct tenderness to palpation is always present. A magnetic resonance imaging (MRI) examination can help differentiate tears of the plantar fascia from tears of the adjacent underlying intrinsic muscles of the foot (Fig. 13.2). Tearing of the latter structures is a less disabling condition and return to play can be anticipated much quicker than if the tear is of the plantar fascia.

Of the fractures seen in the feet of basketball players, stress fractures of the metatarsal and tarsal bones are the most common. Of these, the metatarsal bones are most susceptible. Stress fractures affect the second and third metatarsals most often. Biomechanical studies have suggested that these two metatarsals have more applied stresses to them (2).

The treatment of metatarsal stress fractures should include a well-fitted longitudinal arch support to be worn in the athlete's playing shoes as well as his or her street shoes. The athletes should be asked to stress the foot daily by running or jogging just short of the threshold of unbearable pain. This mechanism of continued repetitious stress stimulates the fracture to heal and results

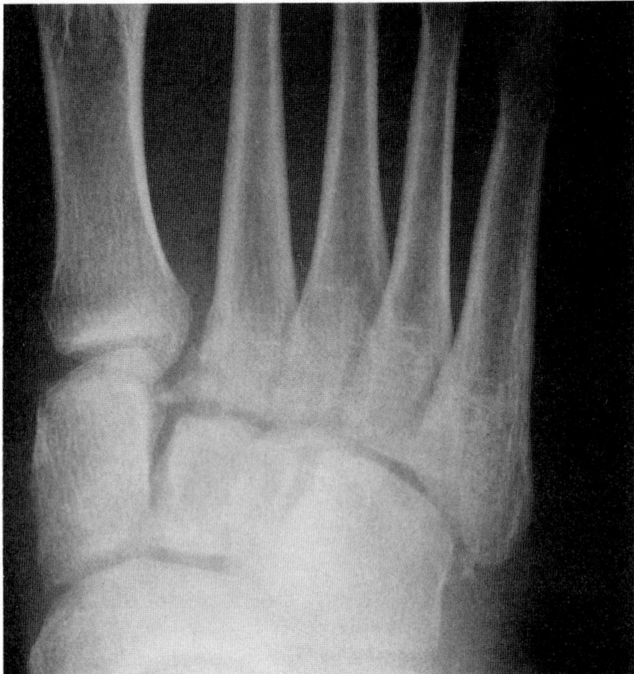

Figure 13.1. AP radiograph of the right midfoot of a collegiate basketball player showing a fracture-dislocation through the tarsometatarsal joints of the second through the fifth metatarsal. Also note the widening between the first and second metatarsal bases and the fracture from the base of the second metatarsal. This occurred while coming down from a rebound off balance.

in increased permanent thickening of the involved cortices and a more prompt return to practice and participation. Occasionally, a complete fracture results (Fig. 13.3). Healing of a complete fracture usually takes only 3 to 4 weeks. Massive callous formation can usually be seen on the radiographs, the result of the prior stimulation from the stress fracture.

Stress fractures of the tarsal navicular bone are less common than stress fractures of the metatarsals and can be much more serious (3). If not promptly recognized, nonunions can result and significant degenerative arthrosis of the talonavicular joint is probable. A stress fracture of the tarsal navicular should be strongly suspected when an athlete presents with walking and running pain on the dorsum of the foot in the region of the tarsal navicular bone. If radiographs do not reveal a sagittal line of decreased density, then technetium scintigraphy will certainly display the increased uptake of the radiopharmaceutical so typical of a stress fracture. Successful treatment can be expected by immobilization in a short leg cast or walking boot. Union can be expected in 4 to 6 weeks. If a nonunion is present, however, open reduction and internal fixation are necessary to prevent or minimize the dread complication of talonavicular arthritis.

Although not totally preventable, the approach to preventing the problem of stress fractures of the foot is to ensure a well-designed preseason conditioning schedule so that the athletes are required to run progressively increasing amounts on a firm surface, simulating the basketball court. Not only is their cardiovas-

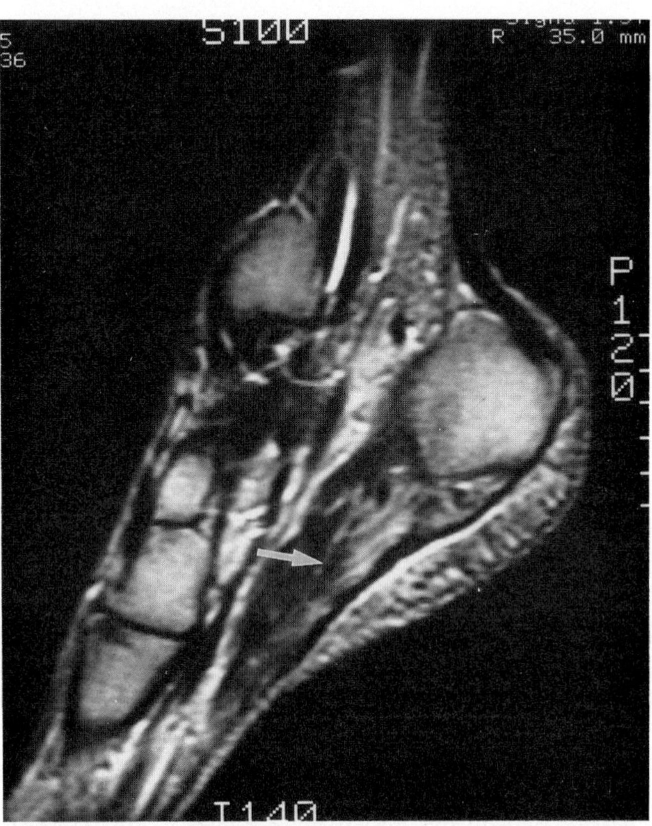

Figure 13.2. Lateral MRI of the right foot of a 22-year-old collegiate basketball player suspected of having an acute tear of the plantar fascia. Note that the plantar fascia (black) is intact but the flexor digitorum brevis muscle demonstrates edema and hemorrhage within its fibers, indicating injury (white). *Arrow* points to area of increased signal density (white) within plantar muscles.

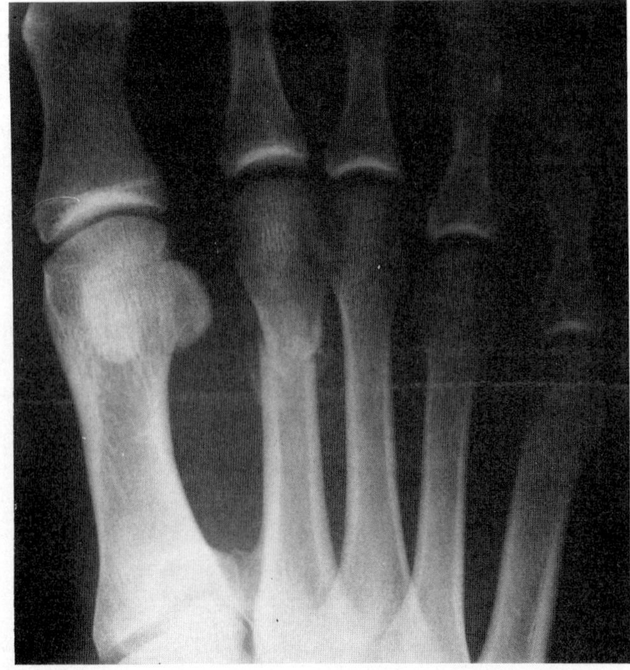

Figure 13.3. AP radiograph demonstrating a complete fracture of the second metatarsal neck at the site of a previous stress fracture. Note the buildup of callus about the fracture site.

cular system conditioned before the preseason practice starts but their skeletal system is also allowed time to strengthen the trabeculae and cortices according to the applied stresses from jumping, rebounding, and running.

Acute fractures of the foot include avulsion fractures of the base of the fifth metatarsal from the pull of the peroneus brevis tendon, fractures of the shafts of the metatarsals from direct and indirect forces, fractures of the neck of the metatarsals, and fractures of the sesamoids of the great toe from hyperextension injuries to the toes or having the foot stepped on by another player (Fig. 13.4). These injuries cannot be anticipated or predicted. Because of the nature of the game, therefore, prevention is impossible. However, prepractice and preparticipation taping of the ankle to minimize inver-

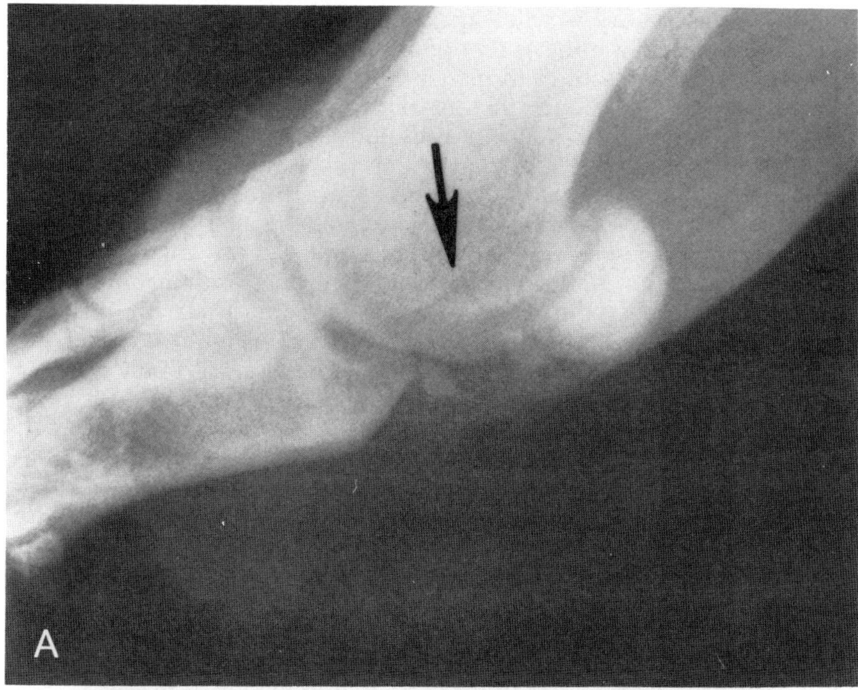

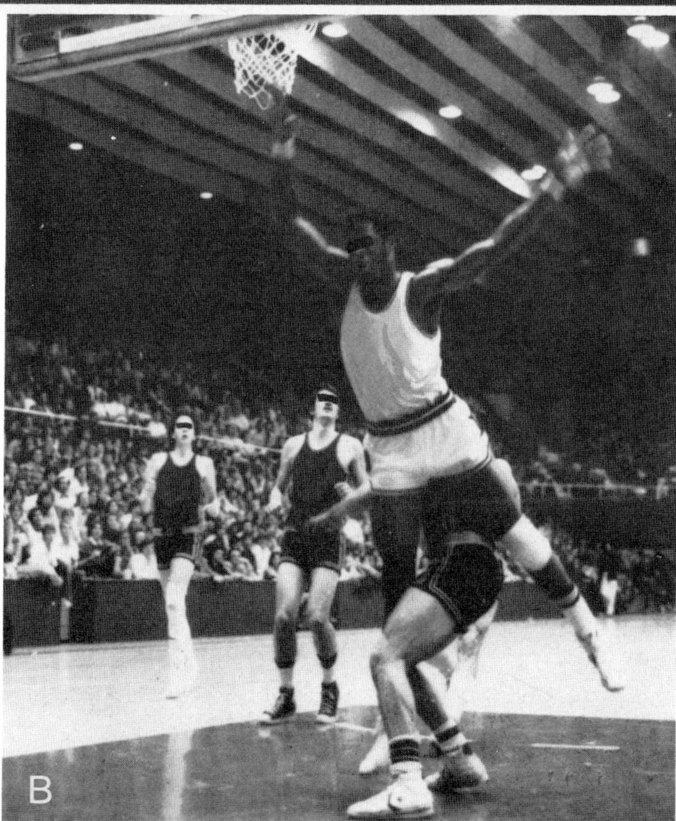

Figure 13.4. A, Lateral radiograph of the right great toe shows a comminuted fracture of the distal portion of the medial sesamoid bone of the great toe. One of the fragments is distracted into the joint *(arrow)*. This injury resulted from a dorsiflexion force to the great toe while the player came down off balance from a rebound. **B.** The mechanism is well-visualized as the player straddling his opponent lands asymmetrically on his right foot.

sion injuries may be of value in decreasing the incidence of avulsion fractures of the base of the fifth metatarsal because this is the result of inversion injury with the foot in the neutral or the dorsiflexed position.

Fractures of the fifth metatarsal distal to the base often result from the inability of the plantar flexed foot to invert at the time of an inversion force to the hindfoot and ankle. It is not unusual for the players to relate a history of prodromal aching in the area of the fracture, which is suggestive of a stress fracture. The superimposed trauma on the already weakened area produces the fracture. This fracture, as well as the other acute injuries of the foot that occur during practice or a game, are painful enough to prevent further competition (Fig. 13.5). The foot should be elevated immediately and ice should be applied to prevent swelling. Crutches will be required for the patient to be transported to the emergency room or an orthopedist's office where roentgenograms can be taken.

If radiographs show signs of chronic stress to the fifth metatarsal in the way of intramedullary sclerosis, then internal fixation with an intramedullary screw and bone grafting often are necessary. However, in the treatment of the acute Jones' fracture with no or little radiographic evidence of a chronic stress situation, immobilization in a short leg cast can produce union (4). If rapid return to participation in expected, then intramedullary screw fixation can permit return as early as 8 to 10 weeks (5).

Ankle

Of all the injuries to the lower extremities in basketball, those of the ankle are the most common. Ankle sprains account for more time lost from basketball practice and games than any other injury. Although this injury is not totally preventable, taping of the ankle before practice and games minimizes the risk of serious sprains and prevents injury altogether in many cases.

Inversion sprains, the most common type of ankle sprain, occur when the ankle is plantar flexed and an inversion force is applied to the foot. Although this can occur while cutting, the most common mechanism of injury is when the player's foot is accidentally placed on another's foot while running or coming down with a rebound. In plantar flexion, the dorsal capsule of the ankle joint, the anterior fibers of the deltoid ligament medially, and the anterior talofibular ligament laterally are under maximum tension. When the limit of excursion of these ligamentous structures is exceeded, tearing of some or all of the fibers results. With inversion, the primary stabilizing ligament of the ankle, the anterior talofibular, is torn. For proper examination of this and other injuries to the foot and ankle, the player's shoes, socks, and tape should be removed, and the player should be taken to the dressing room where a thorough examination can be carried out.

There are three critical parts to the examination. First, the pulses should be palpated and a neurologic examination of the foot and ankle should be done. Although uncommon, stretch palsy of the peroneal nerve can result from traction on the nerve with the plantar flexion and inversion force of the injury. A sensory deficit over the distribution of the superficial and deep peroneal nerves and weakness of the anterior and lateral compartment muscles of the leg should be ruled out. The second critical part of the examination is to palpate the

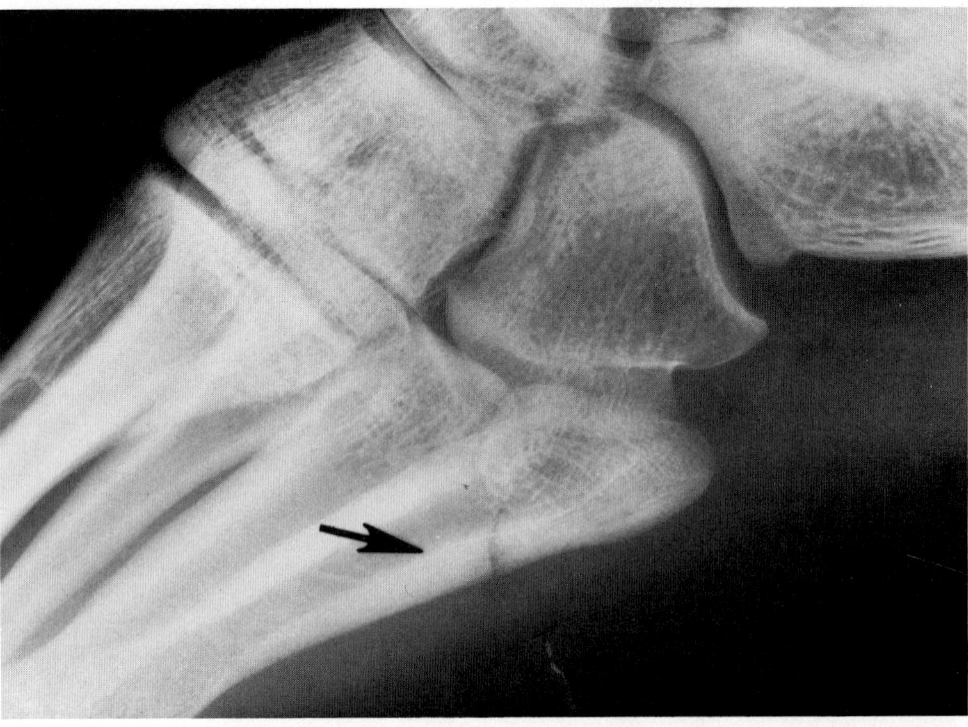

Figure 13.5. Lateral radiograph of the left foot of a college basketball player. Note the fracture through the proximal diaphysis of the fifth metatarsal *(arrow);* this is a slow healing fracture, not an innocuous one.

fibula, medial malleolus, and the other bony prominences about the ankle. If there is tenderness over the bone, then a fracture should be suspected and further diagnostic tests, such as roentgenograms, should be insisted on before permitting the player to resume play. However, if a fracture has been ruled out, ligamentous integrity should be tested. To test for the integrity of the anterior talofibular ligament, the ankle should be slightly plantar flexed to relax the posterior talofibular ligament and capsule, the heel should be cupped in the examiner's hand, with the other hand providing a posterior stabilizing force to the tibia, and anterior subluxation of the talus must be tested by displacing the foot forward. If no anterior subluxation occurs, then the injury to the anterior talofibular ligament is incomplete. If there is a complete tear of the ligament, then the talus can be felt to slide forward and a firm end point will be lacking. A clunk is often felt, and the examiner can see a depression in the skin and soft tissues anterior to the fibula as a result of the separation of the torn soft tissues under the skin in this area.

If the inversion force to the ankle is not dissipated after tearing the anterior talofibular ligament, the calcaneofibular ligament is the next major structure to be torn. The integrity of this particular ligament is difficult to assess by physical examination. Stress inversion roentgenograms of the ankle are usually required. Tilting of the talus in the mortise indicates a tear of the calcaneofibular ligament, in addition to the anterior talofibular ligament.

Major inversion/plantar flexion injuries or sprains often involve the deltoid ligament in addition to the lateral ligamentous tissues. If the predominant force is plantar flexion, then the anterior fibers of the deltoid ligament are stretched or torn and there will be tenderness and swelling in the appropriate area. If the tenderness and swelling is posterior to the medial malleolus, indicating tears of the posterior fibers of the deltoid ligament, this usually indicates that the injury was predominantly an inversion and internal rotation sprain rather than a plantar flexion one. The presence of such medial ligament sprains is simply an indication of the severity of the injury and does not influence treatment or prognosis. Regardless of whether the ankle sprain is a single or double ligament injury, the initial treatment should consist of ice application, a compression dressing to minimize swelling, and the use of some type of rigid support to immobilize the ankle in dorsiflexion. The key to treatment is to maintain the ankle in the dorsiflexed position. This allows coaptation of the torn ends of the ligament. Taping of the ankle or a posterior plaster splint is sufficient initially until roentgenograms can be obtained and a fracture ruled out. Crutches and an elastic bandage are not adequate. An elastic wrap alone does not prevent the foot from dropping back into a plantar flexed position and allowing the torn ends of the ligament to separate.

Syndesmosis sprains of the ankle, as with most injuries occurring on the basketball court, result from close play in and around the basket. With 8 to 10 players fighting for rebounds and jockeying for position for rebounding, falls are not uncommon. Should a player fall or land on the lateral surface of another player's foot and leg, the extremity is forced toward the floor, and eversion and external rotation of the ankle result. Concomitant injury to the medial structures of the knee also may occur. With the foot fixed and with the tibia acting as lever, the stress of the injury is absorbed over the medial aspect of the ankle, tearing the deltoid ligament. The anterior tibiofibular ligament and the interosseous membrane between the tibia and fibula are also torn. This particular sprain, although painful, may seem innocuous at first observation because of the small amount of edema that results. Stress testing, likewise, usually does not reveal an instability. The anterior talofibular ligament is usually not involved, so there is a negative anterior drawer test. Also, it is difficult to detect instability on the medial side of the ankle on physical examination of the syndesmotic sprain. The anterior tibiofibular ligament area is by far the most tender to the palpating finger. Clues to the extent of the syndesmotic sprain can be appreciated by the proximal extent of the tenderness up the interosseous membrane: The farther up the membrane that tenderness is found, the more extensive the injury and the longer it will take for the athlete to return to competition. The more tenderness that is present over the deltoid ligament, the more significant the injury is. Studies have indicated that sprains to the syndesmosis of the ankle take much longer for the athlete to return to competition than inversion sprains (6). Push off and jumping are painful for 6 to 8 weeks. Therefore, comfortable return to play cannot be expected within 4 weeks.

Taping, the liberal use of ice massage to the involved area, and encouragement to walk unaided seem to promote a more rapid return to practice than rigid immobilization. The same emergency and first aid treatment should be provided for this sprain as that provided for inversion sprains. Roentgenograms of the ankle should be obtained after initial application of ice and splinting.

The more serious injuries that result from external rotation and eversion of the ankle are fractures of the distal fibula above the anterior tibiofibular ligament, avulsion fractures of the medial malleolus, and an avulsion fracture of the posterior lip of the tibia. With these injuries, deformity is usually present and roentgenograms are required to determine the exact extent of injury. Ice, elevation, and splinting are effective first aid measures. The goal of treatment, whether it be by external immobilization or by open reduction and internal fixation, is to restore normal anatomic realignment to the ligaments and skeletal structures of the ankle.

Inversion injuries to the ankle and foot that occur when the foot is in a neutral or dorsiflexed position can produce a subtalar dislocation or an isolated tear of the calcaneofibular ligament with instability of the subtalar joint (Fig. 13.6). With subtalar dislocation, gross deformity is obvious and immediate transportation to the emergency room for roentgenographic evaluation and reduction is mandatory. The usual first aid measures should be applied on the side of the basketball court and the player transported immediately.

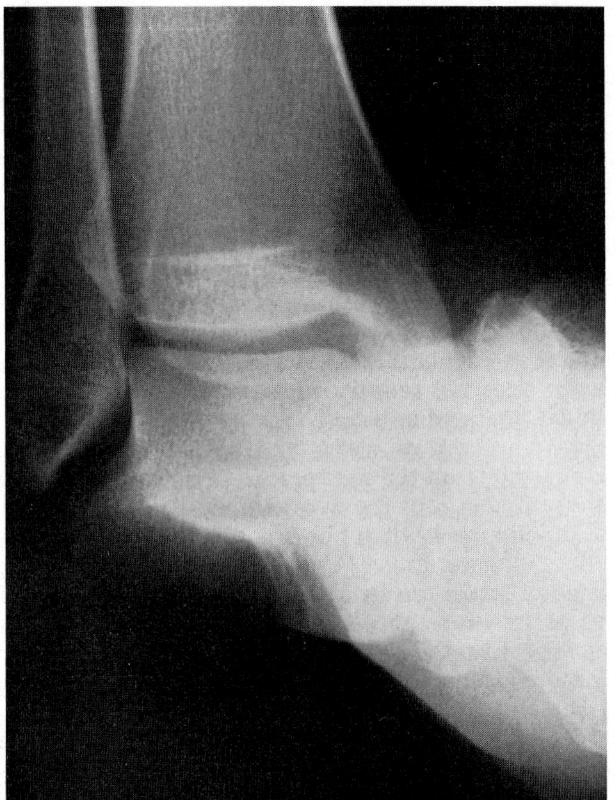

Figure 13.6. AP radiograph of the right ankle of a college basketball player showing complete medial subtalar dislocation.

Following plantar flexion/inversion ankle sprains, chronic, persistent lateral ankle discomfort occasionally is seen. Splitting of the peroneal tendons, usually the longus, occasionally occurs at the time of the original ankle sprain. Persistent popping and retrofibular swelling and pain are indicative signs of this malady. On physical examination of the involved ankle, recurrent popping can be elicited by circumducting the foot and ankle. When the ankle and foot are inverted and the foot is plantar flexed approximately 20°, the split peroneal tendon permits the other tendon to pop into the split, producing the discomfort and the popping noise. A chronic peroneal tenosynovitis almost always accompanies the split tendon. This syndrome should not be confused with anterior subluxation of the peroneal tendon that occurs when the foot is dorsiflexed in contrast to the popping of the split peroneal tendon that occurs in plantar flexion. Surgical repair of the longitudinal split offers correction of the problem (7).

Permanent laxity and incompetency of a stretched-out anterior talofibular ligament occasionally results from a plantar flexion inversion injury. This permits slight anterior extrusion of the talus on dorsiflexion of the ankle. This may cause abrasion or impingement of the anterolateral dome of the talus against the inferior fascicle of the anterior tibiofibular ligament, producing pain and synovitis. Simple resection of the inferior fibers of the anterior tibiofibular ligament fibers will correct the situation (8). This should not be confused with the formation of painful fibrous tissue and scar within the lateral compartment of the ankle joint following ankle sprain. This condition also produces anterolateral ankle pain. Relief of symptoms can be achieved by arthroscopic resection of the fibrous tissue lying along the lateral facet of the talus just anterior to the fibula.

Another cause for persistent symptoms following a plantar flexion inversion sprain is the presence of a chondral fracture of the dome of the talus or a deep bone bruise of the talus and/or tibial plafond. This latter condition, of course, can be appreciated only with magnetic resonance imaging as shown in Figure 13.7. When osteochondral or chondral fragments are free within the joint in the anterior compartment, they easily can be retrieved arthroscopically. Fragments in the posterior compartment of the ankle occasionally cannot be retrieved arthroscopically, and therefore, open surgery is required. A simple posteromedial approach through the posterior tibial tendon sheath exposes approximately 50% of the posterior aspect of the ankle and gives easy access for retrieval of loose bodies in the posterior compartment (9). When a deep bone bruise of the talus or the tibia is seen with magnetic resonance imaging, there is little that can be done other than having the athlete rest the ankle. These fractures usually heal within 2 to 3 months, and no long-term sequelae have been noted.

Leg

Stress fractures of the tibia and fibula, compartment syndromes, muscle and tendon tears, and fascial defects with muscle herniation can all produce chronic discomfort of the leg in basketball players. Because all these conditions can be disabling and prevent high-level performance, accurate diagnosis is essential. Although

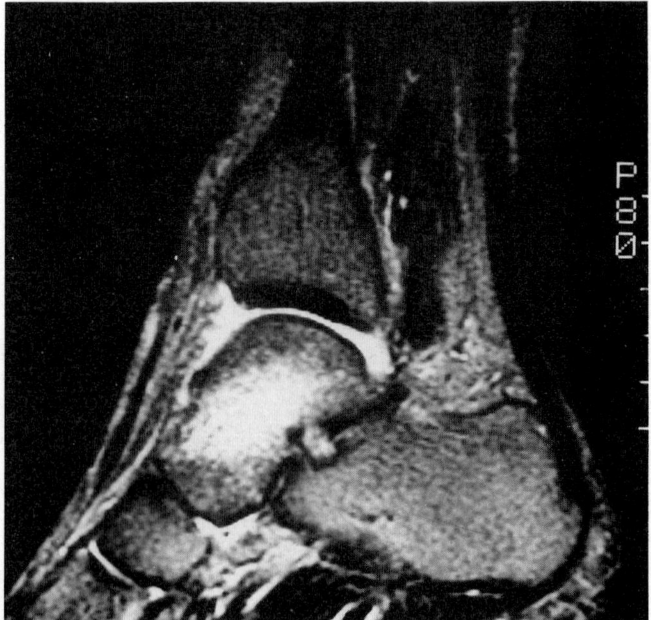

Figure 13.7. MRI of the ankle of a female basketball player who had sustained a severe plantar flexion/inversion ankle sprain 3 weeks previously. Note the effusion (white). Of special note is the increased signal within the body and neck of the talus (white).

these conditions are all commonly assigned the diagnosis of "shin splint," they are distinctly separate entities and respond to distinctly different therapies.

Stress fractures of the tibia and fibula produce a chronic pain, made worse with activity. There may be a painful swelling over the bone; they always produce tenderness to palpation. Early in the onset of the condition, this may be the only positive finding. Although roentgenograms may not demonstrate subperiosteal new bone for 3 to 5 weeks after onset, a bone scan will yield an area of increased uptake. Treatment depends on the intensity of the pain, but the general format of exercise permitted is similar to that prescribed for treatment of stress fractures of the foot. That is, the athlete is allowed to run, always with a soft insert in the shoe, until a threshold of pain is reached. The patient should be requested to run daily, thereby applying relentless stress to the healing stress fracture, stimulating more rapid union and resolution of symptoms.

Exercise produces a physiologic rise of pressure in the compartments of the leg, which promptly returns to normal when the muscles are allowed to rest. When pressure is abnormally high or when the decay of the elevated pressure is abnormally slow, ischemic pain results. The pain is usually localized to one or more of the compartments of the leg, depending on which ones are involved. On physical examination, there is usually some degree of tenderness to firm digital palpation over the involved compartment. Therefore, physically palpating the area of involved pain will usually help differentiate the tenderness of a stress fracture of the tibia from the tenderness of deep posterior compartment syndrome. When a compartment syndrome is suspected, the diagnosis can be confirmed by the absence of increased uptake of technetium on a bone scan and by a measurement of the intracompartment barometric pressures. Correction of a compartment syndrome can usually be achieved by surgical decompression of the compartment by release of the investing layer of fascia of the compartment involved (see Chapter 54).

A defect in the external investing crural fascia with resultant muscle herniation produces a localized area of tenderness at the site of the defect. Although chronic aching in the region of the defect is experienced, the pain usually disappears promptly with rest. Although this can be confused with a compartment syndrome, the presence of tenderness over the fascial defect, the presence of a small bulge at the site of pain that represents a herniation of muscle and the palpable hole or defect in the fascia confirm the diagnosis. Circumferential taping or elastic compression may be of value but usually does not prevent muscle herniation when exercise is resumed. For some reason, surgical closure of the defect usually does not relieve the symptoms. Therefore, the surgical enlargement of the defect, which eliminates the small hole through which the muscle can herniate, is the treatment of choice.

Acute tears at the musculotendinous junction of the gastrocnemius produce a sudden catastrophic sensation to the basketball player, and pain is usually so severe that continuation of play is not possible. Ice to control swelling, a short leg cast to immobilize the tear and 2 to 3 weeks of rest will usually allow firm healing of the tear and permit return to basketball playing. However, a tear of the Achilles tendon itself is a more serious affliction that requires more aggressive therapy and a more prolonged recovery and rehabilitation (see Chapter 54).

Partial rupture of the Achilles tendon is common to athletes in many sports that require a lot of running (10). It produces the syndrome known as Achilles tendinitis. Because the athlete does not have much pain with the initial partial tear, he or she continues to play and firm fibrous healing does not occur. Minor discomfort is experienced initially, but the pain gradually gets worse. Rest is the immediate treatment of choice. Because the pain is experienced predominantly while playing basketball, immobilization in a cast is of no more value than to discontinue basketball playing only; 3 to 6 weeks of not jumping and the elimination of rapid acceleration and deceleration will permit healing.

Complete rupture of the Achilles tendon, on the other hand, requires immobilization in a short leg cast or posterior splint until the decision is made to treat the player definitively. A decision must be made whether to treat the rupture conservatively in a long leg cast with the foot in plantar flexion or to repair surgically the ruptured tendon (see Chapter 54).

Knee

Acute knee injuries in basketball are, fortunately, rare. Although the knee is exposed to the trauma of twisting and collision, incidence of injury is low. Injuries result from other players falling on the athlete's leg or coming down from a jump off balance. Tears of the anterior cruciate ligament, various capsular ligaments, and the menisci can result. When a player describes hearing a pop, a tear of the anterior cruciate ligament should be strongly suspected. A rapidly developing hemarthrosis should alert one to a tear of the anterior cruciate ligament as well as subluxation of the patella with or without osteochondral fracture. First-aid measures such as the application of ice and splinting of the extremity should be done to alleviate pain.

One should be cautious about the injudicious use of ice around the knee, particularly on the lateral side where the peroneal nerve is susceptible to injury from the excessive use of ice. Cryotherapy-induced nerve injury is now a well-recognized entity (11). When applying ice, always consider the location of the major peripheral nerves, the thickness of the overlying subcutaneous fat and the duration of tissue cooling, which should be less than 20 min.

The immediate examination of the knee, before swelling and muscle guarding has developed, is desirable. Look for instabilities of the extensor mechanism of the knee to rule out subluxation of the patella as well as instabilities resulting from injuries to the joint capsule and cruciate ligaments. When instabilities are found or suspected (see Chapter 53) further examination, e.g., under general anesthesia and arthroscopy, is indicated.

Of note is the fact that a high prevalence of noncontact anterior cruciate ligament (ACL) injuries in intercollegiate women basketball players has been observed. Data collected from 29 Division 1 NCAA institutions (from the Atlantic Coast, Big Ten, and Pacific Ten Conferences) have indicated that women basketball players in these conferences were eight times more likely to sustain an ACL injury than their male counterparts. Multiple factors are responsible for this gender difference, including an increase in hamstring flexibility and a decrease in hamstring strength among women and possibly the level or pattern of training techniques (12).

A common painful problem among basketball players is that of "jumper's knee" (13–15). This is caused by a partial tear of the patellar tendon, usually just inferior to the lower pole of the patella. However, it can be seen at its insertion on the tibial tubercle or above the patella in the extensor tendon of the knee. In younger boys and girls, it may manifest itself as Osgood-Schlatter disease or Sinding-Larsen disease. It almost always affects the jump leg, i.e., for right-handed athletes, it affects the left leg. The rapid acceleration and deceleration required in basketball produces repetitive traction on the tendon (Fig. 13.8). When a microscopic or partial tear of the tendon occurs, it usually is insignificant initially, so the athlete continues to play, and his or her symptoms become chronic. Attempts at healing the tear are thereby prevented, resulting in mucoid degeneration or painful scarring.

Examination usually reveals local tenderness, which might be very sensitive, over the patellar tendon just inferior to the patella. It is most easily elicited with the knee in extension and the extensor mechanism relaxed. Tears are always deep within the tendon; therefore, no defects can be felt in the tendon. Minor swelling may be palpable in chronic cases.

Nonsteroidal antiinflammatory agents and icing of the tendon before and after practice and games are of some benefit. In the acute case, one that has been present for less than 3 or 4 months, rest usually is the treatment of choice. In cases for which symptoms have been present for more than 6 months, rest gives relief but once the athlete returns to competition, symptoms usually recur. In chronic cases, when pain is severe enough to limit playing time or to decrease the athlete's efficiency, excision of the scar under local anesthesia usually brings relief.

Sudden deceleration also can produce complete tears of the extensor mechanism, fractures of the upper tibial epiphyses in growing boys and girls, fractures of the inferior pole of the patellae (16), and fractures involving the upper tibia. Some of these are intraarticular (Fig. 13.9). In many cases of fracture or complete rupture there has been a prodromal history of aching about the extensor mechanism, either involving the tibial tuberosity, lower end of the patella, or the patellar tendon.

Another painful condition occasionally affecting the extensor mechanism of the knee in basketball players is that of bipartite patella (17). This produces a chronic recurring pain over the lateral aspect of the patellofemoral joint associated with acceleration and deceleration. Ice before and after practice and NSAIDs may be of benefit. Usually, in the more chronic recalcitrant cases, excision of the separate fragment is needed to obtain permanent relief of symptoms (Fig. 13.10).

Muscle contusions of the thigh are frequent in basketball (18). The thigh is unprotected and is exposed to being struck by other players' knees. A painful hematoma or "charley horse" can result (Fig. 13.11). Initial treatment should consist of the application of ice. Mild compression with an elastic bandage also is of benefit. No heat, forceful stretching, or exercise should be attempted. Massage also should be avoided. Heat, massage, and stretching all tend to aggravate pain, increase blood flow, and may result in myositis ossificans (Fig. 13.12). The treatment of choice is application of ice over the involved area, daily treatment with continuous passive motion machine, and avoidance of further injury. Once pain has been relieved and the player has a full range of motion of the knee, then running, weight lifting, and resumption of basketball can be permitted.

Hip

Injuries about the hip are unusual in basketball players. In the immature athlete avulsion of the lesser trochanter, anterior superior iliac spine, and other epiphyseal growth centers can occur with violent rebounding or deceleration, but these are unusual. Sudden pain about the groin or pelvis should alert one to the possibility. Rest, the use of crutches to minimize pain, and application of cold compresses should be used until roentgenograms can be obtained. Return to basketball is permitted once roentgenograms show union of the displaced epiphysis or symptoms permit.

Although rare, the formation of traumatic bursae over the greater trochanter of the hips have been seen. This injury results from repeated trauma over the lateral aspect of the hip from diving after loose balls on the basketball court. Initially, a hematoma formation is seen. This is associated with tenderness and some discomfort on motion of the hip. The application of ice is beneficial in resolving the discomfort and hematoma formation. With repeated trauma, however, the bursa fills with fluid and occasionally there are round, firm, tender, marble-like masses formed within the confines of the bursa sac. Even light contact with the inflamed bursa is painful, and permanent relief is obtained only by removal of the round masses of infarcted, necrotic fat. This can be done easily under local anesthesia as an outpatient.

Inguinal pain also is occasionally seen in basketball players, the result of inguinal hernias or pubalgia. The cause of the pain may be difficult to diagnose, and other conditions such as osteitis pubis or genitourinary afflictions should be ruled out. An incompetent abdominal wall in the groin and/or a detectible inguinal hernia are the most common causes for the pubic pain. Surgical correction usually yields excellent results (19).

Chest

Serious injury to the chest wall in basketball is uncommon. Contusions are common and usually result

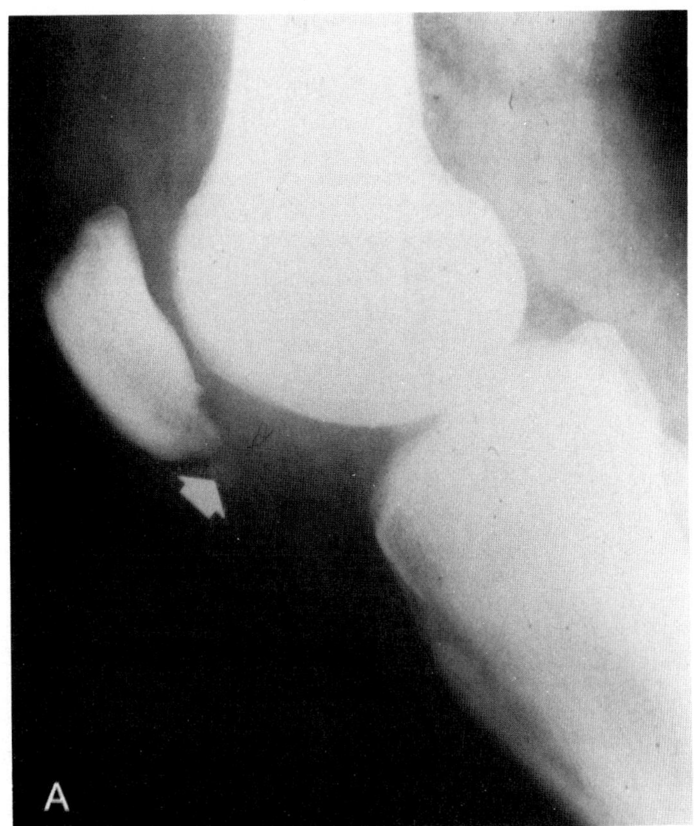

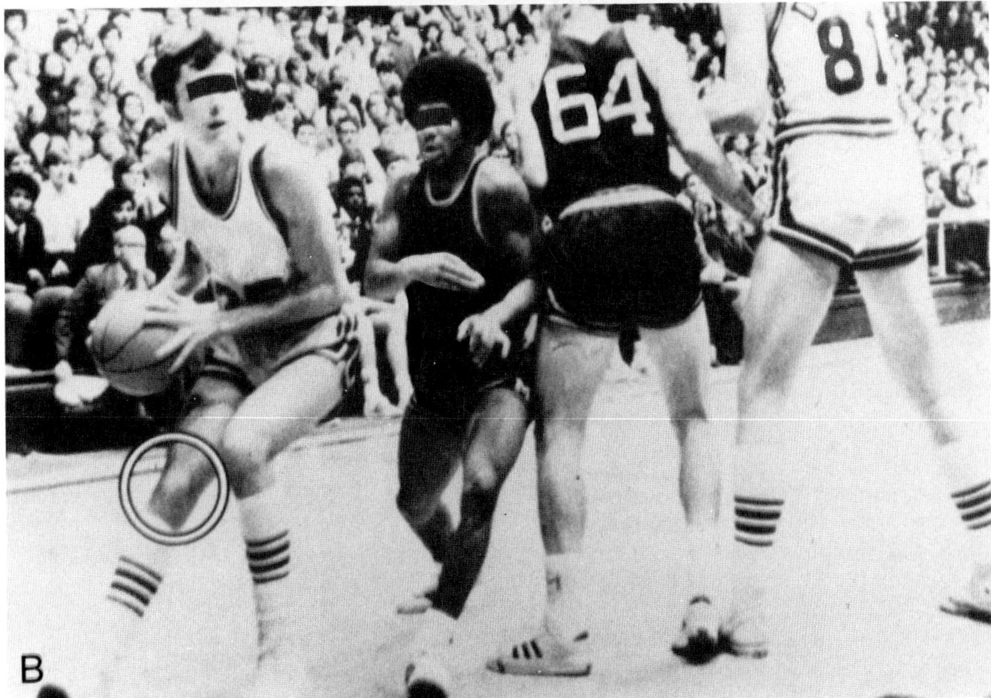

Figure 13.8. **A,** Lateral radiograph of the knee of a professional basketball player with symptoms of jumper's knee of 3 years' duration. Note the area of increased density within the patellar tendon distal to the patella *(arrow).* This represents a focus of cartilaginous metaplasia from a long-standing tear in the patellar tendon. **B,** A basketball player is seen trying to stop suddenly. Such a forceful overload of the extensor mechanism may produce focal partial rupture of the patellar tendon just inferior to the patella. It is important to note that this player is left-handed.

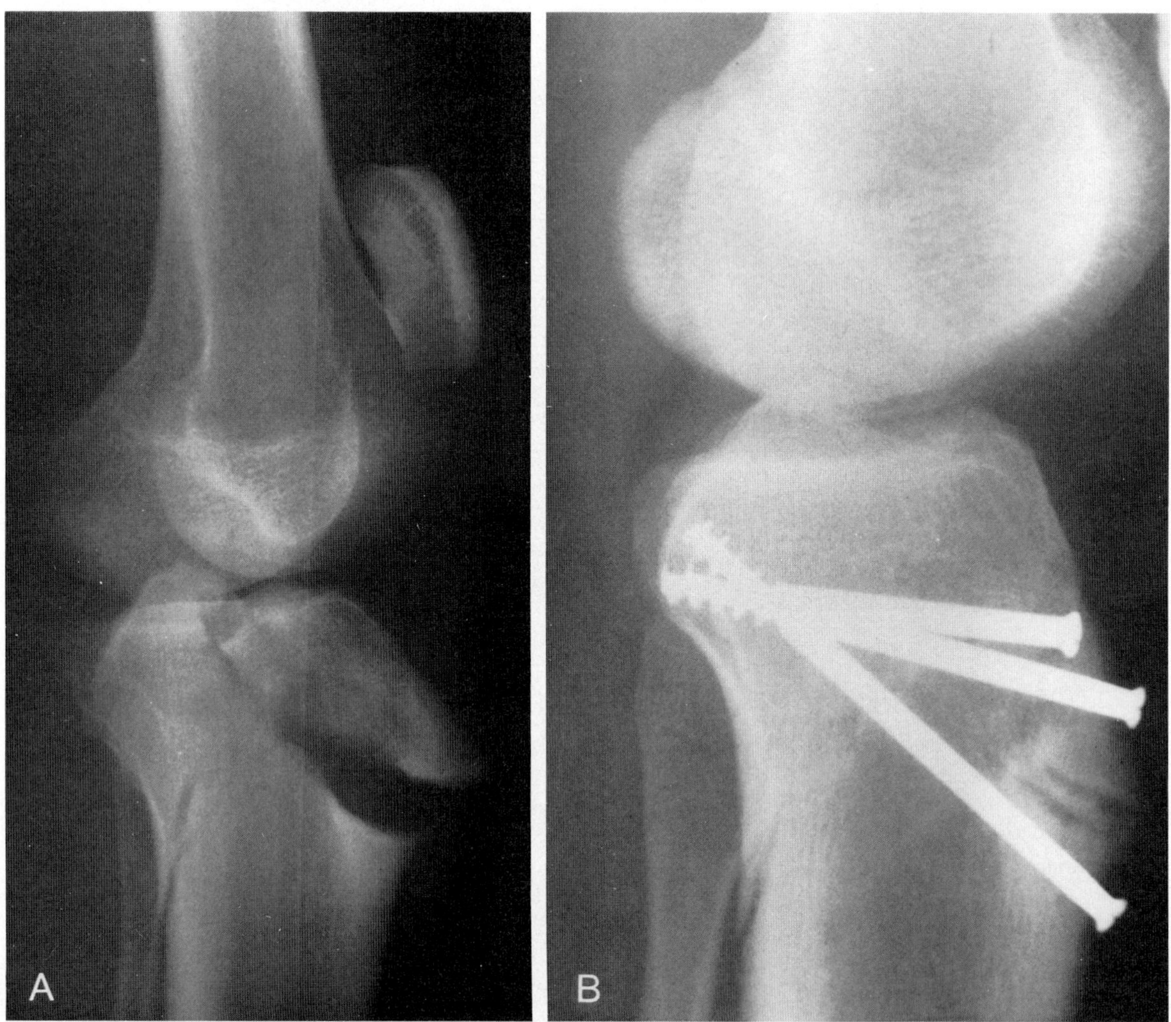

Figure 13.9. A, Lateral radiograph of a 22-year-old basketball player. Note the comminuted fracture of the upper tibia and the proximal displacement of the patella. This was caused by coming down with a rebound and landing on only the ipsilateral foot. This player had noted chronic aching in the region of the tibial tuberosity for 2 to 3 months before the fracture. **B,** Lateral radiograph of the same knee after open reduction and internal fixation. Note the area of cortical thickening with lines of decreased density in the tibial tuberosity, suggesting a preinjury fatigue fracture.

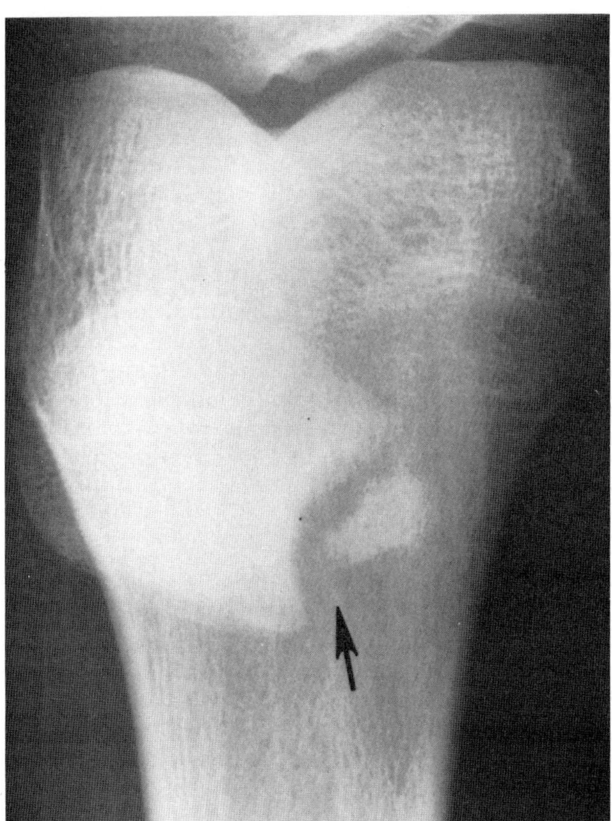

Figure 13.10. AP radiograph of a college basketball player who complained of pain over the lateral patellofemoral joint. The *arrow* is pointing to the symptomatic bipartite patella.

from another player striking the athlete with the elbow. Under the basket, when rebounding players are trying to prevent a member of the other team from grappling the ball away, a trained or reflex jerking of the elbows in a violent manner occurs. Fortunately, the elbows usually are not injured. When this injury occurs to the breast of a female basketball player, pain is usually severe for a short period of time. If any swelling or hematoma formation results, cold compresses and brief periods of ice application should be used. If severe, then a gynecologist should be consulted.

A good supporting brassiere is usually all that is needed to prevent breast injury in women basketball players. Stretching of the breast tissue and injury to the breasts are rare.

Hand

Of the injuries to the upper extremities in basketball, those to the hand are the most frequent. Of these, the most common are jammed fingers or sprains of the interphalangeal joints. These usually result from the basketball striking the tip of the finger. In contrast to finger injuries in baseball and softball where the energy is absorbed at the distal interphalangeal joint, in basketball the energy is transmitted to the proximal joint, which is where most of the sprains occur. Such injuries can produce tears of the collateral ligament or volar capsule, depending on the direction of force. Complete tearing of the collateral ligaments, with instability, is unusual as is dislocation of the joint, but these injuries

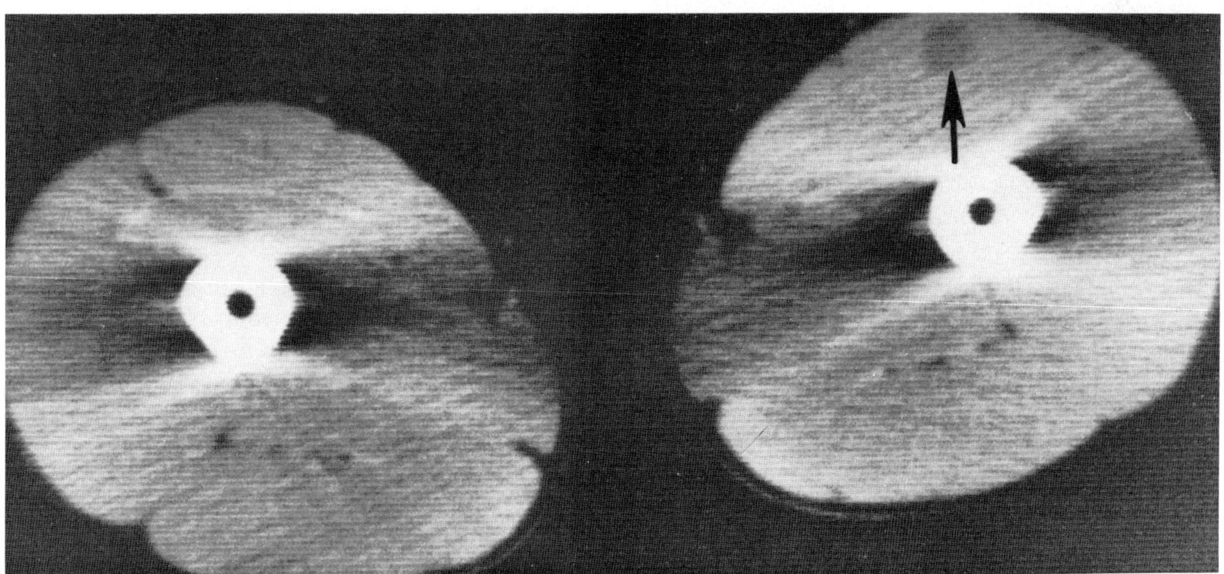

Figure 13.11. Computerized axial tomogram at the midthigh level of a college basketball player who had received a direct blow to the anterior thigh 2 weeks previously. The area of low density *(arrow)* in the right rectus femoris muscle represents an old intramuscular hematoma.

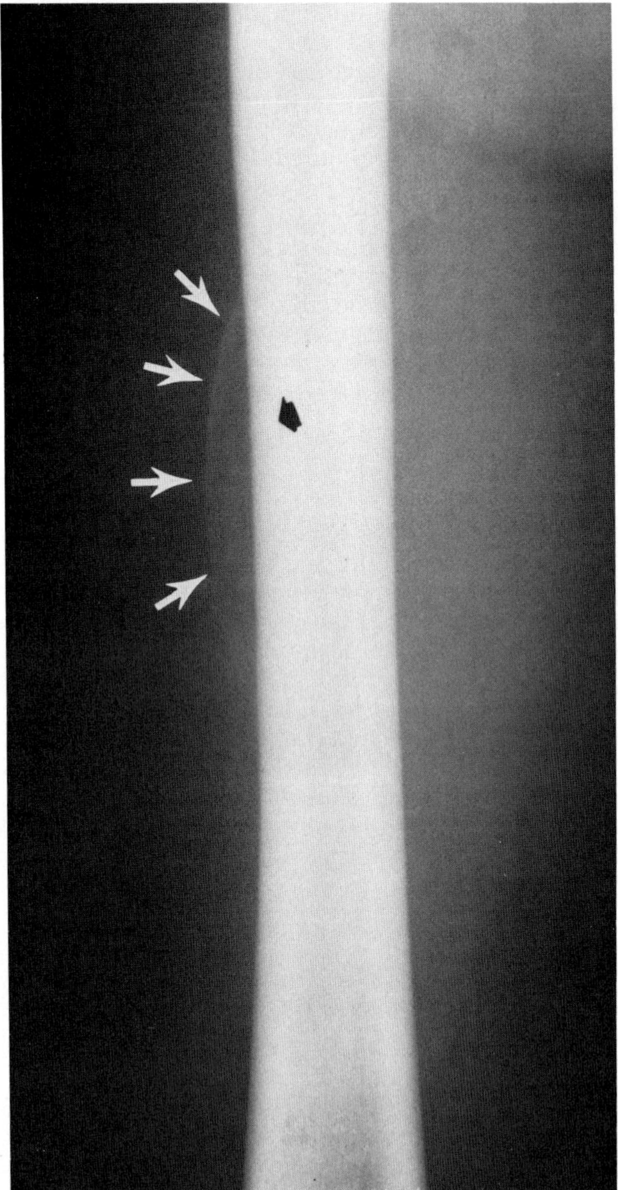

Figure 13.12. AP radiograph of the right thigh of a high school basketball player. He had received a direct blow to the thigh 3 weeks previously. He had only 60° flexion of the knee caused by a myositis ossificans *(arrows)*. He was treated initially with local heat and massage.

can occur. When initially seen, the joint should be tested for stability in all directions, and function of the flexor and extensor tendons should be checked to rule out rupture of either. Icing and aluminum splinting comprise the treatment of choice initially. Roentgenograms should be obtained to rule out a fracture of one of the condyles or avulsion of a small fragment of bone with the volar plate.

Splinting of the digit in slight flexion is occasionally necessary, until pain permits resumption of basketball. Usually, the finger can be taped to the adjacent one for splinting purposes and active motion can be permitted. When fractures are present, additional treatment may be necessary, depending on whether the fragment is displaced or reduction is required (see Chapter 52).

Dislocations of the interphalangeal joint usually result from hyperextension. The diagnosis can be made immediately by the typical deformity of the dorsal step-off at the proximal interphalangeal joint, with the middle phalanx being situated dorsally relative to the proximal phalanx. It is usually safe to attempt immediate reduction of the dislocation by gentle traction on the digit. Once length of the two involved phalanges has been achieved, then flexion at the proximal joint will produce a stable reduction. Roentgenograms are indicated to rule out a fracture at the proximal joint level, and splinting of the digit in flexion is indicated for 1 week to 10 days. When soreness permits, return to basketball is possible by taping the digit to the adjacent one for splint purposes.

Wrist

Injuries to the wrist in basketball players are almost always the result of falling on the outstretched hand. Being undercut while in the air rebounding or shooting can cause the player to land with all his or her force on the outstretched hand, which is the most common cause for injury. In the growing child, a fracture-separation of the distal radial epiphysis is the most common injury. In the mature athlete, a Colles fracture results. If the force is of major proportion, transscaphoid-perilunar dislocations have been seen (Fig. 13.13).

Regardless of the wrist injury, immediate splinting and application of ice are indicated. To assess the extent of injury, the patient should be taken as soon as possible to the emergency room for roentgenograms. Appropriate treatment should be carried out at the earliest convenience, whether it be closed reduction or open reduction and internal fixation (see Chapter 52).

Elbow and Arm

Injuries to the elbow and shoulder are rare in basketball. Falling on the elbow can produce a traumatic olecranon bursitis, which responds promptly to ice and NSAIDs. Fractures of the radial head have been seen, but these are rare. They usually result from running into a wall or a backboard following a lay-up or fast break. If no deformity is present, first aid treatment usually includes the use of a sling or posterior splint for the elbow and ice applications to minimize swelling. If the physical examination reveals tenderness over the radial head or olecranon, roentgenograms should be obtained as soon as possible to rule out a fracture.

Head and Neck

Head and neck injuries are usually the result of falling on the hardwood floor when undercut while rebounding or colliding with the backboard while attempting to block a shot or slam-dunk the basketball. Scalp lacerations and lacerations of the forehead are the most common injuries. If a player is rendered unconscious, a complete neurologic examination and skull roentgenogram are indicated (see Chapter 45). The first

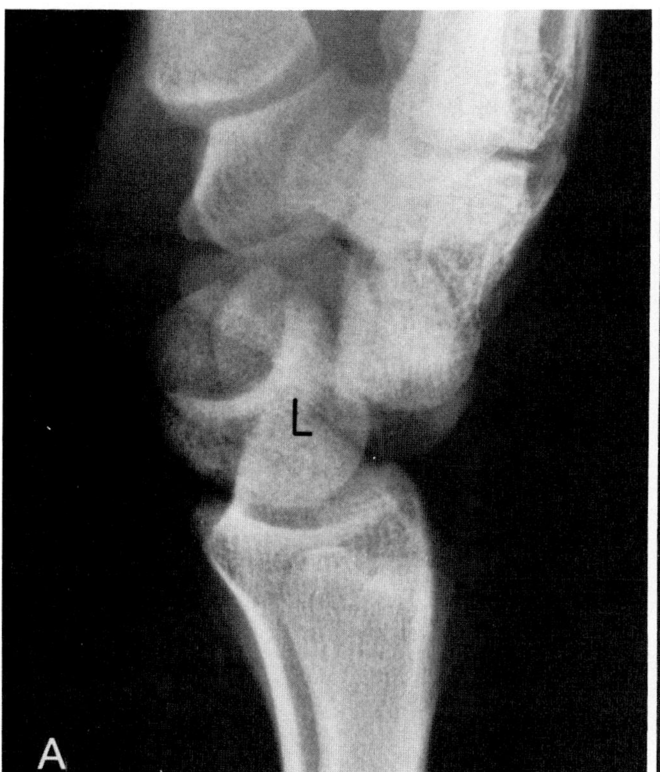

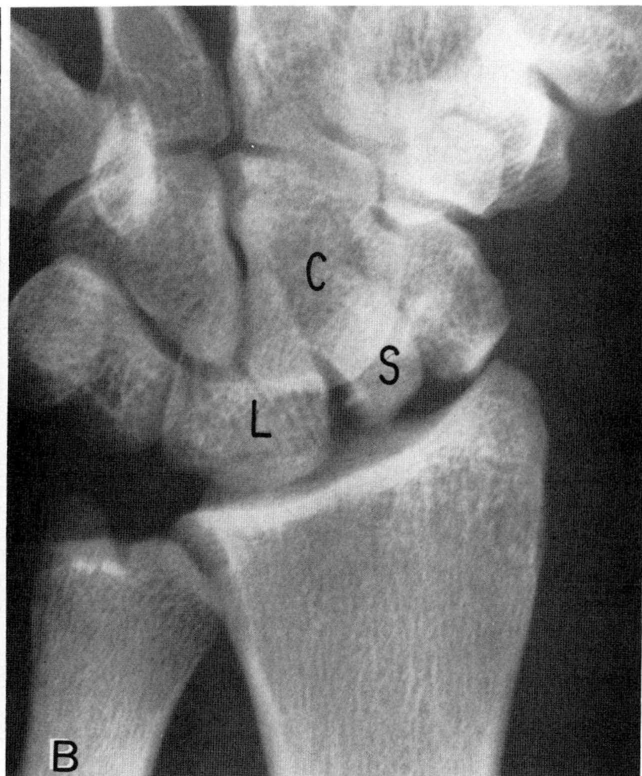

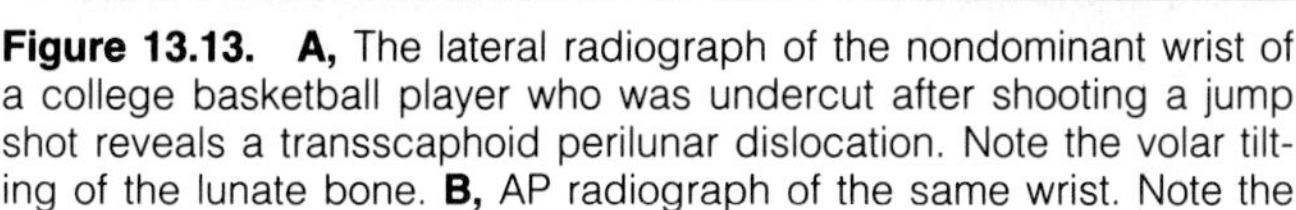

Figure 13.13. **A,** The lateral radiograph of the nondominant wrist of a college basketball player who was undercut after shooting a jump shot reveals a transscaphoid perilunar dislocation. Note the volar tilting of the lunate bone. **B,** AP radiograph of the same wrist. Note the fracture through the waist of the scaphoid *(S)* with rotation of the proximal fragment and the dissociation between the capitate *(C)* and the lunate *(L)*.

aid treatment of scalp lacerations is the same as for lacerations anywhere. Compression dressings to stop bleeding and primary wound closure is indicated at the earliest convenient time.

Maxillofacial injury and injuries to the teeth and lips are common and the result of colliding with other players or being hit by other players' elbows. They make up between 5% and 10% of all the injuries seen in basketball players. Appropriate radiographs and treatment to local wounds should be instituted as soon after the injury as possible.

Fractures of the nose are not rare. They usually result from collisions with another player's head or from being struck on the nose by another player's elbow. The only sign of a fracture initially may be bleeding from the nose. Once this has been controlled by applying ice to the nose and from pressure, the nose should be examined for crepitus or deformity. The nosebleed can usually be effectively controlled by placing a roll of soft material, such as a dental roll, between the front lip and the upper central teeth and having the injured player tighten the lips over it. This applies compression to the majority of the vessels supplying the mucosa of the nose. Occasionally, this does not stop the bleeding completely. Cotton swabs soaked with Adrenalin 1:1000 concentration can be placed up the nose. This causes local vasoconstriction and is of benefit in recalcitrant nosebleeds. Once the bleeding is stopped, palpation over the bridge of the nose should be carried out to check for crepitus or deformity, either of which will indicate a fracture. Roentgenograms of the nose should be obtained and appropriate therapy carried out.

Contact Lenses

With the advent of the soft contact lenses, the risk of eye injury in basketball players having to wear glasses is generally reduced. Hard lenses can result in injury if the eye is struck but very few players wear these at the present time. Soft lenses stay in better (and delay of game from 10 players, 2 referees, and 2 coaches crawling around the floor looking for extruded hard lenses has been greatly diminished), they are less likely to cause injury and are far safer than glasses (see Chapter 47).

Conclusions

Although this chapter has discussed basketball injuries—some serious but most of which are relatively minor—according to anatomic regions, it should be stressed that basketball players are usually in excellent physical condition and have unusually gifted neuromuscular control of their bodies. By their skill, the close scrutiny of officials, and the expertise of the coaches, injuries are kept to a minimum. A preseason conditioning program and proper coaching in regard to physical skills of basketball, particularly for the clumsy and uncoordinated player, also protect against injury. When a player becomes fatigued, he or she should be permitted to rest by substitution. Tired players are more easily hurt than fresh ones.

REFERENCES

1. Bassett FH III. Dislocations of the tarsometatarsal joints. South Med J 1964;57:1294–1302.
2. Gross TS, Bunch RP. A mechanical model of metatarsal stress fracture during distance running. Am J Sports Med 1989;17:669–674.
3. Torg JS, Pavlov H, Cooley LH, et al. Stress fractures of the tarsal navicular—a retrospective review of twenty-one cases. J Bone Joint Surg 1982;64:700–712.
4. Zogby RG, Baker BE. A review of nonoperative treatment of Jones' fracture. Am J Sports Med 1987;15:304–307.
5. DeLee JC, Evans JP, Julian J. Stress fracture of the fifth metatarsal. Am J Sports Med 1983;11:349–353.
6. Taylor DC, Engelhardt DL, Bassett FH III. Syndesmosis sprains of the ankle—the influence of heterotopic ossification. Am J Sports Med 1992;20:146–150.
7. Bassett FH III, Speer KP. Longitudinal rupture of the peroneal tendons. Am J Sports Med 1993;21:354–357.
8. Bassett FH III, Gates HS III, Billys JB, Morris HB, Nikolaou PK. Talar impingement by the anteroinferior tibiofibular ligament—cause of chronic pain in the ankle after inversion sprain. J Bone Joint Surg 1990;72:55–59.
9. Bassett FH III, Billys JB, Gates HS III. A simple surgical approach to the posteromedial ankle. Am J Sports Med 1993;21:144–146.
10. Clancy WG, Neidhart D, Brand RL. Achilles tendinitis in runners: a report of five cases. Am J Sports Med 1976;4:46–57.
11. Bassett FH III, Kirkpatrick JS, Engelhardt DL, Malone TR. Cryotherapy-induced nerve injury. Am J Sports Med 1992;20:516–518.
12. Malone TR, Hardaker WT, Garrett WE, Feagin JA, Bassett FH III. Relationship of gender to anterior cruciate ligament injuries in intercollegiate basketball players. J South Orthop Assoc 1993;2:36–39.
13. Bassett FH III, Soucacos PN, Carr WA. Jumper's knee: Patellar tendinitis and patellar tendon rupture. In: Funk FJ, Jr, ed. Symposium on the athlete's knee. St. Louis: CV Mosby, 1978:96–106.
14. Blazina ME, Kerlan R, Jobe F, Carter V, Carlson G. Jumper's knee. Orthop Clin North Am Rev 1973;4:655–678.
15. Colosimo, AJ, Bassett FH III. Jumper's knee—diagnosis and treatment. Orthop Rev 1990;19:139–149.
16. Tibone JE, Lombardo SJ. Bilateral fractures of the inferior poles of the patella in a basketball player. Am J Sports Med 1981;9:215–216.
17. Weaver JK. Bipartite patellae is a cause of disability in the athlete. Am J Sports Med 1977;5:137–143.
18. Peterson TR. Injuries to the anterior thigh region. In: Funk FJ, Jr, ed. Symposium on the athlete's knee. St. Louis: CV Mosby, 1978:78–95.
19. Taylor DC, Meyers WC, Moylan JA, Lohnes J, Bassett FH III, Garrett WE. Abdominal musculature abnormalities as a cause of groin pain in athletes—inguinal hernias and pubalgia. Am J Sports Med 1991;19:239–242.

14 / BICYCLING

Jack Harvey and Shawn Wotowey

Introduction

The medical care of bicycle racers and recreational riders is not a new topic. Bicycle racing was extremely popular at the turn of the century. Since then there has been a gradual increase in popularity of bicycling, and, recently, recreational, fitness, and competitive use of the bicycle has grown rapidly. With the increasing popularity of the bicycle, the sports medicine physician has been confronted with a "rash" of cycling injuries. Some of these injuries are not unique to cycling. Fractured clavicles and closed head injuries occur in almost epidemic proportions. Other injuries, such as abrasions, affectionately termed "road rash," cover more extensive areas of the anatomy than is seen in other sports. Some injuries, such as saddle sores and nerve palsies of the hand, do seem to be unique to cyclists.

With an increasing interest in fitness, riders participate in training programs that are more intense and more frequent and call for more mileage. This trend has increased the appearance of a variety of overuse injuries. Metabolic problems with body temperature control, dehydration, hypoglycemia, and electrolyte imbalance are seen in citizen races and tours, as well as in stage races and in iron man length triathalons.

The recent popularity of the mountain bike has given cyclists the opportunity to experience a whole new variety of both acute traumatic and overuse injuries. Falls on technical terrain, poor landings on jumps with a trajectory that is too high (too much air), and kamikaze-style descents produce lacerations, concussions, and fractures—care of which is complicated by the remote areas in which they occur.

Knowledge of the technical aspects of cycling and familiarity with the injuries of cyclists will assist the sports medicine physician in effectively treating his cycling patients. Anticipatory counseling may help avert many of the injuries, especially the more serious head injuries. This treatise focuses on cyclists' common injuries, their equipment and training in order to aid the physician care for these patients.

Traumatic Injuries of Cyclists

As anyone who has raced bicycles or provided medical care at a bicycle race can readily attest, the most common injury of cyclists is road rash (Fig. 14.1). This abrasion is a frictional injury that occurs when the falling cyclist lands on a hard surface, such as asphalt. Thin cycling clothing provides little protection to the epidermis, and abrasions of the arms, back, and legs commonly occur. In the case of a racer, this often is taken in stride; the athlete continues in the race to receive first aid after the finish. First aid for this injury is proper cleansing of the wound to remove bits of foreign matter (i.e., gravel, dirt, etc.), debridement of torn skin, and protection of the wound to allow further cycling in the case of a racer in a multiple-day stage race. Generous application of viscous Xylocaine to the wound prior to the first aid gives good anesthesia for the steps that follow. The wound next needs to be vigorously scrubbed with a surgical scrub brush or debrided with a water jet. In the practical surroundings of the medical tent at a bike race, a forceful jet of water from a hose often suffices. The next step is sharp debridement of any nonviable tissue in the wound. Application of a first aid spray is acceptable, but not mandatory. Finally, the wound is covered with a sterile nonadhering dressing. Choices would include Spenco Secondskin, Telfa or similar dressing. This dressing would then be covered by gauze pads and tape. Another tack would to be to use a semi-permeable dressing such as Tegaderm or OpSite. Finally, since many of these injuries occur on elbows, hips, and knees that require movement of the limb, the use of Flexnet or Tubigauze elastic circumferential dressings are critical to holding the dressing in place for the remainder of the race (Fig. 14.2). Wounds need daily care; after the first couple of days, they may be left open to the air if they have good scab formation.

Protection from abrasions can be afforded by wearing more resilient clothing, with long sleeves and legs, when temperatures permit. Careful attention to riding conditions, such as care on high speed turns, or rail-

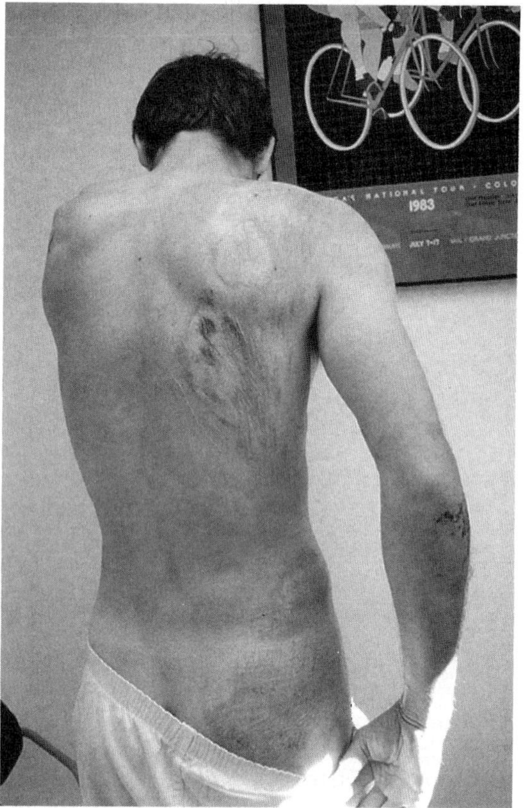

Figure 14.1. Road rash resulting from a high speed fall while descending a mountain road.

road tracks, curbing, and on gravel help prevent falls and injuries. Finally, the care of road rash is facilitated by having the cyclist shave his legs during the cycling season.

Lacerations can also occur when falling against sharp objects such as a competitor's chainring in a crash involving several riders. Lacerations of the head and forehead are also common in cyclists not wearing head protection or wearing just a hat or a leather "hair-net" style protector (Fig. 14.3). These lacerations may not be significant enough to withdraw the cyclist from the race because of bleeding alone; however, the flow of blood down the cyclist's face often obscures vision, putting the injured rider, as well as other competitors, at risk. Adequate closure of a laceration on a sweaty cyclist in a hurry to rejoin the race taxes the physician's first aid skills. If the bleeding can be controlled by direct pressure, the area around the wound can be wiped dry of sweat, prepared with benzoin, and a tight circumferential bandage can be applied over the gauze or semipermeable adhesive dressing. The use of a small surgical staple gun considerably simplifies the procedure, providing hemostasis and secure closure in one quick step. Another field expedient for scalp wounds is to make two small braids of hair, one on each side of the head wound, and then to tie a secure square knot closing the wound. The knot is secured in place by a copious addition of collodion. Often this secures the wound well enough so that suturing or stapling will not be necessary at a later time. As with abrasions, daily wound

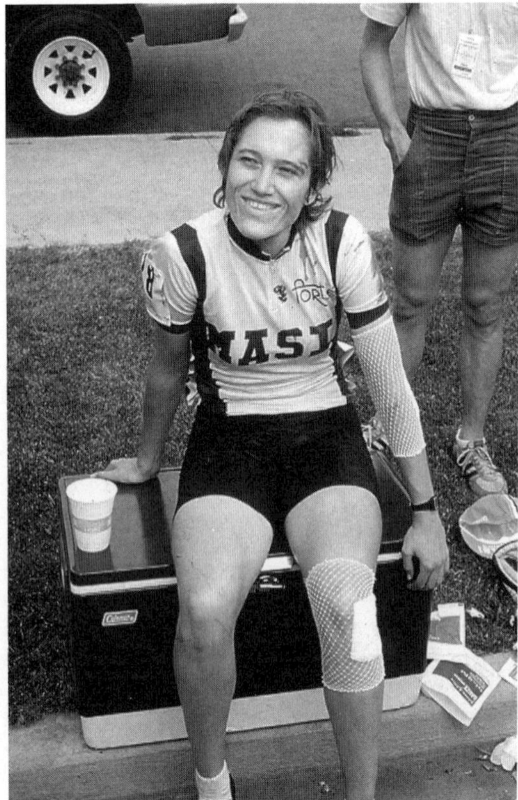

Figure 14.2. The use of flexnet to hold dressings in place.

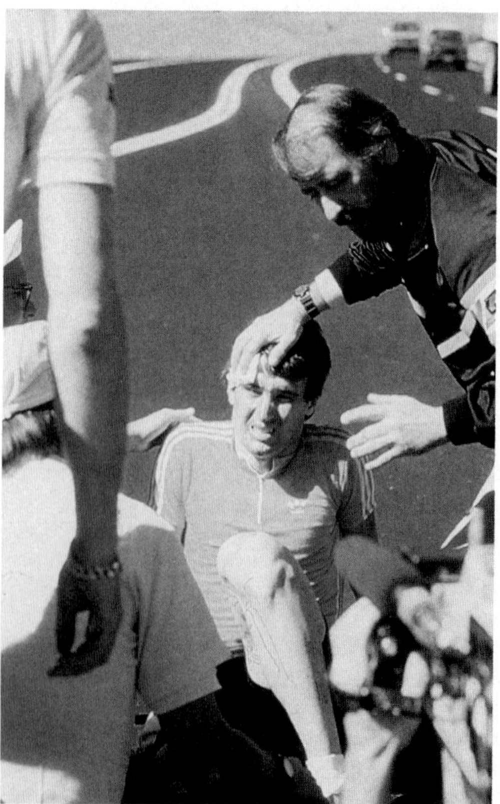

Figure 14.3. Head laceration while wearing the older style "hair-net" head protector.

checks need to be made to ensure that infection doesn't complicate the injury. In addition, if analgesics are required, they need to be limited to those that do not dull the cyclist's mentation or reaction time as well as avoiding positive testing on the postrace doping control.

Contusions and fractures are also the byproduct of a fall and usually affect the outstretched arm, shoulder, or hip. This blunt trauma usually will not prevent a rider from finishing that particular stage in a race, but may cause enough disability to prevent riding the following days. Differentiation of the contusion from a fracture or sprain is necessary. Fracture of the olecranon is an injury frequently sustained by a cyclist whose bicycle slides out from under him on a sharp cornering attempt. The elbow hits the pavement and a fracture results. When going over the handlebars in a fall, the natural reaction is to put out an arm to break the fall. This often results in a fracture of the forearm, or clavicle, or in a separation of the acromioclavicular joint. It is usually better if the cyclist can remain in the cycling position with hands on the bars during such a fall.

In attending a recently downed cyclist during a race, quick assessment of the arm, A-C joint, and clavicle will usually identify the common injuries that will prevent a cyclist from continuing. If these structures are intact and the racer has no evidence of concussion or of a head laceration that would interfere with vision, he may be allowed to reenter the race immediately.

If the rider sustains a clavicular fracture, it is usually about 2 weeks before an exercycle or rollers can be ridden comfortably enough to get any training effect. When the rider becomes proficient on the trainer and when some hard callous has started to form, he may start riding outside, but he must take extra care not to fall and reinjure the upper extremity. In the case of a forearm fracture, a splint or cast can be applied to allow training as soon as pain allows. The final molding of the cast should be done with the cyclist in the riding position to allow the cast to conform to the bars for a more secure positioning of the rider (Fig. 14.4).

Closed head injury is the most serious and life-threatening injury to both the racer and the recreational cyclist (1). Several studies have confirmed the efficacy of hardshelled helmets in preventing serious injury and death (2). One study on recreational cyclists illustrated this by showing 85% of emergency room visits as secondary to head injury in cyclists without helmets (3). The United States Cycling Federation adopted the hard-shell helmet rule in the late 1980s. Today, in the early 1990s, an attempt is being made to institute the rule by the international governing body of racing, International Cycling Federation. Although the safety of the hard-shell helmet is well documented and some aerodynamic advantages have been reported in labs, many riders complain that the helmets are too hot and interfere with cycling efficiency during long races. Nonetheless, the hard-shelled, American National Standards Institute (ANSI) or, Snell Memorial Foundation approved, helmet is the single most important piece of safety equipment a cyclist can wear. A team physician should refuse to provide medical care at any race, tour, or ride where helmets are not mandatory for all riders. Furthermore, all physicians should do everything they can to support and encourage the use of bicycle helmets in daily use by children and adults.

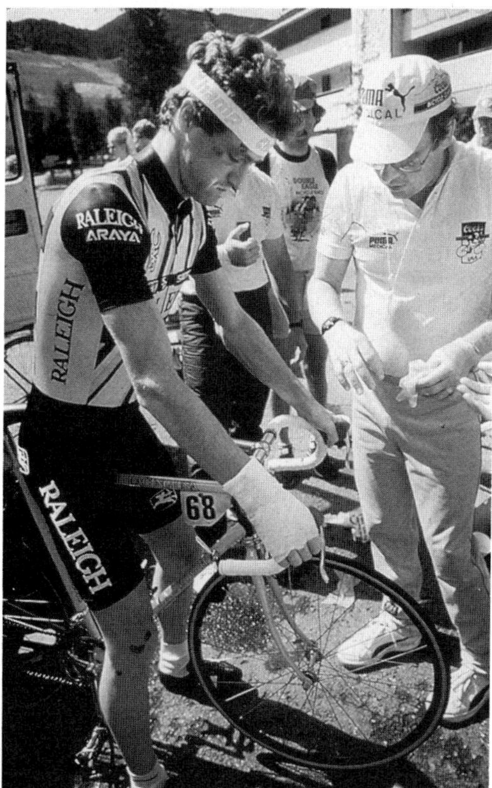

Figure 14.4. Final cast molding is completed while the cyclist grips the brake hoods.

During a cycling race, the assessment of a fallen cyclist must include the evaluation of that cyclist for concussion before allowing that rider to reenter the race (Fig. 14.5). Often the concussed rider is very evident—while other fallen riders are up and straightening their bent bikes or calling for new wheels to replace mangled ones, the concussed rider is standing by, dazed and with little sense of urgency for reentering the race. All downed riders do need a quick neurological check before resuming the race. If there is any doubt about the mental alertness of a cyclist, a period of observation and repeated evaluation needs to be followed. Because of the nature of bicycle racing, any rider with a head injury more severe than the slightest "ding" must be withdrawn from the race. Cyclists with concussion need to have serial evaluation and establishment of the severity of concussion before a decision about when they may race again can be made. Minor concussions may only require a day or two before resolving sufficiently to allow the rider to start riding again. Riders must show they possess the required bike handling skills, demonstrated at speed, prior to being allowed to race again. For more severe concussions, several weeks may be required for recovery especially if postconcussive symptoms are persistent. In such cases, a period of gradually increased intensity and technical difficulty in the training rides will be required before racing is permitted.

Although not lifethreatening, another anatomic part of the cyclist that deserves protection from injury is the eyes (Fig. 14.6). Speeds of 50 to 60 mph can be obtained by elite cyclists during mountainous descents. A rock from a competitor's wheel or an insect can scratch the cornea or even produce a more serious, penetrating injury to the eye. Vision, which is critical to control during downhill also is obscured by the tearing that occurs during fast descents. Therefore, cycling glasses that have a wrapped shape to prevent the tearing are an important protection. If corneal abrasion occurs, treatment is by instillation of a local anesthetic, washing, and patching of the affected eye. Ophthalmologic consultation should be obtained in more serious cases.

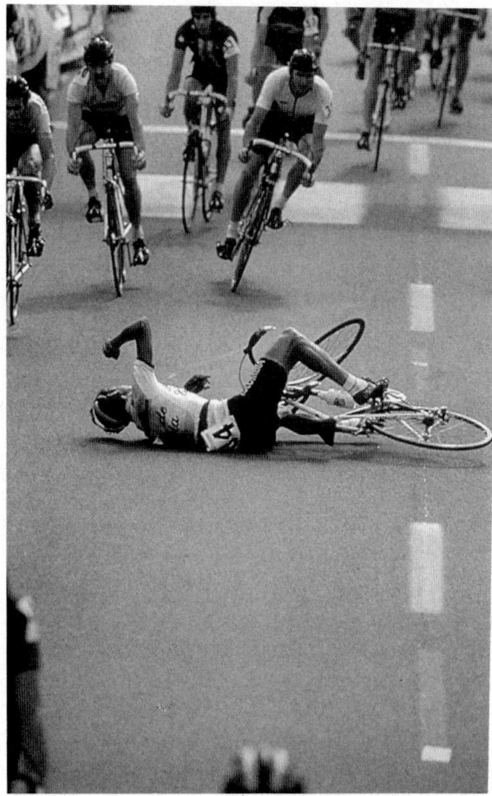

Figure 14.5. The majority of race-related accidents occur in the final sprint, as evidenced here, or in corners during criteriums, and wind directed echelons and descents during road races.

Acute strain of the quadriceps can occur especially during a sprint or hill in a race. Fatigue is also a factor in this injury. As with other strains, this injury is treated with ice, a compressive wrap, and rest. Acutely strapping the knee in a hyperflexed position for 30 to 40 min provides good hemostasis in severe quadriceps strains. Rehabilitation can begin in a couple of days with cryotherapy, gentle stretching, and easy riding. Hamstring strain is unusual and pain in this area is usually secondary to sciatica.

Overuse Injuries in Cyclists

Saddle sores are another common and irritating problem. In their mildest form, saddle sores present as chafing of the buttocks of the novice rider or occur at the beginning of the cycling season. A little rest and careful training usually allow the rider's seat to toughen into accepting the bicycle seat. Properly padded cycling pants, gel seats, and occasional sitz baths usually handle the more advanced cases. The real problem comes with the severe chafing and occasional boil formation seen in the competitive rider. In these individuals, rest from riding is often not an option. Treatment centers around good wound care, frequents changes in pants, application of warm heat (ie., sunlight or a bulb light), and air drying, and avoidance of infection. Antibiotics, and, rarely, incision and drainage are needed in the case of boil or cyst formation. Anticipatory counseling, gradual onset of training, and careful attention to perineal hygiene go a long way in preventing the more advanced cases of saddle soreness.

Nerve compression syndromes of the hand are common complaints in recreational and competitive cy-

Figure 14.6. The use of eyewear is essential in protecting the cyclist's eyes during fast descents, bright sunlight, or inclement weather.

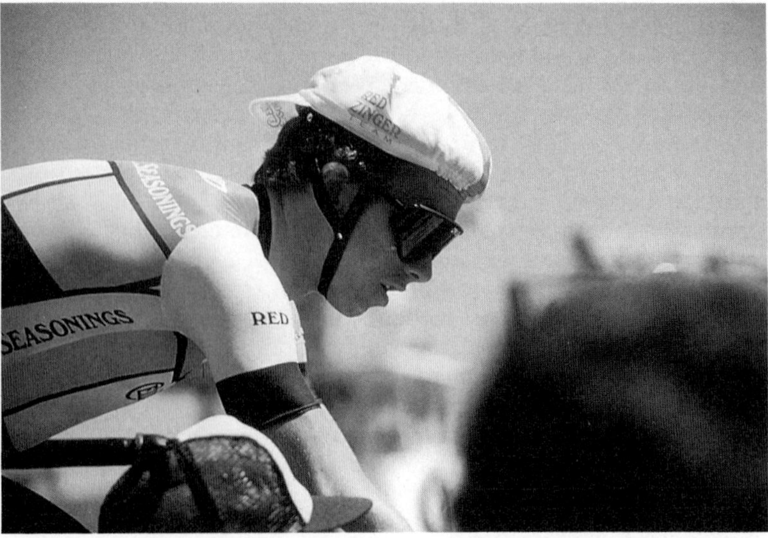

clists. The paresthesias usually appear after riding for a period of time. Ulnar nerve compression at Guyon's canal produces paresthesia and numbness over the fifth finger and the ulnar half of the ring finger. Carpal tunnel syndrome with median nerve compression gives the typical distribution of paresthesia of the remaining fingers of the hand not innervated by the ulnar nerve. Dorsiflexion of the wrist in riding upright handlebars of a mountain bike also serve to aggravate this condition. Finally, compression of the radial digital nerve of the index finger occurs when riding with the hands on the brake hoods. Anything that takes pressure off the nerve, such as padded bicycle gloves, padded or gel-containing handlebar grips, or aero-style bars will accomplish this purpose. Riding for shorter periods of time, changing riding position, and shortening the distance of handlebar to seat all help take pressure off the hands.

The other anatomical site affected by nerve pressure problems is the genital area. Penile and pudendal nerve pressure caused by too upwardly tilted seats or a forward riding position produce these problems. The paresthesias and numbness can last for a considerable period of time, but resolve with rest from the riding position. Prevention centers around proper seat positioning, padded cycling shorts and, occasionally, the use of an innovative seat that doesn't have the forward protruding horn.

Peripheral nerve compressions do occasionally occur in the foot. Tight, narrow toe straps, narrow shoes, and too firm a forefoot sole in the cycling shoe all can contribute to this problem. Solutions involve using wider toe straps, clipless pedals, and properly fitted cycling shoes. Sometimes a padded insole or orthotic device is helpful.

Although cycling provides only concentric exercise, which does not stress tendons and muscles as much as eccentric exercise, there are still episodes of tendonitis during the initial part of training or with heavy training loads. These types of tendonitis affect solely the lower extremity and usually are secondary to high mileage or increased stress on the anatomy from improper bicycle fitting or from pushing too big a gear. The iliotibial band is affected where it crosses the greater trochanter at the hip or at the lateral femoral condyle. This is a friction-type injury, initiated by too tight an iliotibial band, perhaps by some varus positioning of the knee, and by a high training load. The cyclist complains of pain and tenderness at the site where the band crosses the two boney prominences.

Treatment is directed at reducing the inflammation by rest, ice, antiinflammatory medications, and physical therapy modalities. Sometimes an injection of corticosteroid is required for persistent cases and, on rare occasions, competitive cyclists have required the percutaneous surgical division of part of the band to reduce the tension. Once the inflammation is reduced, a program of aggressive stretching exercises is started to decrease the tightness of the band at the sites of friction. Finally, the cyclist's riding position can be analyzed with the bicycle attached to a training stand (Fig. 14.7). A seat height that is too low or a pedal and cleat position that toes in producing varus at the knee are the usual culprits. As the cyclist returns to training, the training load needs to be increased gradually and the stretching program rigorously followed.

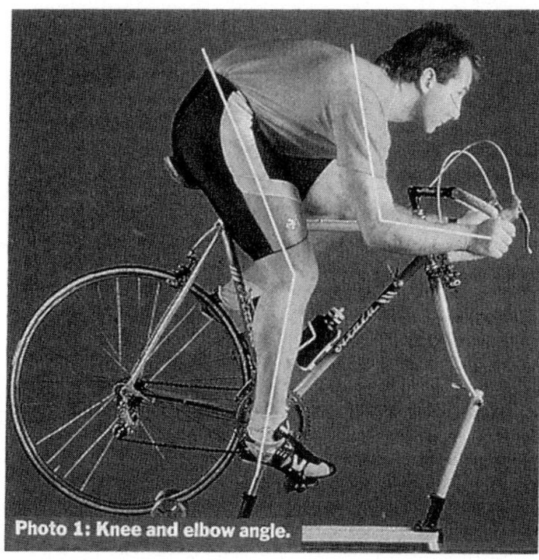

Figure 14.7. Riding position, bicycle fit, and pedaling biomechanics can best be studied while riding a stationry wind trainer or rollers so long as one has ridden rollers previously.

Infrapatellar tendonitis is unusual and must be differentiated from patello-femoral syndromes. Infrapatellar tendonitis presents with pain and tenderness over most of the tendon itself, not just at the tendonous attachment inferior on the patella. This injury is usually secondary to an increased training load or is initiated by some other physical activity the cyclist is involved in, such as weight training or running. Cessation of extraneous activities that aggravate the injury and cycling with a high cadence on short rides is usually well tolerated, while the tendonitis is treated with the usual protocols. Steroid injection is contraindicated in this case as well as in the case of quadriceps and Achilles tendon injury. Weight training is to be resumed carefully, after symptoms have been in remission for a considerable period of time.

Achilles tendonitis can be seen in competitive cyclists who sprint or climb hills in the standing position. Touring cyclists with heavy loads are also quite susceptible to this as well as to patellar problems. Both of these activities load the Achilles tendon more than when the cyclist is pedaling easily in the seated position. Toe clips that are too small and do not allow the cyclist to insert his foot far enough into the clip also produces more stress at the Achilles tendon and gastrocnemius. This increased stress produces the pain and tenderness characteristic of Achilles tendonitis. In very acute cases, crepitance may be noted at the Achilles tendon sheath with plantar and dorsiflexion of the foot. Again, rest, antiinflammatories, heel lifts, or taping the Achilles tendon are of help in arresting this malady. Physical therapy modalities may be adjunctive, while steroid injection is forbidden. After the inflammation subsides, a program of stretching the Achilles tendon and properly positioning the foot over the pedal spindle are necessary.

Posterior tibialis syndrome has been seen on rare occasion. The exact etiology, other than increased training load, is unclear. It readily responds to the usual treatments of rest, ice, physical modalities, and medication. Subsequent stretching and strengthening of the posterior tibialis muscle are indicated.

Patellofemoral problems are common. These are usually the result of the initiation of a too vigorous training program or too high a training load. Touring cyclists are susceptible to this problem because of the loads they carry, often over mountainous terrain. Mountain bikers also have this problem with regularity because of the hills they climb or because of the sand they attempt to grind through. Other activities the cyclist engages in, such as running and jumping sports or weight training, also contribute to this problem. Overdevelopment of the vastus lateralis, common in cyclists, produces lateral subluxation of the patella and increased patellar stresses. Positioning that has the seat too low or has the cleat toe out in order to increase valgus at the knee may contribute to the problem. Finally, the introduction of clipless pedals that did not allow any rotation or angulation at the pedal-cleat interface also produced many patellofemoral problems in competitive cyclists.

Probably the biggest contributor to patellofemoral problems is training error—too many miles, too fast (Fig. 14.8). The addition of interval work and hill work both overload the patella. Setting up the gearing of the bicycle with a small freewheel cluster does not give relief when hills, headwinds, or long rides fatigue the cyclist. A smaller chainring or a third small chainring is often a good idea, especially in mountainous terrain. Unexpected headwinds and long rides aggravate this problem. Keeping a good cadence, 90 to 110 rpm, is one of the most important things a cyclist can do to keep this problem in check. A cyclometer that displays a cadence reading is mandatory for the serious cyclist battling pattelo-femoral problems. Planning for the ride that could unexpectedly turn into an epic is important and, when recovering from a bout of patellagia, a cycle trainer workout will help prevent many of the problems acquired on a road ride.

The cornerstone of treatment is alteration of the training program in order to reduce patellar stresses, and to condition and reeducate the vastus medialis obliquus. This can be done with an endurance exercise program emphasizing minisquats, but it often requires biofeedback training to reeducate the muscles of the thigh. Patellar taping techniques (McConnell technique) to correct abnormal patellar motion are sometimes helpful, as are less restrictive patellar braces. Antiinflammatories and physical therapy modalities also have their place. Patellagia that is resistant to rest and conservative treatment may require further diagnostics, such as MRI, and, sometimes, arthroscopy.

Riding for extended periods of time with racing-style drop bars requires the rider to hold his neck in extension (Fig. 14.9). This is also the case with the newer aerodynamic triathalon-style bars. This neck extension fatigues the extensor muscles of the neck, impinges on neural foramina and may put pressure on nerve roots and cord in the arthritic cervical spine. Older riders especially may complain of neck, shoulder, and arm pain with riding. Paresthesias may be present and the differential diagnosis is between a cervical radiculopathy and a peripheral neuropathy. Riding with upright bars or mountain bike bars allows the rider to hold the head in a more neutral position and often avoids these symptoms. If the drop-style bars are necessary, then a lighter helmet, shorter periods of riding, and physical therapy directed at the radiculopathy may be helpful. Degenerative disc disease and arthritic spurring may require surgical intervention. Postoperatively, the rider with a one or two level fusion may be able to return to the traditional style racing bars.

Low back pain and sciatica are often the reasons athletes take up cycling when they are unable to run or play racquet sports. The bicycle is an excellent means for obtaining the daily 20 to 30 min of aerobic exercise essential to a good conservative program of back care. However, this type of riding places less stress on the

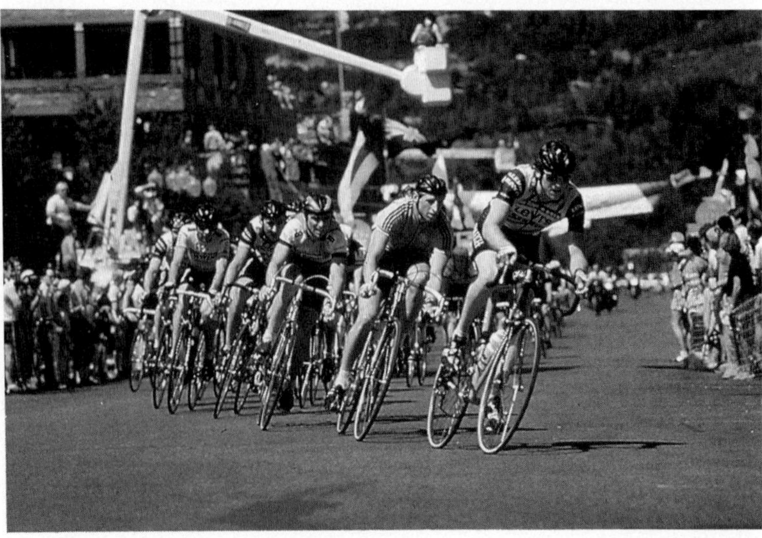

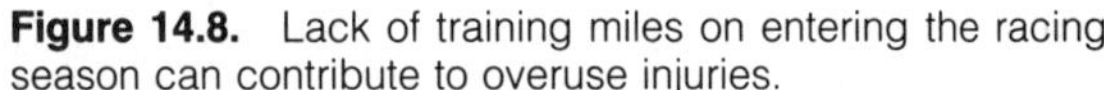

Figure 14.8. Lack of training miles on entering the racing season can contribute to overuse injuries.

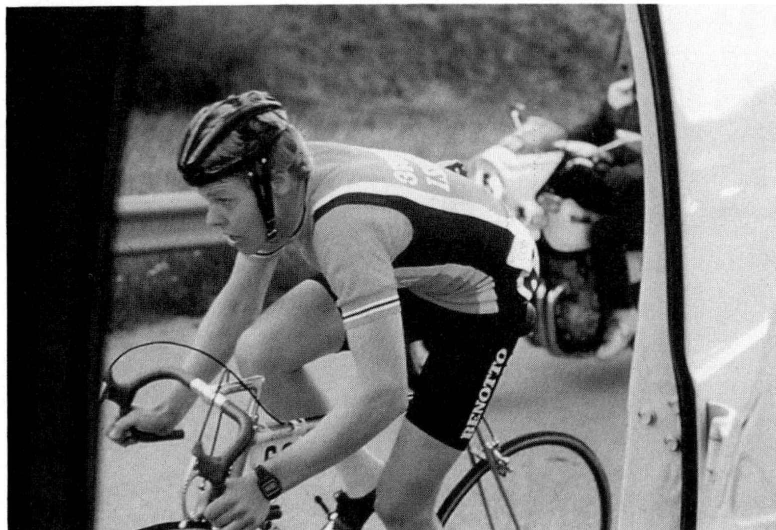

Figure 14.9. Training the neck muscles and correcting bicycle fit and riding position aid in avoiding neck fatigue.

lumbar spine than does racing, extended touring, or mountainous terrain, all of which may result in back pain or sciatica in the cyclist. Treatment of this problem requires careful evaluation by a physician and a treatment program directed by a physical therapist or trainer. Strict adherence to this approach often produces relief from the problem and allows the cyclist to go back to training and racing, at least in a limited manner. Elimination of other activities in the cyclist's day-to-day life that aggravate the lumbar spine is also necessary.

Problems specific to biking and back pain center on bicycle fit and on training program design. A cyclist who has a bicycle with too long a top tube or handle bar stem will find that the extended riding position quickly fatigues the back. This problem is common in female cyclists who have most of their height in their legs; their shorter torsos do not fit the stretched-out riding style required by standard bicycle construction. Many companies are now manufacturing bicycles especially for women. These bicycles have short stems and top tubes and often a smaller front wheel to allow turning clearance. The overall result is a riding position that is not elongated and stretched out, but maintains the back in a stable, rounded configuration. Although aerobars have the rider in a stretched out position, no increase in back complaints has been noted. A mountain bike is a good training alternative for the cyclist with back pain. With the right handle bars, it provides a variety of riding positions, good road shock absorption with the larger tires, and a harder road workout in a shorter riding time.

Cyclists with back pain should alter their training so as not to spend prolonged periods of time in one position, especially a position of sitting flexed forward on the bars. Periods of riding in the upright position or with the low back held in an extended position are recommended. The rider should try to cycle smoothly and proficiently with a cadence of 90 to 110 rpm, not trying to push too big a gear or to ride hills or sprint aggressively when symptomatic. Mountain biking on rugged terrain requiring vigorous bike handling is also sure to aggravate a back problem. Riders should dismount every 40 to 60 min to perform a couple of sets of back extension or similar exercises. If the rider is in a race or tour, these extension exercises can be performed on the bike while sitting upright and forcefully arching backward, holding a firm isometric contraction. After a race or long ride, repeating the extension exercises, applying ice to the low back for 40 to 60 min, and using antiinflammatory medications may be helpful. A transcutaneous electrical nerve stimulation (TENS) unit can be worn during a race; postrace physical therapy often provides considerable relief. Developing back strength through a good back rehabilitation program is necessary. Sometimes a back support may be a helpful adjunct.

Medical Problems in Cyclists

The medical problems relating specifically to cycling involve nutrition and fluids or they are temperature problems that usually are seen in long tours, races, and triathalons. Nutrition problems also may affect a cyclist's training and performance in stage races (Fig. 14.10). Heat problems may cause the cyclist to become light-headed, confused, and disoriented, resulting in a fall off the bike. Race personnel may miss the diagnosis of heat injury thinking the altered mental status is secondary to a concussion. A working knowledge of sports nutrition, training techniques, and the physiology of thermoregulation are important in bicycling medicine.

Nutritionally, cyclists do not have any requirements different from other endurance athletes; however, they do often ride or compete for very extended periods of time, and usually they eat while riding. The training diet should contain 55% to 70% carbohydrates. This diet combined with good tapering off of training prior to a race or long tour provide excellent levels of muscle glycogen storage for the upcoming event, when glycogen will be burned quicker by higher intensity riding (i.e., greater than 70% $\dot{V}_{O_{2max}}$) exhausting the rider who becomes extremely fatigued and virtually unable to complete the event—"bonked" in racing parlance. Levels of muscle glycogen can be preserved by eating or

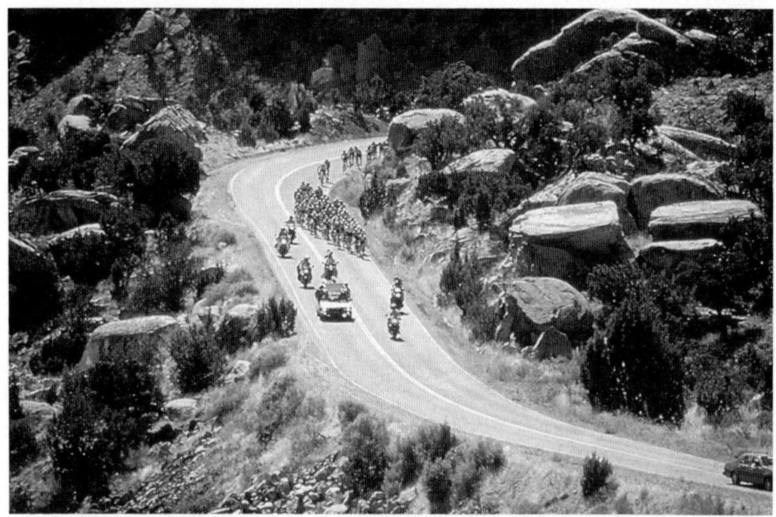

Figure 14.10. Hot, dry, and windy conditions can make fluid and temperature regulation even more critical.

drinking a carbohydrate source during the ride. As little as 26 g of carbohydrate per hr can markedly prolong cycling endurance (5). After the event, recovery for the next day's ride is enhanced by ingestion of 2 g of carbohydrate per kg of the rider's body weight within 30 min postrace. Carbohydrate replacement should then continue throughout the day.

Proper fluid maintenance is essential for good cycling performance as well as necessary for finishing a race or extended tour on a hot day (Fig. 14.11). The rider's circulating volume must be maintained if proper cooling and thermoregulation are to occur. Water bottles containing cold water are best for events lasting less than 90 min. For events lasting from 1.5 hr to 4 hr, a carbohydrate-containing drink should be used. For events on hot days lasting over 4 hr, sodium intake should be increased by using an "ade" drink. Prehydration of the rider by drinking a copious amount is useful in some cases. Riders should maintain a steady regimen of drinking fluids so as not to get behind on fluid requirements. This happens if a cyclist waits until thirst dictates need. Elite riders often expose themselves to heat problems by not drinking in the final stages of a race or by missing a water stop to get bottle refills of needed fluid.

Hyperthermia is the result of not keeping adequately hydrated. When the rider's circulating volume drops from dehydration, his core temperature rises. This makes for a less efficient rider by placing increased demands on the cardiovascular system. It finally results in clinical symptoms of heat injury. Treatment is to stop the exercising and cool the cyclist with cold towels or ice packs. If the cyclist is light-headed, lying supine with the legs elevated is helpful. Cold fluids taken by mouth allow recovery over a period of time. In severe cases or where rapid recovery is needed (such as for preparation for another stage), i.v. hydration is the method of choice. Two to three liters of cold Ringer's lactate with 5% glucose will revive a cyclist in very short order (Fig. 14.12).

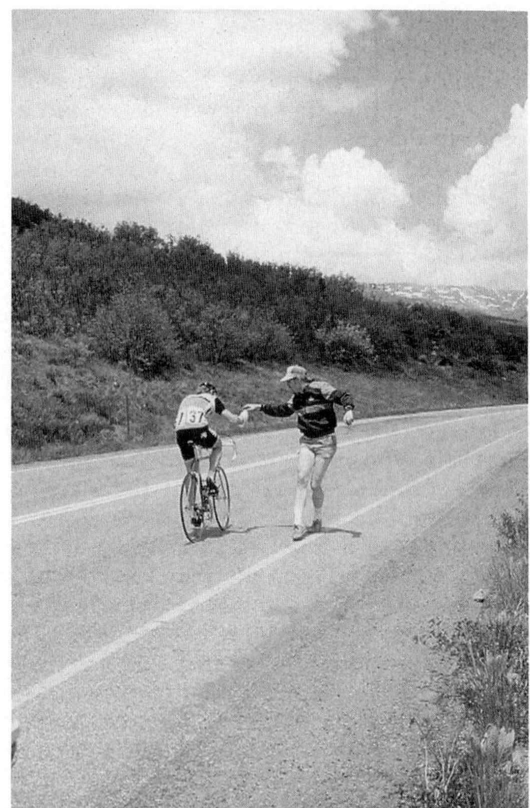

Figure 14.11. Making sure a rider receives adequate fluids while passing through the feed zone.

Hypothermia can result from riding for extended periods of time in cold or cool, inclement weather. Mountainous riding with swift downhills and rain, hail, or snow are often involved in producing hypothermia (Fig. 14.13). Prevention requires selection of appropriate jackets, leggings, gloves, boots, and shell clothing. It is important for the touring cyclist and racer to plan ahead in such an environment because the weather can change quickly and without warning. Nutritional requirements are also elevated by cold weather.

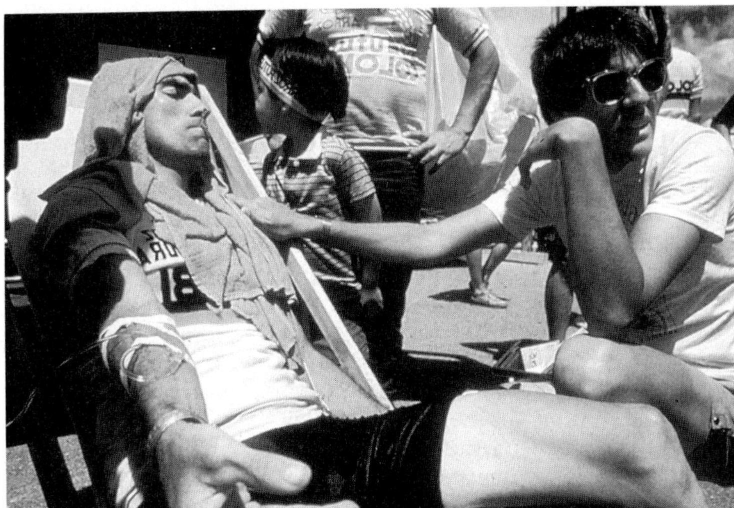

Figure 14.12. Using ice towels and i.v. in the treatment of heat illness.

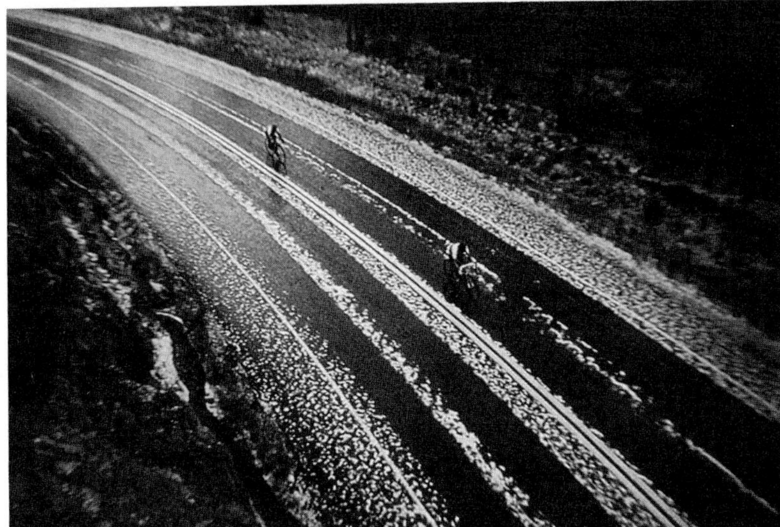

Figure 14.13. Appropriate clothing is paramount while touring or racing in mountainous terrain, as evidenced here by snow and hail during an August race.

Finally, training for competition can be overdone; when it is, the clinical syndrome of overtraining is sometimes encountered. This is usually a cyclist who is training hard with high miles (300 to 450 per week), intervals, and races. The cyclist often thinks of illness or anemia and, in fact, both of these entities need to be excluded from the diagnosis. The symptoms of overtraining include fatigue, lassitude, lack of strength and endurance, and, sometimes, depression. Often, the poor results obtained from the training only prompts the rider to more and harder training efforts, which amplify the syndrome. There are no reliable clinical signs of overtraining syndrome but a careful physical examination and some labwork to exclude organic problems is warranted. Treatment is a prolonged period of absolute rest from the sport. This includes physical and psychological rest from the pressures of training and competing. Only when the athlete is enthusiastically ready to return to training should small and gradually increasing workouts be allowed. During this time, meticulous attention to diet, rest, and other recreation needs to be maintained.

Medical Coverage of Cycling Events

Providing medical coverage at a cycling event is a challenge to the sports medicine team. In some cases, the event may be an out-and-back time trial with little chance of traumatic injury. Circuit races and, especially, criteriums traverse winding courses of varying length with plenty of opportunity for mishaps involving multiple racers in the peleton. Mountain road races, century rides, or tours require medical coverage over courses from 50 to 140 miles in length often with riders spread out over many miles of the course. Each of these events requires a different type of coverage. What they have in common is the need for a comprehensive communication system to summon immediate backup support for medical emergencies that may occur anywhere on the course. The details of this emergency plan, including first aid, advanced life support, and transport of the injured by ambulance or helicopter, must be worked out well in advance (Fig. 14.14). Radio communications with race officials, observers, and medical personnel to identify and locate injured riders is a key aspect of the system.

At the beginning of each event, a medical area must be provided that allows the competitors to deal with prerace problems, such as cleaning and redressing yesterday's road rash (Fig. 14.15). This period also serves as morning sick call for ill riders. Finally, it provides a good opportunity to make decisions on riders who may be in questionable condition for the race that day because of illness (gastroenteritis with dehydration) or injury (minor concussion). Medical personnel need to be alert to which medications they dispense to avoid giving a banned medication in a sanctioned event or giving medication to a rider who may go on to antidoping tests at another event in the near future.

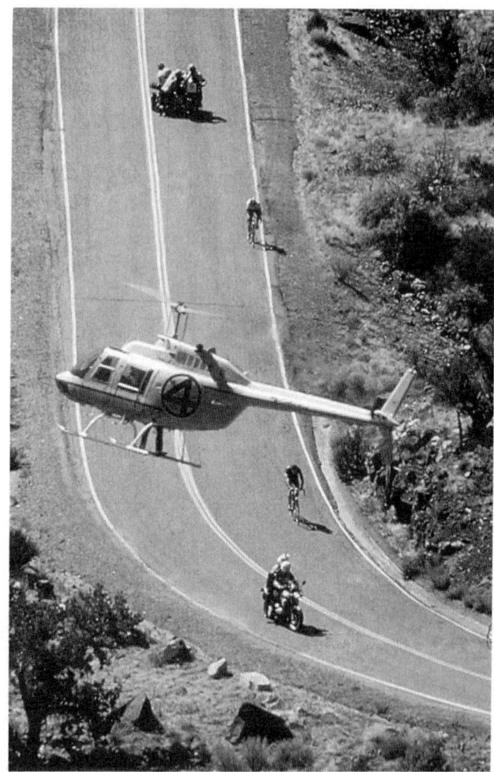

Figure 14.14. In remote areas, transportation may mean the use of a helicopter if necessary. Communication with backup personnel is key.

During the race, it is convenient to station those medical personnel who are well trained to deal with major trauma directly on dangerous corners or other race sites that are hazardous, particularly in the case of time trials, criteriums, and circuit races. Other members of the team and ambulance support can be stationed just off the course but in radio contact with the medical teams at the corners. All personnel need to know that the race does not stop for injured riders so that, when on the course rendering first aid, they know that they must guard their own personal safety as well as that of the fallen riders. The ambulance must have access to enter the course in a manner that is quick, but safe for the remaining riders. In road races, the medical caregivers must travel with the moving peleton. Medical vans, motorcycles, ambulances, and a medical sag wagon (cycling jargon for a van that picks up exhausted riders at the tail end of a race) at the very end of the procession can accomplish this. Again, radio contact among the medical vehicles and race officials is of paramount importance.

After a race, the medical care required is rendered at the prearranged medical site. This site needs to be set up in advance and to be staffed and ready to handle the injuries that show up immediately after the race. This is the time when most injuries will be seen and treated. A key element of this site is a triage area with a physician to assign injured riders to the medical staff members for care. Adequate supplies to deal with road rash, lacerations, contusions, and hypovolemia need to be at hand. Backup support for x-ray, casting, and other diagnostics can be prearranged with the area hospitals.

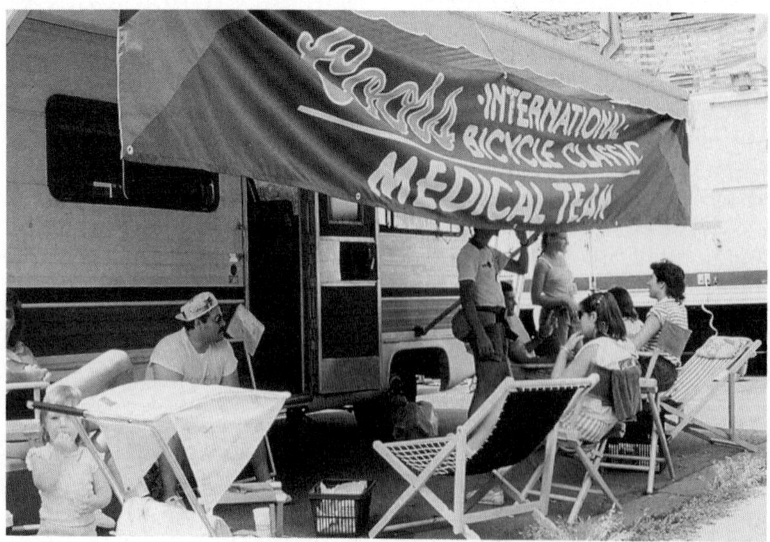

Figure 14.15. The medical area must be easily accessible and large enough to accommodate participant needs while allowing for the privacy of all participants, regardless of gender.

Equipment and Training

The bicycle is obviously the most important piece of equipment for the cyclist; however, safety equipment such as helmets, protective clothing, lights, and mirrors are highly recommended. Several different types of bicycles are available, but only road and mountain bikes will be covered here. Both types of bicycles come in a variety of configurations and components with price ranges from a couple of hundred dollars to several thousand dollars. A good road bike is made of steel alloy, aluminum, or composites and weighs less than 20 pounds. Mountain bikes are made of similar materials; Better bikes weigh between 20 and 25 pounds.

Bike height is the first important consideration in proper fitting. A properly sized road bike should have a top tube that allows the bike to be straddled and 1 to 2 inches of clearance below the rider's crotch. Some racer's even prefer a slightly smaller frame height. A mountain bike frame should have a top tube with a 4 to 6 inch clearance. Again, more aggressive riders prefer an even smaller frame. Top tube length is a second important consideration. A top tube that is too long will stretch the rider out and may aggravate or precipitate back problems. This is especially true for the female rider who often has the leg length to accommodate the taller frame size, but a shorter torso that leaves her stretched out over the bike when in riding position. This problem has been solved by some companies making bikes sized especially for female riders or by the more expensive option of a custom frame. Another solution is to use a shorter stem for the handlebars, which shortens the distance from the seat to the bars.

Seat height is important in order to give the rider a comfortable riding position and to decrease stress to the patello-femoral joint. When the seat height is too low the increased flexion of the knee at the top of the pedal stroke magnifies the patellar compressive forces during the powerful downstroke. For a road bike, the seat adjustment should allow the rider to sit level on the seat with the leg completely extended. A test for this adjustment has the heel lightly resting on the pedal in a full downstroke position; this permits a slight flex in the knee when the foot is correctly positioned on the pedal. Mountain bike seat height is usually lower, allowing the rider to move around or get off quickly while negotiating technical terrain. Some riders raise the seat to a position slightly lower than road bike settings for uphill and lower it 4 to 6 inches for downhill. Many bicycle shops have special kits to help fit the rider to the bike. However, scientific studies are inconclusive regarding seat height and its effect on a rider's physiologic performance (4). The individual cyclist should use the above instruction or fitting kit as a starting point, but not be afraid to experiment with different equipment positioning to obtain the most comfortable riding position.

Handlebar shapes do affect the performance of the cyclist by decreasing drag from the presentation of a more aerodynamic profile in the case of the aero type bars preferred by triathletes and some racers. The 13% to 15% decrease in wind resistance can provide a considerable difference in time during longer races and time trials. The aero-bars may also be a good choice for some patients with chronic back pain. The position they provide is comfortable for many riders and most of the bars provide for a variety of hand positions allowing the rider to move around during the ride. Other riders find that the upright, mountain-bike-type bars provide the most comfort for chronic back pain. Finally, many riders tolerate the conventional drop-style bars, but should get off their bikes on long rides to stretch their backs or do a few sets of therapeutic back exercises. Cyclists with neck pain from arthritis or radiculopathy will almost always prefer the mountain-bike-style bars. However, these bars also may produce an increase in some of the neuropathies of the hand and arm because of the dorsiflexed position of the wrist. Pressure on the hands can be decreased by proper seat-to-bar length, padded bar wraps and cycling gloves. This makes for more comfortable riding as well as for decreased incidence of neuropathy in the hands.

The pedals allow for the transfer of power from cyclist to cycle. Both toeclips and straps used with cycling cleats as well as the newer clipless type pedals accomplish this transfer more efficiently than tennis shoes and platform pedals without straps. Again, science has been unable to establish a clear superiority of clipless pedals over straps and pedals, and the same remains true for the length of the pedal crank arms (4). Some riders do experience an increase in patellofemoral pain when using the clipless pedals. Newer models that allow for rotation and tilt of the foot when clipped in to the pedal have helped alleviate this problem.

Helmets top the list of essential safety equipment for both road bikers and mountain bikers. Several studies attest to the importance of helmets in reducing mortality and morbidity in cycling accidents (5, 6). Today all USCF, ICF, and U.S. Triathalon sponsored races mandate the use of an approved helmet during competition. Physicians providing medical care in local races or rides should insist on such a helmet rule or withdraw from providing medical care at such an event. All recreational riders should receive anticipatory counseling on helmet use when in the physician's office for routine exams or for first aid from a bicycle accident. Encouraging helmet use is the single most important piece of bicycling preventative medicine the physician can practice! Eyeglasses or cycling wraparound glasses should accompany the helmet to protect the eyes from insects and other foreign bodies as well as to prevent tearing and blurring of vision at high speeds.

Other important safety equipment includes a mirror to view traffic approaching from the rear. Clothing should not only protect the cyclist from the environment but should be bright and highly visible to motorists. Bright pink, florescent blues, and other high visibility colors are recommended. Clothing also should be planned to provide adequate warmth and ventilation for long rides. Shell clothing to provide protection from rain and wind needs to be a consideration in preparing for tours. Mountain bikers need long sleeved shirts to protect against brush and falls. Cyclists who ride at night should wear reflective clothing and have lights for both the front and rear of the bicycle.

Cadence of pedaling is probably one of the most important aspects of training and cycling. Recreational riders often ride with a pedal cadence that is too slow, consequently providing increased compressive forces on the patello-femoral joint and subsequent chondromalacea patella. Riding hills, headwinds, and heavily loaded touring bikes as well as many aspects of mountain bike riding, such as hills, sand, or snow, also slow cadence, requiring increased quadriceps effort that produces the same problem. Experienced cyclists should strive for a cadence of 90 to 110 rpm's. On hills, cadence should not fall below 65 rpms. Failure to achieve these cadences requires retraining of the cyclist or changing the gear ratio of the bike. The use of a third chainring, a "granny" or "bail-out" gear for such situations is recommended for riders who cannot maintain proper cadences. A bicycle computer that displays cadence is an aid to all cyclists and is a necessity for the cyclist with patellofemoral problems. Although pedal cadence is an oft-discussed topic in relation to cycling performance, scientific information is not now available to support the anecdotal information regarding performance. (4).

Training programs for cycling should follow the examples set by other endurance sports. Specificity of training is of paramount importance. Nothing improves cycling like cycling. Cross training is only of benefit to the triathlete or recreational rider for whom cycling is just one of the sports he or she enjoys. Furthermore, a well designed and slowly graduated program will help decrease the incidence of overuse syndromes. Length of rides, intensity, terrain, and frequency of training all contribute to the rider's training load. If the rider selects too large a training load or advances the training load too quickly, an overuse syndrome should prompt the rider to decrease the training load while analyzing what actions or patterns in the previous weeks of cycling may have precipitated the problem. After the problem resolves, careful resumption of training and monitoring of the problem will usually allow a return to cycling. Many cyclists make the erroneous assumption that increasing the training load is the only way to become more competitive. Using quality training with adequate rest interspersed during the weekly training schedule is often more successful than just adding more mileage.

Finally, the bike is an excellent rehabilitation tool. It is a good substitute for aerobic exercise in a runner with a lower extremity overuse injury. However, it must be remembered that training is specific—the truly competitive runner would be better served by doing pool running rather than cycling. On the other hand, the recreational rider will certainly enjoy cycling more than hours spent in the boredom of pool running. The lack of impact in cycling also makes it an excellent choice for athletes with arthritis from trauma or aging. It is also an excellent choice for postmenisectomy or chondroplasty patients. The bicycle or exercycle also is good for initiating range of motion and early endurance training in the postoperative lower extremity. Seat height and pedal crank length can be adjusted to allow for a more comfortable range of motion; cadences should be maintained to prevent patellofemoral problems. As the rehabilitation program progresses, specificity can be introduced by tailoring the training load to the upcoming demands of the athlete's specific sport.

REFERENCES

1. Friede AM, Azzara CV, Gallagher SS, Guyer B. The epidemiology of injuries in bicycle riders. Pediatr Clin North Am. 1985;32:141–151.
2. Sachs JJ, Holmgren P, Smith SM, Sosin DM. Bicycle-associated head injuries and deaths in the United States from 1984 through 1988. JAMA 1991; 266:3016–3018.
3. Thompson RS, Rivara FP, Thompson DC. A case-controlled study of the effectiveness of bicycle safety helmets. New Engl J Med. 1989; 320:1361–1367.
4. Gregor RJ, Broker JP, Ryan MM. The biomechanics of cycling. Exer Sport Sci Review 1991;127–169.
5. Wheeler K. Sports nutrition for the primary care physician. 1989;17:106–117.
6. DiGuiseppi CG, Rivara FP, Koepsell TD, et al. Bicycle helmet use by children. Evaluation of a community-wide helmet campaign. JAMA 1989, Oct 27;262(16):2256–61.

15 / BOXING

W. Timothy Ward

History

A historical overview of the ancient origin of boxing has been published by Unterharnscheidt (1) and others (2, 3). Boxing was introduced into the 23rd Olympic games in 688 B.C. Boxers were divided into two classes: either older or younger than 18 years, without consideration of weight or experience. Apparently no ring was used, there was no time limit and no rest period, blows could be landed anywhere, kicking was allowed, and there was no grace period if a boxer was knocked down. Matches continued until one fighter could no longer continue or until he acknowledged defeat. The origin of boxing in ancient Greece and Rome can be divided into three periods. The so-called period of soft thongs extended from Homeric times to the end of the 5th century B.C. Soft thongs were long pieces of leather believed to be made of tanned ox hides that were wrapped around the forearm and hand for protection (Fig. 15.1). Boxing became more brutal with the identification of the second period, called the period of sharp thongs, which lasted from the 4th century B.C. until the 2nd century A.D. during the Roman Empire. Hard thongs consisted of leather gloves extending over the forearm and hand with a hard leather ring encircling the knuckle (Fig. 15.2). While the purpose of a soft thong was to protect the boxer's hand, the purpose of a hard thong was to inflict more punishment. Boxing reached its low point during the third phase, the period of the Roman caestus. A caestus was a type of hard thong that had iron or lead spikes present at the knuckle region (Fig. 15.3). The caestus obviously was intended to inflict great if not fatal punishment to the opponent.

Boxing was apparently banned around A.D. 400 for unclear reasons. It made a brief comeback at the time of the Italian Renaissance only to again fall into obscurity until it was revived in Great Britain in the 18th century. It became popular shortly thereafter in the United States. The modern era of boxing was really ushered in with the Queensbury rules in 1867. These rules included the use of padded boxing gloves, 3-min rounds with 1-min rest periods, banning of wrestling, no hitting of an opponent who had been knocked down, and mandating that a boxer must rise unaided within 10 sec following a knockdown. Other than decreasing the length of a boxing contest in recent years, the nonmedical aspects of the sport have not changed significantly in the last century. On the other hand, significant progress has recently been made in both medical understanding and medical input into boxing. This chapter outlines the current state of boxing from a medical standpoint.

Amateur Versus Professional

Amateur and professional boxing have many similarities but also many significant differences (Table 15.1). Administratively, the amateur sport is much more organized with centralized authority under one national governing body termed USA Boxing, Inc. (4). This organization has a strong central authority with uniform rules and regulations to govern all aspects of amateur boxing nationally. Theoretically, every aspect of the amateur sport should be the same in all states. The detailed amateur organizational structure and working guidelines were developed with boxing safety as a top priority. Professional boxing on the other hand has no centralized authority and, therefore, rules and regulations vary from state to state. In addition, professional boxing is governed by world sanctioning organizations such as the World Boxing Association (WBA) and World Boxing Council (WBC) that have their own rules, which are often in conflict with state regulations. Amateur boxers carry "medical passports" that reflect their prior bouts and any injuries sustained. Professionals have no such document, sometimes leaving state officials without adequate documentation of a boxer's true status.

The optimal result in a professional contest is to ren-

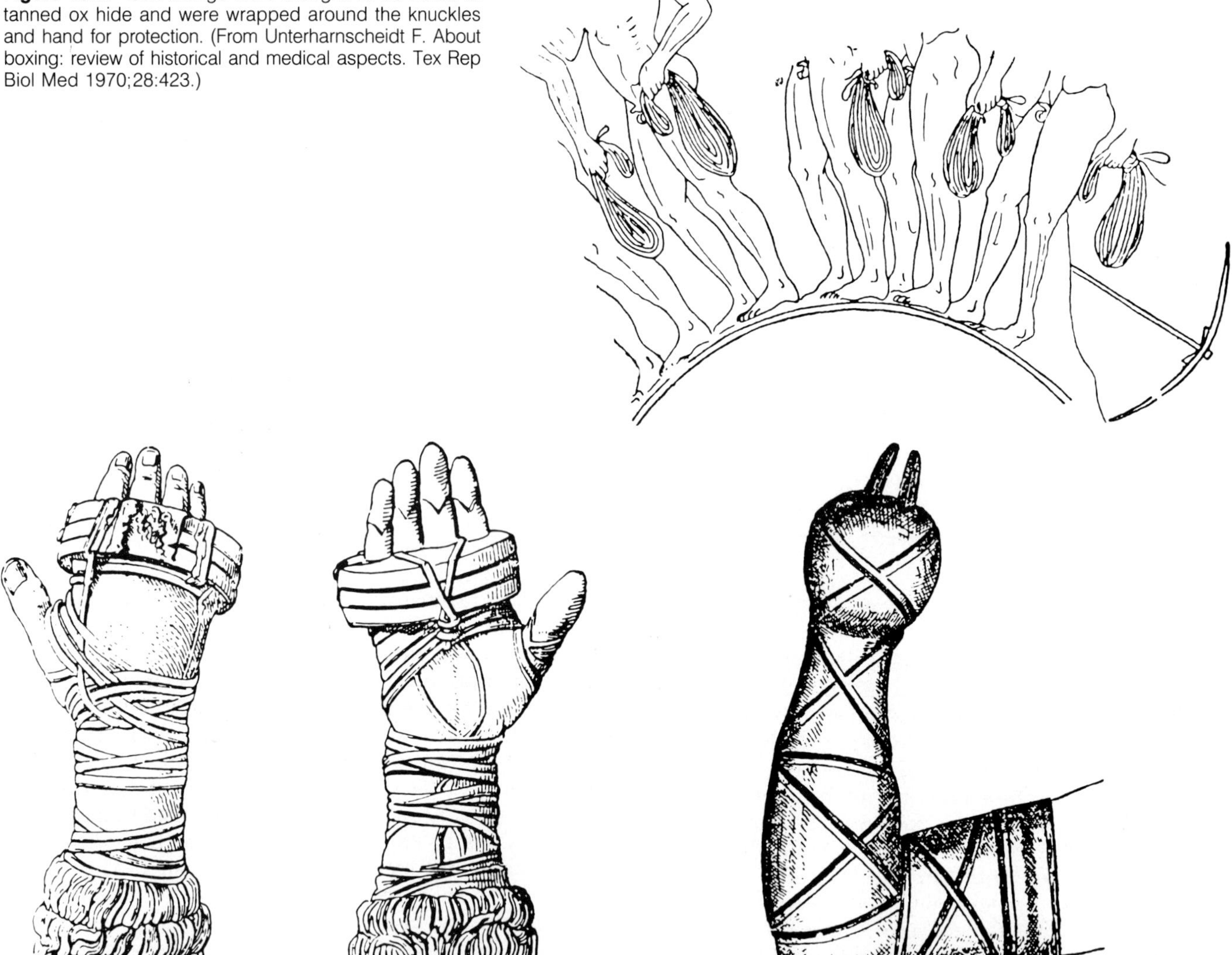

Figure 15.1. Soft thongs were thought to be made of tanned ox hide and were wrapped around the knuckles and hand for protection. (From Unterharnscheidt F. About boxing: review of historical and medical aspects. Tex Rep Biol Med 1970;28:423.)

Figure 15.2. Sharp thongs were hard leather bands that covered the knuckles. They were meant to inflict damage to the opponent. (From Unterharnscheidt F. About boxing: review of historical and medical aspects. Tex Rep Biol Med 1970;28:428.)

Figure 15.3. The Roman caestus was intended to inflict brutal, if not fatal, punishment to the opponent. (From Unterharnscheidt F. About boxing: review of historical and medical aspects. Tex Rep Biol Med 1970;28:429.)

der the opponent neurologically incapable of continuing the match. The scoring system is heavily weighted toward encouraging hard head blows with resultant knockdown or knockout. As a result of this scoring system, it is exceedingly rare for a boxer to be judged the winner of a round if he has been knocked down. In contrast, amateur boxing does not seek to reward a boxer for scoring a knockdown blow. In the amateur ranks, all blows are weighted equally in the scoring system so that landing a knockdown blow does not enhance a boxer's scorecard any more than landing a light body blow. The result is that the amateur competitor tends to emphasize defense and boxing skills over the pursuit of a knockout.

Amateur contests are of considerably shorter duration than are professional contests. Professional contests last between 4 and 12 rounds of 3-min duration, with a veteran professional always scheduled to box at least 10 rounds. In contrast, amateur bouts are limited to 3 rounds of 2- to 3-min duration. On rare occasions, an amateur may box 5 rounds of 2-min duration. The total number of hard head blows landed is presumably less in the shorter amateur contest.

Amateur boxers must always wear headgear, whereas professionals do not. The purposes of the amateur headgear are to reduce the impact force on the head and to reduce the chance of facial cuts and ear injuries. Headgear does appear to decrease the incidence of cuts, but significant reduction in head impact force probably does not occur. The use of a headgear really gives the amateur boxer a false sense of security in terms of blunting the effects of hard head blows.

Amateur officials are much quicker to terminate a contest in which one boxer is out-classed or hurt than

Table 15.1.
Amateur Versus Professional Boxing

Characteristic	Amateur	Professional
Governing body	USA Boxing, Inc.	SBC, WBA, WBC, WBO, IBF, and others
Medical passport	Yes	No
Scoring	All blows equal	Weighted toward knockdown
Competition	3 to 5 rounds of 2 or 3 min each	4 to 12 rounds of 3 min each
Headgear	Yes	Only sparring
Referee	Stops contest early	Stops contest late
Standing eight count	Three in one round, four total	Varied
Cuts	Stop contest	Varied
Medical suspensions	Uniform	Varied
Age limit	32 year (masters)	None
Retinal tear	No competition	Individual decisions
Neurologic risk	Smaller	Larger

are professional officials. Any head blow that stuns an amateur in the slightest is grounds for a standing eight count. Three standing eight counts in one round, or a total of four over the course of the three-round match, automatically terminates the contest in amateur boxing. Professionals, however, are generally allowed to weather the storm, thereby absorbing much more punishment. Any facial laceration will generally be grounds to terminate an amateur contest, whereas a professional contest will generally be stopped only if the laceration is affecting the boxer's vision.

Amateur boxing emphasizes uniform restriction periods for any boxer who has had his match terminated because of hard head blows. Amateur boxing does not recognize the terms *technical knockout* (TKO) and *knockout* (KO) but prefers the euphemisms *referee stops contest due to head blows* (RSCH) and *referee stops contest due to medical reasons* (RSCM). Any amateur sustaining an RSCH is given a 30-day mandatory suspension from any further boxing competition or gym sparring. An RSCM with unconsciousness lasting less than 2 min results in a 90-day suspension, whereas an RSCM with unconsciousness lasting greater than 2 min results in a 180-day suspension. If an RSCH or RSCM occurs a second time within 90 days from the end of the suspension period for the first RSCH or RSCM, the mandatory suspension times are even longer. An RSCH occurring within 90 days after the first RSCH results in an additional 90-day suspension, an RSCH after an RSCM also is an additional 90 days. An RSCM following an RSCH is given a 180-day suspension, whereas an RSCM following a prior RSCM results in a 365-day suspension. These suspensions are noted in the amateur boxers' medical passports, making it difficult for the suspension to be be ignored. Similar initial suspensions are codified by many but not all state boxing commissions for the professional spot.

Because of the absence of national guidelines and communication channels at the professional level, a boxer's suspension in one state may not be known or upheld by another state. All amateur boxers—and professional boxers in most states—are required to provide medical clearance at the end of their suspension periods before resuming boxing. For amateurs, notification of medical clearance is forwarded to the national office. Dissemination of notification of medical clearance is not as structured at the professional level. How well this process really works at the local level for either amateur or professional boxing is unknown.

Many state boxing commissions do not have a codified upper age limit for competition, whereas amateurs have a demarcation point at age 32. After that, an amateur can only compete at the local level in masters competition against similarly aged individuals. Tournament competition past the local level does not exist for masters. This rule effectively serves to discourage amateur boxing after age 32.

Finally, no individual is allowed to compete at the amateur level after having sustained any type of retinal tear or detachment, even if it has been adequately repaired. Further competition at the professional level following successful retinal repair is considered acceptable in many situations.

The amateur boxing establishment feels strongly that the documented neurological sequelae of professional boxing not be extrapolated to include amateur boxing (5–7). There is, however, no randomized study of amateur boxers comparable with Roberts's (8) study of professional boxers (9). The general consensus is that amateur boxing does not involve the same degree of neurologic risk as is present in professional boxing. However, work by Kaste et al. (10) and Casson et al. (11) does cast doubt on the safety of amateur boxing. Similarly, McLatchie et al. (12) studied 20 amateur boxers and noted an abnormal clinical neurologic examination in 7, abnormal EEG in 8, and abnormal neuropsychological testing in 9. No controls were included in this study. Enzenauer et al. (13), in a study of military boxing, noted that 68% of all injuries were caused by head blows and reported one death and one case of unilateral blindness. Most studies that have specifically addressed the neurologic risk in amateur boxing do report much less neurological abnormalities than in the professionals. Thomassen et al. (14) compared the neurological, electroencephalographic, and neuropsychological examinations of 53 amateur boxers and 53 soccer players. They found no significant differences between the two groups, concluding that modern amateur boxing did not lead to serious or permanent brain damage. However, the median age of the boxers in that study was only 36 years. Brooks et al. (15) reported the results of neuropsychological testing in 29 active amateur boxers and also found no evidence of cognitive impairment compared with a matched control group. Heilbronner et al. (16) also reported normal neuropsychological testing following active competition in 23 amateur boxers. Jordan and Zimmerman (17) reported finding no abnormalities on magnetic resonance imaging (MRI) scans of a small group of active amateur boxers examined after a knockout. In a comprehensive look at amateur boxing Haglund et al. (18–20) and Murelius and Haglund (21) studied a group of Swedish amateur boxers and compared them with controls participating in other sports. No differences were noted on neurological examination, computerized tomography (CT) or MRI scanning, or neuropsychological testing. They concluded that no evidence of chronic brain damage could be elicited in modern-day Swedish amateur boxers.

An objective assessment of amateur boxing leads to the conclusion that it probably does not involve the same degree of neurologic risk as seen in the professional sport. This is understandable, because the competitions are much shorter and the likelihood of terminating a contest due to head blows is much greater in the amateurs. The usefulness of other amateur initiatives such as the wearing of headgear and existence of medical passports awaits further proof. Longer follow-up is required before the true risk of current-day amateur boxing can be definitively stated. It seems prudent to accept that some degree of risk for development of chronic traumatic encephalopathy or acute brain injury does exist for amateur boxing but not to the same degree as is seen in professional boxing.

Prefight Examination

The prefight examination is generally performed on the day of the competition. The boxer is asked about any prior history of knockout or concussive episodes in or out of the ring. Any complaints referable to the neurologic, ocular, or musculoskeletal systems should be specifically brought out. The boxer's general demeanor should be scrutinized. Any slurring of words or abnormal movement should be addressed. The physical examination should be conducted in a quiet, well-lit room with a desk or table for the boxer and physician to sit on. On occasion, the promoter or state boxing commissions will expect the physician to conduct the examination in a crowded, noisy environment with boxers qued up waiting to be examined. This type of arrangement should be resisted by the physician. Many boxers are nervous at this time and can be expected to be somewhat tachycardic. However, when relaxed a well-trained boxer may have a heart rate as low as 50 beats per minute. Minor degrees of hypertension do not preclude competition. The physician should be aware of the artificially elevated pressure readings that can be seen in heavier boxers with large arms. Pressures as high as 160/95 are accepted in these individuals. If the boxer's blood pressure is elevated on the initial exam, he should be given an appropriate amount of time to rest and relax in an attempt to lower the pressure. If he is consistently hypertensive, the contest should not take place and referral to an internist for hypertensive evaluation is advised.

Head, Eyes, Ears, Nose, and Throat

Any bruising or swelling about the head or face should be noted. Lacerations that are not well-healed are grounds for failing the examination. A fundoscopic exam should be performed, looking for gross pathology. Unfortunately, many early retinal tears are peripheral and not easily picked up on direct fundoscopy. Scleral hematomas are common and not necessarily grounds for failure. Anisocoria should be noted if present. A tender or swollen nasal septum may indicate a fracture or impending fracture. The tympanic membrane should be examined if any symptoms are elicited.

Cardiopulmonary

Cardiopulmonary symptoms are rare in active boxers. Documentation of any murmurs should be noted, but rarely is this a reason for disapproving a match. An irregular pulse indicates an underlying problem and is reason to cancel a match. Unusual problems such as Wolff-Parkinson-White syndrome are no more common in boxers than in any other individual.

Musculoskeletal

Any swelling or tenderness of the hands, specifically at the knuckles or wrist should be looked for. Metacarpal fracture, extensor tenosynovitis, or capsular synovitis are all capable of limiting a boxer's performance and may be grounds for disapproval in some cases. Shoulder and elbow problems are not common in boxing. Tenderness of the rib cage may indicate a fracture that could result in pneumothorax with further injury.

Abdominal

The abdomen should be examined for organomegaly, although this is unlikely. An enlarged spleen, as might be seen in mononucleosis, will be rarely found. The standard inguinal hernia examination is not necessary in this setting.

Neurologic

All boxers should have a complete neurologic exam consisting of mental status check, cranial nerves, cerebellar testing, and reflex examination. This examination takes only a few minutes but should pick up any obvious focal signs. A neurologic exam may or may not identify early signs of chronic traumatic boxer's encephalopathy.

Musculoskeletal Injury

Musculoskeletal injuries other than the hand and wrist are not very common in boxers but can occur. Occasionally, a rotator cuff tear will be seen. The author also has seen a case of acute rupture of the subscapularis muscle occurring in a boxer. Rarely, anterior cruciate or meniscal knee injuries can be seen if a boxer pivots incorrectly with his foot firmly planted on the canvas.

Hand and Wrist

The most common musculoskeletal injuries in boxing involve the hand and wrist (22). Injury to this area can prematurely end a boxer's career. No studies exist to document the prevalence of hand and wrist injuries in boxing, but they are not uncommon. Considering the nature of this sport, it is surprising that more hand and wrist injuries are not seen. The following are typical injuries.

Thumb

First Metacarpal-Phalangeal Ulnar Collateral Ligament Tear. This injury is analogous to skier's thumb and is caused by forcible abduction of the thumb. The ulnar collateral ligament is stretched or completely torn (Fig. 15.4). Conventional boxing gloves allow the thumb to be abducted, resulting in a potentially injurious situation. Maintaining a secure clenched fist prevents this injury but such concentration is not always possible in the heat of competition. Thumbless gloves, which prevent the thumb from being forcibly abducted, should diminish the occurrence of this injury; however, no studies are available to document this effect. Treatment for incomplete tears is cast immobilization for 4 to 8 weeks. Complete ulnar collateral ligament tears that result in metacarpal phalangeal instability are generally treated with surgical repair, although occasionally closed cast treatment can be successful.

First Carpal-Metacarpal Injury. Injury to the first carpal-metacarpal area represents either traumatic synovitis, subluxation, or fracture of the first metacarpal base. These injuries are caused by striking the opponent's head with the radial side of the fist. Attention to proper punching technique and adequate glove padding will decrease the occurrence of the injury. Traumatic synovitis is treated by avoiding further boxing or heavy bag punching until symptoms subside. Subluxation of the first carpal-metacarpal joint, or a Bennett's fracture, is best treated with closed reduction and percutaneous pin fixation (Fig. 15.5).

Wrist

Second to Fourth Carpal-Metacarpal Injury. Injuries to the second to fourth carpal-metacarpal area can be either a traumatic synovitis, subluxation or dislocation, or fracture of the metacarpal base. The most common site of involvement is at the second and third carpal-metacarpal regions, either alone or in combination. These injuries are caused by direct impact loading at the metacarpal heads. Subluxation or dislocation at the carpal-metacarpal level probably results from landing a direct blow with the wrist in slight volar flexion. These injuries can be diminished by proper wrapping or taping of the wrist region. Synovitis is best treated by rest. Subluxation and dislocation are best treated by closed reduction and percutaneous pin fixation. Fractures in this region are treated closed if nondisplaced and by open reduction internal fixation if displaced. Recurrent injury can lead to a buildup of bone, termed carpal-metacarpal bossing.

Conventional Sprain. This injury is due to stretch or tearing of the dorsal wrist capsule or ligaments. Symptoms include vague pain or swelling in the wrist. No fractures are visible by X-ray. Treatment is rest and proper wrist taping with resumption of boxing activity.

Navicular Fracture and Nonunion. Fracture of the carpal navicular can be either a troublesome or a benign problem for boxers (23). The boxer may or may not recall a specific episode during which the fracture occurred. Symptoms may be mild and indistinguishable from minor wrist sprains. Frequently, the boxer will not seek medical attention for several weeks or months after the injury. An established nonunion may be present by the time a boxer presents for treatment.

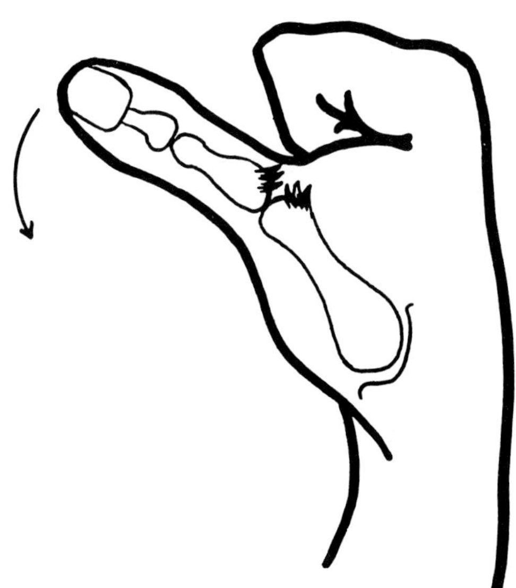

Figure 15.4. Schematic drawing depicting a complete rupture of the ulnar collateral ligament. This is caused by forced abduction of the thumb, which can occur with a standard boxing glove when the thumb is not attached to the remainder of the glove. (From Noble C. Hand injuries in boxing. Am J Sports Med 1987;15:344.)

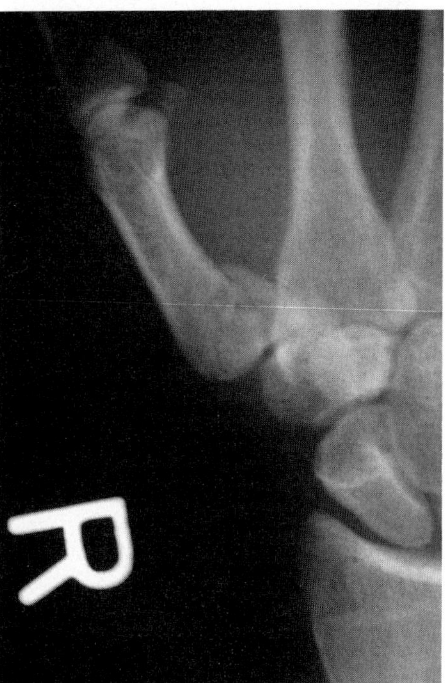

Figure 15.5. Bennett's fracture can occur when the unpadded thumb strikes the opponent's head.

Oftentimes the nonunion will be only minimally symptomatic or completely asymptomatic. If symptoms are not present, the boxer will usually elect not to treat the nonunion so that his career is not interrupted. The long-term consequences of not treating a navicular nonunion are unclear. Symptomatic acute fractures should be treated with a thumb spica cast for 6 to 8 weeks. Symptomatic nonunion can be treated with either cast immobilization, screw fixation, or bone grafting.

Knuckles

Second to Fourth Metacarpal-Phalangeal Sagittal Band Tear. Sagittal band tears in the metacarpal-phalangeal region are common in boxers and are often referred to as boxer's knuckle (24). They are caused by direct impact loading at the knuckle. These tears occur most often at the second metacarpal-phalangeal level, followed by the third and, less frequently, the fourth. Pathology consists of a stretch or tear of the extensor mechanism sagittal bands. Symptoms include tenderness and swelling at the knuckle joint. If the tear is large enough, the extensor tendon may subluxate or dislocate to the side opposite the tear. Minor stretches of the sagittal bands are best treated conservatively, whereas complete rupture requires surgical repair. This injury tends to be recurrent in boxers. Prophylactic avoidance measures include adequate taping and padding of the knuckle region. Increased padding in both sparring and competition gloves also should decrease the occurrence of this problem.

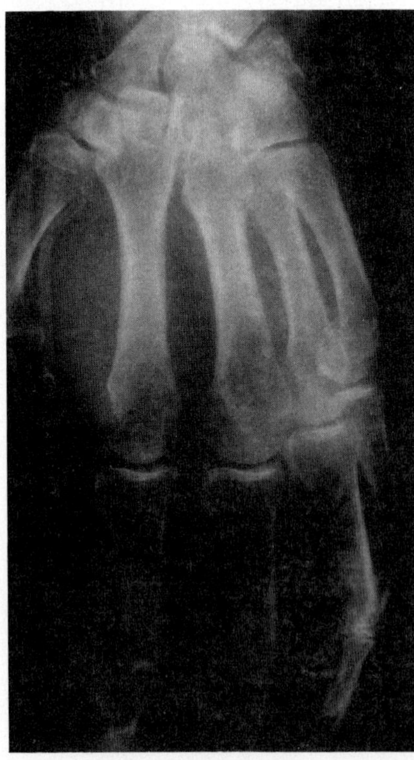

Figure 15.6. The boxer's fracture, a dorsally angulated fracture of the fifth metacarpal neck, is more appropriately titled a street fighter's fracture.

Second to Fourth Metacarpal-Phalangeal Dorsal Capsular Tear. The clinical appearance of metacarpal-phalangeal dorsal capsular tears is similar to that of the sagittal band rupture. Occasionally, a distinct rent in the capsule will be palpable. Rupture of the sagittal band or dislocation of the extensor tendon will always be present in association with a dorsal capsular rupture. Treatment for this injury is direct surgical repair of the defect (24). Prophylactic avoidance mechanisms are identical to those for a sagittal band disruption.

Metacarpal Fracture. Fracture of the neck or shaft of the second or third metacarpals can be seen following properly thrown punches. A direct blow with impact occurring at the prominent second or third knuckle joint can produce this type of fracture, despite the fact that the second and third metacarpals are less mobile than the more ulnar metacarpals and are supported by the thenar eminence (25). These anatomic considerations would tend to diminish the risk of fracture, but generated forces can occasionally overcome these protective features. The commonly labeled boxer's fracture, a dorsally angulated fracture of the fourth or fifth metacarpal neck, is more appropriately termed street fighter's fracture (Fig. 15.6). It is caused by improper punching technique in which the blow is delivered in a roundhouse manner with impact occurring at the relatively unsupported mobile fourth and fifth metacarpal phalangeal joint level (Fig. 15.7). Treatment is either by closed reduction and casting or percutaneous pinning and casting (26–29).

Cervical Fracture

While the fear of cervical fracture is ever present whenever a boxer is knocked down or out its occurrence is actually quite rare. Any unconscious individual should be treated as though a potential neck injury is present, but in boxing the actual presence of cervical fracture is unlikely. To the author's knowledge only three cases of cervical fracture caused by boxing have been reported in the English literature. Kewalramani and Krauss (30) reported one case of a hyperextension injury resulting in a C6 fracture with associated quadri-

UH-
NOW-THE PHANTOM MOVES SWIFTLY AND SILENTLY--
"GHOST WHO WALKS MOVES IN THE DARK LIKE GREAT CAT"-OLD JUNGLE SAYING
UMPH--
PHANTOM

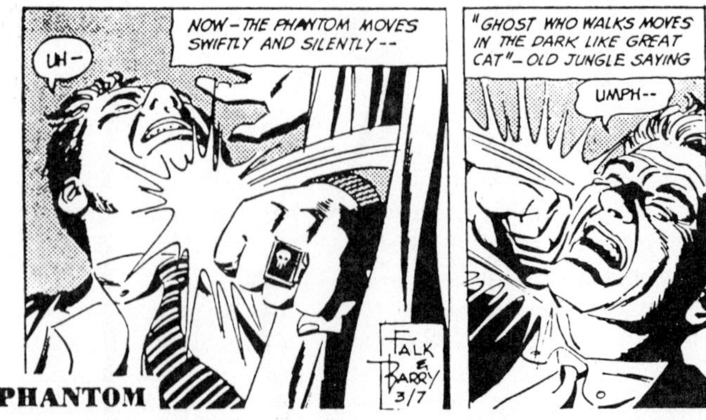

Figure 15.7. Cartoon panel on the *left* demonstrates an improperly thrown punch with forces concentrated at the fifth metacarpal. This type of blow can produce a street fighter's fracture. The panel on the *right* depicts a properly thrown punch, which can fracture the second or third metacarpal. (From Larose JH, Sik KD. Knuckle Fracture. JAMA 1968;206:894.)

plegia. No details of the fracture or of its mechanism of production were given in this report. Strano and Marais (31) reported one case that they believed represented an isolated anterior vertical arch fracture of C1, occurring as a result of long-term boxing exposure. The signs and symptoms were not classic for a C1 arch fracture, and the published CT scan raises the question that the finding may well have been a congenital anomaly rather than a fracture. Jordan et al (32) also reported one boxer who was believed to have sustained a nondisplaced C3 lateral mass fracture from boxing. No mention of neck pain was given in the report, and the boxer received no cervical immobilization as the injury was deemed to be stable.

Ocular Injuries

Earlier authors relying on anecdotal experience have tended to down play the frequency or seriousness of ocular injury in boxing. Blonstein (33) wrote that serious ocular injuries were rare in amateur boxers, noting only four cases of detached retina and making no mention of serious anterior chamber pathology during a 40-year period in which he cared for British amateur boxers. Whiteson (34) also wrote that retinal injury was rare among professional boxers. However, more comprehensive ocular studies in boxers have confirmed that the incidence of minor and major boxing-induced ocular injury is actually quite high (35–38). Elkington (39) surveyed the Ophthalmological Society of the UK and reported that 47% of ophthalmologists had examined at least one boxer with an eye injury. A total of 56% of the survey injuries were said to be retinal detachments. The early lack of awareness of boxing-induced ocular injury was the result of the subtle or nonexistent clinical symptoms of the injuries, failure to perform an adequate ophthalmological examination, and general ringside physician inability to diagnose accurately ocular pathology when present. Giovinazzo et al. (36) pointed out that an adequate ocular examination in a boxer should be performed by a licensed ophthalmologist and should include visual fields and acuity, anterior chamber slit-lamp examination, applanation tonometry, gonioscopy, and dilated examination of the retina, including indirect ophthalmoscopy with scleral depression.

Mechanism of Injury

Blunt trauma to the globe produces ocular injury by one or a combination of mechanisms termed coup, contrecoup, and equatorial expansion (40, 41). Coup injury is that which occurs at the point of impact. Contrecoup injury refers to that occurring at some point distal to the site of a direct blunt trauma. The ocular injuries resulting from a contrecoup force are caused by shockwaves that originate at the site of impact and that transverse the globe, producing injury at the interface of tissue of different densities (Fig. 15.8). Injury from blunt ocular trauma that causes compression of the globe in an anterior-posterior direction with obligatory expansion along the equatorial plane is termed equatorial expansion injury (Fig. 15.9). Equatorial expansion causes traction on the peripheral retina in the region of the vitreous base, leading to tear or detachment of the retina.

Types of Injuries

Both anterior and posterior chamber pathology is seen in boxing. Anterior chamber pathology may included corneal abrasions, injury to the lens, subconjunctival hemorrhage, ciliary body injury and angle recession among others. Posterior chamber injury includes all types of injury to the retina or vitreochoroid complex.

Angle Recession

Palmer et al. (42) examined the anterior chambers in 55 former professional boxers at an average of 33 years from retirement and documented angle recession in 8%. Of note, no boxer demonstrated glaucoma as a consequence of the angle recession. Chronic glaucoma has been reported to occur in 7% to 9% of patients following traumatic angle recession. The onset of the glaucoma may take up to 10 years to be evident after the angle recession. A similar incidence of 9% angle recession also was documented by Giovinazzo et al. (36). In a 1989 study based on the examination of 286 boxers performed by 22 ophthalmologists, angle recession abnormalities were documented in 39% (38). This study by Sills, reported in Jordan (38), included angle reces-

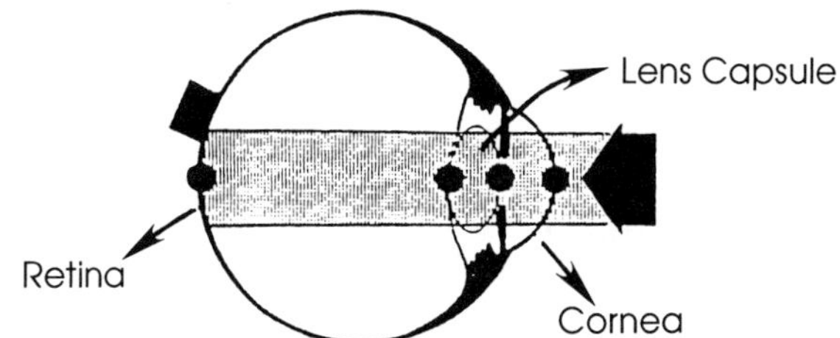

Figure 15.8 Depiction of force transmission with coup and contrecoup sites of injury indicated by the black dots. (From Smith DJ. Ocular injuries in boxing. Int Ophthalmol Clin 1988;28:243.)

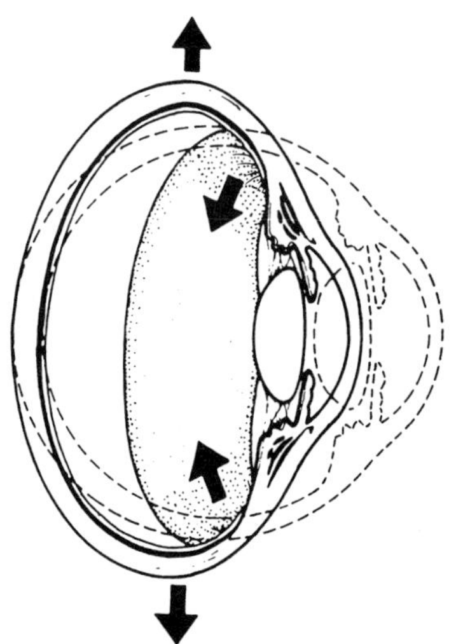

Figure 15.9 Equatorial expansion of the globe caused by compression in the anterior-posterior direction. (From Maguire JI, Benson WE. Retinal injury and detachment in boxers. JAMA 1986;255:2452.)

sions as small as 10%. However, it is generally believed that angle recession must be at least 90% before glaucoma will develop and usually must be 180°. If Sills's data are adjusted to eliminate any angle recession less than 90°, then the incidence of angle recession falls to 4.5°. Interpreted correctly, it would appear that the chance of a boxer developing glaucoma later in life as a result of his occupation is real but low.

Lens Abnormalities

Palmer et al. noted the presence of cataracts in 12 of 55 professional boxers examined. The majority of the cataracts were of the nuclear sclerotic type. Giovinazzo et al. (36) documented a 19% incidence of cataracts in a study of 74 professional boxers. A total of 70% of these cataracts were posterior subcapsular. Only 1 of the boxers in this group had visual impairment because of the cataract, but the possibility exists that vision may decrease as these individuals age. Smith (41) examined a group of 118 professional boxers over an 18-month period and documented a 10% incidence of cataracts with 66% being posterior subcapsular. Smith postulated that the posterior subcapsular cataracts were caused by either transmission of contrecoup forces or equatorial expansion. In addition, Smith pointed out that he had examined other boxers with significant visual impairment as a result of cataract formation. Sills's study of 286 boxers, which was an expansion of the study population used by Giovinazzo et al., documented cataract formation in 10% of the eyes. Only 5% of the eyes with cataracts had uncorrected vision reduced to less than 20/40. Steroid use has been associated with an increased incidence of posterior subcapsular cataracts. Whether the prevalence of posterior subcapsular cataracts in boxers is in any way related to steroid use is unknown.

Retina

Injury to the retina in boxing is common and may result in blindness if not appropriately treated (36, 40, 43). Maguire and Benson (40) reviewed the records of the retina service of the Wills Eye Hospital over a 31-month period and documented seven professional and two amateur boxers with evidence of retinal detachment in eight and retinal tear in one. Symptoms of retinal detachment included decreased visual acuity, peripheral field loss, light flashes (photopsias), and floaters (entopsias). All nine of these boxers had presented because of visual symptoms. Maguire and Benson noted that of the eight retinal detachments, six were secondary to a retinal dialysis, which is a linear tear along the vitreous base. The authors believed that all retinal tears were definitely caused by blunt trauma to the eye. Five of the patients also had evidence of a definite posterior vitreous detachment; three had evidence of vitreous hemorrhage, and two had an avulsed vitreous base, which is know to be pathognomonic for blunt trauma.

Giovinazzo et al. (36) performed a dilated ocular examination on every seventh professional boxer applying for a license within the state of New York over a 2-year period. A total of 74 boxers were examined. None of the boxers had ocular complaints, but 24% showed evidence of a retinal tear. An additional 4% had small atrophic holes in the retina. All of the involved eyes had evidence of vitreous traction, and 2 patients had retinal detachments. The probability of retinal tears correlated with increasing number of bouts and increasing number of losses. Giovinazzo et al. pointed out that after 6 bouts the incidence of retinal tear rises and after 100 bouts nearly all of the boxers in the study had evidence of at least a peripheral retinal tear. In Smith's (41) study of 68 boxers undergoing a dilated retinal examination 13 (19%) had evidence of vitreoretinal pathology and 5 showed evidence of a retinal tear. Sill's study of 286 boxers showed evidence of peripheral retina involvement in the form of either atrophic holes, tears, dialysis, or detachment in a total of 13% (38). The majority of these boxers demonstrated atrophic holes or tears with only three of the group demonstrating a retinal detachment.

Macular Injury

Involvement of the important central retinal macular area may result in severe central visual loss. Four of the retinal injuries in Maguire and Benson's study involved the macular region. Giovinazzo et al. documented macular pathology in 8% of boxers. Sills documented macular pathology in 1.7% of boxers examined.

Safety Measures

Several good measures have been advocated to decrease the incidence of ocular injury in boxing (36, 38, 41), which are listed in Table 15.2 and discussed below.

An annual ophthalmologic examination should be performed on every professional boxer. This examination should include measurement of visual acuity, visual fields, slit-lamp examination, intraocular pressure measurement, gonioscopy, and dilated vitreoretinal examination with indirect ophthalmoscopy. Once an abnormality is documented, its significance must be addressed by the boxer, his manager and the state boxing commissions in conjunction with the treating ophthalmologist. Mandatory yearly ophthalmologic examinations should be performed in all states.

The creation of a national registry to document and follow ocular injuries would be helpful in generating a database concerning the true ocular implications of boxing. The absence of a national database makes it impossible to speak objectively about the real incidence of ocular trauma in boxing.

The use of thumbless gloves may well decrease the

Table 15.2.
Ocular Safety Measures in Boxers

Annual ophthalmologic exam, including visual acuity and fields, slit-lamp, pressure measurements, gonioscopy, and dilated vitreoretinal examination
National ocular database
Use of thumbless gloves
Education of ringside physicians in diagnosing ocular pathology
Mandatory minimal ocular requirements

incidence of ocular injury. The state of New York currently mandates that all nontitle bouts use thumbless gloves. Unfortunately, no evidence currently exists to prove that thumbless gloves decrease the incidence of ocular trauma (37). Because they are seldom used, any impact would be difficult to determine.

More education of ringside physicians in diagnosing ocular trauma is necessary. Most ringside physicians are not qualified or do not possess the requisite equipment to perform an adequate ocular examination. Most attention is paid to periorbital cuts, which are not really serious from an ocular standpoint (44). Temporary visual impairment caused by periorbital bleeding that drips into the eye is easy to appreciate, whereas similar visual impairment caused by retinal injury may elude recognition. It should be the responsibility of the state boxing commissions, working through their medical advisory boards, to educate ringside physicians properly so that ocular injury does not go unrecognized.

Institution of mandatory minimal ocular requirements for state licensure is essential. The state of New York has taken the lead in mandating that all boxers should have an uncorrected visual acuity of at least 20/200 or better in each eye and a corrected visual acuity of 20/40 or better in each eye. The visual fields should be at least 30° centrally in each eye. These minimal requirements seem to be reasonable. No boxer should be allowed to compete if there is evidence of significant angle recession abnormality, lens abnormality, or peripheral retinal or macular abnormalities. Most serious vision-threatening injuries in boxing can be successfully treated if care is instituted early. Unfortunately, this time frame of opportunity is usually over before the boxer experiences clinical ocular symptoms.

The issue of continued boxing participation following successful repair of a retinal tear or detachment is not resolved. Clearly, most boxers who have had successful retinal surgery are able to continue to box. A decision in this regard should be made on a case-by-case basis. Ongoing ophthalmologic evaluation of these individuals is necessary to ensure that no further damage occurs once their boxing careers have resumed.

Rare Injuries

Cases of rare injuries have been reported in boxers (45). Niezgoda et al. (46) reported a case of pharyngoesophageal perforation secondary to blunt neck trauma following a boxing match. Solar plexus knockout, heart knockout (commotio cordis), and carotid sinus knockout also have been mentioned in the literature. Such injuries are exceedingly rare.

Forces in Boxing

Brain injury in boxing results from either linear or angular acceleration of the head or from impact of the boxer's head on the ring mat (47, 48) (Fig. 15.10). All three mechanisms may produce structural coup and contrecoup injury as well as concussion. A direct blow such as a straight jab tends to produce linear acceleration of the head, whereas tangential blows such as hooks or uppercuts produce angular acceleration. Angular acceleration can result in a head force three to four times greater than that produced by linear acceleration. Gurdgian et al. (49) felt that translational acceleration produced a pressure gradient in brain and cerebral spinal fluid, resulting in brainstem shear forces in the region of the foramen magnum. Ommaya et al. (50) stated that similar gradients are produced with angular acceleration. Conversely, Gennerelli et al. (51) used a primate model to suggest that concussive injury was caused by diffuse axonal injury of the entire brain.

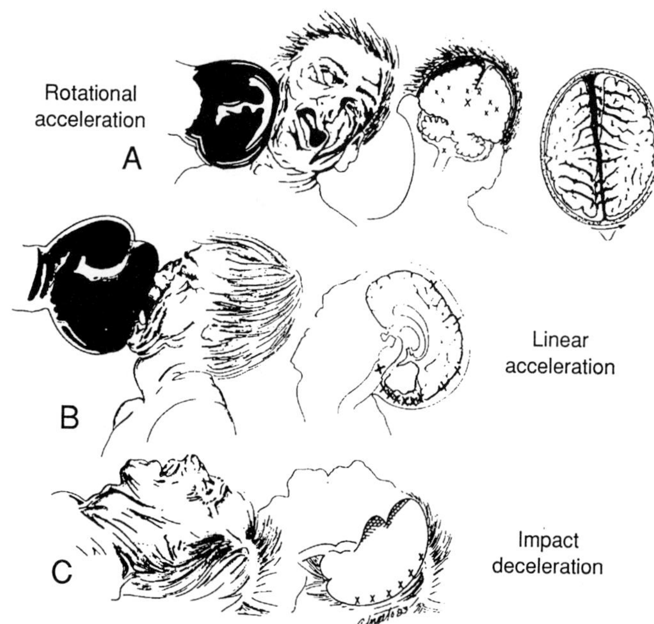

Figure 15.10. Schematic drawings demonstrating **(A)** angular (rotational) acceleration, **(B)** linear acceleration, and **(C)** injury caused by head impact on the mat. (From Lampert PW, Hardman JM. Morphological changes in brains of boxers. JAMA 1984; 251:2677.)

The forces generated by head blows in boxing are revealing. Using the Gadd Severity Index, a measure of the severity of head motion, Johnson et al. (52) showed that in a realistic boxing situation a safe level of force on the head can be exceeded by a factor of four. Schwartz et al. (53) reported that head blows can generate acceleration moments on the head as high as 120 *g*. This force is said to be equivalent to that of an unrestrained passenger striking his or her head on the dashboard in a low-speed auto collision. Atha et al. (54) conducted a particularly revealing study in which a top-rated professional heavyweight boxer punched an instrumented dummy. The peak force on the dummy head reached 0.63 t with 53 *g* of head acceleration. The authors stated that the generated force was equivalent to that produced by a blow from a 13-lb padded wooden mallet swung at 20 mph. Clearly, the force impact caused by boxing head blows is disturbingly high.

The most effective way of diminishing head trauma is to ban head blows in boxing. This approach has been adopted by at least one boxing club in Denmark (55). However, this is currently not a practical solution in North America and would not be accepted on a large scale. More practical potential interventions to decrease head forces have included the mandatory use of headgear and larger gloves. Evidence to support the efficacy of either of these interventions is not available (56). Headgear is mandatory in all amateur competitions and sparring sessions, but professionals use headgear only in sparring sessions. In a study in which small head forces were generated, Schmid et al. (57) demonstrated a 15% to 25% reduction in head acceleration with the use of headgear. However, it is unlikely that a similar reduction in head acceleration can be achieved in an actual boxing match in which there is significantly higher force generation (56, 58). Competition gloves in both amateur and professional boxing weigh 10 oz versus 16 oz for sparring gloves. The increased padding of larger gloves is reported to blunt the forces imparted to the head. Support for this position does exist experimentally. However, concussion and knockdowns are not rare events in the gymnasium, despite the use of headgear and 16-oz gloves. The author believes that concussive blows are primarily related to punch acceleration and to the effective body weight imparted to the punch. When the entire hip region and upper torso are thrown into the punch, force generation is increased (59). The forces generated by hard head blows appear to be higher than the threshold for brain injury. Any potential decrease in force generation by use of bigger gloves or headgear does not appear to be large enough to bring the punch force below the threshold for head injury. Consequently, use of these interventions may provide the boxer with a false sense of security concerning his susceptibility to head injury.

Acute Brain Injury

Death

Contrary to popular belief, the occurrence of death as a direct consequence of acute boxing injury is not as high as in some other sports (60–64). The incidence of boxing fatalities has been reported to be 0.13 per 1000 participants compared with 0.3 in college football, 0.7 in motorcycle racing, 1.1 in scuba diving, 5.1 in mountain climbing, 5.6 in hang gliding, 12.3 in skydiving, and 12.8 in horse racing (54, 65). From 1918 to 1983, there were 645 deaths worldwide reported as an acute result of either professional or amateur boxing. From 1945 to 1983, a total of 353 deaths were recorded, from 1970 to 1981 there were 50 deaths, and from 1979 to 1983 there were 28 deaths (66). These findings appear to show a slight decrease in the acute fatality rate in boxing. Most acute deaths in boxing are the result of the sequelae of acute subdural hematomas with diffuse brain swelling. Whether the deaths are the result of a single blow or multiple blows is not documented, but the author believes that most are secondary to multiple head blows over one or more rounds. High-speed photography has demonstrated that most knockouts occur before the boxer actually falls (3), and further head damage can be sustained when the head strikes the canvas.

Better refereeing should decrease the incidence of acute death. No boxer should be allowed to continue fighting in a groggy or concussed state. It is at this time that a boxer is most vulnerable to further head damage. The referee must appreciate that lack of defense, leaning against the ropes, drowsiness, lethargy, and wobbly legs all signify a concussed state in which the boxer has diminished control over body tone and neck musculature, resulting in the generation of larger coup and contrecoup head forces as the unsupported head is accelerated with each blow.

Hematoma

Subdural Hematoma

Acute subdural hematomas are found in up to 75% of individuals who have died acutely as a result of boxing injury. The subdural hematoma is caused by the tearing of bridging veins connecting the brain with the superior sagittal sinus in the dura mater. The boxer is typically drowsy or unconscious from the moment of impact. Occasionally, a short lucid interval may intervene between the offending blows and onset of symptoms. Clinical signs include stupor, coma, and ipsilateral pupillary dilatation. Brain herniation with resultant death can result without emergency treatment. A CT scan will show a collection of blood. Emergent burr hole drainage is required if the hematoma is large enough. Permanent neurologic damage is common even if the boxer survives.

Subacute Subdural Hematoma

Occasionally, several hours or a few days will pass before symptoms are obvious. The injured boxer will complain of headache, confusion, slowed thinking, or seizure. Coma may develop with a progressively downhill course similar to acute subdural hematoma. Treatment is similar to the acute injury. Any boxer sustaining a knockout should be closely observed for several hours following the knockout. Appropriate instructions should be given to his handlers so that treatment will be rendered if symptoms do occur.

Chronic Subdural Hematoma

Chronic subdural hematoma is seen much less commonly than acute subdural hematoma in boxers. Symptoms are those of headache, confusion, seizure, personality change, or paresis, occurring weeks or months after a bout. Treatment is varied and depends on the size and location of the clot.

Acute Epidural Hematoma

Acute epidural hematoma is rare in boxing and results from rupture of the middle meningeal artery. There is an associated skull fracture in up to 75% of individuals. Symptoms include drowsiness progressing to coma and hemiplegia. Treatment is surgical.

Intracerebral Hemorrhage

Intracerebra hemorrhage is the result of mechanical forces that cause differential movement between the brain and skull, resulting in coup and contrecoup forces propagated through the brain. The hemorrhage may consist of small petechiae or large clots occurring anywhere in the brain (67). In boxers, the injury is more unusual than subdural hematoma, but more common than acute epidural hematoma.

Diffuse Axonal Injury

An unusual injury, diffuse axonal injury caused by widespread disruption of axons, which probably occurs at the time of impact or shortly thereafter (51). The extent of injury may be additive with additional bouts. Prognosis for recovery is not good.

Cerebral Edema and/or Ischemia

The process of cerebral edema and/or ischemia may occur alone or may follow brain contusion or bleeding. It is frequently seen in association with acute subdural hematoma and may lead to death despite drainage of the subdural. Treatment is directed at lowering the intracranial pressure by hyperventilation and intraventricular catheter drainage, if necessary (68).

Concussion

A cerebral concussion is the most common acute neurologic injury occurring in boxing. The definition of concussion remains controversial, because its relationship to structural brain damage remains obscure. Concussion is generally considered to be a clinical syndrome characterized by immediate and fleeting postraumatic change in neural function such as alteration of consciousness, disturbance of movement, or equilibrium. Concussion can be viewed as an acute posttraumatic loss of neural function with rapid and generally complete return of function. Controversy arises concerning its classification and etiology as well as the cumulative effects of multiple concussions and the presence or absence of structural brain damage as a result of concussion (69–71).

Classification

It is important to grade the severity of concussion if it is believed that more severe concussion implies more severe underlying transient or structural brain injury. This correlation would seem to be obvious, but scientific proof is not conclusive. There are several classifications of concussion that can be found in the medical literature. The Congress of Neurological Surgeons define concussion in the following manner:

1. *Mild:* No loss of consciousness.
2. *Moderate:* Loss of consciousness with retrograde amnesia.
3. *Severe:* Unconscious for more than 5 min.

This classification does not appear to be specific enough or encompassing enough to be of much use for boxers. It does not account for different types of amnesia or for amnestic states occurring in individuals without loss of consciousness.

Parkinson, West, and Pathiraja (71) studied slow-motion film strips of 20 boxing knockouts and proposed a classification that is useful for acute boxing-induced concussion.

Stage I: Impairment of memory.
Stage II: Added impairment of somatic motor activity.
Stage III: Motor activity ceases and respirations are impaired.
Stage IV: Respirations cease.

Improvement from stages II to IV to the stage I state generally occurred in a matter of seconds, but recovery from stage I can take minutes to hours. Parkinson et al. stated that most boxing knockouts were stage II concussions, characterized by clumsiness when rising from the canvas, wobbly legs, and/or inability to defend oneself. A standing eight count may allow a boxer time to recover from stage II to stage I, thus enabling him to continue to fight. The referee should either terminate a match or, if permissible, give a standing eight count to any boxer who displays stage II concussive symptoms. Serious additional acute brain injury can occur if a match is allowed to continue while a contestant is in a stage II concussive state. The referee and ringside physician must be able to make this determination.

Jordan (72) has proposed a boxing-specific classification that includes the following grades.

Grade I: Transient neurological impairment without loss of consciousness lasting less than 10 sec.
Grade II: Transient neurological impairment without loss of consciousness lasting more than 10 sec.
Grade III: Loss of consciousness with complete recovery in less than 2 min.
Grade IV: Loss of consciousness with complete recovery taking more than 2 min.

This classification provides a practical working scheme for boxing. For example, a boxer who sustains a grade I concussive blow should be given a standing eight count in an attempt to recover before the match is allowed to continue.

Etiology and Cumulative Effects

The pathophysiologic mechanism by which head blows lead to concussion is not conclusively known. Neuberger et al. (73) proposed a thixotropic cause in which the gel sol equilibrium of the brain is altered as a result of sudden acceleration. Hallervorden (74) also believed that a change produced in the colloid medium of the brain would result in concussive symptoms. Other theories relate to changes in the neural cell membranes or internal cellular components. Whether the responsible alterations are localized to one area, such as the brainstem or limbic system, or more generalized to the entire cortex also is conjectural. Current imaging modalities such as CT and MRI scans do not demonstrate any abnormality in cases of concussion. EEG studies performed shortly after concussive episodes have been documented to be both normal and abnormal. Most, but not all, authors believe that structural brain changes are not present in concussion. The absence of identifiable structural brain change would imply that concussion is caused by a reversible, transient biochemical or mechanical change at the cellular level. Parkinson et al. (71) described a rat model of concussion in which they demonstrated that mild concussion did not result in permanent deficits. However, Windle et al. (75) presented experimental data suggesting that concussion was the result of changes in the neuronal cell bodies of the reticular formation and that measurable changes in memory function and rate of information processing persisted after overt concussive episodes.

It is unclear if multiple concussive blows result in a cumulative effect with manifestations that are more serious than one isolated concussion. Parkinson et al. (71) rat study showed that the effect of multiple concussions was not cumulative. On the other hand, Windle et al. (75) and Gronwall and Wrightson (76) thought that the effects can be cumulative. The unknowns concerning whether concussion is associated with a structural injury to the brain, whether the injury is reversible and over what period of time, and whether multiple concussions are cumulative in their effect are all important in understanding the true implication of boxing-induced concussion. Any definition of concussion probably should imply the potential for cerebral damage with the potential for healing and recovery. Lack of information concerning the true nature of concussion makes it impossible to provide a scientific basis for the recommendation to refrain from boxing for a specified period of time after one or more knock outs.

Chronic Traumatic Boxer's Encephalopathy

The concern relative to chronic neurologic injury occurring subsequent to a career in boxing is the single most divisive issue surrounding any discussion of the medical aspects of boxing. The polemic of this discussion is frequently strident and passionate (77–80). That a distinct constellation of abnormal clinical signs and symptoms can occur following a career in the ring is no longer in question (9, 81–84). Lay expressions used to describe such individuals were common before any medical description of this problem. Boxing afficionados and fans refer to the unfortunate ex-boxer suffering from this syndrome as being cuckoo, goofy, slug nutty, cutting paper dolls, punchy, head case, punch drunk, or stumblebum. The French boxing fan is familiar with the expression *sonnes cloche* ("ringing bells"), the German with *weiche birne* ("soft pair"), and the Italian with *suonato come una campano* ("ringing like a bell") (85). There are an equally large number of terms in the medical literature all describing the same clinical picture (86). Martland (87), in 1928, provided the first medical description of chronic brain damage occurring in ex-boxers with his classic description of what he termed the punch drunk syndrome (88). This syndrome is referred to in the medical literature under several other names: dementia pugilistica (89), chronic progressive traumatic encephalopathy of boxers (90), chronic traumatic encephalopathy of boxers (91), chronic neuropsychosyndrome (91), traumatic encephalopathy (92), and psychopathic deterioration of pugilists (93). The term chronic traumatic boxer's encephalopathy (CTBE) is the preferred term to describe this syndrome.

CTBE is characterized by a varying combination of cortical, pyramidal, extrapyramidal, cerebellar, and psychiatric signs and symptoms (83, 88, 90, 94, 95). The onset of the syndrome is insidious and may first appear after a particularly severe bout, near the end of a boxer's active career, or not until many years after the boxer has retired. This wide range of time of onset as well as varied clinic presentation makes recognition of the early symptoms difficult. It is not possible to give a single, universal description of the CTBE syndrome, because its time of onset, rate of progression, and clinical manifestations are all variable. Rather than attempting to describe a single clinical picture, the researcher should consider the syndrome as a variable combination of cerebral, pyramidal, extrapyramidal, cerebellar, and psychiatric signs occurring in an individual as a result of a career in boxing.

Cortical symptoms include slurred speech, occasional headache, dizziness, and perceived tinnitus, but most important, variable degrees of dementia. An affected individual will demonstrate a decrease in cognitive function, perception, calculation ability, and memory. Short-term memory for nonsignificant events is first affected but may progress to loss of both long- and short-term memory for significant people, events, and places. The ability to perform even the simplest of tasks such as dressing or other activities of daily living can be lost. The dementia of CTBE can be indistinguishable from that of classic Alzheimer's dementia (96).

Cerebellar signs in CTBE include a general disequilibrium, particularly with respect to the lower extremities. A momentary or continuously unsteady gait pattern can develop. Tinnitus and dizziness tends to aggravate the disequilibrium. Pyramidal signs are generally more subtle but tend to occur early, frequently as the first manifestation of CTBE (97). Frequently, a lack of awareness by the affected ex-boxer does not permit him to appreciate early subtle dragging of a leg, or weakness of an upper extremity. Signs of spasticity, including increased tone, hyperactive reflexes, positive Babinski's sign, and clonus may develop.

Extrapyramidal signs are classic in CTBE, explaining the occasional confusion in separating individuals with Parkinsonism from those with CTBE. Extrapyramidal signs seen in CTBE include immobility of the face, slowing or lack of movement, shuffling gait, rigidity, tremors (particularly of the hands and feet), and hypophonia. The occurrence of these symptoms tends to be somewhat later in the course of CTBE.

Psychiatric abnormalities also commonly occur. Affected individuals will show varying degrees of personality deterioration; violent behavior, which can approach momentary periods of rage; a generalized lack of awareness; and intolerance to alcohol consumption. In 1969, Johnson (91) studied 16 ex-professional and 1 ex-amateur boxer. The average age of the sample was

54 and the average time since they last boxed was 22 years. Johnson believed that individuals with CTBE could be grouped into five clinical psychiatric syndromes. The syndromes may or may not be progressive and can overlap; any one individual may show varying degrees of all five clinical syndromes. Johnson's five syndromes are listed below.

1. *Chronic Amnestic State:* Believed to be caused by scarring, neurofibrillary tangle, and plaque formation in the mammilo-thalamic-fornico-hippocampal system in and around the mammillary bodies, at the hippocampal areas, and deep in the midline in and around the third ventricle. The memory loss is typically for short-term impersonal data but can be more global.
2. *Dementia:* A progressive, irreversible disorganization of personality, particularly affecting cognitive function.
3. *Morbid Jealously Syndrome:* Attributed to involvement of the limbic system and typically directed at the boxer's wife in the form of accusations of infidelity. The jealousy may be heightened by sexual impotency, which is seen later as the disease progresses.
4. *Rage Reaction:* Believed to be caused by the involvement of the limbic system and possibly the septum pellucidum. These reactions are manifested as extreme violence, usually of short duration, that may result in emergency psychiatric admission or civil incarceration. Intolerance to alcohol will magnify this problem.
5. *Frank Psychosis:* Generally typified as delirium and paranoia.

Considering the protean manifestations of CTBE, it is difficult to describe a typical case. However, the author believes that the earliest findings consist of subtle slurring of speech with minor disequilibrium such as a momentary or continuous unsteady gait. Inability to perform a tandem gait test may be the first sign of CTBE. Cognitive function is at first only mildly affected but progression can lead to severe dementia. Personality changes and Parkinsonism symptoms tend to develop slightly later in the disease process. End stage involvement results in a severe combined Alzheimer and Parkinsonian picture that can result in permanent institutional placement (Fig. 15.11). There is no agreement in the medical literature concerning the degree of progression in CTBE syndrome. Many individuals will exhibit only minor involvement, without any tendency for progression. On the other hand, there are numerous examples of individuals with relentlessly progressive signs and symptoms However, symptoms are generally progressive if affected individuals are followed long enough.

Although the time of onset and the progressive nature may vary, there is no doubt that a distinct encephalopathy caused by boxing-related trauma does exist. Some authors have actually discounted the existence of a distinct CTBE syndrome, ascribing the pathologic picture to alcohol and drug abuse, genetics, hazards outside the ring, and baseline behavioral states (34). These extraneous factors can exacerbate CTBE symptoms but do not by themselves explain the problem. Attempts by medical apologists to down play the neurologic aftermath of boxing only serve to perpetuate the current inadequate medical understanding of this problem. Analysis of the current body of knowledge allows us to identify significant risk factors, and potentially to effect a change in these risk factors thereby improving boxing safety.

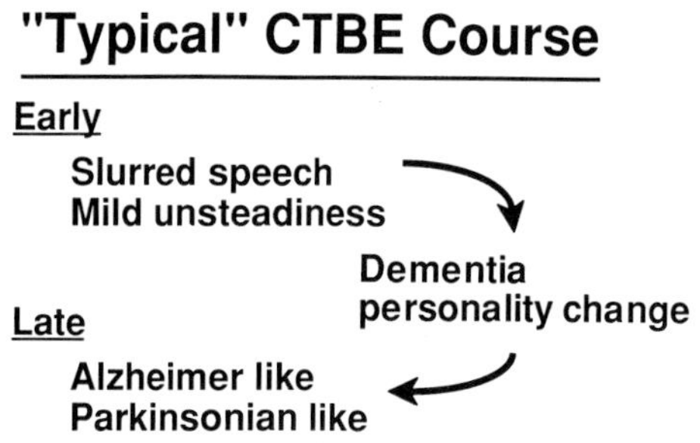

"Typical" CTBE Course

Early
- Slurred speech
- Mild unsteadiness

→ Dementia personality change

Late
- Alzheimer like
- Parkinsonian like

Figure 15.11. CTBE can demonstrate a varied course, but a typical scenario is shown.

Neuropathology

The neuropathologic changes in the brains of selected ex-boxers shed considerable light on the deleterious clinical aftermath sustained in the ring. Most, if not all, of the signs and symptoms comprising CTBE can be explained by these neuropathologic findings. Published literature documenting these neuropathologic changes is not extensive but is sufficient to identify a characteristic picture. Brandenburg and Hallevorden (98) were the first to describe chronic cerebral changes found in ex-boxers. They described the findings in an ex-boxer who had fought as an amateur from age 18 to 29 and who subsequently developed a progressive dementia and Parkinsonian picture beginning at age 38. The brain was grossly atrophied with microscopic vessel degeneration. Wide-spread neurofibrillary tangles and senile plaque formation were noted. The authors interpreted these findings as being consistent with posttraumatic dementia and Parkinsonism, distinct from typical Alzehimer's syndrome. Grahmann and Ule (99) also reported the case of an individual who had boxed as an amateur and in the booth from age 15 to 25 and who subsequently developed dementia and pyramidal and extrapyramidal signs beginning at age 46. Grossly, this brain showed evidence of atrophy and ventricular hypertrophy with a cavum septum pellucidum. Neurofibrillary tangles, without plaque formation, were documented microscopically. In 1959, Neuberger et al. (73) reported on one cortical biopsy and one autopsy specimen obtained from two ex-boxers who demonstrated a severe dementia. Both specimens displayed gross cortical atrophy and gliosis. There were no senile plaques or neurofibrillary tangles.

In 1967 Constantinides and Tissot (100) reported on an ex-amateur boxer who developed progressive clinical signs of dementia, Parkinsonism, and motor weakness. Postmortem examination disclosed brain atrophy and a cavum septum pellucidum with fenestration. Microscopic scarring, neurofibrillary tangles, and a depigmented substantia nigra also were observed. Payne (101) provided the first detailed review of postmortem findings in the brains of six ex-professional boxers. All six specimens showed some enlargement of the ventricular system with an associated cavum septum pellucidum. Three of six cases demonstrated fenestration in the septum. Payne felt that the cavum and fenestration were secondary responses to an internal ventricular enlargement that caused stretching of the corpus callosum and consequent separation of the septal attachments. He believed that injury to septal blood vessels during separation would presumably predispose, or initiate, septal fenestration. All specimens demonstrated a proliferation of the surface layer of the cerebrum, which was interpreted to represent foci of organized subpial hemorrhage. Macroscopic focal scarring was found in four specimens, whereas all six showed evidence of focal microscopic scarring. Scarring was believed to be the result of replacement of nerve cells by hypertrophied and hyperplastic astrocytes. This process was found in both the parietooccipital lobes and cerebellum. In summary, Payne believed that the main pathologic features included an enlarged ventricular system, miniature scars and microscars in the gray matter, focal areas of demyelination in the white matter, and irregular proliferation of the surface layer of the cortex, all of which were believed to indicate small areas of focal brain damage. He did not comment on any possible changes in the midbrain. Critics of Payne's work point out that one subject was old at the time of death, another had malignant hypertension, and two were chronic alcoholics, potentially obscuring the true etiology of these brain changes.

The most comprehensive work documenting the neuropathologic findings in boxers' brains was published in 1973 by Corsellis et al. (102). This eloquent study underscores the anatomic basis for the myriad signs and symptoms present in CTBE (Table 15.3). The study examined the brains of 12 retired professional and 3 amateur boxers, all of whom had boxed between 1900 and 1940. A characteristic pattern of cerebral pathology was documented, consisting of a cavum septum pellucidum with fenestration, cerebellar scarring, cerebral scarring, degeneration of the substantia nigra and locus cerulens, and Alzheimer neurofibrillary tangles without plaque formation.

Normally, the septum pellucidum is composed of two thin sheets of nervous tissue aligned in the midsagittal plane between the under surface of the corpus collosum and the dorsal aspect of the fornix. If these two sheets are separated, forming a cavity, it is referred to as a cavum deformity (103) (Fig. 15.12). Schwiddle (104) studied a general population sample of nonboxers and found a 20% incidence of cavum, most occurring later in life. Corsellis et al. demonstrated a consistent septal abnormality of a cavum septum pellucidum with fenestration. To further confirm the high prevalence of septal abnormalities in boxers, Corsellis et al. then reviewed 500 brains—475 of which were from psychiatrically institutionalized nonboxers in which septal abnormalities would be expected to occur with a greater frequency than in the general population. They found a mean septal cavum width of 1.6 mm in the psychiatric controls compared with 5.17 mm in the boxers. Furthermore, 77% of the boxers demonstrated septal fenestration compared with only 3% of the psychiatric controls. The fornix was found to be almost totally detached from the under surface of the corpus callosum. The two flattened fornical bodies were stretched horizontally over the dorsal surface of the thalamus. The corpus callosum itself was quite thinned. Corsellis et al. believed that repetitive blows to the head caused differential movement at the septal attachments on the ventral corpus callosum and dorsal fornix, resulting in cavum formation and fenestration of the tethered septum. As the ventricles enlarged, the septal tears would further enlarge. However, they did not believe that increased ventricular size alone was enough to cause septal fenestration. Other authors have also commented on the significance of septal changes (105–107).

Cerebellar scarring was particularly marked on the inferior surface of the lateral lobes, especially in the folia of the tonsillar region near the edge of the foramen magnum. As many as one-half to two-thirds of the Purkinje cells in these folia were lost, and the adjacent

Table 15.3.
CTBE Neuropathology

Cavum septum pellucidum with fenestration
Cerebellar scarring
Cerebral scarring
Degeneration of substantia nigra
Alzheimer neurofibrillary tangles with occult plaques

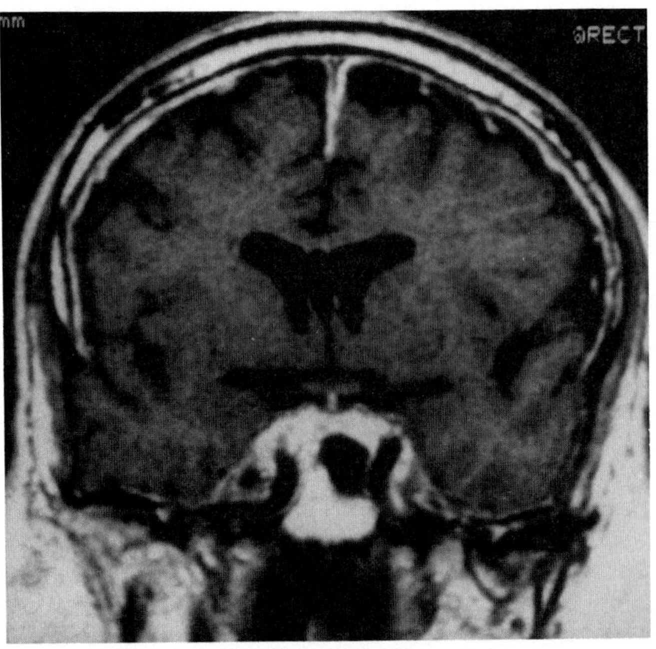

Figure 15.12. A gadolinium-enhanced, T_1-weighted MRI scan demonstrating a large cavum septum pellucidum.

granular layer was thinned with demyelinization of the associated white matter. Purkinje cell loss also extended far beyond the limits of gross scarring. Corsellis et al. postulated that these cerebellar changes could be explained on the basis of multiple bleeds or miniherniations of the tonsils. Corresponding changes, were not seen in the adjacent brainstem. Unterharnscheidt (1) documented similar Purkinje cell and granular layer damage in cats subjected to repetitive low intensity head blows.

Cerebral scarring, particularly in the deep periventricular region, did occur but was not a prominent finding. In 1923, Martland (87) hypothesized that the primary pathology in the punch drunk syndrome was the result of multiple concussive hemorrhages in the deeper portions of the cerebrum, resulting in scarring and atrophy. Martland believed that the hemorrhage and subsequent scarring would be found in the region of the corpora striata and corona radiata but not in the cerebral cortex or cerebellum. Consequently, evidence of old hemorrhage or scarring should be frequently observed in these areas if Martland's hypothesis is correct. Contrary to the findings in Payne's (101) study that do appear to validate Martland's theory, this hypothesis could not be verified by Corsellis et al.'s work; however, they did document decreased brain weight, increased ventricular size, and thinning of the corpus callosum, all of which would be expected as a consequence of decreased cerebral size. Interestingly, subsequent work done by Adams and Bruton (108), using more sophisticated tests for iron deposition, has demonstrated a high incidence of old microscopic hemorrhage throughout the cerebrum.

Degeneration and loss of pigmented nerve cells in the substantia nigra was a common finding in Corsellis et al.'s study. This neuropathologic finding, classically seen in Parkinsonism, readily explains the frequent occurrence of Parkinson-like extrapyramidal signs and symptoms noted in CTBE. The medial nuclear group of the substantia nigra was typically spared while the intermediate and lateral groups were typically involved. In addition, neurofibrillary tangles were common in these areas. Similar depigmentation changes also were documented in the adjacent locus cerulens. How multiple repetitive trauma leads to depigmentation of the substantia nigra is not known (109).

Probably the most striking neuropathologic finding in Corsellis et al.'s study was the documentation of diffuse neurofibrillary tangles without overt senile plaque formation (Fig. 15.13). Neurofibrillary tangles, accompanied by senile plaque formation are a classic finding in Alzheimer's disease. Tangles and plaques are found diffusely throughout the cerebum in Alzheimer's disease but are particularly prominent in the anteromedial temporal gray matter, amygdaloid nucleus, and hippocampus. The periventricular region is generally spared in Alzheimer's. In contrast, neurofibrillary tangles without senile plaque formation are typically seen in the Parkinsonian complex of Guam, postencephalitic Parkinsonism, certain types of chronic encephalitis, and progressive supranuclear palsy. Unlike typical Alzheimer's disease, most of the tangles in these latter conditions are localized to the midbrain, pons, and medulla. In the boxers' brains, tangles were diffusely located throughout the brainstem and cerebral cortex, particularly the medial temporal gray matter, amygdaloid nucleus, hippocampus, and parahippocampal regions. The absence of overt senile plaque formation was similar to the findings of Grahmann and Ule (99) and Constantinides and Tissot (100). How cerebral trauma induces tangle formation is not well-understood.

Roberts (110) later strengthened the neuropathologic relationship between Alzheimer's disease and CTBE. He used immunocytochemical methods in preparing an antisera to the proteinaceous substance found in the tangles of Alzheimer's disease. This antisera gave an identical morphologic and immunoreactive profile to the neurofibrillary tangles seen in CTBE. He postulated that these two conditions shared a common traumatic etiology. The puzzling absence of senile plaque formation

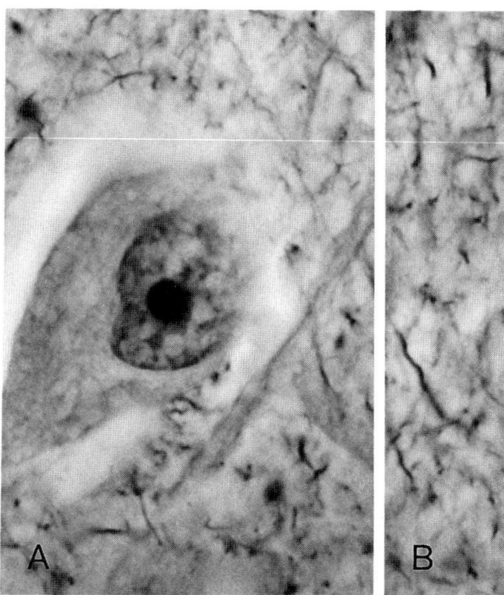

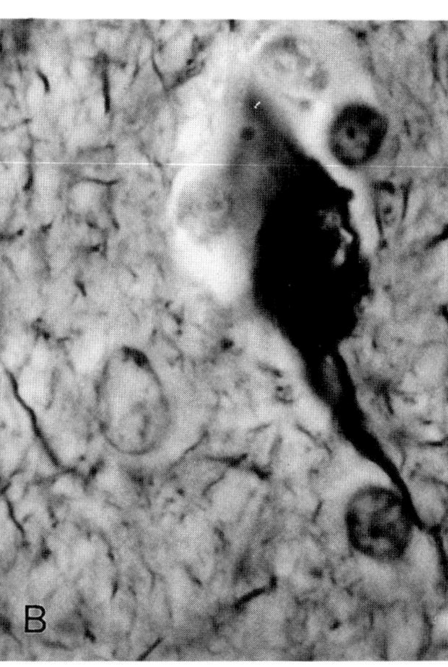

Figure 15.13. **A,** A normal neuronal cell body. **B,** The appearance of a typical neurofibrillary tangle.

observed in Corsellis et al.'s work was eventually explained by additional experiments performed by Roberts. Reinvestigating Corsellis et al.'s original specimens with the help of immunocytologic methods and an antibody to the β-protein present in Alzheimer's plaques, Roberts showed that all CTBE specimens with significant tangle formation also showed evidence of extensive β-protein immunoreactive deposits. These diffuse "occult" plaques were not visible with congo red or standard silver stains, as used by Corsellis et al. but were readily identified when Roberts pretreated the specimens with formic acid and labeled them with antibodies to the β-protein found in Alzheimer's plaques. Roberts postulated that the diffuse occult β-protein immunoreactive plaques of CTBE simply represent a younger version of the diffuse, overt, congophilic plaques seen in classic Alzheimer's disease. Tokuda et al. (111) also demonstrated significant immunocytochemical similarity between the neurofibrillary tangles and plaques found in both Alzheimer's disease and CTBE, providing further proof of a basic connection between the two diseases. In addition, ubiquitin, a protein found in the neurofibrillary tangles of Alzheimer's disease and involved in the degradation of abnormal proteins also has been found in the tangles of CTBE (112). Diffuse tangle and plaque formation are thought to be the hallmark changes resulting in the clinical dementia of Alzheimer's disease and may well explain the analogous signs and symptoms of dementia noted in CTBE. The neurofibrillary tangles in both conditions tend to cluster in the temporal lobe. Current research into the etiology of Alzheimer's disease lists trauma as a predisposing factor. Based on this neuropathologic evidence, it is clear why the clinical signs of Alzheimer's and CTBE are similar (96, 113).

Brain damage in CTBE is thought to result from a combination of mechanical shearing forces on the neurons and breakdown of the cerebral blood-brain barrier. Traumatic damage to the cerebral blood vessels could cause leakage of β-protein into the brain substance, resulting in occult plaque formation. Brayne et al. (14) demonstrated that creatine kinase isoenzyme (CK_1), which is normally found in high concentrations in the brain and low concentrations in blood, rose systemically following amateur boxing competitions. Interestingly, Rodriquez et al. (115) have demonstrated an diminution in regional cerebral blood flow, particularly in the parietal and temporal lobes, of professional but not amateur boxers. Further evidence of diffuse vascular damage in boxers' brains also was provided in a study by Adams and Bruton (108) in which 17 of 22 ex-boxers showed evidence of old hemorrhage either intracerebrally, in the meninges, or in the cerebellum.

The totality of the pathologic changes provide an explanation for the clinical signs and symptoms in CTBE. Memory capability is hypothesized to reside in the limbic areas of the brain, particularly in the medial temporal gray matter and hippocampal formation. Neurofibrillary tangles are numerous in these areas as well as in other limbic areas, which constitute an important control center for memory and cognitive functioning. Extensive cortical scarring, neurofibullary tangles, and plaques would all tend to further diminish cognitive function, thus explaining the Alzheimer-like symptoms seen in CTBE. The macroscopic and microscopic cerebellar changes can easily explain the coordination problems, tremors, and irregular movements. Parkinsonian (extrapyramidal) features, including slowness of movement, rigidity, and blunted facial expression, are all explained by the marked depigmentation noted in the substantia nigra. And finally, the emotional changes noted so frequently in CTBE also can be explained by the limbic and septal changes.

It can unequivocally be stated that although other etiologies such as head injury outside of boxing, alcohol abuse, degeneration due to old age (Alzheimer's), or classic Parkinsonism can each demonstrate selected clinical and pathologic features of the CTBE syndrome, only CTBE displays the constellation of cortical, pyramidal, extrapyramidal, cerebellar, and psychiatric features in association with the five classic pathologic findings of cavum septum pellucidum with fenestration, cerebral atrophy, cerebellar atrophy, depigmentation of the substantia nigra, and diffuse neurofibrillary tangles with occult plaque formation.

Epidemiology

The prevalence of CTBE in professional or amateur boxing varies, depending on the criteria used to make the determination. The syndrome is much more common in professional boxers but not unknown among amateurs (116). Older reports had estimated the prevalence anywhere from 0% to 50%, but documentation of these estimates was not provided. The best study addressing the prevalence of CTBE in professional boxers is undoubtably that of Roberts (83). He examined a random sample of 224 boxers out of a total population of 16,781 registered with the British Boxing Board of Control between 1929 and 1955. The boxers had to be British nationals and have at least 3 years of professional experience to be included in the study. Roberts reported that 37 of the 224 (17%) had definite signs of encephalopathy that were not explainable by other causes. In 13 of those 37, the signs and symptoms of chronic encephalopathy were either of a moderate or severe degree. An additional 11 boxers also demonstrated an encephalopathy, but the etiology could not definitively be attributed to boxing as other relevant factors or diseases also were present. The prevalence of full-blown CTBE was definitely related to the length of the boxers' careers and their age at time of review. Roberts noted that if the boxer was older than 50 years at the time of review and had had a career lasting more than 10 years the incidence of encephalopathy was 47%, compared with 17% if the career was between 6 and 9 years and 13% if the career lasted less than 5 years. Similarly, for boxers less than 50 years old at the time of review with careers lasting greater than 10 years, the incidence was 25% compared with 14% for careers lasting 6 to 9 years and 1% for careers lasting less than 5 years. Of note also were individuals who demonstrated either isolated dysequilibrium, dysarthria, alcohol intolerance, or isolated pyramidal signs but without a full-blown traumatic encephalopathy. Roberts found that one or more of these symptoms were present in 74% of retired boxers who were older than 50 years at time of review and had had careers lasting more than 10 years, compared with a 56% incidence if the career was from 6 to 9 years and 35% if less than 6 years.

Roberts also correlated the prevalence of encephalopathy to the actual number of professional bouts that the boxers were involved in. Similar to length of professional careers, the more professional bouts a boxer had, the higher the prevalence of traumatic encephalopathy. For boxers more than 50 years old at review who had had more than 150 professional fights, the incidence of encephalopathy was 50% versus 19% for those with 50 to 150 fights and 7% for those with less than 50 professional fights.

Criticism of Roberts's work is primarily that his study population is not representative of modern-day boxers who arguably compete under improved medical supervision and better overall supervision. Many of Roberts's boxers had competed before World War II, at a time when careers tended to be much longer and boxers had many more bouts. There was a tendency to allow boxers to absorb far more punishment than is currently deemed appropriate. Matches were frequently longer than is currently permitted, with some bouts lasting longer than 15 rounds. Before World War II an unknown percentage of professional boxers also engaged in unregulated, unlicensed matches, termed booth boxing. In these staged or competitive competitions, weight limits were not observed and varying amounts of head trauma occurred. Professional sparring in which a boxer received payment for services also appeared to be more common before World War II. Neither professional sparring nor booth boxing was considered in Roberts's analysis.

Modern-day studies on boxing encephalopathy have been of a nonrandomized nature, with attention directed to findings on EEG, CT, and MRI. Kaste et al. (10) studied 14 boxers—6 professional and 8 amateur—with neuropsychiatric testing, EEG, physical examination, and CT scanning. They documented evidence of cerebral atrophy in 4 of the professionals and 1 of the amateur boxers. A total of 2 professionals and 7 amateurs showed EEG abnormalities, whereas 2 professionals demonstrated abnormal neuropsychiatric testing; 1 of the boxers, a professional, had obvious encephalopathic symptoms. Overall, structural or functional abnormalities were found in 5 of 6 pros and 4 of 8 amateurs. Kaste et al. concluded that there was no evidence to support the view that modern-day boxing is safe from a neurologic standpoint.

Casson et al. (117) reported the CT findings of 10 professional boxers who had been knocked out a few weeks before their examination. No boxer demonstrated acute pathology, but 5 did have evidence of cerebral atrophy. The presence of a CT abnormality was directly related to the number of bouts fought by the boxer and not to his proficiency. In fact, better boxers tended to have more bouts and more cerebral atrophy on CT scan. Casson et al. concluded that the CT findings were due to multiple subconcussive blows. No boxer demonstrated a clinical CTBE syndrome.

Sironi and Ravagnati (118) performed CT scans and EEG on 10 young professionals and found CT evidence of definite atrophy in 2 and borderline atrophy in 4 as well as definitively abnormal EEGs in 3 and borderline changes in 4. They noted that the CT changes appeared to be related to the number of knockouts sustained by the boxer rather than to the length of career or number of bouts fought. This is in contrast to most other studies that have emphasized number of bouts and length of career.

Ross et al. (119) performed 38 CT scans and 24 EEGs on 40 modern ex-professional boxers. The study was looking for brain atrophy as identified by gyral hypertrophy or ventricular enlargement. A total of 20 of the 38 CT scans showed evidence of brain atrophy. They noted a positive correlation between increasing number of bouts and ventricular enlargement but not with gyral atrophy. The study did find that boxers with more bouts tended to have more EEG changes. Gyral atrophy did not correlate with the number of times a boxer had been knocked out.

Casson et al. (11) studied 18 modern boxers (13 ex-professional, 2 active professionals, and 3 active amateurs) with physical exams, CT scans, EEG, and neuropsychologic testing. All potential causes of brain damage other than boxing were criteria for exclusion from the study. CT scans were reviewed for evidence of generalized cerebral atrophy (increased ventricular size and prominence sulci), central cerebral atrophy (increased ventricals and normal sulci), cerebral cortical atrophy (normal ventricals and prominent sulci), and cavum septum pellucidum. A total of 8 of the professional boxers had an abnormal CT scan, 5 had an abnormal neurologic exam, and 7 had an abnormal EEG. All 18 boxers demonstrated abnormal findings on neuropsychologic testing. Of note, 4 of the 5 professional champions or highly rated boxers in this study demonstrated CT scan abnormalities, and 6 of 8 professionals with greater than 20 bouts had abnormal CT scan findings compared with 2 of 10 with less than 20 bouts. Casson et al. concluded that CT scan abnormalities, EEG changes, and abnormal neuropsychologic tests all correlated with increasing number of bouts. There was no correlation with the number of knockouts. They did not believe that modern-day professional or amateur boxing was safe.

Drew et al. (120) compared 19 young modern professional boxers with 10 nonboxing controls, using neuropsychologic testing and found abnormalities in 15 of 19 boxers compared with 2 of 10 controls. They concluded that modern boxers still suffer brain damage.

The body of evidence shows that overt CTBE was a significant problem for professional boxers who had careers before World War II. Although similar conclusive proof of frequent overt CTBE does not exist for modern-day boxers, much inferential evidence exists to raise the specter that it still may. Almost all recent studies using CT scans and/or neuropsychologic testing demonstrate a high frequency of subclinical abnormalities in professional boxers, with similar but less frequent findings in amateur boxers. Classic cases of overt CTBE continue to be reported albeit not frequently, despite modern-day medical care. Long-term clinical follow-up on the individuals who have been reported to have abnormal CT, EEG, or neuropsychologic findings is necessary to determine if full-blown CTBE will develop. In the meantime, the medical and organizational reform recommendations outlined in this volume should be implemented in the hope that the incidence of CTBE can be reduced in the modern sport of boxing.

Risk Factors

The majority of the medical literature identifies two proven risk factors for CTBE. First, CTBE is much more common following a career in professional boxing than after an isolated amateur career. Second, the longer the professional career, generally translating into more professional bouts, the greater risk of CTBE (83, 121, 122). It is not difficult to understand why professional boxing is riskier than amateur boxing. The contests are longer and much more brutal. The combatants are more skilled, throw harder punches, and absorb far more head trauma than amateur boxers. Sparring sessions are longer with harder and more frequent head blows. A professional boxer's livelihood depends on his ability to absorb head blows. Officiating personnel are much more likely to allow a potentially dangerous bout to continue than are amateur officials. Because multiple subconcussive blows alone can eventually lead to CTBE longer careers are inherently more dangerous. A direct correlation is identified between the number of professional bouts and the likelihood of developing CTBE. There is disagreement concerning the degree of CTBE risk in various boxing weight divisions. Some authors have stated that heavier boxers are at a greater risk because of the harder punches thrown. However, this probably is not true. CTBE is appreciated in ex-boxers of all weight classes. Any boxer, no matter how small, who receives multiple subconcussive head blows is at risk for development of CTBE. Sluggers who are willing to absorb two or three punches to land one are potentially at increased risk. Second-rate boxers and those that frequently work as sparring partners for better boxers are potentially at increased risk. Ironically, boxers with an ability to take a punch and who, therefore, can be expected to win more fights and have longer and more financially productive careers may be at increased risk. Severe CTBE necessitating permanent institutionalization has been seen in many excellent ring technicians including many that have held world titles. Boxing greats such as Joe Louis, Sugar Ray Robinson, Billy Conn, and Fritzi Zivic are prime examples of skilled world champions who had suffered the unfortunate effects of CTBE.

There is no clear correlation beetween the number of knockouts sustained by a boxer and the subsequent development of CTBE. Some authors have observed a direct correlation (123), whereas others refute this claim, instead concentrating on the correlation with multiple subconcussive blows (10, 11, 83). It is clear that CTBE can occur in the absence of repeated knockouts or even one knockout. Although it is argued that the incidence of CTBE has diminished since the inception of stricter medical guidelines after World War II, support for this position is not universal. The studies of boxers whose careers commenced after World War II (described above), raises the specter that significant evidence of both clinical and subclinical CTBE continues to exist.

Preventive Measures

There are many ways to decrease the incidence of CTBE (124, 125) (Table 15.4). Foremost is the belief that better medical supervision will improve all aspects of boxing safety, including decreasing the incidence of CTBE (124, 126, 127). Although there is evidence that acute boxing injuries can be decreased, the effect on CTBE is as yet unproven. Better medical supervision would take the form of better ringside physicians; enforcement of mandatory medical layoffs; serial screening with CT, MRI, EEG, and ophthalmologic examinations; availability of acute life-support measures at ringside; comprehensive evacuation plan for the boxing arena; and available neurosurgical backup support. In addition, significant improvements can be accomplished in other aspects of the sport.

Better Medical Supervision

Ringside Physicians. Having a physician sit at ringside who is knowledgeable in both the medical and nonmedical aspects of boxing is essential. The physician must not only be knowledgeable but also have the authority to intervene without fear of obstruction by state or local boxing officials or from the boxer's corner, if he or she believes that a boxer is in trouble. In many states, the physician is not authorized to stop a match even if he or she feels that a boxer is taking too much punishment. In more progressive states—such as Pennsylvania and New York—the physician can mount the ring apron at any time during a round or rest period to examine the boxer and terminate the contest if deemed medically necessary. In many instances, the physician faces a difficult decision in deciding whether to stop a contest or let it continue. The boxer, his corner, the promoter, and frequently the local governing

Table 15.4.
Potential Preventive Measures against CTBE

Better medical supervision
Ringside physicians
Mandatory medical suspensions
Serial screening
Acute life support
Evacuation plan and neurosurgical support
Decrease length of competition
National boxing commission
State boxing commission
Better trainers, managers, promoters, and referees
Improved gloves, ring, posts, and headgear
Boxer education

body may all want the bout to continue. If in the physician's medical judgment a boxer's well-being is in jeopardy by allowing the contest to continue than he or she must stand firm and terminate the contest. Repeated grade I concussion, or groggy state behavior, is an absolute indication to terminate a contest. Despite their having spent countless years in the sport of boxing, few trainers, promoters, or other lay individual has the physician's medical understanding of the dangers inherent in allowing a boxer to become repeatedly concussed. A situation that has become an obvious and real neuro danger to the boxer may be perceived by the public as mere guttiness, guile, or ability to take a punch. The tendency to repeatedly allow a boxer to weather the storm must be guarded against. It is not necessary for a boxer to be repeatedly knocked down before a bout is halted by the physician. Even though a physician's financial renumeration for working a boxing match is paid for by the promoter, the physician's obligation is first and foremost to protect the medical well-being of the boxer. National sanctioning bodies and state boxing commissions must be supportive of the physician's decision, even if it is unpopular.

The difficulty in deciding to terminate a contest because of excessive head or body blows mandates that the ringside physician have a thorough understanding of the sport of boxing. Boxing is inherently dangerous and seemingly brutal to some individuals. The ringside physician must walk the fine, ill-defined line between accepting this reality and protecting the well-being of the participants. It is only with continued exposure to the sport that the distinction can be appreciated. A ringside physician also must be knowledgeable with respect to the didactic medical aspects of boxing. He or she should be introduced and tutored in the sport by an experienced ringside physician. It is unacceptable for the medical coverage of an amateur or professional boxing show to be provided by a physician who has never attended a boxing match and/or does not understand the risks involved. Refereed journal articles and reviews (66, 85, 128, 129), chapters (130), and even entire books on the medical aspects of boxing are available (38). Unfortunately some physicians who sit ringside for boxing matches do not possess the available knowledge. They are then incapable of knowing when enough punishment is enough. Frequently they will err by either allowing a bout to continue too long or stopping a bout prematurely. Any competent physician can achieve an understanding of boxing and its medical implications. It should be obvious that a professional or amateur boxing competition should never be held without the presence of at least one, and preferably two, competent ringside physicians. Allied health personnel such as chiropractors or physician's assistants are not qualified to sit ringside as the sole providers of medical coverage.

Having two physicians present at a competition allows one to attend to any medical needs in the post-fight dressing room while the other remains at ringside to monitor subsequent bouts. The ringside physician should attempt to arrange appropriate follow-up for suture removal, referral to specialists, and scheduling of tests, if necessary. Facial lacerations should be repaired by the ringside physician in the dressing room if he or she is comfortable with suture repair, otherwise referral to a local emergency room is necessary.

Mandatory Medical Suspensions. Currently if a boxer is under medical suspension in one state there is no guarantee that all other states will know of the suspension or will honor the suspension if the boxer attempts to compete in another state. If a boxer has been knocked out and is medically suspended in one state he may attempt to compete shortly thereafter and risk further injury in another state. While this situation has lessened as state boxing commissions have improved their communication with each other, it is still not ideal. At least four states still lack any boxing commission whatsoever. Medical suspensions by one state boxing commission should be conveyed to all other state commissions and be honored except in rare circumstances.

Many state boxing commissions have regulations regarding medical suspensions but they are not always enforced by the commissions. Enforcement of established medical suspension guidelines should be assiduously performed. Every state should develop and follow guidelines similar to those of New York and Pennsylvania. In Pennsylvania, if a boxer sustains a knockout he is automatically suspended for 45 days. If a boxer loses six straight bouts he must have an examination by a commission-approved physician. Before further competition in New York following a medical suspension a boxer must obtain either an EEG, CT scan, or MRI study. Similar guidelines exist in Pennsylvania.

Currently, if the imaging studies and neuroexams are normal, there is no valid medical rationale that can be used to determine the optimal length of suspension following head trauma sustained in the ring. Empirically, it can be argued that a boxer takes a suspension more seriously if it is for at least 30 days. State boxing commissions should have input from a medical advisory board (composed of physicians with recognized expertise in the medical aspects of boxing) to develop guidelines for medical suspension. The medical advisory board should review the results of all examinations or tests performed at the end of the suspension period before allowing a boxer to enter further competition. A prohibition from further boxing during the suspension period also applies to gym sparring. Practically speaking, enforcement of the sparring prohibition falls completely on the shoulders of the boxer and on his trainer or manager.

Serial Screening. While cavum septum pellucidum and cortical atrophy can be visualized on CT or MRI scans, the presence of an anatomic structural abnormality does not always imply a functional abnormality (103, 105, 131–134). The lack of a direct correlation makes the interpretation of serial imaging studies more difficult in boxers with a normal neurologic examination. If the boxing community were receptive to the concept of baring from competition those individuals with normal exams but with abnormal CT or MRI studies then serial screening would have a significant impact. Unfortunately, this acceptance does not exist for serial imaging studies or for EEGs (135, 136). Yearly screening ophthalmologic examinations also would be quite beneficial to boxers. Subtle retinal changes predisposing to tear and existing peripheral asymptomatic tears can be monitored and the boxer counseled appropriately. The practical concern with any type of serial imagining or ophthalmologic screening is not only boxer compliance but, more important, determining who will pay for the test. Active boxers frequently cannot afford to pay, and managers and promoters are not always willing. Except for New York, state boxing commissions are not presently funded to the level that they can underwrite such an expense.

Acute Life Support. All professional and possibly all amateur competitions should have an ambulance in attendance at the boxing arena. The ringside physician should make a point to speak to the paramedics before the start of the boxing competition and outline a plan for intubation or resuscitation if necessary. Capability to intubate on site and to transport rapidly are essential.

Evacuation Plan and Neurosurgical Support. The ringside physician should arrange with ambulance paramedics and the local hospital for a definite evacuation plan. The hospital to be used should be identified and informed. Proper neurosurgical support should be available or plans should be developed for transfer to the closest facility that has such support. Severe neurologic sequelae or even death following acute boxing head injury is potentially preventable if proper actions are taken immediately.

Decrease Length of Competition

All of the world boxing–sanctioning organizations have enacted a rule that decreases the length of championship bouts from 15 to 12 rounds. This safety feature was presumably enacted in response to public outcry over the dangers of boxing. Although there is no medical evidence supporting the efficacy of this intervention, it does make common sense. The last 3 rounds of a 15-round bout tend to be grueling as both boxers experience fatigue, making them easier to hit and to hurt. Limiting championship bouts to 12 rounds should involve less risk to the boxers, because of fewer head blows landed. This intervention obviously is germane to only a small fraction of individuals who compete as professionals. Consideration should be given to further limiting the number of rounds for all professional bouts. This would not be a popular innovation as both boxers and fans would probably oppose such a rule change.

National Boxing Commission

Currently there is no centralization of boxing authority in the United States. Official sanctioning bodies such as the WBA, WBC, and IBF have not been particularly helpful in leading the movement for boxing safety reform. These organizations propagate their own existence by collecting large sanctioning fees. By virtue of their sanctioning authority, these organizations must take responsibility for many of the inappropriate circumstances that have mired the sport of boxing today. National standards to ensure boxing safety should be enacted. Prefight certification, ringside management, postfight medical suspensions, and yearly screening should be standardized throughout the country and, ideally, the world. The enactment of national safety standards probably would require the institution of some form of federally mandated national boxing commission with real power to enforce and develop guidelines. If uniform safety standards could be enacted nationwide by the existing state boxing commissions, then centralized bureaucracy could be avoided. However, it is doubtful that the existing state boxing commissions will ever be funded sufficiently or can ever work in concert to ensure the type of medical safety guidelines that are necessary. Congressional hearings have been and continue to be held to explore this issue in boxing. The lobby against mandated federal reform in boxing is enormous and consists of a sizable number of promoters, current world sanctioning organizations, and most state boxing commissions. Unfortunately, the boxers themselves have little or no control over this process.

State Boxing Commissions

Most states have a state boxing commission that is empowered to supervise and administrate boxing regulations in that state. Unfortunately, many commissions are underfunded and do not adequately monitor boxing safety. Obvious mismatches as well as poor judging and officiating have been all too standard in boxing. Medical clearance to obtain a boxing license is often capricious and certainly not standardized from state to state. Common rules to govern boxing, ensure its safety, and enforce penalties for violating these rules do not exist. Some state boxing commissions are diligent in their actions while others are either negligent or even nonexistent.

Most commissions have the boxers' best interest at hand but are either underfunded or uninformed. Judging by the display of boxing competition in some states, satisfactory medical input to the commissions is either not provided, ignored, or simply not enforced. Comprehensive national boxing safety reform can only be accomplished via the current state boxing commission system by dramatically increasing each state's budget. This would involve a serious reworking of finances at the state legislative level and would likely be opposed by many groups both in and out of government. Finally, state legislatures need to reexamine the dual roles that they have given to their state boxing commissions, which must encourage and expand boxing as well as provide regulations. These two roles can at times be in conflict. State boxing commissions must at all times keep boxing safety as the primary goal.

Trainers, Managers, Promoters, and Referees

Enlightened understanding of the dangers inherent in boxing head blows and institution of measures to counteract these dangers by trainers, managers, promoters, and referees are paramount to any improvement in boxing safety. Any type of worthwhile mandated safety proposal by either a federal or state regulatory body will be for naught if the boxers' handlers are not brought into the process. Boxing safety awareness must begin with the trainer. Boxing instruction should emphasize tactics to avoid being hit by head blows. The willingness to take two or three blows to administer one must be deterred. Trainers should ensure that sparing sessions are safe, specifically that their boxers do not take undue head punishment, do not routinely spar with bigger boxers, and do not spar while under medical suspension. Trainers should guard against routine lengthy sparring sessions in which the boxers are poorly protected and continually absorb excessive head blows. Amateur trainers should guard against their boxers frequently sparring with professionals. The discrepancy in talent between these two groups is considerable. Trainers should not condone the practice of importing second-rate fighters to act as human punching bags for their charges. A trainer should actively discourage a boxer from continuing with his career if the boxer routinely absorbs undue punishment in either the gym or in competition. Unfortunately, despite having spent their entire adult lives in the sport of boxing, many trainers are ignorant—or worse, indifferent—to the medical dangers that they could potentially deter.

The boxer's manager should work closely with the trainer to ensure the boxer's personal safety. Most professional boxers have signed 1- to 3-year managerial contracts that obligate their professional services to the manager. The manager stands to make a profit by appropriately managing the boxer's career. He or she oversees arrangements to train the boxer and determines who the opponents will be. It is incumbent on the manager not to overmatch the boxer, by purposely offering his or her boxer's services as a mere opponent, playing the role of stepping-stone or trial horse to a younger, stronger, and more-talented competitor. The manager has a moral obligation to protect his or her boxer and even encourage retirement if it is obvious that the boxer is absorbing too much punishment. Unfortunately, the best interest of the boxer and the financial interest of the manager are often in conflict.

The promoter's function is to put together and promote or sell a boxing competition. He or she employs a matchmaker whose job it is to actually put the matches together. The promoter will frequently have legal addenda in the boxer's contract that dictate that a certain number of the boxer's subsequent future bouts be exclusively promoted by this promoter. Such a contractual addendum can give a promoter complete control over a boxer's financial future. It is incumbent on the promoter to treat the boxer fairly. He or she must ensure that the matchmaker has not overmatched the boxer and that the boxer is fairly compensated for his performance. Promoters should instruct their matchmakers to refuse to use boxers who have no chance of winning a match or are known to absorb an excessive amount of head blows.

The referee has a important role in ensuring a boxer's safety (137). He is in the best position to view a boxer's condition and has the authority to terminate a match at any point. The referee must never allow a boxer to absorb repeated, unanswered blows. The referee should stop a bout if the boxer is out on his feet, as manifested by uncoordination, imbalance, and impaired ability to defend himself. A boxer can be in a concussed state without being knocked down. Recognition of this condition by the referee is imperative. Failure to appreciate that a boxer is out on his feet or in a groggy state exposes him to a heightened risk of acute brain injury. If a fighter has lost the ability or will to continue, the referee should stop the contest without regard for fan approval. A referee's primary function is to ensure a boxer's safety. Second-guessing a referee's decision to terminate a contest is rarely helpful. The referee should request a ringside physician's consultation whenever he is in doubt about a boxer's ability to continue. The referee should never disregard a physician's recommendation to stop a contest (138). On the other hand, he should feel free to stop a contest even if the ringside physician would allow the contest to continue. One additional unnecessary blow may be all that it takes to result in serious acute brain injury. It is the responsibility of the state boxing commission to ensure that the referee is competent. Some referees will consistently be a step behind the action or not clearly appreciate that a boxer is in trouble, thereby exposing the boxer to unnecessary risk. Referees such as these should be retired by the state boxing commission.

Managers, promoters, and state boxing commissions should ideally begin discussions toward establishing disability and pension funds for injured or retired boxers. Precedent for such activities certainly exists in other major sports such as baseball and football. Discussions on this issue will obviously be complicated and any enactment expensive, but this certainly would demonstrate a true commitment to improving the lot of the professional boxer.

Gloves, Ring, Posts, and Headgear

Gloves, rings, posts, and headgear are probably more important in preventing an acute injury than in preventing CTBE. Headgear can diminish the incidence of cuts but does not decrease the incidence of acute or chronic head injury. Headgear is mandatory in amateur competition but never used professionally. While some fan attraction with professional boxing would undoubtably decrease if headgear were used, facial lacerations from punches, butts, and elbows would decrease. Proper padding of the ring posts and floor mat should be ensured. While most knockouts occur before the boxer hits the canvas, additional coup and contrecoup forces can be generated if the boxer's head strikes the mat or ring post. Proper padding of these structures can diminish the forces involved.

Boxer Education

An effective way to diminish undesirable medical risks inherent in boxing is to educate the boxer himself. This would seem to be an obvious approach, which is applied to all other aspects of public health but rarely if ever discussed in relation to boxing. The task of educating active boxers about the risks that they subject themselves to will not be easy. Professional boxers generally come from the poorer, less-educated segments of our society. They are too often unaware of the risks inherent in their sport and commonly have inadequate personal or social support systems to help them sort out these risks. Professional and amateur boxers must, in particular, be educated about the acute and chronic neurologic and ocular sequelae of their sport. They should clearly understand the causes, prevention, natural history, and proposed preventive measures with respect to both neurologic and ocular injury. A mature understanding of these risks by the boxer lessens the legitimate argument that the boxer is no more than a pawn in the public's desire for entertainment.

Boxer education should be an objective of both organized medicine, world sanctioning bodies, and state boxing commissions. Trainers, managers, and promoters also should be educated as to the medical risks inherent in the sport. All parties involved should understand that it is likely that better boxing education will lead some professionals to choose to end their careers. Education of parents and teenage children may result in fewer young men choosing to participate in an amateur program. Boxer education will partially offset the argument that boxers are being exploited by denying them information with which they could make informed individual choices. A national boxing commission or unified state boxing commissions could be helpful in disseminating this information.

Pros and Cons of Boxing

The risks inherent in boxing and reported interventions to decrease these risks have been outlined in this chapter. However, any opinion concerning the overall merits or deficiencies of boxing must be made not only on medical but also on sociological, moral, psychological, and financial grounds (139–144). Feelings run deeply about the sport of boxing, from unyielding support to unyielding opposition with a determination to seek its abolition (145–152). Amateur boxing has made a concerted effort to divorce itself from the professional ranks, arguing, with some justification, that their sport is not associated with the same risks as the professional and, therefore, does not deserve the same criticism.

Opponents of all types of boxing argue that even the amateur sport carries undue risks to the brain and is in fact the breeding ground for the professional ranks. Cowart (153) noted that amateur boxing is not an end in itself but a means to get to the pros. Proponents of boxing argue that the sport encourages rigorous training, discipline, resolution, alertness, courage, endurance, and generally builds character. In addition, boxing competition is reported to provide an orderly controlled environment in which the competitors can release innate aggression in a more disciplined framework. Finally, boxing is lauded as one of the few avenues to escape the ghetto for economically disadvantaged minority youths. Opponents of boxing cite its known deleterious cerebral and ocular effects and consider it brutal, atavistic, uncivilized, and inherently discriminatory with predominantly disadvantaged minority youth sacrificing their health for the entertainment and financial remuneration of the more privileged controlling interests and public. Opponents go so far as to liken boxing to earlier outlawed activities such as gun dueling, bullfighting, cockfighting, pit bull fighting, bearbaiting, and feeding Christians to the lions. Sammons (131) eloquently summed up his opposition to boxing: "Most scholarly evidence indicates that boxing success is illusory and short lived, its positive quality greatly overrated. Attracting those who are most dependent on hope, it is, at best, a low percentage proposition, at worst a cruel hoax that discourages tried and tested means to success and legitimates violent behavior.

Organized medicine has clearly voiced its opposition to boxing (77–80, 154–160). Table 15.5 lists organizations that either strongly oppose boxing or have actually called for its abolition. The only medical organizations that have publically supported boxing are the American Academy of Orthopaedic and Neurological Surgeons, the America Association to Improve Boxing, and the American Board of Ringside Physicians. Many medical editorials have called for a physician ban on boxing, citing rationale such as the Declaration of Tokyo that states: "The doctor shall not countenance, condone or participate in the practice of torture or other forms of cruel, inhumane or degrading procedures" (161).

In summary, both amateur and professional boxing are difficult sporting endeavors, requiring significant commitments to dedication and hard work. The participants, particularly at the professional level, expose themselves to significant medical risk with respect to neurologic and ocular injury. The boxing establishment is attempting to reduce these risks, but the effectiveness of these measures is not yet known. Organized medicine generally supports broad condemnation of boxing, primarily on medical grounds, feeling that any libertarian argument to the contrary is either fallacious or provides insufficient justification to offset the inherent medical risks. As is true with most complex social

Table 15.5.
Medical Organizations against Boxing

American Academy of Neurology
American Academy of Pediatrics
American Association of Neurological Surgeons
American Medical Association
American Neurological Association
Australian Medical Association
British Medical Association
California Medical Society
Canadian Medical Association
Canadian Psychiatric Association
New York Medical Society
World Medical Association

issues, and boxing is surely more than simply a medical issue, there is room for compromise. Boxing will simply not be legally outlawed in the foreseeable future because of its inherent medical risks. By refusing to become involved in the effort to reform boxing, medical opponents of the sport may unwittingly be shutting themselves out of the debate. In the meanwhile, diligent medical participants will continue to enhance boxing safety. Ongoing expert care, sophisticated neurologic and ocular monitoring, and high-quality retrospective and prospective medical studies in conjunction with the institution of national administrative reform measures will eventually provide an indisputable database that society can use to make an educated, unemotional decision about whether it chooses to continue to support professional and amateur boxing. Ultimately, it must be society that determines if the objectives of boxing are appropriate and what level of inherent medical risk is acceptable as an unfortunate by-product of this sport.

REFERENCES

1. Unterharnscheidt F. About boxing: review of historical and medical aspects. Tex Rep Biol Med 1970;28(4):421–495.
2. Masterson DW. The ancient Greek origins of sports medicine. Br. J. Sports Med. 1976;10:196–202.
3. Pearn JH. Boxing and the brain. Aust N Z J Med 1987;17:83.
4. U.S. Amateur Boxing, Inc. Official Rules, 1991–93. Colorado Springs: Author, 1993.
5. Blonstein JL. Care of the amateur boxer. J Sports Med 1977;17:79–82.
6. Jordan BD, Voy RO, Stone J. Amateur boxing injuries at the US Olympic training center. Phys Sportsmed 1990;18(2):81–90.
7. Voy RO. Amateur boxing. JAMA 1989;262(4):499–450.
8. Roberts GW. The occult aftermath of boxing. J Neurol Neurosurg Psychiatry 1990;53:373–378.
9. Guny P. Epidemiologic study to examine amateur boxers' potential risks. JAMA 1986;255:2397–2399.
10. Kaste M, Vilkki J, Sainio K, Kuurne T, Katevuo K, Meurala H. Is chronic brain damage in boxing a hazard of the past. Lancet 1982:1186–1188.
11. Casson IR, Siegel O, Sham R, Campbell EA, Tarlau M, DiDomenico A. Brain damage in modern boxers. JAMA 1984;251:2663–2267.
12. McLatchie G, Brooks N, Galbraith S, et al. Clinical neurological examination, neuropsychology, electroencephalography and computed tomographic head scanning in active amateur boxers. J Neurol Neurosurg Psychiatry 1987;50:96–99.
13. Enzenauer RW, Montrey JS, Enzenauer RJ, Mauldin WM. Boxing-related injuries in the US Army, 1980 through 1985. JAMA 1989;261:1463–1466.
14. Thomassen A, Juul-Jensen P, Olivarius B, Bremer J, Christensen A. Neurological, electroencephalographic and neuropsychological examination of 53 former amateur boxers. Acta Neurol Scand 1979;60:352–362.
15. Brooks N, Kupshik G, Wilson L, Galbraith S, Ward R. A neuropsychological study of active amateur boxers. J Neurol Neurosurg Psychiatry 1987;50:997–1000.
16. Heilbronner, RL, Henry GK, Carson-Brewer M. Neuropsychologic test performance in amateur boxers. Am J Sports Med 1991;19:376–380.
17. Jordan BD, Zimmerman RD. Magnetic resonance imaging in amateur boxers. Arch Neurol 1988;45:1207–1208.
18. Haglund Y, Edman G, Murelius O, Oreland L, Sachs C. Does Swedish amateur boxing lead to chronic brain damage? 1. A retrospective medical, neurological and personality trait study. Acta Neurol Scand 1990;82:245–252.
19. Haglund Y, Bergstrand G. Does Swedish amateur boxing lead to chronic brain damage? 2. A retrospective study with CT and MRI. Acta Neurol Scand 1990;82:297–302.
20. Haglund Y, Persson HE. Does Swedish amateur boxing lead to chronic brain damage? 3. A retrospective clinical neurophysicological study. Acta Neurol Scand 1990;82:353–360.
21. Murelius O, Haglund Y. Does Swedish amateur boxing lead to chronic brain damage? A retrospective neurophyschological study. Acta Neurol Scand 1991;83:9–13.
22. Noble C. Hand injuries in boxing. Am J Sports Med 1987;15(4)342–346.
23. Shively RA, Sundaram M. Ununited fractures of the scaphoid in boxers. Am J Sports Med 1980;8(6):440–442.
24. Posner MA, Ambrose L. Boxer's knuckle–dorsal capsular rupture of the metacarpophalangeal joint of a finger. J Hand Surg 1989;14A(2)1:229–235.
25. Larose JH, Sik KD. Knuckle fracture. JAMA 1968;206(4):893–894.
26. McKerrell J, Bowen V, Johnston G, Zondervan J. Boxer's fractures—conservative or operative management? J Trauma 1987;27(5):486–490.
27. Porter ML, Hodgkinson JP, Hirst P, Wharton MR. Cunliffe M. The boxers' fracture: a prospective study of functional recovery. Arch Emerg Med 1988;5:212–215.
28. Vaccaro AR, Kupcha PC, Salvo JP. Accurate reduction and splinting of the common boxer's fracture. Orthopaed Rev 1990;19(11):994–996.
29. Van Demark R. A simple method of treatment of fractures of the fifth metacarpal neck and distal shaft (boxer's fracture). S D J Med 1983;5–7.
30. Kewalramani LS, Krauss JF. Cervical spine injuries resulting from collision sports. Paraplegia 1981;19:303–312.
31. Strano SD, Marais AD. Cervical spine fracture in a boxer—a rare but important sporting injury. S Afr Med J 1983;63:328–330.
32. Jordan BD, Zimmerman RD, Devinsky O, Gamache FW, Folk FS, Campbell EA. Brain contusion and cervical fracture in a professional boxer. Phys Sportsmed 1988;16(6):85–88.
33. Blonstein JL. Boxing injuries. J R Coll Gen Pract 1969;18:100–103.
34. Whiteson AL. Injuries in professional boxing. Their treatment and prevention. Practioner 1981;225:1053–1057.
35. Enzenauer RW, Muldin WM. Boxing-related ocular injuries in the United States Army, 1980 to 1985. South Med J 1989;82:547–549.
36. Giovinazzo VJ, Yannuzzi LA, Sorenson JA, Delrowe DJ, Campbell EA. The ocular complications of boxing. Ophthalmology 1987;94:587–596.
37. Goldsmith MF. Physicians aim to KO boxers' injuries; focus on eyes as title bout nears. JAMA 1987;257:1697–1698.
38. Jordan BD. Medical aspects of boxing. Boca Raton, FL: CRC Press, 1993.
39. Elkington A. Boxing and the eye: results of a questionnaire. Trans. Ophthalmol Soc UK 1985;104:897–902.
40. Maguire JI, Benson WE. Retinal injury and detachment in boxers. JAMA 1986;255(18):2451–2453.
41. Smith DJ. Ocular injuries in boxing. Int Ophthalmol Clin 28(3), 1988;28(3):242–245.
42. Palmer E, Lieberman TW, Burns S. Contusion angle deformity in prizefighters. Arch Ophthalmol 1976;94:225–228.
43. Carter JB, Parke DW. Unusual retinal tears in an amateur boxer. Arch Ophalmol 1987;105:1138.
44. Bartholomew AA. Doctors and boxing contests. Med J Aust 1987;147:212.
45. Lovaas M. Ruptured spleen in a boxer with infectious mononucleosis. Minn Med 1981;461–462.
46. Niezgoda JA, McMenamin P, Graeber GM. Pharyngoesophageal perforation after blunt neck trauma. Ann Thorac Surg 1990;50:615–617.
47. Courville CB, The mechanism of boxing fatalities. Bull L A Neurol Soc 1964;29:59–69.
48. Lampert PW, Hardman JM. Morphological changes in brains of boxers. JAMA 1984;251(20):2676–2679.
49. Gurdgian ES, Lange WA, Patrick LM, Thomas LM. Impact injury and crash protection. Springfield, IL: Thomas, 1970.
50. Ommaya AK, Rockoff SD, Baldwin M. Experimental concussion. J Neurosurg 1964;21:249–267.
51. Gennarelli TA, Thibault LE, Adams JH, Graham DI, Thompson

CJ, Marcincin RP. Diffuse axonal injury and traumatic coma in the primate. Ann Neurol 1982;12:564–574.
52. Johnson J, Skorecki J, Wells RP. Peak accelerations of the head experienced in boxing. Med Biol Eng 1975:396–404.
53. Schwartz ML, Hudson AR, Fernie GR, Hayashi K, Coleclough AA. Biomechanical study of full-contact karate contrasted with boxing. J Neurosurg 1986;64:248–252.
54. Atha J, Yeadon MR, Sandover J, Parsons KC. The damaging punch. Br Med J 1985;291:1756–1757.
55. Frederiks JEP, Jr. Chest boxing. JAMA 1987;257:1050.
56. Schmidt-Olsen S, Jensen S, Mortensen V. Amateur boxing in Denmark. The effect of some preventive measures. Am J Sports Med 1990;18(1):98–100.
57. Schmid L, Hajek E, Votipka F, Teprik O, Blonstein JL. Experience with headgear in boxing. J Sports Med Physical Fit 1968;8(3):171–176.
58. Jordan BD. Letter to editor. Am J Sports Med 1990;18(5)561.
59. Whiting WC, Gregor RJ, Finerman GA. Kinematic analysis of human upper extremity movements in boxing. Am J Sports Med 1988;16(2)130–136.
60. Council on Scientific Affairs. Brain injury in boxing. JAMA 1983;249:254–257.
61. Burns RJ. Boxing and the brain. Aust N Z J Med 1986;16:439–440.
62. Hillman H. Boxing [Editorial]. Resuscitation 1980;8:211–215.
63. Jordan BD, Campbell EA. Acute injuries among professional boxers in New York State: a two-year survey. Phys Sportsmed 1988;18(1):87–91.
64. Lindsay KW, McLatchie G, Jennett B. Serious head injury in sports. Br Med J 1980;281:789–791.
65. Kraus JF, Conroy C. Mortality and morbidity from injuries in sports and recreation. Ann Rev Public Health 1984;5:163–92.
66. Ryan AJ. Intracranial injuries resulting from boxing: a review (1918–1985). Clin Sports Med 1987;6(1):31–40.
67. Cruikshank JK, Higgens CS, Gray JR. Two cases of acute intracranial hemorrhage in young amateur boxers. Lancet 1980;626–627.
68. McQuillen JB, McQuillen EN, Morrow P. Trauma, sport, and malignant cerebral edema. Am J Forensic Med Pathol 1988;9(1):12–15.
69. Beaussart M, Beaussart-Boulenge L. "Experimental" study of cerebral concussion in 123 amateur boxers, by clinical examination and EEG before and immediately after fights. Electroencephalogr Clin Neurophysiol 1970;29:529–536.
70. Breton F, Pincemaille Y, Tarriere C, Renault B. Event-related potential assessment of attention and the orienting reaction in boxers before and after a fight. Biol Psychol 1990;31:57–71.
71. Parkinson D, West M, Pathiraja T. Concussion: comparison of humans and rats. Neurosurgery 1978;3(2):176–180.
72. Jordan BD. Neurologic injury in boxing [Reprint] Hosp Med 1991.
73. Neubuerger KT, Sinton DW, Denst J. Cerebral atrophy associated with boxing. Arch Neurol Psychiatry 1959;81:403–408.
74. Hallervorden J. Hirnerschutterung und thixotripie, zentralbl. Neurochir 1941;6:37–42.
75. Windle WF, Groat RA, Fox CA. Experimental structural alterations in the brain during and after concussion. Surg Gynecol Obstet 1944;79:561–572.
76. Gronwall D, Wrightson P. Delayed recovery of intellectual function after minor head injury. Lancet 1974;2:605–609.
77. Lundberg GD. Boxing should be banned in civilized countries [Editorial]. JAMA 1983;249(2):250.
78. Lundberg GD. Boxing should be banned in civilized countries—round 2. JAMA 1984;251(20):2696.
79. Lundberg GD. Boxing should be banned in civilized countries—round 3. JAMA 1986;255(18):2483.
80. Lundberg GD. Brain injury in boxing. Am J Forensic Med Pathol 1985;6(3):192–198.
81. Anonymous. Boxing and the brain. Br Med J 1973;24:439–440.
82. Corsellis JAN. Boxing and the brain. Br Med J 1989;298:105–109.
83. Roberts AH. Brain damage in boxers. London: Pitman Medical Scientific 1969.
84. Spillane JD. Five boxers. Br Med J 1962:1205–1210.
85. Stiller JW, Weinberger DR. Boxing and chronic brain damage. Psychiatr Clin North Am 1985;8(2)339–356.
86. Sabharwal RK, Sanchetee PC, Sethi PK, Dhamja RM. Chronic traumatic encephalopathy in boxers. JAPI 1987;35(8)571–573.
87. Martland HS. Punch drunk. JAMA 1928;91(15):1103–1107.
88. Hussey HH. Punch drunk [Editorial]. JAMA 1976;256(5):485.
89. Millspaugh JA. Dementia pugilistica. US Naval Med Bull 1937;35:297–303.
90. Critchley M. Medical aspects of boxing, particularly from a neurological standpoint. Br Med J 1957;1:357–366.
91. Johnson J. Organic psychosyndromes due to boxing. Br J Psychiatry 1969;115:45–53.
92. Parker HL. Traumatic encephalopathy (punch drunk) of professional pugilists. J Neurol Psychopathol 1934;15:20–28.
93. Courville CB. Punch drunk. Bull L A Neurol Soc 1962;27:160–168.
94. Charnas L, Pyeritz RE. Neurologic injuries in boxers. Hosp Prac 1986;30–39.
95. Mawdsley C, Ferguson FR. Neurological disease in boxers. Lancet 1963:795–801.
96. McKhann G, Drachman D, Folstein M, Katzman R, Price D, Stadlan EM. Clinical diagnosis of Alzheimer's disease: report of the NINCDS-ADRDA work group under the auspices of Department of Health and Human Services Task Force on Alzehimer's disease. Neurology 1984;34:939–944.
97. Friedman JH. Progressive Parkinsonism in boxers. South Med J 1989;82:543–546.
98. Brandenburg W, Hallervorden J. Dementia pugilistica mit anatomishem befund virchows archiv fur pathologische. Anat Physiol 1954;325:680–709.
99. Grahmann H, Ule G. Beitrag zur kenntnis der chroni schen cerebralen krank heitsbilder bei boxern. Psychiat Neurol 1957;134:261–283.
100. Constantinides J, Tissot R. Lesions neurofibrillaires d'Alzheimer generalisees sans plaques seniles. Arch Suisses Neurol Neurochir Psychiat 1967;100:117–130.
101. Payne EE. Brains of boxers. Neurochirurgia 1968;11(5):173–188.
102. Corsellis JAN, Bruton CJ, Freeman-Browne D. The aftermath of boxing, Psychol Med 1973;3:270–303.
103. Bogdanoff B, Natter HM. Incidence of cavum septum pellucidum in adults: a sign of boxer's encephalopathy. Neurology 1989;39:991–992.
104. Schwidde JT. Incidence of cavum septi pellucidi and cavum vergae in 1,032 human brains. Arch Neurol Psychiatry 1952;67:625–632.
105. Aoki N. Brain damage from boxing. J Neurosurg 1986;64:829–830.
106. Macpherson P, Teasdale E. CT demonstration of a 5th ventricle—a finding to KO boxers? Neuroradiology 1988;30:506–510.
107. Richards PG, Hatfield R, Grant HC. Brain damage from boxing. J Neurosurg 1986;65:723.
108. Adams CWM, Bruton CJ. The cerebral vasculature in dementia pugilistica. J Neurol Neurosurg Psychiatry 1989;52:600–604.
109. Stern MB. Head trauma as a risk factor for Parkinson's disease. Mov Disord 1991;6(2):95–97.
110. Roberts GW. Immunocytochemistry of neurofibrillary tangles in dementia pugilistica and Alzheimer's disease: evidence for common genesis. Lancet 1988:1456–1457.
111. Tokuda T, Ikeda S, Yanagisawa N, Ihara Y, Glenner G. Re-examination of ex-boxers' brains using immunohistochemistry with antibodies to amyloid protein and tau protein. Acta Neuropathol 1991;82:280–285.
112. Dale GE, Leigh PN, Luthert P, Anderton BH, Roberts GW. Neurofibrillary tangles in dementia pugilistica are ubiquintinated. J Neurol Neurosurg Psychiatry 1991;54:116–118.
113. Medical News and Perspective. Is boxing a risk factor for Alzheimer's? [Editorial]. JAMA 1989;261(18):2597–2598.
114. Brayne CEG, Dow L, Calloway SP, Thompson RJ. Blood creatine kinase isoenzyme BB in boxers. Lancet 1982;2:1308–1309.
115. Rodriguez G, Ferrillo F, Montano V, Rosadini G, Sannita WG. Regional cerebral blood flow in boxers. Lancet 1983:858.
116. Harvey PKP, Davis JN. Traumatic encephalopathy in a young boxer. Lancet 1974;928–929.
117. Casson IR, Sham R, Campbell EA, Tarlau M, DiDomenico A. Neurological and CT evaluation of knocked-out boxers. J Neurol Neurosurg Psychiatry 1982;45:170–174.

118. Sironi VA, Ravagnati L. Brain damage in boxers. Lancet 1983;244.
119. Ross RJ, Cole M, Thompson JS, Kim KH. Boxers-computed tomography, EEG, and neurological evaluation. JAMA 1983;249(2)211–213.
120. Drew RH, Templer DI, Schuyler BA, Newell TG, Cannon WG. Neuropsychological deficits in active licensed professional boxers. J Clin Psychol 1986;42:520–522.
121. Lubell A. Chronic brain injury in boxers: is it avoidable? Phys Sportsmed 1989;17(11):126–132.
122. Mortimer JA. Epidemiology of post-traumatic encephalopathy in boxers. Minn Med 1985:299–300.
123. Sironi VA, Scotti G, Ravagnati L, Franzini A, Marossero F. CT-scan and EEG findings in professional pugilists: early detection of cerebral atrophy in young boxers. J Neurosurg Sci 1982;26:165–168.
124. Jordan BD. Medical and safety reforms in boxing. J Natl Med Assoc 1988;80(4):407–412.
125. Ludwig R. Making boxing safer, the Swedish model. JAMA 1986;255(18):2482.
126. Jordan BD. Prevention of neurologic injuries in boxing [Letter to Editor]. Arch Neurol 1988;45:713.
127. LaCava G. Prevention in boxing [Editorial]. Sports Med Physical Fit 1983;23(4):361–363.
128. Morrison RG. Medical and public health aspects of boxing. JAMA 1986;255(18):2475–2480.
129. Ross RJ, Casson IR, Siegel O, Cole M. Boxing injuries: neurologic, radiologic, and neuropsychologic evaluation. Clin Sports Med 1987;6(1):41–51.
130. Guterman A, Smith RW. Neurological sequelae of boxing. Sports Med 1987;4:194–210.
131. Charnas L, Pyeritz RE. Neurological injuries in boxers: the use of tests. JAMA 1990;264:1532.
132. Jordan BD, Zimmerman RD. Computed tomography and magnetic resonance imaging comparisons in boxers. JAMA 1990;263(12):1670–1674.
133. Jordan BD. Boxer's encephalopathy. Neurology 1990;727.
134. Levin HS, Lippold SC, Goldman A, et al. Neurobehavioral functioning and magnetic resonance imaging findings in young boxers. J Neurosurg 1987;67:657–667.
135. Johnson J. The EEG in the traumatic encephalopathy of boxers. Psychiatr Clin 1969;2:204–211.
136. Krejcova H, Cerny R. Vestibular abnormalities in encephalopathia pugilistica. Acta Otolaryngol Suppl (Stockh) 1989;468:209–210.
137. Elia JC. Physicians and boxing [Letter to Editor]. West J Med 1983;139:717.
138. Bernstein H. More on boxing. JAMA 1985;253:2830.
139. Algeo JH Jr, Letter to editor. Milit Med 1988;153:238–239.
140. Finney JL. Boxing in the army. JAMA 1989;262:2089.
141. Patterson R. On boxing and liberty. JAMA 1986;255(18):2481–2482.
142. Pearce JMS. Boxer's brains. Br Med J 1984;288:933–934.
143. Sammons JT. Why physicians should oppose boxing: an interdisciplinary history perspective [Editorial]. JAMA 1989;261(10):1484–1486.
144. Toon PD. Boxing clever. J Med Ethics 1988;14:69.
145. Engel WK. Abolish boxing. N Engl J Med 1982;307(12):761.
146. Enzenauer RW, Enzenauer RJ. Ban military boxing. Milit Med 1987;152:536–537.
147. Piston RE, Boxing. Personal freedom and the right of lions to Christians. JAMA 1986;256:1895.
148. Richards NG. Ban boxing. Neurology 1984;34:1485–1486.
149. Seltzer AP. What should we do about boxing? [Editorial]. J Natl Med Assoc 1967;59(1):64–65.
150. Thomison JB. Addled brains and coffin nails. [Editorial]. South Med J 1989;82(5):941–942.
151. Timperley WR. Banning boxing. Br Med J 1982;285:289.
152. Van Allen MW. The deadly degrading sport. JAMA 1983;249(2):250–251.
153. Cowart VS. Boxing makes more headlines than usual and a lot of the news hasn't been good. JAMA 1989;261:14–15.
154. Committee on Sports Medicine. Participation in boxing among children and young adults. Pediatrics 1984;74:311–312.
155. Anonymous. Health hazards of boxing [Editorial]. Med J Aust 1975;1(Suppl):34, 163.
156. Hudson CJ. Physicians and boxing [Letter to Editor] N Engl J Med 1980:1308.
157. Ioannou S. Should boxing be banned? Can Med Assoc J 1984;131:10.
158. Stening W. Boxing. Med J Aust 1992;156:76–77.
159. Winton R. WMA statements on terminal illness and boxing. Med J Aust 1984;392–393.
160. World Medical Association. Statement on terminal illness and boxing adopted by the 35th World Medical Assembly, Venice, Italy, Oct, 1983. Med J Aust 1984;140:431.
161. Lee NC. Boxing—what should doctors do? [Editorial]. S Afr Med J 1988;74(2):1.

16 / COMPETITIVE DIVING

Richard L. Carter

Diving is one of the most aesthetically pleasing sports. With the possible exception of gymnastics and figure skating, it is unparalleled in terms of rhythm, grace, and beauty. People consider competitive diving to be a dangerous sport; yet, on the contrary, it is generally safe and enjoyable. There are relatively few injuries in the sport, and those that do occur are usually not serious. However, the sport of competitive diving does have some inherent dangers, because the diver is trying to do numerous simultaneous maneuvers off a springboard or a tower and is traveling at a rapid rate of speed when he or she hits the water. With all of the twisting and turning involved, divers put an abnormal amount of stress on their bodies so their muscles need to be strong and flexible and they need to develop this muscle strength by doing exercises or lifting weights. The areas of the body that take the greatest amount of force especially have to be developed. Appropriate conditioning in combination with good teaching and training techniques will help prevent many injuries that can occur, such as those caused by hitting the diving board.

This chapter delineates the various mechanisms of injury in addition to appropriate treatment techniques. Diagnostic modalities will be discussed as they lead to the most effective treatment choice. Conditioning programs and coaching techniques that are important in terms of preventing the more serious injuries will be described.

Mechanisms of Injury

Mechanisms of injury can be categorized into the following groups: blunt traumas, including trauma to the head and neck; joint abuse; injuries to the soft tissues, including myofascial injuries; and injuries to the spine.

Blunt Trauma

There are many injuries that can occur as a result of diving head first into shallow water. The possibility of a head, spine, or shoulder injury from hitting the bottom of a pool is always present. For years, divers were taught to keep their arms over head until reaching the bottom of the pool in an arm stand, but now, divers are "swimming" their arms to the sides or in front on impact with the water to help them into the water with less splash. This technique leaves the head unprotected as the body knives through the water and glides to the bottom. In a deep pool, this is not a problem but in shallow water, the chances of serious injury is ever present. Thus the depth of the pool and the possible presence of an ascending or upwardly sloped bottom must be known to the diver.

Scalp lacerations occur quite frequently. They usually happen during inward and reverse 1½ somersault and 2½ somersault dives (Figs. 16.1 and 16.2). When a diver leans in toward the board on an inward dive or backward on a reverse dive (both of which involve a spinning motion toward the board), it is easy for him or her to be too close, hitting the head on the board. These types of injuries can only be prevented by good board work with many lead-up dives, such as perfecting a reverse-double somersault before attempting to do a reverse 2½ somersault dive.

Case 16.1

A young intercollegiate diver sustained a transfrontoparietal scalp laceration when he struck the edge of a board while performing an inward 2½ somersault dive from a 3-m board. He probably sustained a brief cerebral concussion and on entry into the water developed a convulsive seizure, possibly from the blow to the head or the hypoxia from submersion or both. He was rescued from the water and the hemorrhage from the scalp was controlled by a pressure dressing. He was transported to the hospital in a facedown position. Upon arrival, he was thoroughly suctioned to remove aspirated water from his lungs and the seizure was treated medically. After x-rays showed no cervical spine or skull fracture, the diver was taken to the operating room and the scalp laceration was repaired under local anes-

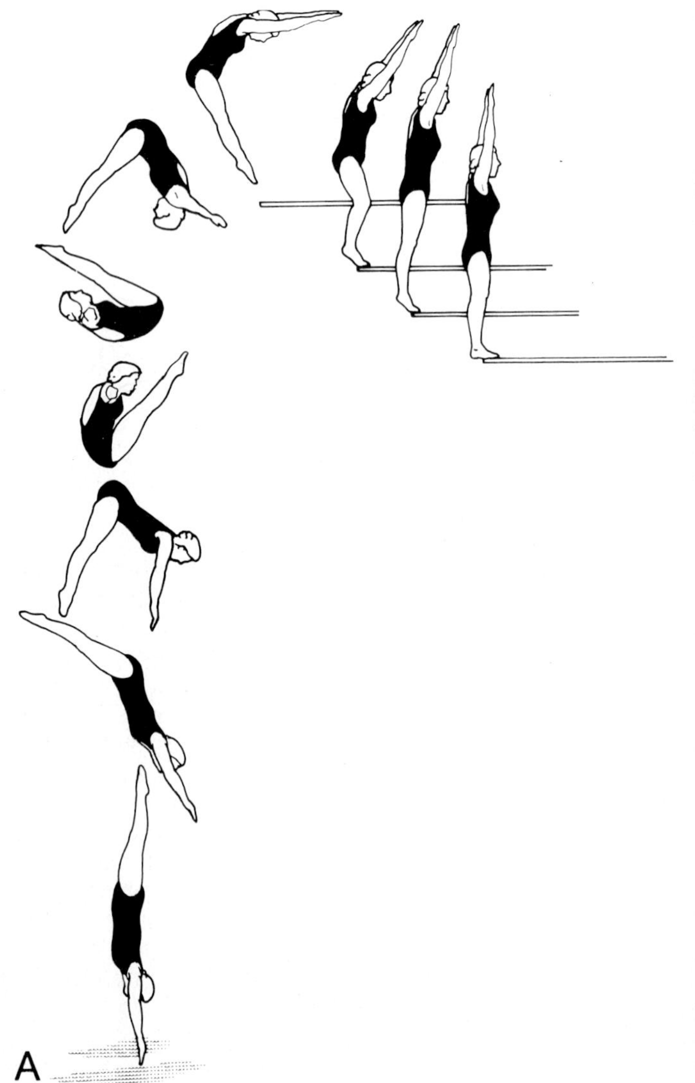

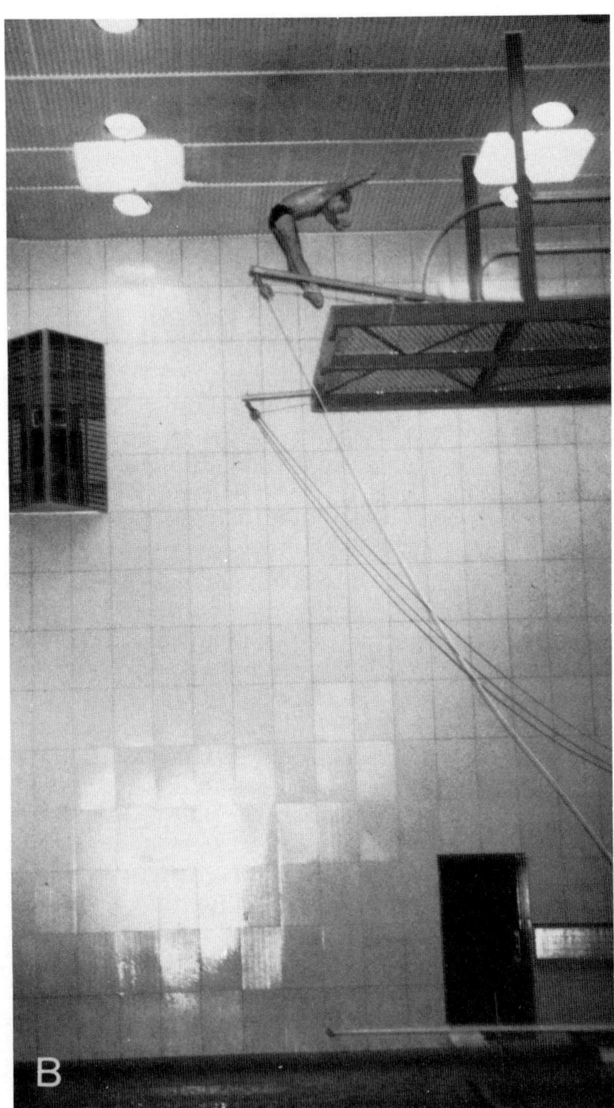

Figure 16.1. The sequence of an inward 1½ somersault platform dive from the pike position is shown. **A,** The diver faces the tower with her hands over head to initiate the inward spinning motion. The ankles are snapped backward while the arms and upward body begin their downward acceleration. After completing the inward revolutions, the diver prepares for entry. **B,** Note the head position originates over the tower, but the force of spinning will ultimately place the diver in a safe position.

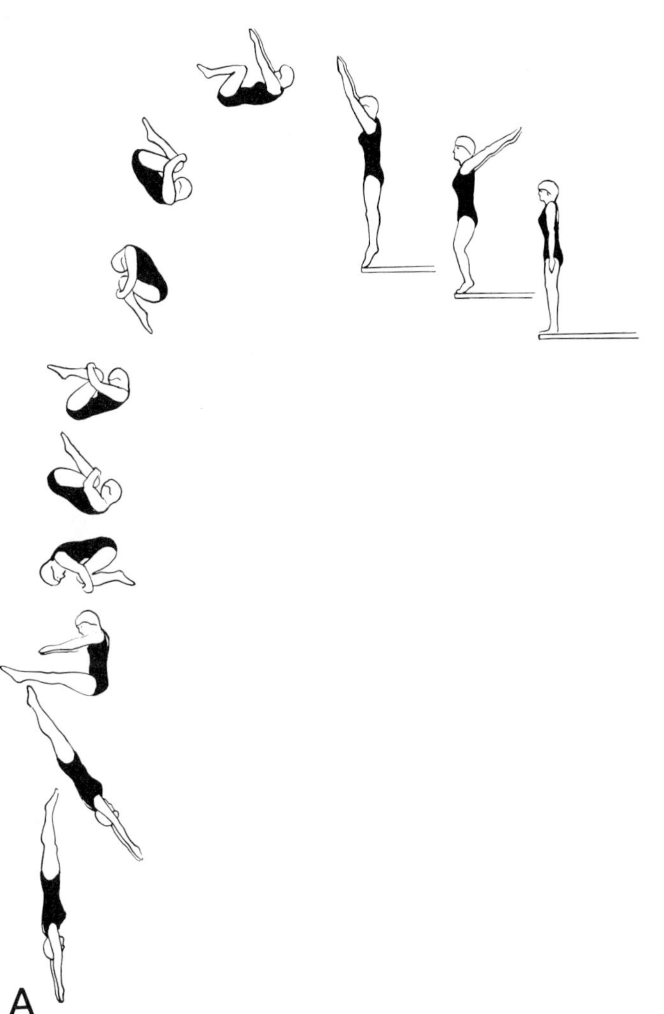

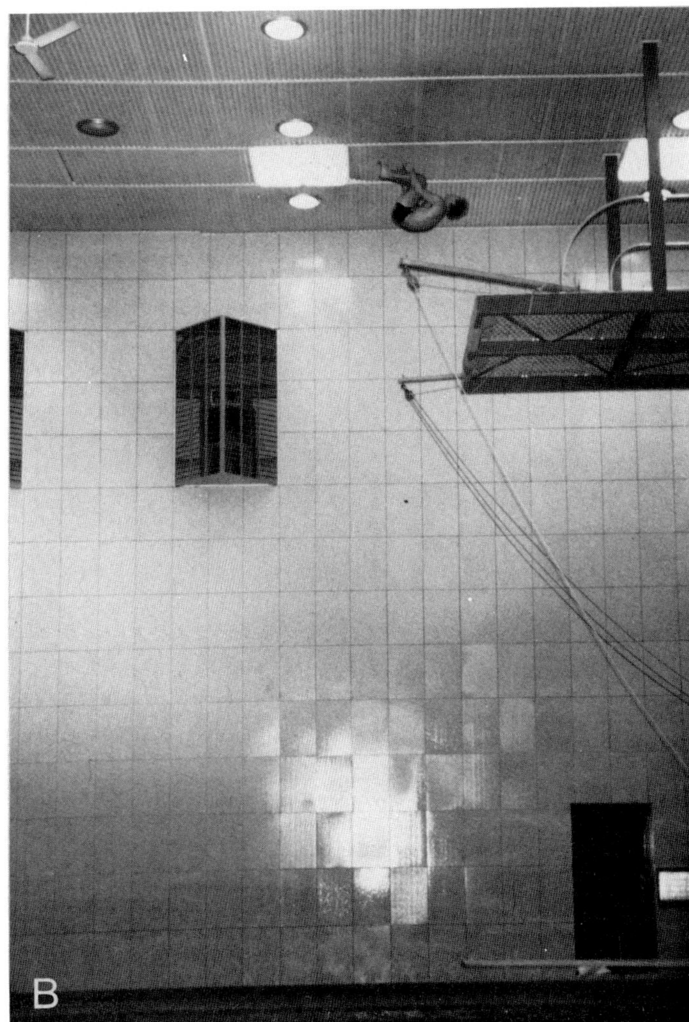

Figure 16.2. The sequence of a reverse 2½ somersault platform dive from the tuck position is shown. **A,** The diver faces the water and initiates the reverse rotation by reaching up into the air while rotating her knees upward into her hands. **B–D,** As the diver finishes the reverse somersaulting action, he tries to visualize a spot on the water, which signals him to initiate the correct body alignment for entry.

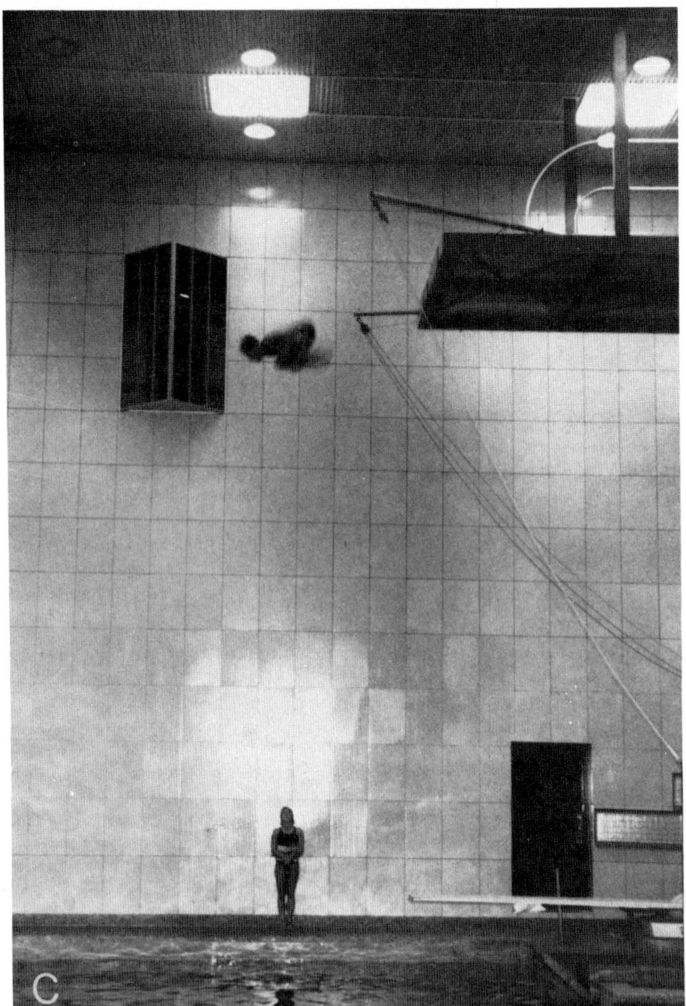

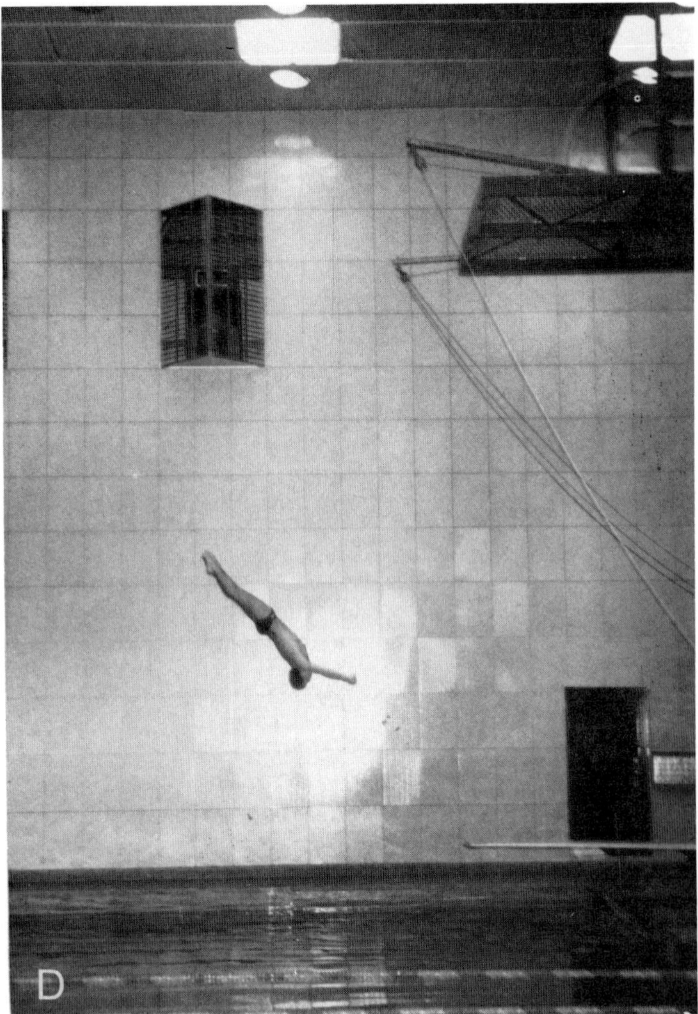

Figure 16.2C and D.

thesia. Recovery was complete without any residual neurologic deficit, and the diver remained seizure free. After a rest period of a number of months, the diver returned for an examination and was found to be physically and neurologically within normal limits, there having been only the initial convulsive seizure. The long buildup of physical, technical, and psychological recovery was started by the diver and culminated a year later with his winning the Olympic gold medal in the 10-m platform event.

Unfortunately, there is an occasional head injury with tragic consequences. The following case illustrates such a tragic event.

Case 16.2

A young diver attempting a standing reverse 3½ somersault in a tucked position struck his head on a 10-m platform (Fig. 16.3). He was rendered unconscious almost immediately and upon arrival at the hospital had dilated, fixed pupils and was unresponsive to painful stimulation. He had brisk bleeding from his left ear and brain tissue was extruding through the nose. These neurologic findings suggested he had a fatal, nonsurgical lesion. The diver was immediately intubated and routine investigative procedures were performed. Shortly thereafter he was taken to the operating room and a right frontal burr hole was made, primarily for the purpose of monitoring intracranial pressure. The patient did not respond to any form of treatment and was pronounced dead a few days after his injury. At autopsy, there was diffuse brain damage with intracerebral hemorrhage, apparently arising from a torn left lateral sinus.

As far as is known, this tragedy is the only one of its kind that has occurred in any international diving meet in the world. Most blunt injuries to the head, eyes, and ears are less catastrophic.

Blunt trauma can affect the eyes. An occasional episode of detached retina has occurred from landing flat in the water while diving from a 10-m tower. Blurring of vision obviously may be transient, but more prolonged symptoms clearly warrant immediate ophthalmologic consultation. The greater the height at which a diver hits the water, the worse the eye lesion could become. Occasionally, this type of injury occurs as the diver loses visual orientation, such as while attempting new dives before maintaining an adequate feel for the complexity of the dive. In addition, any other type of stimulus that causes disorientation such as an inner ear infection could lead to this problem.

Blunt trauma to the eardrum tends to happen when a diver performs a complicated maneuver such as one involving simultaneous somersaults and twisting maneuvers. A good diver can execute a forward 3½ somersault, which calls for a 1260° rotation. Another common dive is a forward 1½ somersault with three twists in which the diver somersaults 540° and twists 1080° (Fig. 16.4) (1). The best divers have begun to perform even more complex feats, such as the forward 2½ somersault with two twists and the reverse 3½ somersault. Rupture of the eardrum is often due to disorientation while performing twisting dives, causing the diver to strike the water directly on his or her ear. The disorientation itself is clearly exacerbated by the lesion. If the

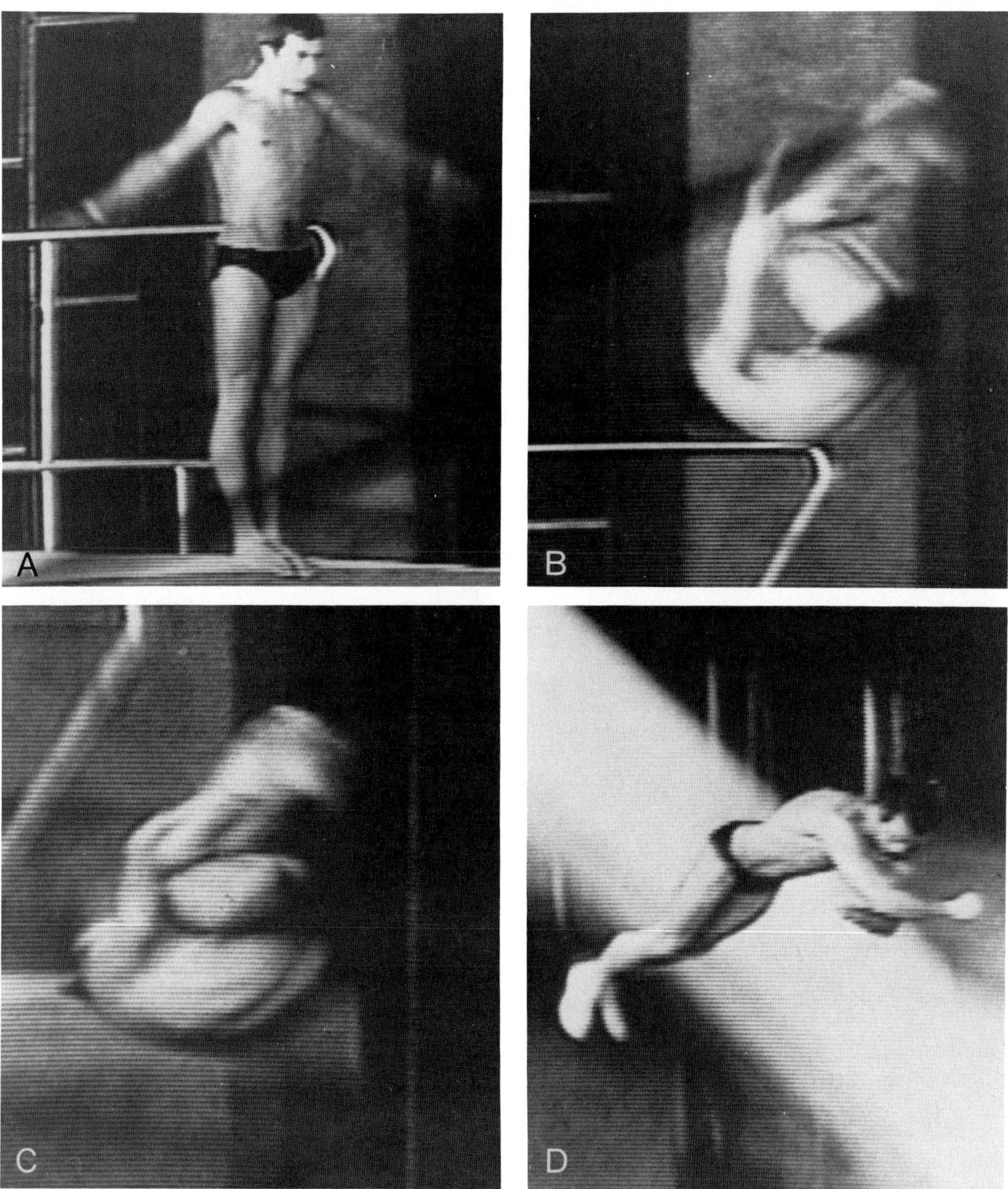

Figure 16.3. An attempted reverse 3½ somersault dive is demonstrated. **A,** The diver begins by swinging his arms behind his back. **B,** He reaches vertically and brings his knees up to his arms to continue the reverse somersaulting motion. **C,** Because of an unfortunate take-off, the diver strikes his head on the platform. **D,** His spinning motion is interrupted and the diver loses his grasp on his legs as he is projected forward in a disruption of his dive. Courtesy of Canapress.

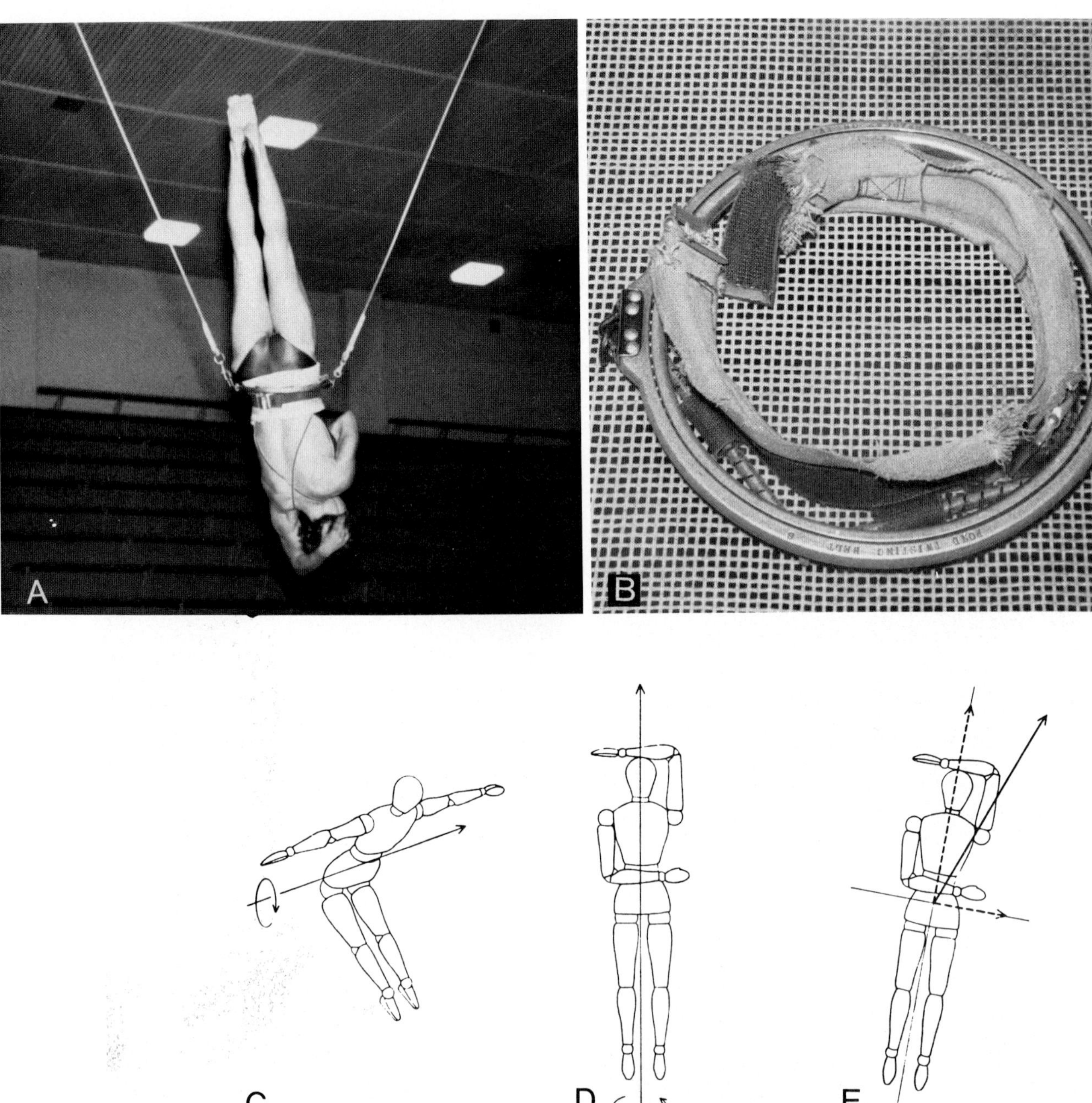

Figure 16.4 Twisting dives are among the most difficult to learn because the diver is spinning in one direction while twisting in a totally different axis. **A,** This diver is shown with the arms in the appropriate position to initiate the twisting movement. **B,** These complex dives are practiced with the aid of the twisting belt, which is composed of an inner ring that is affixed to the diver and an outer ring that is connected to the spotting ropes. This stabilizes the outer ring, permitting the diver and inner ring to twist. **C–E,** The vectors for somersaulting and twisting are indicated. From Frohlich C. The physics of somersaulting and twisting. Sci Am 1980:156.

patient complains of hearing loss, immediate otolaryngologic evaluation is warranted. The patient should refrain from entering the water until there is complete healing of the tympanic membrane, so as to prevent subsequent infections.

Joint Abuse

Shoulder Injuries

Diving injuries frequently involve the shoulder girdle muscles, especially in those divers who perform from great heights. Only occasional episodes of shoulder dislocation actually occur. Most shoulder dislocation injuries occur while diving from the 10-m tower and happen when the diver misses clasping his or her hands before entry, thus the arm is usually severely abducted (pulled back) over the head.

Occasionally, one forgets that the human body is a well-balanced machine and that one corrective action may have a deleterious effect on another body part. An example of such a problem is the development of increasing incidence of shoulder trauma as a result of the entry technique called flat handing. In this maneuver, the palms of the hands are in a position to make impact with the water. To do this, the wrists must be hyperextended as the diver grabs his or her hands (Fig. 16.5). After the surface of the water is broken by the palms of the hands, the diver swims the arms to the side or down the front to displace the water and make less splash on the surface. This technique will work well as long as the entry is done correctly, but too often young divers start to experiment with this technique before their shoulders are strong enough, and they end up having a partial dislocation or at least chronic shoulder trouble. Most of the time, the humerus is dislocated anteriorly as the arm externally rotates. If this happens to a young diver, the incidence of recurrence is high, often necessitating surgical correction of the joint damage (2).

Chronic tendinitis also is a common problem and again is frequently due to a flat handed entry or entering the water while the arm is abducted. To raise the arm to dive, the rotator cuff muscles contract, holding the humeral head against the glenoid fossa while the deltoid muscles contract, thus lifting the arm. If the arm is forcibly abducted and continues behind the back, injury to the rotator cuff occurs. Inflammation involves the subdeltoid bursae and limits the space underneath the acromion process. The next time the arm is raised, the tendon may impinge on the coracoacromial ligament, leading to further inflammation of the tendons. If this process continues, the tendon can become so weak that it will tear (2).

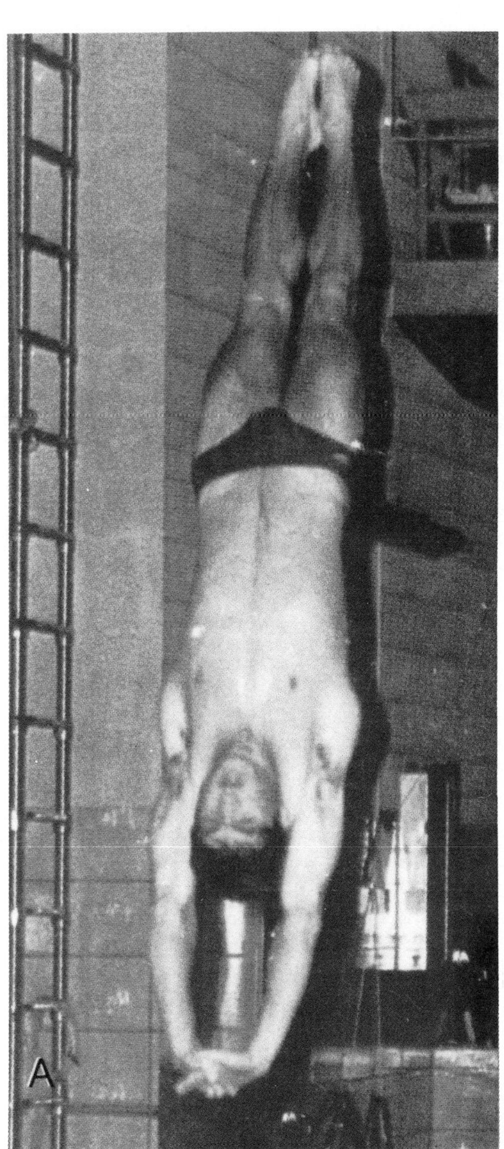

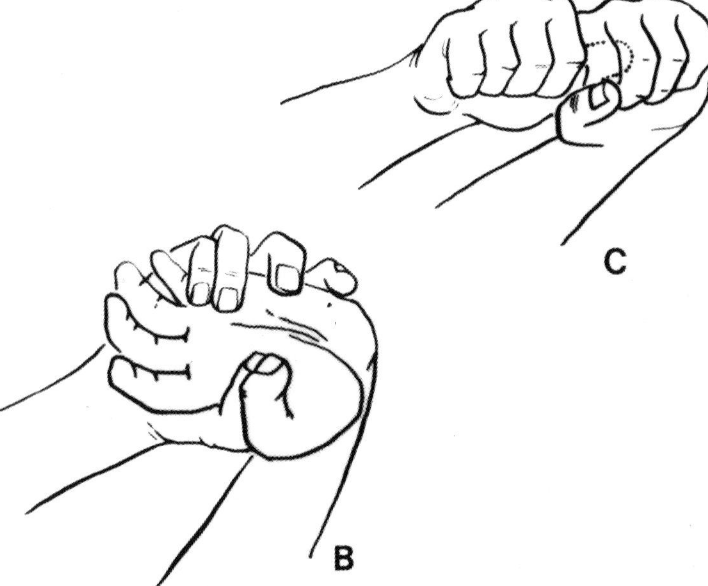

Figure 16.5. **A,** A diver demonstrating the flat handed entry posture. Note his extremely well-developed shoulder muscles, which are essential if this technique is to be used. **B,** The correct position for the multiple finger clasped hand for the flat hand entry. **C,** A less satisfactory solid thumb clasped grip is demonstrated, which may be more rapidly achieved in an emergency.

Wrist and Elbow Injuries

Injuries to the wrist and elbow are fairly common and can only happen when a diver does hundreds of dives per day. The flat hand entry techniques cause a great deal of pressure on the wrist and elbow when the diver makes contact with the water. There is a significant dorsiflexion of the wrist immediately on impact, which can cause an impingement in the distal role of carpal bones. This will frequently result in either a periostitis or a stress fracture of these bones. However, it may not be limited to the bony segment of the wrist but can also involve the capsule and the ligaments surrounding the joints (3). The higher the starting perch, the greater the chance of injury because of the greater speed at impact. As an example, a diver exiting from the 10-m platform is traveling at a rate of speed of approximately 31 mph on impact with the water. At this point, relief can only be achieved by discontinuing the activity until the pain diminishes.

Osteochondritis may be a growth center problem encountered occasionally at the knee joint and rarely at the elbow. It is usually caused by overuse in a young diver. The lesion in the elbow occurs when children go through significant growth spurts at 15 years of age or earlier and especially when diving from the 10-m tower. It is, therefore, often best to keep the diver off the tower during a rapid period of growth.

Spinal Injuries

Musculoskeletal Injuries

Probably the most common type of injury sustained by any athlete, but especially divers, is musculoskeletal. The term *myofascial strain syndrome* is apt and appropriate. In the early portion of the training regimen, it is common to sustain injuries to the neck and low back in addition to other muscle groups. These in and of themselves usually do not cause significant neurologic sequelae and often are treated simply with conservative measures. Most often the mechanism of injury in terms of the etiology of a myofascial strain is either an acute hyperextension of the lumbar spine or rapid rotational motion of the cervical region.

Hyperextension

In many ways, competitive diving is similar to gymnastics. The sport originated when gymnasts began performing stunts on a board over water. Many of the maneuvers are still virtually identical, except that the gymnast finishes his or her maneuvers feet first on solid ground whereas most dives are completed in the head-first position and, of course, always in the water. In terms of training, diving and gymnastics both use the trampoline to learn new stunts. Another similarity is shared with the platform diver. Both the tumbler and the platform diver are subjected to tremendous stress on the vertebral column on initiating their performances. Many of the injuries common to gymnasts are, therefore, often duplicated in divers.

Garrick and Requa in a 1980 study noted that one-third of all gymnastics injuries involved the lumbar spine and one of the more common causes of low-back pack in gymnasts is traumatic spondylolysis (4). This condition is actually a stress fracture that develops in the pars interarticularis, a defect in the vertebrae between the upper joint process and the lower joint process. The pain associated with this condition is usually dull, aching or cramping, and persistent. It is usually the result of repeated stress and is aggravated by movements that involve hyperextension. The pain may initially occur unilaterally and hyperextension may increase the pain only on the affected side. This occurs because the defect in the pars interarticularis may be a unilateral problem. Continued stress to this area can cause subluxation at the site of a stress fracture, the upper vertebrae sliding forward on the lower vertebrae, a condition known as spondylolisthesis (4). The same pathophysiologic response to stress occurs in divers. The exacerbating factor, the hyperextension mechanism, is illustrated in the following case history.

Case 16.3

A 16-year-old high school diver suffered an episode of severe back pain. He had sustained some compression fractures of the upper spine while diving approximately 6 years earlier. This latest episode of severe pain was noted after entering the water with the spine in a hyperextended position after completing a forward 2½ somersault dive in the tuck position. With the pain, there was concomitant, nonlocalized numbness in the right leg, but the patient denied any weakness or bowel or bladder incontinence. Conservative treatment included physical therapy, heat, ultrasound, and muscle relaxants. He experienced only minimal improvement of his symptoms. Because of the persistent low-back pain, the patient was admitted to the hospital. Physical examination revealed no obvious scoliosis, but the patient did have a small amount of tenderness on palpation over his spinous processes in the lumbar region. There was no palpable stepoff. Straight leg raising was positive at 30° on the left side but negative on the right. Complete neurologic testing revealed subtle sensory and motor changes in the distribution of the left L5 nerve root. X-rays of the lumbar spine (Fig. 16.6*A*) revealed a grade I spondylolisthesis of the L5 vertebral body on the sacrum with a defect in the pars interarticularis at this level (Fig. 16.6*B*). Oblique views reveal bilateral spondylolysis at L5. On closer inspection, the defect on the right was old whereas the one on the left was recent. There also appeared to be some changes consistent with old compression fractures of the lower thoracic vertebrae. A bone scan was negative and a myelogram revealed the slippage described above and considerable space at L5–S1 between the contrast medium and the spine, which might conceal a ruptured disc (Fig. 16.6*C*). The patient was treated with immobilization in a cast brace for 5 weeks and ultimately recovered to the point at which diving was again possible after daily stretching exercises and whirlpool treatments.

This case also illustrates one of the typical injury patterns found in diving. Injuries of the lower back frequently are recurrent in nature. Many are simply mis-

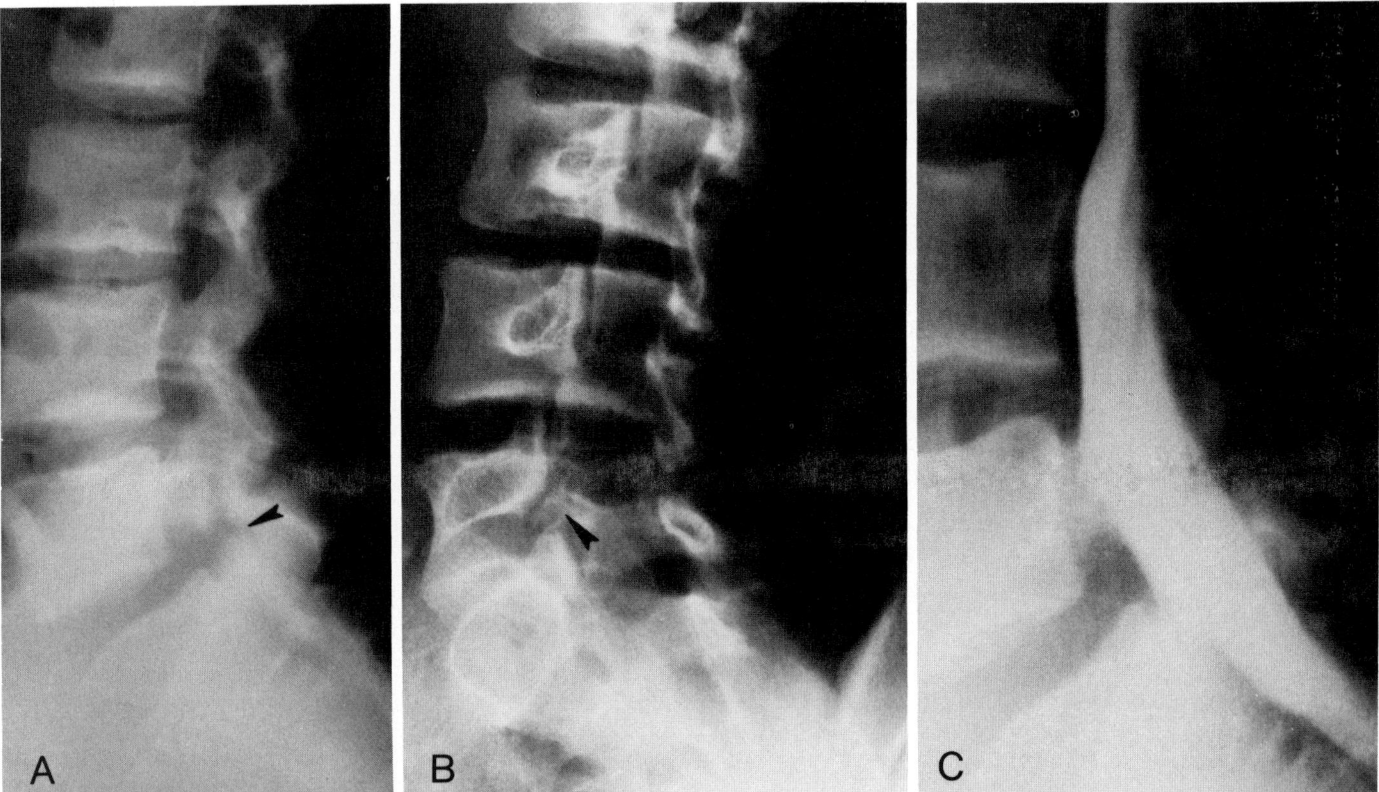

Figure 16.6. **A,** A grade I dislocation of the L5 vertebral body on S1 is exhibited; the *arrowhead* designates the break in the pars interarticularis. **B,** The oblique view accentuates the congenital defect in the L5 pars interarticularis *(arrowhead)*. **C,** This lateral view of the myelogram demonstrates the degree of space between the pantopaque column and the posterior margin of the vertebral bodies in which a herniated disc may be hidden.

diagnosed, being initially attributed to back strain or pulled muscles. Because this is a common initial complaint, it is often ignored by both divers and coaches. Therefore, training can continue to the detriment of the athlete. If minor symptoms do persist, then further evaluation with at least a plain set of spinal x-rays is *always* indicated.

Longitudinal-Directed Stress Injuries

Another common injury involves repeated trauma to the lumbar vertebral column directed in a longitudinal vector parallel to the spine. This type of stress occurs in three situations in diving. First, while performing dives from rigid surfaces, the diver derives all of the spring from a vertically directed push from the tower. An equal and opposite force is thus directed longitudinally through the hips and spine on take-off. Second, when using the trampoline as a training apparatus, the diver is subjected to a similar longitudinal force. Finally, stress is exerted on entry into the water. Dives that are accomplished at a great height such as from a 10-m platform or a 100-foot cliff produce a significant amount of stress on the vertebral column on entry. As a result of these three factors, two common diving related injuries occur: vertebral stress fractures and intervertebral disc space compressions with subsequent herniation of the nucleus pulposus. The following case illustrates both.

Case 16.4

A 20-year-old collegiate diver had experienced multiple episodes of low-back pain over a period of 1 year. These were treated conservatively with heat, massage, muscle relaxants, and bedrest. Lumbosacral spine films on anterior-posterior and oblique views (Fig. 16.7*A,B*) revealed a congenital defect of the right L3 facet and a small T12 compression fracture (Fig. 6.7C). The patient had been performing on the trampoline with the aid of a spotting belt in diving practice for a period of 4 weeks before his initial admission. When he struck the trampoline hard, he noted the instantaneous occurrence of sciatic type pain. The pain radiated posteriorly to the right buttock, thigh, and calf, and to the right lateral aspect of the foot. It was accentuated by coughing, sneezing, and straining.

On physical examination, the diver complained of pain at 20° of forward flexion. Tilting toward the right increased the pain, whereas tilting toward the left caused the pain to diminish in intensity. On straight leg raising, there was pain in the right sciatic distribution when the left leg was at 60° and the left foot was dorsiflexed. Straight leg raising on the right was positive at 35°, and dorsiflexion of the foot caused acute sciatica. There was numbness of the lateral border of the right foot and in the lateral two toes. There was no weakness of the lower extremities and no evidence of impairment of bowel and bladder function. The right Achilles reflex was absent.

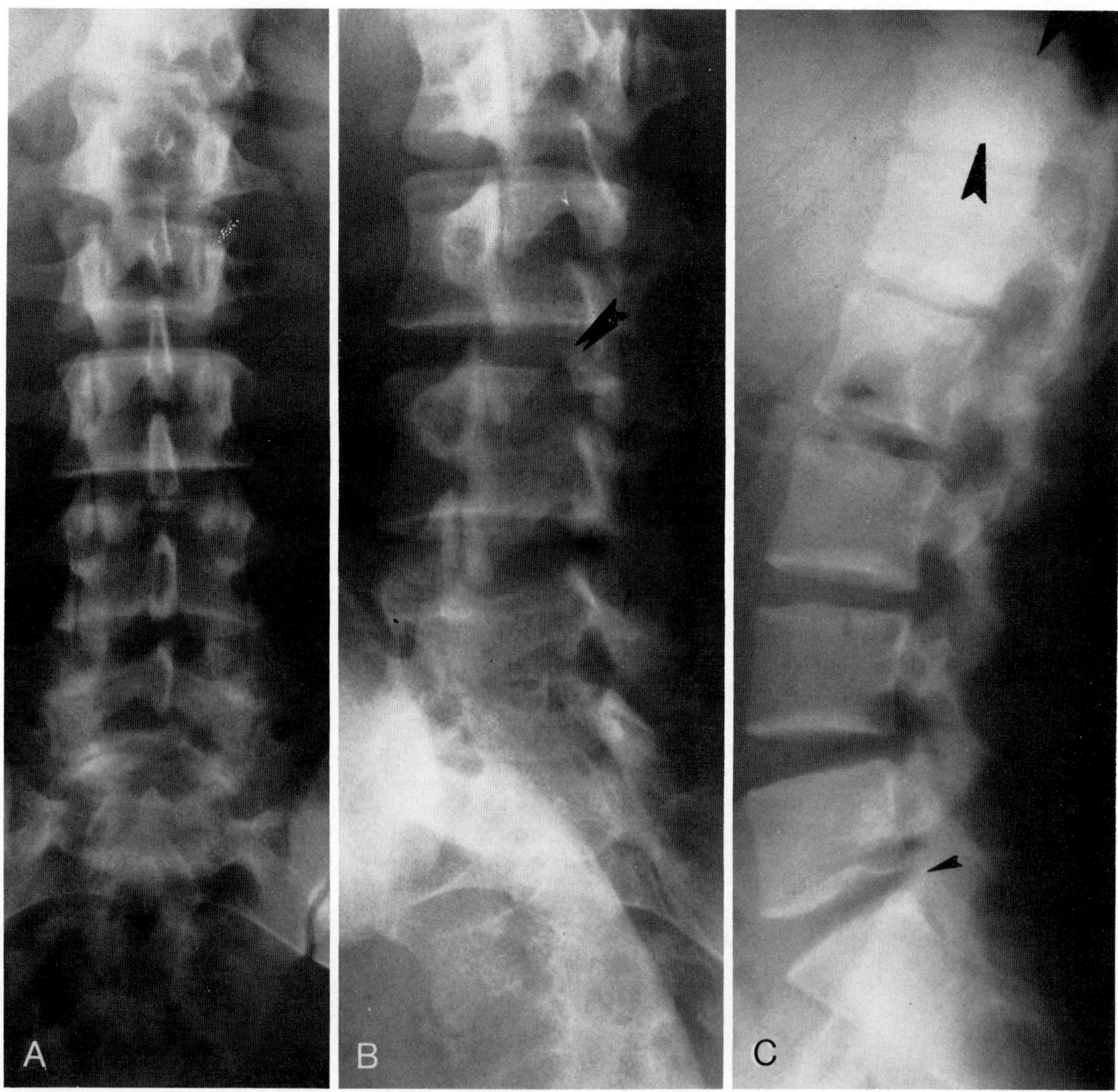

Figure 16.7. A, The anteroposterior view of the x-ray film exhibits a defect in the left articular facet *(arrowhead)*. **B,** The oblique view shows this defect more readily *(arrowhead)*. **C,** The lateral view of the lumbosacral spine x-ray revealed an unsuspected compression fracture of the T12 vertebral body *(arrowheads)*. **D,** The anteroposterior view of the myelogram visualized a right lateral defect in the pantopaque column at the right L5–S1 interspace. **E,** The oblique view confirms this, but **(F)** the lateral myelographic view is not as reassuring; it shows the narrowed L5–S1 interspace posteriorly with slight pantopaque canal impingement.

Myelography demonstrated a large defect in the radiopaque column at the right L5–S1 interspace (Fig. 16.7*D,E*) and a small defect at L5–S1 in the lateral view (Fig. 16.7*F*). Because of the positive contralateral straight leg raising sign, extrusion of the intervertebral disc was probable (3), so the patient was operated on, and the totally extruded disc at the right L5–S1 interspace was removed. The diver recovered nicely and with postoperative exercises was able to return to normal activity level in 4 weeks and diving within 2 months.

Hyperflexion Injuries

Cervical stenosis (a congenitally narrowed spinal canal) is currently receiving more notice in athletic injuries, particularly in contact sports, and it probably should receive more attention in diving. With extreme flexion of the cervical spine, there may be a squeezing of the cervical cord in a tight cervical canal. With cervical stenosis and hyperextension, there is often wrinkling inward of the ligamentum flavum, causing neurologic deficit. A symptomatic congenital atlantoaxial dislocation may occur, which can be detected by viewing the cervical spine in the neutral, flexion, and extension positions or by CT scan.

Often a sudden, acute neck flexion can produce radicular pains in the cervical region with associated numbness and or weakness in a single dermatome or myotome. An appropriate impairment of reflexes also can occur.

Case 16.5

A 26-year-old nationally ranked diver performed a 1½ somersault with a full twist from a 10-m platform but did not have a smooth recovery into the water. She made a flat hand entry into the water with her neck flexed and her hands clasped. Her arms were flung upward and backward over her head (Fig. 16.8*A*) instead of having the normal neutrally extended spine with arms in alignment next to the head (Fig. 16.8*B*). She had pain, numbness, and tingling in her thumb and the index finger bilaterally whenever she would try to bend her head forward and flex her spine. There was tenderness to percussion over the spinous processes of C5 and C6 but no radiating pain. Her neurologic examination was normal. Cervical spine x-rays showed widening of the C5–C6 interspace, and there was a tiny chip fracture of the C7 spinous process. The widening of that interspace was consistent with the C6 nerve root irritation bilaterally, suggesting the possibility of a centrally protruded interverbetral disc at the C6 level. In addition, she had a marginally narrowed spinal canal that measured 13 mm in diameter. The danger of a possible her-

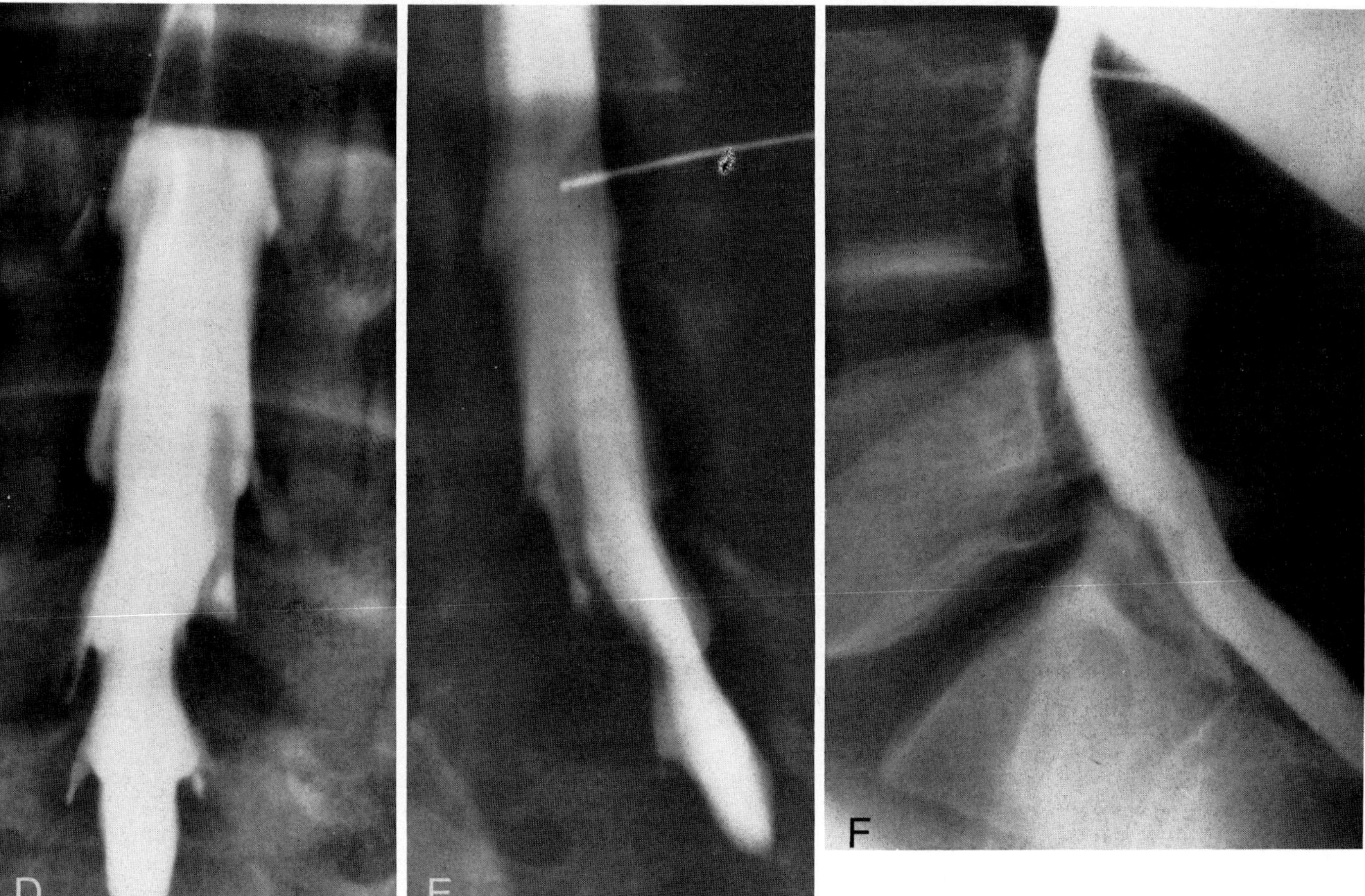

Figure 16.7D–F.

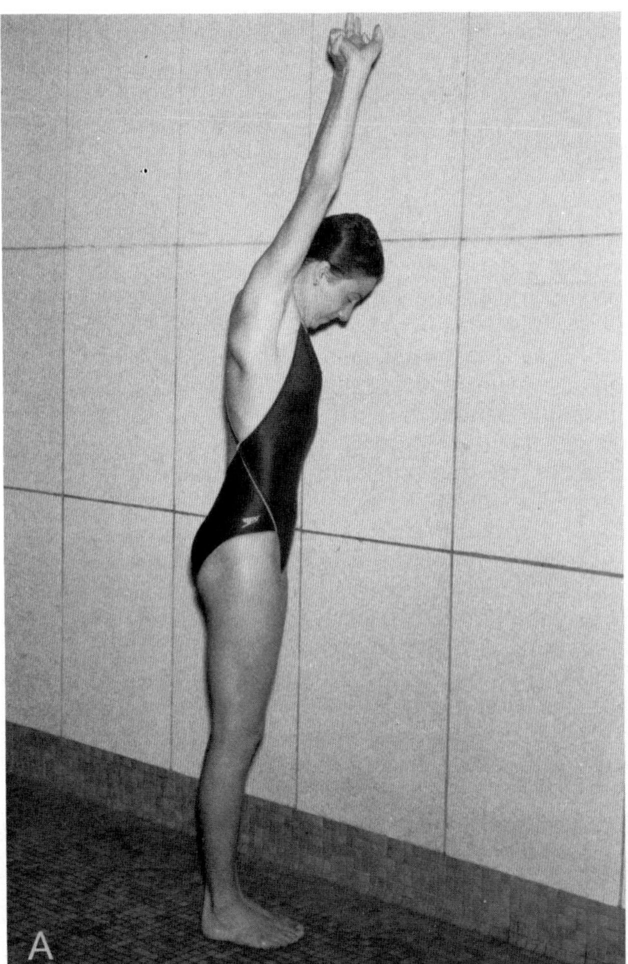

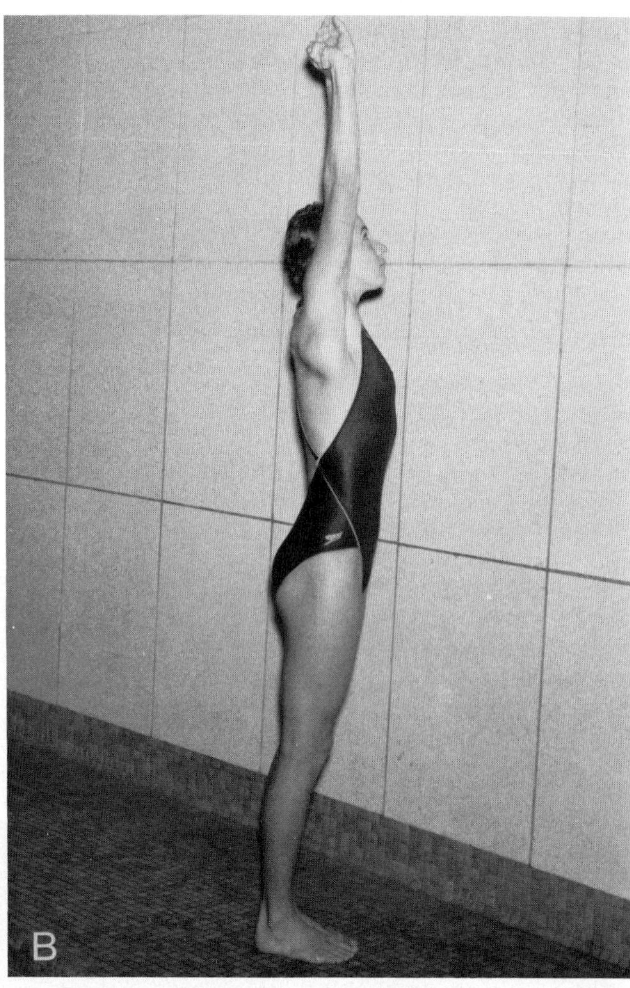

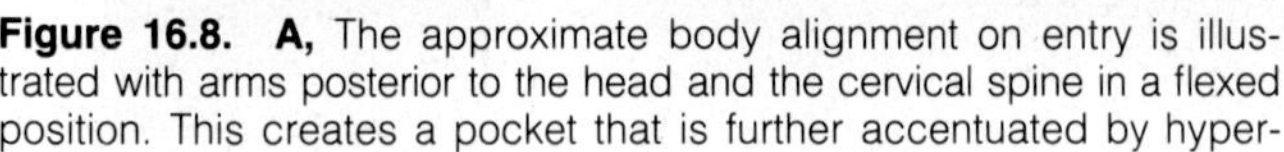
Figure 16.8. **A,** The approximate body alignment on entry is illustrated with arms posterior to the head and the cervical spine in a flexed position. This creates a pocket that is further accentuated by hyperflexion of the neck on entry. **B,** In contrast, this is the appropriate body alignment. The head is in a neutral position, thus protected bilaterally by the arms, and hyperflexion also is prevented.

niated disc striking the cord and causing complete paralysis of all four extremities was explained, and CT scan and myelography were suggested for further measures to determine the diagnosis. In addition, the possibility of a ligamentous injury accompanying a possible disc space abnormality also was suggested as a cause for further concern. The patient, however, refused to undergo the aforementioned studies and signed a release from the orthopedic surgeon and neurosurgeons involved in her care, relieving them of any responsibility. A regimen of neck-strengthening exercises to build up the neck muscles was subsequently advocated. She followed the exercise regimen and later returned to diving, although a poor entry into the water could result in a severe neurologic disability. Fortunately, she has had no further problems.

Finally, although most injuries tend to be acute in nature, it is important to consider the long-term sequela of diving and its effects on the spine. In 1966, Schneider et al. (5) studied the chronic trauma to the cervical spine experienced by Acapulco, Mexico divers. Permission was obtained from the leader of the divers to examine him and five others and to procure cervical spine x-rays with payment for this privilege. The only stipulation in the selection of the divers was that they had to be diving from the 100- or 130-foot perches for many years. The leader picked the group, and the statistics are shown in Table 16.1. The site of the perches from which the divers take off are shown in Fig. 16.9*A*. The divers must project themselves 27 feet outward from the cliff on their dive and then land in 15 to 18 feet of water, depending on the height of the tide. Aside from an occasional stiff neck, they sustained no physical disability and were all neurologically normal. The lateral cervical spine x-rays of the selected six divers are shown in Figure 16.9*B–G*. Case B, the leader, was 33 years old and had a record of 25 years of diving from 130 feet for 25,000 dives and had the best looking spine of all. Two other divers, Cases C and D, had the same x-ray pattern as the leader. Case C had a small compression fracture, but his remaining vertebral bodies as well as those of cases B and D are well-preserved with normal-looking interspaces and spinal canals. In cases E through G, at least two vertebrae are well-fused anteriorly, again with good preservation of the interspaces and spinal canal width. The leader (Case B) and Cases C and D

Table 16.1.
Statistical Data on Mexican Divers Studied for Cervical Spine Abnormalities

Case	Age	Height	Weight (pounds)	Years Diving	Number of Dives
B	33	5′6″	180	25	25,000
C	28	5′5″	125	12	12,000
D	28	5′5″	120	15	15,000
E	35	5′7″	135	18	16,000
F	26	5′7″	138	8	8,000
G	22	5′4″	120	7	5,000

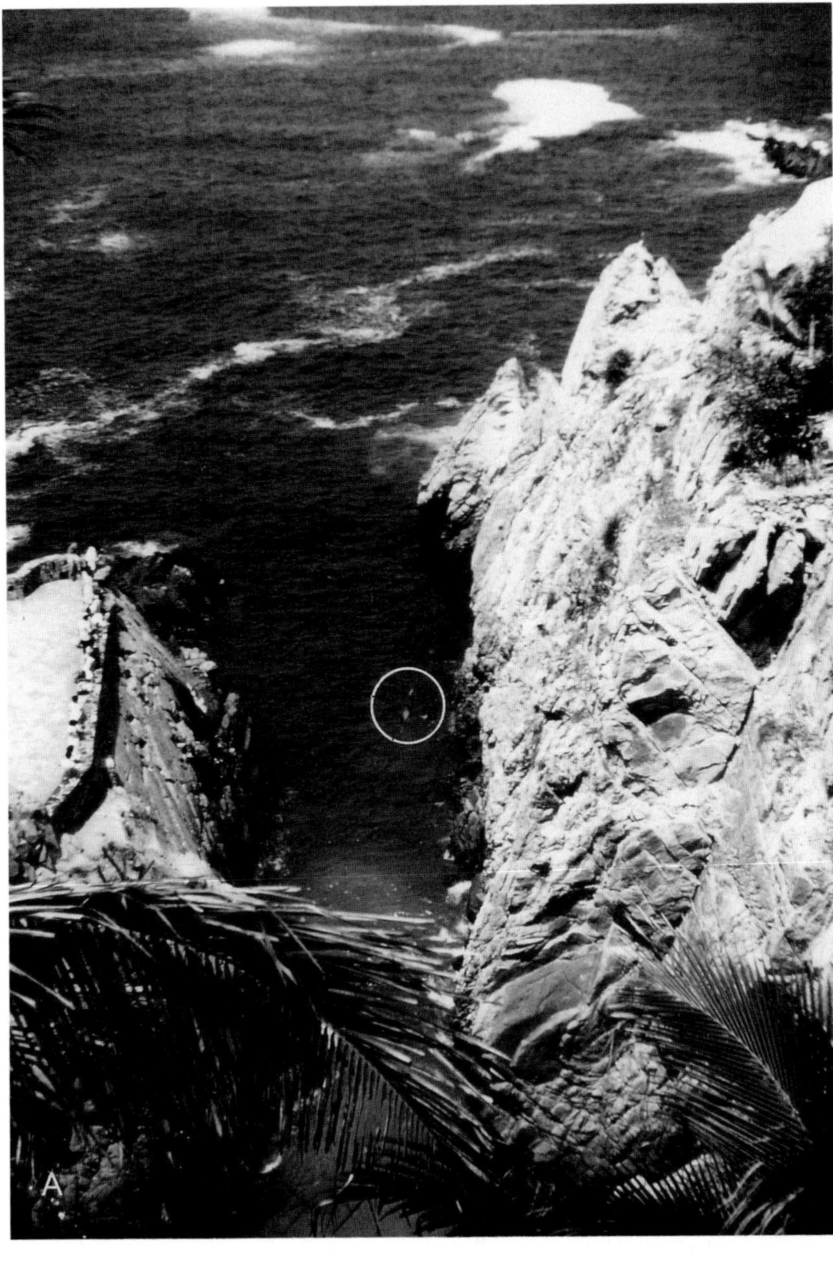

Figure 16.9. A, The Quebrada is shown with the 100- and 130-foot perches on the right cliff from which the divers perform. The diver *(circled)* is shown at a height two-thirds of the way down from the diving platform. **B–D,** The lateral cervical spine x-rays of these three divers generally exhibit preservation of the intervertebral spaces, a normal-size spinal canal, little spurring, and normal vertebral body height, with the exception of **C** who has minimal anterior vertebral body compression. **E–G,** The x-rays of the vertebral bodies of these cervical vertebra showed a spontaneous fusion anteriorly *(white arrows),* but again there was preservation of the intervertebral bodies and the width of these spinal canals *(black arrows).* **H,** The correct method of high diving from these cliffs is to clasp the hands together. The divers whose spines are shown in **B–D** used this technique satisfactorily. The divers whose spine x-rays are shown in **E–G** dove "improperly," with their hands wide apart, as shown in **I,** "punching a hole in the water" and sustaining a blow directly to the head. Courtesy of RC Schneider, M Paop, and R Alverez.

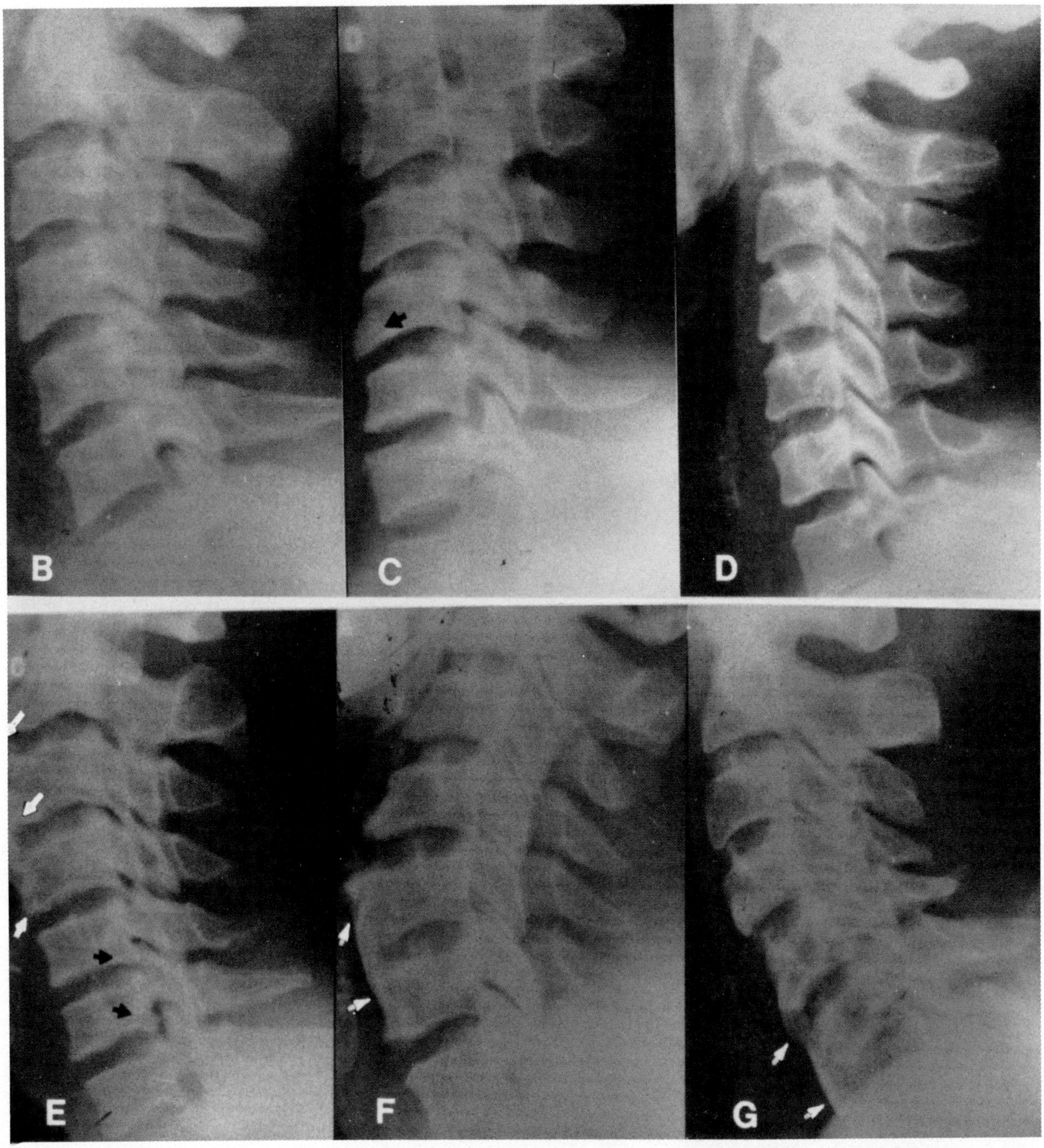

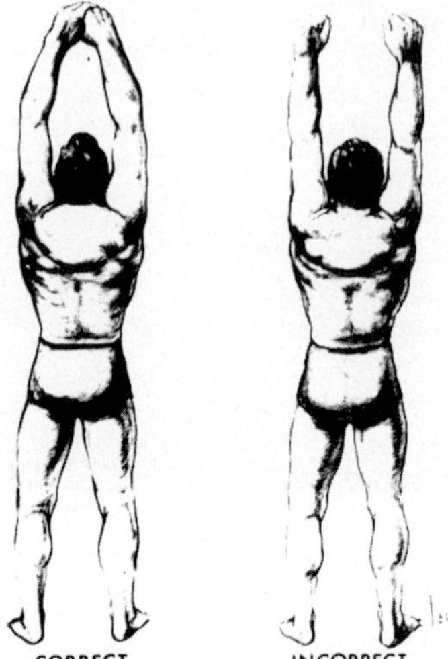

Figure 16.9B–I.

(Fig. 16.9*B–G*) entered the water with their hands locked together in the correct way (Fig. 16.9*H*), whereas cases E, F, and G incorrectly broke the water with their arms shoulder width apart, clutching their fists and striking directly on the vertex of their heads (Fig. 16.7*I*). Although divers E, F, and G showed anterior vertebral body fusion, in none of the spines of the six divers was there any significant loss of intervertebral space, diminution of body height, or narrowing of the spinal canal. This indicates that extensive repetitive cervical trauma had not caused any severe cervical spondylitic arthritic changes.

Although these divers were neurologically normal, it is clear that repetitive trauma to the cervical region can, in time, accelerate the normal aging process of cervical spondylosis. It is not uncommon to see athletes who extensively use neck muscles (football players, wrestlers, and divers) to show some evidence of significant cervical spondylitic problems. In addition, significant changes can occur in terms of cord compression and myelopathy. If any of these problems are present cessation of all types of trauma to the spine is recommended and consultation from a neurosurgeon should be sought.

Treatment

Treatment of most diving-related injuries is usually quite simple and involves minimal medical intervention. Most trauma and soft tissue injuries are treated symptomatically with icing in the initial acute phase; applications of heat can be used later, if necessary. Lacerations tend to be clean injuries because of the chlorinated pool water. However, striking the board should prompt an investigation into the diver's tetanus status.

Treatment of a ruptured eardrum (tympanic membrane) should start with avoiding contamination of the middle ear structures. In addition, diving with a ruptured eardrum can cause significant disorientation, predisposing the diver to further injury. Disorientation in the water itself can be detrimental. Clearly, no diving should continue until a complete otolaryngologic evaluation has been accomplished and the patient has been cleared from that standpoint.

More significant head traumas should immediately be assessed in terms of the ABC's of first aid. Any type of significant head trauma requires neurosurgical consultation, because underlying skull fractures and intraparenchymal brain abnormalities must be considered, especially if there is evidence of loss of consciousness. With significant loss of consciousness, a noncontrasted CT scan of the brain should be undertaken. In addition, a period of observation should ensue and the diver should not return to his or her activities until complete neurologic recovery is documented.

Most joint injuries can be prevented by teaching appropriate techniques. However, if joint trauma does occur, then initial conservative therapy with aspirin or nonsteroidal antiinflammatory drugs (NSAIDs) should be instituted. If pain persists, exacerbating activities should cease until further evaluation, possibly including orthopedic consultation, is complete.

Immobilization techniques are rarely called for. However, with sprains of the ankle and wrist, supports can be used prophylactically and as treatment, so that diving can continue. This might include taping of ankles or placement of foam pads over wrist bony prominences to prevent further trauma. Again, if pain persists, then further evaluation, including the use of x-rays, should be accomplished.

The treatment of myofascial strain syndromes of the cervical or lumbar region is usually self-limiting. It is common to sustain some sort of minor aches and pains when beginning an initial training period. However, divers who have prolonged complaints of low-back pain should undergo further investigation. Presuming the initial evaluation, which should include at least a routine set of cervical and/or lumbar spine x-rays, is negative, then initial treatment with icing techniques and the institution of NSAIDs is warranted. Recent literature suggests that the previous accepted treatment of cervical or lumbar sprains with prolonged immobilization is actually more detrimental in the long run, especially to an athlete. Increased activity levels as a form of treatment of myofascial symptoms, although causing initial pain, can actually produce endogenous endorphins, which can help alleviate the more chronic aspects of myofascial strain syndromes (6). In addition, other evidence suggests that physical therapy with stretching techniques is probably the best treatment for all chronic muscle and ligament injuries (7). Strengthening exercises are an adjunct, but flexibility exercises will treat most injuries and will allow the diver to return to function quicker than any other form of therapy.

A digression is warranted at this time. Correct diagnosis is imperative if adequate treatment is to be rendered. Obviously, a good history and physical examination in reference to an injury is crucial. Appropriate radiographic studies can be valuable. As stated above, in any athlete who has persistent neck or back symptoms, a screening set of spine x-rays is needed. Congenital defects such as congenital spondylolysis and/or congenital stenosis is important in terms of prognosis. In addition, these abnormalities may lead to further neuroradiographic imaging studies.

For most athletes who present with classic neurologic entrapment syndromes, the procedure of choice for the lumbar region would be a plain, noncontrasted CT scan. It is rare at this point to use lumbar myelography, because with an athlete the diagnostic dilemma is usually not present. In addition, the quality of CT scans is markedly improved and most surgical decisions can be made with this excellent modality. If any further imaging studies are indicated, a good-quality MRI has virtually subplanted the myelography for most patients in terms of lumbar and cervical evaluation (Fig. 16.10).

When should the injured athlete return to the sport? Most injuries are minor and little delay is needed before returning the diver to activity. Head injuries, however, deserve a comment. If the patient sustains an episode of loss of consciousness and a noncontrasted CT scan is negative, then the patient can most likely return

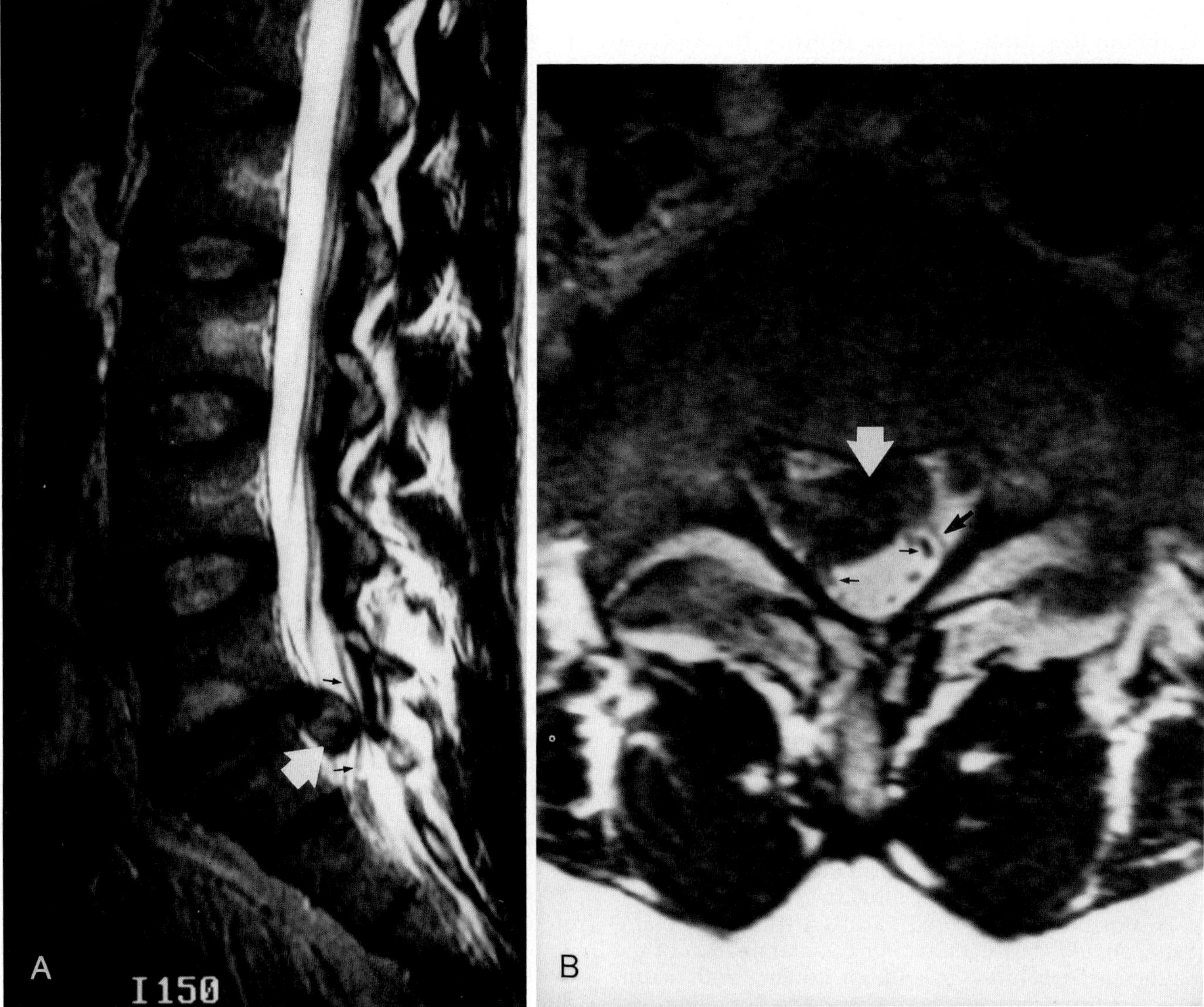

Figure 16.10. T2-weighted MRI scans of a herniated disc. At L5–S1, fast-spin echo sagittal **(A)** and axial **(B)** images demonstrate a large herniated disc *(white arrows)*, the fat-dural interface *(large black arrow)*, compression and posterior displacement of the thecal sac, and compression of the right nerve root compared with the left *(small black arrows)*.

to his or her activities within a few days. If, however, the patient develops evidence of a postconcussive syndrome, described classically as significant head trauma with subsequent chronic headaches, dizziness, fatigue, and depression, then the athlete should not be allowed to dive until complete resolution of the dizziness has occurred.

Musculoskeletal injuries do not necessarily preclude the diver from continuing, which can often be done after 24 hr of rest and ultimate resumption of stretching activities. Once range of motion is returned to normal, the diver should be able to return to the sport without any contraindications.

If a diver sustains an injury that requires surgery (the most common type of procedures would be that of nerve root decompression), adequate wound healing requires 6 weeks. Initial treatment postoperatively should include early activity levels with stretching exercises after 2 weeks of convalescence. During this convalescent period walking should be encouraged. Because of the stress involved with diving, especially from a tower, full activity should be delayed for at least 6 weeks.

With a cervical decompressive procedures, return to the sport should be delayed for a slightly longer period. If the anterior cervical discectomy and fusion procedure is used, then adequate fusion takes anywhere from a minimum of 2 months and probably closer to 3 months for complete fusion. In light of the significant vertically directed stress factors, resumption of complete activities should be delayed until complete fusion has been accomplished. Flexion and extension cervical spine films are needed to assess fusion adequacy. If cervical operations are for nerve root compression only and no evidence of cord compromise exists, there would be no contraindication to allowing the patient to return to diving. If, however, there has been evidence of cord compression, either from acute disc rupture and/or cervical spondylotic changes, then diving should cease in light of the propensity to develop further damage to the spinal cord. In addition, those patients who have congenitally narrow canals should seriously consider leaving the sport, because they have a significant predilection to developing chronic cord compression. Even if no significant deficit initially occurs, prolonged chronic exposure to spinal cord trauma can lead to more debilitating injuries, including evidence of posttraumatic hydromyelia, which has been reported to occur up to 10 years after injuries.

Conditioning

Conditioning for the athlete, including the diver, is an important aspect of training. Many injuries can be prevented with appropriate preseason conditioning. In a 1981 study of 66 divers, a total of 89% suffered from low-back pain, which was usually an isolated event but was sometimes a chronic complaint. From this study came a comprehensive program of exercises. If a program is to be effective, it must be carried out during the off-season as well. Because diving is concerned with precise body alignment, an exercise regimen must stress posture as well as flexibility training (8). Conditioning, therefore, can be broken up into aerobic, flexibility, and strength exercises.

Anthropologic studies have shown that walking and/or running can be preventative in terms of low-back injuries. In addition, walking is a form of therapy for patients with chronic low-back pain. It is believed that walking for 2 to 3 miles/day has maintenance and preventive advantages. For the diver, walking or running should be the hallmark for preseason aerobic conditioning and should be instituted up to 1 month before regular diving practice begins.

Flexibility is the most important portion of preseason training, especially for diving. Because most injuries are musculoskeletal in nature, these can be prevented with flexibility training. Flexibility also is important for many of the maneuvers divers are asked to perform, and having the appropriate flexibility can prevent damage to joints. In regard to stretching, two principal methods include static and ballistic (or dynamic) techniques (8). A dynamic stretch, such as bouncing up and down while attempting to touch one's toes, often does not accomplish as much as a static stretch. In the latter, a certain muscle group is stretched and held between 10 and 60 sec while avoiding sharp, shooting pains. Repeating the stretch three times a day will result in increased flexibility, with minimal chance of muscle injury. Dynamic stretching may place too much stress on the muscle too quickly, leading to injury, and should be avoided. Major muscle groups such as hamstrings, quadriceps, gastrocnemius and soleus muscles, pelvic girdle muscles, and shoulder girdle muscles must be stretched to maximize their flexibility and the function of their respective joints (Fig. 16.11).

Most exercises for posture technique are pinpointed toward the pelvic girdle. This strengthens the pelvis and stomach, which keep the body aligned while it enters the water, preventing low-back pain (Fig. 16.12). Typical conditioning regimens may include running every other day. In addition, stretching exercises should be done before running and also on the alternate days, when running is not involved.

Weights can be used to the enhancement of the diver. Large weights can be somewhat detrimental, because these can cause injury and create too much muscle bulk, inhibiting flexibility. Therefore, it is recommended that low weights be used along with high repetitions. Shoulder girdle strengthening is important. In addition, new advances in biomechanics have led to the development of machines specifically used to isolate the low-back area (Medex). Such machines are recommended for the diver. Unfortunately, these machines are not readily available to the average athlete, especially at the levels below collegiate competition.

Psychological Preparation

The psychological aspects of preparation for diving are intermingled with both conditioning and training. It is difficult, therefore, to talk specifically about this aspect in an isolated fashion. However, certain meth-

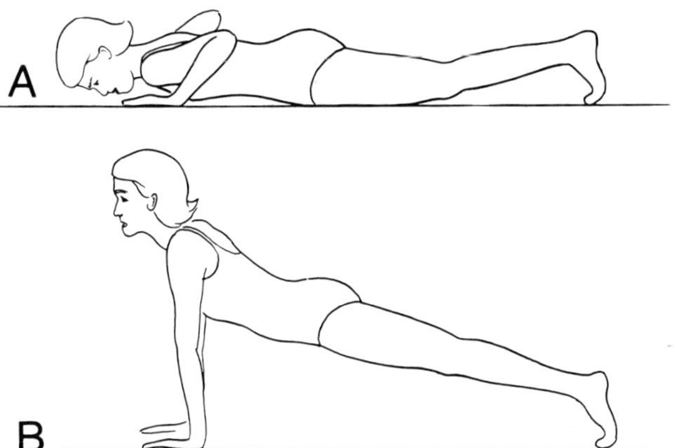

Figure 16.11. Push-ups are the most common exercise for conditioning the chest, arms, and shoulder musculature.

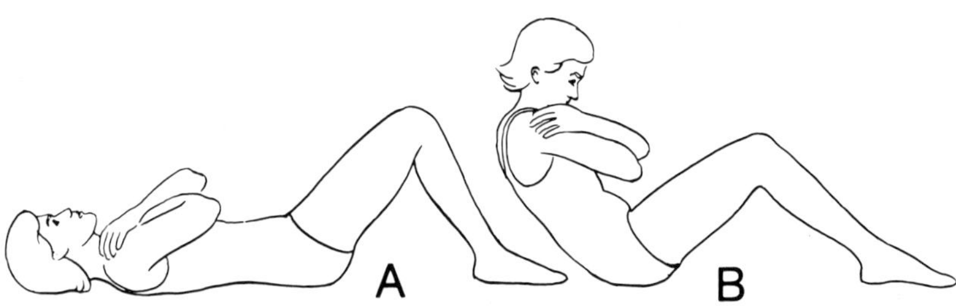

Figure 16.12. A sit-up routine with the hand placed on the shoulders and the knees in a bent position is effective in strengthening the abdominal muscles.

ods are available to help the diver, and less fear leads to more successful attempts at performing maneuvers.

Certain techniques that are crucial with all aspects of diving include the take-off and board work. The appropriate approach can be taught on land drills until adequate balance and coordination can be developed. After this is accomplished, the dive itself can also be practiced with a spotting apparatus. Once the maneuver is repeated often enough, the diver develops a feel for the technique, which enhances not only his or her ability to perform the dive physically but also his or her emotional security. Ultimately, a diver must perform the maneuver the first time without aids. If excellent board work is mastered and spotting techniques have been used, psychologically the transition is extremely smooth. In rare circumstances more difficult dives can be learned by spotting equipment at the pool side to further enhance the transition. A more detailed discussion of training techniques follows.

Prevention

The types of injuries acquired in competitive diving suggests that most injuries can be prevented. Prevention can be divided into five broad categories: primary physical examination, conditioning exercises, midair diving techniques, training techniques, and psychological preparation.

Primary physical examination does not need to be addressed here, although it is crucial to undergo at least a screening examination on a yearly basis for most athletes. Conditioning exercises and psychological components were discussed above.

Midair Diving Techniques

Midair diving techniques are important to the prevention of injuries. Land-based posture exercises can be mimicked in midair to correct positioning or alignment. As already mentioned, many low-back injuries occur because of hyperextension. Hyperextension can be eliminated in midair quite effectively by rotating the pelvis forward while contracting the stomach muscles. The easiest way to do this is to contract the gluteal muscles while performing the Valsalva maneuver. This effectively eliminates the excess curvature of back, aiding not only the alignment and aesthetic value of the dive but also the stabilization of the lumbar spine. By repeatedly performing posturing exercises, this maneuver becomes a conditioned reflex.

The second midair diving technique is use of eyesight. Would you cross a busy street with your eyes closed? Would you drive your car with your eyes closed? Do you close your eyes when you catch a ball? Are you a blind diver? Unfortunately, too many divers must answer yes to the last question. Those who do not open their eyes often do not focus on anything during a dive (9). By using visual cues, the athlete finds diving much easier, because consistency can be reached quite soon after learning a dive. Divers who know where they are in the air can often control the manner in which they enter the water, the point at which most diving injuries occur. After performing a dive hundreds of times, the diver develops an innate sense of timing and thus knows when to finish from a somersault or a twist. If a diver only uses random methods to develop this sense, learning new dives can become difficult and rather painful if he or she consistently lands on the stomach or back. As each person sees different things during a dive, it is not necessary to specify what to look for; it is only imperative that divers open their eyes and look. It seems quite logical that the more senses one uses, the easier it is to perform a task. Trampolinists are excellent examples of those who use repeated visual cues, because they must execute difficult maneuvers in succession while landing on a relatively solid surface (9). It is no secret that many excellent divers were once trampolinists; these divers learn new moves much faster than their peers, because they use their entire sensory systems to program their brains with the movements needed for the new dive.

Training Techniques

The coach must be the one to set up the appropriate team rules. These include forbidding double-bouncing on the board and allowing only one diver on the board at one time. The diver must be informed of the dangers of improper pool depth. The occasional pool bottom slopes upward quickly and may present an unsuspected dangerous feature. The correct techniques for line up and entry must be taught, including hand placement, head placement, and body position.

Coaches should teach basic diving skills on the 1-m board before moving the diver upward to 3 m or greater heights. From the 1-m board, the diver is moving at a relatively slow rate of speed when he or she hits the water, so the body does not get injured nearly as often or as severely.

The divers must do a great number of lead-ups (practicing part of a dive) before attempting to complete the dive or before doing it on a 3-m board. For example, a back double-somersault prepares for the back 2½ somersault, a reverse double-somersault prepares for the reverse 2½ somersault, and a full-twisting somersault prepares for the full-twisting 1½ somersault. The diver should be taught the proper tower take-off technique from the 1-m tower. A diver also must possess skills and strength proportionate to his or her body before attempting tower diving.

Training techniques are as numerous as the number of diving coaches, yet one specific technique is becoming an invaluable aid in teaching the diver. The technique consists of using spotting rigs with trampolines, port-a-pit diving boards, and regular poolside 1-m boards (Fig. 16.13). The trampoline has been used for years for training purposes and is considered a tremendous asset for divers. Spotting equipment is extremely valuable, especially at the junior age group and high school levels. This is the time when the diver is developing the fundamentals. As is often the case, spotting rigs are more frequently available at the places with the least need (e.g., colleges).

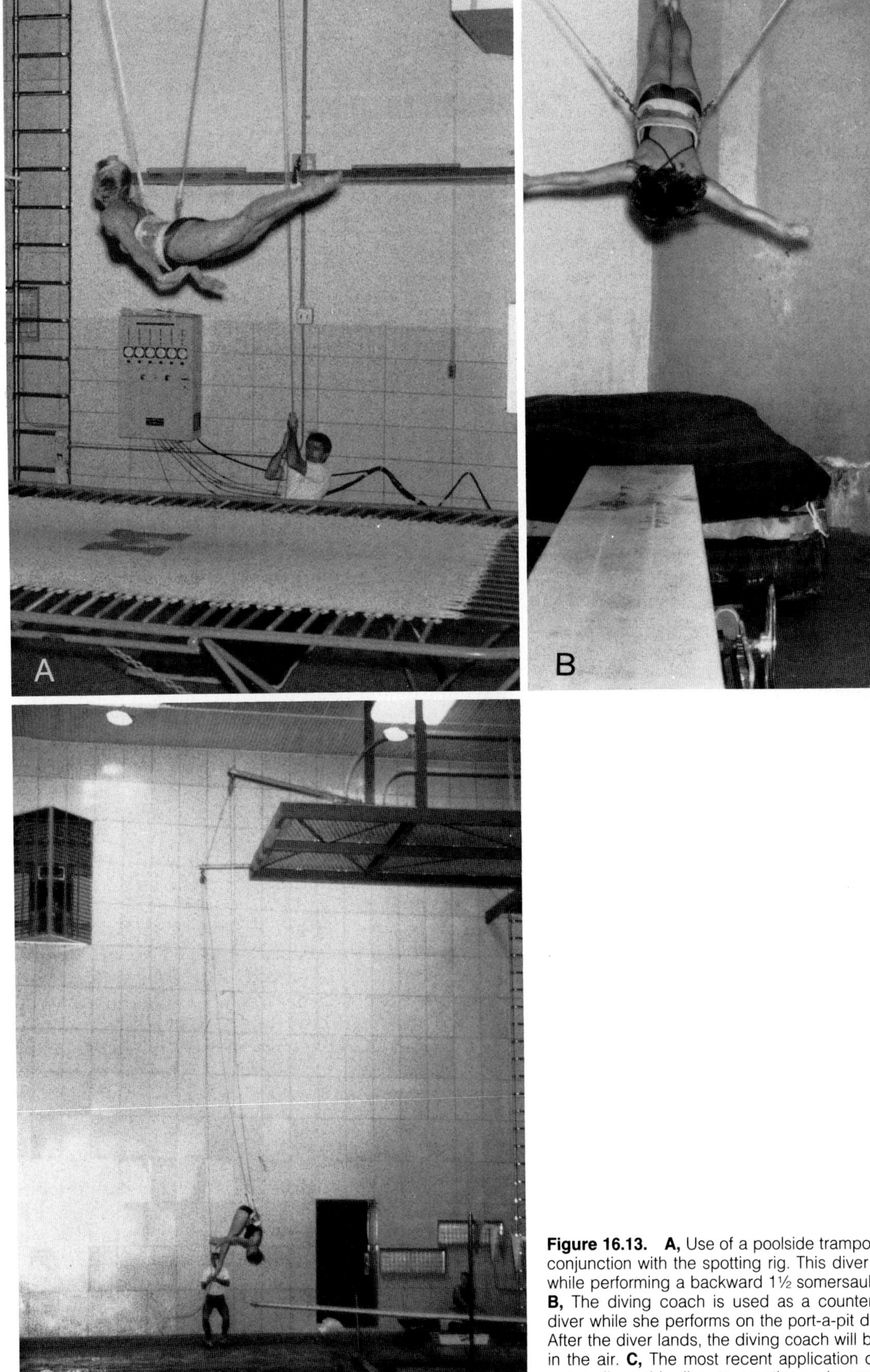

Figure 16.13. A, Use of a poolside trampoline is demonstrated in conjunction with the spotting rig. This diver is supported in midair while performing a backward 1½ somersault in the layout position. **B,** The diving coach is used as a counterweight to support the diver while she performs on the port-a-pit diving board apparatus. After the diver lands, the diving coach will be elevated 8 to 10 feet in the air. **C,** The most recent application of the spotting rig over water allows this diver to practice an inward spinning dive without fear of hitting the board.

Spotting rigs are valuable because new dives can be taught quickly with less fear and danger and with less trial-and-error learning; and visual techniques can also be taught at the same time. Spotting also helps the coach, making it easier to judge accurately whether or not the diver is ready to perform a new dive. It helps to take the guess-work out of coaching (10).

Divers also have made use of a diving board mounted on dry land over a sand pit to practice take-offs and board work. This setup makes it possible for a diver to isolate one aspect of the dive, concentrate on it, and make improvements in a short time span (10). Obviously, with the sand pit, only feet-first landings can be used, and the landing is quite hard. In recent years the port-a-pit has been introduced. This is similar to the "cloud nine" that a high jumper or pole vaulter lands on. This affords the diver a soft landing and allows him or her to land on the back or buttocks. The spotting rig has been combined with the land-based diving board and port-a-pit to eliminate most of the hazards of land-base drills (Fig. 16.13*B*). This apparatus is better than the trampoline for learning and improving spinning dives, because the take-offs are exactly the same as the ones used at the pool. When the diver does reverse or inward take-offs on the port-a-pit board, he or she experiences the same psychological effect as on the poolside board. The trampoline tends to eliminate this effect, because there is no board to contend with (10). However, the trampoline can be a valuable aid, especially when learning the twisting-types of dives. The twisting belt is an excellent aid that can also be used in the poolside setting. It is often used to prevent the disorientation present when learning these dives. Twisting dives tend to be the most difficult to learn because the diver is spinning in one direction while twisting in a totally different axis (Fig. 16.4).

An overhead belt also can be used over a 1-m springboard at poolside (see Fig. 16.13C). This is an improvement over the port-a-pit, because the diver can learn the feeling of the kick out and entry into water while still being protected from injury. After it is clear that a diver has completed the dive and is ready to enter the water correctly, the spotting ropes can be released, allowing a safe entry.

With the recent past, another training apparatus has been used to reduce landing injuries, especially those associated with tower entries. The bubble machine (Fig. 16.14) is composed of a compressor that generates a uniform mixture of air and water in the diving area similar to a foam cushion. Thus the diver can forget the fear of injury and concentrate on the fundamentals of the dive he or she is trying to learn. The bubbler should start before the diver leaves the board and stop after the diver enters the water. This apparatus tends to protect divers on entry, and the localized turbulence makes it easier for the diver to see the water, because there is a break in the homogeneity of the water surface. The bubbler is not readily available, and it is not a substitute for appropriate preparation and teaching with the use of spotting gear.

In terms of preventing traumatic eardrum ruptures, water polo helmets can be helpful, as these consist of strong plastic cups that shield the ear from direct trauma. The use of wet suits can also be used, especially when learning a spinning maneuver from a 3-m springboard or higher platform. The wet suit can absorb some of the punishment of an inappropriate flat landing on the water and prevent soft tissue damage.

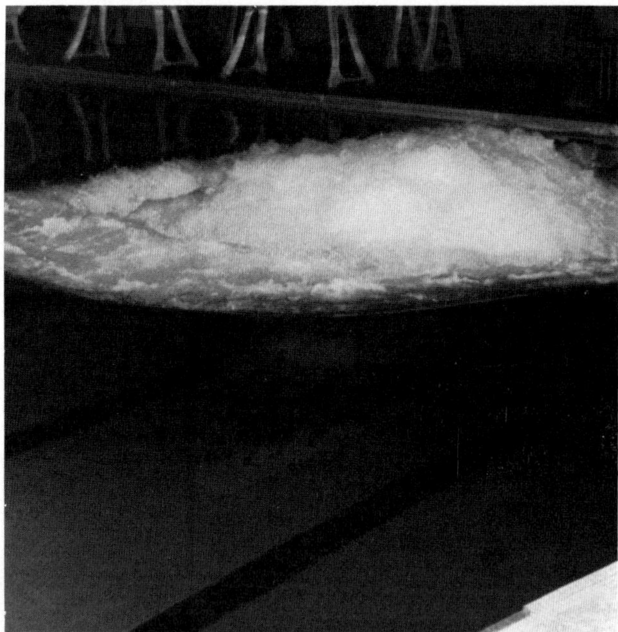

Figure 16.14. The amount of bubbles generated by the bubble machine and the area of distribution is shown here (see text for details).

In addition, in the initial training period for tower maneuvers, it often can be helpful to tape the wrists and perhaps apply pads to the bony prominence of the wrists. When the shoulder girdle muscles are strong enough to prohibit the collapse of the arms on entry (when the head can encounter the hand and soft tissue injuries of the hands can occur) the tape and pads are no longer needed.

Another aspect of training that must be emphasized is the isolation of exercised muscles groups. It is well-known that it is important to exercise muscle groups on an every-other-day basis. Similarly, alternating stressed muscle groups during training is important for diving. Training regimens should, therefore, include springboard work that alternates with tower work. Thus muscle groups are not consistently being fatigued from overuse.

Conclusions

Coaches should work divers into the diving regimen slowly and give the out-of-shape body a chance to become strong again. Workouts should be short and easy at first and the difficulty should increase over a 2- or 3-week period.

Coaches should listen to their divers. If a diver complains about some nagging pain, appropriate medical evaluation should be sought. This may initially be from an athletic trainer, but ultimately a physician may be required for more complicated and persistent complaints. It is important *not* to ignore the diver's complaints, as delayed diagnosis can be detrimental. If there is an injury, it is important to give it time to heal properly. Coaches can learn the difference between normal soreness and real pain or injury, and this experience is invaluable. They must, however, be aware of the danger signs that divers sometimes show when trying to hide an injury. When a diver hits the board with his or her head and it is thought there might be an injury to the neck, back, or head, be sure to use the correct precautions when removing a diver from the water (e.g., using a backboard).

Doctors have an important role in terms of preventative medicine by performing thorough physical examinations. The use of routine spinal screening x-rays may prevent further, more serious injuries. In light of the cost-effectiveness of this relatively inexpensive test, it is recommended that all serious competitive athletes have a baseline set of plain-screening x-rays. If an abnormality exists, then appropriate consultation with a physician should be obtained. A detailed exam by a neurosurgeon should be performed when there is any evidence of spinal trauma and/or head trauma. In this respect, the appropriate consultant can enhance the early diagnosis, and appropriate treatment can be instituted.

REFERENCES

1. Frohlich C. The physics of somersaulting and twisting. Sci Am 1980;242(3):154–156.
2. Clement EL Jr. The shoulder: common problems in athletes [Handout].
3. Mangine RE. Personal communication to RJ Kimball, 1983.
4. Jackson DW. Low back pain in young athletes. Am J Sports Med 1979;7(6):364–366.
5. Schneider RC, Paop M, Alverez R. The effects of chronic recurrent spinal trauma in high diving. A study of Acapulco's divers. J Bone Joint Surg 1962;44A:648–656.
6. Rosomoff HL, Rosomoff RS. Comprehensive multi disciplinary pain center approach to the treatment of low back pain. In: Loeser JD, ed. Special issue. Neuro Clin North Am 1991;2(4):877–890.
7. Khalil TM, Asfour SS, Martinez LM, Waly SM, Rosomoff RS, Rosomoff, HI. Stretching in the rehabilitation of low-back pain patients. *Spine* 1992;17(3):311–317.
8. Mangine RE. Preventive exercises for the back in the competitive diver. Paper presented at the U.S. Aquatic Sport Convention, Memphis, September 1982.
9. Kimball, RJ. Are you a blind diver? [Handout].
10. Kimball RJ. Use of spotting rigs with trampoline, port-a-pit diving board and regular pool one meter diving board [Handout].
11. Chandler WF, Schneider RC. Stenosis of the spinal canal and lumbar and thoracic herniated nucleus pulposus. In: Schneider RC, Kahn EA, Crosby EC, Taren JA, eds. Correlative neurosurgery. 3rd ed. Baltimore: Williams & Wilkins, 1982:1050–1093.

17 / CRICKET

Thomas Crisp and John B. King

Introduction

The Game

Cricket is for the most part an outdoor team game, with 11 players on a side and with some similarities to baseball. The International Cricket Conference was unable to provide numbers for worldwide participation, but the Sports Council in 1986 made available some numbers for the UK. In 1983 0.5% of the UK population—about 650,000 adults—played cricket once a month in the course of the summer, although this number does not distinguish between formal and informal games and school games were not included. Thus cricket is the 10th most popular outdoor sport in the UK, although it may be diminishing in popularity, because it was equal to angling in 1965, which is now the number one sport. On a worldwide basis, there appears to be increasing interest especially in North America; even Holland now has a national team.

A cricket team contains some specialist bowlers (usually four), some specialist batsmen (usually five), one or two "all rounders," and a specialist wicket keeper who stands behind the stumps. Each member of the team must bat, but only the specialist bowlers and all-rounders bowl. Because it is not a contact sport there is a relatively low incidence of injury, but certain aspects of the game carry specific morbidity.

While one side bats with two batsmen in play at any one time, all the players of the other side field. A player from the fielding side bowls the ball overarm six times, attempting to hit a set of three 28-inch-high stumps that are topped with two horizontal rods called bails, which are 22 yards away (the pitch). The batsman protects these stumps with a 4-inch-wide bat. At the same time the batsman tries to hit the ball to a part of the field without fielders and then run to the opposite end of the pitch (changing places with the other batsman), scoring a run. At the end of six balls play switches to the other end of the symmetrical pitch and another bowler delivers six balls. The batsman may be out when the ball hits his or her stumps or when, without first hitting the bat, the ball hits the batsman's leg, which is in front of the stumps, but would have hit the stumps if it had not been stopped (leg before wicket). The batsman is also out if the ball is caught by a fielder before it bounces or if the ball arrives at the stumps from a fielder before the batsman makes his or her ground when attempting a run (run out). The batsman may continue to run until the ball has been returned to one or other end, although if the ball is hit outside the field of play it counts four (or, if the ball did not bounce, six) runs.

The ball weighs approximately 5.5 oz and is propelled at speeds of up to 90 mph. It is circumscribed by a line of stitches called the seam, and this area can be made to bite on the ground as the ball pitches, causing deviation in height and or direction. The ball can be a major source of injury if it hits the batsman and at the top level, where bowling speeds are highest, considerable protection is worn on the head and trunk along with the mandatory pads on the lower legs and the "box," which protects the genital area (Fig. 17.1). Because the game is played outdoors and almost invariably on a grass pitch and because the ball is made to bounce before reaching the batsman, variations in bounce and trajectory are inevitable. It is not, however, approved of to project the ball at the batsman's body full pitch, without it bouncing first (the beamer). Sometimes a bowler will bowl the ball (the bouncer) such that it bounces up toward the head and trunk of the batsman who may fend the ball off, perhaps into the hands of a fielder; this certainly may frighten the batsman, even if it does not cause injury. Repeated use of the bouncer amounts, therefore, to intimidation. Although this is outlawed by the rules, the two umpires do not always enforce this, and the side with the fastest bowlers may use this technique to soften up the batsman who is then more intent on his or her own safety than in scoring runs. The batsman may bat for prolonged periods and may have to attempt many rapid 22-yard sprints to gain runs during the course of a long

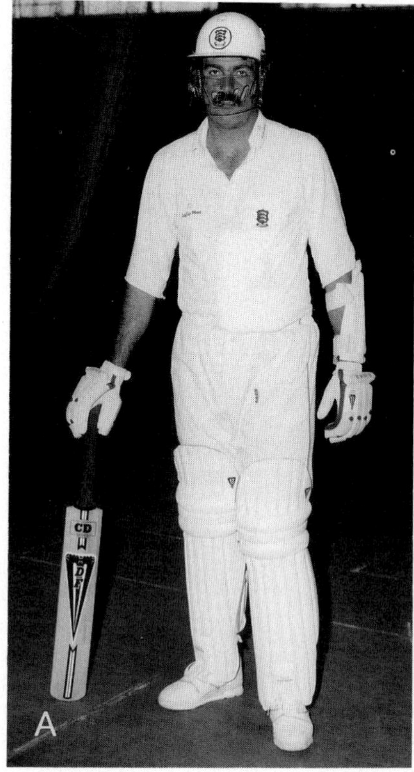

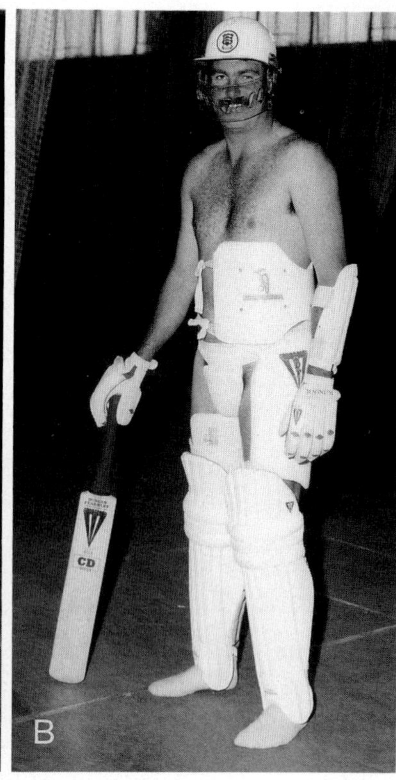

Figure 17.1. A, The dressed batsman. **B,** The batsman's protective gear. Note the helmet with visor, chest protector, forearm guard, gloves, box or genital protector, thigh pads (a larger one is on the leading leg), and the pads protecting the lower legs.

inning. In first-class cricket, it is not unusual in a game that takes place over 3 to 5 days for only one or two batsmen to bat for all three 2-hr sessions held in 1 day.

Bowling

The method of propelling the ball—bowling—hinges on the rule that the elbow must be fully extended at the moment of release of the ball, and thus throwing is not allowed. The standard method of bowling fast involves a run-up of up to 30 yards, as if throwing the javelin, and in the stride before delivery, the bowler arches the back into extension, fully rotating (to the right in a right-handed bowler). In the next step—delivery—the bowler strides rapidly while flexing and rotating the back to the other side (Fig. 17.2). Not surprisingly, this is associated with a high injury rate, especially of the facet joints of the lumbar spine. The straight elbow makes injury in this area rare, but shoulder problems, e.g., rotator cuff strains and impingement, are common. Because a lot of the bowling speed is generated by the trunk, shoulder injuries are much more commonly caused by throwing the ball while fielding. Thus players may participate in the game and bowl freely even though they are unable to throw.

The bowling technique is further complicated by the need to vary the trajectory of the ball. The better bowlers land the ball on its seam, which tends to make the ball deviate as it bounces. Some bowlers also have the ability to make the ball swing in flight as do baseball pitchers. Certain variations in arm and trunk action tend to help the ball to swing either left or right, making hitting the ball more difficult for the batsman but putting more pressure on the bowler's body. There also are slow bowlers who apply spin to the ball, which may then deviate on bouncing. These bowlers may get wear-and-tear injuries to the spinning finger.

Fielding

For the fielder, prolonged periods of relative inactivity may be followed by a sudden sprint to field the ball, which carries a risk of muscle strains. The shoulder may be cold and unstretched before the fielder makes a rapid throw of up to 80 yards. Some fielders are placed very close to the batsman so they can attempt to catch the ball. Unfortunately, these fielders are sometimes hit by the ball, thus they may wear a helmet, shin pads, and a box as do batsmen. This protective gear may provide a false sense of security, causing the fielder to move closer to the batsman than is safe.

A ball that is not stopped by the batsman and does not hit the stumps is collected by the wicket keeper who stands behind the stumps. The wicket keeper wears gloves that are similar to a baseball mitt, they are worn on both hands. The wicket keeper also wears pads on the lower legs to protect them from the ball. This is a specialist position that requires special skills, fitness, and more prolonged concentration than most other fielding positions. The considerable impact of catching a ball may be repeated 200 times or more in a day, which causes much trauma to the wicket keeper's hands. Fractures of the fingers are not uncommon. In addition to taking these balls, the wicket keeper is the most likely person to catch out the batsman when the ball just touches the edge of the bat and is lightly deflected. The agility needed to catch a ball moving an unpredictable direction and changing height at 90 mph is extraordinary.

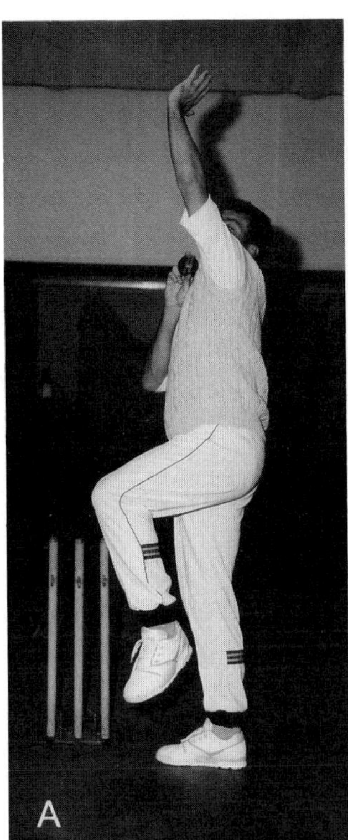

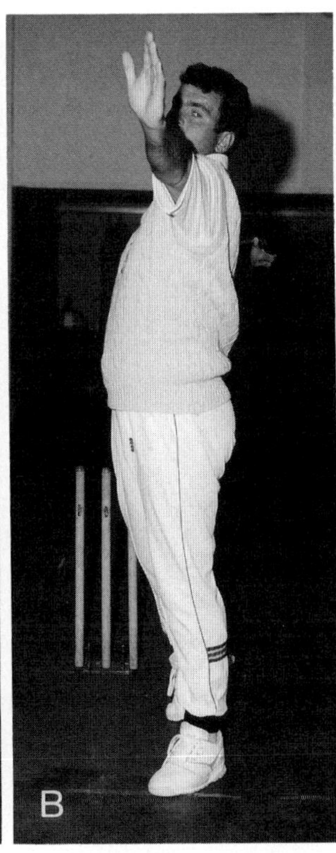

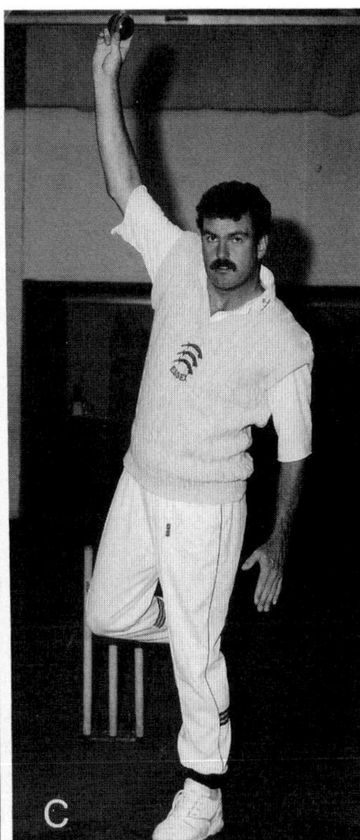

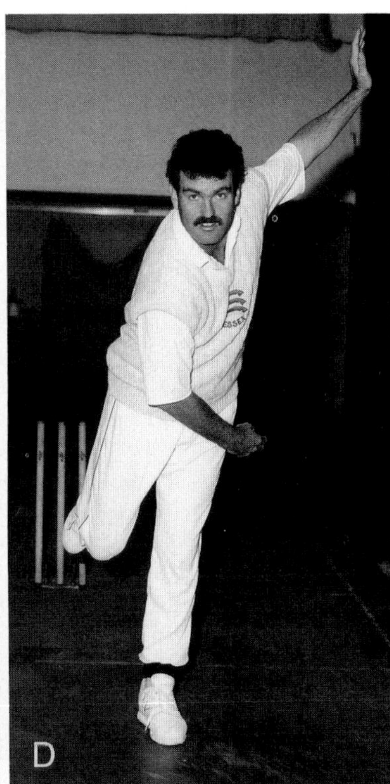

Figure 17.2. The bowling positions from the front during coaching. **A,** The front foot is still to be planted. **B,** The delivery is beginning; note the side on stance in this phase. **C,** The elbow still has to be straightened for the release of the ball, but note the progress to the face on stance. **D,** The ball is released, the trunk has swiveled through nearly 180°, and the back has gone from extension to flexion. The positions more extreme during a real throw.

Knees may be damaged from prolonged squatting, and recently, a wicket keeper lost the sight in one eye after he was struck by a flying bail.

Although it is common practice for cricketers to be less physically fit than many other athletes, they are subject to great strains over a long period. The top-class professionals may play cricket every day for 30 or more days without a break. Thus it may be that the present trend to greater fitness and conditioning in the national teams may reduce injury rates. In recent years, a lot of 1-day cricket has been played. The advantage for the spectators is that they see the final score after 6 to 8 hr of play. However, 1-day play makes swift fielding and the rapid running of single runs more important, which has caused an increase in fielding injuries in particular, for example when fielders throw themselves after the ball to stop it from crossing the boundary of the field of play.

The amateur game is less injury prone than the professional game, but it is played well into middle age and stress on older muscles and tendons can be excessive. The bowling tends to be slower and less dangerous, but the skill and timing of the batsman may be poorer, and sometimes injury occurs.

Foot and Ankle

There may be a great deal of running, and cricketers especially bowlers, can suffer the same foot and ankle injuries as any other runners, including stress fractures of the metatarsals and sesamoids as well as sesamoiditis. Appropriate footwear is important, and it may be necessary to wear different cricket boots for batting and fielding. Furthermore, the condition of the playing surfaces may vary from dry and hard one day to damp and slippery the next. Bowlers may suffer chronic bruising of the big toe and its nail caused by pressure from the shoe; some bowlers even cut a hole in the toe of their shoes to reduce the pressure, although it would seem more logical to wear shoes that fit properly in the first place. In addition there may be chronic bruising of the heel from the repeated trauma of heel plant in the leading foot during the delivery stride.

It is common for a bowler to bowl twenty 6-ball overs in a day, which results in 120 impacts. On occasion, this can cause a chronic bursa within the heel pad, which responds slowly to rest and physical therapy and occasionally requires corticosteroid injection and even surgical excision. Early treatment is easier and involves a good heel pad, but sometimes the problem is only relieved by a molded heel cup made to fit the bowling shoe. The help of the coach may be needed because anything that changes the feel of the impact may interfere with the balance in the delivery stride, causing loss of the essential line and length of the ball.

The toes are at risk while batting from a ball that is delivered fast and to the area of the feet (a yorker). These are difficult balls to play, and they often hit the toes. Despite the protective gear elsewhere on the body, it is common to wear light batting shoes to aid quick running. This results in a high rate of major bruising and fractures; these light shoes often have no protective caps.

The grip of the soles is important and small studs or spikes, similar to those on golf shoes, are usual for fielding, although for batting it is common to wear shoes with a molded ribbed sole to give greater mobility.

Ankle strains may occur in fielding, and lateral ligament strains are the most common. It is unusual to tape cricketers' ankles, and in view of the prolonged play, this may be ineffective anyway. Bowlers with slight weakness of the ankle ligaments may have to wear a support on the ankle, such as an inflatable ankle stirrup. Bowlers are particularly vulnerable because of the rotational and lateral strain to the ankle in the delivery stride. However, most ankle strains respond to physical therapy that has an emphasis on proprioception through wobble board exercises and increasing strength in the peroneal muscles. As in other sports, taping should not be used as a means of getting the player back to competition before he or she has fully recovered.

Fielders rarely do enough running to get Achilles tendon troubles but fast bowlers do get tendonitis as well as bursitis around the Achilles. Usually there is no obvious initiating injury. Instead, there is a gradual onset of pain in the heel, which at first is ignored and often disappears after warming up. However, the pain increases in severity and eventually restricts activity. It is not uncommon for stiffness in the morning to be a prominent symptom in severe cases. It is important to distinguish peritendonitis from tendonitis, when the tendon itself is inflamed, which may be the result of a partial tear. The former usually responds to physical therapy, such as ultrasound and laser, and injections of corticosteroid next to—not into—the tendon. Tendonitis responds more slowly, if at all, and steroid injection carries a risk of rupture of the tendon. In resistant cases, the tendon should be examined via diagnostic ultrasound or computerized tomography (CT) scans. It is important to remember that gout is a possible cause of resistant tendonitis in the age group of recreational cricketers.

Partial rupture and cystic degeneration will, for the most part, require surgery in the form of excision of the paratenon, longitudinal incision into the degenerate area, and removal of obvious cysts. Small tears do not require repair, but large ones do. The ankle need not be immobolized but dorsiflexion should be restricted with a dorsal splint if a repair has been performed. In rehabilitation, it is essential to limit the proportion of the work cycle that is eccentric.

Bursitis is easily detected on examination, and the deep bursa responds well to steroid injection into the area deep to the tendon immediately above the calcaneum. The superficial bursa can cause great problems from contact with the back of the shoe and needs careful treatment (which may benefit from changing the footwear). It may respond to steroid injection, but there is a danger of skin atrophy if the injection is made too superficially; therefore, this should be reserved for failure of physical therapy when a small volume of hydrocortisone acetate is used rather than anything more potent.

In the older age group of cricketers Achilles rupture is not uncommon when running in the field, running between the wickets, or in batting. This happens because the back foot must remain on the ground (Fig. 17.3). Although calf muscle strain can occur in all these maneuvers, complete rupture of the tendon should always be suspected even in the absence of an obvious gap in the tendon. A calf squeeze test that looks for a small amount of plantar flexion on squeezing the bulk of the muscle should be performed.

Lower Leg

Biomechanical abnormalities of the foot such as excessive pronation can lead to lower leg problems in bowlers and runners. Compartment syndromes, periostitis, and tibial stress fractures are well-documented. Stress fracture should always be suspected when the player presents with increasing pain on exercise and tenderness at the junction of the upper and middle thirds of the tibia. Because usual changes on x-ray are late, a bone scan should be performed to confirm the diagnosis. These fractures are more common in the leg impacting on the ground in the delivery stride. Rest is essential, but if there is an underlying biomechanical foot problem it can be corrected as in other sports by orthotics. Compartment syndromes and periostitis—often referred to by the players as shin splints—also usually respond to orthotics. Technique, in particular

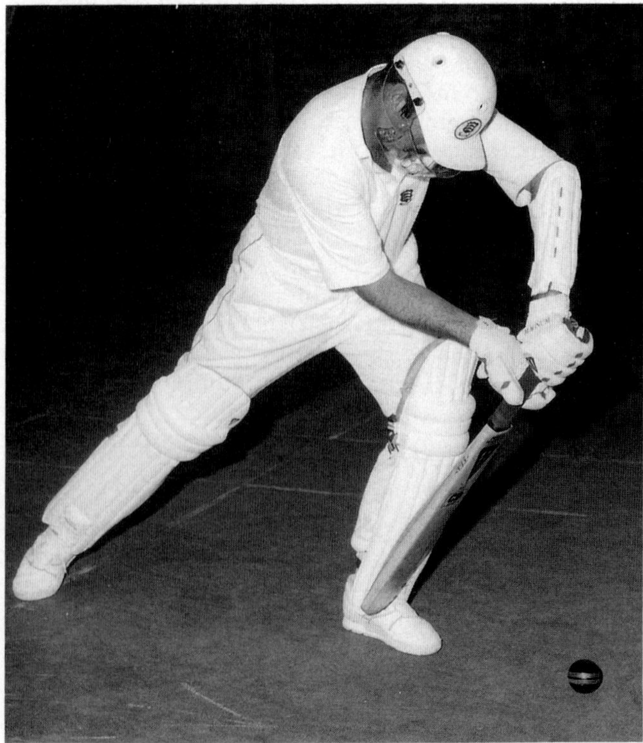

Figure 17.3. The forward defensive stroke with the weight, head, and bat forward but the back foot locked behind the crease, so if the ball is missed, the player cannot be stumped.

the position of the front foot on impact, has a large effect on the stress imposed. The coach must be involved in resistant cases. Keeping the toes of the leading leg pointing forward and not outward helps to keep the body side on to the target, which is associated with a lower injury rate to the back than when the body is more open (front on). However, this means that there is likely to be rotation of the foot after impact as the body follows through. The bowler must immediately swing off the playing areas (the line between the two sets of stumps), causing torsional stress to the lower leg.

Knee

In young bowlers, there is a risk of both Osgood-Schlatter disease and anterior knee pain, arising from the patellofemoral joint. Reducing the level of activity is often enough to cure the pain. The wicket keeper squats for long periods behind the stumps and is at risk to both anterior knee pain and patellar tendon problems. Care is necessary to distinguish these entities. Patellofemoral pain will often respond to rehabilitation of the vastus medialis obliquus muscle by terminal knee extension exercises, except in cases for which symptoms have started in a congenitally bipartite patella. In these cases, surgery is essential if the player is to continue as a wicket keeper. Patellar tendonitis is commonly gradual in its onset, although careful questioning may be necessary to elicit the prodromal history predating an apparently acute episode. If the well-localized pain in the tendon does not settle with 6 weeks of reduction in activity and nonsteroidal antiinflammatory drugs (NSAIDs), the tendon must be investigated with ultrasound, CT, or magnetic resonance imaging (MRI) scanning. Small lesions within the tendon substance close to the bone attachment usually respond to steroid injection. After such an injection, it is important to avoid stressing the tendon for 1 week afterward to avoid any risk of further damage to the tendon. Large lesions, especially those near the middle of the tendon, will only respond to surgery. The paratenon must be excised; if not, there will be a secondary paratendonitis. The tendon is palpated and the pea-like lesions can be easily felt. The fibers are split at that point, and the macroscopically diseased tissue is removed. Because the removed tissue was not functional, rehabilitation can start with skin healing. Full flexion should be regained by 6 weeks, and further return to sport depends on the speed of recovery of muscle strength. Initial return should be to a fielding position some distance from the bat, as the close fielders adopt the alert, bent-knee stance during the bowler's run up.

Twisting injuries causing meniscal and ligament damage occur around the knee from fielding, when a player turns to chase the ball and when a batsman turns at the end of a run to return for a second run. These are not common. On level ground and with no contact, it is rare to damage the cruciate ligaments, but occasionally when diving to stop the ball from crossing the boundary, severe damage is done to the knee. The increasing level of fitness and muscle power of the players may protect the joints from this kind of damage. More common is wear and tear to the articular cartilage of the knee in bowlers, especially in the front leg at delivery when the knee is braced and the leg acts as a pivot for the trunk. This can produce disabling pain, which may be difficult to distinguish from the attritional-type tear of the slightly degenerate meniscus. Technetium bone scan will show a well-localized increase in activity, and for most players, this is the end of the bowling career because the recovery from high tibial osteotomy is so variable that surgery is usually declined, even if it is offered.

Hip and Thigh

The muscles of the upper leg can be strained from fielding or batting, although this can be avoided to a great extent by well-conditioned muscles, a good warmup, and stretching. Unfortunately, the batsman may wait for a long time (perhaps hours) before he or she is called to the center to participate, and he or she then must be able to sprint 22 yards immediately. Clearly, this makes a full warmup impossible, especially when the necessary psychological preparation is included. Not only do batsmen have to run but they may have to stretch their hamstrings suddenly as they put one foot right out in front of themselves to get to the pitch of the ball, while the back foot is locked behind the crease. Even the fielder may find it difficult to remain warm and flexible during long periods of play when the ball does not come near him or her.

Much more common than these intrinsic injuries are hematomas caused by contact with the ball. The shins of the batsman are protected by pads, but even with a thigh pad on the side of the thigh most likely to be hit by the ball, there are large unprotected areas. The most skilful bowlers bowl the ball such that it lands on the seam and can deviate unpredictably, making it difficult for the batsman to make contact with the bat. Furthermore, as with the baseball pitch, the ball may swing in flight and find the body or leg rather than the bat. With immediate ice compression and elevation, such injuries resolve quickly, but if, as is commonly the case, the batsman continues to bat for long afterward, all that can be done at the time is application of analgesic spray, and definitive treatment is delayed.

Adductor strains, traumatic osteitis pubis, stress fractures of the pubis rami, and groin strain with damage to the conjoint tendon occur rather rarely in cricketers. A first-class bowler has recently been invalided with avascular necrosis of the femoral head.

Back

Because cricket at an amateur level is played into or past middle age, there are many overweight cricket players who undergo little or no conditioning. These players are likely to suffer back strains. In these relatively minor injuries, physical therapy such as massage, pulsed microwave and other forms of heating, along with manipulation are usually effective and the batsman may be able to play with a corset or lumbar support, which will reduce mobility only slightly. Emphasis also should be placed on back and abdominal muscle strengthening in rehabilitation, and the role of weight loss in the obese should not be forgotten.

Back problems are common particularly in bowlers (2). As described above, the technique of bowling is stressful. It has evolved as the best way of projecting the ball at speed and with the control necessary to test the batsman. Unfortunately, even with a perfect action, there is the risk of damage to the lumbar spine, in particular from this combination of slight hyperextension then flexion and rotation at speed. The most common injury is to the short ligaments around the facet joints. This presents as stiffness, which may start suddenly and reduce movements in all directions Once the acute episode is past, the bowler may be left with the common symptoms of stiffness, following immobility, easing with gentle exercise, and exacerbated by violent exercise. There is little or no referral of the pain down the leg beyond the buttocks. Examination reveals reduced extension and side flexion and, in particular, reduction in range and pain on performing extension and side flexion together. There is tenderness around the area of the facet joint about 2 inches lateral to the middle on deep palpation.

The acute episode should be treated with physiotherapy aimed at reducing the muscle spasm and increasing movement. Gentle manipulation may be of use at this stage. In the chronic situation, manipulation and other physical therapy should be supported by back and abdominal muscle strengthening exercises designed to give a full range of movement and full muscle power.

Attention to technique is important because recent studies have indicated an increase in incidence of back problems in bowlers who bowl square on, i.e., with the thorax facing the batsman rather than side on, i.e., with the leading shoulder pointing toward the target. Different bowlers use their back more or less than others, who may get more speed from shoulder rotation and thus experience fewer back problems. Input from the coach in the rehabilitation phase may be useful, and prevention requires good education at an early stage.

More severe problems may be caused by spondylolysis in which there is a stress fracture of the pars interarticularis. This injury is relatively common in fast bowlers. Foster et al. (2) showed that 11% of 82 high-performance young male fast bowlers developed a defect in the year of study. The symptoms are similar to those of a facet joint strain, but this problem should always be considered. The diagnosis is traditionally made by oblique views of the lumbar spine, which show the obvious break across the neck of the "Scotty dog." In these athletes, such views may be inadequate and CT scanning with reversed gantry angle must be performed. If a bone scan shows considerable bone activity, the patient should be immobilized and supported. If there is any significant forward slip of the vertebral body or spondylolisthesis and if the symptoms persist surgery may be indicated. Bone scanning is not useful in assessing healing, and repeated CT scans must be performed. Old injuries with no hot spot on a bone scan can be treated like a facet joint strain and are the result of either a congenital defect in the pars or an earlier ununited stress fracture. Rehabilitation is the same as for facet joint strain and includes back and abdominal muscle strengthening exercises.

Shoulder

The most commonly injured joint in cricket is the shoulder, and most injuries occur during throwing. Unfortunately, in coaching little or no emphasis is placed on injury prevention in this area by encouraging strong rotator cuff muscles. In the rehabilitation phase following injury even more attention must be given to strengthening and fine-tuning the rotator cuff muscles, because premature strengthening of the prime movers, e.g., deltoid, trapezius, and pectoralis, may exacerbate the problem. Impingement problems are common.

In cricket a fielder may have to throw the ball up to 80 yards accurately and fast to prevent runs being taken by the batsman. If he or she is not warmed up or if the throw is disordered, there is a risk of injuring one of the rotator cuff muscles, usually the supraspinatus (4). The ball drops short and the fielder experiences severe pain in the shoulder, which will recur when he or she throws again. The shoulder must be rested with the addition of NSAIDs. If this is done promptly, no more than 3 weeks should be lost from the sport. The player may be able to bowl, because this action involves much lower rotational velocities and, consequently, less strain on the rotators. However, the team must accept that he or she is "hidden" in the field and so is not called on to throw.

In a severe injury in the acute phase, there may be restriction of all movements on examination but after 1 or 2 days the pain is principally on abduction, causing a painful arc. If the damage to supraspinatus is severe, initiation of abduction may be lost. Incomplete tears can be differentiated from complete rupture of the tendon by injection of local anesthetic into the subacromial space; the pain of a partial tear or severe tendonitis will be obliterated and the supraspinatus will function normally, whereas no change will be noted if there is a complete tear. There is usually enough damage in these shoulders for abduction to be lost with a complete supraspinatus tear. Strain of the other rotators can be differentiated by detecting pain on resisted external rotation (infraspinatus) and internal rotation (subscapularis); supraspinatus will cause pain on resisting abduction from the neutral position.

The treatment for complete tears is surgical repair. For incomplete tears and tendonitis treatment involves stopping the aggravating exercise (throwing) and physical therapy. As already noted, the rotator cuff must be strengthened before the major muscle groups, and the player should be discouraged from returning to full activity until the recovery is complete.

Chronic cases may be complicated by subacromial space impingement. This condition may respond to rest, strengthening of the rotators, or injection of corticosteroid into the subacromial space. If there is no response to these measures, examination including arthroscopy, if needed, should be performed to rule out instability (which may be multidirectional) in the shoulder joint, which can occasionally present as a chronic thrower's shoulder. Decompression of the subacromial space and excision of the coracoacromial ligament will buy time, but full throwing strength rarely returns.

Elbow and Arm

Injuries to the elbow are not common in cricket, although occasional throwing injuries are seen. There may be traction tears to the flexor mechanism (golfer's elbow) from the acceleration phase of the throw or compression to the lateral aspect of the elbow. More common is a direct blow to the forearm from the cricket balls, which may cause fracture of the radius or ulna. These fractures usually occur in the leading arm, and players often wear a forearm guard on the lower part of this arm to at least soften the blow. The injuries arise when the bounce of the ball is irregular and the ball rises higher than expected, hitting the arm above the bat.

Wrist and Hand

The wrist may be damaged when a player falls on the ground while diving to field the ball. The pressures on the wicket keepers' hands, which suffer repeated microtrauma, acute contusions, and occasionally fractures (particularly when the hard ball is not taken cleanly in the middle of the hand) were already discussed. In the past, wicket keepers apparently were known to put a slice of steak inside their gloves to soften the impact of the ball. These days, gloves are made to withstand the blows, but the 200 to 300 catches made in a day may lead to chronic soft tissue thickening. The gloves need to be flexible for the ball to be taken cleanly and, therefore, must transmit some of the force of the impact. The gloves have webs between the fingers to aid catching as well as to reduce the force separating two fingers if the ball is caught there.

Fielders often stand next to the wicket keeper or in close catching positions to catch any ball that deviates off the edge of the bat. These balls are traveling fast and can cause significant damage. If taken on the end of the finger, the most common injury is a mallet deformity, with or without a segment of bone. Many players choose to do nothing more than tape the finger(s), because the more conventional immobilization of the terminal joint interferes with batting. Intraarticular fractures of the interphalangeal joints and even the base of the proximal phalanges are usually treated by "buddy" taping and early mobilization. Blows to the side of the digits cause ruptures of the colateral ligaments or dislocations. These are again treated by taping and movement.

Balls that wedge between two fingers may cause severe web space lacerations, requiring suture and significant time out of the game. It is important that full mobility is regained as soon as possible after such injuries, because all players may be called on to bat and full-finger function is necessary for proper batting. Bellipia and Barton (5) claim that the fractures of the base of the proximal phalanx are the most likely to be stiff. The authors' experience is more in concordance with that of Sadlier and Horne (6) who report some degree of stiffness and/or deformity in most of these intraarticular fractures. The best prophylaxis for this is practice, to ensure a good hand-eye coordination, and using in these positions only fielders whose reflexes are sufficiently quick.

Batsmen's fingers are at risk from the "lifting" delivery that bounces higher than expected and catches the handle of the bat. Sometimes these balls will trap a finger against the bat. Although batting gloves give good protection most of the time, fractures do occur at the top level of play. Several manufacturers are addressing this problem, but it is difficult to protect the fingers fully without interfering with the grip on the bat. Because of the need to grip the bat, and despite the risk of accelerating possible degenerative changes, it is sometimes necessary to inject the joints that remain stiff after bone healing with a small volume of corticosteroid to reduce inflammation and increase mobility. Exercises to increase range of movement and strengthen intrinsic muscles help in the rehabilitation process. A number of cricket grounds regularly provide a hot wax bath to ease the pain and swelling of such chronically injured fingers.

Face and Head

The bouncer, mentioned above, may not cause the batsman to be bowled out, but it is difficult to score from and may cause bodily harm. At the lower levels of cricket, few bowlers bowl fast enough to make the ball bounce sufficiently high to cause damage; thus this is a problem largely restricted to the professional game. The hook shot necessary to hit the ball aimed at the face involves playing across the trajectory of the ball (Fig. 17.4), and there is thus a higher than usual chance of missing. If the batsman's technique is not good enough he or she is likely to miss the ball completely or to cause the ball to deviate slightly; both result in a hit to the face or body. To avoid such risks, most batsmen wear a helmet and many have a visor of some kind to protect the face, temples, and skull. Despite these measures, head injuries still happen and range from fractures of the nose, facial bones, and teeth to lacerations on the face and ears. Hill et al. (7) suggest that injuries to the face and teeth occur most frequently in rugby, followed by soccer and then cricket in the UK. Recent changes in the rules restrict the number of bouncers that can be bowled at each batsman and have made the game a little safer.

The eye is remarkably vulnerable when the size of the ball is compared with that of a squash ball. Aburn (8) reports that 30% of all sports injuries to the eye were from cricket; this was, however, indoor cricket where the level of protection may be different from that of the outdoor sport. Jones and Tullo (9) describe five serious injuries, including retinal detachment and rupture of the globe, mainly brought about by the rising ball already mentioned. The data do not allow one to estimate the overall incidence of such injuries, but it seems

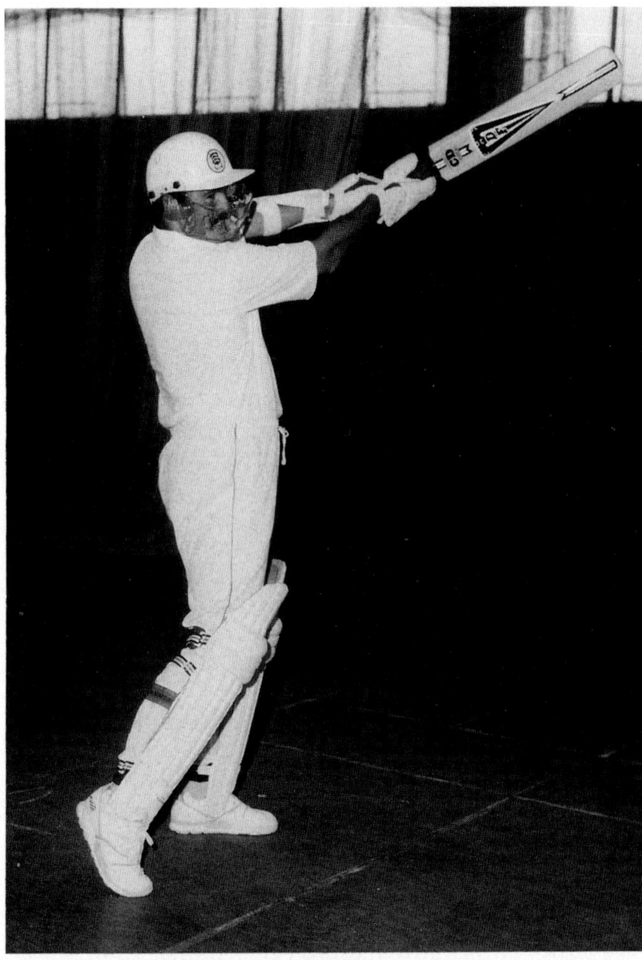

Figure 17.4. The hook shot to a fast ball at face level. If the ball is missed, the consequences are obvious.

as if they have become less frequent with the improved head protection.

Also at risk from head injuries are the close in fielders, but in professional cricket the short leg fielder, who stands within about 8 feet of the batsman, usually wears a helmet similar to the batter's.

Chest and Trunk

The chest and trunk are at risk from impact from the ball, and the area is often protected by padding at the top level of play. A few serious incidents have been reported of a blow on the chest stopping the heart. Fortunately, such occurrences are rare, but they mean that good medical care should be available immediately on site. More common is severe bruising of the ribs with restriction of the full breathing excursion, and it may be necessary to inject the area with long-acting local anesthetic to allow the player to continue the next session.

Conclusion

The game of cricket is not associated with a high level of injury, but certain aspects carry risk. Cricketers are not always in peak condition, and a greater emphasis on physical fitness would reduce some injuries. In other areas, protective equipment is essential and is still being developed to protect batsmen in particular. Correct technique is important and can reduce injury rates; thus coaching can produce cricketers who are not at unnecessary risk. Finally, application of the laws especially about intimidation is essential to minimize risks.

REFERENCES

1. Goodbody J. *The (London) Times.*
2. Hardcastle P. Lumbar pain in fast bowlers. Aust Fam Physician 1991;20(7):946–951.
3. Foster D, John D, Elliott B, Ackland T, Fitch K. Back injuries to fast bowlers in cricket: a prospective study. Br J Sports Med 1989;23(3):150–154.
4. Crisp T. Cricket: fast bowlers back and throwers shoulder. Practitioner 1989;148(11):560–561.
5. Belliappa PP, Barton NJ. Hand injuries in cricketers. J Hand Surg [Br] 1991;16(2):212–214.
6. Sadlier LG, Horne G. Indoor cricket finger injuries. N Z Med J 1990;103(882):3–5.
7. Hill CM, Crosher RF, Mason DA. Dental and facial injuries following sports accidents: a study of 130 patients. Br. J Oral Maxillofac Surg 1985;23(4):268–274.
8. Aburn N. Eye injuries in indoor cricket at Wellington Hospital: a survey Jan 87 through June 89. N Z Med J 1990;103(898):454–456.
9. Jones NP, Tullo AB. Severe eye injuries in cricket. Br J Sports Med 1986;20(4):178–179.

18 / DANCE AND THE ARTS

Ruth Kamenski and Freddie H. Fu

Introduction

In recent years, dance medicine has come into the medical limelight. Attention has been directed toward dance in response to an increased injury rate among both professionals and students. The dancer, like the athlete, has high levels of physical demands related to movement and impact (1). In addition, types of injuries sustained and measures employed to treat such injuries are similar to those associated with other athletic activities. Nonetheless, important differences exist between athletes and dancers. The most obvious is that in dance, aesthetic content and its transmission transcends the athletic aspect of the activity (1). Flexibility, strength, endurance, control, balance, and coordination are essential requirements for expertise in dance. Performance must appear effortless. Because of such demands, to appear graceful and beautiful while performing, the classical dancer will force his or her extremities into awkward anatomical positions, which are potentially injurious (2). Professional dancers must, therefore, be cognizant of the fine line between maximizing versus exceeding their physical limitations. On the one hand, dancers must push to their physical limits to maximize the range and variety of movement available for expression. Yet, on the other hand, dancers must constantly strive to protect themselves against the consequences of stressing their bodies beyond the designed physical limits, thus risking injuries that can interrupt or threaten a career (3).

In an attempt to optimize care, it is imperative that the health care provider familiarize himself or herself with factors that may predispose this population to injury. Recognition and prevention are the keys to a successful rehabilitation and career longevity.

Dance Positions

Five basic foot positions exist in classical ballet. All movements begin, pass through, or end in one of the five positions. One essential requirement for achieving these positions is external rotation (ER), or turnout, of the hips. The five foot positions are as follows (Fig. 18.1) (4):

First Position: Heels are touching, legs are ER so that the feet form a straight line from the toes of the right foot to the toes of the left foot, and both knees are straight.

Second Position: Heels are approximately 12 inches apart with the weight evenly distributed over both feet, legs and feet are ER as in first position, and both knees are straight.

Third Position: Both legs are ER from the hips and the heel of the right foot is placed in front of the arch of the left foot, the feet are touching, weight is evenly distributed over both feet, and both knees are straight.

Fourth Position: Both legs are ER from the hips, the feet are approximately 12 inches apart with the right foot opposite the left and directly in front of it (i.e., the heel of the right foot is in front of the toes of the left), both knees are straight, and weight is evenly distributed over both feet.

Fifth Position: Both legs are ER from the hip, the heel of the right foot is in front of the great toe of the left foot, the feet are touch-

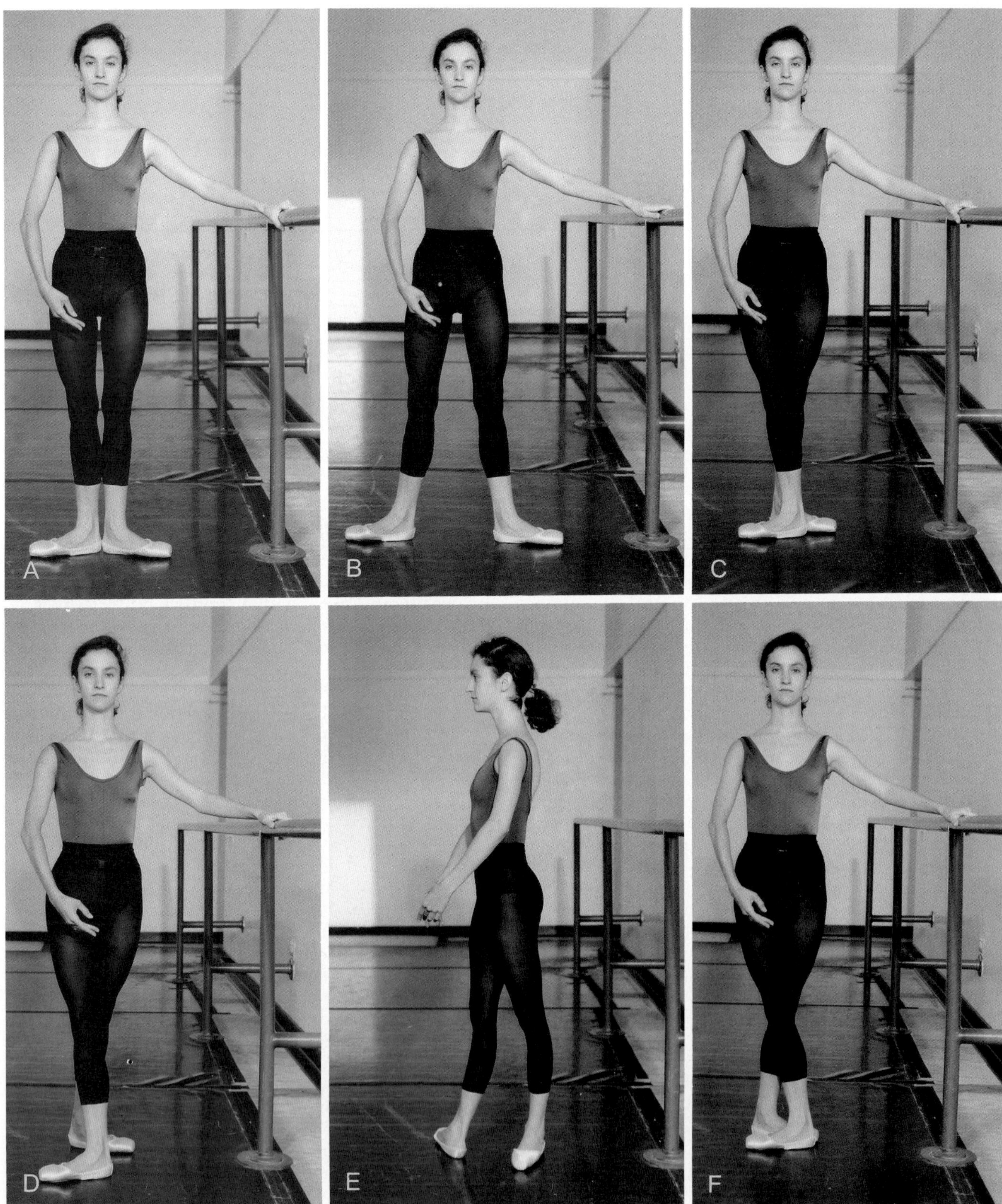

Figure 18.1. **A,** First position. **B,** Second position. **C,** Third position. **D,** Fourth position, anterior view. **E,** Fourth position, lateral view. **F,** Fifth position.

ing at all points, both knees are straight, weight is evenly distributed over both feet.

Dance Movements

Plié involves a simple bending movement of the knees while bearing weight and maintaining ER of the lower extremities. *Pliés* are done in all five positions. There are two types of *pliés, demi pliés* and *grande pliés. Demi pliés* involve a slow partial lowering of the body via a knee bend, keeping the heels on the floor (Fig. 18.2). *Grande pliés,* or full *pliés* are performed in a similar manner, except the bend is deeper and the body is lowered to the floor. The heels are kept on the floor as long as possible while the body is being lowered (Fig. 18.3) (5, 6).

Pointe is another common term. Like *plié, pointe* can be either *demi* or full. *Demi pointe* is when a dancer is dancing on the balls of his or her feet (Fig. 18.4). Full *pointe,* often simply referred to as *pointe,* is reserved for female dancers only and requires the use of a specially designed shoe with a toe box (Fig. 18.5). *Pointe* involves dancing on the extreme tips of the phalanges (5, 6). The maneuver from which the dancer moves from a flat foot position to a *demi pointe* or a *pointe* position is referred to as *relevé* (5, 6).

Arabesque is a maneuver in which the dancer stands balanced on one leg (the supporting leg) while the other leg (the working leg) is extended behind the body, parallel to the floor (Fig. 18.6). The torso is arched forward and the arms extended (6). *Pirouettes* are complete turns of the body while the dancer, balances on one foot (6). *Pirouettes* can be singular or multiple and may rotate either clockwise or counterclockwise relative to the supporting leg (5, 6). A *battement* is a beating movement of the working leg, usually against the support-

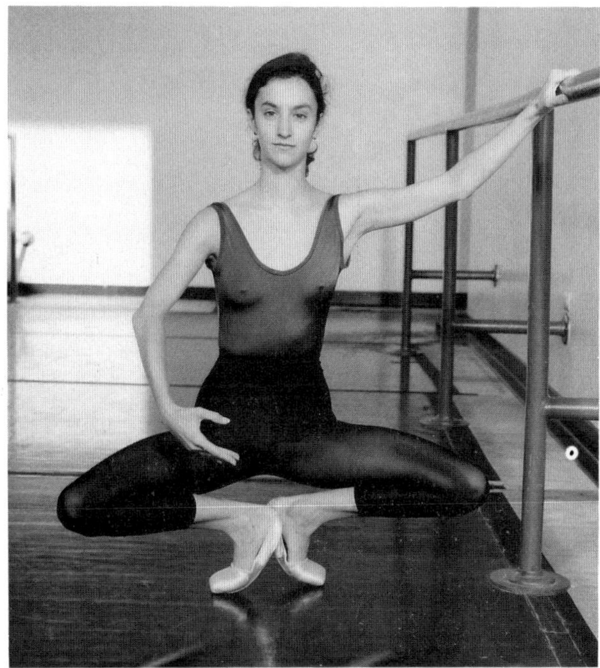

Figure 18.3. *Grand plié* in fifth position.

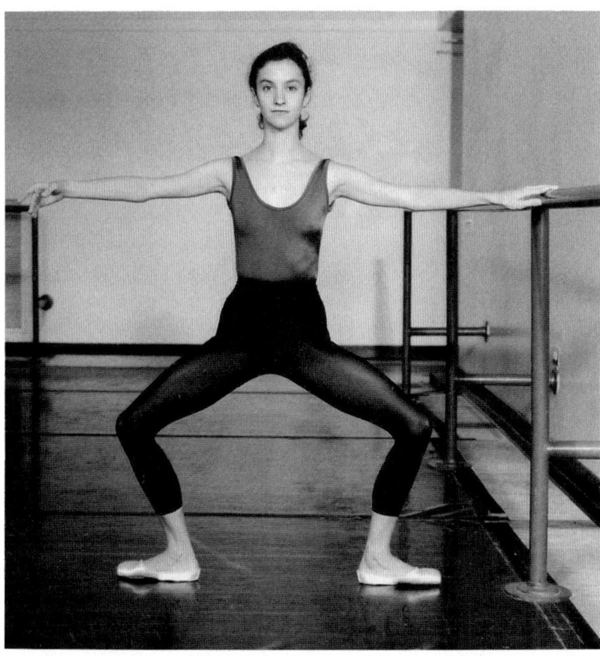

Figure 18.2. *Demi plié* in second position.

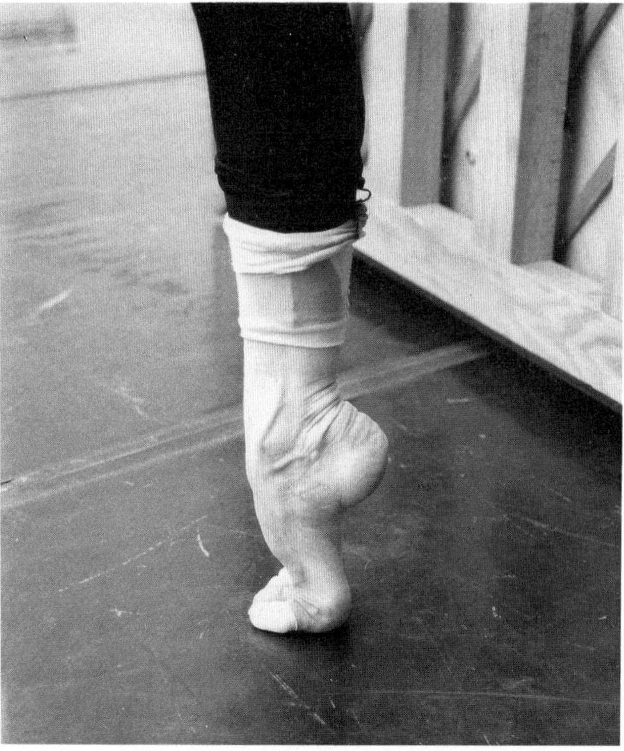

Figure 18.4. *Demi pointe* requires approximately 90° to 100° of dorsiflexion at first metatarsal-phalangeal joint.

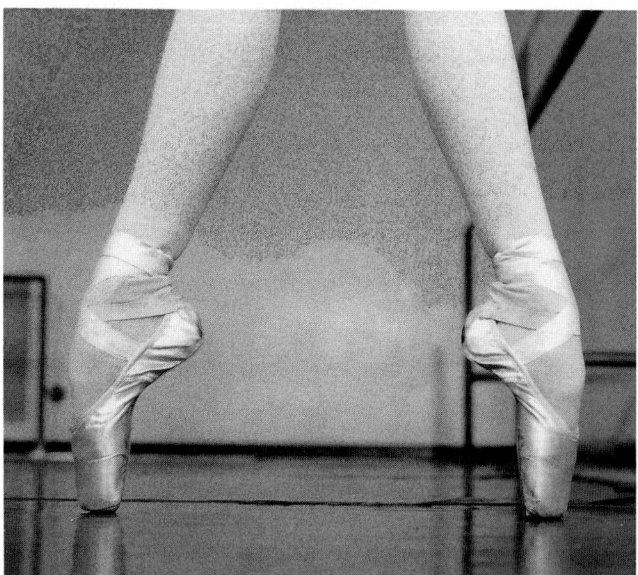

Figure 18.5. Full *pointe.*

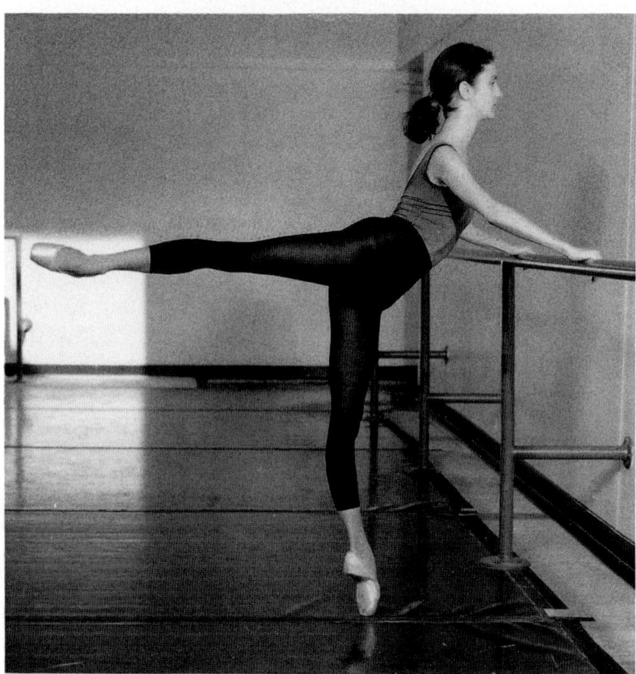

Figure 18.6. *Arabesque* at the *barre.*

ing leg. *Petite battements* are small beating movements of the foot against the ankle of the supporting leg. *Grand battements* involve lifting the entire leg into the air from the hip (6). A jump from one foot to the other when the weight of the body is transferred from the starting foot to the landing foot is known as a *jeté* (Fig. 18.7) (5).

A ballet *barre* is a railing fastened to a studio wall at a height of approximately 3.5 feet to provide hand support for the preliminary exercises of the class. The sequence of exercises that begins every ballet class are referred to as *barre* exercises (5).

Aesthetically, each dancer strives to achieve an acceptable line. Line is the aesthetic conformation or projected image created by the shape and portion of the dancer's body as well as the positioning of the head, shoulders, arms, torso, and legs (6).

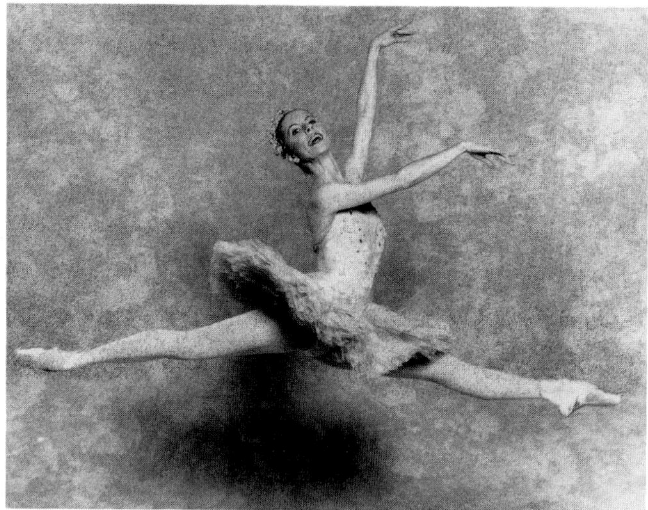

Figure 18.7. *Grand jeté.* Photograph by Susan Cook; courtesy of The Pittsburgh Ballet Theatre.

Several aspects factor into the etiology of ballet injuries. Oftentimes more than one of these factors are responsible for injuries sustained by the dancer. Commonly, these injuries are not acute but are chronic in nature, developing subtly over a period of time. Occupational, training, technique, anatomic, biomechanical, environmental, nutritional, and psychologic factors are among those that contribute to many dance-related injuries.

Occupational Factors

The dance profession is a highly competitive yet private one. Dancers are constantly driven by self-imposed demands and/or those of teachers, staff, colleagues, and the audience (including the critics) to exceed previous standards. In light of this drive, dancers often push to or beyond the point of injury. Dealing with injury is no small task either. Many factors may complicate a dancer's response to injury. Medical services are not often readily available, worker compensation may pose restrictions on the amount of time and/or money available for rehabilitation, and performances and/or castings for upcoming performances may be just around the corner. It is often difficult to slow down goal-oriented, motivated people to prevent further insult or injury. All of these factors may cause the dancer to return prematurely to dance without adequate rehabilitation, which inevitably contributes to the development of chronic injuries (7).

Training Errors

Poor Preseason Conditioning

Dancers are faced with the dilemma of allowing adequate time for healing and rest following the completion of a season and return to dance for conditioning before the onset of a new season. Should the dancer not condition during the off-season, he or she may begin the season in less than optimal physical condition to engage full-time in dance. In such instances, the dancer may predispose himself or herself to overuse injuries as a result of long and demanding rehearsal schedules. If ignored, these injuries may plague the dancer throughout the season.

Inadequate Warmup

In a recent dance survey conducted by Bowling (8), 14% of those surveyed attributed their injuries to insufficient warmup. Dancers should not use class before rehearsals as their primary form of warmup. Adequate flexibility and light exercise before class is encouraged. Nonetheless, dancers can adequately warmup before class and get their bodies warm during class, yet find that the difficulty lies in keeping warm. Some dancers may not rehearse immediately following class as a result of casting and scheduling of rehearsals. On the other hand, some dancers may, in fact, rehearse immediately following class but are active only periodically and then only for short spurts. This problem also arises during performances. Dancers are encouraged to remain active, stretch frequently, and to clothe properly in an attempt to keep warm.

Intensity and Duration of Training

A normal day of dance for most professionals consists of approximately a 1.5-hr class before rehearsal. Rehearsals may run from 4 to 6 hr per day in preparation for upcoming performances. If a dancer is not well-conditioned, this strenuous schedule may result in overuse injuries early in the season. Recovery time during the season may be hindered by contract obligations, dancing roles, or the fear of losing a dancing role. Ideally, dancers should condition during the off-season, and at the onset of a new season, rehearsal schedules should build gradually to a full day. Unfortunately, the ideal is usually not the norm.

Technique Errors

Development of Muscle Imbalances

Good ballet training should develop muscles of the lower extremities symmetrically. However, in some instances, excessive training and/or faulty technique may result in muscle imbalances, especially about the trunk and extremities. Downey et al. (9) conducted a preseason screen of company members of the Pittsburgh Ballet Theatre (18 female, 13 male) to identify trends in flexibility, strength, and posture. Results indicated that dancers had a tendency to lack flexibility in the gastrocsoleus and rectus femoris muscle as well as the tensor fascia latae–iliotibial band. Likewise, strength deficits were noted in the lower abdominal (primarily females) and the middle and lower trapezius muscles (both groups).

Lack of Training Specificity

Often ballet companies in addition to performing the classic full-length ballets such as *Swan Lake* and *The Nutcracker* will incorporate modern pieces into their repertoire. Dancers who do not routinely train in modern technique may find they suffer from uncommon aches and injuries associated with the new movement patterns they must now perform. Injuries sustained during these rehearsals are often short lived, and the symptoms subside with the cessation of rehearsals or once the body has adapted to the new movement patterns.

Compensatory Techniques

Although most professional dance instructors have a good understanding of technique, oftentimes they are unaware of an individual dancer's physical limitations. Therefore, the dancer will try to compensate to appear to execute maneuvers with good technique. Compensation often precipitates faulty technique, which in turn precipitates injury.

Ideal turnout involves 90° of ER at each hip (7). Although this is ideal, it is rarely if ever the norm. Nonetheless, many dancers can achieve adequate turnout for the basic ballet positions. Turnout involves 55° to 70° of ER at the hip, approximately 10° of ER at the knee, tibial torsion up to 12°, and abduction of the forefoot at the midtarsal joint (7).

The tendency to compensate for those who lack adequate turnout can manifest in a variety of ways. Increasing the lumbar lordosis will in effect decrease the tension on the iliofemoral ligament, allowing for increased ER at the hip (Fig. 18.8). This, unfortunately, increases stresses in the lumbar spine, predisposing the dancer to stress fractures and/or possible spondylolisthesis (7, 10–13).

Another method of compensation is known as "screwing the knees," which is accomplished by assuming a *demi plié* position, placing the feet at a 180° angle at the floor and from there straightening the knees (2, 10). Such a maneuver creates a great deal of torque on the knees, producing strain on medial structures that may result in ligamentous injuries, patellofemoral pain, or possible lateral patellar subluxation (2, 10).

Rolling in, or pronation of the foot, is another compensatory technique. Rolling in involves eversion of the hindfoot with forced pronation of the midfoot and forefoot (14). The consequence of rolling in is excessive strain on the medial structures of the foot (10, 14–16). Inadequate length in the Achilles tendon can exacerbate this problem (10). Dancers with inadequate length will roll in, thus decreasing tension in the tendon allowing for increased dorsiflexion at the ankle joint. Although such a maneuver may result in a deeper *plié,* it can often lead to an array of problems involving the medial structures of the foot and the great toe (Fig. 18.9) (17, 18).

Sickling is another faulty maneuver that occurs in *demi pointe* of full *pointe* positions and involves either excessive abduction of the forefoot with valgus at the heel—sickling out (Fig. 18.10)—or excessive forefoot

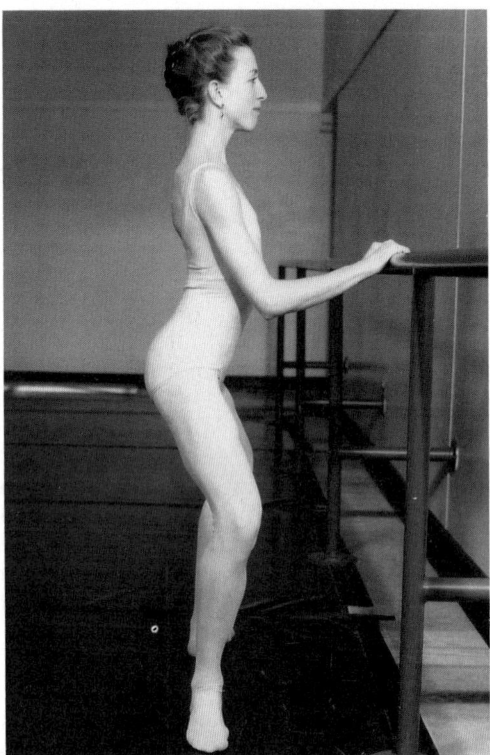

Figure 18.8. Increased lumbar spine lordosis to compensate for inadequate turnout at the hip.

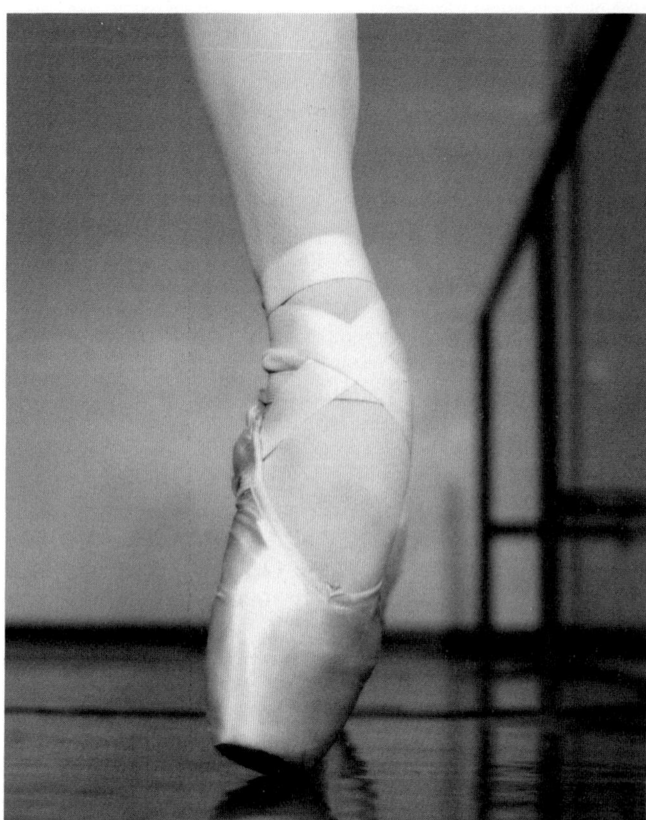

Figure 18.10. Sickling out is a faulty maneuver involving forefoot abduction with calcaneal valgus.

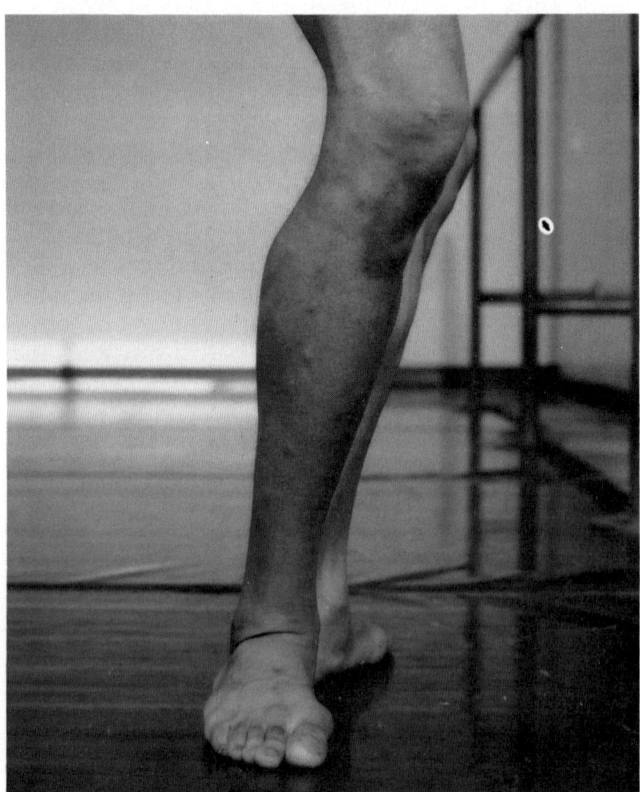

Figure 18.9. Rolling is often associated with inadequate length in the Achilles tendon and can lead to an array of problems involving the medial structures of the foot.

adduction with the heel in varus—sickling in (Fig. 18.11). Sickling may be a result of careless technique, muscular weakness (especially in the peroneal muscle group), and poor balance (15). Some dancers may sickle out as a method of achieving greater turnout of the extremity. Others may sickle in, placing increased stresses on the lateral ligaments. Consequences of sickling out may involve ailments of the medial structures of the foot, whereas sickling in may result in lateral ankle sprains (15, 19).

Certainly other faulty techniques occur that result in inefficient movement patterns and subsequent injury. The ones noted here are simply a few of those commonly seen. The clinician must, therefore, always question technique as a possible causative factor when dealing with the etiology of injury.

Anatomical Factors

In the general dance population, anatomical factors are more likely to contribute to dance injuries. However, as training continues inability to perform adequately without obvious aesthetic variation or painful struggle is almost always a cause of attrition. This allows for natural selection of those more anatomically suitable and likely to succeed as professional dancers. Once a dancer reaches the professional level, anatomical factors may still contribute to injury; however, they may be more subtle and supplementary to other factors such as technique (7).

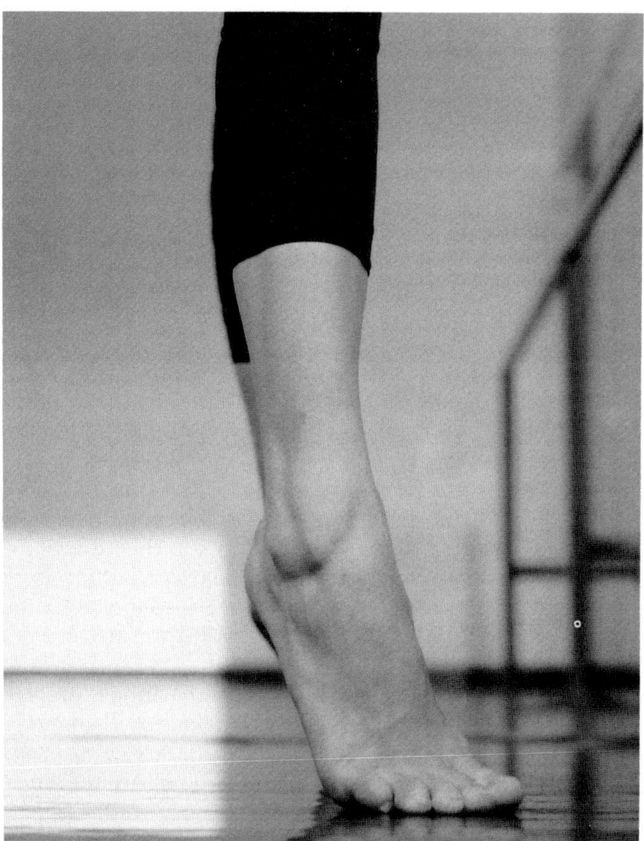

Figure 18.11. Lateral view of sickling in, which is a faulty maneuver involving forefoot adduction with calcaneal varus.

Somatotype

There may be variation from company to company; however, it appears the current aesthetically ideal body projects sleek lines formed by a long neck and long limbs, a slightly short torso, and a small head (2, 10). Likewise, dancers with minimal body fat are preferred. Because of this, the percentage of fat to body weight in female dancers tends to be below the 10th percentile of the normal population. (20).

Femoral Torsion

Femoral torsion will determine the intrinsic amount of external (femoral retroversion) and internal (femoral anteversion) rotation at the hip. A dancer with femoral retroversion may achieve turnout more easily, because this permits ER. Dancers between the ages of 6 and 11 can influence bone modeling to enhance turnout via static stretching into ER or positioning of ER during dance (20, 21). However, after age 11, the femoral neck can no longer be altered by the molding process of continual pressure. Therefore, after this age, subsequent development and maintenance of turnout is achieved primarily by stretching of the soft tissue structures about the hip (20).

Male dancers typically begin dance at a much later age than females and may be into adolescence before the onset of training. These dancers must achieve turnout via natural femoral retroversion and joint flexibility, or they must achieve this rotation by the stretching of soft tissue (20, 21).

Genurecurvatum

Although a slight degree of recurvatum (hyperextension) of the knee is aesthetically desirable in dance, excessive degrees may present problems. For example, in such a position the posterior capsular structures of the knee may become painful, especially when dancing *en pointe* (17). In fact, the dancer *en pointe* may have difficulty maintaining the body weight over the foot when the knee excessively hyperextends. This may lead to overuse injuries of the lower leg and foot (7). Excessive recurvatum may not allow the heels to approximate in first position; thus weight distribution may be more over the heels rather than over the entire foot. A dancer might compensate by increasing his or her anterior pelvic tilt, thereby increasing the lumbar lordosis. This may predispose the dancer to back injuries (7). Excessive hyperextension of the knees also may place greater strain on the triceps surae during repetitive jumping and perhaps contribute to Achilles tendinitis (17).

Tibial Torsion

Normal external tibial torsion is approximately 12°. Excessive torsion (greater than 26°) may result in an inability to align the knee over the foot during dance maneuvers (Fig. 18.12). This is especially true during *pliés* (7). The femur becomes internally rotated over a fixed

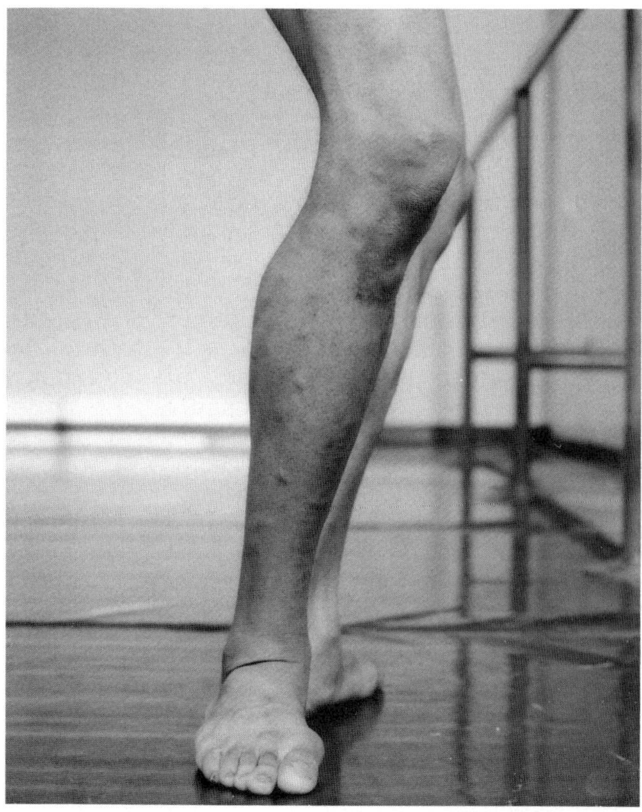

Figure 18.12. Inability to align the knee over the foot during *plié* as a result of excessive tibial torsion and/or inadequate turnout (ER) at the hip.

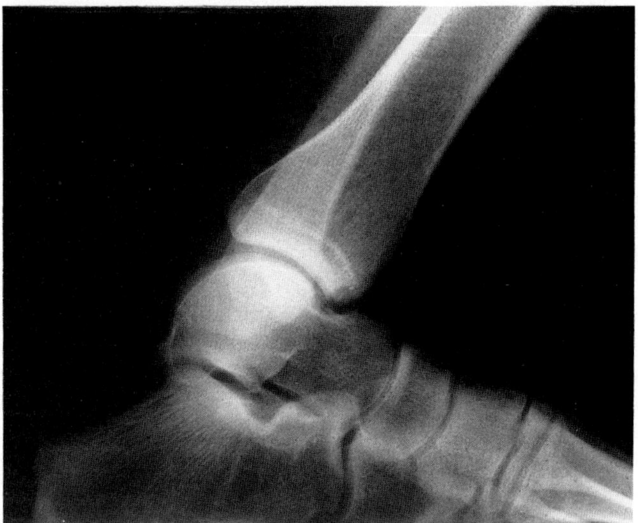

Figure 18.13. Anterior talar impingement during *plié* demonstration by x-ray.

ER tibia. During *pliés* as the femoral internal rotation and the tibial external torsion increase, so does the Q angle, resulting in subsequent patellofemoral and foot problems (22).

Ankle Joint

Impingement syndromes in the lower extremities of the dancer are the natural result of forcing the joints into extreme ranges of dorsiflexion and plantarflexion required for aesthetics and technique in classical ballet (19). Anterior talar impingement syndromes occur during *pliés* and may be a result of years of hitting bottom during *pliés* or laxity in the lateral ligaments secondary to ankle sprains (15, 19). Roentgenographic findings will reveal tibiotalar contact when the foot is in extreme dorsiflexion (Fig. 18.13). An exostosis may be present on the anterior talar neck and/or the anterior lip of the tibia (14, 15). Thus the dancer may lack adequate depth with *pliés* and have pain with such activities.

Posterior talar impingement syndrome occurs with maximal plantarflexion at the ankle as seen with *demi pointe* or full *pointe*. As the foot approaches the extreme range of plantarflexion, an os trigonum (a large posterior-lateral tubercle of the talus) or less commonly a large dorsal process of the os calcis may compress soft tissue structures such as the synovium and joint capsule against the posterior tibia. This may produce a limitation in range of plantarflexion and be associated with pain. Repeated entrapment of the soft tissue will lead to inflammatory changes with eventual thickening and fibrosis (14, 15).

Biomechanical Factors

It is not uncommon for dancers to push to the extremes of their physical limitations to maximize the range and variety of movements available for expression. Unfortunately, this can lead to altered joint mechanics and subsequent injury, especially about the foot and ankle.

Years of dance training and/or faulty technique may result in imbalances of strength and flexibility. Inadequate strength and/or flexibility may alter function and thus lead to inefficient movement patterns. Inefficient movement patterns may manifest in improper muscle sequencing, leading to misuse or overdependence on muscles not designed for the desired action. If training continues in this fashion, it can result in overuse of the inappropriate muscles as well as weakening of those more appropriate for the desired movement (23).

Functional equinus is often seen in dancers secondary to excessive shortening of the plantarflexor muscles. Such tightness will limit the available range of dorsiflexion necessary to achieve adequate depth with *pliés* and landing from jumps. In an attempt to increase dorsiflexion at the ankle in the presence of tight plantarflexors, the dancer will compensate by pronating at the subtalar joint. By virtue of its triplanar axis of motion, the subtalar joint can move in any direction necessary to compensate for deformity of the lower extremity. In the above case, subtalar pronation will provide increased motion at the ankle in a saggital plane, thereby allowing for increased dorsiflexion at the talocrural joint (24).

Unique to *pointe* dancing is the occasional forefoot sprain. Overarching of the foot *en pointe* will increase the amount of stress in the ligamentous and tendinous structures on the dorsum of the foot. This occurs when the line of gravity falls anterior to the dorsum of the foot rather than through the foot (7). Under such conditions, the weak dorsal capsules (now under tension) at the base of the fourth and fifth metatarsals are easily torn, producing the characteristic sprain at the tarsometatarsal joints (19). Likewise, increased dorsal stresses decrease stability over time and may lead to subluxation of the cuboid (16, 17, 19, 25). Marshall and Hamilton (25) tracked dance injuries during two separate 3-week periods and reported that cuboid subluxation totaled more than 17% of foot and ankle injuries. Although the two periods of time examined included 3 weeks of performance and 3 weeks of rehearsal schedules, no significant difference in terms of incidence of subluxation was noted when comparing the two.

Hallux Rigidus

Approximately 90° to 100° of dorsiflexion at the first metatarsal-phalangeal (MTP) joint is necessary to achieve full *relevé* onto *demi pointe* (see Fig. 18.4) (7, 16, 19). Hallux limitus or rigidus is usually an acquired condition in dancers, with an insidious onset leading to gradual stiffening at the joint. Acquired limitus or rigidus may be a result of repeated MTP joint trauma, inability of the first metatarsal to plantarflex, and/or a history of sesmoiditis (16, 24). Impingement spurs are commonly seen in this joint in older dancers and are often a result of direct impingement of bony surfaces in dorsiflexion or from capsular avulsions associated with sprains (19).

Limited hallux motion often results in faulty mechanics when attempting to achieve full *demi pointe.* To accomplish this, the dancer will roll laterally onto the lesser metatarsals, thereby sickling in (see Fig. 18.11). As mentioned previously, this faulty maneuver can lead

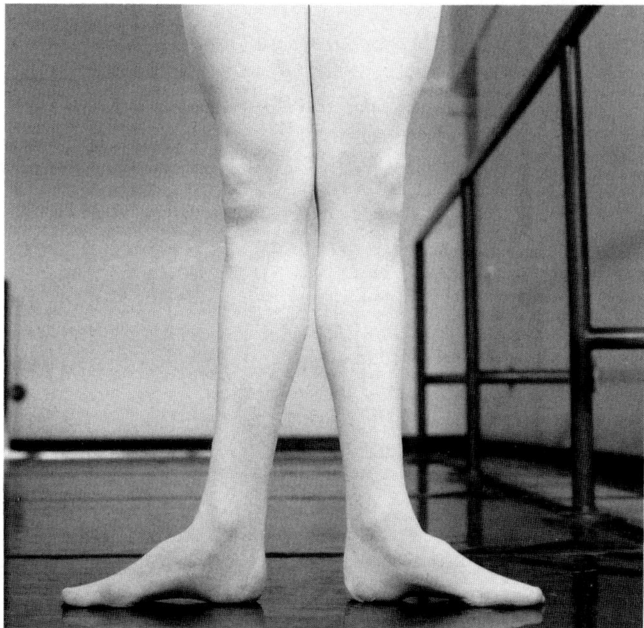

Figure 18.14. Pes cavus foot.

to lateral ankle sprains and malalignment problems (16, 19).

Pes Planus and Cavus

Although aesthetically favorable, the pes cavus foot (Fig. 18.14) is often relatively rigid and proves to be an extremely poor shock absorber (7, 16, 24). A dancer with this condition may have to depend on a forgiving dance surface to assist with shock absorption. In addition, the dancer must ensure proper technique when dancing (i.e., when landing from jumps, *demi pliés,* etc.) to allow the heels to load and contact the floor. Adequate length in the Achilles tendon must be maintained.

Pes planus is a condition often associated with forefoot varus (7). The planus foot allows for excessive pronation. Excessive pronation can lead to a variety of conditions about the foot and ankle as well as up the lower kinetic chain.

Environmental Factors

Environmental factors contribute to dance injury as well. In a survey conducted by Bowling, et al. (8) 25% of those surveyed perceived the cause of their injuries to be related to dancing on unsuitable stages and flooring (i.e., hard, unsprung floors) and 14% attributed injuries to dancing in a cold, drafty environment and being insufficiently warmed up.

Dancers often report dance studios to be cold or drafty, making it difficult to properly warm up or to stay warm. In addition, many dance companies will agree to outdoor performances during the summer months. Cool night air may cause the same problems associated with inadequate warmup. On the other hand, humidity and/or high temperatures can lead to dehydration, heat cramps, heat exhaustion, or heat stroke (7).

The dance surface is another variable that has great bearing on the dancer's ability to perform adequately. The dance surface is often thought to act as a silent partner to enhance performance and confidence (26). Dancing is an interaction between two dynamic systems: the dancer and the floor (27). Dance surfaces must provide adequate shock absorption yet be firm enough to provide sufficient energy return to the dancer to enhance performance and reduce fatigue (27, 28). Surfaces that are too firm with little or no give (such as concrete and asphalt) may lead to early muscular fatigue, because the musculoskeletal system of the lower extremities must act to absorb most of the shock. Once this system fails to absorb shock adequately, afflictions of the feet and legs (e.g., shin splints and stress fractures) may ensue (26, 27).

On the other hand, if a dance surface is too soft, this too can lead to early fatigue. Here there is adequate absorption but inadequate energy return to the dancer, thus requiring considerably more effort to perform the desired movements. An extreme example of such a surface is a sandy beach (27, 28).

Therefore, the most important properties of a dance floor are proper surface friction, resiliency, and shock absorption. For a flooring system to be resilient and shock absorbing, it must perform certain functions. According to Seals (26, 27), a dance floor:

- Should have shock-absorbing qualities.
- Should give under impact to some degree and absorb some of the impact energy in doing so.
- Should not deform permanently or dent under pressure or impact of normal use.
- Should not be so springy that it acts as a trampoline.
- Should not be absolutely rigid or hard and should not give the impression of being so.

To achieve these properties a dance surface must consist of three components: *(a)* a subfloor or base, i.e., concrete, asphalt, or tile; *(b)* a substructure, i.e., rubber pads and sleepers or springs and sleepers; and *(c)* a surface, i.e., hardwood flooring or vinyl sheet flooring. Seals (26–28) provided details of specific substructure designs and floor surfaces.

A final property is surface friction. The friction or traction of the surface is important when the foot is interacting with the flooring surface. There is a delicate balance between the needed slide and traction during performances and rehearsals (27). To ensure dancers will function uninhibited on such a surface, daily care is a must. The surface must be kept free of a buildup of rosin, body oils, cleaning materials, dust, and other foreign materials that may create uneven surfaces or lead to slippage problems (26–28).

Many dance companies encounter difficulties when touring. For this reason, many professional companies tour with portable floors that provide a familiar, uniform surface on which to perform. Still, these floors lack sufficient mass or thickness to mask a rigid stage floor. Nonetheless, portable floors do provide adequate surface traction and friction (26–28).

Dietary and Nutritional Factors

Because of the current aesthetic ideal, a typical dancer's somatotype calls for thinness. Such a demand may be responsible for several nutritionally related health problems. Because ballet is not an aerobic activity, dancing in and of itself does not allow the dancer to reduce and/or maintain weight. Therefore, many dancers resort to improper dieting methods that may result in menstrual irregularities, skeletal abnormalities, and/or serious eating disorders.

A study conducted by Hamilton et al. (29) surveyed 49 female dancers in four national ballet companies in America (65%) and the Peoples Republic of China (35%). Findings showed that all of the groups reported a delay in menarche and weighed approximately 14% below their ideal weight for their corresponding height.

Frusztajer et al. (30) studied 55 female dancers and 59 nondancer controls to investigate the incidence of stress fractures in ballet dancer. Information was gathered via interview questionnaires and medical examination. The authors found that the majority (80%) of the dancers ($n = 10$) with recent stress fracture had weighed less than 75% of their ideal body weight and showed a greater incidence of eating disorders. This group also showed a lower fat intake and a higher intake of low-calorie foods.

Nutritional deficiencies may also contribute to fatigue, anemia, and muscle spasm (31). In the event of injury, those who lack sound nutritional habits may find it difficult to build, maintain, and repair tissue (31).

Given the possibility that quests for ultraleanness by some dancers may precipitate injury, lead to menstrual abnormalities, and/or eating disorders, clinicians and dance instructors alike must attempt to recognize those at risk and seek appropriate professional consultation. Likewise, if the dancer is asked to lose weight, he or she should be directed to a professional source so that weight loss can be achieved in a safe and reasonable manner.

Psychologic Factors

The dance profession is a highly competitive yet private one. The road from childhood training to a professional career can be a long and grueling trip. Many dancers must decide if dance is a career goal at an early age so they can develop their skills. Often young dancers choose to leave home during their formative years to train at certain prestigious schools. The dance school becomes a surrogate parent and most of their lives are consumed with developing enough talent and skill to become a professional. These circumstances may cause some students to become emotionally fatigued or burned out (7). Emotional fatigue can be associated with physical fatigue and inattentiveness, which may lead to injury (7).

For those whose perseverance and talents allow them to capture the professional ranks, competition and pressures may present more barriers. Competition for roles and demands from instructors, other company members, the media, or the dancer himself or herself may lead to self-destruction on a physical and/or emotional level. A total of 38% of those surveyed by Bowling (8) believed their injuries were the result of feeling overtired, rundown, overworked, and under strain and pressure.

Pressure to maintain an ideal versus a realistic somatotype may lead to eating disorders, as discussed previously. Finally, injury and/or age may present an inevitable but possibly premature crossroad for the dancer. Dancers may be presented with a situation in which the instrument of expression—their bodies—cannot function as it used to. The dancers may feel their bodies are "imperfect" instruments trying to perform in a perfect art (7).

Transition from a life of dance to alternative careers can be an anxious time for dancers. A career in dance often begins early in life and may limit formal education. Because of this and their focused career in dance, many dancers are often unaware of their capabilities, talents, and potentials outside of dance (32). The realization that some professional assistance may be needed for such an adjustment has led to the birth of the Dancers Transition Centre of Canada, which addresses the stress of giving up professional dance (32).

Medical Problems

Injuries seen in dance are usually chronic in nature, developing subtly over a period of time. However, on occasion there are acute traumatic injuries. The following discussion will briefly address common injuries seen at specific anatomical regions. This review will in no way be inclusive of all plausible injuries in these areas. It is important to recall the etiological factors that contribute to such injuries, as discussed previously.

Upper Extremities and Spine

Injuries to the neck and upper extremities are less common in dance than those of other regions. Male dancers are more subject to upper extremity injuries because of choreography demands. Males are often required to partner and lift females. Repetitive lifting in the presence of poor technique, poor postural alignment, and inadequate strength or flexibility can predispose one to overuse and/or impingement syndromes, especially at the shoulder. Likewise, ligament sprains of the wrist and hand may ensue when catching their female partners (33). There also exists the possibility of cervical disc disease. Appropriate physical and diagnostic examinations should be used for differential diagnosis.

Spinal injuries in the lumbar area are more common and most often are the result of repetitive microtrauma. Mechanical low-back pain is often seen in dancers and is usually associated with a hyperlordotic posture, both statically and dynamically (11). Such a posture may be a reflection of anatomical alignment and musculotendinous imbalances and is nearly always an acquired posture (11). Poor technique, i.e., hyperlordosis in an attempt to increase turnout or when lifting female partners, must be addressed. Appropriate soft tissue length (especially in the hip flexors and thoracolumbar fascia) and muscle strength (especially in the abdominals) are essential.

Of special consideration is the young dancer. Many young dancers lack sufficient strength and/or are not quite adept in technique. Likewise, the growth spurt of a young dancer can influence flexibility for short periods. Coordination may also be affected if the change in bone length is rapid (34). A study conducted by Kendall and Kendall (35) investigating 5115 children from kindergarten through grade 12 found a decline in flexibility at ages 12 (males) and 13 (females). This decrease in flexibility may translate into improper alignment and faulty technique, thus placing greater stresses on the lumbar spine.

Spondylolysis is another problem associated with dance (Fig. 18.15). The cause is probably a result of the repetitive flexion and extension of the spine, resulting in a stress fracture of one or more pars interarticularis of the lumbar spine (11). Findings on physical examination will include a decrease in lumbar flexion and pain with lumbar hyperextension. Often the dancer complains of pain with unilateral hyperextension (i.e., when performing an *arabesque*) on the affected side (10, 11, 36). One should keep in mind that a dancer who maintains poor alignment (i.e., hyperlordosis) may be predisposed to facet irritation/impingement. Differential diagnosis must, therefore, be made to distinguish facet

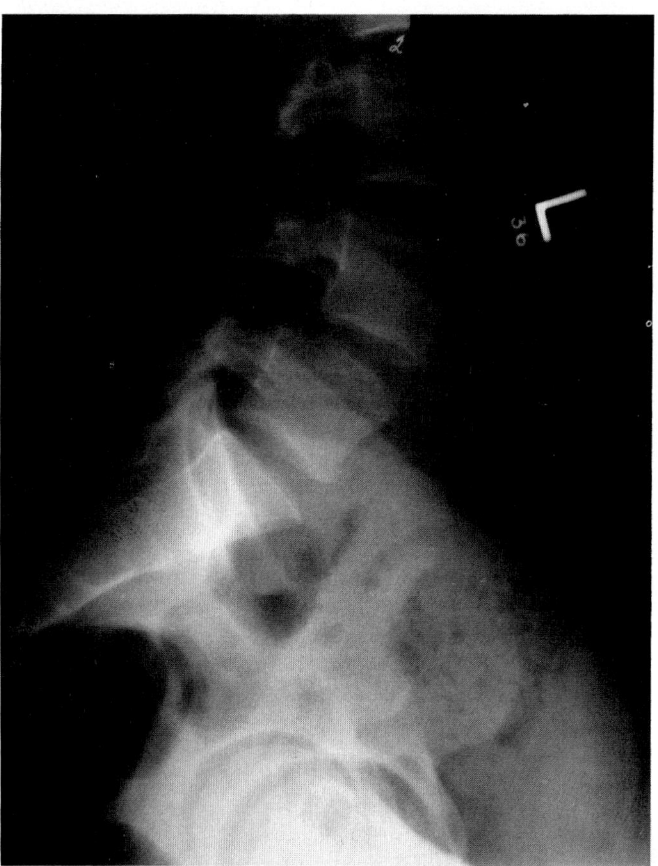

Figure 18.15. Spondylolysis in the professional dancer shown in Figure 18.14.

syndrome from spondylolysis (36). The presence of a pars defect or even a grade I spondylolisthesis does not warrant departure from a career in dance. These defects are often the result of a stress fracture, and the condition is usually a fairly stable one. Dance can continue safely although possibly with discomfort (11).

Discogenic low-back pain in dance, however, appears more prevalent in male dancers, probably caused by lifting (11, 36). Nonoperative management of such a condition is preferred with cessation of lifting and directed exercise. Bracing may be of value, especially on initial return to dance. Nonetheless, bracing is usually not an option for performances because of aesthetics. In the event of disabling pain or progressive neurologic loss, the dancer should be managed like any other patient with a serious herniation (11).

Muscle imbalances also may influence pelvic alignment, leading to sacral and/or innominate rotations, thus causing pain with static and/or dynamic activities. Appropriate exercise, manual therapy, and improved dance technique can assist with correction and maintenance of the correction.

Hip

Anatomic and biomechanical factors at the hip were discussed above. Inadequate turnout can create problems at the hip and elsewhere. Repeatedly stretching the joint capsule with forced turnout can lead to chronic strain and possible calcification at the acetabular attachment of the capsule (20).

Stress fractures of the femoral neck also can be a causative factor of hip pain (20, 37). Nondescript pain is usually found in the groin, with symptoms increasing at the beginning and the end of class, but minimized during class. Rest usually relieves the pain. Early physical examination reveals no limitations of range but groin tenderness is present. Standard x-rays do not show a fracture until several weeks or months later. A bone scan is usually necessary to locate the area of increased activity (20). Progression of symptoms results in decreased hip flexion, abduction, and external rotation secondary to pain. Diagnostic tests may be necessary to rule out other possible conditions such as arthritis, synovitis, infection, or tumor (20). Sammarco (20) believes treatment of a stress fracture requires a dramatic decrease in weight bearing (crutches are recommended). Water *barre* is indicated at this point, using the involved extremity as the working and not the supporting leg. A decrease in symptoms allows for progression to floor *barre* (non-weight–bearing exercise) and initiation of a flexibility program. He feels this should continue 2 or more months before returning to class.

Iliacus tendinitis is often seen in female dancers. This muscle and tendon are in close contact with the inguinal ligament as the hip is brought into flexion, external rotation, and abduction (as in *developpé*). During this motion the tendon becomes U-shaped and irritation may result as the tendon passes beneath the inguinal ligament (20, 37, 38) Crepitus may be noted in the groin. Stiffness may be present, as well as tenderness on palpation of the iliopsoas tendon, especially during *developpé* (20, 37, 38). Resisted hip flexion may elicit pain.

Bursitis may be another affliction in dance. Of the several bursae present in the hip, that which overlies the greater trochanter is most commonly affected. This usually results from irritation of the bursae as the iliotibial band passes over the greater trochanter. Pain is elicited with palpation over the greater trochanter. The examiner may also find crepitus. Pain is accentuated during certain dance steps such as *rond de jambe* and when landing from jumps (20, 39). Bursitis of the anterior hip capsule also may become a problem when the bursae lying between the capsule and the iliopsoas tendon becomes inflamed. Groin pain with active or passive flexion is usually a hallmark of this condition, although crepitus is generally not palpable (20, 39).

Clicks and snaps are frequent complaints of dancers, although such joint noises may be asymptomatic. An anterior click is caused when the iliopsoas tendon passes across the anterior hip capsule as the hip moves from a position of flexion, abduction, and external rotation to first position of ballet, where the hip is in a more neutral position (20, 38).

Schaberg et al. (40) carried out a clinical and radiographic investigation of eight dancers with reports of clicking hips using bursography with cineradiography. Results of this study suggest that the iliopsoas tendon slipping over the osseous ridge of the lesser trochanter or the iliopectineal eminence can be the etiology of the snapping hip.

A snapping hip usually occurs laterally as the iliotibial band passes rapidly over the greater trochanter. This condition often gives the dancer the sensation of the hip going out of place. It frequently occurs when landing from jumps, a time when the load rapidly increases across the hip joint. Upon the initial phases of landing, the hip is flexed, causing the iliotibial band (via contraction of the tensor fascia latae) to move anteriorly. The tendon then snaps backward as the dancer recovers and extends the hip (20, 38).

A study conducted by Jacob and Young (41) set out to identify general characteristics in dancers that manifest with snapping hip problems ($n=11$) when compared with those without such problems ($n=11$). Their results identified the following to be characteristics of those presenting with snapping hip: *(a)* narrow biiliac width; *(b)* greater range of movement (ROM) in hip abduction; *(c)* decreased ROM in external rotation; and *(d)* greater strength in the external rotators.

Hip pain in dancers also may be the result of other conditions such as piriformis syndrome, rheumatoid arthritis, or a disc herniation. Several internal organs also can refer pain to the hip such as the genitourinary system or the female reproductive system (38). Should examination of the hip render negative findings, a complete physical and diagnostic studies should be done to rule out other possible conditions.

Knee

Dancers often encounter knee pain during the course of their careers. Many of these problems are attributed to overuse, muscle imbalances, poorly sprung dance surfaces, and faulty technique (12, 17). Mild hyperextension of the knees, although aesthetically desirable, may result in generalized laxity (17, 39). Posterior capsular structures may become painful, especially in females when dancing *en pointe*. Such a condition may place increased strain on the triceps surae and contribute to Achilles tendinitis (17).

Chronic rotational stresses may be present at the knee in dancers who force their turnout. In such instances, there is increased strain placed on the medial collateral ligament, menisci, and joint capsule. Likewise, patellofemoral disorders may develop, including lateral subluxation, lateral dislocation, excessive lateral pressure syndrome, and/or chondromalacia (38, 39, 42).

Patellar tendinitis, often associated with Osgood-Schlatter disease in the young participant, is commonly seen in dancers. Precipitating factors may include repetitive jumping, unyielding surfaces, and/or an increase in total volume of work (as is often seen during rehearsals for upcoming performances) (10, 17, 43).

On rare occasions, traumatic injuries occur about the knee. These are more often the result of neglect to treat chronic symptoms (i.e., patella tendinitis) rather than a single isolated movement. Nonetheless, traumatic patella subluxation, patellar tendon rupture, knee ligament tears, and meniscal tears do occur.

Knee surgery is rarely a treatment option in dance. However, in the event of meniscal injuries and/or major ligamentous rupture, surgery may be indicated. Some authors reported in earlier literature that it would be almost impossible to get a dancer back to full dance activities after a knee ligament reconstruction (38, 43). However, recent medical advances have provided dancers with a second chance. Doctors at the University of Pittsburgh Medical Center have performed reconstructive surgery for anterior cruciate ligament tears in six professional ballet dancers since 1986. Of those six, two have returned to unrestricted dance in reputable companies and two are employed as full-time university instructors. One returned to dance for a single season following rehabilitation, then self-elected to give up dance in pursuit of a degree in an unrelated field of interest. One dancer never returned to dance because of his belief that he would not able to attain his preinjury level of performance and because he lacked confidence in the ability of his knee to respond adequately to the stresses of dance.

Certainly other ailments plague the dancer such as capsulitis, bursitis, and iliotibial band friction syndrome. Most of the common problems at the knee are self-limiting and can be reversed with appropriate treatment, including medication, modified activity, correction of muscle imbalances, and correction of faulty technique.

Lower Leg, Foot and Ankle

Current belief is that pain associated with shin splints is attributed to a tibial stress fracture, medial tibial stress syndrome, and/or a mild anterior compartment syndrome (28, 40, 44, 45). It has been theorized among dancers, instructors, and medical professionals that shin splints are often the result of dancing on nonresilient surfaces, landing from jumps without placing the heels on the floor, and/or a combination of both (37, 39, 44, 46)

However, a study by Gans (46) investigating the relationship between heel contact and the incidence of shin splints in 16 dancers showed that heel-to-floor contact on ascent or descent from jumps did not appear to be related to the incidence of shin splints in dancers. However, in those with a history of shin splints, Gans noted an increased incidence of what she referred to as double-heel strike—the heel elevated from the floor between landing and pushoff.

The foot and ankle are common sites of injury in dance. Although injury may be acute, chronic injuries usually predominate. Chronic injuries are often the result of repetitive impact loading on relatively unyielding surfaces. Other factors contributing to injury include improper footwear that does not adequately absorb shock, improper technique, anatomical variation, and on occasion, fatigue (14).

Acute injuries at the foot and ankle are most commonly lateral ankle sprains. Injury usually results from forced inversion of the hindfoot when landing from a jump while the foot is in a position of plantarflexion (14, 47). In such a position, the talus is less stable in the ankle mortise and the inversion force places excessive stress on the anterior talofibular ligament, frequently resulting in injury. Should the force continue, injury to the calcaneo-fibular ligament will ensue (47). Fractures of the base of the fifth metatarsal are commonly seen secondary to severe inversion sprains at the ankle (14, 48). Avulsion of the peroneus brevis tendon away from its attachments may carry with it a fragment of bone, resulting in an avulsion fracture (49).

Dance choreography that requires rapid repeated jumps and/or elaborate footwork also can contribute to ankle sprain. Other factors contributing to injury include improper technique (i.e., sickling in), muscular fatigue (especially of the peroneals that provide dynamic stability), and previous history of ankle sprain (47, 48). In addition, the dance surface itself may be a factor in injury. Raked stages, slippery floors, and unusually hard or resilient surfaces might create insecure footing and result in misstep and subsequent injury (28).

Fractures and dislocations also are seen in dance. The most common acute fracture is the spiral fracture of the distal one-third of the fifth metatarsal, occurring when the dancer loses his or her balance on *demi pointe* and rolls over onto the lateral border of the foot (19). Although not commonly seen, high external forces during a *fouetté* (a turn *en pointe* or *demi pointe* away from the supporting leg while the working leg is thrown outward as the body spins) can cause a lateral malleolar fracture or fracture dislocation of the supporting leg (37). Conversely, fracture of the medial malleolus occurs while the foot is forcefully everted such as during the *emboîte* dance step. Here, the dancer jumps rapidly into the air bringing one foot forword in front of the other and lands in a *demi pointe* position (37).

Interphalangeal joint dislocation occasionally occurs in dancers. They are most often the result of direct trauma such as walking into and/or kicking a heavy object or stage equipment while in ballet slippers (19, 48).

Tendon rupture also can occur. Rupture of the Achilles tendon can occur without warning; however, it is typically preceded by tendinitis or degeneration (19). This need not be a career-ending injury. Operative repair ensuring restored physiologic tendon length, prevention of postoperative complications, appropriate rehabilitation, and dedication on the part of the dancer can lead to normal function and safe return to dance. One company member of the Pittsburgh Ballet Theatre sustained a complete rupture of her Achilles tendon during a performance of *Square Dance* in February 1991. She underwent repair several hours after injury and returned to unrestricted dance and performed in October 1991 with no reported loss of function or technical precision. Two cases of partial rupture of the flexor hallucis longus tendon and one case of peroneus brevis rupture in the absence of a peroneus longus muscle have been reported in the literature (49, 50).

Although tendinitis can be an acute condition, the frequency of recurrence and the nature of dance tends to make chronicity more the norm than the exception. Although any tendon about the foot and ankle can be affected in dancers, the Achilles, flexor hallicus, posterior tibialis, and peroneal tendons are most commonly involved (10, 14, 15, 51). Faulty technique, improper dance surfaces, fatigue, the repetitive nature of dance, musculoskeletal imbalances, or a combination of any or all of the above are usually responsible for the onset and persistence of tendinitis.

Stress fractures are not uncommon in the dancer's foot. The proximal shaft of the second and third metatarsals, the sesmoids, the navicular, and the distal tibia are frequently involved (10, 12, 14, 37). Stress fractures are most often the result of cumulative microtrauma rather than a single acute traumatic event. The ability to heal spontaneously is diminished with repetitive impact, as often occurs in dance. Hardaker (14) believes the experienced dancer is less vulnerable than the beginner, because of the gradual adaptive hypertrophy of the bony structures. However, experienced professionals often sustain stress fractures nearing the end of a long tour that required dance on unyielding surfaces. Repeated incidence of stress fracture should be a red flag for the medical practitioner and warrants an investigation of nutritional habits.

Joint bursae and capsules can also become inflamed and irritated in the dancer's foot. Retrocalcaneal bursitis and dorsal capsulitis of the first MTP joint are common sites of involvement.

Plantar fasciitis is another common ailment in the ballet foot. The most likely cause of plantar fasciitis is faulty biomechanics secondary to either a tight triceps surae or an externally rotated lower extremity. As stated previously, one consequence of forced turnout is excessive strain on the medial structures of the foot from resultant pronation. Consequently, normal loading forces are not supported by the primary structures (i.e., bones and ligaments) of the supinated foot and are instead imposed on the secondary structures (i.e., capsules and ligaments). Plantar fasciitis may ensue when the fibrous aponeurosis assumes a greater share of the force than it can physiologically accommodate (52). Fasciitis also may occur in the dancer with a cavus foot secondary to the inability of this foot type to dissipate forces adequately. This too will increase the load on the plantar aponeurosis (52).

A variety of skin and nail problems are encountered by the dancer, especially females required to dance in *pointe* shoes. Dancers are often adept at protective tapings and dressings to minimize problems at the phalanges. When unable to dance because of pain or if there is irritation of the skin or nail bed possibly caused by infection, the dancer should seek the professional consultation of a podiatrist or dermatologist.

Undoubtedly, the dancer can and will incur a multitude of subtle and sometimes less common injuries than those previously discussed as a result of the nature of the dance and its demand for extremes of motion. Therefore, the clinician should not forgo a complete evaluation of an injured dancer, assuming that he or she is afflicted with one of the more commonly seen conditions.

Treatment

Before the onset of treatment, a systematic and thorough evaluation must be performed to allow selection of the most appropriate and beneficial treatment regime. Likewise, it is important to be familiar with the type of dance to which the injured dancer will be returning. Different dance styles impose different physical demands. Regardless of the variance in physical demands, each dancer strives to be a perfect instrument for a perfect art form. Dancers' bodies must allow them to become the creative expression of the choreographer, the visual component of the music, and an ephemeral entity for the audience (53).

With that in mind, treatment goals must be directed towards the following (53):

1. Pain relief.
2. Restoration of full active and passive range of motion.
3. Stability of the joint.
4. Normal muscular strength, endurance, control, and coordination.
5. Proper proprioceptive responses.
6. Restoration of confidence in dancing ability.
7. Patient education in regard to the musculoskeletal system, immediate first aid care, and injury prevention.

The clinician should note that treatment plans should be tailored to meet the specific demands of the dancer, especially during the functional phases of rehabilitation. Pain control must be the first step in treatment. This may simply involve supportive bandages to decrease swelling or undue mechanical stresses, modification (but not necessarily cessation) of dance, appropriate physical and therapeutic modalities, and patient education. Drugs, in particular nonsteroidal antiinflammatory drugs (NSAIDs), are often used as adjuncts to treatment. In the event of an acute injury, the company physician should be notified as soon as possible to rule out serious injury (such as tendon ruptures, fractures, dislocation, or soft tissue tears) and initiate a plan of care.

Once the pain has subsided, treatment is aimed at the restoration of normalcy in terms of range of motion and neuromuscular control. Early in this phase, a pool *barre* may be of great physical and psychologic benefit. It is important to correct for any musculoskeletal imbalances and faulty dance techniques at this time to ensure joint protection and to prevent reinjury. Treatment activities should not be isolated to the specific area of injury, but should be inclusive of a total-body conditioning program to maintain a high level of function while awaiting return to unrestricted dance. Proprioceptive retraining should be incorporated into any treatment regime to elicit appropriate responses before the onset of functional training and return to dance.

Patient education is essential to familiarize the dancer with probable causes of his or her current injury and what measures need to be taken to prevent recurrence. Preventative measures include not only the current exercise program and efforts to correct faulty technique but also adequate rest and adequate nutritional intake. Likewise, in the event of subtle onset of recurrence or full-out reinjury, immediate first aid care should be reviewed (53).

Often after serious injury (i.e., tendon or ligament ruptures) the dancer is apprehensive on return to dance, despite months of postoperative rehabilitation. Introduction to dance should, therefore, be a gradual process incorporated into the treatment plan throughout the course of the rehabilitation, beginning with the basics and progressing to the more technically demanding steps as tolerated. In the event that a dancer cannot overcome a psychological component to return to dance despite his or her physical capabilities to do so, it is often helpful to refer such a dancer to a psychologist who can offer counsel and effectively promote return to dance.

Caution should be taken not to return the dancer too quickly to unrestricted dance after injury, despite his or her seeming urgency to do so because of self-imposed demands or those of the other company members or ballet masters. Inadequate rehabilitation and premature return to dance will likely result in reinjury and/or chronic problems. Open communication with the physician, caregiver, dancer, and the artistic director is imperative to ensure timely and safe return to dance.

REFERENCES

1. Micheli LJ, Gillespie WJ, Walaszek, A. Physiologic profiles of female professional ballerinas. Clin Sports Med 1984;3(1):199–209.
2. Miller EH, Schneider HJ, Bronson JL, McLain D. A new consideration in athletic injuries. The classical ballet dancer. Clin Orthop (111):181–191.

3. Laws K. Physics and the potential for dance injury. Med Prog Performing Arts 1986;(September):73–80.
4. Mara T. First steps in ballet basic exercises at the barre. Princeton, NJ: Princeton Book Co., 1987.
5. Grosser J. Passport to ballet: an illustrated audience prime. San Francisco: San Francisco Ballet, 1990.
6. Ryan AJ, Stephens RE, eds. Dance medicine—a comprehensive guide. Chicago: Pluribus, 1987.
7. Stephens RE. The etiology of injuries in ballet. In: Ryan AJ, Stephens RE, eds. Dance medicine—a comprehensive guide. Chicago: Pluribus, 1987:16–50.
8. Bowling A. Injuries to dancers: prevalence, treatment and perception of causes. Br Med J 1989;18(289):731–734.
9. Downey PM, Irrgang JJ, Fu, FH. Preseason screening of a professional ballet company. Paper presented at the American College of Sports Medicine Dallas, May 1988.
10. Tietz CC. Sports medicine concerns in dance and gymnastics. Pediatr Clin North Am 1982;19(6):1399–1421.
11. Micheli LJ. Back injuries in dancers. Clin Sports Med 1983;2(3):473–484.
12. Medical problems in ballet: A round table. Phys Sportsmed 1982;10(3):98–112.
13. Sohl P, Bowling A. Injuries to dancers—prevalence, treatment and prevention. Sports Med 1990;9(5):317–322.
14. Hardaker WT, Jr. Foot and ankle injuries in classical ballet dancers. Orthop Clin North Am 1989;20(4):621–627.
15. Hardaker WT, Jr, Margello S, Goldner JL. Foot and ankle injuries in theatrical dancers. Foot Ankle 1985;6(2):59–69.
16. Marshall P. The rehabilitation of overuse foot injuries in athletes and dancers. Clin Sports Med 1980;7(1):175–191.
17. Reid DC. Prevention of hip and knee injuries in ballet dancers. Sports Med 1988;6:295–307.
18. Howse J. Disorders of the great toe in dancers. Clin Sports Med 1983;2(3):499–505.
19. Hamilton WG. Foot and ankle injuries in dancers. Clin Sports Med 1988;7(1):143–173.
20. Sammarco GJ. The hip in dancers. Med Probl Performing Arts 1987;(March):5–14.
21. Sammarco GJ. The dancers hip. Clin Sports Med 1983;2(3)485–498.
22. Tietz CC. Patellofemoral pain in dancers. J OPERD 1987;(May–June):34–36.
23. Lauffenburger SK. Bartenieff fundamentals, early detection of potential dance injury. J Phys Educ Recreation Dance 1987;(May–June):59–60.
24. Rour ML, Orien WP, Weed JM. Clinical biomechanics. Vol II. Normal and abnormal function of the foot. Los Angeles: Clinical Biomechanics, 1977.
25. Marshall P, Hamilton WG. Cuboid subluxation in ballet dancers. Am J Sports Med 1992;2(2):169–175.
26. Seals JG. Dance floors. Med Probl Performing Arts 1986;(Septemer):81–84.
27. Seals JG. Dance surfaces. In: Ryan AJ, Stephens RE, Eds. Dance Medicine—a comprehensive guide. Chicago: Pluribus, 1987:321–333.
28. Seals JG. A study of dance surfaces. Clin Sports Med 1983;2(3):557–561.
29. Hamilton LM, Brooks-Gunn J, Warren MP, Hamilton WG. The role of selectivity in the pathogenesis of eating problems in ballet dancers. Med Sci Sports Exerc 1988;20(6):560–565.
30. Frusztajer NT, Dauper S, Warren MP, Brooks-Gunn J, Fox RP. Nutrition and the incidence of stress fracture in ballet dancers. Am J Clin Nutr 1990 S1:779–783.
31. Loosli AR, Benson J, Gillien DM. Nutrition and the dancer. In: Ryan AJ, Stephens RE, eds. Dance medicine—a comprehensive guice. Chicago: Pluribus, 1987;100–106.
32. Greben SE. The dancers transition center of Canada: addressing the stress of giving up professional dancing. Med Probl Performing Arts 1989;(September):128–130.
33. Nixon JE. Injuries to the neck and upper extremities of dancers. Clin Sports Med 2(3):1983;2(3):459–472.
34. Schafle MA. The child dancer—medical considerations. Pediatr Clin North Am 1990;37(5):1211–1221.
35. Kendall MD, Kendall FP. Normal flexibility according to age groups. J Bone Joint Surg 1948;30A(3):690–694.
36. Bachrach RM. Injuries to the dancers spine. In: Ryan AJ, Stephens RE, eds. Dance medicine—comprehensive guide. Chicago: Pluribus, 1987:243–266.
37. Sammarco GJ. Diagnosis and treatment in dancers. Clin Orthop 1984;187:176–187.
38. Sammarco GJ. The dancers hip. In: Ryan AJ, Stephens RE, eds. Dance medicine—a comprehensive guide. Chicago: Pluribus, 1987:220–242.
39. Ende LS, Wickstrom J. Ballet injuries. Phys Sportsmed 1982;10(7):101–118.
40. Schaberg JE, Harper MC, Allen WC. The snapping hip syndrome. Am J Sports Med 1984;12(5):361–365.
41. Jacobs M, Young R. Snapping hip phenomenon among dancers. Am Corr Ther J 1978;32(3):92–97.
42. Quirk R. Knee injuries in classical dancers. Med Probl Performing Arts 1988;(June):52–58.
43. Quirk R. The dancer's knee. In: Ryan AJ, Stephens RE, eds. Dance medicine—a comprehensive guide. Chicago: Pluribus, 1987:177–219.
44. Kleiger B. Foot and ankle injuries in dancers. In Ryan AJ, Stephens RE, eds. Dance medicine—a comprehensive guide. Chicago: Pluribus, 1987;115–134.
45. Jones DC, James SL. Overuse injuries of the lower extremity—shin splints, iliotibial band friction syndrome and external compartment syndromes. Clin Sports Med 1987;6(2):273–290.
46. Gans A. The relationship of heel contact in ascent and descent from jumps to the incidence of shin splints in ballet dancers. Phys Ther 1985;65(8):1192–1196.
47. Hardaker WT, Colosimo AJ, Malone TR, Myers M. Ankle sprains in theatrical dancers. Med Probl Performing Arts 1988;(December):146–150.
48. Robinson MA. Foot and ankle injuries in dance. In: Canto RC, Gillespie WJ, eds. Sports medicine and science—bridging the gap. Boston: DC Health, 1982:143–149.
49. Sammarco GJ, Miller EM. Partial rupture of the flexor hallucis longus tendon in classical ballet dancers. J Bone Joint Surg 1979;61A(1):149–151.
50. Cross MJ, Crichton KJ, Gordon H, Mackie I. Peroneus brevis rupture in the absence of the peroneus longus muscle & tendon in a classical ballet dancer. A case report. Am J Sports Med 1988;16(6):677–678.
51. Sammarco GJ. The foot and ankle in classical ballet and modern dance. In: Jamss M, ed. Disorders of the foot. Philadelphia: WB Saunders, 1982:1626–1659.
52. Kwong PK, Kay D, Voner RT, White MW. Plantar fasciitis: mechanics and pathomechanics of treatment. Clin Sports Med 1988;7(1):119–126.
53. Molnar ME. Rehabilitation of the injured dancer. In: Ryan AJ, Stephens RE, eds. Dance medicine—a comprehensive guide. Chicago: Pluribus, 1987:302–320.

19 / EMERGENCY MEDICAL CARE AT SPORTS EVENTS

Vincent P. Verdile

Introduction

The recent evolutionary changes in out-of-hospital medicine began in the mid-1960s in Belfast with the implementation of mobile coronary care units (1). A nurse and a physician responded by ambulance to patients outside of the hospital who were presumed to be suffering from myocardial ischemia or infarction and who were then administered therapy. Shortly after the 1966 National Academy of Science/National Research Council Report on Accidental Death and Disability as "a neglected disease" was published, federal money was allocated and emergency medical services (EMS) systems blossomed in the United States (2).

Despite the tremendous strides made in the delivery of prehospital care over the last few decades, particularly with the care of cardiac and trauma patients (3–5), sparse attention has been directed to the special circumstances surrounding the emergency medical coverage of sports events. Although most athletic teams have a dedicated team physician, spectators almost uniformly become the responsibility of the EMS system in the locality of the sports event.

If the definition of a disaster from an EMS standpoint is an event that results in a quantity of patients who overwhelm the EMS community, most major sports events in this country attract sufficient numbers of spectators to accomplish this goal. A mass gathering (greater than 1000 people) occurs in many cities every weekend for most professional, college, and high school sports events.

It is fortunate that unexpected tragedy seldom strikes major sports events. To date, most reports in the literature regarding the medical coverage of mass gatherings are retrospective and anecdotal (6–9). Only a few reports have actually addressed sports events (10–13); most describe nonsports or natural disaster medical coverage (14, 15). To discuss the medical coverage of sports events, one must include the potential needs of both participants and spectators.

The purpose of this chapter is to review the current understanding of the state of the art of emergency medical care at sports events and to make recommendations about preparedness for EMS systems.

Emergency Medical Care Experience

Perhaps the simplest means of providing medical coverage at sports events is to follow the traditional disaster model teachings (16, 17). With a contained, finite patient population (spectators plus participants), issues such as medical supplies, transportation needs, and health professional staffing would all be predictable. Unfortunately, although the disaster model is seemingly straight forward, this would clearly not be a cost-effective use of health care providers or EMS systems. On the other hand, to deploy EMS services only when some medical emergency develops would not be serving the public needs effectively. The ideal would be to strive for some middle ground.

Some of the earliest reports concerning the medical coverage of large spectator events centered around nonathletic functions. Several authors (7, 9, 18) reported their experiences with medical coverage of outdoor rock music festivals. While most of the emergencies were minor, a fair number were related to drug or alcohol abuse. The cumulative data from the large, outdoor music concerts suggest that up to 1.5% of the attendees can be expected to require medical attention (7, 9, 18, 19). Levens and Durham (19), based on their rock concert experience, recommend health care professional coverage of one physician and six first aid personnel for every 2000 people.

Another nonathletic event report described the necessary medical coverage for a large indoor convention. While the authors described only a small number of patients treated at the life support station, they justified the deployment of equipment and personnel (one or two physicians and one or two first aid personnel per 2000 people) because three potentially life-threatening conditions were encountered and a total of five patients were transferred to a hospital (20).

Expo '86 held in Vancouver, British Columbia, was another nonsports event that was evaluated for the medical care delivery (21). Weaver et al. (21) reported that an average of 3.93 ± 0.95 per 1000 spectators sought medical care and that the number of patients seen was linearly related to the gate attendance for the day. The authors believed that the vast majority (95%) of the medical problems seen were minor, with only a few necessitating physician intervention. Six cardiac arrests were treated (0.3 per million visitors), all initially seen by security personnel trained in the use of automatic external defibrillators.

Sanders et al. (6) studied the level of medical coverage provided at public gatherings in the state of Arizona. A total of 15 facilities that hosted events such as college and professional sports, rodeos, state fairs, and concerts were surveyed to determine the extent of medical coverage. The authors found that medical emergencies requiring both basic and advanced life support interventions occurred at these facilities. The medical coverage provided, however, was variable and often performed by nurses or emergency medical technicians (EMTs) without physician supervision or input. The authors, based on their findings, developed guidelines for the delivery of medical care at mass gatherings (Appendix 19.A) and generally suggested that EMS must be available for both spectators and participants (6).

Other authors, who by virtue of either the EMS system they were affiliated with or the sports event that occurred in their city, have described specific spectator medical coverage. Pons et al. (13), with the Denver EMS system, described their 1978 experience of covering the football season at the Mile High Stadium, which has seating for slightly more than 72,000 fans. For the 1978 season, 298 patients were treated, 35 were sent to hospitals, and 2 were successfully resuscitated from cardiac arrest. The authors provided medical coverage from three first aid stations and noticed that the greatest number of patients were treated during the warmer months of the season (August 12 through October 1).

Thompson et al. (22) and Baker et al. (8) reported their experiences providing medical coverage for Olympic Games. Thompson was involved with the 1988 Winter Olympic Games in Calgary, Alberta, Canada. His medical team (98 physicians, 161 nurses, 337 first aid attendants) treated 3395 patients at 28 advanced life support clinics. For the 4-week period of medical coverage, there were 1.8 million spectator days in both urban and rural settings.

The medical team encountered 1 emergent (highest acuity) and 40 urgent medical problems, with 50 patients transported by ground and 3 patients transported by rotocraft. The authors proposed, based on the low acuity of patients and the availability of an advanced life support ambulance system in the city limits, that physician-staffed teams were not necessary for urban events, but necessary for the rural events (22).

Baker et al. (8) reported on their experiences at the 1984 Los Angeles Summer Olympic Games. The authors set out to evaluate the spectrum of illness, the use pattern, and the role of physicians and other health care providers. The total attendance at the 15 Olympic sites with medical coverage was 3,447,870. A total of 5,516 spectators were evaluated, with 29% requiring a physician evaluation. Of all the patients cared for, spectators made up 56%; athletes, 12%; and employees, 29%; and 4% of the patients could not be included in any particular group. The use rate (number of patient visits per 1,000 in attendance) ranged from 0.68 to 6.8 with a mean of 1.6.

The most common diagnoses made at the 1984 Summer Olympic Games were minor musculoskeletal and dermal injuries (25%), heat-related injuries (12%), and minor gastrointestinal disorders (8%). A total of 91 patients were transported to a hospital. The authors concluded that physicians at the Olympic sites can decrease the number of hospital transports and that educational programs directed at the spectators could perhaps prevent the frequency of such maladies such as heat illness (8).

Rose et al. (11) have recently described their 6.5-year experience of providing emergency medical services coverage for West Virginia University home football games. The stadium seats 65,000 spectators and 313 patients were treated during the 6.5-year period, which included 38 home games. On-site care was provided by 15 EMTs and EMT paramedics, three advanced life support (ALS) ambulances, and two first aid stations. Two EMS physicians were available by pager within the stadium complex. Of the 313 patients treated in their system, 286 (91.4%) received on-site care and 71 (22.7%) were transported to the local emergency department. An additional 27 patients (8.6%) were not evaluated at the stadium but instead presented to the local emergency department. The largest presenting complaint (20%) was lacerations and abrasions followed by bee stings (9%), heat exhaustion (7.6%), and weakness or dizziness (7%).

The authors conclude that EMS with physician coverage of collegiate football games is required and that one paramedic per 5,000 spectators and one physician per 25,000 spectators were sufficient in their system. Furthermore, most of the care delivered at the stadium was for relatively minor medical emergencies. During their study period, only 25 patients received advanced life support care, which included 7 patients suffering from out-of-hospital sudden death, 4 patients with shortness of breath, and 3 patients with anaphylaxis (11).

Sports Events Coronary Care

Although most of the literature reviewed here has suggested that the medical care delivered at mass gatherings tends to be for the evaluation and care of minor problems, all would agree that every EMS system must be prepared to treat out-of-hospital sudden death. Special attention to the resuscitation of patients with sudden death should be a fundamental aspect of all spectator event medical care planning. Table 19.1 reveals the cardiac death rates for several large public assemblies (21).

Kassanoff et al. (10) describe the life support station that was used at the Atlanta-Fulton County Stadium

Table 19.1.
Cardiac Death Rates for Large Public Assemblies[a]

Event	Attendance (millions)	Cardiac Arrest Deaths[b]
Seattle World's Fair—1963	9.6	1
New York World's Fair—1964–1965	51.6	29
Montreal Expo—1967	53	20
Spokane Expo—1974	5.2	0
Knoxville World's Fair—1982	7.2	12
New Orleans World's Fair—1984	5.3	13
Los Angeles Olympics—1984	3.4	0
Atlanta stadium—1966–1970	9.1	13
Expo '86—Vancouver, 1986	22.1	6

[a]Reprinted by permission from Weaver WD, Southerland K, Wirkus MJ et al. Emergency medical care requirements for large public assemblies and a new strategy for managing cardiac arrest in this setting. Ann Emerg Med 1986;18:155–160.
[b]Average rate, 0.6 deaths/1 million attendees.

for the evaluation and treatment of sudden death during the professional baseball season. All the stadium security personnel were trained in basic cardiopulmonary resuscitation (CPR) and were able to communicate a sudden death event with the life support station via a two-way radio system. An emergency patient transport cart was developed from a standard golf cart to transport patients from the spectator area to the life support station. This transport vehicle was equipped with a defibrillator, monitor, and oxygen.

During the 1970 season, eight patients were treated at a life support station, seven of which were believed to have suffered an acute myocardial event; four patients required resuscitation from either syncope or sudden death. Two of the four patients were successfully resuscitated and were eventually discharged from the hospital, one neurologically intact. The authors had access to the data for sudden death for the first five years of the stadium's operation and discovered that for 27 million hours of fan exposure, 13 episodes of cardiac arrest were documented, including the 1970 season. Overall, 23% of the patients were resuscitated. The authors suggest that the low incidence of cardiac death in the Atlanta-Fulton County Stadium begs the question of the cost-effectiveness of implementing equipment and trained health care personnel. If facilities and personnel are already in place, the authors suggest training them in basic CPR (10).

Weaver et al. (21) offer an excellent solution to the issue of effective mass-gathering coronary care. For Expo '86 held in Vancouver, 15,000 employees were instructed in the proper methods to access 911; 800 security personnel were trained in CPR; and in addition, 160 security personnel were trained in the use of automatic external defibrillators. Of the six cardiac arrests that occurred during the 22-month event, two patients were found to be in ventricular fibrillation, were defibrillated, and survived. The remaining patients had cardiogenic shock, electromechanical dissociation, or respiratory arrests secondary to trauma and were not successfully resuscitated.

The authors suggested, based on their Expo experience and the cumulative cardiac arrest data from other mass gatherings (see Table 19.1), that the use of lay personnel trained in the use of automatic external defibrillators is an ideal approach to managing sudden cardiac death at large public assemblies. This would be particularly true if trained health care professionals are not readily available (21).

An unusual cause of sudden death in youth baseball players is noteworthy in this section dealing with coronary care. Commotio cordis is reportedly the single most common cause of traumatic death in youth baseball players (23). Concussion of the heart as a result of being struck in the chest with a baseball results in cardiac standstill. The heart suffers a functional, nonstructural injury and subsequent dysrhythmia from the blunt force of a baseball striking the thoracic cavity. The true incidence of commotio cordis is probably unknown because of lack of accurate reporting. Several case reports of fatal commotio cordis from sports projectiles, such as baseballs, softballs, and hockey pucks, have been recorded in the medical literature (24–27). The U.S. Consumer Products Safety Commission in 1984 published a 10-year report involving 51 children ages 5 to 14 years who died of baseball-related injuries (28). A total of 23 of these children died of a ball impact to the thoracic cavity. Apparently, resuscitation from cardiac standstill as a result of blunt force to the thoracic cavity from sports objects can be resistant to standard ALS therapy.

Sports Events as Multicasualty Incidents

Although it remains true that most of the literature regarding the medical care delivered at disasters or multipatient incidents centers around nonsports or naturally occurring disasters, there have been some reports related to the medical care response at sports event catastrophes. Although the information provided is anecdotal and the incidents are unique, a review of the medical care response is worthwhile.

In 1985, the Keystone Ski Resort in rural Colorado had a collapse of a chair lift, throwing 60 of the 372 passengers to the ground from heights of up to 50 feet. The remaining 312 people were left stranded on the chair lift for up to 3 hours. The initial medical care was delivered by the ski patrol and 12 volunteer physicians and nurses who were present on the slopes (29, 30).

A total of 49 patients were first triaged to the medical clinic at the base of the mountain once immobilization and oxygen therapy were initiated. Transportation was accomplished by snowcat, snowmobile, or toboggan. Once at the medical clinic, advanced trauma life support measures were carried out, including chest tubes in 6 patients with clinically apparent pneumothorax. The other 11 thrown skiers were assessed to have no injury at the scene (29).

It took 10 rotocraft flights to deliver 16 patients to hospitals, and 17 additional patients were transported by ground ambulance. Of the 33 patients transported to hospitals, 26 were admitted, 8 of which needed emergency operations. A total of 7 skiers were treated and released with minor injuries from the emergency departments, and 20 patients were treated and released from the medical clinic at the ski resort.

The authors suggest that the successful triage, treatment, and transportation of these patients from a remote location was possible only because of advanced planning and the participation of the regional trauma system (29).

Another multiple casualty event that occurred at a major sports event took place in Pittsburgh during the annual Three Rivers Regatta Formula I Boat Race (31). This 3-day event in 1988 attracted 440,000 spectators, and 135,000 were estimated to be present on the day of the boating accident. Spectators generally line up on the riverbanks and bridges and sit in bleachers provided to watch the race.

The City of Pittsburgh EMS System, including river rescue teams, and the EMS medical command physicians were stationed throughout the race course area to facilitate access to both spectators and Formula I drivers. Four river rescue teams made up of 3 EMT paramedics each (two of the four teams also had a physician and two mobile and three stationary EMS teams composed of one physician and 3 EMT paramedics each were strategically placed during the race. A total of seven EMS physicians and 27 paramedics were available for patient care. Communication was coordinated through an on-site command center, which was linked to the citywide communication network, including area hospitals.

During the 50-lap race, one of the Formula I boats traveling at approximately 45 mph veered from the racecourse just after a turn and went into a crowd of approximately 800 spectators. The 1100-lb boat came to rest on the shore after striking 24 spectators.

Once the Formula I boat had crashed, the race stopped, and the closest medical team provided an overall assessment of patients and injuries. The physician-directed triage accomplished the initial treatment and disposition of 24 patients to five hospitals (four of which were level I trauma centers) in 32 min. A physician and paramedic accompanied 6 of the 8 most seriously injured patients to the hospital and used interventions such as intravenous catheters and MAST during transport. A total of nine ground ambulances were employed.

Of the 24 individuals injured, 12 were children. A total of 10 were admitted to the hospital, 6 of which required emergency surgery. The average hospital stay was 11.7 days, and there was one fatality. The authors contribute the success they had in expeditious triage, treatment, and transport of these patients to extensive preplanning; availability of adequate personnel, supplies, and ambulances; integrated communication systems; and the presence of EMS physicians for patient triage and treatment (31).

Ellis et al. (32) described their experience of providing medical coverage for the Pittsburgh Marathon in 1986. The 26.2-mile course had 2,900 runners and an estimated 500,000 spectators on an unusually warm (86°F) day with a wet bulb-globe temperature of 78°F. The medical teams at the 24 field aid stations along the racecourse and at the finish line were composed of 54 emergency and sports medicine physicians, 180 nurses, 141 EMT paramedics, 30 podiatrists, and 86 athletic trainers and physical therapists. The medical team had hundreds of volunteers to support its efforts, including records, escorts, and research assistants.

Each field aid station was equipped with ice, oral rehydration fluids, intravenous fluid therapy, dextrose solutions, and rectal thermometers. The oral fluids, medical therapies, and the weather advisory system were in compliance with the recommendations of the American College of Sports Medicine. Communications for the marathon medical team was coordinated through volunteer ham radio operators.

This sports event, coupled with the unusually warm temperature on race day, accounted for an inordinately high number of patients seen by the medical team. A total of 658 (25%) of the runners required medical attention, with 52 (8%) necessitating transport to a hospital. Of the total number of patients treated, 379 (58%) were cared for at the finish line and the remaining runners were seen out on the racecourse, the majority of which (78%) were seen between miles 16.2 and 22.8. A total of 228 runners dropped out of the race for unknown reasons.

The authors conclude that a marathon provides a unique opportunity to practice disaster management, particularly if the weather conditions are extreme. They recommended having 50% of the medical personnel and equipment dedicated to the finish line area and 80% of the remaining personnel and materials at field aid stations every mile between miles 16 and 23. The health care team must be capable of providing advanced life support therapy, including the determination of hypothermia/hyperthermia and fluid electrolyte disorders (32).

Although the potential for a large-scale disaster is always looming at any mass-gathering sports event, one must not neglect the perhaps more common phenomenon of isolated spectator or athlete injury or illness. There are a fair number of reports in the literature dealing with mostly isolated athlete-related injuries from either projectiles or simply from the playing style (33–35). Occular (36, 37), dental (38, 39), and head and neck (40) trauma are common recurring injuries to athletes; particularly those who play hockey, baseball, or lacrosse. There is little if anything written about isolated spectator injuries for those who attend either high-contact sporting events or sporting events with the potential for projectile-type injuries.

Medical Preparedness for Sports Events

Based on what has been reviewed here, it seems that the vast majority of illnesses and injuries seen at sports events are relatively minor in nature. On the other hand, the prevalence of death from cardiovascular disease and the fact that more than half of these deaths occur outside of the hospital necessitate a well-thought out medical coverage plan for sports events.

While it is difficult to recommend one single plan to fulfill every medical coverage need, there are some mainstay fundamental components that should be included in every plan. Other aspects of medical coverage depend to a large degree on the resources, both staff and pecuniary, available for the medical team or advisers. Preparing for the emergency medical care of sports events must be considered analogous to disaster planning.

Leadership

Just as it is true with most organizations, health related or otherwise, the medical coverage of a sports event needs medical leadership. A physician with experience in out-of-hospital medicine would be the ideal leader, but the head of the medical care team should at least be a physician with expertise in sports medicine. There are training programs that offer experience in EMS and others that offer fellowships in sports medicine (41). The medical leadership, although less ideal, could also take the form of a medical advisory committee, which leads by consensus. The medical leadership of some EMS systems are structured in this fashion.

The physician leadership should determine the optimal way to provide medical care at a sports event; based on experience, the current medical literature, and the resources available. The equipment, personnel, and treatment protocols must all be medically sound and subjected to regular postevent review. Event-day information such as weather conditions, attendance, and potential dangers from the sports event itself should all be taken into consideration and be the impetus for change in the medical coverage plan.

Another responsibility of the medical leadership might be to develop educational programs or materials for spectators and competitors to prevent illness or injuries during the sports event. Factors such as lightning precautions, hot or cold weather precautions, and the location of health care within the stadium or park could all serve to minimize the number and type of injuries encountered during the sports event.

EMS Systems Involvement

Every day, EMS providers respond to emergencies of the acutely ill or injured. Prehospital care providers, acting as physician surrogates, perform lifesaving interventions as part of their routine practice. It is critical to involve the EMS system in the locality of the sports event in the medical care plan. The level of commitment will of course depend on the nature of the sports event and the number of participants and spectators.

For large crowds (greater than 1000 spectators) it would make the most sense to have an ambulance dedicated to the sports event with no other outside patient care responsibilities. This ambulance and crew would be responsible for caring for and transporting the participants and spectators who become ill or injured. If the size of the spectator crowd grew, more EMS crews may be committed to the event.

If it is feasible to have an on-site physician involved with large sports events, then the nurses and EMT paramedics can function under direct physician input. In the absence of a physician, the prehospital providers would need to function from protocols that may or may not require communication with the physician before implementation.

The studies reviewed this chapter nearly all reflected a reliance on the EMS system for the successful operation of the medical care team. Whether it be ground ambulance service, air medical service, or a combination of both, it is imperative to have the support and commitment of the EMS system if any medical care coverage plan for a sports event.

In addition, it behooves the organizers of events and the medical leadership providing the care to familiarize themselves with the local EMS disaster plan. It would be of great mutual benefit to hold mock disaster drills in the stadium or convention hall to test the local disaster response and to familiarize the disaster team members with the sports event facility.

Communications

A common theme in disaster literature is the need for fail-proof communications systems (16, 42). When a disaster occurs, multiple public safety agencies are often involved, along with a potential for a heavier communication load for patient issues. Even if a mass casualty event has not occurred, the ability to promptly report and locate a spectator with sudden death is an essential feature of the medical care provided.

The experience of Ellis et al. (32) using the amateur ham radio operators for the medical team covering the Pittsburgh Marathon has proven over time to have been an excellent way to guarantee communications. The ham radio operators serve as spotters along the racecourse, act as communication links between the medical and operational leadership of the marathon, and serve as the key to the success of the lost runner program. Pittsburgh has continued to use the ham radio operators with its medical team, and I can attest to their importance in making the medical coverage work.

Ham radio operators, cellular telephones, or simple two-way radio systems must be integrated into the medical coverage plan of a sports even for the plan to succeed.

Medical Supplies

It is difficult to speculate on the amount and type of medical supplies that will be needed for any given sports event. It would be nice to have an equation that took into consideration the number of spectators and participants and the incidence of certain types of injuries or illnesses and then provided a medical supply recommendation. Unfortunately, no such formula exists, and the variable nature of sports events and the environments in which they occur make the task of predicting supplies almost impossible.

The provision of ALS medical therapies seems to be essential. Physicians, nurses, and EMT paramedics staffing a sports event without ALS supplies could offer nothing beyond basic CPR. Airway equipment, cardiac resuscitation medications and intravenous catheters and solutions are the minimally essential medical supplies. The quantity of each will obviously depend on the anticipated number of patients. For the 1992 Giant Eagle/City of Pittsburgh Marathon, the EMS team kept a running tabulation of the quantity of supplies put out on the racecourse each year, what was used, and how many runner-patients were treated. In 1992, e.g., 320 patients (less than 10% registered marathon participants) were treated along the racecourse or at the finish line. A total of 15 patients received intravenous crystalloid fluid resuscitation, 2 patients received 50% dextrose and water, and 7 patients received both. This, at least, provides some general idea what will be needed from year to year. Generally, the team has overestimated the medical supplies needed each year by a small percent to be prepared for any untoward events.

Medical Personnel

Several authors have attempted to predict the medical personnel needed based on the number of spectators or participants (11, 22, 43, 44). This method does not take into consideration the different types of sports events, the environmental conditions, or the risk of injury from the different sporting activities. These estimates are a place to start, however, when developing a medical care team. Besides the prehospital providers enlisted, the role of physicians, nurses, or other health care providers must be determined.

The City of Pittsburgh Bureau of EMS and the EMS physicians from the University of Pittsburgh provide medical care for the Three Rivers Stadium and the University of Pittsburgh Football Stadium for the home football season. The stadium medical coverage for each facility is responsible for both spectators and participants, although the football teams usually have preidentified team physicians. Three Rivers Stadium has seating for 59,000 spectators while the University of Pittsburgh football stadium has seating for 56,000 spectators.

The medical team for the Three Rivers Stadium coverage consists of two EMS physicians and 10 EMT paramedics, with two dedicated ambulances at the stadium. The EMS physicians and 4 EMT paramedics are stationed in the single first aid room that cares for the spectators almost exclusively. Another 6 EMT paramedics are on the playing field with the primarily responsibility to care for ill or injured players. All medical personnel share a dedicated radio frequency that can be accessed by the stadium security radio communication system. The City of Pittsburgh EMS system can be called on for additional ambulances and EMT paramedic support as necessary.

The University of Pittsburgh football stadium configuration for medical care is similar to the Three Rivers Stadium coverage. Two or three physicians and eight EMT paramedics and three dedicated ambulances are present for each home football game. The single aid station is staffed with one physician and two or three EMT paramedics. The other EMT paramedics are placed in pairs throughout the stadium in positions that provide optimal access to spectators and the participants. A physician will rendezvous with the EMT paramedics to assist in patient care as needed. All medical personnel share a dedicated radio frequency that can be accessed by the stadium security communications system.

Fortunately, there has not been a mass casualty incident at any of the football games in Pittsburgh thus far. The emergency medical care plan described here has served the needs of the spectators and participants extremely well with both basic and advanced life support care delivered. Furthermore, the integration of the plan into the local EMS system has provided excellent reserve EMT paramedics and ambulances when the need has arisen.

Conclusions

This chapter reviewed the current understanding of emergency medical care at sports events. Unfortunately, most of the medical literature is retrospective and anecdotal, thus making it difficult to propose specific guidelines for medical coverage. The information that can be garnered from descriptive studies is useful; however, the paucity of qualitative research techniques in these reports leaves one with merely suggestions.

Planning medical coverage of a sports event is analogous to disaster preparedness planning and as such should include some of the mainstay features. Leadership, communication, personnel, and supplies must all be detailed in any successful medical plan. The machinations of developing an emergency medical care plan for a sports event offers unique challenges that must be met if the public needs are to be addressed. Organizations such as the National Association of EMS Physicians and the American College of Sports Medicine stand to lead the way to the development of policies and procedures for the emergency medical care of sports events.

REFERENCES

1. Pantridge JF, Geddes JS. A mobile intensive care unit in the management of myocardial infarction. Lancet 1967;2:271–273.
2. National Academy of Sciences/National Research Council, Committee on Trauma and Committee on Shock. Accidental death and disability: the neglected disease of modern society. Washington DC: Author, 1966.
3. Ornato JP, Craren EJ, Nelson NM, et al. Impact of improved emergency medical service and emergency trauma care on the reduction in mortality from trauma. J Trauma 1985;25:575–579.
4. Lewis RP, Stang JM, Fulkerson PK, et al. Effectiveness of advanced paramedics in a mobile coronary care system. JAMA 1979;241:1902–1904.
5. Eisenberg MS, Copass MK, Hallstrom AP, et al. Treatment of out of hospital cardiac arrests with rapid defibrillation by emergency medical technicians. N Engl J Med 1980;302:1379–1383.
6. Sanders AB, Criss E, Steckl P, et al. An analysis of medical care at mass gatherings. Ann Emerg Med 1986;15:515–519.
7. Ounanian LL, Salinas C, Shear CL, et al. Medical care at the 1982 U.S. Festival. Ann Emerg Med 1986;15:520–527.
8. Baker WM, Simone DM, Niemann JT, et al. Special events medical care: the 1984 Los Angeles Summer Olympics experience. Ann Emerg Med 1986;15:185–190.

9. Schlicht J, Mitcheson M, Henry M. Medical aspects of large outdoor festivals. Lancet 1972;1:948–952.
10. Kassanoff I, Whaley W, Walter WH, et al. Stadium coronary care, a concept in emergency health care delivery. JAMA 1972;221:397–399.
11. Rose WD, Laird SL, Prescott JE, et al. Emergency medical services for collegiate football games: A six and a half year review. Prehosp Disaster Med 1992;7:157–159.
12. Cribben D, Olvey S, Edwards S. Acute medical care for championship auto racing. Ann Emerg Med 1985;14:249–253.
13. Pons PT, Holland B, Alfrey E, et al. An advanced emergency medical care system at national football league games. Ann Emerg Med 1980;9:203–206.
14. Orr SM, Robinson WA. The Hyatt Regency skywalk collapse: an EMS-based disaster response. Ann Emerg Med 1983;12:601–605.
15. DeBruycker M, Greco D, Annino I, et al. The 1980 earthquake in southern Italy: rescue of trapped victims and mortality. Bull World Health Organ 1983;61:1021–1025.
16. Waeckerle JF. Disaster planning and response. N Engl J Med 1991;324:815–821.
17. Mahoney LE, Reutershan TP. Catastrophic disasters and the design of disaster medical care systems. Ann Emerg Med 1987;16:1085–1091.
18. Chapman KR, Carmichael FJ, Goode JE. Medical services for outdoor rock music festivals. Can Med Assoc J 1982;126:935–938.
19. Levens LK, Durham JE. Pop music festivals: some medical aspects. Br Med J 1971;1:218–220.
20. Meislin HW, Rosen P, Sternbach JW. Life support system: emergency medical care for conventions. J Am Coll Emerg Phys 1976;5:351–354.
21. Weaver WD, Sutherland K, Wirkus MJ, et al. Emergency medical care requirements for large public assemblies and a new strategy for managing cardiac arrest in this setting. Ann Emerg Med 1989;18:155–160.
22. Thompson JM, Savoia G, Powell G, et al. Level of medical care required for mass gatherings: the XV Winter Olympic Games in Calgary, Canada. Ann Emerg Med 1991;20:385–390.
23. Abrunzo TJ. Commotio cordis: the single most common cause of traumatic death in youth baseball. Am J Dis Child 1991;145:1279–1282.
24. Dickman GL, Hassan A, Luckstead EF. Ventricular fibrillation following a baseball injury. Phys Sportsmed 1978;6:85–86.
25. Green ED, Simson LR, Kellerman HH, et al. Cardiac concussion following softball blow to the chest. Ann Emerg Med 1980;9:155–157.
26. Karofsky PS. Death of a high school hockey player. Phys Sportsmed 1990;18:99–103.
27. Edlich RF, Mayer NE, Fariss BL, et al. Commotio cordis in a lacrosse goalie. J Emerg Med 1987;5:181–184.
28. Rutherford EW, Kennedy J, McGhee L. Hazard analysis: baseball and softball related injuries to children 5–14 years of age. Washington, DC: U.S. Consumer Product Safety Commission, 1984.
29. Ammons MA, Moore EE, Pons PT, et al. The role of a regional trauma system in the management of a mass disaster: an analysis of the Keystone, Colorado chair lift accident. J Trauma 1988;28:1468–1471.
30. Nicholas RA, Oberheide JE. EMS response to a ski lift disaster in the Colorado mountains. J Trauma 1988;28:672–675.
31. Vukmir RE, Paris PM. The Three Rivers Regatta accident: an EMS perspective. Am J Emerg Med 1991;9:64–71.
32. Ellis DG, Verdile VP, Paris PM, et al. Medical coverage of a marathon: establishing guidelines for deployment of health care resources. Prehosp Disaster Med 1991;6:435–441.
33. Meeuwisse WH, Fowler TJ. Frequency and predictability of sports injuries in intercollegiate athletes. Can J Sports Sci 1988;13:35–42.
34. Buckley WE. Concussions in college football: a multivariate analysis. Am J Sports Med 1988;16:51–56.
35. Goldberg B, Rosenthal PT, Robertson LS, et al. Injuries in youth football. Pediatrics 1988;81:255–261.
36. Strahlman E, Sommer A. The epidemiology of sports related occular trauma. Int Ophthalmol Clin 1988;28:199–202.
37. Larrison WI, Hersh PS, Kunzweiler T, et al. Sports related occular trauma. Ophthalmology 1990;97:1265–1269.
38. Sane J, Lindqvist C, Kontio R. Sports-related maxillofacial fracture in a hospital material. Int J Oral Maxillofac Surg 1988;17:122–124.
39. Sane J. Comparison of maxillofacial and dental injuries in four contact team sports: American football, bandy, basketball and handball. Am J Sports Med 1988;16:647–651.
40. Frenguelli A, Roscito P, Bicciolo G, et al. Head and neck trauma in sporting activities: a review of 208 cases. J Craniomaxillofac Surg 1991;19:178–181.
41. Paris PM, Benson NH. Education about prehospital care during emergency education residency training: the results of a survey. Prehosp Disaster Med 1990;5:209–215.
42. Haynes BE, Dahlen RD, Pratt FD, et al. A prehospital approach to multiple-victim incidents. Ann Emerg Med 1986;15:458–462.
43. Gerace RV. Role of medical teams in a community disaster plan. Can Med Assoc J 1979;120:923–929.
44. Whipkey RR, Paris PM, Stewart RD. Emergency care for mass gatherings. Postgrad Med 1984;76:44–52.

APPENDIX

CHAPTER 19/APPENDIX A

Medical Care at Mass Gatherings: Guidelines of Care[a]

Objectives for Medical Care

Mandatory

All mass gatherings should have provisions for emergency medical services to evaluate, treat, and transport patients who develop illness and or injuries that are threats to life or limb. The following objectives must be met at all events:

1. Basic first aid and life support should be provided by someone trained to at least the level of basic emergency medical technician (EMT). Basic aid should be available to anyone at the public gathering within four minutes of being taken ill when the site is at full capacity.
2. Advanced life support resuscitation and immediate treatment of acute medical emergencies should be provided within a maximum of eight minutes of anyone being taken ill when the site is at full capacity. This support could be provided by paramedics under medical control or physicians appropriately trained and equipped.
3. The ability to evacuate the patient to a definitive care facility within 30 min.

[a] These guidelines have been approved by the Arizona Chapter of the American College of Emergency Physicians. They are presented for evaluation and discussion. They have not been approved by the national ACEP Board of Directors. Reprinted by permission from Sanders AB, Criss E, Steckl P, et al. An analysis of medical care at mass gatherings. Ann Emerg Med 1986;15:515–519.

Optional

Those sponsors wishing to have additional care available may provide for the evaluation and treatment of nonemergency illnesses and injuries (e.g., sprains, lacerations). This would allow the spectator to return to the event following evaluation and treatment. The following objectives may be provided for:

4. Medical evaluation and treatment for nonemergency problems should be provided by licensed physicians with attention to appropriate documentation on medical records.
5. Triage and medical evaluation of a presenting complaint involves medical judgment as to whether the complaint is an emergency or a nonemergency and recommendations for follow-up. This should be done by a licensed physician with appropriate documentation on medical records.

In order to accomplish the mandatory objectives, 1, 2, and 3, appropriate planning must be done by sponsors with regard to the following:

a. Communication

Adequate communication must be available

(1) to the public—To understand how to call for medical help and what medical services are available within the facility; and
(2) within the facility—Adequate communications between security, medical, and transport personnel so that they can be dispatched promptly to an area of need within the facility; and
(3) with an areawide emergency medical services (EMS) system—Adequate communication with areawide emergency medical dispatch, base station hospitals, additional paramedic units, and the like.

b. Transportation

Adequate transportation and access must be provided

(1) for medical personnel to get to the injured patients; and
(2) for patients to be transported promptly to a definitive care facility.

c. Emergency Medical Personnel

The number and type of emergency medical personnel to accomplish the objectives will depend on the event and facility involved. Factors to be considered when planning for the number of personnel include age of anticipated audience, length of event, density of crowd, movement of crowd, type of event, design of facility, weather, indoor versus outdoor, availability and use of alcohol or other drugs, location of nearest EMS facilities.

Guidelines for Meeting Objectives

Although the number and type of medical personnel may vary depending on a number of factors, the important point is that they be considered adequately in the planning process to accomplish the stated objectives. The following guidelines are provided as one method that sponsors may use to fulfill the desired objectives.

Mandatory Objectives (1, 2, and 3)

In most circumstances the most practical method of providing emergency medical care for potential threats to life and limb is to ensure that paramedics or paramedic/EMT teams are available within the facility. Two paramedics or one paramedic/EMT team for each 10,000 people is recommended. These teams should be placed strategically throughout the facility so they can promptly respond to a communications system call anywhere within the facility.

Paramedics should be familiar with the EMS services available in the area. They must be state certified. It should be noted that paramedics are not licensed to practice medicine. Therefore, in order to provide advanced life support (paramedic) services at events, appropriate arrangements must be made with paramedic provider agencies and base station hospital. Paramedics are not capable of providing the optional services listed in objectives 4 and 5. They should not be treating nonemergency medical problems or rendering medical judgment regarding patient complaints unless they are under the direct supervision of a physician.

Optional Objectives (4 and 5)

If the sponsor wishes to provide the optional capabilities described, the services of a physician are recommended. It must be emphasized, however, that the provision of these optional services (objectives 4 and 5) alone will *not* necessarily accomplish the mandatory objectives 1, 2, and 3 (emergency services for threats to life and limb).

Mandatory and Optional Objectives (1, 2, 3, 4, and 5)

If the sponsor wishes to provide evaluation and treatment of medical problems (objectives 4 and 5) as well as emergency medical services for threats to life and limb (objectives 1, 2, and 3) teams of physicians and prehospital care providers should be utilized. We recommend one to two physicians for every 50,000 people and two EMTs/paramedics or one paramedic/EMT team for every 10,000 people. These teams should work together as coordinated units to provide both the mandatory and optional services. A system of record keeping and storing of medical records is mandatory. The availability of clinical equipment and designated facilities to care for both emergency and nonemergency problems must be provided in order for health care personnel to adequately utilize their skills.

Physicians should be licensed in the state in which the event occurs. Preferably, they should be board certified in emergency medicine; if this is not possible then they should be advanced cardiac life support (ACLS) and advanced trauma life support certified. They must be familiar with the EMS system and base station hospitals in the area.

Registered nurses may be able to aid in accomplishing these objectives. Whenever possible, they should be certified emergency nurses and ACLS certified.

20 / EQUESTRIAN

John Lester Firth

Introduction

The spectrum of sport with horses stretches from the elegant formality of dressage to pit ponies reemployed in mountain trekking and from therapeutic riding for the handicapped to the boisterousness of point-to-point racing. The art of the equestrian is the product of a long evolution since the fist Scythian adventures 50 centuries ago (1). Since then riding has become a deeply implanted instinct close to the soul of men and women. Riding sports are based on a complex mosaic of emotional as well as physical patterns that have been deliberately fostered, were long essential, and are now exploited—with all that the term implies for good and ill—for sport. The emotions aroused continually defy, often refute, and occasionally confound logic.

Basic Features and Training

Despite the diversity of the equestrian scene, basic common features exist. Horse and rider together comprise an asymmetric couple. Arrest of the former transfers energy to the latter and provides a dynamic opportunity for the accelerated, ballistic ejection of the rider from the pair. Horse weighs up to 500 kg and travels up to 65 kph, while the rider's head is poised up to 4 m from the ground (2). The force of a kick, supplied through a steel-shod hoof, exceeds 10 kilonewtons (kN) (3).

Equus ballus (the horse), by selection and breeding, has become a highly effective, highly specialized, and highly stressed creature (4). Although strong and fast, it is full of Achilles' heels, stumbles, and distractions, often the victim of its own specialization. Less intelligent than the dog, the horse has been likened to an autistic child. A simple mind is backed by good memory but no ability to reason. Clear definition must be provided of what is and what is not allowed, while continuous, firm, and instant discipline is essential to establish and maintain a safe pattern of behavior (5, 6).

In the basic riding unit of mount and rider, the horse always has a separate mind, body, and will of its own. The call of the wild remains part of its mettle. "No horse is a safe horse: though some are safer than others" (7). However well broken-in, an individual horse's training is only the beginning of what may or may not, by familiarity and discipline, become a safe and useful relationship with people. In the rider, enthusiasm necessarily precedes, leads, and often exceeds ability and experience. Herein lies the source of many disasters (8).

The horse/rider bond grows for better or worse with time and mutual familiarity and experience. Its safe and successful development requires tight discipline, continuous schooling, and expert supervision of both parties. The pair progresses at an irregular pace, which depends on the individuals concerned. This one-to-one relationship cannot be hurried and is expensive in terms of time, tuition, and surveillance. Its satisfactory development is essential to avoid the "overmounted menace," a prime cause of serious accidents. Training is the basis of safety (9, 10). Unfortunately, accident avoidance by careful development of each pair is a tradition of the steppes that is ill-translated to large riding schools with occasional riders and at which many mounts and riders intermix.

Riding has evoked a complex technology. Primary control of the animal by reins, bridle, and bit is supplemented by secondary communication through the saddle and above all the stirrup, which has a long history (1, 11). Today the stirrup's effectiveness and safety depend on an exact dimensional and spatial relationship between the individual stirrup and individual heeled boot. The heel prevents prolapse of foot and ankle through the stirrup, converting a potential death trap into a system that is accurately located and quickly disengaged (12). It allows rapid "emergency dismounting," a technique that itself requires specific training (13, 14). All of these components, or tack, are highly stressed and rapidly fatiguing structures (15). Each is a disaster waiting to happen. They place the highest priority on routine maintenance and repeated inspection. Habitual premounting and dismounting checks of all tack are essential (15, 16).

Riding styles vary and change, but essentially the rider is mounted in unstable equilibrium above the horse's centers of gravity and mass. This basic instability is partially compensated by knee/thigh grip and the stirrups acting as outriggers. The currently popular jockey-style forward stance predisposes to a forward roll in response to any sudden change of the horse's direction or velocity (Fig. 20.1). The classic style, with feet thrust out and head held high, is often rewarded by a backward somersault compounded by ensnared boots (Fig. 20.2) (12). Whatever the posture adopted, it is a situation of dynamic imbalance and ballistic opportunity. As in the worst features of motorcycle riding, the rider is mounted outside the vehicle. Worse still, that most fragile and important part of the rider, the brain, is mounted at the point of maximum risk, ballistically and statistically, up to 4 m above the ground. In this situation of real hazard, head protection is central to good riding and horse-handling practice (12, 15, 17). The importance of an adequate helmet to both riders and those handling horses was recognized by the Scythians as soon as they had domesticated the horse (1). It is a recognition that, despite major improvements, is still today often conspicuous by its absence (15, 18).

Statistics

Whether recession will stifle the equestrian renaissance of the 1980s in the industrialized world remains to be seen. If so, it will reverse a steady reemergence of riding as a major human activity from a nadir of interest in the mid-1940s. Today in the United States up to 30,000,000 people ride each year (19, 20). The UK riding community exceeds 3,000,000, half of whom are children (21). This paradoxical increase of a horse-dependent sport as the world becomes more mechanized is not confined to the Western nations and is described on both sides of the former Iron Curtain (22).

Accident statistics are difficult to establish and are often incomplete (13, 14, 23–27). Lumped accident rates tend to be misleading. The British Horse Society is made aware of some eight accidents per day involving horses in the UK. More than 10% involve head injuries. Despite the dangers of generalization, what can be said is that sport with horses carries a high participant morbidity and mortality (8, 29–31). Injury incidence has been increasing by about 10% per year in Germany. Whereas a serious incident can be expected at the rate of one per 7000 hr of motorcycle riding, serious horseback riding injury rates exceeding one per 350 hr have been described, making horseback riding 20 times more dangerous than motorcycling (32). Effectively, riding, motorcycling, and automobile racing have been considered the three most dangerous sports (33–35).

When injury occurs it tends to be serious in detail, in time from work, in total cost, and in key personnel incapacitated (6, 18, 36–46). For planning purposes Western European, North American, and Australian neurosurgical services can expect at least one severe riding head injury per month, per million of local population served (32, 36, 47–49). Published figures only record disasters. Details of success, essential to assessing the performance and development of protective headgear, are unavailable. Figures also reflect overall rates, whereas morbidity and mortality vary widely with age and experience. The highest accident rates occur in young and inexperienced children and teenagers, a group in which girls predominate (32, 36, 50–62). They provide an accident incidence that is out of proportion to the numbers involved (59, 63–66).

Any activity with horses involves risk (4, 67–73). As the Arab proverb says, "The grave yawns for the horseman" (2, 49). Despite this, the major proportion

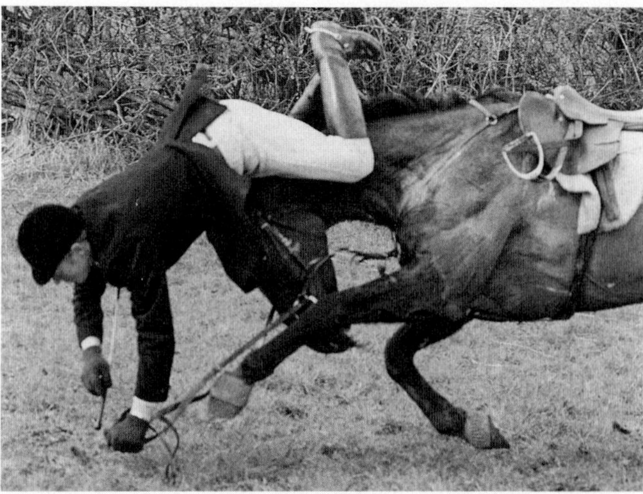

Figure 20.1. A forward role developed from a stumble in forward jockey-style stance. Photo by Stewart Newsham.

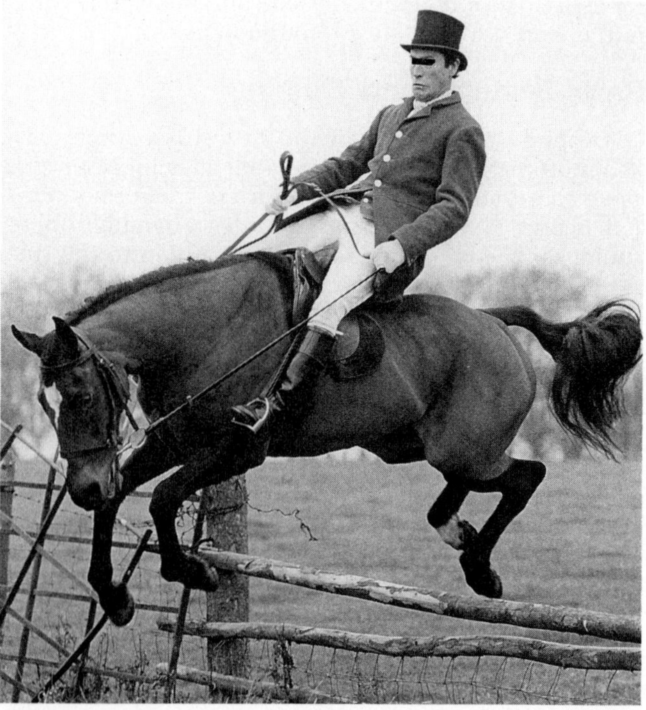

Figure 20.2. The backward roll here develops from a classic-style stance. Well-matched boots and stirrups will prevent dragging by ensuring boot disengagement. Photo by Stewart Newsham.

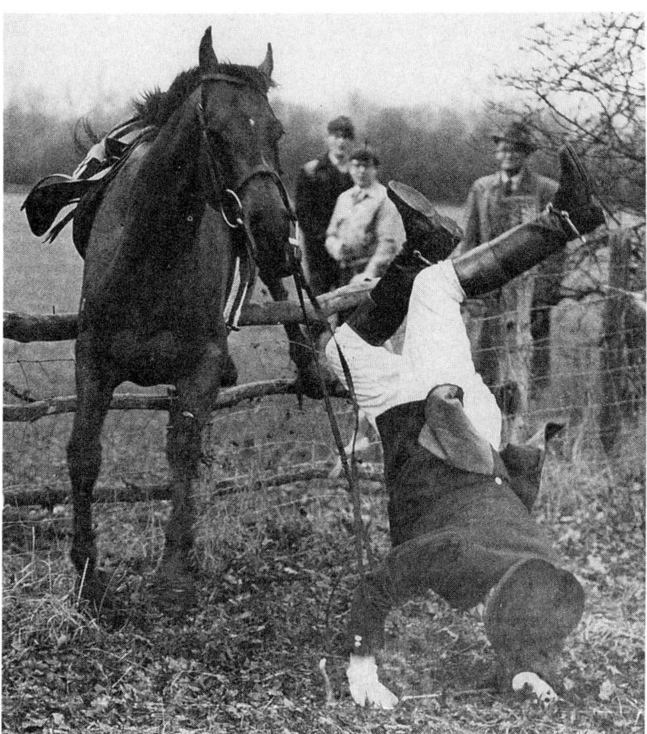

Figure 20.3. This rider is being thrown onto his head and is attempting to protect himself with outstretched arms, a mechanism that frequently results in a fractured clavicle or upper limb. Photo by Stewart Newsham.

of all accidents and severe injuries is avoidable through improved practice and by wearing effective head protection, especially by those in training (15, 56, 58, 59, 64).

Pathology

Trauma

Trauma may be acute or chronic and can be sustained when mounted or on foot. The principal mechanisms of injury are discussed below.

The rider can be thrown onto his or her head and outstretched arm (Fig. 20.3) (2, 36, 64). Secondary spinal—usually flexion—injury is compounded by rotation at the dorsolumbar junction (Fig. 20.4) (74–76). Riders are projected onto and into objects from trajectories starting at 4 m from the ground and at an accelerating initial velocity approaching 65 kph (2).

Rider and horse may behave in Newtonian terms as an asymmetrical couple, abrupt deceleration of the horse occasions simultaneous whole (horse/rider) system energy transfer to the rider who is now provided with an accelerated exit from the situation, accelerating to above the initial whole (horse/rider combined) velocity state. Near-instantaneous increase in rider velocity is imparted about an extended arc or trajectory, which may be tightened with radial acceleration further increased and the vertical (downward) component accentuated by drag from continuing entanglement with horse or tack. This complex, nonaxisymmetric, radial, nonimpact brain acceleration state is further compounded by an unrestrained head on the neck/shoulder in a whiplash motion. Only then does ground strike/head impact occur, the principal interest of head injury studies to date.

The rider may be dragged with repeated, multiple occipital injuries to the head. This is caused by a foot or leg caught in the stirrup, due to failure to wear a matching heeled riding boot (12, 56).

The rider can be crushed or compressed between the horse and ground, with a blunt, or "burst," injury to the chest, viscera, limbs, or head. The injury is caused by the horse's mass of up to 500 kg, which is traveling at variable speed (Fig. 20.5).

The rider may be trampled by iron-shod hooves. The head, ribs, spine, and transverse spinal processes are particularly vulnerable with this type of accident (Fig. 20.6).

Kicks delivered 1 m from the ground by an iron-shod hoof may impact ribs, pelvis, or head. This accident may occur during handling or grooming in confined spaces (77–79). Brown and Silver (3) calculated the minimum forces of such kicks to exceed 10 kN. When 15 cm of shoe contacts the head, it can generate 10 megapascals (MPa) of force, well beyond the breaking strain of most skulls, let alone the brain's energy-transfer envelope (see Fig. 20.6) (80).

The rider may be butted, causing a primary blunt injury to the face and disorganization of the facial skeleton. This may result in mandibular and orbital fractures that require early recognition for successful treatment (81–85). Such injury may be compounded by secondary nasal fracture if corrective eyeglasses are worn; their shattering could cause further facial and ocular laceration. Contact lenses are recommended (86, 87).

An unattractive habit, especially of stallions is biting, which produces compound wounds of the hand, arms, and breasts that are contaminated by *Clostridia* and Gram-positive cocci as well as anaerobes (88–91).

Riders have been scalped while riding without a hat, which is an invitation to entanglement of hair in passing branches (12, 92).

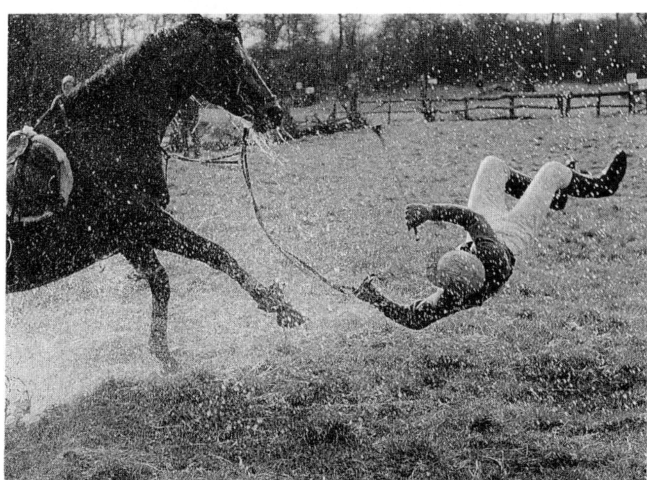

Figure 20.4. When the pelvis and thorax rotate in opposite directions there is rotation at the dorsolumbar junction at impact with the possibility of a fracture dislocation at that site. Photo by Stewart Newsham.

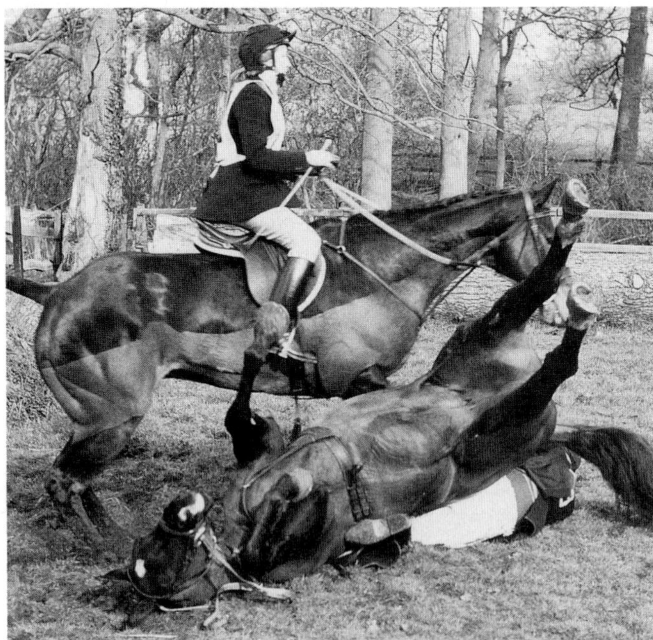

Figure 20.5. A rider is crushed during a race. Note the leg and pelvis of the rider are barely visible under horse. Such crushing is associated with internal injury, pneumothorax, or contusion/laceration of abdominal viscera. Photo by Stewart Newsham.

It is common for riders to have their hands and thighs lacerated and abraded. These injuries rarely call for medical attention (93).

Infection

Pubescent girls who wear nylon and tight pants experience troublesome intertrigo, thrush, and urinary tract infections. Panniculitis occurs in the winter months (94). More serious problems involve tetanus, tuberculosis, brucellosis, anthrax, leptospirosis, histoplasmosis, and salmonellosis. Melioldosis is endemic in Southeast Asia, while rabies poses a hazard to veterinarians during the investigation of its early choking symptoms. As in influenza, humans and horses are end-host targets for the migratory bird-borne group A arboviruses of the equine encephalitides: eastern, western, and Venezuelan. In general, ill-kept stables breed flies. Prevention must be in line with accepted public health practices for tetanus and bacille bilié de Calmette-Guérin (BCG) immunization, stable discipline, and isolation of the horse when practicable, from rodents and other vectors.

Degeneration

Although riding has been blamed for many degenerative conditions, it is likely that the exercise it provides and the restoration and maintenance of the lumbar lordosis that it promotes more than outweigh any deleterious effect on the aged (16). However, spondylosis reduces the mobility of the spine and enhances the risk of spinal injury by focal stabilization and localization of injuring forces and by further reduction of the cross-sectional area of congenitally narrow spinal canals (75).

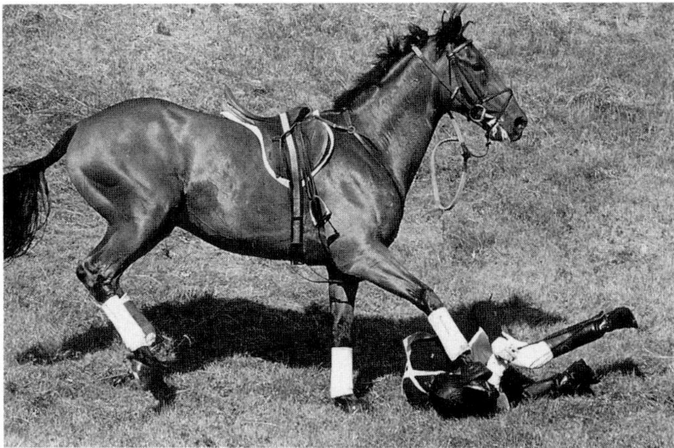

Figure 20.6. This rider was thrown and trampled by the horse while traveling at speed. Note the juxtaposition of hoof and head, guaranteeing serious injury unless protected by helmet shell. Photo by Kit Hughton.

Pathoanatomy

Head

Becker's principal (95) that the proportion of head injuries in a sport reflects the degree of head-forward stance adopted, holds in riding and ensures that head injury complicates much riding trauma (15, 36, 48, 64, 66, 96). Skull penetration and deformation and brain acceleration (linear, radial, and rotational about all three spatial axes), with associated brain tissue shearing, cavitation, and haemorrhage, are all consequences of riding head injury (97). Initial velocities and distances-to-fall in riding accidents provide more than enough energy to exceed all unprotected head tolerances. A fall of <4 m at a 65-kph velocity stretches the capabilities of the most sophisticated head protection systems, as does the kick of an unrestrained hoof to a stationary head. In the past, the cumulative effects of repeated head injury were a major feature of the racing scene, with punch-drunkenness particularly notable among steeple-chasing jockeys (98). Since the early 1960s, aggressive medical surveillance, improved and mandatory head protection, the recording of injuries, and the routine review of the medical status of each rider before each race as well as before the provision of any compensation have greatly reduced this hazard (98–100).

Spine

Spinal injury is traditionally the most feared of riding injuries (41, 86, 98, 101, 102). Racing injuries are usually limited to primary fracturing by direct blows to the spinous and transverse processes, with secondary flexion injuries occasioning stable compression/crush/blowout fractures of the vertebral bodies (41, 74, 75, 100, 103). However, hunting and cross-country accidents can apply any vector to the spine, with hyperflexion, extension, and lateral flexion and rotation (75). In adults, spinal cord injury usually results in actual fracture and dislocation, commonly of the lower cervical segments or the dorsolumbar junction, although spontaneous reduction may have occurred before the time of radiologic examination (75). Odontoid fracture should always be suspect (104). Spondylosis in the elderly enhances these hazards, and spinal stenosis is a complicating factor of acute spinal injury (75). The anatomical peculiarities, mobility, and elasticity of the spine in childhood are reflected by the infrequency of radiologic spinal fracture and the devastating high cervical flexion injuries of those under age 8 (105). Adult-style lower cervical cord injuries occur in the 8-to-16-year-old group, but again, radiologic abnormality may be absent (105, 106). The phenomenon of delayed onset of clinical spinal cord injury is a particular problem in children (105). Initial rapid recovery from immediate motor and sensory symptoms is followed, after a period of apparent normality, by the progressive development of total cord transection. Cord percussion–induced segmental vasoparesis (traumatic local cord blood-flow autoregulatory failure) compounded by sympathoparesis (loss of peripheral sympathetic vasomotor tone due to focal central cord contusion) and consequent systemic hypotension appear to be responsible. Such a child should be kept horizontal until a detailed medical review can be made. Transient, immediate sensory and motor symptoms must be asked for after any child falls from a horse and recognized as of the utmost gravity. As always, it is prudent to presume spinal cord injury after every major incident until proven otherwise.

Systemic

Within the abdomen, ruptured liver and spleen plague the young, while disruption of the aorta and great vessels occurs at any age, although they are uncommon in children. Of intrathoracic injuries, pneumothorax commonly compounds crushing and rib fractures. Of fractures clear of the spine, those of the clavicles (caused by falls on to the outstretched arm) are the most common, limb fractures (arms commoner than legs) are the most painful, and hand and pelvic disruptions are the most troublesome (107). Soft tissue injuries are accepted as commonplace; referral to a physician usually reflects the personality of the individual rider or parents. Skin laceration, abrasion, and superficial cold injury (panniculitis) usually go unreported.

First Aid

Although there are no constant patterns of injuries, there are simple, basic rules of first aid. Good equestrian first aid is founded on a healthy pessimism that each casualty will sustain head, spinal, and visceral injuries compounded by pneumothoraces and internal hemorrhage into both head and abdomen. On-the-spot attention presumes the presence of unstable spinal dislocation and that head, neck, and body must be moved as one unit.

The immediate concerns are

1. *Airway*. To clear and maintain, either by position, jaw protraction, or airway device.
2. *Breathing*. To establish that self-ventilation is adequate and, if not, to institute ventilation promptly by mouth-to-mouth means.
3. *Circulation*. By ECM, external cardiac massage, and/or fluid replacement as indicated with digital control of external hemorrhage.
4. *Detection*. Neurological injuries are the next concern. The level of consciousness is defined and recorded on the Glasgow coma scale (eye opening, speech, and limb movement) (108), and limb motor power (legs as well as arms) is noted on the Medical Research Council (MRC) motor scale (0–5) (109). These are mandatory. Pupil size and reaction and pulse and blood pressure complete the basic recordings required for brain, spinal cord, and systemic injury management. Such injury must be presumed to be present until proved otherwise. Medical Equestrian Association (MEA), Resuscitation Council, and ATLS courses are recommended to provide the basic knowledge and expertise required in initial trauma assessment and management (110–113). A simple observation sheet in the medical officer's bag is invaluable at this stage. Whether megadose steroids or free-radical scavenging should be instituted is a matter of debate.

The next decision is whether the injured rider can be safely left in situ until formal evacuation is arranged or must be moved clear of oncoming danger. In the latter case, the head, neck, and spine are moved as one unit, presuming unstable neck and spinal fractures. Maintenance of the airway and close observation of consciousness level and voluntary limb movement continue. Nothing should be given by mouth, and analgesics should be administered with caution. Any drugs or intravenous fluids given should be clearly recorded on large labels, with details of drug, dose, route, time, and the administrator's identity. The labels are tied to the victim's body and can be used to record serial neurologic observations. Such labels, or better A4 size observation sheets, ensure the immediate availability of this vital information on arrival at admitting hospitals.

That skilled help is available and that casualties can be managed and evacuated promptly to exploit the "golden (first) hour" of injury care require detailed prior planning, a well-practiced organization, adequate personnel, and good communications. In the selection of medical officers, care must be taken to appoint individuals familiar with, prepared for, and practiced in the emergency management of major trauma. The post of chief medical officer is an onerous position with formidable responsibilities (2). Emergency organization for any arranged event has to be defined, agreed on, installed, and practiced from access to potential accident sites to admission to the local neurosurgical unit. The latter should be given long-term warning of arranged events, be alerted of the individual case, and be prepared to receive the potentially disastrous results of equestrian trauma.

The insuperable problem is initial skull penetration, deformation, and acceleration. Here, the key is prior discipline, principally the provision and wearing of effective protective headgear to at least BS4472, BS6473, or equivalent performance level (1, 17, 114). Following head injury, alteration of consciousness, or limb symptoms, no rider should mount again before formal medical review (87, 115, 116). The keeping of individual riding and accident records following the Jockey Club's example, is recommended (87, 100, 115).

Safety

As in automobile use, safety is both passive and active. Prudent riders practice both.

Passive Safety

Passive safety includes tack maintenance, regular inspection, and dress (15). The latter is vital not only for looks and fashion but also for survival. Godiva was culpable in that she did not wear a properly fastened hard hat, although others would add her lack of properly matched boots and stirrups.

Hard Hats: Head and Brain-Protecting Helmets

The purpose of protective headwear is to prevent skull penetration and deformation and to reduce energy transfer to the brain to within the brain's tolerance limits (or envelope). The last is achieved by energy absorption, dispersal, and transfer delay. To be effective, a hard hat must remain properly located on the head at and through impact and remain accurately in position on the head throughout the course of single or multiple head strikes delivered from any direction (17). Movement of the hat on the head may enhance brain injury (117). Loss of the hat before impact leaves no protection at all (118–120). In head injury fatalities caused by riding accidents, many victims wore no head protection at all; in others, the hat was lost before impact because of an inadequate chin strap (Fig. 20.7). In other fatalities, the hat was dislodged or its performance was inadequate. Lack of a well-stabilized, protective hat converts a minor incident into a major disaster. Conversely, the wearing of a fixed effective helmet converts a potentially lethal or maiming accident into a minor embarrassment (10).

The disastrous effects of the lack of head protection are only too obvious (49, 121); the statistics record disasters. Unfortunately, there are few reports of the many successful episodes of head protection from serious injury that can be attributed to the helmet; these events are overlooked and soon forgotten.

To be accepted by the riding community, the hat has to be attractive to the eye; comfortable; convenient to use; cool and lightweight (particularly for children); durable in the face of mechanical, photic, and chemical insult; and relatively inexpensive (18, 107a). Unlike helmets in other situations (such as motorcycling), a riding hat has to be compatible with frequent, rapid head movement, often under considerable acceleration loading. Undistorted hearing and unrestricted vision are essential to the rider, and there should be no fixed protrusions that can snag or catch on passing obstructions, enhancing deceleration, introducing radial head acceleration, and further stressing the cervical spine by forced, head-on-body distortion (107a).

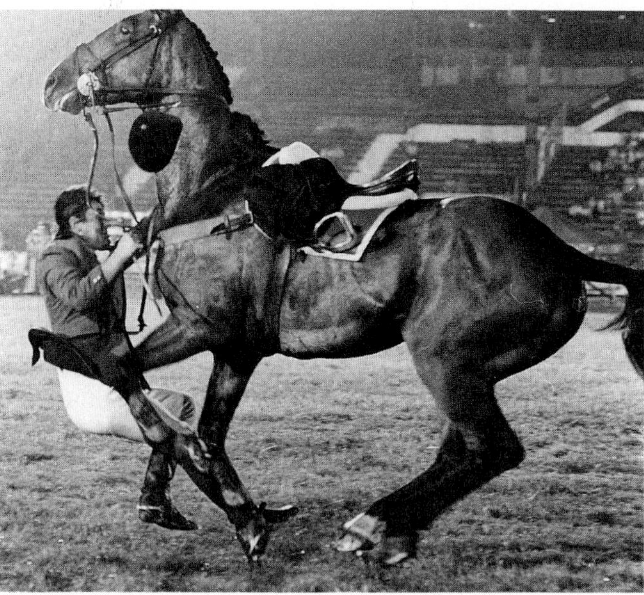

Figure 20.7. Show jumping super ace unhorsed. Note the performance of the "super hat," without benefit of an adequate retention system.

The components of brain-protected riding helmet systems include the following (Fig. 20.8):

1. The nonhomogenous and jellylike brain itself, floating within the cerebrospinal fluid containing subarachnoid space, across which it is irregularly anchored by arachnoidal ligaments, bridging veins, arteries, and cranial nerves to the tough, vascular dura mater that lines the skull and partially divides the intracranial cavity into compartments by its internal reduplication as falx and tentorium cerebelli.
2. The skull, which is a series of hoops and buttresses separated by thin, frangible bone.
3. The suspension system of the hat, ensuring the proper location of the hat on the skull. It must accurately maintain the stability of the geometrical relationship between skull and hat, despite repeated impact, yet be capable of easy release by a third party following an accident. The suspension must transfer energy to the skull buttresses, bridging the intervening pliant sites, and at the same time affording an accurate, comfortable fit for the wearer with adequate cooling in hot weather.
4. The liner may be a structure, a space, or both. It absorbs energy by deformation and reduces acceleration by temporal delay. The transmission of the acute movement of the outer shell to the head is extended in time to reduce peak head acceleration. If the liner is of a progressively collapsible material, then energy also is dissipated by the progressive deformation and destruction of the liner itself. The latter requires replacement of the helmet after such an incident. The continuous introduction of new materials and formats means that liner specification and design deserves continuous review.
5. The shell prevents skull penetration and distortion (45). A contribution to energy dissipation can be

provided by limited shell deformation and partial shell destruction. This should not be to a degree that allows skull deformation and fracture to occur. A smooth, protrusion-free external surface allows the helmet to slide along impact surfaces to allow slow retardation without abrupt arrest, braking, or angular rotation of the head. The area of the head covered by the outer shell should extend down to the level of the superior orbital margins anteriorly, the zygoma and mastoid processes laterally, and the superior nuchal line posteriorly. The last allows for the provision of a posterior cutout to prevent craniocervical or lower cervical fracture dislocation caused by full head extension that impacts the posterior rim of the hat on the cervical spinous processes and provides a fulcrum for head avulsion as was a problem with early American football helmets (Figs. 20.9*B* and 20.9*C*) (122).

6. The outer cover, or "silk," is soft and deformable and allows the provision of an attractive profile and a collapsible peak if required (see Fig. 20.9*A*). The development of collapsible or degradable external

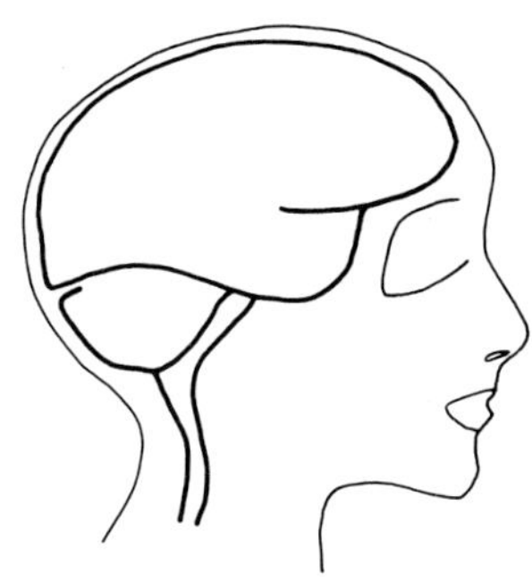

1. Brain : Floating, jelly - like within skull.

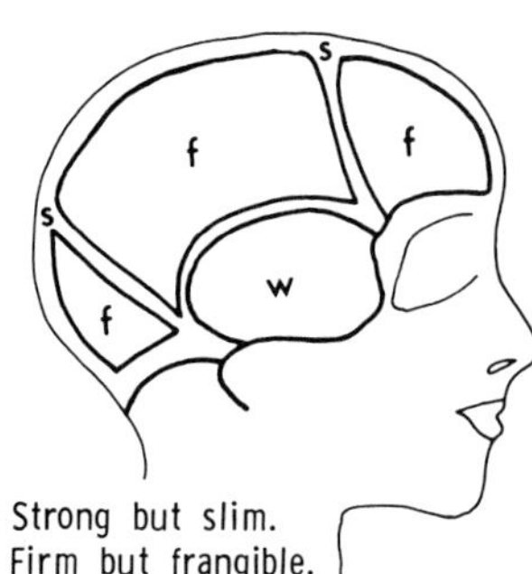

2. Skull : Hoops, buttresses and weaknesses

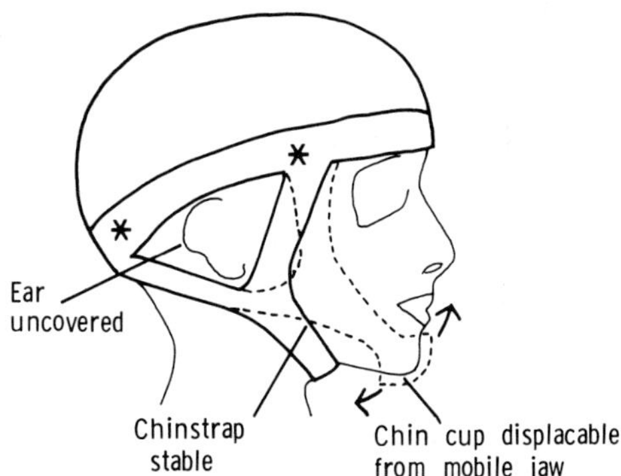

3. Suspension : 4 point system - Accurate, constant yet comfortable location on skull. Ventilation.

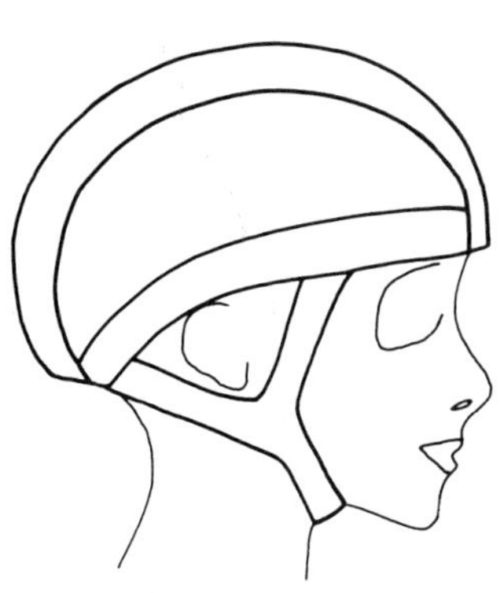

4. Liner : Energy absorption, delay, damping.

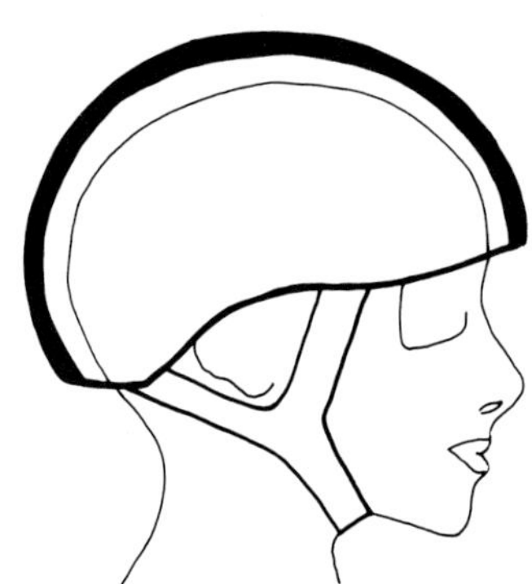

5. Shell : Smooth penetration / deformation resistance. Some contribution to energy dissipation.

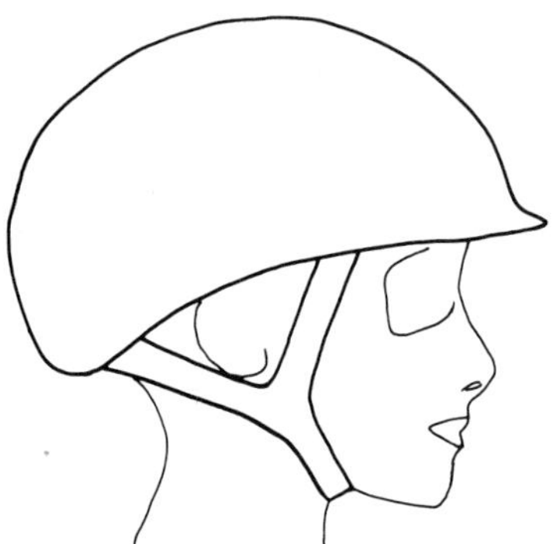

6. 'Silk' or Cover : Aesthetics

Figure 20.8. Components of hard hat and head protection systems. See text for details.

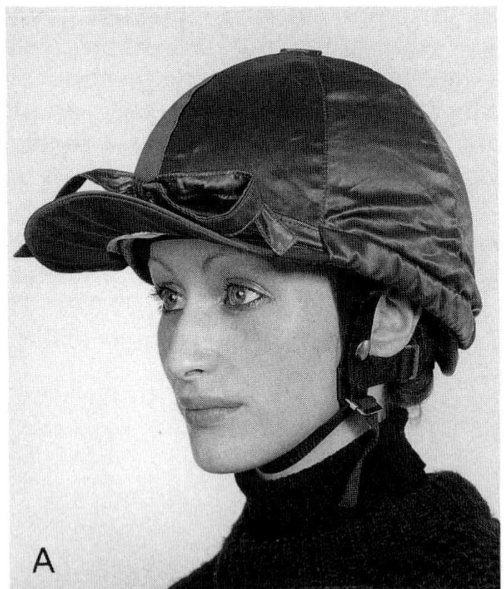

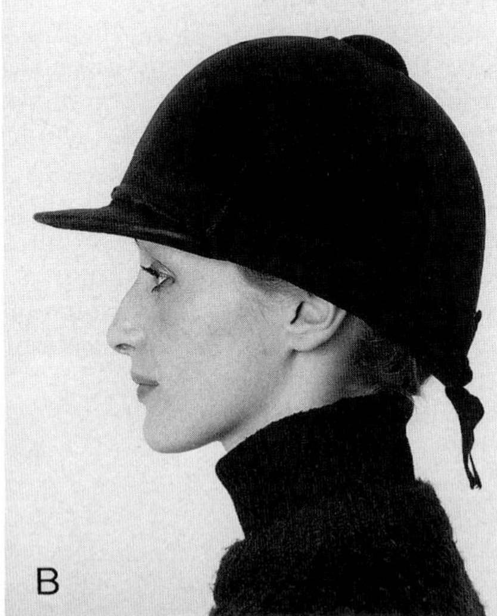

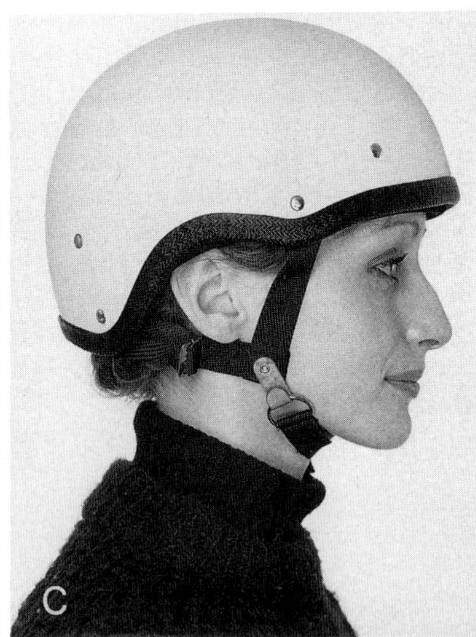

Figure 20.9. **A,** BS4472 complete with silk. This hat remains the state of the art with an at-present acceptable appearance. Note that the suspension is adjusted to maintain auditory acuity. The chin strap is preferred by many, although others favor a chin cup. Photo by Department of Medical Illustration, Derbyshire Royal Infirmary, UK. **B,** BS3686 riding cap. This withdrawn specification provided good protection from vertical blows, but lacked adequate head retention (see Fig. 20.7). **C,** Lateral view of a BS4472 jockey skull without a silk. Note the accurate location by the four-point fixation system and posterior cutout. Photo by Department of Medical Illustration, Derbyshire Royal Infirmary, UK.

outer liners (outside the shell) is under active study in the light of the acceleration protective performance achieved by soft cycle helmets.

The many component variables in helmet systems have led to the availability of a wide range of designs. Unfortunately, appearance is no guarantee of performance. Bitter experience over many years and the initiative of Brigadier Teacher and The Pony Club led to the promulgation of minimum performance specifications by the British Standards Institute (BSI) (2, 98). The original 1963 specification of BS3686 (now withdrawn) provided the popular riding cap that was subsequently modified to remove the rigid peak (see Fig. 20.9*B*) (123). Since July 1, 1983, U.S. Pony Club members have been required to wear a hat approved by the National Organization Sports Committee on Athletic Equipment (NOSCAE) (124, 125).

Further progress and better designs have followed (7, 9, 126). BS4472 produced the higher-performance jockey skull (127), and BS6473 produced the general-purpose, all-day/all-weather hat that in practice has a similar performance (128). Although both designs have their critics, if correctly worn at impact, both provide a high degree of protection, and national and international governing bodies of the equestrian disciplines have introduced appropriate requirements for the use of helmets meeting national and European standards. Regular development means that hats made to BS4472 have reflected the state of the art in the application of head injury biokinetics, available materials, manufacturing techniques, and marketing economics. The BSI committee responsible for helmet specification represents all interests, is sensitive to enthusiasm, and is receptive of new ideas.

Performance is expressed in terms of penetration and deformation resistance, energy transfer through the vertex and superior aspects of the helmet as measured from free fall onto an anvil, and hat retention by the chin strap system. A major area of concern is the frequency of low anterior, posterior, and lateral head impacts in actual practice, a matter not yet addressed adequately by the various specifications (60, 129). This and the need for further shell rim extension laterally (130), the form of cutout posteriorly, improved energy-absorbing materials, designs and composites, and more realistic testing methods are under active review. Protection against lateral impact remains particularly difficult to provide with an at-present aesthetically acceptable shape and size of helmet (Fig. 20.10). As in military practice it is likely that helmets will have to be wider. This in its turn will be a further challenge to fashion and design. Concern over apparent failures of helmets produced to present specifications coupled with changing consumer priorities have fueled a demand for change and a further improvement in helmet performance (44, 58, 60, 119, 131). However, major obstacles to progress persist, including the imperfect, though improving, relationship between head injury computer modeling and clinical experience (132), inadequacies of the Wayne State Trauma Curve (which related head acceleration, time, and brain tolerance to impact, the bases for many present designs) (133), and the still ill-understood brain acceleration–tolerance envelope and its relationship to head injury criteria (HIC) (134–137). It is hoped that rapid progress with echoplanar real-time and fast magnetic resonance imaging may soon add further light to the relationship between brain movement, head injury vectors, and the brain's intolerance of impact.

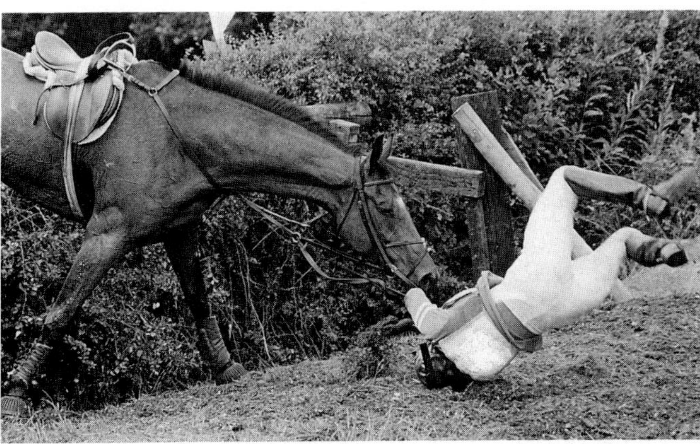

Figure 20.10. A major shortcoming of the present specifications and an area of principal concern and investigation. Photo by Kit Hughton.

Properly Matched Heeled Riding Boots and Stirrups

Riding boots protect feet, ankles, and shins and splint tibiae and fibulae through gates and in collisions. They must accurately fit the individual stirrup used. The heel prevents the foot and ankle prolapsing through and being trapped by the stirrup—the prerequisite for being dragged (12). Although a major innovation in its time, the stirrup, if not matched to the boot, is a death trap (56). Nonslip insteps help, but safety stirrups unlike safety bindings in skiing have yet to prove themselves. In junior events all too often they are tied up and locked by external binding. The requirement that they should not work during competition and times of stress reflects a confusion of priorities in pupil and instructor alike. The principle of detachment beyond a tolerance limit is attractive, but whether this represents a practical improvement over a well-matched stirrup and heeled boot remains to be confirmed.

Other Safety Considerations

Clothing. Appropriate pants reduce chaffing and enhance the comfort and adductor control of the novice. Gloves should be nonslip (often string-based), and a fitted, padded jacket may reduce inadvertent ensnarement in undergrowth and provide cushioning in falls (12, 138). Better still, Kevlar-plated "body protectors" cushion soft tissues and protect ribs and spinous processes when kicked or when falling and rolling clear after being unhorsed (87). They also improve the young rider's confidence to practice and be prepared actively to disengage and roll clear of horse, recognizing the inevitable early on in an emergency, rather than hanging on regardless as an accident develops into a disaster.

Exuberant Hairstyles. The present penchant for exuberant hairstyles provides ready opportunity for being scalped when riding in wooded country. In addition, the rider's attention may be diverted in critical situations by hair in the eyes. Adequate hair restraint, if necessary by a net in either sex, is essential when riding in critical situations, particularly on public roads, near vehicles, or through broken country (12, 92).

Glasses. The wearing of eyeglasses is an open invitation to nasal fracture or facial or ocular laceration by a blow from the horse's neck. Contact lenses are preferable and are mandatory for racing under Jockey Club rules, by which an identity disc recording the fact has to be worn (87, 115).

Active Safety

Active accident prevention begins with sound, basic training and continues with the specialist training of horse and rider (139, 140), responsible course construction (141), and adequate casualty preparation (2, 142).

Now that governments or agriculture rules the steppes and grasslands of the world, few people are raised on horseback. Able horsepeople are trained, not born. Good habits start young. There is no substitute for good example and sound schooling, continuity, and adequate supervision based on a structured syllabus (143). There are many roads to Rome, but each horse/pupil pair proceeds at its own pace. In the West, no legally binding constraint, laws, or regulations exist, but advice and example abound. The growing literature and the formation and activities of the Medical Equestrian Associations are indications of increasing medical interest and concern (7, 110, 144, 145). An international example of constructive education is provided by The Pony Club (116). In France, The École d'Equitation at Saumur serves a similar, if more centralized, function. Its instructor corps, the Cadre Noire, by practice and example provides teaching and training as well as supporting the international competitive activities of the French Equestrian Federation. In the United States, the U.S. Pony Club and instructors' organizations alike provide guidance and leadership (7, 20, 146–148).

For the rider, safe practice (that is, keeping out of trouble) must become automatic. Habitual wearing of a hard hat (17); caution over concussive injury; rapid disengagement; and the ability to fall safely, comfortably, and confidently from any speed, situation, and attitude are most enjoyably learned as a child (101). The need for practiced, rapid, and confident emergency dismounting has been stressed (149). The early recognition of inertia and the inevitable; the use of time; and the technique of discarding the reins, clearing the stirrups, clearing the horse, and rolling clear are again best learned when the individual is small and the acquisition of new motor skills is easy (Fig. 20.11) (138). In Japan the latter is an athletic extension of the martial arts. Sadly, falling practice—using horselike falling machines equipped with reins and stirrups that allow progressive pitch, roll, and yaw at variable heights above foam landing areas—has yet to gain acceptance (41).

Riding schools are the breeding grounds of safety or disaster. They are the foundation of riding's future for good or ill (41). A poor example set by indolent teachers wearing no more than soft caps are all too often the rule (13, 14). No licensing and no legalized supervision

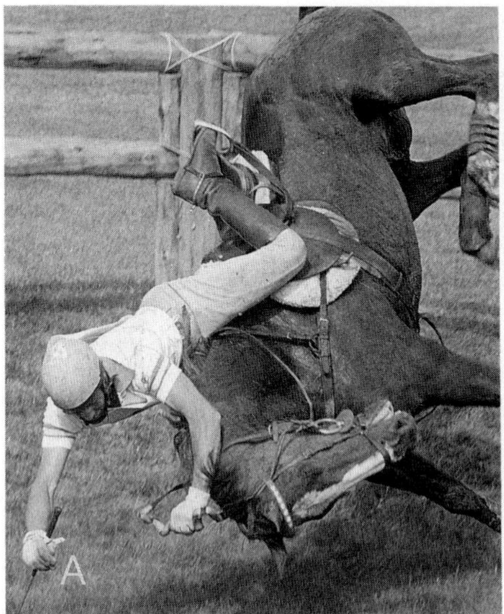

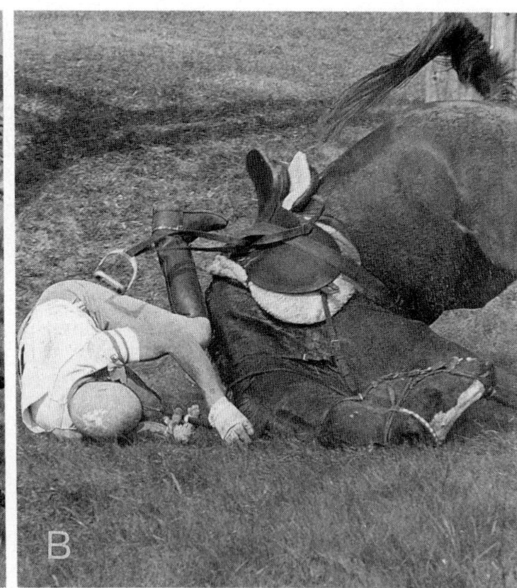

Figure 20.11. **A,** Emergency disengagement from stirrup and horse begins. **B,** Emergency disengagement continues with a roll-clear posture developing. The crown of the BS4472 hat suggests previous incidents. A replacement is recommended after any major incident or helmet impact. Photo by Kit Hughton.

of teaching standards and practice exists. Local government interest is limited to matters of sanitation and building structure. However, change is coming through the courts due to the application of national and European employment legislation on mandatory worker and employee protection. Preparation provided for riding on public roads, where the horse is more dangerous than a sports car or motorcycle, is still inadequate. UK legislation now requires the wearing of protective helmets by children on public roads. In other respects, once out of the paddock, the horse is operated like any other vehicle, yet the rider is untaxed, unlicensed, unrestricted, and untested. This is a position of privilege that is often abused and an invitation to political restriction that the riding community invites at its peril. Unless care is exercised, the efforts of the pony clubs, horse societies, the many excellent schools, and numerous responsible individuals will be jeopardized by the arrogant, ignorant, and irresponsible few.

Equestrian Diversity

Once basically trained, the sport-riding enthusiast is confronted with a confusion of opportunities. Hacking, simple riding for recreation and pleasure, is the commonest practice and also the greatest source of serious injury (46, 56, 59, 64). Children are frequently allowed loose on public roads, often without so much as bicycle training. Compounded by the horse's fear of the mechanical, thoughtless drivers, and worse riders, it is the circumstance in which the unwitting novice is most frequently undone. Youthful inexperience, naïveté, lack of supervision, multiple distraction, and a disinclination to wear hard hats suitably secured have all played their part. Fatalities even among experienced horsepeople have highlighted the problem, and the introduction of mandatory head protection in high-profile, media-oriented disciplines like show jumping has had a beneficial effect. Meanwhile, public incidents have impressed on official circles the need to provide effective head protection in formal headwear for ceremonial occasions. Paradoxically, most ceremonial headwear began as military protection devices, their origins and primary purpose being degraded over the years by fashion. It should not now be beyond the aesthetic wit of the skilled designer to combine appearance with a restoration of protective function.

Trekking combines unknown mount and rider with rough country and long range. Docility of the mount and the progressive adaptation of the rider are basic to success. A walking pace and avoidance of the animal's hindquarters are principal precautions, while the potential medical complications of an unfit population exposed to unaccustomed exercise under arduous conditions have to be kept in mind. Distances are eventually limited by thigh chapping, adductor spasm, ischial bursitis, and lordotic loss.

Racing may be long-range, cross-country, or over formal courses. Long distance (endurance) events involve up to 50 miles at an average speed of 8 mph over designated routes against the clock and under observation. Local competitions culminate in annual national championships. Both sexes are equally represented. British Horse Society Endurance Riding Group Rule 25 requires the wearing of a protective hat to BS4472 or BS6473, securely fastened (150). Despite the progressive extension of distances during a year's events, when fatigue must play a part, the disasters that might be expected have not occurred. This probably reflects the age and experience of competitors and mounts, adequate head protection, the nature of the routes adopted, and low average speeds.

Course racing, "the sport of kings," differs from much else in riding in that large sums of money are involved. High stakes demand fair play and high standards (151). Parliamentary and governmental interest and surveillance are more than a hangover from the enthusiasms of Charles II. Self-regulation is the key within a legal framework in which safety is accepted as being in the interests of all parties concerned. Racing is practiced as two major disciplines: on the flat or over fences and point-to-point. The ruling authority is the Jockey Club. Its famous carpet at Newmarket and its Rules of Racing and Instructions are backed by the services and activities of a full-time medical consultant and a standards inspectorate led by a senior steward of the club. Publications include provisions for medical attention at racecourses and an accident survey. While racecourse authorities are required by act of Parliament to report all serious injuries, the Jockey Club operates an annual licensing system of all individuals professionally involved: trainers; jockeys; and stable hands alike. This is kept under continuous review.

A jockey's license requires an initial medical examination by the individual's general practitioner, reinforced by an annual medical examination by Jockey Club medical officers for jump jockeys who are over 35 years of age and flat-race jockeys over 40. The jockey skull protective helmet made to BS4472 must be worn and appropriately fixed by jockeys and handlers during all events under Jockey Club rules. Lightweight Kevlar body protection against direct injury is recommended.

Each individual jockey, whether professional or amateur, operating under Jockey Club rules has to carry and keep a personal medical record or log in which all accidents are recorded in red. An accident's place, time, and details, together with medical observations and recommendations, which may include suspension for an appropriate period, are all entered. Before each meeting, all intending jockeys' logs are reviewed by the course medical officer. Only then is clearance to ride in the races that day provided. A jockey cannot ride again after an accident without formal medical review, appropriate clearance, and the red entry in his or her record. Suspension for a minimum of 21 days is customary following skull fracture or a period of unconsciousness. All injuries are referred to the various compensation funds, where the individual's records are again reviewed for possible cumulative injury (87, 100, 115, 152).

As well as head protection and good riding practice, perceived safety factors in racing are meteorologic and surface conditions; numbers at and the mechanics of the start; the construction of courses, slopes, fences, and rails; the procedures for saddling up; and returning from the finish. These concern the Race Courses Association as well as the Jockey Club. The provision of ground-aiming lines at fences, their siting, background, construction, and slope and the prevention of horses running under them have all undergone progressive development (153).

Various safety rails (Fig. 20.12) have been introduced (154). The traditional sloped wooden rail was easily splintered on impact by horse and rider. The use of fences, which replaced it, and the metallic gooseneck post provided the disengaged jockey with protected areas. However, the solitary rail barrier often fractured and the Fontana gooseneck rail was developed with a plastic trampoline-style top to throw the jockey into the central field rather than back on to the track. Though plastic rail construction is superficially more attractive than wood or concrete, plastics may suffer low temperature splintering, enhancing their hazard as foreign bodies. However, in initial experience with the Fontana rail, splintering was not a major problem.

Video or film recording, often from several angles, is made of every race run under Jockey Club rules and preserved in a central archive. These allow both instant replay of disputed races and later review of incidents of concern. With many runners, however, precise analysis may be difficult.

In the past paraplegia and tetraplegia, repeated injury, and the specter of the punch-drunk jockey were all features of the racing scene (99, 155). The introduction of the above series of mandatory safety measures has led over the last 25 years to a progressive decline in the incidence of serious injury and disablement, without any decrease in the quality, competitiveness, or excitement of the races (2, 98–100). Racing provides an example of major problems openly recognized, continuously reviewed, and progressively contained that

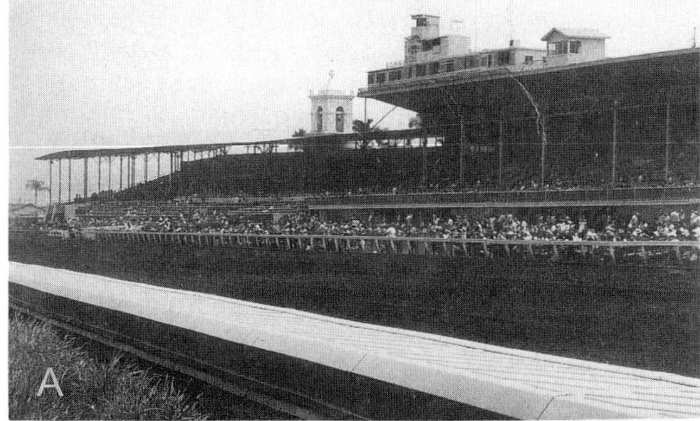

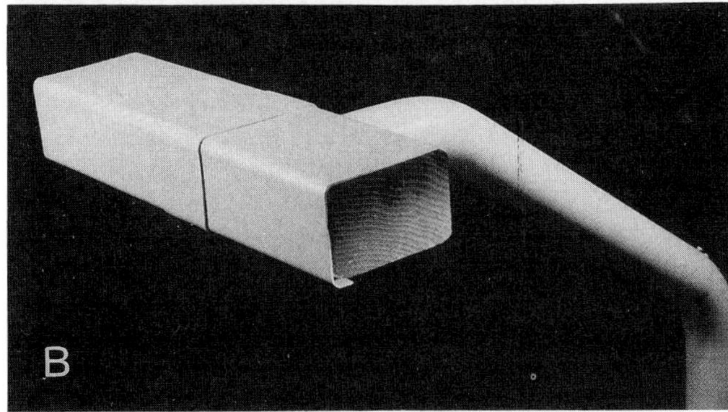

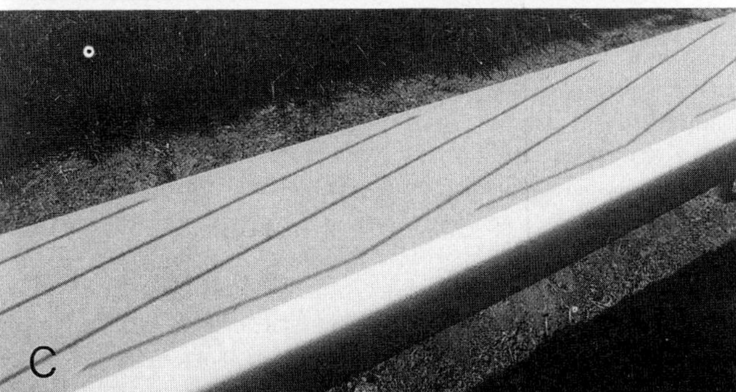

Figure 20.12. Safety rail developments. **A,** Fontana safety rail as introduced. **B,** Patterning to throw jockeys to the in-field section of the track. **C,** Plastic-covered Rovel goosenecked rail.

could be followed with advantage by many other disciplines (100). In the UK, the role of the Jockey Club is now under review. Whether any alternative system or organization could match this record remains to be seen.

Show jumping is variously described as the acme of gilded individualism or the home of the superego. As the art of surmounting any obstacle on horseback in public, it earned a reputation for individual intransigence and irresponsibility through the arrogant and public disdain for head protection displayed by a minority of the leading competitors. Through the mass media and television coverage this exercised a malign influence on those both most susceptible to example and most at risk: young, naive, vulnerable, and inexperienced riders. Within the sport, however, there are >300,000 competitive entries per year. Training, selection, and occasion all produce a high degree of professionalism. Jumps are designed to be jumped, and the raising of the hat in the ring, the excuse for not wearing a chin strap, is not mandatory. In practice, low accident rates reflect the precision, control, and relatively low speeds required, although accidents are not to be expected among those proficient enough to compete. It is among those practicing and those whose ambition is to show jump that the major dangers lie. Several schools of thought on head protection exist within the show-jumping community. Some are concerned with the possibility of involuntary autosuspension by inadvertent head arrest between tree branches, although such an incident has not been reported since biblical times (62). From that report, it appears to be have been just as uncomfortable and certainly more dangerous to be bareheaded. Others insist that chin straps cannot be immediately released by a third party after an accident. However, unlike the relative stasis of the rider's position in dressage, show jumping in particular, like most riding in general, involves continuous head movement, under pronounced head acceleration. This militates for better, not less accurate, hat location. Despite these objections and the difficulties of showground policing, the British Show Jumping Association's Rules 101.3, 101.4, and 267 insist on the wearing of protective headgear, although anomalies persist (156).

The acceptance of major public support, adulation, and the invitation to emulation, which present-day show jumping involves, all bring with them a degree of public responsibility, in the face of which the irresponsibility of a few has rightly been deplored. Nevertheless, their behavior should not deflect attention from the contribution and example of the many leading riders who do wear full head protection and from the many up-and-coming competitors who follow this good example and whose behavior in public is beyond reproach.

Dressage is where sport and art consort to display the full athletic potential of the horse. It is a gymnastic dance form with horse. Of mounted and dismounted forms, the latter is not widely practiced competitively. Mounted dressage involves set patterns of maneuvres on the spot; in a circle; and at the walk, trot, and canter. Relatively low speeds demand the highest precision that, with the habitual wearing of hard hats by grooms, is responsible for the present absence of competition injury. Dressage Group Rules in the UK require a hard hat, but mandatory BSI-standard protection is not compulsory other than in a show jumping phase (157). The result is the impression given through the media that elegance precludes prudence. Although falls and handling injuries are rare, low backache is experienced by a majority of competitors. Poorly described, this is considered anecdotally to reflect the loss of lumbar lordosis, characterized by the riding styles of this discipline and compounded by the continuous demand for extreme pelvic mobility.

Horse trials and eventing involve a series of sections—dressage, speed, and endurance on road and track; steeplechase; cross-country; and show jumping. They are designed to test horse and rider to the limit, both as individuals and as a team in a variety of situations. The intentions of some constructors of international courses in the past has been questioned. Remote and complex cross-country sections are full of distractions and pose hazards to both riders and their medical attendants alike. But best course design and construction aim to provide obstacles with a variety of routes through them from easy but time-consuming to difficult and direct, which are spectacular and demanding but still possible to jump and as safe as is compatible with the spirit of competition. They must be capable of being swiftly dismantled in an emergency. Cross-country course design and fence construction reflect progressive development. A considerable literature is now available from the British Horse Society (158). Grooms and competitors have long worn protective headwear as routine. A significant exception is that while in the British Horse Society's and the riding clubs' horse trials BSI standard hats are mandatory throughout (159, 160), the archaic convention that hard hats may not be worn "where correct dress allows otherwise (i.e., military service dress cap for dressage work only)" lingers on in international competitions, allegedly to facilitate foreign and military participation rather than to foster local dissent. The common aberration is the use of BS4472- and BS6473-style hats for show jumping and cross-country and hard hats without chin straps for dressage, as allowed by the dressage rules (157). The impression given through the visual media is again to promote the social acceptability, even desirability, of unsecured and inadequate head protection. In practice, a high level of individual competence, the widespread wearing of effective helmets properly located and the relatively low speeds involved have limited the traumatic outcome of many spectacular incidents, but fatalities and serious injury continue to occur.

Further progress lies in careful accident review; continuing present policies of development in training and course construction; and in the provision and conspicuous, universal wearing of appropriate helmets of ever-improving performance. Even military personnel are expensive and nondisposable "items" to their countries' taxpayers. The military brain is in no less need of protection, and the elimination of this expression of equivocal attitudes to head protection would make a major impact for good, through press and television, on the young emulators of eventing's stars.

If the "grave yawns" for the rider in general (2, 49), then in hunting the graveyards are wide open and much frequented. In many areas, fox hunting became a fashionable pursuit in which appearance counted for more than reality and rumor more than fact. Imperfect mount/rider bonds; the distraction of numbers, rough country, variable conditions, individual euphoria, and crowd hysteria; the widest variety of rider fitness, age, competence, experience, and practice; opinion tempered with alcohol; and frequent total disregard for the basic tenets of prudence and safety all combined to produce facets of equestrian behavior in comparison with which the more ludicrous excesses of the motorcycle maniacs and rodeo riders appear as sweet examples of good sense (161–163). Hot blood, the primitive thrill of the chase, herd instinct, pride, competition, occasion, and the opportunity to throw every frustration to the wind provide ready explanation for the strength of feeling generated by any hunting matter. The baleful effects of these attitudes can still be seen in the mortality and morbidity rates of a broad socioeconomic group that owes much to and elsewhere has much to contribute to society at large. In hunting, any disaster can and does occur. For the eager and malleable novice, the few poor examples in show jumping are here reinforced by daily exhibition of bad practice and worse sense. Although too often in the past this has been the English scene, it is not universally so. Good hunting is enjoyed in Virginia and the Carolinas where prudence, sense, and habitual effective head protection in no way distract from the furor of the chase, but leave a clinical spectrum of injury incomparably less disastrous than the experience of many British accident departments (15, 47, 164). However, progress in the UK has been made. The Prince of Wales' example, hunting in an effective hard hat appropriately fastened, heralded a new era in which hunting in the UK may yet reflect the best North American practice. Despite this, hunting continues to present a major obstacle to those who counsel progress by consent rather than coercion. The day when a head protective device attractive to the hunter appears will mark a major step forward in the mitigation of equestrian injury.

In polo, prudence promotes enthusiasm. Well-located head protection is mandatory. Knee, knuckle, and shin protection is the rule, and face masks are commonplace. The game and the performance of polo helmets display continuous evolution. The Hurlingham Polo Association (HPA) provides an annual review of the state of the game and the development of its rules, which are published in a yearbook. This is backed by umpiring directions and notes for umpires and officials. Although ferocious to the eye, intelligent and constructive competition has minimized injury while enhancing both competitor enjoyment and spectator excitement. The HPA Rules of Polo frame the various aspects of safety on and off the ground (165).

In tetrathlon, an equestrian cross-country course under Pony Club rules is added to air pistol marksmanship, cross-country running, and distance in set time swimming sections. The rules, as in all Pony Club–associated events, include mandatory head protection and prohibit further competition on the same day following a concussive injury and at any further time without certified medical clearance (116).

Following ancient precedent, riding for the mentally and physically disabled continues to expand and encompasses both recreational riding, in which the disabled individual is in control, therapeutic riding, and equestrian-enhanced physiotherapy or "hippotherapy." Enthusiasm is matched by steadily improving techniques and benefits. From small beginnings in the early 1960s, programs allowed 25,706 disabled individuals (of which 16,183 were children) to ride by the end of 1992 in the UK alone. A total of 723 self-supporting charitable, local groups combine through 18 regions to form the Riding for the Disabled Association. Although nothing can replace local initiative, central organization has a place in this developing field, if only to ensure that each new group has the advantage of building on the communal experience of the rest. All forms of disability are involved, and the basic tenets of this activity are covered in the association's introductory booklet, pamphlets, and annual reports (166).

Of the nonriding equestrian sports, in-hand showing of breed and show classes combine the training dangers of long reins and control from a horse's rear with distraction and assault by the horse when least expected during exhibition (93). Most shows depend on good weather and summer's heat for their success, the least comfortable conditions for presently available, hot and heavy protective hats. A cool, well-ventilated hat is a prime requirement. Horse-driving trials (represented in the UK by the Driving Trials Group of the British Horse Society) are a developing vehicular activity judged on presentation; dressage; cross-country; marathon; and closed arena-based, cone-defined obstacle sections. Events are designed to test driver, groom, trainer, horses, and vehicles alike. The apparent lack of serious injury reflects customary head protection on foot and due caution in the driving of complex and expensive carriages. The emphasis is on skill and precision, rather than brute speed (167). Trotting is a long-established major activity akin to flat racing, to which is added the risk of collision between the light, two-wheeled rigs. Its spectacle combines shades of the Hippodrome with the charisma of Ben Hur. An attitude of anything goes, rig instability, a necessary degree of ruthlessness, and mounting enthusiasm all take their toll (168).

Conclusions

Despite every effort, by their very nature, equestrian sports will always contain an element of risk. However, unnecessary injury discredits any sport (41). Unenviable comparisons with other sporting and vehicular activities should not divert attention from successful examples of trauma control, particularly in racing under Jockey Club rules and in polo. Prevention is always better than cure (139). Avoidable injury is unacceptable injury (41). Most horseback riding trauma is avoidable by active training, discipline, supervision, and example, coupled with passive improvements, particularly enhanced head protection and hat retention in those groups most at risk: the young in training and those involved in general riding and hunting. Public roads, motor vehicles, metaled surfaces, and the novice on a horse represent a highly dangerous combination. All riders, particularly the young, should not abuse their privileged status as untested and unrestricted heavy vehicle operators.

Where equestrianism has fallen furthest behind other sports is in the provision, wearing, and accurate location of head protection (18, 169). Evolved from long and bitter experience, helmets to the present BS4472 and BS6473 are undoubtedly effective if worn, fixed in place, and stable on the head at and through impact. But continuing concern over adequacy of the present specifications (44, 58, 60, 119, 131) and unenviable comparison with head protection progress in other areas, notably cycling helmets (129, 170), call for continuous improvement in specification, design, and manufacture. In the development of new hats the special equestrian imperatives of fashion and fit, comfort, convenience, reasonable cost, ventilation, weight, durability, and auditory acuity must all be considered (18, 107a). Neither the clinical nor experimental analysis of head injury mechanisms, nor their computer simulation, have yet reached a stage in which irrefutable foundations can be provided for further helmet design, engineering, and development.

Real-time echoplanar and other forms of magnetic resonance imaging may soon change this, but for the moment, the extrapolation of progress in other fields, the use of computer simulation, the promotion of further research in brain trauma kinetics, and the review of the basic concepts of the Wayne State curve together with the investigation of new materials, the development of new design concepts and head injury criteria, and the careful analysis of each accident are fundamental responsibilities of those concerned with equestrian safety. The undoubted improvements in racing and polo have already indicated what could be achieved in the general reduction of riding trauma.

Today, the provision, promotion, and use of improved head protection is the first imperative. It poses a challenge and an opportunity to equestrianism as a whole (18). The continued lack of accurate statistics (171) remains unacceptable in a responsible society, particularly when Schneider (122), Torg (172) and their colleagues in North American collegiate sports have achieved so much. Details of incidents, successes and failures, total hours ridden, and local conditions are essential to define problems and assess the effects of induced change (173, 174). A clear reference to horse-related injuries in official returns (175), standardized forms (as popularized by the British Horse Society), and a central registry are all long overdue, while the interest of English coroners is welcome. Not only is fashion a major force in several riding fields but emulation is a characteristic of the age group most at risk. Improved example, training, supervision, and protection must be matched by a greater exhibition of responsible behavior by those in the public eye, especially when recorded through the visual media.

In classic times the Thracians venerated and respected their horses as quasi-divine beings (176). Today veneration has reasonably been replaced by affection, but respect cannot be replaced by complacency or contempt. Many of the lessons of the centuries have been forgotten and must be relearned. Much progress must still be made before sport with the horse has achieved the degree of safety its enjoyment requires. Meanwhile, whatever the psychologic explanation for the love of humans for the horse, few of us are totally indifferent to *Equus*. Equestrian sports in their turn happily, but occasionally tragically, reflect an archaic bond of freedom, mutual understanding, and shared enterprise between people and an old friend, which is never far from our psyche's core.

Acknowledgments

The advice and assistance are gratefully acknowledged of, among many others, Dr. W.M.C. Allen, Mr. Peter Cannon, Dr. David Chapman, Dr. Tom Connors, Anne, Lady Elton, Mr. John Elliott, Major Ronald Ferguson, Mrs. Janette Harrison, Dr. John Lloyd Parry, Mr. Robert Langrish, Dr. James Newman, Dr. N.J. Mills, Mr. Charles Needham, Mr. Hedley Needham, Dr. John Inman, Miss Jocelyn B. Pedder, Professor and Mrs. Howard Pendleton, Miss Jane Wain, Mr. Barry Wilks, and Miss Caroline Cripps for typing the manuscript.

REFERENCES

1. Rice TAT. The Scythians. London: Thames & Hudson, 1957.
2. Miles JR. The racecourse medical officer. J R Coll Gen Pract 1970;19(93):228–232.
3. Brown PN, Silver IA. Personal communication.
4. Anonymous. *Equus caballus*. N Eng J Med 1975;293:665–666.
5. Edwards EH. From paddock to saddle. London: Nelson, 1972.
6. Henggeler J. The riding accident—meaning and prevention. In: Medicine and equestrian sports (Abstracts of the first European and third national conference). 1981:25.
7. Bixby-Hammett DN, Brooks WH. Common injuries in horseback riding. A review. Sports Med 1990;9:36–47.
8. Silver JR, Lloyd-Parry JM. Hazards of horse-riding as a popular sport. Br J Sports Med 1991;25:105–110.
9. American Academy of Pediatrics Committee on Sports Medicine and Fitness: Horseback riding and head injuries. Pediatrics 1992:89(3):512.
10. de Loes M, Goldie I. Incident rate of injuries during sport activity and physical exercise in a rural Swedish municipality: incident rates in 17 sports. Int J Sports Med 1988;9:461–467.
11. Bivar ADH. Cavalry equipment and tactics on Euphrates. Dumbarton Oaks Papers 1972;22:273.
12. Robson SEE. Some factors in the prevention of equestrian injuries. Br J Sports Med 1979;13:33–35.
13. Anonymous. Injuries associated with horseback riding—United States, 1987–88. MMWR 1990;39:329–332.
14. Anonymous. From the CDC. Injuries associated with horseback riding—United States, 1987–88. JAMA 1990;264:18–19.
15. Grossman JA, Kulund DN, Miller CW, Winn HR, Hodge RH, Jr. Equestrian injuries. Results of a prospective study. JAMA 1978;240(17):1881–1882.

16. Barclay WR. Equestrian sports [Editorial]. JAMA 1978;240(17):1892–1893.
17. Brooks WH, Bixby-Hammett DM. Prevention of neurologic injuries in equestrian sports. Phys Sports Med 1988;16:84–95.
18. Condie C, Rivara FP, Bergman AB. Strategies of a successful campaign to preomote the use of equestrian helmets. Public Health Rep 1993;108(1):121–126.
19. Anonymous. Alcohol use and horseback riding associated fatalities—North Carolina, 1979–1989. MMWR 1992; 41(19):335,341–342.
20. Bixby-Hammett DM. Accidents in equestrian sports. Am Fam Physician 1987;36:209–214.
21. Regan PJ et al. Hand injuries from leading horses. Injury 1991;22:124.
22. Fischer P, Elias D. Reitsport ans Medizinischer Sicht. Med Sports 1980;8:248.
23. Bernhang AM, Winslett G. Equestrian injuries. Phys Sports Med 1983;11:90–97.
24. Brote L, Skau A. Horse riding accidents in western Ostergotland—a prospective study 1978–1980. Lakartidningen 1981; 78(24):2356–2357.
25. Consumer Safety Unit. Home and leisure accident research. Eleventh annual report on the home accident surveillance system. 1987 data. London: Department of Trade and Industry, 1989.
26. Edixhoven P, Sinha SC, Dandy DJ. Horse injuries. Injury 1981;12:279–282.
27. Office of Population Censuses and Surveys. Fatal accidents occuring during sporting and leisure activities 1982–8 (DH4 84/3, 85/5, 87/2. 88/3, 88/6 and 89/4). London: HMSO, 1984–1989.
28. Office of Population Censuses and Surveys. General household survey 1986. London: HMSO, 1989.
29. Lennqvist S. Is horseback riding a dangerous sport? Lakartidningen 1977;74(51):4608–4610.
30. Lie HR, Lucht U. Horseback-riding accidents. I. Frequency of accidents in a horseback-riding population. Ugeskr Laeger 1977; 139(28):1687–1689.
31. Lucht U, Lie HR. Horseback-riding accidents. II. A prospective hospital study. Ugeskr Laeger 1977;139(28):1689–1692.
32. Danielsson LG, Westlin NE. Riding accidents. Acta Orthop Scand 1973;44(6):597–603.
33. Clarke KS. Calculated risk of sports fatalities. JAMA 1966;197:894.
34. Metropolitan Life Insurance Co. Competitive sports and their hazards. Stat Bull Metrop Insur Co 1965;46:1.
35. Metropolitan Life Insurance Co. Fatalities in sports 1970–78. Stat Bull Metrop Insur Co 1979;6:2.
36. Barber HM. Horse-play: survey of accidents with horse. Brit Med J 1973;3(879):532–534.
37. Bixby-Hammett DM, Brooks WH. Neurologic injuries in equestrian sports. In: Jordan BD, Tsairis P, Warren RF, eds. Sports neurology. Rockville, MD: Aspen, 1989:Chap 9.
38. Bjornstig U. Skador vid ridsport. Stockholm: Konsumentverket, 1982.
39. Bjornstig U, Eriksson A, Ornehult L. Injuries caused by animals. Injury 1991;22(4):295–298.
40. Dittmer H. The injury pattern in horseback riding. Lagenbecks Arch Chir Suppl 1991:466.
41. Heipertz W, Steinbruck K. Analysis of riding accidents and proposition for their prevention. In: Medicine in equestrian sports (Abstracts of the first European and third national conference). 1981:23.
42. Kricke E. The fatal riding accident. Unfallheilkunde 1980;83:606–608.
43. Lindsay KW, McLatchie G, Jennett B. Serious head injury in sport. Br Med J 1980;281(6243):789–791.
44. Lloyd RG. Riding and other equestrian injuries: considerable severity. Br J Sports Med 1987;21:22–24.
45. Nelson DE, Bixby-Hammett D. Review: equestrian injuries in childhood and young adults. Am J Dis Child 1992;146:611–614.
46. Zachariae L. Hundebid organdre laesioner forarsaget af dyr (Dog bites and other lesions caused by animals). Ugeskr Laeger 1972;135:2817–2819.
47. Gleave JR. The impact of sports on a neurosurgical unit. Paper presented at the British Institute of Sports Medicine, Cambridge, UK, April 1975.
48. Peterson, E, Wenker H. Verletzungen des zentral nerves systems dur Sportunfalle. Beitr Neurochir 1968;15:233.
49. Pounder DJ. "The grave yawns for the horseman": equestrian deaths in south Australia 1973–1983. Med J Aus 1984;141:632–635.
50. American Academy of Pediatrics Council on Child and Adolescent Health. Policy Statement: horseback riding and related injuries. Elk Grove Village, IL: American Academy of Pediatrics, 1980.
51. Avery JG Fact sheet: horse riding accidents in children: London. Child Accident Prevention Trust, 1986.
52. Avery JG, Harper P, Ackroyd S. Do we pay too dearly for our sport and leisure activities? An investigation into fatalities as a result of sporting and leisure activities in England and Wales, 1982–1988. Public Health 1990;104:417–423.
53. Barone GW, Rodgers BM. Paediatric equestrian injuries: A 14-year review. J Trauma 1989;29:245–247.
54. Bergqvist D, Hedelin H. Trends in blunt abdominal trauma among hospital in-patients. Developments in a Swedish rural district over 30 years. Scand J Soc Med 1979;7:33–39.
55. Bixby-Hammett DM. Pediatric equestrian injuries. Pediatrics 1992; 89:1173–1176.
56. Gierup J, Larsson M, Lennqvist S. Incidence and nature of horseriding injuries—a one-year prospective study. Acta Chir Scand 1976;142:57–61.
57. Haller JA. Pediatric trauma: the number one killer of children. JAMA 1983;249:47.
58. Ingemarson H, Grevsten S, Thoren L. Lethal horse-riding injuries. J Trauma 1989;29:25–30.
59. Klasen HJ. Accidents with saddle horses. Ned Tijdschr Geneeskd 1981;125:136–140.
60. McGhee CN, Gullan RW, Miller JD. Horse riding and head injury: admissions to a regional head injury unit. Br J Neurosurg 1987;1:131–135.
61. McLatchie GR. Equestrian injuries—a one-year prospective study. Br J Sports Med 1979;13:29–32.
62. Schmidt B, Hollwarth ME. Sports accidents in children and adolescents. Kinderchir 1989;44:357–362.
63. American Horse Council. Horse industry directory [annual]. Washington, DC: American Horse Council.
64. Dittmer H, Wubbena J. An analysis of 367 riding accidents. Unfallheilkunde 1977;80:21–26.
65. Gratz RR. Accidental injury in childhood: a literature review on pediatric trauma. J Trauma 1979;19:551–555.
66. Schoter I, Wassman H. Der Reitun fallans neurochirurgischer Sicht. Unfallheilkunde 1976;79:443.
67. Goulden RP. The medical hazards of horse riding. Practitioner 1975;215(1286):197–200. Aug.
68. Jones MW. A study of trauma in an Amish community. J Trauma 1990;30:899–902.
69. Seaber AV. Unsafe on any horse. Chronicle Horse 1970;34(17):53.
70. Seaber AV. The human brain: its potential for injury during equestrian events. Chronicle Horse 1978;41(46):55–58.
71. Seaber AV. How hardheaded are we? Chronicle Horse 1979;42(36):12–13.
72. Seaber AV. An intelligent choice. Chronicle Horse 1979;46(27)43–44.
73. Williams LP, Remmenga EE. The blue-tail fly syndrome: horse-related accidents. Paper presented at the 103rd annual American Public Health Association meeting, Chicago, November 1975.
74. Hipp F, von Gumppenberg S, Hackenbruch W, Kircher E. Fracture of the vertebrae due to riding accidents [Abstract]. Fortschr Med 1977;95:1567.
75. Holdsworth F. Fractures, dislocations and fracture-dislocations of the spine. J Bone Joint Surg 1970;52A:1534.
76. Williams JGP. A colour atlas of injuries in sport. London: Wolfe Medical, 1980.
77. Anonymous. A treatise on the blood, inflammation and gunshot wounds. Clin Orthop 1963;28:3–13.
78. Cone TE Jr. Book of Accidents (1830). Excerpt XI: riding a wild horse. Pediatrics 1971;47:947.
79. Reich L. Head and neck injuries in equestrian accidents. HNO 1979;27:416–418.
80. Schneider K, Zernicke RF. Injury tolerance of human skull to

simulation of impact acceleration [English abstract]. Unfallchirurgie 1989;92(2):49–53.
81. Bastian HL. Fractures of the mandible—an analysis of the aetiology and localisation. Tandlaegebledet 1989;93:589–593.
82. Blumel J, Pfeifer G. Injuries caused by horses and their effects on maxillofacial Regions. Analysis of cases in Nordwestdeutsche Kieferklinik from 1970–1975. Unfallheilkunde 1977;80:27–30.
83. Borgogna E, Fogliano F, Re F, Scotto G. Traumatic maxillofacial lesions in rugby, soccer and horseback riding. Minerva Stomatol 1984;33:533–535.
84. Hoehn RJ. Facial injuries. Surg Clin North Am 1973;53(6):1479–1508.
85. Oxsoy Z, Lorber G, Rettig AM. Maxillofacial injuries in riding sports. ZWR 1985;94:818,821–824.
86. Hill CM, Crosher RF, Mason DA. Dental and facial injuries following sports accidents: a study of 130 patients. Br J Oral Maxillofac Surg 1985;23:268–274.
87. Jockey Club. Regulations for point-to-point steeple chases: season 1993. London: The Jockey Club, 1993.
88. Dibb WL, Digranes A, Tonjum S. *Actino bacillus lignieresii* infection after a horse bite. Br Med J 1981;283(6291):583–584.
89. Khaikin GI. Treatment of facial bites. Vestn Khir 1973;109:95–96.
90. McKee R, Bryce G. Animal and human bites as an emergency. Health Bull 1983;41:137–140.
91. Peel MM, Hornidge KA, Luppino M, Stacpoole AM, Weaver RE. Actinobacillus and related bacteria in infected wounds of humans bitten by horses and sheep. J Clin Microbiol 1991;29(11)2535–2538.
92. II Samuel 18:9.
93. Regan PJ, Roberts JO, Feldberg GL, Roberts AH. Hand injuries from leading horses. Injury 1991;22:124–126.
94. Beacham BE, Cooper PH, Buchanan CS, Weary PE. Equestrian cold panniculitis in women. Arch Dermatol 1980;116:1025–1027.
95. Becker T. Das stumpfe Schadel trauma als sportunfall. Mschr Unfallheilkd 1959;62:179.
96. Bixby-Hammett DM. Head injuries in equestrian sports. Phys Sports Med 1983;11:82–86.
97. Doyle D. The nature of head injuries. In: Pedder JB, Mills NJ, eds. Head protection: the state of the art. Symposium proceedings. Burmingham, UK: University of Burmingham, 1983:18.
98. d'Abreu F. Brain damage in jockeys [Letter to the Editor]. Lancet 1976;1(7971):1241.
99. Allen WMC. Brain damage in jockeys [Letter to the Editor]. Lancet 176;1:1135.
100. Allen WMC. Racing accidents in Great Britain—a review of their frequency, nature and the preventative measures for their control. In: Medicine in equestrian sports (Abstracts of the first European and third national conference). 1981:13.
101. Steinbruck K. Spine injuries due to horse-riding Part 1. Unfallheilkunde 1980;83:366–372.
102. Steinbruck K. Spine injuries due to horse-riding Part 2. Unfallheilkunde 1980;83:373–376.
103. Depassio J, Toraldo C, Minaire P, Poison D, Eysette M. Spinal injuries with neurological signs while practising a sport. Semaine Hopitaux Paris. 1983;59(45):3131–3135.
104. Krasuski M, Kiwerski E. Results of the treatment of fracture of the odontoid process of the axis. Ortop Travmatol Protez 1990;(3):52–54.
105. Pang D, Wilberger JE, Jr. Spinal cord injury without radiographic abnormalities in children. J Neurosurg 1982;57:114.
106. Landin LA. Fracture patterns in childhood. Analysis of 8,682 fractures with special reference to the incidence, etiology and secular changes in a Swedish urban population 1950–1979. Acta Orthop Scand Suppl 1983;202:1–109.
107. Flynn M. Disruption of symphasis pubis while horse riding: a report of two cases. Injury 1973;4:357–359.
107a. Firth JL. Equestrian injuries. In: Schneider RD, Kennedy JC, Plant MI, eds. Sports injuries: mechanism, prevention and treatment. Baltimore: Williams & Wilkins, 1985:431–449.
108. Teasdale G, Jennett B. Assessment of coma and impaired consciousness: a practical scale. Lancet 1974;2:81–84.
109. Medical Research Council. Aids to the examination of the peripheral nervous system. London: HMSO, 1976.
110. London: Medical Equestrian Association.
111. Advanced Life Support Working Party of the European Rususcitation Council. Guidelines for advanced life support. A statement. Resuscitation 1992;24:111–121.
112. Basic Life Support Working Party of the European Resusciation Council. Guidelines for basic life support. A statement. Resuscitation 1992;24:103–110.
113. Committee on Trauma. Advanced trauma life support. Chicago: American College of Surgeons, 1992.
114. British Riding Clubs. British Riding Clubs' yearbook 1993. Kenilworth, Warwickshire, UK: The Riding Clubs' Committee, British Equestrian Centre, 1993.
115. British Horseracing Board and the Jockey Club. The orders and instructions of the British Horseracing Board and the rules of racing and instructions of the Jockey Club 1993. London: Authors, 1993.
116. Pony Club. Yearbook 1993. Stoneleigh: British Horse Society, 1993.
117. Maxwell, R, Newcombe RL. Bilateral extradural haematoma in a horse-rider who wore a unfastened helmet [Letter]. Med J Aust 1987;147:623.
118. Mahaley MS, Seaber AV. Accident and safety considerations of horse-back riding. In: Proceedings of the 18th American Meidcal Association Conference on the Medical Aspects of Sports. 1976:37–45.
119. Muwanga LC, Dove AF: Head protection for horse riders: a cause for concern. Arch Emerg Med 1985;2:85–87.
120. Whitlock MR, Whitlock J, Johnston B. Equestrian injuries: a comparison of professional and amateur injuries in Berkshire. Br J Sports Med 1987;21:25–26.
121. Voight J, Delgaard JB. Fatal accidents during riding or other forms of handling horses. Ugeskr Laeger 1970;140(22):1305–1308.
122. Schneider RC. The incidence of head injuries—the potential for protection. In: Pedder JB, Mills NJ, eds. Head protection: the state of the art. Symposium proceedings. Birmingham, UK: University of Birmingham, 1983:5.
123. British Standards Institution. BS3686: specification for protective hats: 1983 for horse and pony riders, as amended (withdrawn). London: British Standards Institution, 1976.
124. American Horse Council. Seal marks approved headgear. Am Horse Council Newslett 1983;10:1.
125. Hammett DB: Safety in horse sports. In: Proceedings of the National Youth Leader. Horse symposium, March 13–15, 1980. Blacksburg, VA: Polytechnical and State University, 1980:97.
126. American Society for Testing and Materials. Standard specification for headgear used in horse sports and horseback riding (F1163-88). Philadelphia: ASTM, 1988.
127. British Standards Institution. BS4472: 1988. Protective skull caps for jockeys. London: British Standards Institution 1988.
128. British Standards Institution. BS6473: 1984 with amendment 1 (AMD 4731 29 March 1985) and amendment 2 (AMD 5423 31 December 1986). London: British Standards Institution, 1984, 1986.
129. Mills NJ, Whitlock MD. Performance of horse-riding helmets in frontal and side impact. Injury 1989;20:189–192.
130. Shanahan DF. Basilar skull fracture in US Army aircraft accidents. Aviat Space Environ Med 1983;54:628.
131. Ilgren EB, Teddy PJ, Vafadis J, Briggs M, Gardiner NG. Clinical and pathological studies of brain injuries in horse-riding accidents: a description of cases and review with a warning to the unhelmeted. Clin Neuropathol 1984;3:253–259.
132. Newman JA. Biomechanics of brain injury—a brief over-view. In: Pedder JB, Mills NJ, eds. Head protection: the state of the art. Symposium Proceedings. Birmingham, UK: University of Birmingham, 1983:32.
133. Gurdjian ES, Roberts VL, Thomas LM. Tolerance curves of acceleration and intracranial pressure and protective index in experimental head injury. J Trauma 1964;6:600–604.
134. Department of Transport. Federal motor vehicle safety standard 208. Occupant crash protection. The head injury criteria score. Federal Register 1989:54(211):s6,2.2.

135. Goldsmith W. Current controversies in the stipulation of head injury criteria. J Biomech 1981;14:883–884.
136. Marguiles SS, Thibault CE. A proposed tolerance criteria for diffuse axonal injury in man. J Biomech 1992;25(8):917–923.
137. National Highway Traffic Safety Administration. Occupant crash protection—head injury criterion (S6.2 of MVSS 571. 208, Docket 69-7, Notice 17). Washington, DC: Department of Transportation.
138. Smythe P. In: Armstrong JR, Tuckers WE, eds. Injuries in sport: the physiology, prevention and treatment of injuries associated with sport. London: Staples, 1964:214.
139. Du Boullay CT, Bardier M, Cheneau J, Bortolasso J, Gaubert J. Sports injuries in children. Epidemiologic study. Chir Pediatr 1984;25:125–135.
140. Sahlin Y. Sports accidents in childhood. Br J Sports Med 1990; 24:40–44.
141. Horse Trials Group. Notes cross-country course design and fence construction. Stoneleigh: British Horse Society, 1993.
142. Hannah HW. The veterinarian's duty to foresee animal-inflicted injury. J Am Vet Med Assoc 1976;169:570–594.
143. Vigouroux RP, Guillermian P, Verando R. Neurotraumatology of sportive origin. neurochirurgie 1978;24:247–250.
144. American Medical Association. Protective headgear for horseback riders: resolution N.107 (A-84). In: AMA, ed. Proceedings of the House of Delegates. Chicago: AMA, 1984:3–60.
145. Waynesville, NC: American Medical Equestrian Assocation.
146. Mount Holly, NJ: American Riding Instructors Certification Programme.
147. Mazomanzie, WI: Horsemanship Safety Association.
148. Westchester, PA: United States Pony Clubs.
149. DeBenedette V. People and horses: the risks of riding. Phys Sportsmed 1989;17:250.
150. Endurance Riding Group. Rules and omnibus schedule 1993. Stoneleigh: British Horse Society, 1993.
151. MacNalty AS. Henry VIII: a difficult patient. London: Johnson, 1952.
152. Gronwall D, Wrightson P. Cumulative effects of concussion. Lancet 1975;2:995–997.
153. Yates JJ. A survey of British racecourses in respect of falls. In: Medicine in equestrian sports (Abstracts of the first European and third national conference). 1991:15.
154. Fontana R. The Fontana rail [videotape]. Aalta Loma: Fontana Products Inc., 1982.
155. Foster JB, Leigurda R, Tilly PJB. Brain damage in national hunt jockeys. Lancet 1976;1:981–983.
156. British Show Jumping Association. The rules and yearbook 1993. Kenilworth, Warwickshire, UK: British Equestrian Centre, 1993.
157. Dressage Group. Dressage rules and official dressage judges panel. Stoneleigh: The British Horse Society incorporating the Pony Club, 1993.
158. Kenilworth, Warwickshire, UK: British Horse Society.
159. Horse Trials Group. Rules 1993. Stoneleigh: British Horse Society, 1993.
160. Riding Clubs Office. Official rules: riding test, equitation, jumping, show jumping, dressage and horse trials competitions. Kenilworth, Warwickshire, UK: British Horse Society, 1993.
161. Griffin R, Peterson KD, Halseth JR. Injuries in professional rodeo. Phys Sportsmed 1984;12:130–137.
162. Myers MC, Elledge JR, Sterling JC, Tolson H. Injuries in intercollegiate rodeo athletes. Am J Sports Med 1990;18:87–91.
163. Morgan RF, Nichter LS, Friedman HI, McCue FC III. Rodeo roping thumb injuries. J Hand Surg [Am] 1984;9:178–180.
164. Harrison CS. Fox hunting injuries in North America. Phys Sportsmed 1984;12:130–134, 136–137.
165. Hurlingham Polo Association. Yearbook 1993. Kirtlington: The Hurlingham Polo Association, 1993.
166. Riding for the Disabled Association. Annual report and accounts 1993. Kenilworth, Warwickshire, UK: Riding for the Disabled Association, 1993.
167. Kiwerski J. Spinal injuries caused by falling from horse carriages. Pol Tyg Lek 1984;39(32):1063–1065.
168. Ives W, Brotman S. A review of horse-drawn buggy accidents [with comments]. Pa Med 1990;93:22–24.
169. Bergman AB, Rivara FP, Richards DD, Rogers LW. The Seattle childrens's bicycle helmet campaign. Am J Dis Child 1990;144:727–731.
170. MacNamara OD. Protective headwear. Med Equestrian Assoc Newslett 1992:3–4.
171. Office of Population Censuses and Surveys. VS3 mortality statistics for England and Wales, Titchfield: OPCS, 1992.
172. Torg JS, ed. Athletic injuries to the head, neck and face. Philadelphia: Lea & Febiger, 1981.
173. Gerberich SG. Sports injuries: implications for prevention. Public Health Rep 1985;100:570–571.
174. Robey JM, Blyth CS, Mueller FO. Athletic injuries: application of epidemiologic methods. JAMA 1971;217:184–189.
175. National Electronic Injury Surveillance System. Reports [annual]. Washington, DC: National Consumer Product Safety Commission.
176. Fol A, Marazov I. Thrace and the Thracians. London: Collier-Macmillan, 1977.

21 / FENCING

Julie A. Moyer, Rebecca Jaffe, and Marlene Adrian

Introduction

General Considerations

Fencing is a sport of European ancestry and has its origins in weapons of war and dueling. The latter could be thought of as a combination of war and sport, because the duelists did not fight to the death but only to save one's honor. A cut across the cheek was a common trademark of dueling with the sword as late as the 20th century. Today, the sport involves blunted weapons and a linear fencing area in which two people attempt to score *touches* (contacts of the weapon to the body) on each other (Fig. 21.1). It is a sport of intense physical and mental activity, the two opponents are within 6 feet of each other most of the time.

The U.S. competitions and rules are governed by the United States Fencing Association (USFA); fencing's National Governing Body (NGB), recognized by the U.S. Olympic Committee (USOC); and the International Fencing Federation, or Federation Internationale d'Escrime (FIE). The USFA was founded as a the Amateur Fencers League of America in 1891. The technical rules established by the FIE are in most cases, the same rules adopted by the U.S. Fencing Association and are, therefore, the rules used to govern fencing in the United States. These rules address such issues as equipment and technique safety, injury time-outs, and drug testing.

The USFA also is the official body that chooses the national teams to represent the United States in international competitions, including world championships. Point awarding competitions (North American circuit and national junior and senior championships) are offered for the purpose of selecting these teams. International competitions include world cups, world championships (junior and senior), the Pan American Games, the World University Games, and the Olympics.

There are three weapons used in fencing: the épée, the foil, and the sabre (Fig. 21.2). Each weapon has its own design and rules of play. All three weapons are fenced by men in international contests, but only the foil is fenced by women in the Olympics and both the foil and épée are fenced by women in the other events. National, sectional, and divisional USFA-sanctioned competitions are offered in all three weapons to both males and females. There are children's events (under 14 years and under 17 years), junior events (under 20 years), open events, and senior events (40 years and older). University and high school leagues also exist and are governed by the appropriate athletic governing body. In the schools, female competitions have been limited to the foil. There have been, however, instances when females have fenced on the male épée and sabre teams, because there were no women's teams with these weapons.

Another form of fencing competition is designed for athletes with physical impairments. National and international wheelchair fencing requires that the individuals fence from a sitting position. These competitions are governed by the relevant national and international disabled sports organizations.

Fencing is offered throughout the United States in many major cities and in some remote towns through recreation programs, private clubs, health/sport clubs, and fencing clubs. The fencing club is known as a fencing *Salle*, and the fencing coach, if a graduate of a fencing school, is known as a fencing master (*maistro*).

Fencing equipment is usually provided by the schools and by the facilities offering novice classes. After the class stage and as the fencers begin to compete and become members of a club, students usually must purchase their own equipment. The mask, weapon, glove, and uniform (exclusive of the shoes) cost approximately $200. If the equipment is certified for international competition, the price is approximately $500, which includes three weapons. All the equipment sold in the United States must meet the fencing standards approved by the FIE for safe fencing. All pertinent equipment must be properly inspected by the technical committee before competition. Most teams and com-

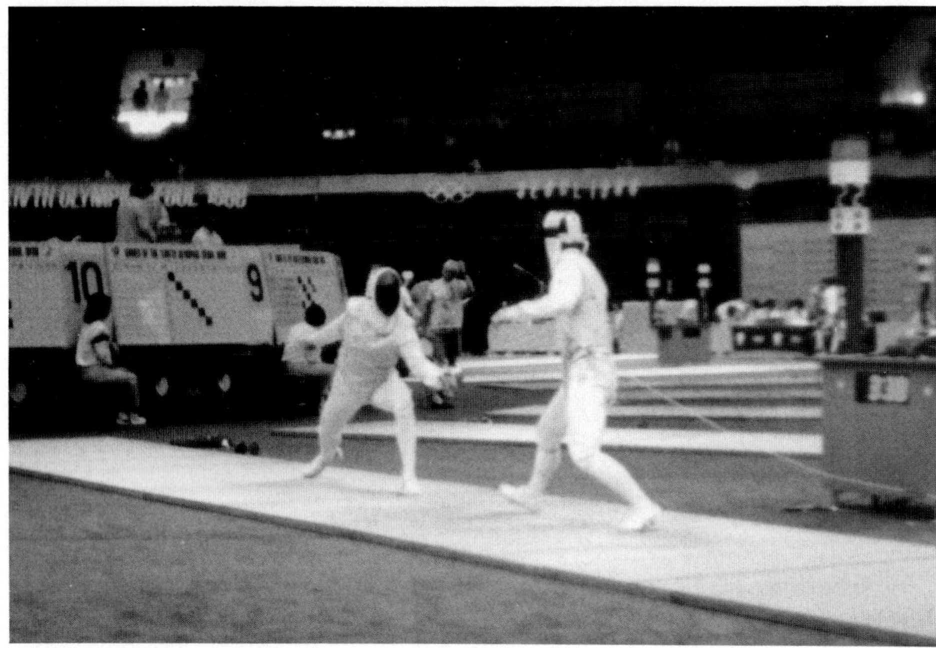

Figure 21.1. Fencing is a sport in which two people attempt to score *touchés* on one another by using blunted weapons on linear fencing area.

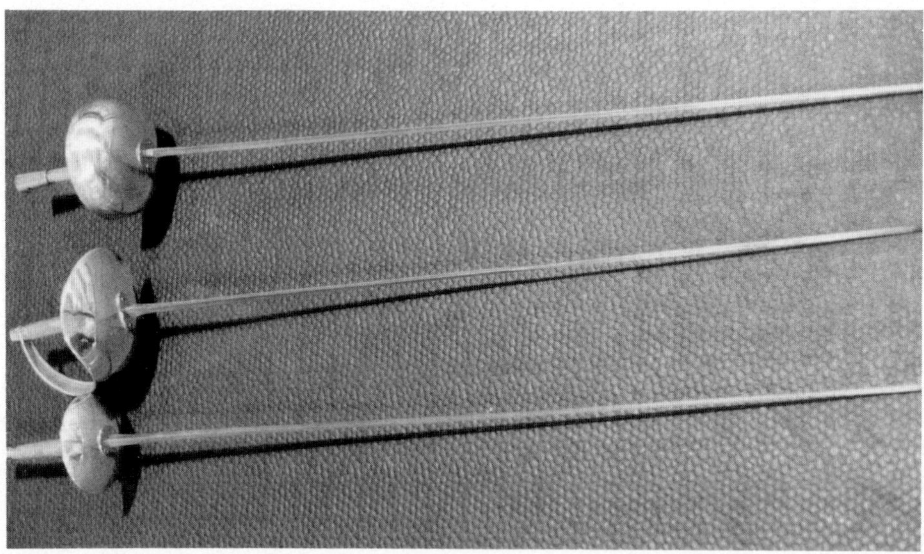

Figure 21.2. The three weapons used in fencing are the épée *(top)* sabre *(middle)*, and foil *(bottom)*.

petition sites have equipment specialists *(armorers)* as part of their entourage to ensure that the equipment meets FIE safety standards (Fig. 21.3). Because scoring is based on electrical contact, the *armorer* also ensures that the equipment has been assembled in such a way as to avoid a malfunctioning or misrepresentation of the electrical scoring system.

Actual equipment design and wear has been made with the athlete's safety in mind. For all three weapons, the protective jacket must overlap the knickers (or uniform of Kevlar-type material), a plastron is mandatory, and females must wear breast protectors. The glove must cover at least one-half of the forearm so that the opponent's weapon cannot enter the sleeve. All masks must be checked, using an instrument with a spring-load point before competition to ensure that the mask cannot be penetrated with the opponent's blade. This instrument must be able to withstand a 12-kg force (1).

To prevent injury, there are rules governing the method by which one fences. It is strictly forbidden for a fencer to perform any abnormal motion, such as severe hits or opponent collision, that may be construed as discourteous and dangerous (1).

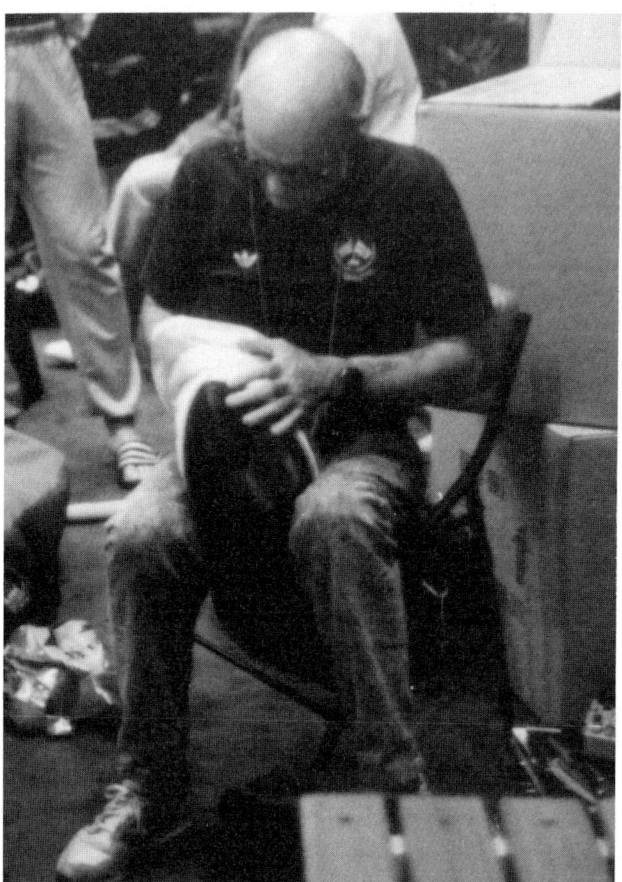

Figure 21.3. The *armorer* is the individual who officially inspects fencing equipment to ensure the athletes' safety.

Rules of Play

Fencing has several courtesies: saluting of the opponent and the director (official) at the beginning of each match and shaking hands with the opponent afterward. The mask, weapon, and clothing of both fencers are evaluated by the director before the start of the bout. The fencers assume the ready position *(en garde).* The director says "Fence," and fencers will fence until the director says "Halt." When there have been five *touches* scored by one fencer, the bout is ended and that fencer is determined the winner. During some competitions and at latter stages of a large competition, fencers must win with a margin of two *touches* in two of three bouts, to a maximum score of six in each bout.

The area of fencing is a linear strip *(piste)* approximately 5 feet wide and 47 feet long (Fig. 21.4). The fencers will exchange a series of offensive attacks and defensive actions, consisting of advances, retreats, lunges, and flèches in which the feet are usually at right angles to each other and the legs are in continual semiflexion or vigorously extending (Fig. 21.5). Defense involves retreats and arm flexion movements. Attack arm actions are primarily elbow and wrist extension and lateral or circular movements of the hand and forearm.

Because of the rules and target area for valid *touches,* the actions of the arm in foil are more restrictive than in the other two weapons. Only the torso is a legal target. Lunges are prominent in the foil strategy. The rule of right of way results in a rather definite pattern of attack–defend–attack–defend before a hit (contact) is made. Right of way refers to the need of a fencer to initiate an attack before the opposing fencer does.

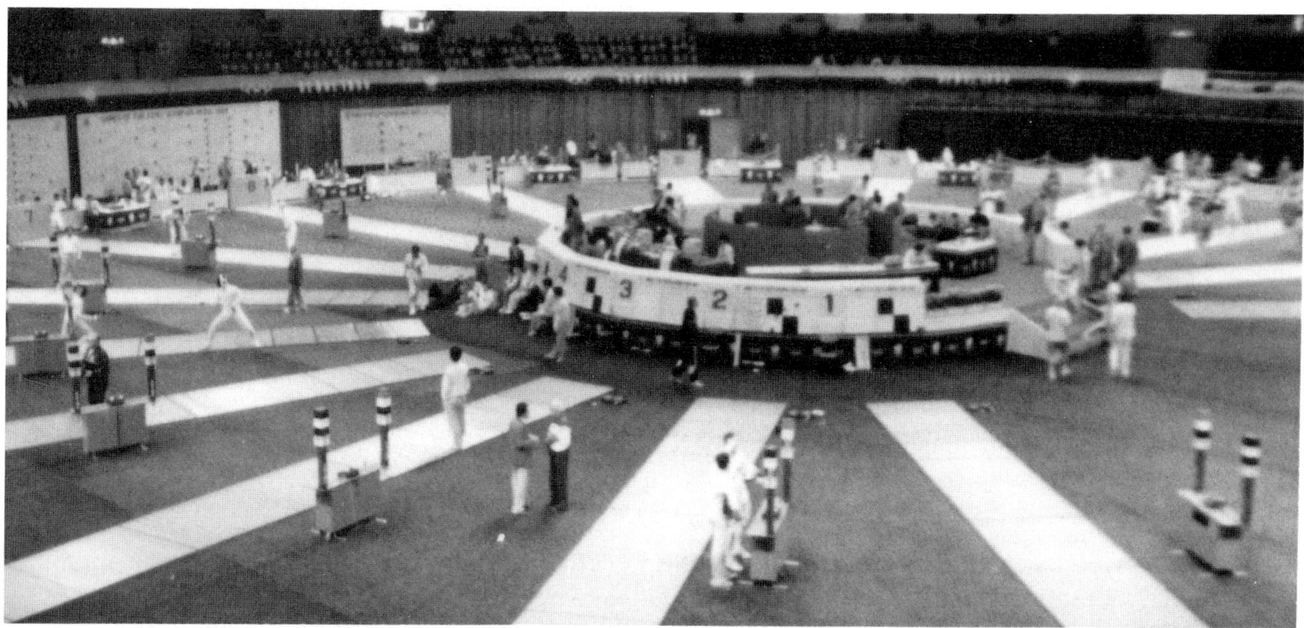

Figure 21.4. The *piste* is the linear strip on which fencers compete.

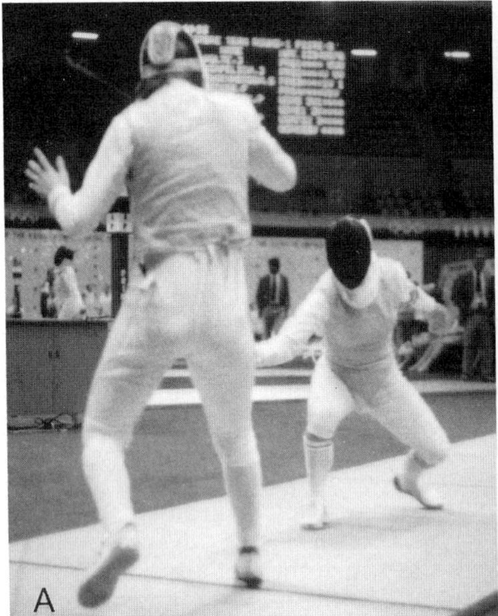

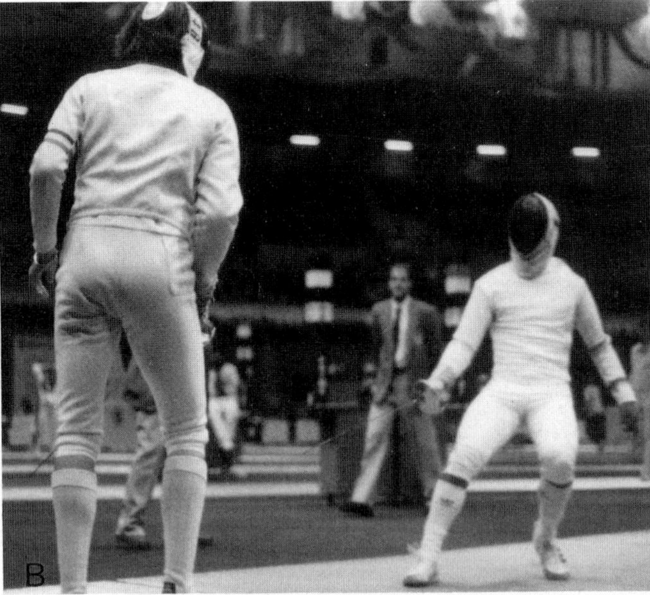

Figure 21.5. A series of attacks and defensive actions produces vigorous extremity movements, and mechanical stresses are common to the sport of fencing.

In the sabre competition, the target is expanded to include the head and arms. In addition, the cutting edge of the blade can be used to score a *touche*. Thus there is a greater variety of arm actions than with the foil. The *flèche* is used more extensively than the lunge. The right-of-way rule also applies to the sabre.

The total body is the legal target in the épée and no right-of-way rule exists. Both fencers can score a *touche* simultaneously as long as it is done within 1/25 sec. As with the foil, only the point of the épée can be used to score a legal *touche*. Lunges and *flèches* are used, but the fencers rely frequently on their quickness or reaction time, and many do not often lunge or *flèche*.

Rules Influencing Medical Care

In international competition, an FIE medical committee or "doctor on duty" is present at all events. If an accident occurs during a fencing bout, the injury must be confirmed by the committee or doctor, and the director of the competition will then allow the athlete an injury break lasting no more than 10 min. The break can be used for treatment of that specific injury only. If the doctor believes the athlete cannot safely continue, the doctor will advise the director of this decision. If the athlete is in an individual competition, the fencer may be asked to withdraw. If it is a team competition, the fencer may be replaced during that event, but may fence other events that same day if approved by the same physician. At no time during the course of that same day can another injury break be taken for the same injury. Muscle and heat cramps are not considered for injury time-outs (1).

Care must also be taken when using tape or other medical supplies and devices. If tape or other devices must be used on the weapon hand, or any other area near the equipment or target area where its use may be interpreted as an attempt to alter the electrical current, interfering with proper scoring, it may be appropriate to have the athlete approved for competition by the director or rules committee before the start of the event (Fig. 21.6).

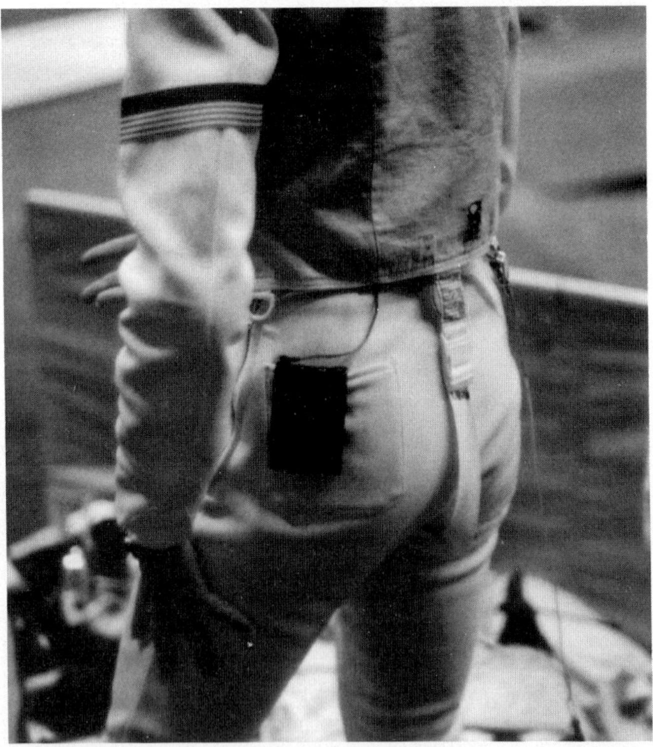

Figure 21.6. Tape or electrical treatment devices, such as this electrical stimulator, should be cleared by the rules committee so that use is not interpreted as an attempt to alter electrical current and hence interfere with proper scoring.

During national events, the USFA recommends that at least a full-time certified athletic trainer and on-call physician be available during the entire competition. Specific duties of the athletic trainer, physician, and local organizing committee (LOC) hosting the event have been outlined by the USFA (Appendices 21.A–21.C). In addition, all athletes are asked to sign waivers of liability and agreement to drug testing (Appendix 21.D).

Mechanisms of Injury

Injuries are a result of many factors relative to the environment, the fencer, and the technique to be performed. In addition, the interrelationships of these components of fencing make the cause of injury complex.

Fencing Environment

The surface on which the fencer will move must be kind to the feet and joints. Sometimes the *piste* is set on concrete, which causes heel bruises and trauma to the joints. If the footwear and the fencing surface are not matched to provide optimum friction (traction) the fencers' feet may slip or stick. In either case, a fall or tearing of soft tissue is possible. Contusions, muscle strains, and ligamentous sprains can result.

The *piste* is often elevated during the final round of a competition. This creates a risk of falling and greater injury can occur. In some cases, the copper strip may be torn, the base may be uneven, and sections may separate from each other. Prevention of injuries caused by these problems rests primarily with the facility director. Adequate standardization of surfaces must be provided so that the fencer can select the proper footwear.

The environment also must have adequate space between *pistes* and between the *piste* and the scorer's table. Weapons, clothing, and other articles must be out of the way of the fencers. Again, proper enforcement of the rules and commonsense behavior will reduce the possibility of injuries.

The Fencer

Injuries are caused by improper training and conditioning. The fencers must develop adequate strength, cardiovascular conditioning, balance, and coordination to compete throughout the tournament. If they do not become fatigued or lose their balance while fencing, they will lower their risk of injury. If in their fencing training and preevent warmup the fencers stretch their bodies to the point needed for their bout, they will have a lower risk of straining the muscles and other soft tissues when going all out on lunges and other movements performed during competition.

The major mechanism of injury is the inability of the fencers to tolerate the forces exerted on their bodies. Their own muscular force, the force of gravity, the acceleration forces of the body segments, and the impact forces (foot to *piste* or weapon to body) must be less than what the human body can tolerate without trauma. There are singular high forces of one action that must be conditioned for, and there are the repetitive lower forces that cause accumulated trauma that also must be conditioned for.

Techniques

The techniques of fencing can be categorized with respect to the sites receiving the greatest forces and being at the highest risk. Fencers, however, do not always perform the techniques exactly the same way. Novices, in particular, may not perform according to the description of the technique. Therefore, a biomechanical analysis of how the fencer moves the body parts is necessary to obtain knowledge of how the technique is being performed. Leg extension mobility at the hip, alignment of the knee over the foot to prevent torsion, extension at the elbow, hand movement about the wrist, and alignment of the trunk are the movements that must be analyzed in each fencer (Fig. 21.7). To reduce the risk of injury, these movements must be performed properly.

Inadequate strength, power, and flexibility will create trauma, because of the high acceleration rates and the repetition of the movements. Balance, agility, and coordination conditioning must be part of a fencer's training so that the movements will be made optimally with a reduction in extraneous forces.

Training and Conditioning

General Concepts

Because of the complexity of the sport, fencing training and conditioning should be divided into three categories: general conditioning, mental exercise, and

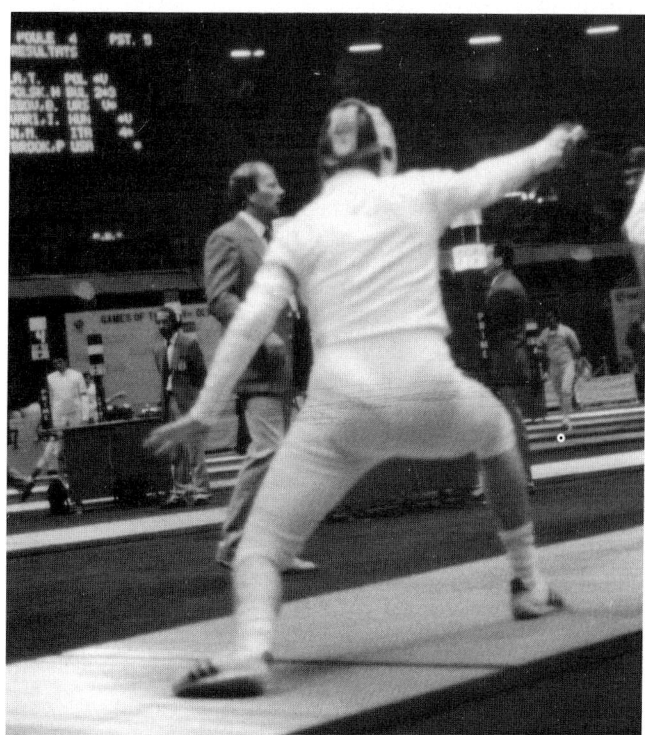

Figure 21.7. There are many upper extremity, trunk, and lower extremity movements in fencing that can be biomechanically evaluated to confirm proper technique and prevent injuries.

sport-specific training. In terms of general conditioning exercises, researchers have shown that cardiovascular fitness and strength influence fencing performance (2–4). Others have suggested that technique, speed, and agility are the essential characteristics for elite performance (5).

A general conditioning and training program is essential not only for good performance but also for injury prevention. This program should include at least several components: (*a*) warmup phase; (*b*) stretching; (*c*) power and strengthening exercises; (*d*) aerobic and endurance activities; (*e*) sport-specific activities; (*f*) warmdown; and (*g*) relaxation techniques to promote mental control and speed fatigue recovery time (6).

As stated previously, the sport-specific skills and mental training components are important and warrant special consideration. Also, strength and endurance workouts are extremely beneficial. The movement pattern in fencing promotes muscular asymmetry, i.e., elbow flexion strength of the weapon hand and strength and muscle mass of the forward leg have been shown to be significantly higher than the contralateral limb (2). Because many injuries are caused by muscular imbalance, it is essential that a total-body strength program, including trail leg strengthening, be implemented.

There are three main types of strength and power exercises that should be incorporated into the program: isometrics; isotonics; and isokinetics. All exercises should be executed both eccentrically and concentrically. The intensity, frequency, and duration of the exercises as well as the age and gender of the fencer should also be considered.

Although power training at a limb speed equal to competition speed would be optimal, this is oftentimes difficult to achieve. Most isokinetic equipment does not exceed a speed of 400°/sec, whereas maximum human limb velocity usually averages between 900° and 1100°/sec (7). Therefore, a suggested protocol for isokinetic power training would be concentric, full-velocity spectrum speeds and one midrange eccentric speed (7–10). The same muscle groups should not be exercised at a frequency of more than every other day, and exercises should be performed until the muscle is at a point of 50% fatigued instead of the traditionally established methods of repetitions and sets (11).

Women and youth should undergo a different weight-training program from men. When training women, it is important to remember that compared with men of equal size and weight women possess approximately 50% of the strength of those men; the difference is primarily in the upper body (12, 13). Because of the musculoskeletal immaturity of youth, modifications should be made in their isotonic training. The following guidelines should be incorporated into a weight-training program developed for youth. Only one to three sets of 6 to 15 repetitions should be performed no more than two to three times a week with at least 1 day of rest between sessions. The program should emphasize full-range, submaximal, concentric lifting. Until the technique is perfected, youth should lift bars or machines without added weight. When 15 repetitions can be properly executed, weight can be added in 1- to 3-lb increments (6, 14).

In fencing, the body must be able to generate quick bursts of high-level energy (anerobic) and maintain submaximal motions for extended periods of time (aerobic). Therefore, to avoid injury from premature fatigue, endurance activities must be included in the conditioning program. A combination of interval training (repetitions of 5- to 10-sec bursts of maximal work with 30- to 60-sec rest periods) with aerobic workouts (minimum of 20 min, 70% to 80% maximum heart rate intensity, 3 to 4 days a week) is suggested (15).

Sport-Specific Training Techniques

Although many injuries occur during competition, some injuries also occur during practice. Often these injuries can be avoided if proper training and conditioning are done. Many fencers do not train in a regular or scientific manner. They do not keep records of their level, frequency, or duration of training or competition. The following training principles and techniques are based on programs that coaches and highly skilled fencers have used. It is believed that participation in such a program will reduce the risk of injury to fencers.

Training intensity, duration, and frequency should be individually prescribed. The training program must be both general and specific, because fencing is a unilateral-type sport. Without general training, the fencer develops asymmetrically. The asymmetrical body does not have the balance and harmony required for intense competition.

Training must be done in an environment that is kind to the body, and the fencer should not train at a level that causes pain or undue discomfort. The training should consist of adequate rest days and hard workouts interspersed with regular workouts. Rests should be given before competitions. Cross-training principles can be used to motivate the fencer and prevent staleness. Cross-training also can be an injury-prevention strategy.

Charting or record keeping is one of the proven ways to evaluate the adequacy of the fencer's training table (Appendix 21.E). For all types of fencing activities, the number of minutes should be recorded as well as the intensity of the activity. The intensity of each activity can be estimated using a perceived exertion scale. This scale can be a three-point (i.e., easy, moderate, hard), five-point (easy, moderate, slightly hard, hard, maximum), or other type of scale. Both general and specific training activities as well as competition results should be recorded. The type of information kept within these categories can follow that shown in Appendix 21.E or can be modified to fit the individual athlete or coach. For example, specific conditioning might include only three categories: footwork; handwork; and total bodywork.

Records of competition identify the limitations of the training program. The number of *touches* scored and the number of *touches* opponents score in competition can be recorded as a ratio. Comments concerning opponents' styles and one's own weaknesses should be recorded. The competition record can be used to modify the training program. If the fencer did not have enough stamina, cardiovascular activities should be increased. If the fencer lost balance and could not perform techniques correctly at the appropriate times, then emphasis should be given to balance and reaction time activities.

Mental Training

Each day time should be spent on mental exercise. These exercises include visual imagery, autogenic training, and relaxation techniques to aid the fencer in improving concentration, reducing stress, speeding injury recovery, and improving overall technical performance. Not only does this training help promote mental conditioning but it helps the elite fencer gain an emotional and physical edge as well.

Acute Injuries

Because of the nature of the sport, fencing produces a wide diversity of acute injuries. A 2-year study was performed by the USFA's medical commission to investigate the actual frequency and distribution of such injuries. This study was conducted from 1988 to 1990 at all North American Circuit Events and two national championships (each weapon has three NAC events and nationals). During this time, 586 injuries were reported by the fencers to official medical personnel, in most cases a certified athletic trainer. Only 323 of the 586 reported injuries were acute injuries, requiring medical attention. (Nonacute injuries included sinusitis and diarrhea.) All acute injuries requiring medical treatment were documented on the Fencing Treatment Form (Appendix 21.B). In addition, for any significant injury that required stabilization, transport, and possible future medical treatment, the Injury Initial Evaluation Form was also completed (Appendix 21.C), which was reviewed by the physician on site or on call whenever possible.

Relationship between Acute Injuries and Weapons

To determine whether the differences in injury ratio (type of injury and body part injured) for each weapon (men's foil, women's foil, men's épée, women's épée, men's sabre, and women's sabre) were the result of chance alone or whether the results were caused by a significant difference between the groups, a statistical analysis using a chi-square and Cramer's V value was performed.

When weapons were compared with body parts injured, a statistical significance was found among the variables ($p = .0177$); however, the Cramer's V value indicated that this relationship was not strong ($V = .32618$). Therefore, a conclusion was made that the body part injured may depend on the type of weapon. When comparing the weapon with the type of injury, researchers found the p value to be .0838 and Cramer's V value to be .18098. Therefore, no statistically significant relationship was found to exist between these two variables.

Distribution and Types

Of all injuries reported during the study, almost 33% were sprains (more than 50% of which occurred during men's épée events). Strains were the second most common injuries at 23.8% of all injuries, followed by heat-related disorders (17.9%), contusions (6.2%), fractures and complete tendon ruptures (1.2%), and other miscellaneous systemic disorders (0.3%) (Table 21.1, Fig. 21.8).

Comparing all six weapons, men's épée accounted for the most injuries, 45.8%. Men's sabre represented 20.7% of all injuries, and men's foil, 10.5%. This may be partially attributed to the fact that épée has a much larger target area than the sabre or foil. Furthermore, the épée is of greater stiffness and weight compared with the other weapons.

Of the three women's events, women's foil represented 15.2% of the total injuries, compared with 6.8% for women's épée and 0.9% for women's sabre. This may be partially because more women compete in women's foil than women's épée or sabre.

Location

In terms of body part, a significantly higher amount of injuries occurred at the ankle (15.8%) compared with the other 23 sites observed. (Table 21.2, Fig. 21.9).

The total body (systemic) was the location for the second most frequently treated acute disorders (usually heat related) at 10.5%, followed by the hand (8.4%) and the knee (8%).

Types

Because of the planted, flexed, and externally rotated/valgus-stressed position of the trail leg, acute injuries such as medial collateral ligament sprains, medial meniscal tears, lateral subluxating patella, groin strains, ruptured Achilles tendons, and eversion ankle sprains have been observed. Quad strains, blisters, and nail contusions have been noted in the front leg. Because the trunk is a target area for all three weapons (and the upper extremities for the sabre and épée), more contusions and lacerations are seen in this area.

Gender Differences

Over one academic year, men's and women's collegiate fencing injuries were monitored and compared. When adjusted for exposure time, no significant gender differences were found. Approximately 0.10 injuries per 100 person-hours were noted in men's fencing, compared with 0.18 injuries per 100 person-hours in women's fencing. There were 0.43 disability days per 100 person-hours associated with these injuries to males, compared with 0.21 disability days per 100 person-hours for females. Overall, 28% of men participating in fencing were injured, compared with 50% of women (16).

Table 21.1.
Types of Acute Fencing Injuries (Percents)

	Type of Injury							
Weapon	Contusions	Open Wounds/ Lacerations	Fractures/ Ruptures	Heat-Related Disorders	Sprains	Strains	Miscellaneous Systemic Disorders	Row Percent (Number)
Men's Foil	0.3	1.9		1.2	3.4	3.7		10.5 (34)
Men's Épée	2.5	9.3	0.6	6.8	18.0	8.4	0.3	45.8 (148)
Men's Saber	0.3	2.5		4.0	5.9	8.0		20.7 (67)
Women's Foil	2.5	2.8	0.3	2.8	4.0	2.8		15.2 (49)
Women's Épée	0.3	0.9	0.3	2.5	1.9	0.9		6.8 (22)
Women's Saber	0.3			0.6				0.9 (3)
Total	6.2	17.4	1.2	17.9	33.2	23.8	0.3	100

Evaluation and Treatment of Emergencies

Management

The fencing instrument is sharp when broken and may inflict lacerations to an opponent's clothing and skin. Basic first aid measures should be employed. Preventing further hemorrhage is paramount.

Foreign bodies in the eye are frequently experienced. One must delineate a scratch from a foreign body that remains inbedded in the cornea. It is wise to numb the eye before evaluating the situation. Next, gross inspection for a foreign body should be done. If one is discovered then thorough rinsing of the eye should be accomplished. If the foreign body remains in place and the facilities are adequate, one may attempt to flick the foreign body out of the cornea with a sterile needle tip. If the foreign body will not move, it would be best to patch the eye and send the athlete to a specialist who will use a slit-lamp for removal. The risk of corneal puncture is real. Fluorescein examination with a blue light would be the next step, looking for a persistent defect in the cornea. If an abrasion is noted, then conservative management with antibiotic cream and patching is appropriate. One must decide on an individual basis if the athlete, with adequate numbing, can complete the competition before definitive treatment is rendered.

Puncture wounds caused by a weapon have been reported. There have been a few cases of brain injury and death from a weapon penetrating the face shield. At least two immediate deaths occurred (17). In these cases, the basic precepts of advanced trauma life support would be the most appropriate steps to follow, managing the patient's airway first and foremost. Case reports of survival after a foil has penetrated the brain, leaving the athlete with a permanent amnesia, have been reported and emphasize the importance of rendering all possible life support to the athlete and transporting seriously injured patients quickly to sophisticated facilities (18).

As with most sports, the support personnel (coaches and referees) are older and under a great deal of stress. These individuals may have cardiac complaints, which should be taken seriously and evaluated and treated quickly. Basic life support (airway, breathing, and circulation) should be immediately initiated if someone is complaining of chest pain and then loses consciousness.

Many of the sporting arenas may be quite warm. The athlete is dressed in gear that makes him or her prone to heat injury. The athlete should be kept well-hydrated and perspiration and weight should be monitored carefully.

Special Supplies

It is important that the physician or ancillary medical staff be properly prepared with additional supplies beyond the usual medical supplies carried by a trainer. An eye kit, including topical anesthetic, fluorescein with a blue light, a fine needle, topical antibiotics, and patches, should be available. A sterile suturing kit with skin and subcuticular sutures should be a part of the medical supplies; this should include topical antibiotics. A hand-held electric cautery device is helpful for subungual hematomas. Intravenous fluids, oral rehydration, and ice should be available for the possibility of heat problems. A vacuum splint kit may be helpful for the stabilization of fractures.

Overuse Injuries

Because of the nature of the sport and its unique positioning, fencers are prone to sprains and strains as well as overuse injuries in multiple body parts. Fencers must maintain balance while holding their weapons in a prepared position for extended periods of time. Thus inflammatory syndromes, usually tendonitis about the

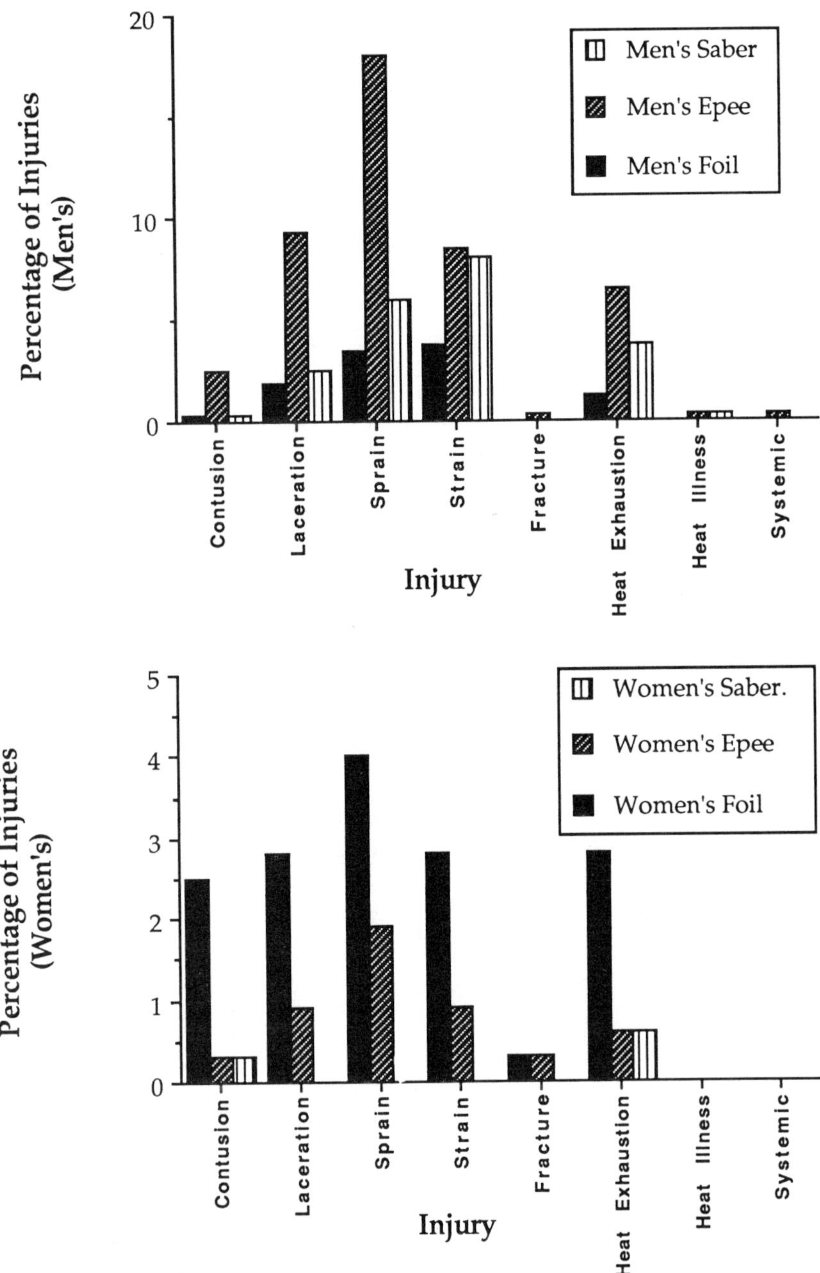

Figure 21.8. Percentage of acute injuries in men's and women's fencing. Numbers are based on men's and women's fencing combined. Graphs drawn by D. Grygo.

Table 21.2.
Location of Fencing Injuries (Percents)

Weapon	Head	Neck	Shoulder	Clavicle	Upper Arm	Elbow	Forearm	Wrist	Hand	Thumb	Finger	Upper Back	Lower Back	Hip	Groin	Thigh	Knee	Shin	Calf	Ankle	Foot	Heel	Toe	Systemic	Row Percent (Number)
Men's Foil	0.6	0.3				0.6		0.9	0.6	0.9	0.9	0.3	0.6	0.3		0.3	0.9		0.3	1.2	0.6	0.3		0.6	10.5 (34)
Men's Épée	1.2	0.9	3.7		1.2	0.3	0.6	2.2	3.7	0.9	2.5	0.3	2.2			2.2	3.7	1.9	0.3	9.0	2.8	0.3	0.6	4.6	45.8 (148)
Men's Saber	1.9	0.6	0.3			0.3		0.6	1.9	0.3	0.6	0.6	1.9	0.3	0.3	1.9	2.5	0.3	0.3	3.7	0.6			1.9	20.7 (67)
Women's Foil	0.6	0.3	0.9		0.3	1.2		0.6	1.5		1.5	0.3	0.3	0.3		0.6	0.9			1.5	0.3	0.6	0.3	2.5	15.2 (49)
Women's Épée	1.5		0.6	0.6		0.3	0.6	0.3	0.3		0.3							0.3		0.3	0.9			0.3	6.8 (22)
Women's Saber									0.3															0.6	0.9 (3)
Total	5.9	2.2	5.6	0.6	1.5	2.8	1.2	4.6	8.4	2.2	5.9	1.5	5.0	0.9	0.3	5.0	8.0	2.5	0.9	15.8	5.3	1.2	0.9	10.5	100

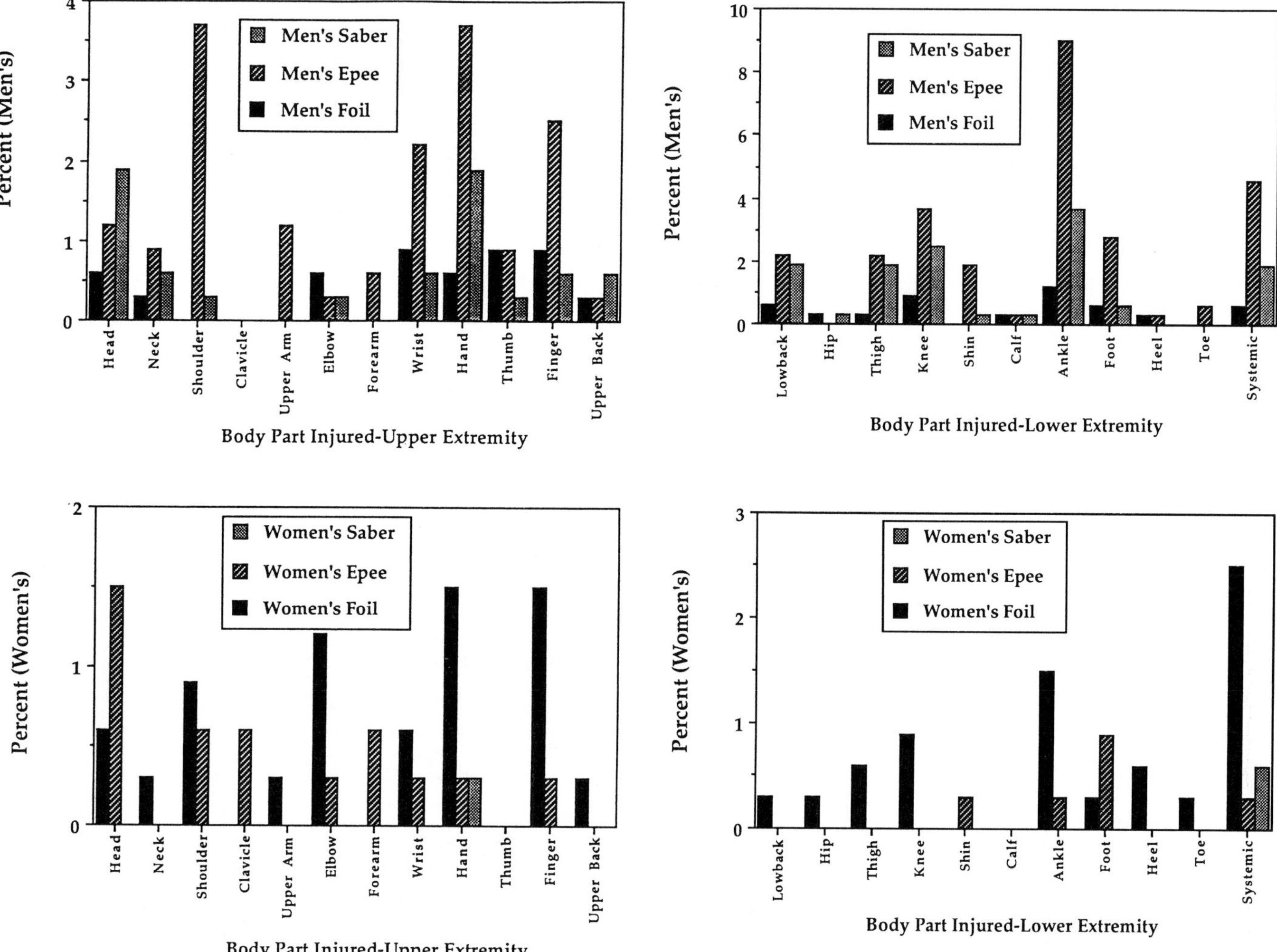

Figure 21.9. Percentage of acute injuries by body part in men's and women's fencing. Numbers are based on men's and women's fencing combined. Graphs drawn by D. Grygo.

wrist and hand, are often seen. Fencers may experience muscle cramping when they are forced to compete several times in a short period of time. Whether this is caused by muscle fatigue or electrolyte disturbances from sweating is unclear.

Fencers also suffer from back problems. Most of these involve the trunk extensor musculature. Lumbosacral strains are seen. It is important to emphasize a strengthening program for the back to avoid unnecessary injuries.

Lower extremity injuries are most frequently seen. These may occur in many different circumstances. When competing on a raised *piste*, the fencer is at risk for ankle sprains caused by imbalances and falling off the platform. Iliotibial band syndromes result from the stance required. There have been reports of cases of osteochondritis dissecans of the patella attributed to the angle at which the knee must be maintained and the repeated microtrauma caused by the trail leg in valgus stress while the leg is externally rotated (19). One must keep this is mind if an athlete presents with anterior knee pain. The diagnosis is made by magnetic resonance imaging (MRI) or arthroscopy.

The fencing footwear is not supportive, and therefore, the legs are prone to lower-extremity overuse injuries. The hyperpronated stance leads to an increase in plantar fascitis, posterior tibialis tendonitis, shin splints, stress fractures, and possibly periostitis of the navicular.

The asymmetry of the fencer's body may make him or her prone to non–sport-related injury. Both the weapon side upper extremity and forward lower extremity test stronger isometrically and dynamically (2).

Rehabilitation

Rehabilitation of fencing follows the same general guidelines as rehabilitating other sports-related injuries. Naturally, the specific adaptations to imposed demands (SAID) principle is imperative. Rehabilitation and functional tests before return to play must be specifically geared toward the athlete's sport, weapon, and age.

The two basic treatment regimes used in sports rehabilitation are therapeutic modalities and exercise. Modalities are primarily used in the early stages of rehabilitation to enhance the fencer's exercise program (20). The therapeutic exercise program actually helps restore injured tissue to its previous level of function (21). Rehabilitation should include exercising uninvolved body parts while treating the involved body part. This will minimize the chance of injuring deconditioned areas when the athlete returns to his or her sport.

The athlete must undergo functional testing before he or she is allowed to return to fencing. Normally, sport-specific activities can begin during the rehabilitation program when the athlete has 70% of the strength and 75% of the balance and proprioception of the contralateral limb. However, because of the pronounced asymmetry usually found with fencers, this may be difficult to access. These functional activities should encompass all aspects of the sport such as jumping, hopping, lunging, and squatting.

Actual return to sport should not be allowed until the athlete: *(a)* has passed a funcational test at least 90% of the contralateral limb; *(b)* has 100% proprioception of the contralateral limb; *(c)* has 90% of the peak strength, total work, and average power of the contralateral limb; *(d)* uses proper protective equipment as indicated; and *(e)* passes a clinical examination.

Conclusions

Proper conditioning is a key to injury prevention in fencing, especially because pronounced muscular imbalances are common to the sport. Proper techniques and mechanics as well as equipment are important for injury prevention. The positions and techniques involved in fencing contribute to some of the sport's common injuries such as medial collateral ligament sprains of the trailing knee, ankle sprains, plantar fascitis, and stress fractures.

There is a variety of acute injuries, which can occur throughout the body. More injuries are seen with men's épée compared with all other weapons. Sprains are the most common type of injury, and the ankle is the body part most frequently injured.

It is essential to have qualified medical personnel at all fencing events. At least 1 full-time athletic trainer and 1 part-time/full-time, on-call physician should be present. All health care providers working at fencing competitions should be well-versed in the management of medical emergencies, including puncture wounds, fractures, and eye injuries.

Rehabilitation of fencing injuries is similar to the rehabilitation of other sports-related injuries. The SAID principle applies, and sport-specific activities must be incorporated in the exercise regime. Functional tests before return to fencing are essential.

Acknowledgments

The authors would like to acknowledge D. Hammond, D. Grygo, and C. M. Richards for their assistance in the preparation and review of the manuscript.

REFERENCES

1. U.S. Fencing Association. USFA rules. Colorado Springs: USFA, 1990.
2. Nystrom J, Lindwall O, Ceci R, et al. Physiological and morphological characteristics of world class fencers. Int J Sports Med 1990;11(2):136–139.
3. Roi GS, Fasci A. Survey of requests for medical assistance during fencing matches. Ital J Sports Trauma 1988;10(1):55–62.
4. Stewart KJ, Perecto AR, Williams CM. Physiological and morphological characteristics associated with successful fencing performance. J Hum Ergol 1977;6(1):53–60.
5. Vander LB, Franklin BA, Wrisley D, et al. Physiological profile of national class NCAA fencers. JAMA 1984;252(4):500–503.
6. Grana WA, Lombardo JA, Sharkey BJ, Stone JA, eds. Advances in sports medicine and fitness. Chicago: Year Book Medical, 1990.
7. Parker MG. Characteristics of skeletal muscle during rehabilitation: quadriceps femoris. Athletic Train 1981;4:122–124.
8. Hageman PA, Gillaspie DM, Hill LD. Effects of speed and limb dominance on eccentric and concentric isokinetic testing of the knee. J Orthop Sport Phys Ther 1988;10:59–65.
9. Thomee R, Renstrom P, Grimby G, et al. Slow or fast isokinetic training after knee ligament surgery. J Orthop Sports Phys Ther 1987;8:475–479.
10. Weltman A, Tippett S, Janney C, et al. Measurement of isokinetic strength in prepubertal males. J Orthop Sports Phys Ther 1988;9:345–351.
11. Timm KE. Investigation of the physiologic overflow effect from speed-specific isokinetic activity. J Orthop Sports Phys Ther 1987;9:106–110.
12. Klafs CE, Arnheim DD. Modern principles of athletic training. St. Louis: CV Mosby, 1977.
13. Kuland DN. The injured athlete. Philadelphia: JB Lippincott, 1982.
14. Duda M. Prepubescent strength training gains support. Phys Sportsmed 1986;14:157–161.
15. Rothman J, Levine R, eds. Injury prevention and rehabilitation. Philadelphia: WB Saunders, 1992.
16. Lanese R, Strauss R, Leizman D, et al. Injury and disability in matched men's and women's intercollegiate sports. Am J Public Health 1990;80(12):1459–1462.
17. Crawford AR. Death of a fencer. Br J Sports Med 1984;18(3):220–222.
18. Squire LR, Amaral DG, Zola-Morgans S, et al. Description of brain injury in the amnesic patient N.A. based on magnetic resonance imaging. Exp Neurol 1989;105(1):23–35.
19. Gray WJ, Bassett FH. Osteochondritis dissecans of the patella in a competitive fencer. Orthop Rev 1990;19(1):96–98.
20. Torg JS, Vegso JJ, Torg E. Rehabilitation of athletic injuries—an atlas of therapeutic exercises. Chicago: Year Book Medical, 1987.
21. Allman FL. Rehabilitation of sports injuries: a practical approach. In: Ryan AJ, Allman FL, eds. Sports medicine. San Diego: Academic Press, 1989.

APPENDICES

CHAPTER 21/APPENDIX A

Personnel Responsibilities for Medical Coverage

The duties of the local organizing committee shall include the following.

1. Coordinate medical coverage through the assistance of the USFA's Medical Commission.
2. Notify the area hospital when and where the fencing event is going to be held.
3. Provide food, housing, and transportation reimbursement for the trainer and physician. If a local athletic trainer and/or physician cannot be obtained or if the USFA/local organizing committee chooses to bring in a trainer/physician from outside the area, the trainer/physician must also be supplied with a vehicle for local transportation and medical purposes.
4. Mail the completed treatment report forms and initial evaluation forms to both the USFA Headquarters and the Medical Commission.
5. If the trainer or physician engaged is not familiar with fencing, the local organizing committee along with a fencing official shall instruct the medical personnel as to their duties.
6. Events with a higher number of entrants require additional staffing. Each event should have at least 1 physician and 1 trainer present at all times (Nationals = 3 trainers, 2 physicians, minimal).
7. Notify USFA headquarters of all serious injuries or injuries requiring hospital transport.
8. Notify the trainer and physician of the ambulance response time, transportation time, and give the medical staff a map of the area including competition site, hotel, and hospital.
9. Find a suitable training room area in close proximity to the actual competition. Communication devices between the training room, physician, and committee are recommended.
10. Medical personnel should be provided with adequate medical supplies. An example of supplies used for a 4-day tournament follows:

    80 rolls (2 cases 1½″ white tape)
    8-oz. can tape spray
    4 ace wraps (4″)
    8 oz. hydrogen peroxide
    box 100 knuckle Band-Aids
    pack 100 sterile 3″ × 3″ gauze
    1 bottle (100) aspirin
    1 bottle (100) Tylenol
    4-oz. tube bacitracin
    rubber gloves
    eye wash
    crutches
    5 rolls prewrap
    pack (minimum 100) mid-size supermarket plastic bags and biohazard bags
    400 cups
    2 10-gallon water coolers
    ice
    20 treatment report forms
    20 initial evaluation forms

11. Contact the local medical groups and licensure committee to confirm temporary medical practice of out-of-state medical personnel.

The duties of the athletic trainer shall include the following:

1. Provide prevention and immediate care of injuries to athletes and supportive staff.
2. Arrange for transportation of injured persons to the hospital.
3. Make necessary referrals to the physician.
4. Bring their own standard trainer's kit.
5. Maintain treatment reports and initial evaluation forms.
6. Notify the local organizing committee of all serious injuries or injuries requiring hospital transport.
7. All medical personnel (including physicians) are responsible for their own malpractice insurance; however, because the services are of a volunteer nature, in some states the Good Samaritan Law may cover emergency care of injuries.

The duties of the physician shall include the following:

1. Fulfill the role as described in the rules and regulations involving the determinations if an injury is a result of trauma (i.e., rule out cramps).
2. Determine and make a record of all interruptions of combat granted.
3. If a 10-min request is denied, the physician must issue a warning and subsequently notify the bout committee, as a repetition of the offense will result in exclusion.
4. In addition to the above requirements in the rules of fencing, the physician must provide emergency treatment of injuries as necessary or as requested by the athletic trainer.

CHAPTER 21/APPENDIX B

USFA Fencing Treatment Form

				Clinical Impression		Treatment										
Date	Name	Weapon[a]	Injury Location[b]	Code[c]	Describe	Ice	Heat	Massage	Exercise	Mobilization	Dressing	Tape	Modalities (spec.)	Medication (spec.)	Stabilize and Transport	Treatment by

[a] 1 = MF, 2 = ME, 3 = MS, 4 = WF, 5 = WE, 6 = WS.

[b] 1 = head, 2 = face, 3 = neck, 10 = shoulder, 11 = clavicle, 13 = upper arm, 14 = elbow, 15 = forearm, 16 = wrist, 17 = hand, 18 = thumb, 19 = fingers, 22 = upper back, 33 = lower back, 36 = hip, 37 = groin, 38 = thigh, 39 = meniscus, 40 = knee, 41 = patella, 42 = tibia/shin, 43 = fibula/calf, 44 = ankle, 45 = foot, 46 = heel, 47 = great toe, 48 = toes, 50 = systemic conditions.

[c] 51 = abrasion, 52 = contusion, 53 = puncture, 54 = laceration, 55 = blister, 56 = heat illness, 57 = heat exhaustion, 58 = sprain, 59 = strain, 60 = fracture, 70 = systemic.

Fencing Event:
Medical Coordinator:
Dates:
Comments:
Page ________ of ________

CHAPTER 21/APPENDIX C

USFA Injury Initial Evaluation Form

Name ______________________ Age ______ Telephone No. ______________

Competition ______________________ Weapon ______________________

Date of Onset ______________________ Date Reported ______________________

Nature of Injury ______ Acute ______ Chronic ______ Complication ______ Recurrence

Mechanism of Injury ____

____

S:

O:

A:

P:

Clinical Impression:

Cleared for Competition:

____
Signature

____
Date

CHAPTER 21/APPENDIX D

USFA Injury Waiver and Drug Testing Form

ENTRY CANNOT BE ACCEPTED UNLESS STATEMENTS BELOW ARE SIGNED

DOPING CONTROL AGREEMENT: I understand that the drug testing program is implemented at all USFA point events. Any athlete competing in these events is subject to drug testing during the competition. I understand that the detection of use of banned drugs would make me subject to suspension by the USFA and the USOC for at least six months. By registering for this competition, I am consenting to a drug test if selected and am subject to penalties if declared positive for a banned substance. If selected, I am aware that failure to comply with the drug test will be cause for the same penalties for those who are positive for a banned substance. I know that I may call the USOC Drug Hotline (800) 233-0393 for any questions about medications and banned substances or practices.

FENCER'S SIGNATURE________________________

PLEASE BE AWARE THAT MANY NON-PRESCRIPTION MEDICATIONS HAVE BANNED SUBSTANCES. ANY ATHLETE WHO IS TAKING ANY MEDICATION VERIFY WITH THE USOC HOTLINE 1-800-233-0393 THAT THE MEDICATION DOES NOT CONTAIN A BANNED SUBSTANCE. THE USOC MAINTAINS A CURRENT LIST OF RELATED MEDICATIONS.

WAIVER OF LIABILITY: Upon entering this North American Circuit tournament, sponsored by the USFA, I agree to abide by the rules of the USFA, as currently published. I understand and appreciate that participation in sport carries a risk to me of serious injury, including permanent paralysis or death. I voluntarily and knowingly recognize, accept, and assume this risk and release the USFA, their sponsors, event organizers, and officials from any liability. The undersigned certifies that the individual for which this entry is submitted is a current competitive member of the USFA or another recognized Fencing Federation from which the fencer has a current FIE card.

________________________ __________

FENCER'S SIGNATURE DATE

ATHLETES UNDER-18 YRS. OLD: I have explained to my son/daughter the aforementioned stipulated conditions and their ramifications and I further consent to his/her registration for this USFA competition under the above-stipulated conditions.

________________________ __________

SIGNATURE OF PARENT/GUARDIAN DATE

MEDICAL PROBLEMS: Please indicate any significant or special medical problems that you have (e.g., diabetes, asthma, etc.) that the organizers should be aware of:

CHAPTER 21/APPENDIX E

Fencing-Specific Training Chart

Month: ________________ Fencer: ____________

Date

General[a]					
cvr[d]		s		rom	

Specific[b]													
foot		blade		rt		test		theme		bout		mp	

Competition[c]			
w/l		s/r	

Comments

[a] cvr = aerobic, s = strength, rom = flexibility, range of motion.
[b] foot = footwork, blade = bladework, rt = reaction time activities, test = intense practices in which testing is done (score may be written here), theme = bouting with a theme (one fencer practices specific techniques), bout = intense bouting (wins and losses are recorded and *touches* scored and received are recorded), mp = mental practice.
[c] w/l = wins and losses, s/r = *touchés* scored and received.
[d] Each space has two columns—one to record time and one to record intensity.

22 / FOOTBALL

James J. Irrgang, Mark D. Miller, and Darren L. Johnson

Introduction

Football has become the most popular collision sport in the United States. Football has its share of unusual and distinct injuries related to contact, although some injuries occur without contact. The player's position may predispose him to different types of injury and may affect return to participation. What may be a significant injury for one player might be a minor inconvenience for another. For example, a fractured finger may prevent a wide receiver from playing for 4 to 6 weeks, whereas a lineman can continue to participate with his finger immobilized.

During the past two decades football equipment has improved significantly. Protective padding, helmets, and shoulder pads are becoming lighter, more durable, less restrictive, and more shock absorbing. These factors allow the game to be played at a faster pace, which unfortunately may make the athletes more susceptible to injury. Artificial turf also has increased the speed of the game and affected the incidence of injury.

Epidemiology of Football Injuries

It is estimated that there are 1.3 million high school and 75,000 college football players in the United States (1). The number of injuries related to football has been estimated to be 600,000 per year (2, 3). The injury rate has been reported to vary widely between 11% and 81% (1, 4–6). Statistics from the National Football League indicate an injury rate of 1.5 injuries per player per year. The variation in the injury rate among studies is the result of differences in the definition of injury and severity, the identification of the population at risk, and exposure time. DeLee and Farney (3) reported an overall injury rate of 0.509 per athlete per year in high school football players. In their study, injury was defined as any episode that caused the football player to miss time from a practice or game, that required treatment by a physician and/or any head injury. Their sample consisted of 100 randomly selected class 4A and class 5A high schools in Texas. Over one season 2,228 injuries were documented. Even though the majority of time was spent in practice, 56% of the injuries occurred during games. The risk of injury in a game is reported to be 3 to 20 times higher than during practice (7). Furthermore, the majority of deaths and catastrophic football injuries occur during a game. Similar injury rates were reported by Prager et al. (8) (42.1%) and McLain and Reynolds (9) (62%). Lowe et al. (10) reported a slightly lower injury rate (32.1%). Their lower injury rate was probably the result of their definition of injury as any event that caused the athlete to miss a game or practice. Mild injuries occurring during a game on Friday or Saturday that allowed the athlete to recover before practice on Monday would not have been included as an injury in their study. DeLee and Farney (3) calculated exposure to practices and games and found an overall rate of 0.003 injuries per hour of exposure per athlete.

DeLee and Farney (3), defined a severe injury as one that required hospitalization and/or surgery. The injury rate for a severe injury was determined to be 0.031 per athlete per year. The incidence of hospitalization for injury in a sample of 871 males aged 15 to 18 enrolled in a health care plan in San Antonio, Texas, was 0.0149. The rate of hospitalizations per year in the sample of football players was 0.0311. This indicates that football players are almost twice as likely as the age-matched general population to sustain a severe injury. If only knee injuries requiring hospitalization and surgery are considered, the incidence in the general population was 0.0023 knee injuries per year compared with 0.0134 knee injuries per year in the sample of football players. This indicates that a football player is 5.8 times more likely to sustain a knee injury than the general population.

The type and location of injuries occurring in football players has been consistent among the studies that have been reported (7, 8, 11–15). Approximately 50% of injuries occurring in football players involve the lower extremity and 30% involve the upper extremity. The knee is the most common area injured and accounts for approximately 20% of all injuries (3). The ankle is the next most common area injured and accounts for approximately 18% of all football injuries. Sprains and strains are the most common types of injuries that occur and account for 40% of all injuries. Contusions account for 25% of injuries; fractures, 10%; concussions, 5%; and dislocations, 5%. The remaining 15% consist of a variety of other types of injuries.

Andresen et al. (16) and Prager et al. (8) described the frequency of injuries by player position. They found the greatest percentage of injuries were sustained by running backs (43%) followed by tackles (18%), guards (12%), and ends (10%). Quarterbacks (6%), safetys (5%), and centers (5%) accounted for the lowest percentage of injury. However, in terms of relative risk, the highest risk for injuries was found for running backs (3.0), quarterbacks (2.5), tackles (2.0), and centers (2.0). The lowest relative risk for injury was found for ends (1.1) and guards (1.2). The number of injuries are equally distributed between offensive and defensive players.

The activity at the time of injury was described by Andresen et al. (16). The greatest percentage of injuries occurred during tackling (32%), followed by blocking (26%), carrying the ball (19%), and being blocked (10%). Running, receiving, and passing each resulted in less than 3% of the injuries.

As noted above, the highest risk for injury occurs during a game. The distribution of injuries during a game has been evaluated (5, 11, 16, 17). The greatest number of injuries occur in the second and third quarters (29% and 31%, respectively) (16). The fewest number of injuries occur in the first quarter (13%). The injury rate is not equally distributed throughout the season. More injuries occur in the first half of the season and the peak injury rate occurs at mid-season. Fewer injuries occur in the final weeks of the season (16).

Risk Factors and Prevention

There have been a number of studies conducted in an attempt to identify risk factors for injuries in football. Several of these studies have lead to equipment and/or rule changes that have reduced the frequency of injuries. The large number of ankle and knee injuries implicates playing surface and shoewear as possible risk factors. Mueller and Blyth (1) randomly selected nine high schools in North Carolina, resurfaced their fields, and maintained them in good condition throughout the season. The resurfacing and maintenance of the fields resulted in a 30.5% reduction in ankle and knee injuries compared with schools that did not play on resurfaced and well-maintained fields. They demonstrated a further reduction in injuries when shoes were changed to the soccer-style shoe. Andresen et al. (16) demonstrated a lower injury rate on wet, slippery fields. A wet, slippery field was defined as a field that had a normal grass cover with the addition of rain. Interestingly, the highest injury rate was found with good field conditions. They postulated that the lower injury rate on wet, slippery fields was related to reduced speed of game and decreased friction between the shoe–playing-surface interface. The risk for injury on an artificial surface also may be reduced when the surface is wet (2). Several studies have evaluated the effects of artificial turf on football injuries. These studies have been reviewed by Skovron et al. (18) who concluded that investigations on the risk of injury on artificial surface are incomplete; however, there is probably a relative increase in the risk of injuries to the lower extremity. They noted that more well-controlled studies are needed.

Shoes also have been implicated as a source for injury. In the 1970s, football shoes typically had seven cleats that were 0.5 to 0.75 inch long. It was hypothesized that longer cleats fixed the foot to the ground, making it noncompliant to intrinsic and extrinsic forces and resulting in a greater risk for injury. Torg and Quedenfeld (19) demonstrated a reduced incidence and severity of injuries when football shoes with long cleats were replaced with soccer-style shoes. This resulted in a change in the type of shoes worn by football players. Currently, the standard football-style shoe has seven cleats that are 0.5 inch long and 0.375 inch in diameter. Soccer-style shoes have a number of small rubber cleats on the sole of the shoe. These shoes tend to be flexible and have lead to an increased incidence of turf toe. In the last 10 years, a number of lineman and other players not concerned with speed have begun to use high-top shoes in an attempt to reduce ankle injuries.

Activities during practice also have been found to influence the rate of injury. Mueller and Blyth (1) studied 6 schools in North Carolina that consented to limit the amount of contact practices. The schools that had limited contact practices had a lower injury rate compared with schools that had regular contact practices. Similar results were seen by Cahill and Griffith (20) in a study involving football teams from the Big 10. Noncontact and controlled practices resulted in a lower risk for injury compared with contact practices. Contact practices were found to have 4.7 times greater risk than controlled practice activities. The highest risk for injuries was found during preseason practices, which were 5.4 times more likely to produce injuries than in-season practices. Coaching also influences the risk of injury. The risk of injury is increased for coaches with less experience as well as for those staffs that have fewer assistant coaches (5).

A number of rule changes have been implemented to reduce the risk of injury. An example of this is the change in rules related to spearing and initial contact with the head for blocking and tackling (21). In 1976, the NCAA and the National Federation of High School Athletic Associations (NFHSAA) implemented rules to eliminate spearing and initial contact with the head. Between 1976 and 1987 the number of serious and catastrophic neck injuries documented by the National Football Head and Neck Injury Registry decreased compared with the previous decade. In 1976, the rate of fractures, dislocations, and subluxations of the cervical spine was 7.72 per 100,00 and 30.6 per 100,000 for high school and college football, respectively. These injury rates decreased to 2.31 per 100,000 and 10.66 per 100,000 for high school and college, respectively, in the subsequent 12 years. Similar results were noted for the incidence of quadriplegia. Other rule changes such as elimination of the crack back block and penalties for grabbing the face mask have been implemented to help reduce the number and severity of injuries.

Protective Equipment

Over the last 20 years, improvements in material and design have made protective equipment lighter, more comfortable, and more protective. However, without proper fit and maintenance, equipment may not only fail to protect the athlete but may actually cause injury. The National Operating Committee on Standards for Athletic Equipment (NOCSAE) is responsible for establishing guidelines for equipment maintenance and reconditioning. NCAA rules state that players must wear a NOCSAE-approved helmet, soft knee pads at least 0.5-inch thick, shoulder pads, hip pads, thigh pads, and a mouth piece. All helmets used in high school, college, and professional football must have a NOCSAE seal of approval, indicating that the helmet has met the requirements established for safe use. Helmets also carry a warning sticker from NOCSAE that must be placed on the outer shell of the helmet; it states, "Do not use this helmet to butt, ram, or spear an opposing player. This is in violation of football rules and can result in severe head, brain or neck injury, paralysis or death to you and possible injury to your opponent. There is a risk these injuries may also occur as a result of accidental contact without intent to butt, ram or spear. No helmet can prevent all such injuries" (Fig. 22.1).

Correct selection and fit of a football helmet are essential for the safety of the athlete. An improperly fitted helmet increases the likelihood of injury to the head and neck. Helmets are classified by the type of suspension system or padding within the shell. The types of suspension systems include air- and fluid-filled cells, a combination of air and pads, pads alone, and suspension type (Fig. 22.2). The outer shell of the helmet is made of polycarbonate that is an alloy polymer plastic called Kralite II. This polymer is lightweight yet able to withstand high impact.

Proper fitting of the helmet is important to ensure proper use and function. The helmet should be fit when the athlete has a hair length that he will wear throughout the season. Before fitting the helmet, it should be inspected to ensure that it does not have any cracks in the hard outer shell or soft inner padding. All air pockets should be filled to normal levels as recommended by the manufacturer. The soft inner pads and air cells should be checked for cracks and punctures. The attachment sites for screws and rivets should be checked to ensure that they are tight and that there are no stress cracks in the helmet at these points. The athlete's head should also be inspected for any obvious variations such as a slanted forehead or a large occipital bone.

When fitting the helmet, the athlete should be instructed in proper donning and doffing of the helmet. The helmet should be placed on the athlete's head by spreading the ear holes apart with the thumbs. Once the helmet is in place, it should be inspected to make sure that it is not rotated to one side. An attempt should be made to rotate the helmet while having the athlete hold his head still. The helmet should only turn slightly

WARNING
Do not strike an opponent with any part of this helmet or face mask. This is a violation of football rules and may cause you to suffer severe brain or neck injury, including paralysis or death.
Severe brain or neck injury may also occur accidentally while playing football.
NO HELMET CAN PREVENT ALL SUCH INJURIES.
YOU USE THIS HELMET AT YOUR OWN RISK.
Riddell

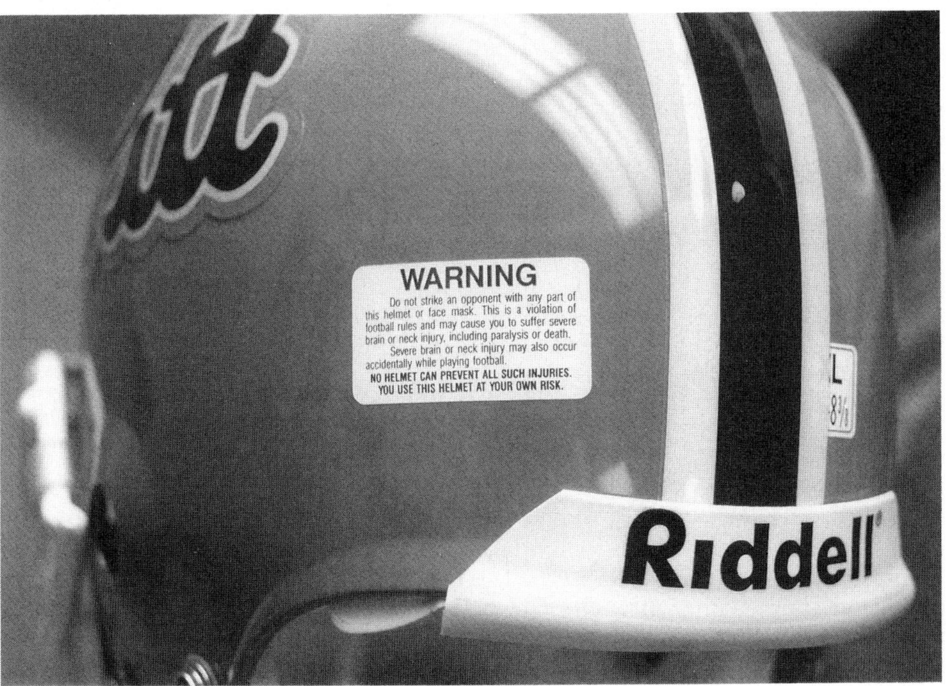

Figure 22.1. NOCSAE label on helmet warns players that improper use of the helmet to butt, ram, or spear an opposing player may cause severe injury to the head, brain, or neck and paralysis or death.

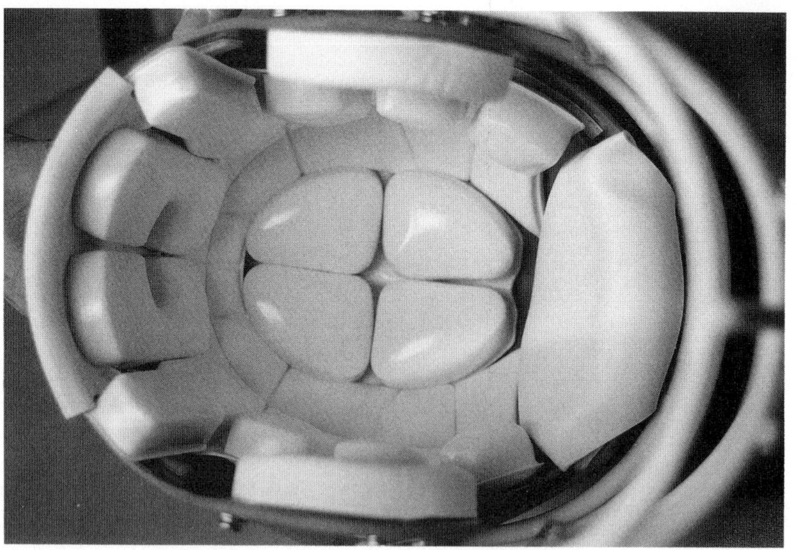

Figure 22.2. Suspension and padding inside helmet.

if it fits correctly. The anterior rim of the helmet should be one to two finger widths or 0.75 inch above the eyebrows. Air cells can be inflated or deflated to adjust the height of the helmet. The athlete should feel an even pressure on the top of the head when pressure is applied to the top of the helmet. If pressure is felt on the forehead, the helmet may be too low. The posterior rim of the helmet should cover the occipital bone, but not pinch the neck when the neck is extended. There should be no gap between the forehead and the anterior rim of the helmet when the examiner presses on the back of the helmet and the athlete holds his head still.

Jaw pads should fit snugly against the cheeks and are available in different thicknesses to provide proper fit. The chin strap should fit tightly with equal tension on both sides. For increased safety, a four-point chin strap should be used to restrict forward and backward movement of the helmet. When the helmet is properly fitted, the person fitting the athlete should not be able to place his or her thumb between the lining and the front or back regions of the helmet.

Shoulder pads are designed to absorb large forces and protect the athlete from injury to the shoulder and upper trunk. Serious injury may result from poorly fitted shoulder pads. The model and type of shoulder pads may need to be varied according to the player's position.

To fit the shoulder pads correctly, the distance from shoulder to shoulder should be measured. This measurement should be compared with the manufacturer's chart to determine the correct shoulder pad size. Once the correct size has been selected, the shoulder pads should be placed over the athlete's head. The elastic straps under the axilla should be attached to the front of the shoulder pads and should be adjusted so that the pads fit snugly. Loose straps often cause chaffing of the axilla. The shoulder pads should be laced in front so that the pads meet but do not overlap.

To ensure proper fit, the athlete should stand with his arms at his sides. There should be one to two finger widths between the neck and the padding on the inside rim of the shoulder pads. The padding should extend slightly beyond the lateral aspect of the shoulder (Fig. 22.3). The front of the shoulder pads should cover the chest to below the nipple. The posterior aspect of the shoulder pads should cover approximately 1 inch below the scapula. The individual fitting the athlete

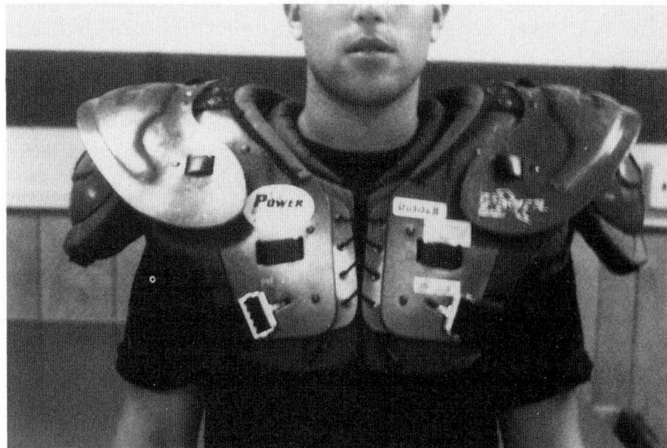

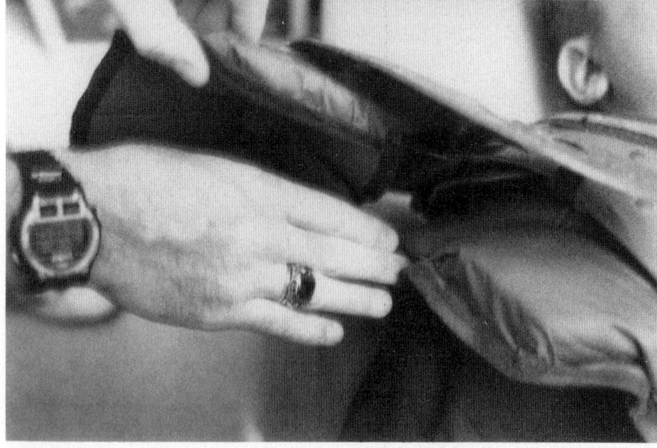

Figure 22.3. Properly fitting shoulder pads. There should be one to two finger widths between the player's neck and the inside rim of the shoulder pads. The padding should extend slightly beyond the lateral aspect of the shoulder.

should grasp the shoulder pads and attempt to slide them from front to back and side to side. There should be minimal movement. The athlete should be able to raise his arms over his head comfortably.

Other equipment worn by football players includes hip pads to protect the iliac crest and tail bone. Often these pads are inserted in a girdle. Thigh and knee pads are inserted in the pants. The pants should fit snugly to prevent slippage of these pads. All players should use a mouthpiece to reduce dental and head injuries. The mouthpiece should be form fitted to the athlete's teeth.

Players at particular positions may wear additional protective equipment. Quarterbacks may use a flack jacket to protect their ribs. Linemen typically use sparring gloves to protect their hands.

Head and Neck

Concussion

In the United States, American football causes more minor head injuries than any other single sport. The incidence is estimated to be 250,00 per year or approximately 20% (22). There is no universal agreement on the definition of a concussion or the various grades and severity of closed head injuries. One of the most commonly used definitions accepted by both the medical and surgical communities, is "a clinical syndrome characterized by immediate and transient post-traumatic impairment of neurological function, such as alteration of consciousness, disturbance of vision, equilibrium, etc., due to brain stem involvement" (22a). Cantu (22a) developed a useful system for grading the severity of a cerebral concussion that uses duration of unconsciousness and/or retrograde or posttraumatic amnesia (Table 22.1).

In a grade 1 cerebral concussion, which is the most common (90% of concussions), there is no loss of consciousness and the period of posttraumatic amnesia is less than 30 min. This is the most difficult to recognize and requires the greatest amount of clinical judgment. Retrograde amnesia for this condition is less than 30 min in duration and often lasts only a few fleeting minutes. It is not uncommon for a player to be "dinged" or to "have his bell rung" and continue playing. The only way players, coaches, and medical staff know who has been dinged is when they realize that the player can no longer remember the plays. Treatment of this type of injury involves removal of the athlete from competition and observing him on the bench. When the athlete has no headache, dizziness, or impaired concentration after a brief period and has full recall of events without any persistent retrograde amnesia, then return to the contest may be considered in selected cases (23, 24).

Table 22.1.
Severity of Concussion is Graded in Terms of 1, 2, and 3 and Characterized by the Loss of Consciousness or Posttraumatic Amnesia

Grade	Loss of Consciousness	Duration of Posttraumatic Amnesia
1 (mild)	None	$<$30 min
2 (moderate)	$<$5 min	30 min–$<$24 hr
3 (severe)	$\geq$5 min	$\geq$24 hr

Reprinted by permission from Cantu RC. Cerebral concussion in sport management and prevention. Sports Med. 1992;14(1):64–74.

A grade 2, or moderate, cerebral concussion is usually associated with loss of consciousness for less than 5 min or a period of posttraumatic amnesia that lasts more than 30 min but less than 24 hr. Initial management of a grade 2 concussion is similar to a grade 3 concussion (described below) except clinical judgment may dictate that if the period of unconsciousness is brief and if the athlete has no neck or peripheral extremity complaints, removal on a fracture board (recommended for grade 3) may not be necessary.

A grade 3, or severe, concussion is one in which the period of unconsciousness is greater than 5 min or in which the patient's posttraumatic amnesia lasts more than 24 hr. Any unconscious athlete should be treated as though he has a concurrent cervical spine injury. The neck should be immobilized until the athlete regains consciousness and clearly indicates he has no neck pain or until cervical spine x-rays eliminate the possibility of a cervical fracture. The patient should be assumed to have a cervical spine injury and be treated accordingly. It is often recommended that all athletes with a grade 3 concussion should be admitted to the hospital for observation and neuroradiologic evaluation for possible intracranial bleeding. The longer the period of unconsciousness or retrograde amnesia, the greater the likelihood of diffuse axonal injury and possible permanent brain injury.

As long as the airway is adequate, the helmet should not be removed. If there is any question, the patient should be log rolled to the face-up position while carefully supporting the head and neck on a spine board (Fig. 22.4). The face mask should be removed with a bolt cutter or a knife, depending on how it is fixed to the helmet (Fig. 22.5). If there is any concern about the airway or if breathing is impaired, the helmet should be removed with the neck in a neutral position, neither flexed nor extended (Fig. 22.6). When the helmet is removed the shoulder pads also must be removed to maintain the cervical spine in a neutral position. Opening the airway of a victim who is unconscious and suspected of having a neck injury is best performed using the jaw/thrust technique. This technique is accomplished by grasping the angles of the victim's lower jaw and lifting with both hands, displacing the mandible forward while tilting the head slightly backward (25). If this technique is not successful, the head-tilt jaw-lift should be substituted and care taken not to overextend the neck. As soon as possible, radiographs should be taken of the cervical spine, while the athlete is still on the spine board, using a cross-table lateral technique and taking care to visualize all cervical vertabrae. In most situations, a computed tomography (CT) scan of the head should be done and repeated if symptoms of headache, nausea and vomiting, visual impairment, or

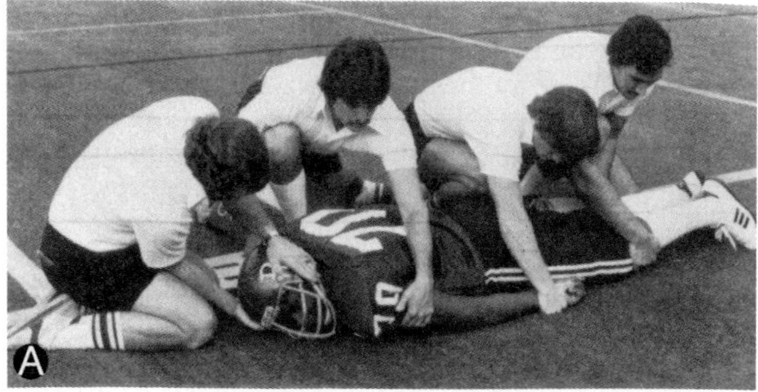

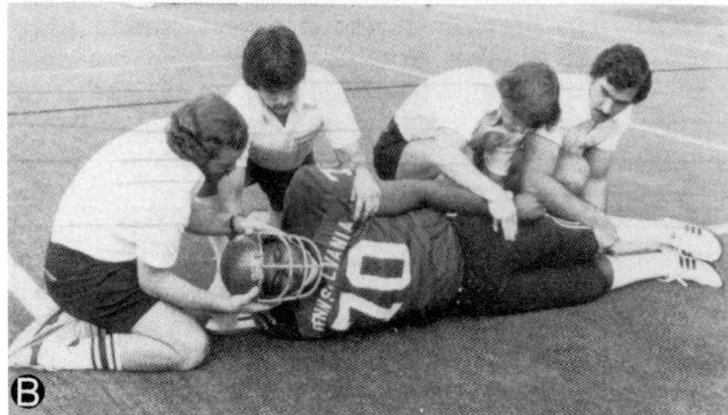

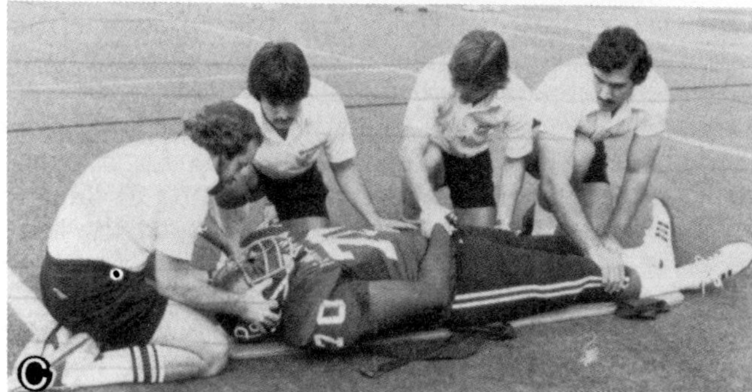

Figure 22.4. Log roll to a spine board. **A,** Chief of the team immobilizes the head and neck, while the support team concentrates on the lower body. Members of the support team should be positioned at the shoulder, hips, and lower legs. **B,** The chief initiates the move while immobilizing the head and neck at all times as the injured player is turned. **C,** The player is positioned on the center of the spine board while the chief continues to immobilize the head and neck. Reprinted by permission from Vegso JJ, Lehman RC. Field evaluation and management of head and neck injuries. Clin Sports Med 1987;6(1):1–15.

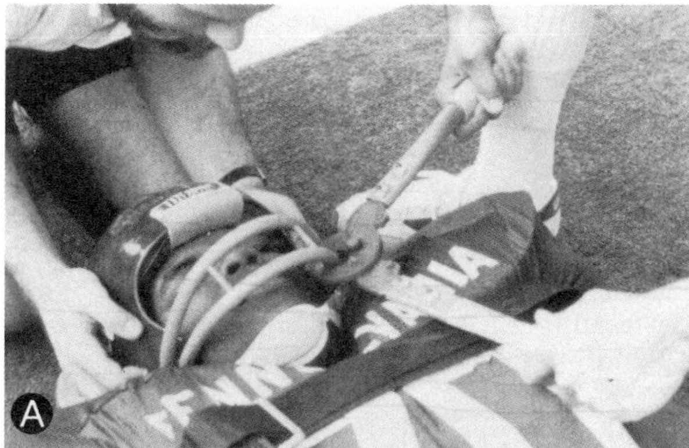

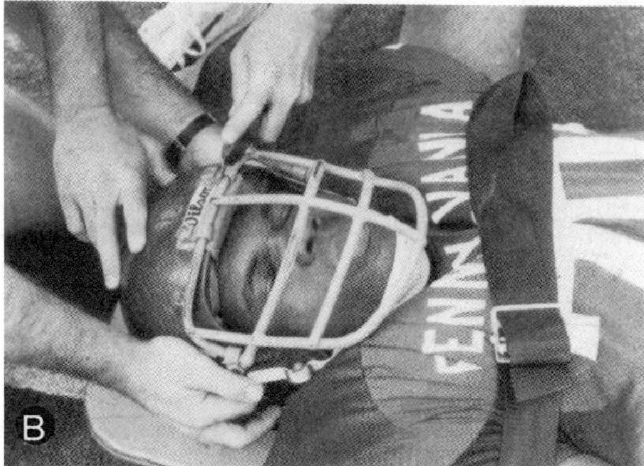

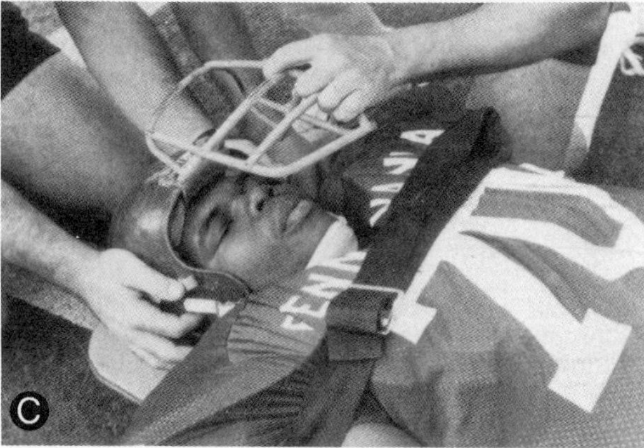

Figure 22.5. **A,** Remove single-bar and double-bar face masks with bolt cutters. **B,** The face mask also can be removed by using a utility knife. **C,** The entire face mask whether it be a double-bar, single-bar, or cage type must be completely removed from the helmet so that it does not interfere with further management of the patient. Reprinted by permission from Vegso JJ, Lehman RC. Field evaluation and management of head and neck injuries. Clin Sports Med 1987;6(1):1–15.

disequilibrium have not abated within the first 12 to 24 hr.

Incidence

In football, concussions most commonly occur while the player is making a tackle (43%), being tackled (23%), blocking (20%), or being blocked (10%) (22). Head injuries are twice as frequent as neck injuries, with nearly 9 out of 10 being a cerebral concussion (26). One in five high school and university football athletes can anticipate receiving a cerebral concussion each season (22).

Return to Competition after a Concussion

Just as there is no accepted definition of concussion, there are no established criteria for when to allow the athlete to return to competition. Treatment recommendations are summarized in Table 22.2 but should be based on clinical judgment. The physician can never be faulted for being too conservative, especially when return to play can result in second impact syndrome (27). Second impact syndrome is a variant of malignant brain edema syndrome seen in children. The syndrome occurs when an athlete sustains a second head injury—often a concussion or a worse injury, such as a cerebral contusion—before symptoms associated with the first concussion have cleared. Symptoms include visual, motor, or sensory changes and difficulty with thought and memory processes. This syndrome has a mortality rate approaching 50% and a morbidity rate nearly 100%, which is why prevention is of utmost importance. Once a player has sustained a concussion, the chance of a second concussion is four times greater than for the athlete who has never sustained a concussion (22). The following recommendations for return to competition following a cerebral concussion are *based* on the grade of concussion and prior incidence of concussion.

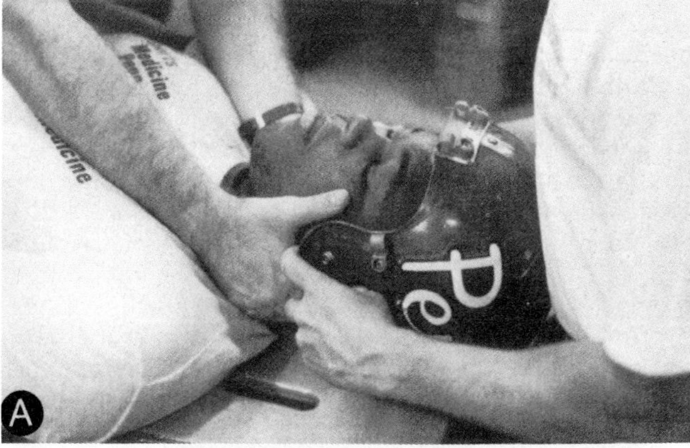

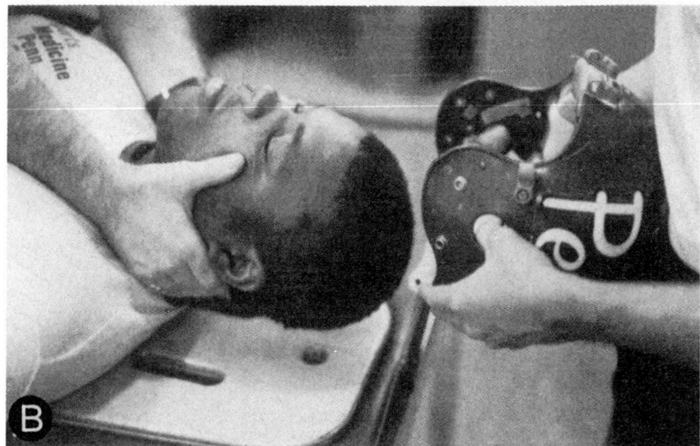

Figure 22.6. Two people should be involved in removal of the helmet. **A,** The helmet should be removed only when permanent immobilization can be instituted. One person supports the oxiput and posterior aspect of the neck while the other person spreads the helmet by pulling the ear holes apart and pulls off the helmet in a straight line with the cervical spine. **B,** Support of the oxiput and neck posteriorly must be performed during and after the removal. Reprinted by permission from Vegso JJ, Lehman RC. Field evaluation and management of head and neck injuries. Clin Sports Med 1987;6(1):1–15.

Grade 1 Return following an initial grade 1 concussion may be as soon as 1 week if the individual remains asymptomatic both at rest and on exertion during that week.

Grade 2 Following a grade 2 cerebral concussion, the athlete may return to competition within 2 weeks if asymptomatic at rest and exertion for the preceding 7 days.

Grade 3 Following a grade 3 concussion, the athlete should be held out of competition for at least 1 month and then may return to play only if asymptomatic at rest and on exertion for the preceding 7 days. Two grade 3 concussions should raise considerable doubt as to whether the individual should be allowed to return to any contact or collision sport.

Postconcussion syndrome consists of headache, dizziness, fatigue, irritability, and in particular impaired memory and concentration. This syndrome is not uncommon. If symptoms persist for a significant length of time, the athlete should be evaluated with a CT scan and/or magnet resonance imaging (MRI) and neuropsychologic testing. Return to competition in collision or contact sports must be deferred until all symptoms have abated to reduce the risk of second impact syndrome. An athlete who is symptomatic from a head injury must not participate in contact or collision sports until all cerebral symptoms have subsided, and preferably not for at least an additional week. Whether it takes days, weeks, or months to reach the asymptomatic state, the athlete must never be permitted to practice or compete while he or she has postconcussion symptoms.

Prevention of Head Injuries

There are five principal aspects of care that have effectively reduced the incidence of head injuries. First, is in the area of improved medical care, especially in on-the-field recognition and treatment of head injuries.

Table 22.2.
Guidelines for Return to Play after Concussion[a]

Grade	First Concussion	Second Concussion	Third Concussion
1 (mild)	May return to play if asymptomatic[b] for 1 week	Return to play in 2 weeks if asymptomatic at that time for 1 week	Terminate season; may return to play next season if asymptomatic
2 (moderate)	May return to play if asymptomatic for 1 week	Minimum of 1 month; may return to play then if asymptomatic for 1 week; consider terminating season	Terminate season; may return to play next season if asymptomatic
3 (severe)	Minimum of 1 month; may then return to play if asymptomatic for 1 week	Terminate season; may return to play next season if asymptomatic	

[a]Reprinted by permission from Cantu RC. Cerebral concussion in sport management and prevention. Sports Med 1992;14(1):64–74.
[b]No headache; dizziness; or impaired orientation, concentration, or memory during rest or exertion.

Understanding when it is safe to return to competition following a head injury lessens the risk of catastrophic injury and the possibility of second impact syndrome. The second area involves improved conditioning, especially of the neck. A strong neck and wise use of the head in blocking and tackling will prevent many catastrophic injuries. Improved protective head gear, properly fitted and maintained, can reduce the incidence of head injury. Analysis of videotape by the coaches, trainers, and physicians after all documented head injuries can demonstrate improper placement of the head and faulty technique. Changes in rules and coaching techniques also are important for the reduction of head injuries. In 1976, a rule change was made when it became clear that the use of the head as a battering ram in tackling was the cause of the most serious head and neck injuries. As a result of this rule change, the incidence of serious head and neck injuries has dropped approximately 50% since the 1970s (26).

Nasal Fractures and Cuts to the Bridge of the Nose

Football has seen a significant decrease in injuries around the facial region (28–30). Soft tissue injuries around the face—including abrasions, contusions, and lacerations—are frequently encountered and should be evaluated to rule out fracture or other significant underlying injury. Repair of facial lacerations should be performed immediately. They usually heal quickly with minimal scar formation. Absorbable or nonabsorbable skin sutures can be placed in a meticulous fashion with little tension on the skin edges. They can be removed in 5 to 7 days to avoid leaving permanent suture marks on the face. Lip and mucosal lacerations that present through-and-through defects from the skin to the oral mucosa should be closed by first suturing the mucosal surface with chromic catgut or other absorbable suture. Closure of the muscle layer is then performed followed by closure of the subcutaneous layer. Finally, the skin is closed with monofilament suture, if necessary.

Ocular injuries in football are not as common as in basketball; however, when they occur they should be investigated fully, including a visual acuity test, pupillary responses, extraocular movements, and fundoscopic examination. Ophthalmology referral may be necessary.

The position and projection of the nose make it a common site of injury for team sports such as football. The parent nasal bones are thick and narrow superiorly and are rarely fractured; however, the lower portion of the nasal bones are broad, thin, and subject to fracture (31). Fractures of the nose may vary with location of impact, direction, magnitude of force, and the age of the subject. Fractures and dislocation of the anterior (cartilaginous) septum often accompany nasal fractures. Cartilage has a degree of flexibility and bends on moderate impact but can fracture with more severe injuries.

In examining a player with a nasal fracture, crepitus and mobility of the fracture segments are noted. External nasal deviation may be present but can be absent or masked by swelling. The intranasal structures should be thoroughly examined after shrinking the mucosa with a 0.25% phenylephrine hydrochloride spray. In particular, septal hematoma should be ruled out. A septal hematoma is a collection of blood between the cartilage and the mucoperichondrium and presents as a bluish red bulging in the nasal vestibule. Players who cannot breath through the nose following a nasal injury should be promptly referred for evaluation. Treatment of nasal fractures is similar in adolescence and adults. Under intravenous sedation or general anesthesia, nasal bones are realigned, and if necessary, an osteotomy is performed to improve symmetry. If the septum is fractured, the segments are straightened. If there is displacement, the septum is realigned and septal splints may be used for approximately 2 weeks to maintain proper position during the initial healing process. Even if proper treatment is rendered at the time of injury, children and adults who have nasal fractures may develop deformed noses later. It is important to counsel patients and parents that long-term follow-up and further surgical intervention may be required. In general, it takes 6 weeks for a fracture of the nose to heal; however, return to sports can be before then as long as protective gear is worn. Care should be taken to confirm proper fit and design of the nose-protection device.

Cervical Sprains

Acute strain of the musculotendinous structure of the neck is probably the most common cervical injury in football. Strain occurs when the musculotendinous unit is overloaded or stretched. Cervical muscles that are the most commonly involved are the sternocleidomastoid, trapezius, rhomboids, erector spinae, scalenes, and levator scapulae. The clinical picture is similar to other musculotendinous injuries. There will be pain at the time of injury that may subside after a few minutes, thus permitting the athlete to return to full participation. As local bleeding occurs in the torn muscle fibers, pain, swelling, and tenderness become apparent. Neck motion becomes painful and reaches a peak after several hours or the next day. Initial treatment is with ice followed by rest, antiinflammatory medications, heat, massage, and other modalities to increase the range of motion and decrease pain.

Diagnosis of a cervical sprain implies that there has been damage to the ligamentous and capsular structures connecting the facet joints and vertebrae. It may be difficult to distinguish between a strain and a sprain in this area. Usually, compressive-type injuries that result in neck pain without severe muscle tenderness are classified as sprains. There is limitation of motion and pain in the area of injury. Radiation of the pain along muscle groups in the area can occur. However, no neurologic symptoms should be present. Ligamentous disruption can be extensive enough to result in instability, resulting in associated neurologic involvement. Therefore, routine cervical radiographs, including flexion and extension views, are recommended. Treatment consists of immobilization, rest, support, and antiinflammatory medications. Return to athletic participation is permitted when motion is normal and muscle strength has been reestablished. Chronic inflammatory changes seen radiographically may occur as a result of recurrent sprains or return to participation before complete healing has occurred.

Fractures and Dislocations of the Cervical Spine

Injuries to the cervical spine resulting in fractures or dislocations with subsequent paraplegia or quadriplegia are infrequent but catastrophic events in football. In 1976, the National Football Head and Neck Injury Registry was established to evaluate epidemiologic factors leading to fracture, dislocation, and subsequent quadriplegia (32, 33). This study looked at cervical spine injuries from 1971 to 1975 and compared them with data complied by Schneider (34), who conducted a similar study between 1959 and 1963. In comparing injuries incurred from 1959 to 1963 with those from 1971 to 1975, a 204% increase in cervical spine fractures, subluxations, and dislocations, and a 116% increase in cases of cervical quadriplegia were seen. Although the rates of head injuries had decreased, the rates of cervical spine injuries with or without quadriplegia had increased dramatically from the data previously reported by Schneider (34). From this study, it was concluded that improved protective capabilities of modern helmets accounted for the decrease in head injuries between the two studies. The improved protection of the head led to the development of playing techniques that used the top or crown of the helmet as the initial point of contact and these head-first techniques placed the cervical spine at risk for serious injury. It was postulated that the athlete's cervical spine was exposed to excessive axial loads, making the spinal cord particularly susceptible to injury in that area. As a result of this study, NCAA football rules were changed in February 1976. At that time, intentionally striking a runner with the crown or top of the helmet, spearing, or the deliberate use of the helmet in an attempt to punish the opponent and use of the helmet to butt or ram an opponent were outlawed. These changes were the result of the determination that axial loading was the primary mechanism of injury responsible for producing severe spinal injuries in tackle football through a review of epidemiologic, biomechanical, and cinematographic data compiled by the National Football Head and Neck Injury Registry.

Between 1976 and 1987, fractures, subluxations, and dislocations of the cervical spine have progressively declined (21). These rates represent a 70% reduction in high school injuries and a 65% reduction in college injuries. Cervical spine injuries resulting in quadriplegia declined from a total of 34 cases in 1976 before the rule change to 5 cases in 1984. Axial compression was identified as the mechanism causing the highest percentage of football cervical fractures, dislocations, and subluxation with and without quadriplegia. Torg et al.'s (21) classic study demonstrated that in the 51 films reviewed it was possible to observe the mechanism of injury. Axial loading was determined to be the primary cause in every instance. It is usually seen in the case of a defensive back who makes a tackle by striking his opponent with the top of his helmet. Other potential mechanisms of injury include hyperflexion and hyperextension along with axial loading, which places the cervical spinal cord at risk for nonreversible injury.

Because the neck is what allows the player to see what is happening around him, it is quite vulnerable in any position, not simply flexion, extension, or rotation. The intrinsic and extrinsic neck muscles are generally small with poor strength. As such, all football players should be taught to strengthen the neck in hope of stabilizing the spine during contact.

The mechanisms of injury to the cervical spine should be kept in mind by all individuals who take care of football players. These include flexion with anterior compression and posterior distraction, lateral flexion or rotation that will stretch the convex side and impinge on the concave side, extension with distraction anteriorly and compression posteriorly, and direct axial compression. Flexion and rotation injuries are commonly found in players who are running down field and following the flight of the ball, such as offensive linemen, receivers, and defensive backs. They may block or tackle an opposing player with their head in an offset position and with the neck muscles relaxed. On-the-field examination of a player with a suspected neck injury, neck or radicular pain is mandatory (Fig. 22.7). The on-field evaluation begins by determining if the patient has or had motor or sensory loss. Did he have neck pain? Was he unconscious? Is there neck or arm pain? Is there spine and leg pain? If the player has significant neck tenderness, it is usually best to transport him as if he had a spinal cord injury and to conduct further evaluation. If there are any neurologic findings, the patient should be transported as if they had a spinal cord injury. Temporary quadriplegia must be differentiated from a loss of consciousness from a head injury. Changes in reflexes, muscle strength, sensation, and a positive Spurling's test are all criteria for transport of the athlete as if he had a spinal cord injury. When in doubt, do not take chances. To evaluate a player laying on his stomach a log roll with one person monitoring the head and neck at all times is appropriate. The most common error in this technique is not having enough people to assist (Fig. 22.8). The key to this technique is to have one person control the head and shoulders and not be responsible for the transfer of weight. This person should be the chief and direct the movements of the team. The chief should position himself or herself to immobilize the head by clasping the trapexius, clavicle, and scapula and cradle the athlete's head under his or her forearms. The player can be rolled onto a backboard that is placed under him. The patient usually can be moved very safely. Do not remove the helmet on the field. If there is any question about adequacy of the airway, the face mask can be removed quickly by using either a bolt cutter or a utility knife.

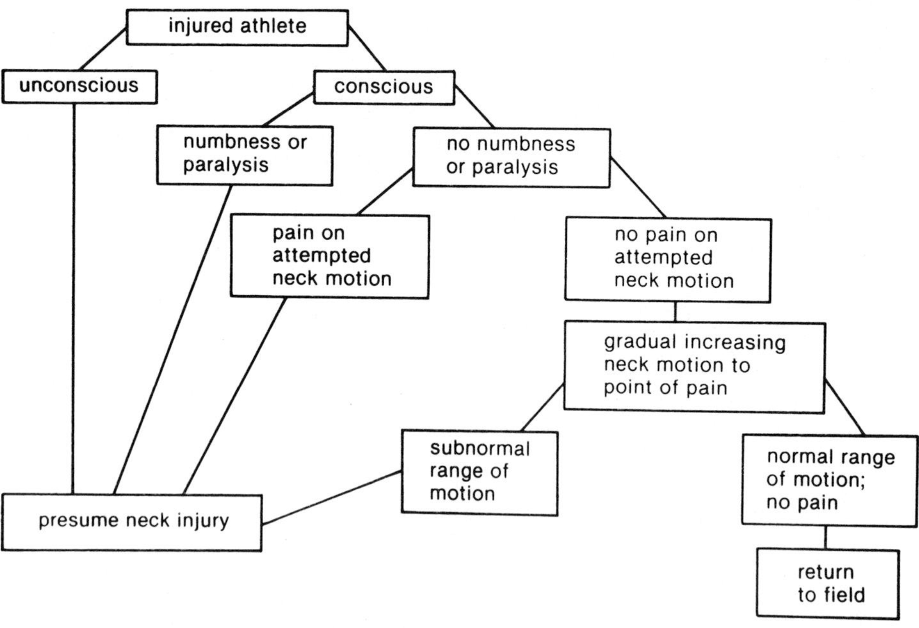

Figure 22.7. Algorhythm for evaluation of an athlete with a cervical injury. Reprinted by permission from Jackson DW, Lohr FT. Cervical spine injuries. Clin Sports Med 1986;5(2):373–386.

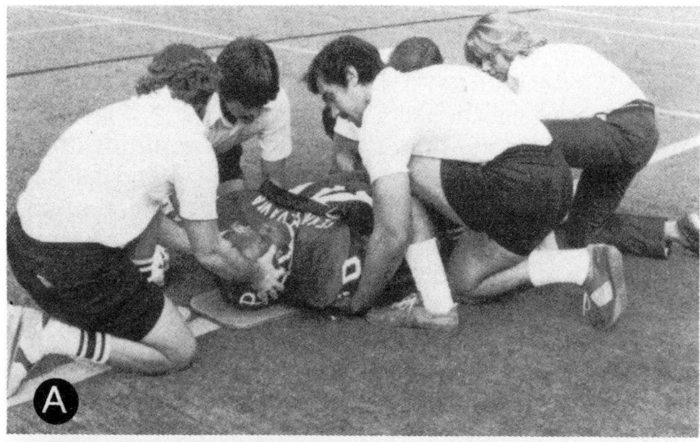

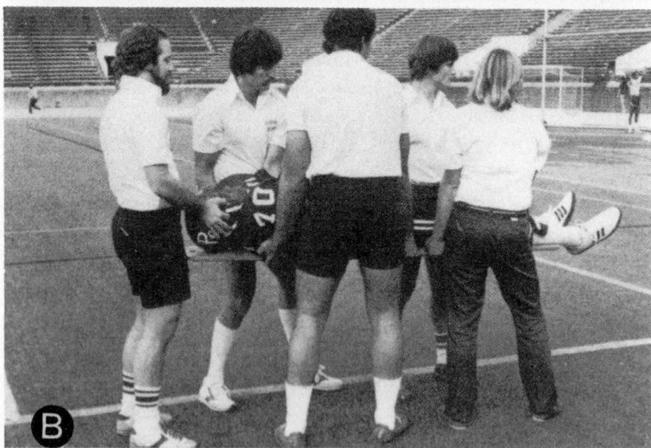

Figure 22.8. It is important to have a complete medical team available to avoid potential complications in transport. **A,** The chief maintains control of the head and neck while the support team centers the body on the spine board. **B,** The player is in position on the spine board, ready for transport. Reprinted by permission from Vegso JJ, Lehman RC. Field evaluation and management of head and neck injuries. Clin Sports Med 1987;6(1):1–15.

Physical Examination

Physical examination consists of a complete neurologic examination, head compression test, Spurling's and Adson's maneuvers, resistive head pressure, and cervical range of motion. If there is any question of a cervical spine fracture, dislocation, or instability, the patient should be transported to the hospital with his helmet in place and a lateral x-ray should be obtained first before the helmet is removed. If there is an unstable spine or cervical spine injury documented radiographically, the helmet must be removed in the hospital where definitive treatment facilities are at your disposal. To remove the helmet, the jaw pads should be removed. One individual should reach inside the shoulder pads and helmet to stabilize the head and neck. Two assistants should then separate the ear holes of the helmet and remove it in a posterior direction. The athlete's head and neck must be stabilized during this procedure to prevent further injury.

Two criteria should be used for removing a player from the game. The first is radiating arm pain and loss of function, such as paresthesias and weakness. The second finding is the loss of cervical range of motion. Until complete diagnostic evaluation is carried out, the player should not play.

Radiographic Evaluation

Radiographic evaluation of the suspected cervical spine injury patient includes AP, lateral, oblique, and flexion/extension films and an open-mouth odontoid view. At no point should an inadequate radiograph be accepted. If radiographs are ordered and C7 is not visualized, an unstable cervical spine cannot be ruled out. Further radiologic tests should be ordered to clear the patient. Review of these films will show potential sites of fractures. Review of the flexion/extension views should alert the examiner to potential areas of instability. If there is an angle of 11° or greater than the sum of the angles measured at the levels above and below, it should be considered an area of potential instability. Greater than 3.5 mm of horizontal translation also is indicative of ligament instability (21). If the athlete has symptoms that suggest spinal cord involvement, such as transient quadriplegia, burning hands syndrome, or other bilateral motor or sensory symptoms, the physician should consider obtaining a magnetic resonance imaging scan.

In summary, understanding neck injuries in football players begins with an appreciation of how the game is played and the potential mechanisms of injury. Neck injuries are an unavoidable part of the game. Preventative measures, treatment techniques, and criteria for return to play following a neck injury must be clear. Torg et al. (33) have shown that 1.25 million football players are exposed to injuries annually. Tackling is the leading cause of neck injury, and being tackled is the second most common cause. Cervical spine injuries leading to permanent paralysis are usually caused by playing techniques that use the crown of the helmet as a primary point of contact in high-impact situations (spearing). All surveys have shown that injuries in football can occur if the recommendations involving head blocking and tackling are not carefully observed. The team physician is responsible for recognizing and determining the nature of injury. Radiographs should be carefully reviewed to identify abnormalities. Criteria for return to football include no pain, full range of motion, and a normal neurologic examination, including restoration of all strength and power of the neck and extremity musculature. The use of horseshoe neck rolls to provide support for extension and lateral bending forces have not been scientifically proven to prevent injuries. However, they are frequently used in individuals who have a stiff, sore neck without any other pathology demonstrated on radiographic studies.

Shoulder

Shoulder injuries are common in football; in fact, in one study the frequency of shoulder injuries was found to be second only to the knee (35). There are a variety of injuries about the shoulder that can occur in football players. These injuries are not peculiar to football, but there are certain injuries that occur more commonly in football players. Included among this group are brachial plexus injuries, acromioclavicular injuries, contusions and exostoses, glenohumeral instability, and rotator cuff injuries. Some of these injuries are position specific. For example, brachial plexus injuries and proximal humeral contusions are more common in defensive players, whereas rotator cuff injuries are more frequently encountered in quarterbacks. A more detailed discussion of some of these specific injuries and their treatment is provided in the chapter on shoulder injuries.

Brachial Plexus Injuries

Brachial plexus injuries—also known as stingers, burners, or pinched nerves—are quite common in football players. They are usually related to forced lateral deviation of the neck when tackling an opposing player. The injury is often associated with pain and numbness or paresthesias in the ipsilateral extremity. Burners are probably the most common neurologic injury in football. In one study, approximately 50% of the players on a NCAA Division I football squad indicated that they had suffered a suspected injury of the brachial plexus during their careers (36). Another recent study indicates that 65% of Division III football players surveyed suffered this injury during their college careers. Of these injuries, 70% were not reported (37). Because of its high association with cervical spine disorders, careful evaluation of the spine and neurologic testing is indicated (38).

As with all injuries, the history and physical examination is critical. The exact mechanism of injury can usually be obtained from discussion with the athletic trainer and/or team physician or review of game films. Usually the athlete's head is forced laterally, stretching the brachial plexus (39) (Fig. 22.9). Occasionally, there may be a visible contusion to the area over the plexus. The player will often complain of numbness, pain, and tingling in the affected extremity that usually resolves in a short period. During physical examination, the patient may feel pain radiating from the scapulae with or without associated clavicular pain. Careful evaluation of the neck also is important. This should include range of motion, assessment of tenderness along the spinous processes, and careful neurologic examination. Thorough assessment of motor strength, particularly in the C5 to C6 distribution, may reveal weakness of the deltoid, biceps, or rotator cuff muscles (36). Transient numbness in the radial forearm and hand also may be noted. Documented paresthesias and weakness in the other arm or in the legs raises the possibility of transient quadraplegia, anterior cord syndrome, or more

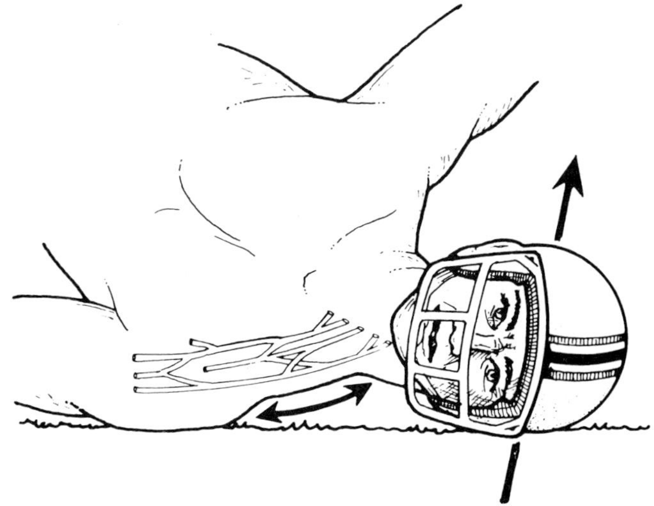

Figure 22.9. Mechanism of injury to the brachial plexus (burners). Reprinted by permission from Zarins B, Prodromos LC. Shoulder injuries in sports. In: Rowe CR, ed. The shoulder. New York: Churchill Livingston, 1988:411–433. The shoulder. New York: Churchill Livingston, 1988:419.

severe cervical injury (40). *Radiographs should be obtained if there is any significant neck pain, limited motion, or weakness and for all players with initial episode of a burner.* Radiographs should include AP, oblique, lateral flexion and extension, and odontoid films. These films should be reviewed for congenital fusions, instability, degenerative changes, evidence of acute trauma, and cervical stenosis (38). Cervical stenosis can be assessed on the lateral radiograph based on Torg's ratio (41). An abnormal Torg's ratio (<0.80) should suggest the need for further workup. Though the ratio overestimates the presence of spinal stenosis, if a player has spinal stenosis, the ratio is almost always abnormal. Brachial plexopathy should not be confused with the "dead arm" syndrome that occurs with anterior shoulder subluxation (42).

Because the symptoms are transient, the patient is anxious to resume play following the episode. If there are no neck complaints, the player has full cervical motion, and all neurologic findings are normal, then he may return to competition with the addition of a neck roll or other device (Fig. 22.10). However, if any of the above findings are positive or if the symptoms are more significant, then a complete workup including cervical films and neurologic testing may be indicated. Rigid interpretation of electromyographic (EMG) changes in patients with brachial plexopathy is probably not indicated. One follow-up study of players with transient brachial plexus injuries noted a high percentage of persistent EMG changes several years after injury (43). Careful attention to blocking and tackling techniques also is appropriate. The use of high shoulder pads and soft cervical collars may help decrease the recurrence rate of brachial plexus injuries (see Fig. 22.10).

Of particular concern is the prolonged burner syndrome. Despite the obvious concern to the team physician, one study noted that there was no difference between this subgroup of players and those with shorter periods of symptoms (44). The authors recently treated a patient with a severe burner with complete paralysis of the affected upper extremity that persisted almost 24 hr. Complete workup, including cervical radiographs, MRI, and neurologic testing, revealed no significant difference between this patient and others with shorter periods of symptoms. Although it was of significant concern to the authors, the patient's symptoms gradually resolved, and he has a completely normal examination at this point. He has returned to play without any recurrent symptoms.

Acromioclavicular Injuries

Acromioclavicular (AC) joint injuries are quite common in football. In one study of acromioclavicular injuries in athletes, 41% occurred as a result of football injuries (45). Acromioclavicular injuries in football, as in other sports, are usually caused by a direct blow from a fall on the point of the shoulder. The severity of acute separations depends on whether the coracoclavicular ligaments are disrupted. This is the basis for the classification scheme described by Rockwood (46) (Fig. 22.11).

Again, discussion with the trainer or team physician and review of game films will reveal the typical mechanism of injury, usually a fall directly onto the shoulder. Physical examination is characterized by point tenderness directly over the AC joint, and in more significant injuries, there may be a stepoff between the clavicle and the acromion. Patients may have limitation of abduction and horizontal adduction with grade 2 injuries and significant limitation of motion with grade 3 and higher injuries. Radiographs are normal for grade

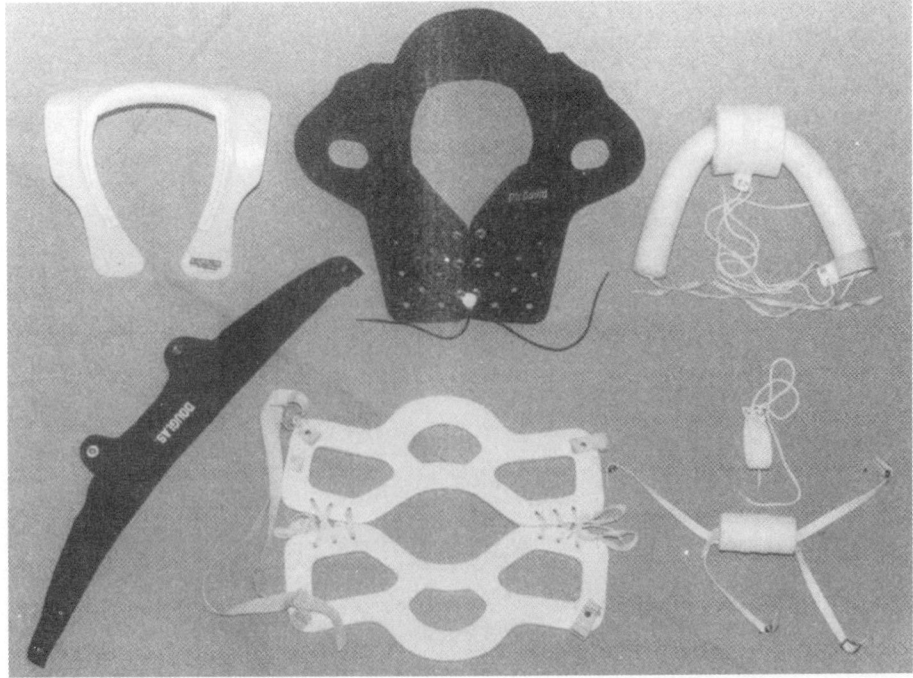

Figure 22.10. Devices that can be used to help reduce the incidence and recurrence of burners. *Top (left to right):* La Porta cervical collar; cowboy collar; bike neck roll. *Bottom (left to right):* Douglas neckroll; shoulder injury pad (elevates shoulder pads); neck flexion chin strap. Reprinted by permission of McGraw-Hill, Inc., from Sallis RE, Jones K, Knopp W. Burners: offensive strategy for an underreported injury. Phys Sportsmed 1992;20:47–55.

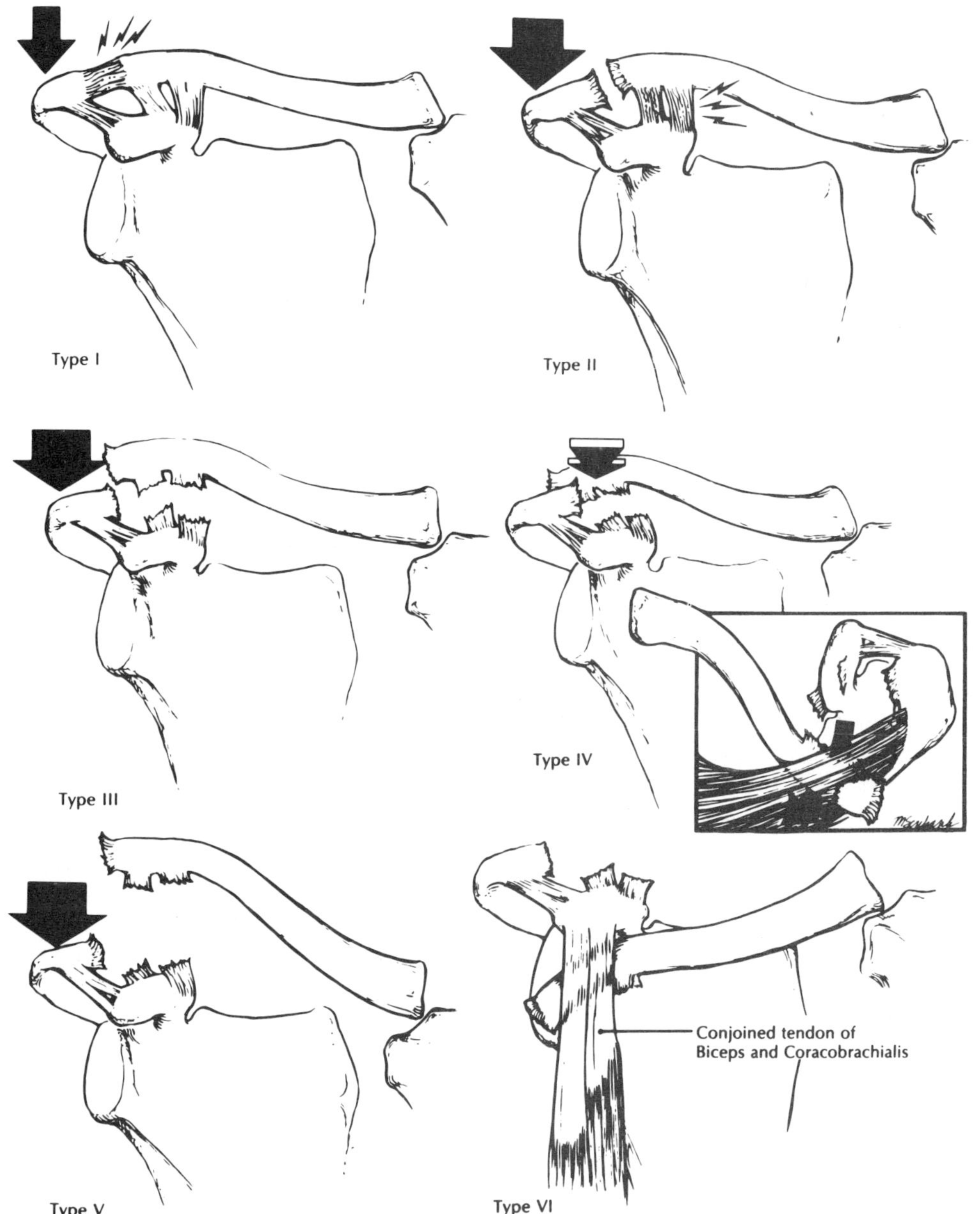

Figure 22.11. Classification of acromioclavicular injuries. Note that type III and above are associated with coracoclavicular disruptions. Reprinted by permission from Rockwood CA. Injuries to the acromioclavicular joint. In: Rockwood CA, Green DG, eds. Fractures in adults. 2nd ed. Philadelphia: JB Lippincott, 1984:871.

1 injuries, may show a slight stepoff in grade 2 injuries, and show a more significant separation of the acromion and clavicle in grade 3 and higher injuries. Treatment of grade 1 and 2 injuries typically involves rest and activity modification, with the addition of a modified Kenny-Howard sling for grade 2 injuries. Treatment of grade 3 injuries is somewhat controversial, with most surgeons currently favoring nonoperative management of these injuries (47). Nonoperative management necessarily results in a residual deformity of the AC joint; however, there is little correlation between the final radiograph, clinical appearance, and the incidence of significant pain and disability (48). Nonoperative management consists of the use of orthotic devices such as the modified Kenny-Howard sling for a period of 1 to 2 weeks and the use of isometric exercises while in the sling, followed by range-of-motion and progressive-resistance exercises. Surgical treatment is reserved for significant grade 3 injuries in quarterbacks, and grade 4 and higher injuries. Open reduction of the AC joint; coracoclavicular repair; and temporary stabilization with a screw, wire, or absorbable sutures/tape to maintain reduction of the coracoclavicular space for approximately 8 to 10 weeks postoperatively is usually favored.

Chronic acromioclavicular separations may be best managed with a modified Weaver-Dunn procedure (49). This procedure uses the intact coracoacromial ligament, which is detached from the acromion and transferred to the end of the transacted distal clavicle through drill holes and tied over the superior cortex of the clavicle. The repair is supplemented with a temporary fixation device as described for acute treatments above.

Contusions

Soft tissue injuries to the shoulder girdle are quite common in football players, particularly in linebackers. These are usually caused by direct blows, and the injury is analogous to the iliac crest contusion, or hip pointer (50). Repetitive contusions over the subcutaneous part of the anterior lateral humerus just distal to the edge of the normal shoulder pads can result in tacklers' exostosis. In this condition, repetitive blows damage the deltoid insertion or the brachialis origin, resulting in periosteal tearing and new bone formation. Radiographs may demonstrate a "dotted veil" in the region that later develops into a mature exostosis. Treatment, if recognized early, consists of icing, compression wraps, and possible aspiration of a hematoma. Late recognition occasionally necessitates surgical removal of a symptomatic mature exostosis.

Myositis ossificans, which occurs in the younger football player (51), can be differentiated from tacklers' exostosis by its radiodense cleavage plane between the lesion and the humeral cortex. Additional padding below the level of the shoulder pads can be preventative. Both lesions can result in a flexion contracture of the elbow, necessitating surgical intervention.

Glenohumeral Instability

Improper tackling techniques such as demonstrated in Figure 22.12 have been implicated as a cause of anterior shoulder instability (50). Instability represents a spectrum from a simple sprain to a frank dislocation. Several classification schemes have been devised, based on the direction of the instability, degree of instability, and chronology. Rowe classifies shoulder dislocations in five categories: traumatic; atraumatic; voluntary; transient subluxation; and involuntary subluxation (50). Management of acute dislocations consists of immediate reduction, immobilization for approximately 3 weeks, and rehabilitation. The role of arthroscopy in the management of acute shoulder dislocations is controversial. One recent study suggested that acute arthroscopic shoulder stabilization may be more successful than immobilization and rehabilitation (52). Arthroscopic stabilization in a competitive football player, however, may not be the most efficacious form of treatment.

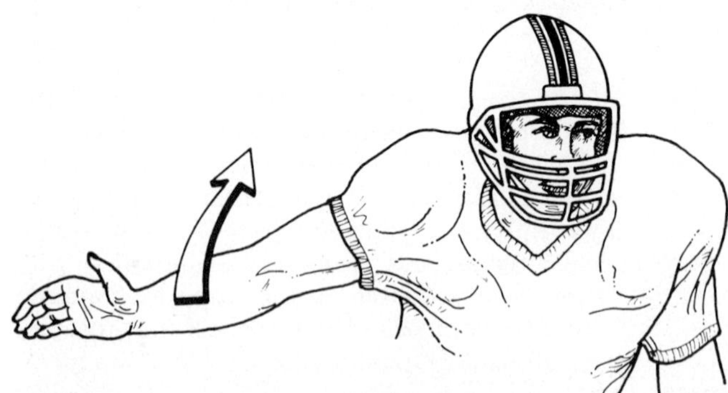

Figure 22.12. Improper tracking technique can result in anterior shoulder dislocation. Note the position of the arm, which is completely abducted, creating a lever that can result in a large moment across the shoulder. Reprinted by permission from Zarins B, Prodromos LC. Shoulder injuries in sports. In: Rowe CR, ed. The shoulder. New York: Churchill, Livingston, 1988:411–433.

Recurrent instability has been subclassified by Matson (53) into two types: traumatic unidirectional Bankart lesion surgery, or TUBS (often necessary), and atraumatic multidirectional bilateral rehabilitation (encouraged) and inferior capsular shift, or AMBRI (if necessary). The typical football player would usually fall into the TUBS category and may ultimately require a change in sport or surgery for recurrent instability. Open Bankart repair, usually with a capsular shift, is currently the authors' procedure of choice, with the possible exception of arthroscopic stabilization for the elite quarterback.

Posterior shoulder instability can result from a fall on an internally rotated adducted arm or a direct blow to the anterior aspect of the shoulder (54). Physical findings are notable for presentation with the arm abducted and internally rotated with a prominent coracoid process and an empty glenoid fossa medially and bulging posteriorly. In addition, the patient may be unable fully to supinate his forearm with the arm forward flexed (55). AP and physician-assisted axillary lateral radiographs are essential to make this often-missed diagnosis. Treatment consists of reduction with lateral and distal traction, immobilization, and rehabilitation. Recurrent posterior instability is a difficult problem because surgery, even in the most experienced hands, is associated with a high recurrence rate (56).

Rotator Cuff Injuries

Rotator cuff injuries typically occur in middle-aged individuals; however, overhead-throwing athletes, such as quarterbacks, may be susceptible to these injuries at an earlier age. Players may complain of pain with throwing and with overhead activities. Physical examination should include a careful evaluation for anterior instability, which can lead to secondary impingement. Examination maneuvers specific for impingement include the impingement sign (flexion of the arm causes pain in approximately the 90° to 120° arc of motion), Hawkins test (forward flexion and internal rotation of the arm causes impingement pain), and the impingement test (injection of lidocaine subacromially allows the patient to perform these maneuvers without pain). Weakness with abduction and external rotation also are consistent with rotator cuff pathology. Radiographs should include both a 30° caudal tilt (57) and a supraspinatus outlet view (58) to evaluate the presence and type of subacromial spurring. Studies to evaluate the rotator cuff itself such as ultrasonography, arthrography, and magnetic resonance imaging, may also be necessary. Although still in its infancy, shoulder arthroscopy may have a role in the treatment of impingement and partial thickness rotator cuff tears in the athlete. Initial results of arthroscopic subacromial decompression have been encouraging (59, 60). Debridement of partial thickness (incomplete) tears resulted in a favorable clinical outcome in 85% of one series (61). Full-thickness rotator cuff tears are distinctly unusual in the younger athlete. Treatment of these injuries necessitates an open or an arthroscopically assisted procedure and will probably result in the end of that player's career.

Elbow Injuries

Throwing athletes are at risk for a variety of elbow disorders (62–64). Elbow instability is covered in detail in the chapter on baseball injuries; however, it is important to note that this condition can exist in quarterbacks as well. Injuries are caused by repetitive valgus forces that are generated during the late cocking and acceleration phases of throwing (65). A history of repetitive overhead throwing activities is seen with localized pain on the medial aspect of the elbow, tenderness, and instability with valgus stressing. Treatment consists initially of rest, nonsteroidal antiinflammatory drugs, and supervised stretching and strengthening. Reconstruction of the ulnar collateral ligament with a graft placed through tunnels has been recommended by some authors (64).

Elbow dislocations can occur as a result of hyperextension (66), usually as a result of a fall on a hand or wrist. Elbow dislocations are classified by the position of the ulna relative to the humerus. Most elbow dislocations are posterior and involve both the radius and the ulna (67). A careful neurovascular examination is critical before manipulation of the dislocated elbow because of a high association with neurovascular injury (68). Reduction with distraction followed by anterior translation usually results in a stable reduction. Although the period of immobilization following reduction is controversial, most authors recommend less than 1 week. Therapy is individualized based on the extent of the injury. Other injuries of the elbow are covered elsewhere in this volume.

Injuries of the Forearm, Wrist, and Hand

In football, the forearm, wrist, and hand are particularly vulnerable to injuries because they are used against rigid objects such as the helmet, face mask, and shoulder pads. The forearm is prone to contusions, particularly when used for blocking. Forearm pads can be used to protect the forearm; however, the pads must comply with the rules for the particular level of play. Generally, use of hard or unyielding surfaces below the level of the elbow are prohibited. Fractures of the bones of the forearm are uncommon, but they can occur with direct blows such as when arm tackling. Forearm fractures are more common when falling on the outstretched arm and often result in a spiral fracture.

Contusions over the dorsum of the hand are particularly common. They occur as a result of a direct blow such as contact with an opponent's face mask or after being stepped on. Players with a contusion will present with pain, tenderness, and marked swelling of the dorsum of the hand. Ecchymosis may also be present. Fractures of the metacarpals must be ruled out. Contusions are treated with ice and compression in the acute phase. Padding should be used to protect the hand from further injury with return to football.

Fractures of the metacarpals can occur as a result of a direct blow or a fall on the outstretched hand. A boxers' fracture of the fifth metacarpal may occur as a result of a poorly executed punch with the closed hand. Individuals with a metacarpal fracture will present with symptoms similar to that of a contusion, including pain, tenderness, and swelling. Crepitus at the fracture site may be elicited with passive flexion and extension of the metacarpophalangeal joint. Obvious deformity is rare. Most metacarpal fractures are undisplaced or minimally displaced and are considered to be stable. In football, metacarpal fractures are evenly distributed among the fingers (69). Most metacarpal fractures occurring in football can be treated with the application of a cast and/or splint. A hard cast may be used during the week for practice. It can be replaced with a special cast constructed of silicone rubber for games (Fig. 22.13). At the completion of the game, the hard cast should be reapplied. Use of a cast should be maintained until there is radiographic evidence of healing. After healing, the hand should continue to be protected for the remainder of the season. Fractures that are displaced should be treated with internal fixation. This allows early motion and return to football with protective padding. Rettig et al. (69) described metacarpal fractures occurring in football players. Average loss of practice or game time for metacarpal fractures treated with simple immobilization was 12 days. Those requiring internal fixation averaged 22 days of lost practice or game time. Follow-up of these injuries revealed no residual subjective or objective limitations. Displacement of the fracture with return to football is not expected.

Fractures of the scaphoid are common in football.

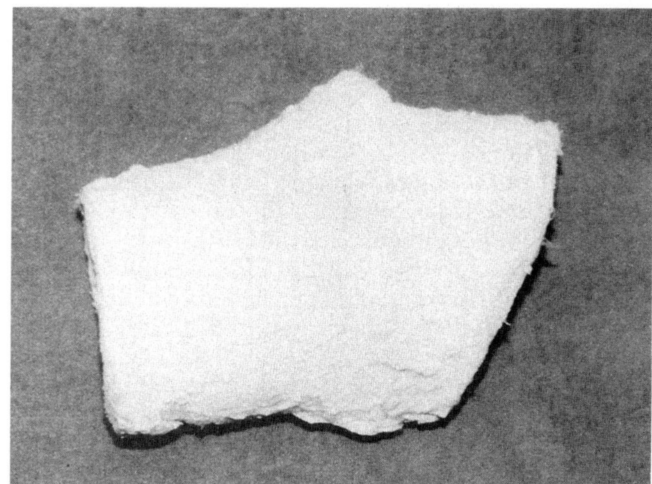

Figure 22.13. A silicone rubber cast can be constructed of General Electric RTV-11 and gauze. The silicone rubber cast is pliable and conforms to the rule that bans hard, unyielding surfaces below the elbow.

They occur when the player falls on the outstretched arm with the wrist in the extended position. The athlete will present with pain and tenderness in the anatomic snuff box. Pain can be increased with extension and radial deviation of the wrist. Radiographs may initially be negative. The fracture line may become evident with serial x-rays several weeks later. A high index of suspicion is needed to diagnose these injuries in the absence a positive radiograph immediately after injury. A bone scan may be used to confirm this suspicion. Fractures that have a stepoff or gap of less than 1 mm are considered to be nondisplaced. Most fractures involving the scaphoid in football are nondisplaced or minimally displaced and are considered to be stable (70). Treatment consists of application of a short arm-thumb spica cast with the wrist in neutral position. The thumb should be included to the level of the interphalangeal joint. Athletes in unskilled positions who do not need to handle the ball can return to playing with a padded cast. Because NCAA and high school rules do not allow use of hard and unyielding surfaces below the elbow, the cast should be removed before competition and replaced with a custom-made silicone rubber cast. This can be worn during the game but must be approved by the officials. Following the game, the silicone rubber cast should be removed and a new short arm-thumb spica cast should be applied. Fractures that are detected and treated early can be expected to heal; however, the length of immobilization may be up to 6 months (70). Some fractures involving the scaphoid, particularly those for which diagnosis and treatment is delayed, may develop into a nonunion and require bone grafting. Nonunion may be more likely with those fractures that involve the proximal pole because of the retrograde nature of the blood supply to the scaphoid.

Football players are prone to injury of the ulnar collateral ligament of the first metacarpophalangeal joint, which is called game keepers' thumb. The injury usually results from forced abduction of the thumb. It can also occur as a combination of abduction and hyperextension and less frequently as a combination of abduction and flexion (71). Football players are particularly prone to this injury. It can occur as a result of the player's thumb becoming entangled with the opposing player's jersey, or as the player falls on his outstretched hand. The injury involves a partial or complete tear of the ulnar collateral ligament. It is imperative to distinguish between a stable and unstable injury as this may affect treatment. The player may complain of pain and weakness with use of the thumb, particularly when attempting to pinch between the thumb and forefinger. There is usually localized tenderness over the ulnar collateral ligament. Pain can be elicited by radially deviating (abducting) the first metacarpophalangeal joint. Stability of the joint must be determined with the thumb in flexion and extension and should be compared with the uninvolved side to assess for individual differences in laxity. Partial tears of the ulnar collateral ligament are stable with radial stressing of the joint and have a good end point. Complete tears will demonstrate instability with radial deviation and will not have a firm end point. In a complete tear, laxity is at least 30° greater than that present on the uninjured side (71). Radiographs should be determined to rule out an associated fracture. Fractures associated with this type of injury most commonly involve an avulsion from the base of the proximal phalanx. Bilateral stress views may be used for comparison when it is difficult to determine the difference between complete and partial tears by physical examination.

Treatment depends on whether the injury is stable or unstable. If the injury is stable, indicating a partial tear of the ulnar collateral ligament, it may be successfully treated by placing the thumb in a spica cast. Immobilization should be maintained for 3 weeks, followed by protection for an additional 2 weeks (71). During immobilization, the thumb should be placed in the mid-position of abduction/adduction and flexion/extension to minimize stress on the ulnar collateral ligament. Following immobilization, exercises are used to reestablish range of motion and use of the hand. Nonskill players may return to activity during the period of immobilization, with a padded or silicone rubber–type cast. Football players who require use of their hands such as quarterbacks and receivers may not be able to return to football until the injury has healed.

For unstable injuries (indicating a complete tear of the ulnar collateral ligament), repair of the ulnar collateral ligament is indicated to restore stability to the ulnar side of the thumb (71). These ligamentous injuries often do not spontaneously heal because of soft tissue interposition (Stenner's lesion). Stability of the ulnar side of the joint is important to allow functional use of the thumb, particularly during activities that require pinch. Following surgical repair, the thumb is placed is a spica cast or a thumb spica splint for 3 weeks. After 3 weeks of immobilization, the patient should be instructed in an exercise program consisting of active isolated joint motion as well as active exercises to increase composite flexion and extension of the thumb. Protective splinting should be continued for up to 6 weeks from the date of surgery.

Following partial or complete tear of the ulnar collateral ligament, the player's thumb should be protected when he returns to activity. Protection may be provided by use of a splint or adhesive tape. For skilled players, the tape should be applied in a figure of eight around the thumb. For nonskilled players that do not handle the ball, taping may be used to hold the thumb against the second finger or to anchor it to the index finger (Fig. 22.14).

Fumich et al. (72) reported two cases involving dorsal dislocation of the metacarpophalangeal joint of the thumb in offensive linemen. This injury was caused by use of improper blocking technique in which the player dorsiflexed his wrist and drove his closed fist into the opponent's chest, using his thumb to push against the inferior border of the opposing player's shoulder pads. A dorsal dislocation of the phalanx occurred when the thumb was hyperextended. The radial collateral ligament was torn when the thumb was flexed, driving the radial border of the thumb against the shoulder pads.

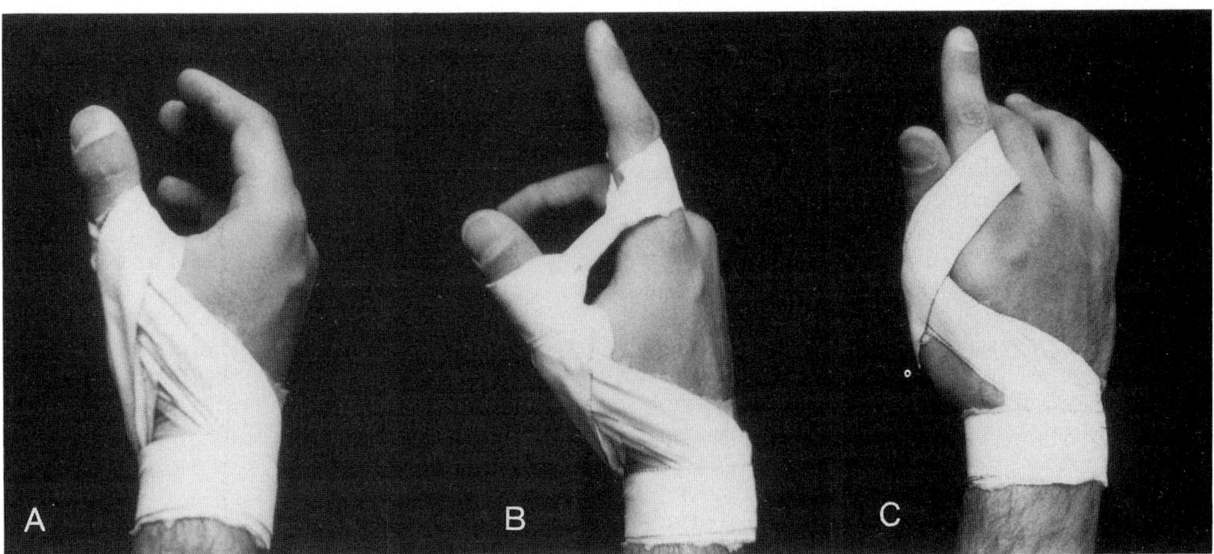

Figure 22.14. Taping to protect the thumb. **A,** The figure eight applied to the thumb is used for skilled positions. **B,** The thumb is taped to the index finger. **C,** The figure eight is used with the thumb anchored to index finger. **B** and **C** are used for players who are not required to handle the ball.

Offensive linemen should be taught proper blocking techniques to avoid these injuries.

Injuries to the fingers are common in football players. Sprains of the interphalangeal joints may occur as the player's fingers become entangled with the opposing player. Injuries to the interphalangeal joints may be caused by the ball. If these injuries are ignored and improperly treated, loss of motion and deformity may occur. Players will typically report that they jammed or stoved their fingers. Assessment will reveal pain and localized tenderness to the involved joint, which will typically be swollen and have limited motion. Stability should be assessed by applying an abduction/adduction force to the joint. Radiographs should be taken to ensure that a fracture has not occurred. Occasionally, these injuries involve an avulsion fracture or an intraarticular fracture. Treatment for most sprained fingers involves buddy taping and range-of-motion exercises. When taping the injured finger to an adjacent finger, material such as a gauze pad or foam rubber should be placed between the two fingers to minimize maceration of the skin. Injuries involving a complete tear of the ligament or a fracture may require immobilization and/or internal fixation. Intraarticular fractures should be carefully reduced and internally fixated to ensure restoration of the normal geometry of the articular surface.

Tendon injuries such as avulsion injuries of the flexor digitorum profundus may occur as the player grasps an opponent's jersey (jersey finger). Players presenting with this injury will be unable to flex the distal interphalangeal joint. Surgical repair should be performed to restore use of the finger.

Lumbar Spine Injuries

The lumbar spine is resilient and resistant to serious injury; however, mild injuries can be disabling. Some of the activities intrinsic to football, e.g., repetitive flexion, extension, and torsional stresses to the lumbar motion segments, predispose the lumbar spine to injury. Studies suggest that 30% of college football players will lose playing time because of a lumbar spine problem (73). In the NFL, players reported a 12% incidence of spine injuries, resulting in lost playing time (73). Most low-back injuries will respond promptly to conservative care, including modalities and therapeutic exercise. The patient whose symptoms persist or has multiple recurrences deserves a more in-depth investigation.

A review of common injury patterns in football reveals lumbar contusions or strains are the most common injuries (74). These are generally managed by modification of athletic activities, or restriction of participation, followed by conditioning and strengthening of the lumbar muscles. The main goal of rehabilitation is to attain adequate musculoligamentous control of lumbar spine forces to reduce the risk of repetitive injury. Gradual resumption of athletic activities is allowed once symptoms subside and as improved conditioning and muscle support develops.

Spondylolysis, a common and controversial condition of the lumbar spine of football players, has caused indecision among physicians and trainers on the treatment modalities and the ability of the athlete to participate. An incidence of 21% was reported in a survey of 677 male high school and university athletes (75). A study of college football players noted a 15% incidence of lumbar spondylolysis, which did not significantly increase during their college years (76). The incidence in college linemen has been reported to be 50% (77). Spondylolysis is thought to be the result of repetitive loading of the posterior lumbar elements that occurs when the linemen come out of their stance into the blocking posture while excessively extending the lumbar spine. It is generally now well-accepted that spondylolysis is an acquired defect of the pars interarticularis secondary to repetitive extension and loading of the posterior elements of the lumbar spine (78, 79). Many football players are involved in an active weight-lifting program that involves repetitive extension maneuvers. It is felt that improper technique while attempting squats using free weights may contribute to spondylolysis as much as any other factor (80, 81). The actual number of athletes who participate in football with a spondylolysis or spondylisthesis is unknown, because the condition often remains asymptomatic. The presence of spondylolysis in an asymptomatic individual does not preclude him from active participation; however, the player with back pain with radiographically demonstrated spondylolysis should be held out from playing, and conservative treatment should be rendered until he becomes asymptomatic (82). Return to play may be allowed once symptoms have completely subsided and physical exam fails to reveal any neurologic findings or signs of nerve root irritation. If conservative treatment modalities fail or findings of the physical examination suggest neurologic involvement, further investigational studies, including MRI, CT, or bone scintigraphy, are warranted to evaluate further the pars defect.

Treatment of the football player that presents with spondylolisthesis is generally similar to that for spondylolysis (83, 84). Spondylolisthesis is most commonly seen at the L5 to S1 junction and is graded by the amount of slippage of the L5 vertebral body on S1. L5 nerve root involvement can be seen with this type of slip (i.e., the nerve root is closely attached to the L5 pedicle). Any player with back pain, radicular symptoms, or neurologic deficits in the lower extremities should be held out from participation. Spondylolisthesis greater than 50% of the vertebral body width (grade 3/4) or radiographic evidence of progression of the spondylolisthesis during a season should be closely evaluated and operative intervention considered.

Disc herniation is not uncommon in football players. These injuries are generally seen acutely with the onset of back pain and radicular pain to the lower extremity. If a herniated disc is suspected, an MRI is indicated. Once a herniated disc is confirmed, conservative treatment is the preferred treatment (85). If neurologic symptoms or findings fail to improve or if they progress, operative intervention may be necessary. Operative intervention will not reverse neurologic deficits, only decrease chances of further neurologic progression and pain. Current operative techniques using a microscope and a small incision with minimal soft tissue disruption are still controversial. Exact time to return is player/position specific; however, in general, the physical exam must show return of normal lumbar motion, strength, and absence of nerve root tension signs.

Hip Injuries

Because of the inherent stability of the hip and pelvis region, fractures and dislocations about the hip are unusual in football, generally representing less than 3% of football injuries (11, 12). Perhaps the most common of these injuries is the so-called hip pointer. This is actually a contusion over the iliac crest. Much like contusions of the proximal humerus, these can occasionally result in periostitis or exostoses. Complete avulsion of the iliac apophysis can occur in the adolescent athlete. Acutely, these injuries are managed with ice and progressive range-of-motion exercises. Nonsteroidals and occasionally injections can be helpful. Protective padding is the mainstay of prevention and treatment and may include the addition of a doughnut pad or custom-made thermoplastic pad to the area of injury (Fig. 22.15). Treatment of fractures to the apophysis includes 4 to 6 weeks of activity limitation.

Contusions in the groin can have serious consequences, including traumatic phlebitis, phlebothrombosis, and femoral neuropathy (86). The most common injury around the groin, however, is the strain of the iliopsoas tendon. Radiographs are important to rule out an avulsion of the lesser trochanter (87). Treatment of

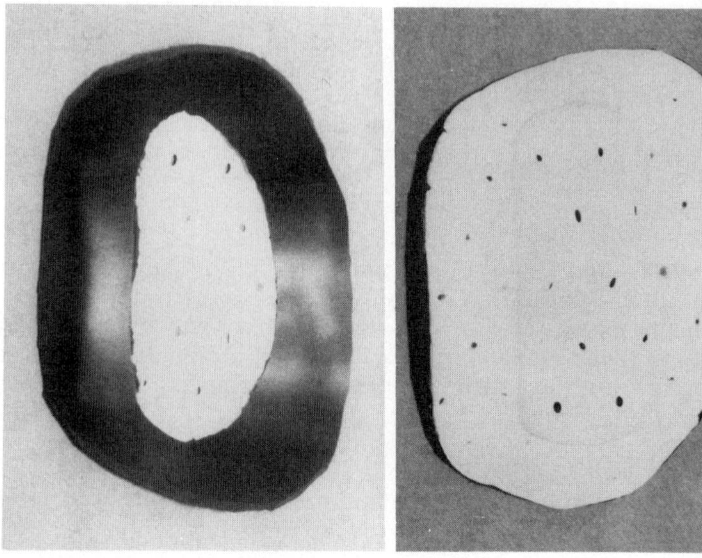

Figure 22.15. A thermoplastic pad is fabricated to protect against hip pointer.

these injuries consists of limitation of activities followed by gradual physical therapy and limited athletic participation. The use of modalities such as ultrasound may also have a role in treatment.

A recent hip injury in a premiere professional football running back (88) highlighted another problem that is unusual but may be more common than previously recognized (89). Osteonecrosis occurring as a result of a traumatic hip injury can be devastating and terminate a professional athlete's career. The etiology of this injury is interruption of the blood supply to the femoral head (90). Although this may commonly occur following a posterior dislocation of the hip, these two recent cases apparently represented a subluxation alone. Early recognition of this disorder may help avoid some of the disastrous sequela of this injury.

Thigh Injuries

Injuries to the thigh in football include quadriceps contusions and muscle strains. Quadriceps contusions occur as a result of a direct blow, usually caused from an opposing player's helmet or knee. The quadriceps muscle lies in contact with the femur throughout the full length of the thigh and is particularly vulnerable to external compressive forces. Blunt trauma causes transmission of force through the fluid compartment of the muscle and damage occurs only in the layer next to the bone. Major muscle injury is associated with capillary damage, hemorrhage, and fiber disruption (91). This may lead to formation of scar tissue that may calcify to form myositis ossificans.

Quadriceps contusions are characterized by localized pain and tenderness in the quadriceps with associated swelling. The degree of swelling depends on the degree of injury. Swelling should be documented by serial girth measurements of the thigh. Jackson and Feagin (92) described a classification scheme for quadriceps contusions. Mild contusions were characterized by localized tenderness in the quadriceps with more than 90° of knee flexion with no alterations in gait. A moderate contusion was characterized by an antalgic gait and less than 90° of knee flexion. A severe contusion was marked by a severe limp and less than 45° of knee flexion. Frequently, the individual with a severe contusion of the thigh will have an associated effusion of the knee. The knee must be carefully evaluated to rule out an intraarticular lesion.

Acute treatment of quadriceps contusions consists of cold and compression to minimize hemorrhage. The athlete should be encouraged to rest with the injured knee in as much flexion as possible. Assistive devices should be used for weight bearing if the individual has an antalgic gait. Use of assistive devices should be continued until the athlete has at least 90° of flexion, has good quadriceps control, and is able to walk normally without use of assistive devices. Early passive pain-free range of motion, emphasizing flexion, should be initiated once swelling has stabilized. Once range of motion has been restored, the athlete should undergo rehabilitation to increase quadriceps strength and prepare the individual for return to football. The thigh should be protected from further injury when the athlete returns to football. Additional padding can be added to a standard thigh pad to protect the area (Fig. 22.16). The thigh pad should be held in place with the use of an elastic bandage or tape to ensure that it does not slip.

The results of quadriceps contusions in West Point cadets was reported by Ryan et al. (94). Average disability for mild contusions was 13 days. For moderate contusions average disability was 19 days, and for severe contusions average disability was 21 days. A possible consequence of a quadriceps contusion is development of myositis ossificans, which is heterotopic bone formation in the layers of muscle along the bone. In the West Point study, myositis ossificans developed in 4% of the mild contusions, 18% of the moderate contusions, and 13% of the severe contusions (93). No cadet with a range of knee flexion greater than 120° at initial

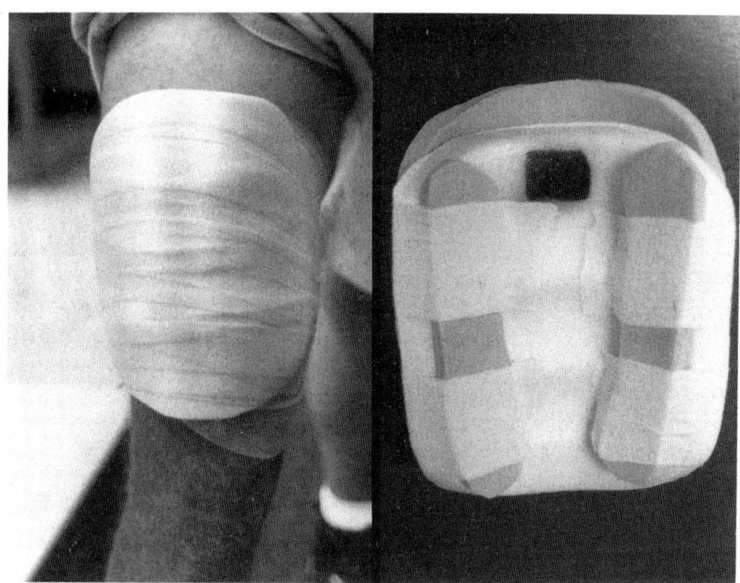

Figure 22.16. A thigh pad is modified to protect against thigh contusion.

evaluation developed myositis ossificans. It is the authors' experience that myositis ossificans will develop if treatment in the early phase is too aggressive or if the athlete is reinjured. These conditions perpetuate the inflammatory process and make it more likely that myositis ossificans will develop.

A severe thigh contusion can result in development of a thigh compartment syndrome. Development of thigh compartment syndrome should be considered when an athlete suffers a direct blow to the anterior thigh with subsequent swelling, unrelenting pain, and loss of knee motion (94). Classic signs for compartment syndrome include pain out of proportion to the injury, pain on passive motion of associated joints, pulselessness, paresthesia, and pallor (95). Thigh compartment syndrome occurs as a result of significant trauma and bleeding that cause soft tissue swelling within a finite osteofascial compartment. Swelling within a finite compartment results in increased compartment pressures and can lead to muscle ischemia and necrosis as well as compromise to the nerves within the compartment. This diagnosis requires a high index of suspicion. Patients with a compartment syndrome present with a tense, hard anterior thigh on palpation with a significant loss of knee motion. The injury is extremely painful and may demonstrate neurovascular compromise distal to the compartment. The definitive diagnosis is made by monitoring intracompartment pressure. Treatment of a thigh compartment syndrome requires immediate fasciotomy.

Football players are susceptible to a variety of thigh muscle strains, including strains of the quadriceps, hamstrings, and groin muscles. Most groin muscle strains involve the hip flexors. Players at positions that required speed—receivers, running backs, and defensive backs—are prone to hamstring strains. Kickers and punters are prone to strains of the rectus femoris. Muscle strains occur as the muscle is lengthened while it is in the contracted state. Inadequate warmup and muscle fatigue have been implicated as predisposing factors (96). Strains are characterized by pain and localized tenderness. A palpable defect may be detected in severe cases. Pain can be reproduced by stretching or by resisted contraction of the involved muscle.

The degree of disability depends on the degree of injury. Treatment consists of cold and compression in the early phase to limit bleeding and inflammation. As pain subsides, stretching and resisted exercises should be performed to restore flexibility, strength, and endurance of the involved muscle. Mild strains may disable the athlete for 1 to 2 weeks, while severe strains may disable the athlete for 6 to 8 weeks. Prevention of muscle strains in the thigh region involves proper warmup and conditioning. Maintenance of a normal hamstring: quadriceps strength ratio may also help minimize the incidence of thigh muscle strains. Heiser et al. (96) demonstrated a reduction in the incidence of hamstring injuries with a stretching and year-round weight-training and running program. Isokinetic testing was used to identify deficits in the hamstrings, quadriceps, and hamstring:quadriceps ratio. Athletes with isokinetic deficits were placed on a specific strength-training program to eliminate the strength deficits.

Knee Injuries

The knee is the most frequently injured joint in football. Knee injuries account for 22% to 36.5% of all football injuries (2, 3, 7). Other than catastrophic head or neck injuries, knee injuries are the most common reason that the athlete cannot return to participation. Football is a high-demand sport that requires running, cutting, pivoting, jumping, and deceleration combined with contact and noncontact injury mechanisms, placing ligamentous structures around the knee at significant risk. Medial collateral ligament injuries of the knee are the most common, followed by meniscal and anterior cruciate ligament injuries. Over the last 10 years, the authors have seen an increase in both the size and speed of the athlete participating in football that when superimposed on the contact mechanisms can lead to more serious ligamentous injuries.

Types of injuries seen in football players can often be predicted by player position and the mechanism of injury at the time of injury. For example, offensive and defensive linemen hit from the lateral aspect of the knee, sustain a valgus force and injure the medial collateral ligament (MCL). Wide receivers running down the field plant their foot to decelerate and rotate their upper leg, injuring the anterior cruciate ligament (ACL). A force applied to the anterior aspect of the proximal tibia with the knee flexed as in a running back who is tackled and falls to the ground with a lineman on his back, will have a posterior force directed at his proximal tibia, which could lead to a tear of the posterior cruciate ligament (PCL). The mechanism of injury can help lead the clinician to the correct diagnosis and determine if the player has the ability to return to competitive play at that time or not.

Prevention of knee injuries in football remains a controversial subject (97–99). The relationship between the foot and the playing surface contributes to the incidence and severity of knee ligament injuries. If the foot is able to move with contact, the forces on the knee ligaments are reduced dramatically. If the foot is planted firmly, small external forces could potentially damage knee ligaments. The consequences of this relationship are made obvious by comparing football and hockey. Both are contact sports, but because of the relative frictionless surface, hockey players suffer fewer knee ligament injuries and often play with ACL-deficient knees. A football player, however, may find a knee ligament injury to be disabling and may result in functional instability. Shoes matched to the playing surface can also reduce the incidence of knee ligament injuries. Long cleats that provide increased traction on a grass surface increase the likelihood of injuring the knee. The most appropriate type of cleat is a low (less than 0.5 inch) and wide (0.375-inch diameter) cleat. Such a shoe can provide adequate traction for running, cutting, and turning but also tends to give way and slide with strong external forces. For artificial turf, Torg et al. (97) recommend a multicleat shoe with a polyurethene sole.

Prevention of injuries related to noncontact forces has been directed at strengthening of the quadriceps and hamstring muscles about the knee while ensuring flexibility of the hamstrings and the iliotibial band. The use of a prophylactic knee brace in football remains controversial. A review of the current literature includes a number of different studies with uncontrolled variables that, unfortunately, leaves the reader without a simple answer to the question of whether to recommend the use of a brace. At this time, it seems that the main advantage of prophylatic knee braces is to prevent MCL injuries that occur from a contact mechanism in offensive and defensive linemen and linebackers. Two studies, a small high school study and a large collegiate study, have found that braces may be hazardous rather than protective (98, 99). A study from a military academy strongly supports the concept that the use of braces prevent MCL injuries in defensive players (100). Subjects who wore the prophylactic knee brace while on defense had significantly fewer knee injuries than nonbraced subjects who served as the controls. This was not seen, however, in offensive players. The severity of injuries to the MCL and ACL, however, were not statistically significantly reduced. The most frequent mechanism of injury in that study was attributed to a direct lateral blow to the knee that produced a valgus force. There was no significant differences between the braced group and the control group in the frequency of ankle injuries. Based on these and other studies, the decision to use a prophylactic brace should be left to the player and not be recommended by the team physician. However, further well-controlled studies may lead to the recommendation of certain specific prophylactic knees braces, depending on player size and position and the playing surface.

Ligament Injuries

Treatment

Treatment of knee ligament injuries in football players requires a careful thought process incorporating substantial data, including position, size, strength, age, level of competition, previous knee injury, and structures injured. The decision-making process should involve the trainer, coach, physician, and player. A careful history including previous injury to the knee, a thorough physical examination outlining the specific anatomical structures that are injured, and the athlete's ultimate goals are important considerations. One has to remember that there are both primary and secondary stabilizers of the knee. An isolated injury to one ligamentous structure often may be well-tolerated by a player at a certain position but not by another player playing a different position. Treatment of knee ligament injuries is player and position dependent.

Medial Collateral Ligament Injury

Injuries to the medial collateral ligament are the most common ligament injuries around the knee in football.

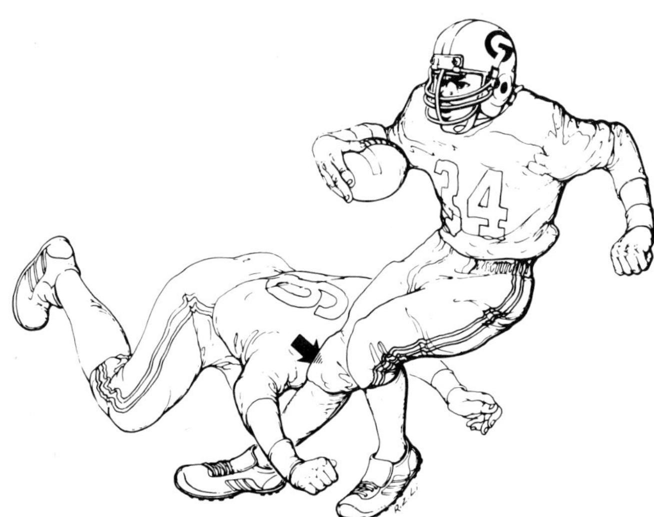

Figure 22.17. The most common mechanism of injury to the medial collateral ligament is seen when a player gets struck by an opposing player on the outside lateral aspect of the knee, which produces valgus force with tearing of the medial collateral ligament. Reprinted by permission from Tria AJ, Hosea TM. Diagnosis of knee ligament injuries: an illustrated guide to the knee. New York: Churchill Livingston, 1992:87–99.

The injury is usually a contact-induced valgus stress to the knee with the foot fixed (Fig. 22.17). MCL injuries are divided into grades 1, 2, and 3. In a grade 1 injury tenderness is palpable along the length of the ligament; however, there is no increase in laxity on physical examination and there is no disruption of ligamentous fibers. The knee is treated symptomatically and the player is allowed to bear weight as tolerated. Once the athlete has full range of motion and strength, he may return to play. Grade 2 and 3 injuries are more serious. In a grade 2 injury, partial disruption of the ligament fibers has occurred; however, the ligament is still intact. Increased laxity on physical examination is noted, but there is a firm end point at the extreme of valgus stress. In a grade 3 injury, there is a complete disruption of the ligament, discontinuity of fibers, and no end point on stress testing. If a grade 3 injury is suspected on physical examination, careful attention must be paid to the other secondary stabilizers preventing valgus force, including the anterior cruciate ligament, menisci, posterior oblique ligament, and capsule. Isolated grade 2 and 3 injuries should be treated nonoperatively with a double upright knee brace and range-of-motion and rehabilitation exercises as soon as the athlete can tolerate them (101). In both grade 2 and 3 injuries, players may return to participation when there is no swelling or tenderness and full range of motion and muscle function has been restored. Exact timing for return to play is athlete and position specific.

Anterior Cruciate Ligament Injury

Treatment recommendations for anterior cruciate ligament injuries in football players is complicated with many variables. These include previous injuries about the knee, player age and position, leg strength, and long-term career goals. The presence or absence of injury to the secondary stabilizers, including the medial and lateral ligamentous structures and menisci, has important ramifications on treatment. Players at certain positions who cover a limited area (offensive/defensive linemen) may be able to participate with an isolated ACL-deficient knee. However, players such as running backs who require the ability to accelerate, decelerate, and change direction quickly may have unacceptable symptoms and be unable to participate.

For those individuals whose physical examination demonstrates only increased anterior laxity with no associated increased medial, lateral, or posterior laxity and minimally positive Lachman's and pivot-shift tests and who have to perform a low-demand position such as tackle or center may be able to return without operative intervention. Nonoperative treatment consists of an aggressive rehabilitation program focusing on hamstring strengthening and the use of a functional knee brace to return to athletic competition. If laxity of secondary restraints eventually occurs along with symptoms of instability, reconstruction can then be performed.

The indication for primary anterior cruciate ligament reconstruction in a grossly unstable knee is a player with functional instability. Wide receivers, defensive backs, and linebackers require the ability to plant their feet and cut and will rarely tolerate a complete anterior cruciate ligament injury associated with functional instability. These players usually require operative intervention.

Details of operative choice of anterior cruciate ligament reconstructions will not be discussed in this chapter; however, the current gold standard includes autogenous bone-patellar tendon-bone reconstruction of the anterior cruciate ligament. Using arthroscopic techniques, greater than 90% good to excellent results have been reported in the literature (102). At the time of the operative procedure, it is important to examine the knee carefully under anesthesia to detect any subtle rotary instabilities and treat them accordingly. Failure to detect combined instability patterns will result in surgical failure. In general, the level of performance after ACL reconstruction is player and position specific. The use of a functional knee brace after surgical reconstruction of the anterior cruciate ligament is generally recommended. However, objective tests supporting their use have not been performed. It may be that a functional knee brace provides proprioceptive feedback to the quadriceps-hamstring mechanism that helps prevent recurrent injuries to the ACL.

Posterior Cruciate Ligament Injuries

PCL injuries are relatively uncommon. Recently, the National Football League predraft physical examinations have consistently revealed that 2% of the players have isolated posterior laxity (103). The mechanism of injury for 80% of posterior cruciate ligament injuries is hyperflexion with a direct force applied to the anterior aspect of the proximal tibia. Other potential mechanisms include direct trauma to the anterior aspect of the proximal tibia (Fig. 22.18). Detailed examination of

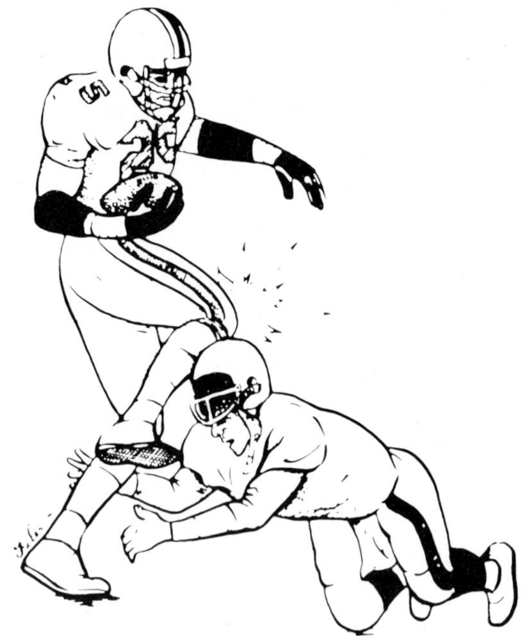

Figure 22.18. Potential mechanism of PCL injury includes direct contact with an anterior force applied to the proximal tibia.

these patients should be done to determine if the injury is isolated to the PCL or is combined with an injury to other ligaments. Isolated injuries (with minimal posterior laxity) generally do well with nonoperative management, whereas multiple ligament injuries that result in combined instabilities generally need operative intervention. Nonoperative treatment for PCL injuries emphasizes quadriceps-strengthening exercises to help reduce posterior laxity. If operative reconstruction is required for pain and/or functional instability, current arthroscopic techniques using autograft or allograft tissue have demonstrated fair to good results in greater than 70% of cases (104). However, the player should be carefully counseled that results from this operation are currently not as successful as those for anterior cruciate ligament reconstruction.

In summary, treatment of the knee ligament injuries should be based on player and position. In football players, knees can deteriorate with time by delays in diagnosis, surgical indications, poor surgical technique, a willingness to rely on an inadequate examination, and failure to modify expectations for both the player and the physician. The earlier the player is seen after the original injury, the greater the chances for successful treatment. Over the last 10 years, the authors have seen advances in arthroscopic techniques used for surgical reconstruction of knee ligament injuries. This has led to improved results following knee ligament reconstruction; however, some great athletes have played with significant ligamentous injury treated nonoperatively for many years with minimal arthritis. With careful history, diagnosis, and player counseling, decisions regarding operative or nonoperative treatment can be made successfully in these high-performance athletes.

Meniscal Injuries

Meniscal injuries are common in football players. The mechanism of injury usually involves internal/external rotation of the knee over the foot planted. Arthroscopic surgery should be performed early in those patients with symptomatic tears with the hope of getting the athlete back to competition quickly. Isolated repair of a meniscal tear in a football player without ligamentous reconstruction is debatable. Evidence has shown, however, that removing part of the meniscus leads to increased stress on the articular cartilage and an increased chance of degenerative arthritis at a later date. However, performing partial meniscectomy versus an arthroscopic meniscal repair can mean the difference between returning to the playing field in the current season as opposed to the following one (i.e., season-ending injury). This can present the physician with a dilemma. DeHaven (105) noted, "When viewed from the standpoint of the potential for normal knee function and absence of degenerative problems, participation in a particular season may be an inordinately high price to pay for undergoing partial meniscectomy rather than repair." Decisions such as these need to be carefully made between physician and player.

Patella-Femoral Problems

Patella Dislocation

The mechanism for patellar dislocation usually involves external rotation of the leg, active contraction of the quadriceps, and extension of the knee. These are often self-induced injuries occurring without contact. A football player usually presents with an acutely swollen knee and may be unable to bear weight. Physical exam may demonstrate a tense hemarthrosis and tenderness over the medial retinaculum and superior aspect of the adductor tubercle. Pain and swelling will make it difficult to assess the integrity of the ligaments, but this is important because dislocation of the patellofemoral joint may occur in conjunction with sprains of the MCL, the ACL, or both. Radiographs, including the merchant view, must be reviewed to rule out intraarticular fractures. Initial treatment involves the application of ice, local compression, immobilization, rest, and elevation. Definitive treatment for a first-time dislocation is generally conservative with range-of-motion and quadriceps-strengthening exercises. It is generally 6 weeks before the athlete is able to return to competition. At that time, the authors recommend that the athlete wear a knee sleeve with a lateral buttress.

Patellar Tendinitis (Jumpers' Knee)

Patellar tendinitis is a common overuse injury in football players and other athletes whose sport requires jumping. It is an inflammatory tendinitis of the patellar tendon as it comes off the inferior pole of the patella. The patient often complains of anterior knee pain that increases with the use of stairs and with jumping activities. Physical exam reveals tenderness located at the inferior pole of the patella. Treatment of this condition is conservative and includes oral antiinflammatory medication, a patella-restraining brace, and hamstring and quadriceps stretching and strengthening. A brace to limit proximal movement of the patella or to decrease tension on the patellar tendon may be beneficial. In some cases, patellar tendinitis may lead to rupture of the patella tendon; however, this is an uncommon injury in football players. In refractory cases, surgical intervention may be required. MRI or ultrasound can be used to delineate areas of degeneration. The patient is asked to locate the area of maximal tenderness, and it is marked with a pen. This part of the patellar tendon is excised under local anesthesia. Often myxoid degeneration of the fibers can be demonstrated in the patella tendon. The authors' experience indicates that the outcome from a surgical procedure is usually good with return of the athlete to the previous level of competition.

Fat Pad Syndrome (Hoffa's Disease)

Fat pad syndrome is occasionally seen in football players, especially in linemen who have repeated trauma to the anterior aspect of the knee. On physical examination, there is tenderness medial and lateral to the patella tendon. It is often associated with thickening of the capsular area around the patella tendon. Usually, conservative management of this syndrome is successful and consists of antiinflammatory medicine, a patella-restraining brace, and a rehabilitation program focusing on quadriceps and hamstring flexibility. Refractory cases may be treated arthroscopically, and findings typically include a thickening of the fibers in the anterior fat pad.

Ankle Injuries

The ankle is a frequently injured joint in football (3). Lateral ankle sprains are the most common injury; however, a significant number of medial and syndesmosis sprains also occur in football. Injury to the lateral ligaments occurs when the foot supinates with internal rotation of the talus on the tibia. This produces successive injury to the anterior talofibular ligament, calcaneofibular ligament, and posterior talotibial ligament (106). These injuries are common when cutting and changing direction. They also can occur when a player steps on another individual's foot.

Pronation of the foot with external rotation of the talus relative to the tibia results in successive injury to the anterior tibiofibular ligament, interosseous ligament, posterior tibiofibular ligament, and deltoid ligament (106). This occurs when the foot is fixed to the ground and the athlete's body is twisted away from the injured side, producing external rotation of the foot relative to the leg. Alternatively, this injury can occur when a downed player's foot is externally rotated and he receives a direct blow to his leg, which forces the foot into further external rotation (Fig. 22.19).

Individuals with ankle sprains present with pain, swelling, and loss of function. There is tenderness over

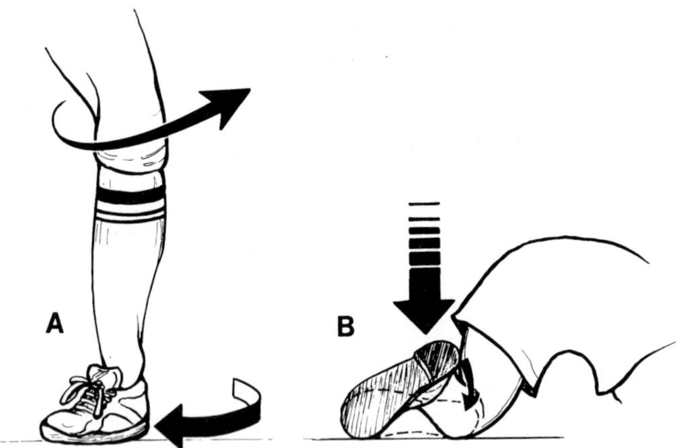

Figure 22.19. Mechanism for external rotation injuries to the ankle. **A,** With the foot fixed to the ground, the athlete's body is twisted away from the injured side. **B,** The player's foot is externally rotated when he receives a blow to the lower leg. Reprinted by permission from Boytim MJ, Fischer DA, Neumann L. Syndesmotic ankle sprains. Am J Sports Med 1991;19:294–298.

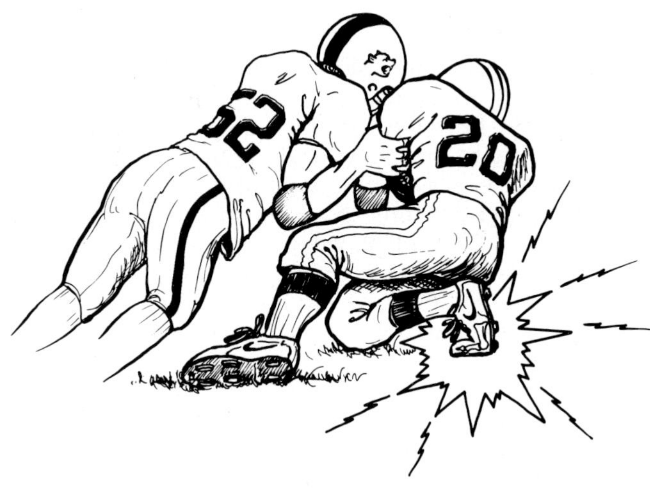

Figure 22.20. Mechanism of injury for turf toe. Forced dorsiflexion of the first metatarsophalangeal joint commonly occurs when a player falls across the posterior aspect of another player's leg. Reprinted by permission from Rodeo SA, O'Brien S, Warren RF, Barnes R, Wickiewicz TL, Dillingham MF. Turf toe: an analysis of metatarsalphalangeal joint sprains in professional football players. Am J Sports Med 1990;18:280–285.

the involved ligament. Stability of the ankle should be assessed. The anterior drawer test in 30° of plantar flexion is used to assess the anterior talofibular ligament. The talar tilt test can be used to assess the calcaneofibular ligament. The external rotation stress test should be used to assess syndesmotic and deltoid ligament sprains (107). The external rotation test is performed by applying an external rotation stress to the involved foot and ankle with the knee held at 90° of flexion and the ankle in the neutral position. A positive test produces pain over the anterior or posterior tibiofibular ligaments and interosseous membrane. Determination of the specific nature and severity of the sprain is important to establish prognosis. Syndesmotic ankle sprains result in significantly more missed and/or limited practices and games. In addition, they require more extensive treatment compared with lateral ankle sprains (107).

Treatment of acute ankle sprains includes protection, rest, ice, compression, and elevation (PRICE). An ankle orthosis may be useful to allow plantar and dorsiflexion while preventing medial and lateral motion. Limited immobilization may be used for severe ankle sprains. As range of motion improves, strengthening and proprioception exercises should be initiated to develop dynamic stability for the ankle. Return to activity should include a series of position-specific activities that are required for the player's position. Ankle braces, taping, and/or high-top shoes can be used to provide protection to the injured ankle when the athlete returns to sport. Surgery for acute ankle sprains is rarely indicated, because the majority of football players with ankle sprains do well with nonoperative treatment. Reconstruction of the ankle may be considered for those who develop chronic ankle instability.

Sprains involving the distal tibiofibular syndesmosis may develop heterotopic ossification or a tibiofibular synostosis. These can occur following a severe internal rotation sprain followed by recurrent stress and injury to the ankle. In addition, they also can occur following external rotation injury to the ankle. Patients with a synostosis have limited ankle dorsiflexion and disabling pain with running. Excision of the synostosis usually relieves the pain and restores ankle dorsiflexion (108).

The advent of artificial surfaces and lighter more flexible shoes have led to development of turf toe, which is a sprain of the plantar capsular ligament of the first metatarsophalangeal joint (109). This injury occurs with forced dorsiflexion of the first metatarsophalangeal joint, with the foot in a slightly dorsiflexed position. Commonly, this occurs as a player falls across the posterior aspect of another player's leg forcing the first metatarsophalangeal joint into dorsiflexion (Fig. 22.20). Turf toe can also occur as a result of forced plantarflexion of the great toe (109). This occurs as the ball carrier is tackled from behind, forcing the ankle and toe into plantarflexion. Valgus stress to the first metatarsophalangeal joint, such as when a lineman pushes off from his stance, may also give rise to turf toe. Forced dorsiflexion is the mechanism of injury for 85% of the players who suffer turf toe. Forced plantarflexion (12%) and valgus stress (4%) are less common mechanisms for developing turf toe (109). Patients with turf toe complain of pain in the first metatarsophalangeal joint that occurs during push off in gait. The joint is often warm and swollen. The pain is increased by forced dorsiflexion. Often mobility of the first metatarsophalangeal joint is limited. Plantarflexion of the first ray (first metatarsal and medial cuneiform) also may be limited.

Treatment includes rest and protection from further injury. Ice is used to control pain and swelling. Joint mobilization techniques can be used to increase range of motion. The first ray should be mobilized if plantarflexion is limited. Tape can be used to limit motion and protect the joint. Use of a stiff-soled shoe can provide additional protection. The football shoe can be modified by placing a 1/32-inch spring steel plate in the midsole of the forefoot of the shoe. This increases stiffness of the shoe and protects the joint from further injury.

REFERENCES

1. Mueller FO, Blyth CS. North Carolina high school football injury study; equipment and prevention. J Sports Med 1974;2:1–10.
2. Adkison JW, Requa RK, Garrick JG. Injury rates in high school football. A comparison of synthetic surfaces and grass fields. Clin Orthop 1974;99:131–136.
3. DeLee JC, Farney WC. Incidence of injury in Texas high school football. Am J Sports Med 1992;20:575–580.
4. Backx FJG, Erich BM, Kemper ABA, et al. Sports injuries in school-aged children. Am J Sports Med 1989;17:234–240.
5. Blyth CS, Mueller FO. Football injury survey. Part III. Injury rates vary with coaching. Phys Sportsmed, 1974;2(11):45–50.
6. Robey JM, Blyth CS, Mueller FO. Athletic injuries: application of epidemiologic methods. Phys Sportsmed 1984;12 (9):79–84.
7. Olson OC. The Spokane study: high school football injuries. Phys Sportsmed 1979;7(12):75–82.
8. Prager, BI, Fitton WL, Cahill BR, Olson GH. High school football injuries: a prospective study and pitfalls of data collection. Am J Sports Med 1989;17:681–682.
9. McLain LG, Reynolds S. Sports injuries in a high school. Pediatrics 1989;84:446–450.
10. Lowe EB, Perkins ER, Herndon JH. Rhode Island high school athletic injuries 1985–1986. R I Med J 1987;70:265–270.
11. Hal RW, Mitchell W. Football injuries in Hawaii in 1979. Hawaii Med J 1981;40:180–812.
12. Culpepper MI, Niemann KMW. High school football injuries in Birmingham, Alabama. South Med J 1983;76:873–878.
13. Pritchett JW. High cost of high school football injuries. Am J Sports Med 1980;8:197–199.
14. Moretz A, Rashkin A, Grana WA. Oklahoma high school football injury study: a preliminary report. J Okla State Med Assoc 1978;71:85–88.
15. Canale ST, Cantler ED, Sisk TD, et al. A chronicle of injuries of an American intercollegiate football team. Am J Sports Med 1981;9:384–389.
16. Andresen BL, Hoffman MD, Barton LW. High school football injuries: field conditions and other factors. Wis Med J 1989;28–31.
17. McClelland M. High school football injuries. JAMA 1965;193:628.
18. Skovron, ML, Levy IM, Agel J. Living with artificial grass: a knowledge update. Part 2: epidemiology. Am J Sports Med 1990;18:510–513.
19. Torg JS, Quedenfeld T. Effect of shoe type and cleat length on incidence and severity of knee injuries among high school football players. Res Q 1971;42:203–211.
20. Cahill BR, Griffith EH. Exposure to injury in major college football: a preliminary report of data collection to determine injury exposure rates and activity risk factors. Am J Sports Med 1979;7:183–185.
21. Torg JS, Vegso JJ, O'Neill MJ, Sennett B. The epidemiologic, pathologic, biomechanical and cinematographic analysis of football-induced cervical spine trauma. Am J Sports Med 1990;18:50–57.
22. Greberich SG, Priest JD, Boen JR, et al. Concussion incidences and severity in secondary school varsity football plays. Am J Public Health, 1983;73:1370–1375.

22a. Cantu RC. Cerebral concussion in sport management and prevention. Sports Med 1992;14(1):64–74.

23. Maroon JC, Steele PB, Berlin R. Football head and neck injuries: an update. Clin Neurosurg 1980;27:414–429.
24. Yarnell PR, Lynch S. The 'ding' amnestic states in football trauma. Neurology 1973;23:196–197.
25. American Heart Association. Textbook of advanced cardiac life support. 2nd ed. Dallas: AHA, 1990.
26. Cantu RC, Mueller F. Catastrophic spine injury in football 1977–1989. J Spinal Dis 1990;3:227–231.
27. Cantu RC. Second impact syndrome, immediate management. Phys Sportsmed 1992;20(9):55–66.
28. Castaldi CR. Sports-related oral and facial injuries in the young athlete: a new challenge for the pediatric dentist. Pediatr Dent 1986;8:311–316.
29. Stenger J, Lawson E, Wright J, et al. Mouthguards: protection against shock to head, neck and teeth. J Am Dent Assoc 1964;69:273–281.
30. Stevens O. Prevention of traumatic dental and oral injuries. In: Andreasen JO, ed. Traumatic injuries of the teeth. 2nd ed. Copenhagen: Munksgard, 1981:419.
31. Manson PN. Facial injuries. In: McCarthy JG, ed. Plastic surgery: the face. Philadelphia: WB Saunders, 1990;2:867–1141.
32. Torg JS, Quedenfeld TC, Burstein A, et al. National football head and neck injury registry report on cervical quadriplegia 1971–1975. Am J Sports Med 1977;7:127–132.
33. Torg JS, Truex R, Quedenfeld TC, et al. The national football head and neck injury registry. Report and conclusions 1978. JAMA 1979;241:1477–1479.
34. Schneider RC. Serious and fatal neurosurgical football injuries. Clin Neurosurg 1966;12:226–236.
35. Shields, CL, Zommar VD. Analysis of professional football injuries Contemp Orthop 1982;4:90–95.
36. Robertson WC, Eichman EL, Clancy WD. Upper trunk brachial plexopathy in football players. JAMA 1979; 241:1480–1482.
37. Sallis RE, Jones K, Knopp W. Burners: offensive strategy for an underreported injury. Phys Sportsmed 1992;20:47–55.
38. Hu R, Burnham R, Reid DC, Grace M, Saboe L. Burners in contact sports. Clin J Sports Med 1991;1:236–242.
39. Chrisman OB, Snook GA, Stanitis JM, et al. Lateral flexion neck injuries in athletic competition. JAMA 1965;192:117–119.
40. Warren RF. Neurologic injuries in football. In: Jordan BD, Tsairis P, Warren RF, eds. Sports neurology. Rockville, MD: Aspen, 1989:235–244.
41. Torg JS, Pavlov H, Genuario SE, et al. Neuropraxia of the cervical spinal cord with transient quadriplegia. J Bone Joint Surg 1986;68A:1354–1370.
42. Rowe CR, Zarens B. Recurrent subluxation of the shoulder. J Bone Joint Surg 1981;63A:863–872.
43. Bergifeld GA. Brachial plexus injuries. Paper presented at the American Academy of Orthopedic Surgeons Winter Sports Injury Course, Steamboat Springs, CO, March 1987.
44. Speer KP, Bassett FH. The prolonged burner syndrome. Am J Sports Med 1990;18:591–594.
45. Cox JS. The fate of the acromioclavicular joint in athletic injuries. Am J Sports Med 1981;9:50–59.
46. Rockwood CA Jr. Injuries to the acromioclavicular joint. In: Rockwood CA, Green DG, eds. Fractures in adults. 2nd ed. Philadelphia: JB Lippincott, 1984:860–910.
47. Bergfield JA. Acromioclavicular complex. In: Nicholas JA, Hurshman FB, Posner MA, eds. The upper extremity in sports medicine. St. Louis: CV Mosby, 1990:169–180.
48. Glick JM, Milburn LJ, Haggerty JF, Nishimoto D. Dislocated acromioclavicular joint: follow up study of 35 related to acromioclavicular dislocations. Am J Sports Med 1977;5:264–263.
49. Weaver JK, Dunn HK. Treatment of acromioclavicular injuries: especially complete acromioclavicular separation. J Bone Joint Surg 1972;54A:1187–1197.
50. Zarins B Prodromos LC. Shoulder injuries in sports. In: Rowe CR, ed. The shoulder. New York: Churchill Livingston, 1988:411–433.
51. Husk CD, Puhl JJ. Myositis ossificans of the upper arm. Am J Sports Med 1980;8:419–424.
52. Arciero RA, Wheeler JH, Ryan JB, McBride JT. Arthroscopic bankart repair for acute initial anterior shoulder dislocations. Paper presented at the 60th annual meeting of the American Association of Orthopedic Surgeons, February 1993.
53. Matsen FA, Thomas SC, Rockwood CA. Anterior glenohumeral instability. In: Rockwood CA, Matsen FA, eds. The shoulder. Philadelphia: WB Saunders, 1990:526–622.
54. Norwood LA, Terry GC. Shoulder posterior subluxation. Am J Sports Med 1984;12:25–30.
55. Rowe CR, Zarins B. Chronic unreduced dislocations of the shoulder. J Bone Joint Surg 1982;64:A494–505.
56. Grassi F, Chun JM, Groh GI, Rockwood CA. Surgical treatment of posterior glenohumeral instability. Paper presented at the 60th

annual meeting of the American Association of Orthopedic Surgeons, February 1993.
57. Ono K, Yamamuro T, Rockwood CA Jr. Use of a 30° caudal tilt radiography in the shoulder impingement syndrome. J Shoulder Elbow Surg 1992;1:246–252.
58. Bigliani LU, Morrison D, April EW. The morphology of the acromion and its relation to rotator cuff tears. Orthop Trans 1986;10:228.
59. Altchek TW, Warren RF, Wickiewicz TL, et al. Arthroscopic acromioplasty technique and results. Bone Joint Surg 1990;72A:1198–1207.
60. Gartsman GM. Arthroscopic acromioplasty for lesions of the rotator cuff. Bone Joint Surg 1990;72A:169–180.
61. Snyder SJ, Pachelli AF, Del Pizzo W, et al. Partial thickness rotator cuff tears: results of arthroscopic treatment. Arthroscopy 1991;7:1–7.
62. Bennett JB. Articular injuries in the athlete. In: Morey ER, ed. The elbow and its disorders. 2nd ed. Philadelphia: WB Saunders, 1993:581–595.
63. Morry BF. The elbow and its disorders. Philadelphia: WB Saunders, 1985.
64. Jobe FW, Kvitne RS. Elbow instability in the athlete (Instructional Course Lecture No. 40). American Academy of Orthopaedic Surgeons, 1991.
65. Glousman RE, Barron OJ, Jobe FW, Perry J, Pink M. Electromyographic analysis of the elbow in normal and injured pitchers with medialcollateral ligament insufficiency. Am J Sports Med 1992;20:311–317.
66. Wheeler DK, Linscheid RL. Fracture-dislocations of the elbow. Clin Orthop 1967;50:95–106.
67. Linscheid RL, Wheeler DK. Elbow dislocations. JAMA 1965;194:1117–1176.
68. Hotchkiss RN, Green DP. Fractures and dislocations of the elbow. In: Rockwood CA, Green DP, Buchloz RW, eds. Fractures in Adults. Philadelphia: JB Lippincott, 1991:739–841.
69. Rettig AC, Ryan R, Shelbourne KD, McCarroll JR, Johnson F, Ahlfeld SK. Metacarpal fractures in the athlete. Am J Sports Med 1989;17:567–572.
70. Riester JN, Baker BE, Mosher JF, Lowe D. A review of scaphoid fracture healing in competitive athletes. Am J Sports Med 1985;13:159–161.
71. McCue FC, Mayer VI, Moran DJ. Gamekeeper's thumb: ulnar collateral ligament reupture. J Musculoskeletal Med 1988;5(12):53–63.
72. Fumich RM, Fink RJ, Hanna GR. Offensive lineman's thumb. Phys Sportsmed 1983;11:113–115.
73. Powell JW. Summary of injury patterns for seven seasons 1980–1986. San Diego: San Diego State University, Department of Physical Education, 1987.
74. Halpern B, Thompson N, Curl WW, Andrews JR, Hunter SC, Boring JR. High school football injuries: identifying the risk factors. Am J Sports Med 1987;15:316–320.
75. Hoshina H. Spondylosis in athletes. Phys Sportsmed 1980;8:75–79.
76. McCarrol JR, Miller JM, Ritter MA. Lumbar spondylolisthesis in college football players: a prospective study. Am J Sports Med 1986;14:404–406.
77. Ferguson RJ, McMaster JH, Stanitski CL. Low back pain in college football linemen. J Sports Med Physical Fit 1974;2:63–69.
78. Cyron BM, Hutton WC. The fatigue strength of the lumbar neural arch in spondylolysis. J Bone Joint Surg 1978;60B:234–238.
79. Jackson DW. Low back pain in young athletes: evaluation of stress reaction and discogenic problems. Am J Sports Med 1979;7:364–366.
80. Saal JA. Rehabilitation of football players with lumbar spine injury (Part 1). Phys Sportsmed 1988;16:61–74.
81. Saal JA. Rehabilitation of football players with lumbar spine injury (Part 2). Phys Sportsmed 1988;16:117–125.
82. Semon R, Spengler D. Significance of lumbar spondylolysis in college football players. Spine 1981;6(2):172–174.
83. Wiltse LL, Widell EH Jr, Jackson DW. Fatigue fracture: the basic lesion in isthmic spondylolisthesis. J Bone Joint Surg 1975;57A:17–22.
84. Wiltse LL, Newman MD, MacNab I. Classification of spondylolysis and spondylolisthesis. Clin Orthop 1976;117:23–29.
85. Saal JA, Saal JS. Nonoperative treatment of herniated lumbar intervertebral disc with radiculopathy: an outcome study. Spine 1989;14:431–437.
86. Renstom PAHF. Tendon and muscle injuries in the groin area. Clin Sports Med 1992;11:815–833.
87. O'Donoghue DH. Treatment of injuries to athletes. Philadelphia: WB Saunders, 1984.
88. Stenger A. Bo's hip dislocates stellar athletic career. Phys Sportsmed 1991;19(5):17–18.
89. Cooper DE, Warren RF, Barnes R. Traumatic subluxation of the hip resulting in aseptic necrosis and condrylolysis in a professional football player. Am J Sports Med 1991;19:322–324.
90. Stewart WJ. Aseptic necrosis of the head of the femur following traumatic dislocation of the hip joint case reported in an experimental studies. J Bone Surg 1933;15:413–438.
91. Ciullo JV, Zarins B. Biomechanics of the musculotendinious unit: relation to athletic performance and injury. Clin Sports Med 1983;2:71–86.
92. Jackson DW, Feagin JA. Quadriceps contusions in young athletes. J Bone Joint Surg 1973;55-A:95–105.
93. Ryan JB, Wheeler JH, Hopkinson WJ, Arciero RA, Kolakowski KR. Quadriceps contusions. West Point update. Am J Sports Med 1991;19:299–304.
94. Colosimo AJ, Ireland ML. Thigh compartment syndrome in a football athlete: a case report and review of the literature. Med Sci Sports Exerc 1992;24:958–963.
95. Whitesides TE, Haney TC, Morimoto K, Harada H. Tissue pressure measurements as a determinant for the need of fasciotomy. Clin Orthop 1975;113:43–51.
96. Heiser TM, Weber J, Sullivan G, Clare P, Jacobs RR. Prophylaxis and management of hamstring muscle injuries in intercollegiate football players. Am J Sports Med 1984;12:368–370.
97. Torg JS, et al. The shoe surface interface and its relationship to football knee injuries. Am J Sports Med 1974;2:261–270.
98. Grace TG, Skipper BJ Newberry JC, et al. Prophylactic knee braces and injury to the lower extremity. J Bone Joint Surg 1987;70A:422–427.
99. Teitz CC, Hermanson RK, Kronmal RA, et al. Evaluations of the use of braces to prevent injury to the knee in collegiate football players. J Bone Joint Surg, 1987;69A:2–9.
100. Sitler M, Ryan J, Hopkinson et al. The efficacy of prophylactic knee brace to reduce knee injuries in football: a prospective randomized study at West Point. Am J Sports Med 1990;18:310–315.
101. Indelicato PA, Hermansdorfer J, Huegel M. Nonoperative management of complete tears of the medial collateral ligament of the knee in intercollegiate football players. Clin Orthop 1990;256:174–177.
102. Noyes FR, Barber SD. The effect of a ligament-augmentation device on allograft reconstructions for chronic ruptures of the anterior cruciate ligament. J Bone Joint Surg 1992;74A:960–973.
103. Bergfeld JA. Diagnosis and nonoperative treatment of acute posterior cruciate ligament injury. Paper presented at the American Association of Orthopedic Surgeons Instructional Course, 1990.
104. Maday MG, Harner CD, Millder MD, et al. Posterior cruciate ligament reconstruction using fresh-frozen allograft tissue. Orthop Trans, in press.
105. DeHaven KE. Meniscus repair in the athlete. Clin Orthop 1985;198:31–35.
106. Guise ER. Rotational ligamentous injuries to the ankle in football. Am J Sports Med 1976;4:1–6.
107. Boytim MF, Fischer DA, Neumann L. Syndesmotic ankle sprains. Am J Sports Med 1991;19:294–298.
108. Whiteside LA, Reynolds FC, Ellsasser JC. Tibiofibular synostosis and recurrent ankle sprains in high performance athletes. Am J Sports Med 1978;6:204–208.
109. Rodeo SA, O'Brien S, Warren RF, Barnes R, Wickiewicz TL, Dillingham MF. Turf toe: an analysis of metatorsalphalangeal joint sprains in professional football players. Am J Sports Med 1990;18:280–285.

23 / GOLF

John R. McCarroll

Epidemiology

The person who has never played golf may imagine that it is a harmless activity that is less taxing than other sports. However, bad backs, sprained wrists, and aching shoulders lead the list of ailments affecting the golfer. Unfortunately, golf injuries have received little attention in the literature. There have been isolated reports of carpal fractures (1), ulnar and median tendinitis in various areas (2), skin rashes (3), nerve injuries (2), and eye injuries (4–6).

Two studies (7, 8) have reported on injuries in the professional and amateur golfer. In the professional golfer, the most common injury is to the wrist, followed closely by the back, hand, shoulder, and knee. In the amateur golfer, the most common injury is to the lower back, followed by the elbow, wrist, shoulder, and knee (Table 23.1). Most of these injuries were caused by frequent play or practice, resulting in overuse syndromes. The other causes such as poor swing mechanics, hitting an object other than the ball, and poor warmup are summarized in Table 23.2. These injuries received various forms of treatment from rest to surgery. Specific injuries and their treatment will be discussed later in this chapter. It is important to note that 44.6% of the amateur and 53% of the professionals included in these studies are still bothered in some degree by their injuries (7, 8).

There have been isolated reports of injury, death, physiologic aspects of golf, and oculophysical problems experienced by the golfer (3, 5, 9, 10). In one case, a man broke his tibia in two places after executing a golf swing (11). Excitement on the golf course has also led to injuries unique to golf. One woman threw her putter into the air after making a long putt, fell over her bag, and broke both her wrists. Another golfer threw his club into the air and knocked out his playing companion (10, 11).

Many deaths have occurred on the golf course. Causes of death include lightning strikes, heart attacks, heat stroke, and electrocution after striking power lines (12). Likewise, anger has led to death on the golf course. One man broke his club on a tree; the broken shaft subsequently rebounded off of another tree, and the jagged end plunged into his body. One golfer was charged with attempted murder after engaging in a bloody, club-swinging brawl with a faster foursome that tried to overtake his group (12). Finally, in 1939 a Philadelphia golfer was convicted of involuntary manslaughter for killing his caddy while swinging his club in anger after missing a shot (12).

There is a golfing disease known as the "twitch" or "yipps" that seems to be such a ridiculous disease that nonsufferers rarely credit it (10). It attacks the victim almost always on short putts and occasionally on chip shots. The golfer becomes totally incapable of moving the putter head to and fro without giving at the critical moment of impact a convulsive twitch. Some players simply strike the ground, whereas others move the ball only a few inches. Bobby Jones, Henry Varden, Sam Snead, Ben Hogan, and Henry Longhurst have been afflicted with this disease. There may be some basis to the idea that yipps is actually a psychological disease. However, the many attempts to find a cure, using hypnotism and changing putters, putting grips, and putting styles, have been to no avail.

Finally, there appears to be a paradox in golf: Many excellent players have poor eyesight yet cannot play with glasses. The long game seems to depend on pure, physical action rather than oculophysical coordination. On the other hand, the short game depends more on the visual component, and it is in this aspect of the game in which the high refractive errors such as astigmatism and muscle imbalance may take their toll (5).

The Golf Swing

To evaluate, treat, and prevent golf injuries, it is important to understand the biomechanics of the golf swing. For the purpose of this chapter, the golf swing will be broken down into three parts: take-away; impact; and follow-through. The golf swing occurs in two

Table 23.1.
Frequency of Injuries

Body Part	Professional Golfer (*N* = 393)	Amateur Golfer (*N* = 908)
Lower Back	93 (23.7%)	244 (34.5%)
Wrist	105 (26.7%)	142 (20.1%)
Elbow	26 (6.6%)	234 (33.1%)
Shoulder	37 (9.4%)	84 (11.7%)
Knee	26 (6.6%)	66 (9.3%)
Neck	12 (3.1%)	28 (4%)
Hip	4 (1.0%)	22 (3.1%)
Ribs	12 (3.1%)	22 (3.1%)
Ankle	8 (2.0%)	18 (2.5%)
Foot	13 (3.3%)	12 (1.7%)

Table 23.2.
Mechanisms of Injury

Injury	Professional	Amateur
Too much play or practice	270	204
Poor swing mechanics	0	150
Hit ground (divet)	40	171
Overswing	0	85
Poor warmup	0	60
Twist during swing	18	22
Grip or swing change	0	26
Fall	2	24
Bending over putt	5	8
Injury caused by the cart	0	18
Hit by ball	3	36

planes: the plane of the backswing and the plane of the downswing. The swing evolves around three dimensions: vertical; lateral; and rotatory (13).

Take-Away

Take-away consists of the setup and movement to the top of the backswing (Fig. 23.1). This phase starts when the golfer addresses the ball. The golfer rotates the knees, hips, and lumbar and cervical spine while the head remains relatively stationary and the weight shifts to the right side. As the backswing continues, the left arm (for a right-handed golfer) is raised and swings across the trunk. The only substantial electromyogram (EMG) activity in the upper extremities during this phase of the golf swing is that of the subscapularis of the left arm (14). There is hyperabduction of the left thumb, radial deviation of the left wrist, and dorsiflexion of the right wrist. However, less than 25% of all golf injuries occur during this part of the swing (Table 23.3).

Impact

Impact consists of the downswing and the impact of the club with the ball (Fig. 23.2). Table 23.3 shows that there are more than twice as many injuries during impact than there are during take-away. This is easy to believe, because the club during downswing covers the same range of motion as does the backswing but moves about three times as fast.

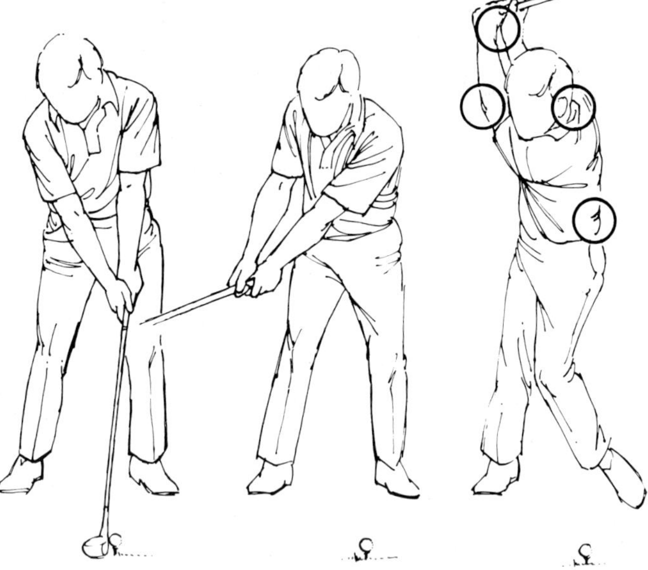

Figure 23.1. The golfer at take-away is removing a club from the set position to the top of the backswing. The circles indicate areas of stress.

Table 23.3.
Relationship of Injury to Swing

Swing Phase and Body Part	Total Injuries
Take-Away	
Back	28
Wrist	25
Elbow, neck, knee	9
Hand	7
Shoulder	6
Total	75
Impact	
Wrist	73
Back	50
Elbow	22
Hand	16
Shoulder	9
Knee	7
Upper back	2
Total	179
Follow-Through	
Back	43
Shoulder	18
Ribs	12
Knee	10
Wrist	9
Neck	6
Hand	4
Elbow	4
Total	106

As the downswing begins, the golfer shifts his or her weight to the left side by moving the hip toward the target. Good golfers actually begin this hip movement about 0.1 sec before the downswing starts (15, 16). To develop maximum acceleration in the downswing phase, the golfer applies the stretch reflex principle. When the whole muscle is stretched, the stretch of the muscle spindles causes a reflex contraction of their host muscles. As a result, the contractile force of the muscle increases and facilitates the recoil of elastic tissue. This principle can be further developed by increasing the flexibility of the major muscle groups. Thus the farther a person can rotate his or her shoulders away from the target, the greater the club head speed that can be generated, thus increasing distance.

This counterclockwise torque in the upper body is generated by the buttocks, quadriceps, hamstrings, and lower-back muscles. The torque causes moderate levels of activity in the pectoralis major, latissimus dorsi, and rotator cuff muscles in both shoulders (14). During the downswing, the wrists apply a negative torque by remaining cocked. At this time, the right wrist is in maximum dorsiflexion; the left thumb is hyperabducted; and the left ulnar nerve, elbow, and forearm muscles are under tension. When the club is approximately horizontal to the ground, the wrists uncock, and this uncocking of the wrists accelerates the club into the ball. These movements are powered by the pectoralis major, subscapularis, and latissimus dorsi of both arms (14).

The impact stage of the golf swing begins the instant before contact when the club head has attained its maximum velocity to the instant that the ball has completely left the club. From a performance aspect, the purpose of impact is to hit the ball as far as possible in the proper direction. From the safety aspect, the purpose of the impact stage is to have a smooth transition from acceleration to deceleration.

At impact, the weight is shifted to left side so that 80% to 95% of the weight has been transferred (17). This is true of both low- and high-handicap golfers. The skilled golfers, however, generally have their weight supported toward the heel of the foot, whereas the less-skilled golfers tend to support themselves right in the middle of the foot (15). This implies that skilled golfers probably get more counterclockwise rotation during their swing.

Valgus stress occurs on the right knee. Furthermore, both wrists are under compression and the left elbow extension mass contracts. The left wrist, hand, and elbow are often hurt during the compression of impact.

Follow-Through

About 25% of all golf swing injuries occur during follow-through (Fig. 23.3). After impact, the left forearm supinates, the right forearm pronates, and the lumbar and cervical spines rotate and hyperextend, in the right-handed golfer. Hip rotation also is completed. The subscapularis along with reduced levels of the latissimus dorsi and pectoralis muscles of both arms continue to be active, decelerating the swing (14). Both knees rotate: the right knee flexes and the left knee everts. At this point, all the weight should be transferred to the left side. As the club decelerates, the golfer extends his or her back into a reverse C position (Fig. 23.4). This

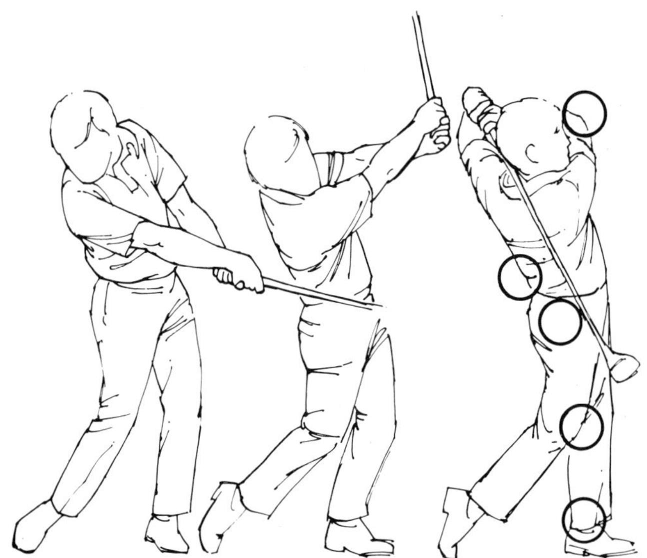

Figure 23.3. Follow-through, showing completion of impact through completion of the golf swing. The circles show areas of stress.

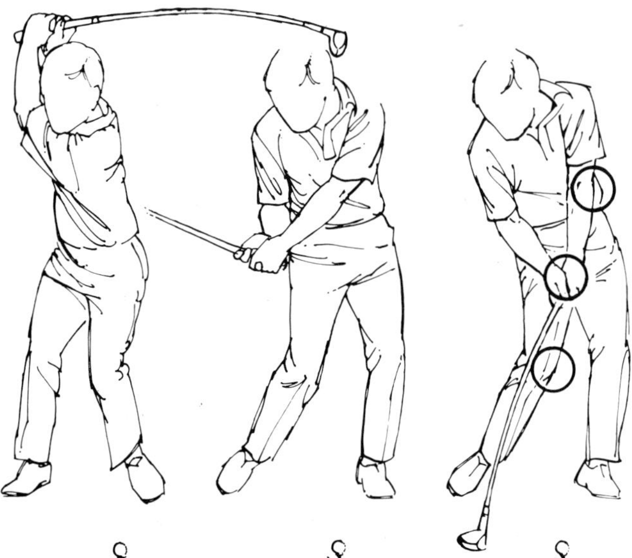

Figure 23.2. A golfer starting from the top of the backswing through impact. The circles show areas of stress.

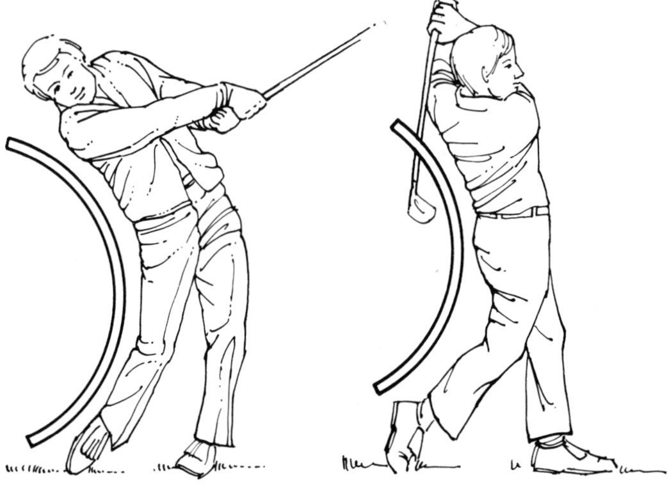

Figure 23.4. *Left*, The golfer is in the reverse C position. *Right*, This golfer has much less stress placed on the lower back, because he is more erect. The golfer on the *left* experiences more torque and more risk of spinal injury then the golfer on the *right*.

position was once taught as essential to playing golf; this is not necessarily true of the more modern golf swing. Most injuries in this phase occur in the back caused by the reverse C position.

The golf swing is the cause of many golf injuries. The physician can certainly treat many of the medical problems, some of which will be discussed in the next section. However, to correct the cause of the injuries, the golfer must correct the faulty swing mechanics. Professional golf instructors, using years of experience with equipment such as video recorders, can correct the mechanics of the golf swing to prevent injuries and change the abnormal stresses applied to various body parts. Also, there are many different types of clubs, shafts, and other equipment, about which the golf professional should be consulted before the golfer make a final decision on what equipment to use.

Injuries and Treatment

Hand and Wrist

Hand and wrist injuries accounted for 37% of the total in a study of golf injuries (7, 8). Tendinitis is the most common problem seen in the wrist and forearm of the golfer. This is the result of the repetitive motions of the wrist and forearm during the swing and the stress at impact. Tendinitis may involve any of the tendons about the wrist. The pain is usually aching or burning in nature. On physical examination, there may be tenderness on the specific tendon or tendons, especially with resisted motions of the wrist. There may be crepitus felt along specific tendons associated with motion.

Tendinitis is treated with rest and/or modification of activity, antiinflammatory mediation, ice, or other modalities such as phonophoresis with 10% hydrocortisone cream and ultrasound, the use of electroacuscope (18), and physical therapy programs as described by Standish et al. (19). The golfer is then returned to a functional progression golf program (Table 23.4) before returning to full activity.

Table 23.4.
Interval Golf Rehabilitation Program[a]

Week	Monday	Wednesday	Friday
1	5 min Chip & Putt 5 min Rest 5 min Chip	5 min Chip & Putt 5 min Rest 5 min Chip 5 min Rest 5 min Chip	5 min Chip & Putt 5 min Rest 5 min Chip 5 min Rest 5 min Chip
2	10 min Chip 10 min Rest 10 min Short iron	10 min Chip 10 min Rest 10 min Short iron 10 min Rest 10 min Short iron	10 min Short iron 10 min Rest 10 min Short iron 10 min Rest 10 min Short iron
3	15 min Short iron 10 min Rest 15 min Long iron 10 min Rest 15 min Long iron	15 min Short iron 10 min Rest 15 min Long iron 10 min Rest 15 min Long iron	15 min Short iron 10 min Rest 15 min Long iron 10 min Rest 15 min Long iron
4	Repeat Friday of week 3	Play 9 holes	Play 18 holes

[a] Do flexibility exercises before hitting and use ice after hitting.

De Quervain's disease is a common condition; the author has seen at least five professional golfers who developed this disease as a result of repetitive practice. De Quervain's disease is a tenosynovitis of the first dorsal compartment of the wrist. The diagnostic sign is Finkelstein's test, which is performed with the thumb and hand forced and deviated toward the ulnar side of the wrist. There is exquisite pain over the radial styloid process and the common sheath of the first compartment. This test is similar to the mechanisms that are involved in hitting the golf ball, especially at preimpact and impact. Conservative treatment of de Quervain's disease usually involves splints, ice, and medication. Only in resistant cases is injection or operative treatment considered.

The hook of the hamate is a long, thin bone that is subject to injury as it projects toward the palmar surface of the hand (1). Fractures occur in golf when the grip of the club strikes the hook of the hamate. Clinical exam shows tenderness over the hook of the hamate. Roentgenograms should include anterior-posterior, lateral, oblique, and carpal tunnel views of the wrist. If these views do not show a fracture but the injury is still suspected, then a bone scan or computerized tomography (CT) may be helpful. In the acute nondisplaced fracture, the treatment is a short arm cast and rest for 6 weeks. The incidence of nonunion of this fracture is high. In a badly displaced fracture or in a nonunion, the excision of the hook of the hamate is indicated.

The golfer may suffer from other miscellaneous hand and wrist conditions, including ligamentous sprains, carpal tunnel syndrome, Guyon canal syndrome, impaction/impingement syndromes (20, 21), occult or overt ganglia (21), ulnar compression syndromes (22–24), and distal radial ulnar joint syndrome (21). All of these occur during the golf swing and must be considered when treating hand and wrist injuries.

Elbow

The golfer may suffer two common elbow injuries: medial and lateral epicondylitis (6). These may be caused by faulty swing mechanics or by strain placed on the elbow during repetitive swinging throughout the season. Tennis and golfer's elbow develop similarly, with essentially the same symptoms, treatment, and prognosis; they differ only in the site of inflammation. In the author's experience, medial epicondylitis occurs more in golf than in tennis, but lateral epicondylitis is the most common injury.

Epicondylitis results in varying degrees of disability. In mild cases, some pain is felt only when the golfer swings the club. In more severe cases, sufferers may find themselves unable to perform even simple, everyday tasks. The diagnosis of epicondylitis can usually be determined by a series of simple tests. Tenderness to palpitation over either epicondyle and pain with resisted dorsi or volar flexion of the wrist are symptoms. Tendinitis is by far the most common of all elbow injuries, but one must consider radial tunnel syndrome and ulnar nerve entrapment as a cause of these symptoms. Furthermore, radiating pain caused by degenerative changes in the cervical spine in the region of C5 and C6 may be the cause.

Treatment is divided into four stages. *(a)* Relief of acute or chronic inflammation, which is accomplished by rest, ice, antiinflammatory medication, and splinting (25). *(b)* Increased forearm muscle strength, flexibility,and endurance (25), which is accomplished through physical therapy that stresses flexibility of the muscles and eccentric exercises to increase strength of the muscles in conjunction with cross-friction massage. *(c)* Decreased movement of force at the wrist, which may be done by altering the swing mechanics. One must correct poor technique to ensure that the injury will not recur. Equipment changes also may be necessary to correct the force that is placed on the forearm muscles. Few equipment changes are available to golfers to alleviate symptoms of tendinitis in the elbow; however, one change that might help is to try a larger grip size. Graphite shaft clubs cause less torque and may relieve some of the stress in the epicondyle area. The use of curved grips has been shown to reduce pain in some injuries of the hand and wrist, but they are not approved by the U.S. Golf Association. Elbow supports also can be helpful; they provide a reactive force against the contractile muscles and either spread the force over a wider area or decrease the contractile pull of the epicondyle. *(d)* Steroid injections are used if nothing else has made a difference. If injections do not help and all other conservative treatment fails, surgery must be considered.

Shoulder

Repetitive overuse syndromes are the most common cause of shoulder pathology in golfers. However, previous insults, incomplete recovery from those insults, and degeneration of general body strength and lack of conditioning by nonuse or extended time of play may be less-recognized causes of problems. Inflammation of the rotator cuff musculotendinous units initiates a clinical pattern that, at first, is reversible. With continued repetitive insults, soft tissue structures microscopically tear, articular cartilage degenerates, osseous tissue produces osteophytes, and the labral rim erodes. At this stage, spontaneous reversibility is doubtful. When scarring, decreased range of motion (or instability), and impingement occur, surgical intervention and rehabilitation are usually necessary for recovery.

Total body conditioning before playing golf is advisable. However, special attentions should be given to the shoulder joint. Here strengthening and proper swing mechanics must be stressed to prevent overuse injuries.

Back

Injuries to the back, especially of the lumbar spine, are some of the most common injuries in both professional and amateur golfers (see Table 23.1). The repetitive and increased rotational and compression forces placed on the back during the golf swing affect the bony structures, intervertebral discs, ligaments, and muscles of the lower back. The reverse C position (see Fig. 23.4) was once thought to be essential to the player. By holding this position through impact, the golfer promotes correct ball trajectory, better body leverage, and solid impact. Many players exaggerate this position in an effort to hit the ball farther, and through repetitive practice, such golfers have paid the penalty of severe back problems. It is now thought that the more upright finish (see Fig. 23.4) puts less stress on the lower back.

Hosea et al. (26) have done a study on the kinematic and myoelectric analysis of the golfer's back. They found that the period from initiation of the backswing to the end of follow-through averaged 1.55 sec for professional golfers compared with 1.86 sec for amateur golfers. The backswing averaged 49% of the total swing (0.76 sec) for the pros compared with 53% (nearly 1 sec) in the amateurs. The professionals took 0.23 sec from the top of the backswing to ball impact, and the amateurs covered the same portion of the swing in 0.37 sec. Yet both groups achieved nearly the same club-head velocity at impact (23.17 + 3.52 m/sec for the pros versus 20.02 + 1.84 m/sec for the amateurs); the professional group generated more than 34% greater peak club-head acceleration, which occurred just before impact.

The golf swing produced a complex loading pattern, involving large shear, lateral bending, compression, and axial torsional loads with rapid changes in directional forces. The amateurs generated an average of 596.74 + 514.01 N in peak shear load at the L3 to L4 segment after impact, yet the large standard deviation indicated the variation in golf mechanics present in this group. The professionals averaged 329.36 + 141.27 N or 80% less peak shear load. Furthermore, the amateurs generated 81% greater peak lateral bending force than professionals. This is well-demonstrated by the fact that the professional golfer exhibits a classic weight shift from right side to left side when changing direction from takeaway to follow-through, whereas the amateur golfer reveals the common problem of swinging from the top, or reverse pivoting, causing the upper torso actually to lean away from the ball at impact.

Although the professionals generated a greater peak compression load than the amateurs, both groups generated more than eight times their body weight at the peak in the lower back. There were two peaks of compression forces: at the top of the backswing and during follow-through (see Figs. 23.1–23.3). The amateurs generated a peak torsional load of 85.4 + 34.21 N, while the load of the professionals was 50% less. Yet despite the lower torque force, the professionals generated 34% greater club-head acceleration at impact, indicating that they use the arms and wrists instead of the trunk unlike most amateurs.

The myoelectric analysis revealed that the left external oblique and, to a lesser degree, the left rectus abdominous and the left L3 paraspinal initiate the takeaway, whereas the right-sided muscles lead from the top of the backswing through to impact. It is during this period that the peak muscle forces occur. Anterior muscles continue to fire during the follow-through, while the paraspinals are essentially inactive. The right-sided external oblique and rectus muscles of the abdomen develop a higher peak activity than the left, while the paraspinals are nearly symmetrical. The amateurs who demonstrated higher shear, lateral bending, and torsional loads, also generated a higher peak total overall activity of the tested muscles.

This study demonstrated that the magnitude of force on the lumbar spine during the golf swing are sufficient enough to produce pathologic changes over time. These changes would most likely occur at the intervertebral disc, pars intraarticularis, and/or the facet joints.

In the diagnosis of lower-back problems, besides the physical exam, one must consider the use of routine x-rays, CT scans, bone scans, and magnetic resonance imaging (MRI). To treat lower-back problems, the patient should be place on antiinflammatory medications and should undergo physical therapy. It also is important that the golfer's swing be analyzed, because in Hosea et al.'s (26) study, swing deviations—especially in the amateur golfer—resulted in greater stress in the lower back. The presence of rapid and intense loading of the lumbar spine in what was previously considered not to be a strenuous sport, indicates the need for preparticipation conditioning, reasonable practice patterns, and thorough warmup before play.

Lower Extremities

The lower extremities are important in the golf swing for they are the foundation around which the swing takes place. Proper leg action promotes good rhythm, balance, and tempo. Injuries to the lower extremities, although not as frequent as upper-extremity injuries in golf, can be bothersome. McCarroll and Gioe (7) and McCarroll et al. (8) found, in studies on amateur and professional golfers, that the knee was injured in 6.6% of the professional and 9.3% of the amateur golfers (Table 23.5).

The most common hip problem seen in the author's clinic is trochanteric bursitis. This inflammatory condition of the bursa overlying the greater trochanter is most often seen in the female golfer. This condition is usually caused by rotation of the hip during practice or by overuse in the golfer who plays frequently and does a lot of walking on uneven terrain. Treatment includes rest, ice, antiinflammatory medication, and physical therapy, which may include cross-friction massage, ultrasound, and stretching of the tight tensor fascia latae or iliotibial band.

The author has seen five male golfers from 35 to 40 years of age who have osteoarthritic changes of both hips. These golfers complain of loss of hip motion, especially with abduction and internal rotation, and experience aching following or during a round of golf. None of these golfers had any past medical reasons for this condition. X-rays revealed early arthritic changes about the hip, with narrowing of the joint space. Four of the five responded to antiinflammatory medication and physical therapy. One, however, continued to deteriorate and eventually had to undergo a total hip joint replacement. He has returned to golf, but his opposite hip is developing similar problems.

Other common injuries to the lower extremity are meniscus tears, usually of the degenerative type; patellofemoral syndrome; calf strains; Achilles tendinitis; and plantar fascitis.

Table 23.5.
Injuries in the Lower Extremity (Percent)

Body Part	Professional	Amateur
Knee	6.6	9.3
Hip	1	3.1
Ankle	2	2.5
Feet	3.3	1.7
Thigh	1.2	1.1
Calf	0	0.6

Conditioning

Golf is an activity demanding a high degree of refined motor skills. There are many frustrated golfers who are not in good physical shape. The weekend golfer, and even the professional golfer, must condition his or her body before going to the course or assume the risk of injury. Injuries, sore muscles, and frustrating days on the golf course can be eliminated by a preseason, regular season, and off-season conditioning program.

There are four types of exercises that the golfer should do to maintain his or her fullest ability to avoid injuries. Stretching exercises (27) are used to maintain complete range of motion of the hamstrings, back, and shoulders. Without complete range of motion and flexibility, the golfer will put abnormal stress on the various body structures during the golf swing.

Golf is not a strength game like other sports. Strength in itself will not enable the individual to hit the ball farther or longer. However, it will allow the skilled player to strike shots with more consistent, explosive power

Table 23.6.
Nautilus Workout Program for Golfers[a]

Exercise[b]	Muscles	Skills
Hip and back	Buttocks, lower back	Driving power, walking endurance
Leg extension	Quadriceps	Driving power, walking endurance
Leg curl	Hamstrings	Hip turn, driving power
Double shoulder (lateral press)	Deltoids	Club control, impact velocity
Double shoulder (seated press)	Deltoids, triceps	Shoulder turn, club extension
Pull over	Latissimus dorsi	Shoulder turn, club extension
Wrist curl	Forearm flexors	Club head control, impact power, acceleration
Reverse wrist curls	Forearms extensors	Club head control, acceleration

[a]From Peterson J. Conditioning for a purpose the West Point way. West Point, NY: Leisure Press, 1977.

[b]Perform one set of 8 to 12 repetitions of each exercise. Take no more than 60 sec to perform each set. Rest no more than 30 sec between each set.

over extended periods. Any golfer with a weak area, especially the knee and/or back is at risk for a golfing injury. One can use equipment such as Nautilus (Table 23.6), Universal gyms, or home devices such as free weights or weighted clubs to increase strength (25).

These workout programs also develop the endurance strength needed to walk long distances, climb hills, and repeat the swing over and over during the game. There are various muscles that must be strengthened to improve basic golf skills. Table 23.6 reviews the Nautilus workout program for golf. For the golfer who does not have access to specialized exercise equipment, an excellent reference book is available that describes home exercises (27).

Cardiovascular exercise for endurance is another essential part of conditioning. Climbing hills and walking 18 holes is impossible without a cardiovascular system that will respond to strenuous exercise. The golfer should follow a preseason conditioning program that includes jogging, riding a bike, walking and/or using a stair machine to get into cardiovascular shape for the sport.

In many sports, such as football, basketball, and baseball, the athletes are put through a functional progression rehabilitation program before returning to their sport. The same should be true for golf. Table 23.4 shows an example of an interval golf rehabilitation for the injured golfer to return safely to his or her sport.

Golfers are athletes, because golf is a sport. To play it well, one must have athletic ability, strength, agility, coordination, and endurance. The golf swing is physically demanding and can contribute to various types of injuries. The wrist, back, and shoulder are the most frequently injured body parts. These injuries may be prevented or reduced by a combination of proper conditioning, treatment, and correct swing mechanics.

REFERENCES

1. Torisu T. Fracture of the hook of the hamate by a golf swing. Clin Orthop 1972;83:91–94.
2. Stover CN, Wiren G, Topaz SR. The modern golf swing and stress syndromes. Phys Sportsmed 1976;4:42–47.
3. Mattikow MS. The ubiquitous golfer. Cutis 1977;19:471.
4. O'Grady R, Shock P. Golf-ball granuloma of the eyelids and conjunctiva. Am J Ophthalmol 1973;76:148–151.
5. Vallottow W. The ocular aspect of golf. South Med J 1965;58:44–47.
6. Weston PA. Injury from a disrupted golf ball. Lancet 1977;1:375.
7. McCarroll JR, Gioe TJ. Professional golfers and the price they pay. Phys Sportsmed 1966;10:64–67.
8. McCarroll JR, Shelbourne KD, Rettig AC. Injuries in the amateur golfer. Phys Sportsmed 1990;18(3):122–125.
9. Roberts J. Injuries, handicaps, mashies, and cleeks. Phys Sportsmed 1978;6:121–124.
10. Shulenberg C. Medical aspect and curiosities of golfing. Practitioner 1976;217:625–627.
11. Everard A. Golf. J R Coll Gen Pract 1970;3:2930–2935.
12. *Indianapolis Star,* 1982.
13. Maddalozzo, GF. An anatomical and biomechanical analysis of the full golf swing. Natl Strength Coaches Assoc J 1990;9(4):6.
14. Jobe FW, Moynes DR, Antonelli DJ. Rotator cuff function during a golf swing. Am J Sports Med 1986;14:388–392.
15. Hay JG. The biomechanics of sports techniques. Englewood Cliffs, NJ: Prentice-Hall, 1973.
16. Cochran A, Stobbs J. The search for the perfect swing. Heinemann Educational, 1968.
17. Richards J, Farrell M, Kent J, Kraft R. Weight transfer patterns during the golf swing. Res Q Exerc Sport 1985;56(4):361–365.
18. Gieck JH, Saliba EN. Application of modalities in overuse syndromes. Clin Sports Med 1987;6:448–449.
19. Standish WD, Rubinovich RM, Arwin S. Eccentric exercise in chronic tendinitis. Clin Orthop 1986;2080:65–68.
20. Linscheid RL, Dobyns JH. Athletic injuries of the wrist. Clin Orthop 1985;198:141–151.
21. Dobyns JH, Sim FH, Linscheid RL. Sports stress syndromes of the hand and wrist. Am J Sports Med 1978;6:236–253.
22. Coleman HM. Injuries of the articular disc of the wrist. J Bone Joint Surg 1960;42B:522–528.
23. Joseph RB, Linscheid RL, Dobyns JH, Bryan RS. Chronic sprains of the carpometacarpal joints. J Bone Joint Surg 1981;6:1720–1729.
24. Roth JH, Peohling GC, Whipple TL. Arthroscopic surgery of the wrist. Instr Course Lect 1986;37:183–194.
25. Standish WD. Tendinitis: its etiology and treatment. Lexington, MA: DC Heath, 1986.
26. Hosea TM, Gatt CJ, Calli KM, Langrana NA, Zawadsky JP. The golfer's back: a kinematic and myoelectric analysis. Paper presented at the American Orthopaedic Society for Sports Medicine Meeting and the First Scientific Meeting of Gold Science, Edinburgh, Scotland, 1991.
27. Jobe FW, Moynes DR. 30 exercises for better golf. Inglewood, CA: Champion Press.

24 / GYMNASTICS

Jeffery R. Weiss

Introduction

Although gymnastics has been traced to ancient Egypt (1), gymnastics in the United States officially began only in 1848, when the Turners Gymnastic Club, derived from the Turnverin Club in Germany, was founded in Cincinnati (1). At about this same time, the Sokol organization from Czechoslovakia began to establish private gymnastic clubs in America. The Sokols believed in the motto Strong mind and a strong body, and the gymnastics by the Sokol organization was a combination of dance and acrobatics with calisthenics.

Enthusiasm for gymnastics as a sport continued to grow until the mid 1940s, when most gymnastics took place in large public schools and men's athletic clubs in larger cities. From the end of World War II until about 1980 interest resurged mainly as the result of strong collegiate support and televised gymnastic events (2). Budgetary demands subsequently brought a second decline in collegiate and high school gymnastic programs, but over the past 25 years, private gymnastic facilities have increased, in part because of the growing popularity of the sport after the 1972 Olympics, in Munich (3). Televised gymnastic events in Europe and America fueled this second wave of popularity and highlighted the increasingly complex skills and tricks. The private gymnastic clubs grew more popular, and specialized coaching was needed to learn the skills necessary to compete.

In June 1991, there were approximately 2,600 private gymnastic clubs with more than 45,000 gymnasts registered (4). By June 1993, over 3,000 private clubs were registered with the U.S. Gymnastic Federation, and the current number of gymnasts totals approximately 35,000 females and 10,000 males. Before 1990, gymnastics skills were divided into five levels—elite and classes I–IV—and most epidemiologic studies were performed using this system. Currently, skills are divided into 10 levels, with the top level referred to as elite. As a result of the reclassification, elite became level 1, class I became levels 8 and 9, class II was divided into the levels 6 and 7, class III was divided into levels 4 and 5, and class IV was divided into levels 1, 2, and 3. There are currently about 300 elite-level gymnasts. Most are found at the lower competitive levels, level 1 includes some 15,000 participants (Table 24.1)

College and high school programs seem to be losing gymnasts. For example, from 1979 to 1983, the number of southern California high schools offering boys' gymnastics decreased 62%. An even greater decrease had occurred by 1984 when 82% of the schools still offering gymnastics dropped the sport. The number of female high school gymnasts decreased by 63% between 1973 and 1984 (5). By 1990, the National Federation of State High School Associations (6) reported that there were 23,367 female gymnasts and 3,865 male gymnasts across the United States, representing a 50% decrease in participants between 1985 and 1990. The number of female gymnasts at the high school level has undergone a smaller decline (35%) from 35,440 in 1985 to 23,367 in 1990. The reasons for the decline in school programs were as follows: *(a)* the level of tricks grew more and more intricate; *(b)* injury rates and law suits increased; *(c)* overall student enrollment decreased, even though participation in all sports increased; and *(d)* smaller teams were disbanded to funnel money into larger, revenue-producing teams (5). According to a recent National Collegiate Athletic Association (7) report, 1,493 female gymnasts and 663 male gymnasts participated in the 1989–1990 season. There were less than half as many male gymnastic teams (45) as female teams (108).

Gymnastics demands that athletes have total control of their bodies at all times. They must train themselves physically and mentally as they climb from level to level, because the tricks become more demanding and complex.

A good gymnast begins a career by choosing a suitable program. The coach is an important consideration. Coaches should possess a thorough knowledge of the sport and be honest in their communication with the athlete. As athletes climb up the ladder of competition, they should be referred elsewhere if the coach does not

Table 24.1.
Gymnastic Participants 1990

Club	
Male	300
Female	15,000
High School	
Male	3,865
Female	23,367
College	
Division 1	
Male	594
Female	937
Division 2	
Male	24
Female	291
Division 3	
Male	46
Female	265

Table 24.2.
Practice Schedules for Private Clubs

Levels	Days a Week	Hours per Session
Elite	5	4
9–10	5	4
7–8	4	4
4, 5, and 6	3	4
1, 2, and 3	2	4
Pre	1	4

feel qualified to teach or spot the advanced-level tricks. Recently, the U.S. Gymnastics Federation instituted a course for coaches on safety and proficiency in spotting, with the goal of providing certification in these areas. Coaches must possess proof of certification in order for their gymnasts to compete on a regional level.

Gymnasts begin to participate at increasingly younger ages (1). It is not uncommon to find participants beginning preparatory classes at age 5 (8). In private gymnastics clubs, the sport generally continues year round with a 2-week break. The number of hours spent in practice will vary with the level of competition. Approximate hours are listed in Table 24.2.

Equipment Considerations

Understanding gymnastics injuries requires familiarity with gymnastics equipment and techniques. Women's gymnastics is composed of four events: floor exercise; balance beam; uneven parallel bars; and vault. Male gymnasts compete on the rings, floor exercise, vault, parallel bars, pommel horse, and horizontal bar.

Although both men and women participate in vault and floor exercise, they perform them differently. The key differences in vaulting are the height and positioning of the horse. Men place the horse at a height of 5.5 feet; women at 4.5 feet. For men, the horse is placed in the line of direction of the run, hence the name long-horse vaulting. For women, the horse is placed perpendicular to the run, hence the name side-horse vaulting. Over the years, the height of the horse has been raised because the spring boards used to propel the gymnasts have improved (Fig. 24.1). This makes for the achievement of greater heights and increasingly difficult tricks (3).

While the same floor dimensions are used in male and female floor exercise, the time of the event differs; men compete for 50 to 70 sec, and women, for 70 to 90 sec. Women's routines are performed to music. For both men and women, floor exercise is now performed on either metal springs under plywood or, more common, a material called Ethafoam (9), which provides a softer, more forgiving surface for landing after tumbling passes (Fig. 24.2). This surface has significantly reduced the number of injuries associated with floor exercise. The spring floor does not increase the height that a gymnast can obtain.

The balance beam is 16.5 feet long, slightly less than 4 inches wide, and 4 feet off the floor. It is most often made of hardwood with a thin rubber coating for shock absorption. The gymnast must perform both dance and tumbling skills on the beam. This event is the most stressful to the gymnast, because she must be in total command of her body during this routine (3).

Uneven parallel bars grew out of the mens' parallel bars. The uneven bars compensated for the lesser upper extremity strength in females, incorporating swinging into the routine. Although the two rails are adjustable, the lower rail is approximately 4.5 to 5 feet from the floor, and the upper rail is 7 to 7.5 feet from the floor. The rails are now made of Fiberglas to avoid splitting and cracking. They are 7 feet, 9 inches long

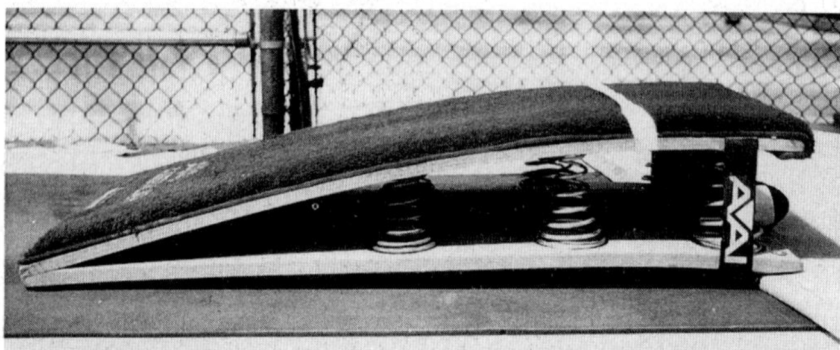

Figure 24.1. Design of the modern spring board.

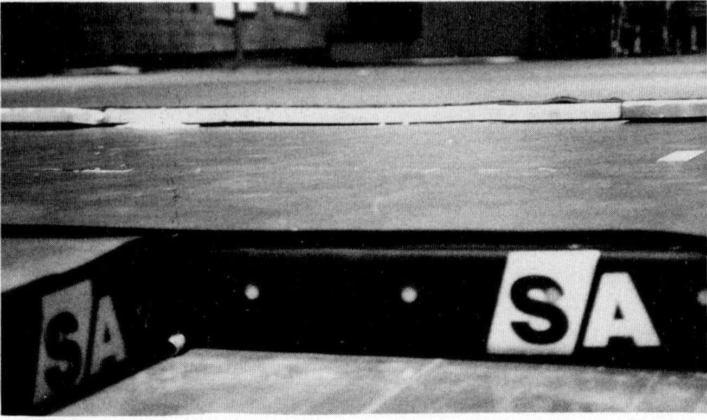

Figure 24.2. A gymnastics floor is sprung and padded with Ethafoam.

and provide for some spring. The routine consists of a series of grasp and release moves as well as large swings (3).

The parallel bars consists of two 11-foot-long rails, 5 feet, 9 inches off the floor. The horizontal width of the bars is adjusted to each individual gymnast (3). The event requires great upper extremity strength, because the upper extremity functions mainly as a closed kinetic chain throughout a series of swinging and support moves.

The pommel horse stands approximately 3 feet, 8 inches from the floor; the pommels add 5 inches to the height (8). The gymnast must maintain himself on the horse while performing both support and swinging moves. He must complete a routine on all sections of the pommel horse. Good form and body control along with physical strength are necessary to maintain oneself on the pommels.

The still rings and the horizontal bar require the gymnast to begin a routine from a hanging position. The still rings are 8.5 feet from the floor and are supposed to be hung from a distance of 18 feet from the floor; shorter distances make the event easier for support moves. The gymnast maintains contact with this apparatus until dismount. As with the pommel horse, the rings combine both swing and support moves (3). Although the gymnast swings the rings should remain relatively still.

The horizontal bar is made of tempered steel and is 8.5 feet from the floor. The gymnast is mainly concerned with grasping, releasing, and regrasping the bar, making the event one of timing and strength. The gymnast must control as much as 5 to 7 times body weight while swinging (3).

Equipment as well as coaching are important in the prevention of injuries. The gymnast must be able to have trust in the coach/spotter who can play a direct role only during practice sessions to ensure that injury does not occur. During competition, the spotter may not touch the gymnast or the gymnast is disqualified from that event. When teaching new tricks, some coaches use belts and harnesses around the waist of the gymnast to provide more protection than is possible by simply standing below the gymnast. Pits made of foam rubber and foam matting are sometimes used during practice to ensure safe landings.

Epidemiologic studies have been conducted to determine the site, frequency, and type of injuries that occur on each apparatus. Most of these studies have focused on females at the club level. All the epidemiologic studies were conducted before gymnastics was reclassified into 10 levels.

Snook (10) conducted a 5-year study to determine the frequency of injury in collegiate women's gymnastics. Injury was defined as any event that required the gymnast to see a physician. A total of 66 injuries were recorded in 70 participants, most involving the lower extremities. In 1980, Garrick (11) reported injury rates of female gymnasts at college, high school, and club levels. Injuries most often occurred in the lower extremities, with sprains being the most common type. The greatest number of injuries occurred during the floor exercise (45%), followed by the balance beam (12%). Among male and female collegiate-level gymnasts, Whiteside (12) found that the majority of injuries occurred during practice. Lower extremity injuries were more common in women, and upper extremity injuries were more common among men. Sprains were the most common type of injury for both male and female gymnasts. Locations of sprains were not specified.

Most of the more recent studies have involved female gymnasts (13–15), with a mean age ranging from 9.8 to 12.6 years. Injuries to the lower extremity predominated. The most common acute injury was an ankle sprain, and the most common chronic injury was patellofemoral pain. Floor exercise was responsible for approximately 35% of the injuries (15). Between 75% and 85% of the injuries occurred without a spotter. Class 1 (elite) gymnasts were often injured and this was attributed to the intensity of training involved with learning higher-level tricks (13, 15).

The NCAA Injury and Illness Surveillance Systems (16) reported on gymnastic injuries that were followed up for 5 years. The most common injury to the collegiate female gymnast (29%) was a sprained ankle. In womens' gymnastics, floor exercise was responsible for the largest number of injuries (432, or 33%) followed by the uneven parallel bars (261 injuries, or 20.6%). Average practice time lost per injury was 1 to 2 days. However, if the gymnast was not able to return within 2 days, the time between injury and return to practice was 10 or more days.

Floor exercise also was the most common cause of injury in male gymnasts, accounting for 26.7% of all injuries; The horizontal bar was second (20.8%). The most frequently injured areas were the ankle, knee, shoulder, and wrist. The return to gymnastics for men was similar to that for women, 40% being able to return within 2 days and 27% of the remainder within 3 to 6 days. The others took more than 10 days to return.

Over the past 5 years at the collegiate level, there have not been any fatal accidents in men's or women's gymnastics. There has been only one nonfatal catastrophic accident in women's collegiate gymnastics in the last 5 years.

Upper Extremity Injuries

Although less common than lower extremity injuries in both men's and women's gymnastics, upper extremity injuries are difficult to protect and frequently delay the return to practice and competition (Fig. 24.3).

Hand Injuries

Skin tears are a common problem and usually occur as the gymnast begins to resume a workout schedule after taking some time off. They usually result from friction that builds between either the skin and the apparatus or the skin and the grips. They also can occur with a new set of grips.

The tear should be kept clean and well-lubricated, and further ripping should be prevented by gradually

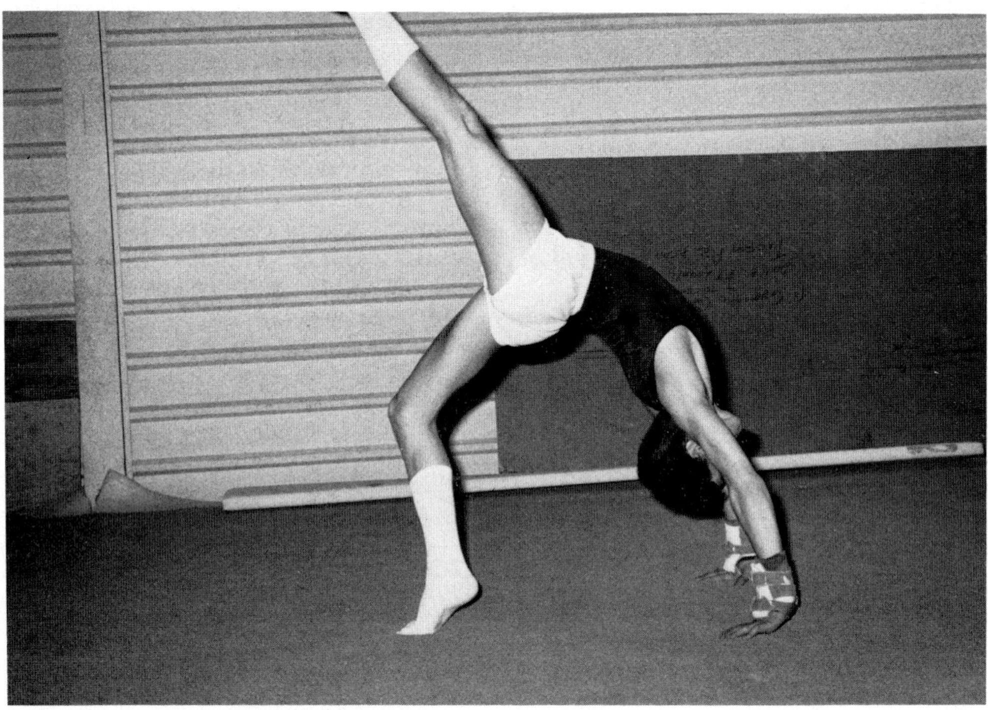

Figure 24.3. In gymnastics, all four extremities are weight bearing. Wrist and elbow hyperextension can cause medial epicondyle strains, fractures, and avulsions.

retoughening the callous located at the metacarpophalangeal (MCP) joints. Fresh chalk should be used before starting work on any apparatus. Cleaning the apparatus periodically avoids buildup of caked chalk.

The most common mechanism for wrist injuries involves a combination of compression, hyperdorsiflexion, and torsion (17, 18), which result from use of the upper extremity as a weight-bearing structure. Common injuries at the wrist include dorsal wrist pain, distal radius stress fractures, carpal stress fractures and wrist ganglia.

The pommel horse has been implicated as the main contributor to wrist injuries in male gymnastics (18). During the pommel horse exercise, the gymnast uses his wrist as a rigid structure of support for his body weight. The wrist is subjected to the high intensity of impact and the stress of repetition. During a front scissors maneuver, the wrist may bear loads averaging 1 to 1.5 times body weight. The duration as well as the force generated to support this maneuver increase the risk of injury (19).

Dorsal wrist pain is described as an intense pain on the lower lateral region of the wrist. Most likely it is capsulitis. The onset of dorsal wrist pain is usually insidious and tends to increase with activity (20). Pain usually occurs with vaulting, floor exercise, and pommel horse, for which the wrist is forced into hyperdorsiflexion with compression or torsion (21). The treatment for dorsal wrist pain involves the use of modalities, flexibility, and strengthening of the wrist musculature as well as the use of a dorsiflexion block. Blocks placed around the dorsal aspect of the wrist just distal to the midcarpal junction prevent the wrist from moving into full extension.

Distal radius stress fractures can occur in either a weight-bearing or a non–weight-bearing position. In a weight-bearing position, sudden-impact loading in a hyperextended position may cause the distal radial epiphysis or metaphysis to fracture (21). Dobyns (17) also attributes a stress fractures of the distal radius to a traction injury. The traction causes an increase in compressive forces on the radial styloid, which in turn cause a fracture. Dobyns suggests that the dowel grip, often used to increase the speed of the gymnast around the high bar, increases the force on the wrist. Other events in which a traction injury can occur are the still rings and the uneven bars.

Scaphoid fractures are uncommon in gymnastics, but the usual mechanism of injury is repeated compression force with the wrist held in hyperextension; though the forces applied in this position are usually subthreshold, their continued application results in a stress reaction (17). Scaphoid fractures also can occur from a fall on an extended wrist and an extended arm, such as when a gymnast falls off an apparatus and does not tuck and roll from protection (21, 22).

Another source of wrist pain is ulnar impaction syndrome. Mandelbaum (18) discovered that the location of this pain was different in male and female gymnasts, the males having pain on the dorsal aspect of the wrist toward the ulnar side, and females, on the ulnar side of the wrist but not on the dorsal or the palmar aspect. Both men and women felt pain during compression of the wrist, but none complained of pain with distraction. Pain was most prevalent in males during the pommel horse and was related to weight bearing on the wrist. Females had pain primarily while vaulting.

Treatment of these injuries initially focuses on activity modification along with ice and nonsteroidal antiinflammatory drugs (NSAIDs). After the pain cycle has been eliminated, stretching and strengthening can be initiated. A graduated return to sports with cryotherapy after completion of practice is most beneficial. During practice, the gymnast may be taped as shown in Figure 24.4. This type of strapping provides the forearm with compression and support. It may be difficult to devise a splint or brace without involving the palmar surface of the hand. This can create significant problems from the gymnast, as it may prevent him or her from obtaining an accurate feel for the apparatus. In addition, the use of a brace that includes the palm of the hand will make grasp difficult and interfere with the use of grips.

During the acute stage, it is important to minimize swelling and pain. Early active range of motion in the pain-free range should begin as quickly as possible. Musculotendinous injuries of the wrist respond well to rest, ice, compression, and elevation (RICE) and gentle stretching exercises. The wrist flexors and extensors should be stretched. Sustained static stretching is preferred over bouncing or ballistic stretching, which will only increase the insult of the injury. Sustained stretches should be held for a minimum of 30 sec. The gymnast must be encouraged to stop at the point of pain and then release so that only a mild stretch is felt along the muscle. As the injury becomes subacute and the pain lessens, treatment may be progressed to include the use of heat modalities such as hot packs, paraffin, whirlpool, and ultrasound. Care must be taken during this phase of rehabilitation to prevent the athlete from regressing to the acute stage of inflammation. Full pain-free active range of motion is emphasized during this stage of rehabilitation. The athlete is progressed to submaximal isometric contractions throughout the range of motion, and the force of the contractions is then progressed to patient tolerance.

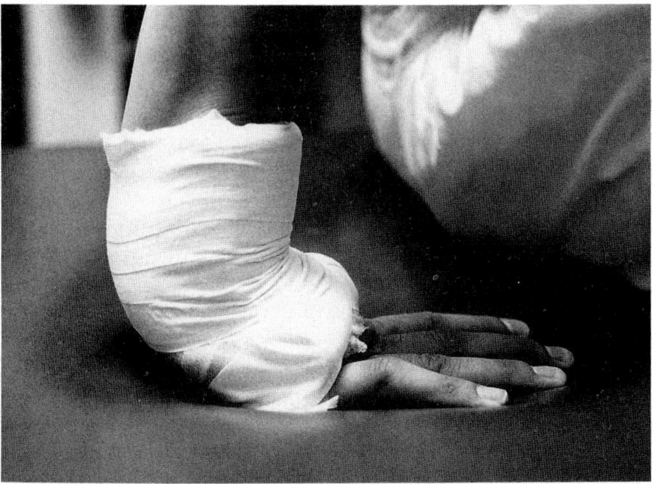

Figure 24.4. Dorsal wrist block prevents full wrist extension.

If range of motion does not improve, the use of joint-mobilization techniques may prove to be of benefit. Before joint mobilization is used, it is important to assess each of the individuals' carpal joint bilaterally. Joint mobilization should only be performed to those joints that demonstrate hypomotility. The force used to mobilize the joint depends on the grading of the restriction as well as the irritability of the athlete. Each of the joint-mobilization techniques should be held 5 to 10 sec and for approximately 8 to 10 repetitions. Range of motion and stretching should be assessed, and if motion improves at least 10°, mobilization should be halted for the session. After the joint-mobilization techniques, active and passive range of motion should be performed to preserve the new ranges of motion. The athlete should be cautioned that he or she may feel soreness after the first trial application of joint strength and that repeated injury may result. Scaphoid fracture treatment is detailed in Chapter 53. Average time to return to gymnastics is 3 months.

Shoulder Injuries

Shoulder injuries are more common in male than female gymnasts. In one study of mens' college gymnastics injuries between 1986 and 1991, the shoulder was the most commonly injured joint (16).

The most common shoulder injury is a supraspinatus strain (10). Events such as the still rings produce stress on the shoulder musculature. The use of the dowel grip always increases the forces across the shoulder by allowing the gymnast to reach higher velocities. These forces are controlled by eccentric rotator cuff contractions. Muscle strains of the rotator cuff are particularly common in the younger gymnast because upper body strength, especially the rotator cuff, may not be adequate.

Impingement syndrome also occurs frequently in both males and females. Impingement can be primary or secondary to either glenohumeral or functional scapular instability (23). Gymnasts often demonstrate excessive ranges of motion in multiple joints. Primary instability, however, is rare (21). The complaints of instability are often related to hypermobility combined with poor technique and poor muscle tone. Subluxation and dislocation are usually the result of missing a trick and falling from the apparatus.

Gymnasts also can develop bicipital tendinitis or subluxation of the biceps tendon from the bicipital groove. This occurs more frequently in males. The onset of pain is commonly felt as a sensation that "something is moving" when the gymnast is performing on the rings, pommel horse, or parallel bars. As the arm becomes extended and fully supinated, the biceps tendon may override a shallow bicipital groove. The gymnast complains of swelling, pain, and discomfort about the bicipital groove.

Elbow Injuries

Elbow injuries in gymnastics are rare. Caine (15) noted that elbow injuries only accounted for 4.8% of the total injuries in gymnasts. The total number of elbow injuries incurred during that study was seven: three acute and four of gradual onset. Lindner (14) confirmed these findings, noting that the usual mechanisms were missed moves, falls from an apparatus, or incorrect dismounts. The most common acute injuries are fractures and dislocations. The most common chronic problems are triceps tendinitis, medial and lateral epicondylitis, and osteochondritis dissecans. Priest (24) found 41 separate elbow injuries in 30 acute traumatized elbows. A total of 41% of these injuries were fractures to the medial epicondyle and 39% were dislocations. These two types of injuries make up 80% of the total elbow injuries. During further analysis, Priest found that 60% occurred without a spotter present. There were twice as many injuries sustained on a thin mat or on a bare floor compared with the thicker mats. Priest (24) was unable to determine which apparatus caused the most injuries or to determine which tricks caused elbow injuries. Only 12% of all elbow injuries occur during a dismount maneuver.

Upon contemplating return to the gymnasium, the gymnast should be able to demonstrate full range of motion at the elbow joint as well as full strength of the surrounding musculature. The gymnast should also be able to support his or her body weight for an adequate length of time without pain. It may be of benefit to provide supportive strapping. The athlete should be progressed slowly back into his or her regular gymnastic routine, first by concentrating on support moves and then working up to the more difficult tricks.

Overuse problems also can occur at the elbow joint. Medial epicondylitis is common in both male and female gymnasts, because weight bearing on the upper extremity places a significant amount of force on the common flexor mass (25). Female gymnasts are more likely to contract medial epicondylitis, because women have a greater valgus angle of the elbow joint, which in turn causes a higher traction force on the medial flexor mass during weight-bearing maneuvers (21). The main mechanisms of medial epicondylitis in male gymnasts are power moves, such as the iron cross on the rings and grasping the high bar with the wrist in a flexed position. Both of these maneuvers increase the force needed in the flexor muscle mass. A gymnast also may suffer medial epicondylitis while performing the floor exercise. Most tumbling passes are performed with the wrist in maximal hyperextension, thus fully stretching the flexor mass.

Triceps tendinitis, sometimes termed "jumper's knee of the elbow" (21), can develop after a gymnast irritates the triceps tendon as it attaches distally into the olecranon process. The most frequent mechanism of injury is the repeated exertion of great force in the triceps to propel the body. This usually occurs with vaulting and floor exercises in which the gymnast flexes and then rapidly extends the elbow, thus creating large forces on the triceps tendon. In vaulting, gymnasts commonly produce force on the their upper extremities in excess of 2.5 to 3.5 times their body weight (21). Osteochondritis dissecans may also become an overuse problem for the gymnast. It generally presents with pain in the posterior aspect of the elbow. The bone fragments from the olecranon can be forced into the olecranon fossa during hyperextension, creating inflammation, pain, and fractures in the distal radius (20). Treatment of this type of injury should rely mainly on early detection and correct technique. If pain does occur, modalities can be used for symptomatic relief as well as strengthening of the elbow musculature. If nonoperative treatment fails, then the gymnast may be forced to undergo arthroscopic debridement of the elbow joint.

Knee Injuries

Epidemiologic studies generally indicate that the lower extremity is the most common area affected in gymnastics (13, 15, 26). There is some discrepancy as to whether the knee or the ankle injuries are more commonly injured joints. Weiker (13) sites a high rate of overuse injury in the knee, with chondromalacia patella as the most common.

Acute injuries to the knee are often linked to dismount maneuvers, because the forces are many times greater than other landings (15). Because scoring procedures in gymnastics award the highest scores to complicated dismounts, attaining a higher score involves increased risk. During dismounts, the gymnast should be educated not to land on a fully extended or hyperextended knee, which may result in an isolated tear of the anterior cruciate ligament (ACL) injury or the extensor mechanism (Fig. 24.5). Instead, the knee should be in slight flexion (27). Rotation on the mat or floor can also cause an ACL injury. The menisci may also tear with torsional stress, most often during floor exercise or from a fall from an apparatus.

Patellar dislocations or subluxations also occur. Andrish (28) followed 28 male gymnasts and 142 female gymnasts for a 78-month period. During this time, there were a total of 170 knee injuries recorded. A total of 9.4% of these injuries were patellar subluxation or dislocation, and the most common mechanism was a twisting injury with the femur internally rotated on a fixed tibia followed by a sudden burst of quadriceps activity. This injury was usually seen during a dismount procedure or a vault. Predisposing factors to patellar subluxation are lateral patellar posture and patellar alta, weakness in the vastus medialis, and lateral concavity or shortening of the lateral retinaculum. The young female gymnast often presents with genu valgum, medial femoral rotation, proximal tibial vara, and external tibial torsion (29), and this combination produces an increased Q angle, resulting in lateral riding of the patella (29).

Patellar tendon ruptures are a rare injury. Donati (30) reported on a 21-year-old college gymnast who ruptured both patellar tendons simultaneously while vaulting. Before this injury, she had no symptoms. Patellar tendon rupture is uncommon in young athletes.

Chronic knee injuries in gymnastics are patellofemoral pain, jumper's knee, and Osgood-Schlatter disease (13). Weiker followed 873 gymnasts for a 9-month

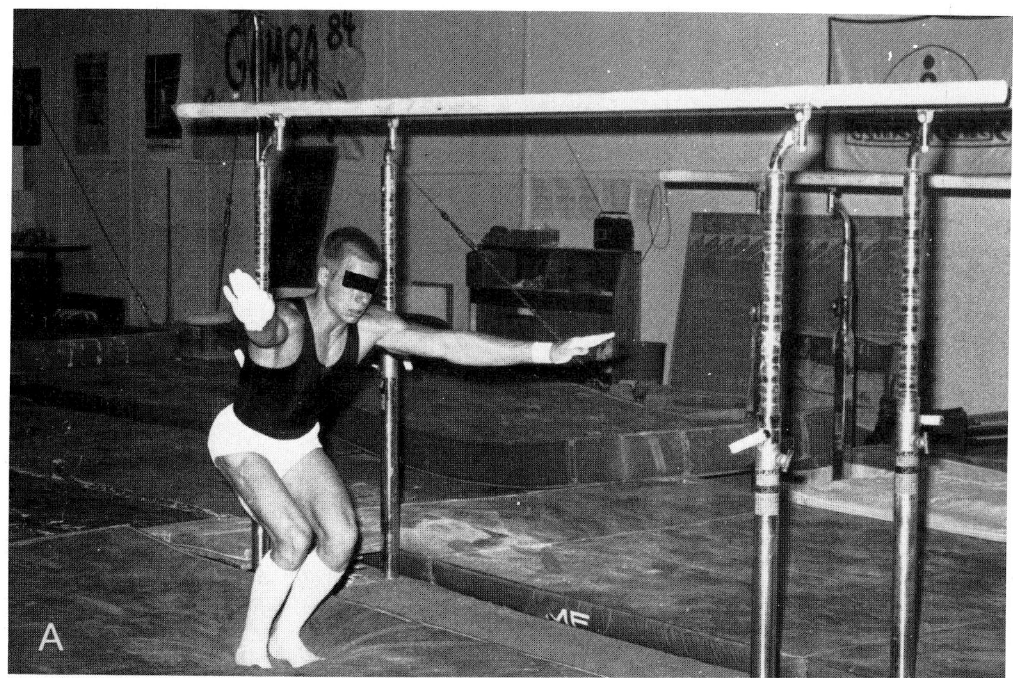

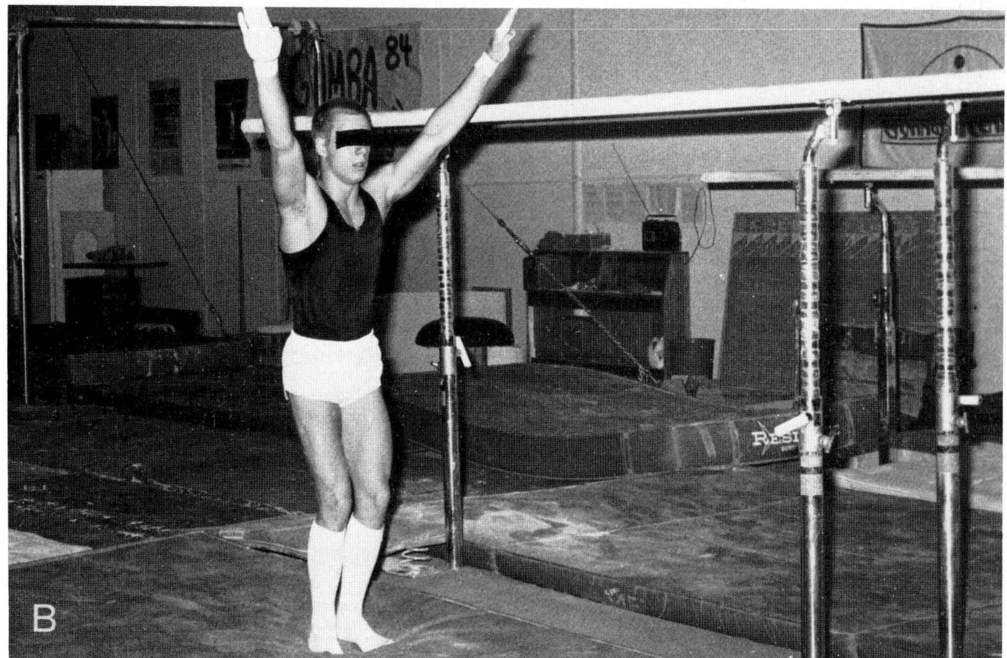

Figure 24.5. Proper dismount includes slight knee flexion. The dismount is the most dangerous and most difficult part of the gymnast's routine.

season and found that the most common problem was patellofemoral pain, most often the result of forceful leaping from a hyperflexed knee. Patellar femoral pain in a young female gymnast can be brought on simply by postural positioning (31). Short falls and the repetition of practices also predispose the gymnast to patellofemoral pain.

Osgood-Schlatter disease is common among both male and female gymnasts and frequently occurs during rapid growth. Long practice sessions and increasing repetitions during practice adds to the stress placed on the patellar tendon. It is usually self-limiting (32), and in most instances, flexibility exercises, the use of an infrapatellar strap, and postpractice cryotherapy are adequate treatment. Patellar tendinitis, or jumper's knee, is also a common finding in gymnastics, caused by repetitive jumping (30). It also can accompany Osgood-Schlatter disease. Treatment should include modalities as needed, transverse friction massage across the patellar tendon, flexibility exercises, and eccentric exercises.

During acute episodes, the gymnast should be encouraged to rest. Infrapatellar straps may be of benefit.

In Weiker's (13) study, strains were the second most common type of injury, although specific locations were not given. Caine (15) found that strains accounted for 17.7% of all injuries recorded, most often in the lower extremities. He also found that the frequency increased during the 1st hr of practice. He attributed this to improper warmup and stretching before practice. Gymnasts possess increased flexibility. Compared with normals during a toe-touching exercise, gymnasts were able to out reach a control group by approximately 20.8 cm (33). A gymnast's lead leg in a split possesses greater flexibility than the trail leg.

Most common strains occur during a vault run or floor exercise. During the sudden burst of energy, the hamstring is placed under maximal stretch when the hip is forced into flexion and the knee then is forced into extension during forward striding movements. The hamstring acts to try to decelerate the extension of the knee. If the muscle is not adequately stretched, a strain may result (34). Treatment of hamstring strains starts with good prevention techniques. The gymnast should be required to warm up adequately and stretch before practice and competition. If a hamstring injury does occur, the use of modalities and stretching should take place as tolerated. Transverse friction massage may reduce scar tissue. Strengthening of the hamstrings should emphasize endurance and low-weight activities. Return to gymnastics should be controlled so that reinjury does not take place. The athlete initially should not undergo any activities that require a sudden burst of energy. Dismounts should not be performed until the athlete is pain free.

Low Back Injuries

Low back pain is a common entity in gymnastics and can arise from either macrotrauma or repeated microtraumas (Fig. 24.6). As the level of competition increases in gymnastics, practice time to learn more intricate skills increases (35). Sward (35) used magnetic resonance imaging (MRI) to female gymnasts and found as the level of gymnastic competition increased so did the amount of injury. A total of 9% preelite, 43% elite, and 63% Olympic-level gymnasts had low back pain with positive MRI testing. He concluded from this study that there was a positive correlation between the hours spent in training per week and the MRI results. Athletes spending more that 15 hr a week in training were more likely to have a positive MRI than those who spent less time in training (36).

Because flexibility is a judge characteristic in gymnastics, gymnasts attempt to gain greater and greater ranges of motion. Performing at these end ranges of motion may predispose gymnasts to injury. Injury to the low back is associated with decreased flexibility (33). Low back pain in gymnasts is usually symmetric and affects the floor exercise or balance beam the most. It is usually brought on by maneuvers involving extension of the lumbar spine.

Gymnasts often present with hyperlordosis and flexibility losses of the low back, hip, and knees. Abdominal weakness also is often present. Failure to correct

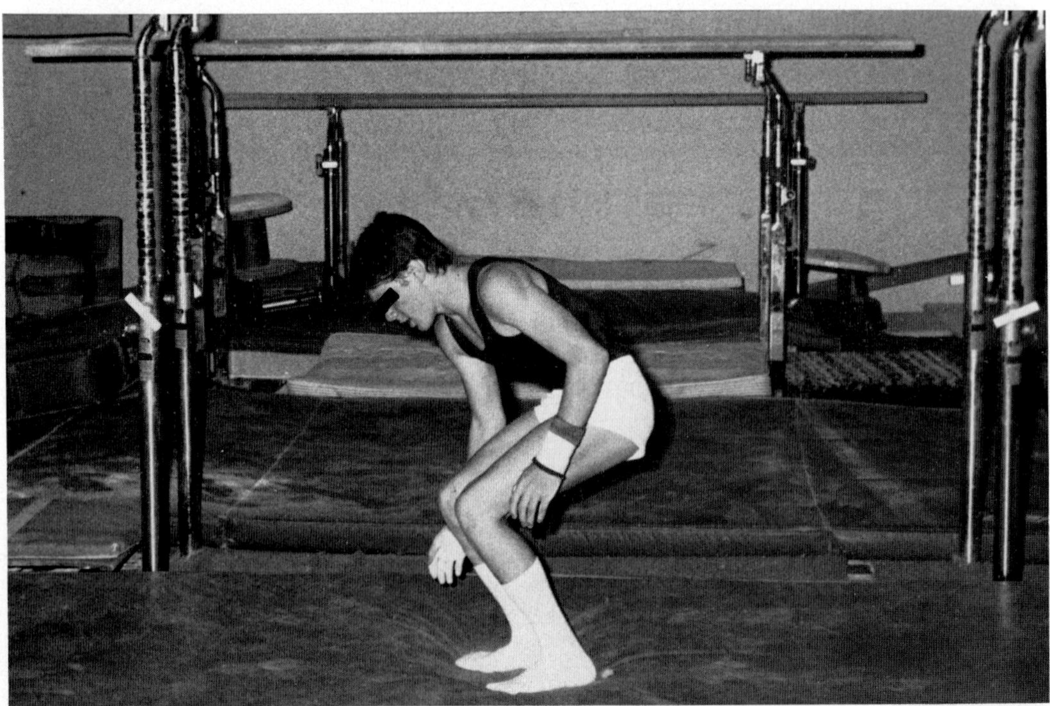

Figure 24.6. The dismount stance upon footstrike is usually one of flexion at the thoracolumbar spine, hips, and knees. This position repeated many times over the active life span of a gymnast can cause chronic vertebral changes at the thoracolumbar junction.

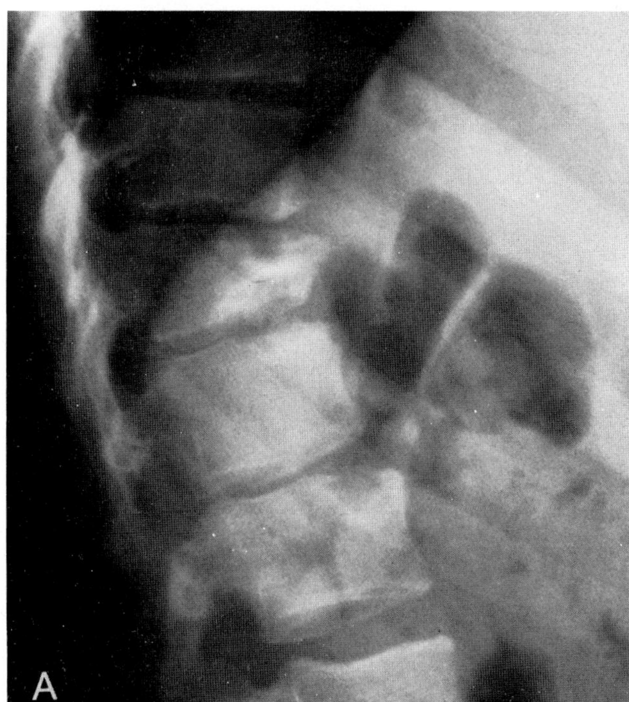

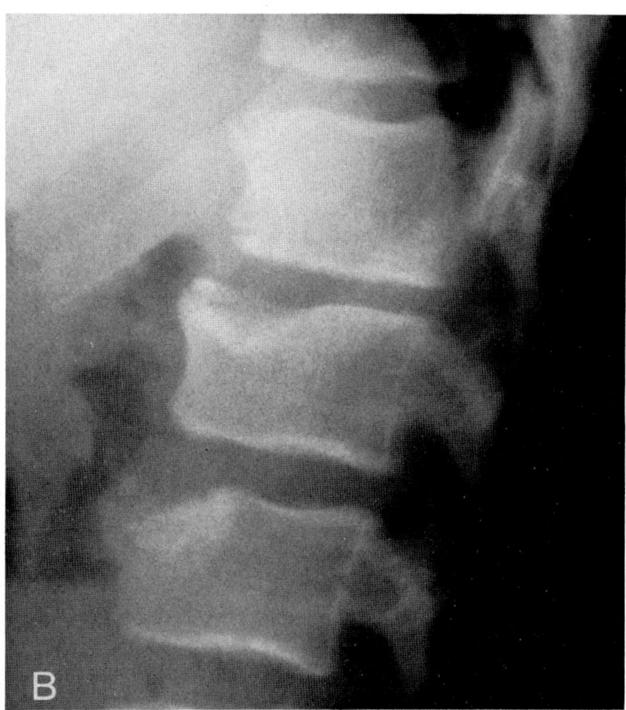

Figure 24.7. A, Lateral radiograph of a class 1 gymnast, showing marked superior and inferior collapse of the body of T12 and superior changes in the body of L2. **B,** Lateral radiograph of class 1 gymnast with destructive change in the upper body of L3.

these muscle imbalances can result in low back pain (37). A major contributor to mechanical low back pain in the adolescent gymnast may be rapid growth spurts in which the bony elements grow more quickly than the muscles, predisposing to inflexibility and altered kinematics at the vertebral end plate, creating Schmorl's nodes, a common finding in gymnasts (35).

Scheuermann disease is usually associated with hard physical labor in adolescents. There may be a failure of the disc, resulting in a decrease in the disc height and abnormalities of the vertebral body or fractures through the growth plate of the vertebral body, secondary to repetitive flexion and extension activities. It is most often found in the thoracolumbar area and is more common in athletes than in nonathletes (35, 37). Athletes may also have associated lumbar lordosis and thoracic kyphosis (Fig. 24.7).

Gymnastics places high demands on the spine with increased risk of disc injuries (37). Herniated nucleus pulposus has been reported in the adolescent population, and the probable mechanism is repetitive torsional forces in a flexed position. The greatest segmental risk for disc herniation is at L3–L4, and L4–L5. Actual loading and repetitive flexion would cause greater disc herniation between the L5 and S1 levels (38).

In the acute onset of low back pain, disc injury must be considered. Sward (35) used MRI to study male elite gymnasts and found a higher incidence of disc degeneration in them than in nonathletes. Because nonathletes were used as the control group and were slightly older, the effect of gymnastics on the spine may be underrated. Of the gymnasts surveyed, 79% had a history of low back pain and approximately 50% had back pain at the time of the study. None of the nonathletes had reported any type of back pain at the time of the study.

Spondylolysis (9), the stress fracture of the pars intraarticularis, results from repeated loading of the pars as the spine moves from full flexion to hyperextension. Athlete's have a higher rate of spondylolysis than the general population, and gymnasts and football players have the highest rate among athletes (35, 37). The pain is usually midline and unilateral but can be bilateral (Fig. 24.8).

Spondylolythesis usually occurs at L5. The athlete usually presents with low back pain, aggravated by standing, walking, and running and relieved by flexion or lying down. Examination often reveals increased lumbar lordosis and tight hamstrings. Associated nerve root irritation may produce lower extremity pain (39) (Fig. 24.9).

Treatment can be split into two phases. Initially, pain relieving modalities and rest are employed, but a lumbar support with a thermoplastic insert to block hyperextension may be helpful. The athlete should be given instructions to have the brace properly in place at all times. In the second phase after acute pain has subsided, the brace can be used during increased activity. The second phase involves active rehabilitation.

The goal of rehabilitation should be good trunk stability, flexibility, and a solid base of support. Hip strengthening should take place in cardinal planes of movement. Care should be taken not to cause an increase in pain in either the low back or the extremities. Proper positioning should be attained so as to make certain that the athlete gets the maximum recruitment of the particular muscle targeted for strengthening.

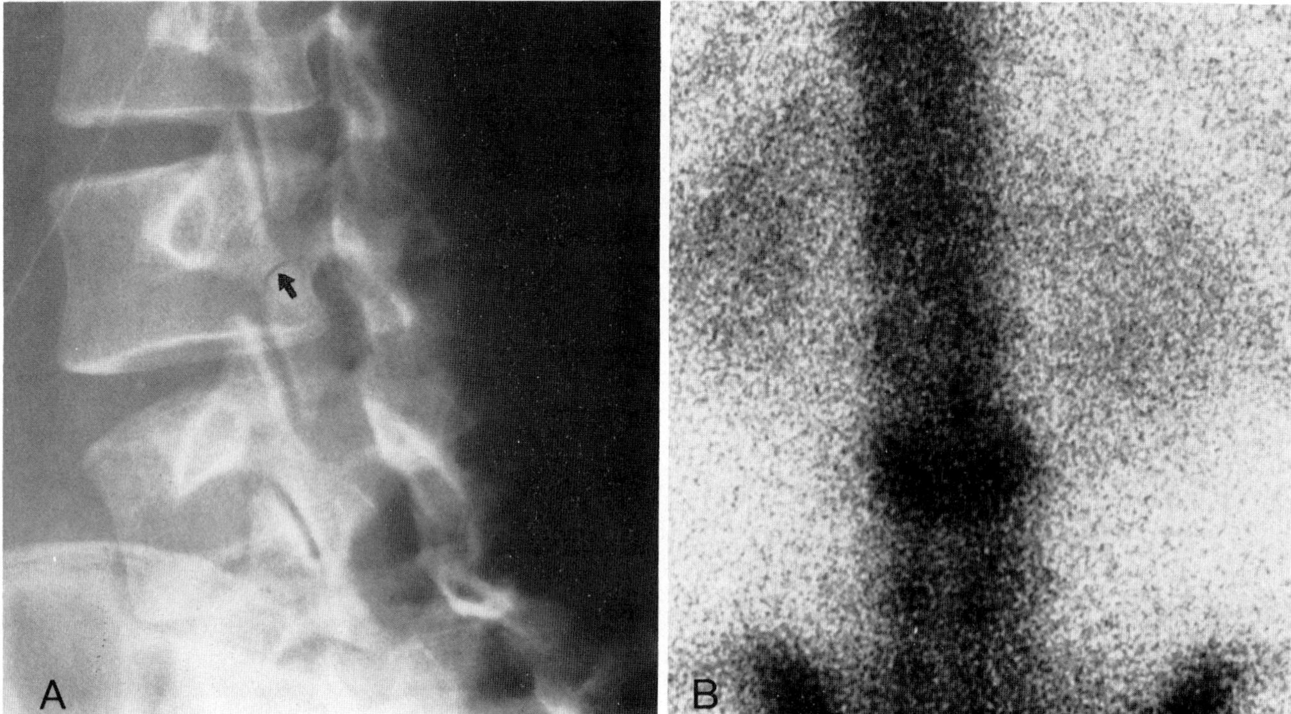

Figure 24.8. A, Oblique radiograph of an 18-year-old gymnast with an acute pars fracture of L3 *(arrow).* **B,** AP bone scan of same gymnast. This young woman participates in strenuous gymnastics with a new acute onset of back pain upon dismount.

Functional strength can also be achieved by performing manually resisted trunk and lower extremity proprioceptive neuromuscular facilitation patterns. Lower extremity patterns include non–weight-bearing diagonals, resisted crawling, bridging, and plantigrade movements. Resisted trunk movements may include lifts for the upper extremities, alternating isometrics while hook lying, low trunk rotations, and rolling.

Extension of the lumbar spine must be progressed without introducing pain. Gentle grade 1 and 2 PA mobilization can be performed to free up the stiff lumbar segments. Press-ups while the pelvis remains on the plinth and in the prone position can also be used.

Once pain free in the prone progression, the gymnast should be encouraged to attempt increased extension in standing. The ultimate goal is to achieve a back walkover. The athlete is asked to extend just shy of pain, then gradually continue until he or she reaches certain plateaus, usually established by using a plinth. The progression should stop at a specific height agreed on by coach, therapist, and athlete or until the gymnast can reach the floor. During this phase of the rehabilitation, the gymnast should be reeducated about the importance of maintaining correct posture both during static and dynamic positioning. Once back walkovers can be completed without any exacerbation of pain, the athlete is progressed to handsprings and then gradually back to full participation. Weaning from the brace usually takes place in this phase.

It is important that the coach be involved in the final return to sport. Coaches must be educated about bringing gymnasts back slowly, beginning with tricks that the gymnast feels comfortable performing. It is always easier to restore the gymnast's confidence level by allowing the opportunity to prove to himself or herself that tricks can be completed without reinjury.

Ankle Injuries

In some studies, the ankle has been the most frequent site of injury (11, 14, 26), with the inversion/plantar flexion sprain being the most common injury (10, 11). Most of the injuries occur with twisting motions during floor exercise, vaulting, and dismounts from the beams and the uneven parallel bars. Sprains also can be the result of falling from an apparatus or missed moves while practicing. Ankle sprains are the most common injury that is not a direct result of practice on any of the apparatus (14).

Capsulitis can be a direct result of the ankle sprain and frequently involves the anterior ankle. Anterior ankle impingement syndrome, secondary to osteophytes, may develop on the anterior aspect of the talus. The osteophytes were thought to be a direct result of traction placed on the capsule when working with the foot constantly in plantar flexion. When an osteophyte develops, dismounts and tumbling may be difficult. If a gymnast lands "short," causing the ankle to be placed in a position of hyperdorsiflexion, the osteophyte then impinges on the capsule, causing pain and swelling (40).

Anterior impingement syndrome is better prevented than treated, and emphasis on good coaching and spotting techniques is important. The coach must teach the athlete how to stick dismounts and landings cor-

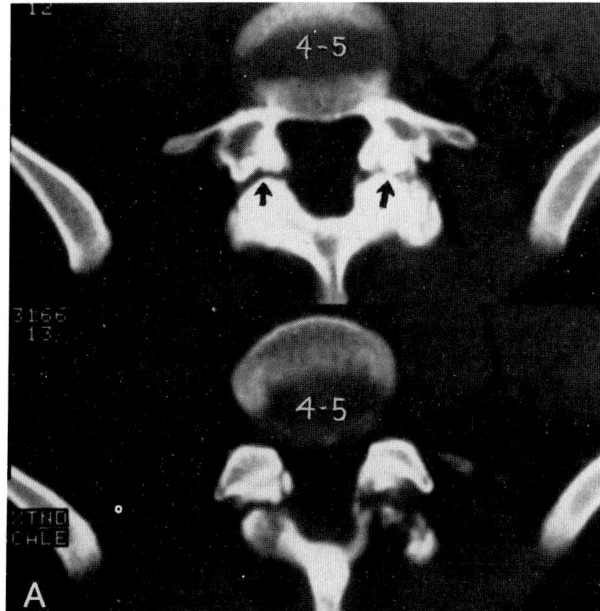

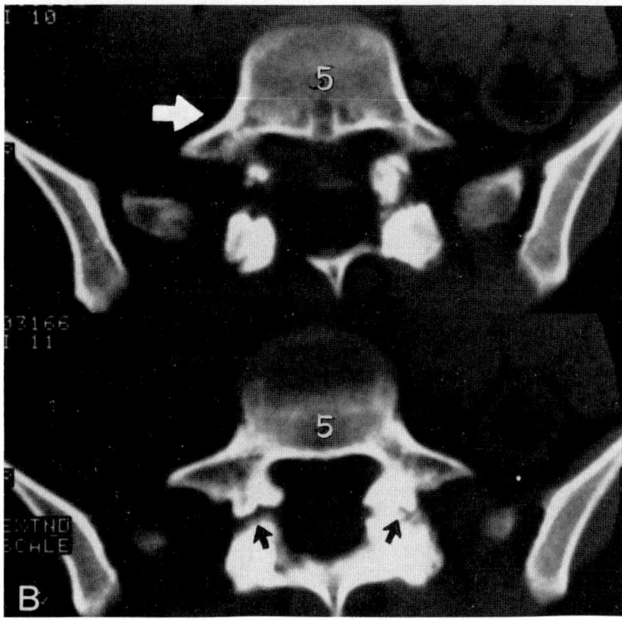

Figure 24.9. **A,** Computed tomography (CT) scan of the lumbosacral junction of a 22-year-old gymnast who ignored her low back pain for 5 years. A grade 1 spondylolisthesis is present. **B,** The "Darth Vader" *(large arrow)* sign is exhibited by the CT appearance of the slip *(small arrows)*.

rectly, alleviating the problems of landing short. If pain does occur, however, initial treatment is symptomatic. The use of athletic taping with the ankle preset in slight plantar flexion may be effective by restricting ankle dorsiflexion (Fig. 24.10). If taping is inadequate, the use of an Ethafoam block may be necessary to act as a bumper and limit dorsiflexion. During painful periods, avoidance of dismounts and hard tumbling passes is frequently necessary. Modalities, NSAIDs, and occasionally, injections to decrease swelling may also be of benefit. Stretching and strengthening exercises to the ankle musculature should follow.

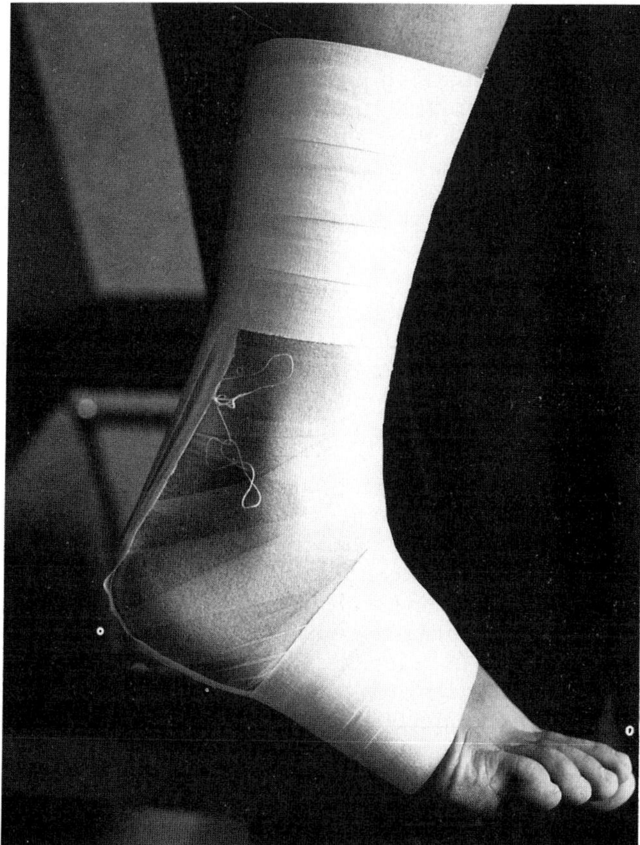

Figure 24.10. Taping the ankle helps prevent the athlete from falling short.

Problems with Achilles tendinitis are relatively common in gymnastics. Gymnasts perform most of their maneuvers with a pointed toe, which leads to decreased flexibility of the tendon (40). The repetitive nature of the sport, especially during practice, also increases the risk of injury. Usually, problems with the Achilles tendon may be attributed to dismounts and tumbling (25). Acute rupture of the Achilles tendon is rare, and most Achilles tendon problems are of gradual onset (15). Achilles tendinitis should be taken seriously. Absolute rest from the sport may be the indicated treatment of choice (40). A gentle, pain-free, non–weight-bearing stretching program progressing to weight-bearing stretches should be encouraged. Strengthening also should be started, and coaches should review from and technique. Before full return to the sport, the gymnast must be pain free and show adequate flexibility and strength. Gradual return is necessary with an adequate amount of time spent stretching before and after each event.

Plantar fasciitis may also be difficult to treat. Gymnasts have approximately three times the normal population's incidence of plantar fasciitis, ostensibly the result of the repetitive nature of practice, in particular tumbling and the vault run (33). During the vault run, the gymnast places excessive force on the plantar fascia and calf muscles for propulsion off the spring board to create the height to complete the vault. The posterior calf musculature may be tight simply because the foot and ankle are held in the plantar flexed position throughout routines. If a gymnast lands short, he or she forces the ankle into extreme dorsiflexion, potentially injuring the plantar fascial insertion. Biomechanical deficiencies may also increase plantar fasciitis. Excessive pronation may increase the stress placed across the plantar fascia. The tightness in the posterior calf musculature makes disseminating force appropriately difficult. Finally, the tightness in the posterior musculature may create a valgus heel position, which in turn can restrict the midfoot and cause pain from midstance to early pushoff (41).

Rehabilitation of plantar fasciitis may be quite difficult. The normal course of rehabilitation would include modalities and rest, night splint, flexibility and strengthening, and functional return with the use of orthotics to correct biomechanical deficiencies. However, in gymnastics there is little if any true rest period, because the sports is conducted 12 months a year. The use of an orthotic device may not be an option, as most gymnasts perform in their bare feet. A small orthotic placed in a pair of beam shoes for practices can be used. The use of low-dye arch tapping may also be of great benefit. The best treatment is to screen athletes for possible deficiencies before beginning practices. The coach must insist that all athletes take the proper time to stretch before the start of practice sessions and competitions.

Sever disease is an apophysitis of the os calis. It is usually associated with the growth spurt or increased in muscular activity. The symptoms are aggravated by increased running and also may be associated with abnormal foot biomechanics. The treatment of choice is increased flexibility of the Achilles tendon, increased strength of the dorsiflexors and rest. Heel cups and foot orthotics may be of benefit. However, with gymnastics these may not be an option during practice and competition. The use of low-dye arch tapping may help with control of excessive pronation (42, 43).

Ankle Rehabilitation

Rehabilitation begins with RICE. Cold with compression can be performed with a Cyro/Cuff (Aircast, Summit, NJ), which allows the gymnast to recirculate cold water every hour through a specially designed cuff that surrounds the joint and thus applies firm compression. If the injury is severe enough or if the gymnast's gait is antalgic, crutches may be used. The immediate goal is to reduce inflammation and pain. Normal gait should be encouraged at all times. Early weight bearing should be encouraged so long as it is well-tolerated.

Passive stretching for the entire lower extremity should be encouraged a well as submaximal isometrics in all planes of movement about the ankle. During the early stages of rehabilitation, it is important to maintain cardiovascular fitness as close to preinjury status as possible. This can be done by using an upper body ergometer or by allowing the gymnast to run in a pool. It will be necessary to use the deeper end of the pool and a wet vest (Sport Support, Dallas, TX). While the gymnast is in the pool, range of motion and strengthening exercises can be performed a well as gait training, and water pressure can help control swelling. Strengthening is performed by having the gymnast increase the speed at which range of motion exercises are being performed. The faster the individual moves the more resistance will be felt. Flippers can be used to increase resistance.

In addition to aquatic therapy, the gymnast should be encouraged to continue to stretch and progress other aspects of rehabilitation. It is important to remember that as the athlete enters the subacute phase of the healing process caution must be exercised not to over stress the tissues and reenter the acute stage. During this phase of the rehabilitation process, emphasis should be on reducing edema; mobilizing scar tissue; increasing flexibility, strength, and function; and improving proprioception. Contrasting cold and heat may be of benefit to control pain while decreasing swelling. Scar mobilization should take place so that the athlete will not have a feeling of stiffness. Early mobilization of the scar will result in less stiffness, strong bonding, and increased range of motion.

Strengthening during this phase of rehabilitation should emphasize low weight and high repetitions and should encompass the full range of motion, without causing an increase in pain. The author generally uses either Theraband (The Hygienic Corp., Akron, OH) or manual resistance that offer both a concentric and an eccentric mode of exercise. Manual resistance allows the therapist to control the amount of resistance placed on the ankle. This also affords the therapist valuable information regarding the athlete's physical status. The therapist can assess pain, range of motion, strength, and smoothness of contraction.

Functional strengthening and proprioception may take place toward the later part of this phase. Strengthening may be performed in the closed-chain position by using a Biomechanical Ankle Platform System (BAPS; CAMP, Jackson, MI). The BAPS board can also be used to increase range of motion and create proprioceptive awareness. The author uses the larger balls to improve range of motion and the smaller balls to gain proprioceptive control. The BAPs board is initially performed in the sitting position and progressed to the standing position.

As painless full range of motion and strength return, the rehabilitation can begin to focus on increased flexibility, endurance, and function. Jogging in the pool with the water at chest level should be encouraged, progressing to a waist-high water level. The gymnast should also perform balancing in the water on the affected lower extremity. Functional return can be started in the pool as well. The buoyancy of the water decreases the effects of gravity and thus decreases stress across the ankle. The gymnast should begin to perform leaps and jumps in chest-high water and, if pain free, move to waist-high water. The last stage of jumping and leaping before working on the apparatus involves use of the spring floor or a mat.

Strength training should consist of free weights as well as machines. Proprioceptive neuromuscular resistance using manual resistance makes good use of the entire lower extremity for carryover and neural adaptation. A BAPS board can be used with weights on a circuit program. The circuit program uses weights placed at different locations on the board and will enable the gymnast to stress all the muscle groups surrounding the ankle.

Proprioception should be aggressively worked as well. Initially, the gymnast can simply be asked to perform a one-legged stance with the eyes open, progressing to eyes closed. The next progression consists of balancing exercises on a minitrampoline. Machines currently available to help improve proprioception include the Balance System Dynamic (Chattecx Corp., Chattanooga, TN) and the KAT Balance Platform Breg, Vista, CA). The Balance System Dynamic has a movable platform and provides the athlete with an immediate visual feedback via computer tracking of the force platform. The system also can be used to quantify sway, which is useful in determining progress. The KAT makes use of an air bladder that can be filled to a specified pressure. The greater the pressure the more stable the platform, however, KAT will not provide any quantifiable data on how the athlete is performing.

Once the athlete is pain free and strength has returned to normal, the athlete is weaned from formal rehabilitation toward total functional return, using the SAID principle, which stands for specific adaptations to imposed demands. The athlete may now begin to perform watered-down routines. The ankle should be taped during practice sessions, which provides proprioceptive input more than support to the ankle joint. Initially, the gymnast should be encouraged to perform low-impact maneuvers, such as dance routines, which will enable him or her to gain confidence while placing only minimal stress on the ankle. Gradually, the athlete may be progressed to tumbling. All tumbling should begin in the AP plane of motion. Twisting should be avoided initially to reduce stress placed on the ankle joint upon landing.

Criterion for full return to practice and competition should rest more heavily on the gymnast's ability to demonstrate that functionally they are capable of all the demands imposed by the sport. Strength and range of motion testing are simply not enough to determine the athlete's preparedness. The athlete's ankle must be stressed functionally and should be able to perform all tricks and dismounts safely. There should be no pain at the end of the functional testing period. In addition, the athlete must be encouraged to perform exercises regularly to maintain ankle strength and flexibility.

REFERENCES

1. Weiker GG. Introduction and history of gymnastics. Sports Med 1985;4(1):3–5.
2. Schenk B. History of gymnastics. Unpublished manuscript, 1991.
3. Sands B. Everybody's gymnastics book. New York: Scribner's, 1984.
4. Maskovitz D. Personal communication, 1991.
5. Johnson KM. Where have all the gymnasts gone? J Phys Ed Rec Dance 1985;3:28–29.
6. National Federation of High School Associations. Personal communication, 1991.
7. National Collegiate Athletic Association. 1989–90 NCAA participation study. Women's gymnastics, March 1991.
8. Weiker GG. Club gymnastics. Clin Sports Med 1985;4(1):39–43.
9. Warbutton, D. Personal Communication, 1991.
10. Snook GA. Injuries in women's gymnastics: a 5-year study. Am J Sports Med 1979;7(4):242–244.
11. Garrick JG. Epidemiology of women's gymnastic injuries. Am J Sports Med 1980;8(4):261–264.
12. Whiteside PA. Men's and women's injuries in comparable sports. Phys Sportsmed 1980;8(3):130–140.
13. Weiker GG. Injuries in club gymnastics. Phys Sportsmed 1985; 13(4):63–66.
14. Lindner KJ. Injury patterns of female competitive club gymnastics. Can J Sport Sci 1990;15(4):254–261.
15. Caine D. An epidemiologic investigation of injuries affecting young competitive female gymnastics. Am J Sports Med 1989;17(6):811–820.
16. National Collegiate Athletic Association. NCAA injury surveillance system: men's & women's gymnastics, April 1991.
17. Dobyns JH. Gymnastic's wrist. Hand Clin 1990;6(3):493–504.
18. Mandelbaum BR. Wrist pain syndrome in the gymnast. Am J Sports Med 1989;17(3):305–317.
19. Markolf KL. Wrist loading patterns during pommel horse exercises. J Biomech 1990;23(10):1001–1011.
20. Aronen JG. Problems of the upper extremity in gymnastics. Clin Sports Med 1985;4(1):61–70.
21. Weiker GG. Upper extremity gymnastic injuries. In: Nicholas JA, Hershmann EB, eds. The upper extremity in sports medicine. St. Louis: CV Mosby, 1990:861–882.
22. McCue FH. Rehabilitation of common athletic injuries of the hand and wrist. Clin Sports Med 1989;8(4):731–775.
23. Fu FH. Shoulder impingement syndrome. Clin Orthop 1991;269:162–172.
24. Prist JD. Elbow injuries in women's gymnastics. Am J Sports Med 1981;9(5):288–295.
25. Dziobd RB. Gymnastics. In Schneider RC, Kennedy CJ, Plant MJ, eds. Sports injuries prevention, and treatment. Baltimore: Williams & Wilkins, 1985:139–162.
26. McAuley E. Injuries in women's gymnastics. Am J Sports Med 1987;15(6):558–565.
27. DeHaven KE. Injuries to the menisci of the knee. In: Nicholas JA, Herschman EB, eds. The lower extremity and spine in sports medicine. St. Louis: CV Mosby, 1986.
28. Andrish JT. Knee injuries in gymnastics. Clin Sports Med 1985;4(1):11–121.
29. Hughston JC. Knee injuries in gymnastics. Clin Sports Med 1989;8(2):153–162.
30. Donati RB. Bilateral simultaneous patellar tendon rupture in a female collegiate gymnast. Am J Sports Med 1986;14(3):237–239.
31. Goldberg MJ. Gymnastic injuries. Orthop Clin North Am 1980;11(4):717–726.
32. Dunn JF. Osgood-Schlatter disease Am Fam Pract 1990;41(1):173–176.
33. Kirby RL. Flexibility and musculoskeletal symptomatology in female gymnasts and age matched controls. Am J Sports Med 1981;9(3):160–164.
34. Fox JM. Injuries to the thigh. In: Nicholas JA, Herschman EB, eds. The lower extremity and spine in sports medicine. St. Louis: CV Mosby, 1986:1087–1117.
35. Sward L. Thoracolumbar spine in young elite athletes. Sports Med 1992;13(5):357–364.
36. Goldstein JD. Spine injuries in gymnast and swimmers. Am J Sports Med 19(5):463–468.
37. Micheli LJ. Low back pain in the adolescent: differential diagnosis. Am J Sports Med 1979;7(6):362–364.

38. Saal JA. Lumbar injuries in gymnastics. In: Hochschuler S, ed. The spine in sports. Philadelphia: Hanley & Belfus, 1990:192–206.
39. Salter RB. Textbook of disorders and injuries of the musculoskeletal system. 2nd ed. Baltimore: Williams & Wilkins, 1983.
40. Teitz CC. Sports medicine concerns in dance and gymnastics. Clin Sports Med 1983;2(3):571–593.
41. Chandler TJ. A biomechanical approach to the prevention, treatment and rehabilitation of plantar fasiciitis. Sports Med 1993;15(5):344–352.
42. Jahgg MH. Disorders of the foot. Philadelphia: WB Saunders, 1987.
43. Micheli LV. The traction apophysitises. Clin Sports Med 1987;6(2):389–404.

25 / ICE HOCKEY

Jeffrey Minkoff, Gerard P. Varlotta, and Barry G. Simonson

A Brief History of Ice Hockey

Ice skating appears to have originated in Northern Europe during the Renaissance; animal bones served as skate blades (1). Although the precise origins of ice hockey are obscure and mired in controversy, it is at least clear that the game was conceived and played originally in Eastern Canada near the midportion of the nineteenth century (2). Pashby (1) cites Sagard (1939) as having reported that the origins of ice hockey are traceable to 17th century Huronia (Ontario, Canada) where a wooden ball was pushed along the ice with curved sticks. Derivatively, hockey is probably a homonymic descendant of the old French word "hoquet," meaning "Shepherd's Staff." Like its cousin of North American origin, basketball, ice hockey saw the creation of professional leagues within a few decades of its conception and entered the registry of Olympic Games prior to the outbreak of World War II (Antwerp in 1920) (2).

The Nature of the Game

Pashby (1) explains that sequential changes in the evolution of the game increased risk to the players. The introduction of the forward pass and a center red line increased the speed of the game and its collision energies. The center red line is a part of the "icing" rule, whereby opposing players are made to race each other to the end boards trying to reach the puck first, often with collision. In Olympic hockey, there is no red line and there is "nontouch" icing (Personal communication P. Flatley and J. Norton, NY Islanders and former Olympians, 1991).

Curved sticks appeared (*see* Fig. 25.39) and begat the slap shot (1950) (3), driving pucks at speeds well over 100 mph; the curved stick also taunted the goalies with rising, dropping, and curving pucks, adding danger to the unprotected faces and throats of the net-minders. Recognition of the progression of dramatic injuries evolved slowly; measures to reduce their severity began nearly 70 years after the Ontario Hockey Association, 1890, forerunner of the National Hockey League (NHL), was founded. In 1959, a professional goalie began to use a molded mask for protection in games (*see* Fig. 25.34*A*). Although not completely effective, it was a beginning. Today, ice hockey is an aggressive contact sport in which opportunity for injury derives from numerous sources.

The Mechanics of Skating

Components of Skating

The kinematics of the skating motion are evident in all the ice skating sports, such as ice hockey, speed skating, figure skating, as well as in nonice skating activities, such as cross country skiing, rollerblading (inline skating), and skateboarding. Ice hockey is unique among all these activities by virtue of its combination of forward power skating, frequent stops and starts, lateral agility, and backwards propulsion.

The ice, the skate, and the technique of skating are among the factors that must be scrutinized in a discussion of skating dynamics. The quality and composition of the ice surface impacts on skating resistance and energy expenditure. Ice may vary in topographical smoothness, surface water, and density, each with a potential influence on speed, power movements, and agility.

Assessment of the skate is important since it is the moderating link between the power generator (lower extremity of the skater) and the ice surface. In order to attempt alteration of a technique to maximize performance, the biomechanics and kinematics of an individual's skating characteristics must be analyzed. Skaters of different body types and training demonstrate great variability in skating efficiency.

Variability of the ice surface can have an impact on the mechanics of skating since the coefficient friction of an ice surface (if fresh) can be as low as 0.004 or as high as 0.02 (on a well-used surface) (4, 5). The temperature of the surrounding environment may also have an impact on density, resistance, and coefficient of friction of the skating surface. High air temperature and humidity can result in as much as a 0.001–0.0002 change in the ice friction coefficient with the possible consequence of reduced velocity or greater fatigue (5). The authors could locate no studies evaluating the effect of the ice surface density on the power output of the skater.

As indicated, the skate is a vital and moderating link between the ice surface and the skater. Technology and design modifications have improved the skate boot, blade, and assembly. The skate consists of a leather or composite material boot, ankle support, toe box, heel counter, rigid sole, skate blade housing, and blade (Fig. 25.1). Each of the components have an effect on comfort and efficiency of skating.

Historically, the first ice skates evolved from a blade attached to a walking boot. The first skate blades were made of bones from animals endemic to Scandinavia (6). By the late 1880s, the metal blade was attached to the boot by means of a wooden support. Eventually, a pure metal blade assembly was used, adding considerable weight to the skate and reducing skating speed (*see* Fig. 25.39). With the progression of technology, a tubular skate blade was developed around 1975. This evolution considerably lightened the weight of the skate, facilitating an increase in skating speed.

While the evolution of blade design had unburdened the work of skating by the 1970s, acral promontories remained which could lacerate or puncture players. In 1977, stimulated by the North American hockey community to develop a safer blade, the Association of Standardization and Testing Materials (ASTM) worked towards development of an appropriate standard for skates. After several years of diligence, standards were developed (in 1981 and 1986) that reduced the potential for skate blade injuries (*see* Fig. 25.38). As an aside to the improved safety design, a very lightweight plastic and metal blade assembly was developed that improved skating speed and maneuverability even more than had its predecessors.

Recently, at the international level, the International Olympic Committee (IOC) has supported research by the ICE (Ice Skating Conditioning Equipment Corporation) to investigate the blade and boot design of figure skates (7). This research has led to a confirmation of variables in skate design that impact on performance. These include: edge sharpness, blade geometry, (including thickness and taper of the blade and rocker radius), and the boot-to-blade angle.

In cross-section, the skate has 2 edges separated by a hollow (Fig. 25.2). The depth of the hollow can span the gamut between shallow or deep in accordance with the sharpening technique. The deeper hollow results in a sharper blade edge that cuts deeper into the ice thereby increasing push-off while compromising smooth stops.

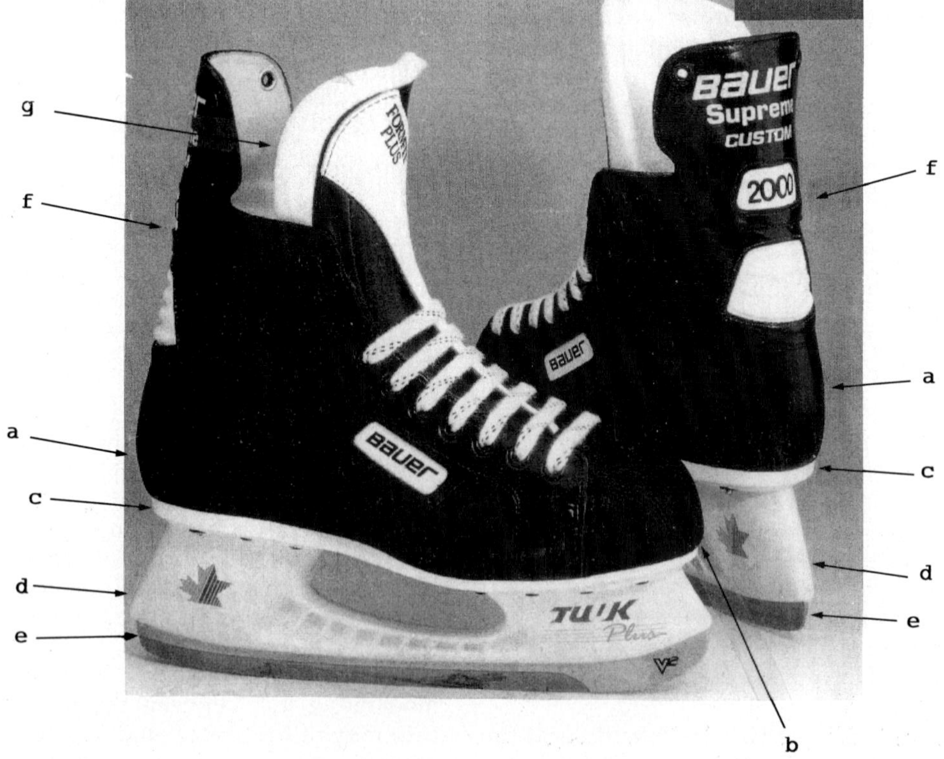

Figure 25.1. Bauer hockey skate boot with Tuuk V2 Blade. Note the narrow blade from the distal one-third of the blade proximally. Key: *a* = heel counter; *b* = toe box; *c* = rigid plastic sole; *d* = skate blade housing; *e* = metal blade; *f* = Achilles guard; *g* = padded tongue (Courtesy of CanStar, Toronto, Canada).

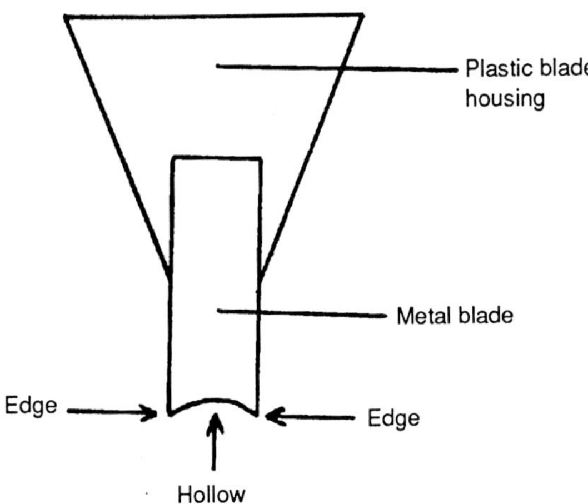

Figure 25.2 Skate blade in cross-section with 2 edges (inner and outer) and hollow.

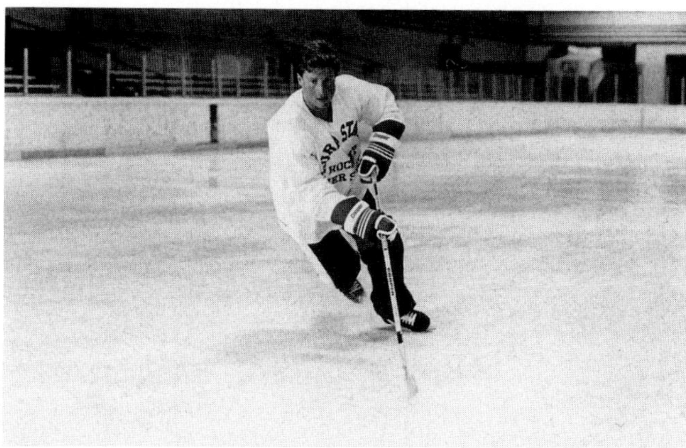

Figure 25.3 Skater using left inside edge for push-off. Used with permission—Laura Stamm.

Conversely, the more shallow hollow compromises the skater's ability to engage the ice surface, thereby reducing agility and push-off power.

Skaters are perpetually mindful of their blade "edges." Edges influence the stability, agility, and power of the skater. The inside edge contacts and penetrates the ice during the push-off and glide phases (Fig. 25.3). The outer edge of the skate blade is used predominantly in effecting stops and turns (Fig. 25.4). A dull or angled edge will not penetrate the ice effectively and the loss of an edge during turns or an ineffective stop would occur (Fig. 25.5).

In a recent geometric modification of the skate blade, (see blade in Fig. 25.1), its width was narrowed to increase the amount of force per unit area in contact with the ice; the force increase facilitates penetration of the ice by the blades and thereby increases the power of the stroke, while reducing the frictional resistance of the blade (Personal communication, A. Mullen, CANSTAR Corp, Division of Research and Development, 1991). This design modification is theoretically sound, but there remains a technical difficulty in sharpening the skates to create an adequate hollow flanked by edges of appropriate height (Personal Communication, M. Pappas, former NHL Equipment Manager, 1991.).

The skate blade is created with a radius of curvature (the rocker), which may be modified by skate sharpening (Fig. 25.6*A*, *B*). The rocker radius has reciprocal influences on the ability and stability of the skater. Elite and professional players have reported anecdotally an increase in their agility when using decreased radius (7 foot or 9 foot) of the rocker ("greater rocker") (Fig. 25.6*A*); increased stability has been reported when using an increased radius (11 foot or 13 foot) of the rocker (flatterblade) (Fig. 25.6*B*). The magnitude of the rocker varies among skate models and manufacturers. It may be questioned whether there is a "critical" radius whereby stability is compromised in the quest for agility. Centering of the rocker is critical for optimal skating performance. If the center line is too far anterior or posterior, then turning, starting, stopping, passing, and shooting abilities may be variably effected. To date, there are no published design manuals and guidelines, or test reports by manufacturers, or scientific papers delineating the functional benefits of the various aspects of blade design.

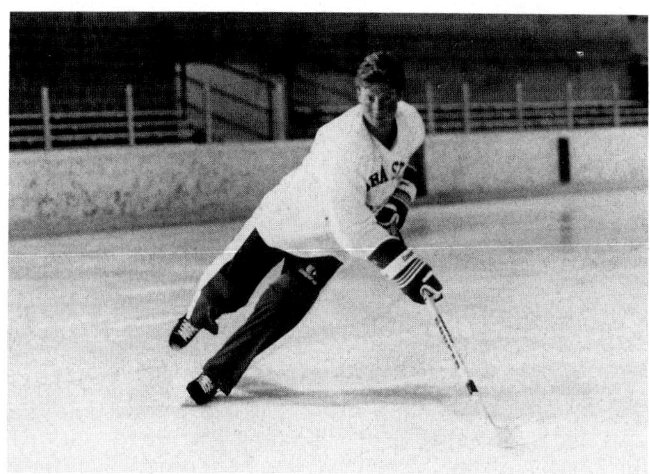

Figure 25.4. Skater using left outside edge for agility (turns and crossovers) Used with permission—Laura Stamm.

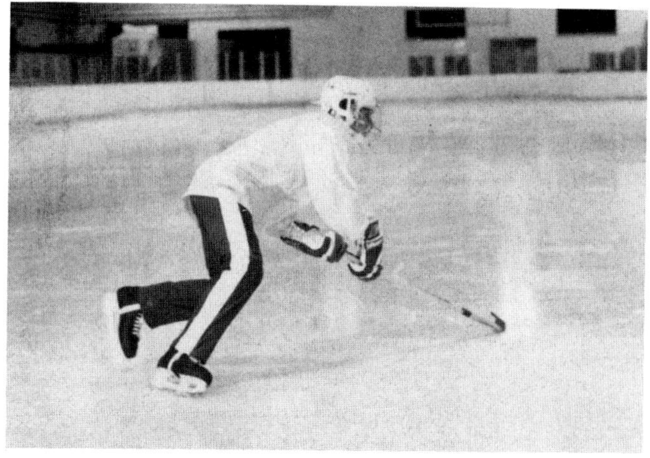

Figure 25.5. Skater losing right inside edge. Used with permission—Laura Stamm.

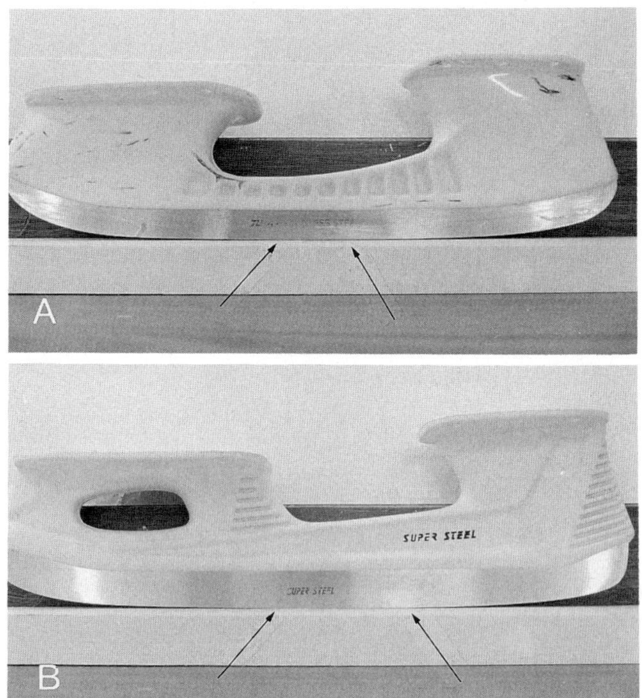

Figure 25.6. **(A)** Photo of skate blade with a 7 foot radius rocker ("greater rocker"). **(B)** Photo of skate blade with a 13 foot radius rocker (flatterblade, *arrows*, ice contact).

Kinematics and Kinesiology of Skating

The biphasic skating motion in ice hockey is illustrated in Figure 25.7 *A–J*. The nomenclature identifying the phases of the skating cycle varies among authors. The terminology used by Stamm (8) includes the wind-up, the release, the follow-through, and the return (recovery) phases. The glide phase (single support) occurs during the return (recovery) phase of the contralateral leg (Fig. 25.7 *G, H*). At a comfortable skating speed, the single support (glide) constitutes 82%, and the double support (wind-up, release, and follow-through) constitutes 18% of the "skating" cycle. Acceleration occurs throughout the double support phase and for 50% of the single support (glide) phase (9). The precise demarcation in the skating cycle between acceleration and deceleration has not been determined and is probably variable among skaters.

Ice skating differs from other types of human locomotion, specifically in the push-off phase. In skating, the direction of the push-off skate is perpendicular to the direction of travel of the opposite glide skate (Figs. 25.7 *I and J*, and 25.8 *A, B*). There is a decrease in plantar flexion force developed at this phase of the cycle as compared with bipedal terrestial gait (5, 10). The push-off action of skating has been correlated to a catapult-like action with the power output being generated from the muscular action of hip (adductors and extensors), and from knee extension. The overall force of the muscle contraction of the lower extremity (in the form of a leg press) is summated during propulsion (Fig. 25.9) (5, 7, 10–13). Peak forces during the push-off phase reach values up to 140% of body weight (5) and have a bearing on the frequency of observed hip muscle strains. The kinematics of skating is summarized in Table 25.1.

The wind-up phase (Fig. 25.7 *A–C*) follows the end of recovery phase with touchdown of the swing skate to the ice. The center of gravity is located directly in line with the ipsilateral ankle joint in the sagittal plane. In the frontal plane, the center of gravity is just anterior to the ankle joint and fosters dorsiflexion of the ankle and flexion of the knee and hip.

During the release phase (Fig. 25.7 *D–E*), the contraction of the gluteus maximus and medius, semitendinosis, biceps femoris, and triceps surae result in a progression of the hip and knee towards full extension, abduction, and external rotation. The ankle is in the neutral position. The center of gravity shifts towards the contralateral (glide) extremity. The skate is fully on the inside edge.

The follow-through phase (Fig. 25.7 *F*) completes the powerful push off with full extension of the hip and knee and a final forceful plantar flexion of the ankle.

During the recovery phase (Fig. 25.7 *G, H*), the hip and knee flex to about 40° and 90°, respectively. The hip rotates internally and the ankle is maximally dorsiflexed. The end of recovery of the ipsilateral leg should correspond to the release phase of the contralateral lower extremity.

The push-off phase (wind-up, release, and follow-through) in skating is handicapped by the absence of rapid, powerful plantar flexion developed by the triceps surae that occurs in other bipedal activities, such as running and jumping (5). The reduction of muscularly controlled ankle motion takes its toll in maneuverability and speed. The precise contribution of plantar flexion to skating power and speed has not been determined. Many players at all levels do *not* tape their skateboot to their skin pads to avoid a reduction in their final thrust, thereby sacrificing safety for performance. See discussion below under Injury. Technical modifications of the skateboot allowing an increase in the dorsiflexion and plantar flexion of the ankle have the potential for greater propulsion and an increase in skating velocity.

Acceleration and Skating Velocity

Acceleration relates to the location of the center of gravity, which varies throughout the skating cycle. During the glide phase, it is located above the ankle joint of the stabilizing leg and then moves anteriorly as acceleration is generated by the push-off leg (5). The lateral trajectory of the center of gravity follows a sine wave pattern as it does in ambulation. The amplitude of displacement is about 25 cm with higher stroke frequencies, and it increases up to 50 cm at lower stroke frequencies as the result of a prolonged glide phase (Fig. 25.10) (5, 10, 14). Acceleration in skating occurs when the center of gravity is anterior to the support foot and when the push-off lower extremity is externally rotated to establish an appropriate blade/ice surface angle (Fig. 25.11) (13). The skate blade-to-ice angle, is considered

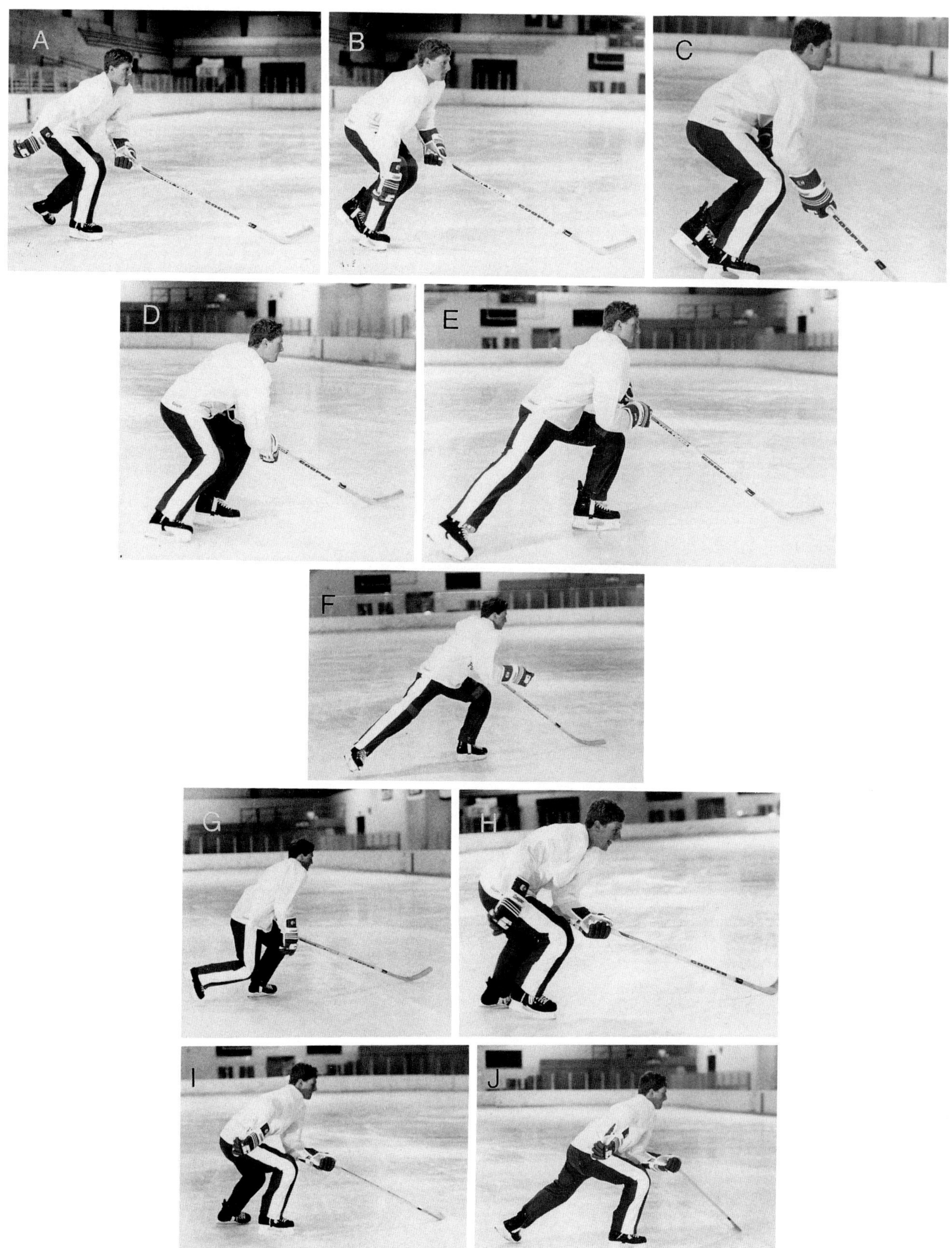

Figure 25.7. Skating motion for right lower extremity. **(A, B, C)** Wind-up Phase; **(D, E)** Release Phase; **(F)** Follow-Through Phase; **(G, H)** Recovery Phase; **(I, J)** Glide Phase. Used with permission—Laura Stamm.

to be of importance. In fact, it has been suggested (8) that the application of the blade to the ice at precisely 45° is critical to the achievement of maximum skating thrust. Not only blade design, but freedom of ankle and subtalar motion would influence the contact angle (15, 16). In addition, Marino and Weese, (9), determined that the achievement of a maximally accelerated velocity without a compromise in skating balance was accomplished with a quick internal rotation of the push-off lower extremity during the recovery phase and a quick propulsive thrust during the push-off phase.

An increase in velocity has been shown to be directly related to an increased stride rate (17, 18). Stride length does not have an effect on velocity (5, 14, 17). Hence, the power and acceleration of skating is the product of the stroke frequency and the mechanical work per stroke.

The highest rate of acceleration and shortest skating time to cover a 6 m distance correlated highly with factors other than increased stride rate alone (19). They include an increased forward lean of the torso at the touchdown of the swing skate, a reduction of the single support phase of the skate cycle, and the precise placement of the swing skate directly below the hip joint

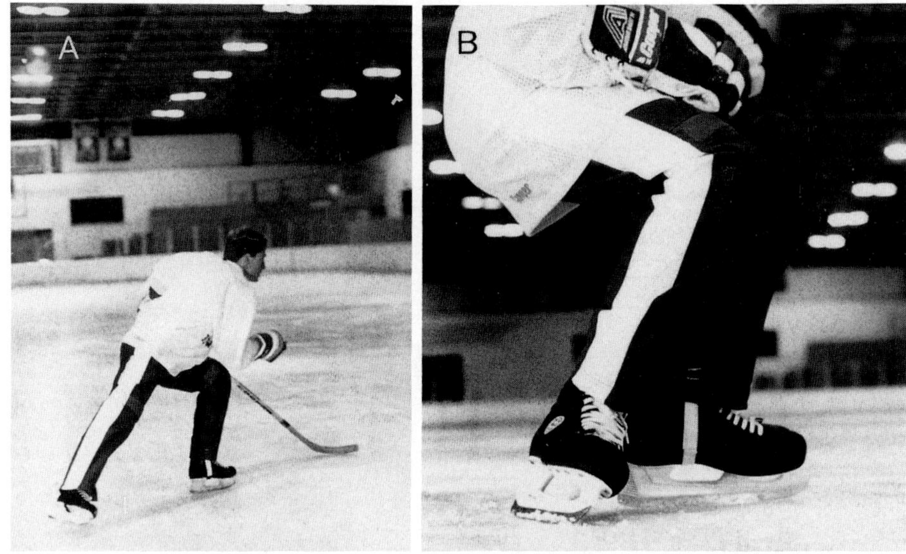

Figure 25.8 Push-off skate (**A,** right foot); perpendicular to glide skate (**B,** left foot).

Table 25.1.
The Kinematics of Skating

	Wind-Up	Release	Follow Through	Recovery
Support:	Double	Double	Double	Single
Center of Gravity:				
Frontal Plane:	Anterior to Ipsilateral Ankle	Further Anterior to Ipsilateral Ankle	Anterior to Contralateral Ankle	Anterior to Contralateral Ankle
Sagital Plane:	Ipsilateral Ankle	Center of body	Contralateral ankle	Contralateral ankle
Hip Angle:	40° to 45°	100°	180°	180° to 40°
Knee Angle:	90° to 100°	160°	180°	180° to 90°
Ankle Angle:	Dorsiflexion	Neutral	Plantarflexion	Dorsiflexion
Muscle Activity (Action):				
Gluteus Maximus:	Active Concentric (hip extension)	Active Concentric (hip extension)	Inactive	Inactive
Biceps Femoris & Semitendinosis:	Active Eccentric (hip and knee extension)	Active Eccentric (hip and knee extension)	Inactive	Active Concentric (knee flexion)
Quadriceps:	Active Eccentric (knee extension)	Active Eccentric (knee extension)	Active Eccentric (knee extension)	Active Concentric (hip flexion)
Triceps Surae:	Active Eccentric (knee extension)	Active Eccentric (knee extension)	Active Concentric (ankle plantar-flexion)	Inactive
Anterior Tibialis:	Inactive	Inactive	Inactive	Active Concentric (dorsiflexion)

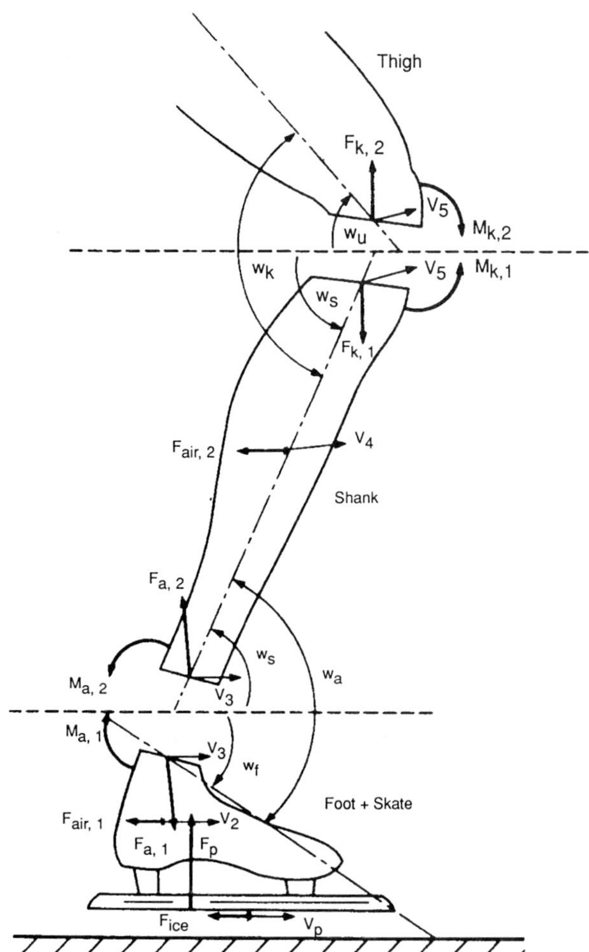

Figure 25.9 Power sources per segments are the external movements and forces (except gravity) per link. From Van Ingen Schenau GJ, Cavanaugh PR. Power equations in endurance sports. Biomechanics, 1990, 333 (9):865–881.

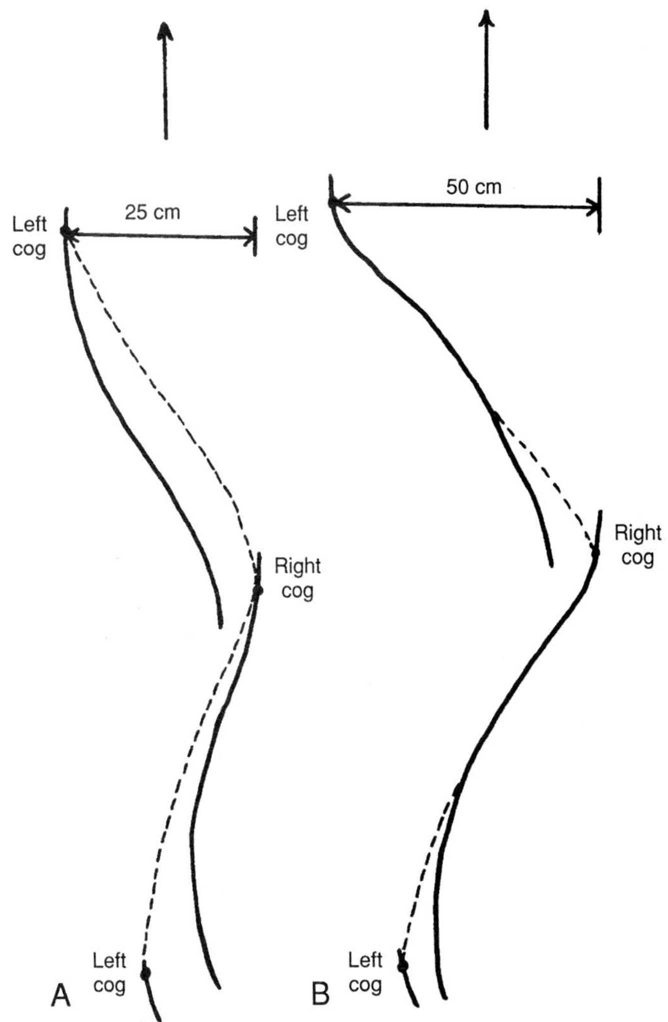

Figure 25.10 Ice cuts *(solid line)* and trajectory of the center of gravity *(broken line)* for higher stroke frequency **(A)** and lower stroke frequency **(B).** Direction of travel is noted *(arrow).*

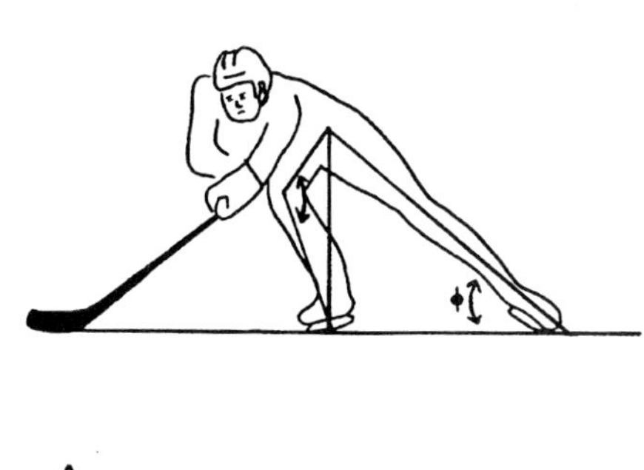

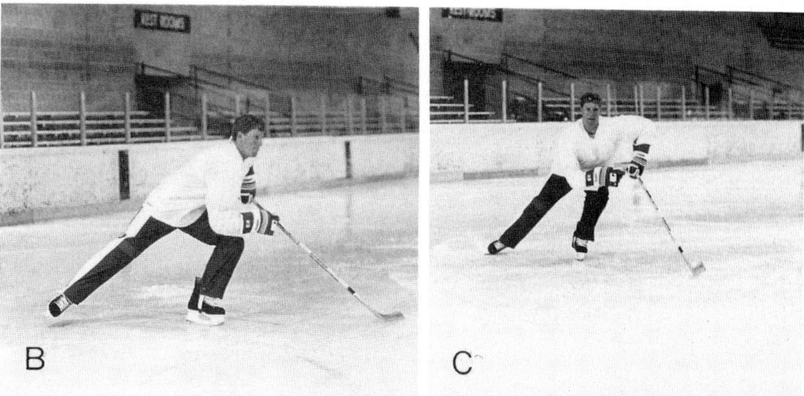

Figure 25.11 **A** Drawing of angle between push-off leg and the ice (0) determines the effectiveness of the push-off. From Van Ingen Schenau GJ, deBoer RW, DeGroot G. Biomechanics of speed skating. In: Vaughan CL, ed. Biomechanics of sport. Boca Raton, FL: CRC Press, Inc., 1989. **B,** Side view of the push-off angle. **C,** Front view of the push-off angle. (**B** and **C** With permission—Laura Stamm).

at the start of the wind-up phase. Increased acceleration is the result of a decreased leg angle at takeoff of the skate blade (Fig. 25.11*A, B*) (approximately 45°) at the end of the follow-through phase, a decreased hip flexion angle at touchdown of the skate, and an increased stride rate (5, 8, 20, 21). The variables that contribute to increased acceleration are summarized in Table 25.2. Double support time, stride length, hip and knee angle at push-off, the lower extremity push-off angle, the hip flexion angle at touchdown, and the angle of the skate blade at push-off did not correlate with increased acceleration (13, 18). When considering all kinematic parameters, elite skaters differ from skaters at lesser levels by achievement in the following categories:

1. Smaller knee angle early in the wind-up phase of push-off. (approximately 90°)
2. Significantly greater amount of work per stroke and a slightly higher stroke frequency.
3. Greater knee extension velocity.
4. A rapid, but powerful push-off.
5. A push-off angle at 45°.

Table 25.2.
Summary of Acceleration Variables

1. Increased stride rate (5, 9, 17)
2. Increased truncal lean (decreased hip flexion angle) (40°) at touchdown of recovery skate (5, 8, 13, 18, 21)
3. Short double support phase (13, 18, 19)
4. Skate under hip at beginning of push-off (18)
5. Decreased leg angle at take-off of skate blade (follow through phase) (45°–52°) (5, 8, 18, 21)
6. Center of gravity anterior to support foot (8, 9)
7. Decreased blade/ice surface angle (45°) (5, 8, 9)

The best of the elite performers can be identified by the ability to achieve superior scores in categories 2, 3, and 5 (5). The ability to accelerate distinguishes the elite hockey skater from those of lesser skating ability. Overall, faster skaters show more precise push-off mechanics with an effective glide perpendicular to the push-

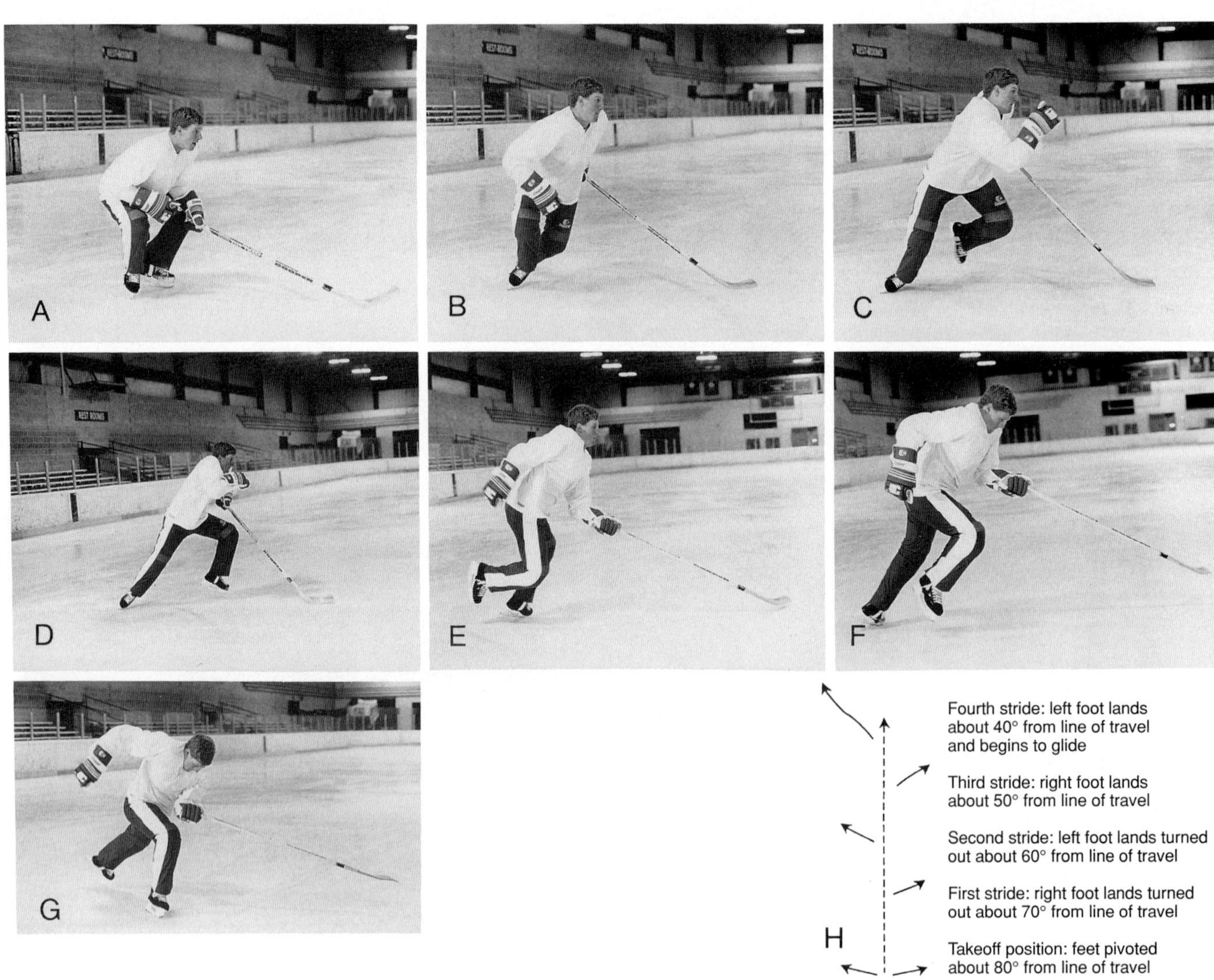

Figure 25.12*A-H*. Forward start sequence **(A-G)**. Note the precise blade to ice angle at push-off and the quick powerful knee extension. **H,** Forward start ice cuts *(solid arrows)* and direction of travel *(broken arrows)*. With permission—Laura Stamm.

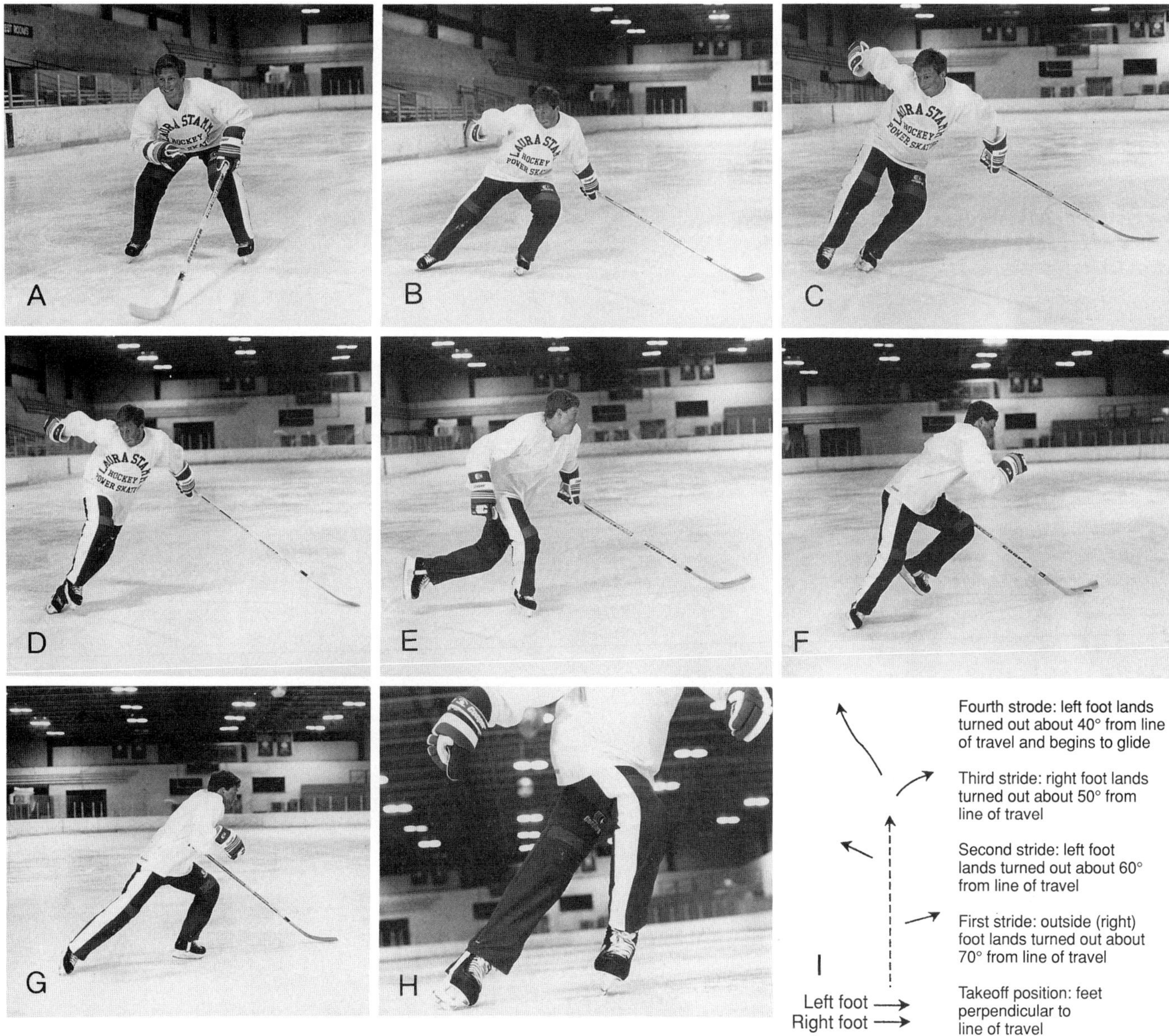

Figure 25.13A–I Crossover side start sequence **(A–G)**. Note the precise use of the left outside and right inside edges. **H,** Close-up of Crossover side start. **I,** Ice cuts for crossover side start *(solid arrow)* and direction of travel *(broken arrow)*. With permission—Laura Stamm.

off direction. These factors will maximize the power output of the skaters' lower extremity.

A specific category of skating acceleration is the start. Few studies have evaluated the effectiveness of the hockey start. There are three basic ice hockey starts: standing forward start (Fig. 25.12*A, B*), crossover side start (Fig. 25.13*A, B*), and thrust and glide start. Disagreement in the published literature exists as to the most effective start. The backwards skating stride and start, the forward skating crossovers and backwards and forward starts have not been evaluated in the academic literature. Descriptions of each can be found in detail in Stamm's Power Skating (8).

Epidemiology of Injury and Contributing Implements and Forces

Among the 21 colleges participating in the National Collegiate Athletic Association (NCAA) Injury Surveillance System (ISS), injuries were recorded twice as often in games as in practices despite the fact that there were approximately four practices for each game (22) (Fig. 25.14). This bears testimony to the aggressive intensity manifested in games.

While most recorded injuries were new, about 25% were recurrences or complications of prior injuries (Fig. 25.15). Nearly 70% of all injuries were contact injuries, the majority of which were due to contact with another player (Fig. 25.16). The most frequently injured body parts were the knee, shoulder, and groin, where contusions, sprains, and strains were the predominant injuries. Surgery was an infrequent sequel.

In a report of injuries sustained in international competition, Lorentzon et al. (23) reported an injury rate of about 80 per 1000 game hours. Contusions and sprains were the most common injuries. The primary causes of missed games and practices were checks (31.6%) and contact with other players (42.1%). As in the NCAA study, forwards were injured more often than defensemen, and goalies the least. In Thomson's survey of amateur hockey in Ontario (24), forwards and defensemen were at equal risk from the atom to the senior level, but the former were more likely to be injured by a stick and the latter by a puck.

Players skating at speeds of up to or more than 20–25 mph may collide with each other, the hard side boards of the rink, the ice, or the goal posts (which were immovable until the mid 1980s). Impact injuries also may be sustained from implements of the game,

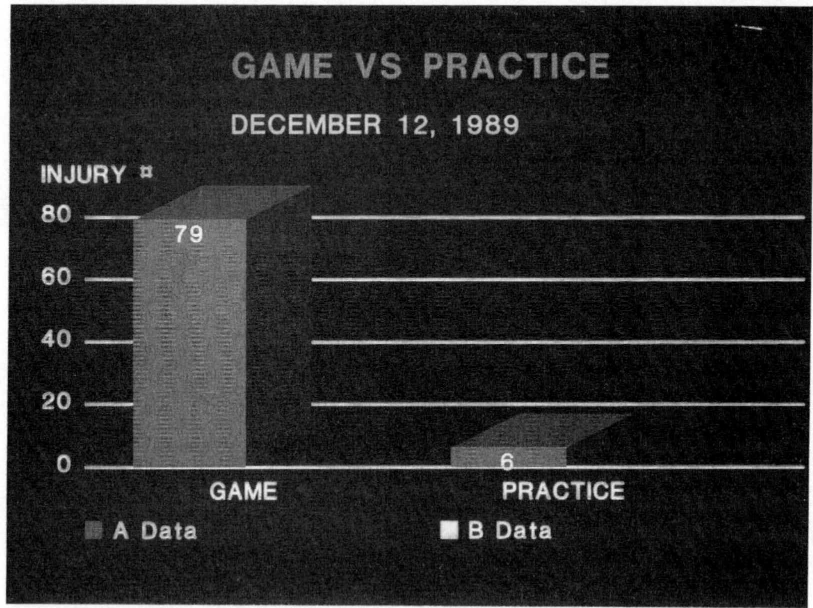

Figure 25.14. Injury incidence for games vs. practices during a 12 week period of an NHL hockey season.

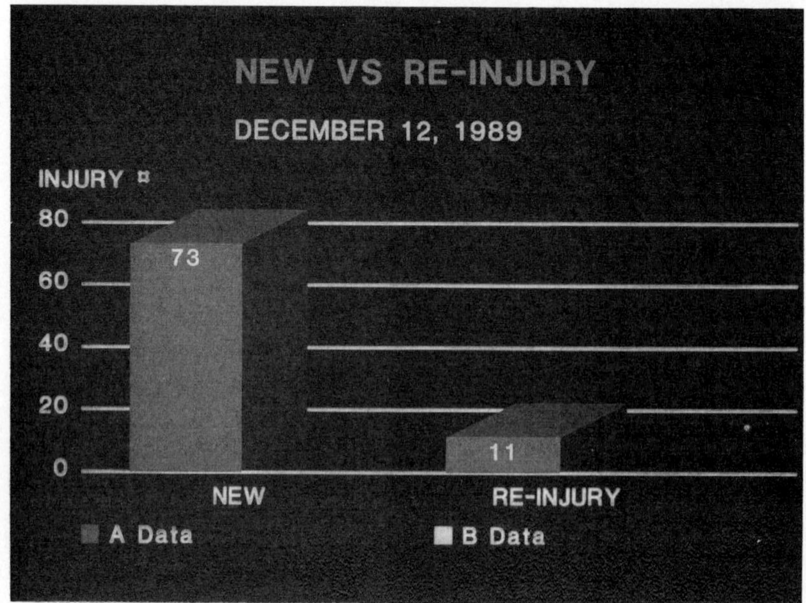

Figure 25.15. Injury incidence for new vs reinjuries in a 12-week period of an NHL hockey season, representing a 15% reinjury rate vs a 25% reinjury rate in the NCAA.

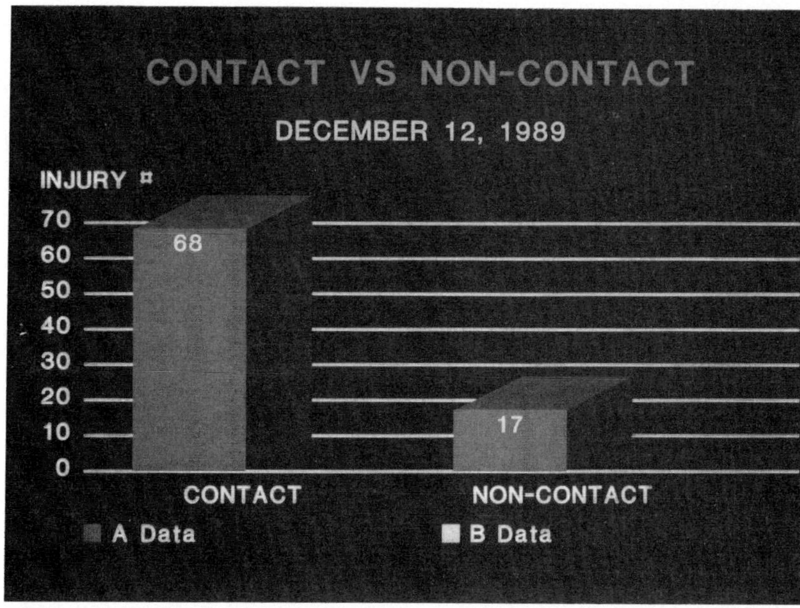

Figure 25.16. Injury incidence for contact vs noncontact in a 12-week period of an NHL hockey season.

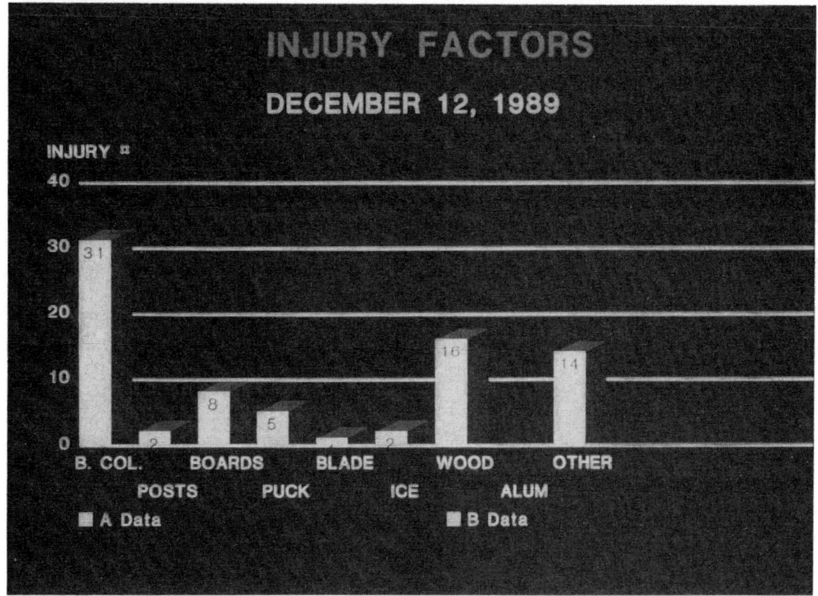

Figure 25.17. Causes of injury: A distribution of causes of contact injuries in a 12-week period of an NHL hockey season. (B. COL., body collision; ALUM, aluminum stick; WOOD, wood or wood composite stick; BLADE, skate blade.)

from the frozen, 6 ounce, vulcanized-rubber puck to the blades, heels, and handle butt ends of the hockey sticks and skate blades (Fig. 25.17).

Rink Design and Injury

Rink design is an issue in relation to the flow of the game and the injuries which may occur. The end and side-boards are critical components in concussions, cervical spine fractures and dislocations, and numerous other injuries. The goal is situated close to the end boards, and the lane between them is a haven of congestion and injuries (Fig. 25.18). Amateur rinks have moved the goal further from the end boards to create a wider lane than the 10 feet or so customary in NHL hockey rinks.

In a discussion of rink design Keating and Norris (12) explain that two basic rink designs have evolved worldwide. One is the North American variety, small in size (85 by 200 feet), and characterized by tight corners. A second design predominates in Europe with larger dimensions (98 by 197 feet) and corners with a large radius of curvature. Commensurate with their respective dimensions, the North American rink is better geared for tight checking games and many spectators, while the European is geared for wide open skating.

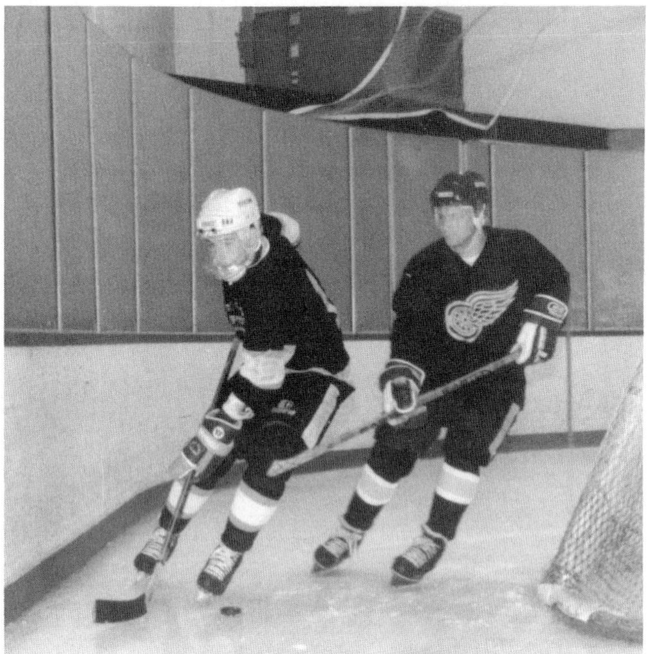

Figure 25.18. Narrow lane (in NHL especially) between end boards and the goal net.

Keating and Norris have concluded on the basis of videotape reviews that most injuries occur along the rink's end boards and in the corners (or at least the majority of severe injuries). On this basis, the authors propose that the corners be modified to form a continuous, smooth curve, that the goal be moved further away from the end boards, and that the blue line also be moved farther out. A national standard for rinks has been established in Germany (The standard is defined under the German standards code DIN 32 927), and a provincial one has been established in Ontario by the Ontario Hockey Association (OHA).

Kinesiology and Injury Potential

As already suggested, the speed achieved by players is an important contributor to injury potential. Sim et al. (21) used high speed cinematographic methods to determine that senior amateur players achieved velocities of about 30 mph. Fallen players can achieve velocities of up to 12 mph while sliding. If deceleration occurs by cranial impact upon the boards, for example, the impact can cause serious injury to the cervical spine (*see* Fig. 25.52).

The puck has been measured at velocities of as much as 90 mph for senior amateurs and up to 120 mph for professionals (21). Puck impact forces have been estimated as capable of exceeding 1200 lbs., underscoring the need for adequate protective equipment (21, 25).

According to Sim et al. (21), stick angular velocities during puck shooting are in the range of 20–40 radians/sec, which not only can drive the puck to impact forces in excess of 1200 lbs., but which can inflict significant injuries to players in its path. As the result of assertions of many player and trainers of NHL teams, the aluminum stick, recently introduced and suspected as the cause of more dramatic slashing injuries, was subjected to scrutiny. Studies undertaken by Haas (25), however, revealed no greater amount of force was delivered by aluminum sticks than by conventional (wooden) sticks.

Forces generated by power skating per se, even in the absence of contact, can predispose to musculotendinous injuries (usually of the groin) or to knee sprains. Dynamic force plate analysis during simulated power push-off demonstrated a vertical thrust reaction in the 300 lb range, a posterior thrust in the 150 lb range, a lateral thrust in the 80 lb range, and vertical twisting forces in the 40–80 inch-pound range (21). These forces help explain the incidence of groin pulls. An excellent synopsis of the relative contributions of the implements and forces of ice hockey to injuries, collated from several studies, is listed in Table 25.3.

It can be seen from Table 25.3 that the skate was responsible for between 3% to 5% of injuries. The authors would agree with this relatively low incidence. In nearly 20 years experience with NHL teams, the senior author (JM) witnessed only two significant skate blade injuries. One was a partial amputation of the distal segment of a little finger and the other was a deep laceration of the popliteal fossa, just superficial to the popliteal vessels and nerves. Certainly, the potential for more serious injuries is present.

The fiercely competitive and contact nature of ice hockey leaves room only for the intrepid and for those with physical makeup that can withstand incessant pounding. There are few injury-prone elite participants. However, there are many whose styles of play predispose them to higher rates of injury (accident

Table 25.3.
Mechanisms of Ice Hockey Injuries[a]

Mechanism	Biener and Muller (Switzerland)	Hayes (1972) (Canada/USA)	Hanzo et al. (1973) (Czechoslovakia)	Mathe (1967) (USA)
Stick	25%	29.1%	18%	8%
Puck	17%	15.2%	20%	16%
Skate	5%	3.5%	6%	5%
Collision	17%	38.3%	14%	33%
Misc.	36%	13.9%	42%	38%

From Sim et al. (37, 54, 74). By permission of Mayo Foundation.
[a] It should be noted that all studies cited above antedated any mandates for the use of helmets and/or shields.

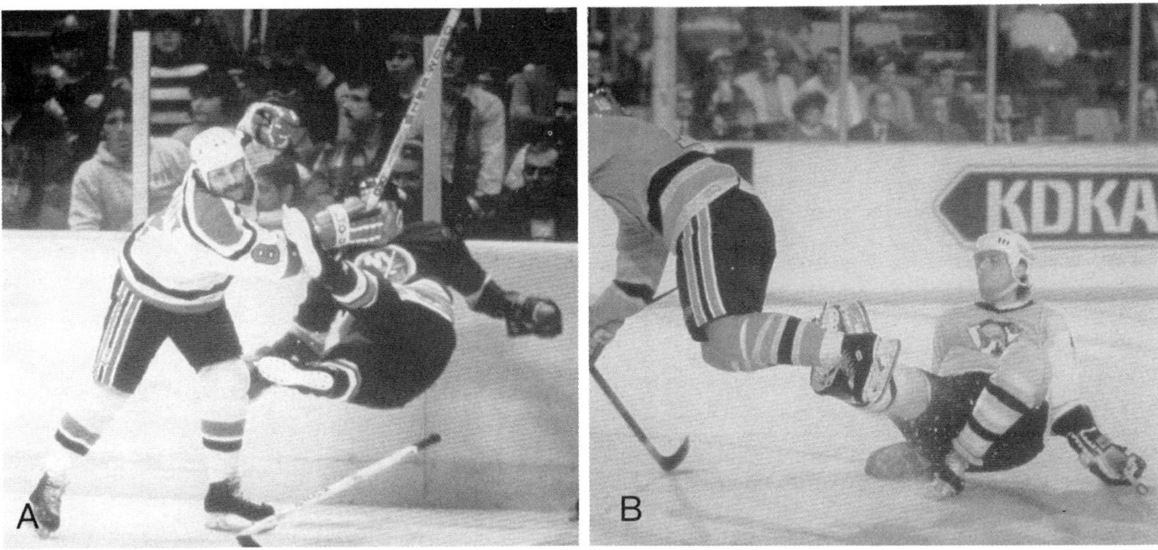

Figure 25.19. A, B. Purposeful collisions (shoulder checking). (Courtesy of Paul Bereswill.)

proneness). This style is often hard to characterize or alter, even under the observant eye of an experienced coach. Game strategy incorporates purposeful collisions of one player into another, otherwise known as "checking." Body-checking is a vital component of the game. It may be instigated with any magnitude of force as long as it is done from a position at the front or side of the recipient using the torso (including the shoulder) (Fig. 25.19) or the hip (known as a hip check) (Fig. 25.20).

In North American hockey, fisticuffs are a common and accepted (although penalized) aspect of the game. With the exception of occasional nasal, zygomatic, malar, and hand fractures, fighting rarely results in injuries more severe than facial lacerations.

A first offense for fighting in the NCAA results in a one game suspension; a second offense results in a two-game suspension, and a third offense costs the player the remainder of the season. Fighting in the Olympics results in disqualification from the tournament (Personal Communications, P. Flatley & J. Norton, New York Islander, & former Olympians).

Hastings (1974) reported that fighting produces only 3% of the injuries in his series (26). The present authors have observed that the majority of fighting injuries are facial lacerations, but facial and tooth fractures as well as hand (Fig. 25.21) and wrist fractures are not unknown. (See Chapter 15 on boxing). Lacerations on the knuckles of the hand are usually sustained from the opponent's teeth penetrating the skin. Naturally, these wounds are dirty; they should be thoroughly irrigated, painted with antiseptic, and not sewn closed; antibiotics should be administered.

Clearly, many of the injuries sustained in ice hockey may be attributed to the violent nature of the sport. The North American style of hockey has been traditionally distinguished by its more physical, choppy movements from the more gracile style of European hockey. In fact, the notoriety of hockey violence in North America was such that the U.S. Senate actually undertook an investigation of violence in the sport, barely a decade ago.

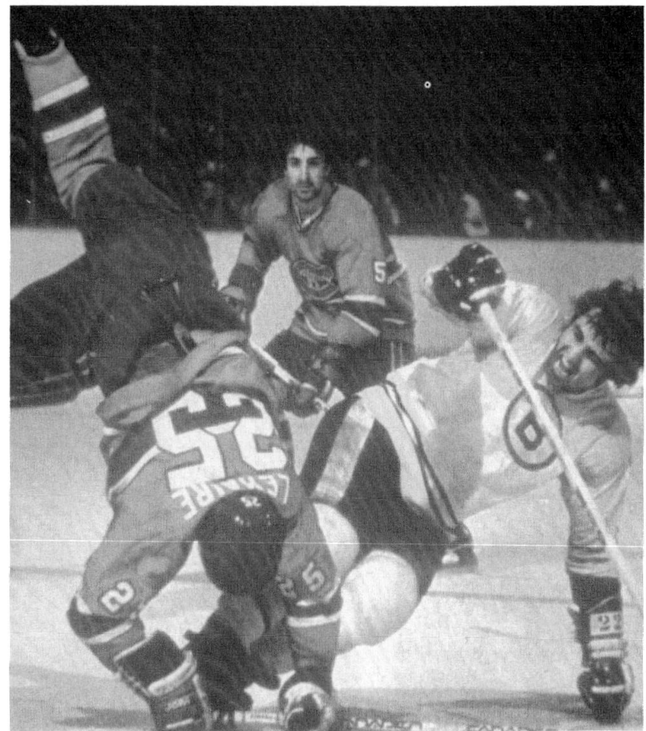

Figure 25.20. Hip check. (Courtesy of Paul Bereswill.)

Hockey Participants and Injury Epidemiology

It is well known to most sports enthusiasts that hockey has both professional and amateur participants. Among amateur associations worldwide, divisions of players are made according to age, citizenship, checking and non-checking participation, and geography. This is true of the Amateur Hockey Associations of the United States and Canada (AHAUS, now USA Hockey, and

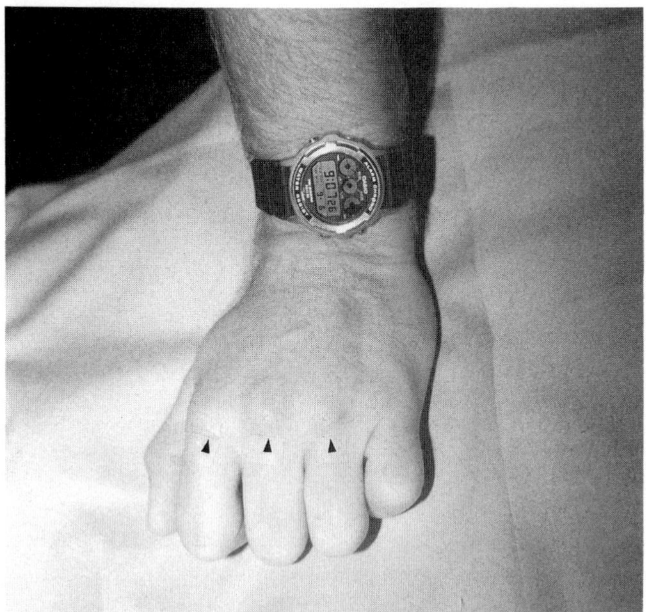

Figure 25.21. Photo of professional player's fist. Note the numerous old lacerations over the knuckles *(Arrowheads).*

CAHA). These organizations have senior groupings (over 30 years of age and under 30 years of age, checking and non-checking) and Junior groupings (19 years of age and younger). The latter is divisible into multiple groupings for boys by age: Midget (15 to 17), Bantam (13 to 15), Pee Wee (11 to 13), Squirt (9 to 11), Mite (7 to 9), Mini to Mite (5 to 7). Girls have fewer groupings (senior, 19 and under, 15 and under, and 12 and under), and there is a women's grouping; neither the girls' or women's groups have checking. In Canada, the smallest participants are designated atoms, (equivalent to the minimites and mites), and they have no checking. There are numerous regional affiliate organizations, industrial leagues, college and high school classifications adding to the complexities of groupings (Personal Communication, M. Rudolf, Director of Officials, Amateur Hockey Association of the U.S. [USA Hockey], 1991).

The divisional breakdown by age is an important procedure for avoiding catastrophic mismatches in size and weight and for surveying injury patterns, which can be used to alter the game towards increased safety.

Among the earliest comprehensive studies of hockey injuries was that of Marchant et al. (27). It reviewed a 10-year experience (1963–1973) of the British Columbia Amateur Hockey Association in the pre-helmet and face mask era. Over the ten years studied, injury rates per 1000 participants declined: from 0.874 to 0.199 for Pee Wees, from 3.64 to 0.610 for Bantams, from 4.37 to 0.784 for Midgets, and from 16.72 to 4.03 for Juniors. As might be expected in the absence of helmets and face protectors, 70% of injuries were lacerations, dental injuries, and fractures. Concussions were not uncommon and primarily a result of board and ice collisions (80% combined). Protective equipment evaluation revealed many difficulties with quality, fit, and condition. Poor fit was

Table 25.4.
Yearly Injury Rate[a]

Class	Players Injured (%)
Atom/below	1.7
Pee Wee	9.6
Bantam/Midget	14.7
Junior	38.1
University	66.9
Industrial/Recreational	12.1

[a] Adapted from Thomson (24)

particularly noted in helmets (42.2%), mouthguards (38.2%) and skates (14.8%).

The revelation of injury formats by studies such as that of Marchant et al. (27) stimulated the creation of annual injury reviews. The annual reviews began in 1975 just as helmets and face masks were introduced. The Amateur Hockey Association of the United States (AHAUS, now USA Hockey) annual reports revealed a reduction of the injury rate from 8.9% in the 1975–76 season to 6.5% in the 1987–88 season. However, the anatomical distribution of injuries had changed with an expected reduction of injuries above the shoulders. Unfortunately, the incidence of spinal injuries, often with paralysis, had risen to epidemic proportions, and the incidence of ocular injuries in older players for whom there is no mandate with respect to face protection (27).

There are other excellent recent, comprehensive surveys of injury patterns in amateur hockey. One such study was undertaken by Thomson (24) as a representative of the Hockey Development Center of Ontario. Using detailed questionnaires, injury information was gleaned from 1558 amateur teams with injury details on 1025 injuries.

The study showed an average of 2.1 injuries per team per season which involved 11.4% of the players, and that the injury rate was 55% greater in games than practices. However, analysis by player division painted a more enlightening picture. (Table 25.4).

Despite the apparent alarming rates for Junior and University players, the Industrial/Recreational group players had the highest injury rates when exposure is factored into the analysis (3.6 times higher than the average).

Bruises, contusions, and muscle pulls represented about 40% of injuries, fractures represented 15%, and dislocations and separations, 13%. The most often injured body areas were: shoulder (22%), knee (16%), and the head/face, arm/wrist/hand, and leg (8% each). Specifically, shoulder separations and/or dislocations and knee sprains were the most common entities (22%). These injuries were caused by body checks (26%), collisions (16%), hitting the boards (12%), being hit from behind (11%) and sticks (11%).

Returning to the point, it was clear that the above-described patterns are to some extent a function of the level of the player. Of the factors considered (e.g., dislocation/separation of the shoulder, 9 of 22 were of value in discriminating levels of play. By way of example, the

Atoms class of player had negative correlation to shoulder dislocation while Juniors had a positive correlation. Both groups had positive correlations for equipment failure. Further development of such analyses may result in level-specific reductions in injuries.

Overall, Thomson's analysis pointed the hockey world toward the trail of prevention. It showed that ice quality and officials played no significant role in injury predilection when the current rules are used. Being hit from behind caused 11% of injuries despite the illegality (as of a 1985 ruling) of such actions. The boards accounted for 12%, raising the issue of board alteration discussed below under spine fractures. Body checks accounted most for injury production by collision (26%) and injury rates were substantially higher for checking versus nonchecking teams. Of the more than 50 concussions, 84% were due to checking, being hit from behind, and other collisions. About 30% were attributed to helmet failure (despite the use of Canadian Standards Association (CSA) approved helmets). Equipment failure was implicated in 20% of all injuries, primarily due to poor quality (either of manufacture or design). In-depth research of this type on equipment must be continued.

Surgical Consequences of Hockey in the NHL

A sport with as much contact, violence, and ballistic movement as is seen in ice hockey is bound to produce injuries requiring more than conservative treatment. In a survey of NHL players (28), 80 of 213 respondents (38%) had undergone surgery for injuries sustained subsequent to joining the NHL. Of players who had been in the league for less than 5 years, 20% had required surgery. For those who had played 6–10 years, the incidence of surgery had risen to 60%, and then to 76% for those who had played between 10 and 17 years (28).

Psychological Considerations in Aggression and Injury

The introduction of protective equipment has been a blessing with respect to head and face injuries. The helmet and face mask, however, have been implicated in the creation of additional violence within the game of ice hockey. Players wearing this gear feel confident and invincible and charge with abandon, having no respect of the possibility that their opponent, armed with similar protection, can be seriously hurt by high sticks, slashes, or cross-checks (29). Nevertheless, this attitude must be one that is cultivated, for the same violence that marks North American hockey is not so much a part of the European game, where the same type of protective gear is available and worn. Paraye (29) indicates that many of the "old Guard" coaches, mentors, and TV sports commentators wean the young players on phrases that die hard:

"Take him out of the play."
"Protect the goalie at all costs."
"Don't let them intimidate you."

In the spirit of these teachings, an aggressive attitude, disrespectful of injury, replaces propriety. According to Walsh (30), the US College Hockey Coaches' Association rendered a unanimous opinion at its 1988 annual meeting that the use of the full face protector has promoted excessive violence in the sport. Walsh, however, claims, "There is a lack of respect by the player for himself as well as his opponent. It is human nature . . . to consider himself as a battering ram." As indicated above, the authors, however, believe that this is culture and training dependent. The learning of aggression is begun at a very tender age.

In the study of Pee Wees, comparing participation with and without body-checking, Regnier et al. (31) reported that "hostile penalties" (such as for charging and cross-checking) were more numerous when checking was permitted (7.7 penalties per game) than when checking was not permitted (4.8 penalties per game). High sticking penalties were twice as frequent in the presence of checking. A comparison of checking and nonchecking Pee Wee leagues in Quebec (1985–86) revealed a fracture rate 12 times greater of the former than the latter. Body-checking caused 88% of fractures, the majority of which (58%) involved the clavicle. Body-checking was again banned in Quebec for Pee Wees in 1987.

Gerberich et al. (32) studied high school players in Minnesota, asking each to prioritize their reasons for playing. When "ridding of tension" was selected as either the first or second choice, the player ran a fourfold risk of concussion (32).

An interesting psychosocial statement about hockey was made by the study of Frank and Gilovich (33). Based on the socially accepted premise that black is bad (e.g., "blacklist" or "blackball"); these researchers undertook to study the potential influence of black uniforms in the NHL and discovered a strong correlation between blackness of uniforms and the numbers of team penalties. Teams that switched to black uniforms from other colors began to register more penalties. Assuming a validity to the trends demonstrated, it remains unanswered whether the uniform instills aggression into the player, whether the referee calls more penalties on black-uniformed players, or whether the management selecting black has an aggressive attitude, which it then instills into its members.

Widmeyer and Birch (34) studied hockey performance and its relation to "aggressive penalties" (those involving stick and/or body contact) in the NHL over 4 seasons spanning 15 years. It was discovered that a significant correlation existed between points accumulated per game and aggressive penalties incurred during the first period of play. The study implied (without statistical significance) that aggression was often employed as a reaction to losing. Widmeyer and Birch cite Cullen and Cullen's 1975 findings, that winning college hockey teams were more aggressive both when the score was close or very disparate.

It is evident that there are multiple psychosocial elements of aggression affiliated with the game of hockey. To reduce serious injuries, these elements must be altered in the formative years, or the game itself must be dramatically altered.

The Role of Fitness: Relation to Performance and Injury

Muscular, Cardiovascular, and Visual

Ice hockey is practiced with a skating format known as "power skating" as opposed to "speed" or "figure" skating. The long, flat blade of the speed skater is ill-suited to maneuverability while the short, front ratcheted blade of figure skating is designed for grace and maneuverability. The hockey blade evolved as a compromise of these functions, offering both speed and maneuverability.

Muscle test profiling of sports and teams generally characterizes strength or work performed by an isolated joint or the ratios of muscles controlling that joint. Recognizing the combined importance of explosive knee extension and hip flexion, extension, abduction, and adduction, Minkoff (35) sought to pursue ratios not previously considered for correlations to performance. The results of these correlations are reviewed in Table 25.5.

Minkoff noted the cinematographic work by Holt in 1977, which revealed that faster skaters had a wider left leg stride and a longer right leg stride. Also, the early training of many skaters involves primarily counterclockwise skating (35). Agre et al. (36) found none of the right-to-left strength differentials (lower extremity) reported by Minkoff (35). However, Minkoff found no obvious differentials of significance when evaluating isokinetic strength about a given joint, only when working with strength ratios of one joint to another.

With respect to standard ratios about a given joint, Minkoff (35) found that the hamstring:quadriceps ratios of hockey players are similar to those of other athletes (about 0.6). However, the ratio of knee extension to hip flexion distinguishes hockey players and accents again the importance of the hip in this sport. For almost two dozen American League baseball players, this ratio averaged 0.62, while for the professional hockey players it averaged 0.79, and for hockey All-Stars, 0.89 (35).

The subject of fatigue is important in hockey, a game which is intermittently continuous, and in which much energy is expended in leverage, checking, and inefficiency of style in addition to that expended by skating alone.

Fatigued players commit more errors, predisposing to injury, and defensemen, in particular, "chase the play," committing more penalties (hooking and tripping) in an effort to thwart the puck carrier.

In his study of professional hockey players, Minkoff (35) concluded that their $m\dot{V}_{O_2max}$ levels were lower than those of endurance athletes, and that they correlated poorly with performance success. He further concluded that the $\dot{V}_{O_2max}$ breakpoint of these players was a more significant evaluator of their function.

Sim et al. (37), drawing on the studies of several workers, disclose that the mean oxygen consumption of ice hockey players is 55%, which is 10–15% lower than that reported for endurance athletes, but that their anaerobic capacity is increased to fairly high levels (though less than in sprinters and swimmers).

Citing Green et al. (21), Sim et al. (37) indicate that forwards play about 20 min per game. The time is divisible into 14–21 shifts, each with just under 40 sec of continuous playing time at an average speed of 8.5 mph.

Montgomery (6) phrased these demands of the game somewhat differently. He indicated that hockey shifts last from between 30–80 sec with 4–5 min of intershift rest. The obvious implication of these figures is that hockey is neither a wholly aerobic, nor a wholly anaerobic sport. "Players must enter into a season conditioned rather than playing into shape," is a commonly practiced myth; once the season is under way, strengthening, cardiovascular training, and skills development activities must not be abandoned. There is evidence that shorter shifts would reduce lactate buildup and allow for restoration of the high energy phosphate bonds with preservation of valued glycogen reserves (6). Glycogen is often depleted significantly after a game. Back-to-back games can lead to severe energy problems, especially in the absence of nutritional counseling (6).

In his study of a championship NHL team, Minkoff (35) found several tests of visual function that correlated significantly to success in hockey. Composites of eye test scores related strongly to shooting accuracy as did tests of visual span. Visual span correlated strongly to face-off success. Only 3 players of those studied scored the maximum in both tests, of the 3, 2 were goalies, while the third player was the team's leading scorer. Concurrent testing of a professional baseball team (a slower sport visually) revealed no maximum scores among those tested. Furthermore, maximum stereoscopic scores were found among all past and present hockey All-Star players (35).

Table 25.5.
Correlations of Skating Attributes to Muscle Testing[a]

Parameter	Skating Speed	Skating Smoothness	Skating Agility
Time to Peak Torque-Knee Extension	Positive-Left only: Significant	Positive-Left only: Significant	—
Ratio of Knee Extension to only Hip Flexion	Positive-Left only: Significant	Positive-Left only: Significant	Positive-Left
Ratio of Knee Extension to Hip Abduction	Positive-Left only: Significant	Positive-Left: Significant	—

[a] Adapted from Minkoff (35)

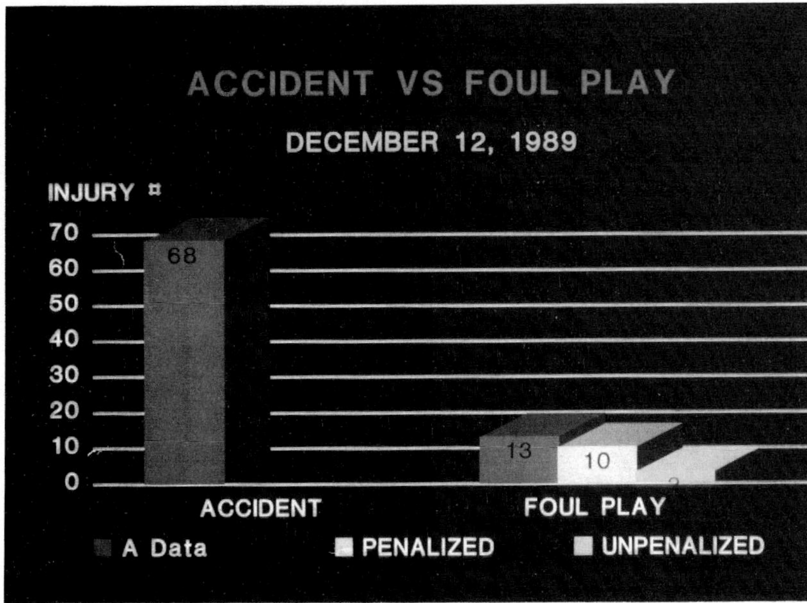

Figure 25.22. Injury incidence over a 12-week period of an NHL hockey season. 30% of injuries are a result of foul play (penalties).

Hockey Penalties

In a large epidemiological study of all levels of amateur hockey in Canada, Thomson (24) determined that 17% of injuries were associated with penalties. This is in accord with Sutherland's report (6) in which 25% of injuries were associated with penalties (Fig. 25.2).

These penalties are photographically represented in Figure 25.23 *(A–Q)*. It is considered by some that the consequences of many of the penalties are insufficient to adequately allay violence.

The Rink and Collision Injuries

Peculiarities of the hockey rink may ultimately contribute to injuries. Contrary to general expectation, there are limited standards for design and construction of professional rinks. In North America rinks need only meet a size requirement minimum of 160 feet long and 60 feet wide (2). The goal cage must be at least 10 feet away from the end of the backboards (Fig. 25.18). Depending on the width of this passageway, the frenzy of activity and the numerous collisions that occur behind the goal increase the potential for injury (6) (Table 25.6).

Moore noted that scrambles behind the net resulted in 7% of injuries (6). Montgomery referred to a report by Sutherland that activity (around the net, not just in front of the net) accounted for 42% of injuries in his study (6). The material and yield characteristics of the boards also have potential for modifying the character and severity of injuries due to collision. The height of the boards has not been designed by scientific intent to reduce injuries (Fig. 25.24). In many rinks today, there are plexiglass extensions of the boards that ascend several feet above them. These extensions permit abutment of the face or head into their rigid panels by boarding and cross-checking maneuvers (Figs. 25.25,26).

Protective Equipment in Hockey

Hockey is a sport in which injuries are sustained by virtually every body part. At the inception of the sport, equipment was scant and the thrust for the development of protective wear did not accelerate until the 1970s, after the initial epidemiological studies began to elucidate vulnerabilities and injuries. The manufacturers and organizations that test and approve equipment around the world have responded by producing progressively better equipment that offers not only greater protection, but, in many instances, products with better function (Fig. 25.27). Other factors of importance include fit, weight, ventilation, motion, durability, unimpeded vision & hearing, and economic reality (38, 39). To equip a child for amateur hockey could cost from $100–200 US per year (considering the child's rapid growth and the importance of maintaining proper fit). Failure to replace outgrown or poorly maintained equipment risks a tradeoff between parsimony and the risk of serious injury. The maximum protective equipment available for skaters and goaltenders can be seen in Figure 25.28. Areas of incomplete protection can be seen in Figure 25.29*A,B,C*.

Helmet

An awareness of severe head injuries received in hockey in Sweden in the 1950s prompted the Swedish Hockey Association to conduct surveys which led ultimately to compulsory use of helmets in 1963 (40). The early helmets were flimsy in construction and deficient in protection. In the late 1950s, for example, leather helmets lined with felt were in vogue. These were followed by compression-moulded plastic and leather helmets and then by injection-moulded plastic (41) (Fig. 25.30).

In 1965, the Canadian Amateur Hockey Association

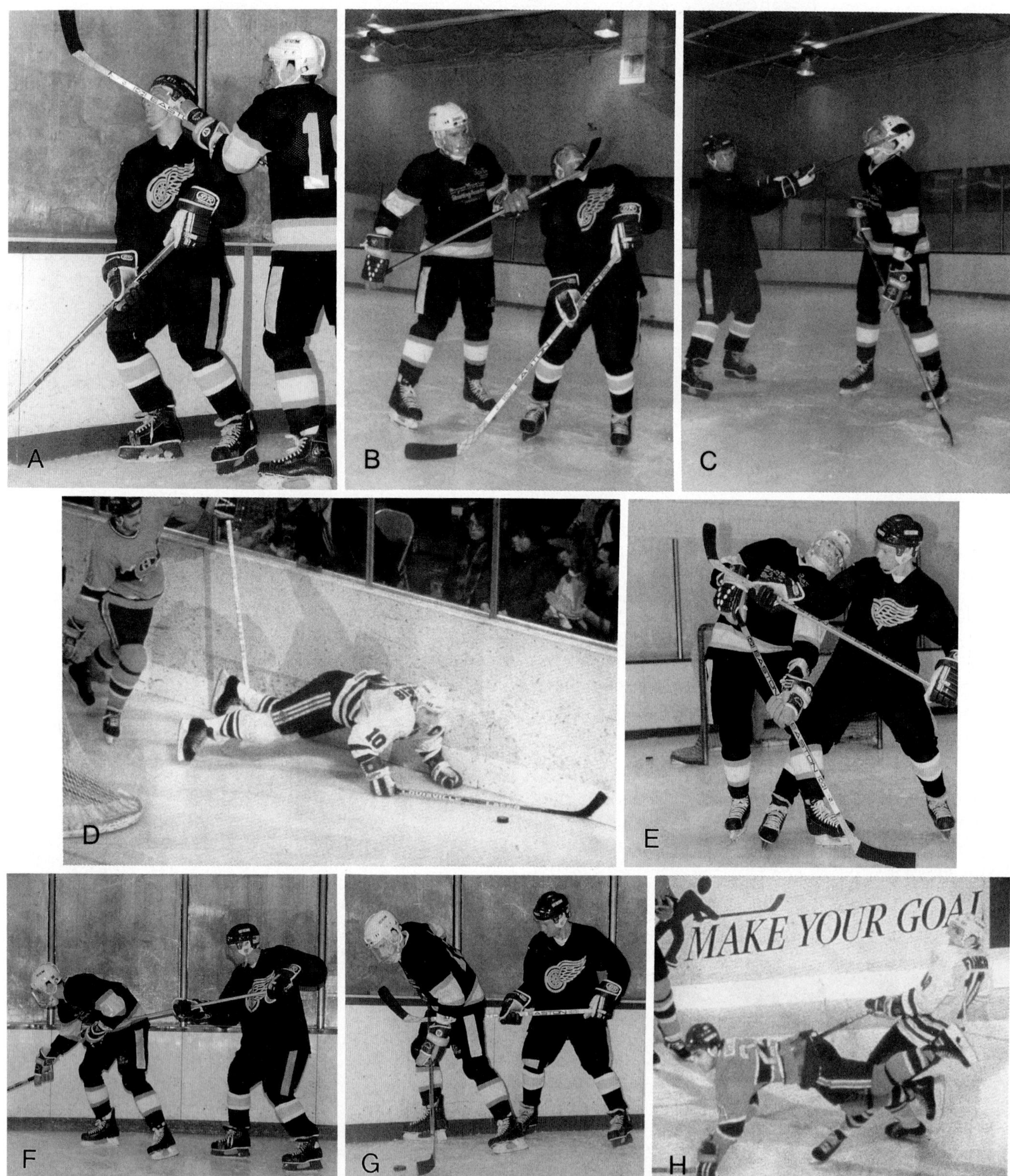

Figure 25.23. Representation of penalties which produce injury: **(A, B, C),** high sticking; **(D),** tripping; **(E),** combination high sticking/tripping; **(F, G, H),** hooking; **(I, J, K),** crosschecking; **(L, M),** butt-ending; **(N),** elbowing; **(O),** spearing; **(P),** kneeing; **(Q),** holding.

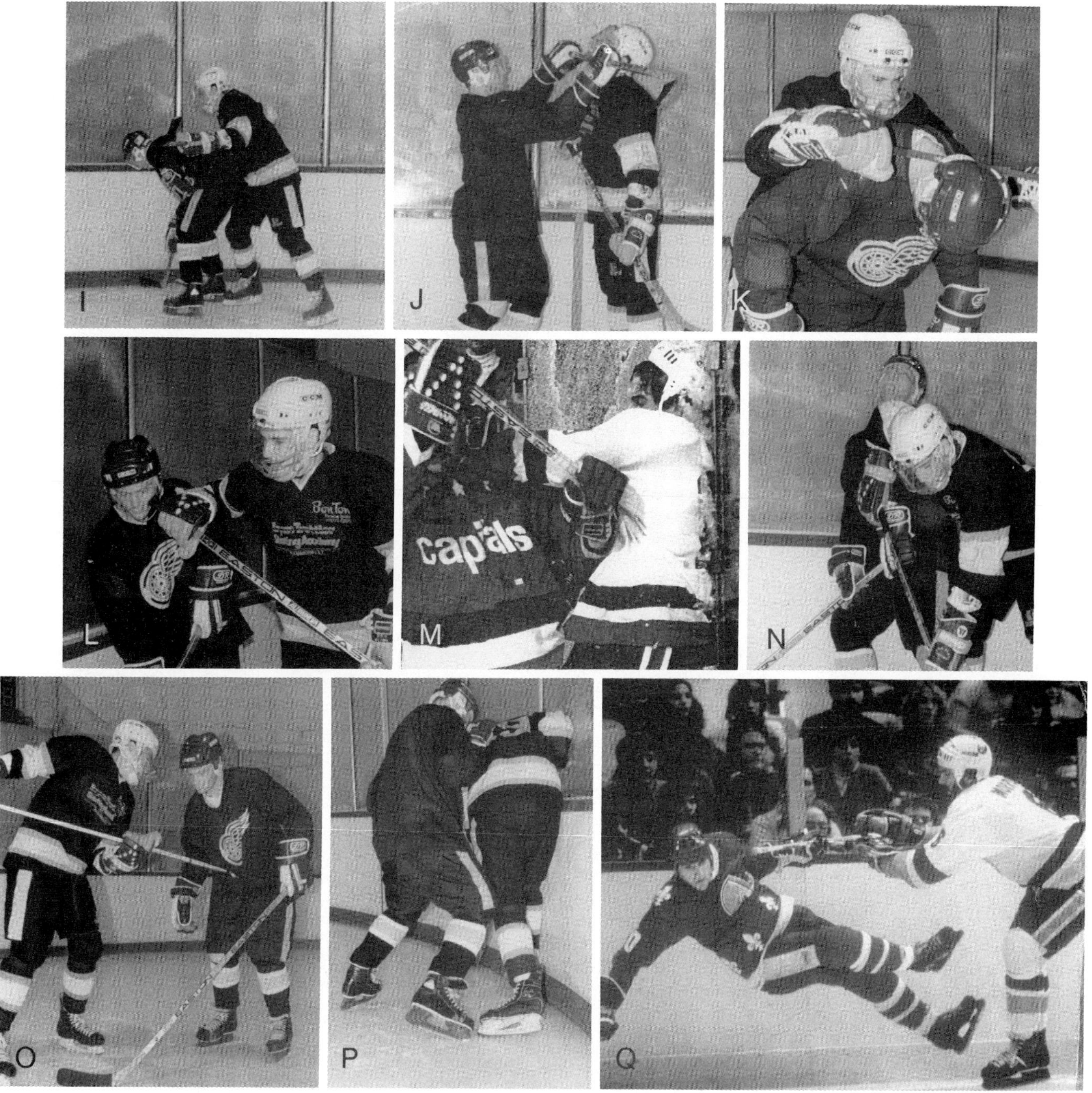

Figure 25.23 *(cont.)* **D, H, Q** courtesy of Paul Bereswill; **M** courtesy of Sports Illustrated, 12/31/90.

(CAHA) mandated the use of helmets for all juvenile and younger players. In 1969, CAHA requested the Canadian Standards Association (CSA) to establish a standard for helmets (42).

In 1973, responding to outcries about head injuries, the CSA published a standard for the manufacture of hockey helmets (43). In the 1970s, modern plastic helmets with suspension liners met the early CSA standards (41). While there was general accord that the CSA standard was a safety improvement over preexisting helmet designs, there were questions about its merits. Many design factors had to be considered: peak forces, peak acceleration, kinetic energy absorbed, as well as other factors. Organizations responsible for testing, such as the CSA and NOCSAE (National Operating Committee on Standards for Athletic Equipment) perform testing using different methods (43). Countries other than Canada have their own testing protocols and standards. Bishop et al. (43) explains the two basic components needed for "safe" helmets: first, a firm outer shell is needed to diffuse forces from the site of impact; second, an energy-absorbing liner is required to decelerate impact forces to a tolerable level.

On the issue of impact testing for helmets, Johnson (44) states that the Gadd severity index (GSI), which is based on the Wayne State Curve (gravitation accelera-

Table 25.6.
Causes of Injury In Ice Hockey[a]

Cause	Frequency (%)
Skater being checked	21.9
Player trying to gain possession of puck	15.2
Carrying or passing the puck	17.8
Checking	14.8
Scrambles in front of the net	7.0
Blocking a shot	4.0
Skating without interference	3.0
Miscellaneous causes (incl. fighting)	16.3

[a]Adapted from Moore, 1980. In: Montgomery DL. Physiology of ice hockey. Sports Med 1988; 5:99–126.

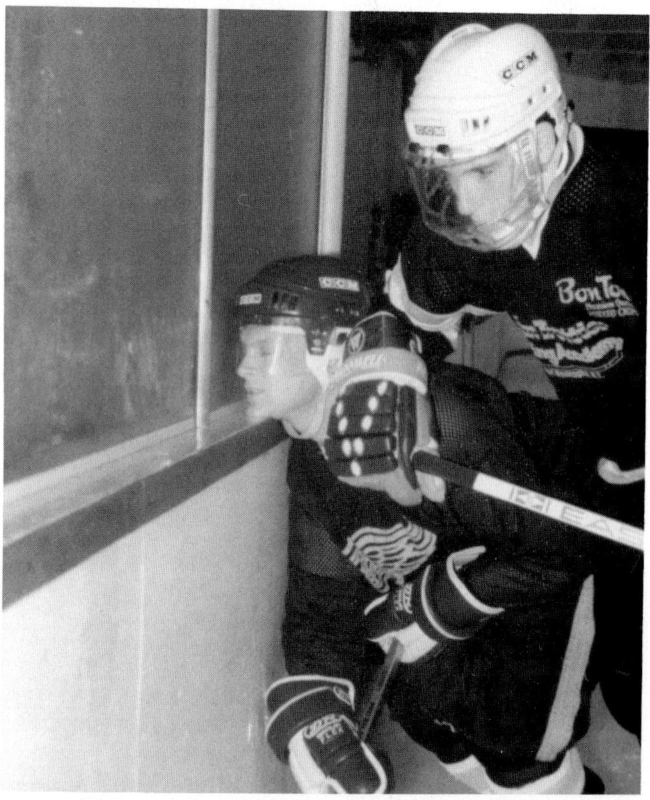

Figure 25.24. Ledge of the side boards—glass interface is an area of potential serious injury.

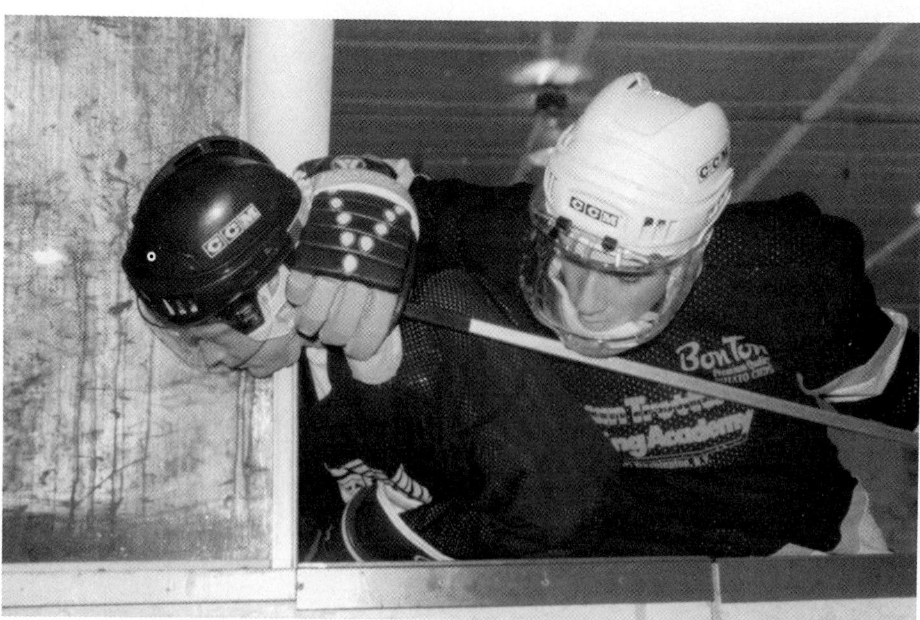

Figure 25.25. Plexiglass abruptly ends at the penalty box and players' bench areas, leaving an area of potential serious injury (viewed from players' bench).

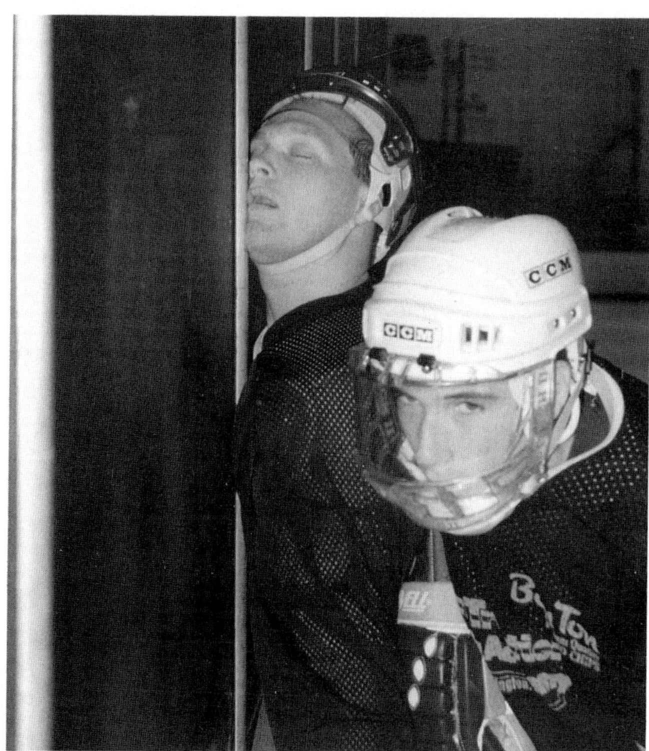

Figure 25.26. Injury can occur while being checked from behind into the rigid plexiglass panels.

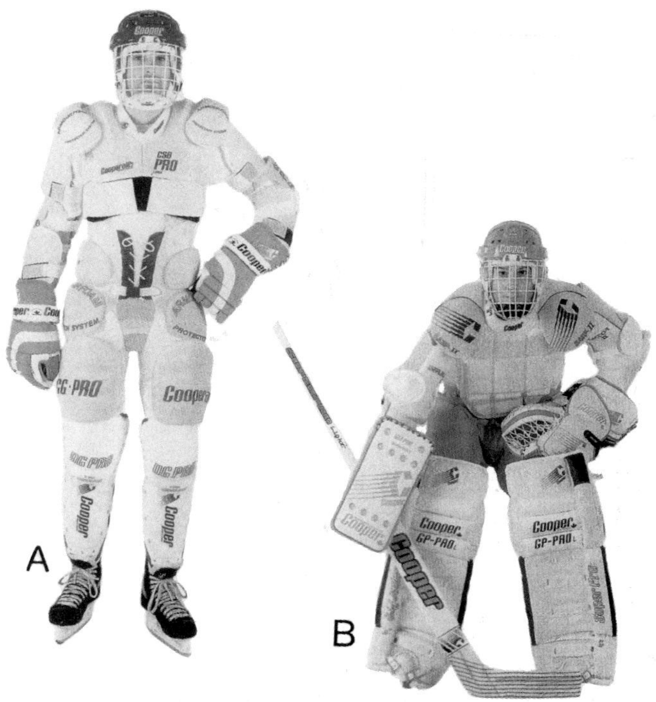

Figure 25.28. Maximum protective equipment for skaters (A) and goaltenders (B). Note the junction of the shoulder pads, elbow pads and gloves in the upper body. Pants, shin pads and skates are confluent. Cooper Canada, Ltd, Toronto, Canada

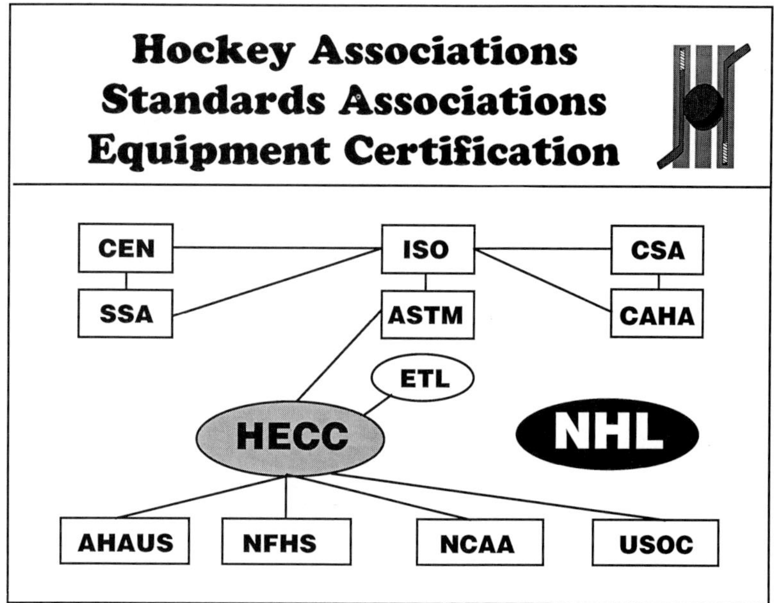

Figure 25.27. Graphic representative interaction of Standards Associations (ISO, CEN, SSA, ASTM, HECC, CSA) and Hockey Associations (CAHA, NHL, AHAUS, NFHS, NCAA, USOC) for equipment certification. (Note that the NHL presently does not directly interact with the Standards and equipment certification organizations.) [ISO = International Standards Organization; CEN = European Standards Organization; SSA = Swedish Standards Association; ASTM = Association of Standardization and Testing of Materials; CSA = Canadian Standards Association; CAHA = Canadian Amateur Hockey Association: HECC = Hockey Equipment Certification Council (USA); ETL = Equipment Testing Laboratories (Independent) (USA); NHL = National Hockey League; AHAUS = Amateur Hockey Association of the United States (now USA Hockey); NFHS = National Federation of High Schools; NCAA = National Collegiate Athletic Association; USOC = United States Olympic Committee.]

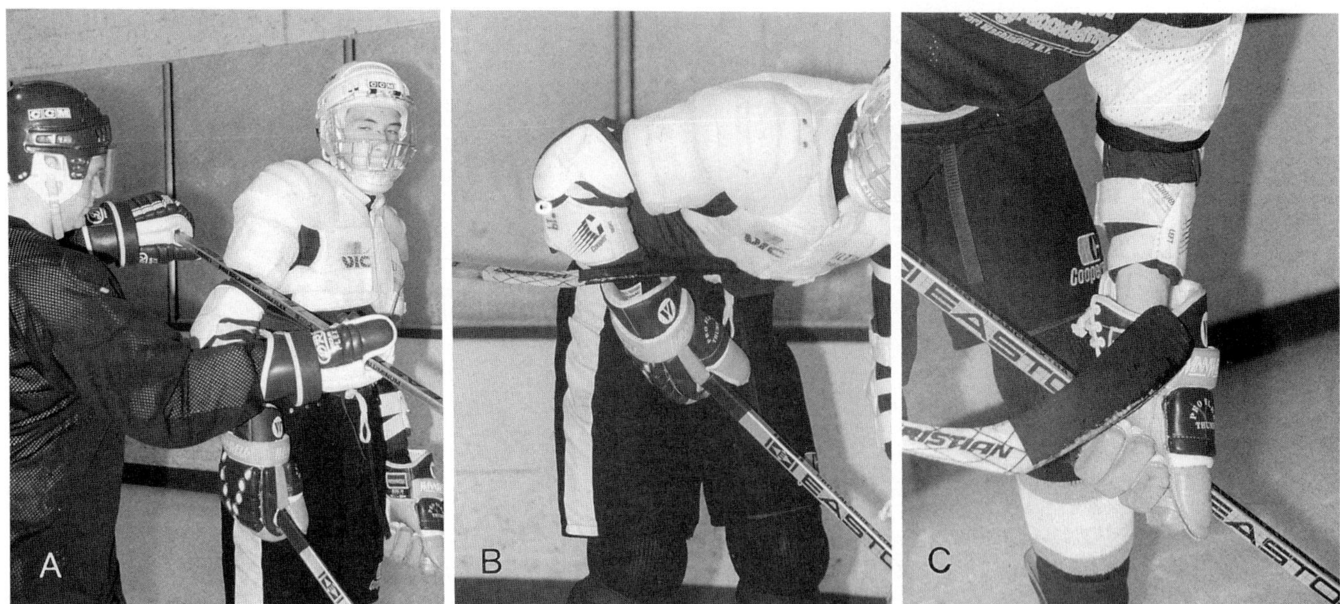

Figure 25.29 Incomplete protection of the lateral arm. **(B)** Incomplete protection of the dorsal forearm. **(C)** Incomplete protection on the volar surface of the elbow and forearm.

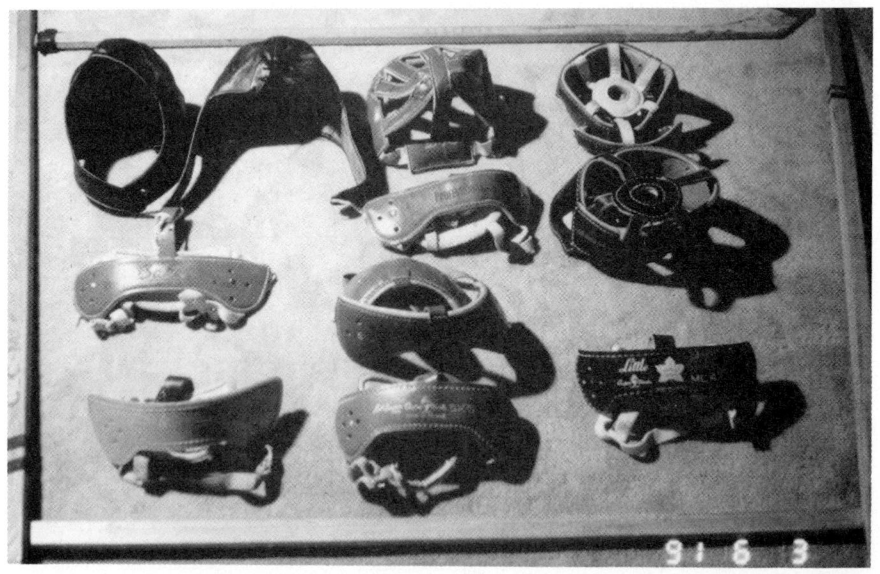

Figure 25.30. Early Helmets: Sears sports helmet circa 1890 *(upper left)*. Leather helmets circa 1940's with minimal protection *(upper right and middle row)*. Compression-moulded plastic helmet *(lower left)*. Courtesy of Dave Beaune, Toronto, Canada.

tion as a function of time), is among the most popular methods of evaluating injury hazard. This index, as well as other popular ones (e.g., the head injury criterion (HIC)), address only frontal blows. There are no corresponding indices for rotational acceleration. Johnson, in Sweden, and investigators in North America utilize head forms with triaxial accelerators to record impact phenomena, which they then relate to the indices to ascertain danger levels. Johnson contends that dropping the head form onto an anvil (Fig. 25.31) is a more physiologically realistic test format than that used by others in which an object is dropped on to the head form (44). The Association of Standardization and Testing of Materials (ASTM) Performance Specification for Ice Hockey Helmets (specification F 1045-87) in the U.S. also utilizes an evaluation in which head forms are dropped (45). Instead of the wooden head form used by Johnson (44), Moorehouse (45) selected a magnesium alloy (Z-90) for its reliability. This points up the complexity of considerations entering into the evaluation of safety levels of hockey products worldwide today. Moorehouse explains that Gadd derived a maximum safe level of 1500 units (effective acceleration/time), beyond which there is a risk of concussion. The ASTM standard deals with "G max" rather than the Gadd Severity Index. However, Moorehouse (45) cites the work of Calvano and Berger that established a correlation between the two, whereby a Gadd Severity Index of 1500 corresponds to a G max of 225. The ASTM has selected a G max of 275 for its helmet standard (45). Tested helmets must comply this protection value by testing multiple sizes, multiple times with impacts at each of 6 designated sites on the helmet. Chin straps are also tested by loading them with suspensory weights. They must not break prior to adding 50N and must release before 550N; elongation must not exceed 25 M (45) (Fig. 25.32).

Hoerner (39) makes the point that hockey helmets must be able to absorb kinetic energies ranging from a player's high mass (weight) and low velocity (speed) to the puck's low mass and high velocity without compromising defense at either of these extremes or at levels between the extremes. This principle is partly exemplified by motorcycle crash helmets. These helmets are lined with polystyerene beads within a Styrofoam pad to absorb the energy of high mass, high speed collision. However, for lower energy impacts, such as those occurring in hockey, Schneider reported an increased incidence and degree of concussion with the use of this type of helmet (46).

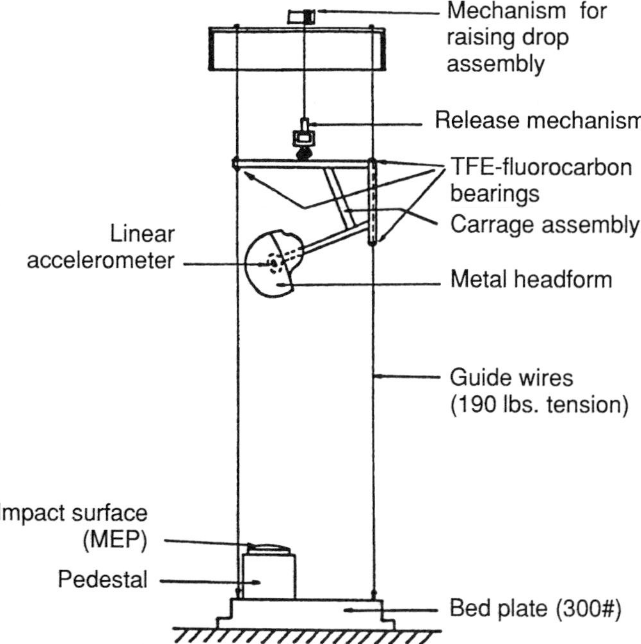

Figure 25.31. Helmet impact test apparatus of drop-head type. From Dixon, ISO Draft, 1991.

Drafts for an international standard for headgear under ISO (International Standards Organization) supervision and with the cooperative efforts of standards organizations from various nations (44, 47, 48) are under way. Unlike the headforms of Johnson's studies (wooden), and of the Moorehouse's ASTM studies (magnesium alloy), the headform for the international standard is made of a rubberized epoxy. This standard (unlike that of the ASTM) calls for the use of the Gadd Severity Index limit (1500). The gravity-drop form of testing has been adopted. Chin strap testing has a format similar to that described above (48) (Fig. 25.33).

Face masks

Puck speed can exceed velocities of 100 mph and generate impact forces of up to 1200 lbs (37). Thus, the need for face protection in hockey is apparent. Nevertheless, almost 70 years of professional hockey had been played before an NHL goalie sought to protect himself by using a moulded face plate (Fig. 25.34*A*, *B*). These face plates were better than no protection, but they allowed facial contact when hard shots were fired. Some of the early polycarbonate face plate models had large windows for the eyes. Sticks and/or pucks could enter these windows even with wire-mesh face protectors. In Sweden, some standards for faceguards were finally approved in 1972. New, more elaborate standards awaited the creation of the Swedish Hockey Association in 1978 (40). In North America, there were no stan-

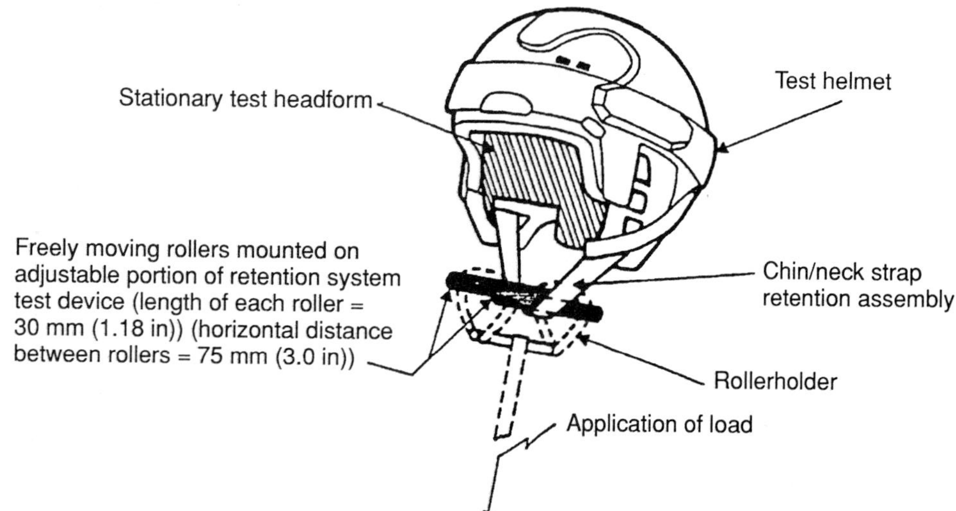

Figure 25.32. Chin strap loading apparatus with suspension weights. From Dixon, ISO Draft, 1991.

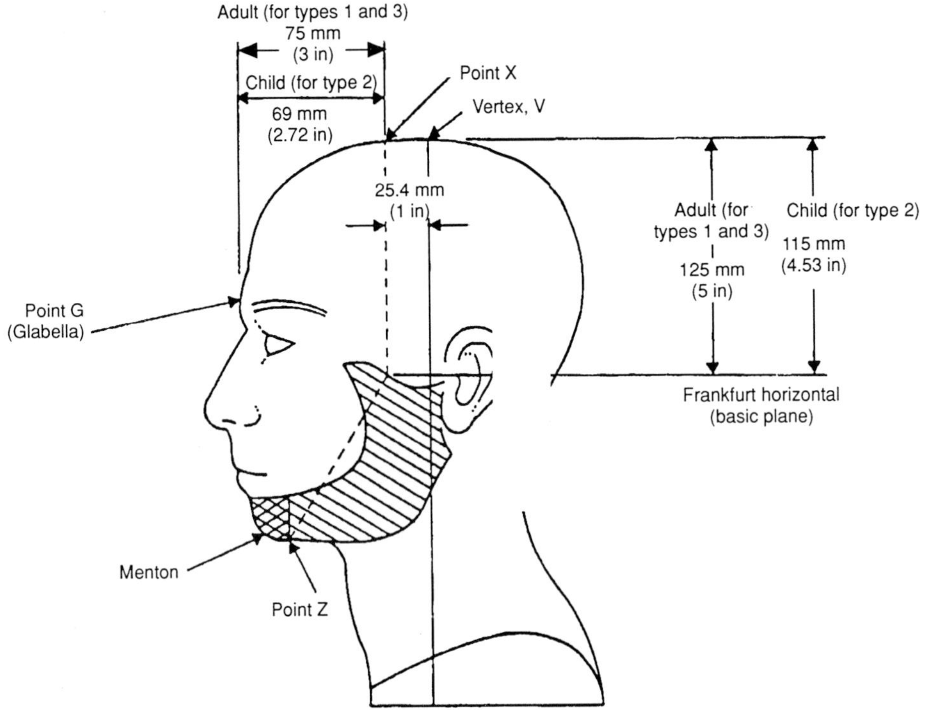

Figure 25.33. Areas of concern and dimensions for helmet design. (From Dixon, ISO Draft, 1991)

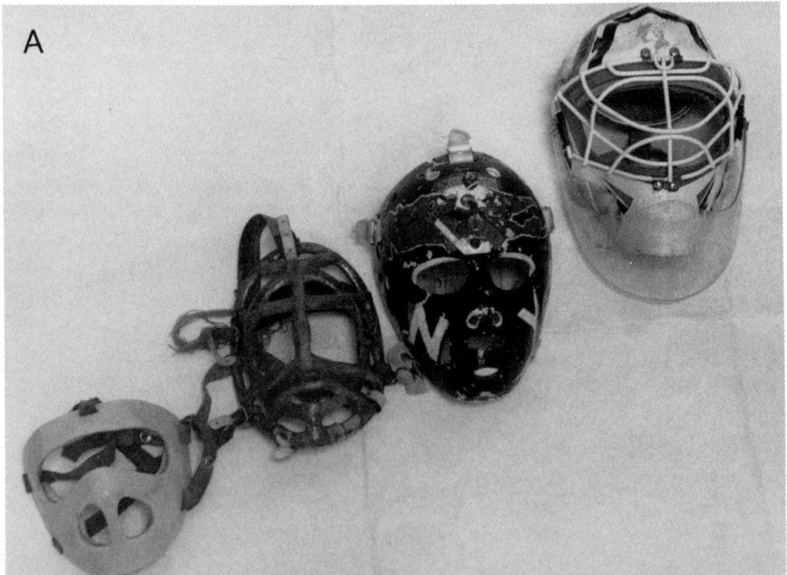

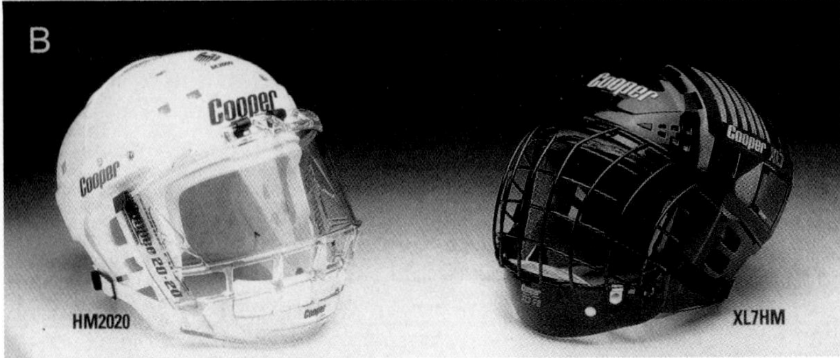

Figure 25.34 A, B. *(A)* Face masks in evolution from 1960's *(left)* to early 1980's *(right)*. Courtesy of Chico Resch. *(B)* HECC and CSA approved helmet with faceshield *(left)* and metal cage *(right)*. Cooper Canada, Toronto, Canada.

dards for face masks prior to 1977, but after a preliminary standard was established in that year, modifications have occurred several times (42, 49).

Presently, ISO drafts are under consideration for ISO-approved face masks (Fig. 25.35) (49). See Table 25.7 for face mask categories for types of masks and description of function.

Performance tests for face masks must ascertain the following: areas of facial coverage, penetratability (through orifices), impact tolerance, and preservation of vision (through a complicated battery of visual tests) (42, 44, 49).

Half-Face Visor

The American College Hockey Coach's Association voted unanimously (1988) in favor of half shields rather than full-face masks, claiming that the latter serve as an instigation to increased violence and result in more dangerous injuries (30). Walsh (30) points out that half shields are used in European hockey and in Canadian College and Major Junior Hockey. Smith and Bishop (50) tested visors as well as full-face protectors. They found that polycarbonate visors allowed facial contact at puck impact velocities of 50 mph or 22.4 m/s. The findings of Roy and Dore cited by Smith and Bishop assess mean and expected maximum puck velocities for different age levels (Table 25.8) (50).

It is evident that the visor will permit facial contact

Table 25.7.
Types and Functions of Face Masks

Type	Description of Function
1A	Large full face, for players older than 10 years
1B	Medium, full face; for players older than 10 years
1C	Small, full face; for players through 10 years
2A/B	Large/medium, full face; for goaltenders
3	Visor (partial face)

Dixon JL, ed. Face protectors and visors for ice hockey players. CSA May, 1990.

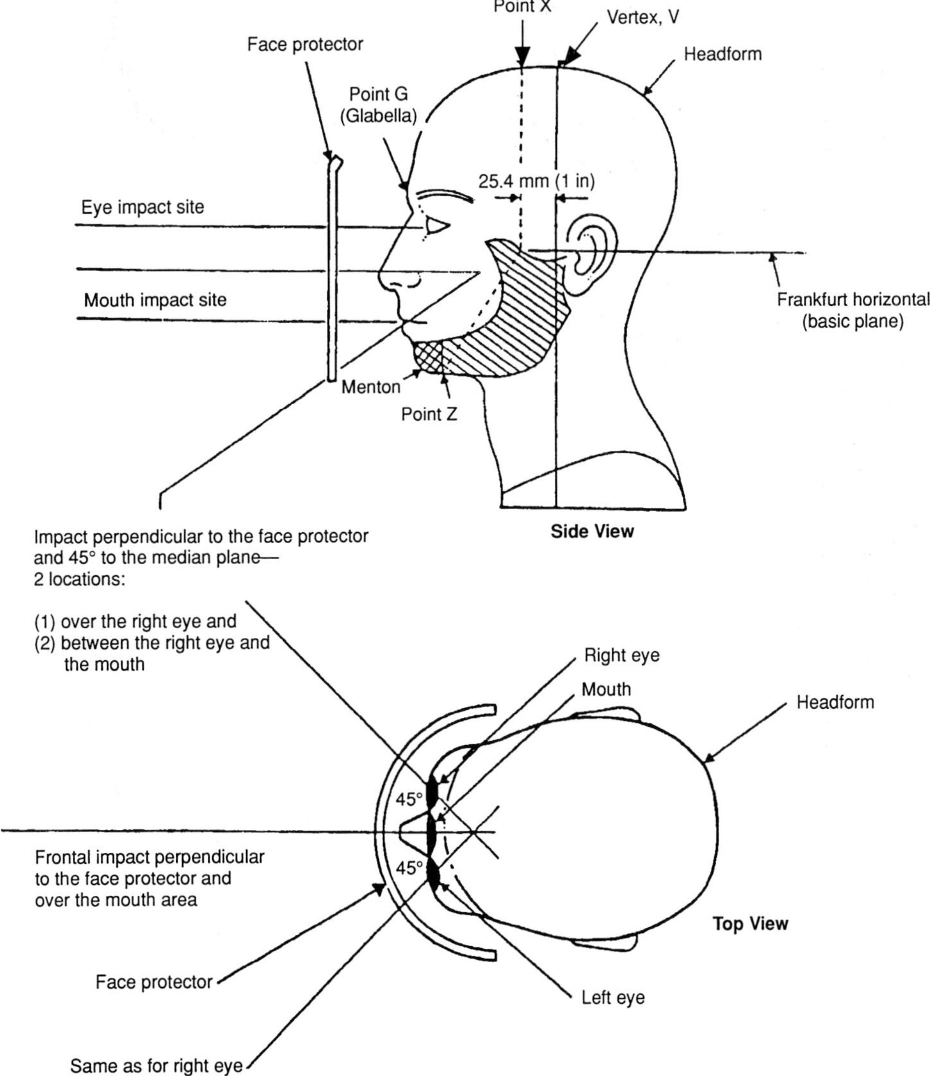

Figure 25.35. Impact methodology for facemasks including impact sites perpendicular and at 45° from center. Visual fields (laterally—90°, superiorly—45°, and inferiorly—60°) must be unimpaired. From Dixon, ISO Draft, 1991.

at the expected maximum velocity achieved by a 13-year-old player, and certainly at the mean velocity achieved by a 14-year-old (wherein 50 mph equates to 22.5 m/s).

While visors may not be wholly protective of the eyes and face for all consequences of impact, it is, at least, of value in reducing the incidence of facial lacerations (Fig. 25.36). Reporting on observations of elite Swedish players, Lorentzon et al. (23) noted that those who used a visor had 52% fewer lacerations about the face. The use of visors is currently increasing among collegiate players and many industrial and recreational league players. Furthermore, players wearing a visor have suffered *no* blinding injuries thus far (51).

Table 25.8.
Shooting Speeds of Ice Hockey Players[a]

Age	Mean Velocity (m/sec)	Expected Maximum Velocity (m/sec)	Expected Maximum Velocity (mph)
13	19.4	29.79	66
14	21.7	31.14	69
15	24.0	32.49	72
16	25.7	31.14	69
17	27.1	42.42	94
18–25	28.9	32.94	73

[a] Smith TA, Bishop PJ. Impact of full face and visor type hockey face guards. In: Castaldi CR, Hoerner EF, eds. Safety in ice hockey (Philadelphia: ASTM, 1989 (STP 1050): 235–239).

Neck Protectors

The use of neck protectors has become increasingly popular. In the past decade, neck protectors have been used fairly routinely by goalies and, more recently, by forwards and defensemen to prevent skate cuts around the neck (see section below on neck injuries) (Fig. 25.37). A movement to create standards for neck protectors has been started. Standards for throat protectors were set by the Swedish Hockey Association in 1987 (40). The area to be protected is demonstrated in Figure 25.37.

Skates

By the beginning of the twentieth century, metal had replaced wood and the blade was attached permanently to a boot (Fig. 25.38 *A, B*). The solid metal blades and runner were heavy and clumsy. Within a few decades the metal runners and blades had been streamlined for increased skating speed and made taller so that the puck would less likely contuse the feet within the boots. By the midtwentieth century, the blade had become tubular (hollow), allowing greater speed by vir-

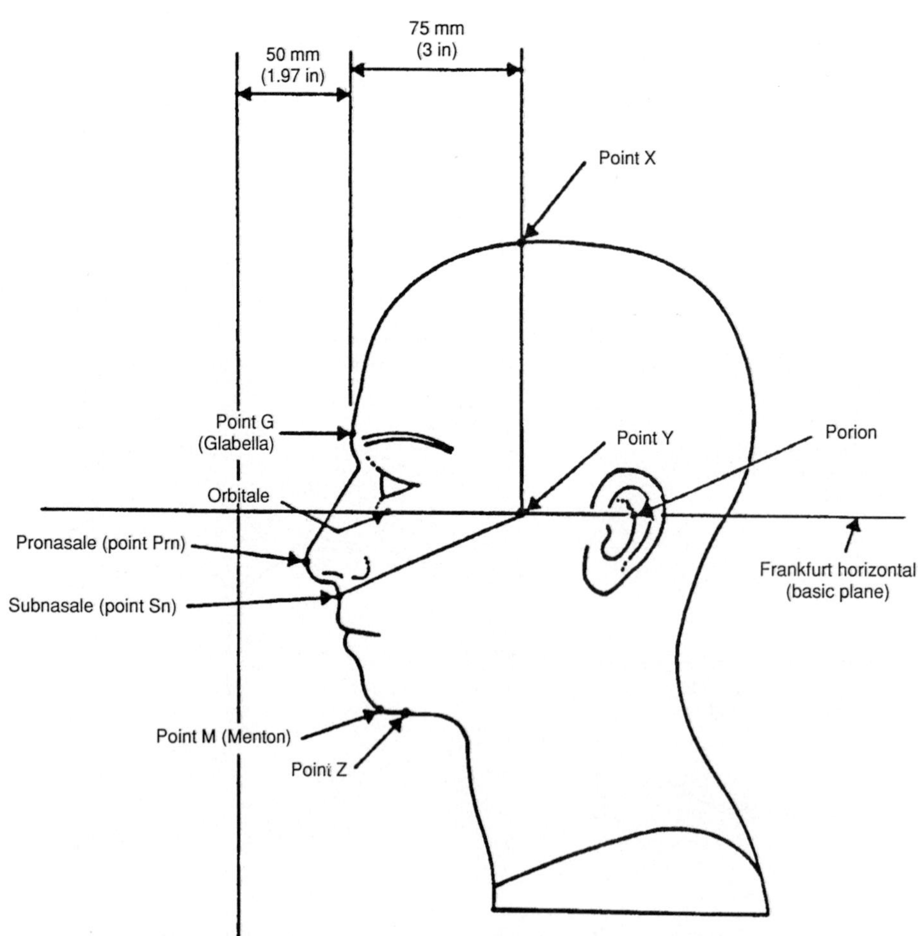

Figure 25.36. Areas of coverage for protective visors. From Dixon, ISO Draft, 1991.

tue of its reduced weight (Fig. 25.38*C*). Later, tubular models were also canted for improved acceleration. These skates, however, had a special liability, in that the exposed back end of the blade acted as a weapon, especially after repeated sharpenings of the blade. By 1960, bumpers had been designed to cap the pointed blade end to avoid some of the fatalities (quite literal throat-cutting fatalities) known to have occurred (52). Today, skates have either a safety guard (if the skate blade is open in the back) or a heel guard (when the skate is totally closed in the back) (Fig. 25.38*D*). By the early 1970s, the all-metal blades and runners were giving way to plastic assemblies into which blades were fixed (Fig. 25.38*E*). These models were even lighter than those before them, thus fostering another escalation in skating velocity. Unfortunately, many of the assemblages broke, representing a measure of danger. The ASTM was requested to create guidelines for quality and safety. They did, and, in 1986, the new guidelines included a mandate that the plastic portion of the blade assembly must extend 3 mm beyond the front and rear of the runner for safety.

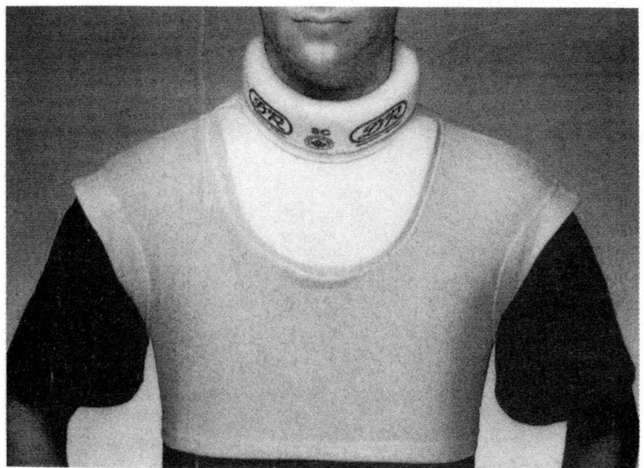

Figure 25.37. Neck protector recommended to reduce cut injuries, not presently designed to prevent impact injuries.

With respect to skates, there are two basic concerns. The first is their ability to protect the foot from lacerations and impacts. This has been accomplished to some extent by elevating the boot adequately above the ice and by the creation of molded skate boots with various guards (such as one for the Achilles tendon). The second basic concern is the achievement of comfort and support, while allowing an adequate range of motion of the ankle for maximum performance. Hoshizaki evaluated motion and stability of the ankle for several power skating activities by testing a variety of molded skates as well as other skates and concluded that the type of skate used can, in fact, limit ankle and hindfoot range of motion, reducing acceleration, although the molded skates did not substantially restrict motion in these areas. The fit of the skate is, naturally, of critical importance.

Sticks

From hockey stick forerunners made exclusively of wood, hockey sticks have evolved into eclectic instruments, combining wood, fiberglass, aluminum, and plastic in various combinations. Certain dimensions of the sticks have been standardized, but certainly not all

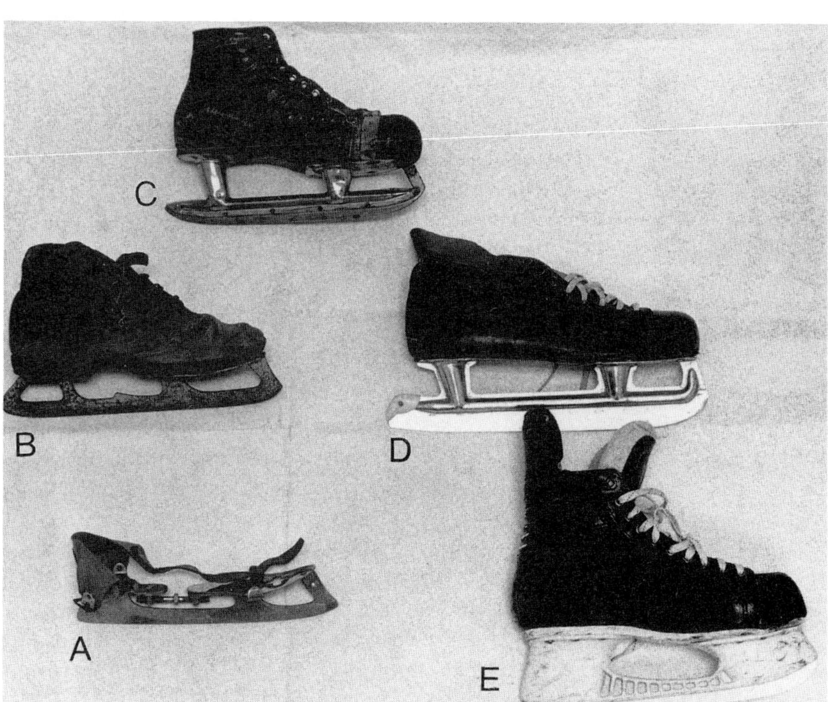

Figure 25.38. Evolution of ice hockey skates *(clockwise from lower left):* **(A)** skate circa 1910; **(B)** skate permanently mounted to a leather boot circa 1920; **(C)** "tube skates" with pointed back of the blade; **(D)** tube skate circa 1950 with plastic over the back of the blade; **(E)** modern skate with plastic blade holder. Courtesy of Chico Resch.

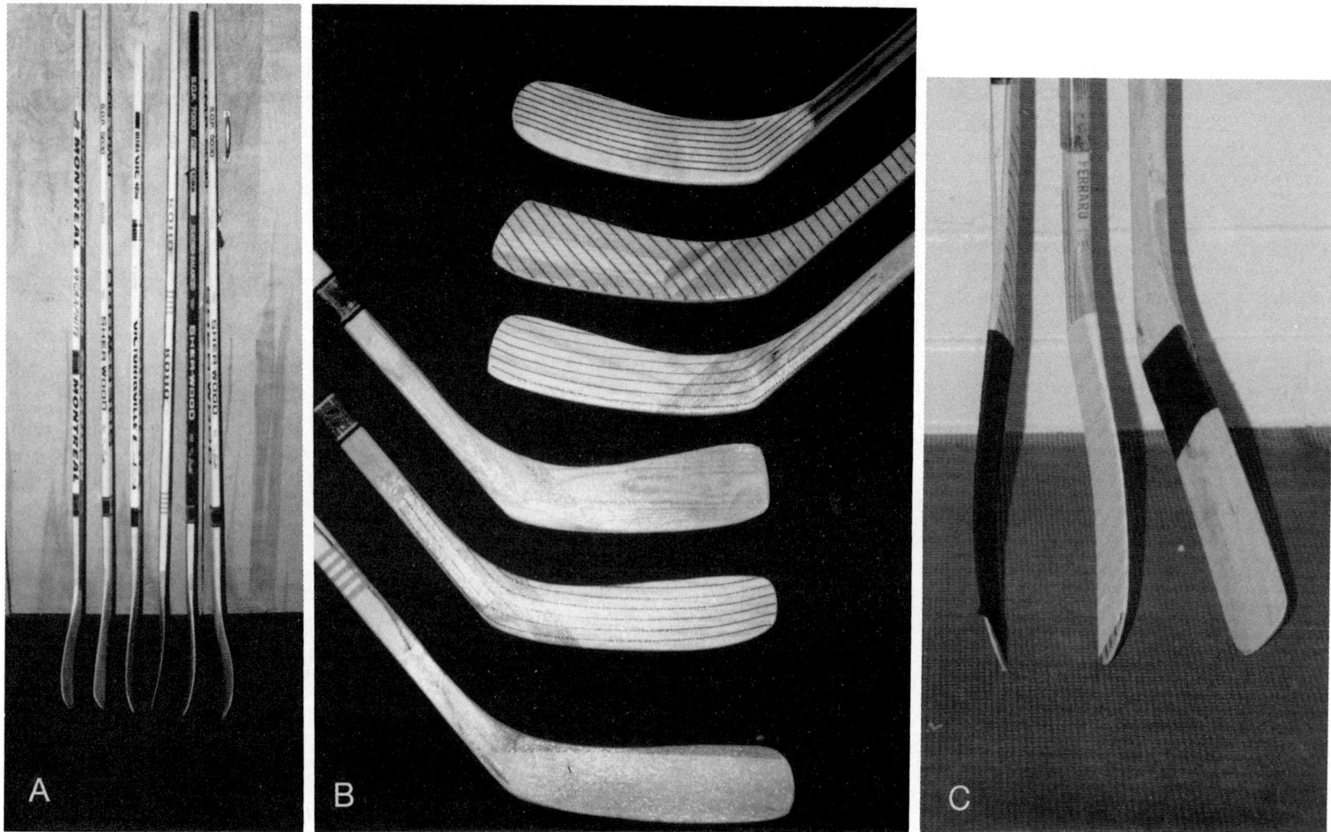

Figure 25.39. Right and left curved sticks showing variability in *(A)* blade curves, *(B)* geometry, and *(C)* blade taping.

(Fig. 25.39). Many players wrap tape around the blades of their sticks, claiming it assists their effectiveness. No studies have been done to ascertain the merits of taping.

Sticks have figured significantly in the production of injuries. Sticks represent a danger when use above the shoulder (high sticking) (Fig. 25.23 *A, B, C*), for slashing (Fig. 25.23*C*), for tripping (Fig. 25.23*D*), or for cross-checking (Fig. 25.23*I, J*). They also represent a danger because of breakage (mostly at the angle of the shaft and blade), thus allowing the loose, jagged segment to become a missile when a break occurs in the act of shooting. Players must immediately drop a broken stick, so that the handle cannot act as a pointed lance.

Other Equipment

Because much of the early equipment, such as pants and gloves, was adapted from lacrosse and cricket, the specific protective value as equipment for hockey was deficient. The evolution of hockey equipment can be seen in Figures 25.40–25.48. The evolution of modern hip, pelvis, and thigh protection, as exemplified by Cooperalls (Cooper Canada, Ltd, Ontario, Canada), took several decades (41) (Fig. 25.48*A* and *B*).

Testing the resilience of protective material today is done by automatic puck-delivery systems with impacts recorded by special video systems (41). Such sophisticated testing methods are expected to increase the protective nature of equipment in order to avoid catastrophic injuries as depicted in Figure 25.49.

Injuries

There are several injury categories of particular concern. They include:

1. Head and brain injuries.
2. Spinal injuries (especially cervical spine injuries).
3. Ocular injuries.
4. Groin strains—by virtue of their frequency, not their severity.

Head and Face

In the 1989–1990 NCAA ice hockey season, only about 6% of injuries involved the head, face, eyes, ears, or nose; most of these were concussions. Face guards, almost evenly divided between plastic and metal, apparently served a great protective function (22).

Lacerations are frequent about the head and face. Studies have clearly demonstrated that face shields will prevent many of them (23).

With the exception of lacerations, the most commonly occurring serious traumatic head injuries are concussions (53). In accordance with criteria listed by Sim et al. (54), any evident loss of consciousness exceeding 10 sec indicates a grade IV concussion, and implies brain damage. Any player unconscious from a head

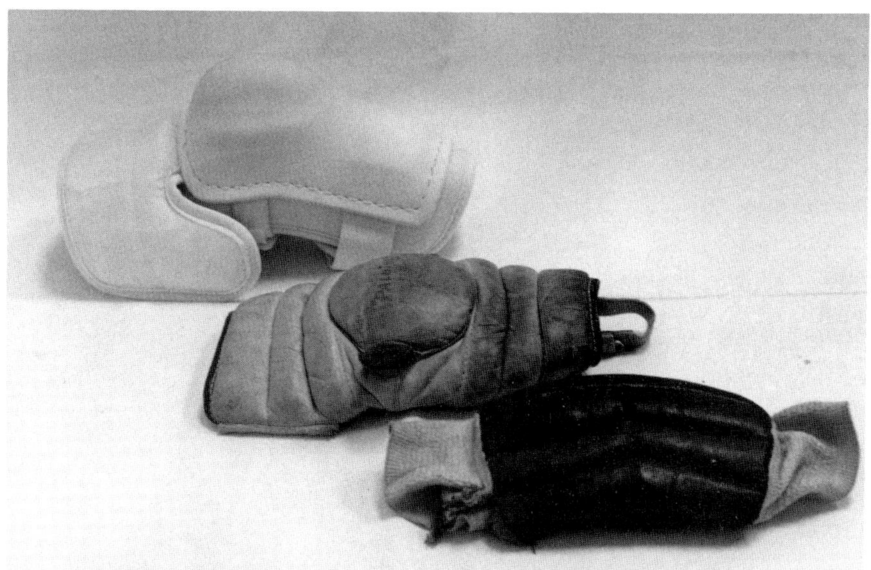

Figure 25.40. Elbow pads from the 1920's *(lower)* made of horse or deer hair rolled and sewn into the leather; 1940's *(middle)* elbow pads with protective olecranon cap; 1980's *(upper)* elbow pads with a short forearm protector made of plastic and foam. Courtesy of Chico Resch.

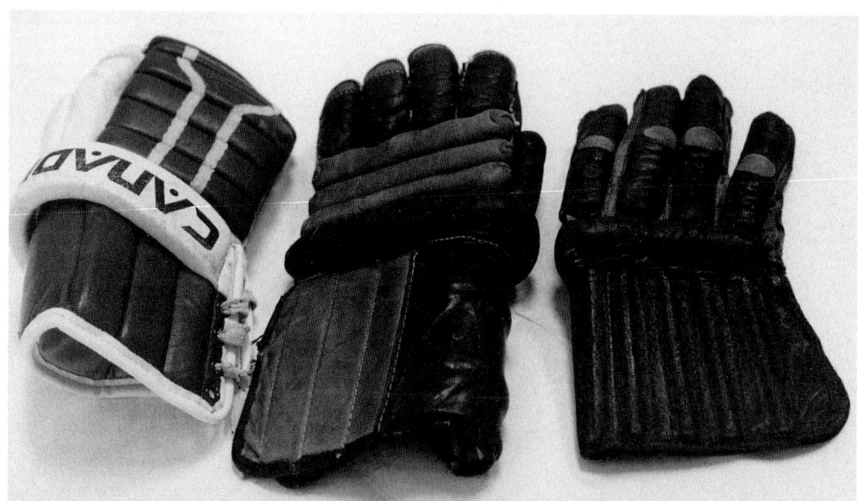

Figure 25.41. Hockey gloves in evolution from 1930s model *(right)* with deer hair and dried sugar cane sewn into the leather. Palms were sewn flat onto the glove. 1940s glove *(middle)* made with plastic forearm protector. The palm is better contoured to hold the stick. Modern glove *(left)* is made of lightweight dense foam. Courtesy of Chico Resch.

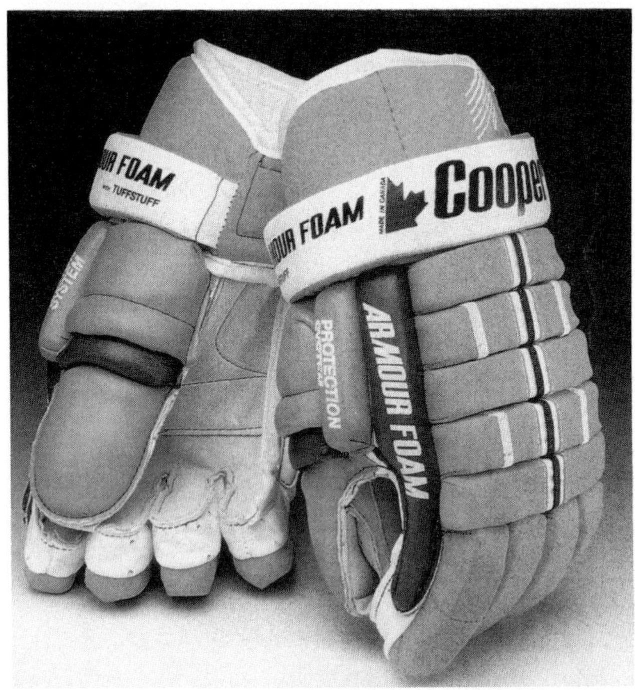

Figure 25.42. 1990s hockey glove with shortened forearm protection (should be used in conjunction with an elbow pad with an extended forearm piece). Cooper Canada, Ltd., Toronto, Canada.

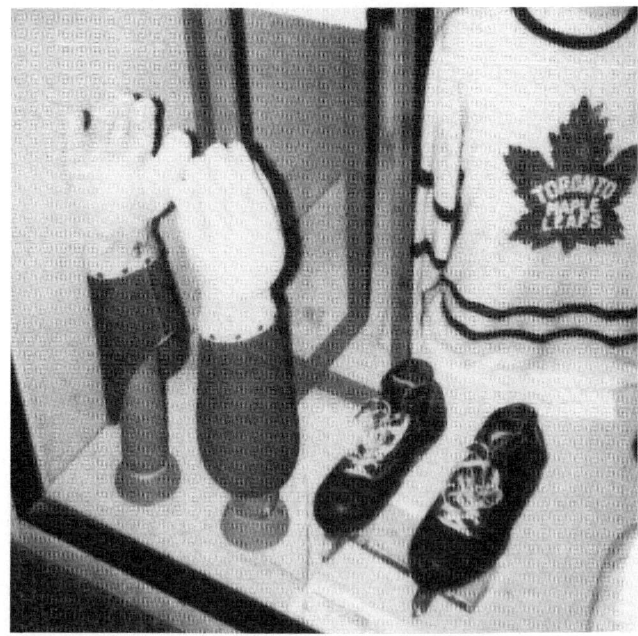

Figure 25.43. Forearm protectors circa early 1900s made of metal riveted to non-protective glove. Courtesy of Philip Pritchard, Hockey Hall of Fame, Toronto, Canada.

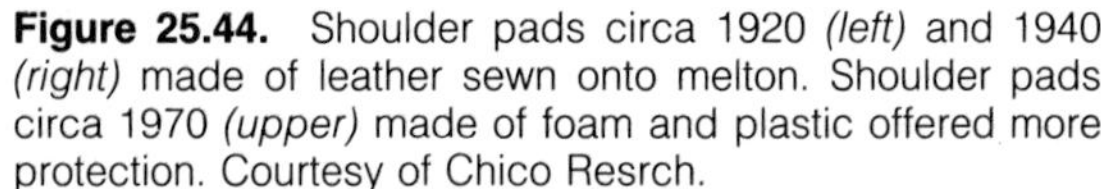

Figure 25.44. Shoulder pads circa 1920 *(left)* and 1940 *(right)* made of leather sewn onto melton. Shoulder pads circa 1970 *(upper)* made of foam and plastic offered more protection. Courtesy of Chico Resrch.

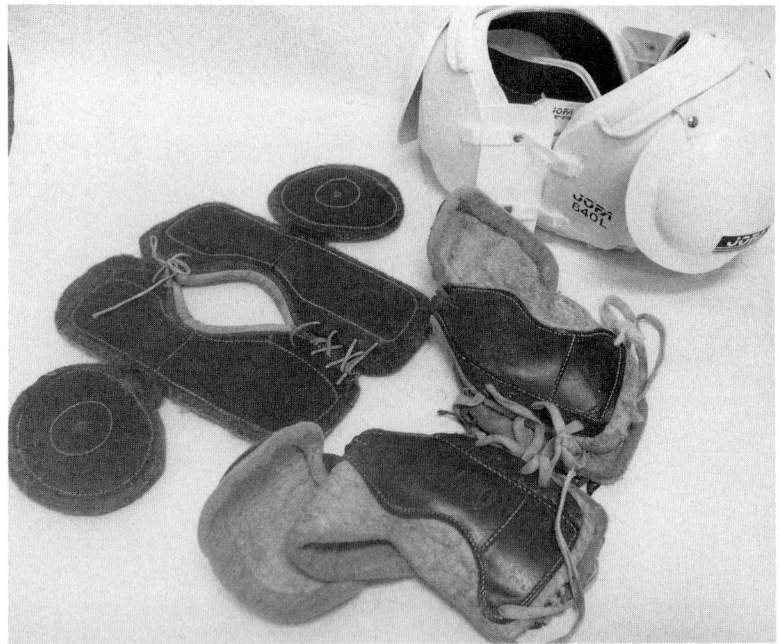

injury should be presumed to have a cervical spine injury (54).

Nagobads' unpublished studies of the early 1970s were the first formal ones on head injuries in ice hockey cited by Sims (37). Of nearly 100 injuries primarily caused by sticks, pucks, and collision (in that order), 30% were concussions or fractures despite the fact that helmets were worn by 87 of the 97 injured players.

Bull (53) describes numerous fatal and near fatal catastrophes in nonhelmeted players of yesteryear caused by impacts with ice, sticks, and boards that resulted in skull fractures and/or epidural and subdural hemorrhages. According to Bull (53), fractures and head injuries resulting in sudden or near sudden death have been curtailed in the era of the helmet (mandated even in the NHL for all players entering the League since

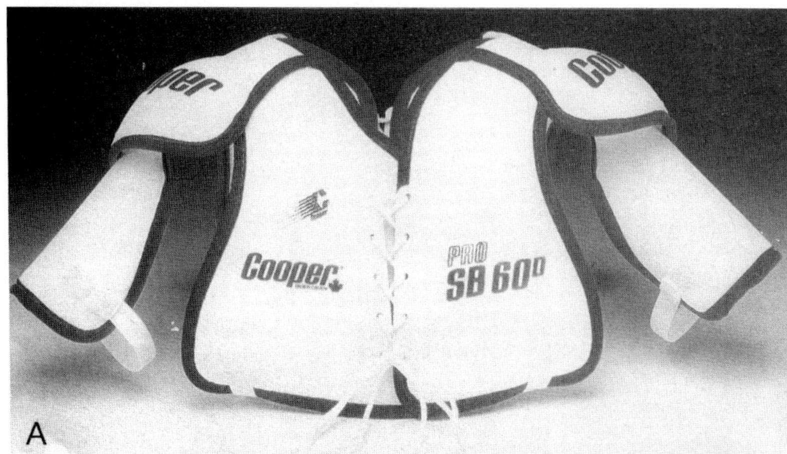

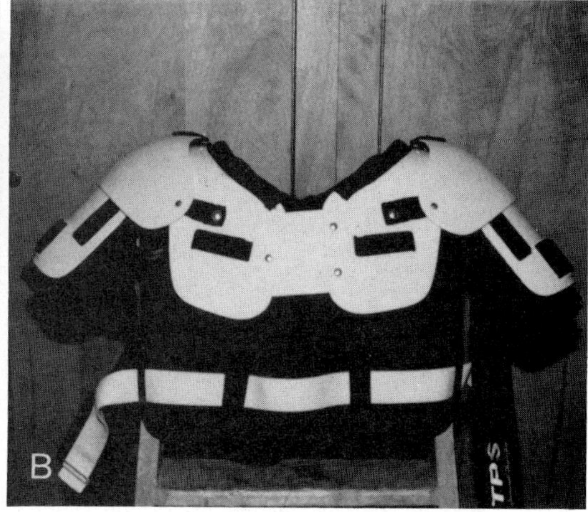

Figure 25.45. **(A)** Modern shoulder pads made of lightweight plastic and foam providing adequate shoulder and chest protection. Posteriorly, the shoulder pad should be continuous with the pant. **(B)** Modern shoulder pads made of thin foam and plastic with adequate coverage but inadequate protection. Cooper Canada, Toronto, Canada.

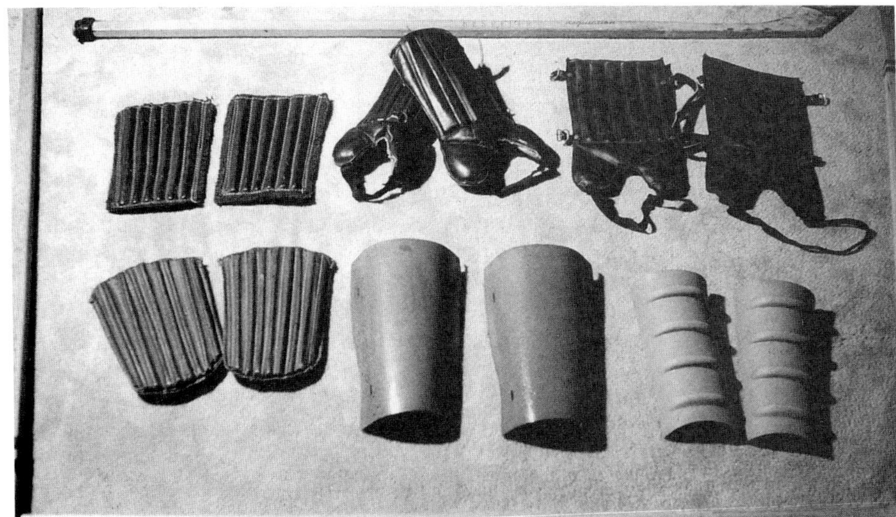

Figure 25.46. Cricket shin guards circa 1920 used for ice hockey. Courtesy of Dave Beaune, Toronto, Canada.

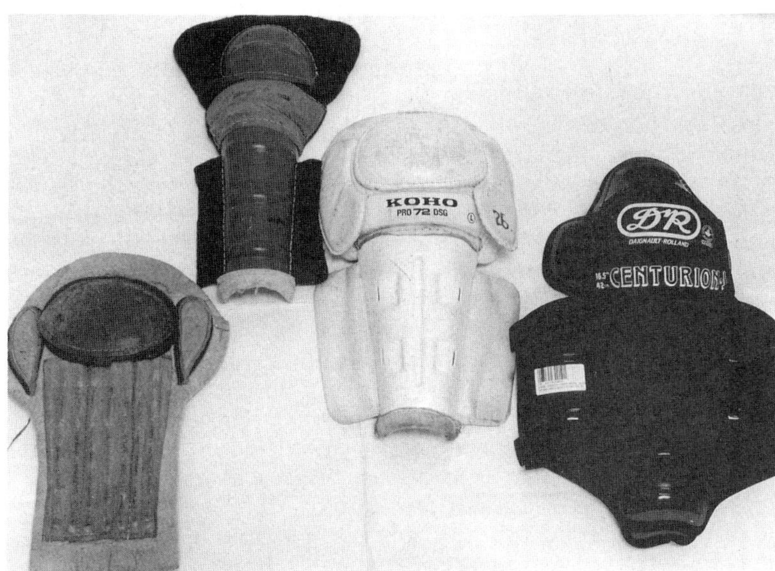

Figure 25.47. Shin pads circa 1930s *(left)* made for hockey with leather sewn onto melton. Dried sugar cane was used as struts for tibial protection. Evolution to the modern shin pads *(right)*. Note the increased protection of the patellar tendon, patella, peroneal nerve area and calf. Courtesy of Chico Resch.

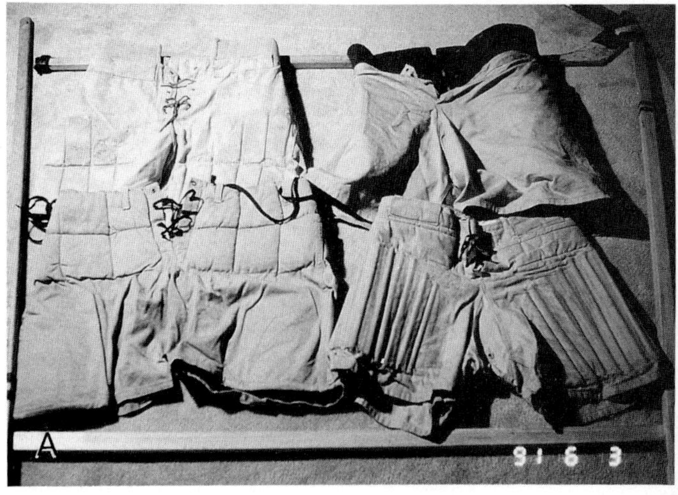

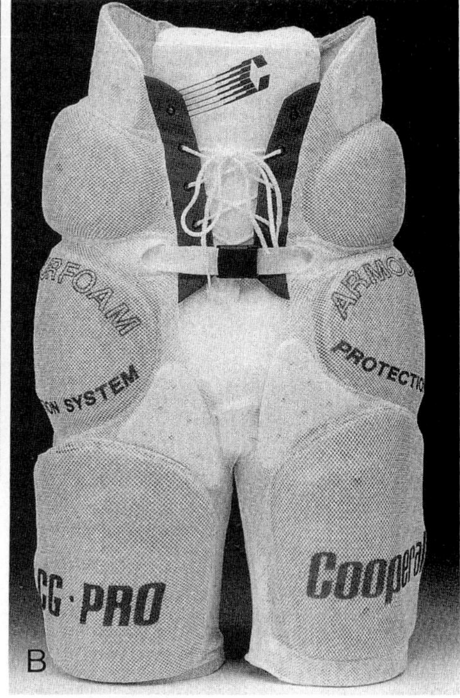

Figure 25.48 (A) Pants *(lower right)* circa 1930s with dried sugar cane struts sewn into pants **(A)** Courtesy of Dave Beaune, Toronto, Canada. **(B)** Modern pants with maximum protection. **(B)** Cooper Canada, Ltd., Toronto, Canada.

1980). Bull also cautions, however, that even helmeted players are subject to these injuries, particularly when poorly designed helmets are worn. Even the most effective helmet is of limited value if improperly fitted, or cross-matched with different manufacturer's face shield.

The attending physician must have a view of play that allows observation of injuries and their mechanism, easy access to the ice to facilitate emergency treatment, and a full array of the medical equipment needed to carry out treatment. Logistical issues, such as the availability of ambulances, hospitals, and special consultants, should be settled at the outset of the season. In instances of choking or apnea, it must be remembered that false teeth or even gum may have been dislodged from the mouth into the trachea (53). In one instance of loss of consciousness with apnea and cyanosis (experienced by one of the present authors) a video replay revealed that the mechanism was not a head injury, but a collision which drove the handle of the player's own stick into his solar plexus. In another personal experience of the author, a player hitting the boards with his face and chest lost consciousness for a moment and became dyspneic. Absent breath sounds presaged x-ray findings of a complete unilateral pneumothorax (in conjunction with a clinical concussion).

Sim et al. (54) state that hockey helmets are less tightly fitted than football helmets, and hence, their removal to maintain an airway is less risky than their being left in place.

The Face, Mouth, and Mandible

Initiation of protection against injury in hockey (as well as in other sports) took place in 1969 when the F-8 Committee of ASTM was formed to set standards for protective equipment; it antedated by 4 years the creation of the Committee of Safety and Protective Equipment USA Hockey (formerly AHAUS). Also, in the early 1970s, CR Castaldi proposed a mandatory mouthguard rule to AHAUS, and in 1974 face protector designs were undertaken for adoption as standard equipment (55).

Bull (53) makes the important point that behind every facial laceration is a potential fracture. Lacerations over the cheek area may overlie malar, zygomatic, or even orbital fractures.

Mandibular fractures are not uncommon in hockey, and most often require surgical treatment with internal fixation. A sense of malocclusion is often a clue in addition to whatever pain is present. While the "toothless" hockey player is a fading visual cliche, dental injuries have been a hockey tradition.

Sane et al. (56) studied maxillofacial and dental injuries in all registered ice hockey players in Finland between 1979–1982 (108,921 players) and between July, 1984 and December, 1985 (62,182 players). Full face masks were made mandatory beginning with the 1979–1980 season. In the first study period, 11.5% of 6885 injuries involved the maxillofacial and dental regions. Sticks were the primary culprits (54.1% of cases) and pucks were the second major cause (14.2% of cases). About 65% of these maxillofacial and dental injuries required prosthetic or endodontic treatment. Crown fractures were the most common injuries (51.7%) and serious bone fractures represented 7% of the series. Full face cages substantially reduced the incidence of injuries to the areas in discussion (56).

With head and face trauma, three particularly serious sequelae are of concern. The first is brain damage. The second is cervical spine pathology; this includes

Hockey Death Raises Gear, Rules Issues

Researcher Hopes It Will Spur New Testing

Hard-Hit Puck Caused Fatal Heart Attack

Central High School Students Shocked

By JOHN CLAYTON
Union Leader Staff

Although sporting goods manufacturers are held to demanding quality standards for most athletic equipment, there is no industry standard for hockey chest protectors like that worn by Kevin Charbonneau when he was killed last Saturday by a hockey puck.

And despite recent studies that show impact injuries to the heart to be the most common cause of sudden death in athletes, there are no efforts underway in amateur hockey circles to standardize body protection equipment.

Thus, even though the 15-year-old bantam player was encased in $500 worth of protective gear when he skated onto the ice at the West Side Arena last Saturday, the chest protection he wore was not regulated by the Hockey Equipment Certification Council (HECC) or the American Society of Testing and Materials (ASTM).

"They have standards for everything — helmets, face masks, mouth guards, shoulder pads, shin pads, even skate blades — but there is no standard on body protection equipment, which is far more imperative," said Dr. Blaine Hoshizaki, vice president for research and development for Canstar, manufacturer of Cooper and Bauer hockey gear.

In his Quebec testing labs, Hoshizaki fires hockey pucks into pads at speeds up to 100 miles per hour, but he admits that his firm is one of the few developing procedures to test body equipment.

"What happened in Manchester is a tragedy," Hoshizaki said, "and we can only hope that it will push the industry further to develop standards for body protection."

News of Charbonneau's death has spread quickly through the sporting world.

Information has already been forwarded to

HOCKEY, Page 12A

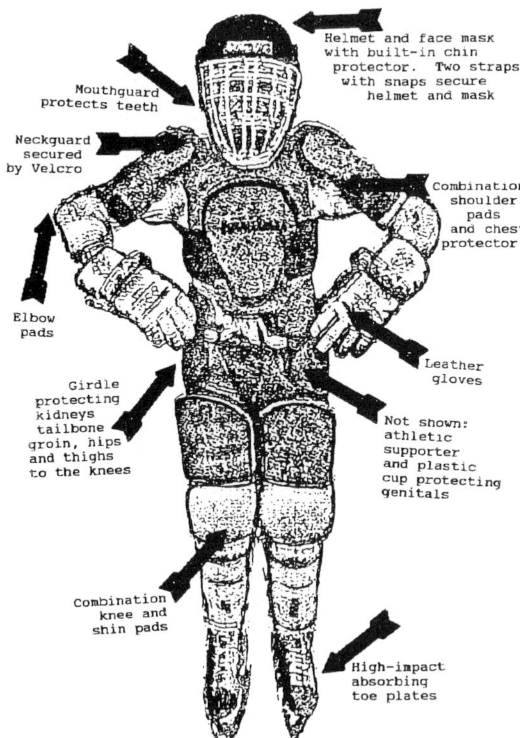

Equipment is key to youth hockey safety

By BARRY SCANLON
Democrat Staff Writer

By all accounts, the death of a 15-year-old Manchester youth hockey player last Saturday night was a freak accident.

Kevin Charbonneau, a member of a Hitchcock Clinic team, was struck in the chest by a slap shot during a Bantam League championship game at West Side Arena in Manchester.

An autopsy has revealed that the puck bruised Charbonneau's heart, causing it to beat irregularly and setting off a fatal heart attack.

His death has stunned the New Hampshire hockey community. It has also prompted safety directors and league officials to investigate how a similar accident can be prevented in the future.

The sobering fact is — outside of possibly waiting for technology to upgrade hockey equipment, which is already quite advanced compared to even a few years ago — it appears little can be done.

Figure 25.49. Newspaper reports of a fatality of a 15-year-old male who sustained a traumatic cardiac arrest as the result of a puck impact to the chest. Reports such as these underscore the need for the regulation of equipment.

fractures and dislocations (with paralysis). The third is permanent loss of vision due to an ocular injury.

The Neck and Spinal Fractures

In the experience of the authors, serious spine fractures are a rare occurrence. In nearly twenty years of an association with NHL teams, the authors have encountered several fractures of the transverse processes of the lumbar spine and a single instance of a fracture-dislocation of the cervical spine with quadraparesis.

Despite this relative paucity of spine trauma, Reid and Saboe (57) reported on just over 200 sport-related spine fractures collected over a 7 year period. Hockey accounted for 3% of these injuries, but just under 70% of the hockey-related fractures were associated with a permanent paralysis. Of the fractures diagnosed 50% were of the cervical spine. The mechanism of injury was consistently the same: the player either hit the boards or, prior to displaceable posts, the goalposts. Checks from behind often enhanced the impact (Fig. 25.50). Helmeted individuals were protected against severe concussion, but not from axial loading of the cervical spine with the neck in neutral or slight forward flexion (the usual fracture positions) (Fig. 25.50*B*).

The magnetic breakaway fixation introduced in the latter part of the 1980s, then abandoned in 1991 for flexible rubber posts, have reduced the threat of goalposts (Fig. 25.51). To reduce board injury, the boards

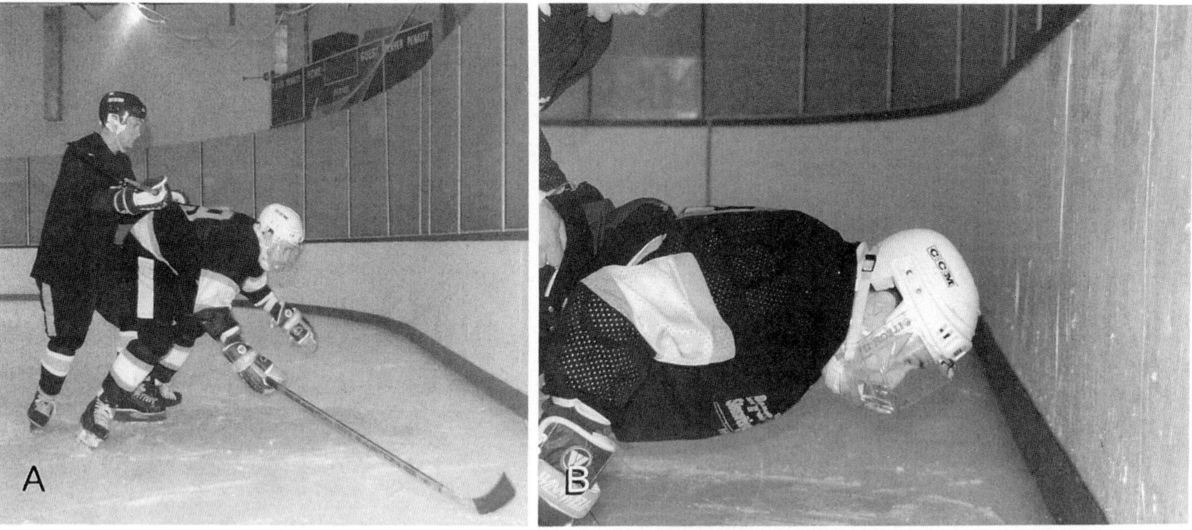

Figure 25.50. Checking from behind (illegal) with potentially catastrophic results. **(B)** A helmeted player striking the boards with axial loading of the cervical spine.

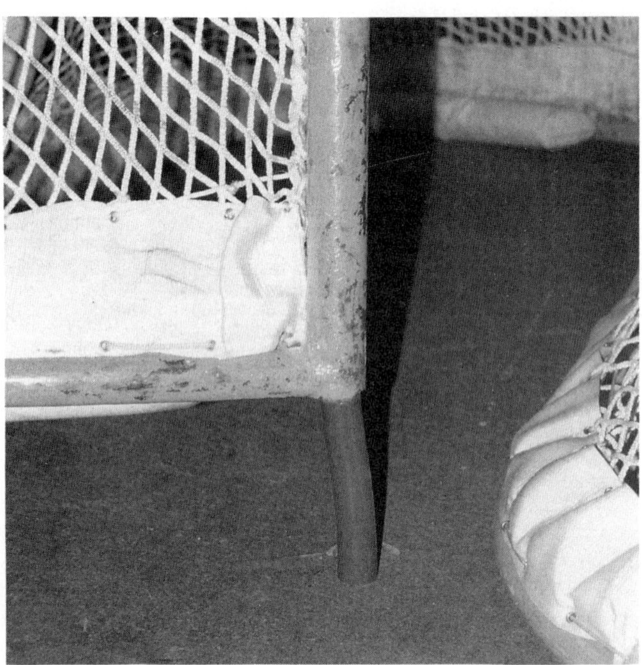

Figure 25.51. Flexible rubber posts used beginning with the 1991 season.

might be better padded or made more resilient; the development of a potential space between the boards and the plexiglass extension could inhibit face and head collisions. Reid and Saboe (57) did not confirm the contentions of those who blame face-mask pulling for a rising trend of cervical fractures in ice hockey. However, according to Sim et al. (37), Tator et al. fear that helmet and face-mask protective apparatus may be associated with an increasing frequency of cervical spine injury based upon an increased number of cases noted, starting in 1980.

Tator et al. (58) report that there had been no reports of spinal injury due to hockey in the English-speaking medical literature prior to 1984. Nevertheless, the Committee on Prevention of Spinal Cord Injuries due to Hockey was formed in 1981. By March, 1987, 117 hockey-related spinal injuries had been registered. The preponderance of victims (64%) were in the 11–20-year-old age group; 80% of the incidents involved the cervical spine. Just over 50% of those with injury to the spinal cord (52.1%) suffered a permanent sensory or motor loss, and 5 players died. Nearly 65% of the injuries were sustained as a result of a collision with the boards. The predominant causes were being pushed, checked, and/or tripped, with over 20% of episodes accounted for by players' having been pushed or checked from behind. In 1985, the CAHA initiated a prohibition against pushing and checking from behind. Almost all players in Tator's series were helmeted, and the majority were wearing face masks (58).

About 50% of the cervical spine injuries in the study of Tator et al. involved the region between C4 and C6, with burst fractures and fracture-dislocations predominating (Fig. 25.52). Bishop and Wells (59) indicate that the top of the crown of the head striking an immovable object results in axial compressive loading of the cervical spine. They studied this phenomenon using anthropometric test dummies (AIDS) propelled in free flight against a rigid barrier and used high speed photography to record the results. The protocol was performed with bareheaded and with helmeted (multiple types of helmets) AIDS and with the AIDS neck in neutral and in slight forward flexion. It was determined that once the head came to rest, inertial movement of the torso continued, thereby causing an "S"-shaped inflection of the cervical spine. Helmets did little to alleviate loads upon the neck. Using the formats represented in Figure 25.53 and computing the expected influences of anticipated spinal ligament tension and spinous process compression, Bishop and Wells determined the high probability of lower cervical vertebral failure (Table 25.9).

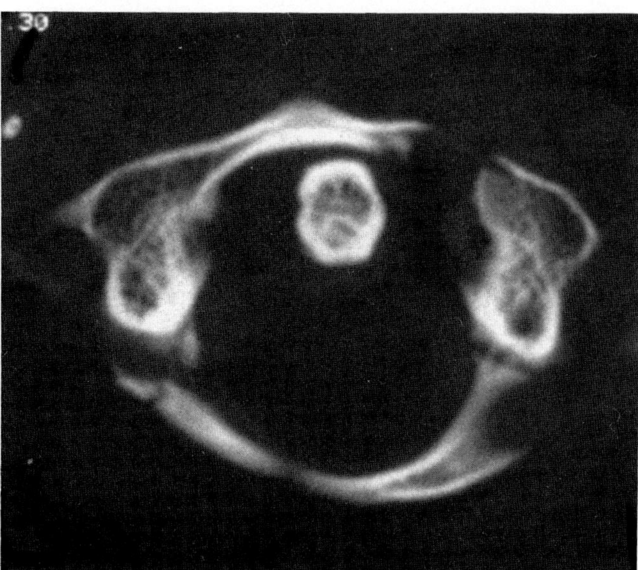

Figure 25.52. Relatively uncommon burst fracture of C1 (Jefferson Fracture) in a junior hockey player.

Table 25.9.
Dynamic Failure Loads in Compression for Cervical Vertebrae[a]

Aid	Level	Failure Loads Compression (N)	Peak Compressive Loads Axial (N)	Peak Compressive Loads Flexed (N)
2	C2	5750	4621	3859
3	C3	6125	5372	4677
4	C4-5	6875	5789	5005
5	C6	8000	6100	5119
6	C7-T1	9300	6055	5126

[a]N = Newtons; "Axial" and "Flexed" refer to AID neck postures. Adapted from Bishop PJ, Wells RP. Cervical spine fractures: mechanisms, neck loads, and methods of prevention. In: Castaldi CR, Hoerner EF, eds. Safety in ice hockey. Philadelphia: ASTM (STP 1050) 1989: 71–83.

These calculations were made on the basis of impact at 1.8 m/sec, knowing that impacts at 3.1 m/sec always cause cervical fracture and that hockey impacts can exceed 1.8 m/sec. Note the risk to failure with axial loading at the C5 level where fractures are most frequent.

While padded helmets effectively protect the brain from serious injury with the collision types in discussion, it would require padding several inches thick to prevent or deter cervical fractures, an obviously impractical consideration.

In seeking clues that would help prevent spinal catastrophes, Tator et al. (58) made some keen observations. These are excerpted in Table 25.10 in the left column.

Table 25.10.
Causes of Cervical Spine Injuries in Ice Hockey

Excerpted from Tator et al.[a]	Authors' Comments
1. Present size and weight of players increase forces of impact.	Unlikely major contributor since most injuries were in the 11–20 year old group.
*2. Sense of invincibility due to protective equipment.	Most players in the 11–20 age group wear helmets and shields.
3. Rules—often not enforced.	Unreasonable to assume refereeing quality has declined since 1980. Officials can only enforce rules after the fact.
*4. Coaching—Poor instruction in neck strengthening. Almost no reports of spinal injuries in Europe.	Not appropriate and/or ineffective in pre- or early adolescence. The issues of style and preventive coaching are serious considerations.
5. Rinks/Equipment—Small rinks implicated. Board rigidity implicated. Helmets and shields implicated.	Rink sizes have not changed; boards are rigid in Europe also. Helmets and shields in widespread use in the 1970s, also in Europe.

[a]Tator CH, et al. Spinal injuries in ice hockey players, 1966–1987. 1990.
*Major factor.

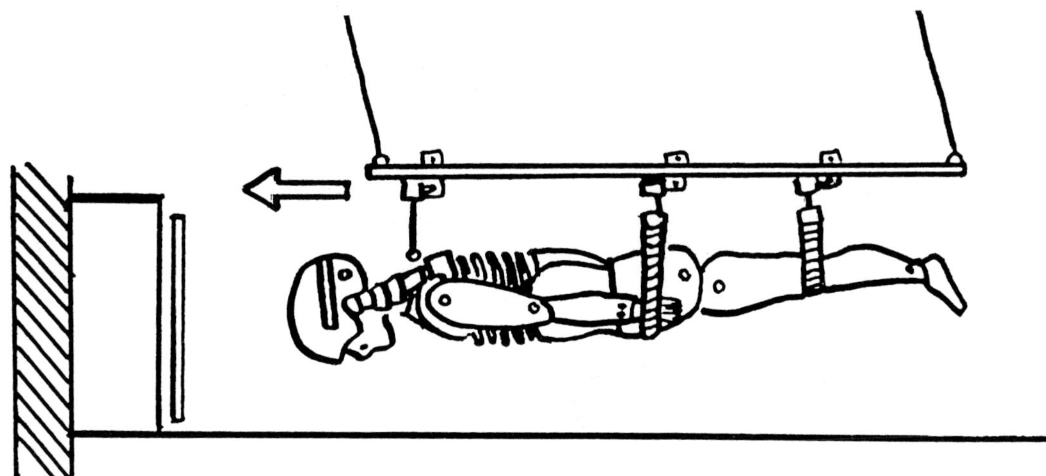

Figure 25.53. Loading apparatus testing cervical spine impact with test dummies. Adapted from Bishop PJ, Wells RP. Cervical spine fractures; Mechanisms, neck loads, and methods of prevention. In: Castaldi CR, Hoerner EF, eds. Safety in ice hockey. Philadelphia: ASTM 1989:71–83.

Helmets and shields have been implicated as causative agents by virtue of their widespread acceptance just prior to the onslaught of spinal injuries. However, their role in injury production is more likely psychological, producing a sense of invincibility for the North American style of hockey. In Europe, spinal injury is apparently less prevalent, despite the use of protective gear. This raises the issue of instruction in learning the game and in developing an attitude of play that is respectful of spinal trauma. In 1988, the Committee on Prevention of Spinal and Head Injuries produced a videotape for universal distribution entitled: *Smart Hockey*. A neck strengthening protocol, detailed in a brochure entitled: *Neck and Spinal Conditioning for Hockey Players* has also been disseminated by the Committee. Professional players, who wear a minimum of supracervical protective equipment, have suffered little in the way of spinal trauma, perhaps by virtue of their neck strength, or their know-how. Neck strengthening for females and younger (preadolescent) males is likely not to be productive from a protection standpoint. Bishop et al. (59) warn that the evolution of approval criteria to be met by helmet-mask protectors has resulted in a relatively heavy apparatus designed to avoid a foreward offset; this weight may predispose to cervical spine injuries. The weight of the apparatus on a weak young neck will foster fatigue of the neck muscles, adding a flexion moment to the neck.

"Uncrowding" rinks by altering their dimensions may help prevent these injuries to a degree, but it may be more practical and productive to concentrate on the padding, height, and/or shape of the sideboards. The several inches of padding that is excessive weight for helmets might be applied to the boards (if puck caroming can be controlled). If the boards are lowered, sloped away from the ice from bottom to top, and are curved for helmet deflection, cervical risk might be reduced. If the plexiglass is recessed away from the boards, there would be more potential space to allow dissipation of impact velocity. In any case, the foci of preventive efforts should be directed at the attitude and gamesmanship of players and at altering the energy absorption properties of the collision surfaces.

If a spinal fracture and/or dislocation should occur, proper control of neck movements is imperative, although no consensus has been reached (Table 25.11).

It is important in transporting the player to avoid manipulation of the disrupted area. Having assured an airway by whatever means is necessary, including tracheotomy, the spinal segment should be immobilized with the use of sandbags or support by immediately available implements, such as hockey gloves and cerclage taping. It is best *not* to implement traction in the absence of x-ray control. To get the player off the ice (Fig. 25.54), the authors recommend the scoop stretcher which separates longitudinally into two parts, each with a shovellike scoop. The two shovel-like portions are then slid beneath the player and closed without the need to lift the player at all.

Probably the best preventatives for soft tissue and bony injuries to the neck include a major program of neck strengthening (Fig. 25.55), avoidance of lowering the head anywhere near the boards to avert skeletal catastrophes, and the use of a neck protective device to prevent puck impacts and skate lacerations.

Table 25.11.
On-Field (Ice) Treatment of Cervical Spine Injuries

References	Suggested Treatment
75	". . . . . the single most important point to remember is: prevent further injury. Be sure that whatever action is taken does not cause further harm. Therefore, immediately immobilize the head and neck by holding them in the neutral position. . . ."
76	". . . . . his neck should be supported manually in a neutral position with his head and neck aligned with his spine. Forceful traction is unnecessary, and a pillow should not be placed under his head. If he holds his head in a fixed position, he may have locked the facets: no attempt should be made to straighten the neck out, maintaining it instead in a position in which he is holding it."
77	". . . . . working as a unit with the head and neck held neutrally, neither flexed nor extended, and with gentle traction applied, the patient is slowly turned onto the headboard or other flat surface. If the player is helmeted, the helmet is left on to take advantage of this excellent traction device."
78	". . . . . gentle traction for stabilization purposes is applied directly in line with the thoracic and cervical vertebrae."
79	". . . . . prevention of further injury is the most important objective in initial care of the victim. The team should not take any action that could possibly cause further damage. The first step should be to immobilize the head and neck by supporting them in a stable position . . . . at this point, simply maintain the position and monitor vital signs until transportation is available or until the athlete regains consciousness."
80	". . . . . when the unconscious athlete is approached on the field, the leader must be certain that no movements are initiated that could result in additional damage to the patient. The prevention of further injury must be the primary objective in management . . . the head and neck should be initially immobilized in a neutral position simply by manual stabilization."

Cervical fractures and dislocations are not the only serious neck injuries. Laryngeal fractures are also potentially life threatening. Stridor, hemoptysis, subcutaneous crepitus, and a loss of the "Adam's Apple" promontory ar the most flagrant signs of this fracture. A tracheotomy is sometimès necessary. A cross-check at the cervical level (Fig. 25.23 *J*, *K*) or garotting from behind (Fig. 25.56), with the stick across the front of the neck, are causes that are preventable by rule application or neck protectors. Bull (53) refers to the personal experience of McGrail who reported 6 laryngeal fractures over an 18-year period with an NHL team.

Eye Injuries and Protection

Eye damage with visual loss or compromise is one of the most worrisome consequences of sports accidents. It is among the greatest current concerns among NHL physicians. In the absence of face protectors, pucks and sticks inflict all-too-frequent eye injuries, which either compromise vision or blind outright (Fig. 25.57). Avoidance of such damage may only be accomplished with the use of eye protection devices. 1977 was a banner year of the advancement of eye protection in ice hockey. In that year, the ASTM Committee F-8 on sports equipment issued a standard for face protection in hockey, as did the CSA; the net result was a subsequent dramatic decrease in the incidence of eye injuries in amateur and professional hockey (11). Nevertheless, ocular pathology attributable to hockey has remained an epidemic that has been underappreciated by its participants. Progress toward ocular safety in ice hockey has been made grudgingly over the past two decades; improvements have come largely through the crusading efforts of two ophthalmologists, Tom Pashby in Canada and Paul Vinger in the United States, who have pioneered protective reforms in their respective countries.

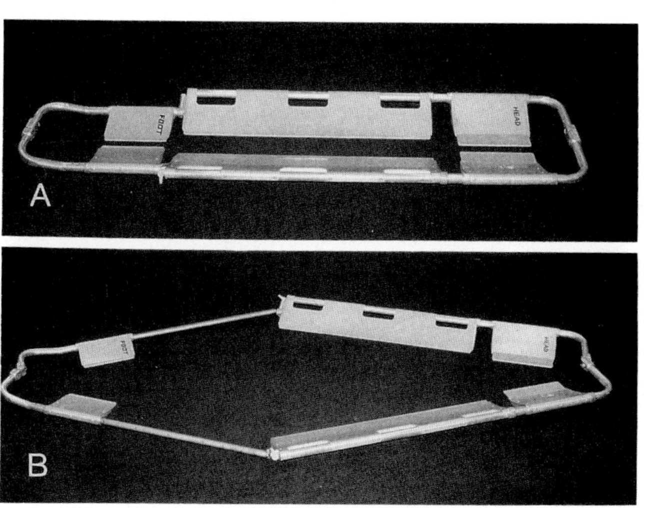

Figure 25.54. Scoop Stretcher; *(a)* closed, *(b)* open.

In 1974, statistics of an eye injury survey in hockey were presented by Pashby (1, 60), demonstrating that eye injuries in hockey had become an unchecked epidemic. Twenty eyes had been blinded, primarily from sticks and mostly in the age range of 11 to 15.

In 1975, Pashby and Vinger joined forces. Polycarbonate and heavy wire mesh face protectors were produced. Face masks were mandated 2 years later by AHAUS for all but Junior A and B players. And the CAHA issued a similar mandate (1977). The Hockey Equipment Certification Council (HECC) was also formed in 1977 (55). Results of the ongoing eye injury

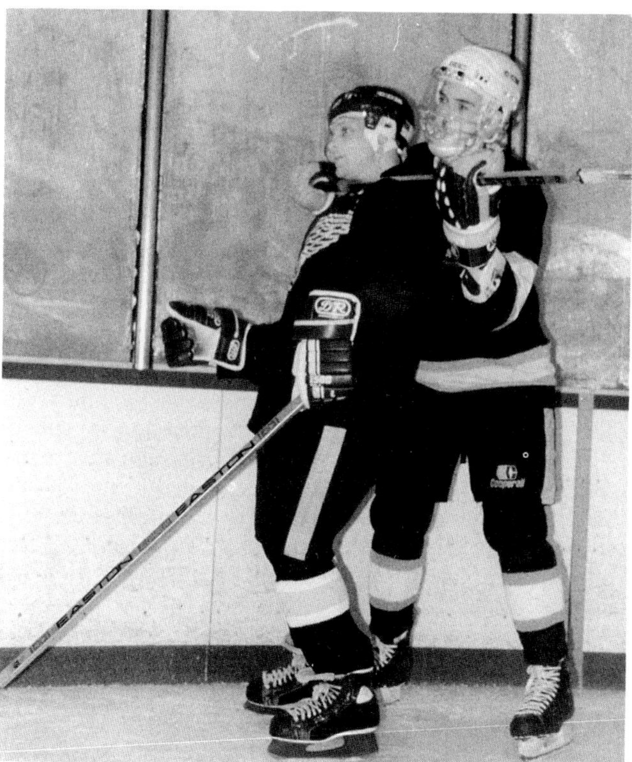

Figure 25.56. Garotting from behind.

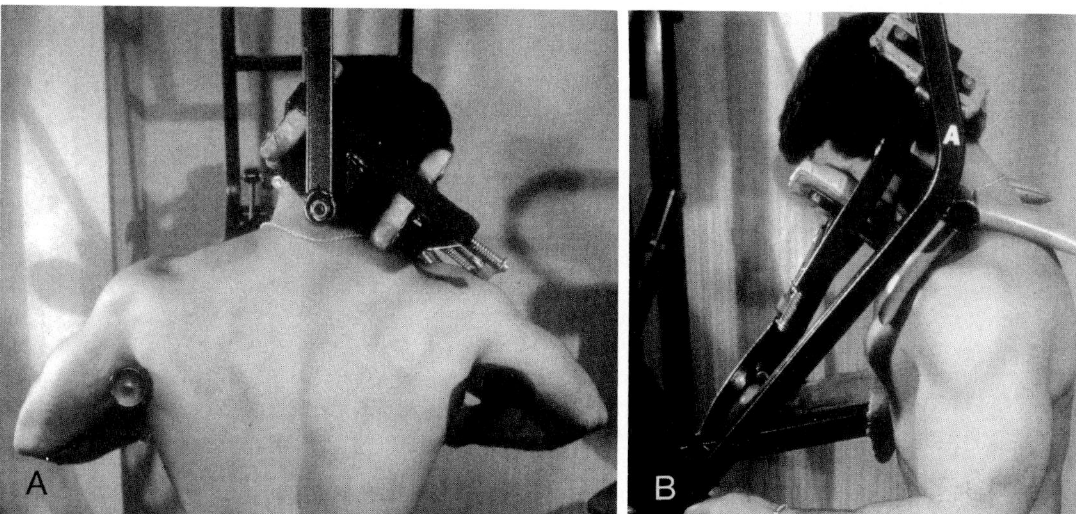

Figure 25.55. A, B. Neck strengthening exercises.

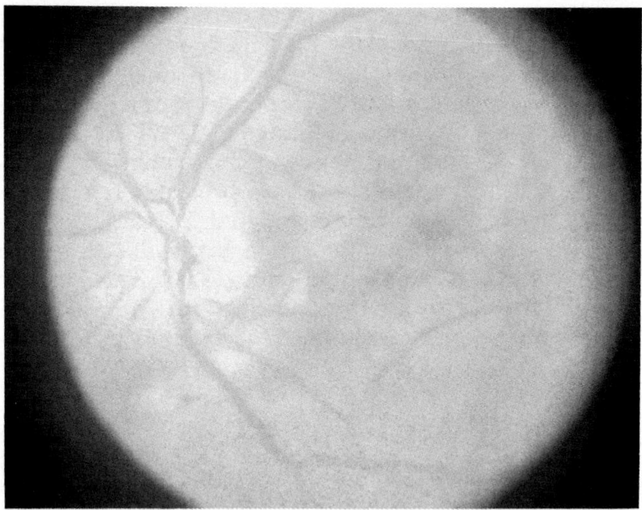

Figure 25.57. Professional hockey player without face mask was hit in the right eye by a puck sustaining a hyphema. Retinal hemorrhages and partial loss of central vision were the consequences. The player may go on to develop secondary glaucoma as a result of damage to the ciliary body.

Table 25.12.
Ocular Injuries and Blinded Eyes Among Canadian Hockey Players[a]

Season	Number/Injuries	Number/Blind Eyes
1972–1973	287	20
1974–1975	258	43
	Face Masks Introduced to Canadians	
1976–1977	90	12
1977–1978	52	8
1978–1979	43	13
1979–1980	85	21
1980–1981	68	20
1982–1983	119	18
1983–1984	124	12
1984–1985	121	18
1985–1986	123	22
1986–1987	93	18

[a]With permission from Pashby TJ. Ocular injuries in hockey. Int Ophthalmol Clin 1988; 28;3:229.

survey in Canada for the 1976–1977 season demonstrated an altered pattern. The 12 cases of blind eyes occurred only in players who wore no masks, and were older, mostly over 16 years of age. Studies in subsequent years of the decade persisted in showing a trend of reduced blindness and a rising average age of the afflicted; those with face protectors remained essentially immune. The predominance of stick-inflicted serious injuries decreased as puck-induced injuries increased (1, 60).

Vinger (55) made the statement that prior to the institution of mandatory eye and face protectors, two thirds of all injuries in hockey were a result of eye and face injuries As of the end of 1980, the CAHA and AHAUS had each mandated full face protectors fastened to helmets for all players including goalies. At about the same time, new players entering the NHL were required to wear helmets, but without specifications and without a requirement to wear face shields.

A chronological summary of ocular injuries in relation to blindness is seen in Table 25.12.

Jones (46) states the issue of the eye injury with cynical accuracy: "The belief that 'it will never happen to me' is common. . . ." Wilson et al. (1977) surveyed players at all levels of play and determined that only 3% of college players and 9% of professionals considered a mask acceptable (61). They concluded a mandate was needed.

An epidemiologic survey questionnaire was distributed to the players at the NHL in 1987 (28). The players were asked to prioritize their concerns about injuries to various body parts. Of the players (90 of 225) responding, 40% ranked knee ligament injuries their primary concern. Remarkably, only 14% of players ranked head and face injuries in first place; and only 0.5% placed their concern for their eyes first. From a medical standpoint, the priority concerns are in inverse proportions to those expressed by the players. Two important conclusions result from this study. The first is that players are undereducated about the import of such injuries and about treatment results when injuries to these areas occur. The second is that the failure of education has been a major obstacle to the routine donning of helmets and face protectors, when not specifically mandated by rules governing the hockey organization of which the player is a member (e.g., the NHL and amateur leagues for older players).

Pashby (1, 60) offers the following suggestions to reduce the sequelae of hockey violence in general and of eye injuries in particular. He asserts that rink sizes should be standardized and that the end-board-to-goal distance should be lengthened from 10 to 13 feet to obviate collisions due to congestion. These parameters, including rink dimensions of 200 × 100 feet, are stipulated in the rulebook of the International Ice Hockey Federation (IIHF) (62).

Based upon more than 30,000 responses to questionnaires answered by parents of hockey-playing children in Canada, the following excerpted summation of feelings is presented:

1. Skills only taught prior to age 10.
2. No all-star hockey prior to age 11.
3. No slap-shooting prior to age 12.
4. No body-checking prior to age 13.
5. More appropriate leadership in prevention should be demonstrated by junior and professional teams.
6. At least one practice should take place for each game.
7. Referees should be less inhibited in calling penalties.
8. Players should serve out all penalties and not be released even when a goal is scored.

An additional recommendation offered by the Minister of Fitness and Amateur Sport of Canada (1980) is to give full responsibility for player conduct to the

Table 25.13.
Risk Level for Eye Injury in Certain Sports, and Recommendations for Protective Wear

Risk	Sport	Protective Wear
Unacceptable	Boxing	Not Applicable
Very High	Ice Hockey Basketball	Helmet with full visor
Protector		Polycarbonate Sports

[a]Adapted with permission from Jones NP. Eye Injury in Sport. Sports Med. 1989;7:178.

coaches, as an inducement to mellow any thoughts of teaching aggression (1).

The goal in developing prophylactic eye devices is the dissipation and diffusion of potentially damaging forces away from the soft ocular structures and toward the less vulnerable bony orbit and periocular soft tissues. Recommended sports eye protection is listed for three sports in Table 25.13.

There are those in the NHL who would argue not only that the introduction of helmets and face masks is an invitation to increased use of the stick and to other violence directed toward the head (see discussion on neck trauma and equipment), but also that the wearer has an increased sense of invulnerability and may demonstrate increased aggression in charging the goal and elsewhere in the game. An increased risk of cervical sprains and fractures has also been ascribed to face masks, when upward leverage on the mask results in hyperextension injuries. The absence of any mandate to wear face protection in the NHL has initiated the creation of special rules governing their use, e.g., an instigation penalty for player with protection who taunt unprotected players into aggressive retaliatory acts.

The Lower Extremity

The Knee

Hockey players sustain the full gamut of knee injuries, ranging from torn menisci to torn cruciate and collateral ligaments. It is the mechanisms by which these injuries are commonly caused that are characteristic of ice hockey. As indicated by Bull (53), the basic mechanism in ice hockey is almost invariably contact, whereas in sports with greater degrees of foot fixation (as with cleats), many meniscal and ligament injuries are sustained in the act of cutting (without contact). Paradoxically, it is the absence of foot fixation that often enables hockey players to function with moderate instabilities not withstood in other sports. In any case, the hockey player skating with the knee in flexion (which is the case for most of the stride), has his knee exposed to collisions by the knees or thighs of opponents. A hit is usually received on the lateral aspect of the knee, spraining the medial side of the joint and often tearing the anterior cruciate ligament as well as the medial capsule (Fig. 25.23*P*). Derotational braces and strengthening suffice for lesser degrees of disruption, but surgical reconstruction is needed for severe ligament disruptions. Sometimes a player's knee is hit from the front, causing a hyperextension injury. Although an effusion and missed playing days are the rule, ligamentous disruption is rare. Magnetic resonance imaging (MRI) often shows bone bruising on the anterior aspect of the femoral condyle(s). A hyperextension-blocking brace and physical therapy are the usual treatments.

The knee-shin protective apparatus is not always efficient in preventing injuries. The authors have witnessed a variety of patellar fractures despite the protection. These have been caused by pucks, falls against the ice, and by hitting the boards knee-first (Figs. 25.58 and 25.59).

The flimsy hinge between the knee and shin shells allows pucks to hit the interval overlying the patellar tendon (Fig. 25.47). Traumatic tendinitis ensues and can result in a loss of playing time.

Ankle and Foot

Ankle sprains are infrequent in ice hockey by virtue of the rigidity of the skate boot. However, entrapment of the skate blade by the ice or against the boards, as the pronated ankles is abducted and externally rotated by the player's inertia, will not infrequently produce a low grade syndesmosis rupture. McConkey (63) indicates that ankle syndesmosis injuries occur by a different mechanism than do common ankle sprains. They result from pronation-external rotation or pronation-abduction displacements, which may produce a sequence of injuries beginning with rupture of the distal tibiofibular syndesmosis and progressing to ruptures of the interosseous membrane and/or the deltoid ligament, or even fracture of the fibular neck.

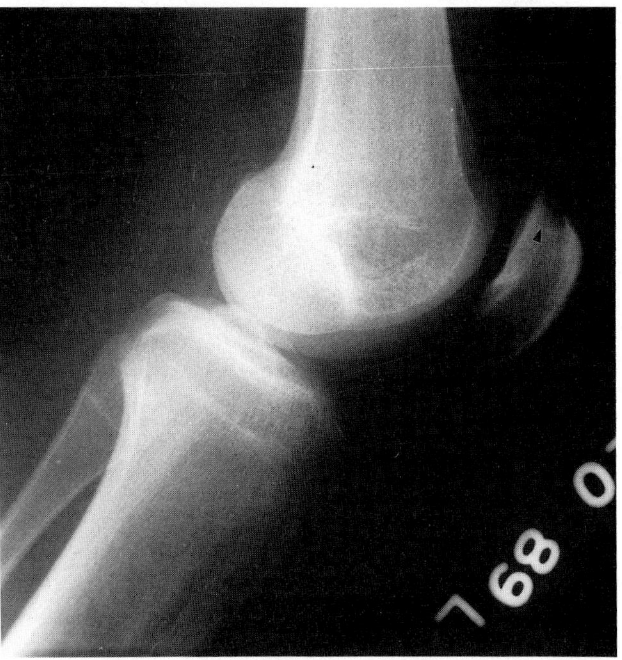

Figure 25.58. Division I collegiate hockey player who sustained a direct impact of the knee against the ice resulting in a superior pole avulsion type fracture *(arrowheads)*.

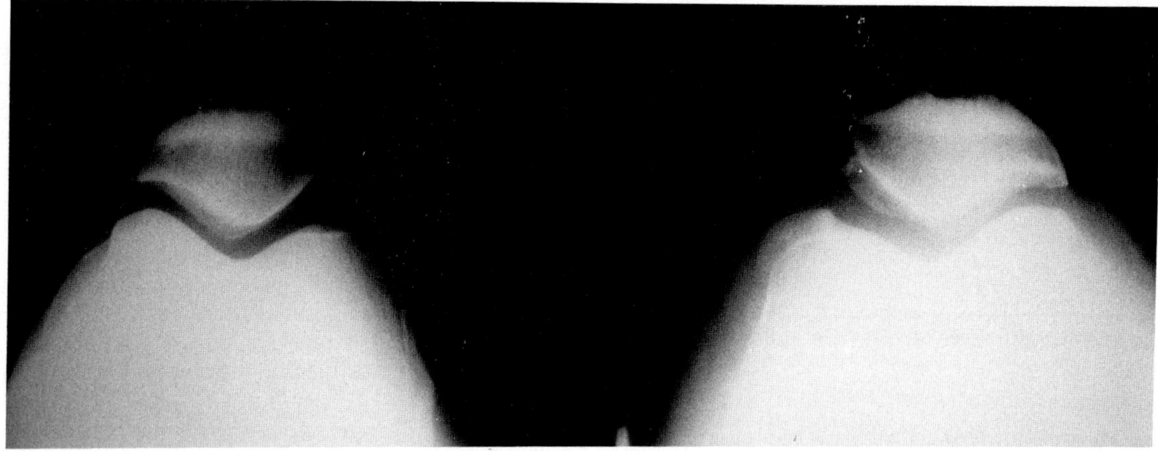

Figure 25.59. Patellar irregularities in a retired NHL "Hall of Fame" defenseman who sustained multiple contusions to the knees during his career.

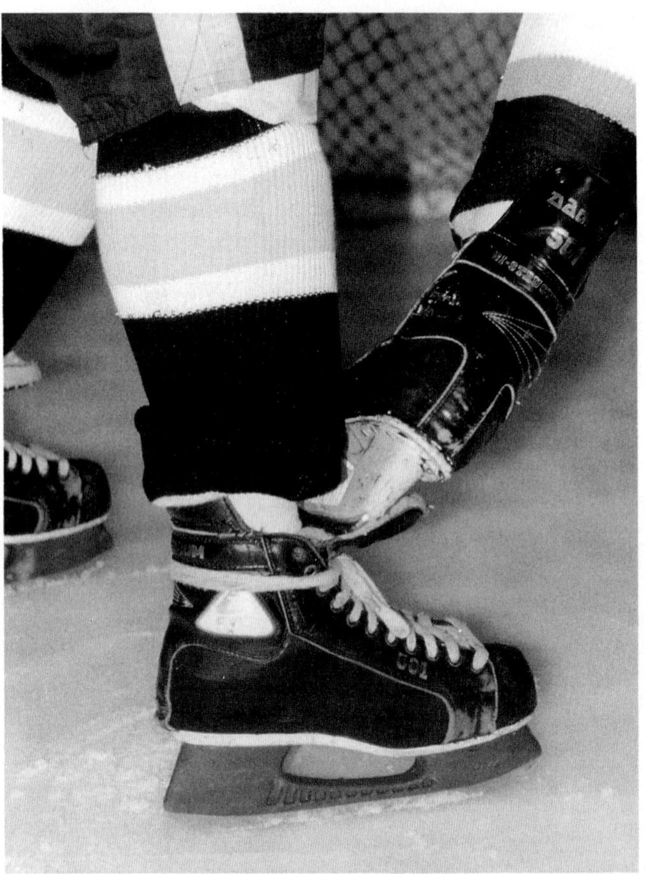

Figure 25.60. Representation of the mechanism of extensor tendon laceration. Note the top 2 eyeholes of the player's skates are not laced and the tongue is not taped to the anterior shin pad.

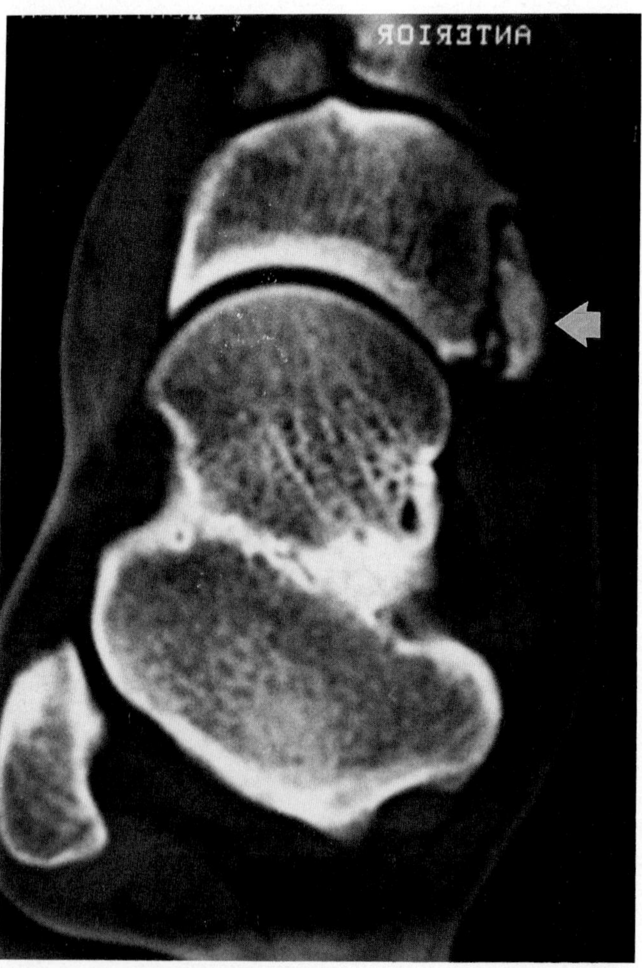

Figure 25.61. Fracture of the medial side of the navicular *(arrowhead)* due to puck impact.

Fractures of the ankle are relatively uncommon but bursal enlargements over the malleoli, which have been repeatedly impacted by pucks, are common.

In lacing skates, it is usual to make the distal and upper laces very tight while leaving the throat area lacing looser for flexibility. The tightness of the upper boot lacing sometime cause extensor tenosynovial reactions and even painful venous thromboses of the superficial veins. Some players leave the skate tongue everted for greater flexibility. This has led to an incidence of lacerated extensor tendons from skate blades (Fig. 25.60).

Fractures of the feet are relatively common, almost invariably the result of the puck. The most commonly fractured bone is the navicular (Fig. 25.61). If nondisplaced, players will often play through the pain.

On occasion, a player may slide and hit the boards with the blade portion of the boot. While severe injuries are uncommonly encountered, Figures 25.62*A–G* demonstrates, a dramatic consequence. Such injuries stimulate thoughts about modifying the design of the boot.

The Upper Extremity
Common Shoulder Afflictions

Acromioclavicular (AC) separations are among the most common injuries sustained by postadolescent and adult hockey players. In an NHL locker room, finding

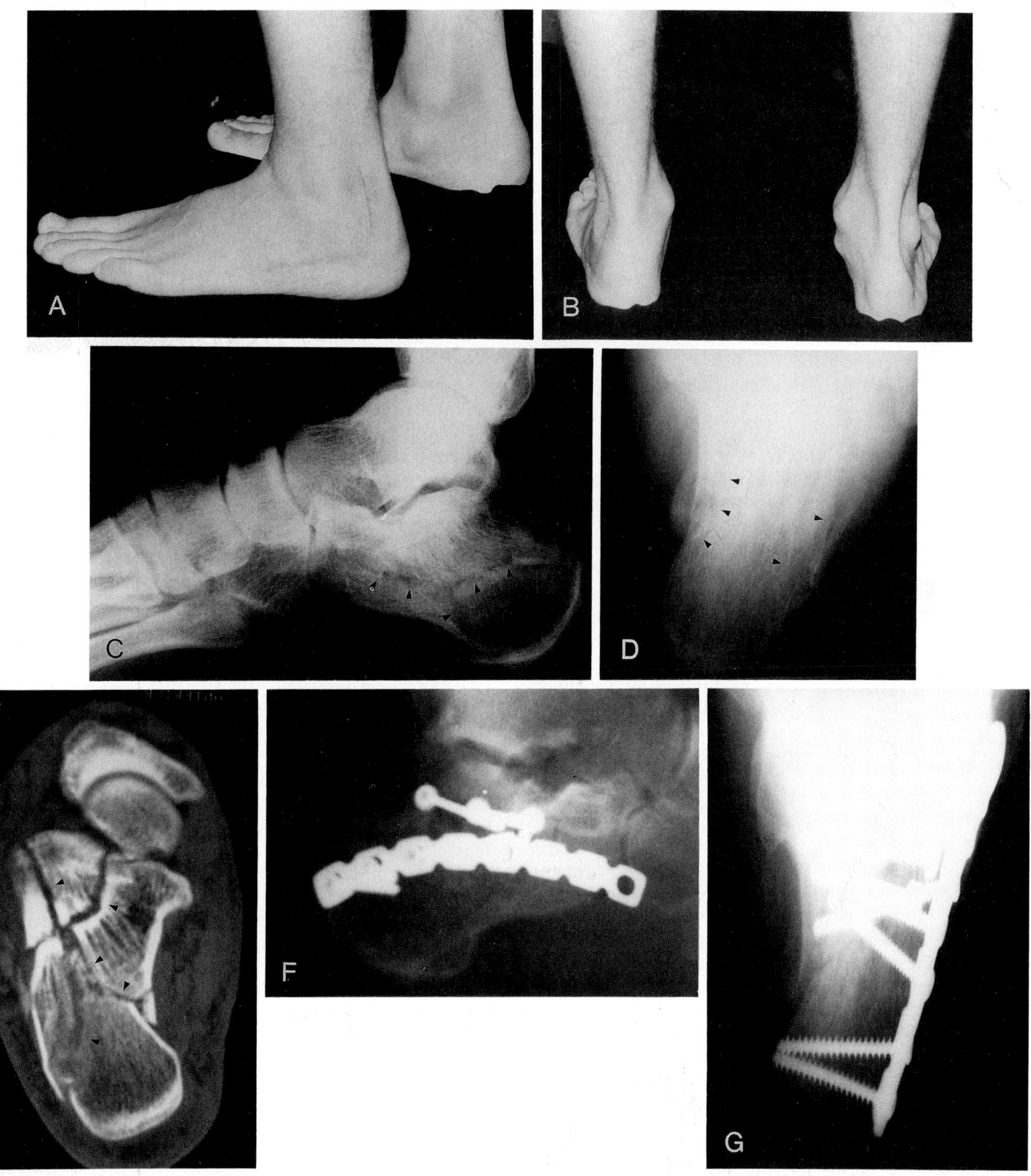

Figure 25.62. Professional hockey player with a comminuted and displaced fracture of the left calcaneus. **(A** and **B),** Clinical postoperative photograph; **(C** and **D),** preoperative radiograph; **(E),** preoperative CT scan; **(F** and **G),** postoperative radiographs.

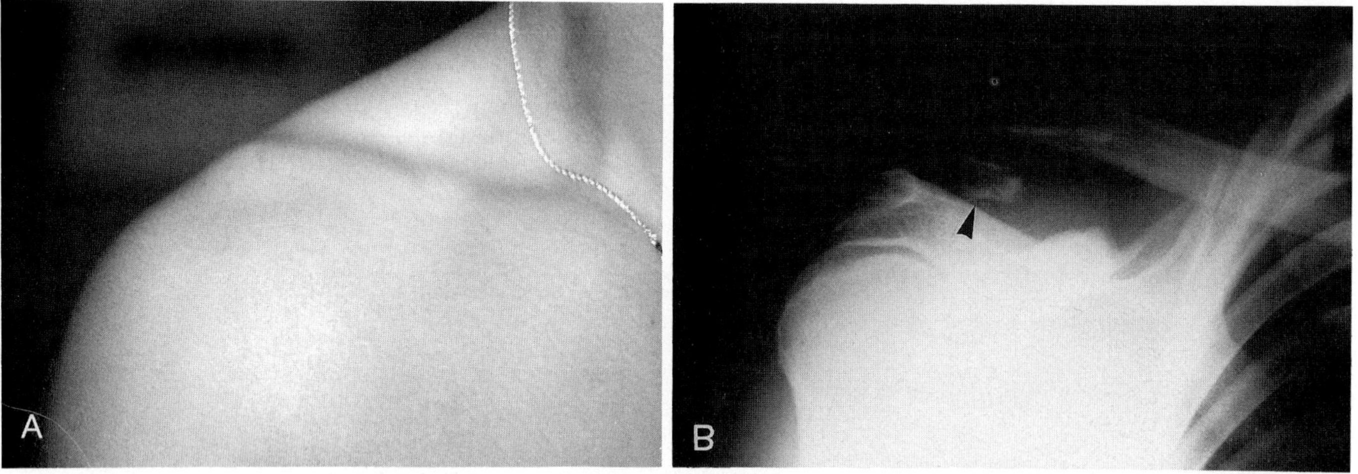

Figure 25.63. **(A)** Professional hockey player who sustained an acromioclavicular separation with an associated fracture of the distal end of the clavicle (**B,** *Arrowhead*).

players with two normal AC joints is the exception rather than the rule (Fig. 25.63).

In testimony to the common involvement of the acromioclavicular joint in hockey is the study by Norfray et al. (61). Professional and amateur hockey players were evaluated radiographically. It was determined that 35 of 77 evaluated professional players (or 45.5%) demonstrated radiographic abnormalities of the clavicle and/or acromioclavicular joints; 31% of the abnormalities were confined to the AC joint. Clavicular fractures were more common than ligamentous disruptions among young teenage amateurs while the reverse was true in amateurs between 18 and 21 years of age. The injury is commonly caused by the transmission of force to the AC joint due to impact of the outstretched abducted arm or the point or back of the shoulder against the ice or the boards. The AC joint may be separated with or without an associated fracture of the portion of clavicle or acromion adjoining it (Fig. 25.63*B*). Almost regardless of the grade of the separation, operative intervention as a primary treatment is rarely, if ever, needed. This is in accord with the study of Glick et al. (65) in which 35 unreduced AC dislocations in athletes (more than 50% of which were in football players) were followed for an average of 3 years. Of these, 70% returned to their specific sport within 4 weeks, and the majority were uninhibited by symptoms other than weakness. A tardy excisional arthroplasty (with resection of the distal end of the clavicle) can be performed if severe pain and/or significant restriction of arm elevation in abduction results from the impinging hypertrophy of the dislocated clavicular head. The senior author of the present text (JM) has operated on no acute AC dislocations and found the need to perform two tardy joint arthroplasties in 20 years with an NHL team. Pain with use and restricted arm elevation were the indications for surgery.

In the cases of many grade I dislocations, players miss none to a few games due to pain and disability. In mild grade II dislocations, players miss 10 to 14 days, and with grade II-III dislocations, they miss 3 to 6 weeks due more to the delay in restoration of adequate strength than to actual pain. Traditionally, the last range of motion to be restored to adequate strength is horizontal abduction, an important range used by players to push their opponents away in struggles along the boards (Figs. 25.19*A* and 25.64). Since the mechanisms by which the injury is sustained are by transmitted forces rather than by direct impact to the joint, protective equipment is not preventive despite the marketing statements of some manufacturers. Upon return to play after recovery, larger protective shoulder pads (Fig. 25.45*B*) help withstand the pain of direct blows, but recurrences of dislocation symptoms are observed on occasion. Subcutaneous dislocations (severe grade III) should be operated, if for no other reason than to reattach the muscles bridging the joint area (the deltoid and trapezius, in particular). Over the past two decades, the once popular trend of operating on AC dislocations, by any of the numerous techniques available, has waned. The once equally popular use of acromioclavicular separation harnesses has also been abandoned because of the limited success (and value) of the reductions they effected and because of the pressure sores they often produced in the skin beneath the shoulder strap and overlying the bony deformity. It is now more popular among sports orthopedists to initiate a strengthening and motion program as soon as tolerance permits (often immediately).

Shoulder (glenohumeral) dislocations and subluxations are common in ice hockey, but they are an infrequent cause of missed player days. Thomson (24) reported shoulder dislocations and separations to be among the 3 most frequent groupings of injuries in his analysis of more than 1000 amateur player injuries. Hovelius (66) reported an 8% incidence of recurrent dislocation among the most elite of Sweden's divisions. Taking into consideration that most hockey players are "left handers" (the left is the bottom hand on the stick), Hovelius (66) undertook to study the relevance of this fact to dislocation. He concluded that 80% of the oper-

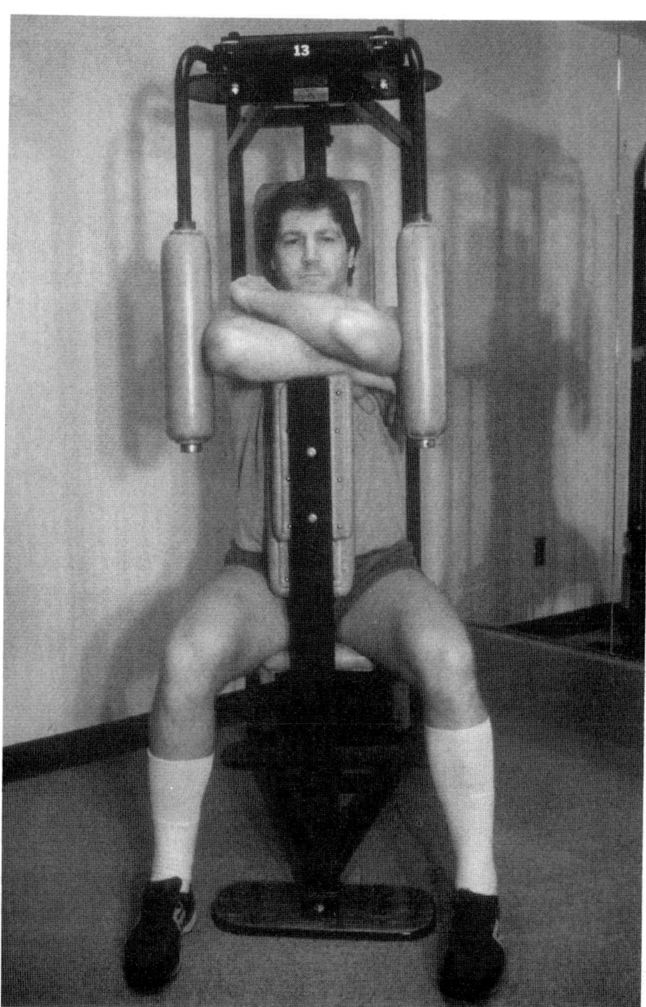

Figure 25.64. Horizontal abduction used frequently in hockey to push opponents during interactions along the boards.

ative repairs were performed upon the left shoulder, but that this is not a representation of the distribution of unstable shoulders (dominant versus nondominant).

The present authors have not observed this skew in an NHL team. In nearly 20 years with an NHL team the senior author (JM) has had occasion to pursue surgical reconstructions in only 4 players with 2 reconstructions in the right, and 2 in the left shoulder. Many player have unilateral or bilateral subluxability evident in preseason examinations, but few players have frank dislocations during the season. The occasional player with a history of chronic recurrence often shrugs off his periodic dislocations, allowing or assisting them to reduce and then returning immediately to play. The advent of arthroscopy and MRI permit detailed evaluations of labral, cuff, and Bankart lesions after acute dislocations. The "modern" player, being more concerned about a progression of damage, may use the information from these tests to decide to pursue reconstruction, partly as prophylaxis but also as a means of eliminating the current disability. In other instances, the dislocations are so disabling that a decision to operate need not be predicated upon an elucidation of existing

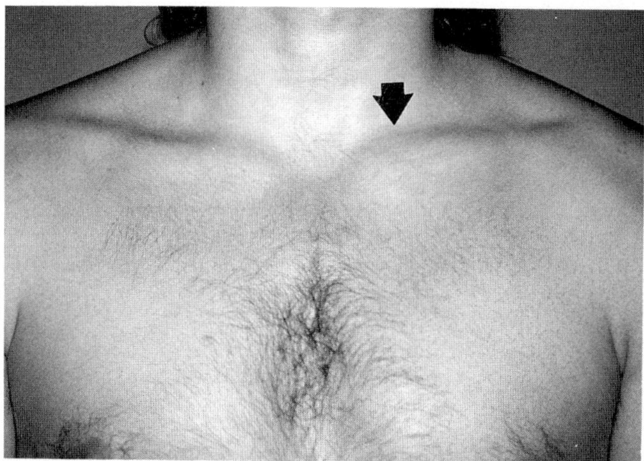

Figure 25.65. Sternoclavicular injury *(arrowhead)* in a professional hockey player. Pain and swelling was noted after being checked into the boards chest-first.

pathology. In many instances, players determine that they will tolerate their instability, either until the end of the season, or sometimes, indefinitely. Dislocation harnesses may help inhibit the tendency to dislocation, but players complain about the severe inhibition of functional motion they create. Overall, for those electing to play, the most effective potentiator of shoulder function is a continuing program of strengthening, emphasizing the internal rotators.

The Sternoclavicular Joints and Ribs

Not as frequent as AC joint injuries are sternoclavicular injuries (Fig. 25.65). These are sustained by hitting the boards chest-first, while experiencing a sudden retraction of the shoulders from a hit to the back. These injuries and injuries of the ribs and costochondral junctions are treated by abstinence from play as well as by supportive and symptom-relieving measures, after ascertaining that the underlying viscera are unimpaired. Special protection, such as a flack jacket, on return to play is recommended.

Elbow

Apart from simple contusions and impact injuries to the elbow, the more common significant afflictions are olecranon bursitis and hyperextension and/or valgus injuries to the capsule. Either may be caused by falls on the ice or elbow-first collisions into the boards. In addition, leveraged forces through the player's stick by an opponent can cause capsular injuries. Standard elbow pads are not always helpful in preventing concussive damage and are of no help in leverage injuries.

Olecranon bursitis is sometimes acute, but more often chronic. The pressure from an enlarged, tense bursa can be painful, but rarely precludes play. Aspiration should only be considered for severe pain and/or restricted motion or to rule out the presence of infected contents. In most cases, the bursal inflammation subsides after the season without a need for surgical excision.

Hyperextension and/or valgus injuries can be disabling enough to cause a loss of playing days. Shooting the puck, pressing the stick against the ice, and pushing opponents away are painful. Hyperextension blocking braces with hinges or strappings are often helpful in providing stability and allaying pain. Modalities and strengthening exercises accelerate a return to function. Surgery has never been necessary in the authors' experience.

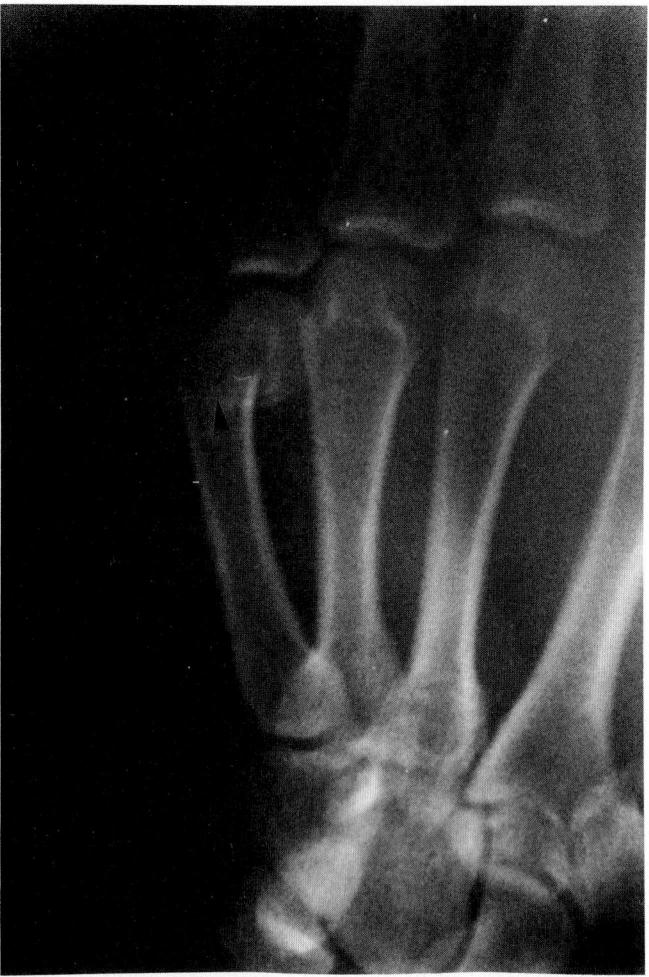

Figure 25.66. Fracture of 5th metacarpal neck (boxer's fracture). The unwanted result of fisticuffs.

Hand and Wrist

The variety of hand and wrist injuries in hockey is too large to cover. Fractures of the metacarpals occur from slashes and fisticuffs (Fig. 25.66). Carpal fractures and dislocations derive from falls on the flexed or extended wrist. But perhaps the most traditional hand injury is the "gamekeeper's thumb." Bull (53) indicates that this can come from fighting, but more particularly, from falls with stick in hand, whereby the stick imparts a radially directed force that ruptures the ulnar collateral ligament of the metacarpophalangeal joint (MPJ). Surgery is frequently necessary to restore maximum function, but spica immobilization is sometimes adequate for partial tears and when there has been no concurrent bony avulsion. Specially contrived splints of plastic or fiberglass may be used to permit the player to continue performing.

Dermatologic Disorders

Contact dermatitis is a relatively common entity among hockey players. It is manifested as either an acute or chronic inflammatory disorder of the skin secondary to irritation. Such irritant skin reactions in athletes are usually secondary to physical and mechanical agents. In hockey players, the excessive sweating beneath protective equipment results in an eczematous dermatitis (Fig. 25.67), fondly referred to as "the gonk" (67).

Soft Tissue Injuries

Musculotendinous Strains

The incidence of strains in NCAA hockey was 54 per 1000 exposures, or about 17% of injuries for the 1989–1990 season (22). In the NHL, the predominant strain is the groin or adductor pull. In the 1986–1987 NHL season, with 21 teams and nearly 400 players, 4470 player days were lost to injury, 12% of which were at-

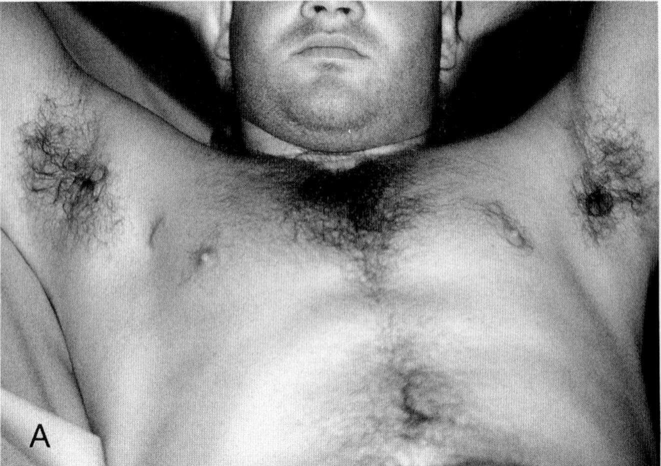

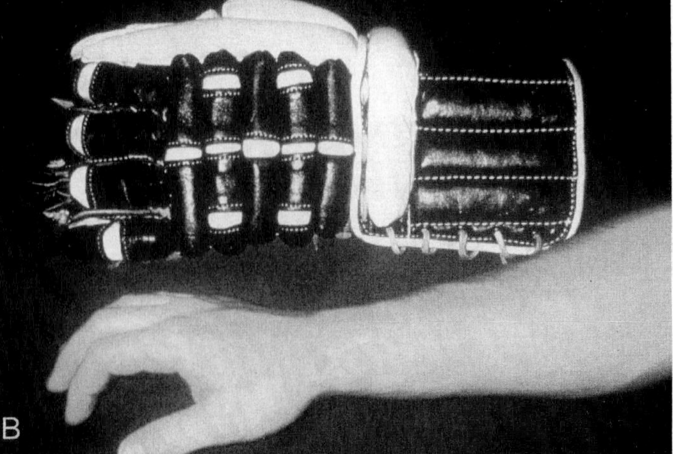

Figure 25.67 A, B. Dermatitis caused by excessive sweating under protective equipment.

tributable to lower extremity strains. Of these, approximately 80% were groin strains. Groin pulls produced an average of 7 player days missed per injury, with a range from 1 to 49 days (68). Strains of the hip flexors, hamstrings, quadriceps, and abdominal muscles combined accounted for only 63 player days missed.

What is not accounted for in the "injury statistics" are players who have missed a season or who have undergone surgery related to groin strain. A morbid pattern, observed with all-too-frequent regularity, is a progression from an apparently routine groin pull into a chronic and recalcitrant disability. Symptoms progress proximally toward the pubis (as in osteitis pubis) and thence more proximally to the lower abdominal wall. This progression is an apparent result of the recruitment of contiguous proximal musculature and tissue to perform the tasks normally incumbent upon the adductors. R. Davidson in Vancouver (personal communication, 1991) reports having performed a number of modified herniorrhaphies of the suprainguinal abdominal fascia for these conditions, with reasonably good success as measured by the return of players to competitive hockey without recrudescence of symptoms. These more dramatic sequelae of groin strains undoubtedly would not have become manifest, had the players interrupted their participation (thereby precluding a recruitment progression) and undertaken a therapeutic and prophylactic course of physical therapy.

The groin muscles are critical force generators for the power starts of ice hockey, making them particularly susceptible. The occurrence of a pull has been thought to be instigated by factors including tight muscles, inadequate warm-up, weakness and/or fatigue, and muscle imbalances. The player typically experiences a pop or tearing sensation and for one to several days is unable to use the muscle effectively. Work by Nikolau et al. (69) would suggest that muscle strength returns rapidly, but that pain and inflammation impede its functional usage. For this reason, some physicians prescribe antiinflammatory drugs, which may actually delay regeneration of injured muscle tissue (70). Generally, within a few weeks, most symptoms have dissipated, but there is a high susceptibility to recurrence of strain by virtue of progressing immature collagen within the injured site and weakness and inflexibility of the recovering muscle.

Before a player is allowed to return to competition, he must have restored the preinjury level of strength (if the preinjury level was normal) of the muscle and the extremity as well as full flexibility (Fig. 25.68). Ekstrand and Gillquist demonstrated that persistent muscle weakness will result in a higher rate of strain recurrence (71).

The role of strength (or a strength ratio) as a protector was implied by the study of Merrifield and Cowan (72) who had performed preparticipation Cybex tests on players and related the results to subsequent injury. All players who sustained groin pulls were among those who had demonstrated strength deficits of the hip muscles of at least 25% in the involved versus the uninvolved extremity.

Restoration of strength is not as simple a concept as first it might appear. It must be appreciated that the entire extremity often becomes deconditioned in the wake of (or as a predisposition to) injury. Restoration of general strength as well as specific ratios (35) is the goal of the rehabilitation program. Common formats of abductor-adductor strengthening are not wholly adequate for rehabilitation of groin pulls in ice hockey players. Common abductor-adductor variable resistance machines, for example, work the muscles with the only hips flexed, and only through limited arcs. The use of the adductors in hockey is often with the extremity extended and widely abducted relative to the plane of the body. This movement format is often best simulated by pulley systems, the Eagle multi-hip machine, and other closed kinetic chain formats. Once recovery has been achieved, and, in general to prevent such injuries, the following practices should be maintained:

1. Maintenance of strength for reasons provided above.
2. Maintenance of general conditioning to achieve increased blood flow, enhanced delivery of nutriments, and resilience to fatigue.
3. Warm-ups prior to participation, including low intensity activity and nonballistic stretching. The re-

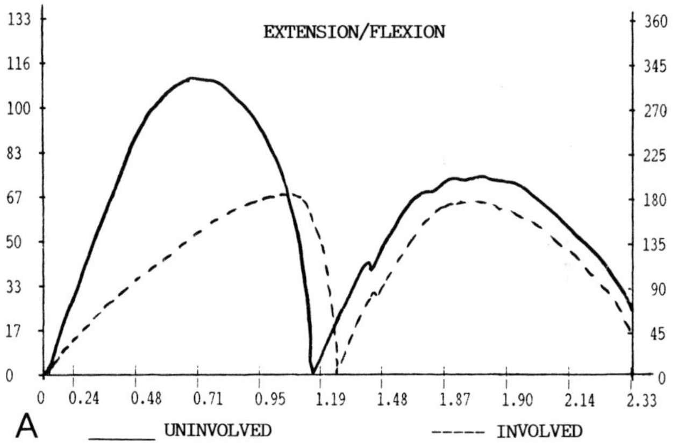

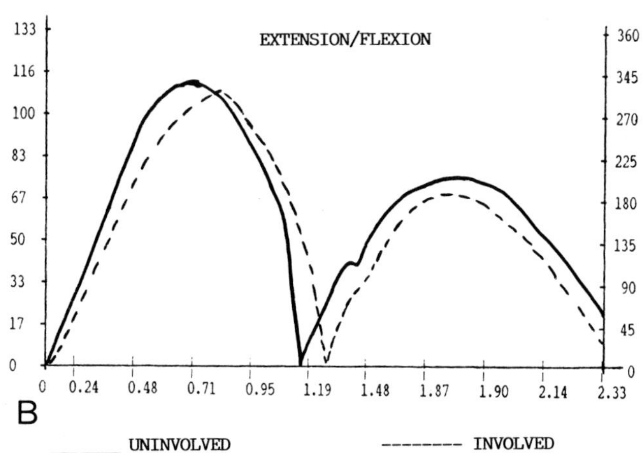

Figure 25.68. Graphs depicting relationship of extension/flexion of uninvolved/involved extremities. **(A),** Postinjury; **(B),** postrehabilitation.

sult is increased muscle heat with greater viscosity of muscle elements and an associated stress relaxation requiring greater forces to tear the muscle. (73).

Other Soft Tissue Injuries

With the number of collisions in ice hockey, it is no surprise that hematoma, in one form or another, is a common injury, despite use of protective pads over the predilected sites (Fig. 25.69). The two most characteristic and disability-producing sties are the anterior or lateral thigh (the Charley horse) and about the iliac crests (the hip pointer). The former is usually a result of an opponent's knee hitting the thigh, the latter a result of slashes or impacts of the hip against the ice or boards. When a hematoma in the thigh is small, it is common to hear trainers refer to a Charlie horse as a "Chuck's pony." When large, thigh pain is moderate and knee flexion is severely curtailed.

Immediate rest, ice, compression, modalities, antiinflammatory medication, and gentle active range of motion are usual early treatment formats. When defiant of a program of relative rest, youths are particularly prone to develop myositis ossificans, especially if repeated blows to the thigh are sustained over a period of time. On occasion, a player will complain of vague discomforts in the hip, associated with stiffness, but have no obvious Charlie horse. By placing a hand on either side of the thigh (medial and lateral) a shock "fluid wave" initiated by the sudden movement of one hand will be subtly detected by the other hand. Repeating the test on the contralateral thigh will reveal virtually no sensation of a fluid wave in the "receiving hand."

Hip pointers, or collections of blood within or around the periosteum of the iliac crest, are quite painful, especially from collision contact. It is common to see players wearing large foam rubber sheets or pads beneath their standard hip pads to avert or protect against hip pointers. Because of the level of pain, it has been an all-too-frequent practice to inject the site with steroids so that the player can resume participation. Sometimes these collections can be aspirated to gain relief. Both the Charlie horse and hip pointer are indicators of the inadequacy of the existing protective equipment.

Visceral Injuries

Of the viscera, the spleen is the most vulnerable in ice hockey. The left upper quadrant is unprotected from elbows and from the blades and butts of sticks. The spleen can also be injured by crushing blows to the rib area. Injuries to the spleen range from subcapsular hematomas (Fig. 25.70) to the surgical emergency of rupture with massive bleeding. Splenic rupture is a life-threatening injury. There is virtually no professional team physician of tenure who has not known at least one player to require a splenectomy.

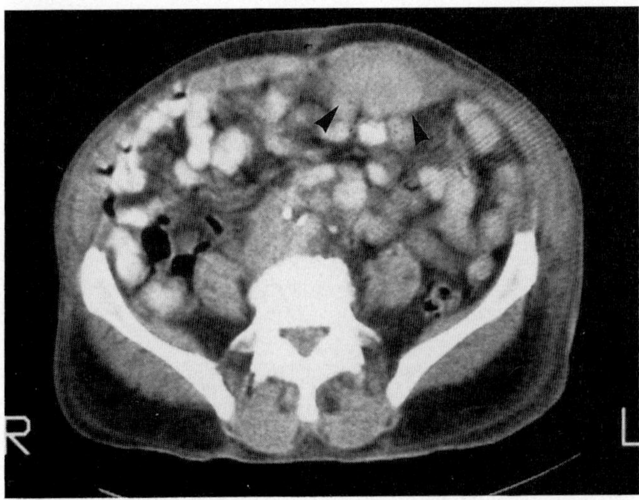

Figure 25.69. Left rectus abdominus hematoma on CT scan *(arrowheads)* in a junior hockey player.

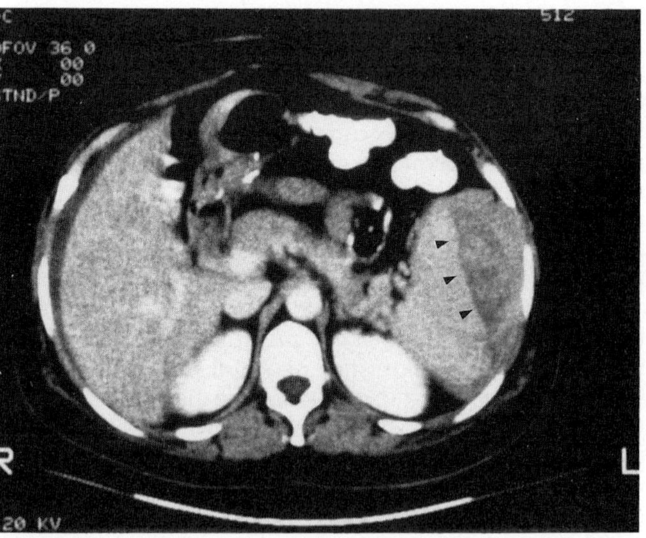

Figure 25.70. Subcapsular hematoma on CT scan *(arrowheads)* in an adult men's hockey league player.

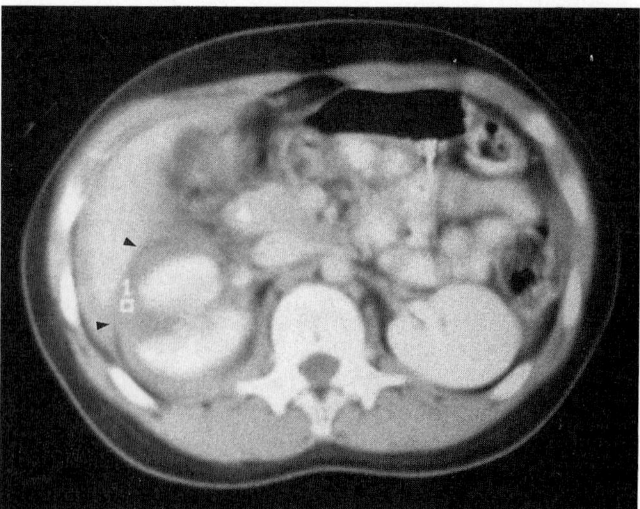

Figure 25.71. Perinephric hematoma on CT scan *(arrowheads)* in a junior hockey player after being cross-checked from behind. Initial complaints were of back pain and hematuria.

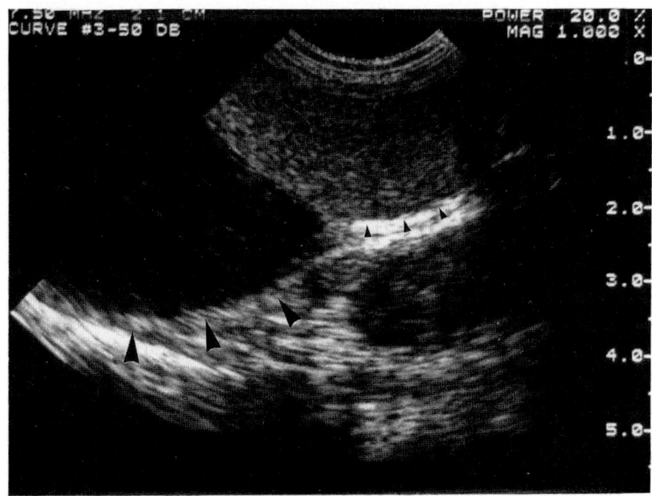

Figure 25.72. Testicular hematoma *(large arrowheads) (testicle, small arrowheads)* demonstrated on ultrasound in a Midget hockey player after being struck by a puck.

Less often, perinephric bleeding is diagnosed (Fig. 25.71). Injury of a kidney is usually heralded by frank hematuria. Serial urinalysis, abdominal x-rays, and an excretory urogram are among the diagnostics that may be implemented to rule out damage (54). Preexisting splenomegaly, as from mononucleosis, predisposes to rupture. When suspected, splenic abnormalities are best evaluated by a CT scan. Players with a history of mononucleosis or whose preseason physical examination reveals splenomegaly, may be screened and followed by sonography (52). Hemoptysis and dyspnea have been observed after chest contusions that produced bleeding within the lungs. Testicular hematomas (Fig. 25.72) have been witnessed after puck or stick contact.

REFERENCES

1. Pashby, TJ, Eye injuries in hockey. Ophthalmol Clin 1981;21(4):59–81.
2. Menke, F., The Encyclopedia of Sports, 6th Edition, Doubleday and Co., Inc., Garden City, New York, 1977.
3. Nagobads VG, Head injuries and protective face masks for goalies in ice-hockey. Presented, IIHF Medical Congress. Fribourg, Switzerland, April 21, 1990.
4. Terjung RL, ed. Exercise and sport science reviews. American College of Sports Medicine Series. Massachusetts; Collamorem Press, 1984:406.
5. Van Ingen Schenau GJ, de Boer RW, De Groot G. Biomechanics of speed skating. In: Vaughan, CL, ed. Biomechanics of sport. Boca Raton, FL: CRC Press, Inc, 1989.
6. Montgomery DL, Physiology of ice hockey. Sports Med 1988;5:99–126.
7. Broadbent S. Skateology: The science and technology of the edge/ice interface. USOC/SETC Conference, Colorado Springs, CO, December 8–9, 1989.
8. Stamm L. Laura Stamm's Power Skating. Champaign, IL: Leisure Press, 1989.
9. Marino GW, Weese RG, A kinematic analysis of the ice skating stride. In: Terauds, Gros, eds. Science in skiing, skating and hockey, 65–74. Del Mar, CA: Academic Publishers. 1979.
10. Van Ingen Schenau GJ, Cavanaugh PR. Power equations in endurance sports. J Biomechanics 1990;1333(9):865–881.
11. Diamond GR, Quinn GE, Pashby TJ, et al. Ophthalmologic Injuries. Clin Sports Med 1982;1(3):469–82.
12. Keating M, Norris R. Design of hockey rinks and the development of standards, in safety in ice hockey. ASTM, 1989;187–201.
13. Marino GW, Analysis of selected factors in the ice skating strides of adolescents. CAHPER J 1984;50(3):4–8.
14. Van Ingen Schenau, GJ, de Groot G, de Boer RW, The control of speed in elite female speed skaters. J Biomechan 1985;(18)91–96.
15. Hoshizaki TB, Kirchner GJ. A kinematic description of the ankle during acceleration phase of forward skating. Proceedings of the International Symposium of Biomechanics in Sports, 1987.
16. Hoshizaki TB, Kirchner G, and Hall K, Kinematic analysis of the talocrural and subtalar joints during hockey skating stride. In: Safety in ice hockey, Philadelphia: ASTM. 1989;141–49.
17. Marino GW. Kinematics of ice skating at different velocities. Res Q 1977;48:93–97.
18. Marino, GW, Selected mechanical factors associated with acceleration in ice skating. Res Q Exerc Sport 1983;54(3):234–238.
19. Marino GW. Acceleration—Time relationships in an ice skating start. Res Q 1979;50(1):55–59.
20. de Boer RW, Calori J, Vaes W, et al. Movements of force, power, and muscle coordination in speed-skating. Int. J, Sports Med 1987;8:371–378.
21. Green NL, Dillman CJ. Acceleration of elite ice hockey players. In: Terauds J, ed. Sports biomechanics. Proceedings of the International Symposium of Biomechanics in Sports, Colorado Springs, CO, 1984.
22. Anonymous. Men's Ice Hockey. In: NCAA Injury Surveillance System, 1989–1990.
23. Lorentzon R, Wedren H, Pietila T, et al. Injuries in international ice hockey, a prospective, comparative study of injury incidence and injury types in international and Swedish elite ice hockey. Am J Sports Med 1988;16(4)389–91.
24. Thomson DH, Analysis of data obtained from sport-specific injury studies. Study by LGL, Environmental Research Associates for the Hockey Development Center of Ontario (HDC), Nov. 16, 1989;1–82.
25. Haas S. Biomechanical evaluation of forces produced by the aluminum hockey stick. Presented, NHL Physicians Association, annual meetings. Pittsburgh, 1990.
26. Hastings, DE, et al. A study of ice hockey injuries in Ontario. Ontario Med Rev 1974; 686–98.
27. Marchant L, Roy E, Warshaw Shi, Jr. British Columbia Amateur Hockey Association: Hockey Injury Study. Department of Physical Education, University of British Columbia, Vancouver, British Columbia, Canada, 1974.
28. Minkoff J, A survey of injury statistics and player mentality in the NHL. Presented, NHL Physicians' Association. 1989.
29. Parayre R, The effect of rules and officiating on the occurrence and prevention of injuries, in safety in ice hockey, Philadelphia: ASTM, 1989;37–42.
30. Walsh S., A proposal for the use of the half face, clear plastic visor for National Collegiate Athletic Association Hockey. In: Safety in Ice Hockey. Philadelphia: ASTM, 1989:55–57.
31. Regnier G, Boileau R, Marcotte G, et al. Effects of body-checking in the Pee Wee (12 and 13 year olds) division in the Province of Quebec. In: Safety in Ice Hockey. ASTM 1989;84–103.
32. Gerberich, SG. An epidemiological study of high school ice hockey injuries. Childs Nerv Syst 3:59–64, 1987.
33. Frank MG, Gilovich T. The dark side of self and social perception: Black uniforms and aggression in professional sports. J Pers Soc Psychol 1988;54(1)74–85.
34. Widmeyer WN, Birch JS, Aggression in professional ice hockey: A strategy for success or a reaction to failure?. J Psychol 1984;117:77–84.
35. Minkoff J. Evaluating parameters of a professional hockey team. Am J Sports Med 1982;10(5)285–292.
36. Agre JC, Casal DC, Leon AS, et al. Professional ice hockey players: Physiologic, anthropometric, and musculoskeletal characteristics. Arch Phys Med Rehabil 1988;69:188–192.
37. Sim FH, Simonet WT, Melton LJ, Lehn TA, Ice hockey injuries. Am J Sports Med 1987;15(1):30–40.
38. Hoerner EF, Ice hockey protective equipment—Its value, capabilities, and limitations. In: Safety in ice hockey. Philadelphia: ASTM, 1989;150–153.

39. Hoerner EF, The dynamic role played by the ice hockey stick. In: Safety in Ice Hockey. Philadelphia: ASTM, 1989;154–163.
40. Odelgard B. The development of head, face, and neck protectors for ice hockey players. Philadelphia: ASTM, 1989;220–234.
41. Clement L, Jones D. Research and development of hockey protective equipment—A historical perspective, In: Safety in ice hockey, Philadelphia: ASTM 1989;164–183.
42. Dixon JL, The Canadian Standards Association and the evolution of head and face protection in Canadian hockey. In: Safety in ice hockey. Philadelphia: ASTM, 1989:207–219.
43. Bishop PJ, Norman RW, Pierrynowski M. The ice hockey helmet: How effective is it? Phys Sportsmed 1979;7(2):97–107.
44. Johnson, GI, Development of an impact testing method for protective helmets, in safety in ice hockey. Philadelphia: ASTM 1989:240–261.
45. Morehouse CA, The ASTM F 1045-87 Standard Performance Specification for Ice Hockey Helmets. In: Safety in ice hockey. Philadelphia: ASTM, 1989:262–273.
46. Jones, NP. Eye injury in sport. Sports Med 1989;7:163–181.
47. Dixon JL. ed. Ice Hockey Helmets. Canadian Standards Association. May, 1990.
48. International Standard on Protective Headgear for Ice Hockey Players, a draft for the creation of a standard. Philadelphia: ASTM, Jan., 1991.
49. Dixon, JL. ed. Face protectors and visors for ice hockey players. Canadian Standards Association, May, 1990.
50. Smith TA, Bishop PJ. Impact of full face and visor type hockey face guards. In: Safety in ice hockey. Philadelphia: ASTM, 1989;235–239.
51. Dixon J. A letter to members of the CSA technical committee on protective equipment for ice hockey players. April, 1990.
52. Couture G. Safety factors in the modern ice hockey skate blade. In: Safety in ice hockey. Philadelphia: ASTM, 1979:117–140.
53. Bull C. Hockey injuries. In: sports injuries: mechanism, prevention, and treatment. Baltimore: Williams & Wilkins, 90–113.
54. Sim FH, Simonet WT, Scott SG. Ice hockey injuries: Causes, treatment, and prevention. J Musculoskeletal Med Mar, 1989;15–41.
55. Vinger, PF, Eye and face protection for United States hockey players: A chronology. Appendix. Ophthalmol Clin 1981;21(4):83–86.
56. Sane, J, Ylipaavalniemi P, Leppanen H, Maxillofacial and dental ice hockey injuries. Med Sci Sports and Exercise, 1988;20(2):202–207.
57. Reid, DC, Saboe L; Spine fractures in winter sports. Sports Med 1989;7:393–399.
58. Tator CH, Edmonds VE, Lapczak L, Tator IB. Spinal injuries in ice hockey players, 1966–1987. 1990.
59. Bishop PJ, Wells RP. Cervical spine fractures: Mechanisms, neck loads, and methods of prevention. In: Castaldi CR, Hoerner EF, ed. Safety in ice hockey. Philadelphia: ASTM, 1989:71–83.
60. Pashby TJ, Eye injuries in Canadian amateur hockey. Opthalmol Clin, 1988;28,3:228–231.
61. Wilson, K., Cram B, Rontal E, et al. Facial injuries in hockey players. Minn Med 1977;60:13–19.
62. Pashby, TJ, Ocular Injuries in Hockey. Int Ophthalmol Clin 1988;28;3:228–231.
63. McConkey JP, Ankle sprains, consequences and mimics. Med Sport Sci 23, 39–55. Karger, Basel, 1987.
64. Norfray JF, Tremaine MJ, Groves HC, Bachman DC, The clavicle in hockey. Am J Sports Med 1977;5(6)275–280.
65. Glick JM, Milburn LJ, Haggerty JF, et al. Dislocated acromioclavicular joint: Follow-up study of 35 unreduced acromioclavicular dislocations. Am J Sports Med 1977;5(6)264–70.
66. Hovelius L, Shoulder dislocation in Swedish ice hockey players. Am J Sports Med 6(6)373–377.
67. Bergfeld WF, Dermatology problems in athletes. Clin Sports Med 1982;1(3):419–30.
68. NHL Injury Analysis; 1986–1987. Courtesy of the National Hockey League Executive Offices.
69. Nikolau PK, MacDonald BL, Glisson RR, et al. Biomechanical and histological evaluation of muscle after controlled strain injury. Am J Sports Med 1987;15(1)9–14.
70. Almekinders LC, Gilbert JA, Healing of experimental muscle strains and the effects of nonsteroidal anti-inflammatory medication. Am J Sports Med 1984;12(5):368–70.
71. Ekstrand J, Gillquist J. The frequency of muscle tightness and inquiries in soccer players. Am J Sports Med 10:75–78, 1982.
72. Merrifield HH, Cowan RFJ, Groin strain injuries in ice hockey. J Sports Med Jan/Feb, 1973;41–42.
73. Safran MR, Seaber AV, and Garrett Jr, WE, Warm-up and muscular injury prevention—An update. Sports Med 1989;8(4):239–249.
74. Sim FH, Chao EY, Injury potential in modern ice hockey. Am J Sports Med 1978;6(6)378–384.
75. Torg, JS, Athletic injuries to the head, neck, and face. Philadelphia: Lea & Febiger, 1982.
76. Kulund DN, The injured athlete. Philadelphia: JB Lippincott, 1982.
77. Vinger PF, Hoerner EF, Sports injuries: The unthwarted epidemic. Littleton, MA: PSG Publishing Co, 1981.
78. Scott WN, Nissonson B, Ncholas JA, Principles of sports medicine. Baltimore: Williams & Wilkins, 1984.
79. Torg, JS, and Gennarelli, TA, Head and neck injury. In: Grana WA, Kalenak A, eds. Clinical sports medicine. Philadelphia: WB Saunders Company, 1991.
80. Gersoff W. Head and neck injuries. In: Reider B, ed. Sports medicine: The school-age athlete, Philadelphia: WB Saunders, 1991.

26 / ICE SKATING: Figure, Speed, Long Distance, and In-Line

David L. Muller, Per A. F. H. Renström, and John I. B. Pyne

Overview and History

Figure skating and speed skating have gained increased popularity in recent times, especially with widespread media attention to events such as the Winter Olympics. These sports have traditionally been popular in countries with naturally occurring ice. In recent decades, they also have become popular in countries that have built artificial ice tracks and skating rinks. Now, with the advent of in-line skating, skating injuries once exclusive to colder climates are being seen and treated in areas previously not exposed to these sports. The types and frequencies of injuries seen vary among different skating events as well as between recreational athletes and competitive skaters. The development of highly technical training programs has led to better understanding of skating biomechanics and injury risk and prevention.

Figure, speed, long-distance, and in-line skating involve different equipment and techniques and, therefore, expose skaters to unique patterns of injuries. Figure skating involves several different events, including singles, pair skating, and ice dancing. Both singles and pairs events emphasize acrobatic jumps, placing great torque on the landing leg, leading to both overuse and acute traumatic injuries. Ice dancing emphasizes foot work and coordination and does not generate high levels of rotational forces. Speed skating involves great strength, endurance, and technique. Speed skating has been a relatively safe sport, because the skating motion is biomechanically sound and falls are infrequent. This has been changing with the introduction of short-track racing; its explosive pack starts and tight turns have led to many falls.

Long-distance skating, most common in Scandinavian countries and Holland, involves traveling long distances on lakes and canals (Fig. 26.1). Skating is a popular sport in countries with ice on lakes during the winter season. In a national survey in Sweden, 33% of the population had skated during a 6-year period (1). Most were recreational skaters and 50% had participated in long-distance skating. Long-distance skating injuries are usually related to poor ice conditions and harsh climate.

Although traditional roller skating is dwindling in popularity, in-line skating is rapidly growing in the United States and Europe. Most participants are recreational skaters who use bike paths and roads for general fitness and fun. In-line skating in the summer is well-suited for cross-training for a number of winter sports. More recently, racing events and roller hockey have been organized. Roller hockey was a demonstration sport in the 1992 Summer Olympics in Barcelona; Spain won the gold medal. The smooth motion of in-line skating is believed to place little stress on joints, but frequent falls on hard pavement cause many injuries. Padding and prophylactic bracing appear to be crucial in in-line skating to decrease the incidence of fall-related injuries.

Many theories exist regarding the origin of skating. One possibility is that skating originated from skiing, and that skates evolved merely as miniature skis. Another theory suggests that an accidental slip on a piece of bone across the ice led to the development of skating (2). Nevertheless, the origins of skating have been noted in archaeological discoveries in Asia and Europe and from Scandinavian and Icelandic legends that date back more than 3000 years. Drawings depict prehistoric hunters traveling on snow and ice with pieces of bone and wood on their footwear.

Primitive forms of skates were made of shank or leg bones that were fastened to the feet by leather straps. The word *skate* is derived from the Dutch word *schaats*, which can be further traced to old German and French

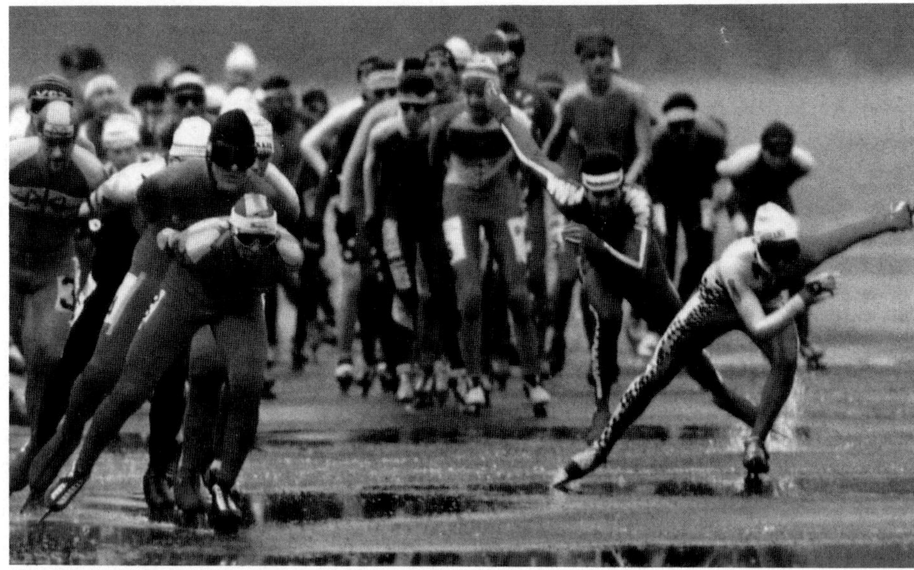

Figure 26.1. Long-distance skating is both a recreational and competitive sport in Scandinavian countries. Pack-style races are common in this sport.

words meaning "shank bone" or "leg bone." Eventually, animal bones were replaced by wood and finally by iron, a true advance in skating technology. A wood carving from the 15th century shows that iron skate blades have existed for at least 600 years (3). The most significant advance was the invention of all-metal skates in Philadelphia in 1848. These provided superior fixation to a persons' foot by eliminating the wooden foot plate that was often too loose and fell off or was too tight and cut off circulation.

Initially used as a form of travel, early skating did not entail a push-off and glide technique. Apparently, this technique is from Holland and was characterized by a sideward push-off technique using sharp "whetted iron blades."

Skating competition started before the 17th century. The famous Elfstedentocht in Holland was first held in 1763; it is a long-distance race that visits 11 cities and is more than 250 km long. In 1985, a total of 16,176 skaters participated with nearly 75% completing the race (3).

The first skating club was formed in Edinburgh, Scotland, in 1742. Individuals had to prove various technical skating skills to gain membership (2). The first speed skating world championships were held in 1891 in Amsterdam.

Since the development of artificial ice, colder climates, still water, and minimal snowfall are now no longer prerequisites for a strong skating community. Therefore, many nationalities are now evident in elite skating competitions. The first artificial ice rink was built in 1876 in London. Madison Square Garden, which opened in 1879 in New York City is the oldest American skating rink.

The oldest known skating injury is recorded in *The Life of Saint Lidvinia,* written by Brogman in 1498. Saint Lidvinia suffered a fracture while skating, and according to the book, was confined to bed for the rest of her life (2).

Roller skating dates back to the 1700s. Myth has it that a Dutch skater, frustrated by the hot summer months, strapped wheels onto his shoes (4). The old steel rollers were popularized in the United States in the 1860s and remained essentially unchanged until 1965 when polyurethane wheels and precision bearings were introduced. These provide a quiet, smooth ride with better traction, speed, and maneuverability, and their introduction was responsible for the increased popularity of roller skating in the 1970s. By 1979, approximately 57% of teenagers and 12% of adults participated in roller skating in the United States (5). Participation has decreased through the 1980s coincident with a rise in popularity of in-line skating.

In-line skates were developed in 1980 for off-season training for ice hockey. In 1984, marketing was directed at the general fitness crowd, resulting in 4 to 5 million in-line skaters in 1991.

Biomechanics and Technique

Most recreational skaters have little concern for power, work per stroke, center of gravity, and hip and knee angle. However, proper biomechanics and technique are crucial to the success of a competitive skater. Speed skating has been the most extensively studied, because improvements in times by fractions of seconds can drastically alter race outcomes. The skating technique of speed skaters and figure skaters is remarkably different. Recognizing these differences can help in the understanding of injury patterns related to these sports.

A knowledge of the different techniques used in the three events of figure skating is necessary for proper care of the injured skater. These events are singles, pairs skating, and ice dancing and each event stresses different skills and exposes the skater to different types of injuries. Singles skating involves forward and backward maneuvers, footwork, jumps, and spins. More and more emphasis in competition has been placed on difficult and dangerous jumps. Now, skaters even at the novice level spend a significant amount of time practicing triple jumps. These jumps require great rotational speed to complete the revolutions. Rotational speed must be decreased before landing. This is done by extending the arms and nonlanding leg away from the axis of rotation to decrease the moment of inertia just before landing. Opening out a fraction of a second too early or late on a landing can place significant rotational forces on the landing leg. This can lead to single fall injuries or overuse syndromes from repeated microtrauma.

Pairs skating requires similar skills as singles skating, except that the jumps and spins must be precisely coordinated with a partner. Spins can be done side by side or about a common axis of rotation. Pairs skating also involves lifting maneuvers and throws. In the lifts the male lifts the female high above the ice. Both spins and lifts increase the risk for skate blade lacerations. In the throw jumps, the male throws the female into the air where she completes two or three revolutions. Greater heights and distance in throws will improve scores in competitions. This leads to even greater axial loading and rotational forces on the landing leg and is responsible for the high incidence of injuries in the female pairs skater. The lifts and throws require upper extremity strength in the male, who is at risk for overuse injuries, including rotator cuff strains and tendinitis.

Ice dancers concentrate on speed, precision, coordinated footwork, and body lean. The spins are shorter and the lifts are smaller than pair skating, and there are no throws. Couples are judged on artistry, form, symmetry, and music interpretation. The rotational forces encountered in the lower extremities are much less than in pairs skating. The dancers are still at risk for injuries caused by contact between partners.

Techniques in speed skating are related to the event. Olympic or metric-style races use time trials in which two skaters race at once against the clock. The races are carried out on 400-m long outdoor tracks, and the races vary from 500 to 10,000 m for men and 500 to 5,000 m for women. Collisions and falls are infrequent as are acute traumatic injuries. Recently, short-track skating has been introduced, in which there are four to seven skaters per heat who are competing on an 111-m oval indoor track. These races are characterized by explosive pack starts and tight, crowded turns. Short-track speed skating has become popular because special outdoor tracks are not needed. The races are run in standard indoor rinks. This has broadened the accessibility of speed skating.

Speed skating involves a powerful start and long skating strokes with constant repetition. The body position of a speed skater is illustrated in Figure 26.2. The goal of a speed skater at any level is to improve his or her efficiency and speed by maintaining the trunk position as parallel to the ice as possible throughout a race. Variations in body position and anthropometry measurements have been shown to exist between less competitive skaters and elite skaters; the less competitive skaters are more upright (6, 7) (Fig. 26.3). Multiple factors are important for efficiency in speed skating. Factors such as air friction, ice friction, weather, and air pressure will influence times and, thereby, drastically influence race outcomes (3). Air pressure and resistance are reduced at high altitudes. The air pressure at the Medeorink in Alma Ata, Kazakhstan, which is at 1700 m, is reduced by 20%. Maximum oxygen consumption has been shown not to be drastically altered at this altitude in the shorter race distances (8). These near-optimal climatic conditions coincide with the high number of world records set at the Medeorink.

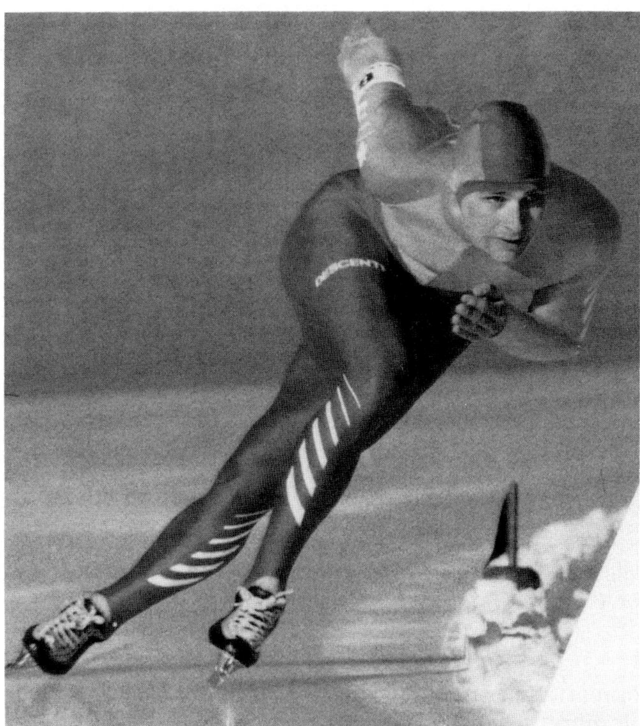
Figure 26.2. Elite speed skaters maintain a parallel trunk position during the entire race. Skins are worn to minimize wind resistance.

As mentioned earlier, in-line skating was developed as an off-season training tool for ice hockey. In-line skating techniques can be modified to resemble various winter sports such as speed skating, figure skating, ice hockey, cross-country skiing, and downhill skiing. This allows winter athletes to customize their off-season training to optimize the benefits for their specific sport. In this fashion, in-line skating can be used to improve both technique and conditioning.

Using in-line skating to cross-train for nordic skiing has become more popular as the skating technique has emerged in that sport. Ski poles can be used with the double-pole push-off technique to more closely simulate nordic skiing. The weight transfer, edging, and turns of alpine skiing can be practiced with in-line skates on sloped surfaces. Some ski areas now have paved trails serviced by ski lifts for skiing with in-line skates in the summer. Recreational in-line skating has undergone a

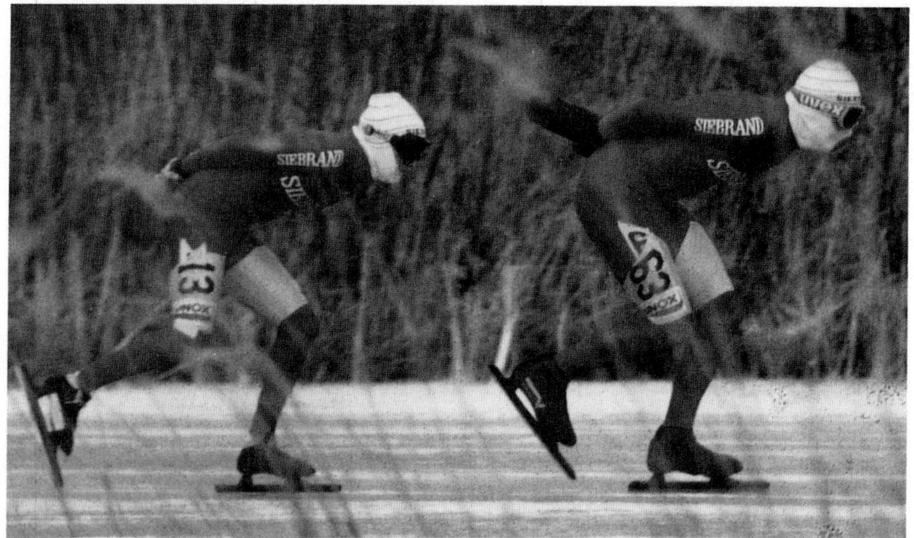

Figure 26.3. The trunk position of these long distance competitive skaters is more upright then that of an elite Olympic skater. Hats, gloves, masks, and goggles are worn for protection from cold weather.

popularity explosion in the United States and is now a common form of general fitness training.

During the off-season, skaters may train on roads, streets, or bike paths using in-line skates. Most injuries are caused by uneven skating surfaces. Stones, pot holes, sand, and wet pavement cause many falls. Downhill terrain can be challenging, as high speeds can be obtained and braking is more difficult than with ice skates. The skaters stop by using friction bumpers on the back of the skate that are pushed against the pavement with the hip flexed and the knee extended in front of the skater (Fig. 26.4). Many skaters prefer to use a T-stop when traveling at faster speeds. To T-stop, the braking leg is dragged behind the skater with the skate perpendicular to the direction of travel. Both breaking techniques are difficult and cannot stop the skater suddenly. In-line skate manufacturers are trying to develop better breaking systems. Almost all injuries are related to collisions or falls on hard pavement, so in-line skaters require more padding and prophylactic bracing.

Long-distance skaters in Scandinavia travel on unfamiliar ice surfaces over lakes, seas, and canals. The technique involves a more upright body position, often using a pole or stick for balance, support, and speed. These skaters often carry ice spikes and rope in case they fall through the ice.

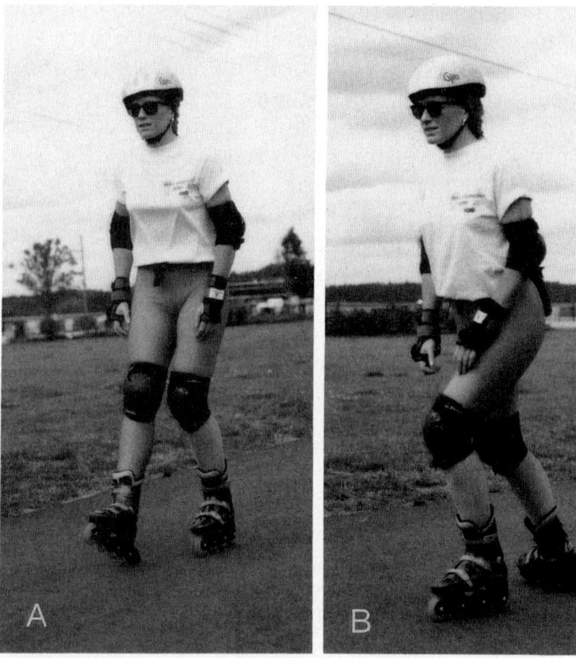

Figure 26.4. Stopping with a friction bumper **(A)** or by a T-stop **(B)** requires practice to help avoid high-speed falls and injury.

Equipment

Improperly fitting equipment can lead to injury. The myth of weak ankles is probably an equipment-related phenomenon. Figure skates, speed skates, long-distance skates, and in-line skates are all quite different.

Figure skating boots provide good support and a snug fit (Fig. 26.5). The boot is in slight plantar flexion with a raised heel. The skate blade is approximately 4 mm wide and has a slight crown or rock along its entire length. The inner and outer edges are sharp with a slight hollow between them (9). The front of the blade is molded with a toe pick for starting and spins.

The leather boots of speed skates are low cut and provide less ankle support than other skates (Fig. 26.6). The speed skate blade is designed for maximal contact with the ice and is 15 to 16 inches long and flat along the length of the blade. The blade is 2 to 3 mm wide and is sharpened without a hollow. Competitive speed skaters wear tight suits, called skins, for minimum wind resistance during a race (see Fig. 26.2). The skins are thin, and there is a risk of exposure to cold weather.

The introduction of short-track skating has necessitated changes in the design of the speed skate. The short-track skate has a rock or crown along the length of the blade. The blade is not centered under the boot, but is positioned just to the left of center in both the right and left foot. The heel post is higher, which allows a more acute skate-to-ice-surface angle for tight turning. These two adaptations ensure that the boot does not contact the ice, resulting in a fall. Elite skaters will bend both blades to the left to allow tighter cornering. In short-track skating protective equipment is essential. A helmet is required as are leather gloves, knee pads, and often shin pads. Recently, neck guards have been introduced to prevent lacerations. Short-track skating races are performed in indoor hockey rinks equipped with standard corner padding to cushion the falls of the skaters.

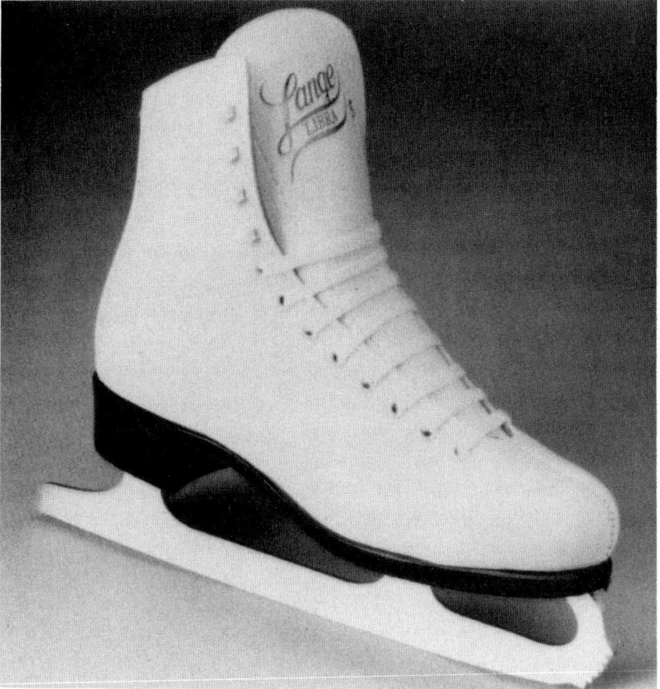

Figure 26.5. A properly fitting figure skate can prevent many of the foot and ankle injuries to which figure skaters are susceptible.

The long-distance skater often wears a winter boot on which he or she straps the blades of a skate. As noted, long-distance skaters carry ice spikes and rope. These skaters should wear helmets and elbow and knee pads for injury prevention.

The boots of in-line skates are either leather or molded plastic and are similar to hockey skate boots. Special racing skates are made that have a low-cut boot and a longer blade, similar to speed skates. The wheels are approximately 1 cm in width and are arranged in a single line. Recreational skates have three or four wheels (depending on the shoe size) and racing skates have five wheels (Fig. 26.7). Because of uneven wear, the wheels should be rotated every 40 to 50 miles and should be replaced when worn out. The hard plastic brake extends from the heel behind the wheels and needs to be replaced when worn down. Protective equipment is an essential part of in-line skating (Fig. 26.8). Although the incidence of head injuries is low, the risks are great, and helmet use is recommended. Wrist guards are recommended at all times because of the high incidence of wrist fractures. The guards have internal metal splints that attempt to prevent wrist dorsiflexion. No studies have been published to prove their efficacy. Anecdotally, the authors have seen wrist fractures in patients who wore wrist guards, but these have been minimally displaced. Distal radius fractures seen in patients not wearing wrist guards are usually displaced and are occasionally open fractures. Knee pads and elbow pads also are considered routine protective gear.

Epidemiology and Incidence of Injuries

Several reports have been published on the epidemiology of figure skating injuries. Various results have been reported, depending on the skating population studied. These studies indicate that competitive, recreational, and novice skaters are at risk for different types of injuries.

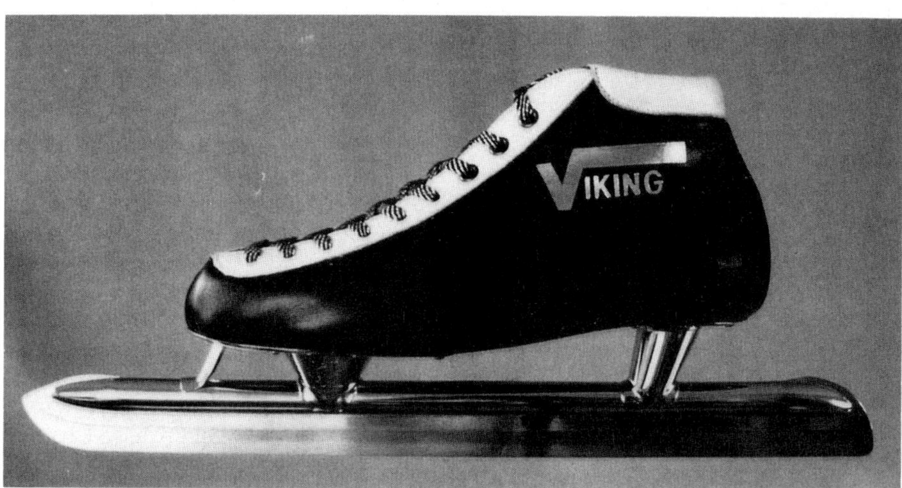

Figure 26.6. The speed skate boot is low cut, providing minimal ankle support. The long blade is designed for speed.

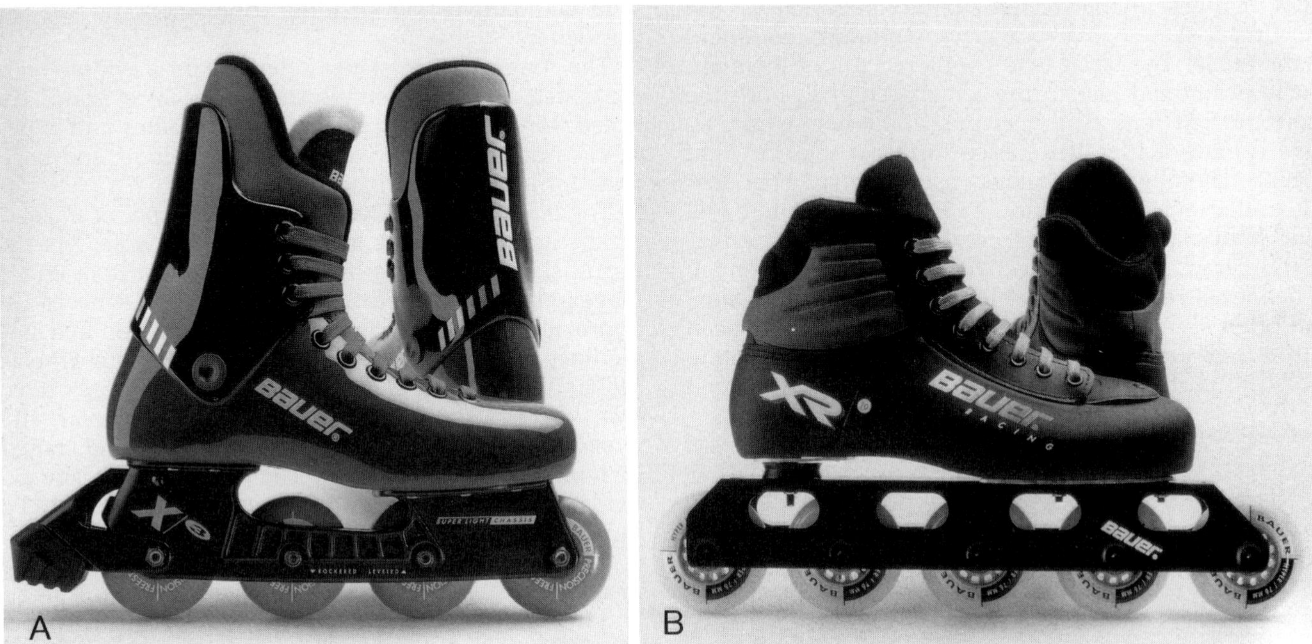

Figure 26.7. **A,** In-line skates are usually made of molded plastic and provide good ankle support. **B,** Racing skates are lower cut and have an additional wheel for speed.

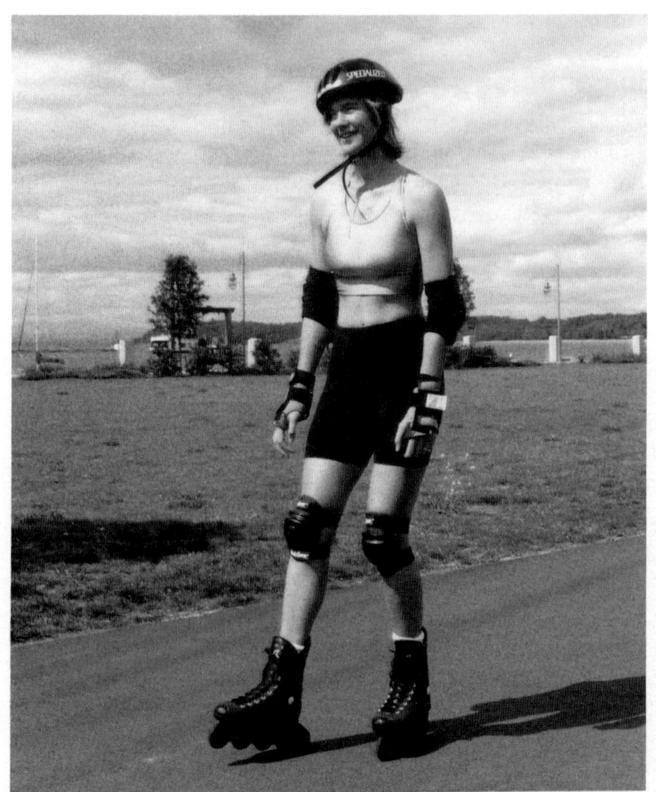

Speed 26.8. The in-line skater should be adequately equipped with protective gear. A helmet, wrist guards, and elbow and knee pads can prevent serious injury.

Williamson and Lowdon (10) reported the injuries seen in the local emergency department during the 2-month period following the opening of a public skating facility in an area previously without a rink. They found an injury risk of 1 per 1000 visits. A total of 60% were fractures, of which 80% involved the upper extremities and 50% were distal radius fractures. The rest of the injuries were lacerations, 66% of which involved the hand. Approximately 75% had skated less than 10 times, and only 8% had received formal instruction.

Garrick (11) reported on the population of injured athletes referred to his clinic, which deals primarily with recreational athletes. Figure skating was the ninth most common sport seen. Approximately 85% of the figure skating patients were female and 63% were between 13 and 18 years old. Overuse injuries slightly outnumbered acute injuries, and fractures represented only 8% of the injuries. The knee (30%), ankle (25%), and back (10%) were most commonly injured.

Several studies have looked specifically at competitive figure skaters. It has been observed that there has been an increased incidence of injuries in these skaters because of the increased demands of training time and the increased difficulty of maneuvers practiced. These athletes skate up to 6 hours per day for 50 weeks per years. Emphasis has shifted to triple jumps, which are performed at all levels. Missed triple-jump landings can cause tremendous rotational forces on the landing leg. Repeated practicing of the same maneuver leads to repetitive microtrauma and overuse injuries.

Brock and Striowski (12) looked at the injuries in 64 nationally ranked Canadian skaters and found that 45% sustained a significant injury over a 1-year period. Overuse and acute injuries were equally seen; 60% of the acute injuries occurred during jumps. The overuse injuries were believed to be caused by the minimal time spent stretching. Smith and Micheli (13) looked at injuries throughout the careers of 19 competitive skaters and found 52 overuse injuries and only 8 acute injuries. The most common problem seen was low-back pain, which is believed to be secondary to tight lumbar fascia from an overgrowth syndrome. Both studies found few serious injuries, especially compared with sports with similar training demands, such as gymnastics. The authors believed that the majority of overuse injuries could be prevented with better warmup and flexibility exercises.

Ice dancers and pairs skaters are exposed to additional risks because of the potential for contact with their partners. As noted the demands of ice dancing are different from the demands of pairs skating. Smith and Ludington (14) looked at injuries in elite pair skaters and ice dancers in a prospective study. They found 33 significant injuries in 48 skaters over a 9-month period. The female pair skaters were at highest risk, with a rate of 1.9 significant injuries per skater per year.

No epidemiologic studies have been published on speed skating injuries. By competing two at a time in time trials, the sport has remained relatively safe from acute injury. Collisions are rare, and falls are infrequent and usually well-padded. However, the popularity of short-track pack racing may change this. The potential for collisions and lacerations is much greater, and protective equipment will play an important role in injury prevention. The speed skating motion is thought to provide little stress to the bone and joints of the lower extremities, but the sustained forward flexion trunk position is a cause of back pain. Boot-related problems of tendinitis and callouses are common overuse injuries. The violent movement during a sprint can cause adductor strains or skate blade lacerations. However, most injuries seen in competitive speed skaters occur during off-season training with weight lifting, running, or cycling.

Injuries among long-distance skaters are not uncommon. In a study in Sweden (15), an injury incidence of 2.2 injuries per 1000 skater days was found, which is similar to that reported in downhill skiing. In an interview with the 4000 members of a skating club in Stockholm, it was found that 20% had sustained an injury during long-distance skating. The upper extremities and head were the most common locations. A total of 18% were head injuries, indicating that a helmet should be worn. Femoral neck fractures were otherwise the most common serious injury. Most of the skaters were 30 to 65 years old, with a mean age of 55 years, which explains the high number of hip fractures. Most injuries are sustained during falls because of poor ice conditions. The most common causes are related to cracks in the ice and overice, a phenomenon in which a thin surface layer of ice has not bonded to the underlying ice. A skater's blade can penetrate the thin surface layer leading to falls. These can cause severe hand and facial lacerations from the sharp shards of ice.

No epidemiologic studies have been published on in-line skating injuries. However, following the increase in popularity of roller skating in the late 1970s, a number of studies were published on the epidemiology of roller skating injuries. These retrospective studies looked at skaters with injuries presenting to the emergency room and noted that 65% were fractures, 10% sprains, 10% contusions, and 8% lacerations (4, 16–18). A total of 75% of the fractures in roller skaters involved the upper extremities, and 75% of these were caused by falls onto the outstretched hand. Of the wrist injuries, 90% were distal radius fractures and 10% were scaphoid fractures. Both bone forearm fractures were common in children under 9 years of age but rare in adults. The elbow was the second most common site injured, and 65% of these injuries were radial head fractures, 10% were olecranon fractures, and 7% were capitellar fractures. Upper extremity injuries were usually caused by falls on irregular or sloped surfaces, whereas lower extremity injuries were often caused by collisions as the result of overcrowding. Approximately 10% of all injuries were ankle injuries, with 80% of these being fractures. Of these ankle fractures, 65% required surgery. Patella fractures, tibia fractures, and knee ligament injuries are occasionally seen. In-line skating injuries appear to follow similar patterns. It is not unusual for the injured in-line skater to have been skating for the first time, often with borrowed skates and little protective equipment.

Orthopedic Injuries and Treatment

Both acute and chronic injuries are noted in skaters of all types. The recreational skater is more apt to sustain an acute injury in a fall or collision rather than an overuse injury, whereas competitive figure skaters are susceptible to an equal number of both acute and overuse injuries. Speed skaters are less likely to sustain acute injuries related to falls, as noted previously. The following is a representation by anatomical area of the types of injuries that plague skaters.

Foot

All skaters are aware of the problems poorly fitting skates can cause. Toe numbness and foot pain may simply be related to narrow boots. Outdoor skaters may be more susceptible to frostbite with skates that are too tight. Bursitis and callosities are common in skaters. Well-fitting and often custom-made boots are necessary to prevent these painful and annoying injuries. Doughnut-shaped pads and boot modification can distribute pressures over bony prominences. Davis and Litman (19) evaluated 45 competitive figure skaters and found that 40% had intermittent foot pain severe enough to limit training, and 69% had hammertoe deformities. These were usually multiple and bilateral. Hard corns were noted in most skaters.

Stress fractures are the most common foot injuries. Pecina et al. (20) reported seven foot stress fractures in

42 competitive skaters. Two involved the tarsal navicular; two, the base of the fifth metatarsal; two, the fourth metatarsal; and one, the second metatarsal. Most healed with rest, one underwent open reduction internal fixation (ORIF), and two were successfully treated in short leg casts. The tarsal navicular stress fracture is often overlooked. The diagnosis is secured with a bone scan and tomograms. Smith (21) reported that most figure skaters do well with decreasing jumping activity until the stress fracture heals; some skaters, however, may need to be forced to rest from skating, if they are not willing to modify their skating regimen. Orthotics can occasionally help redistribute forces within the skate boot to help prevent further injury.

Lower Leg and Ankle

The lower leg and ankle are common areas of injury in all types of ice skaters. Problems include stress fractures, tendinitis, tendon subluxation, bursitis, shin splints, compartment syndromes, sprains, fractures, and dislocations.

Stress Fractures

Pecina et al.'s (20) series of 42 world-class figure skaters reported a total of nine stress fractures. Of these one involved the fibula and one, the tibia. The skater with the tibial stress fracture noted a sudden increase in training jumps associated with the occurrence of this injury. Stress fractures usually heal well with rest; some need immobilization and time. The exception is the "dreaded black line" type of fracture on the shaft of the tibia, which can be resistant to usual treatment methods (22). These fractures should be taken seriously and treated aggressively, i.e., up to 12 weeks in a cast, and may sometimes require surgery. Although not proven, electrical stimulators may improve healing.

Tendinitis

Poorly fitting skates can lead to inflammation over the tibialis anterior and extensor hallucis longus tendon. If left untreated, this may progress and lead to chronic tendinitis. This initially presents as "lace bite" and can be treated effectively with padding taped both medial and lateral to the tendons at the ankle joint to relieve the pressure caused by the skater's boot (23). This condition usually resolves quickly if treated early.

Achilles tendon injuries are common in skaters. Figure skaters are at high risk, because tremendous forces are generated in the Achilles tendon as it works eccentrically in the landing of jumps. Older figure skaters are at increased risk for partial tears as the tendon degenerates and weakens with age. Adequate stretching and warmup are helpful in preventing these injuries. A heel wedge can often improve symptoms.

The plantar flexed nature of the skate can lead to Achilles peritendinitis. Pain is often located at the insertion of the tendon into the tuberosity of the calcaneus. Pain may be relieved by activity. Tenderness often radiates proximally several centimeters up the tendon. Retrocalcaneal bursitis should be considered in the differential diagnosis. Treatment includes rest initially, then muscle stretching and strengthening, and antiinflammatory medication. Casting for a short time may be necessary. Occasionally, ultrasound and electrical stimulation may be used.

Although rare, peroneal tendon subluxation has been reported in figure skaters. Conservative treatment is preferred, but surgical reconstruction of the tendon sheath, in combination with deepening of the groove in fibula, may be necessary.

Speed skaters are at risk for medial tibial stress syndrome (shin splints). Treatment includes decreased training until symptoms improve, followed by gradually increasing stretching and strengthening program.

Bursitis

Fluid-filled bursas can develop over prominent areas such as the medial or lateral malleolus, or anterior tibial tendon and can contain up to 30 ml fluid (21). These are usually caused by excessive pressure from tightly fitting boots. Boot modifications are usually successful in improving these painful areas.

Exertional Compartment Syndrome

Compartment syndrome occasionally occurs in competitive skaters. Individuals usually complain of severe pain after a heavy workout, often in the anterior compartment of the leg. These can occasionally present acutely and should then be treated as a surgical emergency by performing compartment releases following measurement of elevated pressures. In the nonacute setting, increased pressure can be caused by muscle hypertrophy or thickened muscle fascias. In these patients, it is necessary to measure pressures in the office after an exercise routine that creates typical pain. Compartment releases may be necessary if elevated pressures correlate with symptoms and conservative treatment has failed.

Sprains, Fractures, and Dislocations

Garrick reported an incidence of one ankle sprain in 36 competitive figure skaters (11). Davis and Litman found that skaters using heavier and stiffer boots were more prone to ankle sprains (19). It is not known if this is a cause-and-effect relationship.

Ankle fractures and dislocations can occur in competitive skaters but are infrequent. More commonly these injuries are seen in beginner skaters, in-line skaters, and those with poorly fitting equipment. These should be managed with appropriate radiographs and treatments not discussed in this chapter.

Knee

Knee pain is common in all types of skaters. Acute injuries such as ligamentous disruption and meniscal injuries do occur, but overuse syndromes are by far more common. Injuries such as osteochondral fracture or osteochondritis dissecans should be in the differential diagnosis. These should be ruled out with careful physical examination and radiographs.

Patellar tendinitis or jumper's knee is the most frequently seen overuse injury in the competitive figure skater. Its course can develop quickly and lead to lengthy lost training time. In the adolescent, a high incidence of Osgood-Schlatter disease is evident. Patellofemoral pain or anterior knee pain, patellar subluxation, and bursitis also should enter the differential diagnosis of these athletes. Smith et al. (24) studied 46 junior elite figure skaters and showed that adolescent skaters with anterior knee pain, jumper's knee, Osgood-Schlatter disease, or isolated patellofemoral pain had less quadriceps and hamstring flexibility than similar skaters without knee pain. A stretching program designed for these individuals decreased the presence of knee pain in 9 of 14 skaters. Approximately 75% of all adolescent skaters evaluated needed improved flexibility, regardless of the presence of knee pain.

Speed skaters frequently develop knee pain related to dry-land and off-season sports, including cycling, running, and weight lifting. Meniscal tears can occur in speed skaters from twisting falls. This may become more prevalent in short-track speed skating, caused by catching an edge during falls into corners of the hockey rink.

Hip and Groin

Cramer and McQueen (25) identified four causes of groin injuries in figure skaters, which are related to muscle imbalance between hip adductors and gluteus medius, forcible push-off adducting the hip, forced external rotation of the adducted leg, and forced adduction of the hip. The differential diagnosis includes strain or tendinitis in rectus femoris, adductor longus, iliopsoas, or gracilis muscles. The most common site is the adductor longus. A detailed physical exam and history will often lead to the proper diagnosis of these injuries. Prevention by stretching during warmup is imperative for all types of skaters.

As reported by Garrick (4) and Smith and Micheli (13) overuse injuries of the hip are rare. Femoral neck fractures are a rare but serious injury, more frequently seen in recreational skaters than in competitors.

Back

Both figure skaters and speed skaters have a high incidence of back pain. Smith and Micheli (13) noted 6 of 19 competitive figure skaters reporting back pain in a retrospective analysis. This study found 5 of 15 girls with scoliosis by physical exam, an unusually high incidence compared with the general population (15%). The question of joint laxity and scoliosis arises in this group of athletes known for flexibility. Low-back pain is related to repeated jumping, hyperextension, and lifting and twisting in pairs skaters and is a problem for dancers and gymnasts as well. The authors believed this was related to tight lumbodorsal fascia as a result of an overgrowth syndrome in which soft tissues become taut secondary to skeletal growth. They also noted that most of these skaters had no stretching regimen in their training routines.

Speed skaters, because of the repetitive movements and the extreme forward flexed position of the skater's trunk, are prone to chronic low-back problems. Specific strengthening of the lumbar musculature is important in prevention. Speed skaters occasionally use heat retainers to keep lumbar musculature warm during outdoor training and competition.

Shoulder

Shoulder injuries are infrequent in skaters. Lifting injuries in pairs skaters can lead to rotator cuff strain and tendinitis, but again these are uncommon. Clavicle fractures are reported in the recreational skater (26).

Elbow and Wrist

Almost all injuries to the elbow and wrist are fractures. These are caused by direct trauma to the elbow or a fall onto the outstretched hand. Direct trauma to the elbow may cause traumatic olecranon bursitis or olecranon fractures. Most olecranon fractures require surgical treatment. Falling onto an outstretched hand with the wrist and elbow extended is the most common mechanism of injury in the inexperienced skater. The position of the wrist at the time of impact can determine whether the wrist or elbow is injured. If the wrist is dorsiflexed more than 40°, then a distal radius fracture or scaphoid fracture is produced. If the wrist is dorsiflexed less than 40%, then a radial head or capitellar fracture is produced (27). The incidence of these injuries could be decreased by instruction for beginning skaters, protective gear, and avoidance of crowded facilities and poor skating surfaces.

Hand

Most hand injuries in ice skating are lacerations caused by a skate blade. These are usually seen in a recreational skater who was skating a crowded public facility. Competitive skaters at risk for these injuries are short-track speed skaters and pairs skaters. Protective gloves would prevent many of these lacerations. In-line skaters are at risk for abrasions from a fall onto pavement. Most of these problems can be prevented by routine use of wrist guards, which protect the palm.

Nonorthopedic Injuries

Competitive and recreational ice skaters are exposed to cold weather conditions. Training and conditioning can be compromised in cold weather. Bergh (28) showed that lowering muscle temperature between 2° and 6° will decrease maximum aerobic effort as well as maximal isometric and dynamic muscle power. Hixon (29) showed that Olympic athletes perspire during training and competition despite subzero temperatures. Dehydration and decreased blood volume in muscles can be a contributing factor in acute and overuse injuries. Adequate fluid replacement is important for the competitive skater in outdoor conditions.

Frostnip is a superficial blue-white discoloration of the skin with associated insensitivity, usually found on exposed skin such as the face. Often the athlete does not recognize its presence. Treatment includes rewarming the affected area. Frostbite, however, is a deeper affliction of the skin layers and is painful. Initial treatment is rewarming and increased activity. Blisters can result from frostbite and involve tissue loss. Clear blisters indicate a superficial injury and can be debrided. Hemorrhagic blisters indicate a deeper injury. These should be left intact as debridement can lead to progression of the zone of injury.

Conclusions

Speed skaters, figure skaters, long-distance skaters, and in-line skaters are at risk for numerous overuse and acute injuries. Most overuse injuries can be prevented by proper warmup, stretching, and conditioning. Skaters should gradually increase training duration and intensity. Properly fitting skates are crucial to avoiding foot and ankle injuries. Many acute injuries can be prevented by wearing protective equipment in appropriate circumstances. Skating for a well-trained, well-equipped, and experienced individual is a rewarding, enjoyable, and relatively safe sport.

REFERENCES

1. Eriksson E. Langfardsakning pa skidsko [Long distance skating]. Stockholm: Konsument Verket, 1979.
2. Brasch R. *How did sports begin? A look at the origins of man at play.* New York: David McKay, 1970:224–234.
3. van Ingen Schenau GJ, DeBoer RW, De Groot G. Biomechanics of speed skating. In: C. Vaughan, ed. Boca Raton, FL: CRC Press, 1989:121–167.
4. Ferkel RS, Mai LL, Ullis KC, Finerman GA. An analysis of roller-skating injuries. Am J Sports Med 1981;10(1):24–30.
5. Bregenzer RJ. AC Nielson Company News—international mar-aketing research. Northbrook, IL: AC Nielson, July 30, 1979.
6. van Ingen Schenau GJ, De Groot G. On the origin of differences in performance level between elite male and female speed skaters. Hum Movement Sci 1983;2:151.
7. De Boer RW, Schermerhorn P, Gademan J, De Groot G, van Ingen Schenau GJ. Characteristic stroke mechanics of elite and trained male speed skaters. J Sport Biomech 1986;2:175–185.
8. Malhotra MS, Gupta JS. Work capacity at altitude. In Jokl E, Anad RL, Stoboy H, eds. Medicine sport. Vol. 9, Advances in exercise physiology. Basel: S Karger, 1976:165–177.
9. Smith A. Figure skating. In: Schneider RC, Kennedy JC, Plant ML, eds. *Sports injuries, mechanisms, prevention and treatment.* Baltimore: Williams & Wilkins, 1985:516–531.
10. Williamson DM, Lowdon IMP. Ice-skating injuries. Injury 1986;17:205–207.
11. Garrick JG. Characterization of the patient population in a sports medicine facility. Phys Sportsmed 1985;13(10):73–76.
12. Brock RM, Striowski CC. Injuries in the elite figure skaters. Phys Sportsmed 1986;15(1):111–115.
13. Smith AD, Micheli LJ. Injuries in competitive figure skating. Phys Sportsmed 1982;10(1):36–47.
14. Smith AD, Ludington P. Injuries in elite pair skaters and ice dancers. Am J Sports Med. 1989;17(4):482–488.
15. Eriksson E, Lofström B, Räf L, Sartok T. Injuries from long distance lake skating. Nord Idrettsmedisinsk Kongress Proc Beitostolen Norway. 1977:142–149.
16. Schwarzman PS. Rollerskating injuries. Ann Emerg Med 1980;9(4):193–195.
17. Sedlin ED, Zitner DT, McGinniss G. Rollerskating accidents and injuries. J Trauma 1984;24(2):136–139.
18. Inkelis SH, Stroberg AJ, Keller EL, Christenson PD. Rollerskating injuries in children. Pediatr Emerg Care 1988;4(2):127–132.
19. Davis MW, Litman T. Figure skater's foot. Minn Med 1979;62:647–648.
20. Pecina M, Bojanic I, Dubravcic S. Stress fractures in figure skaters. Am J Sports Med 1990;18(3):277.
21. Smith AD. Foot and ankle injuries in figure skaters. Phys Sportsmed 1990;18(3):73–86.
22. Micheli LJ. Stress fractures in athletes. Paper presented at the Sports Symposium. Burlington, VT, 1991.
23. Cummings T. Lace-bite padding. Phys Sportsmed 1984;12(2):166.
24. Smith AD, Stroud L, McQueen C. Flexibility and anterior knee pain in adolescent elite figure skaters. J Pedratr Orthop 1991;11(1):77–82.
25. Cramer LM, McQueen CH. Overuse injuries in figure skating. In: Casey MJ, ed. *Winter sports medicine.* Philadelphia: FA Davis, 1990:254–268.
26. Murphy NM, Riley P, Keys C. Ice-skating injuries to the hand. J Hand Surg 1990;15B(3):349–351.
27. Frykman G. Fracture of the distal radius including sequelae—shoulder-hand-finger syndrome, disturbance in the distal radioulnar joint, and impairment of nerve function: a clinical and experimental study. Acta Orthop Scand Suppl 1967;108:1–26.
28. Bergh U. Human power at subnormal body temperatures. Acta Physiol Scand (Suppl) 1980;478:1–39.
29. Hixson E. Injury patterns in cross-country skiing. Phys Sportsmed 1981;9:45–53.

27 / JUDO AND KARATE-DO

Joseph F. Fetto

Introduction

The prevention of injuries is the ideal toward which sports medicine strives. It is through the identification and control of factors that cause injuries that this goal can be achieved. It is in this context that this chapter will discuss the sports of judo and karate-do.

Although the array, prevalence, and incidence of injuries vary from sport to sport, the analysis of injuries occurring in a specific sport such as judo or karate-do can be performed in a logical and standardized, rather than anecdotal, manner. The result of such analysis is a better understanding of the etiology of the specific sport's injuries. As a corollary of such an understanding comes a more efficient means of identifying a given athlete's potential for injury, a potential that represents a mismatch of that athlete's physical attributes versus the demands of performing a given sport activity.

The concepts on which this analysis is predicated are as follows (Fig. 27.1). Injuries are an unavoidable aspect of sports participation. They occur for a variety of reasons. Some injuries go on to recovery; others go on to chronic disability. The critical questions are *(a)* Why do injuries occur? *(b)* Can they be anticipated? *(c)* Can one prepare for their occurrence? *(d)* Can their incidence be reduced? *(e)* Can their consequences be modified? *(f)* Can injuries be prevented?

Temporarily setting aside from consideration psychological factors such as motivation, discipline, etc., sports injuries can be studied as events occurring within a mechanical system. This system, although organic, alive, and able to respond, is still subject to the same laws of physics and mechanics as inorganic systems. As such, injuries represent mechanical failure of the system. This failure may occur in one of two modes. It can be either the result of a single event in which acute, excessive stress is applied to an otherwise normal system, i.e., fracture or sprain, or the result of repeated submaximal stresses that produce a fatigued state within the system, i.e., stress fracture or tendinitis (Fig. 27.2). In either type of failure, the organic system will attempt to respond. The intensity and extent of this response are determined by the magnitude of the injury. This inflammatory response is the system's attempt to initiate healing of the injury. It relies on multiple events at the chemical, hormonal, and cellular levels. These events may be modified by immediate medical intervention, with general medical modalities such as rest, ice, elevation, and compression as well as definitive, specific treatment choices dictated by the nature of the injury at hand. In any case, the outcome of a period of injury-imposed rest (removal of stress) will be a lowered tolerance and, therefore, increased vulnerability to reinjury. If nothing is done to restore or increase the system's tolerance limit to its preinjury state, the injured athlete has a significant likelihood of going on to reinjury and chronic disability. (Fig. 27.3*A*). This pattern has been described as a vicious circle of injury.

A corollary of this model is the effect of training (stress) on injury prevention and postinjury recovery. Unlike the inorganic system, (an airplane wing) which is destined to ultimate failure, the organic system, if given the opportunity, can adapt to applied stresses. Stress, in this way, can be considered a stimulus. When it is applied at a frequency, intensity, and duration so as to permit adaptation before fatigue failure occurs, the result will be a raised level of tolerance (conditioning) and hence a reduced vulnerability to injury (Fig. 27.3*B*).

This model has two important consequences. First, it provides a methodology by which training techniques can be evaluated and refined in terms of the desired goal. Second, this model encourages an appreciation for and consideration of individual variability (age, sex, body type, anatomy, etc.) when evaluating the appropriateness of various training techniques and routines for a given individual or group of individuals. It permits the identification of potential areas of vulnerability to injury. Therefore, a specific activity (sport, level of play, or position) can be analyzed for its prerequisites (strength, flexibility, or cardiovascular endurance), which will create a composite of what specific

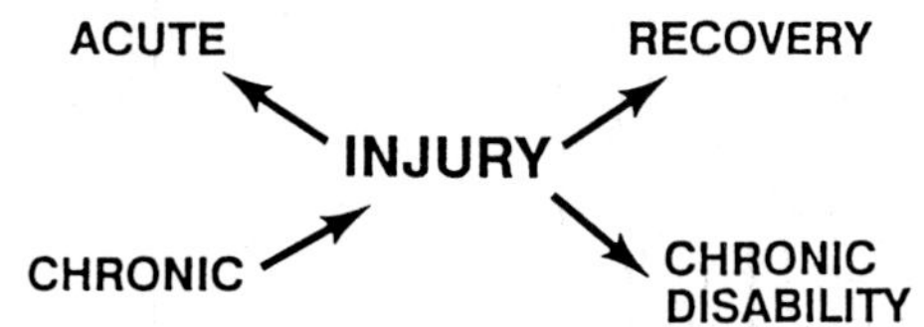

Figure 27.1. Types of trauma and their possible outcomes.

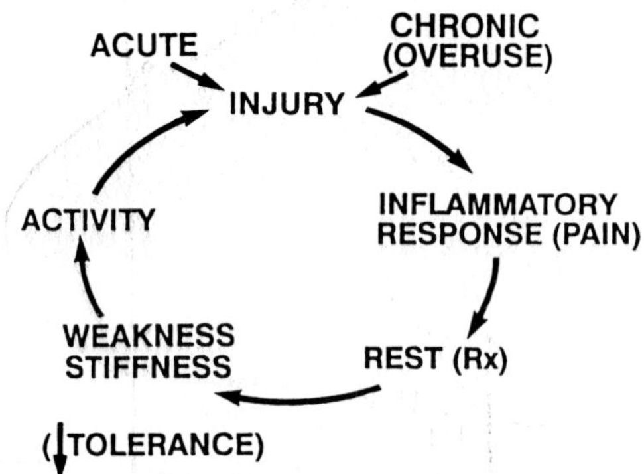

Figure 27.2. The vicious circle of injury brought on by system failure as a function of either acute overload or repetitive submaximal stress.

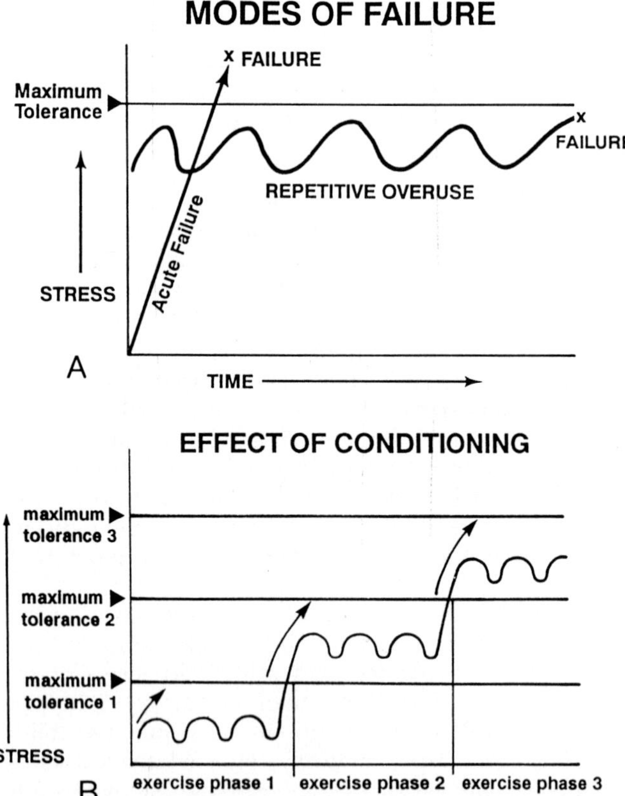

Figure 27.3. A, Increased risk of reinjury is a direct consequence of reduced tolerance caused by rest of the injured part. **B,** Conditioning is the result of the controlled application of stress at a frequency, intensity, and duration that can be tolerated by the system, permitting adaptation and increasing the maximum tolerance level achieved before the onset of fatigue.

attributes may be required to permit successful participation and lessen the likelihood of injury. This concept of comparing the individual against the anticipated demands of the chosen activity has been referred to as profiling. This model lays the logical foundation for injury prevention as well as an accurate foundation for exercise prescriptions.

With this preamble, a more productive discussion will be undertaken of judo and karate-do injuries and their prevention.

Origins

To have a thorough understanding of the traditional and technical aspects of a sport, it is necessary to have an appreciation of its cultural and historical origins as well as its evolution. Judo, karate-do, and sumo are combat techniques that evolved in Japan in a unique way. All of them were derived and developed from individual fighting techniques used in historic times. Judo, originally called *jujitsu,* was initially developed in the latter half of the 16th century, when samurai knights grappled with each other in battle. At that time, Japan was in the midst of civil wars. In the early 19th century, the *Teno* (emperor) system was established in Japan after a series of civil wars, and Jigoro Kanoh (1860–1939) rose to became the master of *jujitsu.* At the same time, he made a comparative study of the techniques of *jujitsu* as taught in the various schools. He picked out what was best among those schools and developed a technique that enables the most effective mental and physical training. Kanoh called his technique *judo* and his training *odokan,* meaning that the disciplinary principles should be extended and highly respected. Karate-do is a martial art that was developed in the Okinawa Island area at the southern tip of Japan. Since ancient times, the Okinawa has had a fist combat technique called *te* (hand). During the latter half of the 14th century, there was an interchange of information on the fist-fighting arts with the Chinese via trade routes. This contact was said to have had an important influence on the conventional *te* arts of Okinawa. About the time that the *Teno* system was established on the mainland of Japan, previously unknown Okinawan martial arts were introduced and spread gradually all over Japan. It was in 1901 that the name *karate* was first formally used. However, like judo, it is officially called karate-do, meaning that it should not merely be interpreted as a form of combative technique, but emphasis should be put on self-defense, which aims to develop a mentally and physically mature person by mastering the integral arts used to defend oneself.

Today, judo and karate-do are played throughout the world. Judo is recognized Olympic sport. Through Western involvement in Southeast Asia, it has become popular in Europe (especially France) and the United States. It has, as a result of this Western involvement, expanded to include a significant number of female participants. Karate-do, unlike judo, is usually considered more of a fighting and self-defense activity than a competitive sport. This is reflective of its greater emphasis on contact through strikes, blows, and kicks as opposed to the grappling techniques of judo.

Differences between Judo and Karate-Do

Judo and karate-do are similar combative sports in the sense that two players who wear a training suit stipulated in the rules stand facing each other and fight to win the match. However, there is a fundamental difference in the essentials of the respective arts (1–5). Judo requires grappling, and karate-do involves contact from a distance, employing strikes, kicks, and blows.

The natural posture in judo is as follows. The distance between the ankles is approximately 1 foot, and the body weight is equally distributed on both feet. No particular strain is applied to the four extremities. The participants should look and stand straight. Either the left or right leg may be put forward by one sole length when the participant moves in any direction. He or she walks smoothly, rubbing the floor lightly with the sole of the foot. In contrast, the natural posture of karate-do can vary. The feet may be placed shoulder width apart, with the knees flexible. The player faces forward and stands straight. The player may also stand with the feet touching lightly or with the feet double shoulder width apart. In accordance with the distance between the players, the whole body will bend, extend, rotate, or propel at an accelerating speed. The purpose of such motion is to increase the attacking or defending effect.

Basic Forms of Grappling

In judo, the players grapple with each other by gripping the uniform of the opponent with one hand, with the other hand at the middle of the sleeve (Fig. 27.4). By doing this, the player can perform a pushing, pulling, or turning action most effectively. According to the present form of judo, each player grapples with his or her partner with both hands and tries to apply the attacking technique or to dodge the attack. The player throws the opponent, keeps the opponent on his or her back for 30 sec, or strangles the opponent just short of falling into unconsciousness, or applies damaging stress to the opponent's joints. Therefore, the action consists of throwing, pressing, strangling, or joint-attacking techniques.

In karate-do, two players face each other standing at a distance. They never grapple with each other (Fig. 27.5), but there may be many patterns of how to hold the arms. In one case, the hand is closed to form a fist, and in another, it is open and loose. There are many kinds of winning techniques in karate-do. Basically, the sport consists of thrusting and hitting with the upper extremities, kicking with the lower extremities, and striking with the elbows as well as receiving techniques for defense against an enemy attack. Except for the receiving techniques, karate-do essentially aims to strike a sensitive area of the other player while moving swiftly from the confronting posture. Such a technique requires a bending and jumping movement with the whole body. The winning technique is judged effective when

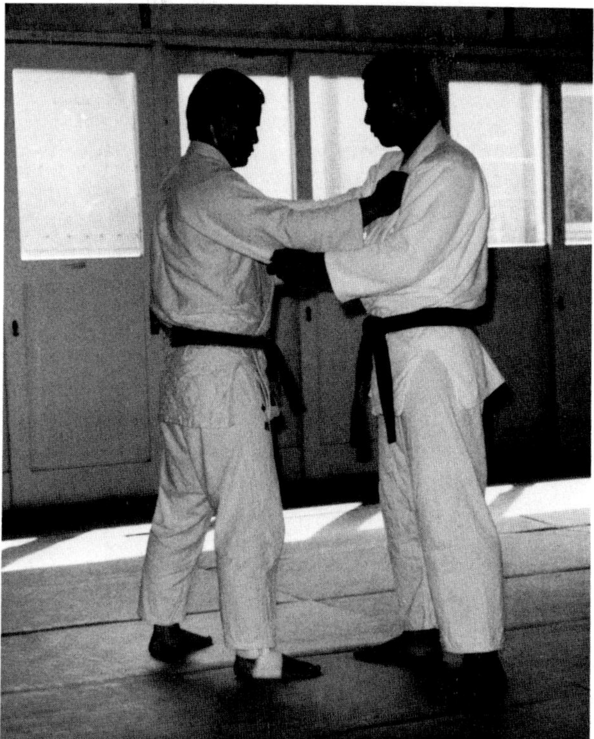

Figure 27.4. The players demonstrate the basic form of grappl used in judo.

the strike is made at the aimed-for spot on the otl player. There is no throwing, pressing, strangling, or joint-damaging techniques in karate-do.

Injuries

Every sport and activity has an inherent risk of injury. No study to date reports the absolute incidence of injury among judo and karate-do players. It is noted in Japan that judo ranks after skiing, baseball, karate-do, field athletics, and skating in frequency of injured athletes reporting to hospitals (6). This is similar to the American experience, which ranks judo far below contact sports such as football, rugby, and hockey and similar to that of wrestling. The latter has an expected incidence of significant injury occurring in approximately 10% of participants (significant injury is defined, according to the American College of Sports Medicine, as one causing absence from sport participation for 24 or more consecutive hours). The types of injury reported in judo and their frequency are sprains (56.5%), dislocations (21.7%), fractures (19.2%), and other (3%). The regions of the body most frequently reported injured, in order of incidence, are the knee, ankle, shoulder, elbow, lumbar spine, wrist, neck, toes, and fingers. The incidence of toe and finger injuries is believed to be highly underreported by most individuals familiar with the sport (Fig. 27.6). The remaining injuries include chest and abdominal contusions, concussions, and rare intracranial hemorrhages.

The limited available data on karate-do demonstrate a greater than 50% incidence of injuries occurring among

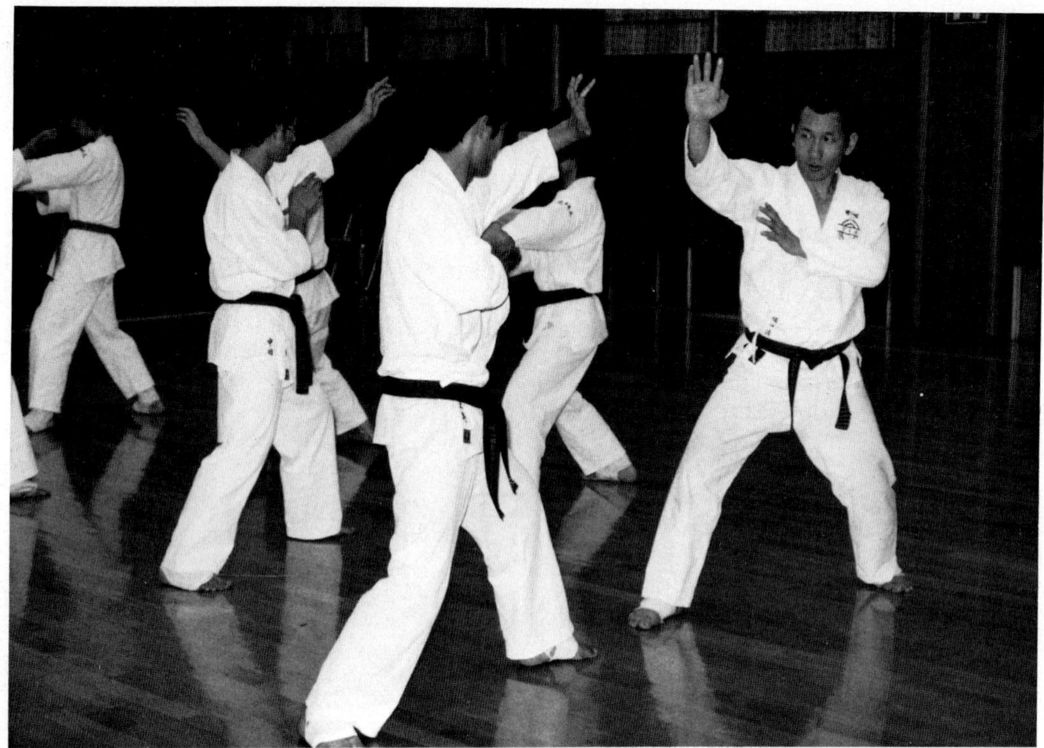

Figure 27.5. The basic form of karate-do is shown; players face each other at a regulation distance.

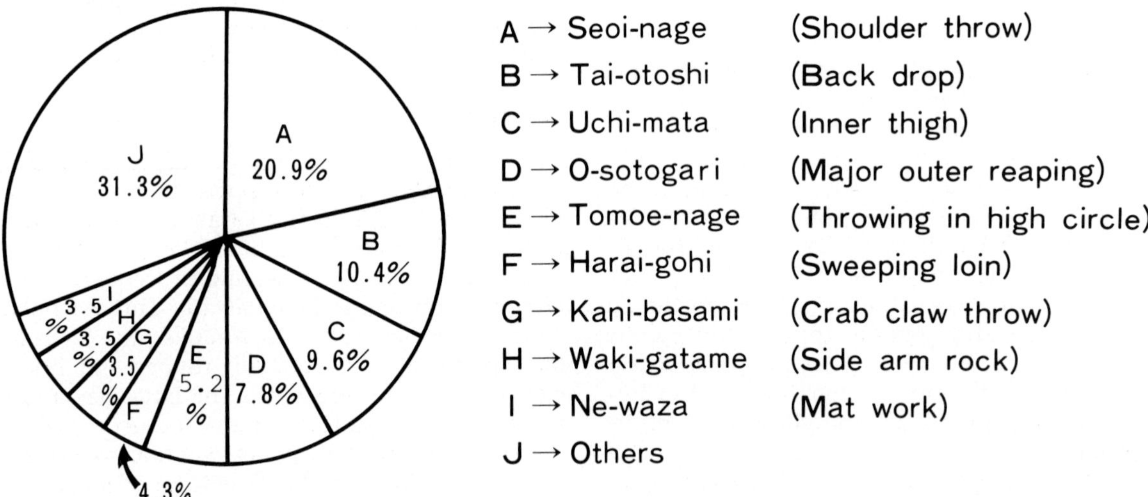

Figure 27.6. The nine judo techniques most frequently responsible for causing injuries. From Mifune T. Canon of judo. Tokyo: Seibundo-Shinkosha, 1956. Courtesy of Horiyasu.

tournament participants, an obviously experienced group (7). In one tournament, injuries occurring among 70 participants were extremities, 18; head and neck, 11; trunk, 8; thigh and leg hematomas, 8; hand and fingers, 5; concussion, 2; and eye, 1. (6) Both judo and karate-do have reports of hematuria and myoglobinuria after competition and from training sessions.

These injury profiles reinforce the fact that judo and karate-do are dissimilar sports, in both the type and the frequency of injuries that they engender. More data exist on injuries as a function of specific techniques for judo than for karate-do. The incidence of injuries in judo as a function of specific techniques is illustrated in Figure 27.6. When comparing matches against free exercise, injuries in judo occur somewhat more frequently during match competition. The defense techniques in judo usually cause more injuries than the attacking techniques (Fig. 27.7). The defending player in karate-do also is more frequently injured. Injuries are a commonly caused by throwing techniques. The attacking players using the shoulder throw *(seoi-nage)* and back drop *(tai-otoshi)* techniques sustained more injuries when they were unsuccessful and were subsequently crushed under the defending players (Figs. 27.8 and 27.9). The defending players were most often injured when subjected to the attacking techniques of the inner thigh *(uchi-mata)*, major outer reaping *(o-sotogari)*, or sweeping loin *(marai-goshi)* (Figs. 27.10–27.12). These injuries were the result of the defending player being thrown or the extremity being caught between the two players.

When throwing in the high circle *(tomoe-nage)*, both attacking players, as they were crushed, and the defending players, as they were thrown, suffered a similar number of injuries (Fig. 27.13). The crab-claw throw *(kani-basami)* showed a smaller percentage of injuries (Fig. 27.14). It should be noted, however, that this particular technique has recently been under vigorous discussion as one to be prohibited from being a legitimate technique. The basis for this discussion has centered around the severity of lower extremity injuries (triad lesions: complete anterior cruciate; medial collateral ligament; and medial meniscus tears) caused by this throw even when it is executed properly.

Groundwork techniques (mat work, or *ne-waza*) produce few injuries except for occasional severe muscular strains of the torso. During exercise and training, olecranon, acromioclavicular, and minor trochanteric bursitises have occurred in connection with forward rotation of the body, whereas cervical strains are generated by backward rotation.

Depending on the skill of the receiver, contusions of the hypothenar aspect of the hand; compression-disruption of the ankle mortises, the calcaneus, and the talus; and contusion of the lateral malleolus also have been observed.

Stand-up throwing *(tachiwaza)* can frequently cause strain, fracture, and dislocation of the toes and the foot. A difficult problem occurs when actual rotation movement is applied to the half-bent knee, resulting in a serious ligament sprain or subluxation/dislocation of the patellofemoral joint.

When a judo player is thrown and falls to the floor onto the shoulder, an acromioclavicular separation can occur. If body distortion is involved, the player may also suffer a clavicular or rib fracture. If a judo player takes a violent fall backward, he or she may hit the occipital region, resulting in concussion or acute subdural hematoma. This was seen in the neurosurgical department at the University of Tokyo.

The strangling technique is often applied during mat work. The player being strangled can fall into temporary unconsciousness. This mechanism is explained by the sudden oxygen deprivation of the brain caused by compression of the common carotid artery bilaterally. In the articular technique (usually applying a hyperextension force), disruption of ligaments with resultant dislocation is caused by excessive application of force. According to Norton and Cutler (8) serious injury of this sort is most likely to occur at the knee and shoulder. The elbow is directly attacked quite often, but the defenders usually yield before dislocation of the elbow occurs. This is because of the continuous, rather than sudden, manner in which correct technique applies stress to the elbow joint. Frequently, the toes suffer minor injuries, and contusions, sprains, fractures, and dislocations are significantly underreported. The rare

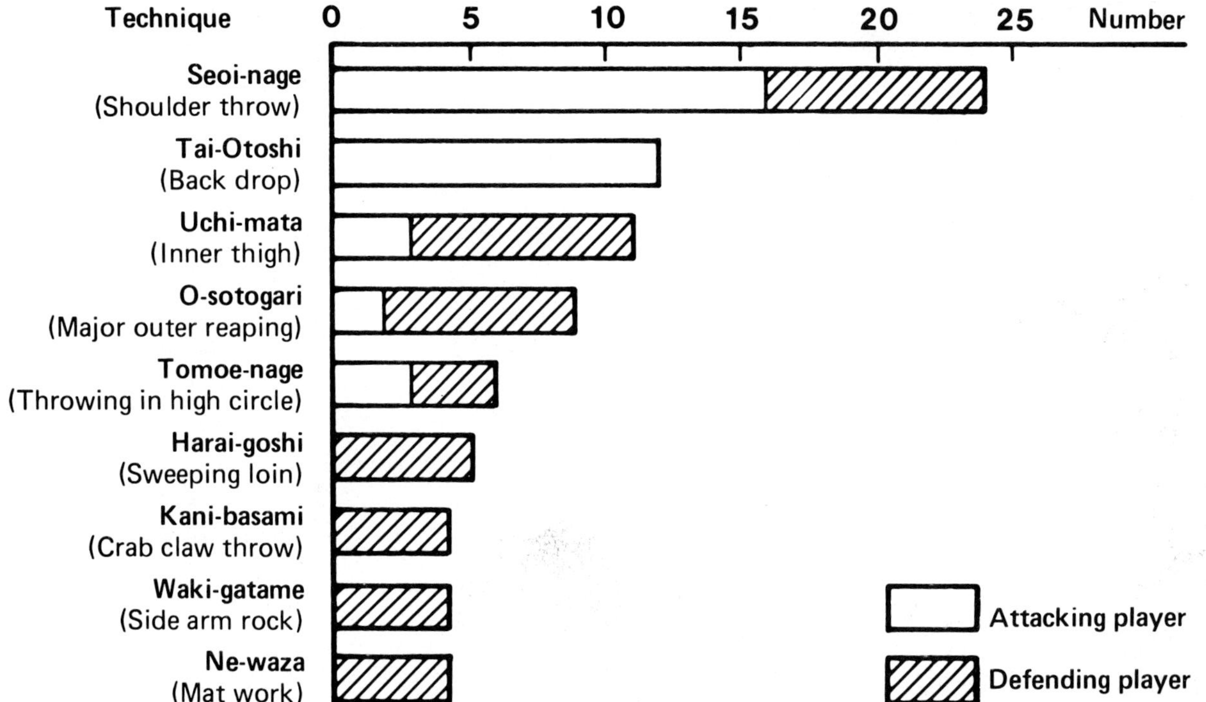

Figure 27.7. The nine judo techniques most frequently responsible for causing injuries, depending on whether the player is using an attacking or defense technique. From Mifune T. Canon of judo. Tokyo: Seibundo-Shinkosha, 1956. Courtesy of Horiyasu.

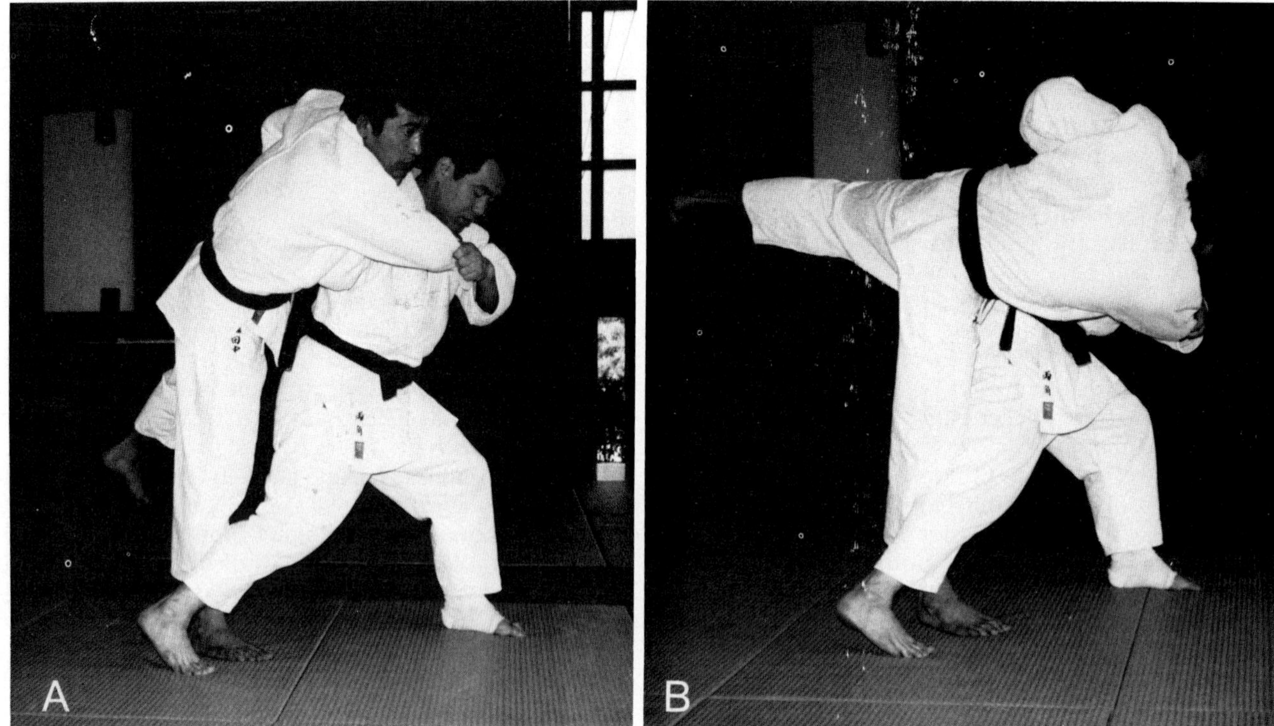

Figure 27.8. The shoulder throw *(seoi-nage)* is the technique responsible for the highest number of injuries in judo (20.9%).

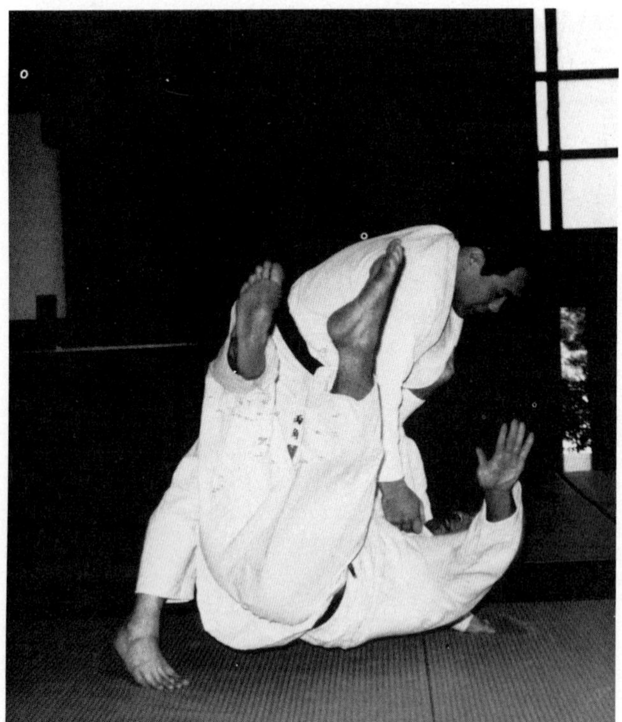

Figure 27.9. The back drop *(tai-otoshi)* is the second leading cause of judo injury (10.4%).

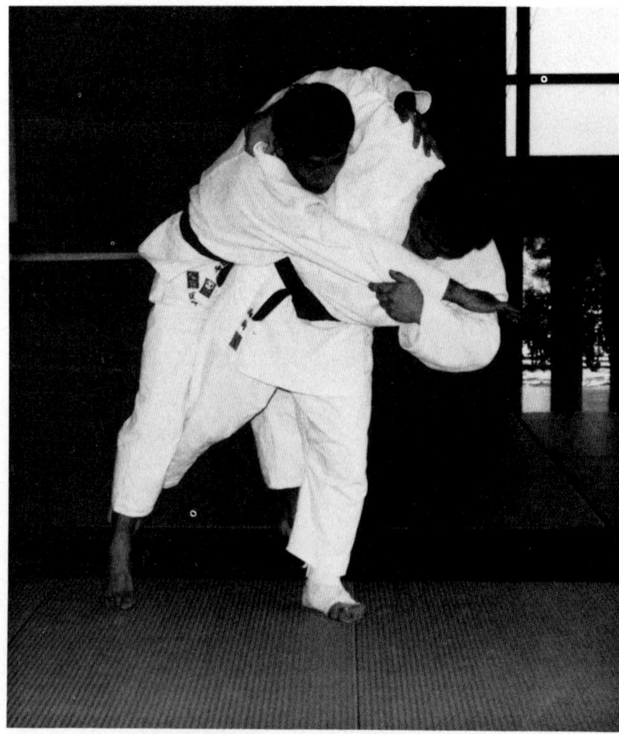

Figure 27.10. The frequency of judo injuries from use of the inner thigh *(uchi-mata)* technique (9.6%) is close to that of the back drop.

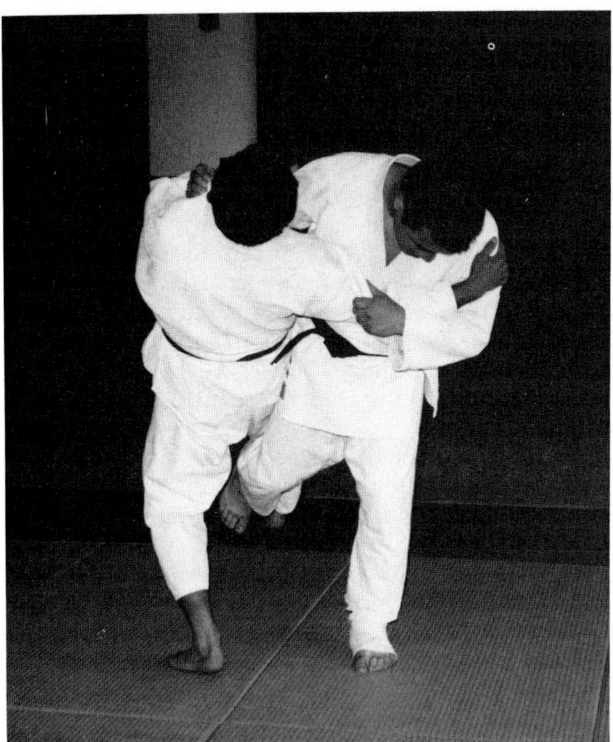

Figure 27.11. The major outer reaping *(o-sotogari)* approach of judo is demonstrated.

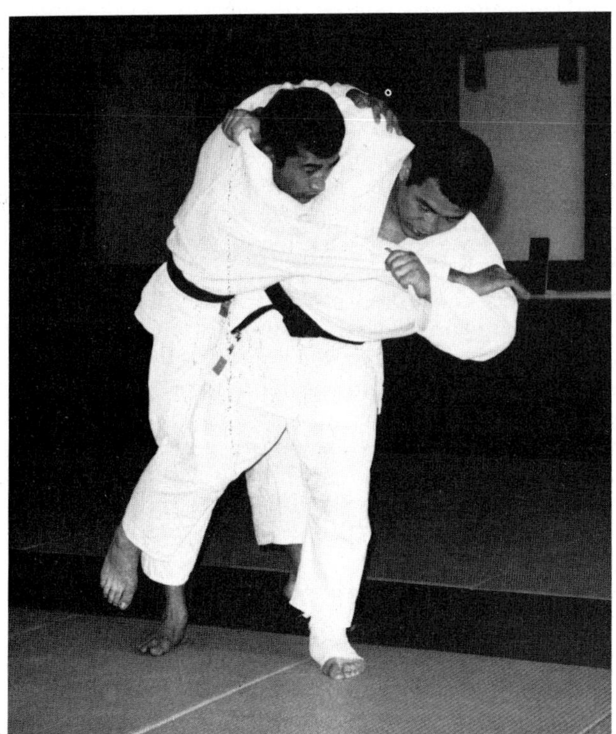

Figure 27.12. The initial phase of the sweeping loin *(harai-goshi)* technique of judo is demonstrated.

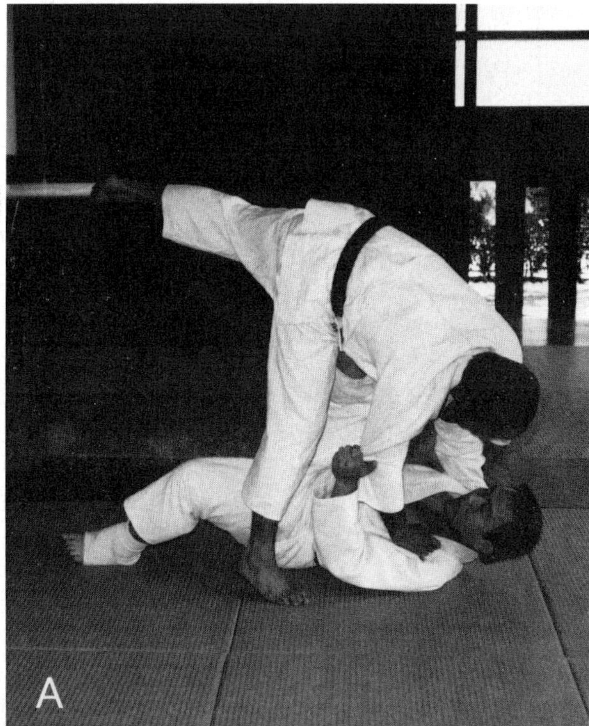

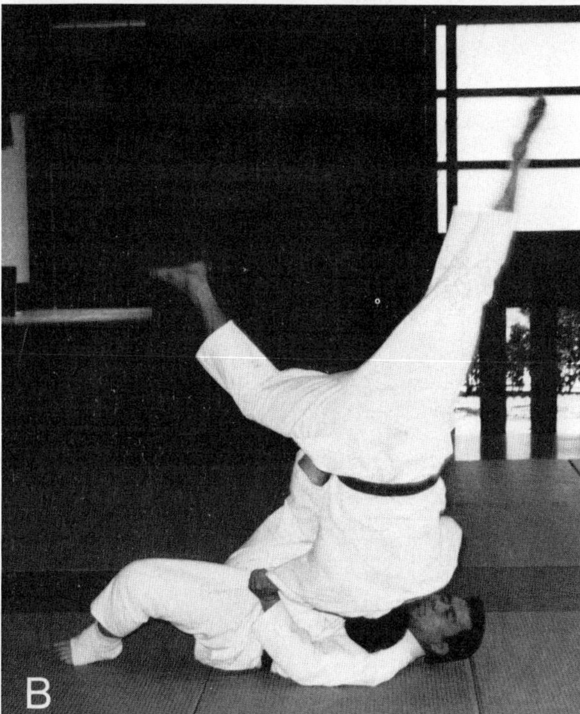

Figure 27.13. The rigors of the judo move of throwing in the high circle *(tomoe-nage)* are demonstrated.

cases of reported fatalities caused by strangling have involved players with preexisting heart conditions and/or liver dysfunctions.

Studies have attributed judo injuries to several factors (1): *(a)* poor technique with excessive force (61.7%); *(b)* inexperience with the technique employed (17.4%); *(c)* insufficient physical strength and/or conditioning for the level of activity attempted (14.8%); and *(d)* inadequate equipment, environment, and supervision (6.1%). These statistics are used to explain the occurrence, causes, and mechanisms of injuries that occur in the sport of judo. A such, attention has traditionally been concentrated on training methods that will enhance technical skill, particularly in defense techniques.

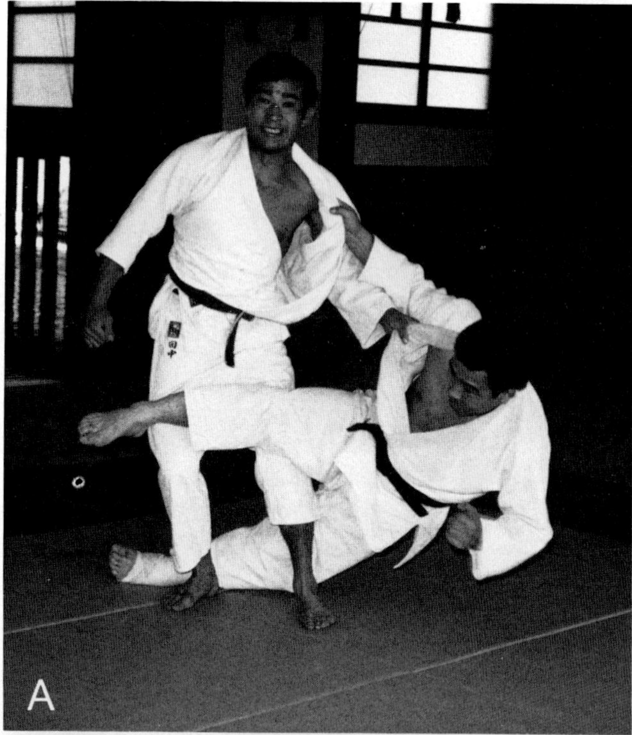

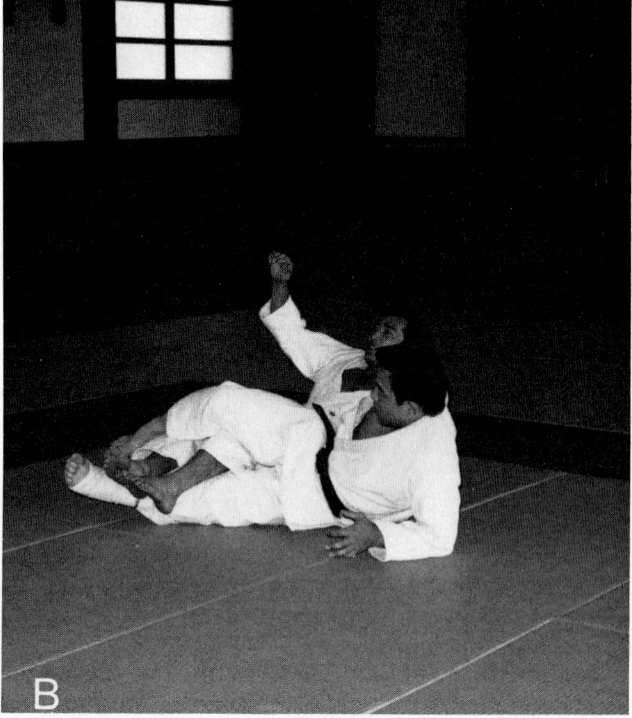

Figure 27.14. The crab-claw throw *(kani-basami)* technique is responsible for a small percentage of judo injuries (3.5%).

The receiving technique is a defensive move against a good throw executed by the opponent. Norton and Cutler (8) concurred with this analysis of injuries in judo. According to their explanation, the receiving, or defensive, technique is the absolute essential first step in judo training. It is *indispensable.* Notwithstanding these reports, the fact remains that many players become discouraged early in their experience with judo as a result of suffering injuries that occurred because of not only poor technique but also because of fatigue and/or inadequate physical condition. Both judo and karate-do require quickness and repetitive movements over an extended period of time.

In addition to acute trauma, overuse syndromes are frequently encountered. Because overuse conditions are not dramatic—although incapacitating—they are grossly underreported by judo and karate-do participants. These injuries include tendinitis of the lateral extensor musculature of the forearm (secondary to sustained grip activity), rotator cuff and shoulder girdle strains, paraspinal strains (secondary to throwing and lifting techniques), and hamstring strains (secondary to sweeping and rapid extension moves involving the lower extremities). Each of these conditions are brought on by the explosive, repetitive loading of the muscle group. Thus preparation of the athlete must emphasize sufficient flexibility (stretching) and aerobic conditioning along with strengthening exercises so he or she can withstand the sudden and sustained output of energy and effort required by the sport. Experience has shown that proper and successful execution of the movements requires quickness, agility, and flexibility.

In 1978, comparison of the anthropomorphic data of judo veterans versus that of average adult Japanese males showed three points of variance: strength of back muscles, girth of the chest, and side-step quickness. A similar attempt to profile karate-do players seemed to show a bias in favor of their having shorter reaction times. These data are of interest but cannot be relied on to predict success. However, DeMeersman and Ruhling (9) evaluated the physiologic effect of a specific training regime. Their conclusion was that judo training enhanced cardiorespiratory function. This result, although also observed in Canada by Taylor and Brassard (10), did not clearly show an advantage over the results achieved in other sports. More data are required before a more complete profile for judo and karate-do can be constructed. Because of the explosive and sustained output of energy and effort required by judo and karate-do, the player must have adequate stamina to avoid premature fatigue and increased vulnerability to injury.

Prevention and Treatment

Prevention depends on anticipation, environment and equipment, supervision, and preparation.

Anticipation

Understanding how winning is accomplished in a given sport aids in the anticipation of injury-producing situations. Winning in judo is determined by the accumulation of a greater number of points than the opponent or ending a match by pinning or choking out the opponent. Points are awarded by performing specific techniques of bringing the opponent to the mat, performing near-pinning movements, or successfully executing escape or reversal maneuvers. The number of points awarded also is reflective of the technical excellence with which the execution of a given maneuver is performed, in adherence with specific defined parameters of the sport. Therefore, success in judo depends on a combination of technical skill, endurance throughout the match, and sufficient strength to execute attack and defense maneuvers well.

In karate-do, winning is determined in a similar manner of point accumulation. Points are awarded according to the specific style of karate-do being performed (noncontact, limited contact, or full contact). Here, quickness and agility are paramount, endurance is important, and strength is a lesser prerequisite for success.

Judo techniques consist of overthrowing, holding, strangling, and joint articular. Each of these can be divided into a large number of subtechniques. The common general training methods are as follows. The beginner must first become accustomed to the atmosphere of judo and get rid of excessive tension. Furthermore, he or she must learn the manners of judo. When the athlete stands, he or she must master the natural posture without fail. Then, the player must repeatedly practice the smooth and quick movements in any direction, while keeping the sole of the foot in contact with the floor. The overthrow must be started with a simple movement. Its series of steps must be understood fully by the analysis of the motion in detail. This exercise must be done repeatedly, because the mastering of these basic actions is indispensable to safety in the contact training that comes later. One-on-one training with players who do not know the basic techniques well is highly dangerous and frequently ends in injury. This must be strictly prohibited. The remaining aspects of beginning training for judo players are concerned with the aggressive method of overthrow and the receiving technique. The properly executed receiving technique protects the player who is being overthrown from injury. For the holding technique, the application and evading methods must be practiced.

When the correct technique has been learned from solitary practice, the player may practice the attack and receiving techniques with a partner, after they have agreed on the exercise contents. At the beginning, the player should avoid performing the techniques with full strength. The free practice *(rando-ri)* must be done with a partner. It is recommended that this free practice exercise be done with a more experienced player to help with learning the correct technique. After the basic action has been learned, other kinds of overthrow and holding techniques must be mastered in the way. The player tries to distort the opponent's posture and simultaneously to apply his or her own technique in response to the opponent's movement. In this way, the forte or special technique of a player is developed. Free practice with a partner becomes the mainstay of the exercise, and the full-force practice is repeated. At the same time, the technique is perfected through the practice matches.

The art of karate-do is theoretically identical to that of judo. However, the technical aspects are different. Roughly speaking, there are three schools of karate-do. In the first school, a technical motion must be stopped shortly before it comes in contact with the opponent. In the second school, only the thrust technique against the face is prohibited. Otherwise, contact with the body of the other player is allowed. In the third school, the player must wear protective gear during the match while technique is applied directly by the other player (Fig. 27.15). Various standard postures and footwork must be learned, and the purposes and advantages of each must be considered. Then, the motions of the hand and foot must be learned. After all these steps are mastered, the self-practice must repeat the respective techniques such as the thrust, strike, hit, kick, and receiving movements. In karate-do, the throwing and strangling are prohibited in principle. While receiving, however, a player may try tripping or throwing to attempt to thwart the opponent. After repeated practice, players become accustomed to the techniques, after which the following two practice methods are applied. First, the various movements are carried out in succession by one player alone. This is the practice of *Kata* form. If two players try to apply the karate-do movements against each other with full force, there is a danger of causing injury. Therefore, it is indispensable to learn fully a series of *kata* forms. The second practice method is called *jumite* and involves the combination of techniques employed by two players. Here, the players agree in advance on which moves to practice. For the free technique, combinations of movements are used, and the players make no agreement in advance. The latter is equal to the free practice method *(randori)* of judo.

Environment

The traditional training facility of judo and karate-do is called the *dojo.* The training and matches for judo are carried out on straw mats *(tatami)* put down over a wooden floor, whereas karate-do is usually performed without mats. These setups have obvious hazards inherent to them. As such, Western programs usually use padded mats (4×6 feet or 4×8 feet) connected by velcro on four sides. A training hall floor should be founded on a sprung base. The standard allocation is three *tatami* mats per player. In all cases, both judo and karate-do are performed in bare feet. Thus, to avoid foot trauma, the need for meticulous care, maintenance, and cleanliness of the exercise facility is obvious. The *dojo* should be well-lit and well-ventilated. Proper recommended lighting is 150 to 300 lux for training, and 200 to 500 lux for match purposes.

The training uniform is called the *gi.* It is composed of a loose-fitting jacket and pants fastened by a cloth

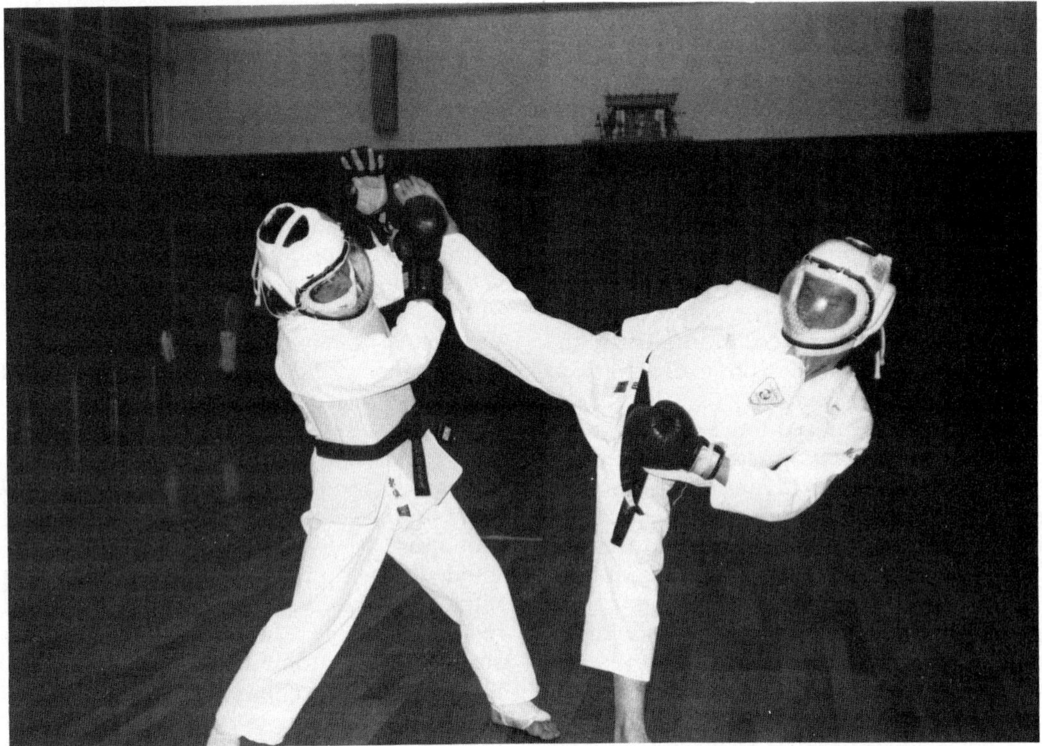

Figure 27.15. Two karate-do players are pictured in action wearing full protection.

belt. The belt color is used to designate the level of proficiency of the athlete.

These seemingly reasonable prerequisites have led, however, to a philosophical schism among advocates of these sports. For example, in karate-do, devices should be used in one-on-one practice to protect the face, abdomen, hands, back and ankles. Purists who adhere to the need to enhance "total effect of training" through the use of the environment encourage severe surroundings for training and practice.

At present, both judo and karate-do are popular internationally as sports for physical education and the art of self-defense. Women are increasingly engaged in these traditional male activities. Both these sports were developed from martial arts, thus, even when handled as sports, the original military spirit remains. However the names of judo and karate-do are applied, they are not to be thought of as simply military combat activities. *Do* means "the way" or "disciplinary principle." Through the practice of politeness, fraternity, calmness, modesty, seriousness, courage, and other human qualities, judo and karate-do attempt to address the total person. Together with the aesthetics of the sport, importance is given to the development of mental skills such as the powers of observation, patience, and the ability to focus attention. Above all, good manners are emphasized as an essential part of both sports' traditions. The player is taught always to respect the senior or more experienced player. At the match, the player must wear the training uniform *(gi)* correctly. Before and after the match, the players sit down formally and make a bow to each other, expressing mutual respect.

The Oriental philosophy that human integrity must be maintained while learning and practicing the techniques is strongly evident. The overt and intentional inclusion of these concepts gives a greater dimension to the sports of judo and karate-do than are usually encountered in general physical education or Western sport activities. Unfortunately, this spirit of commitment to the whole person sometimes leads to dangerous or, at best, unwise training environments. To foster patience and self-control, some have suggested that winter practice be carried out in the frigid early mornings, whereas summer practice should be performed in the heat of the midday sun. It is alleged that in both cases, the mental discipline to overcome these unbearable environments and the strength and positive spirit gained are more important objectives than the mere improvement of the techniques.

The positive physiologic effects of athletic participation have been reported on numerous occasions in Western medical literature. However, a tremendous amount of evidence also exists concerning the adverse effects of severe climatic conditions on physiologic systems and their performance. Therefore, the enthusiastic adherence to the Oriental philosophy must be tempered with the judicious management of environmental conditions in the training hall. In this way, injuries arising from the environment itself and those that may occur as a result of impaired performance as a consequence of suboptimal training hall climatic conditions (such as excessive heat, cold, and/or humidity) will be avoided.

Supervision

Because injuries do occur and the goal is to minimize their occurrence, frequency, and consequences, supervision of sport activities is a critical factor in establishing a safe environment for the athletes. Supervision has three aspects: preseasonal, intraseasonal, and interseasonal. Supervision is mandatory for training and competition, and it requires a multitude of skills and expertise. This section outlines an ideal program of supervision. Limitation of resources and personnel will obviously force choices to be made in executing an individual program. An attempt will be made to underscore the relative importance of each factor to assist the reader in selecting optimal choices when faced with the reality of a limited amount of available resource on which to draw.

It is absolutely imperative that there be a clearly designated person to direct the program. This person may also embody other responsibilities outlined below. Supervision responsibilities may be delineated between those concerned with medical issues and those pertaining to specific issues of training, training techniques, and competition (Fig. 27.16). Certainly, these are complementary and not mutually exclusive areas of concern. Thus both areas must be serviced by individuals with not only a thorough knowledge of their specific area of responsibility but also a familiarity with the areas to the other members of the supervisory team. For optimal function, open, frequent, and candid communication among these individuals is an absolute necessity.

A complete medical program requires, at the barest minimum, involvement of a person or persons who have completed a certified first aid course through a recognized agency (e.g., American Red Cross, local medical center educational program, or American College of Sports Medicine). This person should be present at all training sessions and *must* be present at all competitions. He or she must be designated as a central figure responsible for identification, management, and triage of injuries. Ideally, the person responsible should be a physician, certified athletic trainer, or someone with established, recognized competence in the area of sports medicine. He or she should have an established and posted plan for the management of medical situations (emergent, urgent, and follow-up), including *(a)* steps to be taken in the event of an emergency; *(b)* location of first aid equipment; *(c)* name, location, and phone number of program supervisor; *(d)* name, location, and phone number of local emergency transport service (i.e., 911); *(e)* name, location, and phone number of local emergency room or emergency treatment center; and *(f)* name, location, and phone number of physician affiliated with the program or telephone number of local emergency room director.

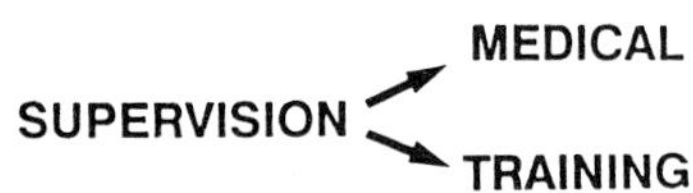

Figure 27.16. The two components of sports supervision.

In the preseason, the supervisory personnel are responsible for preparticipation evaluation of the players. They will organize preseason physical fitness assessments and obtain appropriate medical record documentation on all players. These data (anthropomorphic as well as medical history) should be filed in a secure and central location for easy access and referral. This information will form the basis for player profiles, from which specific training prescriptions and modifications can be formulated. Intraseasonally, the medical supervisor (not necessarily a physician) will arrange on-site coverage for training and match sessions. The supervisor's responsibilities include monitoring environmental and equipment issues, injury assessments, proper administration of first aid, and triage of injured athletes; he or she must maintain complete and accurate injury data, including number of incidences and follow-up records. The supervisor also is responsible for establishing a mechanism for appropriate transportation of injured players to the local treatment center. This includes a personal, on-site review of the referral center facility and evaluation of transportation service, equipment, and personnel. There should also be an in-person and written communication with these support services and their staff personnel.

The training hall must be fully stocked with first aid supplies. A complete list of recommended supplies and equipment can be obtained from the American College of Sports Medicine, the America Athletic Trainers Association, the American Red Cross, or regional medical centers and departments of sports medicine. The extent of this equipment will obviously be limited by available financial resources; however, as an absolute minimum, it should include a commercially available prepared first aid box with Band-Aids, ace bandages (3-inch, 4-inch, and 6-inch), sterile gauzes and dressing materials, disinfectant solution, eye patches, eye wash solution, sling, oral airway, smelling salts, splint material, cervical collar (two-piece), and back board (two-piece preferred). More sophisticated additional equipment and supplies should be available, if possible.

At the end of the competition season, the medical supervisor must prepare an off-season maintenance program (including individualized flexibility, endurance, and strength activities) for each player. References have been published (11, 12) and information can be obtained for the American College of Sports Medicine to help the supervisor create these programs.

Preparation

Knowledge and familiarity with judo and karate-do assists in the anticipation of injuries. A proper and adequate environment as well as high-quality equipment will prevent unnecessary injuries. Good supervision will encourage safe participation. Injury prevention must be taken care of before attention can be focused on preparation of the player.

Training for judo and karate-do is traditionally divided into three distinct phases—*kata* (learning), *randori* (free practice), and *kumite* (advanced practice)—each of which should be further broken down into warmup, play, and cooldown periods. Match competition be attempted only after training has been established and techniques have been learned. The key tenet of judo and karate-do training is that defense (receiving technique) must be mastered before offense training can be started.

The learning of form includes understanding the intent and proper application of the specific techniques. It starts with the repetitive practice of basic movements. Then a training partner is introduced onto the mat. Movements are then repeatedly practiced with the partner. Next, the players agree on what techniques to practice and actual execution is attempted. Overthrowing and pressing are carried out with the partner only after *kata* has been completed. In karate-do, this phase does not always involve a partner.

The free practice of judo and karate-do is a training method by which well-rehearsed and mastered basic forms are tried freely on a partner. After the combination of various techniques is learned, practice matches are conducted to master the entirety of the sport.

Advanced practice involves two players who have agreed on what moves to practice; they then engage in learning through mutual execution of the techniques. This also is referred to as the agreed combination technique. More advanced training involves the free combination technique, which is, in effect, mock competition.

Each of these levels of practice has the express purpose of mastering techniques. To minimize injury during training, players must learn warmup and cooldown routines. The warmup must be performed before initiation of the formal practice session. It involves flexibility as well as light aerobic (cardiovascular) exercises. Every player should be analyzed in regard to his or her inherent musculoskeletal flexibility or lack thereof. Accordingly, the athlete should be guided through a logical, formal program of stretching movements for the torso and lower extremities (11). It is important to give special attention to individual needs and to keep in mind any previous trauma. Nonimpact or low-impact aerobic activity (calisthenics) provides cardiovascular preparation for a training session.

At the conclusion of a training session, it is equally important for the athlete to engage in a cooldown period, which includes cardiovascular and stretching components. Usually, the warmup and cooldown segments should consist of 10 to 15 min of stretching and 5 to 10 min of cardiovascular exercise.

Specific Traumas

Head and Neck

Even if the head sustains an impact from throwing in judo or being kicked in karate-do, it is not necessarily an emergency, unless the player is unconsciousness or shows evidence of brain damage, including violent headache or vomiting. A concussion or blood clot must be suspected for players who cannot stand, have impairment of their state of consciousness, respond slowly, or do not respond to their name. In such cases, the patient must be lain down with the head turned laterally and positioned lower than the feet to encourage draining from the bronchial tree during the observation and transportation. Pulse rate, blood pressure, and respiration must be checked. If the athlete's condition is found to be stable, then he or she should be moved to a room where he or she can lie quietly and observation should be continued for a time. If the base of the tongue drops backward and respiration is impaired due to a disturbed state of consciousness, the mouth must be opened, the tongue pulled forward, and an oral airway inserted. The patient must then be transported to a medical facility. Even when consciousness has been regained, transportation to the hospital should be considered if the patient complains of violent headache or if vomiting occurs. Of course, if convulsion or unconsciousness lasts more than 10 min, rapid transfer to the hospital must take place. Generally, if the initial state of unconsciousness continues for more than 10 min, some type of brain damage, which is demonstrable in 25% of the cases on a scan, has probably occurred. A fracture of the skull seldom happens when the head strikes a *tatami*. However, an acute subdural hematoma sometimes does occur from the rupture of a parasagittal bridging vein.

If choking is caused from the strangling technique, followed by unconsciousness, cerebral hypoxia results from the circulatory disturbance. The patient should be placed on the back with the head in a lower position than the feet. Usually, there is recovery of consciousness in about 10 sec.

A blow to the head is often accompanied by trauma to the cervical vertebrae and neck region. A cerebral vertebral fracture causes violent pain. If pain is distributed over the upper extremities, a cervical fracture is quite likely. It also is necessary to check for any spinal cord damage involved in these fractures; symptoms include diaphragmatic respiration, numbness in the region below the upper extremities or chest, trouble in stretching out or bending the forearm, and paralysis of the lower extremities. The patient should be lain down and carefully transferred to a stretcher. Then the position of the head and neck should be fixed by sandbags or cervical collar before transfer to the hospital.

Face and Teeth

In karate-do, trauma to the face and teeth and laceration to the oral cavity are frequently sustained. Fractures of the nasal cartilage, zygomata, and upper and lower jaws need surgical treatment. Local treatment is not possible. However, resultant nasal hemorrhage with bleeding in the oral cavity must be treated at the injury site. This hemorrhage may occur with a blow to the nose or face, even without fracture or damage to the teeth. For a severe nasal hemorrhage, the patient should be lain in the lateral posture at the site to prevent blood flow into the larynx, which could block the respiratory pathway. If available, clean gauze soaked with epinephrine diluted to about 100,000 times and 1% lidocaine solution should be inserted into the nostrils to compress the region, thus stopping the bleeding. The nasal membrane is rich in small vessels and is prone to bleeding. Most nasal hemorrhages occur at Little's area in the external nasal region; thus pieces of clean gauze should be applied at that point. If no medication is available, gauze packing can be used alone. If nasal hemorrhage is slight, the patient should lie down quietly. A towel should be placed on the upper face, including the base of the nose. Bleeding in the oral cavity, fractures of the jaw, broken teeth, and laceration of oral membranes, can be caused by a hand blow to the lower face. The blood caught in the oral cavity and mixed with viscous saliva may eventually move into the upper respiratory passage and cause blockage; pieces of broken teeth can also block respiration. Therefore, the injured patient should be lain down in a side-face position, and foreign material should be removed from the oral cavity. A piece of gauze soaked with epinephrine and Xylocaine may be packed at the bleeding site. The medical supervisor may have the patient gargle with a hydrogen peroxide solution. After the acute condition is somewhat abated, the patient should be transported to an oral surgeon. It is imperative that all loose or broken teeth be saved and transported with the patient.

Chest

Rib fractures may occur in karate-do practice performed without chest protection and occasionally in judo practice. Local pain will be strong at the region of the fracture, particularly during respiration. Therefore, the injured person should be lain on his or her back in a suitable place. Pain is usually alleviated by slight elevation of the upper body. Do not bandage the chest.

Abdomen

Trauma to the abdomen may occur in karate-do matches. If the player is hit severely in the abdomen, impairing the state of consciousness, or if the player is found in a shock-like state with complaints of violent pains in the abdomen, damage to internal organs must be suspected. Pain in the right abdominal region leads to suspicion of liver damage. Left abdominal pain may indicate splenic damage or rib fracture. The patient should be placed in the most comfortable position and then transported to the hospital at once. Oxygen inhalation therapy and intravenous drip infusion are desirable on such occasions, if available.

Testes

In karate practice, the testes are sometimes kicked in error. Violent pain occurs instantaneously, which spreads to the upper abdominal region. Furthermore, there is accompanying nausea and vomiting, and the patient suffers, in some cases, from transient shock conditions. However, it is seldom that the testes or ancillary area is burst open. Some bleeding at the scrotal region and edema are usually observed. The prompt recovery from shock is usually achieved by keeping the patient in a quiet, head-down position. Cooling of the affected area is recommended. If the scrotum has swelled significantly, a hematoma may be present. The patient should be sent to a urologist for further evaluation.

Lumbar Vertebrae

Trauma to the lumbar vertebrae often occurs in judo practice, because players must lift or throw their opponents while also twisting their bodies. During mat work, the body has to be bent in forced postures. Fracture dislocation of the lumbar vertebrae rarely happens, but a lumbar sprain can occur during preliminary exercises or matches. Therefore, violent and severe lumbosacral discomfort may present during these activities. It is recommended that the patient be placed supine on a solid surface with a pillow behind the knee and the hips flexed approximately 45°. This position gives the most pain relief. If there are symptoms of spinal cord injuries, such as paralysis of the lower extremities, the sides the trunk must be fixed with pillows or sandbags and immediate transport, with a back board, should be undertaken.

Extremities

If the player complains of intense pain in the joints in any of the extremities, it is safe to assume that dislocation or fracture has occurred. Accurate diagnosis and treatment must be made at a local emergency facility. The basic treatment is the application of splint, protecting and fixing the injured area in the position in which it is found. Restoration of alignment is to be undertaken only by people competent to do so. For this purpose, the practice hall or athletic facility should be equipped with various sizes of splints, triangular cloths, and slings. An inflatable air splint is useful for handling fractures of the extremities or severe ligament injuries. It is recommended one should be prepared in advance and readily available. After the injured region has been fixed in a proper fashion, the patient should be promptly transferred to hospital for further evaluation and treatment.

Conclusions

Judo and karate-do are dissimilar sports. However, their training and supervision can be managed with common logic. These sports encourage and reward flexibility, endurance, and agility. As such, they are excellent tools for achieving fitness. However, they also engender potentially injurious activities. Learning of the techniques of these sports must be well-supervised. Their mastery requires rigorous adherence to a formalized program of training, which does not allow competition until mastery of techniques has been well-demonstrated.

REFERENCES

1. Matsumoto Y. Coaching of judo. Tokyo: Daishudan-Shoten, 1975.
2. Nakamura R. Judo. In: Japan Amateur Sports Association, ed. The report of researchers on sports medical science in Japan. No. 2. Tokyo: Author, 1981:167–184.
3. Oyama M. This is karate. Tokyo: Japan Publication Trading, 1974.

4. Roth J. Black belt karate. Rutland, VT: CE Tuttle, 1974.
5. Smith RW. A complete guide to judo. Rutland, VT: CE Tuttle, 1958.
6. Kodama T. Sports injuries and their prevention. Int Congress Sports Sci 1964:1–50.
7. McLatchie G, Davies JE, Caulouey JH. Injuries in karate: a case for medical control. J Trauma 1980;20:956–971.
8. Norton NL, Cutler C. Injuries related to the study and practice of judo. J Sports Med Physical Fitness 1965:149–173.
9. DeMeersman RE, Ruhling RO. Effects of judo instruction on cardiorespiratory parameter. J Sports Med Physical Fitness 1977;17:169–183.
10. Taylor AW, Blassard L. A physiologic profile of the Canadian judo team. J Sports Med Physical Fitness 1981;21:160–174.
11. Anderson, B. Stretching. New York: McGraw-Hill, 1974.
12. Glover B. Family fitness guide. New York: McGraw-Hill, 1988.

28 / LACROSSE

Leslie S. Matthews and Roger H. Michael

Introduction

Known as the "fastest game on two feet," lacrosse is a sport now enjoyed by many men and women. Organized lacrosse is played at the interscholastic, intercollegiate, club, and professional levels throughout the United States and Canada. The international form of the game also has flourished and is now played in Australia, England, and most recently Japan.

This chapter reviews the history of the sport and briefly describes its most popular forms (men's and women's field and box). Recognition, treatment, and prevention of those injuries most commonly encountered in lacrosse are discussed. Consideration is given to factors relating to the sport's equipment as well as to conditioning techniques specific to lacrosse.

History

Lacrosse is said to the oldest American sport, having originated with American Indian groups (1–3). Its early form was called *baggataway,* which was a regular feature of American Indian life. It had definite religious significance and was played by several different tribes. The players often dressed in full regalia of feathers and paint, and the game was preceded by days of celebration and preparation. Games could be played over hundreds of miles of prairie. The first reference to the game was made in 1636 by Jesuit missionary John de Brebeuf, who watched the Huron Indians play near Thunder Bay, Ontario. The Algonquin Indian version was described in detail by another Jesuit missionary, Pierre de Charlevoix, in 1721.

The original game was rough and required endurance, because it was often played for a 2- or 3-day period without rest. From the beginning, the game was played with a stick with a netted loop at one end, which resembled a crosier (*la crosse,* a symbol of pastoral office); hence the name of the game. The original ball was about the size of a modern tennis ball and was made of a firm, durable substance such as wood or deerskin. American Indian players were skilled enough with their lacrosse sticks that the ball seldom touched the ground.

A more organized form of the game developed among the six nations of the Iroquois Confederacy and the Hurons, who settled in the Montreal area in the early colonial days.

After the Revolutionary War, the game underwent a number of changes. Teams became limited to 60 men, and fields were standardized to about 500 yards in length. The game remained truly a Native American sport. By 1825, the game was played with 7-men teams on fields 50 yards long. To be skilled enough to make the traveling team was a great tribal honor. These American Indian players were later to challenge and help train the early collegiate teams.

More changes in the game occurred in 1856 at the Montreal Lacrosse Club. Members of the club used a longer stick with a wide triangular netting, which was tightly strung with gut. This helped to establish Montreal as the cradle of modern lacrosse. In 1867, the year the Dominion of Canada was created, the game of lacrosse was declared its national sport. Within a year, 80 clubs had formed. Later that same year, an American Indian team traveled to England, Ireland, France, and Scotland, generating considerable interest in Great Britain. Clubs were formed near London and Liverpool, and in the following year, an English lacrosse association was formed.

At the same time, widespread interest in lacrosse in the United States was engendered as a result of American newspaper coverage of games played between Canadian Indian and U.S. Indian teams. In 1868, the first lacrosse club in the United States—the Mohawk Club of Troy—was formed, and soon there were clubs in the Midwest, North, and East. Later that same year, the *New York Tribune* called it "a madman's game, so wild that it is," and the *New York World* called it "the most exciting and at the same time the most laughter provoking among the whole range of outdoor sports." (2).

In 1874 and 1878, the game was introduced into Australia and New Zealand, respectively. An exhibition game was played for Queen Victoria at Windsor Castle in 1876. She was quite pleased with the game and presented each of the players with an autographed picture of herself. As a result of this royal interest, the teams were invited to play at the Westchester Polo Club in Newport, Rhode Island to demonstrate lacrosse to the vacationers at that exclusive resort. A crowd of more than 8000 people attended, and the *New York Herald* reported that "the immense popular success of the game caused lacrosse to be the talk of Newport. The universal verdict is that lacrosse is the most remarkable, versatile and exciting of all games of ball." In 1880 and 1881, interest spread to colleges and universities. Harvard, New York University, Princeton, Columbia, and a number of clubs in the New York area became active. In the following year, the Intercollegiate Lacrosse Association was formed.

Around the turn of the century, several innovations greatly improved the game. Netting was added to the goal, and lacrosse sticks were modified so they were shorter and lighter. World War I temporarily interrupted the lacrosse schedule. A major change in lacrosse occurred in 1921. For the first time, the field was divided in half by a center line. Each team was required to keep at least three men, exclusive of goalies, in each half of the field. In 1926, the U.S. Intercollegiate Lacrosse Association (USILA) was organized with unlimited membership to accommodate more teams interested in the sport. In 1928, the United States sent a Johns Hopkins team to Amsterdam to participate in the Olympic Games. Lacrosse also was an Olympic sport played in the 1932 Los Angeles games. Johns Hopkins beat the Canadians in two of three games for the Olympic Championship.

In subsequent years, the sport of lacrosse was dropped as an Olympic event because of lack of participatory countries. In the 1960s, an international competition that included teams from the United States, Canada, the UK, and Australia was organized and called the World Games. This competition, which occurs every 4 years, continues to flourish today. The games were last played in 1990 in Perth, Australia, and will be played in Manchester, UK, in 1994.

Probably the most influential changes in the game of modern lacrosse were enacted in 1933. Rules were included to speed up the play of the game and to give it more wide open play. The number of players on a side was reduced from 12 to 10. The distance between the goals (which had been 110 yards since 1922) was reduced to 80 yards and the playing area in the rear of each goal was fixed at 20 yards. Furthermore, although total playing remained at 60 min, the game was divided into four quarters, with teams changing goals after each quarter.

Following World War II, the game continued to gain in popularity. In 1953, a new rule went into effect that allowed for freer movement of players when play was stopped. (4) Before this, a player had to freeze in position at the sound of a whistle. In 1959, the Lacrosse Foundation (originally founded as the Lacrosse Hall of Fame Foundation) was formed in dedication to the sport and development of the game throughout the United States. A new freestanding facility has recently opened on the campus of Johns Hopkins University, which houses the Lacrosse Foundation as well as the Lacrosse Hall of Fame. The first year of NCAA Lacrosse Championship Tournament play was in 1971, and Cornell University was the first champion. In 1974, the NCAA inaugurated a Division II and III Championship, which replaced the USILA tournament. NCAA Division I and III Women's Championships are now also sanctioned.

Intercollegiate lacrosse grew from 4 teams in 1881 to 227 teams in 1990. Historically, the game has been played mainly in the East; however, through the 1980s clubs and collegiate teams were formed throughout the country. Expansion at the high school level has also been impressive. Great interest has been shown, particularly in high schools in Maryland, New York, New Jersey, Pennsylvania, Massachusetts, and Connecticut. During the 1980s the sport was one of the fastest growing interscholastic sports in the United States. More than 805 high schools and prep schools have lacrosse teams, and there are youth teams, women's teams, and club teams as well as numerous summer camps and lacrosse leagues.

Box Lacrosse

Box lacrosse (5, 6) is a direct outgrowth of the original game of lacrosse as played by the early American Indians and still exists today. It is a wild swinging and hitting sport that differs significantly from men's field lacrosse. Each team has six players on the field, which is an enclosed area the size of an ice hockey rink with a concrete or artificial turf playing surface. The sticks are shorter and narrower than those used in field lacrosse. The goal is 4×4 feet. The sport is played most prominently in Canada, although a professional box league has recently become established in the United States.

Women's Field Lacrosse

Women's field lacrosse (7, 8) had its inception in the 1890s in England as an offshoot of the men's lacrosse game. It was introduced to schools and colleges in the United States in the 1920s. It is similar to the original American Indian game but is not as rough. The goals are 100 yards apart. The playing area has no measured boundaries but is recommended to be approximately 120×70 yards. As in the men's game, the stick used by women players is usually made of fiberglass or wood with a wood or aluminum handle, the head of which cannot be more than 9 inches in width. There are 12 women on each team, and only the goalie wears protective equipment, which includes helmet, face mask, padded gloves, chest protector, and leg guard (Fig. 28.1). Substitution is allowed only for an injured player and no deliberate physical contact is allowed but sticks can be checked. The U.S. Women's Lacrosse Association (USWLA), founded in 1931, controls the affairs of the game, and through its initiative and efforts, the game

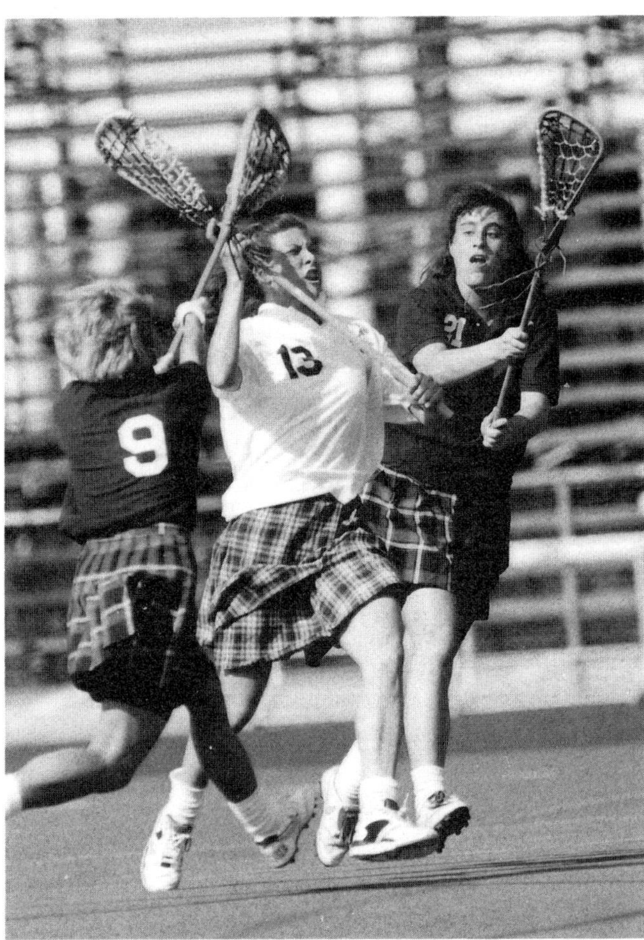

Figure 28.1. Women's lacrosse is played without use of protective equipment, with the exception of the goal keeper. Courtesy David Preece.

has made great strides in the late 20th century. The women's game has become a Division I scholarship sport at many universities across the country. Specifics regarding conditioning and injuries commonly encountered in the women's game will be discussed later.

Rules

Field and Goals

The playing area for men's field lacrosse is 110 yards long and from 53⅓ to 60 yards in width. The goals are 80 yards apart, and there is a playing area of 15 yards behind each goal, permitting more action behind the goal than is seen in ice hockey. The field is divided in half by a midfield line. A circle with a 9-foot radius is drawn around each goal and is known as the crease. A rectangular box, 35×40 yards, surrounds each goal and is called the goal area. It is formed by marking a line 40 yards in length centered on the goal parallel to and 20 yards from the center line. A wing area is formed on each side of the field by marking a line parallel to the sidelines and 20 yards from the center of the field. The line extends 10 yards on each side of the center line. A point on the center line an equal distance from each sideline is marked with an X and is designated as the center of the field (Fig. 28.2).

There is a special substitution area on the sideline next to the timer's table and marked by two lines that are 2 yards from the center line. The goals consist of two 6×6-foot vertical posts joined by a crossbar, also 6 feet in length, resulting in a goal area of 36 square feet. A line is drawn between the goal posts to indicate the plane of the goal and is designated the goal line. Attached to the goal is a pyramid-shaped cord netting which is fastened to the ground at a point 7 feet behind the center of the goal. A goal is scored when a loose ball passes from the front completely through the imaginary plane formed by the goal line, goal post, and top crossbar. A goal counts as one point.

Players

There are 10 players on a men's field lacrosse team and a number of substitutes. There are four positions: goal, defense, midfield, and attack. The goal keeper, or goalie, guards the goal and receives primary support from three defensemen. They are normally in the proximity of the goal and also are known as close defense. Three midfielders cover the entire field, operating as both offensive and defensive players. One of the midfielders handles the face-offs and is called either the center or the face-off man. Three attackmen spend most of their playing time around the opponent's goal and are referred to as the close attack.

Balls and Sticks

The lacrosse ball is solid rubber, white or orange in color. It is slightly smaller than a baseball but just as hard. The ball may not be touched by the hands except by a goalie while he is in the crease. It is legal to kick the ball with the foot or bat it with the stick; however, most of the action takes place with the ball being controlled in the pockets of the players' sticks. The lacrosse stick may be of an overall length of between 40 and 72 inches with the exception of the goalie's stick, which may be of any length. The inside measurement of the head of every stick, except the goalie's, is between 6.5 and 10 inches. Attackmen usually use sticks with the smallest dimensions to aide them in ball control and dodging. Close midfielders will also use relatively small sticks, whereas close defensemen prefer sticks of longer length and wider head to enhance reach and blocking ability.

Virtually all sticks used in the men's field game today have heads constructed of plastic or other synthetic material and replaceable handles made of wood or aluminum. The uniformity, balance, and lightness of the plastic stick gives it a decided advantage over the wood sticks used before the early 1970s. The net of the stick (crosse) is generally constructed of gut, rawhide, cord, or nylon or other synthetic material and is roughly triangular in shape. The pocket of the stick may not sag to such a depth that it becomes unreasonably difficult for an opponent to dislodge the ball. This is determined by placing a ball in the pocket; if the top surface of the ball is below the bottom edge of the wall, the pocket is deemed too deep and must be adjusted. This

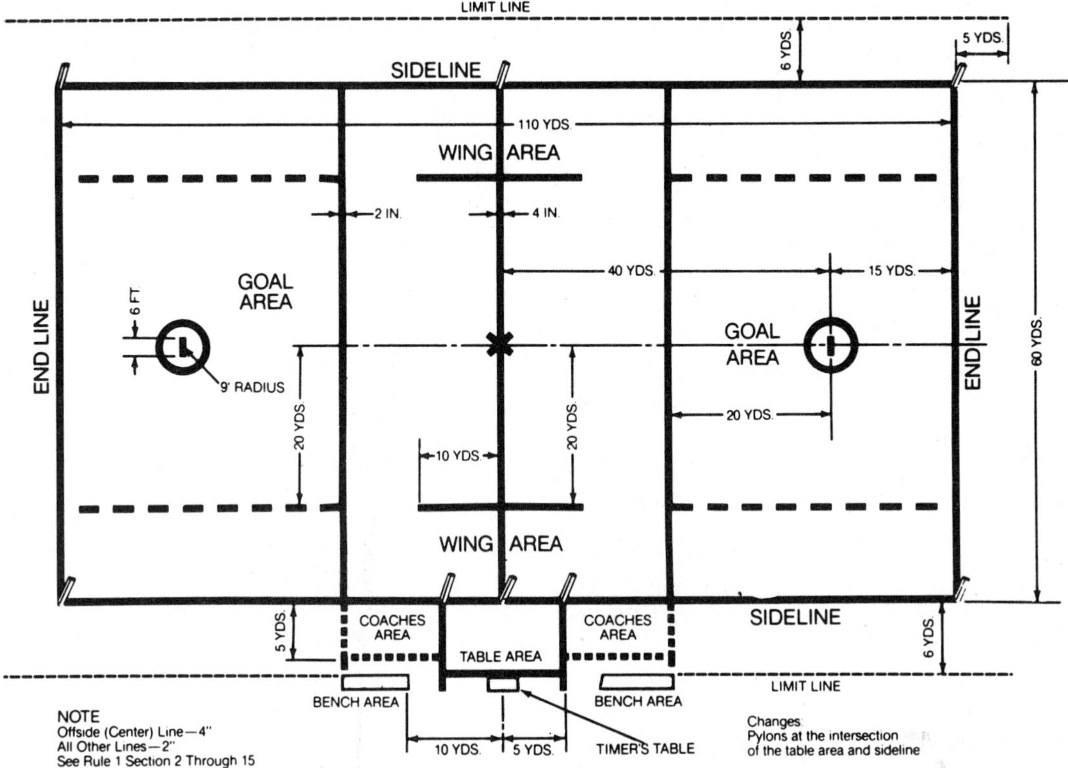

Figure 28.2. Diagram of the field of play for men's lacrosse.

rule, however, does not apply to the goalie's stick. The end of the handle is known as the butt.

Personal Equipment

All players are required to wear gloves and a helmet equipped with a face mask. The face mask must have a chin pad, which acts as a cushion in the event the mask is pushed into the facial area. Brightly colored mouth guards are required of all players. The chin strap must be fastened on both sides of the helmet, and a four-point chin guard fixation is now required. A throat protector attached to the lower end of the mask is a required piece of equipment for the goalie, as is a chest protector. The lacrosse helmet is considerably lighter than a football helmet but lacrosse helmets must meet standards set forth by the National Operating Committee on Standards for Athletic Equipment (NOCOSAE). The helmet is designed principally to provide protection from the ball or blows from the opponents' sticks. Gloves are worn for the same reason and are quite similar to ice hockey gloves but somewhat more flexible. Alterations of the gloves, including removal of palms or fingers to enhance tactile sensation is prohibited. Shoulder pads are required equipment for all players except the goalie. Arm pads are not required. Most offensive players choose to wear arm or elbow pads for protection from stick checks. The remaining pieces of equipment used in men's field lacrosse are standard and include shoes, jerseys, and shorts.

Play of the Game

Regulation playing time in a college varsity lacrosse game is 60 min divided into four periods of 15 min each. High school teams generally play 10-min periods. If the score is still tied at the conclusion of the game, a sudden-death playoff will begin, with the winner being the team that scores the first goal.

The game is controlled by two officials: a referee and an umpire. If both teams agree, a third official—the field judge—may be used. The referee has the final word in all decisions. The officials start the game at the beginning of each period and after each goal with a face-off. The players on each team are assigned to a specific area of the field for the face-off: the goalie and three players are in the defensive goal area, three players are in the offensive goal area, one player is in each of the wing areas, and the face-off man is in the center of the field. When the whistle sounds to start play, the players in the wing area are released, but all other players are confined to their respective areas until a player on either team gains possession of the ball or the ball goes out of bounds or crosses either goal line area.

After gaining control of the ball, the team moves it toward the opponent's goal and tries to score. The offside rule, peculiar to the game of lacrosse, requires each team to have three players located in its offensive half of the field and four players in its defensive half of the field at all times. This rule prevents all 10 players from congregating in front of the goal in an effort to prevent scoring as is done in the game of hockey. These rules enable lacrosse to be more wide open and free wheeling, providing ample opportunity for scoring.

When a player throws or carries a ball out of bounds, the opposing team gains possession. One exception to this rule occurs when a loose ball goes out of bounds as a result of a shot taken at the goal. In this situation, the ball is awarded to the team whose player is closest to it at the exact time it crosses the boundary line. This gives the offense an opportunity to maintain control of the ball after a missed shot goes out of bounds, because an attackman is normally responsible for backing up a shot at the goal.

There are two methods for substituting players in lacrosse. The regular method follows that used in basketball, with the player entering the game whenever play has been suspended by an official. The other method is known as substitution on the fly and is similar to ice hockey, with substitution of players occurring while the game is in progress. One player at a time may enter the game after a teammate leaves the playing area through a special substitution area at the center line.

To the uninitiated spectator, lacrosse may appear to be a wild, stick-swinging game, but it is not nearly so rough as that first impression might indicate. Even though body and stick checks are part of lacrosse, there are definite limitations that help prevent injury. Body checking of an opponent is legal as long as he has possession of the ball or is within 5 yards of a loose ball. Contact must be from the front or side and above the knees only. A player can check his opponent's stick with his stick when the opponent has possession of the ball or is within 5 yards of a loose ball. The opponent's gloved hand, while on the stick, is considered part of the stick and can be legally checked. No other part of his body may be checked, however.

Penalties

Penalties in lacrosse are similar to ice hockey in that players who violate the rules must, under most circumstances, serve time in a penalty box. This forces the violator's team to operate with one less player than the opponent, giving the opponent a decided advantage. During this time, the team with the manpower advantage attempts to achieve a close-range shot at the opponent's goal. There are two types of penalties in lacrosse: personal fouls and technical fouls.

Personal Fouls

Personal fouls are the more serious and consist of the following:

1. *Illegal Body Checking:* Hitting an opponent from the rear, at or below the knees, or when he is not in possession of the ball or within 5 yards of a loose ball.
2. *Slashing:* Striking an opponent on his arm, shoulders, head, or any part of his body except the gloved hand that is holding the stick. Slashing may also be called when, in the opinion of the referee, a swing is malicious or uncontrolled.
3. *Cross-Checking:* Using the portion of the handle between the player's hands to check or push the opponent.
4. *Clipping:* Obstructing an opponent below the knee with the stick, hand, arms, feet, legs, or body.
5. *Unsportsmanlike Conduct:* Using threatening, profane, or obscene language to an opposing player or official or an act considered unsportsmenlike by the official.

The penalty for a personal foul is suspension of the offending player from the game for a period of 1 to 2 min, depending on the official judgment regarding severity and intention of the foul. Most personal fouls call for only a 1-min suspension. An expulsion foul can be levied against a player who deliberately strikes or attempts to strike a player with his fist or stick. Such a player receives a 3-minute penalty and is not allowed to return to the game. Players having committed a foul may otherwise return to the game after completion of the penalty time or after the opposing team scores a goal.

Technical Fouls

Technical fouls are less serious than personal fouls and consist of the following:

1. *Interference:* Interfering in any manner with an opponent who has not had possession of the ball, thus preventing his free movement on the field.
2. *Holding:* Grasping an opponent's stick or any part of his body in any manner.
3. *Pushing:* Shoving an opponent with the hand, arm, or any other part of the body, unless he has possession of the ball or is within 5 yards of a loose ball. A player may never push an opponent with his stick or push him in any part of his body from the rear.
4. *Illegal Action with the Stick:* Throwing the stick under any circumstances or taking part in the play of the game in any manner without a stick.
5. *Withholding the Ball from Play:* Lying on a loose ball on the ground or trapping it with a stick longer than necessary to control the ball and to pick it up with one continuous motion.
6. *Illegal Procedure:* Checking the goalie's stick when he has possession of the ball in the crease when the ball is in the attacking half of the field, defending player with the ball in his possession and running through the crease.
7. *Offsides:* Having less than three men in the offensive half of the field or less than four men in the defensive half of the field.

The penalty for a technical foul is a suspension of the game for 30 sec if the offending team does not have possession of the ball at the time the foul is committed. If the offending team has possession of the ball at the time the technical foul is committed, it simply loses possession to the opposition. This is also the case if neither team has possession when the foul is committed. Checking the goalie is penalized by a free clear (positioning the ball on the opposing team's offensive half of the field).

Each player and coach should have a complete understanding of the rules of the game. These are updated and published annually by the NCAA.

Injuries

Men's Field Lacrosse

Lacrosse shares with other high-speed contact sports a significant incidence of injury. Mueller and Blyth (9) studied 20 NCAA lacrosse teams over a 1-year period and determined an overall lacrosse injury rate of 52.5%. Other studies, however, have shown a low incidence of serious injury resulting from lacrosse, despite the aggressive nature of the sport (10–12). Nelson et al. (13) studied the injuries that occurred within one team over a season and found that although only 15% of athletes played an entire season without injury, only 20% of the injuries that did occur were serious enough to cause players to miss game or practice time. The NCAA's Injury Surveillance Committee monitors men's lacrosse injuries, and data have been made available for seasons extending from 1984 through 1990 (11). The injury rate for men's collegiate lacrosse as defined by a simple ratio between the number of injuries relative to the athlete's exposure has been compiled for a representative sample of U.S. men's lacrosse teams at all levels of competition. The overall injury rate per 1000 athlete exposures for men's collegiate lacrosse is reported to be 14.08 for Division I, 19.47 for Division II, and 17.22 for Division III. The injury rate per 1000 exposures was found to be lower for postseason competition (3.63) than for preseason (6.21) or regular season (6.51) competition.

Combined game and practice playing surface injury rate also was analyzed for men's lacrosse and was found to be slightly higher for artificial playing surfaces (6.77 per 1000 athletic exposures) than for natural playing surfaces (5.75). Interestingly, despite a much higher practice exposure than game exposure, the NCAA survey found a greater injury rate per 1000 athletic exposures in game competition (16.15) than in the practice setting (3.93).

When analyzed by anatomical location, the majority of men's lacrosse injuries occurred to the lower extremities (ankles, knees, and upper legs, with shoulder injury occurring next most commonly). The vast majority of injuries encountered have been classified as nonserious, including contusion, strains, and sprains. The combined game and practice injury rate for men's field lacrosse ranks the sport seventh compared with other NCAA sports. Lacrosse places behind spring and fall football, wrestling, men's and women's soccer, and women's gymnastics (11).

Women's Lacrosse

The NCAA has published the results of a survey of injuries in women's lacrosse (12). The survey includes data obtained from representative programs competing at all collegiate levels for the period of 1986 through 1990. For women's lacrosse, the injury rate per 1000 athletic exposures averaged 7.47 for Division I athletes, 4.04 for Division II athletes, and 6.85 for Division III athletes. As in men's lacrosse, the larger percentage of injuries occurred in preseason and regular season competition.

Playing surface injury analysis was also analyzed. While exposure to artificial playing surfaces were significantly less for women athletes, the overall incidence of injury was 4.13 injuries per 1000 athletic exposures for natural surfaces and 4.06 injuries for artificial playing surfaces. As in men's lacrosse, the incidence of women's lacrosse injuries was found to be higher in game play than in practice. Women's injury rates were 3.46 per 1000 athletic exposures in practice verses 6.85 for game exposures. The overall injury rate for women's lacrosse was 4.12 injuries per 1000 athletic exposures.

As in men's lacrosse, the most frequently injured anatomic regions for women were the lower extremities, including the knees, ankles, and upper legs. Notably absent from the women's lacrosse injuries were injuries to the shoulder. This is assumed to be related to the reduced level of contact in women's lacrosse compared with men's field lacrosse. The overall injury rate for women's lacrosse compared with other NCAA sports was remarkably low; it ranked 15th of the 16 sports surveyed. Baseball was the only sport demonstrating a lower injury rate than women's lacrosse. As in men's lacrosse, the majority of injuries seen in women's lacrosse have been categorized as minor, including contusions, strains, and sprains.

Types of Injuries

Virtually every study performed on the incidence and location of injuries occurring in lacrosse has demonstrated lower extremity injuries to be most common (9–13). This fact has been attributed in part to the high velocity nature of the sport, which involves high-speed running and quick change of direction combined with the potential for stick, ball, and body contact. In addition, although the face, head, shoulder girdle, and upper extremities are relatively well-protected, no protective equipment is generally worn on the lower extremities, perhaps further contributing to this pattern of injury.

A noted, NCAA survey of 20 teams found an overall injury rate of 52.2%. The body parts most frequently injured were the knees, ankles, clavicles, and upper legs. More than 70% of the injuries were found to be contusions, sprains, or strains. Fractures accounted for 9% of injuries and concussions, 2%. Of eight head injuries reported in this study, six were concussions and two were fractures of the mandible. The majority of upper extremity injuries were categorized as soft tissue in nature. Injuries of the shoulder girdle tended to be the most severe upper extremity injuries and included clavicular fractures, acromioclavicular joint separation, and shoulder dislocations. In addition, hand and finger injuries were frequent, probably related to the rules that allow for stick contact with the gloved hand and to the tendencies for the players surveyed to modify their gloves. Glove modification is no longer allowed by NCAA rules. Midfielders were found to be the most vulnerable players, thought to be attributable to their open field play, similar to that occurring in football players who are heavily involved in the action. Midfielders in this study found to sustain not only the greatest number of injuries but also the most severe. Remarkably, goalies sustained the fewest number of injuries.

Nelson et al. (13) also noted a high incidence of back strain among midfielders and attackmen. This was attributed to the twisting and dodging movement required of these offensive players.

To the authors' knowledge no similar such studies have been performed to analyze types of injuries in women's lacrosse. It has been the authors' experience that women's lacrosse teams suffer fewer and less severe injuries than men's teams. This is supported by the NCAA survey (12). Women's lacrosse injuries tend to occur in the lower extremity and consist of contusions, sprains, and strains. Shoulder and upper extremity injuries have been notably lacking in women lacrosse players. Because women players do not wear protective gloves, occasional hand and finger injuries are seen. In addition, the incidence of laceration in women's lacrosse appears anecdotally to be somewhat higher than that seen in men's lacrosse, probably because no protective head or facial equipment is worn by women.

The potential for injury to officials and spectators of the game of lacrosse must also be mentioned. A lacrosse ball shot on goal by an experienced player may travel up to 100 mph. Errant shots have been known to strike inattentive spectators and several occurrences of serious eye injuries to spectators of lacrosse are known to have occurred. Organizers of lacrosse events should be careful to erect barriers behind the goals to protect spectators or to prohibit seating in these locations. In addition, injury to officials caused by inadvertent contact with the sticks of players and by being hit by passed or shot lacrosse balls have also occurred.

Mechanisms of Injuries

To better analyze the types of lacrosse injuries most commonly encountered, it is convenient to group them into noncontact and contact injuries. Lacrosse shares with other stick sports, such as ice hockey and racketball, the fact that contact injuries may result not only from body-to-body contact but also from stick-to-body contact. This fact creates a potential for certain injuries to be more prominent in stick-related sports such as lacrosse. The hard rubber construction of the lacrosse ball also creates another subgroup of contact injuries, which can be called ball-to-body contact injuries. The classification of lacrosse injuries used in this chapter is as follows:

- Noncontact Injuries
- Contact Injuries
  - Body to body
  - Stick to body
  - Ball to body
  - Body to playing surface

Noncontact Injuries

Noncontact injuries may vary greatly in their mechanism, severity, and anatomical location and are certainly not unique to lacrosse. All field sports that require quick acceleration and deceleration of speed and sudden changes of direction will carry a certain incidence of noncontact injuries and lacrosse is no exception. The overall incidence of noncontact injuries in women's lacrosse appears to be higher than that of men's lacrosse, because of the rules governing the two sports. The type of noncontact injury seen in women's lacrosse does not seem to vary significantly from those encountered in men's lacrosse. Mueller and Blyth (9) reported that approximately 30% of all injuries encountered were noncontact in etiology. It has been the authors' experience that the incidence of noncontact injury overall is somewhat higher than that reported, with the majority of these injuries affecting the lower extremities and consisting of ligamentous injuries of the knees and ankles, muscle strains, shin splints, and stress fractures. Nelson et al. (13) also found a high incidence of ankle sprains occurring in lacrosse players.

Prevention of these various forms of noncontact injury center around proper coaching, conditioning, and preventative measures. The importance of proper strengthening, conditioning, flexibility, and prophylactic taping when appropriate cannot be overemphasized.

In any discussion of noncontact lacrosse injuries, the relative lack of overuse injuries afflicting the upper extremities should be noted. Unlike other throwing or racket sports, lacrosse appears relatively free from the problems of epicondylitis, bicipital or rotator cuff tendinitis, and other inflammatory conditions. This is because of the great leverage afforded by the lacrosse stick, which in turn allows the ball to be thrown at a relatively high rate of speed without subjecting the shoulder or elbow joint to extreme arcs of motion, acceleration, deceleration, and the stresses attributable thereto. The concern over prolonged or repetitive play among small and growing children appears less justified in lacrosse than in other sports such as baseball or tennis because of this apparent lack of overuse-type syndromes, which may have significant deleterious effects on growing children.

Contact Injuries

Body-to-Body Contact

Body contact is allowed in men's field lacrosse and box lacrosse but is prohibited in women's lacrosse. As a result, the incidence of body-to-body contact injuries in women's lacrosse is almost nonexistent. Body contact occurring in men's lacrosse can vary from simple shield blocking to high-velocity body contact (Fig. 28.3). Despite the potential for high-velocity contact injuries, the equipment used by the lacrosse player is not necessarily designed to protect the athlete from these high-speed injuries. As a result, injuries of a significant nature may occur not only to the player receiving the blow but also to the player rendering the blow.

While lower extremity injuries predominate statistically, upper extremity injuries seem to be more commonly the result of a contact mechanism. Injuries to the shoulder girdle in particular frequently occur as a result of body-to-body contact. Although shoulder pads are now mandatory for all players except goal keepers, these are not designed to protect the shoulders from body contact as football shoulder pads are. Contact shoulder injuries have been found to outnumber other upper extremity injuries by a ratio of at least two to one. Clavicle fractures and acromioclavicular joint separations have been the most commonly seen shoulder girdle injuries resulting from body contact.

Stationary "picks" such as those allowed in basketball are allowed in lacrosse but cross-body–type blocking in which a player leaves his feet is illegal. As a result, the lacrosse player is forced to pick in a more upright and exposed position, using the head, neck, and shoulder regions predominantly. As a result, neck and upper torso injuries may be more likely to occur. There is some anecdotal evidence of cervical spine fractures occurring in lacrosse players. As in all other contact sports, concerns over the potential for this devastating type injury must exist. Concussions are the most frequently encountered head injury resulting from body contact (14). The design of the helmet undoubtedly contributes to this type of injury. The lacrosse helmet is designed to protect the cranium from blows by the lacrosse stick and appears to be quite effective in this role. It is loose fitting, vented, and constructed of a much more flexible material than is a football helmet. Despite the requirement for NOCOSAE approval, the helmet provides less adequate protection from high-speed body collisions occurring to the head region.

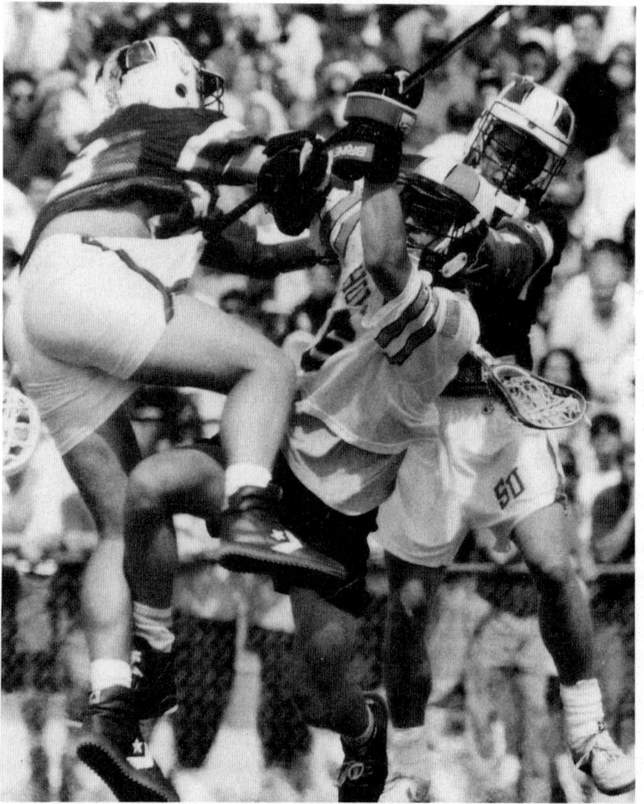

Figure 28.3. Typical form of body contact occurring in men's lacrosse. Courtesy David Preece.

Noncontact mechanisms produce meniscal and ligamentous injuries of the knee in lacrosse with greater frequency than do contact mechanisms. When knee injuries result from body contact, they are almost invariably the result of an illegal block. This factor alone seems to account for the relatively low incidence of posterior cruciate ligament injuries and the relatively high incidence of anterior cruciate and medial ligamentous injuries found in lacrosse players. When seen, however, contact injuries about the knee region are often serious and frequently involve multiligamentous injuries for which surgical intervention is usually necessary.

For reasons that are not entirely clear, abdominal injuries appear to be rare in lacrosse. Because blocking is done in a more upright position, it can be postulated that blows resulting from blocking injuries are taken about the shoulder girdle, head, and thorax region rather than the abdomen. One case of pancreatitis (9) occurring in a lacrosse player has been reported that was thought to be the result of a direct blow to the abdominal area. Injuries to the spleen appear to be rare. Chest and rib cage injuries seem to occur with greater frequencies than do abdominal injuries. As a result of body contact, fractures of one or multiple ribs is not an infrequent finding, as little if any protection is afforded the rib cage by standard lacrosse equipment and upright blocking rules seem to predispose to injuries in this area. The authors are aware of one case of a pulmonary contusion and hemothorax occurring in an All-American attackman as a result of body contact.

Stick-to-Body Contact

Fractures of the hand and shoulder girdle regions are the most serious type of trauma encountered as a result of stick-to-body contact. While the protective equipment used in lacrosse to shield the shoulder girdle and hand is specifically designed to shield the exposed body parts from this type of injury, injuries to these areas still seem to occur with regularity. Fractures in the shoulder girdle region are most commonly the result of illegal checks, resulting in violent stick-to-body contact. Fractures of the clavicle as well as the rare first rib fracture have been seen, despite the use of standard lacrosse shoulder pads.

Fractures of the forearm may also occur from direct stick-to-body contact. While controlling the ball, an offensive player will routinely carry the stick in one hand and use and place the opposite forearm in a protective posture as a shield in front of the body to ward off blows from a defensive player (Fig. 28.4). In this position, particularly if arm pads are not used, either or both forearm bones may be fractured. Isolated ulnar shaft fractures have been seen as have the generally less common isolated radial shaft fractures as a result of these mechanisms.

Fractures of the hand are usually the result of stick-to-body contact (Fig. 28.5). It has been the authors' impression that since rules restricting alteration of the palms and fingers of protective gloves have been enforced, hand injuries are less common. Hand and finger fractures are seen in women lacrosse athletes because no protective gloves are worn. For fractures of the metacarpal, an orthoplast playing splint, fabricated to fit inside a lacrosse glove, can be used to allow players to return to competition at an early date.

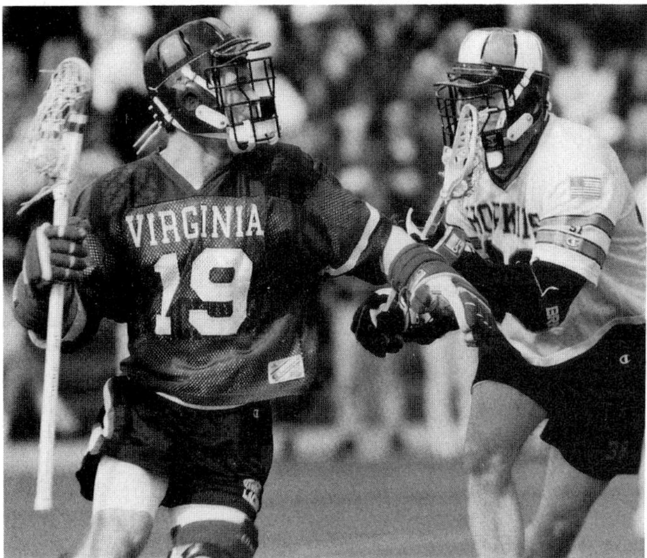

Figure 28.4. Typical protective posture of an attackman using his forearm to protect himself from opposing blows, predisposing this area to injury. Courtesy David Preece.

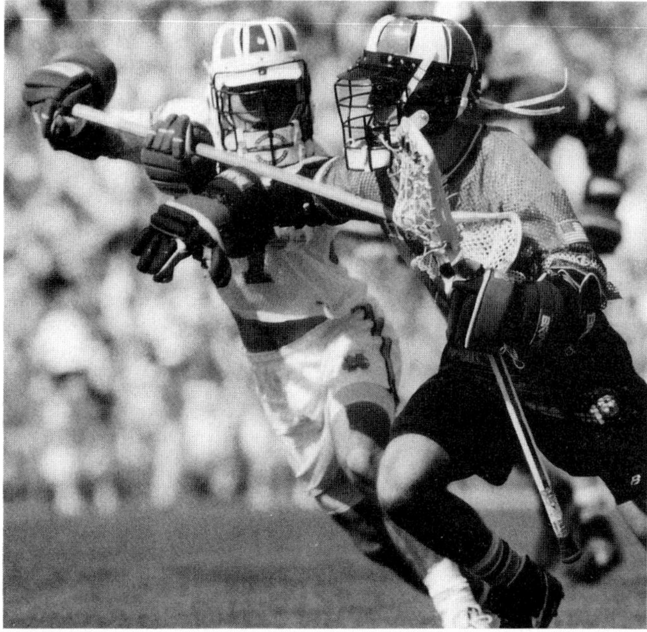
Figure 28.5. Stick-to-gloved-hand contact may result in fracture, although rules prohibiting glove modifications seem to have helped greatly.

Eye and facial injuries resulting from stick-to-body contact are less frequent in men's lacrosse than in women's, because of the men's protective helmets and face masks. On occasion, the edge of the cross or the butt of the stick, as a result of an illegal check, can slip between the bars of a face mask and inflict this type of injury. Rimel et al. (14) have reported a stick injury to the parietal area of the skull resulting in an epidural hematoma that required parietal craniotomy and hematoma evacuation. This occurred in a player who was wearing a lacrosse helmet, albeit at a time before regulations required the use of NOCOSAE-approved protective helmets.

NCAA rules now mandate the use of brightly colored mouth guards for all players. Bright colors are specified so that compliance may be more readily monitored by officials. Compliance with this rule and extension to interscholastic and club competition will undoubtedly serve to reduce the risk of dental injuries.

Soft tissue injuries occur with regularity as a result of stick-to-body contact. Soft tissue injury may result from one severe blow to an unprotected body part, such as the thigh or upper arm, or from chronic repetitive trauma. Chronic repetitive injury is most commonly seen in attack players who routinely use one arm in a protective posture to ward off defensive blows. Several players have developed myositis ossificans in the humeral region as a result of chronic repetitive blows to this area; these players missed significant playing time as a result of the condition (Fig. 28.6). With the frequency of soft tissue injuries encountered as a result of stick-to-body contact, mandatory use of protective arm pads that extend from the deltoid to the cuff of the lacrosse glove should be implemented.

Ball-to-Body Contact

The hard rubber composition of a lacrosse ball combined with the high velocity at which it is propelled (often in excess of 90 mph) and the large body area that is exposed make ball-to-body contact injuries relatively frequent and potentially serious. It is estimated that 10% of all lacrosse injuries result from this mechanism.

Injuries to the neck and throat area are potentially the most serious. Nelson et al. (15) described one player who suffered syncopy, bradycardia, and hypertension following a blow to the neck. An injury to the carotid sinus mechanism was postulated in this player, who recovered fully with conservative treatment. The authors emphasize by virtue of this occurrence, the importance of basic life support instruction for coaches and trainers who are regularly in attendance at games and practices. Since 1983, it has been mandatory for all goal keepers to wear a protective throat shield, which is suspended from the lower portion of the face mask of the helmet.

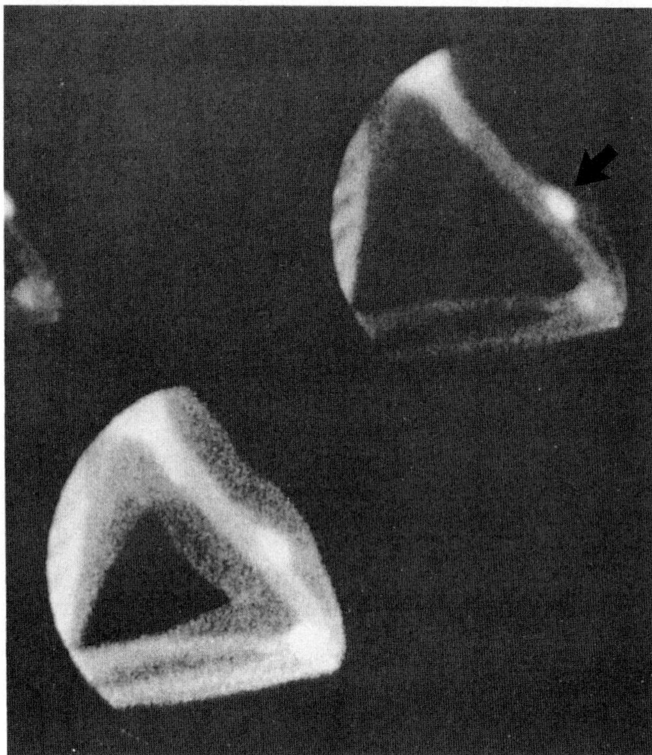

Figure 28.6. Bone scan showing intense focal activity *(arrow)* at the site of myositis ossificans of the distal humeral region in a lacrosse midfielder.

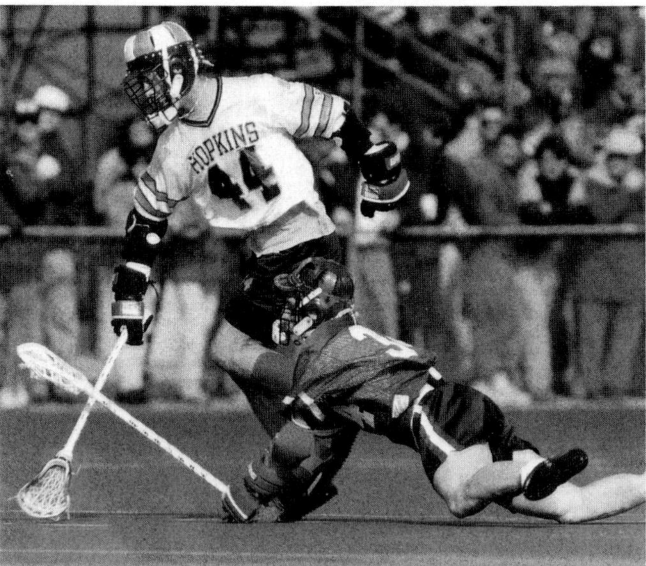

Figure 28.7. High-velocity contact between unprotected body regions and the playing surface can result in significant injury. Courtesy David Preece.

Facial lacerations and eye injuries occur in men's lacrosse despite the use of a protective helmet and mask. The somewhat loose-fitting nature of the helmet may, on certain occasions, allow a shot that strikes the face mask to displace the mask forcefully against the face, causing the mask itself to lacerate the facial region. Use of a four-point chin strap mechanism will help prevent such displacement of the helmet and reduce the risk of this injury.

In women's lacrosse where no head or facial protection is worn, ball contact injuries are more common. In the women's game, however, the velocity at which the ball travels is generally much less than that in men's lacrosse, making these injuries less severe.

Testicular injuries can occur as a result of a blow to the groin area by a lacrosse ball. A protective cup is required to be used by the goal keeper but is not required of other players. Much of the offensive and defensive play in lacrosse occurs in front of the goal, thereby placing both offensive and defensive players at risk for being hit while defending or attempting to screen the goal keeper. Protective cups should be worn by close defensive and offensive players who are at the greatest risk to be inadvertently hit by a shot ball.

Body-to-Playing-Surface Contact

Lacrosse shares with all other field sports the potential for players to fall or be knocked to the playing surface, resulting in a variety of injuries (Fig. 28.7). Lacrosse is increasingly being played on artificial playing surfaces, and this factor has led to new types of problems. As described previously, despite a greater exposure to natural playing surfaces, the incidence of reported injuries was higher for artificial turf.

Abrasions, or turf burns, have the potential to be significant problems in lacrosse. Lacrosse is generally a warm-weather sport in which the players wear shorts. No protection of the lower extremities is afforded by the standard lacrosse uniform. Falls and skids on artificial turf can result in deep abrasions, which if improperly treated can readily go on to secondary infection.

Preventative measures can be extremely helpful in minimizing the risk and severity of these types of injuries. Application of relatively thin layers of petroleum gel to areas of bony prominence such as the elbows or knees has been helpful in decreasing friction and thereby decreasing the severity of turf burns. In addition, thin tube gauze and stocking-like material over elbows and knees also have been used to protect against such injuries. Proper maintenance and routine cleaning of the artificial surface also is important to minimize the risk of secondary infection. Proper local treatment once a turf abrasion occurs is essential and must include prompt and thorough cleansing and debridement of the wound.

The authors have noted that play on artificial surfaces has increased the incidence of traumatic prepatellar and olecranon bursitis in lacrosse players. Again, the fact that standard lacrosse equipment does not afford protection to these areas combined with the speed at which the game is played, predispose to this form of injury. Standard treatment for a traumatically induced olecranon or prepatellar bursitis is aspiration of the inflamed bursa. Frequently, the first aspiration will reveal a bloody bursal effusion. This is then combined with a pressure dressing, institution of antiinflammatory medication, and supplemental padding. When treating a lacrosse player with such an injury, there also is the potential for an associated abrasion to have led to a septic bursitis. Cultures of aspirated bursal fluid should be obtained if such a diagnosis is considered.

Players falling or being blocked to the playing surface can also result in a wide variety of upper extremity injuries. Wrist fractures, elbow dislocations, acromioclavicular joint separations, and glenohumeral dislocations can result from a player falling onto an outstretched arm. These are perhaps the most unavoidable type of injuries in lacrosse. This type of injury is not significant in the women's game, because of the lack of body contact.

Conditioning

Lacrosse is a fast-moving field sport for which speed, agility, and endurance are essential attributes. Conditioning for lacrosse strives to foster each of these athletic attributes. Endurance, strength, and agility are generally emphasized in preseason conditioning programs. Most Division I NCAA lacrosse teams now participate in a year-round strength-training program that emphasizes the shoulder girdle and lower extremities. Endurance training is generally accomplished through aerobic conditioning by long-distance running.

Most lacrosse coaches require an off-season running program for endurance of 20 to 25 miles/week combined with three weight-training sessions a week. Goal keepers must also train to improve foot speed and hand-eye coordination. Off-season conditioning, therefore, includes participation in sports such as racketball as well as jumping rope.

Once the season begins, endurance training is frequently fostered by practice participation and full-field scrimmaging on a regular basis. Strength training continues with at least two weight-training sessions per week. Speed conditioning increases with regular use of short-distance (40- to 60-yard) sprints and interval training on the part of the team.

Conditioning for women's lacrosse follows similar lines, although most Division I women's teams do not seem to place the same emphasis on strength training as do their male counterparts. Endurance is fostered through running long distances in the off-season and is supported by scrimmage time during the season. Speed training also is accomplished by short-distance sprints and interval training.

Conclusions

Significant changes have recently occurred in the rules governing the game of lacrosse that have made positive strides toward reducing the tendency for injuries. Many of these rule changes were suggested by the authors earlier (16), such as mandatory use of mouth guards and shoulder pads and prohibition of alteration of gloves, and are now being enforced. The fact that lacrosse has been shown to be a relatively safe sport compared with other contact field sports should not reduce enthusiasm for continuing to strive for better equipment; modification of rules, and improved coaching, officiating, and conditioning techniques, which will all reduce the incidence of injury. The meaningful dialogue and degree of cooperation between the coach, the athletic trainer, the team physician, and the governing bodies determining the rules of the sport should continue to strive to further reduce the risk of lacrosse injuries.

REFERENCES

1. Morrill WK. Lacrosse. New York: Ronald Press, 1966.
2. Scott B. Lacrosse: technique and tradition. Baltimore: Johns Hopkins University Press, 1976.
3. Weyand AM, Roberts MR. The lacrosse story. Baltimore: Herman, 1965.
4. Hartman PE. Lacrosse fundamentals. Columbus, OH: CE Merrill, 1968.
5. Ginsburg B. You think hockey is rough? Take a look at box lacrosse. Phys Sportsmed 1975;3:100.
6. McCue FC. Box lacrosse. In: Larson LA, ed. Encyclopedia of sport sciences and medicine. New York: Macmillan, 1971:325–326.
7. Brackenridge C. Women's lacrosse. Woodbury, NY: Barron's, 1978.
8. Miller S. Women's lacrosse: the name's the same. Lacrosse 1978;1:15.
9. Mueller FO, Blyth CS. A survey of 1981 college lacrosse injuries. Phys Sportsmed 1981;9:94.
10. Kulund DN, Schildwachter TL, McCue FC, Gierk JH. Lacrosse injuries. Phys Sportsmed 1979;7:82.
11. NCAA. Injury surveillance system, 1989–90: men's lacrosse. Mission, KS: NCAA.
12. NCAA. Injury surveillance system, 1989–90: women's lacrosse. Mission, KS: NCAA.
13. Nelson WE, DePalma B, Gieck, JH, McCue FC, Kulund DN. Intercollegiate lacrosse injuries. Phys Sportsmed 1981;9:86.
14. Rimel RW, Nelson WE, Persing JA, Jane JA. Epidural hematoma in lacrosse. Phys Sportsmed 1983;11:140.
15. Nelson WE, Crampton RS, McCue FC, Gieck JH. Syncope, bradycardia, and hypotension after a lacrosse shot to the neck. Phys Sportsmed 1981;9:94.
16. Michael RH, Matthews LS. Lacrosse. In Schneider RC, Kennedy JC, Plant ML, eds. Sports injuries. Baltimore: Williams & Wilkins, 1985:178–191.

29 / NORDIC AND ALPINE SKIING

Lars-Gunnar Elmqvist, Robert J. Johnson, Michael J. Kaplan, and Per A.F.H. Renstrom

HISTORICAL PERSPECTIVE

Skiing has been used as a means of transportation in Scandinavia for more than 5000 years (1). The oldest skis in the world were discovered in 1924 outside a small village of Kalvträsk in Västerbotten in the northern part of Sweden. They dated to about 3200 BC. A total of almost 200 different prehistoric skis made and used before 1050 AD and 2000 to 3000 years old, have been discovered in the Nordic countries of Sweden, Finland and Norway. Drawings of prehistoric skis used for hunting and dating back to 2000 BC have been found in Norway and Russia.

One of the first ski races in history took place in Sweden in 1521 when Gustav Vasa tried to escape the Danes. Two Swedes pursued him on skis for approximately 90 km before they overtook him bringing an offer to become king of Sweden. The so-called Vasa Race changed Swedish history. Eventually it also gave rise to the oldest ski race—and one of the most popular long distance races (89 kilometers)—in the world. This race was started in 1922 and now attracts nearly 20,000 participants from several different countries (2). Cross-country ski racing has increased in popularity all over the world for top level and recreational athletes. Today long distance races are held in many countries around the world.

In 1722, the Norwegian army organized ski races for both cross-country and downhill events, the latter termed "slalaam" (3). These slalaam races were designed to challenge the soldiers to stay upright for the duration of the slope rather than to compete for time. The first actual timed race took place in Telemark, Norway in 1848. Soon after, ski jumping had its first competition, also organized in Norway in 1866 (4). The first organized competition including all three types of skiing events occurred in Huseby, Norway in 1879. After this many cross-country and ski jumping events developed. These events increased in popularity, prevailing in the Scandinavian countries, while the downhill events flourished in the Alps. Today, all three types of skiing are popular throughout the world.

SKI JUMPING

Ski jumping is a spectacular sport. It is not surprising that there is the expectation that associated accidents are also sensational, with severe injuries not infrequently sustained. However, Nordic ski jumping is by nature a competitive sport with a limited number of participants. This contrasts with cross-country and alpine skiing, which are practiced by large numbers of recreational and competitive skiers. While the general public may view the daring jumps of Nordic aerial jumpers as a dangerous sport with a correspondingly high incidence of injuries, the ski jumpers themselves and the event officials view it as a safe sport with a rather low injury frequency. They point to the very strict regulation of the ski jumper and ski-jumping facilities by national and international (Federation International de Ski or FIS) ski organizations.

Technique and Equipment

Nordic ski jumping is a high-speed sport with take-off velocities of 100 km per hr (60 miles per hr). Downhill racers can reach 125 km per hr (80 miles per hr) (5). The ski jump begins at the top of the inrun, which is a tower and ramp construction (6). On the inrun, the skier crouches to decrease wind resistance and maximize the take-off speed. The take-off edge is 2 to 4 m above the ground, which is called the knoll. The jumper has to make the take-off at exactly the right moment, pushing the body forward over the skis to generate life and to reach proper air flight position. The ski jumper maintains this forward lean for as long as possible. At the end of the jump, the jumper straightens the body somewhat to land half-crouched with one foot ahead of the other in a so-called telemark landing. The skis are traditionally kept parallel during the flight. Recently, however, a top Swedish ski jumper began jumping with

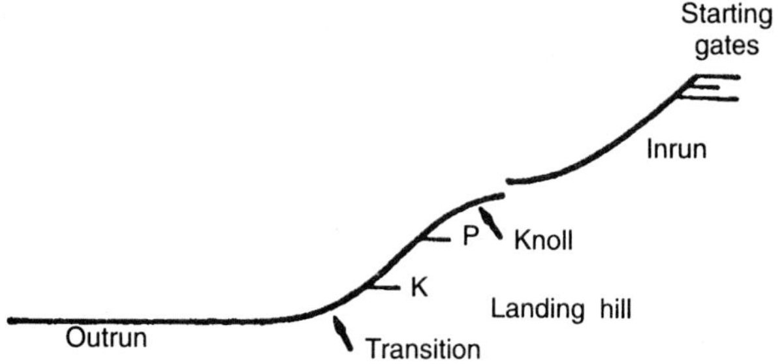

Figure 29.1. The landing hill is convex near its top, the knoll, and is concave near its bottom, the transition. The height of the starting gate at the top of the inrun is set so that the majority of jumpers will land on the straight, (i.e., steep) portion of the landing hill (between the normal point [P] and the critical point [K]) and so that the best jumpers will not land beyond K, the point at which the transition begins. When jumpers fail to land on the steep middle portion of the landing hill, they land with greater impact and risk a serious fall, whereas jumpers falling on the steep portion of the landing hill merely slide down the hill dissipating their kinetic energies. In a ski-jumping competition, the winner is determined on the basis of total style and distance points awarded for each of two official jumps. If jumpers exceed the critical point (i.e., "outjump" the hill) during one of these two rounds of jumping, the starting gate is lowered and that round is restarted. Reprinted by permission from Wright JR, McIntyre L, Rand JJ, et al. Nordic Ski Jumping Injuries, A survey of active American jumpers. Am J Sports Med 1991;19:615–619.

his skis in a V-shape and lengthened his jump by 5 to 7 meters. After landing, the skier continues down the slope to the bottom of the hill and onto the deceleration area, or outrun. The jumping hill is usually 70 to 90 m from the take-off point to the landing area, reflecting the length of the jump that can be performed (Fig. 29.1).

Jumping skis are much wider and thicker than downhill skis and are up to 9 feet in length. They have 4 to 6 shallow longitudinal grooves and no metal edges. This diminishes the risk of the ski catching in the snow and twisting the lower extremity. The boot is generally soft with a low top, which theoretically might predispose for ankle fractures. However, the cable binding system used to attach the foot to the ski is not very firm. This makes rotation torques of the lower extremity less likely to occur than in downhill skiing (7).

Ski Jumping Injuries

Rate of injury

Ski jumping as an official event is still limited in the number of participants so that the rate and type of injuries and the circumstances in which they occur are infrequently cited in the literature.

In a nationwide survey during the 1973 to 1974 ski season in Sweden, Eriksson (8) reported only 22 ski jumping injuries out of a total of 1199 injuries; 885 injuries occurred during downhill skiing and 98 during mountain touring, while the remaining 140 occurred during cross-country skiing. The only other information given about ski jumpers was that 27% of the injuries were fractures compared to 46% in downhill and 12% in cross-country skiing. No injury rate was calculated.

Sandelin et al. (9) in Finland reported on 39 ski jumping injuries as recorded by the insurance company that covered all competitive jumpers in Finland from 1976 to 1978. The annual injury rate was 4.7% for the 275 licensed competitive ski jumpers of Finland. This figure was significantly higher than the corresponding figures found for competitive cross-country (0.3%) and downhill (1.8%) skiers.

Wright et al. (10) analyzed the accident reports at the Intervale Ski Jumping Complex in Lake Placid, U.S., during a 5-year period beginning with the 1980 to 1981 season. Forty-seven injury reports were analyzed. Of 40 jumpers, only 1 sustained an injury, 2 jumpers sustained 2 injuries, and 1 sustained 3 injuries. The mean age of the injured jumpers was 21.7 years with a wide range from 6 to 57 years of age. In the last two seasons of the time period studied, plastic mats were installed for summer training on two of the hills, resulting in a higher number of injuries during the summer seasons (n = 20) than during the winter seasons (n = 9).

Because there was no registration of the practice jumps performed, the injury rates at Lake Placid were only estimated for the number of competitive jumps on a "per skier day" basis. There were a total of 8 injuries recorded for the competitive events of the Juniors, Seniors, Masters, and unclassified jumpers during the 5 years (1881 skier-days), giving an injury rate of 4.3 injuries per 1000 skier-days. During World Cup competition, both training and competitive jumps were calculated, giving a total of 2233 jumps and 864 skier-days. The only injury was scapular contusion and acromioclavicular separation recorded during a training jump. This yielded an injury rate of 1.2 injuries per 1000 skier days of World Cup Competition.

In 1991, Wright et al. (7) further investigated the injuries of American ski jumpers by asking all jumpers registered by the United States Ski Association to fill out a questionnaire detailing any jumping-related injuries sustained that required examination by a physician. Nearly half, 46.5% or 133 out of 286 jumpers, responded to the inquiry. However, several of the questions were left unanswered, suggesting a potential underestimation of the injury rate. A total of 211 injuries in 151 accidents were recorded, but only 81 (60.9%) of the injured jumpers sought an examination by a physician. Of these 81 injured jumpers, 39 sustained an injury serious enough to prohibit them from jumping the rest of the season. The risk of injury was calculated in this study to be 9.4 injuries per 100 skier-years. Of the 96 jumpers who had participated in summer jumping, 65 believed that summer jumping was more dangerous than winter jumping, and this sentiment reflects the contention of Wright et al. (10) in their retrospective Lake Placid analysis (Table 29.1). A summary of the injury rates found in the different investigations is made in Table 29.1.

Type and Severity of Injuries

In a survey of Finnish competitive ski jumpers carried out during the period of 1976 to 1978 (9), fractures and dislocations were the most common injuries, comprising 37% of the total number of injuries. One-third

Table 29.1
Injury Risk According to Different Ski Jumping Injury Investigations[a]

Investigator/Country	Injury Risk
Sandelin et al., (9)/Finland	4.7/100 ski jumper/year
Wright et al., (10)/Lake Placid, USA	
Non World Cup jumpers	4.3 injuries per 1000 skier days
World Cup jumpers	1.2 injuries per 1000 skier days
Wright et al., (7)/USA	9.4/100 ski jumper/years
Wester (11) (disabling injury)/Norway	0.54/100 ski jumper/5 years
Wester (12) (disabling injury)/Norway	0.12/100 ski jumper/5 years

[a]From Johnson et al. Skier injury trends—1976–1990. Skiing trauma and safety: Ninth International Symposium 1993;11–22.

Table 29.2.
Frequency of Various Types of Ski Jumping Injuries[a]

Injury	No. of Injuries	Percent of Injured Jumpers (N=47)	Percentage of Total Injuries (N=72)
Contusions	19	40.4	26.4
Fractures	11	23.4	15.3
Abrasions	10	22.1	13.9
Concussions	7	14.9	9.7
Dislocations	7	14.9	9.7
Visceral injuries	5	10.6	6.9
Sprains	5	10.6	6.9
Muscular strain	4	8.5	5.6
Lacerations	3	6.4	4.2
Epistaxis	1	2.1	1.3
Total	72		

[a]Injuries sustained at the Intervale Ski Jump Complex in Lake Placid from 1980 to 1985. From Wright JR, Hixson EG, Rand JJ. Injury patterns in nordic ski jumpers. A retrospective analysis of injuries occurring at the Intervale ski jump complex from 1980 to 1985. Am J Sports Med 1986;14:393–397.

(33%) of the injuries involved ligaments while the muscle-tendon units and wounds/abrasions comprised 15% each. Of the injuries studied, 33% involved the head and neck, 30%, the lower extremity; 25%, the upper extremity; and the remaining 12%, the trunk. Only one of the injured jumpers sustained an injury that resulted in permanent disability.

The 47 injured jumpers in the Lake Placid study (10) had a total of 72 different injuries of various types (Table 29.2).

As shown in the table, the most common type of injury was a contusion (40.4%) involving the shoulder, elbow, or knee. Eleven fractures occurred in 23.4% of the injured jumpers. The upper extremity was involved in 6 fractures, with 4 in the lower extremity; there was 1 vertebral fracture. The majority of the fractures were nondisplaced and were treated conservatively. Abrasions, usually facial, were sustained in 22.1% of the jumpers while 14.9% had concussions of a mild degree (two jumpers had to remain in hospital for overnight observation). Five shoulder dislocations and two acromioclavicular joint separations were found in 14.9% of the injured jumpers. Visceral injuries and sprains of the medial collateral ligament of the knee joint each occurred in 10.6% of the injured ski jumpers. Although 8 of the jumpers required hospitalization, the longest for 16 days, no follow-up is noted that mentions further disability.

In the questionnaire investigation of all registered American ski jumpers Wright et al. (7) found a fracture rate of 21.8%. This is similar to the 23.4% frequency of the Lake Placid analysis (10). The upper extremity fracture was the dominant injury type with 60.9%, compared to the 26.1%, for lower extremity injuries and 13% for the rest of the body. After fractures, the most common types of injuries were sprains with 14.2%, dislocation/separation 13.3%, concussion 8.5%, and contusion 7.6%. The number of contusions is quite low compared to the retrospective Lake Placid investigation and might be due to an underestimation of the less serious injuries or to different definitions of what constituted a reportable injury. The anatomical distribution of these injuries is shown in Figure 29.2.

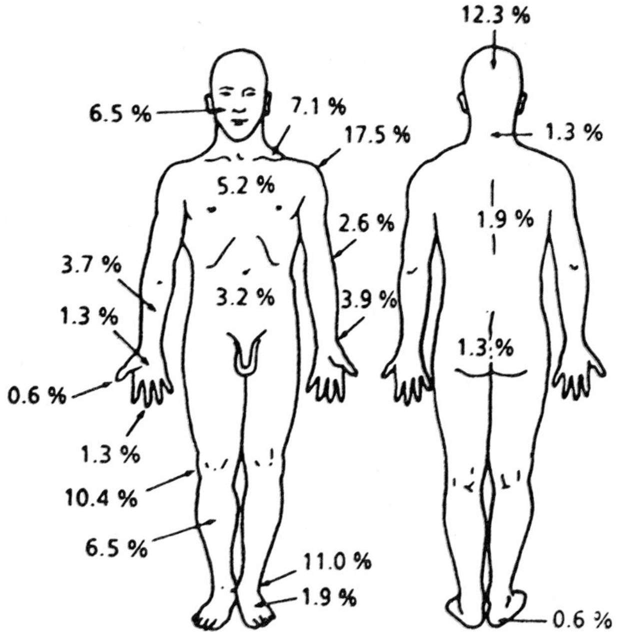

Figure 29.2. Anatomical distribution of nordic ski jumping injuries. Reprinted by permission from Wright JR, McIntyre L, Rand JJ, et al. Nordic Ski Jumping Injuries, A survey of active American jumpers. Am J Sports Med 1991;19:615–619.

Wester (11, 12) studied serious ski jumping injuries in Norway in two separate series; the first (I) covered the 5-year period from 1977 to 1981 and the second (II) from 1982 to 1986. Their definition of a serious injury implied a permanent medical disability of at least 10%. This definition rules out those injuries that initially were considered serious, but progressed to healing without permanent sequelae or complications. The data were collected from three sources—the insurance company covering all licensed jumpers in Norway, the ski clubs, and all Norwegian hospitals. Twelve persons with disabling injuries were identified during period I. Because only those injuries acquired during competition, and not during practice, were recorded during period I, the data were not comprehensive. The second series (II) recorded injuries occurring during competition and training with only 3 disabled ski jumpers found. During the last season of the first series, the exact number of licensed ski jumpers was 2238 in Norway. Assuming that each jumper performed 400 jumps each year, Wester (12) calculated a total of 5 million ski jumps over the 5-year period. The risk of suffering a serious disabling injury in 1 ski jump is therefore very low, 0.0003%. During the second series, 2593 licensed ski jumpers were involved. Similar calculations lead to a calculation of 5.2 million jumps while the risk quotient becomes 0.00006% risk of suffering a disabling injury in 1 ski jump. Thus, the risk to jumper of suffering a permanent, disabling injury during the second 5-year period was 0.12% compared to 0.54% during the first period. Wester concluded that the safety in ski jumping had improved by a factor of almost 5 between the 2 periods studied.

Of the disabling injuries recorded in series I by Wester (11), 7 were classified as very serious (CNS lesions, leg amputations and blindness of one eye) and 5 as slightly or moderately disabling (all were sequelae following lower leg fractures) (Table 29.3). In the second series, only 1 of the injuries was classified as very serious (blindness of one eye), while the other 2 were moderately disabling (head injuries with mild neurological symptoms).

In reviewing the Norwegian series, it was clear that serious injuries occurred at the beginning and at the end of the season, usually during the first two jumps of the day. During the inrun before takeoff, 4 of the jumpers fell and landed on a knoll, which was typically ungroomed loose snow. This type of fall resulted in the most serious injuries (spinal cord lesions and leg amputation), while the rest occurred during the landing phase and resulted in less severe injuries (ankle fractures). Poor snow conditions were frequently implicated as a reason for the accidents.

Table 29.3.
Serious Injuries Caused by Ski Jumping[a]

Injury	Medical Disability (%)	Age/Sex (Years)
Cervical fracture with complete spinal cord lesion at level:		
C6	100	17/M
Th6	100	16/M
Th7	100	14/F
Intracerebral hematoma/contusion with subsequent resection of the right temporal lobe	70	28/M
Leg amputation:		
Poor prosthesis function	45	14/M
Good prosthesis function	25	23/M
Blindness, one eye	18	23/M
Ankle fracture leading to arthrodesis	20	28/M
Fracture of collum femoris with later complications	20	12/M
Not finally evaluated	(>15)	15/M
Tibia/fibula fracture with shortening	10	15/M
Ankle fracture w/severely limited ROM	10	32/M

[a]From Wester K. Serious ski jumping injuries in Norway. Am J Sports Med 1985;124–127.

Wright (13) supplied some interesting facts about the dangers of ski jumping in a retrospective survey of all ski jumping fatalities in the U.S. during a 50-year period ending in 1988. He found only 6 known fatal ski jumping accidents, with 4 of the 6 jumpers having suffered cervical fractures or closed head injuries. The number of participants in ski jumping during this entire period is postulated to be only 1000 per year. A rough estimate of the fatality rate for Nordic ski jumping would be 12/100,000 participants annually. This is higher than the figures mentioned for both recreational (0.1/100,000) and competitive alpine skiing (2.5/100,000), but well below the figures for driving an automobile (26.6/100,000), based on National Safety Council figures from 1974 (14). Estimates for cross-country skiing are difficult to find, but in the Vasa Ski Race, there were six nontraumatic deaths between 1923 and 1985 giving a fatality rate of 0.05/100,000 participants annually (15).

In conclusion, most of the injuries in ski jumping are to the upper body with fractures, dislocations, and wounds being the most common types. The risk of injury has steadily declined as rules have become more strictly enforced and jumping conditions have improved. Nevertheless, the risk of injury is still higher for ski jumping than for cross-country and downhill skiing.

Prevention of Injuries

Weather and snow conditions are important causative factors for ski jumping injuries. Although weather cannot be controlled, postponement or delays of the competitions can be made to accommodate bad conditions. The fact that many of the accidents occur during the very first jump and mostly at jumping facilities familiar to the jumper, suggest that unexpected snow conditions may confront the jumper. Grooming and snow conditions should be optimized in order to obviate a deceleration or fall before take-off on the inrun or after landing on the transition or outrun where the hill flattens out.

Ski jumping technique has improved over the years into a more aerodynamic style that allows the jumper to fly further without gaining too much height. The jumping hills have also been modernized with the transition and outrun zones not as flat as they had been previously. These changes decrease the injury risk when landing. Removal of obstacles such as rocks or light towers reduces the risk of collisions. Equipment has also improved and the mandatory use of helmets has presumably prevented a number of serious head injuries.

The risks of summer jumping are high and because many of the risk factors are material-dependent, good maintenance of the summer ski slopes seems to be of utmost importance. Because many of these summer jumping injuries occur when the jumper falls outside the landing area, an expansion of the plastic surface might prevent several of these injuries.

CROSS-COUNTRY SKIING

Cross-country skiing is one of the most demanding sports because it involves a majority of the muscles in the body and stresses the cardiovascular system for a sustained period of time. Cross-country skiing typically involves skiing in prepared tracks, but can also include skiing on mountainous and rough terrain. It is considered an ideal recreational sport that can be enjoyed by people of all age groups and physiologic makeups. Development of new skating techniques and the overall increase in the popularity of the sport has resulted in changes in the type, severity, and number of injuries sustained.

Technique and Equipment

Cross-country skiing has traditionally been performed by three different classic techniques all involving skiing in a set of parallel tracks. The three techniques are termed diagonal stride, kick double pole and double pole (16) (Fig. 29.3). The first two rely solely on the friction generated between the snow and the ski in order to move the skier forward. This involves pulling and pushing of both the upper and the lower extremities. The third technique, double pole, relies entirely on the arms and trunk for forward motion. The stride is divided in three phases: the kick, the free glide, and the pole phase, all 3 of which are used in the first two techniques, while double poling uses only the glide and the pole phases. In the first two classic techniques, the ski comes to a complete stop during the kick phase when it is driven against the snow at which point the kick wax grips the snow making it possible to perform the forward kick. This is why cross-country skis need to be waxed with both kick and glide wax.

The skating techniques originated in the mid-1970s when the marathon skating technique was developed by a Finnish skier in an effort to increase speed. It was popularized in 1982 by the American skier Bill Koch who used this technique in the World Cup races (16). By the 1985 season, it was used by an estimated 10% of all recreational skiers (17). Currently there are three different skating techniques in use: the original marathon skate and two newer and faster techniques called the V1 skate and the V2 skate (Fig. 29.4). These techniques require a well-packed snow trail, but do not require parallel tracks. In skating, the skis never stop moving over the snow in contrast to the classic cross-country techniques. One ski is always angled obliquely to the forward direction, under these circumstances, there is need for glide wax, but not for kick wax. The poles can be utilized in numerous combinations; there is no proven advantage of one technique over another.

The maximum speed obtained on a level surface for diagonal stride is about 6 m/sec; for double poling, 6 to 7 m/sec; and for double poling with skating, 8 to 9 m/sec (18). The hip extensors, knee flexors, and ankle plantar flexors are the most active muscle groups involved in cross-country skiing that uses the classic techniques. For skating, more strain is put on the hip adductors and external rotators. Since cross-country skiing is an endurance sport, all of these muscles are suspectible to overuse injuries.

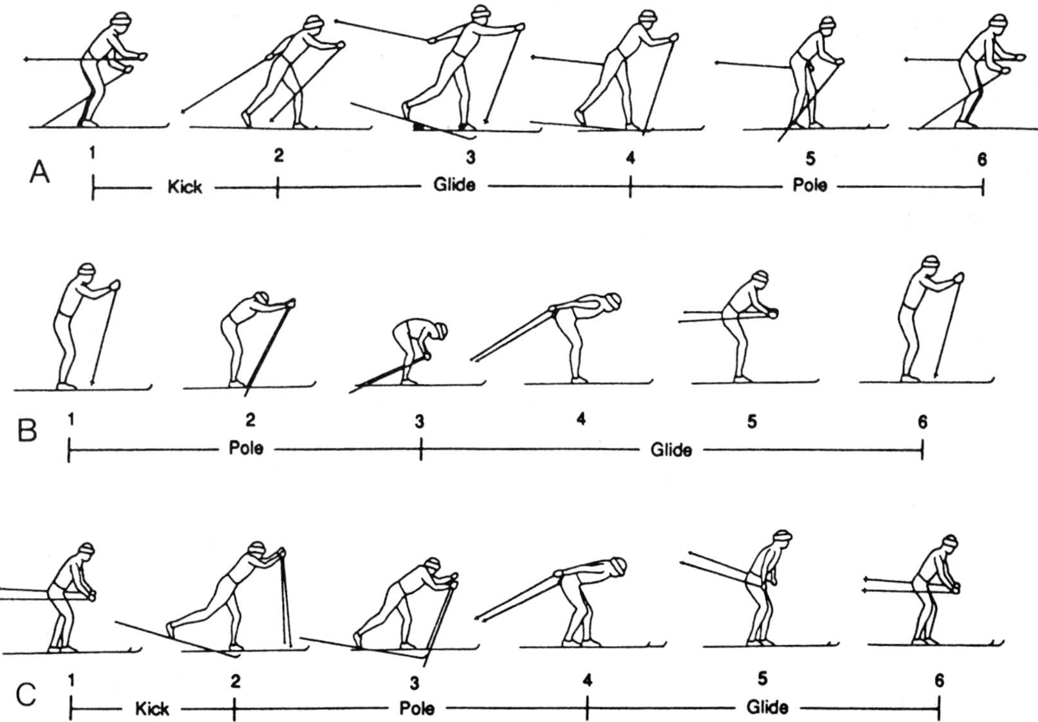

Figure 29.3. General movement pattern for **(A)** the classic or diagonal stride, **(B)** for the double pole technique, and **(C)** for the kick-double pole technique. Reprinted by permission from Casey J, Foster C and Hixon EG, eds. Winter sports medicine. Philadelphia: 1990.

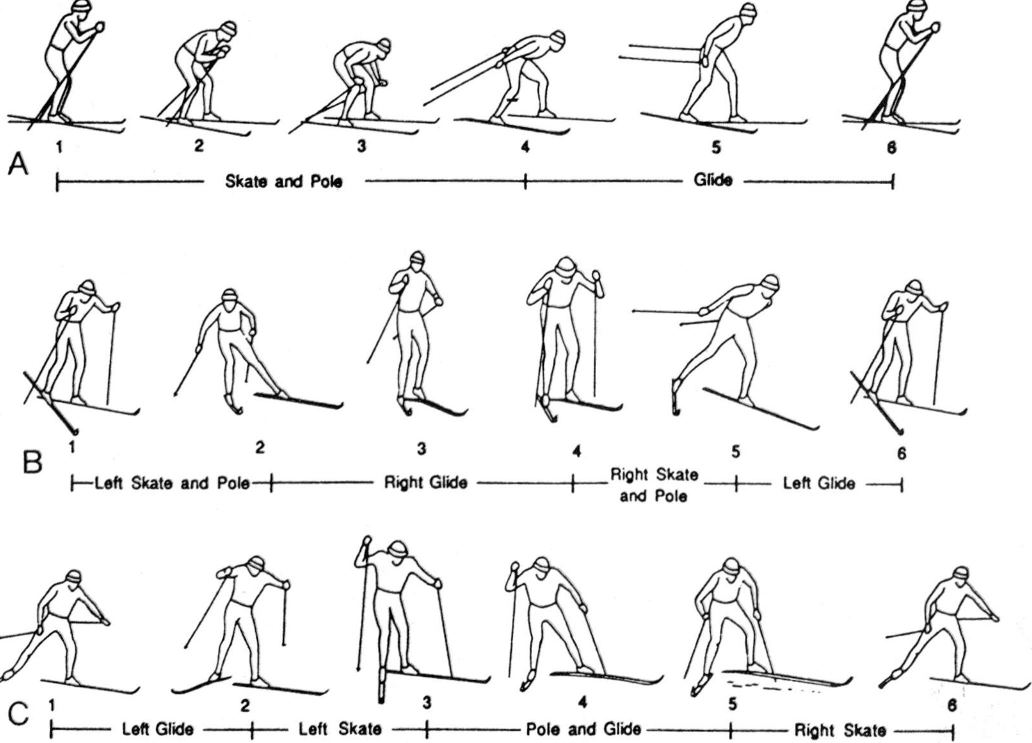

Figure 29.4. General movement patterns in the recently evolved ski-skating techniques, including **(A)** the marathon skate, **(B)** the V2 skate, and **(C)** the V1 skate reprinted by permission from Casey J, Foster C, and Hixon EG, eds. Winter sports medicine. Philadelphia: 1990.

The traditional wooden skis were replaced by fiber glass skis between 1973 and 1974. This brought about a revolution in cross-country skiing. These new skis have considerably greater strength and less weight than their wooden predecessors. Today, racing skis weigh approximately 500 g per ski. The fiber glass skis are divided into one kick area and two gliding areas, making the waxing procedure more complicated than for wooden skis, which were waxed over most of the surface for traction as well as for gliding. The new skating technique has fostered the development of shorter and stiffer skis. For these skis, the role of waxing has also changed in that gliding wax is only necessary on the skating skis.

The ski bindings in cross-country skiing must allow for an unrestricted range of motion of the toes and ankles. The forward tip of the boot is fixed in the binding while the heel is free to elevate from the ski. (Fig. 29.5) Since there is a need for the heel of the boot to achieve fixation during turning on the downhill parts of a track, different heel fixation devices have been developed (Fig. 29.5).

This heel fixation increases the risk of injuring the lower leg in a weighted, twisting fall because the heel then cannot be released from the ski. The development of a releasable binding has been suggested for cross-country skis because the bindings and skis of cross-country equipment have a strength in bending and torsion that is 2 to 5 times higher than the recommended values for alpine release (19).

Skiers involved in ski touring or mountaineering are encouraged to use skis and bindings that are more reliable in ungroomed terrain. Their skis are typically wider, and they have metal edges and cable bindings that can fix the boot to the ski when necessary. In the heel-fixed configuration, many of these bindings become nonreleasable.

The ski boot used in traditional cross-country skiing is usually a low top with a very flexible forefoot. The boots recommended for the skating technique are higher with a stiffer ankle allowing only plantar and dorsi flexion of the foot. Boots for ski touring are a bit heavier, more insulated, and inherently more weather-durable than racing boots.

The poles are important because as much as 30% of the forward thrust of a top-level cross-country skier comes from poling (20). As with skis, there has been a trend toward light, durable poles.

Cross-Country Ski Injuries

Rate of Injury

Because cross-country skiing can take place wherever snow is available and because the population at risk is unknown, it is difficult to calculate an accurate injury rate. In contrast, alpine ski areas with associated lift systems are well defined, thus making epidemiologic studies more feasible. Nevertheless, studies do exist, and, in Sweden, Westlin (21) found 290 injuries caused by cross-country skiing out of a total of 951 ski-related injuries treated in a hospital located near a large ski area over a three-year period. Eriksson and Danielsson (22) estimated the cross-country injury rate in Sweden to be 0.2 per 1000 skier-days. Garrick et al. (23)

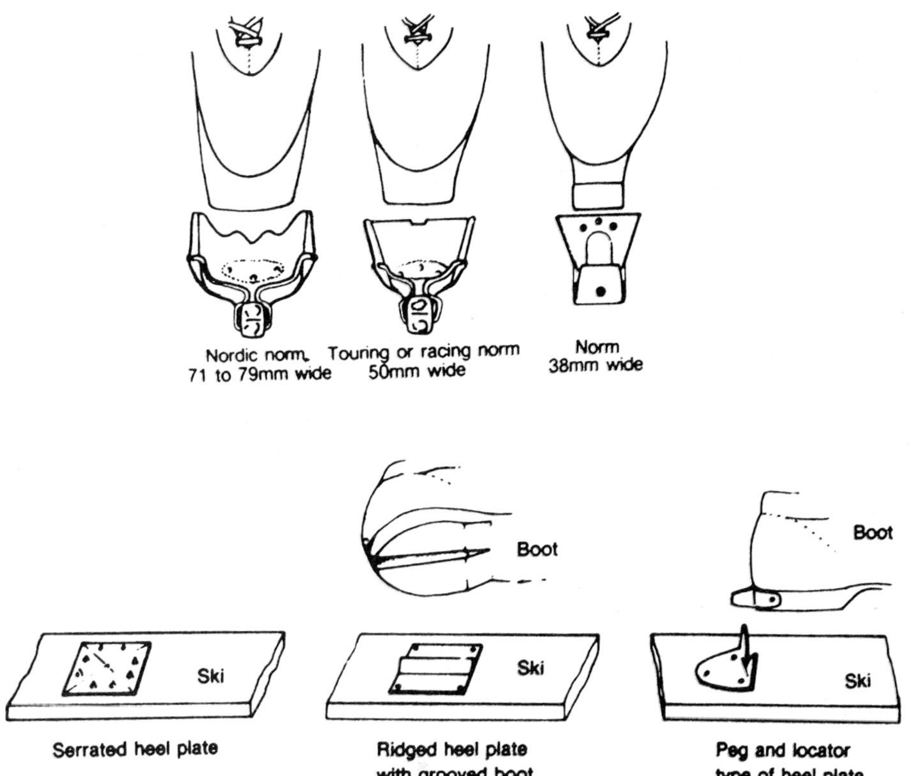

Figure 29.5. Examples of typical cross-country ski bindings and heel fixation devices presently in use. Reprinted by permission from Renström P, Johnson RJ. Cross-country skiing injuries and biomechanics. Sports Med 1989;346–370.

found the rate of injuries to be 1.5 to 2.0 per 1000 skier-days. Hemborg et al. (24) in 1982 found only 77 injuries from cross-country skiing that needed hospital care in an estimated at-risk population of 200,000 skiers per year. These last figures certainly represent an underestimation of the total number of injured skiers because many of the skiers with minor injuries presumably did not seek medical attention at the hospital.

Because of this uncertainty about the real population at risk, an attempt to carry out a controlled prospective study of cross-country injuries was performed in northern Vermont by Boyle et al. (25). To the author's knowledge, this investigation is still the only prospective study available. Five ski touring centers participated during the 1979 to 1980 and 1980 to 1981 seasons. The first season was atypical because of warm temperatures and less than average snowfall, which resulted in only 14,000 skier-days in comparison to a normal season of 60,000 skier-days. Twenty-one injured skiers with 24 injuries were reported during this season resulting in an injury rate of 1.5 injury per 1000 skier days. The next season had more normal snow conditions, which resulted in 22 injured skiers with 25 injuries and 45,000 skier-days. The injury rate was 0.48 per 1000 skier-days for this second season. The combined rate for both seasons was 0.72 per 1000 skier-days. In 1987, Sherry and Asquith (26) reported an injury rate from Australia of 0.49 per 1000 skier-days for recreational cross-country skiing during the 1984–85 season.

Sandelin et al. (9) reported the number of injuries from all competitive skiers in Finland during the seasons 1976 to 1978. From the records of the insurance company that insures all competitive skiers, the authors found 57 injured cross-country skiers out of a total of 21,156 competitive skiers. Accounting for the three seasons, this correlates with an injury rate of 3 per 1000 skiers per year.

In a group of elite Swedish skiers (either on the national ski team or the level just below) investigated during the 1983 to 1984 season, Hemmingsson and Ohlsén (27) found an injury rate of 76% and 66% respectively. For this series, an injury was defined as absence from skiing for more than 2 days. In a one-year study of young elite skiers (mean age, 19 years), training with the V-skating technique, only 4% had a similar absence from skiing, while 20 out of 182 (11%) had recurrent problems (28). During the Vasa Ski Race (89 km) in 1983 and 1984 344 skiers ceased skiing for medical reasons; thus, only 1.75% of the 19,623 skiers who started the race (15) had to quit. In only 6% of these was the reason for interrupting the race an injury, which was usually caused by a fall or collision. The remainder stopped skiing because of diffuse muscular pain or cramps (29%), exhaustion (21%), infections (20%), gastrointestinal problems (11%), and assorted other complaints (13%).

Shealy and Miller (29) published a comparison of 1018 recreational downhill and 119 recreational cross-country skiing injuries in the U.S. between 1979 and 1983. The data were based on an analysis of ski injury reports gathered by the Consumer Product Safety Commission (CPSC), which in turn gets its data from approximately 100 hospital emergency rooms, supposed to be statistically representative of the U.S. This reporting system is called the National Electronic Injury Surveillance System (NEISS). According to the CPSC weighing procedures, the reported 1018 alpine and 119 cross-country injuries represent over 50,000 downhill injuries and 7000 cross-country injuries in the U.S. during this period. Thus, the ratio of downhill to cross-country injuries was 7 to 1. A 1984 study of the skiing population estimated 13 million US skiers with a ratio of 2 downhill skiers to every 1 cross-country skier. Downhill injuries are usually seen, and occasionally treated, at first-aid stations located at the ski areas, whereas the cross-country injuries take place where there is no organized first-aid facility. Thus, the data for downhill skiing in this investigation will show a decreased number of injuries compared to the data for cross-country skiing. Since the NEISS database does not contain any control groups or exposure to risk information, it was not possible to calculate an injury rate. However, one advantage of Shealy and Miller's data was that diagnoses are always made by medically qualified people. There is a distinct difference in the age distribution of the injuries sustained by cross-country skiers compared to downhill skiers. In the data from Sherry's investigation (26), the average cross-country skier was 31 years of age compared to 22 years for the alpine skier. Boyle et al. (25) found the same mean age for the injured cross-country skiers in the Vermont ski areas. Slightly more than half of the injured Vermont skiers were males. In Shealy and Miller's investigation (29), the median age for the cross-country skiers was 27 years compared to 20 years for downhill skiers. The relative frequency of males to females was 44 to 56% in cross-country and 62 to 38% in downhill skiing injuries.

An analysis of the outpatient orthopedic sport injury patients at two clinics in Germany over a period of 15 years showed that 70% of the injured downhill skiers were under 30 years of age while 87% of the injured cross-country skiers were above 30 years of age (30). Unfortunately, the injury rate could not be calculated in this study because the number of skiers at risk was unknown.

Type and Severity of Injury

Shealy and Miller's investigation (29) showed that strain and sprain injuries are the most common in both downhill and cross-country skiing (Table 29.4). The second most common cross-country skiing injury is a fracture, while, for downhill skiing, the next leading injury is an abrasion.

The injuries in cross-country skiing have been located to the upper body in a higher percentage than in downhill skiing. This was obvious in the statistics in two separate investigations from the same Swedish ski area (21, 24). The distribution of injuries to the different body parts in Shealy and Miller's four-year investigation (29) from the U.S. showed that knee injuries have the same proportion in both types of skiing and that cross-country skiing has a higher percentage of shoulder, hand, wrist, arm, elbow, ankle, foot, and toe injuries than downhill skiing (Table 29.5).

Table 29.4.
Distribution of Injury Types in Downhill versus Cross-country Skiing[a]

Injury Type	% Downhill	% Cross-country
Strain/sprain	42.7	42.9
Abrasion/bruise	23.4	17.7
Fracture	21.7	25.2
Laceration	5.0	7.6
Dislocation	2.6	5.0
Concussion/head injury	2.6	1.7
All others	2.1	0.0

[a]Based on 1018 downhill and 119 cross country skiing injuries. From Shealy JE, Miller DA. A relative analysis of downhill and cross-country ski injuries. In: Mote CD, Johnson RJ, eds. Skiing trauma and safety. Eighth International Symposium, ASTM STP 1104. Philadelphia: ASTM 1991:133–143.

Table 29.5.
Distribution of Injuries by Body Part in Downhill versus Cross-country Skiing[a]

Part of Body	% Downhill	% Cross-country
Head, face, and trunk	9.5	5.9
Shoulder	7.7	10.1
Hand, wrist, arm, elbow	7.5	13.4
Finger, thumb	17.0	10.9
Torso	7.8	10.1
Upper leg	1.7	0.8
Knee	26.5	26.1
Lower leg	11.2	4.2
Ankle	9.0	11.8
Foot and toe	2.1	6.7

[a]Based on 1018 downhill and 119 cross-country injuries. From Shealy JE, Miller DA. A relative analysis of downhill and cross-country ski injuries. In: Mote CD, Johnson RJ, eds. Skiing trauma and safety. Eighth International Symposium, ASTM STP 1104. Philadelphia: ASTM 1991:133–143.

Heuman et al. reported (31) that 15% of all ski injuries seen in their hospital, which is close to a major Swedish ski area, were caused by cross-country skiing compared to 85% sustained in downhill skiing. They further investigated the two seasons of 1979 and 1983 and found a tendency towards more severe injuries in the 1983 season. In the following table (Table 29.6), it can be seen that during the 1983 season there were instances of cross-country skiers with fractures of the hip joint, femur, tibia, and vertebral column that were nonexistent in the 1979 season.

The authors attribute the increase in serious injuries to newer and faster skis as well as to the hard packed ski tracks that allow higher speeds. The heel fixation devices and the no-release ski bindings together with the stiffer and unbreakable skis are other factors that may account for this increase.

In the prospective study of Boyle et al. (25) it was noted that a background in downhill skiing appeared to reduce the risk of injury, but that ski lessons per se did not reduce the likelihood of injury. They found that approximately 90% of the injuries occurred in downhill terrain and 63% on tracked trails, while the rest injured

Table 29.6.
Cross-country Skiing Injuries during the 1979 and 1983 Seasons[a]

Injury Location	Number of Injuries	
	1979 (n = 43)	1983 (n = 89)
Ankle	6 (14%)	6 (6.7%)
Tibia fractures	0 (0%)	3 (3.4%)
Knee	7 (16.3%)	16 (18.0%)
Femur	0 (0%)	4 (4.5%)
Hip joint	0 (0%)	3 (3.4%)
Spinal	0 (0%)	3 (3.4%)
Upper extremity	19 (44.2%)	34 (38.2%)
Head	0 (0%)	3 (3.4%)
Other	11 (25.6%)	17 (19.1%)

[a]Conducted in a Swedish hospital close to a major ski area. From Heuman R, Sten J, Tidermark J. Ski injuries in Northern Dalecarlia during the seasons 1979 and 1983. (Swedish). Läkartidningen 1985;82:584–586.

themselves on untracked but prepared trails. Most of the accidents were caused by falls, and the injuries sustained resulted mostly from impact (32 out of 43), with the snow or other objects. They also found an overrepresentation of skiers using heel plates with the ridge and groove design among those who had sustained injuries. The distribution of the recorded injuries in this prospective study of cross-country skiing injuries is shown in the following table (Table 29.7).

Frost and Bauer (32) reported in 1991 on 10 proximal femur fractures sustained in 4 female and 6 male cross-country skiers in order to point out that some of the cross-country skiing injuries can be quite severe. They suggested that the injury mechanism was not a rotational trauma, but a fall with a direct impact force on the trochanteric region. This was evidenced by the frequent massive soft tissue hematoma observed in this region. Because no rotational trauma was involved, the use of releasable bindings would not have had any preventive effect on this type of injury. One of their explanations for this injury was the same as Heuman (31) had suggested, that is, high speed achieved on well-prepared tracks together with lightweight equipment. They also suggested that awareness of injury risks and proper training in the use of the sophisticated equipment together with good judgement and adaptation to the surroundings can reduce the risk of injury in cross-country skiing. Because this injury seems to involve cross-country skiers with a typical injury mechanism, they suggested that this should be called a "skier's hip," much as the skier thumb injury involving the ulnar collateral ligament of the metacarpophalangeal joint was named.

In cross-country skiing, overuse injuries are common. In competitive cross-country skiers of Finland (9), muscle and tendon injuries were the most frequent injury (35%), followed by ligament injuries (33%), fractures (25%), and wound and abrasions (7%). The lower extremity was injured in 44% of the cases and the upper in 35%. Hemmingsson and Ohlsén (27) found in their investigation of Swedish elite skiers that more than 50% of the injuries that caused absence from skiing were

Table 29.7.
Cross-country Ski Injuries for the 1979/80 and 1980/81 Seasons[a]

Type of Injury	Number of Injuries
Upper Extremity (40.8%)	
Thumb sprains	6
Shoulder dislocations	3
Shoulder contusions	3
Colles fractures	2
Finger sprains (proximal interphalangeal joint)	2
Elbow contusions	2
Elbow fracture/dislocation	1
Hand contusions	1
Total	20
Lower Extremity (48.9%)	
Knee contusions	4
Ankle sprains	3
Hip contusions	2
Knee ligament total disruptions (medial collateral ligament and anterior cruciate ligament)	2
Knee ligament partial ruptures	2
Leg contusions	2
Subtrochanteric femur fracture	1
Patellar tendon open rupture	1
Tibia and fibula fracture	1
Ankle fracture	1
Patellar subluxation	1
Hamstring strain	1
Knee laceration	1
Knee abrasion	1
Hip massive subcutaneous hematoma	1
Total	24
Head, Face and Trunk (10.2%)	
Fracture of sacrum	1
Concussion	1
Mandible fracture	1
Skull contusion	1
Ear laceration	1
Total	5

[a]Study conducted in ski touring areas in northern Vermont (43 patients with 49 injuries). From Boyle JJ, Johnson RJ, Pope MH, et al. Cross-country skiing injuries. In: Johnson RJ, Mote CD, eds. Skiing trauma and safety. Fifth International Symposium, ASTM STP 860. Philadelphia: ASTM 1985:411–422.

overuse injuries. The most common overuse injuries in descending order were medial tibial stress syndrome (shin splint), Achilles tendon problems, and low back pain.

Kannus et al. (33) studied cross-country skiers who were treated at the Tampere (Finland) Research Station of Sports Medicine during the period of 1985 to 1987. By that time the classic diagonal stride technique had been replaced almost completely by the skating technique in competitive skiing. The number, types, and sites of acute injuries remained unchanged, but the number of overuse injuries fell by about 50% during this time period. The knee was still the most frequent site of overuse injuries, but the number had decreased by half. Nonspecific synovitis, meniscus degeneration, and extensor tendinitis were the most common overuse injuries found to involve the knee. The most common sites of injury in the lower limb besides the knee were the shin, the ankle and the Achilles tendon. There were no overuse injuries of the lower and upper back, the neck-shoulder region, and the upper limb during the last 6-month observation period. The authors concluded that "there appears to be no sports traumatological reason why the skating technique should not be recommended as an equivalent alternative to the diagonal technique."

There have been very few reports of increased problems related to the new skating technique, but there is at least one report of an elite Swiss skier who after starting with this technique developed a lower leg compartment syndrome that hampered his performance and finally required a fasciotomy (34).

Hemmingson (28) had, in an earlier investigation, specifically addressed the problems of the skating technique and found that there was a low frequency of overuse injuries that caused disability and that 66% of these were caused by low back pain. Frymoyer et al. (35) showed that the compressive forces applied to the disc during the kick phase of the diagonal stride were calculated to be almost 2900 N while the shear forces were lower, approximately 1000 N. In the double poling technique, the compressive forces were 109 N and the shearing forces, 233 N. The calculated shear failure occurs at a force of 2000 N, which is twice the kick phase force mentioned above. Frymoyer believes that, used repetitively, these forces can be of importance in developing low back problems. In one investigation of young Finnish cross-country skiers with low back pain (36), functional scoliosis was found in 49% and radiological spinal anomalies in 23%. However, none of the radiological findings had any effect on the therapy of these skiers. All continued skiing without major back problem after undergoing a specific exercise program. Kannus et al. (33) found a decrease in low back pain problems between 1985 and 1987 when the skating technique had been adopted by most of the cross-country skiers. The skating technique probably implies less mechanical load on the back since more static work and slower rotational motion of the spine is involved in the skating technique compared to the classic diagonal stride.

Prevention of Injuries

The idea that specific cross-country ski instructions could reduce the number of injuries at first seems credible. However, Boyle (25) found in his prospective investigation that more injured skiers (51.2%) had taken ski lessons than the control skiers (27.1%) during the 1980/81 season. These findings are similar to what has previously been reported for downhill skiing (23, 37, 38). Instruction is given about skiing technique and not about safety or improper equipment. Also, very few ski schools teach the students how to fall in a "controlled way" to avoid injuries. Because the skier wants to be able to control turning and edging of the skis in downhill parts of the tracks, different heel fixation devices (see above) have made this possible. However, this also increases the risk of injury, which should be pointed out to the skier. Boyle et al. (25) found that more than 33% of all injured skiers wore the ridge and groove design heel plate in comparison to 11% of the control skiers. This finding supported the view of Ekström (19), who suggested that a new cross-country ski binding with release in toe-up and toe-side directions could reduce the number of cross-country skiing injuries. However, as Frost and Bauer (32) pointed out, such a release binding will not protect the skier from direct impact forces, but only from rotational trauma. They suggest that some form of protective padding could prevent injuries caused by a direct fall, but they also doubt that many skiers would use this padding.

Keeping the tracks wide and removing all obstacles close to the prepared tracks are obvious preventative measures that have merit. Because many skiers want to explore nature on their own, there will always be unexpected obstacles, trees, or weather conditions that may cause injuries. The only way to avoid many of these injuries is to provide information about skiing safety to all cross-country skiers. They should be urged to keep their equipment in good condition, adapt themselves to current weather conditions, and not to overestimate their own ability. In the Vermont investigation, over 81% of those injured were beginner or intermediate skiers, a fact that reflects the increasing popularity of cross-country skiing in the U.S. (25). In the Scandinavian countries, cross-country skiing has always been a popular winter sport, and the majority of the population has been skiing since early childhood. However, this does not rule out the need for safety instructions.

Good fitness makes skiing more enjoyable. Cross-country skiing itself is, as already mentioned, a very efficient means for getting into good shape after various injuries and illnesses.

There is need for a new type of ski school that teaches the cross-country skier not only skiing technique, but also how to deal with equipment problems, how to fall properly under different conditions, and how to account for weather or track conditions.

Telemarking

Telemarking is a way of descending slopes that has recently become popular. The equipment is a specific type of cross-country or long distance ski with metal edges and a rather sturdy toe binding. The heel is left free. Specific release bindings are available. The skier uses leather boots that are higher and stiffer than ordinary cross-country boots. The skier descends downhill slopes with the skis parallel and one ski slightly in front of the other, in a deep knee bend position. Turning is performed by shifting the leading ski and also by using the poles almost like a jump turn.

Jørgsholm et al. (39) have, in their Swedish investigation, found 46 injured telemark skiers out of a total of 1364 injured skiers. The population at risk is not known. The average age for the injured telemarker was 24.2 years (in an age range of 14 to 36), and 63% of them were male. In contrast to the snowboarders, only 33% considered themselves beginners, while 52% had a great deal of experience in this type of skiing. Of all injuries, 31% were thumb injuries (ulnar collateral lig-

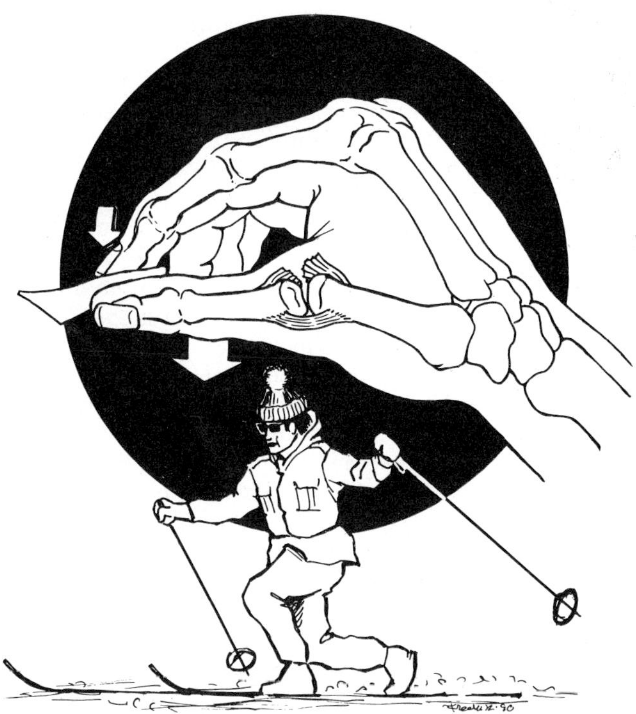

Figure 29.6. A telemark skier with the most common injury type—ulnar collateral ligament rupture of the thumb. Reprinted by permission from Jorgsholm P, Bauer M, Ljung BO, et al. Downhill skiing is developing—snowboard and telemark skiing give new injury pattern. Läkartidningen 1991;88:1589–1592 and by permission of Fredrik Johansson, medical artist.

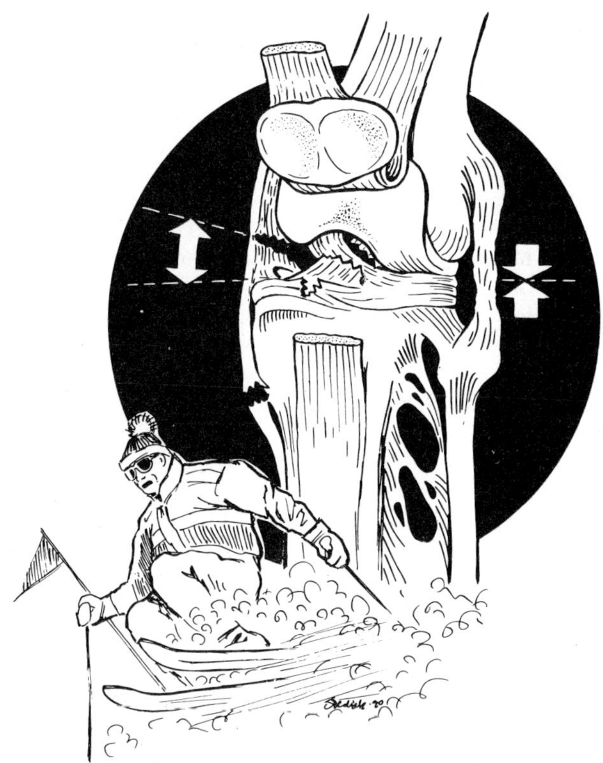

Figure 29.7. An alpine skier with the most common injury type—grade III knee ligament sprain. Reprinted by permission from Jorgsholm P, Bauer M, Ljung BO, et al. Downhill skiing is developing—snowboard and telemark skiing give new injury pattern. Läkartidningen 1991; 88:1589–1592 and by permission of Fredrik Johansson, medical artist.

ament injuries of the metacarpophalangeal joint). This was twice as many as the authors had found in their downhill skiers (Fig. 29.6). This is probably because the telemark binding permits the skier to fall forward more easily than the downhill binding, thereby causing the skier to try to break the fall with the hand holding the ski pole. The 25% frequency of knee injuries reflected the risk of sustaining too much external rotational force in the valgus while making telemark turns. Thirty-five percent of the downhill skiers had sustained knee injuries. The difference could, according to the authors, be explained by the soft and lower ski boot in telemarking. The particular type of binding in conjunction with the soft boot also might explain why as many as 15% of the telemark skiers had ankle distortions compared to 2 to 3% among the downhill skiers.

Prevention of Injuries

The preventive measures suggested for this specific type of skiing are similar to the other categories of "downhill skiing," that is, use of release bindings, instructions on how to fall, avoidance of bad weather, and proper estimation of one's own capability.

DOWNHILL SKIING

Downhill, or Alpine skiing, is among the most popular of winter sports worldwide. It is enjoyed by all age groups, from the novice to the most talented individual. While musculoskeletal injuries are the frequent sequelae of falls and collisions, the nature of these injuries has changed recently, reflecting in large part changes in equipment and style.

Technique and Equipment

The simplest form of downhill skiing is sliding down a slope on skis while avoiding obstacles and moving in a controlled fashion. Competitive downhill skiing is characterized by four disciplines: downhill, super g, giant slalom and slalom. The ultimate speed reached by a skier reflects the length of the course and the number of turns typical for each of the events.

The basic skiing position begins with the feet placed a hip-width apart. The knees are flexed in a forward lean to absorb bumps (40). The trunk is slightly bent at the waist and the arms are held in front of the body. The hip flexors absorb bumps actively by pulling the knees upward or passively by allowing the bumps to push the knees up (Fig. 29.7).

By transferring weight from the inside to the outside ski, a technique known as unweighting, the turn is initiated. The pole is planted in front to help unweighting and for balance. As the upper body faces downhill and the speed increases, the angulation of the skis continue to increase. The skier then points back from the fall line and the turn is complete. The pressure on the skis is decreased as the skier returns to the neutral position.

This technique requires strong activation of the quadriceps muscles, which are considered the most important muscle group in downhill skiing. Hip rotators are employed during turns, while the hip flexors and extensors are important for unweighting and absorbing the moguls or bumps. The lower leg muscles are used a great deal to shift the body weight forwards and backwards and to control the edges of the ski. Thus, both strength and endurance of the lower leg muscles are important for downhill skiers. As mentioned above, the pole plant is used to help in turning and consequently strains the shoulder joint and its surrounding muscles. Downhill skiers need to have strength, coordination, balance, and endurance to be able to perform on the recreational as well as at the top level.

The ski becomes an extension of the leg by a system that couples skier to boot to binding to ski, acting as a lever to inflict high loads on the lower leg. The bindings have traditionally played a major role in causing lower extremity skiing injuries with as high as 44% of these injuries attributed to binding malfunction in the 1970s (41). More recently, this figure has been remarkably reduced as skiing equipment has improved during the last 10 to 15 years (42).

The ideal ski binding should be able to release the boot from the ski when the loads are getting close to the threshold of injury to the lower extremity. It should also ignore forces not dangerous to the leg, but that are generated during "normal" maneuvers. The setting of the bindings is based on biomechanical studies of the torsional and bending strengths of the tibia. However, these studies are meant only to prevent tibial fractures. They do not address knee ligament injuries.

Ski bindings can be classified into two types based upon their release capabilities: two-mode and multimode (Fig. 29.8). The two-mode release bindings release in an outward and inward twist at the toe and in a forward lean at the heel. Multimode bindings have an additional one or more directions of release. Most of the current bindings fall into the two-mode category, but many major manufacturers have offered models with an upward release at the toe in recent years. In theory, it would be useful to devise bindings that release in all possible directions, but, in the past, such bindings as were available had the reputation of frequently releasing inadvertently. Such bindings with omnidirectional release have not yet been devised.

The release settings are very important. It has been shown that the settings for all groups of skiers are usually too high. Only 41% of the bindings in competitive downhill skiers in Norway released in accordance with the indicated setting, and only 77% were correctly mounted on the skis (43). The majority of both child and adult racers from a New England ski area were found to have their settings well above the values recommended by the manufacturer (44). In a prospective study, there was a significant decrease in the number of reported injuries in one skier group with bindings that were correctly installed, set, and functionally tested (17.6%) versus a control group which had given no special attention to their bindings (24.5%) (45). The author has found that the risk for lower-extremity, equipment-related (LEER) injuries was 3.5-fold lower with properly adjusted bindings compared to the average setting found on the ski slopes.

Antifriction devices function as a fulcrum for the forward release mechanism, and they prevent friction in twists and forward leans. The maintenance of the binding is also often overlooked. Johnson et al. (46) and Young et al. (47) reported that the number of skiers who lubricated their bindings was much lower among injured skiers than in the control population. The classic ski boot has a fixation buckle placed anteriorly, which opens anteriorly by spreading the sides. Ski boots were originally made of leather, but plastic materials are now dominant. The rear entry boot has become popular during the last few years. It has one anterior and one posterior part, with the foot entering from the top. The boot is closed with a cable device on the back of the boot. The boots have become higher and stiffer, almost eliminating injuries to the ankle and the lower leg. However, the incidence of severe knee sprains has markedly increased as a result of the changes in the boot and the inability of bindings to protect the knee ligaments.

The ski poles have been considered important in causing thumb injuries, and various grips have been constructed to minimize this risk.

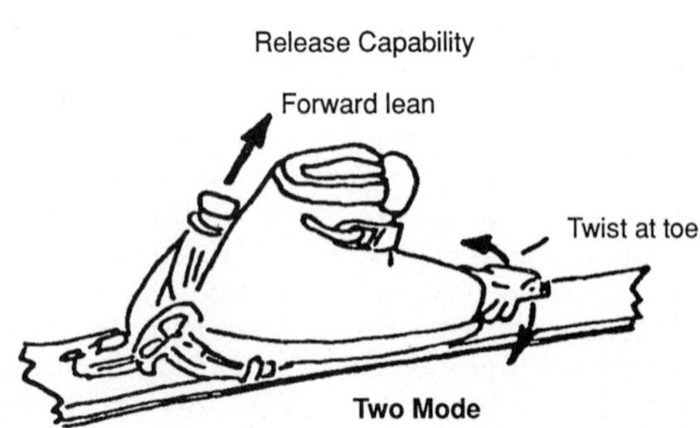

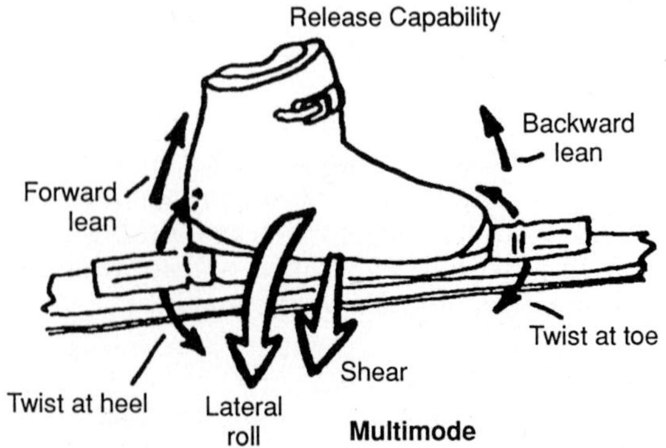

Figure 29.8. Representing the most common ski binding, two-mode release capability releases in twist at the toe and forward lean at the heel. Multimode release capability releases in additional directions, including backward lean at the toe, twist at the heel, and lateral shear, and lateral roll. Reprinted by permission from Eriksson E and Johnson RJ. Exercise and Sports Medicine Sciences Reviews. Philadelphia: Franklin Press, 1981.

Downhill Ski Injuries

Rate of Injury

Compared to other types of skiing, the injury rate of downhill skiing is easier to calculate. Alpine resorts utilize a lift system, allowing tabulation of the number of skiers at risk. Moreover, it is frequently possible to estimate the number of injuries from a ski area from their first-aid station. Using parking lot interviews, Johnson et al. (48) found that 27% of the injuries sustained at a Northern Vermont ski area went unreported, and noting that at least 66% of these were of minor significance. This compares favorably with other studies (23, 37).

Eriksson (8) published a one-year inventory of skiing injuries in Sweden during the 1973 to 1974 season with a total of 1199 registered injuries. This was further estimated to be only 60 to 70% of the total number of injuries. The majority of the injuries, or 885 (75%), took place during downhill skiing. Of all the injured, 42% were under 15 years of age; 17 skiers were over 70 years of age; the range was 3 to 79 years of age. Of the injured skiers, 63% were male. Unfortunately, it was impossible to estimate the population at risk and, thus, no real injury rate can be calculated from these figures.

In another investigation published the same year by Young et al. (47), data were collected over an eight-year period and a total of 4458 injuries were found. A control group of 659 skiers was sampled during one season. The ski population was determined by the number of day tickets sold at the ski area. It was found that the injury rate declined from 4.2 to 2.8 per 1000 man-skier-days during the period of the 1966 to 1973 seasons. Three times as many injuries took place during the weekends than the rest of the week. The number of injuries occurring during each hour of the day showed an increase at the end of the day. Also, the average time skiing before injury occurs was more than three hours. These two findings support the suspicion that fatigue as a contributory factor has an important role in ski accidents. The injured skiers were slightly younger than the control population, with a median age of 21 to 22 years compared to 24 years for the uninjured skiers. Therefore, the inexperienced skier was more at risk than the experienced skier. This was especially dramatic for the first-year skier, who, in this investigation, accounted for 7% of the population and for 16% of the injured skiers.

Young et al. (49), in an update of their ski injury statistics from the same ski area (Waterville Valley, New Hampshire) found an injury rate of 3.37 per 1000 skier-days. A new and faster chair lift had been introduced during the 1988 to 1989 season, so the time spent skiing on the slopes probably had increased. The result suggested a slight correlative increase, but the authors did not identify the increased exposure caused by the new lift as a factor in the increase.

In a retrospective analysis of skiing injuries in Australia from 1962 to 1988, Sherry and Fenelon (50) found that the injury rate had dropped from 10.9 per 1000 skier-days in 1962 to 3.22 in 1988 with a statistically significant annual decline of 2%.

At one Swedish ski area, turnstile registration at each ski run was introduced during the season of 1987/1988, thus making the injury rate calculations more accurate (51). The number of runs was 5,940,000 with 840 registered ski injuries seen by a doctor at the ski clinic during that season. This gives an injury rate of 0.14 injuries per 1000 ski runs. The length of the different ski runs is not mentioned in this study nor have the number of runs an average skier makes per day been estimated. This makes it difficult to evaluate this injury rate in relation to the more common method of injury rate calculation (injuries per thousand skier-days). Johnson et al. (52) reported a thorough study of all skiing injuries for 18 seasons in a moderate-sized northern Vermont ski area, from the 1972/1973 through the 1989/1990 seasons. They found 6671 injuries sustained by 6139 skiers. There were approximately 2,032,000 skier-days at the ski area during the eighteen-year period. The injury rate has declined by 48% from 5 per 1000 skier visits to 2.5 at the end of the study period; lower extremity injuries had also declined from 67% to 53%.

Most studies have used injuries per thousand skier days to indicate the injury rate in skiing. Instead of changing the base for relatively rare injury groups to 10,000 or 100,000 Johnson et al. (48) have chosen to indicate the incidence in terms of "mean days between injuries" (MDBI). This is defined by the following equation:

$$MDBI = \frac{Skier\ Visits}{Number\ of\ Injuries}$$

The change in MDBI between year one (YR1) and year eighteen (YR18) is determined by the following equation:

$$\%\ change = 1 - \frac{MDBI\ (initial)}{MDBI\ (final)}$$

Figure 29.9 shows the injury rate change in MDBI reported by Johnson et al. (52).

Type and Severity of Injury

The Swedish investigation by Eriksson (8) reported that 72% of the 885 downhill injuries involved the lower limb, 20% the upper limb and that 46% were fractures of the leg. No more specification of the severity of the injuries was made.

In the 8-year study of ski injuries from Waterville Valley in New Hampshire by Young et al. (47), both the number of knee (21%) and ankle (26%) injuries far exceeded the number of lower leg injuries (13%). Thumb injuries made up about 8% of the total number. During the study period, a fairly constant 25% of the injuries were fractures. An equal percentage of cases was classified as muscle injuries without any further details. The high stiff ski boot was introduced between the years 1968 to 1972 and influenced the type and the severity of the injury. The number of ankle injuries decreased, while lower leg injuries increased; knee injuries remained the same in the years before 1968 as compared to the years after 1972.

In the 1989 update of the ski injuries from the same ski area, Young et al. (49) reported a higher percentage of knee injuries—25% of all injuries—than in 1976; the rate was even higher during the 1985/1986 season (30%). The percentage of lower leg injuries has continued to decline from 13% to only 5% of the total. Thumb injuries have leveled off at around 10%, and head and shoulder injuries have reached the 10% level (Fig. 29.10).

In an Australian ski injury analysis (50), significant changes were found in 4 of 6 injury types over the 27 years that this retrospective study covered. The knee injuries had an annual increase in incidence by the order of 3.8%, while tibial fractures, ankle injuries, and lacerations decreased in frequency. Upper body and thumb injury rates were noted to have an upward but still not significant trend. In the study by Johnson et al. (52), injuries were divided into fracture and soft tissue categories. The soft tissue group was then further subdivided into laceration, strain, contusion, sprain, and other soft tissue groups. These were further subdivided by part of the body. In this study, tibia and ankle fractures showed significant improvements with a decrease of 88% and 92% respectively over the 18-year period while fractures of the clavicle showed the only negative trend in the fracture group with an increase by 179%. In the soft tissue group, boot top contusions were down by 88%, ankle sprains by 89%, knee sprains grade I and II by 70%, while the serious grade III knee sprains normally involving the anterior cruciate ligament (ACL) were up by 209% (Fig. 29.11). This is the most significant negative trend discovered in this study. The grade III knee sprains have increased from 17% to 73% of all knee sprains over the 18-year study period. In terms of MDBI, grade III knee sprains now occur once in every 2111 skier visits; this is a higher incidence than for tibia fractures 18 years ago when it was 1 in every 3247 skier visits. Currently, at 19% of all reported injuries, serious knee sprains represent a larger proportion of injuries than any other soft tissue group, larger even than the all fracture group. Skiers sustaining ACL injuries are older, heavier, more often female, and they have more experience than other skier groups. These skiers used both state of the art bindings and boots.

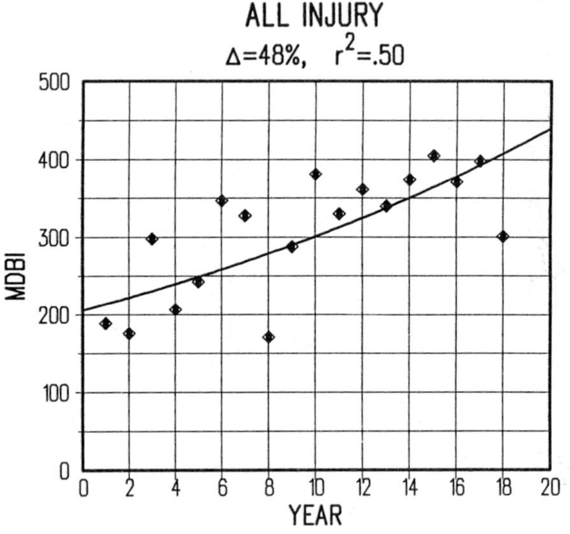

Figure 29.9. This figure illustrates the overall injury rate change (increase in MDBI) found in the Vermont study of 18 seasons of ski injuries. Reprinted by permission from Johnson RJ, Ettlinger CF, Shealy J. Skier injury trends—1976–1990. In Mote CD, Johnson RJ, eds. Skiing Trauma and Safety: Ninth International Symposium, ASTM STP 1182. Philadelphia: ASTM 1193;11–22.

In Great Britain there is a paucity of snow, which has led to the construction of artificial ski slopes. On this type of slope, the major difference in injury pattern is the higher ratio of arm to leg injuries, 4.2:1, with thumb injuries making up 32% of all injuries (53). The range and incidence of other injuries correspond closely to those sustained during skiing on snow.

Recently, there have been reports of increased numbers of serious injuries occurring on the ski slopes. A

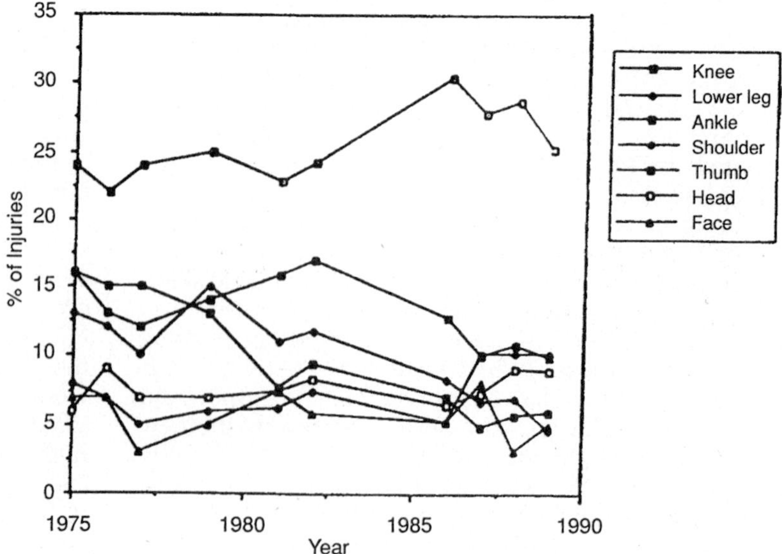

Figure 29.10. Comparison of incidence in ski injuries of different parts of the body registered at Waterville Valley, NH over a 15 year period. Reprinted by permission from Young LR, Lee SM. Alpine injury pattern at Watterville Valley—1989 update. In: Mote CD, Johnson RJ, eds. Skiing Trauma and Safety: Eighth International Symposium, ASTM STP 1104. Philadelphia: ASTM 1991:125–132.

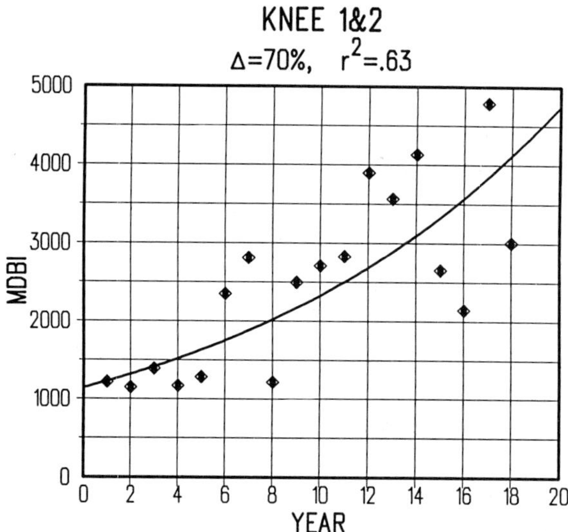

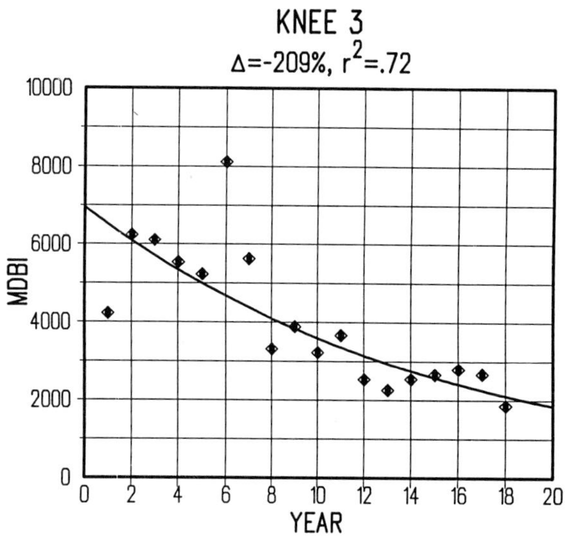

Figure 29.11. This figure illustrates the injury rate decrease (increase in MDBI, mean days between injuries) found for grade I and II knee sprains *(left)* and the increase (decrease in MDBI) for grade III knee sprains *(right)* in the Vermont study of 18 seasons of ski injuries. Reprinted by permission from Johnson RJ, Etlinger CF, Shealy J. Skier injury trends—1976–1990. In: Mote CD, Johnson RJ, eds. Skiing Trauma and Safety: Ninth International Symposium, ASTM STP 1182. Philadelphia: ASTM 1993;11–22.

recent Swedish investigation from the only hospital in a county having approximately 30% of the downhill market in Sweden, studied all the ski injuries examined at that hospital during the ski season of 1989 to 1990 (54). Of the total of 395 injured patients, 146 were admitted to the hospital and were included in the study. Downhill skiing was the cause of injury in 118 of the 146 patients. The total number of injuries sustained by these 118 downhill skiers was 135 injuries—35 head injuries (2 lethal injuries), 4 injuries to the thorax, 7 to the spine, 10 pelvic or abdominal injuries, 17 upper limb injuries, and 62 lower limb injuries. The mean age of the injured skiers was 22.7 years with 66% of the injured skiers being male. Almost 80% considered themselves good or expert skiers. More than 90% had injured themselves while skiing on a groomed slope. The most serious injuries (including the fatal head injuries) occurred while skiing off the groomed area and colliding with an obstacle. Since the population at risk was unknown in this study, no injury rate could be calculated. The findings from this study show that most of the injuries requiring hospital admittance happened to experienced male skiers traveling down the slopes at high speeds. Simply falling, not colliding with other skiers or obstacles was the usual mechanism of injury.

Stanley et al. (55), in a retrospective study from a Canadian ski area, studied all serious injuries defined as "life- or limb-threatening injuries requiring immediate stabilization and transfer to a tertiary care facility" during the 1989 to 1990 ski season. A total of 50 serious ski injuries were recorded in a predominantly male (73%) population with a mean age of 38 years. Twelve patients had multiple injuries. The incidence rate was calculated at 4.1 in 100,000 skier-days. The injury rates for the different categories are summarized in the following table (Table 29.8).

Fatalities in downhill skiing have been reported as part of general ski injury reports and more specifically by Shealy (14), looking at data from the Consumer Product Safety Commission (CPSC), and by Morrow et al. (56) from the state of Vermont. Shealy went through the CPSC files and found 117 death certificates relating to skiing for the period of 1973 to 1983. The actual rate of death in skiing, exclusive of heart attacks, avalanches, and lift-related deaths, is on the order of 20 to 30 deaths per year in the U.S. The number of skier visits is estimated to be around 50 million annually, which means that the rate of fatal injuries probably is less than 0.5 deaths per 1 million skier visits or 0.2 deaths per 100,000 participants annually. Shealy found the fatally injured skier to be predominantly male (83.1%) and older (27.4 years) than both the control group (25.8 years) and the typical, injured ski population (21.2 years). A fatal injury involves a head trauma in 60% of cases, and, although massive brain and internal injuries are quite rare in the typical ski injury, they accounted for 93% of all fatalities. Impact with a tree was the cause

Table 29.8.
Rate of Serious Injuries in Downhill Skiing[a]

Injury Category	Number of Patients	Injury Rate Per 100,000 Skier Days
Head	11	0.9
Cervical	6 (3 in combination with head injuries)	0.49
Chest	9	0.74
Fracture/dislocation	26	2.1
Hypothermia	1	0.08
Total	50	4.1

[a]From Stanley RL, Meeuwisse WH. Life and limb threatening injuries in Alpine skiing. Clin J Sports Med 1991;1:162–165.

of death in 76% of the cases. Jenkins et al. (57) studied collision injuries and found only 18.5% of all injuries resulted from collisions. He also found that, as a group, these injuries were actually less severe than the non-collision injuries. However, some of the most severe injuries were associated with collisions with trees.

Morrow et al. (56) found very similar figures during the 1979 to 1980 through 1985 to 1986 ski seasons in Vermont. They observed 16 deaths, 13 (81%) of which were males, with a mean age of 29.7 years. During the study period, 24.17 million skier-days were logged for an estimated rate of 0.66 deaths per million skier-days. Fourteen cases involved a collision between the skier and a stationary objects such as a tree, rock, or lift tower. High speed and loss of control were the major factors in these collision injuries. Blood ethanol testing associated with 13 fatalities detected no alcohol in 12 and only a very low concentration (less than 0.01%) in one case. The visibility was good in all cases, the terrain adequately covered by snow, and most were skiing on trails equal to their ability when the accident happened. Blunt trauma to the head was the cause of death in 14 instances, while the remaining 2 died of trauma to the chest or abdomen. This study suggested that fatigue was one factor in the cause because the accidents tended to occur in the afternoon. The general injury risk in skiing has been found to be higher for the beginner skier, but, when looking at the skiing ability in these fatal injuries, only 2 were beginners while 9 were advanced skiers.

Sherry and Clout (58) examined the ski-related deaths over 32 years from 1956 to 1987 in an Australian ski area providing both downhill and cross-country skiing. They found 29 deaths of which 8 were trauma-related, 15 cardiovascular-related and 6 hypothermia-related. The incidence for trauma-related deaths was calculated to be 0.24 per million skier-days. At least 4 of the trauma-related deaths occurred during activities other than downhill skiing, and, hence, the incidence was in fact lower than is stated in their article. In this study, 7 of the 8 trauma-related deaths were male and 7 were caused by head and neck injuries.

A summary of some of the data from these three studies is made in the following table (Table 29.9).

From these studies, one might conclude that the seriously or fatally injured skier is usually an experienced male skier with an average age above that of the typical injured skier. The skier is typically moving at a high speed, loses his balance, falls and collides with a stationary object, such as a tree, receiving a massive head injury that often results in death. However, the annual incidence of deaths in downhill skiing (0.2 deaths per 100,000 participants) is low in comparison to other sporting activities, such as water sports (2.8/100,000), or in comparison to firearm-related deaths (1.3/100,000). These figures are put into perspective with knowledge of the figures of automobile-driving-related deaths (26.6/100,000), based on National Safety Council figures from 1974 (14).

Table 29.9
Fatal Injuries Occurring during Downhill Skiing

Rate Per Million Skier Days/ Skier Visits	% Male	Mean Age (Years)	Reference
0.5	83	27.4	14
0.66	81	29.7	56
0.12	100	31.5	58

Prevention of Injuries

In recent years, considerable effort has been made to diminish risk factors inherent in the Alpine techniques. Specific safety prevention measures include information about ski equipment and binding design, standards for the preparation of slopes, and skier-responsibility codes. It is commonly agreed that the development and use of modern ski equipment, especially release bindings, and plastic ski boots have contributed to the decline in injury in downhill skiing (59). All of the earlier mentioned investigations show a marked decline of the lower extremity injuries to approximately 50% of the incidence of 15 to 20 years ago. However, upper body injuries have changed very little (52). In a prospective study of German skiers with an experimental group (n=460) and a control group (n=690), it was found that proper binding setting and mounting reduced lower extremity equipment-related injuries by a factor of 3.5 compared to the control group (45). It was also found, that by using a ski pole specifically designed to prevent the thumb from being inserted into the snow during a fall, the frequency of skier's thumb injuries was reduced from 4.0% to 2.8%. Using the data from his investigation, Hauser (45) estimated that approximately 30,000 of the annual 80,000 ski injuries in Germany that required medical treatment could have been avoided by using correctly mounted and properly adjusted ski equipment. Equipment ought to be designed ergonomically and be easy for the skier to handle, mount, and adjust. Well-qualified technicians and pertinent information to the skier concerning equipment are also necessary measures to accomplish a reduction in equipment-related ski injuries. Because many of the ski injuries in this estimate were considered to be the result of the skier's behavior, ski resorts now insist on a basic code of skiing safety rules, which, if infringed, result in ticket revocation.

While the overall incidence of lower extremity injuries has decreased, the frequency of severe knee injuries continues to rise (52, 60). The ski equipment presently available is incapable of providing the same protection to the knee that it does for the rest of the lower extremity (52). Bindings are designed to protect the tibia from injury, but not the knee joint. Upward release at the toe and boots that allow plantar flexion at the ankle may represent equipment changes that can deter ACL injuries in skiers, but it appears that even these options will not significantly reduce the risk of severe knee sprains. Ettlinger and Johnson (61) have suggested a fall-training program as another solution to the problem of knee injuries and ACL tears in particular. However, no specific recommendations can yet be made for an effective injury-prevention program for knee and ACL injuries.

To prevent head injuries, helmets are mandatory in all downhill events except the slalom and occasionally the giant slalom. Many of the most severe injuries sustained during Alpine skiing involve closed head trauma (14, 55), which may be prevented by a protective helmet. The most common injury (18%) in the 15- to 19-year-old age group in Norwegian recreational skiers involved the head (62, 63). Because helmets are seldom used in this age group, the Norwegian Alpine Skiing Safety Council has launched a campaign to increase their use among teenagers. In Sweden, wearing of helmets, has been widely encouraged. In a nationwide registration of ski injuries in Sweden, it was found that during the 1985 to 1986 season, there was a statistically significant lower rate of head injuries among those skiers wearing a helmet as compared to a group which wore no helmets (64). Tree collisions were the second most common type of injury in the collision investigation by Jenkins et al. (57). The removal of all trees is impossible, but widening the slopes enough for safe skiing may be an important measure. Manmade objects should either be placed well off the ski trails or be made more visible and padded to minimize the risk of injury. Skiing at high speed contributes to the magnitude of ski injuries and efforts to lower a slope's danger potential should be considered. Shealy (14) suggested leaving some moguls or gentle undulations which serve as speed control devices.

Ekeland et al. (62) found that beginners had an injury ratio 4 times greater than the intermediate skier. They also had a higher frequency of LEER injuries than expert skiers, who suffered more shoulder injuries. Those attending ski school had fewer and less severe injuries. Jenkins et al. (57) found that skiers involved in collisions had greater skills than those injured in noncollisions. It seems that skill alone is not enough to protect the skier and that the talented athlete is not necessarily immune to injury. The majority of severe or fatal ski injuries result from high speed accidents of predominantly experienced male skiers who lose control (14, 55, 54). Shealy (14) noted that males are typically more inclined to risk-taking than females.

Ski safety campaigns have been launched in many countries. In Sweden, the frequency of ski injuries decreased after a campaign for safer skiing was launched (22). The injury risk was reported to diminish by almost 20% as a result of the promotion of binding testing alone. Five times the amount of money that was spent on the campaign was saved by the Swedish community from the reduction in medical and social expenses (65).

In conclusion, the skier has the ultimate responsibility to educate himself or herself about ski safety measures, to avoid injuries by skiing according to his or her ability, and to adapt to the conditions present on the ski slopes while using well-maintained and reliable ski equipment. There are several important ways of preventing ski injury in downhill skiing. But, regardless of the safeguards provided on the slopes and regardless of the individual efforts made to exercise caution and good sense, downhill skiing will retain its reputation as a high-risk sport. Inherent to the thrill of speed and the challenge of trail navigation is the ever present element of danger.

SNOWBOARDING

Snowboarding is the world's fastest growing winter sport. The number of snowboards in 1991 was 290,000 according to manufacturing sources. Where it is allowed, snowboarding can now be found at every ski area where downhill skiing is practiced. The requirements for slopes and lifts are similar for both sports.

Technique and Equipment

The first primitive boards were manufactured in the 1920s. The design was improved in the 1970s by enthusiasts both on the West Coast and in New England. A snowboard is a 30 to 40 cm wide and 140 to 190 cm long ski on which the skiers stands sideways. There are now three major types of snowboard (alpine, all-around and freestyle). The boot consists of two types, either a soft shell (Sorell-type) boot with a specific binding or a hard shell boot with a corresponding binding. The soft shell system is less expensive. Most of the bindings are nonreleasable, in contrast to ordinary downhill ski bindings. The boots are fixed at different angles to the horizontal axis of the board and with different distances between the feet depending on the type of snowboard. The typical stance in snowboarding is with the left foot forward (Fig. 29.12). No ski poles are

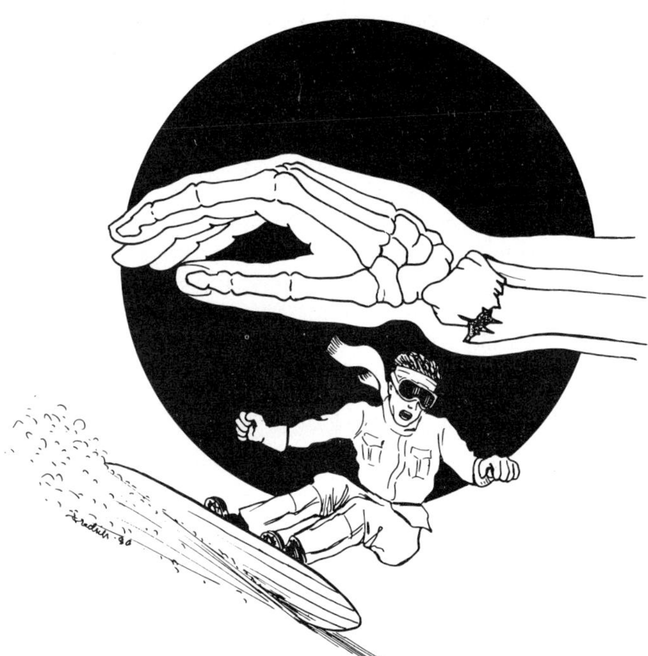

Figure 29.12. A snowboarder with the most common type of injury—fracture of the wrist. Reprinted by permission from Jorgsholm P, Bauer M, Ljung BO, et al. Downhill skiing is developing—snowboard and telemark skiing give new injury pattern. Läkartidningen 1991;88:1589–1592, and by permission of Fredrik Johansson, medical artist.

used. Turning is performed by changes in weight distribution achieved by moving the hips and knees and by foot pressure.

Different kinds of protective equipment are available to the snowboarder: helmets, wrist pads, knee pads, and layered clothing. These, however, are rarely used by snowboarders (66).

Snowboarding Injuries

Rate of Injury

Investigation of snowboarding injuries has only been undertaken during the last 5 to 6 years. Shealy and Sundman reported (67) data from the 1985 to 1986 season from three ski areas in New England and Colorado. They found 51 injuries in 12,000 snowboard days giving an injury rate of 4.2 injuries per 1000 days. The vast majority (90%) were young (average age 19.6 years) males and more than half (55.3%) considered themselves beginners.

Another investigation from the U.S. West Coast (68) showed that 90% of the 267 interviewed snowboarders were male with a mean age of 21 years. In this study, the majority considered themselves to be intermediate (49%) or expert (36%) snowboard riders. In an investigation of 460 snowboard injuries after 1986 conducted in two major ski areas, the rate of injury was estimated to be 1.7 per 1000 snowboard days (66). The authors also tried to estimate the number of injuries requiring more than minor care. Incorporating this estimate lowered the rate to 0.7 injuries per 1000 snowboard-days. In this study, 90% of the injuries occurred in young males (average age, 19 years), with minimal instruction and experience (80% having less than 2 years experience). Most of them (70%) used soft boots and only 10% used helmets and 20% used wrist or knee pads.

In one Swedish investigation (39) of skier injuries during the season of 1989 to 1990, at a fairly large ski area with approximately 500,000 tourists per season, 1311 skiers out of a total of 1439 injured skiers were injured during downhill skiing. Seventy-seven of these injuries occurred to snowboarders. Their mean age was 19 years and 82% were male. Of these 77 snowboarders, 71% were beginners compared to 24% of the downhill skiers. The conclusion that can be drawn from these figures is that the average snowboarder sustaining an injury is a 19-year-old male who has just started snowboarding.

Type and Severity of Injury

Since snowboarding is practiced with both feet attached to the board and usually with the left foot forward, the lower extremity injuries occur twice as often on the left as compared to the right (67). The injury type was directly related to the type of boot and binding. The soft boot was associated with more ankle injuries, while the hard boot put more stress on the knee joint. Because poles are not used, the snowboarder has to stick out an arm or hand to break a fall, and, thus, the injury mechanism to the upper extremity usually involves impact from a fall or collision. The same trend of an increased number of injuries in the forward leg is also true for the forward arm.

Table 29.10.
Different Injury Types in Snowboarding vs. Alpine Skiing[a]

Injury	% Snowboarding	% Alpine
Strain/sprain	64.4	48.4
Fracture	13.6	19.1
Contusion	11.9	11.9
Laceration	1.8	14.6
Dislocation	5.1	5.5
Other	3.6	0.5

[a]From Shealy JE, Sandman PD. Snowboarding injuries on alpine slopes. In: Johnson RJ, Mote CD, Binet M-H, eds. Skiing trauma and safety. Seventh International Symposium, ASTM STP 1022. Philadelphia: ASTM 1989:75–81.

The distribution of reported injury types has been quite variable from one study to another. Shealy and Sundman (67) compared snowboarding with alpine skiing and found a different distribution of injury types (Table 29.10).

They found more strain and sprain type injuries in snowboarding compared to alpine skiing. The percentage of fractures was similar, 13.6 versus 19.1. Similar numbers for snowboarders were found in McLennan and McLennan's study (66) with 19% fractures, 55% sprains, and 16% contusions. A different distribution was found in a Swedish investigation (38), which reported almost 41% fractures, 33% sprains and dislocations, and 26% contusions and lacerations.

The localization of the injuries in the study by Shealy et al. (67) was 35.6% to the upper body and 59.3% to the lower body with the ankle and foot being the most injured parts (36.9% of all injuries). Compared to alpine skiing, there was a lower percentage of injuries to the knee joint (15.8% versus 27%) Pino and Colville (68) reported similar figures with 29% ankle and 13% knee injuries. McLennan and McLennan (66) also found the ankle to be the most common site of injury, accounting for 21% of the sprains and 40% of the fractures in their report of 460 snowboard injuries.

Jørgsholm et al. (39) found quite different localization figures compared to the other studies; 37% hand and wrist injuries and 15% in the ankle and knee joints, respectively. A total of 70% of the hand injuries were distal radius fractures. One explanation for the high number of wrist fractures that the authors present was that the majority of the injuries occurred in beginners (71%). Kannus and Johnson (69) and McLennan and McLennan (66) have reported that 80% of the injured skiers were beginners. Further explanations are that 87% of the injured snowboarders used soft boots and that most of the injuries occurred on hard and well-prepared slopes. Johnson et al. (70), in a case-controlled study from a New England ski area, also found that arm and hand injuries dominated, comprising 52% of all snowboarding injuries; 58% of the arm and hand injuries were distal radius fractures. One observation common to most of the studies has been the very low frequency of reported thumb injuries compared to that for alpine skiing.

Johnson et al. (70) reported that more than 50% of the snowboarding injuries were classified as severe, while in alpine skiing only 22% were severe. However, 81% of the injured riders in McLennan and McLennan's study returned to snowboarding within 4 weeks (66).

Prevention of Injuries

The development of snowboarding has also resulted in specific safety equipment, but, for various reasons, not many of the snowboard skiers care to use it. McLennan and McLennan (66) found the number of riders using safety equipment to be very low. Only 10% used helmets, and 20% used wrist and knee pads. The increase in the use of hard boots seems to decrease the number of ankle injuries but gives a relative increase in knee injuries (67, 68). Shealy and Sundman also suggested that a binding release of both feet at the same time might decrease the number of lower extremity injuries.

Since many of the upper extremity injuries result from the skier's loss of balance and effort to catch himself or herself before falling, the use of poles has been suggested at least in the beginning of the learning process (67). Instruction in the technique of falling might also prevent some of the injuries.

Treatment of Ski Injuries

The treatment of ski injuries is predicated on an accurate diagnosis using the traditional techniques of clinical acumen. The gamut of extremity and trunk pathology resulting from impact, torsion, and shear moments cannot be reasonably covered in this chapter. So, too, it is inappropriate to give specific treatment recommendations for those injuries typically associated with skiing accidents. Suffice it to say, that the fundamentals and principles of sound orthopedic practice pertain to skiing injuries with the goals being return of function, alleviation of pain, and restoration of anatomy to mirror the original biomechanical architecture and physiologic morphology.

REFERENCES

1. Åström K, Norberg O. Förhistoriska och medeltida skidor Västerbotten (Västerbottens läns hembygdsförening) 1984:82–88.
2. Martinell V. Längdlöpning Västerbotten (Västerbottens läns hembygdsförening) 1984;117–136.
3. Forsberg L: Utförsåkning Västerbotten (Västerbottens läns hembygdsförening) 1984:144–157.
4. Petersson SP. Backhoppning Västerbotten (Västerbottens läns hembygdsförening) 1984;137–144.
5. USA Weekend. January 31–February 1992, p. 20.
6. Bland PT. Ski jumping injuries. Phys Sportsmed 1975;3(1):63–66.
7. Wright JR, McIntyre L, Rand JJ, et al. Nordic ski jumping injuries. A survey of active American jumpers. Am J Sports Med 1991;19:615–619.
8. Eriksson E: Ski injuries in Sweden: A one year survey. Orthop Clin North Am 1976;7:3–9.
9. Sandelin J, Kiviluoto O, Santavirta S. Injuries of competitive skiers in Finland: A three-year survey. Ann Chir Gynecol 1980;69:97–101.
10. Wright JR, Hixson EG, Rand JJ. Injury patterns in nordic ski jumpers. A retrospective analysis of injuries occurring at the Intervale ski jump complex from 1980 to 1985. Am J Sports Med 1986;14:393–397.
11. Wester K. Serious ski jumping injuries in Norway. Am J Sports Med 1985;13:124–127.
12. Wester K. Improved safety in ski jumping. Am J Sports Med 1988;16:499–500.
13. Wright JR. Nordic ski jumping fatalities in the United States: A 50-year summary. J Trauma 1988;28:848–851.
14. Shealy JE: Death in downhill skiing. In: Johnson RJ, Mote CD, eds. Skiing Trauma and Safety: Fifth International Symposium, ASTM STP 860. Philadelphia, ASTM 1985:349–357.
15. Hållmarker U, Aronsson D. Exhaustion and muscle pain: The most common causes to discontinue the Vasa Ski Race. Läkartidningen 1985;82:582–583.
16. Street GM. Biomechanics of cross-country skiing. In: Casey MJ, Foster C, Hixon EG, eds. Winter sports medicine. Philadelphia: Davis Company, 1990:284–301.
17. Oja P, Vuori I. Luistelu hiihdossa—hiihtäjien kokemuksia talvelta 1985. (Skating style in cross-country skiing—skiers' experience in winter 1985). Sport and Science 1985;5:226–231.
18. Ekström H. Future developments in cross-country skiing equipment. In: Johnson RJ, Mote CD, eds. Skiing Trauma and Safety: Sixth International Symposium, ASTM STP 860. Philadelphia: ASTM 1985:433–441.
19. Eckström H. The force interplay between the foot, binding and ski in cross-country skiing. In: Johnson RJ, Mote CD, eds. Skiing Trauma and Safety: Sixth International Symposium, ASTM STP 938. Philadelphia: ASTM 1987:109.
20. Renström P, Johnson RJ. Cross-country skiing injuries and biomechanics. Sports Med 1989;8:346–370.
21. Westlin NE. Injuries in long distance, cross-country, and downhill skiing. Orthop Clin No Am 1976;7:55–58.
22. Eriksson E, Danielsson K. A national ski injury survey in Skiing Safety II. In: Figueras JM, ed. International series on sport sciences, Vol 5, Baltimore: University Park Press, 1978:47–55.
23. Garrick JG, Requa R. The role of instruction in preventing ski injuries. Phys and Sports Med 1977;5:57.
24. Hemborg A, Edlund G; Gedda S. Skiing injuries in Jämtland 1977—an overview. Läkartidningen 1982;79:116–118.
25. Boyle JJ, Johnson RJ, Pope MH, et al. Cross-country skiing injuries. In: Johnson RJ, Mote CD, eds. Skiing Trauma and Safety. Fifth International Symposium, ASTM STP 860. Philadelphia: ASTM 1985:411–422.
26. Sherry E, Asquith J. Nordic cross-country skiing injuries in Australia. Med J Aust 1987;146:245–246.
27. Hemmingsson P, Ohlsén P. Injuries and diseases in elite cross-country skiers. Idrottsmedicin (Journal of Swedish Society of Sports Medicine) 1987;2:14–15.
28. Hemmingsson P. Injuries in cross-country skiing using the skating technique. Idrottsmedicin (Journal of Swedish Society of Sports Medicine) 1984;4:21–22.
29. Shealy JE, Miller DA. A relative analysis of downhill and cross-country ski injuries. In: Mote CD, Johnson RJ, eds. Skiing Trauma and Safety. Eighth International Symposium, ASTM STP 1104. Philadelphia: ASTM 1991:133–143.
30. Steinbrück K. Frequency and aetiology of injury in cross-country skiing. J Sports Sci 1987;5:187–196.
31. Heuman R, Sten J, Tidermark J. Ski injuries in Northern Dalecarlia during the seasons 1979 and 1983. Läkartidningen 1985;82:584–586.
32. Frost A, Bauer M. Skier's hip—a new clinical entity? Proximal femur fractures sustained in cross-country skiing. J Orthop Trauma 1991;5:47–50.
33. Kannus P, Niittymäki S, Järvinen M. Cross-country skiing injuries: Has the change of skiing style affected the frequency and types of skiing injuries treated at an outpatient sports clinic? Scan J Sports Sci 1988;10:17–21.
34. Gertsch P, Borgeat A, Wälli T. New cross-country skiing tech-

nique and compartment syndrome. Am J Sports Med 1987;15:612–613.
35. Frymoyer JW, Pope MH, Kristiansen T. Skiing and spinal trauma. Clin Sports Med 1982;1:309–318.
36. Mahlamäki S, Soimakallio S, Michelsson J-E. Radiological findings in the lumbar spine of 39 young cross-country skiers with low back pain. Int J Sports Med 1988;9:196–197.
37. Shealy JE, Geyer LH, Haden R. Epidemiology of ski injuries: An investigation of the effect of method of skill acquisition and release binding used on accident rates. Industrial engineering research report, State University of New York at Buffalo, 1973.
38. Johnson RJ, Pope MH, Ettlinger C. Ski injuries and equipment Function. J Sports Med 1974;2:299.
39. Jorgsholm P, Bauer M, Ljung BO, et al. Downhill skiing is developing—snowboard and telemark skiing give new injury pattern. Läkartidningen 1991;88:1589–1592.
40. McMurtry JG. Biomechanics of alpine skiing. In: Casey MJ, ed. Winter sports medicine. Philadelphia: Davis Company, 1990:344–350.
41. Johnson RJ, Pope MH, Weisman G. Knee injury in skiing. Am J Sports Med 1979;7:321–327.
42. Eriksson E, Johnson RJ. The etiology of downhill ski injuries. In: Hutton RS, Miller DI, eds. Exercise and Sports Sciences Reviews. Philadelphia: Franklin Press, 1981;8:1–17.
43. Ekeland A, Lund Ø: On-slope evaluation of alpine release bindings. In: Mote CD, Johnson RJ, eds. Skiing Trauma and Safety: Sixth International Symposium, ASTM STP 938. Philadelphia: ASTM 1987:169–179.
44. Young L. Elevated racer binding settings and inadvertent release. In: Johnson RJ, Mote CD, Binet M-H, eds. Skiing Trauma and Safety: Seventh International Symposium, ASTM STP 1022. Philadelphia: ASTM 1989:222–227.
45. Hauser W. Experimental prospective skiing injury study. In: Johnson RJ, Mote CD, Binet M-H, eds. Skiing Trauma and Safety: Seventh International Symposium, ASTM STP 1022. Philadelphia: ASTM 1989:18–24.
46. Johnson RJ, Pope MH, Ettlinger C. The interrelationship between ski accidents, the resultant injury, the skier's characteristics and the ski-binding-boot system. J Sports Med 1974;6:299–307.
47. Young LR, Oman CM, Crane H, et al. The etiology of ski injuries: An eight year study of the skier and his equipment. Orth Clin North Am 1976;7:13–29.
48. Johnson RJ, Ettlinger CF, Shealy JE. Skier injury trends. In: Johnson RJ, Mote CD, Binet M-H, eds. Skiing and Trauma Safety: Seventh International Symposium, ASTM STP 1022. Philadelphia: ASTM 1989:25–31.
49. Young LR, Lee SM. Alpine injury pattern at Waterville Valley—1989 update. In: Mote CD, Johnson RJ, eds. Skiing Trauma and Safety: Eighth International Symposium, ASTM STP 1104. Philadelphia: ASTM 1991:125–132.
50. Sherry E, Fenelon L. Trends in skiing injury type and rates in Australia. A review of 22,261 injuries over 27 years in the Snowy Mountains. Med J Aust 1991;155:513–515.
51. Linden B, Berg R, Balkfors B, Engkvist O. Decreasing number of skiing accidents in the Swedish mountains. Läkartidningen 1991;88:308–309.
52. Johnson RJ, Ettlinger CF, Shealy J. Skier injury trends—1976–1990. In: Mote CD, Johnson RJ, eds. Skiing Trauma and Safety: Ninth International Symposium, ASTM STP 1182. Philadelphia: ASTM 1993;11–22.
53. Steedman DJ: Artificial ski slope: a 1-year prospective study. Injury 1986;17:208–212.
54. Ljung BO, Bauer M, Edlund G. Severe ski accidents—the skier's own responsibility is crucial. Läkartidningen 1991;88:1583–1586.
55. Stanley RL, Meeuwisse WH. Life and limb threatening injuries in Alpine skiing. Clin J Sport Med 1991;1:162–165.
56. Morrow PL, McQuillen EN, Eaton LA, et al. Downhill ski fatalities: The Vermont experience. J Trauma 1988;28:95–100.
57. Jenkins R, Johnson RJ, Pope MH. Collision injuries in downhill skiing. In: Johnson RJ, Mote CD, eds. Skiing Trauma and Safety: Fifth International Symposium, ASTM STP 860. Philadelphia: ASTM 1985:358–366.
58. Sherry E, Clout L. Deaths associated with skiing in Australia: A 32-year study of cases from Snowy Mountains. Med J Aust 1988;149:615–618.
59. Bouter LM, Knipschild PG, Volovics A. Binding function in relation to injury risk in downhill skiing. Am J Sports Med 1989;17:226–233.
60. Howe J, Johnson RJ. Knee injuries in skiing. Clin in Sport Med 1982;1:277–288.
61. Ettlinger CF, Johnson RJ. Can knee injuries be prevented? Skiing March 1991:120–123.
62. Ekeland A, Holtmoen Å, Lystad H. Skiing injuries in Alpine recreational skiers. In: Johnson RJ, Mote CD, Binet M-H, eds. Skiing Trauma and Safety: Seventh International Symposium, ASTM STP 1022. Philadelphia: ASTM 1989:41–50.
63. Ekeland A, Holtmoen Å, Lystad H. Alpine skiing injuries in Scandinavian skiers. In: Mote CD, Johnson RJ, eds. Skiing Trauma and Safety: Eighth International Symposium, ASTM STP 1104. Philadelphia: ASTM 1991:144–151.
64. Sandegård J, Eriksson B, Lundkvist S. Nationwide registration of ski injuries in Sweden. In: Mote CD, Johnson RJ, eds. Skiing Trauma and Safety: Eighth International Symposium, ASTM STP 1104. Philadelphia: ASTM 1991:170–176.
65. Danielsson K, Eriksson E, Jonsson E, et al. Attempts to reduce the incidence of skiing injuries in Sweden. In: Johnson RJ, Mote CD, eds. Skiing Trauma and Safety: Fifth International Symposium, ASTM STP 860. Philadelphia: ASTM 1985:326–337.
66. McLennan JC, McLennan JG: Snowboarding. What injuries to expect in this rapidly growing sport. J Musculoskeletal Med 1991;8(11):75–89.
67. Shealy JE, Sundman PD. Snowboarding injuries on alpine slopes. In: Johnson RJ, Mote CD, Binet M-H, eds. Skiing trauma and safety. Seventh International Symposium, ASTM STP 1022. Philadelphia: ASTM 1989:75–81.
68. Pino EC, Colville MR. Snowboard injuries. Am J Sports Med 1989;17:778–781.
69. Kannus P, Johnson RJ. Downhill skiing injuries: Trends to watch for this season. J Musculoskeletal Med 1991;8(1):13–31.
70. Beskind D, Johnson RJ, Ettlinger CF. Snowboard Injuries. presented at Skiing Trauma and Safety: Ninth International Symposium, Thredbo, Australia, June 1991.

30 / PARAGLIDING AND HANG GLIDING

Douglas H. Hildreth, Linda L. Hildreth, Mark W. Shipman, and Robert P. Wills

PART 1
Paragliding

Mark W. Shipman and Robert P. Wills

Introduction

It is difficult to imagine a more exhilarating experience than that of flying off a mountain that one has climbed, soaring around for 1 or 2 hours, and landing in the valley below (Fig. 30.1).

Paragliding or parapenting (the French and the Spanish word) is the most recent form of gliding sport to hit the American scene. If the European experience is any indication, there should be well over 100,000 active participants in the sport in the United States by the mid-1990s. Many ski areas in Europe now remain open year round to accommodate paragliding enthusiasts.

Modern paragliding owes its existence to a long history of dreamers, scientists, and engineers and encompasses many different countries. Leonardo da Vinci's work, data from military experiments conducted during both World Wars, Lillianthal's work in the 1800s, and the Wright brothers' work at the turn of the century form the basis on which Harbot, Crowley, Neumark, and the British Association of Parascending Clubs worked in the 1950s. Neumark is credited with the first ground-launched flight of a nonrigid canopy in 1962. In the 1980s, the French, particularly Jean-Claude Betemps, Andre Bohn, and Gerard Bosson, began modifying parachutes so one could run down a steep slope near a mountaintop and glide gently down to the valley below. Early participants in paragliding were often moutaineers who simply added a new dimension to their sport. *Enchainment* became a buzzword among world-class climbers in the late 1980s, as it became possible to carry a lightweight canopy up a difficult route, fly from the summit to the base of another route, and in this way climb multiple difficult north face routes in the Alps in a single day. Within a few years, there were more than 30 manufacturers of paragliders worldwide, and canopies with glide ratios of greater than 6:1 and sink rates of as low as 1.1 m/sec became available. With the development of these more advanced gliders, soaring became possible and paragliding took off as a sport in its own right.

The sport continues to develop rapidly, yet in many ways it is still in its infancy. Leaders in the sport are trying desperately to avoid some of the problems experienced in the early development of hang gliding.

Paragliding is a self-regulated sport. It comes under the jurisdiction of the Federal Aviation Administration only so far as FAR 103 relates: No flight is allowed at night or into restricted air space; right-of-way rules give hang gliders and paragliders the lowest priority, generally. The U.S. Forest Service's current policy prevents paragliding in designated wilderness areas, although it is hoped that this may change in the future. The American Paragliding Association (APA) does accident investigation, disseminates information about the sport (including safety information), and is the clearinghouse for certification of instructors and pilot rating in the United States.

Equipment

The canopy itself has both an upper and lower surface connected by ribs of nylon cloth. With few exceptions, paragliders have no rigid parts. Ports at the lead-

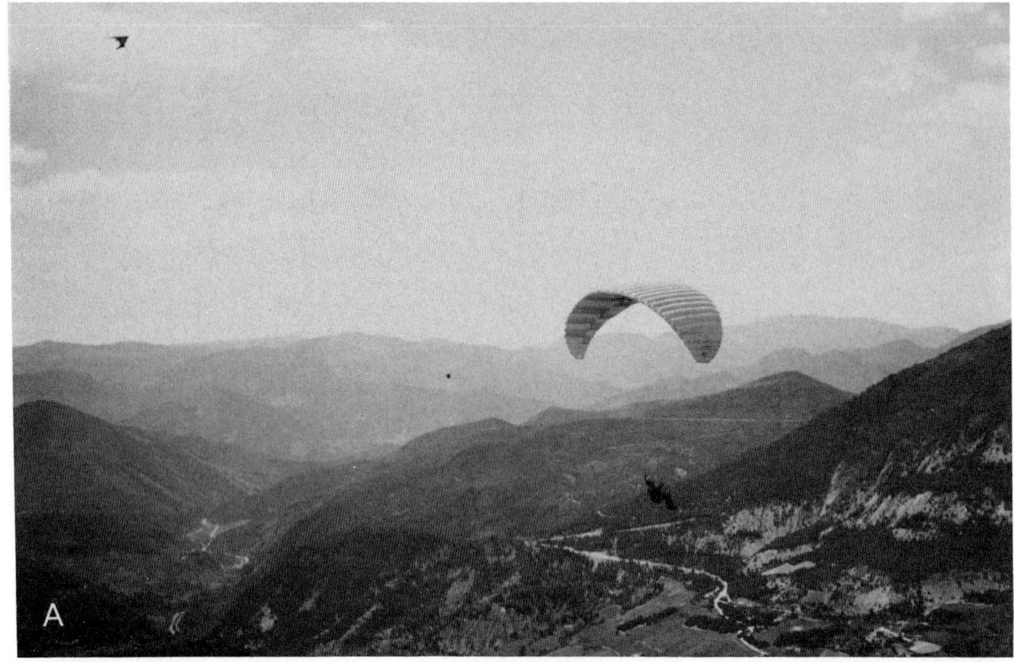
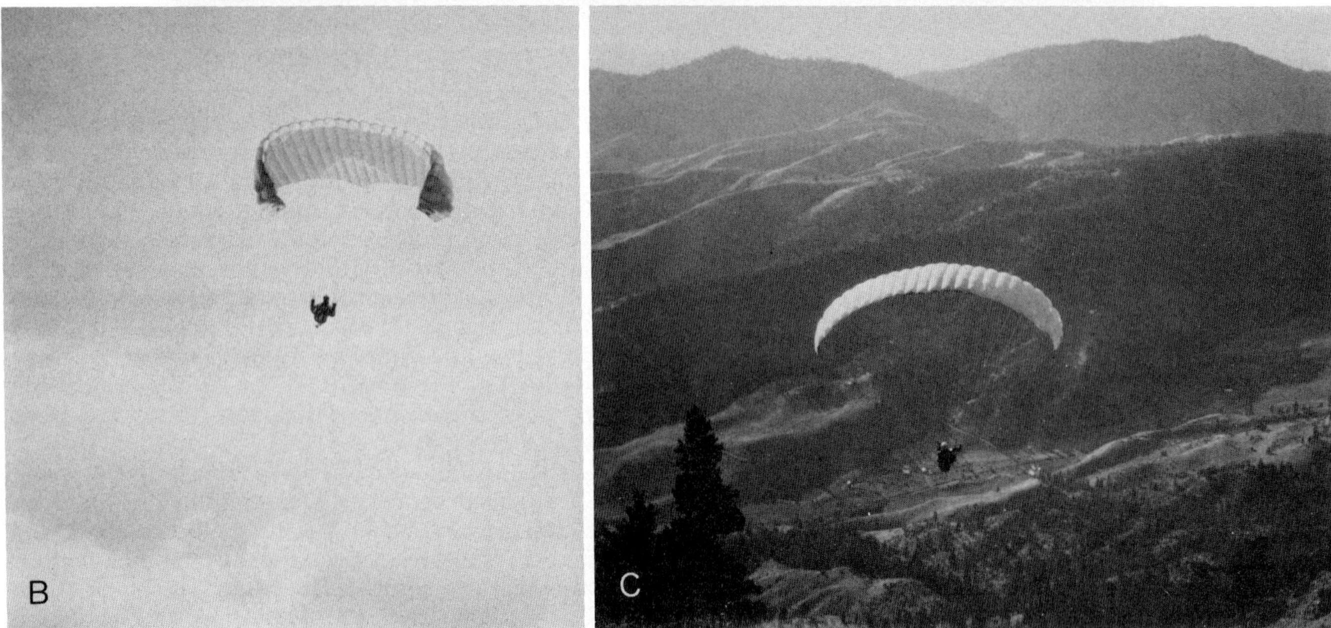

Figure 30.1. A, Sharing the air with the birds in southern France. **B,** "Dog earing" a canopy for a more rigid descent. **C,** Paragliding in the central Cascades of Washington.

ing edge allow air to enter for inflation and serve to keep the canopy full. Cross-ports in the ribs allow side-to-side flow of air to keep all parts of the canopy pressurized equally. Paraglider canopies are made of rip-stop polyester or nylon with various coatings, depending on the manufacturer. They are, therefore, less porous than parachutes. Attachment lines are made either of sheathed Kevlar, sheathed Spectra, or nylon. They are not made to withstand the forces to which parachutes are subjected.

A sagittal section of the canopy creates a shape of a wing, and the aspect ratio (relationship between the wing span and its cord, or measurement front to rear) is higher than that of a parachute. Therefore, a paraglider behaves more like a wing than a parachute. From this comes its increased efficiency and also its increased danger. Of course, because there are no rigid parts paragliders will collapse in turbulence. They will also stall and can spin. They can enter deep stall or parachutage, a condition in which the canopy is open but traveling straight down at a rate of 15 feet/sec or more, because there is no air passing over and under the wing to produce lift. Paragliders also have a much narrower speed envelope than hang gliders, with takeoff and stall air speeds of 11 to 12 statute mph and top speeds ranging from 19 to about 28 mph.

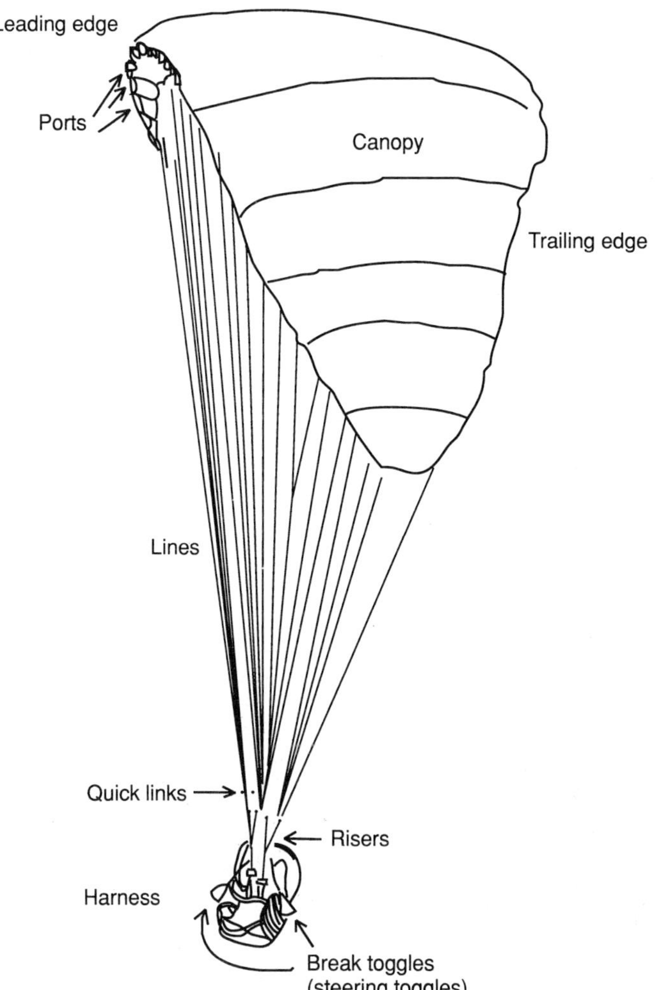

Figure 30.2. Components of a paraglider.

The pilot wears a harness that is attached to risers that are in turn attached to the lines from the canopy via quick links, which are small locking carabiners (Fig. 30.2). There are, of course, many types of harnesses. One French manufacturer has patented a popular harness system in which the risers are attached to the seat so that the pilot can control both pitch and roll by his or her position on the seat (see Fig. 30.2).

All paragliders have directional control via lines attached to the trailing edge of each side of the canopy just like that of a square parachute. These allow the glider to be flown faster or slower, to turn, and to flare on landing.

A paraglider can be folded into a pack, hiked to a takeoff zone, and readied in minutes to carry the pilot aloft. The basics of flying a paraglider can be taught in a couple of days. The simplicity of the sport is appealing to instructors and students alike.

However, paragliding is truly a high-risk sport and as in all aviation endeavors, nature is horribly unforgiving of any mistake. In fact, it would appear from Swiss, French, and American paragliding accident statistics that participation in paragliding has about the same risks of morbidity and mortality as that of hang gliding.

Accidents

Most of the trends from U.S. and European data are consistent:

1. Low-time pilots (less than 40 flights) are at greatest risk for both major and minor injury.
2. As experience is gained by the pilot, the incidence of accidents drops off but rises again after 100 to 150 flights, probably because of willingness to fly more advanced paragliders in more difficult conditions.
3. Ankle injuries, wrist injuries, and spinal column compression fractures are the most common injuries reported.
4. The incidence of head injuries in paragliding has significantly decreased probably as a result of the increased use of helmets.

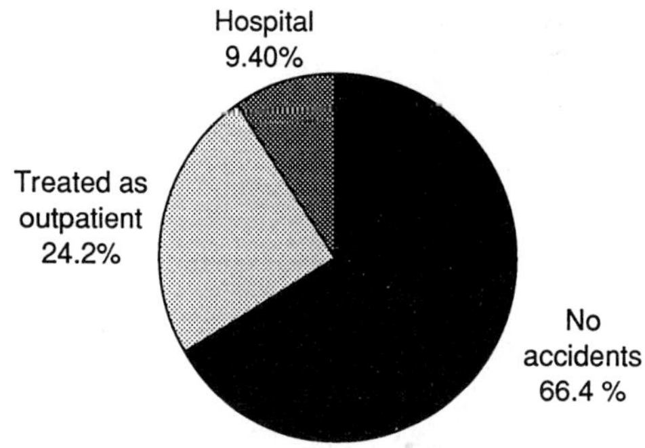

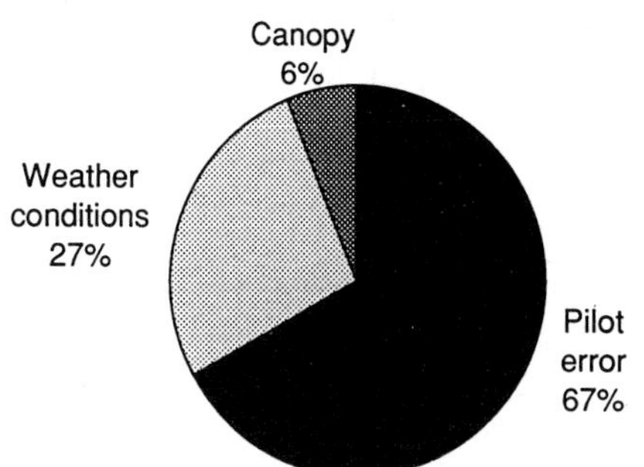

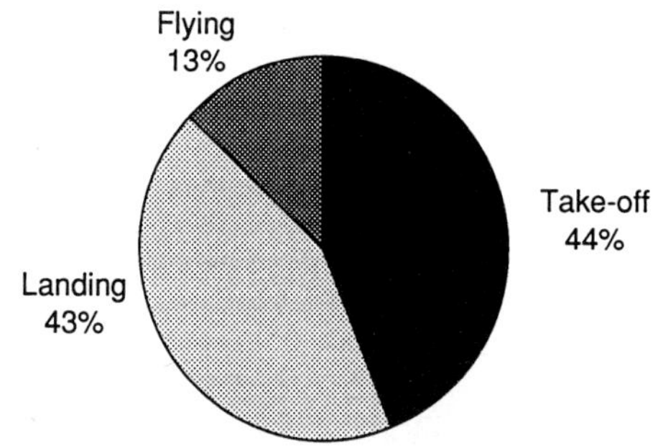

Figure 30.3. Swiss statistics for paraglider accidents.

In a reader survey conducted by the Swiss paragliding magazine *Gleitschirm*, 519 (33.6%) of 1546 respondents had had at least one accident and 145 (9.4%) had been hospitalized as a result (Fig. 30.3).

Statistics from the Commission Securite Parapente in France for 1989 demonstrate major accident trends for the sport in France, which are probably transferable to the rest of the world (Table 30.1). Types of injuries reported are shown in Figure 30.4.

The preponderance of lower extremity injuries and lumbar compression fractures probably simply reflect the fact that most injuries result from falls. Paraglider harness systems allow the pilot to land on his or her feet. Upper extremity injuries, especially wrist injuries, are usually the result of a fall onto an outstretched hand, particularly on landing.

Injuries

Overuse injuries are, of course, uncommon among paraglider pilots. Medial epicondylitis (flexor origin syndrome of the elbow) is occasionally seen among competition pilots because of continuous and repetitive use of the brake toggles over long periods of time.

Table 30.1.
French Statistics for Paraglider Accidents[a]

Estimated participants in the sport	25,000 to 30,000
Total accidents reported	465
Women	95
Men	370
Fatalities	8

[a]Approximately 66% of accident victims have less than 40 flights. Minor accidents are often unreported.

Lower Extremity Injuries

Abduction mechanism of injury to the forefoot can occur if wearing soft or loose-fitting shoes. Lis-Franc fractures, talar neck fractures, and lateral subtalar dislocations were occasionally seen early in the development of the sport. Later on more rigid footwear was developed, which protected the foot and transferred energy into the ankle and leg.

Ankle Injuries

Ligamentous sprains of the medial and lateral ankle ligaments occur commonly as a result of rotational mechanisms of injury. A fall onto a hillside will put a rotational load onto the medial or lateral ankle stabilizing ligaments. Tears of the anterior talofibular ligament, calcaneofibular ligament, and deltoid ligament complex are common. Tibiofibular syndesmosis injuries caused by a pure external rotation mechanism also will occasionally occur.

Ankle fractures are the most common surgical injury suffered by paragliding enthusiasts. External rotation of the ankle up on the lower leg is the most common mechanism of injury. The falling pilot usually has a forward velocity of 20 to 50 km/hr and a vertical velocity of between 1 and 3 m/sec. The lower extremities are dangling from the pelvic harness with hip and knee at approximately 45° of flexion, and the ankle in 20° to 30° of plantar flexion and variable external rotation. Impact with the ground forcibly externally rotates and abducts the ankle and foot on the leg, producing medial bony or ligamentous injury, tibiofibular syndesmosis disruption, and fibular fracture above the level of the ankle joint. Pure axial compression injuries such as pilon fractures of the ankle are much less common than ro-

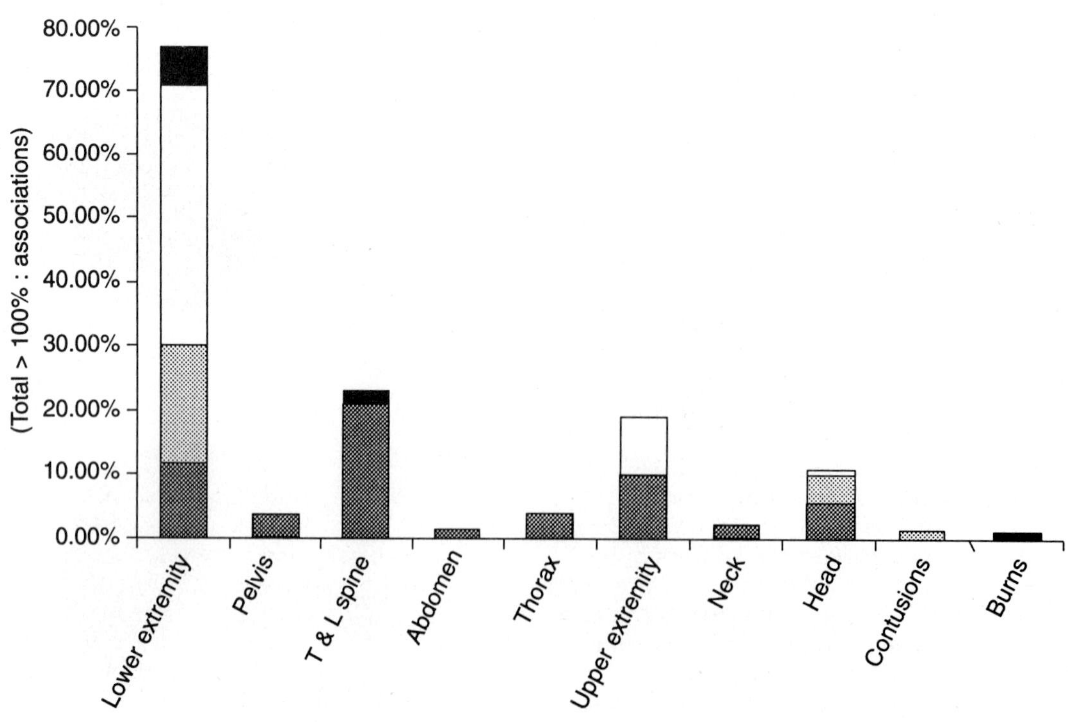

Figure 30.4. Paraglider accidents by category.

tational injuries, because the pilot is usually falling forward as well as downward.

Knee Injuries

Knee injuries are fairly uncommon in paragliding. Occasionally, mild medial collateral ligaments sprains are seen.

Spinal Column

Thoracolumbar spine fractures are the second most common type of injury among paraglider pilots. The relaxed, flexed lower extremities usually absorb little of the impact load during the fall. Pelvis and buttocks usually impact the ground with significant force, producing axial compression fractures of the thoracolumbar spine, such as anterior vertebral body wedging and thoracolumbar burst fractures. Cervical flexion or extension injuries also are occasionally seen. Elite paraglider pilots often loose 2 to 5 cm of height because of multiple thoracolumbar spinal compression fractures.

Wrist

A fall on the outstretched hand commonly produces carpal ligament fractures, dislocations or fracture-dislocations. Transscaphoid and transstyloid perilunate dislocations are common injury patterns. Medial epicondylitis caused by overuse of the flexor origin is occasionally seen among elite pilots.

Prevention

Proper Training

Sound judgment is, of course, the most important component of the injury prevention formula for paragliding. It also is the most difficult to test for and to acquire. Proper training and adequate experience are extremely important. Training should only be taken under the tutelage of an APA-certified instructor. Teaching should include thorough training in parachute landing fall (PLF), which has been used and refined over many years by parachutists.

Certification of Equipment

Most paragliders now for sale in the United States are certified by one or the other European certifying agency. It is important for the pilot buying a new glider not only to know the glider has been certified but also to understand how the certification level was obtained and exactly what it means.

Reserve Parachutes

Use of reserve parachutes among paraglider pilots is becoming more common both in the United States and abroad. In Germany, as of January 1991, reserve parachutes are required. There are now enough reports of main canopy irreversible malfunctions that carrying a reserve clearly should be recommended.

However, it also has been shown that if a reserve parachute is deployed and the main canopy resumes flight, disaster can result from a phenomenon called downplaning. Simply carrying one is not enough. The proper knowledge of how and when to use a reserve parachute is perhaps more important in paragliding than in other aviation sports.

Helmets

Head injury was a common cause of morbidity and mortality from paraglider accidents a few years ago in Europe. This has been changed substantially by nearly universal use of helmets in the sport.

For obvious reasons most pilots prefer a lightweight helmet, and newer materials such as carbon fiber and Kevlar are being used more commonly in their manufacture. The French are now encouraging the use of helmets with facial protection in an attempt to decrease the incidence of facial injury.

The religious use of helmets, preferably with facial protection, is to be encouraged among paraglider pilots.

Clothing

Minor abrasions and contusions can often be avoided by simply wearing long-sleeved shirts, long pants, gloves, etc. A lightweight wind suit (without loops or buckles that can catch on lines) is recommended. If the participant is likely to ascend to a significant altitude or is ridge soaring in cold conditions, plenty of layered insulation and wind protection are important. The actual flying of the paraglider takes little energy, so heat is not produced.

Boots

The degree of cushioning in the heel and sole as well as ankle protection are probably important factors when shopping for paragliding footwear. Boots made specifically for paragliding are available from several different European manufacturers. Medial and lateral polyethylene or metal ankle stays may be useful in protecting the ankles from low-energy injuries. The use of this type of footwear is encouraged, although the authors are unaware of any studies that show their value in injury prevention.

Communication

Good quality two-way radios are now available and affordable. Their use by all paraglider pilots should be strongly encouraged.

Treatment

Emergency and Trauma Care

The most important piece of emergency equipment on the scene of a paragliding accident is a good two-way radio or cellular telephone. In the case of severe or multiple trauma, appropriate advanced life support (ALS) transport must be arranged expeditiously. The physician on the scene in such a situation can stabilize the victim as much as possible, arrange appropriate transport, and discuss the case with emergency department and other personnel at the nearest trauma center.

Emergency physicians, family physicians, general surgeons, orthopedic surgeons, and others appropriately trained in trauma care are all qualified to act as covering physician at a paragliding competition. He or she should be advanced trauma life support (ATLS) certified or have equivalent training and experience.

Emergency transport arrangements should be thought out well in advance of any large paragliding event. Pilots are often unable to evacuate themselves from their back-country crash sites. Vehicular evacuation also is frequently not possible. If helicopter evacuation is likely to be used, a mechanism for warning all pilots must be available so that the approaching aircraft does not endanger other competitors.

Because neck and back injuries are particularly common among these pilots, special attention must be paid to stabilizing the spinal column at the scene, once the airway has been attended to. The emergency department physician on duty at the receiving hospital must also be aware of the likelihood of spinal column injury in these patients, which may be easily overlooked in the presence of other more obvious orthopedic injuries.

Discussion of ATLS protocol is beyond the scope of this chapter. Please refer to the ATLS manual published by the American College of Surgeons.

Lower Extremities

Feet and Ankles

Foot fractures and fracture-dislocations, when isolated, usually require non–weight-bearing ambulation and splinting for evacuation. Long-distance non–weight-bearing back-country travel over hilly terrain is impractical. Two-way radio communication is recommended to plan evacuation. Ankle sprain patients can be evacuated with partial weight bearing if the injury is isolated. The usual treatment with rest, ice, elevation, and compression is helpful. Because of the preponderance of high-energy external rotation injury patterns, an x-ray and musculoskeletal consultation is usually recommended if the injury is severe. The syndesmosis is more frequently disrupted in paragliding ankle injuries. This injury pattern usually requires operative fixation of the bony injuries and screw fixation of the tibiofibular syndesmosis. Tibiotalar alignment must be within 1 mm of normal to produce a reliably good outcome.

Knees

Mild MCL sprains usually respond well to partial weight-bearing ambulation and/or splinting, wrapping, and ice.

Spinal Column

Spinal compression fractures, thoracolumbar compression fractures, and cervical fractures are a common sequel to landing injuries. These often require helicopter evacuation if the injured pilot is not ambulatory. Immobilization of the spine should be performed in a routine fashion and x-ray and possibly a computerized tomography (CT) evaluation of the spine should be performed. Particular attention should be paid to the interpedicular distance on the A-P radiograph of the thoracolumbar spine. Unstable thoracolumbar burst fractures will commonly increase the interpedicular distance by 2 to 3 mm compared with adjacent levels. This will alert the physician to the need for CT scanning at the appropriate levels. Posterior instrumentation and fusion is usually needed following unstable thoracolumbar burst fractures.

Cervical hyperextension injuries and hyperflexion injuries occasionally occur but rarely produce a neurological deficit. Nonoperative treatment in a cervicothoracic orthosis or HALO brace is usually sufficient.

Upper Extremities

Hyperextension injuries of the wrist with a fall on the outstretched hand, produce carpal disruption, including scapholunate dissociation, transscaphoid perilunate dislocation and transstyloid perilunate dislocation. These complex injuries often require treatment of both the bony and the ligamentous injury with pinning or internal fixation.

Medial Epicondylitis

The medial epicondylitis (flexor origin syndrome) occasionally seen in professional or competition pilots responds to the usual measures. Tennis elbow straps should be avoided during flight, because the pilot's hands are elevated most of the time and circulatory compromise might occur. Adjusting the length of the brake lines also may help.

General Information

Little is available yet in the medical literature about this exhilarating sport and its associated injuries. As paragliding grows in popularity in North America, so will knowledge in dealing with its injuries and, more important, the ability to help in their prevention.

The American Paragliding Association is located at 25 Goller Place, Staten Island, NY 10314. Since November 1992, the U.S. Hang Gliding Association has assumed all official communications and operations of what had been the APA.

PART 2
Hang Gliding

Douglas H. Hildreth and Linda L. Hildreth

Introduction

In ancient Crete, a man named Daedalus had a dream of being able to fly with the soaring birds. His aspirations have been shared throughout history, but it is only in the last 20 years that we have been truly able to achieve that legendary vision. Today's hang glider pilots can attach their harness to the glider, run down a mountain slope, be lifted gently by the rising thermals, and soar for hours in the peaceful serenity of which their ancestors could only dream.

Icarus, Daedalus's son, is like the modern hang glider

pilot in yet another way. Displaying a typical error in pilot judgment, he was overcome by his enthusiasm, ignored the manufacturer's warning, and exceeded the safe operating limits of his craft, which sustained structural failure and caused the unfortunate Icarus to fall from the sky.

Hang gliding developed in the late 1800s through the efforts of Otto Lillienthal in Germany, John Montgomery in San Diego, and Octave Chanute in Indiana. These men simultaneously conducted independent flights from 50 to 200 feet in altitude and several hundred feet in length. The Wright brothers, too, were primarily hang gliding enthusiasts, and spent several summers gliding at Kitty Hawk, North Carolina. As an afterthought, they added an engine. With their historic flight in 1903 powered aviation took off and hang gliding disappeared for half a century.

Frances Rogallo, in 1951, designed a reentry airfoil for the National Aeronautics and Space Administration (NASA). In the 1960s the Rogallo wing became the template for modern hang gliding. These early hang gliders were made from bamboo poles, plastic sheeting, tape, and string and were affectionately nicknamed "bamboo bombers." But with them, one could run down a sand dune into the strong steady sea breezes, be lifted into the air, and land gently on the beach below. In the 30 years since then, significant advances have been made in hang glider design and technology, allowing precision handling, 15,000-foot altitude gains, and 300-mile cross-country flights.

Hang gliders are now constructed of tubular aluminum frames that are held in flying position by cables. The air frame is covered with a Dacron sailcloth, which is shaped with aluminum battens. Gliders weigh 60 to 70 pounds and have a 30- to 35-foot wingspan. The pilot lies in the prone position, cradled in a harness that is attached to the glider. (Approximately 3% of pilots fly supine.) The pilot's hands rest lightly on the triangular-shaped control bar, allowing the shifting of weight to control precisely the flight path of the glider.

Students taught by the United States Hang Gliding Association (USHGA) certified instructors learn hang gliding in a slow, progressive manner. After ground school and glider assembly instruction, students begin running with the glider on level ground, then down a gradual hill without leaving the ground. Next, by running faster the students are able to "fly" for a few feet. After many repeated flights, students gradually increase their distance and altitude by working their way farther up the training hill. Turns and airspeed control are learned so that corrective weight shifts become conditioned reflexes. After many weeks, students move to an intermediate hill 50 to 500 feet high. As the students' skills advance over several months, they will fly at higher altitudes at sites that allow soaring flight in either ridge or thermal lift. These prolonged periods allow the pilots to fine-tune their flying skills.

Here is a summary of the flight sequence. The pilot stands in an erect position with the glider supported on his or her shoulders. Running down the hill, into the wind, the glider quickly flies, lifting its own weight. As the pilot runs faster, the wing reaches an air speed of 18 to 20 mph, which generates enough lift to raise the pilot off the ground, still in an upright position. The pilot then rotates into the prone position for the duration of the flight, but as the pilot approaches the landing area he or she once again rotates into the upright position to land. At 2 to 3 feet above the ground, as the glider slows to stall speed (the same 18 to 20 mph), the pilot briskly pushes out on the control bar, which raises the nose abruptly. This "flare" allows the wing to become an airbrake; the glider stops, and the pilot lands softly on his or her feet.

Statistics

The Federal Aviation Administration (FAA) has rather broad guidelines for hang gliding (FAR part 103). No license, no physical examination, and no federal aircraft certification are required. The voluntary regulation of the sport by the USHGA includes an accident reporting system that has been extremely effective. The USHGA's concern for safety and accident review has been evident since its birth in 1970. Accident and safety information have been published monthly and summaries of fatality and injury information has been published since that time annually (1–14). Few, if any, recreational sports have such a database. The data in Tables 30.2 and 30.3 are extracted from the 1981–1990 accident reports and represent the current state of the art of hang gliding. There have been well over 2500 accident reports analyzed and 113 fatalities in this decade.

The news media's presentation and the public's perception of the fatality risk of hang gliding have been grossly exaggerated. It has been given "the highest 'kill-ratio' in all of sports" (15) and called "the dying sport." (16) Most physicians in the United States continue to believe that the sport is risky and maintain a highly negative and judgmental attitude toward its participants who become patients (17). Only a few articles, dealing with subset populations, have appeared in the medical literature (15–24).

In fact, the statistical data on hang gliding fatalities are extremely favorable. As can be seen in Table 30.3, deaths have decreased to a fairly steady state of 6 to 8 per year. Careful analysis results in a denominator of at least 35,000 participants per year. This computes to a ratio of 18 to 24 fatalities per 100,000 participants per year, which is considerably better than general aviation, ballooning, rock climbing, power-boat racing, all-terrain vehicles, and the Peace Corps. Compare hang gliding to driving an automobile, which reports 24 to 29 fatalities per 100,000 participants.

Causes of Accidents

In all of aviation, the takeoff and landing are potentially dangerous because both occur near stall speed and in close proximity to the ground. When flown at stall speed, the wing will loose its ability to generate lift (fly) and will become uncontrollable; the nose will fall toward the ground in a dive (an attempt to regain flying speed). If, as frequently happens, one wing stalls first, the re-

Table 30.2.
Incidence of Hang Gliding Accidents and Injury by Cause and Type

Causes of Accidents	Percent per Year
Crash on launch	25
Crash on landing	35
Inflight stall	9
Flew into something	10
Adverse weather	8
Aerobatics	2
Midair collision	1
Improper assembly	0.5
Harness problems	1
Failure to hook-in	3
Landed in surf	0.5
Parachute saves reported	13
Injury Pattern	**Percent per Year**
Head	11
Face	11
Neck	7
Chest	7
Shoulder	9
Arm	10
Elbow	5
Forearm	9
Abdomen	2
Back	4
Pelvis	2
Thigh	5
Knee	3
Leg	7
Ankle and foot	8

Table 30.3.
Fatality Statistics for Hang Gliding

Year	Foot Launch	Tow	Tandem	Total
1970	0			0
1971	2			2
1972	4			4
1973	9			9
1974	40			40
1975	32			32
1976	38			38
1977	24			24
1978	23			23
1980	22	1		23
1981	16	5		21
1982	11	1		12
1983	11	3		14
1984	4	4		8
1985	6	1	2	9
1986	5			5
1987	17	1		18
1988	10	2	(2)[a]	12
1989	6			6
1990	5	3		8
1991	5	2	2	9
1992	7	2		9

[a]A single accident involving towing a tandem glider. Both pilot and passenger died.

sultant uncontrollable turn compounds the dive. If the glider has adequate altitude, it will recover speed and resume flying. But during takeoff and landing, the glider usually hits the ground before flying speed can be regained.

Crashes on Launch

For the glider to fly, the pilot launching must create an airspeed over the wing of at least 18 to 20 mph. In no wind conditions, the pilot must run this fast with the glider. If a wind is blowing toward the pilot as he or she launches (or lands) the speed at which the pilot must run to affect the relative airspeed over the wing is reduced (and conversely).

There are a number of possible components involved in launch accidents: the nose of the glider may be too high (angle of attack); there may be a run too weak for the wind conditions or the pilot may jump into the glider before it is going fast enough to fly; the wings may not be level; there may be no wind, a crosswind, or worse yet, a downwind or tailwind. The universal result is that the glider is not flying (i.e., is stalled) and thus falls to the ground.

Crashes on Landing

Like crashes on launch, the final event for crashes on landing is the glider and pilot hitting the ground. The causative factors usually start long before that final event. A proper setup and approach to a landing before that final event. A proper setup and approach to a landing zone require considerable forethought and attention. The glider should be 20 to 50 feet above the ground at the downwind edge of the open field and flying straight and level, well above stall speed. The final glide brings the pilot, with wings level, headed directly into the wind, 2 to 4 feet off the ground, ready for a correctly timed and vigorous flare. Errors in any part of this sequence may result in a crash to the ground or into a tree or other obstruction. This event usually occurs with significant foreword momentum, thus the pilot falls forward. Occasionally, the glider is stalled at a higher altitude (10 to 40 feet), stops flying and drops straight down to the ground, simulating a fall from a height (25).

Inflight Stall

Stalling while flying at altitude tends to be less serious than stalls near the ground, because there is adequate room (altitude) for the recovery dive. Students, particularly during their first several altitude flights, are usually closer to the hill and have immature stall recognition and recovery skills, often leading to serious injury or death. Inflight stalls are a leading cause of accidents in students.

Flying into Things

The pilot usually flies into things on landing, but this can occur anywhere at anytime. The most common targets are trees, fences, vehicles parked in the landing area, other gliders on the ground (training hill), buildings, spectators (rarely), and power lines. Only one or two midair collisions between two gliders occur each year.

Adverse Weather

To be optimally performed, hang gliding (as sailplane soaring) demands unstable weather. Stronger winds and strong thermal lift results in higher flights and longer cross-country distances. But with stronger conditions comes the risk of overpowering weather. Usually, adverse weather can be predicted and avoided, but sometimes weather changes arrive unexpectedly. Occasionally, aggressive pilots seek such conditions, flying the fine line between great conditions and too strong.

Aerobatics

A small number of pilots pursue aerobatics. They can be performed safely, but the margin for error—both for structural integrity and for judgment and execution flaws—is very narrow.

Structural Failure

Most structural failures are directly related to exceeding the design specifications by aerobatic flying or are related to weather-induced tumbles. Fewer failures still are related to old, improperly maintained gliders. All types of structural failures combined result in two or three accidents a year.

Improper Assembly and Inadequate Preflight

Murphy's Law notes that if something can be done improperly, incorrectly, or mistakenly, someone will do it. Two or three times a year, a glider is improperly assembled; something is not properly put together or is forgotten completely. Coupled with haste and an inadequate preflight check, the glider will fly abnormally or come apart completely.

Failure to Hook In

The final act a pilot must complete before launching is to attach his or her harness to the hang loop of the glider. Unfortunately, about a dozen people a year forget. Because most of the launches around the country are gradual slopes, the glider flies away and the pilot rolls down the hill. Occasionally, in a cliff launch situation, the pilot is left hanging from the control bar. Fast thinking and prior practice can still save the day, but every other year or so, someone falls and dies.

New Conditions

New conditions include a new site to fly, unique wind conditions, a new glider, and a new harness, and anytime there is a change, a new factor, or a different set of circumstances, there is a greater risk of accident. This is particularly true for pilots with little experience, for whom everything tends to be new. The more "news" at one time, the greater the danger. It is recommended that pilots add only one new thing at a time; but this advice is not always followed.

Attitude

There are three attitudes that cause danger in hang gliding. They also cause accidental injury in other sports and daily activities. The first is complacency, which is typically seen in experienced, seasoned pilots who have done it so often that they do not have to think about it—so they don't. The second, called the intermediate syndrome, is manifest by the pilot who, having gained some knowledge and skill, develops the attitude that he or she knows more and can do more than he or she can. Such pilots attempt flights and maneuvers that are beyond their abilities and that result in injury or death. The third attitude, and perhaps most difficult to deal with, is the know-it-all. Reaching these accidents-waiting-to-happen folks is extremely difficult.

For a few pilots who cannot admit their fears of flight, an accident is the only ego-acceptable mechanism to exit the sport. Infrequently, someone buys an ancient glider at a garage sale and jumps off a cliff. Unfortunately, he or she is still counted as a fatality for the sport. Although drug and alcohol use by hang glider pilots does occur and has been known to cause or contribute to accidents, the incidence is low.

Towing

In many parts of the country, particularly in the flatlands, towing is a popular method of launching a hang glider. The glider and pilot are placed on the bed of a pickup truck and attached with a rope to a winch drum. The truck accelerates to 30 mph, the glider releases and rises up as the line is paid out (just like a kite on a fishing reel). When an altitude of 1000 to 3000 feet is reached, the pilot releases the tow line and flies off in search of a thermal. Boat towing, fixed-winch towing, and aerotowing (with an ultralite aircraft) also are practiced.

Most towing accidents are directly related to the towing process: the pilot's angle of attack leaving the truck bed may be too high; the pilot may deviate too far off to one side of the tow vehicle (lock-out); the pilot may accidentally release from the tow line at a low altitude; the tow line may break or become tangled; and a wind gust or strong thermal may buffet the glider. Towing does add an additional element of risk but can be done safely and may be the only method of flying available.

Types of Injuries

Almost all injuries are a direct result of violent deceleration of the pilot's body. This is similar to injuries seen in automobile and motorcycle accidents, crashes in general aviation, and falls from heights. Bodily damage occurs when the pilot hits the ground or a part of the glider. In those instances in which the glider happens to absorb the shock and decelerates the pilot more slowly, even severe crashes can leave the pilot uninjured. Alternately, the pilot's body may be the first thing to hit the ground at speeds between 15 and 50 mph, which causes severe deceleration and contusion injuries.

Head

Because the hang glider pilot is prone, injuries tend to involve the "leading points"—head, neck, chest, and upper extremities. Closed head injuries with or without basilar skull fractures are the most common cause of death. The head usually strikes the ground (Fig. 30.5). Helmets are universally worn and numerous anecdotal testimonials confirm their value. But a helmet can only dissipate so much energy. Helmets with face guards are becoming more popular and will, it is hoped, reduce the severity of facial and dental injuries that are frequently associated with these major head traumas.

Spine

Cervical

Of the nonfatal injuries, cervical spine fracture with resultant paraplegia or quadriplegia bestows the most severe sequelae on the hang glider pilot. The direct axial load mechanism is similar to those of other sporting injuries, and the type of fracture depends on whether the spine is flexed, extended, or neutral at the time of impact. It seems that frequently a neutral position, with resultant central body burst fracture does occur. Most paraplegia quadriplegia is complete and permanent. Several central cord injuries with predominant upper extremity paralysis have been reported.

Thoracolumbar

After the cervical spine, the T7 to T10 level holds a distant second in the frequency of vertebral fractures. When such fractures occur, they may or may not result in corresponding paraplegia. Lumbar fractures are uncommon, even in the supine pilot.

Thoracic

After head injury and high cervical cord transection, the most common cause of immediate death is aortic arch disruption. This injury is classic for massive decelerate trauma and is seen in a wide variety of trauma. Fractured ribs, pneumothorax, hemothorax, pulmonary contusion, ruptured diaphragm, and rarely cardiac rupture also are seen.

Abdominal

Intraabdominal injuries are uncommon. When present, they are usually a component of multiple systems deceleration injuries. Ruptured liver, lacerated spleen, mesenteric tears, perforated viscus, and pancreatic contusion/transection are seen. Retroperitoneal hematomas and renal contusion can occur. Bladder rupture is distinctly uncommon, because most pilots empty their bladder before flying in the hopes of soaring for hours.

Upper Extremities

Colles Fracture of the Wrist

Distal forearm and wrist fractures during landing are common injuries, particularly in students. One or both forearm bones may be broken. During the accident, the pilot extends the wrist and/or arm to break the fall or, more commonly, the student freezes with a "death grip" on the control bar with elbow and wrist locked in extension (Fig. 30.6). As pilots gain experience they learn how to crash by reconditioning themselves not to hold onto the control bar or extend their arms. Women, perhaps because of lesser bone strength and/or muscle mass and perhaps because of a greater concern for physical injury than their male counterparts, seem to have a high incidence of upper extremity fractures. It has been speculated that their lack of experience on the athletic field with tuck-and-roll, falling-down type sports may also be a factor.

Elbow and Distal Humerus

The most prevalent fracture of the upper extremity is fracture of the supracondylar humerus (see Table 30.2). One mechanism is identical to that described earlier for Colles fracture. When the force is transmitted up the forearm to the humerus in the presence of slight flexion of the elbow, this fracture results. The second mechanism is that of the pilot (often a student) falling

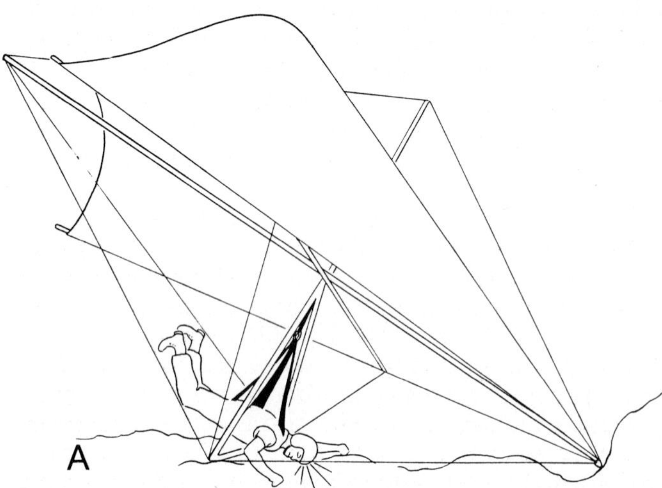

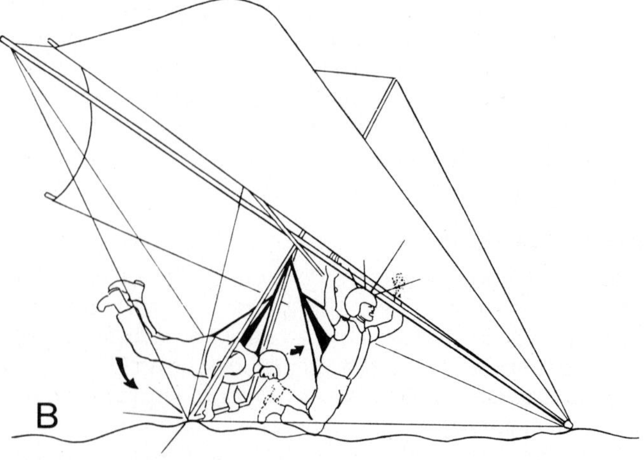

Figure 30.5. When the control bar and nose hit the ground, the glider stops abruptly and **(A)** the pilot's head may strike the ground or **(B)** the pilot may strike a part of the glider; usually, he or she hits the aluminum keel spur.

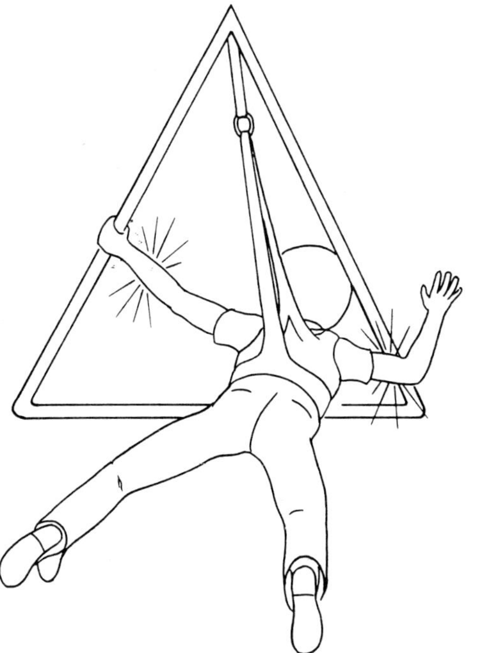

Figure 30.6. With accidental impact on the ground, the extended left arm may sustain a Colles fracture or the right humerus may be fractured.

forward, his or her hand and forearm slipping off the outside of the upright tubing of the control bar, while the body goes through the inside of the control bar. The upright tubing then strikes the distal humerus just above the elbow (see Fig. 30.6). Rotational forces are involved in both these mechanisms, and this frequently results in a spiral fracture of the distal humerus; usually, the elbow joint is spared. Fractures at higher levels of the humerus can occur but are less frequent as are dislocations or fracture-dislocations of the elbow. Major shoulder injuries, including clavicular or scapular fracture and acromioclavicular separations are unusual, but contusions and shoulder (glenohumeral) dislocations are more common.

Five cases of spontaneous humeral fracture have been reported. These occur in flight when vigorous and forceful pilot weight shift corrections are done. Because the pilot is pulling and pushing the body from side to side, considerable force is applied to the humeral shaft. In each instance of this "spontaneous" fracture, a prior injury or fracture to the humerus had existed. For this reason, extra healing time should be given before returning the pilot with a humeral fracture to flying.

Lower Extremities

Sprained ankles and contusions and abrasions of the thighs, knees, and calves do occur, but lower extremity fractures are distinctly less common than those of the upper extremity. Usually, the glider has forward momentum and the pilot falls forward with his or her legs trailing, which is a less vulnerable position. But if the glider stalls at 10 to 50 feet and falls straight down, the pilot is in an upright position for landing and will hit with the lower extremities first. Ground skimming at high speed while still in the prone position may result in femur fracture if the thigh strikes a rock or other object hidden in the grass.

Pelvic Fracture

Pelvic fractures are usually a part of multiple injuries and are frequently a result of the above-described stall and vertical descent. These injuries approximate injuries that occur in a fall from a height, with lower extremity, intraabdominal, and urethral injury potential.

Multiple Injuries

Most of the severely injured pilots will have multisystem damage. Emergency physicians must remember the magnitude of the forces involved in any aircraft accident, and hang gliding is no exception. Expect and anticipate head and cervical spine injuries, pneumothorax, aortic transection, intraabdominal bleeding or contusion, and upper and lower extremity and pelvic injuries. Paraplegia or quadriplegia may mask other injuries.

Miscellaneous

One or two pilots land in the surf each year. Once the heavy surf covers the sail, the pilot and glider are at the complete mercy of the waves. The only chance of escape is for the pilot to use a knife to cut free from the glider. Once every 2 or 3 years, someone drowns.

Electrocution or burns result from landing on power lines. The uncommon tree landing can be done safely, but pilots have been known to fall attempting to climb down from the tree.

At least a dozen pilots have reported carpal tunnel syndrome, presumably related to hyperextension of the wrists during prolonged flights. Temporary sciatic symptoms have been experienced by the seated/supine pilot (even without a billfold).

Fatalities

Most fatalities result from head injury (65%), high cervical spine fracture (10%), or ruptured thoracic aorta (9%). Most pilots die instantly. A very few live a short time and die at the scene. Only 4% of those who die reach the hospital alive, and subsequently die there. The types of injuries sustained by pilots who die are the same as those who survive; the difference is in the extent of injury (how badly the head gets smashed) and in luck.

The causes of fatal accidents and the causes of all accidents are identical. Preventing hang gliding fatalities rests on reducing all types of accidents. The decline in hang gliding fatalities is related to a number of developments. The parachute, which is worn by 94% of pilots, originally was hand thrown but now is rocket deployed (full deployment in 2 sec). There has been an average of 13 reported saves each year and probably some additional unreported ones. Helmets are now used universally. Glider certification ensures that all current gliders are certified by a voluntary testing program. Glider inspection and maintenance services keep older gliders airworthy. Teaching methods are better. USHGA certified instruction includes the use of training wheels, radios, good equipment, and modern teaching techniques. Safety information dissemination continues on a national (USHGA) and local levels.

Areas for future improvement include a hook-in warning device, an audible stall warning system, glider- or harness-mounted airbags, and the continued development of gliders that are easier to launch and land but still retain excellent performance. Safe flying sites need to be preserved.

First Aid

Hang gliding accidents can occur anywhere. Although they often happen in the designated landing area, they may occur in remote locations. First aid requires common sense, clear thinking, and improvisation (26).

1. Secure and stabilize the glider so that no further damage to the pilot occurs from the wind moving the glider.
2. Rapidly assess the pilot's condition—breathing, pulse, bleeding, and the need for cardiopulmonary resuscitation.
3. Do not move the pilot unless leaving the pilot where he or she is poses a great immediate threat.
4. When adequate help arrives, support and protect the pilot's head and neck, and cut the hang strap holding the harness to the glider. *Do not* remove the helmet. *Do not* remove the harness (unless CPR or other specific torso treatment is needed).
5. Carefully move the glider away from the pilot. Do not move the pilot. At all times assume that a cervical spine injury is present.
6. Reevaluate all systems for injury.
7. Send someone for help, making sure he or she can give accurate directions to the ambulance of how to reach the pilot. If possible, send someone to an obvious place to meet and guide the ambulance.
8. Remember that parts of the glider and harness can be used for splints, dressings, stretcher, etc.
9. In addition to a basic first aid kit, desirable equipment includes a backboard, cervical collar, air splints, knife, and rope.
10. Even pilots who appear unhurt may have significant injuries. Keep them lying down and quiet. Encourage injured pilots to seek a medical evaluation.

Here is advice that a physician might give to patients considering taking up the sport of hang gliding:

1. Hang gliding is a mature sport that can be done safely.
2. Be sure you are of sound mental and physical health.
3. Be aware that some people can play basketball and others cannot. Some individuals were born with the talent, coordination and athletic ability to be pilots and some do not have the necessary physical, mental or judgmental gifts to be a safe and skilled hang glider pilot.
4. There are certain inherent unavoidable risks involved in hang gliding. You can be killed or injured.
5. Discuss the risks and dangers and costs of the sport—are you and your significant others willing to accept the consequences?
6. Make sure you are comfortable with your level of life and disability insurance. It is generally easier to obtain these before you begin hang gliding rather than after.
7. Choose an experienced and respected USHGA certified instructor.
8. Start out with one or two lessons to see if you like it. Admit it to yourself if you do not.
9. Take lots of instruction.
10. Ask your instructor to tell you honestly if he or she thinks you do not have the natural ability and skills to be a safe pilot.
11. Join the USHGA and read all you can about the sport.
12. Join the local hang gliding club and learn from the other pilots.
13. Ask advice from your instructor and fellow pilots about your first equipment purchases—glider, harness, parachute, gear, etc.
14. Advance gradually, mastering each step before progressing on to the next.
15. Beware of the intermediate syndrome—when you get a little experience and think you know everything.
16. If the sport becomes stressful or no longer fun, reevaluate the type of flying you are doing and modify it, or give it up completely.

Conclusions

Hang gliding is a spectacular sport that allows humankind at long last to fulfill the age-old dream of joining the birds in the silent beauty of flight. Although tremendous advancement has occurred in glider design, instruction, information dissemination, and safety, accidents will continue to happen, and the predicable injury patterns of the past will continue. If the physician and paramedical personnel understand the mechanisms of hang glider accidents, are aware of the injury patterns, remember the magnitude of the forces involved, and care for the patient in a nonjudgmental manner, the patient will be the ultimate benefactor.

Physicians and paramedical personnel are encouraged to participate in voluntary accident reporting to the USHGA at P.O. Box 8300, Colorado Springs, CO 80933-8300.

REFERENCES

1. Hildreth D. Accident review. Hang Gliding 1981;99:40–42.
2. Hildreth D. Accident review. Hang Gliding 1982;110:40–42.
3. Hildreth D. Accident review. Hang Gliding 1982;111:39–41.
4. Hildreth D. Accident review. Hang Gliding 1983;122:35–37.
5. Hildreth D. Accident review. Hang Gliding 1984;14:34–36.
6. Hildreth D. Accident review. Hang Gliding 1985;15:35–37.
7. Hildreth D. Accident review. Hang Gliding 1986;16:17–19.
8. Hildreth D. Accident review. Hang Gliding 1987;17:12–13.
9. Hildreth D. Accident review. Hang Gliding 1988;18:12–14.

10. Hildreth D. Accident review. Hang Gliding 1989;19:38–39.
11. Hildreth D. Accident review. Hang Gliding 1990;20:20–21.
12. Hildreth D. Accident review. Hang Gliding 1991;21:27–30.
13. Wills RV. Accident review. Hang Gliding 1979;82:20–22.
14. Wills RV. Accident review. Hang Gliding 1980;92:42–45.
15. Imperato PJ, Mitchell G. Acceptable risks. New York: Viking, 1985.
16. Wahe JW, Nolte KB, Zumwalt RE. Hang gliding: the dying sport [Abstract]. Am Soc Forensic Sci, in press.
17. Anonymous. Hazards of hang gliding [Editorial]. Br Med J 1978;1:388.
18. Bell M. Hang gliding injuries. Injury 1976;8:148–150.
19. Davidson CS. Hang gliding injuries. NC Med J 1983;44:439–440.
20. Krissoff WB. Follow-up on hang gliding injuries in Colorado. Am J Sports Med 1976;4:222–229.
21. Krissoff WB, Eiseman B. Injuries associated with hang gliding. JAMA 1975;233:158–160.
22. Margreiter R, Lugger LJ. Hang gliding accidents. Br Med J 1978;1:400–402.
23. Tongue JR. Hang gliding injuries in California. J Trauma 1977;17:898–902.
24. Yuill GM. Icarus' syndrome: new hazards in flight. Br Med J 1977;1:823–825.
25. Reynolds BM, Balsano NA, Reynolds FX. Falls from heights: surgical experience of two hundred consecutive cases. Ann Surg 1971;174:304–311.
26. Nelson L. The first thirty minutes. Hang Gliding 1983;120:28–30, 40.

SUGGESTED READINGS

American College of Surgeons Committee on Trauma. Advanced trauma life support course. Lincoln, NE: Author, 1980.

Aupetit H. ABC of paragliding. Paris: Editions Retine, 1989.

Banks, G. Statistics accidents analysis. Paragliding Magazine 1990;1(2):44.

Commission Securite Parapente. Report. Crolles, France: Author, 1990.

Gordon D, Koerner M. NW paragliding accident survey. Unpublished data.

Hildreth D. 1990 accident review, the first 20 years. Hang Gliding 1991;21:27–30.

Pagan D. Walking on air! Paragliding flight. Mingoville, PA: Author, 1990.

Shipman M. APA 1990 accident statistics. Paragliding Magazine 1991;2(4).

31 / POWER LIFTING, WEIGHT LIFTING, AND BODYBUILDING

Thomas C. Namey and Peter J. Carek

The use of weight training, whether training for the specific sports of weight lifting, power lifting, and bodybuilding or as part of the overall conditioning regimen of athletes of other sports, has steadily increased in the United States over the past several years. Strength training is being used not only in an attempt to excel in the chosen sport but also as an adjunctive modality in the rehabilitation and prevention of injuries. The numerous benefits of a solid weight-training program need to be defined and potential uses have yet to be discovered.

As with any other sport, specific injuries occur with regularity in the weight lifting sports. Although the true frequency of injuries that occur while training and competing for these sports has not been well-documented, the incidence of injuries occurring during general strength training is surprisingly low and comparable with several other sports (1–3). With the increased popularity, the primary care physician as well as the sports physician will undoubtedly be presented with a growing number of weight-lifting associated injuries. To treat these injuries effectively, the physician must be familiar not only with sports injuries in general but also with the injuries commonly seen in the strength athlete.

Historical Perspective

Competitions involving weight lifting and demonstrations of strength have been present since the beginning of humankind. Using various forms of strength development, early humans used rocks, stones, or irons to determine who was the strongest. A "scientific" approach to weight training was begun by Milo of Crotona (6th century B.C.), a six-time Olympic champion, who used a growing calf in a form of progressive resistance training, lifting it on his shoulders every day until it was full grown.

Until the late 19th century, weight lifters were delegated to act as strongmen in shows and circuses where they could demonstrate their strength and skill. During the late 1800s, weight lifting as a sport was born in Europe with the organization of the first European Championship in Rotterdam (1896) and the first World Championship in Vienna (1898). Weight lifting also was included as a competition during the first modern Olympic Games (1896).

Since the establishment of the International Weightlifting Federation (IWF) in 1905, numerous weight-lifting associations have formed and several other sports involving demonstrations of strength and muscular hypertrophy have been created (i.e., power lifting and bodybuilding). The popularity of these newer forms of strength sports has surpassed that of the original form of weight lifting.

In recent history, the superiority of the Eastern European countries and the former Soviet Union in international weight-lifting competitions was used as a psychological weapon during the Cold War as a gauge of political and ethnic supremacy. Furthermore, several Third World countries have used their citizens who excel in international competitions as a means to increase the country's exposure and, possibly, prominence in the world.

The international popularity of the strength sports remains significant and appears to be increasing. Historically, these sports have been popular in the Eastern European community and the former Soviet Union. Whether the changing political climate in that area of the world affects participation is yet to be seen.

Definition of the Specific Sports

The goal of these sports is to demonstrate strength in a controlled and regulated manner, whether lifting a one repetition maximum or exhibiting muscular hypertrophy. The rules and regulations associated with these sports are determined by the specific governing bodies, who also determine the eligibility of the participants and the levels of competition (Table 31.1).

The sports that demonstrate strength and power by lifting one repetition at maximum weight within three

Table 31.1.
Governing Bodies and Levels of Competition of the Specific Strength-Training Sports

Governing Bodies	Levels of Competition
Weight lifting	Weight lifting[a]
IWF	Junior (up to and including age 20)
USWF[b]	—
AAU	Senior
	Veteran (age 40+)
Power lifting	Power lifting
IPF	teenage (ages 14 to 19)
USPF	senior (age 14+)
APF	master (age 40+)
	special Olympians (juniors and seniors)
Bodybuilding	Bodybuilding
IFBB	

[a] The minimum age for the Junior Word Championships is 15 years; for the Senior World Championships and Olympic Games, 17 years.
[b] USWF registration is at 12 years.

Table 31.2.
Comparison of Barbells and Machines

Characteristic	Free Weights	Weight Machines
Cost	+	+
Safety		+
Time efficiency		+
Technique	+	
Beginner athletes		+
Power development	+	
Versatility	+	
Motivation	+	
Muscle isolation		+
Variety	+	
Rehabilitation		+
Space efficiency	+	
Constant resistance through entire range of motion		+

Adapted from Weltman A, Stamford B. Strength training: free weights vs. machines. Phys Sportsmed 1982;10(11):1970.

attempts (i.e., weight lifting and power lifting) consist of the successful completion of specific lifts. The participant is allowed to set the weight at the level at which he or she will begin to compete, similar to high jumpers and pole vaulters setting the height of their initial attempt. Each lift has specific guidelines for approved completion and each is associated with sites susceptible to injury.

Olympic weight-lifting competitions consist of the completion of two lifts: the snatch and the clean-and-jerk. To perform the snatch, the weight is lifted from a position in front of the lifter's legs to above the head with the elbows in full extension. The bar must pass with a continuous movement along the body. This lift may be accomplished with either a split or squat move as the lifter maneuvers himself or herself underneath the lifted weight.

The clean-and-jerk consists of two distinct moves. The weight is pulled from the floor to the shoulders, while either squatting or splitting the legs. The bar may rest on the clavicles, on the chest above the nipples, or on the fully bent arms. After recovery to a standing position, the weight is then lifted over the head until the arms are vertical and the elbows are fully extended.

Power-lifting competition consists of three lifts: bench press, squat, and dead lift. For the bench press, the barbell is held with the elbows fully extended while the athlete lies supine on the bench. The lifter lowers the weight to the chest and raises it again to the elbow-extended position. The squat involves supporting the barbell, while standing, on the shoulders posterior to the neck with the top of the bar not more than 3 cm below the top of the deltoid. The weight is lowered by flexing the knees and hips until the thighs are parallel to the floor. Once cleared by the referee, the lifter must recover to an upright position with the knees locked. During the dead lift, the barbell is lifted from a position in front of the lifter's legs as the individual stands, without raising his or her hands, until the knees are locked in a straight position and the shoulders held in an upright position.

Although each specific lift predisposes several anatomical sites to injury, the bench press and its mandatory equipment is associated with an increased risk of serious injury. A significant number of injuries and deaths occur during the performance of bench pressing, especially in the unsupervised, home setting (4, 5).

Equipment

Although the equipment used for training varies considerably among individual athletes, the equipment used for the strength sports in competition is standardized. The purpose of the modifications is to allow for safe, effective, and fair means of demonstrating strength and power.

The free weights and bars have several unique design features. The plates have a larger caliber hole and the bar has smaller caliber ends compared with nonstandardized equipment, allowing for a rapid exchange of plates and ease of balance. The grip area is knurled to create a secure, nonslip surface.

Designed more for athletes not involved with a specific weight-lifting sport, the numerous weight machines (e.g., Universal and Nautilus) do offer several advantages over the free weights (Table 31.2). A theoretical advantage to using weight machines is that the supporting musculature used during the balancing of the barbell is not given the opportunity to develop if machines are used exclusively.

Accessory equipment, including lifting belts, joint wraps, lifting shoes, proper clothing, and hand protection (gloves, chalk, and wrist straps) are often used during training to reduce the risk of injury and allow maximal work. Many of these items are legally used during competition as long as they meet specific criteria.

Weight-lifting belts have been shown to support indirectly the spinal column and musculature of the lower back by maintaining or even increasing intraabdominal pressure (6, 7). The effect may reduce back muscle and disc compressive forces while improving lifting safety

(8). This additional support is especially pronounced during squatting moves and in lifters without optimally conditioned torso musculature. A competitive lifting belt is 12 cm wide and one layer thick. The benefits in terms of improving performance are not well known and several world records have been set by individuals who have opted not to use one.

Joint wraps, allowed only around the knee and wrist joints under IWF rules, are usually composed of inexpensive, thin material of specific width and length wrapped circumferentially around the specific joint. Though limited data exist as to their effectiveness, justifications for their use include keeping the joint warm, providing external support to the joint, preventing skin-to-skin sticking around the knee during squatting, limiting the range of motion of the wrist joint, and providing comfort and confidence to the weight lifter (9). Joint wraps may be partially responsible for the formation of hematomas and varicosities of the lower extremities. In addition, they may cause the development of blood pooling and vascular collapse, hemodynamic changes that when combined with the other physiologic changes that occur with weight lifting could ultimately result in acute complications, such as syncopal episodes.

Weight-lifting shoes need to provide a firm, snug, nonslip foundation. The shoes should have a small, wide heel to prevent side movement, providing better balance than a continuous incline wedge-type shoe. A thin, solid sole does not provide an exaggerated platform from which to lift tremendous weights. The presence of a solid heel counter with the addition of a strap around the arch are modifications that create additional support.

Proper clothing, in addition to being a marker of team membership, is essential for comfort and safety. The weight-lifting suit, which must adhere to the specific rules of the sport, should be lightweight, firm fitting, and supportive. T-shirts, worn under the suit, are both popular and legal under most rules. The use of athletic supporters or approved lifting briefs is essential, although the use of garments with legs or ones that act as girdles, are illegal.

Gloves and chalk are used in an effort to improve the security of the grip during a lift attempt and to protect the hands from blister and callus formation. Chalk, usually in the form of baby powder, pool hall chalk, liquid chalk, resin, talc, or magnesium carbonate, maintains a dry grip and is often added to the body and attire to dry extra moisture. The effectiveness of these items is not known.

Straps are used during training sessions to improve the grip, especially while attempting heavier weights. These straps are wrapped around the hand, wrist, and bar to assist in securing a strong grip. Excessive training with straps may be deleterious and result in a weakened grip strength, adversely affecting performance in competition, during which they are not allowed. Straps also may disrupt proper position of hand-wrist-elbow-shoulder during clean-and-jerk movements and cause delay when the athlete attempts to move out from under the weight during a missed lift.

Science of Strength Training

Many variables are involved in the successful completion of a weight-lifting movement. Two basic variables, strength and power, are commonly considered to be similar terms, yet each has a specific definition and a vital role in weight-lifting sports.

Strength is defined as the ability to develop force against an unyielding resistance of unrestricted duration (10). It is the maximal amount of weight that can be lifted during one complete repetition of a particular movement, using the force generated by a specific muscle group (11). To lift maximal weight, the individual consciously and unconsciously performs several neurophysiological actions to increase the amount of force he or she is able to generate: *(a)* recruitment of additional motor units and muscle fibers; *(b)* initiate movement while the muscle is at an optimal length; *(c)* fire involved motor units in a synchronous fashion; and *(d)* relax the antagonistic musculature (11, 12). Strength is the variable that is probably measured to a greater extent during a power-lifting competition.

In contrast to strength, *power* is defined as the amount of work performed during a specific period of time, i.e., work rate (11). It is a function of both the amount of muscular force exerted and the rate of body or limb movement (13). If the work performed is mechanical and the force applied is constant, power simply equals force times the first derivative of distance with respect to time, or force times speed (1). Power is important in Olympic-style weight lifting as an element of quickness and speed is present as the participant attempts quickly to lift and lunge under the bar as it is raised. The element of power is demonstrated as weight lifters have the highest power outputs and vertical jumps of all athletes (14). Power also is an important factor while training for sports other than the strength-training sports. Power as an important variable in power lifting has not been demonstrated. During the action of weight lifting, isometric and isotonic contractions of involved muscle groups occur (10). Isometric action is a contraction of muscle that occurs without a change in the total length of the muscle. Because no movement occurs, no work is performed. In regard to strength development and injury risk, this form of muscular contraction is the most efficient in terms of repetitions per yield of strength development and has minimal risk of injury. This form of exercise is specific for the muscle length and joint angle at which it is performed.

Isotonic contraction is a contraction of the muscle that is associated with changes in total muscular length; therefore, work is performed (10). If relevant loads are chosen, a frequency of five to six repetitions per session appears to provide the best results in terms of strength development. Muscles performing isotonic exercises do not encounter constant resistance through the entire range of motion and most of the improvement noted with training or limitation of maximal lifts occurs at the weakest point along the strength curve for the particular muscle group and joint.

Isokinetic contraction, an additional form of muscle

action, is a contraction that occurs at a constant velocity. An isokinetic exercise is an accommodating resistance type in which the muscle experiences the same relative resistance at all points in the range of motion to maintain a constant speed (10). This form of exercise is used primarily during rehabilitation and may be associated with submaximal strength gain.

In addition to these forms of muscular actions, muscle contractions may be considered either concentric or eccentric. Concentric weight training refers to a muscle contraction that causes a shortening of muscle length, and positive work is performed. Eccentric muscle contraction refers to an increase in muscle length during contraction. This form of action produces negative work and is usually associated with an increased risk of injury and muscle soreness.

Nutrition and Diet

Strength-training athletes, as a result of their unique body composition and rigorous training schedule, have specific nutritional and dietary requirements (14). To maintain a positive energy balance, weight lifters require a larger amount of caloric consumption per day than would be expected of individuals of similar size and weight (2500 to 8000 kcal/day). This added caloric intake takes into account the obligatory increased energy demand required by these athletes who possess a greater lean body mass, with its associated increased amount of muscle tissue, which requires a greater amount of total calories at rest than fat.

The increased caloric consumption is achieved through ingestion of various amounts of carbohydrates, proteins, and fats. Carbohydrates are the preferred metabolic fuel used during anaerobic exercise and should constitute approximately 50% to 60% of total caloric intake. Proteins provide a minimal amount of the total energy requirement during training if a regular diet is followed. Athletes in a heavy weight-training cycle or in the process of losing weight may require additional protein (1.5 to 2.0 g/kg body weight/day compared with a maintenance intake of 0.8 g/kg/day) to account for tissue injury (breakdown) that requires repair and resynthesis. Fats are concentrated aerobic fuel (9 kcal/gm of fat compared with 4 kcal/g of both carbohydrates and proteins) and should constitute 20% to 30% of total caloric intake.

Minerals and vitamins, which function as coenzymes, enzyme cofactors, and structural material and in gas transport and muscle contractions, are often used and abused by athletes. The scientific basis for mineral and vitamin supplementation remains unclear, and specific recommendations depends on individual needs. The intake of supplements ensures adequate intake. No proven benefit has been demonstrated from the ingestion of megadoses of vitamins and minerals and, in reality, may be associated with adverse effects. An example of such an adverse effect is the deposition of oxalate with increased intake of ascorbic acid, which may lead to nephrolithiasis if dehydration occurs. A significant problem with most athletes is maintaining an adequate volume status, especially during times of unusual environmental conditions or intense training. To maintain an appropriate level of hydration and electrolyte balance, especially in lieu of an obligatory plasma volume expansion associated with some forms of training, the weight-training athlete should consume sufficient fluids that are supplemented with the appropriate minerals, especially potassium.

In addition to vitamins and minerals, other medications and chemicals are used on a regular basis as ergometric aids in an attempt to improve performance. Amino acids and proteins are taken in large quantities to increase synthesis of lean body mass, particularly muscle. This action is based on anecdotal evidence and myths, with no supportive data present. Although banned by most competitive associations, anabolic steroids and growth hormone are used to promote protein synthesis. Though data support the enhancement of strength using one repetition maximum measurement, these chemicals are associated with numerous adverse side effects, including alterations in the blood lipid profile and changes in psychological mood; their use should be strongly discouraged (15, 16). Furthermore, the use of drugs used to counteract the short-term side effects of anabolic steroids could lead to additional complications (17).

Medical and Physiologic Adaptations to Weight Training

Several physiologic parameters are influenced by weight training, and numerous misconceptions exist pertaining to possible harmful effects on such measurements as blood pressure and body composition. During dynamic resistive exercises, both systolic and diastolic blood pressures rise, with recordings reaching 450/310 mm Hg during a double-leg press (18). In contrast, normal or even slightly lower blood pressures result with prolonged training, even in individuals who initially had elevated blood pressures (19). The use of an appropriately sized blood pressure cuff in these disproportionally large individuals is mandatory to ensure reliable and reproducible measurements. Increase in blood pressure may be the result of other factors unrelated to the physiologic response to resistive training (Table 31.3). Increases in stroke volume, muscle mass and strength and insulin sensitivity and decreases in heart rate and body fat are possible mechanisms by which resistive exercises lower blood pressure (20)

Although elevated during the strenuous activity of training and composition, the heart rate of weight lift-

Table 31.3.
Factors Causing Significant Blood Pressure Increases in Weight Lifters

Hypertension (primary or secondary)
Gains in body mass
Overtraining
Drug use
Error in measurement (usually too small cuff size)

ers is typically lower at rest than the average adult. When calculating the double product during acute resistive exercise, using the increased heart rate and markedly elevated systolic blood pressures, the result indicates a significantly increased oxygen demand on the myocardium.

Aerobic fitness or power, usually measured by maximum oxygen consumption in liters of oxygen per minute or milliliters of oxygen per kilogram per minute, may demonstrate small to moderate increases with high-volume weight training compared with sedentary individuals (14, 21–23). Training specifically to improve aerobic power and endurance using typical methods such as jogging and stationary bicycle ergometer will compromise maximum anaerobic power and, subsequently, will reduce weight lifting performance (24, 25). On the other hand, interval training programs or high-volume weight training can increase $\dot{V}_{O_2max}$ with little or no compromise in strength and power compared with typical aerobic endurance training (26).

Beneficial alterations in blood lipid profiles, with declines in total cholesterol, low-density lipoprotein (LDL) cholesterol, and the ratio of total cholesterol to high-density lipoprotein (HDL) cholesterol, have resulted from high-volume weight training, such as performed by bodybuilders (27–29). These favorable effects may be altered with anabolic steroid use (28).

The body composition of most weight lifters and, as would be expected, most bodybuilders, appears to demonstrate an average or increased lean body mass with an associated decrease of percent body fat (14, 22, 23, 30). This characteristic of strength-training athletes, although needing further study, indicates that a program of intense resistive exercise maintains and may decrease the percentage of body fat in addition to increasing muscle mass.

Weight training results in changes in measures of pulmonary functioning. Weight lifters have group mean values for vital capacity (VC) and maximum breathing capacity measures of 10% to 20% greater than the values predicted from height and age tables (14). In particular, individuals suffering from exercise-induced asthma (EIA) (also known as exercise-induced bronchospasms) usually are able to train and perform competitively in weight lifting because the symptoms associated with EIA have a longer duration of exercise demand before onset than the time required to perform the necessary lifts. Pulmonary problems, such as spontaneous pneumothorax, are more associated with running and only infrequently reported with weight lifting, despite the increase in intrathoracic pressure that occurs (13).

Considerations for Health and Disease

Weight lifting and weight training are associated with several specific medical problems. These problems arise from the exaggerated demands placed on the internal organs and external structures during training and competition. Many of these conditions actually reflect an appropriate physiologic response to conditioning rather than a pathophysiologic process.

The incidence of hypertension among competitive weight lifters and bodybuilders is well-known but may be related to risk factors separate from the sport itself (Table 31.4). Hypertension is a relative contraindication to weight training. Once controlled, hypertension should not pose a threat to the health of an individual who chooses to lift weights and may act as an adjunctive therapy, actually reducing blood pressure (19, 32).

The athletic heart, a condition associated with increased diastolic dimensions of the left ventricle, thickness of the left ventricular wall, and calculated left ventricular mass, commonly occurs with long-term athletic training. It is often difficult to distinguish from pathologic forms of hypertrophy, such as hypertrophic cardiomyopathy, a leading cause of sudden death in young athletes (33). An increase in the thickness of the left ventricle results from hypertrophy of cardiac muscles and is thought to be a compensatory mechanism caused by an increased vascular resistance (afterload) that occurs during resistive-type exercises. In comparison, endurance-trained athletes have increased left ventricular dimensions (i.e., end-diastolic volume) caused by an

Table 31.4.
Contraindications to Weight Lifting and Weight Training

Cardiac
- Angina pectoris
- Aortic stenosis (gradient greater than 40 mm Hg across the valve)
- Pulmonary stenosis (RV pressure greater than 75 mm Hg)
- Cardiac arrhythmia, uncontrolled
- Congestive heart failure, uncontrolled
- Cystic medial necrosis of aorta (Marfan's syndrome)
- Myocardial infarction, acute or recent
- Myocarditis or cardiomyopathy
- Obstructive hypertrophic cardiomyopathy
- Other significant valvular heart disease

Endocrine
- Adrenal insufficiency
- Diabetes mellitus, uncontrolled
- Electrolyte abnormality
- Hypothyroidism or hyperthyroidism, untreated

Infection
- Acute, febrile infectious disease

Metabolic
- Hypatic or renal insufficiency, severe

Orthopedic
- Fracture or recent dislocation
- Lumbosacral disc disease, symptomatic
- Sprain or strain, recent and symptomatic

Pulmonary
- Chronic obstructive pulmonary disease, untreated
- Cor pulmonale
- Pneumonitis, acute or untreated

Rheumatic
- Degenerative arthritis, acute and symptomatic
- Rheumatoid arthritis, acute and symptomatic

Vascular and circulatory
- Anemia, severe or unknown etiology
- Aneurysm, large or dissecting
- Cerebrovascular disease, acute or symptomatic
- Embolism, acute
- Hypertension, acute
- Thrombophlebitis, acute

Adapted from McKeag DB. Preparticipation screening of the potential athlete. Clin Sports Med 1989:8(3)373–397; Taylor. 1983; and Puffer JC. Management of over use injuries. Am Fam Physician 1988;38(3):225–232.

increase in plasma volume (preload). In mild forms, the increased wall thickness is a natural result of athletic training. Markedly elevated measures of wall thickness, especially septal wall thickness and mass:volume ratio, are present in such conditions as asymmetric septal hypertrophy (ASH) and idiopathic hypertrophic subaortic stenosis (IHSS) (34). These conditions are noted on physical exam by the presence of an enlarged heart, an S_4 gallop, or a systolic murmur that is accentuated by standing or the Valsalva maneuver. Weight lifters, as a population, do not experience as great an increase in echocardiographic-measured left ventricular wall thickness as athletes in the endurance sports of rowing and cycling or in individuals with ASH or IHSS (34, 35). Although left ventricular hypertrophy is noted, it is accompanied by normal relative diastolic volume and function, consistent with physiologic hypertrophy (36).

Weight lifters also experience difficulties associated with the exaggerated demands placed on the venous vascular system, including lower extremity varicosities, phlebitis, and hemorrhoids. Hemorrhoids, a complication of the increased venous pressure occurring during a Valsalva maneuver, are best treated symptomatically and can be improved with a diet rich in fiber and an adequate fluid intake.

In addition, headaches (also known as weight lifters cephalgia) and syncope occur commonly. The headaches, which appear to be a variant of the exertional headache, also may be associated with other forms of intense physical activity. These headaches have an abrupt onset, are of brief duration (4 to 6 hr), and begin during periods of exertional activity (37, 38). The etiology of these episodes has yet to be delineated. Though potentially serious etiologies are only occasionally present, other causes of severe headache have been reported and should be considered (37–39). Treatment usually consists of cessation of activity and use of a nonsteroidal antinflammatory drug (NSAID).

Syncopal episodes appear secondary to a seemingly mandatory Valsalva maneuver performed while attempting maximal lifts. The decrease in venous return of blood associated with the use of several pieces of ancillary equipment may exacerbate the dramatic decline of cardiac output that causes these episodes. The abrupt loss of consciousness may be associated with severe injuries as a result of the falling weight and are best prevented by attempting to continue regular breathing throughout the entire performance of the lift.

Dermatologic problems, including hematomas, abrasions, and calluses, occur because of the need for a firm, nonslip grip and various maneuvers required to lift immense weights. These problems are usually treated on a symptomatic basis, but are best dealt with by avoiding them initially through proper preventive measures such as the use of gloves while training.

Several other medical conditions have been noted to occur in weight lifters, but only through anecdotal reports. These problems include aortic dissection (40), rhabdomyolysis (41), chest wall deformities (42), and posttraumatic syringomyelia (43). The incidence of these injuries is not well-documented.

As with other sports, the preparticipation examination for weight lifting must be sport specific. A comprehensive medical history should be performed, including questions concerning previous medical problems, unusual symptoms (i.e., episodes of syncope, dyspnea with exertion and chest pains), and previous injuries. A family history must include questions pertaining to the occurrence of sudden death or other congenital heart disease in close relatives. The physical examination should highlight areas of concern noted in the history as well as the shoulders, lower back, and knees. Contraindications, both absolute and relative, are similar to those found in other strenuous sports (see Table 31.4).

Specific event coverage consists of proper preparation to ensure prompt and effective medical treatment of the injured athlete. Proper preparations include adequate supply of medical equipment (Table 31.5) and prepared medical personnel, alert local medical consultants, authority pertaining to medical disqualifications, and clearance from participants to allow emergency medical treatment.

Strength-Training Injuries

Training for weight lifting and the other strength sports of power lifting and bodybuilding is truly sport specific, unlike other sports that use strength training in an attempt to improve performance in a dissimilar activity. As training is sport specific, the incidence of weight-training injuries is less than in many of the other sports.

Injuries that occur with weight training, like with most sports, can be divided into acute (i.e., sprains and strains) and chronic or overuse (i.e., tendinitis). A strain is a stretching or tearing of a musculotendinous unit, and a sprain is a similar type injury occurring to a ligament or other stabilizing connective tissue structure. A sprain will generally result in pain with passive movement of the involved joint, whereas a strain pro-

Table 31.5.
Categories of Medical Supplies Required for Adequate Event Coverage

Medications
Antiinflammatories
Antiallergic/asthmatic medications
Cardiac medications
Gastrointestinal medications
Intravenous fluids
Local anesthetics
Muscle relaxants
Ophthalmic injury kit
Pain-relieving medications
Topical agents, including corticosteroids, antifungals, antiseptics
Equipment
Airway maintenance
Diagnostic equipment (i.e., ophthalmoscope, stethoscope)
Pocket equipment
Splints, including knee immobilizer, slings, and crutches
Surgical equipment (suturing equipment)
Miscellaneous

Adapted from Ray RL, Feld FX. The team physician's bag. Clin Sports Med. 1989;8(1):139–146.

Table 31.6.
Classifications and Immediate Care of Sprains and Strains[a]

Severity	Symptoms	Immediate Care
First degree	Minimal microscopic injury, mild pain within 24 hr of injury, local tenderness may or may not be present	Active rest,[b] ice massages (apply ice for 20 min, rest for 20 to 30 min, and repeat), begin range of motion exercises
Second degree	Macroscopic injury, though structure remains contiguous; pain during activity; pain and local tenderness are moderate to severe, especially when injury is stressed	Same as first degree including compression and elevation (may require short-term immobilization if motion or weight bearing causes discomfort)
Third degree	Complete or near complete rupture or avulsion of at least a portion of the structure with severe pain and loss of function, palpable defect may be present, stressing the structure may cause minimal or no discomfort	Same as above, usually requires immediate immobilization and referral

[a]Adapted from Kellet J. Acute soft tissue injuries: a review of the literature. Med Sci Sport Exer 1986:18(5):489–500; and Webb DR. Sprains and strains. Paper presented at the National Sports Medicine Conference, April 1991.
[b]Movement that causes worsening or onset of discomfort should be discontinued.

duces pain with active movement of the joint. The classifications, symptoms, and initial therapy of sprains and strains is similar (Table 31.6). Sprains of varying severity display differences in the amount of laxity and prescence of an end point on physical exam when the structure is stressed (Table 31.7).

Numerous underlying mechanisms have been incriminated as etiologies to these types of injuries and include inadequate warmup and/or stretching; improper technique; trying out an untested new technique; maximum effort, usually during competition, far exceeding that previously attempted; losing concentration; not completely rehabilitating from a previous injury; or coaching failure (44, 45). The risk of these injuries can be significantly decreased if the proper preventive measures are taken: proper warmup; flexibility training; balanced strength training, using simultaneous development of agonist-antagonist muscle groups; and proper coaching.

Chronic or overuse injuries, usually seen as tendinitis, occur as a result of repetitive microtrauma to a specific structure that accumulates with time until a threshold is surpassed, resulting in macroscopic injury with symptoms and dysfunction. Overuse injuries frequently occur as a result of overtraining; a sudden increase in training frequency, duration, and/or intensity; inadequate training, leading to muscular imbalance between agonist-antagonist muscle groups; poor technique; a decrease in flexibility; and failure to rehabilitate fully after an injury. These injuries require accurate diagnosis not only to target the symptomatic problem but also to determine underlying abnormalities that may leave the athlete vulnerable to further injury or reinjury. Treatment of overuse problems usually consists of active rest, continued aerobic training of some form, and correction of the underlying mechanism (Table 31.8). These injuries are best treated by adequate prevention, which includes proper warmup, flexibility training, appropriate coaching, periodization of training, and restoration of proper technique.

Table 31.7.
Ligamentous Injuries[a]

Severity	Laxity	End Point
First degree	None to mild[b]	Present
Second degree	Mild to moderate	Present
Third degree	Severe	Absent

[a]Adapted from Garrick JG, Webb DR. Sports injuries: Diagnosis and management. Philadelphia: WB Saunders, 1990.
[b]Examination of the uninjured joint on other limb must be performed to determine extent of physiologic laxity present.

Table 31.8.
Classification and Management of Overuse Injuries

Classification	Characteristic	Management
Type 1	Pain only after activity	Reduce workload by 25%, ice massages after activity, stretching program, physical therapy and rehabilitation
Type 2	Pain during activity, not restricting performance	Reduce in workload by 50%, ice massages after activity, stretching program, physical therapy and rehabilitation, NSAIDs
Type 3	Pain during activity, restricting performance	Rest affected area, physical therapy and rehabilitation, NSAIDs, local injections of corticosteroids
Type 4	Chronic, unremitting	Same as type 3, surgical intervention may be necessary

Adapted from Puffer JC, Zachazewski JE. Management of overuse injuries. Am Fam Phys 1988;38(3):225–232.

The NSAIDs prescribed for both acute and chronic injuries are some of the most frequently prescribed medications in the United States. Although the superiority of clinical efficacy of any of these medications is difficult to distinguish, the differing pharmacologic properties provide some rationale for specific choices. As the antiinflammatory dose is greater than the dosage needed for analgesia, an adequate yet safe dosage must be prescribed, depending on the goal of therapy. In addition to the well-known side effects of this group of drugs, specific NSAIDs differ in their effects on the repair rate of tissue, with some increasing the strength of healing ligaments with short-term administration (46, 47). Therefore, the drug of choice to be used in a majority of these conditions provides both analgesic and antiinflammatory action at safe dosages, can be taken on a simple dosing schedule (no more than twice daily), has a low frequency of adverse effects, and has a favorable effect on healing.

The return of the injured athlete to activity depends on several variables: presence of symptoms, with and without activity; adequate rehabilitation of injured structures; and improvement in any preexisting biomechanical abnormalities, including increased flexibility and correction of muscle-strength imbalances. During the rehabilitation process, the athlete may continue to remain active and continue aerobic conditioning, if possible, and strength training on unaffected muscle groups.

Back

The lumbosacral spines of weight lifters are often asked to support a tremendous amount of weight not only acutely but also cumulatively over an extended period of time during training sessions and competitive seasons. Competitive weight lifters have been shown to have a greater incidence of radiographic changes to their lower spine than athletes in other sports. Except in the case of fractures, no correlation between these radiographic changes and lower back pain could be found, because the incidence of lower-back pain is less than the incidence of radiographic changes (48–50). Many of these x-ray findings were noted in asymptomatic male weight lifters who had normal physical exams (50).

The true incidence of lower back injuries in competitive weight lifters is not well-known, although it may be less than previously reported (51, 52). Studies suggesting an increased rate of injuries to the lower back were noted in adolescents (2, 53) and the rate was comparable with that of high school football players (2).

Sprains, strains, and other soft tissue injuries of the lower back are the most common cause of lower-back pain in weight lifters (2). These injuries usually result from a sudden reaching or twisting motion associated with sharp, stabbing, localized pain. The neurologic exam is unremarkable, and radiographs demonstrate no acute findings. Other causes of lower-back pain, including discogenic and nondiscogenic, should be excluded (54, 55). Initially, these injuries are treated with rest and ice for the first 24 to 36 hr and mild NSAIDs. Physical therapy is initiated immediately and emphasizes improvement or maintenance of a full range of painless motion followed by a program of stretching

Table 31.9.
Incidence of Spondylolysis by Plain Radiographs in Selected Sports

Sport	Incidence (%)
Diving	63.2
Weight lifting	36.2
Wrestling	33.0
Gymnastics	32.0
Athletics (mainly track and field)	22.5
College football	15.2
General population	5 to 6

Adapted from Rossi F. Spondylolysis, spondylolithesis and sports. J Sports Med Phys Fittness 1978;18:317–340; and McCarroll JR, Miller JM, Ritter MA. Lumbar spondylolysis and spondylolithesis in college football players. Am J Sports Med 1986;14(5):404–406.

and strengthening exercises. Chronic low-back problems result from improper rehabilitation following prior injury, weak abdominal musculature, increased lumbar lordosis, tight hamstring muscles, and leg length discrepancies.

Weight lifting, along with several other sports that require repetitive hyperextension of the lumbosacral spine, has an increased incidence of spondylolysis (Table 31.9) (56, 57). Spondylolysis can either be a congenital or acquired defect of the pars interarticularis related to a stress-type reaction or a stress-fracture (also described as a fatigue fracture of the pars interarticularis (58–60). It develops following microtrauma caused by repetitive hyperextension of the lumbar spine. This problem often presents as subacute, unilateral, well-localized low-back pain, which is exacerbated by activity and hyperextension. It is often associated with the hyperlordotic position, although not as frequently as is spondylolithesis. On physical exam, the pain is reproduced with lumbar hyperextension and the one-leg lumbar extension test. Tight hamstrings and decreased flexibility are found in up to 80% of these individuals (61). This defect usually occurs at the level of the fifth lumbar vertebrae (62). Lumbosacral radiographs that include obliques are necessary to ensure accurate diagnosis, because a significant number of these lesions are not seen on regular A-P or lateral views (62). If symptoms persist despite normal plain radiographs and conservative therapy (i.e., active rest, antiinflammatory medications, and physical therapy), a bone scan may be necessary to assist with the diagnosis. In addition, a bone scan will help differentiate an acute defect from an old lesion (63).

If a defect is detected, the treatment consists of restricting activities that exacerbate symptoms, especially ones that result in compressive loading of the lumbar spine; selective bracing; and an individualized exercise program. Return to activity is determined by symptoms and progression of muscular development and flexibility. The bone scan may remain positive for several months after adequate healing secondary to remodeling. A fibrous union is common. The long-term significance of a spondolytic defect has yet to be defined, although a recent review implies that a fairly benign course with an incidence of low back pain no more frequent than the general population (64).

Spondylolithesis is the favored displacement or slipping of one vertebra over another and is usually associated with either a pars defect or elongation. This defect usually occurs at the junction of the fifth lumbar vertebrae and sacrum. Spondylolithesis and spondylolysis usually have similar presentations and mechanisms of injury, although the epidemiology of spondylolithesis is not as well-known. The classification of this defect determines the treatment (65). Grade I and II lesions (less than 50% of the A-P diameter of the vertebral body and no neurologic symptoms) can be treated with a conservative exercise program and careful observation for progression of symptoms. The exercise treatment should include an emphasis on flattening of the lumbar lordosis, stretching of the hamstrings and strengthening of the abdominal musculature. Conservative therapy in this group of individuals, especially adolescents, has results similar to those who underwent surgical stabilization (66). When the athlete is asymptomatic he or she is allowed to return to full activity without restrictions, because there is no definite evidence that athletic activity increases the risk of further slippage, especially following an adequate rehabilitation program.

Grade III through IV lesions (slippage over 50% of the A-P diameter of the vertebral body) mandates a discontinuation of sports that require repetitive hyperextension or axial loading, specifically weight lifting. The athlete may engage in sports that do not require axial loading or repetitive hyperextension (e.g., bicycling and swimming). Progressive slippage and/or continued low-back pain in spite of a conservative rehabilitation program, neurologic symptoms that are not cleared by physical therapy, and cosmetic deformity that is unacceptable are indications for surgical referral.

Although the incidence of intervertebral disc problems occurring in weight lifters is not well-known, the frequency of radiographically demonstrated reduction in disc height is increased (49). These problems are the result of extreme loading and abnormal rotational forces, usually occurring in the lower lumbar spine. Disc degeneration occurs with aging as the disc loses hydration and elasticity, becoming more fibrotic (67). The greatest changes occur between the ages of 25 and 35 years of age, a period of life when most lifters are constantly increasing the peak compressive forces applied to their spines (68). The most common cause of this degenerative process is thought to be mechanical (68).

Symptoms of degenerative disc disease and an associated bulging or herniation of the nucleus pulpolsus include lower-back pain exacerbated by coughing, radiation of pain into the lower extremity, paresthesias and neurologic deficits. On physical exam, a pattern of specific dermatome involvement, symptoms (i.e., paresthesias and radiation of pain) reproduced or exaggerated by stretching of the sciatic nerve (some form of a positive straight leg test), and loss of spinal reflex of appropriate level are found. The differential diagnosis of these findings include lumbar spinal stenosis and nondiscogenic causes of sciatica, such as piriformis syndrome, sacroiliitis, iliolumbar syndrome, facet syndrome, quadratus lumborum syndrome, trochanteric bursitis, and ischiogluteal bursitis (54, 55). These causes of nondiscogenic low-back sciatica often accompany pain associated with intervertebral disc disease.

Conservative treatment may be begun if symptoms are stable and of recent onset. Aggressive conservative treatment, including adequate pain control and physical therapy, has been shown successfully to treat herniated nucleus pulposus of the lumbar intervertebral disc compared with surgical intervention, even when a radiculopathy is present (69). Following initial presentation there should be a period of relative rest in which no overhead lifting or axial loading exercises are attempted until symptoms dissipate. Once asymptomatic, the athlete may begin rehabilitative exercises that concentrate on back flexibility, focusing on extension and abdominal muscle strengthening isometrically or in short arc crunches without contracting the hip flexors (70). Biomechanical factors, such as poor resting and lifting postures and muscular imbalances, are corrected. If symptoms progress or are unrelieved with conservative therapy, referral for further diagnostic evaluations and treatment is warranted.

Shoulder

Most injuries of the shoulder in strength-training athletes are the result of strains and overuse problems of the musculature, which include the rotator cuff, biceps, and deltoid. These injuries are usually secondary to poor flexibility, muscle-strength imbalances, and overtraining. Power lifters, as a group, especially demonstrate less flexibility in shoulder movements (71). Unless a complete, macroscopic tear of a muscle has occurred, treatment mainly consists of relative rest, proper medication, and rehabilitative exercise, as has been previously discussed.

Impingement syndrome occurs in weight lifters and involves the rotator cuff musculature (i.e., strains and tendinitis) and associated structures (i.e., bursitis). This syndrome is related to muscular insufficiency or imbalance between the anterior and posterior muscle groups of the rotator cuff and/or glenohumoral instability. Symptoms occur when flexion of the shoulder as the arm is internally rotated causes the muscles of the rotator cuff to rub against the inferior aspects of the acromion process and coracoacromial ligament, resulting in both chronic and acute injury, from tendinitis and bursitis to an acute rupture. This particular movement is replicated during the physical exam in an attempt to elicit symptoms and are the commonly performed tests of impingement.

The rotator cuff muscles may be individually injured by specific mechanisms (44). Subscapularis injury is usually the result of forced or repetitive abduction and external rotation. Injury to the posterior musculature, mainly the teres minor and the infraspinatus muscles, is secondary to forced or repetitive adduction and internal rotation. These muscles are often neglected during strength-training regimens, leading to muscle-strength imbalances. Resisted abduction or forced adduction, which occurs with the snatch maneuver, causes injury to the supraspinatus.

These injuries present with a deep, aching shoulder pain exacerbated by overhead activity. Localization of the pain is often difficult and occasional radiation to lateral shoulder and arm may occur. Further radiation of symptoms may indicate a nerve compression. Duration of symptoms vary and the incidence of chronic shoulder pain is not infrequent.

On physical exam, point tenderness may be present over the involved musculotendinous unit or bursa. The pain of tendinitis or muscle strain is reproduced with specific muscle testing, as in the use of the supraspinatus, or empty can, test to isolate tension in the supraspinatus muscle. Glenohumoral joint instability is demonstrated by documenting passive subluxation of the humeral head on the glenoid fossa and reproducing symptoms by performing apprehension tests. Weakness of the posterior musculature may be present. A positive impingement sign, either Neer's impingement test or Hawkin's sign of impingement, may be present. Plain radiographs are performed to demonstrate suspected fractures or dislocations, although they usually provide little additional information to a thorough physical exam. Magnetic resonance imaging (MRI) may be helpful if a completer tear of the musculature is suspected.

Conservative treatment is usually instituted before obtaining the more elaborate diagnostic studies. If therapy, active rest, NSAIDs, and rehabilitative exercises that concentrate on flexibility and correcting muscle-strength imbalances fail to improve symptoms, further diagnostic studies and possible referral are indicated. Return to activity is determined by resolution of symptoms, return of full range of painless motion, and acquisition of balanced strength.

Condensing osteitis is a dense thickening of the clavicle caused by inflammation and overuse that frequently occur in weight lifters (45). On plain radiographs, sclerosis and enlargement of the medial end of the clavicle is apparent with a normal sternoclavicular joint. Conservative therapy is indicated with activity as limited by pain.

Osteolysis of the distal clavicle has been associated with weight lifting and weight training (72). This injury probably results from excessive stresses being concentrated on the distal part of the clavicle and the acromial process during weight lifting, leading to microfractures of the subchondral bone and subsequent repair. It presents as pain and tenderness of slow onset in the area of the acromioclavicular joint and is usually first noted while bench pressing. Pain worsens without loss of glenohumoral motion. Subluxation of the acromioclavicular joint does not occur. Characteristic radiographic signs include osteoporosis, loss of subchondral bone detail, and cystic changes in the distal part of the clavicle in varying degrees (72–74). Joint scintigraphy may be necessary to confirm the diagnosis. Treatment is conservative with antiinflammatory medication and physical therapy. Surgery is indicated if initial therapy fails to improve symptoms but generally not before 6 to 12 months of treatment.

Elbow

The elbow, because of its importance in the proper execution of several of the major lifts, is the site of numerous reported injuries, though epidemiologic data are limited. Documented injuries involving the elbow and associated structures include ulna neuritis, ruptured biceps (distal) and triceps, and other undefined elbow pains, including brachialis and anconeus injuries, intraarticular difficulties, and nerve impingement (74). Depending on the specific injury and severity, early range of motion exercises are important to maintain full functioning of the joint.

Medial and lateral epicondylitis result from heavy repetitive forearm activity, causing microtrauma to either the extensor or flexor conjoined tendons of the wrist, leading to inflammation and pain. The classic signs of these conditions on physical exam include tenderness over the involved epicondyle and pain exacerbated by either active flexion or extension of the wrist against resistance. This injury is best treated with relative rest, NSAIDs, and a proper strengthening and flexibility program with postexercise cold application. A proximal forearm brace may offer some relief. Surgical release of the conjoined tendons is rarely necessary.

Complete tendinous ruptures of the biceps and triceps are fairly uncommon injuries but have been reported in weight lifters (74, 75). Rupture of the triceps insertion on the olecranon process has been seen primarily during the snatch and the bench press, with its deceleration stress and eccentric contraction. The mechanism of injury that causes rupture of the biceps tendon is probably similar. Complete ruptures usually are fairly apparent on physical exam with dependent ecchymosis; the defect is noted along the musculotendinous unit and there is little or no resistance on specific muscle testing. These injuries frequently require surgical repair.

Repeated or old trauma to the ulnar nerve as it traverses just lateral to the medial epicondyle may result in an ulnar neuropathy. Significant trauma to the nerve may occur secondary to compression of the nerve between the heads of the flexor carpi ulnaris muscle, subluxation of a taut nerve over the medial epicondyle (hypertrophied triceps further promote subluxation of the nerve across the medial epicondyle), lack of full flexibility, partial rupture of the surrounding tissue, and direct trauma to the nerve itself (45, 76). The individual usually presents complaining of medial elbow pain, radiating distally along the ulnar aspect of the forearm and paresthesias along the distribution of the ulnar nerve. A Tinel's test at the elbow may be present (44). Weakness of grip, atrophy of the hypothenar eminence and adductor pollicus muscle, and a positive Wartenburg sign also may be present (76).

If diagnosed early, an ulnar neuropathy may be treated nonsurgically with rest (immobilization if needed), NSAIDs, vitamin B_6, and a thorough rehabilitative exercise program. If problems persist despite conservative therapy, surgical release may be necessary. Full recovery and return to previous level of activity is expected.

Compartment syndromes of the arm, although rare, occur as a result of overuse, usually involving the triceps and biceps muscles (77). These problems present as significant pain along the length of the muscle, representing expansion of the tense facial tissue as a result of the swelling of underlying tissue. Neurologic changes may occur, including paresthesias and motor weakness secondary to ischemic muscle and compression of peripheral nerves. This syndrome is associated with severe pain and muscle weakness on passive stretch of the muscles involved (78). Compartment syndromes can be adequately treated if diagnosed early with rest, ice, NSAIDs, and physical therapy; otherwise, release by fasciotomy, often emergently, is required.

Violent dislocations of the elbow occur often in the weight-training sports. An acute dislocation should be quickly reduced to prevent further soft tissue and neurovascular damage, which are commonly associated with this type of injury. Before reduction, neurovascular exam should be well-documented and radiographs should be taken to determine the presence of coexisting fractures.

Forearm, Wrist, and Hand

Proper forearm, wrist, and hand functioning are an integral part of proper weight lifting technique. With their importance, they lend themselves to be particularly susceptible to injury, especially when lifters fail to get their elbows around in the clean maneuver, forcing the elbow into the knees while the wrist is hyperextended and loaded (45).

The wrist sprain is the most common injury to these structures and is usually the result of hyperextension. Although it is occasionally difficult to distinguish a sprain from a strain, initial management is the same for both: rest, ice, immobilization, and NSAIDs. Radiographs are usually recommended to detect possible fractures and dislocations, particularly scaphoid features and scaphoulnate dissociations.

Fractures and dislocations of the ulna and radius have been reported in weight lifters, although the incidence of such injuries is unknown (79–81). Many of the reported fractures are stress fractures involving the ulna. If a fracture is suspected (well-localized tenderness, palpable periosteal elevation, pain with distant stress of the bone, no improvement of symptoms following a short-term period of rest) and plain radiographs are normal, a bone scan is indicated. These fractures can be treated with restricted activity and immobilization until healing occurs.

Forearm compartment syndromes, which have been noted in the weight-lifting sports, are the result of repetitive use and activity (82). This injury is associated with forearm pain, especially noted with passive dorsiflexion. Treatment consists of rest, ice massages, immobilization, and NSAIDs. If symptoms worsen or are associated with neurovascular compromise, fasciotomy may be required.

Nerve entrapment syndromes, caused by a mechanical compression within a confined anatomic space and/or unusually thick peritendinous tissue pressing a nerve against bone or ligament, occur within several anatomical tunnels of the wrist (45). These tunnels are the radial, pronator, cubital, carpal, and ulnar at the wrist (Guyon's canal). The sport's techniques require tremendous weight to be placed on the extended wrist, increasing risk of developing these problems. Following prompt and accurate diagnosis, this condition is best treated with rest, immobilization, ice massages, and NSAIDs. If symptoms persist with prolonged or worsening neurovascular compromise, surgical decompression is indicated.

Wrist ganglions are considered to be herniations of the joint capsule or synovial sheath of the tendon and frequently occur about the wrist joint. Ganglions usually develop following a sprain on the dorsal aspect of the wrist. Unless symptomatic, treatment of wrist ganglions is not necessary.

The most frequently encountered problems of the hands occur as the result of callus formation. Calluses are the result of the shearing forces produced while gripping the knurled bar. They are vulnerable to tears and cracks, with subsequent exposure of the underlying dermis and infection of the surrounding tissue (83). Treatment of torn calluses consists of properly protecting the underlying skin. As lack of elasticity predisposes the callus to tearing, the best preventive measure against this complication entails the use of an emery file to reduce the callus, especially following bathing, and the application of a lanolin hand lotion to help maintain the skin's elasticity.

Groin and Thigh

Acute injuries to the large musculature associated with the hip and knee occur with weight lifting. The hamstrings are particularly susceptible to acute strains for several reasons: lack of flexibility; strength imbalance between quadriceps and hamstrings; strength imbalance between hamstrings in both legs; and activities that cause excessive fatigue of the hamstrings (45). Initial treatment consists of rest, ice massages, elevation, and compression, with additional treatment targeted at correcting the underlying abnormalities. Firm-fitting shorts, such as used by cyclists, may provide additional support during rehabilitation.

In dealing with such sites of susceptible injury, it is important to perform the proper preventive measures: attention to balanced strength; proper flexibility exercises; adherence to the principle of specificity of training to acclimate the muscular to specific demands; biomechanical abnormalities; and proper warmup and cooldown. Recurrent injuries to these muscle groups probably reflect a combination of the above abnormalities in addition to inadequate rehabilitation of previous injuries.

Knee

Contrary to commonly held beliefs and previous recommendations (84), weight lifting is not commonly associated with an increased risk of knee injury (2, 85).

In fact, proper strength training maintains (and may increase) the stability of the joint and its ligaments (86, 87). Compared with athletes of other sports who demonstrate increased ligamentous laxity following a period of their selected activity, performing a session of squats resulted in no change in the anterior-posterior laxity noted in the knee joint as measured by a mechanical device (88). When knee injuries do occur, they are usually the result of factors other than the biomechanical aspects of the lifts themselves: inadequate warmup and/or stretching; improper technique; poor flexibility; attempting new or unfamiliar techniques; performing maximal efforts; or participating in other activities besides weight lifting (45, 74). The initial treatment of knee injuries, as with other soft tissue problems, consists of rest, ice, elevation, and protection of the area from further injury. After the initial phase of therapy, treatment is aimed at correcting underlying abnormalities.

Patellar tendinitis results from excessive, repetitive contractile forces of the quadriceps, causing microscopic tears of the musculotendinous unit. This repeated stress and loading, which also inhibits the healing process, ultimately leads to inflammation, pain, and dysfunction. This condition is worsened by activities that encourage full range of active motion of the knee joint, which places immense stress on the tendon and associated structures, e.g., squats, squat snatches, and squat cleans.

Patella tendinitis usually presents as pain just below the inferior aspect of the patella. The pain initially is present following activity, and may progress to pain at the onset of activity that diminishes with warmup. Severe tendinitis is distinguished by the presence of constant pain and swelling. Treatment is similar to that described for patellofemoral problems, with the possibility of an increased benefit of using eccentric exercises early in the strengthening problem. The use of a patellar-tendon band may provide further support and relief.

The patellofemoral syndrome, with the associated arthroscopic diagnosis of chondromalacia patellae, is a degenerative process that results in the softening of the hyaline cartilage on the undersurface of the patella and the articulating condyles of the femur (articular cartilage). Several factors predispose the weight lifter to this condition: *(a)* malalignment of the thigh and the lower leg, resulting in an increased Q-angle; *(b)* abnormally small or high-riding patella; *(c)* deformity of the patella or femur; and *(d)* tight hamstrings or iliotibial band. This condition symptomatically presents with anterior knee pain with active flexion, weakness, subjective feelings of apprehension associated with subluxation, tenderness about the patella and the patellar facets, hypermobile patella, and patella crepitus. Treatment of this condition consists of rest and ice during the acute phase, followed by active rehabilitation including stretching and strengthening, specifically in arcs of motion that do not produce symptoms, and selective bracing (89). Isokinetic rehabilitative strengthening programs afford a definite advantage in patellofemoral syndromes.

Bursitis, true inflammation of one or more of the bursae that surround the knee joint, is caused by either the repetitive compressional forces created by the large muscle groups during flexion and extension, instability of the knee joint secondary to osteoarthritis and previous internal derangement, or direct trauma to the bursae. Localized treatment with ice massages and protection from further injury in addition to NSAIDs are the therapies of choice. Local injection of a corticosteroid and anesthetic provide almost immediate relief and is indicated for both severe bursitis or more prolonged pain refractory to physical modalities and oral agents. The bursa most often overlooked is anserine bursitis, a cause of chronic or acute medial compartment pain. The pes anserine bursa is inferior and slightly anterior to the inferior insertion of the medial collateral ligament. Pes anserine bursitis is a common sequala of improper technique in performing both squats and repetitive power cleans.

Ligamentous injuries about the knee primarily involve the medial and lateral collateral ligaments and usually are the result of excessive knee rotation, abnormal valgus or varus stress, hyperflexion, or hyperextension. These injuries present as localized pain, swelling, and tenderness over the involved structure. Stress placed on the ligament may or may not exacerbate the symptoms, depending on the presence of a partial versus a complete tear of the ligament. These injuries are treated initially with rest, ice massages, and protected motion. Complete tears of these structures require evaluation by a specialist. Complete return to previous level of activity is expected and with proper rehabilitative exercises, these structures are strengthened with weight training and aerobic exercises such as bicycling.

Meniscal and cruciate ligament injuries (also known as internal derangements of the knee) are usually the result of a direct blow to the knee, forced hyperextension, or an abnormal twist. They also may develop secondary to chronic but repetitive minor injury. These injuries commonly present as acute onset of pain (especially following an audible "pop" or "snap"), swelling that occurs immediately or within a few hours of the injury, inability to fully extend or flex the knee, pain with walking or standing, or the sensation of joint instability. Injuries of this type are usually associated with a significant effusion which if immediately aspirated reveals a hemarthrosis; they should be radiographed to assist with the diagnosis and determine the presence of possible fractures. Arthrocentesis and joint fluid analysis assists in the differentiation of possible etiologies of the effusion, because rheumatic syndromes, such as Reiter's syndrome, may also present with acute onset knee with effusion. The presence of a hemarthrosis is highly correlated with the tearing of the cruciate ligaments. Initial therapy includes protecting the joint from additional injury and providing adequate relief, usually with a NSAID. Partial anterior cruciate tears are frequently rehabilitated successfully without surgery. Complete or recurrent tears usually require surgical intervention, but significant rehabilitation must follow, and current surgical technique for repair will almost always preclude competitive lifting for 12 months.

Particular attention to strengthening the hamstrings is one important goal and a strength ratio with the quadriceps femoris of 2:3 or even 3:4 is desired. Musculotendinous tears and ruptures of the patella tendon, gastrocnemius tendon, and distal insertions of the hamstrings have been reported in weight lifters. These injuries are often believed to occur at sites in the tendon weakened by overuse. Partial tears can usually be treated conservatively, whereas complete tears require surgical evaluation.

Ankle and Foot

Fortunately for weight-lifting athletes who require a solid foundation from which to lift the tremendous amount of weight, ankle and foot injuries in their sports are rare. The incidence of ankle sprains is rare, contrary to the incidence of this injury in other sports. A number of injuries occur from dropped weight plates or from wearing of overtight shoes, which causes entrapment of the peroneal nerve.

Children and Strength Training

Although recent research has demonstrated short-term programs in which prepubescent athletes can increase strength without risk of significant injury (90–92), studies on long-term weight training; weight training in less-supervised programs; and the effects of weight training on strength, injury prevention, and improved performance are lacking. Anecdotal reports on strength training in pubescent athletes often detail significant musculoskeletal injuries, including epiphyseal fractures, ruptured intervertebral disks, and low-back bony disruptions, especially when performing the major lifts (53, 80, 93). The true incidence of these significant injuries is not well-known, even though several studies have attempted to quantify the injury rate. Considering the flaws associated with the limited data on the incidence of injuries in adolescent weight lifters, the incidence of injury in this group of athletes compares favorably with the incidence of injuries in other sports (1).

The sports of weight lifting, power lifting, and bodybuilding are gaining increased popularity among teenagers. The number of teenagers joining established associations is increasing, with the USWF reporting close to 600 teenage members and the USPF reporting more than 3000 teenage members. Approximately 8500 adolescents are formally involved in the sport of bodybuilding.

With the increased popularity of these sports among the pediatric population, the American Academy of Pediatrics has established the following recommendations (94):

1. Strength training programs for prepubescent, pubescent, and postpubescent athletes should be permitted only if conducted by well-trained adults. The adults should be qualified to plan progress appropriate to the athletes' stage of maturation, which should be assessed objectively by medical personnel.
2. Unless good data become available that demonstrate safety, children and adolescents should avoid the practice of weight lifting, power lifting and bodybuilding as well as the repetitive use of maximal amounts of weight in strength-training programs until they have reached the Tanner stage 5 level of developmental maturity.

Women and Strength Training

Women participating in weight training and competing in weight lifting and bodybuilding has become a common occurrence, despite the outdated notion that strength is solely a masculine quality. The involvement of women in the strength-training sports has created an interest in the relative strength of females compared with males. If static measures of strength are used, absolute strength in females is less than that of males (95). These differences in strength decrease if anatomic and physiologic variations are considered (96). Gains in strength and hypertrophy of musculature is expected with training in females, although not to the extent found in males (97).

Although the benefits of a successful weight-training program in males is well-documented, the benefits of such a program in females are not as well-known. Some of the benefits females appear to gain from weight training are increased lean body mass and improved psychological profile, including being somewhat less anxious, neurotic, depressed, angry, and confused and more extroverted, vigorous, and self-motivated than the general public (98). Furthermore, the density of bone in weight lifters is increased and whether this alteration results in a decreased incidence of osteoporosis in later life is not known.

Intense weight training may have several deleterious effects on female physiology, particularly to normal menstrual functioning. Exercise-associated amenorrhea (EAA) is associated with several endurance sports. Although the exact incidence is unknown, EAA also has been associated with competitive female bodybuilders and is probably found in other strength-training women involved in intense training (99).

Elderly and Strength Training

National and international weightlifters usually obtain their maximal lifts between the ages of 28 and 34 years. As a seemingly dependent variable of the aging process, a decline in measurable strength occurs (100). Although total strength may decrease, the ability to increase strength and of the muscle to hypertrophy through a proper program of resistive exercises appears to be maintained, even in the very old (101, 102). Gains in strength during a power-lifting training program were demonstrated by a 50-year-old retired competitive, Olympic-style weight lifter (103). The effect of a regular, long-term program of strength training on the decline of strength with age is not known but may similar to the slower decline in aerobic fitness with aging noted in individuals who maintain a regular program of endurance exercise (104).

REFERENCES

1. Webb DR. Strength training in children and adolescents. Pediatr Clin North Am 1990;37(5)1187–1210.
2. Risser WL. Musculoskeletal injuries caused by weight training. Clin Pediatr 1990;29(6):306–310.
3. Garrick JG, Requa R. Medical care and injury surveillance in the high school setting. Phys Sportsmed 1981;9(2):115–120.
4. George DH, Stakiw K, Wright CJ. Fatal accident with weight-lifting equipment: implications for safety standards. Can Med Assoc 1989;140:925–926.
5. National Injury Information Clearinghouse. 1990.
6. Harman EA, Rosenstein RM, Fryman PN, Nigro GA. Effects of a belt on intra-abdominal pressure during weight lifting. Med Sci Sports Exerc 1989;21(2):186–190.
7. Lander JE, Simonton RL, Giacobbe JK. The effectiveness of weight-belts during the squat exercise. Med Sci Sports Exerc 1990; 22(1)117–126.
8. Lander JE, Bates BT, Devita P. Biomechanics of the squat exercise using a modified center of mass bar. Med Sci Sports Exerc 1986;18(4):469–478.
9. Garhammer J. Safety equipment in weightlifting. In: Chandler J, Stone MH, eds. United States Weightlifting Federation Safety Manual. 1990:57–78.
10. Atha J. Strengthening muscle. Exerc Sports Rev 1981;91–73.
11. Powers SK, Howley ET. Exercise physiology: theory and application to fitness and performance. Dubuque, IA: Brown, 1990.
12. Smith MJ. Muscle fiber type: their relationship to athletic training and rehabilitation. Orthop Clin North Am 1983;14(2):403–411.
13. Deleted in pages.
14. Stone MH. Physical and physiological preparation for weightlifting. In: Chandler J, Stone MH, eds. United States Weightlifting Federation Safety Manual 1990:79–101.
15. Haupt HA, Rovere GD. Anabolic steroids: a review of the literature. Am J Sports Med 1984;12(6):469–484.
16. Elashoff JD, Jacknow AD, Shains SG, Braunstein GD. Effects of anabolic-androgenic steroids on muscular strength. Ann Intern Med 1991;115(5):387–393.
17. Hill JA, Suker JR, Sacks K, Brighman C. The athletic polydrug abuse phenomenon [A case report]. Am J Sports Med 1983;11(4):269–271.
18. MacDougall D, Tuxen D, Sale D, Sexton A, Moroz J, Sutton J. Direct measurement of arterial blood pressure during heavy resistance training. Med Sci Sports Exerc 1983;15:158.
19. Hagberg JM, Ehsani AA, Goldring D, Hernandez A, Sinacore DR, Holloszy JO. Effect of weight training on blood pressure and hemodynamics in hypertensive adolescents. J Pediatr 1984;104:147–151.
20. Goldberg, AP. Aerobic and resistive exercise modify risk factors for coronary heart disease. Med Sci Sport Exerc 1989;21(6)669–674.
21. Saltin B, Astrand P. Maximal oxygen uptake in athletes. J Appl Physiol 1967;23(3):353–358.
22. Fahey TD, Akka L, Rolph R. Body composition and $\dot{V}_{O_{2max}}$ of exceptional weight-trained athletes. J Appl Physiol 1975;39(4):559–561.
23. Spitler DL, Diaz FJ, Horvath SM, Wright JE. Body composition and maximal aerobic capacity of bodybuilders. J Sports Med 1980;20:181–188.
24. Dudley GA, Djamil R. Incompatibility of endurance- and strength-training modes of exercise. J Appl Physiol 1985;59(5):1446–1451.
25. Deleted in pages.
26. Deleted in pages.
27. Deleted in pages.
28. Hurley BF, Seals DR, Hagberg JM, et al. High-density-lipoprotein cholesterol in bodybuilders v powerlifters: negative effects of androgen use. 1984;JAMA 252(4):507–513.
29. Goldberg L, Elliott DL, Schutz RW, Kloster FE. Changes in lipid and lipoproteing levels after weight training. JAMA 1984;252(4):504–506.
30. Katch VL, Katch FI, Moffatt R, Gittleson M. Muscular development and lean body weight in body builders and weight lifters. Med Sci Sport Exerc 1980;12(5):340–344.
31. Simoneaux SF, Murphy BJ, Tehranzadeh J. Spontaneous pneumothorax in a weight lifter. Am J Sports Med 1990;18(6):647–648.
32. McKeag DB. Preparticipation screening of the potential athlete. Clin Sports Med 1989;8(3)373–397.
33. Maron BJ, Roberts WC, McAllister HA, Rosing DR, Epstein SE. Sudden death in young athletes. Circulation 1980;62(2):218–229.
34. Menapace FJ, Hammer WJ, Ritzer TF, et al. Left ventricular size in competitive weight lifters: an echocardiographic study. Med Sci Sports Exerc 1982;14(1)72–75.
35. Pelliccia AM, Maron BJ, Spataro A, Proschan MA, Spirito P. The upper limit of physiologic cardiac hypertrophy in highly trained elite athletes. N Engl J Med 1991;324:295–301.
36. Pearson AC, Schiff M, Mrosek D, Labovitz AJ, Williams GA. Left ventricular diastolic function in weight lifters. Am J Cardiol 1986;58:1254–1259.
37. Rooke ED. Benign exertional headache. Med Clin North Am 1968;52(4):801–808.
38. Perry WJ. Exertional headache. Phys Sportsmed 1985;13(10):95–99.
39. Carswell H. Headaches: a weighty problem for lifters? Phys Sportsmed 1984;12(7):23.
40. deVirgilo C, Nelson RJ, Milliken J, et al. Ascending aortic dissection in weight lifters with cystic medial degeneration. Ann Thorac Surg 1990;49:638–642.
41. Doriguzzi C, Palmucci I, Mongini T. Body building and rhabdomyolysis. J Neurol Neurosurg Psychiatry 1990;53(9)806–807.
42. Hodgkinson DJ. Chest wall deformities and their correction in bodybuilders. Ann Plast Surg 1990;25:181–187.
43. Balmaseda MT, Wunder JA, Gordon C, Cannell C. Posttraumatic syringomyelia associated with heavy weightlifting exercises: case report. Arch Phys Med Rehabil 1988;69:970–972.
44. Garrick JC, Webb DR. Sports injuries: diagnosis and management. Philadlphia: WB Saunders, 1990.
45. Herrik R, Stoessel L. Prevention, diagnosis, and treatment of common weightlifting injuries. In: Chandler J, Stone MH, eds. United States Weightlifting Federation safety manuel. 1990;30–45.
46. Tornkvist H, Lindholm TS, Netz P, Stromberg L, Linholm TC. Effect of ibuprofen and indomethacin on bone metabolism reflected on bone strength. Clin Orthop 187:255–259.
47. Dahers LE, Gilbert JA, Lester GE, Taft TN, Payne LZ. The effect of a nonsteroidal anti-inflammatory drug on the healing of ligaments. Am J Sports Med 1988;16(6):641–646.
48. Aggrawal ND, Kaur S, Mathur DN. A study of changes in the spine in weight lifters and other athletes. Br J Sports Med 1979;13:58–61.
49. Granhed H, Morelli B. Low back pain among retired wrestlers and heavyweight lifters. Am J Sports Med 1988;16(5):530–533.
50. Niethard FU, Gussbacher A. Weight lifting and the spine. Back Lett 5(6):6.
51. Kuland DN, Dewey JB, Brubaker CE, Roberts JR. Olympic weightlifting injuries. Phys Sportsmed 1978;111–119.
52. Davies JE. The spine in sports–injuries, prevention and treatment. Bri J Sports Med 1980;14:18–20.
53. Brown EW, Kimball RG. Medical history associated with adolescent powerlifting. Pediatrics 1983;72(5):636–644.
54. Namey TC. Diagnosis and treatment of nondiscogenic low back pain and sciatica: part I. J Pain Manage 1990;207–213.
55. Namey TC. Diagnosis and treatment of nondiscogenic low back pain and sciatica: part II. J. Pain Manage 1990;328–333.
56. Kotani PT, Ichikawa N, Wakabayashi W, Yoshii T, Koshimune M. Studies of spondylolysis found among weight lifters. Bri J Sports Med 1971;6:4–7.
57. Rossi F. Spondylolysis, spondylolithesis and sports. J Sports Med Phys Fitness 1978;18:317–340.
58. McCarroll JR, Miller JM, Ritter MA. Lumbar spondylolysis and spondylolithesis in college football players. Am J Sports Med 1986;14(5):404–406.
59. Deleted in pages.
60. Deleted in pages.
61. Hensinger RN. Spondylolysis and spondylolithesis in children and adolescents. J Bone Joint Surg 1989;71A(7):1098–1107.
62. Libson E, Bloom RA, Dinari G, Robin GC. Oblique lumbar spine

radiographs: importance in young patients. Radiology 1984;151:89–90.
63. Namey TC. Nuclear medicine and special radiologic imaging and technique in the diagnosis of rheumatic disorders. In: Kelley, Harris, Sledge, eds. Textbook of rheumatology. 2nd ed. Philadelphia: WB Saunders 1986:622–650.
64. Seitsalo S. Spondylolithesis, often benign. Back Lett 5(2):2.
65. Weiker GG. Evaluation and treatment of common spine and trunk problems. Clin Sports Med 1989;8(3):399–417.
66. Seitsalo S. Operative and conservative treatment of moderate spondylolithesis in young patients. J Bone Joint Surg 1990;72B(5):908–913.
67. Urban JPG, McMullin. Swelling. Pressure of the lumbar intervertebral discs: influence of age, spinal level, composition, and degeneration. Spine 1988;13(2):179–187.
68. Miller JAA, Schnatz C, Schultz AB. Lumbar disc degeneration: correlation with age, sex, and spine level in 600 autopsy specimens. Spine 1988;13(2):173–177.
69. Saal JA, Saal JS. Nonoperative treatment of herniated lumbar intervertebral disc with radiculopathy. Spine 1989;14(4):431–437.
70. Feeler LC. Weight lifting. Spine 1990;4(2):366–376.
71. Chang DE, Buschbacher LP. Edlich RF. Limited joint mobility in power lifters. Am J Sports Med 1988;16(3):280–284.
72. Cahill BR. Osteolysis of the distal part of the clavicle in male athletes. J Bone Joint Surg 1982;64(7):1053–1058.
73. Seymour EQ. Osteolysis of the clavicular tip associated with repeated minor trauma to the shoulder. Radiology 1977;123(56):56.
74. Herrick RT, Stone M, Herrick S. Injuries of strength–power athletes with special reference to the knee. Am Med Athletic Assoc 1986;1(4):12–14.
75. Bach BR, Warren RF, Wickiewicz TL. Ticeps rupture: a case report and literature review. Am J Sports Med 1987;15(3):285–289.
76. Dangles CJ, Bilos ZJ. Unlar nerve neuritis in a world champion weightlifter. Am J Sports Med 1980;8(6):443–445.
77. Segan DJ, Sladek EC, Gomez J, McCoy J, Cairns DA. Weight lifting as a cause of bilateral upper extremity compartment syndrome. Phys Sportsmed 1988;16(10):73–76.
78. Braddom RI, Wolfe C. Musculocutaneous nerve injury after heavy exercise. Arch Phys Med Rehabil 1978;59:290–293.
79. Francobandiera C, Maffulli N, Lepord L. Distal radio-ulnar joint dislocation, ulna volar in a female body builder. Med Sci Sports Exerc 1990;22(2):155–158.
80. Gumbs V, Segal D, Halligan JB, Lower G. Bilateral distal radius and ulnar fractures in adolescent weight lifters. Am J Sports Med 1982;10(6):375–379.
81. Hamilton HK. Stress fracture of the diaphysis of the ulna in a body builder. Am J Sports Med 1984;12(5):405–406.
82. Bird CB, McCoy JW. Weight-lifting as a cause of compartment syndrome in the forearm. J Bone Joint Surg 1983;406.
83. Deleted in pages.
84. Klein KK. The deep squat exercise as utilized in weight training for athletics and its effect on the ligaments of the knee. 1961;15(1):6–23.
85. Kulund DN, Tottossy MS. Warm-up, strength, and power. Orthop Clin North Am 1989;14(2):427–448.
86. Chandler TJ, Wilson GD, Stone MH. The effect of the squat exercise on knee stability. Med Sci Sports Exerc 1989;21(3):299–303.
87. Tipton CM, Matthes RD, Maynard JA, Carey RA. The influence of physical activity on ligaments and tendons. Med Sci Sports 1975;7(3):165–175.
88. Steiner ME, Grana WA, Chillag K, Schelberg-Karnes E. The effect of exercise on anterior-posterior knee laxity. Am J Sports Med 1986;14(1):24–29.
89. Brunet ME, Stewart GW. Patellofermoral rehabilitation. Clin Sports Med 1989;8(2):319–329.
90. Rians CB, Weltman A, Cahill BR, Janney CA, Tippett SR, Katch FI. Strength training for prepubescent males: is it safe? Am J Sports Med 1987;15(5):483–489.
91. Servedio FJ, Bartels RL, Hamlin RL, Teske D, Shaffer T, Servidio A. The effects of weight training, using Olympic style lifts, on various physiological variables in pre-pubescent boys. Med Sci Sport Exerc 1985;17(2):288.
92. Sewall L, Micheli LJ. Strength training for children. J Pediatr Orthop 1986;6:143–146.
93. Brady T, Cahill B, Bodnar LM. Weight training related injuries in the high school athlete. Am J Sports Med 1982;10(1):1–5.
94. American Academy of Pediatrics. Strength training, weight and power lifting, and body building by children and adolescents. Pediatrics. 1990;86(5):801–803.
95. Laubach LL. Comparative muscular strength of men and women: a review of the literature. Aviat Space Envirn Med 1976;47(5):534–542.
96. Holloway JB, Baechle TR. Strength training for female athletes. Sports Med 1990;9(4):216–228.
97. O'Shea JP, Wegner J. Power weight training and the female athlete. Phys Sportsmed 1981;9(6):109–120.
98. Freedson PS, Mihevic PM, Loucks AB, Girandola RN. Physique, body composition, and psychological characteristics of competitive female body builders. Phys Sportsmed 1983;11(5):85–93.
99. Elliott DL, Goldberg L. Weight lifting and amenorrhea [letter] JAMA 1983;249(3):354.
100. Deleted in pages.
101. Frontera WR, Meredith CN, O'Reilly KP, Knuttgen HG, Evans WJ. Strength conditioning in older men: skeletal muscle hypertrophy and improved function. J Appl Physiol 1988;64(3):1038–1044.
102. Fiatarone MA, Marks EC, Ryan ND, Meredith CN, Lipsitz LA, Evans WJ. High-intensity strength training in nonagenarians. JAMA 1990;2639(22):3029–3034.
103. O'Shea JP. Masters power weight training. Phys Sportsmed 1981;9(8):133–137.
104. Deleted in pages.

32 / RACQUET SPORTS

W. Benjamin Kibler and T. Jeff Chandler

Tennis

Tennis is the widest played of all the racquet sports. Several million people play tennis on a regular basis. Of these, 5000 to 8000 play in tournaments sanctioned by the United States Tennis Association, while approximately 800 play tennis professionally. Only recently have concerted efforts been made to understand the sports science of tennis. However, within the last five years, great strides have been made in understanding the biomechanics, physiology, psychology, and sports medicine of tennis, largely through research funded by the U.S. Tennis Association. On this base of information, programs can be developed for better identification of injuries, for preventative conditioning programs, and for better skill acquisition programs.

Model for Sport Evaluation

To better evaluate the demands of a given sport, a model was developed to show how the inherent demands of the sport interact with the individual athlete to produce "results," either performance and/or injury (Fig. 32.1). This model is certainly not unique to tennis, but provides a good method of assessing "intrinsic" factors (those related to the athlete that can be modified and improved) and "extrinsic" factors (those associated with playing the game that usually must be dealt with rather than modified). Physicians and players are usually too concerned with the right-hand side of the equation, looking at performance or injury. Actually, improvement in performance and decrease in injury risk can be more effectively handled by more attention to the left-hand side of the equation. The knowledge collected in each of these areas is presented below.

Tennis-Specific Demands

Anatomic and Biomechanical Demands

Shoulder. Tennis imposes large demands on the shoulder area, including the glenohumeral, acromion-clavicular, and scapulo-thoracic joints (Fig. 32.2) in terms of motion, loads, and velocities. The scapula moves on the thorax from full retraction in the "backscratch" position of cocking, to full protraction around the curve of the thorax in follow through, a distance of up to 18 cm. It also rotates through an arc of 65° to allow the rotator cuff to move under the acromion in shoulder abduction (Fig. 32.3). The glenohumeral joint moves through an arc of around 130°, from 50° external rotation to about 80° internal rotation. This rotation must stay centered in the glenoid on a rapidly moving scapula.

The loads on the anterior aspect of the glenoid in the throwing motion have been estimated to be two times body weight (1). In unpublished data collected on three elite male tennis players at the University of Kentucky Biodynamics Laboratory (2), the peak velocity of a tennis racquet in the serve ranged from 62 to 72 miles per hour. Corresponding ball velocities were measured at 83 to 125 miles per hour on the serve. This speed is achieved approximately 0.2 to 0.3 seconds after the near zero velocity of the "back scratch" position of cocking. The shoulder was internally rotating at 1140° to 1715° per second to achieve these velocities. Even in the ground strokes, the racquet achieves velocities of 52 to 56 miles per hour in the forehand and 40 to 47 miles per hour in the backhand. Ball velocities were 80 to 85 miles per hour and 65 to 70 miles per hour in the forehand and backhand, respectively.

These motions and forces are generated and controlled by coordinated muscle contraction. At the shoulder, the forces are the summation of the kinetic chain activity that starts with the ground reaction force in the legs and proceeds to the shoulder. At the shoulder, the forces are transmitted through a graded coordinated muscular firing pattern (Fig. 32.4) to the arm and then to the racquet. The firing pattern allows early scapular stabilization, early acromial elevation, rotator cuff firing, anterior force generation, and posterior force regulation in follow through. It is interesting to note that many muscles contribute to force generation to achieve high velocities, but relatively few muscles contribute to force regulation. The work of Jobe and asso-

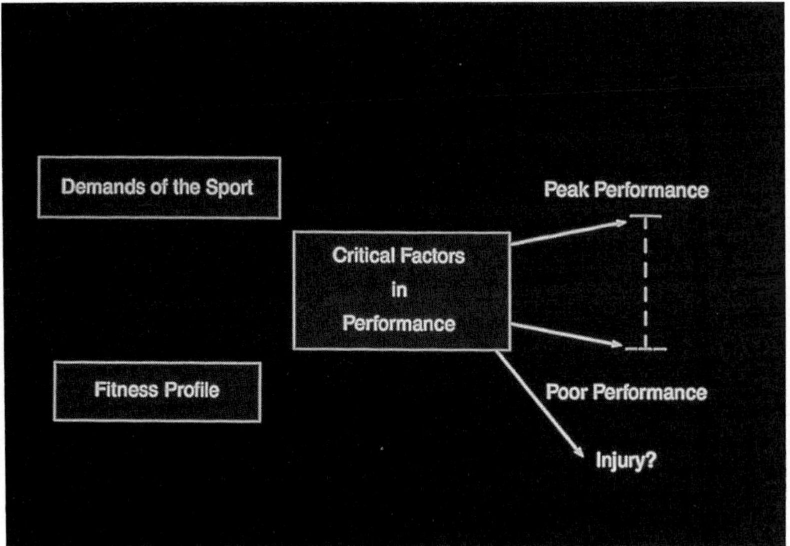

Figure 32.1. Critical Point Model.

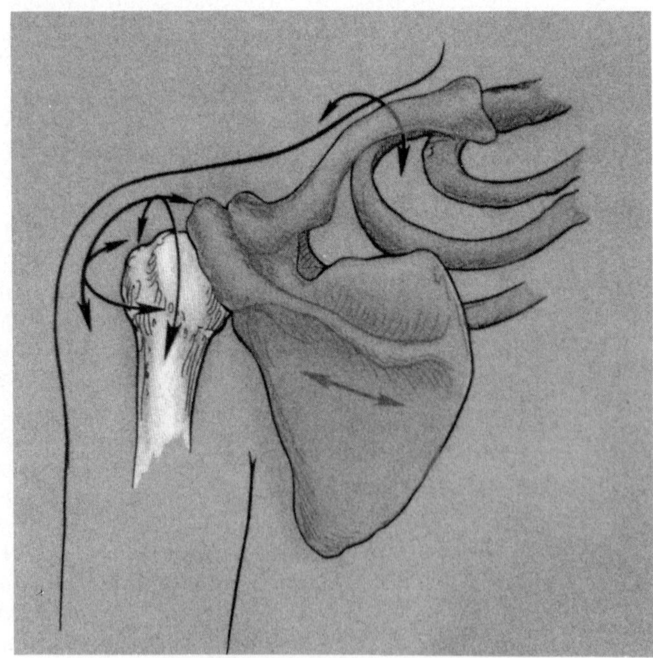

Figure 32.2. Shoulder joint complex.

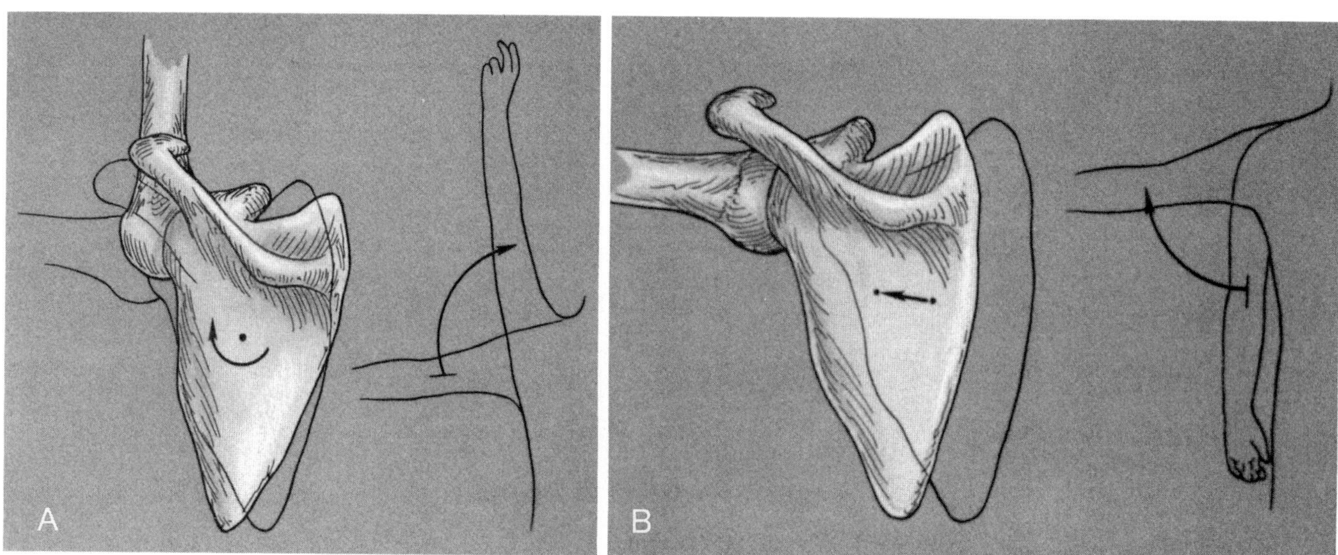

Figure 32.3 A,B. Scapular rotation.

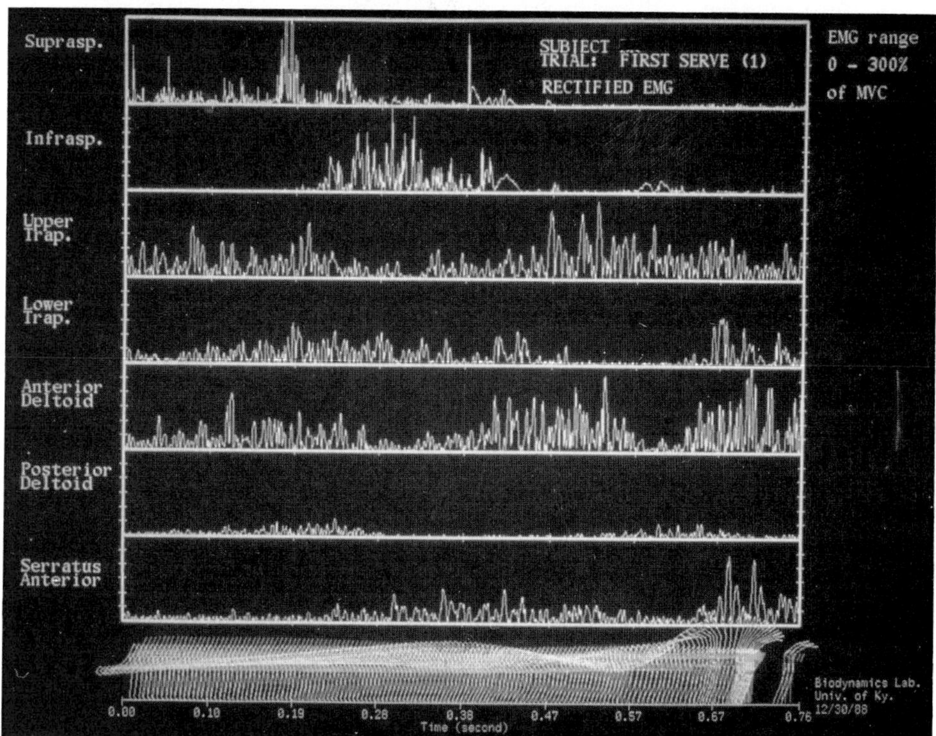

Figure 32.4. Muscle firing pattern. High speed video and integrated EMG of tennis serve. The scapular stabilizing upper trapezius, lower trapezius, and serratus anterior muscles work concentrically to stabilize the scapula. Later, they work eccentrically to regulate and dissipate the generated forces. In each phase of the motion, the muscles are coordinated to maximize the effort and stabilize the joint. Reprinted by permission from Contemp Orthop 1991;22(5):525–532.

ciates (3–5) should be consulted for a more in-depth discussion of the firing patterns in normal and abnormal injured throwing motions.

Arm. The elbow, forearm, and wrist have demands placed on them because they must absorb most of the rotational torque transmitted from an off-center hit. In addition, they have extra stress applied to them as a result of the "power game" that is the dominant style practiced and taught at this time. In this style, more extreme positions of the racquet in the hand (full "western" grip) and limitation of shoulder motion in favor of an "open" stance and "windshield wiper" stroke, create more velocity of the ball, but put extra stress on the elbow and forearm (Figs. 32.5, 6).

The elbow has a lot of motion in the serve, flexing to around 120° in cocking and extending to around 15°–20° at ball impact. Extension velocity in the serve is around 900° per sec. The elbow does not have much motion on the ground strokes in accomplished tennis players (2). Acceleration and deceleration of the elbow in the serve, forearm pronation in the serve, and elbow flexor and extensor muscle load absorption in ground

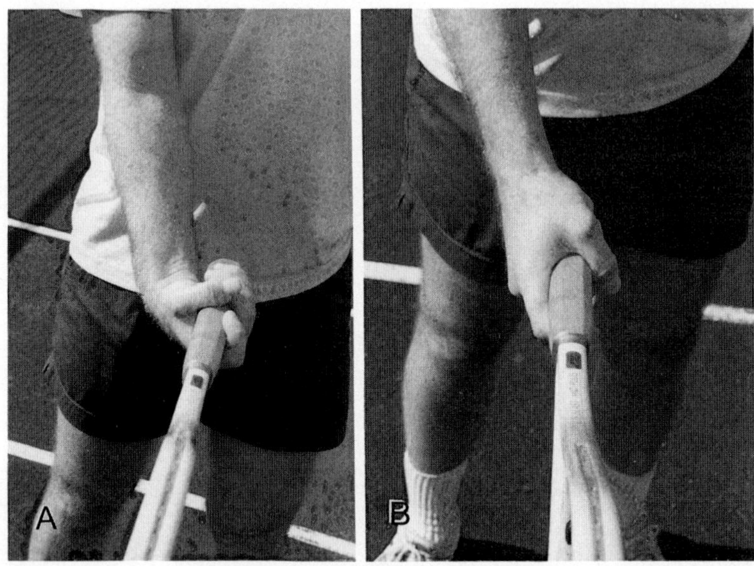

Figure 32.5. **A,** Western grip; **B,** Eastern grip.

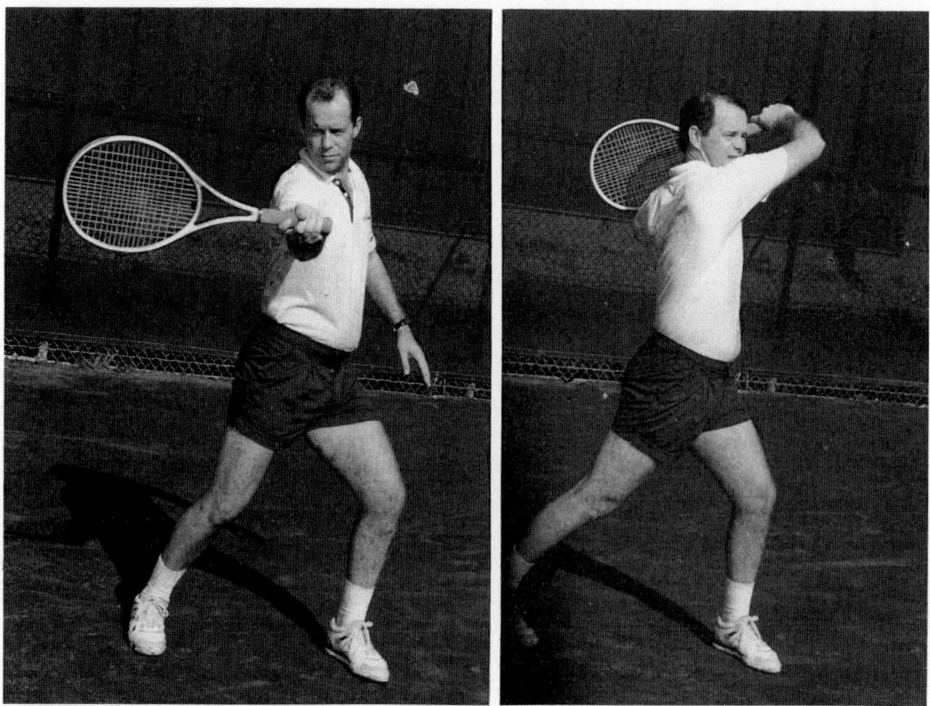

Figure 32.6 A, B. "Windshield wiper" forehand.

strokes are the major ways that muscles act around the arm.

Back, Trunk, and Hips. This large area is vitally important as a center of rotation and as a transfer link for the large forces generated in the legs to be passed on to the shoulder and arm. Rotations of the hips and trunk are large in all of the tennis strokes. This rotation is around 300° per sec on the serve, is as high as 500° per sec on the forehand, and is around 200° per sec on the backhand. Trunk rotational arcs are about 80° on the serve, 60° to 90° on the forehand (depending on foot position), and 60° on the backhand. Muscular activity is important in guiding these motions and stabilizing the hips so that trunk rotation can occur. The oblique abdominal muscles, the rectus abdominis, and the intrinsic trunk rotators are most active.

Leg. The legs are subject to demands specific to tennis and also to the demands inherent in running, stopping, and cutting. The leg contralateral from the serving arm undergoes slight flexion in cocking, then rapid extension in acceleration. Ground reaction forces peak with maximal flexion of the front leg. Muscular contractions in the quadriceps are most important in eccentric work, absorbing the load as the front knee flexes. The "sprint, stop, and cut" nature of running in tennis puts repetitive demands on the bones, ligaments, and muscles to absorb the shear forces.

Metabolic Demands

The metabolic demands in the sport of tennis have been characterized by Fox (6) as being approximately 70% alactic anaerobic, 20% lactic anaerobic, and 10% aerobic. Of course this varies with the age of the player, the skill level, the skill level of the competition, and the style of play. Metabolic specificity in the sport of tennis dictates that the alactic anaerobic energy system is the primary system used in the sport.

The relative duration of each of the three primary energy systems indicates that the first 10 to 15 seconds of maximal exercise is alactic anaerobic. Because tennis is not a sport of constant maximal exertion, much of the energy in a tennis match comes from the alactic component. Recovery from this alactic anaerobic work, particularly alactic oxygen debt, can take place during low intensity exercise or short rest periods. Within 20 seconds, 50% of the depleted ATP is replenished; in 40 seconds 75% is replenished; and in 60 sec, 87% is replenished (7).

It is likely that playing tennis confers some degree of cardiorespiratory fitness (8). There is an increasing body of data to suggest that repeated short bursts of energy, such as the metabolic work patterns in tennis, may improve aerobic endurance (9). Particularly for the recreational tennis player, this would depend on whether the individual plays singles or doubles, the level of competition, the initial fitness level of the individual, and the style of play.

Work/Rest Intervals

Table 32.1 presents the results of a time study analysis of the 1988 Men's and Women's Finals of the U.S. Open (10). These results indicate that a large majority of the points in tennis are of relatively short duration. Results indicated that over 80% of the points lasted 20 seconds or less. These data depict only 4 professional players and are not necessarily reflective of all tennis players. In the accomplished recreational player, our data indicate the average work/rest ratio on clay is 16.7/29.2 sec in males and 15.8/33.6 sec in females. On hard courts, the average work rest ratio was 12.7/28.4 sec and 14.2/32.5 sec in males and females, respectively. These results suggest that most metabolic demands in tennis are alactic anaerobic.

Table 32.1.
Summary of Time Study Analysis, U.S. Open 1988, Men's and Women's Finals

Lendl vs Wilander—1988 U.S. Open Men's Finals	
Average point	12.2 secs
Rest between points	28.3 secs
Rest on out/net serves	12.1 secs
Rest between games	
With court change	128.2 secs
Without court change	42.3 secs
Total points	325
Match time	294 min. (4 hrs. 54 min.)
Work/rest interval within games	1:2.3
Overall work/rest interval	1:3.4
Summary of Point Durations	
<10 secs.	59%
10–20 secs.	22%
>20 secs.	19%
Graf vs Sabatini—1988 U.S. Open Women's Finals	
Average point	10.8 secs
Average rest between points	16.2 secs
Rest on out/net serves	10.7 secs
Rest between games	
With court change	100.1 secs
Without court change	24.1 secs
Total points	151
Match time	101 min (1 hr, 41 min)
Work/rest interval within games	1:1.5
Overall work/rest interval	1:2.7
Summary of Point Durations	
<10 secs	62%
10–20 secs	25%
>20 secs	13%

Athletic Fitness Demands

Few can argue about the importance of speed, power, and quickness in most all athletic events, especially in tennis. Strength is an important component of power and short-term anaerobic endurance. For this reason, in addition to the factor of injury prevention, a weight training program would be advisable to improve performance in the sport of tennis. For tennis players, gains in athletic fitness can be accomplished through weight training, sprint/interval running, footwork and foot speed drills, and plyometrics.

Role of Equipment and Surfaces

Racquet. Most of the advances in tennis high technology have come in racquet size, composition, and playing characteristics. These changes have had a sizable impact on the nature of play at all levels.

Most racquets are now made in "midsize" or "large size" head sizes. Both of these versions create larger maximal hitting zones. There has been a fair amount of research that supports the advantages of each version, but no clear-cut performance advantage or injury disadvantage has been demonstrated. Similarly, there has been no demonstrated protective benefit from injury solely by the use of these racquets. There are as many anecdotes about tennis elbow and sore shoulders being caused by the racquets as there are about these conditions being cured by the racquets.

Grip size is important. Nirschl (11) has recommended that the grip size on the racquet should correspond to the length of the long finger measured from the tip to the distal palmar crease. A size too small makes the player grip the handle too firmly, and may cause muscle fatigue from overuse. A grip size too big causes the player to have less "feel" for and control over the racquet.

String tension is an area of much debate. The "best" string tension has varied from the extremely high tension of the Bjorn Borg era to a more moderate tension favored by most players now. Although there is laboratory evidence that slightly looser strings produce more velocity in the ball, the difference in terms of demands on the tennis player is negligible. Similarly, there has been no demonstrated evidence that string tension is a variable in cause or prevention of tennis-related injuries.

The latest generation of racquets plays a major role in creating demands on the tennis player by the power that they can deliver. As a result, players of all ages and abilities are trying to play the "power game," which emphasizes topspin, large motions on wind-up and follow through, swinging hard on all shots, and playing offensively. These racquets also allow players to remain competitive in this type of game for a longer number of years. In this situation, the player's musculoskeletal base must be properly prepared for the extra demands on flexibility and strength that this style dictates.

Shoes. The sports shoe industry has been revolutionized by the many types and designs of shoes that have been developed. A lot of the innovations, such as the sole cushioning systems and lacing patterns, have no research basis to prove the superiority of one type over another. However, tennis players may benefit from wearing shoes that are made specifically for tennis. Regardless of price, the shoes should have a fairly wide heel and good heel counter for rearfoot control, medial arch support that is appropriate for the individual's arch, and good lateral support for the forefoot. Very seldom are custom-made orthotics necessary for the average player. Their shock absorption functions are not high, and foot control can be better maintained by flexible joints and muscular strength in the legs.

Court Surface. Surfaces can alter the demands that are placed on the tennis player. In general, clay courts and some synthetic courts slow the ball down, allowing for longer points and longer matches. Because more strokes are hit in trying to impart more speed to a slower ball, there may be extra strain on the arm and back. The softer surface cushions the knees and legs, but the extra running may put more demands on the legs, and there may be more muscle pulls from sliding on the soft surfaces. Most synthetic courts and hard courts speed the ball up, creating shorter points. However, because of the speed of the ball, more impact forces may be placed on the racquet and arm. Similarly, the quick pace of the points on the harder surface may cause increased stress on the legs. Some physical characteristics, such as chronic knee trouble or either fast or slow running speed, may dictate the surface on which a player feels most comfortable and has the least demands. The musculoskeletal base should be prepared for the different demands of the different playing surfaces.

Musculoskeletal Base of the Tennis Player

Tennis players of all ages and abilities enter the sport with different musculoskeletal bases. As the individual continues to participate in the sport of tennis, the musculoskeletal base adapts to the sport altering flexibility and strength. Some studies propose that these adaptations to the musculoskeletal base may increase the individual athlete's chance of injury. Each athlete enters a sport with a quantifiable musculoskeletal base in terms of strength, flexibility, muscle balance, and endurance. If the musculoskeletal base is adequate for the specific sport, there will be a decreased chance of overload injuries. If the musculoskeletal base is exceptional for the specific sport, improved performance may well be the result, assuming an adequate skill level in the sport or activity. If the musculoskeletal base is inadequate for the sport, overload injury, fatigue, and decreased performance may well be the result. As the season progresses, injury and decreased performance become more likely.

Preparticipation Fitness Evaluations

The evaluation of sports specific adaptations or sports-specific preparedness with a sports-specific exam is best accomplished in a preseason fitness exam. Data on the preseason evaluation of tennis players demonstrates a pattern of musculoskeletal adaptation (or maladaptation) that could perhaps be corrected to alter the incidence of injury and improve performance. In performing a preparticipation evaluation of tennis players, relevant sport-specific fitness parameters should be chosen specific to the sport of tennis.

Flexibility Adaptations to Tennis

Studies of tennis players have demonstrated areas of inflexibility in musculoskeletal structure that are in high demand in the sport. In one study (12), flexibility measurements were obtained on 139 nontennis athletes and compared to the flexibility measurements of 86 junior elite tennis players. Tennis players were significantly tighter in sit and reach, dominant shoulder internal rotation, and nondominant shoulder internal rotation. Tennis players were significantly more flexible in dom-

Table 32.2.
Rotational Range of Motion Measurements at the Hip and Forearm

Area	Musculoskeletal Base Flexibility Deficits Dominant	Nondominant
Hip Internal Rotation	49	34
Hip External Rotation	53	57
Forearm Pronation	55	75
Forearm Supination	67	80

inant shoulder external rotation and nondominant shoulder external rotation. Unpublished data from the authors' clinic has demonstrated tightness in both pronation and supination of the dominant forarms and tightness in the nondominant hip internal rotation (Table 32.2). All of these areas are where high-tensile stresses are applied over short periods of time, and where rotational velocities have been shown to be high. The flexibility differences in tennis players suggest adaptations to the repetitive, short-duration, high velocity musculoskeletal demands of the sport of tennis.

Strength Adaptations to Tennis

Muscle weakness patterns and muscle imbalances have been identified in "throwing" athletes, including tennis players (13, 10). In one study on tennis players (14), 24 male and female college tennis players were tested for bilateral shoulder internal/external rotation strength on a Cybex 340 isokinetic dynamometer. Subjects produced significantly ($p < 0.01$) more torque in internal rotation at 60° and 300°/sec in the dominant arm compared to the nondominant arm. The increase in internal rotation strength may be related to the plyometric action of the tennis stroke (15). By significantly increasing the strength of the dominant shoulder in internal rotation without subsequent strengthening of the external rotators, muscle imbalances may be created in the dominant arm that could possibly affect the tennis player's predisposition to overload injuries of the shoulder joint.

These flexibility and strength adaptations are important for several reasons. First, they have been demonstrated in players as young as 12 to 14 years of age (16), indicating that age is not a protective factor. Second, these adaptations are in the exact anatomic places that show high incidences of injury—the shoulder, elbow, and back. Third, posterior shoulder inflexibility has been implicated in possible shoulder injury (17–19), and elbow inflexibility has been shown to be a risk factor in lateral epicondylitis (11).

It may be that these adaptations are local efforts to control the high forces applied. However, these adaptations appear to be deleterious to the entire kinetic chain. These appear to create biomechanical inefficiencies and cause functional alterations, so that injury risk is higher and optimum performance requires more energy. The demonstration of these adaptations in a large number of active tennis players may raise the question of whether these are "normal" adaptations and should be left alone. We feel that these are statistically "average" but not "normal." Improvement in these adaptations can alter injury risk by improving anatomic stability and movement and improve tennis performance by improving biomechanical efficiency (20). These adaptations should be sought during a comprehensive preparticipation exam, and should be aggressively corrected.

Common Injuries in Tennis Players

Epidemiology

There are few good epidemiologic studies that accurately show the incidence of injuries in tennis players. Kibler (8) looked at elite International and American Junior Tennis Players, and found that 100 total injuries occurred in 63 out of 97 junior tennis players over the 18 months prior to the study (Table 32.3). Similarly, a U.S. Tennis Association Survey (unpublished data) of the 27 players on its national team showed that 45 injuries occurred in 23 players over the 18 months prior to the study. The anatomic areas of injury were similar in both studies, with the shoulder and back having the highest incidence, followed by elbow, knee, and ankle (Table 32.4). When the injuries were analyzed by type (Table 32.5), it was found that overload injuries, representing a failed body response to chronic repetitive tensile microtrauma, were present in 63% of the cases. Examples of these injuries include rotator cuff tendinitis, lateral epicondylitis, chronic muscle strain, plantar fasciitis, and stress fractures. Traumatic injuries, representing acute responses to one time microtrauma, were present 37% of the time. Examples of these are acute ankle sprains, torn menisci, or fractures.

Evaluation Process

The evaluation process for acute injuries that occur in tennis should be the same as for any acute injury. Proper early evaluation, stabilization, protection, and early treatment should be carried out. In the evaluation of overload injuries, several additional points should be observed. This is necessary for the evaluation of overload injuries in any sport, but it is especially relevant in tennis because of the high preponderance of this type of injury.

Since overload injuries are the product of long-term repetitive microtrauma overload, these injuries are the result of a *process* rather than an *event* (21). The kinetic chain of which the injured area is a part will adapt to

Table 32.3.
Injuries in Junior Elite and Recreational Tennis Players[a]

	Elite Juniors (%)	Recreational (%)
Overload	63	62
Sprains	25	22
Fractures	12	14
Other		2

[a] Reprinted by permission from Kibler WB et al. Fitness evaluations and fitness findings in competitive junior tennis players clinics. Sports Med 1988; 7:2.

Table 32.4.
Tennis Injury Site

	US Tennis Assoc			English			Swedish			Bollettieri		
	O	S	F[a]	O	S	F	O	S	F	O	S	F
Shoulder	4	0	0	4	0	0	3	0	0	3	0	0
Elbow	1	0	0	2	0	0	0	0	0	4	0	0
Wrist	3	0	1	1	0	0	2	0	0	0	0	1
Back	2	0	0	1	0	0	2	1	0	1	2	0
Hamstrings	2	0	0	1	0	0	0	0	0	2	0	0
Knee	2	3	0	0	0	0	1	3	0	4	3	0
Achilles	2	0	0	2	0	0	1	0	0	0	0	0
Ankle	0	3	2	0	1	0	0	2	0	0	4	0
Foot	0	0	0	1	1	0	1	2	0	3	0	0

	Players Reporting Injuries	Number of Injuries
US Tennis Assoc	22/34	26
English	11/17	14
Swedish	12/13	18
Bollettieri	18/33	27

[a]O = Overload S = Sprain F = Fracture. Reprinted by permission from Kibler WB et al. Fitness evaluations and fitness findings in competitive junior tennis players clinics. Sports Med 1988; 7:2.

Table 32.5.
Tennis Injury Type[a]

	Total	Male	O/S + F	Female	O/S + F
Shoulder	20	7	7/0	13	13/0
Elbow	7	4	4/0	3	3/0
Wrist	8	3	2/1	5	4/1
Back	9	6	5/1	3	1/2
Hamstrings	5	4	4/0	1	1/0
Knee	16	10	4/6	6	3/3
Achilles	5	2	2/0	3	3/0
Ankle	12	6	0/6	6	0/6
Foot	8	5	4/1	3	1/2
			32/15		29/14

[a]O = Overload S = Sprain F = Fracture. Reprinted by permission from Kibler WB et al. Fitness evaluations and fitness findings in competitive junior tennis players clinics. Sports Med 1988;7:2.

this gradual process. Some of these adaptations, such as increased tendon or muscle size, may be beneficial. Some, such as joint or muscle inflexibility, muscle strength imbalance, or alterations in throwing or running mechanics, are not beneficial. Identification of these adaptations must be part of the evaluation process in these injuries.

A framework for this evaluation process is available for use (22). It is in the form of a negative feedback vicious cycle (Fig. 32.7) and relates how chronic overload interacts with inflexibilities, strength deficits, and mechanical alterations to create further chance of overt injury. It also shows how the actual clinical symptoms are a rather small part of the entire injury presentation. Finally, it creates five "complexes" that may be looked for to make a complete and accurate diagnosis of each overload injury (Table 32.6).

These five complexes correspond to the different stages of the vicious cycle. They are:

1. Tissue injury complex—that group of anatomic structures that is disrupted.
2. Clinical symptom complex—that grouping of overt signs and symptoms that characterizes the injury.
3. Tissue overload complex—that group of tissues that is subject to tensile overload.
4. Functional biomechanical deficit complex—inflexibilities and\or muscle strength imbalances that create altered athletic mechanics.
5. Subclinical adaptation complex—the substitute ac-

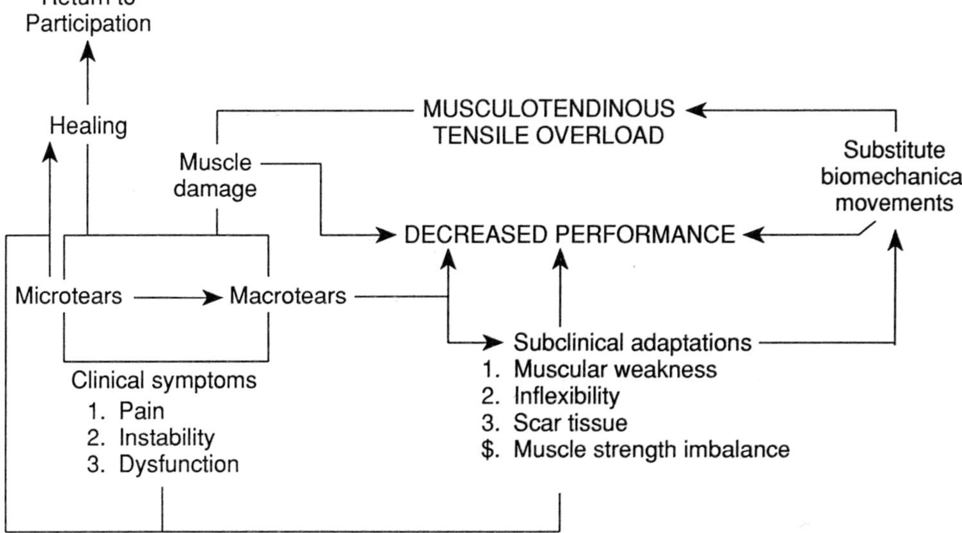

Figure 32.7. Overload vicious cycle.

Table 32.6.
Vicious Cycle Complexes

Tissue injury
Clinical symptoms
Tissue overload
Functional biomechanical deficit
Subclinical adaptation

tivities that the athlete uses to compensate for altered mechanics.

The examination process incorporates standard sports medicine evaluation tools, but places special emphasis on looking at the entire kinetic chain in which the injured area is one part. Examples of pertinent examination points are given with each specific injury, and categorization of each injury by the vicious cycle complexes is also done.

Specific Injuries

Rotator Cuff Tendinitis. This specific injury is one of the most common injuries at all activity levels in tennis players. However, recent investigations have pointed toward an alteration of the normal concept of this tendinitis. Although the classical symptoms and signs of crepitus and point tender pain over the anterior and lateral aspects of the shoulder upon overhead motion, which are relieved with the arm at the side, are usually present in most cases, there are probably two separate etiologies for these symptoms and signs.

In the athlete under 35 years of age, most of these symptoms are due to subclinical or mildly overt instabilities of the glenohumeral joint due to anterior inferior or anterior superior capsular and labral deficiencies (11). These rotator cuff injuries have been termed "secondary tensile overload injuries" (1), because they occur as a result of deficits in muscular strength and balance and of muscular inflexibility, which predispose to the capsular and labral deficiencies (5, 23). Treatment in this group starts off with evaluation of flexibility and strength deficits that may be present, proceeds with anterior, superior or multidirectional instability evaluation, and includes tests for competence of all rotator cuff muscles. Conservative treatment that consists of decreased activity, range of motion exercises, and gradual muscle strengthening exercises which start at the scapula and work out to the shoulder should be instituted first. In addition to the clinical symptom complex that has been described, treatment should be based on the complete analysis of all of the identified deficiencies. Analysis of this problem usually shows the following:

Tissue overload—Posterior capsule, shoulder external rotator muscles, scapular stabilizers;
Tissue injury—Rotator cuff impingement or tensile stretch, glenoid labrum, anterior capsule;
Clinical symptoms—Pain over anterior lateral acromion, impingement upon abduction and rotation, glenohumeral subluxation, positive "clunk" or anterior slide test;
Functional biomechanical deficit—Functional "lateral scapular slide," consisting of inflexibility in internal rotation, muscle strength deficits in shoulder external rotators and scapular stabilizers; in more advanced cases, superior or anterior glenohumeral translation occurs;

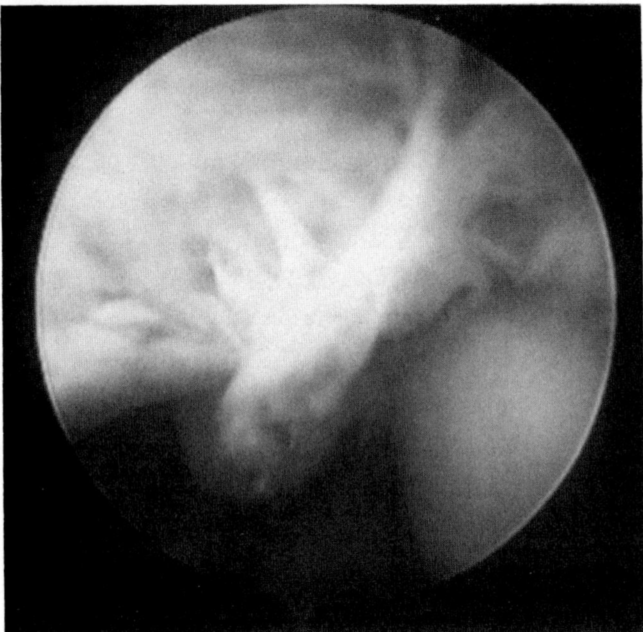

Figure 32.8. Undersurface tear of the rotator cuff in association with a labral tear (tear not shown).

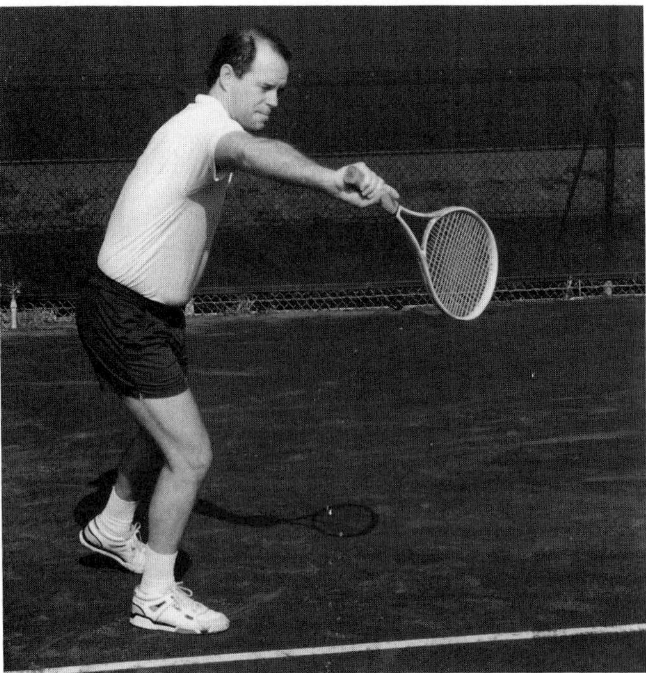

Figure 32.9. Leading with the elbow on the backhand stroke.

Subclinical adaptations—"Short arming" the throw, alteration of arm position during throwing or lifting, muscle recruitment from anterior shoulder, forearm, or trunk.

Treatment of the symptomatic tendinitis may be limited by the anatomic instability, so if conservative treatment is not successful in progressing the athlete by 6 to 8 weeks, further evaluation by computed tomography (CT) arthrogram or magnetic resonance imaging (MRI) should be considered, to evaluate possible surgical cases. In these cases, the superior surface of the rotator cuff and subacromial space is usually not involved. The pathological problem will be found in the glenohumeral joint and on the undersurface of the rotator cuff (Fig. 32.8).

In the older tennis athlete, the signs and symptoms are more commonly based on actual rotator cuff impingement and degeneration. In these patients the tendinitis has been described as "primary compressive" because it is caused by damage directly to the cuff (1). A high percentage will show plain x-ray changes in the acromioclavicular (AC) joint, subacromial area, or greater tuberosity consistent with chronic wear. Tests for instability will usually be normal, but a pattern of strength imbalances similar to younger athletes may be present. Conservative treatment may be instituted, especially if there are few indications of muscle tears. However, more complete diagnosis of the anatomic problem by arthrogram, CT arthrogram, or MRI should be considered early in the treatment process, so that accurate information about diagnosis, prognosis, treatment options, and return to play can be given.

Actual tearing of rotator cuff is the end stage of the tendinitis spectrum. In most cases, there is a definite history of a painful episode after hitting an overhead or extending the arm. The pain may range from mild to severe, but the condition is usually functionally disabling. Early accurate diagnosis and institution of definite treatment is important to minimize functional deficit. Some small tears may be rehabilitated nonoperatively, but most tears are incompatible with vigorous overhead function. Surgical evaluation and repair should be considered if vigorous activity is contemplated. Even with early surgery, results are often disappointing, especially in the large tears.

Lateral Epicondylitis. "Tennis elbow" is a very common problem in recreational athletes, but a rather infrequent problem in more accomplished tennis players. This injury occurs almost exclusively as a result of repetitive overload. Pathologic change is seen in the extensor tendon attachments around the lateral epicondyle, especially in the extensor carpi radialis brevis. The clinical symptoms and signs are point tenderness in this area, pain upon resisted finger or wrist extension or forearm supination, pain upon gripping objects, and, most commonly, pain on the backhand stroke.

Mechanical factors are thought to play a major role in the pathogenesis of this problem. Relatively unskilled players may have alterations in stroke technique or strength that place extra stress on the elbow as the racquet moves through the hitting zone. Examples of this are "leading with the elbow" (Fig. 32.9), which places tensile load on the stretched extensor muscles, attempting to play with underspin by excessively pronating the forearm, or decreased strength in shoulder external rotators, which cause the elbow extensors to work harder in the hitting zone. Some of these problems can be identified in the office exam by having a racquet available for patients to demonstrate their strokes.

Complete analysis of musculoskeletal assessment will show, in addition to clinical symptoms, the following:

Tissue overload—lateral muscle mass, mainly extensor carpi radialis brevis, wrist pronators and extensors, shoulder external rotators
Tissue injury—same as for tissue overload, plus annular ligament and joint capsule
Clinical symptoms—point tender pain over extensor muscle mass, swelling in varying degree, pain on hitting backhand (usually in recreational athlete)
Functional biomechanical deficit—extensor inflexibility and muscle weakness, decreased range of motion (ROM) in pronators and supinators, decreased shoulder external rotation strength
Subclinical adaptations—hitting "behind the body," hitting with wrist movement, recruitment of triceps or alteration of position of elbow

Treatment should be pursued both from the point of view of improving mechanics and of reducing symptoms. A good tennis teaching professional can be of major help in improving mechanics. Rehabilitation starts with decreasing painful activities to reduce stress, and antiinflammatory medications in the acute phase. Strengthening exercises should start at the shoulder and proceed distally, with special emphasis on all of the deficits of strength, strength imbalance, and flexibility noted in the exam. Rubber tuning has been found to be a good way to start the strengthening process. Early use of a counter force brace (Fig. 32.10) will decrease the load applied at the site of injury and allow more vigorous rehabilitation. In addition, its use allows earlier return to play.

Steroid injections have been used as treatment in many cases of "tennis elbow." It certainly should not be the first form of treatment, unless there is an extremely tender, inflamed area. The only major benefit of corticosteroid injections is the antiinflammatory action, so its use should be confined to those situations where active inflammation is present. After injections, the patient should refrain from tennis for 10 days. A physical therapy program should be instituted after injection. Repeated injections are deleterious to the tendon and subcutaneous tissues, and they are not recommended.

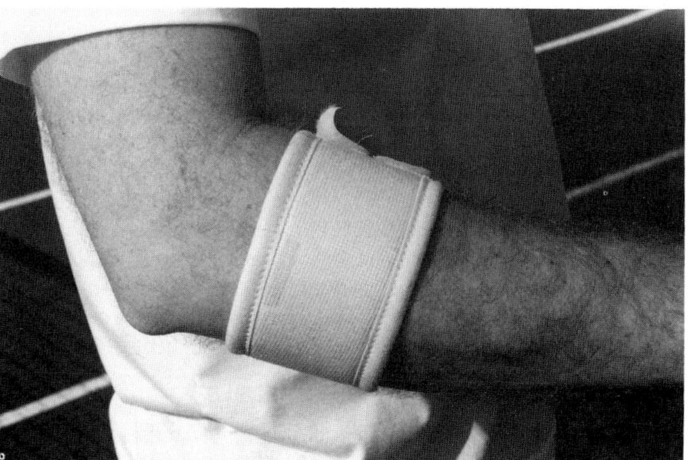
Figure 32.10. Elbow counterforce brace.

Failure to respond to conservative treatment will make surgery necessary to regain athletic function. Six to eight weeks of a properly devised and supervised program should be enough to identify those patients who do not respond. If the symptoms and signs remain the same, further modality or rehabilitative treatment is not going to be beneficial in healing the injury. The patient will continue to be in the overload vicious cycle with more deficits and adaptations. Most commonly, the surgical procedure will remove the degenerative granulation tissue and will repair the tendon either side to side or back to bone. Postoperative care includes a period of protection of the repair and gradual rehabilitation along the same lines advocated for nonoperative treatment. Return to play averages 3 months.

Medial Epicondylitis. "Medial tennis elbow" is not as common as lateral epicondylitis, but is more commonly seen in advanced and competitive players. The pathology appears to be the same, with repetitive tensile microtears eventually giving rise to clinical tears and symptoms. The pain is usually felt more on the forehand stroke or serve and is localized to a point tender area just anterior and distal to the medial epicondyle.

The mechanical factors operating to produce this injury are excessive racquet velocity, exaggerated racquet position, and desire to create heavy topspin. All of these factors place an absolute overload on the muscle tendon area.

Complete analysis of medial epicondylitis includes the following:

Tissue overload—Forearm flexor mass, biceps, pronator tests, usually absolute overload;
Tissue injury—Same as for tissue overload, ± medial collateral ligament, ulnar nerve, and/or posterior medial olecranon ("valgus overload complex");
Clinical symptoms—Point tender over flexor muscle mass, medial collateral ligament, posterior medial elbow, ± ulnar nerve symptoms;
Functional biomechanical deficit—Functional pronation contracture, consisting of elbow flexion and pronation inflexibility, and tight and weak flexors;
Subclinical adaptations—Hitting "behind the body," more overhead throwing motion, more wrist snap, more use of shoulder in throwing motion.

Treatment of this problem more commonly involves surgical repair. Surgery consists of excision of all degenerative tendon tissue, fasciotomy and debridement of damaged muscle, and either side-to-side or tendon-to-bone repair. Failure of this entity to heal nonoperatively probably reflects the larger peak forces generated by the advanced player that can result in more tissue disruption. Conservative treatment should be employed first, with rest, alteration of mechanics, and antiinflammatory medicine or modalities. Medial counterforce braces may be beneficial.

Prior to surgery, it is important to differentiate "epicondylitis" from the "valgus overload" syndrome, which is common in baseball players but less common in tennis participants. This syndrome is caused by medial collateral ligament deficiency and is characterized by valgus instability, ulnar nerve irritation, and posteromedial bony impingement. The evaluation process for the injury is described in detail in the section on racquet ball.

After surgery, the repair is protected in a splint for 10 to 14 days, after which gradual range of motion exercises are instituted with protection in a functional brace. Rehabilitation should include muscle strengthening, as advocated for lateral epicondylitis, and restoration of normal flexibility. Before returning to play, the athlete either should have adequate muscular strength to withstand the demands of the "power game" or should alter the mechanics of the forehand strokes.

Wrist Tendinitis. This uncommon injury is usually seen either in very advanced players, who may use more wrist motion to create shots or to respond to hard shots, or in beginners, who use more wrist motion because of poor mechanics. The pain is usually in the wrist extensors, either at their insertion or in the extensor retinaculum. Flexor tendons may be involved on the ulnar side of the wrist. Distal radioulnar joint symptoms may accompany flexor tendon injury.

Treatment is almost always conservative; it involves rest, ice, oral antiinflammatories, and mechanical corrections. Wrist braces that leave the palm free are helpful. There are usually no associated biomechanical deficits or substitute patterns.

The differential diagnosis of flexor tendinitis should also include fractures of the hook of the hamate, ulnar nerve injury in Guyon's canal, and ulnar artery thrombosis, all of which can occur as a result of the pressure of the butt of the racquet in the palm. "Carpal tunnel view" plain x-rays, Tinel's sign testing, and/or EMG and nerve conduction velocity studies as well as digital subtraction angiography are the tools used to help in the diagnostic evaluation of these rarer conditions.

Low Back and Trunk Pain. This anatomic area is the site of many tennis related injuries. Three main types of injuries are seen. The first is located in the posterior midline, and is usually associated with the service motion or with straight-ahead activities, such as running to the net or hitting a low volley. The second is in the peripheral musculature of the quadratus lumborum or oblique abdominal muscles; it is associated with change in service motion or with ground strokes. The third is a tear of the rectus abdominis anteriorum, which is associated with hitting overheads or many serves. The symptoms usually present as a sudden onset of sharp, muscle-tearing-type pain after a shot. There is usually immediate athletic disability. There are no radicular signs or symptoms.

In the first two cases, the same set of underlying musculoskeletal base deficits render the back and trunk unable to accept the demands of the activities mentioned above. The difference in presentation is in how the demands are made. These deficits cause the relative overload to the muscles and can be identified by the physical exam.

Tissue overload—Posterior back musculature, hamstrings, and hip rotators;
Tissue injury—Same as for tissue overload, with the addition of facet joints or S-I joints;
Functional biomechanical deficit—Tight hamstrings, tight hip rotation and decreased trunk rotation;
Subclinical adaptations—Alteration of arm motion, excessive thoracolumbar motion, and excessive hip and leg rotation.

Treatment starts, as usual, with rest. This is especially important in these injuries, because as players try to "play through" the pain, they may further injure this area. This area is notoriously slow to return to normal function, and further insults slow the process down even more. Also, if this vital area of force transfer is impaired, alteration in the mechanics of the strokes is inevitable, leading to decreased performance and increased injury risk.

Further treatment emphasizes short-term protection with a light lumbosacral corset for pain relief, ice, and modalities. Early range of motion exercises are encouraged, with special emphasis on trunk rotation. Strengthening of both the flexor/extensor muscles and the trunk rotators must be complete before return to play.

If proper recognition and correction of the underlying musculoskeletal deficits is not accomplished as part of the rehabilitation process, the acute back strain may become chronic, with much more difficulty in returning to top performance.

Some tennis players will present with acute back pain and radicular symptoms. These should be managed as any nerve impingement. Leadbetter (24) has reported success with lumbar discectomy in selected patients in returning them to tennis activity.

Leg Muscle Strains. Acute muscle strains or acute exacerbation of chronic muscle strains may occur in any of the leg muscles, but they seem to be most common in the adductors (groin strain), the medial head of the gastrocnemius ("tennis leg"), and the hamstrings.

Adductor strains usually occur when the player changes directions quickly. The pain is felt at the proximal tendon-bone or muscle-tendon area. It is functionally incapacitating because of the need to powerfully push off in the serve, in ground strokes, and in the net game.

Gastrocnemius tears occur during explosive activation of the leg, such as in sprinting to the net or jumping for an overhead. There is usually simultaneous ankle dorsiflexion and knee extension, putting stress on both ends of the muscle. MRI studies have conclusively shown that this injury is in the gastrocnemius, not in the plantaris. Most patients will describe a feeling of being kicked or hit in the calf. Pain will be localized on the medial aspect of the calf, close to the muscle tendon junction.

Hamstring injuries occur in sprinting, either to the net or side to side. The pain may be in the proximal or distal aspects of the muscle, but it is always associated with a muscle tendon disruption (25).

All of these may be acute injuries, but a substantial proportion of them are acute exacerbations of chronic injuries (26). The chronic injury may be mildly symptomatic or overtly asymptomatic but still capable of creating a functional biomechanical deficit. Before initiating treatment, it is important to inquire about previous injuries or prodromal symptoms and to check for anatomic deficits.

The difference between examining for acute hamstring strains and chronic hamstring strains may be seen in the evaluations. In the acute hamstring strain, the following complexes are observed:

Tissue overload—Origin/insertion of hamstring or muscle tendon junction;
Tissue injury—Medial or lateral hamstring, secondary to mechanical disruption, varying degrees of inflammation;
Clinical symptoms—Point tenderness, swelling and/or bruising, mass;
Functional biomechanical deficit—None;
Subclinical adaptations—None.

In the chronic hamstring strain, the following complexes are observed:

Tissue overload—Same as acute;
Tissue injury—Same as acute plus fibrosis;
Clinical symptoms—Point tender, diffuse over leg, reinjury;
Functional biomechanical deficit—Hamstring inflexibility, quadriceps/hamstring muscle imbalance, adductor inflexibility;
Subclinical adaptations—Shortened stride, shortened kick, use of hip extensors and gastrocnemius.

Chronic adductor strains show the same general patterns as hamstring strains. Gastrocnemius strains show the pattern of Achilles tendinitis, to be discussed below.

Treatment of all the strains follows the same pattern. Ice should be used for early edema control. Support with conforming neoprene wraps helps to decrease further injury, and allows early muscle use. Severe tears with large muscle damage, especially in the gastrocemius, quadriceps, or hamstrings, should be splinted in a stretched position for 7 to 10 days, as this position has been shown to maintain maximal muscle tension and decrease scar contracture. Early massage will reduce edema and fibrous adhesions. Stretching exercises are instituted as soon as pain allows, followed by strengthening. Concentric power usually returns early, but eccentric power returns more slowly. Return to play should occur only after eccentric power has returned and any deficits have been corrected.

Internal Derangement of the Knee. These injuries have been adequately covered in other sections. Although tennis does not put the same intensity of stress to the knee that football and basketball do, the start/stop, cutting, and pivoting that are inherent demands of tennis require a stable knee for optimum performance. Most young or active tennis players are not able to perform well with a cruciate ligament deficient knee, but can perform well after a reconstruction. It may be well to recommend that tennis players with patellofemoral chondromalacia or with a partial or complete meniscectomy play on softer surfaces such as clay.

Achilles Tendinitis. This injury is not very common in tennis players, but is disabling when it occurs. It usually occurs when playing surfaces are changed, such as going from hard courts indoors to soft courts outdoors in the spring. It may also occur when playing intensity increases, such as when attending a tennis camp. There may be swelling anywhere along the tendon, sometimes accompanied by a palpable knot of paratendinosis. These almost always occur as acute exacerbations of chronic underlying conditions. The accompanying deficits are as follows:

Tissue overload—gastrocnemius/soleus muscle, or muscle tendon junction.
Tissue injury—Achilles tendon, along its course or at its distal tendon bone attachment.
Clinical symptoms—point tender, ± knot, stiffness after rest.
Functional biomechanical deficit—inflexibility in dorsiflexion, weak plantar flexors.
Subclinical adaptations—shortened stance, less push-off.

This injury is often prolonged in its treatment. In addition to standard antiinflammatory modalities, brace protection, and stretching are advocated. Soft court surfaces may actually exacerbate the symptoms upon return to play if the gastrocnemius is still tight and unable to absorb the applied load.

Achilles tendon rupture is relatively common in tennis players, especially among older players. Unfortunately, this is often underdiagnosed. Classically, patients feel a "pop" or feel that they have been struck in the leg. Plantar flexion may still be present due to tibialis posterior activity, but the patient cannot stand on the toes and cannot "power off" the foot. The most sensitive test is the Thomas test, in which manual compression of the calf fails to produce passive plantar flexion of the foot (Fig. 32.11).

Treatment of Achilles tendon ruptures may be surgical or nonsurgical. In active tennis players, surgical treatment allows secure repair, accurate coaptation of tendon tissue, minimal immobilization, and earlier onset of rehabilitation. This set of circumstances usually leads to earlier and more complete return to athletic function.

Ankle sprains. Just as in other sports in which running, cutting and stopping and starting are major demands, ankle sprains are the most common macrotrauma injury in tennis players. Twisting forces, especially in plantar flexion, account for most of the injuries.

Precise diagnosis of the anatomical disruption, both in terms of degree and in terms of which ligaments or bones are injured, is important to ascertain before treatment is started. Severe second degree and third degree injuries take longer to heal, and are more prone to residual functional deficits or reinjury. Similarly, ti-

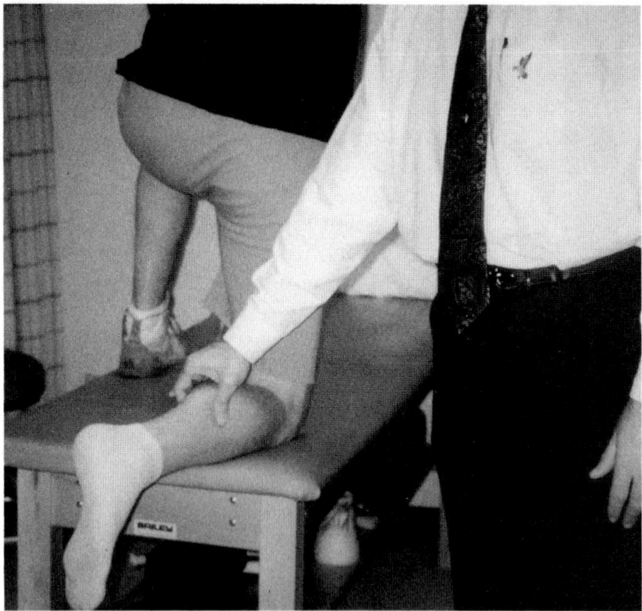

Figure 32.11. Thomas test.

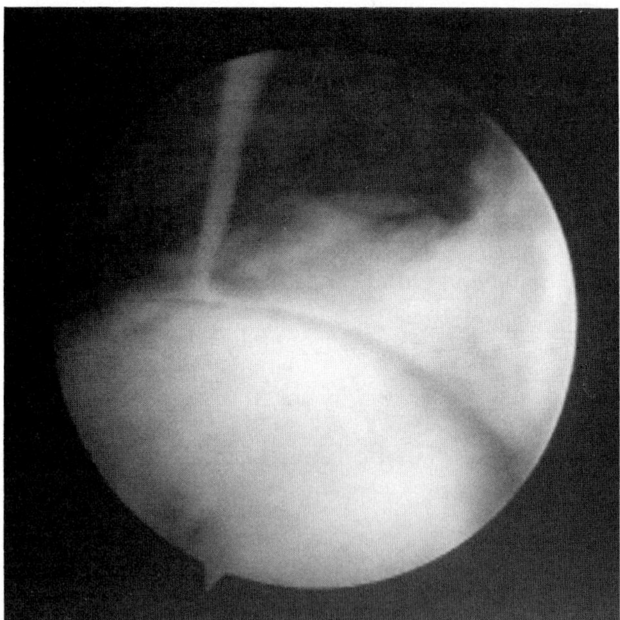

Figure 32.12. Meniscoid and soft tissue of the ankle.

biofibular ligament injuries, alone or in combination with anterior talofibular ligament injuries, take longer to heal. X-rays can help delineate any bony avulsions or talar dome osteochondral defects.

Treatment for the large majority of acute ankle sprains should be conservative. Relative rest, protection, commonly in a pneumatic splint and only rarely in a cast, and ice are first line modalities. Early protected range of motion and strengthening can be started as symptoms abate. Most ankle sprains tend to be treated too nonchalantly, with return to play when symptoms are gone. The reinjury rate within 1 year in these circumstances is around 70% (27). Inadequate treatment of the acute ankle sprain leads to the chronic ankle sprain syndrome, which has a more complex evaluation and which is more difficult to rehabilitate. Therefore, treatment should ensure good ligamentous stability, full flexibility, and good plantar flexion and eversion strength before return to play.

Acute Ankle Sprain
Tissue overload—None;
Tissue injury—Anterior talofibular, fibulocalcaneal ligaments;
Clinical symptoms—Pain, swelling, point tender area;
Functional biomechanical deficit—None;
Subclinical adaptations—None;
Chronic Ankle Sprain
Tissue overload—Plantar flexors, evertors;
Tissue injury—Same as above, plus ankle capsule;
Clinical symptoms—Recurrent sprains, locking of joint;
Functional biomechanical deficit—Plantar flexion inflexibility and weakness;
Subclinical adaptations—Running on heels, decreased stride length.

Surgical treatment of ankle sprain problems is recommended in three special cases. One case is the loose or detached osteochondral fragment from the talar bone. Arthroscopic techniques are usually adequate to remove this piece of bone. The second case is soft tissue impingement in the anterolateral gutter. This impingement may take the form of "meniscoid" tissue, or other types of scar tissue that may get trapped between the bones (Fig. 32.12). Arthroscopic debridement has been very successful in this case as well. The final case is the chronically unstable ankle with functional instability, a positive anterior drawer test, some varus instability, and a failure of conservative treatment. A combination of an arthroscopic debridement of intraarticular scar and a modified Bronstrom-type repair of the lateral ligaments and retinaculum works well in most cases. In those cases in which the lateral ligaments are too thin for plication, reconstruction with a portion of the peroneus brevis does well.

Plantar Fasciitis. Plantar fasciitis is common among athletes who run as part of their sport. The classical findings are of pin point tenderness over the insertion of the plantar fascia into the calcaneus, pain upon first arising or after sitting, and return of symptoms during activity. Differential diagnostic possibilities include stress fractures of the calcaneus and impingement of the posterior tibial or medial calcaneal nerves. X-ray demonstration of an inferior calcaneal "heel spur" is not necessary for the diagnosis and is actually often misleading. In most cases, the spur is of secondary importance, since it is not the cause of the pain.

Treatment is directed toward relieving the painful symptoms with the use of "arch aid" counter force braces, modalities, rest and medication. Athletes with plantar fasciitis have been shown to have deficits in flexibility and strength in the ankle plantar flexors that affect the onset of the symptoms and the outcome of the treatment (28). These deficits can be categorized into the following deficits:

Tissue overload—Plantar flexor muscles, plantar fascial; insertion at heel, foot intrinsic muscles;
Tissue injury—Some plantar fascial attachment at heel;
Clinical symptoms—Point tenderness at base of calcaneus, worse in and/or after running;
Functional biomechanical deficit—Plantar flexor inflexibility and weakness, creating functional pronation;
Subclinical adaptations—Running on toes, shortened stride length, foot inversion.

Correction of these deficits speeds the recovery process and allows for normalization of strength for running and jumping.

Surgical treatment, consisting of debridement of the damaged tissue and releasing the involved plantar fascia, is necessary in 10% to 15% of the cases. Recovery after such surgery is good but can be prolonged because of the important role of the heel pad and the plantar fascia in absorbing loads about the foot.

Heat Illness. Of all of the relatively infrequent nonorthopedic problems that afflict tennis players, heat illness should be mentioned. It is potentially the most devastating problem that may occur.

Conditions conducive to heat illness abound in tennis. Matches are frequently played in the heat of the day, are often prolonged, are in areas with little or no shade, and players may have limited access to water. In tournaments, several matches may be scheduled for the same day.

Preventative precautions include playing in cooler times of the day, "water loading" by drinking fluids the day before the match, drinking water or electrolyte solutions during the match, wearing light, cotton-based clothing, seeking shade whenever possible, and stopping if symptoms of light-headedness, dizziness, nausea, weakness, cramps, or automatic behavior occur.

Players should not be allowed to return to play until they have replaced the weight lost through perspiration water loss and are completely recovered from their symptoms.

Principles of Rehabilitation

Adequate rehabilitation is the key to restoration of athletic function after injury. Most of the common tennis injuries can be successfully treated by nonsurgical means. In some athletes' and coaches' minds, this implies that little rehabilitation must be done. To the contrary, this group of repetitive microtrauma overload injuries (Table 32.7) requires the most precise rehabilitation due to the nature of the pathogenesis of the injury. The outline of this process has been presented for each of the injuries. Several other points need to be emphasized.

The negative feedback vicious cycle may be used to guide rehabilitation as well. As has been demonstrated, there may be significant abnormalities in surrounding and supporting tissues in addition to the abnormalities causing symptoms. A complete and accurate diagnosis of all of the abnormalities by the process that has been outlined above is the first prerequisite for proper rehabilitation (Table 32.8).

The second prerequisite is satisfactory completion of all phases of rehabilitation (29). The first is the acute phase (Table 32.9), in which new clinical symptoms are reduced and tissue injury is controlled and started towards healing. The second is the recovery phase, where tissue injury is healed, tissue overloads are reduced, and the functional biomechanical deficits are normalized (Table 32.10). The third is the maintenance phase, in which all of the previous gains are directed towards elimination of the subclinical alterations, and functional progressions for sports-specific and kinetic chain-specific activities are instituted (Table 32.11).

The final prerequisite is a clearly defined set of criteria for return to play. This should include normalization of all of the parts of the negative feedback vicious

Table 32.7.
Leadbetter's Tendon Injury Classification

Name	Definition and Histology	Clinical Presentation
Tendinosis	Intratendinous degeneration due to repetitive microtrauma. Noninflammatory intratendinous collagen degeneration	Palpable nodule with no tendon or sheath swelling
Tendinitis	Symptomatic degeneration with vascular disruption and inflammatory repair. Inflammation is major characteristic, superimposed on acute or chronic injury	Symptoms are of classical inflammation and proportional to vascular disruption

Table 32.8.
Prerequisites for Proper Rehabilitation

Complete and accurate diagnosis
Completion of phases of rehabilitation
  Acute
  Recovery
  Maintenance
Criteria for return to play
  Normalization of deficits
  Functional progression

Table 32.9.
Acute Phase of Rehabilitation

Complexes Involved
  Tissue injury
  Clinical symptom
Therapeutic Activities
  Active rest
  Conditioning of other areas
  ANSAIDs
  PT modalities
  Protected ROM
  Muscle activity
    isometric
    isotonic
Criteria for Advancement
  Resolution of swelling
  Decreased pain—Level II
  Tissue healing
  Improved ROM

Table 32.10.
Recovery Phase of Rehabilitation

Complexes Involved
Tissue overload
Functional biomechanical deficit
Therapeutic Activities
Appropriate loading
Protected ROM
Resistive exercise
Local
Balance
Kinetic chain
Functional exercises
Criteria for Advancement
No pain
ROM equal to opposite side
No remaining pathology
Strength 75% of normal
Smooth kinetic motion

Table 32.11.
Maintenance Phase of Rehabilitation

Complexes Involved
Functional biomechanical deficit
Subclinical adaptations
Therapeutic Activities
Strength and flexibility balance
Plyometrics
Functional progressions
Throwing
Running
Kicking
Criteria For Return To Play
Essential full ROM
Normal strength and balance
Normal mechanics
Sports specific progression

cycle and completion of functional progression for that activity (Table 32.11).

In the specific case of lateral epicondylitis of the elbow, the acute phase addresses the symptoms of pain, soreness, and athletic dysfunction with rest, ice, antiinflammatory modalities and medications; it also protects the tissue injury with a counterforce elbow brace and a decrease in playing activities as well as other activities that cause stress to the area. The recovery phase completes the tissue-healing process with continued protection, but it also starts to improve flexibility of the biceps, wrist extensors and supinators, to thereby reduce tissue overload. In addition, strengthening exercises are started to improve the shoulder external rotators, wrist extensors, pronators, and supinators. When strength and flexibility are obtained, the maintenance phase allows hitting, with emphasis on proper biomechanics, and correction of any adaptations that have occurred. Strengthening continues during this phase. Full return to play is allowed when normal strength and flexibility are measured and good hitting patterns can be demonstrated.

Intervention Strategies for Injury Prevention

It is an enticing thought that since many of these injuries proceed through a rather long process of gradual damage before producing clinical symptoms, recognition of athletes in the preclinical stages could be accomplished and adequate steps could be undertaken to prevent further progression. It is also enticing to think that if all the sports-specific demands could be identified, then skill training programs could be designed to stay within certain limits, or "doses," and conditioning programs could be designed to optimize the musculoskeletal base for a particular sport. Research along these lines is proceeding, and early evidence points to support for these thoughts. Most of the research concerning tennis has already been presented. Several concepts concerning the "shoulder at risk" have recently been presented (20, FW Jobe, personal communication, 1991). Reviews of the role of subclinical adaptations in injury causation and the role of strengthening in injury prevention point to positive results from improvement of these important parameters (29, 30). Because of these findings, interventional strategies should be actively pursued in tennis injury work.

Identification of muscle weaknesses and inflexibilities can best be approached through a sports-specific preparticipation examination (12, 15, 17). By testing specific anatomic areas with tests relatively specific for the sport or activity, a profile of musculoskeletal "readiness" for play can be identified. Conditioning programs based on correcting deficits and strengthening areas of high demand can then be constructed. These have shown promise in decreasing injury (30). "Fine tuning" of both the examination process and the conditioning programs will allow better results in the future.

This process of "prehabilitation," or prospective conditioning, is also important in young elite athletes who have the prospect of more intensive play as they get older. Studies have shown that adaptive changes occur as a result of playing sports in tennis players as young as 12 to 13 years of age (16). Injuries are not prevalent in this age group, but are seen with high incidence in the 15- to 18-year-old group (U.S. Tennis Association, unpublished data). It is surmised that the younger athlete's adaptive changes may be creating biomechanical deficits that predispose the athlete to injury with continued, increased use. The areas of injury in the players, (the shoulder, back, and knee) correspond with the areas of demonstrated inflexibility and weakness. In the young athlete, much work is now being directed toward defining the proper exercise dose to prevent such adaptations and defining the most appropriate conditioning programs, given the age and physical limitations in these athletes.

Conditioning for Tennis

Due to factors such as the length of the season, the musculoskeletal maladaptations that occur with the sport, and the sport-specific injury patterns, it is necessary to discuss the sport-specific aspects of conditioning for tennis. A conditioning program for tennis can be divided into the following areas: prehabilitation (the correction of musculoskeletal maladaptations that may predispose the tennis player to injury), resistive training, and, finally, sprint/interval, footwork, and speed training.

Prehabilitation

Prehabilitation exercises would consist of exercises to correct musculoskeletal deficits found in a preparticipation evaluation of the tennis player. At the elite level, such exercises are important both to prevent injury and to improve performance. At the recreational level, these exercises are important to prevent injury and to allow the player to continue to enjoy and benefit from the sport of tennis. Typical goals of a prehabilitation program might be:

1. To improve internal rotation range of motion on the dominant arm;
2. To improve external rotation strength and endurance;
3. To improve the strength of the scapular stabilizing musculature;
4. To improve low back and hamstring flexibility; and
5. To correct any individual weaknesses in terms of strength and range of motion.

Resistive Training

Resistive training for the tennis player is an important goal if the player is interested in preventing injuries and improving performance. Resistive training includes not only weight training, but also drills for abdominal strength, medicine ball drills for total body strength, and calisthenic exercises. By improving strength, power is increased, which is becoming an increasingly important component of tennis. Also, short term endurance is increased, which is of tremendous importance to the tennis player. Conditioning with medicine balls has the advantage of conditioning the entire kinetic chain in a way that promotes improved power in the tennis stroke.

Sprint/Interval, Footwork, and Speed Training

As previously mentioned, the sport of tennis is generally played in short bursts of activity. Interval training in the off-season progressing to shorter bursts of activity as the tennis season approaches is likely the best way to train for tennis. Interval training can provide an aerobic base that can be maintained by sprint training during the season. It is possible that extensive aerobic training during the season would interfere with the production of strength and power (31). Particularly for competitive tennis players, training in 10 to 20 second bursts is more specific to tennis performance than running long distances. By training in shorter bursts for long periods of time, the aerobic energy system will be utilized during the recovery process between exercise bouts, which is the same way it is used in a tennis match, i.e., recovery between points.

One problem that often arises with competitive tennis players is that there is no off-season in which to condition. The best answer is found in the concept of periodization. By carefully planning the competitive year and by choosing the times of the year when the player wants to be at his or her best, a schedule of conditioning can be incorporated into this plan. Typically, there will be an off-season, pre-season, and an in-season leading to a peak. After a peak, there should be some time of active rest, where the athlete is allowed time to recover from intense competition. An athlete who would like to peak twice in a period of 4 to 6 weeks will not likely have the opportunity for active rest or for going into an off-season phase.

Racquetball and Squash

There is less research on the musculoskeletal aspects of racquetball and squash than on tennis. However, analysis of the demands of these two sports shows many similarities to tennis. This section concentrates on the musculoskeletal aspects of the differences, in particular, a brief review of the major difference—eye injuries.

The major musculoskeletal demands in racquetball and squash are to the shoulder, elbow and wrist in the arm, and the knee and ankle in the leg. In addition, contusions occur more frequently, due to contact with the racquet, the ball, or a wall.

Common Injuries

Shoulder Problems

The overhead service motion is not needed in racquetball or squash, but overhead shots are needed. Rotator cuff impingement or rotator cuff tendinitis are less frequent problems. However, when they are present, the presenting complaints and findings are the same as in tennis players. The evaluation profile is also similar to tennis players. Treatment should include attention to mechanics and to strengthening the scapular stabilizers and rotator cuff.

Medial Elbow Strain

This is a common problem in racquetball and squash, due to the snapping mechanism of the kill shots and to the lighter racquet. Contact with the wall also may cause some extra valgus overload. Evaluation of medial elbow symptoms must include muscle-tendon and tendon-bone pathology of epicondylitis and ulnar collateral ligament strain, ulnar nerve irritation, and posterior medial bony impingement of the valgus overload syndrome. The two entities—medial epicondylitis and valgus overload syndrome—can certainly coexist, but differentiation between the two is important, since different treatment strategies are necessary.

Medial epicondylitis is characterized by pain in the flexor-pronator muscle group, just anterior and distal to the medial epicondyle. The exact location may vary, depending on whether the lesion is in the tendon-bone area or in the muscle tendon area (Fig. 32.13). The pain is experienced during athletic activity, especially during the forehand stroke, but it also may occur in nonathletic activities that require muscle activity, such as shaking hands or opening doors.

Valgus overload syndrome is characterized by pain in the medial and posterior medial areas of the elbow (Fig. 32.14). Palpation for pain in the ulnar collateral ligament starts just anterior and inferior to the medial epicondyle and proceeds obliquely to the ulna. Ligamentous instability should be checked by valgus stress testing at 10° and 30° of flexion. The ulnar nerve should be palpated along its entire course in the groove posterior to the medial epicondyle. The posterior medial bony impingement is discovered by eliciting pain over the medial part of the olecranon when the elbow goes into full extension as a valgus force is applied (Fig. 32.15). Valgus overload pain is experienced during athletic activity, especially during the forehand stroke, and may occur in nonathletic activities that put a valgus stress on the arm, such as reaching over a car seat or holding an object at arm's length. In addition, ulnar nerve impingement may give rise to ulnar neuropathy findings, such as numbness, tingling, or shooting pains into the little and ring fingers.

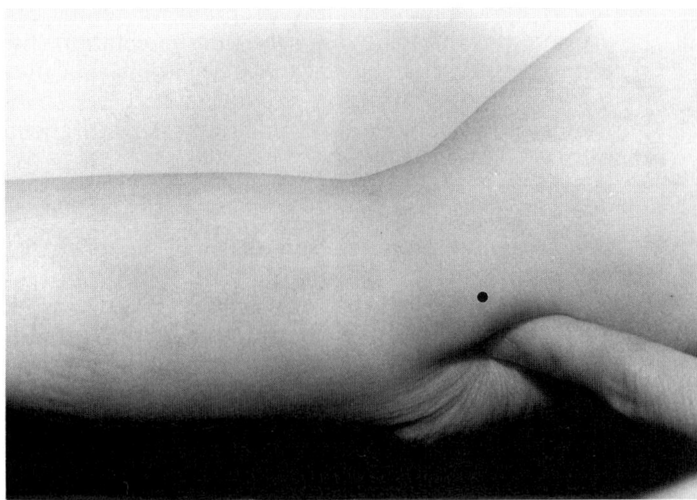

Figure 32.15. Valgus force bony impingement.

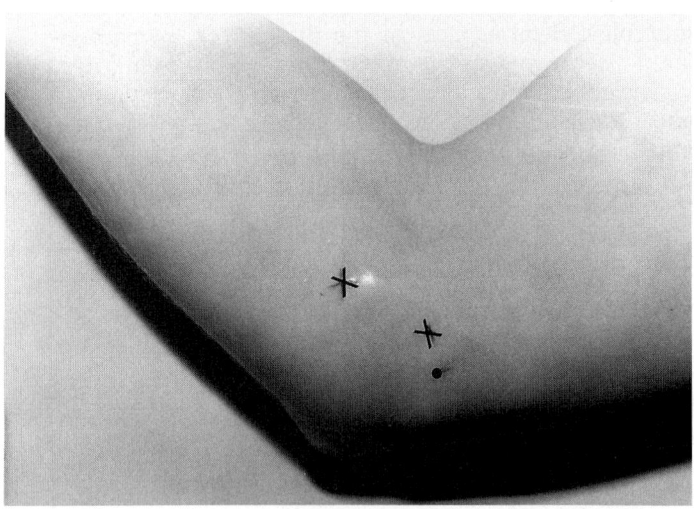

Figure 32.13. Medial epicondylitis. **X** shows points of tenderness; • shows medial epicondyle.

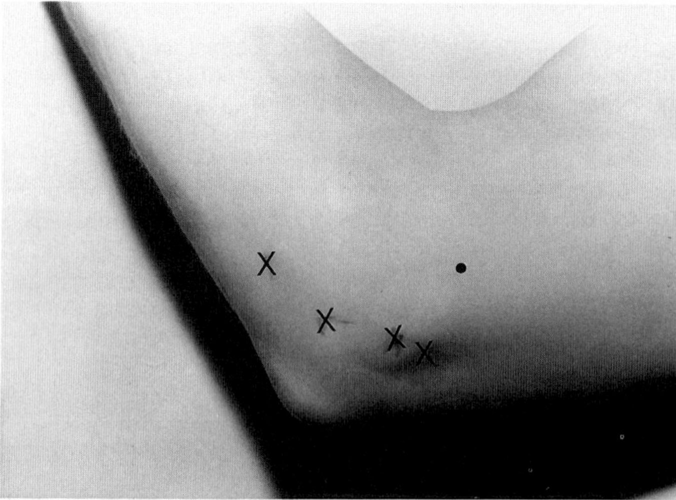

Figure 32.14. Points for valgus overload. **X** shows points of tenderness over ulnar nerve, ulnar collateral ligament, and posterior medial spur; • shows medial epicondyle.

It is important to recognize the presence or absence of any or all of these anatomical abnormalities (Fig. 32.16), so that effective treatment can be rendered. In addition to the physical examination, plain film, arthrograms, with or without CT images, and MRI scans are helpful imaging tests for differentiating the pathology.

Nonoperative treatment should be used first. It should help to resolve the tendinitis inflammation and promote healing of the injured muscle and tendon. Correction of inflexibilities of the elbow flexors and forearm pronators helps relieve valgus stress in activities.

Significant, persisting valgus overload or recurrent tendinitis problems require surgical correction. Correction of the valgus overload starts with medial collateral ligament stabilization, usually with a palmaris longus graft, anchored distally through drill holes in the ulna or with a Mitek anchor and brought proximally through drill holes in the epicondyle. In addition, posterior medial arthrotomy for excision of hypertrophied synovium, bony spurs, loose bodies, and hypertrophic articular cartilage is done. Finally, ulnar nerve decompression is carried out, with or without transposition depending on the amount of scar in the groove and the stability of the nerve after neurolysis. Treatment of the tendinitis problem is the same as was outlined in the section on tennis.

Wrist Problems

Tendinitis can be seen in all of the wrist extensor tendons, either in the dorsal compartments or at distal insertions, once again due to the extra snapping motion that is present as a normal part of the racquetball and squash stroke. Nonoperative treatment, with rest, ice, antiinflammatories, and proper wrist support, either with taping or a splint, will result in good relief of symptoms. Symptom resolution should then be fol-

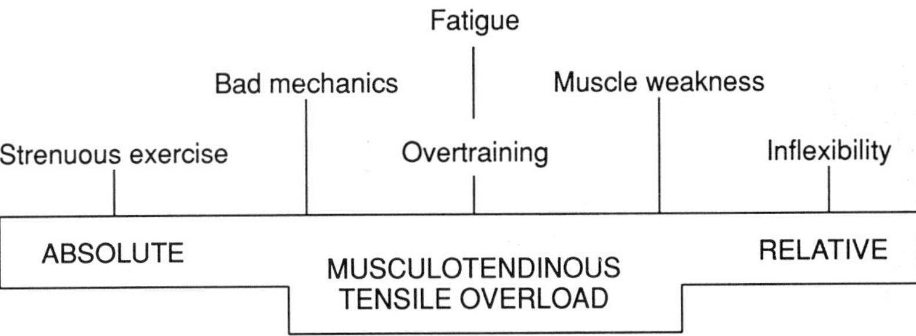

Figure 32.16. Potential causes of tensile overload injuries to soft tissue.

lowed by strengthening exercises for both flexor and extensor muscles before return to play.

Contusions

Contusions that occur to the trunk or extremities due to the impact by the ball are painful but usually superficial. Local swelling is usually small, and can be controlled by ice application. Early return to activity is the rule. Contusions that occur due to racquet impact may, however, have more damaging consequences. These may involve deeper structures and may actually involve muscle tears. Pain may be significant enough to stop athletic activity. Any swelling, which may be immediate, must be controlled. Ice, a light compression dressing, and protection are necessary in the acute phase. The injured muscle should be kept in as much stretch as possible in this phase. Gradual return to normal use should be advocated, since experimental work on direct-blow muscle contusions shows that optimum healing takes place by regeneration of muscle tissue. This process may take 3 to 4 weeks and will result in excessive scar tissue if too much tension is placed on the repair site early in recovery.

Shin Splints

Overload-induced shin splints, both anterior and posterior, are seen in racquetball players. Evaluation will usually show diffuse areas of increased tenderness over the anterior or posterior bony attachments of the tibialis anterior muscles to the tibia. Swelling may accompany the tenderness in acute cases. There is usually a history of extra use (such as a tournament or increased frequency of athletic activity) or a change in shoes. Range of motion may be decreased. This relatively mild condition must be distinguished from its two more disabling cousins, tibial stress fracture and chronic exertional compartment syndrome. The similarity in causative conditions and frequency of association give rise to the possibility that these conditions are points along a spectrum of overload problems in the tibia. Plain x-rays, bone scans, and compartment pressure measurements are all diagnostic aids to be used in distinguishing the conditions.

Treatment should start by alleviating the aggravating problems with decreased activities and corrections in shoes or surface. Most athletes will demonstrate dorsiflexion or plantar flexion inflexibility, which needs to be normalized. Neoprene sleeves may give support while therapy is progressing and may allow earlier return to play.

Eye Problems

The most dangerous injury that occurs in all racquet sports is damage to the eye, either by contact with the ball or the racquet. It is much more common in racquetball and squash than in tennis, because of the confined nature of the court. Hyphemas, which result from direct contact between the racquet or ball and the eye, may be effectively treated in the acute stage, but also may be associated with cataract, retinal detachment, or retinal hemorrhages. Increased risk of future glaucoma is present with these conditions (32). Both the racquet ball and squash ball have been shown capable of conforming tightly into the orbital cavity on direct impact, creating tremendous direct and concussive forces on the fragile eyeball. With high ball speeds and limited room for player movement, even experienced players may be injured.

The most effective treatment of this problem is prevention. Eyeguards have gone through several stages of evolution (32), so that effective prevention is available by a combination of polycarbonate lenses, a wraparound configuration so that eyegard rims are posterior to the orbital rim, antifog coating, and secure posterior stabilization to the back of the head. Regular glasses or open-lensed protectors have been shown to be totally ineffective in preventing eye injuries, and may actually increase the injury because of shattering.

Eyeguards now are mandatory in most tournaments and should be advocated for all levels of play at all times.

REFERENCES

1. Andrews–Wolffe Lecture, Keynote Lecture. American College of Sports Medicine. Salt Lake City UT, 1990.
2. Shapiro R. Unpublished Data The University of Kentucky Biodynamics Laboratory, Lexington, KY.
3. Glousman RE, Jobe FW, Tibone JE. Dynamic electromyographic analysis of the throwing shoulder with Glenerohumeral instability. J Bone Joint Surg. 1988;70:220–226.
4. Jobe FW, Tibone JE, Perry J. An EMG analysis of the shoulder in throwing and pitching. A preliminary report. Am J Sports Med 1983;11:3–5.
5. Jobe FW, Moynes DR, Tibone JE. An EMG analysis of the shoulder in pitching: A second report. Am J Sp Med 1984;12:218–220.
6. Fox EL, Matthews DK. Interval training. Philadelphia: Saunders, 1974.
7. Fleck SJ, Kraemer WJ. Designing resistance training programs. Champaign, IL: Human Kinetics Books, 1987.

8. Kibler WB, McQueen C, Uhl TL. Fitness evaluations and fitness findings in competitive junior tennis players. Clin Sports Med 1988;7:403–416.
9. Pollock ML, Fox JH, Fox SM. Health and fitness through physical activity. New York: Wiley and Sons, 1990.
10. Chandler TJ: Work\rest intervals in world class tennis. Tennis Pro 1991; January\February:4.
11. Nirschl RP. Shoulder impingement syndromes. Instructional Course Lecture, Chicago: AAOS, 1989.
12. Kibler WB, Chandler TJ, Uhl TL, et al. A musculoskeletal approach to the preparticipation physical examination. Preventing injury and improving performance. Am J Sports Med 1989;17, 525–531.
13. Alderink GJ, Kuck DJ. Isokinetic shoulder strength of high school and college-aged pitchers. J Orthop Sports Phys Ther 1986;163–172.
14. Chandler TJ, Kibler WB, Stracener EC. Shoulder strength, power, and endurance in college tennis players. Am J Sports Med. 1992;20(4):455–458.
15. Warner JD, Micheli LJ, et al. Patterns of flexibility, laxity, and strength in normal shoulders and shoulders with instability and impingement. Am J Sports Med 1990;18:336–375.
16. Kibler WB, Chandler TS. Musculoskeletal adaptations and injuries associated with intense participation in youth sports. In: Cahill BR, Pearl AJ, eds. Intensive participation in children's sports. Chicago: AOSS, 1993.
17. Chandler TJ, Kibler WB, Uhl TL, et al. Flexibility comparisons of junior elite tennis players to other athletes. Am J Sports Med 1990;18(2):134–136.
18. Harryman DT, Sidles JA, Clark JM, et al. Translation of the humeral head on the glenoid with passive glenohumeral motion. J Bone Joint Surg 1990;72a(3):1334–1343.
19. Kibler, WB. Motions Around the Shoulder, Symposia, American Orthopedic Society for Sports Medicine, Orlando, FL. 1991.
20. Silliman JF, Hawkins RJ. Current concepts and recent advances in the athlete's shoulder. Clin Sports Med 1991;10(4), 693–705.
21. Leadbetter W. An introduction to sports induced soft tissue inflammation. In: Sports induced inflammation. Chicago: Am Academy of Orthop Surg, 1990.
22. Kibler, W.B. Concepts in exercise rehabilitation. In: Leadbetter W, Buckwalter JA, Gordon SL. Sports induced inflammation. 1990:759–769.
23. Kibler WB: The role of the scapula in the throwing motion. Contemporary Orthop 1991;22(5):525–532.
24. Leadbetter WB. Back surgery in tennis players. First world congress for medicine and science in tennis, New Haven, CT: Yale University, 1991.
25. Garrett WE. Muscle strain injuries: Clinical and basic aspects. Medicine and Science in Sports and Exercise. 1990;22(4):436–443.
26. Kibler WB. Clinical aspects of muscle injury. Medicine and Science in Sports and Exercise. 1990;22(4), 450–452.
27. Herring SA. Rehabilitation from muscle injury. Med Sci Sports Ex 1990;22:4.
28. Kibler WB, Goldberg C, Chandler TJ. Functional biomechanical deficits in running athletes with plantar fasciitis. Am J Sports Med 1991;19(1):66–71.
29. Kibler WB, Chandler TJ, Pace BP. Principles for rehabilitation after chronic tendon injuries. Clin Sports Med 1992;11(3):661–671.
30. Chandler TJ, Kibler WB. Sport specific screening and testing in the prevention of injury. In: Per Renstrom, ed. The Encylcopaedia of Sports Medicine. London: Blackwell Scientific Publications, 1993.
31. Hickson RC. Interference of strength development by simultaneously training for strength and endurance. European Journal of Applied Physiology. 1980;215:255–263.
32. Easterbrook M. Eye protection in racquet sports. Clin Sports Med 1988;7:253–266.

33 / RUGBY

J.P.R. Williams

Rugby union is played by two teams of 15 players each who are allowed to carry, pass, and kick the ball to another player who is on side, i.e., behind the player who last played the ball. The ball is oval in shape and somewhat larger than that used in American football. The team who scores the greater number of points is the winner. The players score by placing the ball on or over the opposite goal line (try) or by kicking it over the cross-bar between the goal posts, either as a conversion of a try, a penalty (field goal), or a drop goal.

The game is usually played on a grass surface on a rectangular field, slightly shorter, but wider than American football (Fig. 33.1). It is controlled by a referee who may be assisted by a touch judge on each side line. The referee blows a whistle to signal the start of play and time-outs for infringements and scores. The game is played in two 40-min periods, with a 5-min break at halftime during which the players remain on the field of play.

The players must not wear any item of clothing that may have dangerous projections, such as buckles and rings, or harness-type shoulder pads, unless they have special dispensation from the referee. A soft pad of cotton wool or sponge rubber may be worn, again with the referee's approval, for protection following injury. The spikes of the players' boots must be of an approved material and size. Players are encouraged to wear fitted mouth guards to prevent dental injuries and concussion.

Replacement of players may be allowed in trial matches, but in all other matches players are replaced only if injured. The number of players that are replaced varies, but at international level, there are generally six substitutes. If an injured player does not request substitution, the referee may, on the advice of the medical personnel, require the player to leave the field if continued play could be harmful, e.g., after concussion. The captain also has the authority to ask one of his or her players to leave the field. Once the player has been replaced, he or she cannot return.

Apart from injuries, all players remain on the field throughout the game. Each team has eight forwards and seven backs. The forwards' essential function is to win possession of the ball from set plays, such as scrums and line outs, and in the loose from mauls and rucks. The backs, whenever possible, run the ball toward their opponent's line or try to gain ground by tactical kicking. Accordingly, forwards tend to be bigger and more muscular to engage in the physical contact in tight play, whereas backs need to be fast with ball handling and kicking skills.

Rugby league is a variant of rugby union. The rugby league was formed in an attempt to allow players who had missed work to be able to reclaim money (broken time payments). At the top level it is a professional game and is played mainly in Australia, northern England, and France. New Zealand and New Guinea also play. Rugby league teams have 13 players on a side. There are no line outs, and there are different rules for playing the ball when tackled. This removes the element of mauling and rucking, and scrums are modified. Many of the top rugby union players are highly sought after by rugby league. When a player signs for a professional rugby league team he forfeits his amateur status and no longer is allowed to play rugby union. However, recently the rules regarding amateurism have been relaxed, and perhaps rugby league players will eventually be allowed to return to rugby union. It is only recently that former rugby league players have been allowed to coach rugby union.

Incidence of Injury

Studies have shown that rugby is a relatively safe sport. Unfortunately, comparison of these studies is difficult because they used different methods to assess risk and examined the sport during different time periods. Available data on the rate of injury are shown in Table 33.1 (1–9). Allemando's (1) statistical review of injuries in France is based on data supplied by the

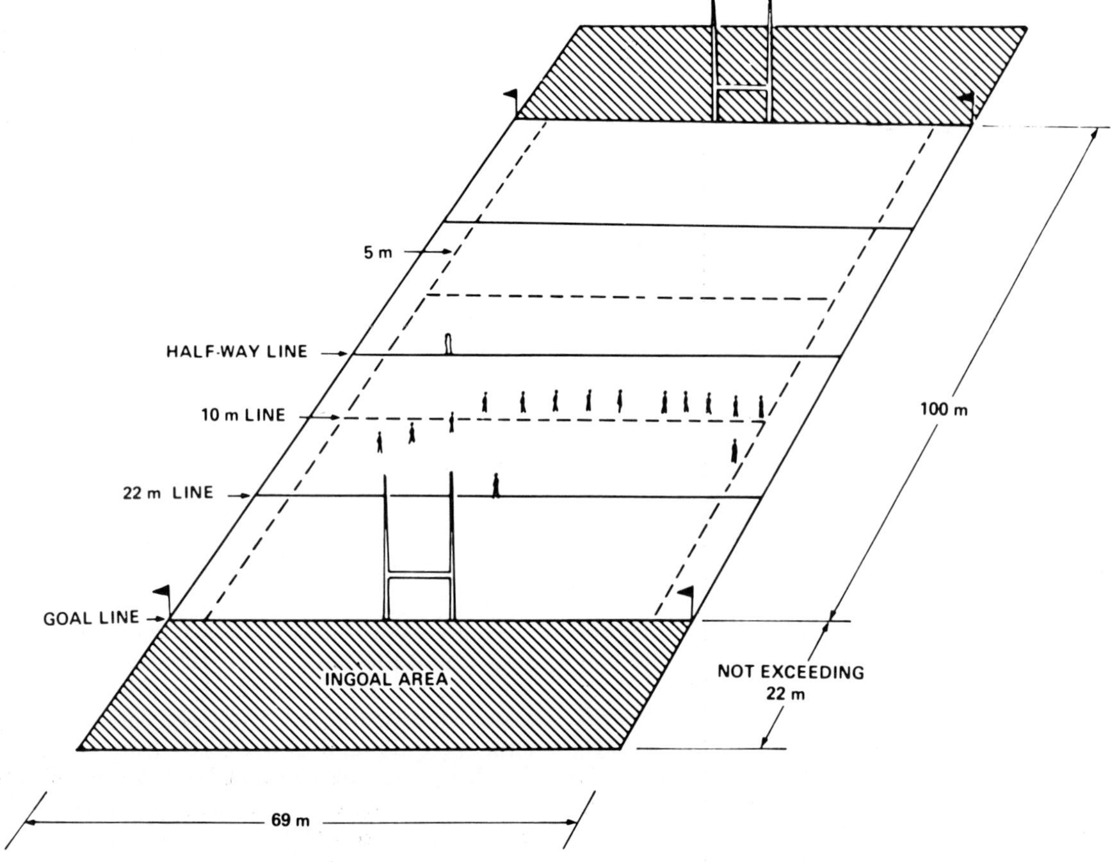

Figure 33.1. Plan of a full-size rugby field, which is not to exceed 100 m in length and 69 m in width. The players of one team are in position for kickoff from center field. The referee stands at the halfway line.

Table 33.1.
Injury Rate per 10,000 Player/Games

Population (year)	Rate	Reference
France (1971)	36.8	1
Clubs in northern England (1974)	30.5	2
U.S. colleges and clubs (1975)	110.5	3
Gloucester, New Zealand (1980)	52.4	4
Rugby school in England (1981)	197.7	5
Newington College, Sidney, Australia (1982)	132.0	6

French Insurance System, which is imposed on all players. For the year studied, 75,238 players of all ages were involved, each playing an average of 40 games. There were 11,349 accidents, and of these 10,524 were fully investigated. The overall risk was low: 1 accident in 256 appearances. The study revealed that 12.5% of the accidents occurred during training and fewer accidents were reported by schoolboys.

More recently, in a smaller, comparable epidemiologic study in Canterbury (New Zealand), Dalley et al. (7) found 1 injury in 191 appearances, i.e., 52.4 per 10,000 playing games. They attributed some of the apparent increase in injury rate to the maul and subsequent pileup of the modern game. They also noticed 14.87% of the injuries involved illegal play away from the ball. The peak age group for injury was 16 to 20 years.

For schoolboys the risks of serious injury were lower, although minor injuries were more likely to be recorded, especially in boarding school. Sparks (5), medical officer to a rugby school, recorded a somewhat higher injury rate in a survey over 30 seasons and stated that few of the injuries had been serious. Davidson et al. (6) also found a low incidence of severe injuries at Newington College, Sidney, Australia. They found only 75 severe injuries in 71,340 player/games, i.e., only 9.9 per 10,000 players/games. A study (5) of 25 Australian school rugby union teams, covering more than 45,000 player/games demonstrated a somewhat lower incidence of injury in boys aged 9 to 19.

Type of Injury

Walkden (8) honorary medical officer of the Rugby Football Union, diagnosed and classified injuries for 12 years at Twickenham, UK. His statistics indicated a player risk of minor injury of 0.1 per game and 0.017 for serious injuries (concussion, fractures, and conditions that ultimately required orthopedic opinion or kept the player from competition for 3 weeks). Data by type of injury are shown in Table 33.2. He noted that 50% percent of the lacerations required suturing and 66% of these were in the head and neck area. The knee followed by the shoulder and ankle were most frequent joint injuries.

Mechanisms

Understanding the modes of injury in rugby requires involvement of qualified personnel who have the ability to appreciate the interplay of the factors that may result in injury. Little hard data have been collected, perhaps because there was generally not thought to be any need for extensive investigation of rugby injuries. However, some indication of risk factors can be gained from the surveys that have been conducted.

Circumstances of Accident

The aspects of rugby play in which injuries can occur are as follows.

Table 33.2.
Analysis of Injuries (Twickenham, 1964 to 1976)

Tissue Injured	Percent
Skin	38.5
Musculotendinous	22.0
Joint	21.0
Head	6.5
Bones	6.0
Miscellaneous (eye, ear, oral, etc.)	6.0

Tackle

The tackle is the most frequent cause of injury, accounting for at least 33%. The injury may be sustained by the tackler or the tackled. A running tackle from behind may cause an injury to either player, usually affecting the hands, wrists, shoulders, and legs; these injuries can be severe (Fig. 33.2). A tackle from front on is likely to be dangerous to the tackler, especially if the tackler's head is in the opponent's hip area, where the lifted thigh can cause a head or neck injury (Fig. 33.3); the tackled player may land on the tackler's head as they hit the ground (Fig. 33.4). To avoid head-on contact the tackler should try to maneuver the opposing player to one side and use the shoulder. The head should then finish uppermost (see Fig. 33.2). Neck-high and stiff-arm tackles are illegal, and referees have been encouraged to be stricter on penalizing these types of tackles.

Maul, Ruck, and Pileup

The maul, ruck, and pileup are also frequent causes of injury. A maul is formed by one or more players of each side, on their feet and in physical contact, closing around the player who is carrying the ball. A maul ends when the ball is on the ground or the ball carrier emerges (Fig. 33.5). A ruck ensues when the ball is on the ground and one or more players from each team, on their feet, are in contact and are contesting it (Fig. 33.6). These situations involve twisting and straining of the upper body and stresses on the knees. When the ball is on the ground it can be played with the foot, adding the risk of players being kicked. It is illegal to collapse the

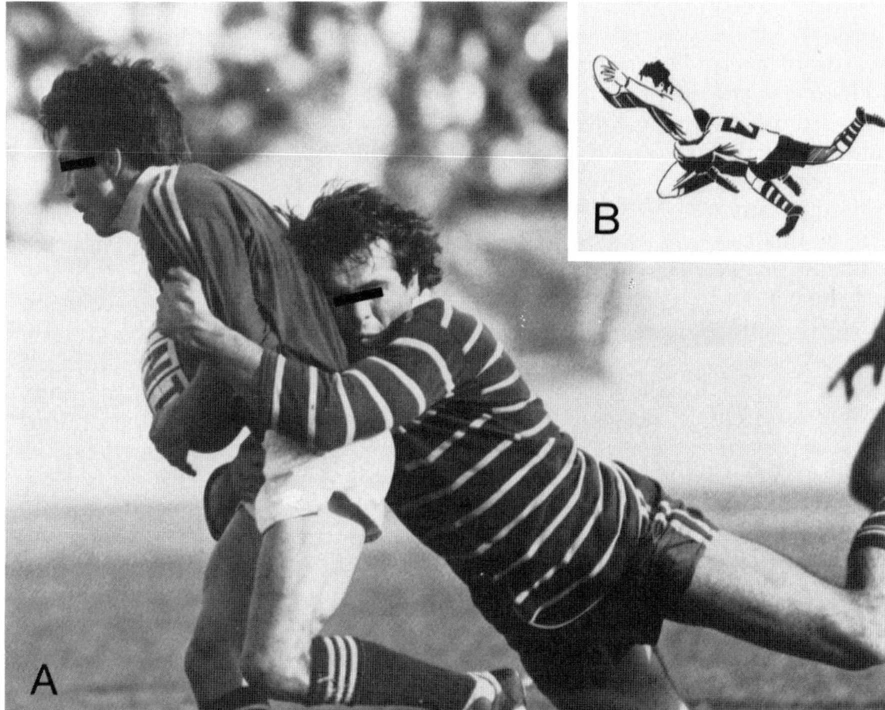

Figure 33.2. A, The running tackle correctly executed. **B,** The head will finish uppermost.

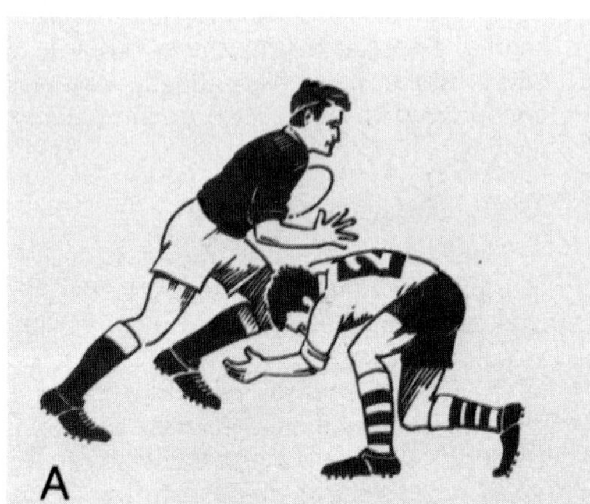

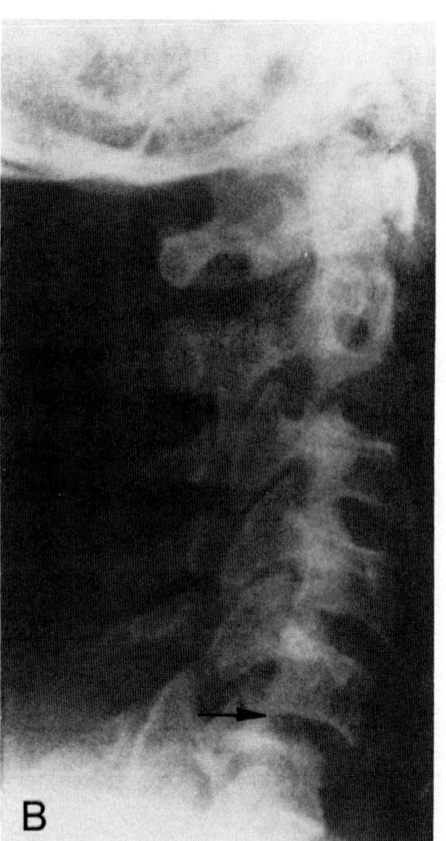

Figure 33.3. A, The player is tackling with the head to the lifted knee; the thigh or hip has been identified as a cause of serious neck injuries. **B,** This anterior dislocation of the C5 on C6 vertebral body *(arrow)* with bilateral locking facets resulted from a tackle with forced neck flexion.

maul. If this happens, a pileup follows (Fig. 33.7), and the referee should promptly stop the game to prevent injury.

Scrum

When the scrum is set the eight forwards of each team pack together, usually in a three-four-one information. The three players making up each front row should not illegally charge, and the scrum should not collapse. The correct method of binding is illustrated in Figure 33.8. If a scrum should collapse it is imperative that the players be prevented from pushing as this can lead to severe neck injuries (Fig. 33.9). These severe neck injuries involve flexion and rotation of the cervical spine.

Line Out

Because players are relatively stationary and on their feet, injuries in the line out are not common for players away from the ball (Fig. 33.10). In rugby, physical contact should only occur between players who are contesting the possession of the ball, but sometimes other players may suffer injuries. Leg injuries may occur with sudden stopping, starting, or swerving and running at full speed, especially if the athlete is cold, fatigued, or has a weak hamstring. Injuries may occur from accidental collisions or from illegal interference (e.g., from early or late tackles or other maneuvers). Dalley et al. (7) found illegal involvement in 15% of reported injuries.

Sites of Injury

Sites of injury will be analyzed according to the anatomical region of the body involved (Table 33.3). Injuries to the lower limbs are most frequent, followed by injuries to the head, including neck and face, and then the shoulder and arms.

Head and Face

Most injuries to the head and face are slight and superficial, requiring no more than a dressing or a few skin sutures. They may result from contact or collision with another player, an indiscriminate boot, the ground, or even a goal post. In a small proportion, fractures of the facial bones may occur, most frequently of the nose. These are rarely serious and most often happen to forwards playing in the front row of the scrum. Concussion may occur accidentally because of the contact nature of the sport. The blow causing a concussion is usually glancing and mild compared with boxing, in which there is a deliberate intention to inflict damage to the head, and American football, in which vertex or head-on tackling is used.

Many of these injuries are slight, and estimating the incidence is difficult. Adams (9) recorded 3.1%, but concussions possibly constitute up to 5% of the injuries

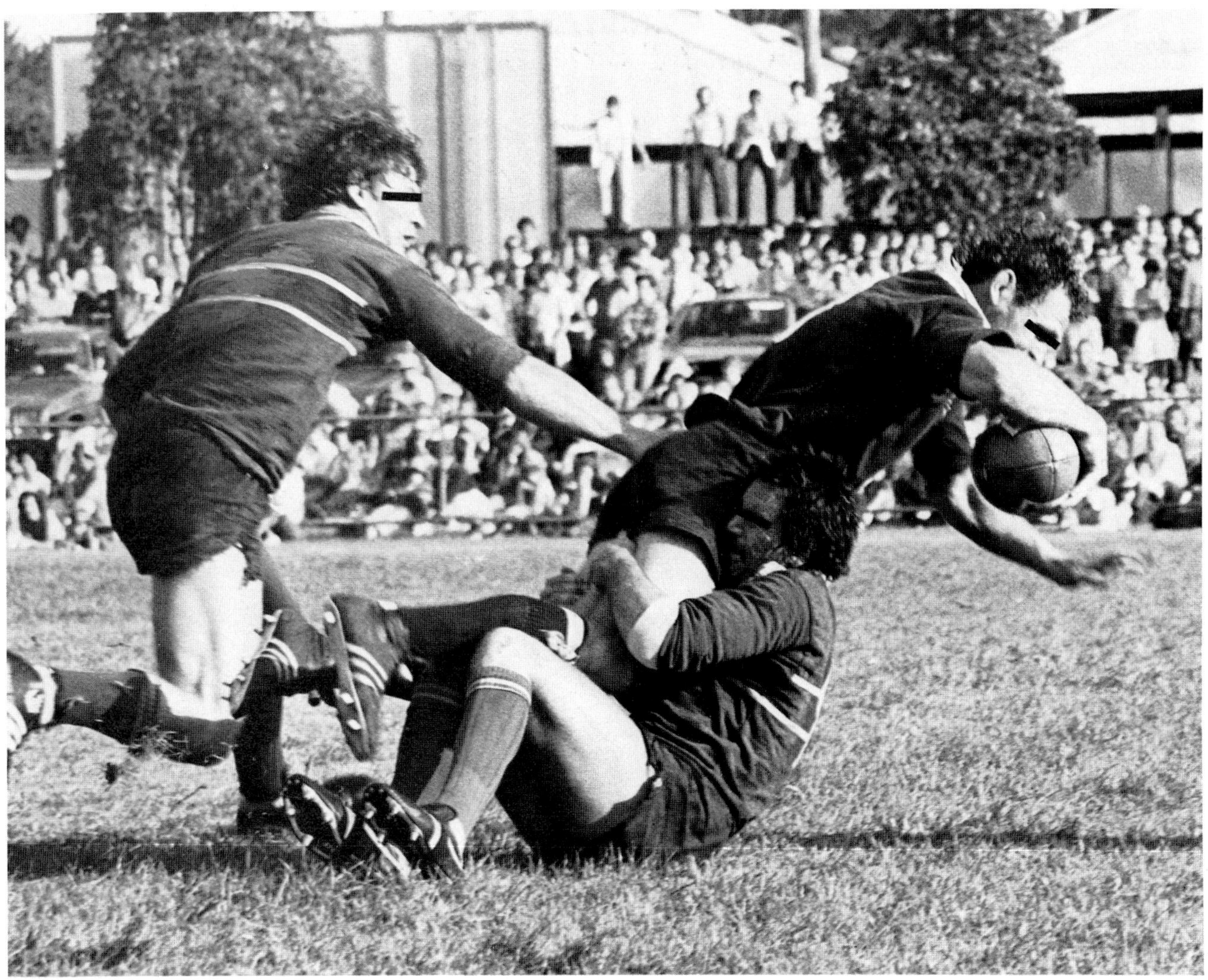

Figure 33.4. An incorrect tackle is being made from in front. The ball carrier's momentum will probably force the tackler's head backward so it strikes the ground.

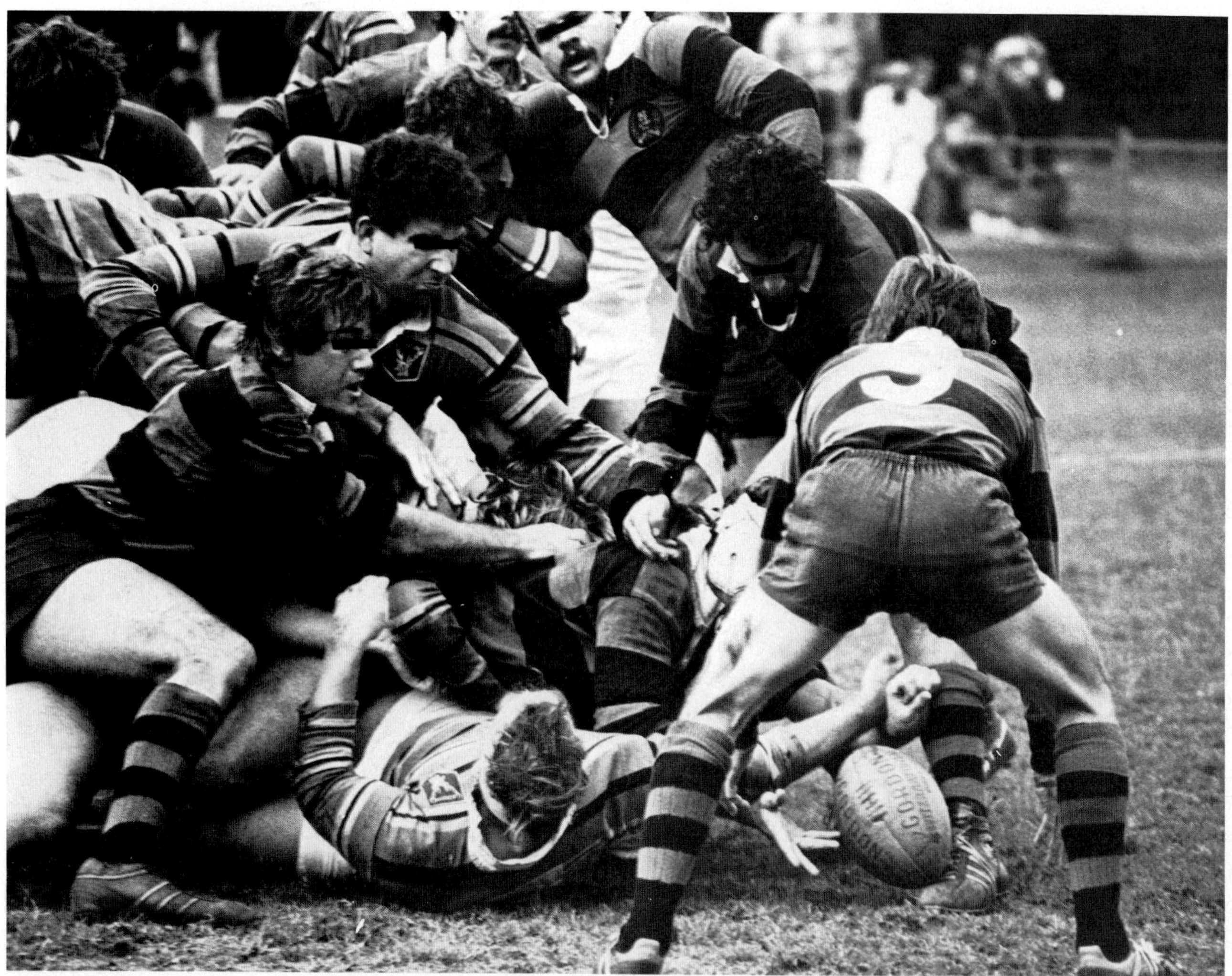

Figure 33.5. The pressures and strains are evident in this maul.

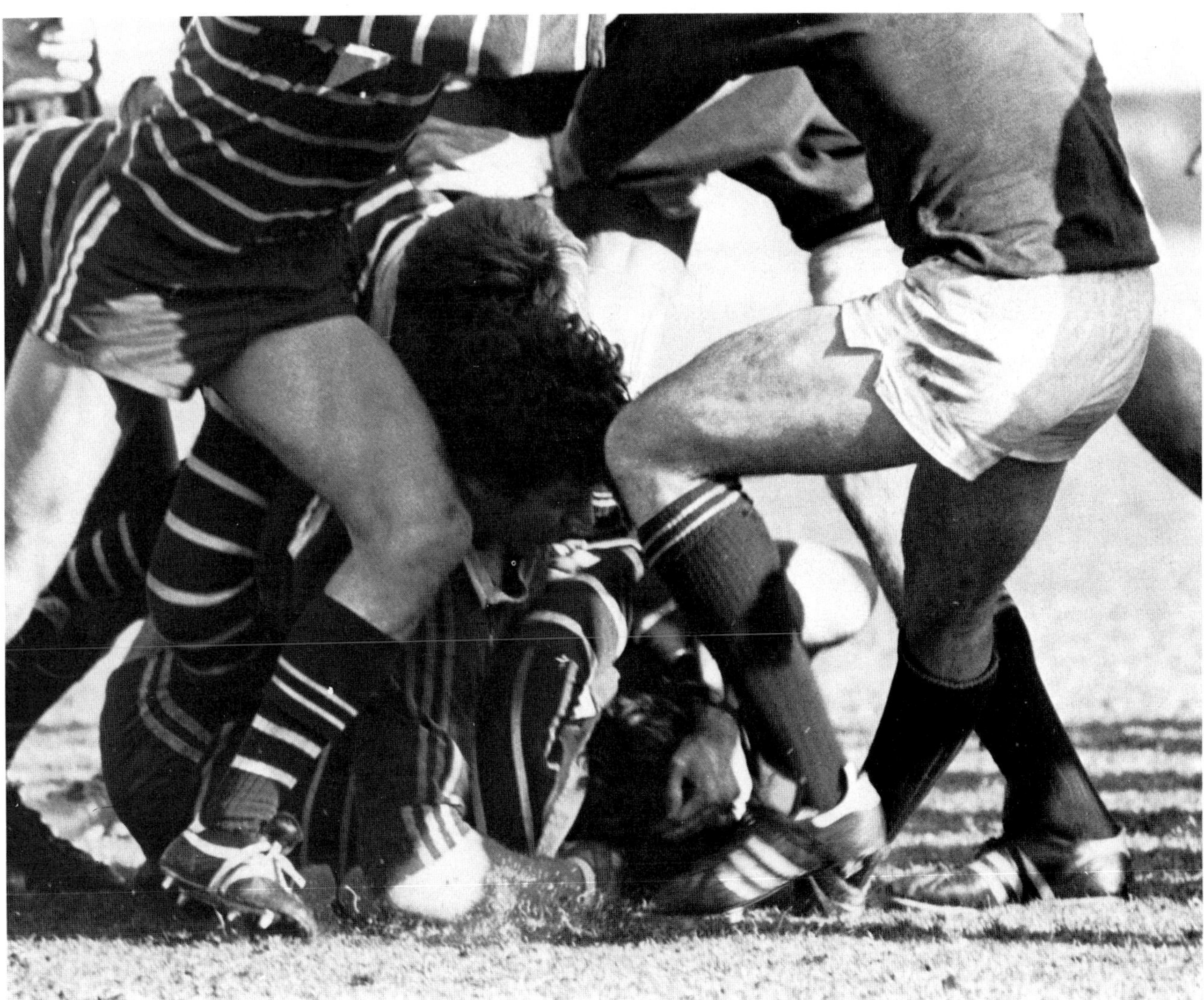

Figure 33.6. A ruck has formed around the ball on the ground. The players are at risk to injuries from boots unless play is stopped quickly.

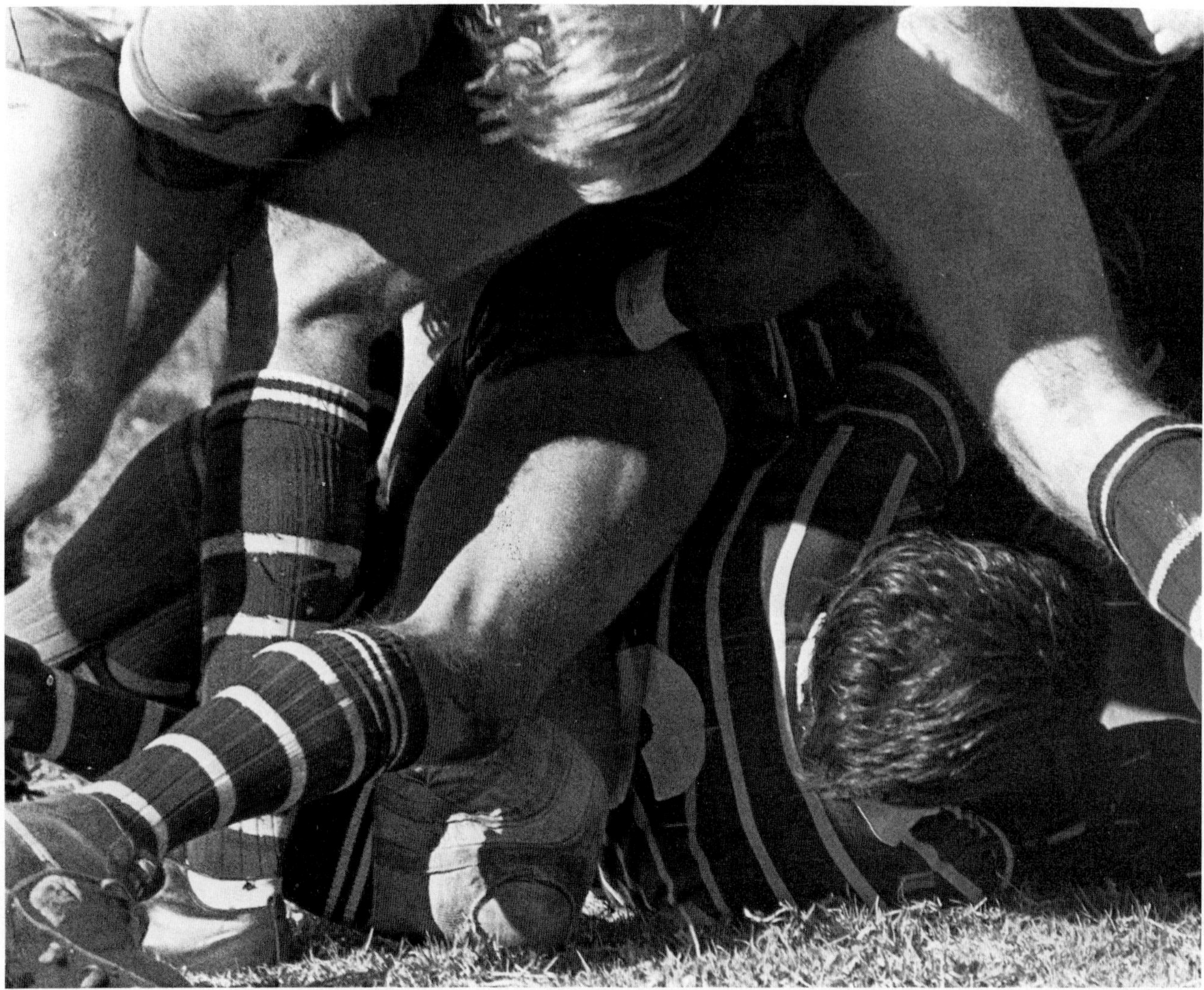

Figure 33.7. A pileup causes obvious stresses and strenuous contacts.

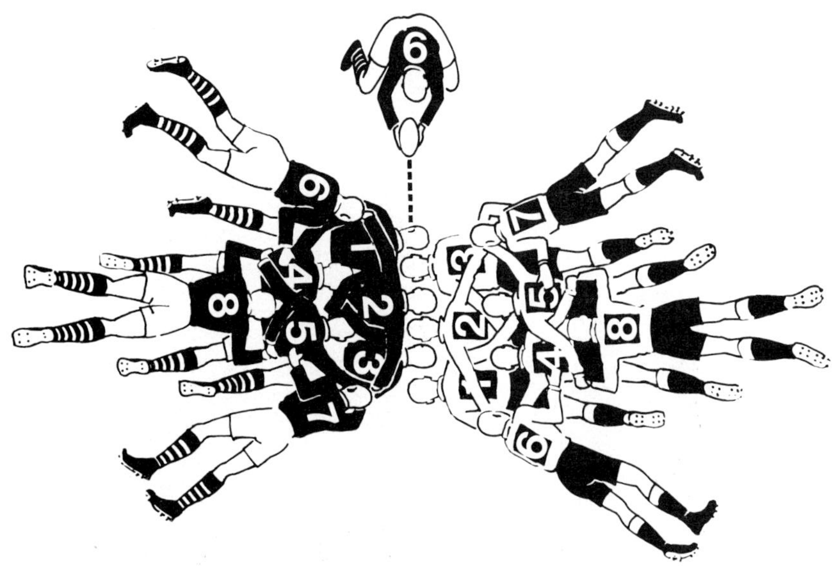

A

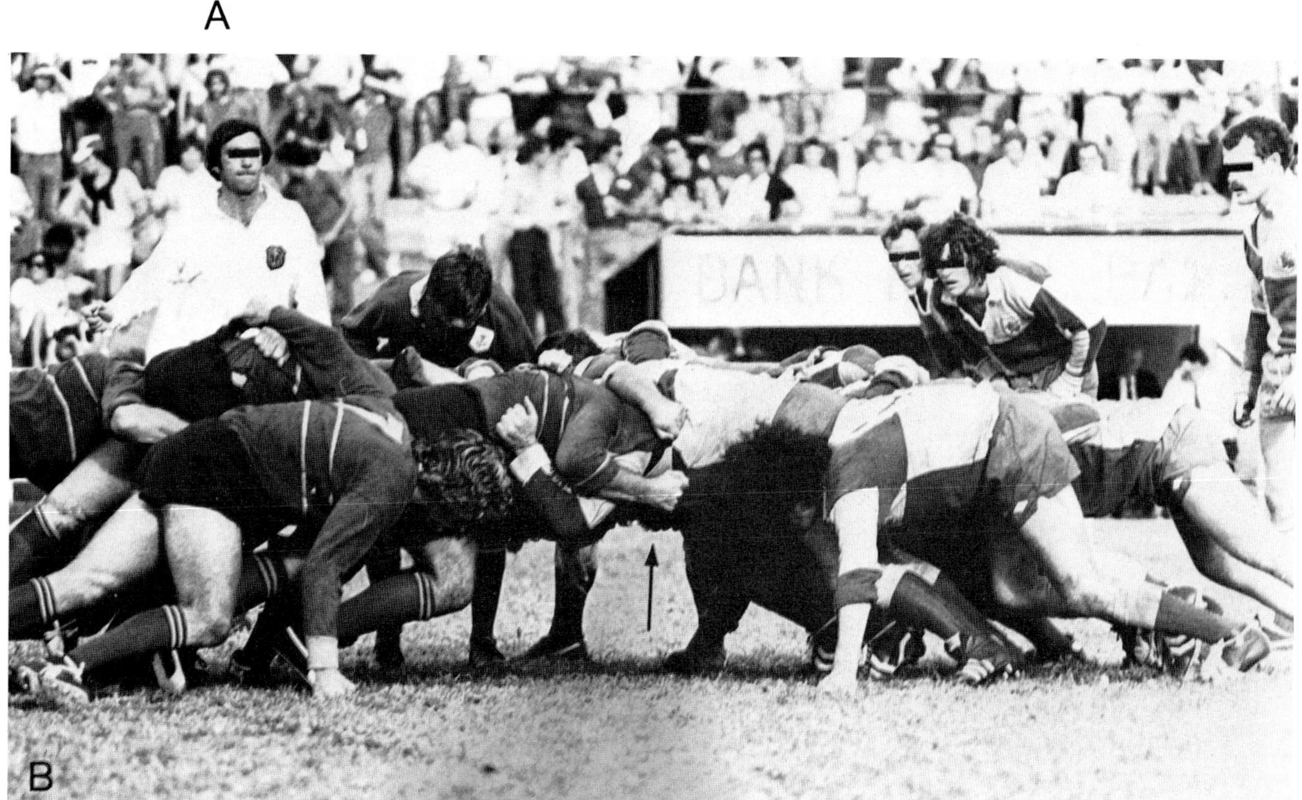

Figure 33.8. A, Diagram of set scrum is shown from above. The half back (no. 9) is about to put in the ball. At this point there is a concerted push to assist the strike going forward, thus getting a good ball. **B,** A scene of the scrum which is properly formed, stable, and safe. The *arrow* shows the binding of arms in the front row.

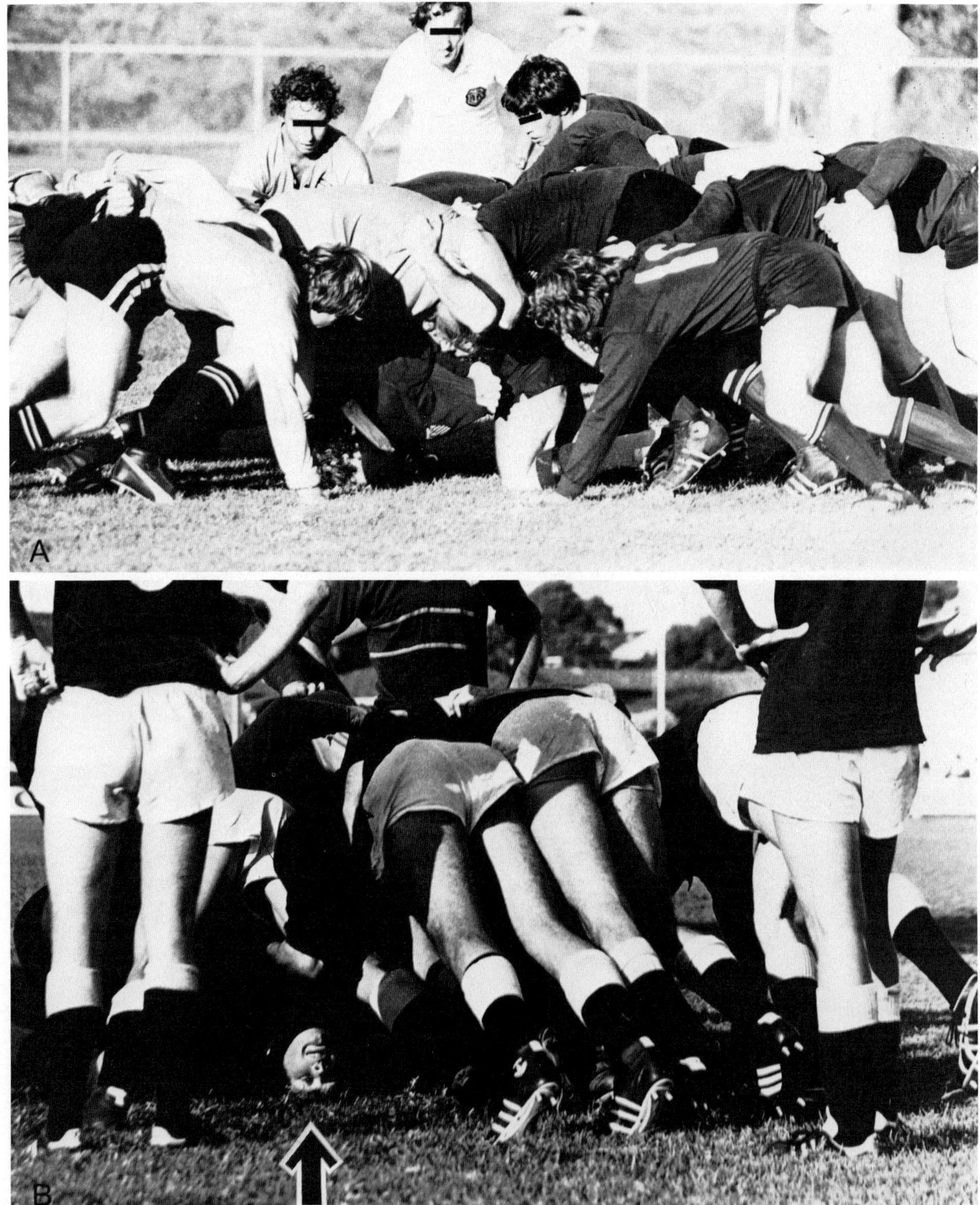

Figure 33.9. A, The scrum is beginning to collapse and become dangerous. **B,** The head of the front row forward *(arrow)* has been forced into an acutely fixed position in the collapsing scrum. This has been recognized as the mechanism most likely to account for cervical fracture dislocations in scrums.

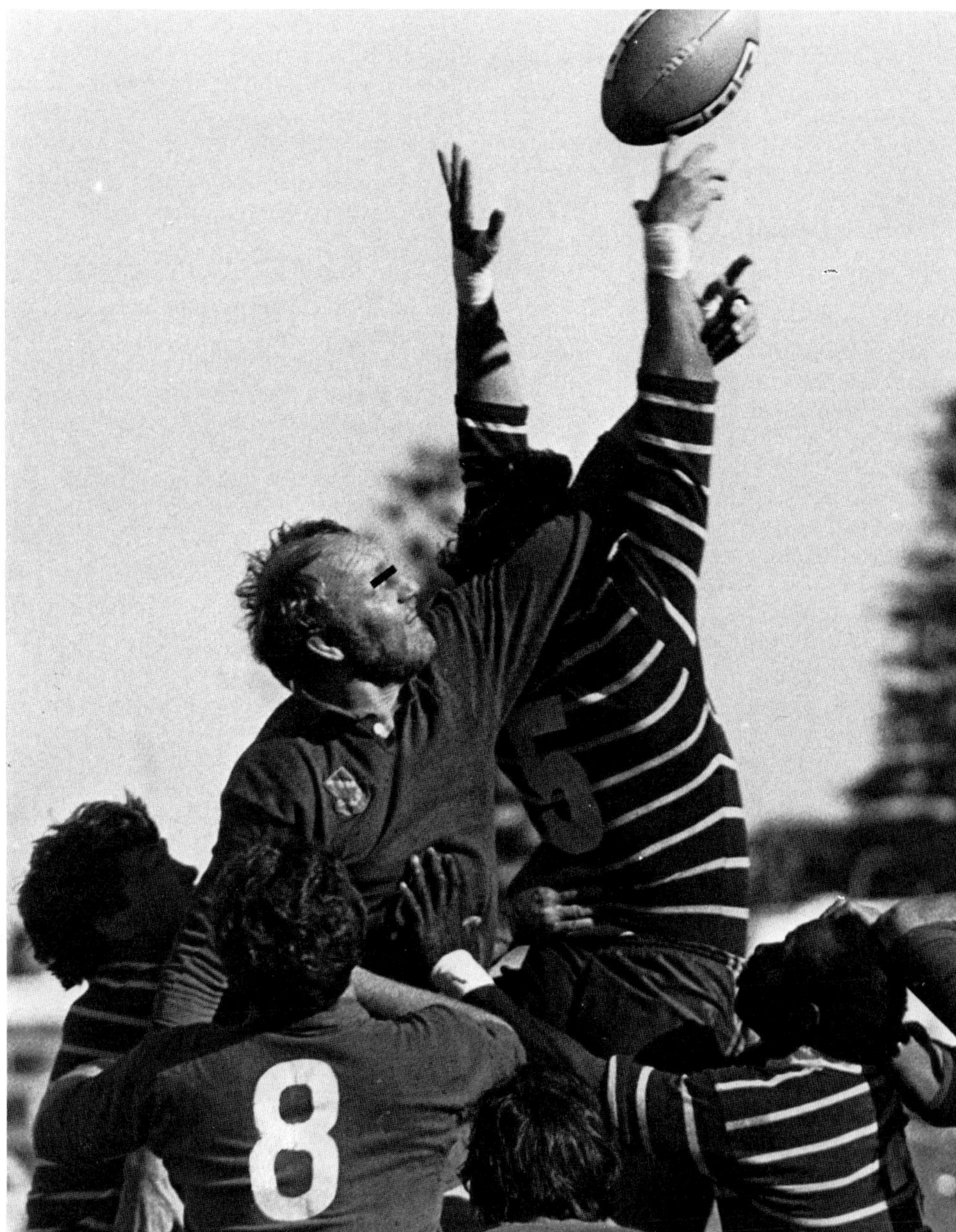

Figure 33.10. Players striving for the ball being thrown in at line out to restart play after the ball has gone into touch.

Table 33.3.
Site of Injury (Percent)

Region	Reference 10	1	2	7
Head	23.9	16.3	30.6	30.2
Shoulder/arm	31.2	29.4	22.1	18.3
Trunk	11.2	15.6	11.8	11.8
Lower limbs	33.8	33.8	35.7	39.7

calling for medical treatment. Concussive injuries must be taken seriously because of the occasional severe sequelae. Concussion is usually of a mild nature. There has been a tightening up of medical treatment of concussion, and it is now mandatory for the player who has been lost consciousness for any length of time to be removed from the field and prevented from training or playing for 3 weeks. This is in line with the rules for amateur boxing, and there has been good progress on behalf of the rugby medical community in complying with this law.

Neck

Most neck injuries are mild to moderate strains of the musculotendinous structures that occur in scrummaging, mauling, and rucking. Occasionally, serious injuries occur during a scrum tackle or maul. Cervical injuries and fracture-dislocation appeared to be on the rise during the 1970s, and this was generally attributed to the increasing frequency of scrum collapse. The mechanism of injury is flexion and rotation (4).

Scher (11, 12) reviewed 20 cervical cord injuries in rugby players admitted to a spinal unit between 1964 and 1976 and found 40% had resulted from fracture-dislocation caused by the scrum collapsing. Scher identified that high tackles were the cause of some serious neck injuries, and this tackling technique has since been outlawed.

Shoulder and Arm

Shoulder injuries are common in rugby. The most common being that of an acromioclavicular sprain. This is caused by the player falling on the point of the shoulder, and results in a characteristic bump at the junction between the acromion and the clavicle (Fig. 33.11). Fractures of the clavicle and shoulder dislocations also occur. Dislocations in young rugby players are potentially serious, because they frequently lead to recurrent anterior instability and ultimately the need for surgical shoulder stabilization. Tackling efficiently and falling correctly are important in reducing shoulder injuries.

Trunk

There are times when internal bleeding is suspected, but serious injury to the abdomen is uncommon in rugby. If increasing dyspnea and chest pain follow an injury, the player should be referred for x-ray to check out rib fractures and pneumothorax.

Musculotendinous strains of the lower spine are quite common, particularly in forwards because of the demands in scrummaging. Occasionally, chip fractures of the transverse process of the lumbar spine may occur when a player is down on the ball as might happen in a ruck. Haematuria may result from an inadvertent blow to the loin. This needs proper investigation and usually involves observation in hospital for a day or so.

Training and Personnel

Rugby's popularity is growing. However, it is a physical contact game, and because there is little protective gear, there is naturally concern among parents in allowing their children to play this game. It is, therefore, important that players, coaches, administrators, first aid providers, and doctors are all aware of the dangers inherent in the sport. Ideally, a doctor should be present at every game, although logistically this is impossible in most countries. Educating players, coaches, and referees is important so that dangerous sequelae can be prevented.

Treatment

If a player is injured, it is important to prevent any further injury, and this involves cessation of playing with treatment of rest, ice, compression, and elevation (RICE). Any suspicion of concussion in a player should be taken seriously, and the player should be taken off the field of play. If the player has been knocked out, 24 hr neurologic observation in a hospital is necessary. Facial injuries should be seen in the local casualty or emergency room, and adequate x-rays should be taken to exclude facial fractures.

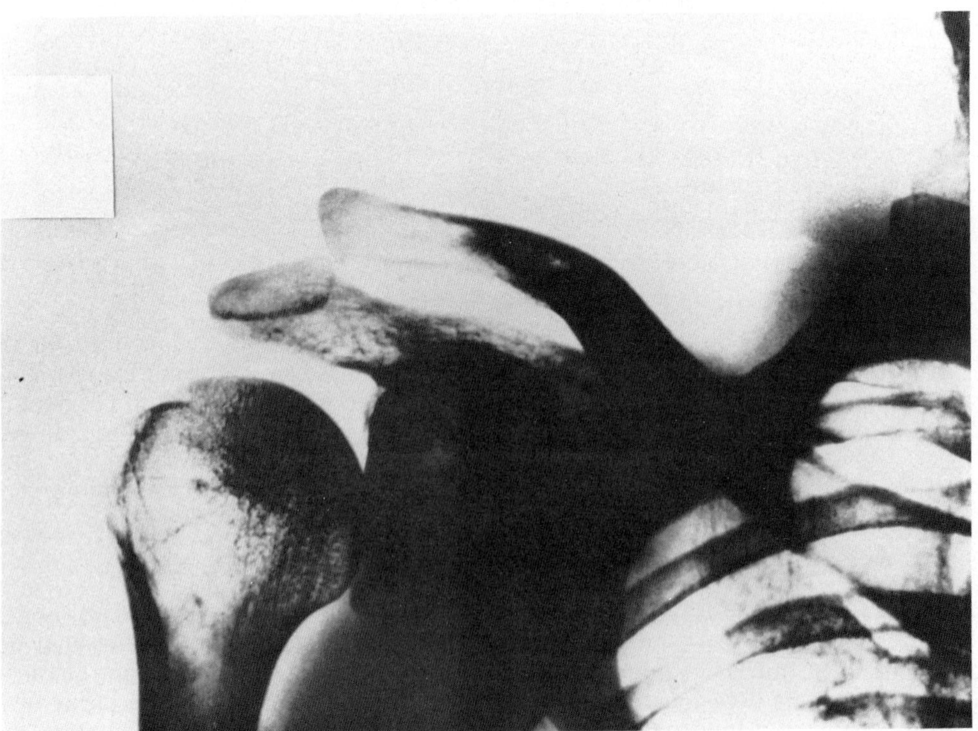

Figure 33.11. An acromioclavicular dislocation after a fall on the shoulder tip is shown.

Head, Neck, and Shoulder

A high index suspicion should be the norm for all neck injuries. These are the most serious of all rugby injuries and need hospital investigation and treatment. Neurologic examination and x-rays are mandatory, and if any doubt exists as to the presence of cervical fracture or instability then specialist opinion should be sought. Generally, neck injuries should be immobilized for short periods, and then aggressively rehabilitated.

Williams and McKibbin (13) reported on nine cervical spine cases treated in four seasons in Cardiff and found scrum injuries predominant, but others had occurred during and after a tackle. They noted that these injuries were more likely early in the season and pointed out the importance of fitness and strength in the neck muscles.

Bury and Gowland (14), in a survey in New Zealand, confirmed that scrum was a danger area for cervical injury but also noted that the danger in the formation of the scrum seemed to be greater than previously thought. They thought that young players were particularly vulnerable in scrums. Because of the nature of scrummaging it is vital that young players undergo special exercises to strengthen their neck muscles. Learning correct technique is also important. Players should be aware of the potential dangers of the scrum. Injuries to the acromioclavicular joint and fractures to the clavicle are treated with rest for 2 or 3 weeks, followed by active mobilization. Anterior dislocation of the shoulder is treated with relocation under sedation as soon as possible. Recurrent dislocation may need surgical stabilization. For this, the modified Bristow procedure is preferred. Mostly rugby injuries are of the soft tissue variety and can be adequately treated by RICE.

Lower Extremities

Davies and Gibson (15) confirmed general experience when they reported that the leg was the most common site of injury in a prospective study of 95 rugby players attached to 10 British rugby clubs. Leg injuries were more likely when the player was running than when he was static. The knees were the predominant site of injury. Davies and Gibson noted that diagnostic information was often lacking, particularly for injuries affecting joints such as the knee and the ankle.

The most common knee injury is that of sprain of the medial collateral ligament (MCL) in the knee caused by a valgus stress, frequently occurring when the tackled person is hit from the side. Meniscal injuries may also occur, particularly if the spikes of the boot are caught in the ground and rotation of the limb ensues. However, muscle injuries may follow direct trauma to the leg, particularly quadriceps contusions. Muscle tears are an occasional result of indirect trauma. These injuries can occur early in a game in a player who has not warmed up or late in a game when fatigue leads to muscle strains.

Injuries of the knee associated with immediate swelling are usually those causing bleeding into the knee (haemarthrosis). The common causes are anterior cruciate ligament (ACL) tears, meniscal tears, intraarticular fractures, and synovial bleeding. These require arthroscopic evaluation. It is important that arthroscopic washout is performed to relieve this condition, although aspiration is often the only initial treatment, and all hemarthroses do not need arthroscopic treatment. Generally, the injury is aspirated in the initial phase and followed up on an outpatient basis. If there is continued giving way or locking, then arthroscopy is indicated. The ACL tear is not always operated on in the initial phase and remains a somewhat controversial subject. Because standard derotational braces are illegal in rugby, the ACL-deficient knee can only be treated with rehabilitation and support. MCL sprains of the knee are generally adequately treated with rest, immobilization, and a functional rehabilitation program. MCL braces are illegal in rugby, and thus cannot be used. Lateral ligament sprains of the ankle are common and are treated with physiotherapy and functional rehabilitation.

Table 33.4.
Prevention of Rugby Injuries

Level of fitness
Mouth guards (gum shields)
Knee guards
Correct boots
Correct spikes
Correct clothing
Bandaging joints
Shin pads
Electrolyte solutions
Warming up and cooling down
Psychological preparation

Prevention

It is important for players to warm up well before a game to get the muscles prepared for physical contact. It also is important for all players to have a high level of fitness, which helps protect against injury. Psychological preparation also is necessary as well as the application and adherence to the rules of the game.

It is important for players to wear mouth guards (gum shields) to protect their teeth and to help prevent concussion. Mouth guards lessen the transmission of pressure to the temporomandibular joint. The importance of neck muscle exercises has already been stressed. The correct technique in tackling and scrummaging is of vital importance in avoiding these potentially catastrophic injuries.

The proper equipment also helps prevent injuries. This includes boots, spikes, jerseys, shorts, and socks. Bandaging of joints including the knee and ankle are of benefit, and knee guards prevent friction burns when the game is played on hard surfaces. The use of petroleum jelly also is important when playing on hard ground and should be applied to shoulders, elbows, and knees. Shin pads worn by the front-row forwards guard against trauma to the front of the lower legs.

When playing in warm climates the use of electrolyte solutions helps prevent cramps and muscle fatigue. Dehydration is usually considered the most common reason for muscle cramps and proper hydration before and during matches is imperative. Table 33.4 summarizes the prevention of injuries in rugby.

REFERENCES

1. Allemandou A. A statistical review of injuries. In: Injuries in rugby football and other team sports. Dublin: Irish Rugby Football Union, 1975:80–83.
2. Weightman D, Browne RC. Injuries in association and rugby football. Br J Sports Med 1974;8:183.
3. Micheli LJ, Riseborough ED. The incidence of injuries in rugby football. J. Sports Med 1975;2:93.
4. Durkin TE. A survey of injuries in a 1st class rugby union football club from 1972–1976. Br J Sports Med 1977;11:7.
5. Sparks JP. Half a million hours of rugby football: the injuries. Br J Sports Med 1981;15:30.
6. Davidson R, Kennedy M, Kennedy J, Vanderfield G. Casualty room presentations and schoolboy rugby union. Med J Aust 1978;1:247.
7. Dalley DR, Laing DR, Rowberry JM, Caird MJ. Rugby injuries: an epidemiological survey, Canterbury Rugby Football Union (Inc), 1979–1980. Christchurch, NZ, 1981.
8. Walkden I. Immediate postinjury consideration in rugby football proceedings. Br J Sports Med 1978;12:39.
9. Adams ID. Rugby football injuries. Br J Sports Med 1977;11:4.
10. O'Connell TCJ. A statistical review of injuries. In: Injuries in rugby football and other team sports. Dublin: Irish Rugby Football Union 1975:83–91.
11. Scher AT. Rugby injuries to the cervical spinal cord. S Afr Med J 1977;51:473.
12. Scher AT. The high rugby tackle—an avoidable cause of cervical spinal injury. S Afr Med J 1978;53:1015.
13. Williams JPR, McKibben B. Cervical spine injuries in rugby union football. Br Med J. 1978;2:1747.
14. Burry HC, Gowland H. Cervical injury in rugby football—a New Zealand survey. Br J Sports Med 1981;15:56.
15. Davies JE, Gibson T. Injuries in rugby union football. Br Med J 1978;2:1759.

34 / RUNNING

David N. M. Caborn, Larry J. Grollman, John A. Nyland, and Tony Brosky

PART 1
Evaluation and Treatment of the Injured Runner

David N. M. Caborn, John A. Nyland, and Tony Brosky

The effect of running on contemporary society has become ubiquitous. As humans evolved from a quadruped to a biped, bipedal running became a natural progression from walking. However, it was not until the mid-1970s with Frank Shorter's memorable Olympic marathon victory that the running boom evolved. This growth has occurred as a result of easy accessibility, low cost, and lack of ethnic or cultural boundaries. The busy schedules and time constraints of modern lifestyles have increased the importance of running as an integral part of many individuals' lives for both psychological and physiologic reasons. Unfortunately, in addition to these benefits there is an increased risk of developing microtraumatic overuse injury to the musculoskeletal system. It has been estimated that 37% to 56% of the 30 million recreational runners in the United States sustain an annual injury (1–3). Approximately 2.5 to 5.5 injuries per 1000 hours of running have been reported (4, 5). Injured male (52%) and female (49%) runners will eventually visit a health care professional (5). Although running injuries occur approximately 2 to 2.5 times less frequently than injuries from other sports, this represents a multimillion-dollar annual expenditure (4). It is hoped that through preventative education this can be reduced (2, 3).

Running injuries occur because of the repetitive stresses that are placed on the musculoskeletal system. During running, midstance ground reaction forces are equivalent to a vertical force of approximately 1.5 to 5 times body weight (6). These forces are generated over the 110 foot strikes that occur on average per mile and the 5000 foot strikes that occur in 1 hr of running (7). During running, joint shear forces increase to approximately 50 times that of walking (7). Taking this into consideration it is easy to appreciate how musculoskeletal dysfunctions caused by small intrinsic or extrinsic abnormalities can be significantly amplified when pro-amplified when progressing from a walk to a run.

As alluded to earlier, running is a normal progression from walking, but certain key factors must be appreciated. During running, stance phase comprises less than 50% of the total gait cycle. Another major distinction is the presence of a double-float period during running, which represents approximately 10% of the total gait cycle (8). The double-float period occurs when both feet are off the ground (Fig. 34.1). Upon heel strike, the rear foot is inverted, and as the foot becomes loaded, the tibia starts to rotate internally while the foot is converted from a rigid body support (supinated position) to a shock absorber (pronated position) (7). Pronation refers to a normal combination of rear-foot eversion, ankle dorsiflexion, and fore-foot abduction. Supination refers to a normal combination of rear-foot inversion, ankle plantar flexion, and fore-foot adduction. Pronation or supination that demonstrates excessive displacement or velocity during stance phase may contribute to running injuries. The subtalar joint functions as a vertical-to-longitudinal torque converter. As the body is propelled forward, the foot again becomes supinated and rigid to provide the maximum propulsion lever effect. Throughout the running gait cycle, the talus follows a cyclical movement pattern. Compared with walking, running normally presents an increased rate of subtalar pronation, diminished pronation time, and diminished pronation range.

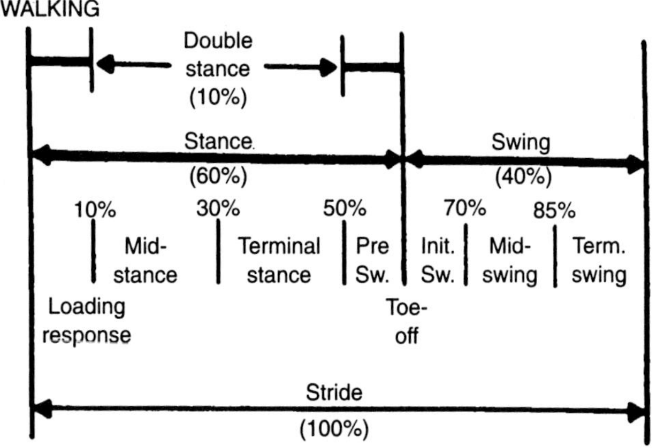

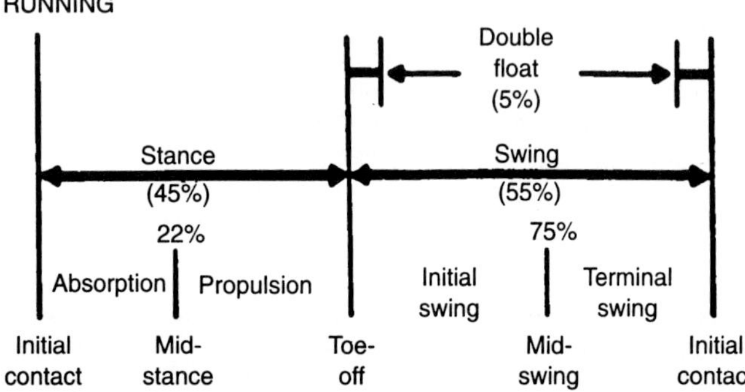

Figure 34.1. Walking and running gait cycles. Reproduced by permission from Ounpuu S. The biomechanics of running: a kinematic and kinetic analysis. In: Green WB, ed. Instr Course Lect 1990;39:305–318.

All major muscle groups show an increase in electromyographic (EMG) activity during running (9–11). Quadriceps EMG activity increases approximately 172%; hamstrings, 86%; tibialis anterior, 56%; and gastrocnemius-soleus, 95% (8). Concurrently, the major joints of the lower extremity also show increased motion during running. The hips and knees become eschewed toward flexion, and the ankle demonstrates increased range of motion and specific modulation changes related to landing strategy; 80% of distance runners are rear-foot strikers, and 20% are midfoot strikers (12). During the stance phase of running, the major site of power generation is the ankle. The ankle performs 1.5 times the work of the knee and 3 times the work of the hip. In other words, the ankle is responsible for 60% of the running power generation, whereas the knee and hip are responsible for 40% and 20%, respectively. The knee, however, is the principal power absorber, performing approximately 2 times the work of the ankle and the hip.

Understanding the energy transfer and power generation concepts of the running gait cycle helps improve the recognition of the underlying etiology of injury. Power generation during the swing phase is contributed primarily from the hip. Power from hip flexion during the initial swing phase, power for hip extension during the terminal swing phase, and all other motions are the result of inertia. Energy transfer at the knee and the hip occurs through concentric rectus femoris action during the initial swing phase and hamstring action during the terminal swing phase, with some evidence of balanced concentric activity proximally and eccentric activity distally (8). The majority of running injuries occur during stance phase at which time there is maximal eccentric muscle activation and power absorption within the musculoskeletal system.

If abnormal pronation occurs during midstance, musculoskeletal stresses from this hypermobility may become manifested, primarily on the medial aspect of the extremity. In contrast, if abnormal supination or rigidity, as seen with a cavus foot, occurs during midstance, poor stress absorption will occur within the musculoskeletal system and associated injury patterns will be seen on the lateral side of the foot and knee (13) (Figs. 34.2 and 34.3) (Table 34.1).

Etiology

Runners display an estimated 70% of all overuse injuries and of these an extrinsic or intrinsic etiology is subsequently identifiable (1, 14–16). The majority of overuse injuries in runners are the result of extrinsic factors such as training errors, running terrain, running surfaces, and running shoes.

Primary Extrinsic Factors

Running shoes can affect the type and frequency of injury (17). When running shoes become wet or if the midsole has been worn for greater than 400 km, the shock absorption capability decreases approximately 30% to 50% (18). In addition, the proficiency in which running shoes provide effective heel pad containment is important (19). Proper heel pad containment in the normal foot can increase shock absorption by 29.5% and in the traumatized heel pad can increase shock absorption capability by as much as 48.5%.

Running terrain refers to the topography of the course. Downhill running causes significant knee stress, because the line of action of gravitational forces is positioned posterior to the knees. In addition, downhill running increases the magnitude of knee flexion, patellofemoral contact forces, the net extensor moment, power absorption, and EMG activity of the knee extensors as they attempt to maintain dynamic stability (8). Studies of the effect of running terrain on biodynamics, however, are somewhat conflicting. While certain studies have shown hill running to increase overuse injury incidence, others have found no association (20, 21). However, downhill running has demonstrated injury trends toward increased incidence of patellofemoral pain and iliotibial band syndrome. In addition, uphill running has shown trends toward increased incidence of Achilles peritendinitis and plantar fascitis.

The importance of running surface in the etiology of running injuries may as much as quadruple the frequency of injury in certain sporting activities (16). Increases in mechanical loading because of frequent running on asphalt or concrete surfaces may subsequently overload joints, muscles, and tendons, promoting greater

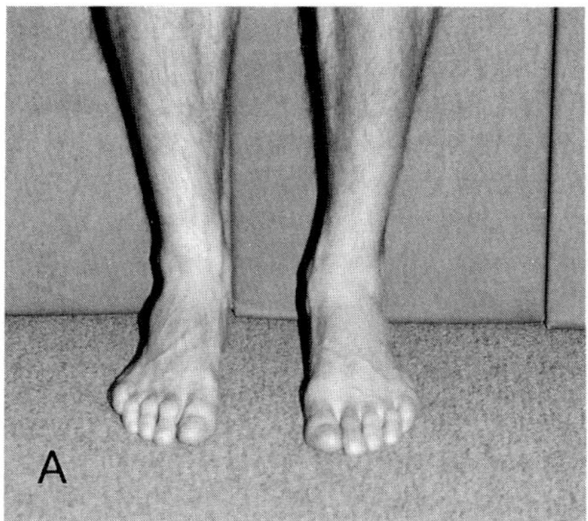

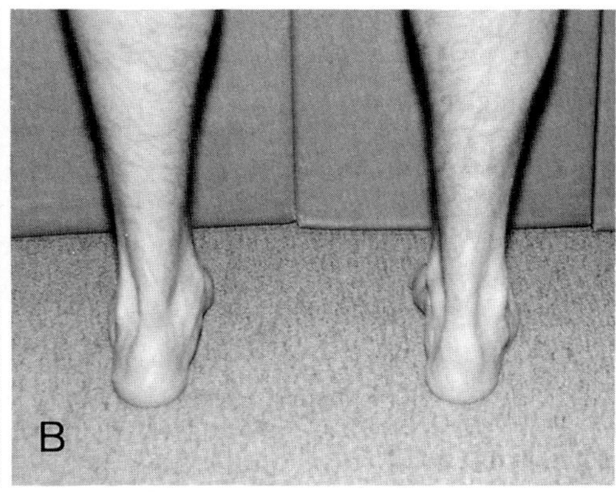

Figure 34.2. Anterior and posterior views of habitus varus.

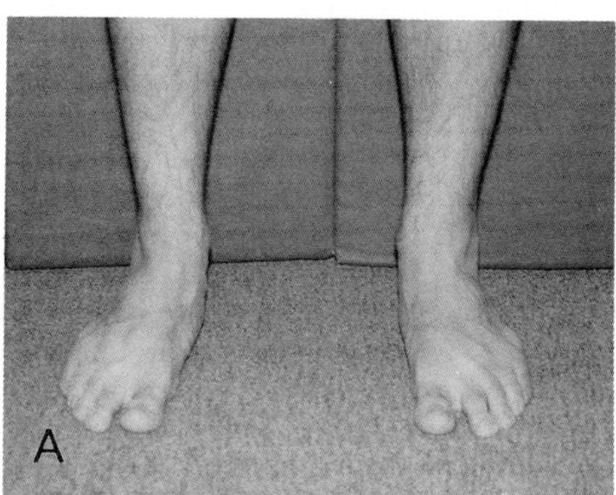

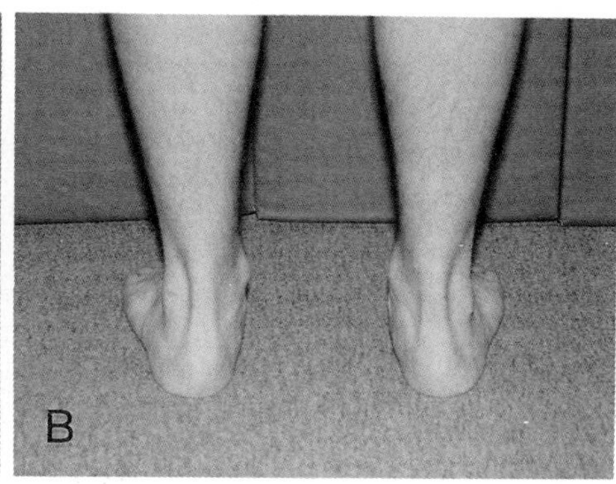

Figure 34.3. Anterior and posterior views of habitus valgus.

Table 34.1.
Specific Injuries Seen in the Running Population

- Lower Back
  - Spondylosis
  - Hyperextension facet syndrome
  - Pars stress fracture
  - Sciatic nerve irritation
- Hip
  - Pyriformis syndrome
  - Sacroiliac joint dysfunction
  - External rotator tightness
  - Gluteus medius syndrome
  - Iliotibial band syndrome
  - Stress fracture of the femoral neck
- Knee
  - Patellofemoral pain
  - Iliotibial band syndrome
  - Popliteus tendinitis
  - Pes anserine bursitis
  - Patella tendinitis
  - Intraarticular abnormalities
- Lower Leg
  - Stress fractures
  - Medial tibial stress syndrome
  - Chronic compartment syndrome
  - Achilles tendinitis
  - Posterior tibial tendinitis
  - Popliteal artery entrapment syndrome
- Ankle
  - Ligamentous sprains
  - Fractures
  - Osteochondral lesions
  - Impingement syndrome
- Foot
  - Rear Foot
    - Central heel syndrome
    - Plantar fascitis
    - Calcaneal stress fracture
    - Achilles bursitis
      - Retrocalcaneal
      - Retrotendinous
    - Tarsal tunnel syndrome
  - Midfoot
    - Navicular stress fracture
    - Accessory navicular
    - Cuboid dislocation
    - Extensor tenosynovitis
  - Fore Foot
    - First Metatarsal
      - Hallux valgus
      - Hallux limitus/rigidus
      - Keratosis
      - Sesamoiditis
      - Sesamoid fracture
      - Ingrown toenail
    - Second to Fourth Metatarsals
      - Morton's neuroma
      - Stress fracture
      - Crossover of second toe
      - Nonspecific synovitis

injury rates (18). In contrast, running on too soft a surface may cause a hypermobility within the joints, tendons, and muscles and as such could cause overuse injuries (13). Running on uneven surfaces, slippery roads, and banked roads or tracks may cause a functional leg length discrepancy. This could cause excessive loading on the long leg and a resultant iliotibial band syndrome or trochanteric bursitis.

Errors in training are by far the greatest extrinsic cause of running injury. These may include too much volume or too much intensity, with inadequate recovery. Clement et al. (20) described four categories of training error: (*a*) persistent high-intensity training without lower intensity (easy days); (*b*) sudden increases in mileage and intensity without adequate rest; (*c*) single, severe training or competitive sessions; and (*d*) repetitive uphill-downhill training.

Running experience or speed of training has not been shown to alter the propensity for running injury (22). The need for an individualized balance between training volume, intensity, and recovery must be recognized and maintained.

Intrinsic injury factors are categorized as basic, primary, or secondary. The key intrinsic factors are malalignment, muscle imbalance, inflexibility, and leg length discrepancy. Secondary acquired factors such as kinetic chain dysfunction and prior history of injury also are important. When considering gender, it is important to determine an accurate menstrual history, because amenorrhea may be a cause of recurrent stress syndromes involving not only the bones but also the soft tissues (23).

Although there are physiologic and metabolic musculoskeletal system changes associated with aging, there does not appear to be a significant predisposition to injury among this group. Konradsen et al. (24), in examining subjects with 30 to 40 years of distance running experience, failed to discover an increased incidence of osteoarthrosis of the hip. Similar findings have been noted at the knee and ankle (25, 26).

In childhood and adolescence, bone growth rate exceeds the rate of growth of the musculotendinous unit. This can result in secondary inflexibility with resultant apophysitis. These factors provide further justification for the importance of optimal musculotendinous flexibility. Height appears to have no association with running injury, and reports about weight are conflicting (27).

Primary Intrinsic Factors

Malalignment

The relationship between abnormal pronation/supination during the gait cycle and predisposition to injury has already been discussed. It should be further emphasized, however, that on initial ground impact a minimal injury effect is seen. As the runner moves into midstance and push off, however, higher forces are generated from increased muscle activity, resulting in a secondary greater peak load on the tissues (28). The important distinction between total pronation displacement and the rate of pronation will be discussed later.

The so-called malicious malalignment syndrome can be seen in certain runners (29, 30). This is a combination of a broad pelvis, increased femoral anteversion, genu valgum with or without genu recurvatum, squinting patellae, excessive Q-angle, tibial varum, and excess pronation of the foot.

Leg Length Discrepancy

Leg length discrepancy can be related to sacroiliac (SI) dysfunction, lumbar paravertebral muscle spasm, poor musculotendinous flexibility, muscle imbalance, and unilateral abnormal pronation or supination (31). Leg length discrepancy can result in pelvic tilt with secondary lumbar convexity toward the shorter extremity as well as increased hip adduction, hip internal rotation, and supination. In the longer extremity, excessive pronation, increased knee valgus, genu recurvatum, hip abduction, and hip external rotation also may be noted. Leg length discrepancy may result in iliotibial band friction syndrome, trochanteric bursitis, low-back pain and stress fractures. A 20-to-30-mm leg length discrepancy may be acceptable in a low-demand population. In the running population, however, the repetitive high loading forces may require that a leg length discrepancy as small as 5 mm be compensated (13, 32).

Structural variations around the foot and ankle that create impingements, traction effects, or decreased mobility can subsequently predispose the runner to injury. Examples of structural variations include Haglund's deformity, tarsal coalition, and an accessory navicular bone.

The importance of the overall muscular condition remains contentious; however, it is believed that neuromuscular coordination and ligamentous laxity may be important factors in hypermobility etiologies. Dysfunctions in musculotendinous strength, flexibility, or coordination may result in increased impact loading forces.

Acquired or Secondary Factors

Steindler (33) and, more recently, Gray (34) have discussed the concept of the kinetic chain. The kinetic chain concept defines the body as a series of interrelated linkages. Anything interfering with the progression and mechanics of force transfer can lead to compensatory changes in motion within one segment or in a subsequently balancing segment within the kinetic chain. For example, the individual with a history of an untreated hamstring strain may subsequently develop problems in the Achilles tendon as the gastrocnemius compensates for the dysfunctional proximal linkage in the kinetic chain.

Dysfunction of the mobility and orientation of the SI joint is frequently seen (35). This joint remains somewhat enigmatic and should be carefully evaluated in the static and dynamic states (36).

Obtaining a thorough athletic and nonathletic injury history may also be of considerable importance to understanding soft tissue healing and the potential for complete recovery. In the area of soft tissue healing, however, researchers are just beginning to obtain a greater working knowledge. In examining specific injuries, certain biodynamic parameters should be noted. When considering the effect of downhill running on knee and ankle kinematics, it is easy for one to understand why certain overuse injuries occur. During downhill running, knee flexion, peak extensor moments, patellofemoral compressive forces, power absorption, and eccentric activation of the knee extensors are increased. Ankle dorsiflexion, net plantar flexor moments, power absorption, and eccentric activation of the plantar flexors also are increased. Downhill running by runners with anterior knee pain results in increased select kinematic and kinetic parameters. Examples of this include doubled knee flexion angles, tripled peak knee extensor moments and patellofemoral compressive forces, quadrupled peak power generation, quintupled peak power absorption, and increased eccentric muscular activity (8). The runner with iliotibial band syndrome may present increased hip adduction, peak hip abductor moments, peak hip power absorption, peak hip power generation, and increased lower extremity muscular activity.

Knee

MacIntyre et al. (37) conducted a survey of 4173 running injury cases in 1991. They found that the knee was the most common site of running injury, comprising 48% of all of the injuries, followed by the lower leg, 20.4%; foot, 17.2%; hip, 6%; upper leg and thigh, 4.2%;

and lower back 4.1%. When these injuries are further broken down into specific conditions, anterior knee pain, which made up 24.3% and 29.6% of the total running injuries in men and women, respectively, was the most common injury. The following frequencies of injuries are presented for men and women, respectively: iliotibial band syndrome, 7.2% and 7.9%; patellar tendinitis, 5.1% and 3.1%; medial tibial stress syndrome, 7.2% and 11.4%; Achilles tendinitis, 4.7% and 27%; and metatarsal stress syndrome, 3.1% and 3.8%.

When considering running injuries to the knee, medical personnel must remember that the knee is the major power absorber, accomplishing this primarily through eccentric muscle activation. The knee performs twice as much work as the ankle or the hip in this capacity. The majority of knee problems seen in runners will be extraarticular in nature, with occasional complaints of mechanical intraarticular irritation secondary to a plica, an osteochondrotic lesion, degeneration of the chondral surface of the patella, or in the older population a degenerative meniscal tear (37).

Extraarticular anterior knee pain or patellofemoral pain syndrome is the most common knee problem. Hypermobility of the foot and ankle and malalignment of the hip, knee, ankle, and foot relationships can become manifested in altered biodynamics with secondarily increased patellofemoral compression or traction effects in the muscles, tendons, and ligaments. The necessity for a comprehensive static and dynamic biomechanical evaluation has been reviewed. Frequently, extraarticular knee pain will be seen in runners with a malicious malalignment syndrome. In addition, it is often observed if the runner presents a tight lateral retinaculum; poor vastus medialis obliquis tone; and poor flexibility of the hamstring, quadriceps femoris and gastrocnemius-soleus musculature. Furthermore, examination may reveal divergent insertional levels of the vastus medialis obliquis and the vastus lateralis obliquis muscles, with the more distal vastus lateralis obliquis insertion creating a fulcrum-type effect, thereby affecting patellar orientation.

When examining the patella, the physician should pay attention not only to patellar height and tracking but also to the assessment of superior, medial, and lateral patellar glide. Patellar tilt; J-tracking; and functional Q-angle at 0°, 60°, and 90° of knee flexion should also be noted. The best functional test for isolating the patellofemoral joint is the single leg squat at approximately 45° to 60° of knee flexion, as described by Drez (38). Anteroposterior and lateral radiographs while weight bearing in addition to Merchant views at 30° and 60° of knee flexion should be obtained to evaluate patellar subluxation and tilt (Fig. 34.4).

Specifics of treatment for patellofemoral conditions should include the correction of static and dynamic imbalances through rehabilitation and conditioning programs and the addition of a neutral orthosis if excessive static pronation is present. Runners who are experiencing an acute patellofemoral syndrome may also benefit from the McConnell patellar taping protocol (39) (Fig. 34.5). Various patellar tendon straps and open patellar neoprene sleeves, with and without buttresses and dynamic straps also may be effective. These devices may enhance proprioception at the patellofemoral articulation (40).

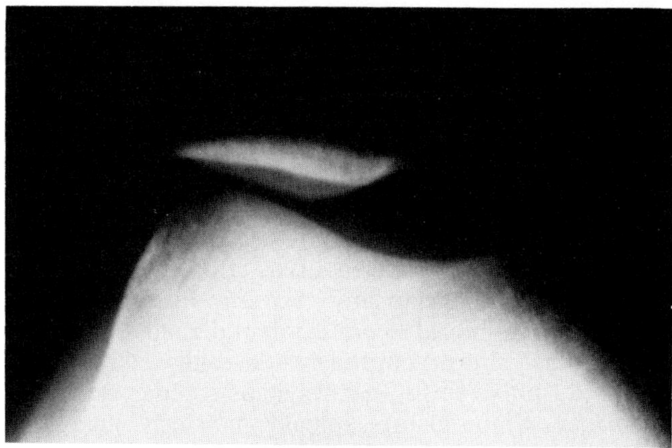

Figure 34.4. Lateral patellar compression.

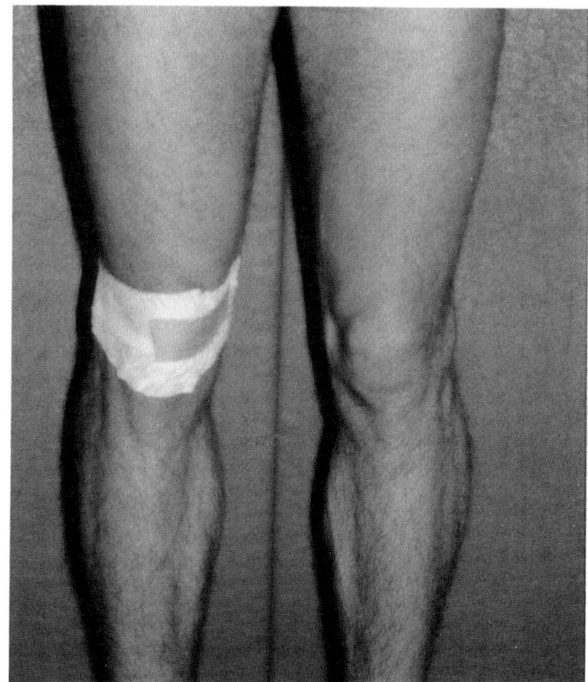

Figure 34.5. McConnell taping method.

The second most common overuse condition of the knee is iliotibial band syndrome (ITBS). Runners frequently complain of pain while running downhill, because the iliotibial band impinges on the lateral femoral condyle when the knee is flexed approximately 20° to 30°. This friction may result in tenderness over the condyle, the bursa that is located midway between the condyle and Gerdy's tubercle, the tibia, or Gerdy's tubercle itself. Excessive lateral shoe wear and functional rear-foot varus are often seen in runners with ITBS. These runners also will present with a positive Ober test, weak hip abductors, and poor hamstring flexibility.

The presence of diffuse pain in this region, however, requires careful evaluation to rule out the presence of lumbar disc pathology. As with any overuse injury condition, it should be emphasized that the entire kinetic chain requires evaluation as ITBS may occur in combination with excessive genu varum, decreased pronation and functional supination, cavus feet, heel varus, and compensatory fore-foot abduction.

The treatment for ITBS involves strict counseling regarding running terrain and running surface choices. These runners should avoid cambered roads and hills. Rehabilitation should emphasize flexibility of the iliotibial band, hamstrings, gastrocneius-soleus, and gluteus maximus musculature. Initially, a ⅛-inch lateral heel wedge may help alleviate symptoms. Iontophoresis can provide a local antiinflammatory and/or anesthetic effect. Ultrasound (US) over this region should be avoided, because it may exacerbate symptoms. Occasionally, injection or excision as described by Martens et al. (41) is performed.

Proximal medial tibial pain is the next most common overuse condition at the knee. This condition is often confused with other pathologies at the medial knee, and may precede a medial tibial stress fracture. This condition will be discussed later with stress fracture syndromes.

Pes anserine bursitis has a similar presentation to proximal medial tibial pain; however, the pain is located more posteromedially near the insertions of the medial hamstring group. This condition often occurs in conjunction with excessive pronation. Iontophoresis, hamstring stretching, posterior tibialis strengthening exercises, and functional drills that emphasize eccentric hamstring muscle action are often beneficial. The presence of a medial stress fracture must be ruled out if any doubt is present.

Quadriceps tendinitis is not usually seen in the running population. If this condition does occur, it should be managed in a similar manner as anterior knee pain.

A rare condition in runners is popliteal artery entrapment syndrome. This is caused by the presence of an anatomical variation of the gastrocnemius muscle that constricts the artery. Runners with this condition present with intermittent claudication and decreased pulses of the dorsalis pedis, posterior tibial, and popliteal arteries. Diagnosis is performed by biplanar arteriography, although magnetic resonance imaging (MRI) may be helpful in evaluating the specific entrapments. Treatment is surgical release versus arterial grafting.

Lower Leg

Styf and Kormer (42) used microcapillary infusion ^{133}Xe clearance studies on 98 patients with chronic, exercise-induced, anterior lower leg pain. They reported that 26 had a documentable chronic compartment syndrome, 25 had anterior compartment tenderness, 16 had posteromedial compartment tenderness, and 13 had a compression of the superficial peroneal nerve. A total of 42% of these subjects also experienced tibial periostitis. Chronic compartment syndromes most frequently involve the anterior and anterolateral compartments and less commonly the posterior tibial compartments (43). Evaluation criteria using the slit-catheter method are considered to be positive when intracompartmental pressures are >15 mm Hg preexercise, >30 mm Hg 1 min postexercise, and >20 mm Hg at 5 min postexercise. More sophisticated catheter systems are currently available; however, the criteria for diagnosis remains the same (44). Amendola et al. (45) employed MRI on 4 patients with chronic compartment syndrome and noted that the T_{-1} signal increased in 30% of chronic compartment syndrome cases. This method, however, was only 80% sensitive, with high variability. This technique allows simultaneous visualization of all of the lower leg compartments. As MRI techniques become more sophisticated, this method may become an impressive diagnostic tool. The use of EMG in biodynamic testing for chronic compartment syndrome is currently being evaluated.

Runners with a chronic compartment syndrome present a history of a nonspecific lower leg fullness and painful pressure in the region of the involved lower leg compartment that occurs at a specific moment during the training session. These runners also will complain of weakness and/or paresthesia along the distribution of the involved nerve. Anterior compartment compression is associated with paresthesia over the dorsum of the foot, whereas posterior compartment compression is associated with paresthesia over the instep. Treatment, if the diagnosis is conclusive, is surgical; however, stretching activities and the use of an air-stirrup with an anterior tibial pad may help reduce compartmental pressure changes caused by periosteal traction. D'Ambrosia (46) attempted a nonoperative approach for approximately 15 weeks; however, surgical intervention was generally inevitable. Martens and Moeyersoons (47) found a 100% failure rate in compartment syndrome patients that they treated nonoperatively. Rorabeck (48) reported similar results.

Before surgical intervention, the runner should be carefully evaluated for an occult involvement within the deep posterior or posterior tibial compartments. The omission of this diagnosis is the most common cause of failure following the surgical release of the anterior or anterolateral compartments. Surgical release of chronic compartment syndromes are generally performed through a single lateral approach or a combined lateral and medial approach. The lateral approach provides easy access to the anterior and anterolateral compartments, whereas the medial approach can be used for easier access to the superficial posterior, deep posterior, and tibialis posterior compartments. When using the lateral approach, the surgeon may use a relatively large single incision or smaller double incisions to avoid injuring the superficial peroneal nerve.

Following surgical intervention, Rorabeck et al. (49) reported approximately a 92% success rate for pain relief and improved function. Detmer et al. (50) reported a 90% rate of cure, and Martens and Moeyersoons (47) reported a good to excellent score for 85% of their patients who underwent fasciotomy. A portion of these positive results may represent the surgical denervation of the periosteum in addition to the actual fascial compartment release.

Postoperatively, patients should receive ice, compression, and elevation to the involved extremity for approximately 48 hr. A gradual return to full weight-bearing ambulation generally takes 2 to 4 days. By the 5th postoperative day, the patient may begin aquatic therapy, emphasizing range of motion exercises, and progressing through closed kinetic chain functional activities. A dry land functional rehabilitation progression is initiated shortly thereafter, terminating with the return to full activity by approximately 4 to 6 weeks following surgery.

The shin splint conundrum can be considered to be two distinct etiologies: *(a)* medial or posteromedial tibial stress syndrome (MTSS), which is seen generally in those who pronate excessively, and *(b)* anterior or anterolateral stress syndrome, which is more common among runners who have diminished dynamic shock absorption capability.

Runners with MTSS present pain over the distal third of the posteromedial tibia. Through cadaveric dissection, Michael and Holder (51) located this area of tenderness in the soleus and in the investing fascia of the soleus. This finding was substantiated by bone scintigraphy. Michael and Holder also reported a strong association between excess pronation of the foot and MTSS. Cadaveric dissections demonstrated that the soleus is medially rotated 90° to its insertion on the calcaneus. This suggests that the soleus is a primary invertor of the subtalar joint in addition to being a primary plantar flexor of the ankle (51). This information adds to the appreciation of the traction effect it undergoes in the presence of excess subtalar pronation. D'Ambrosia et al. (52) believed that MTSS was attributable to hypermobility in the posterior tibial musculature, which was most evident with manual muscle testing of the posterior tibialis muscle. Garth and Miller (53) noted that runners with MTSS may develop a concomitant flexor digitorum longus overuse condition and weakened intrinsic muscles of the foot secondary to keeping the toes in greater flexion at push off. Radiographs of runners with MTSS may show hypertrophy of the medial tibial cortex. Scintigraphy may show myositis and tendinitis, which are differentiated by an increased blood pool phase.

Conservative treatment is generally aimed at improving flexibility, correcting biomechanical deficiencies, improving shock absorption, and increasing the eccentric strength of antagonistic muscles. Nonsteroidal antiinflammatory drugs (NSAIDs) should generally be avoided, because these may mask the progression to a definitive stress fracture. Occasionally, iontophoresis with Dexamethasone and Xylocaine may alleviate symptoms. Garth and Miller (53) mentioned the use of a special orthosis with a metatarsal pad attachment that facilitates toe down during push off. This may be indicated if atrophy of the intrinsic muscles of the foot is noted. Surgical intervention for this condition is infrequent in the United States, but common in Scandinavia. A 2-mm posterior tibial margin surgical release probably serves to denervate the periosteum. This surgical approach provides 80% to 100% pain relief (51).

Achilles tendinitis, although decreasing in frequency remains a relatively common presentation among runners. The plantar flexors of the ankle are the major power generators of the lower extremity during running. During running, dorsiflexion range of motion increases, peak concentric work or power generation more than doubles, and peak eccentric work or power absorption may quintuple (8). The initial clinical exam should rule out any friction of the Achilles tendon on the heel counter of the running shoe. Runners who experience Achilles tendinitis often complain of pain that is exacerbated by uphill running. Two contrasting etiologies may be factors in the occurrence of this condition among runners: (*a*) greater shock transmitted through the Achilles tendon because of subtalar hypomobility and (*b*) greater torque at the medial soleus because of subtalar hypermobility. Approximately 50% of runners who experience Achilles tendinitis will present bilateral symptoms, primarily at the musculotendinous junction region of the Achilles tendon, which is several centimeters proximal to the calcaneus. Initially, a "creaking" peritendinitis may be palpated with dorsiflexion and plantar flexion of the ankle. Over time, this progresses to a tendinosis with mucolipid degeneration and fibrinoid necrosis (Fig. 34.6). Frequently, runners with

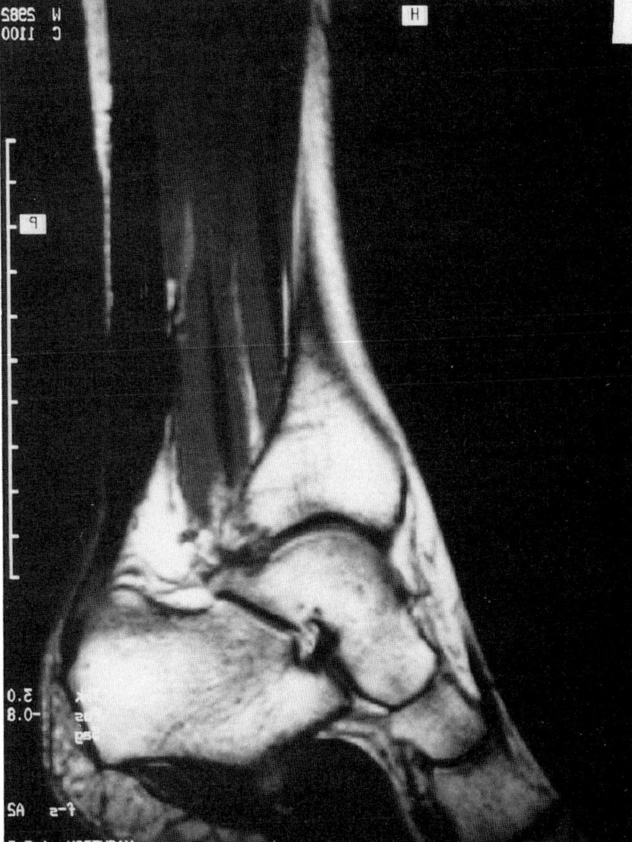

Figure 34.6. MRI view of Achilles tendon degeneration.

Achilles tendinitis will complain of increased symptoms when getting out of bed in the morning, difficulty with stair climbing, and decreased push off while ambulating. Partial tears of the Achilles tendon are often missed during the initial clinical exam and are characterized by a sudden onset of pain, distinct tenderness, and localized swelling. These findings help distinguish partial tears from peritendinitis and tendinosis. Allenmark et al. (54) reported that 82% and 73% of runners with US- or MRI-verified partial Achilles tendon tears continued to have problems at 5 and 10 years postinjury, respectively.

Treatment for acute peritendinitis includes flexibility and eccentric strengthening activities, NSAIDs, iontophoresis, ice massage, 15-mm heel lifts, and a resting night splint. Furthermore, the runner is counseled regarding training and activity modifications to diminish stresses at the injured area. If symptoms persist for more than 6 months, surgical intervention is recommended. Surgery for a partial tear of the Achilles tendon includes excision of scar tissue and granulation tissue as well as an osteotomy of the calcaneal tuberosity if a Haglund's deformity (Fig. 34.7) is viewed on a lateral x-ray.

In cases in which a Haglund's deformity is present, it is common to locate pain and swelling anterior to the Achilles tendon from the retrocalcaneal bursa. Retrocalcaneal bursitis may respond to conservative local treatments such as iontophoresis or the injection of a corticosteroid/local anesthetic combination. When retrocalcaneal bursitis is present in combination with Achilles tendinitis, a surgical approach as described by Leach and Hammond (55) is recommended. This approach involves a medial incision bursectomy and excision of the posterior-superior angle of the calcaneus. Leach and Hammond reported an excellent to good rating for 88% of peritendinitis cases, as opposed to in situ suture (73%), flap (88%), and retrocalcaneal bursal excision (71%). However, a 6% incidence of skin necrosis was reported with this technique. A posterior longitudinal incision should only be used if there is substantial degeneration within the tendon or if a medial or lateral approach would not provide adequate visualization of the injured area.

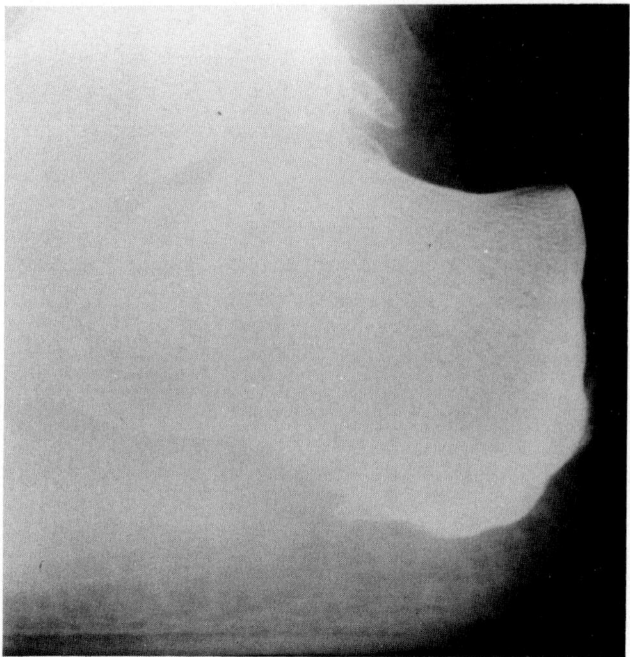

Figure 34.7. Haglund's calcaneal deformity.

Postoperative management begins with a walking cast locked at 10° of plantar flexion for 2 weeks and progresses to a shoe with a 1-cm heel lift for 3 weeks. Flexibility exercises and progressive functional training are begun judiciously following the 2nd postoperative week; however, this varies with the amount of tissue that was excised.

Runners account for 69% of all stress fractures either through high stresses on normal bone or normal to high stresses on weakened bone. Grimston et al. (56) reported that the development of stress fractures was not associated with reduced bone mineral density. Leg length discrepancy, gait abnormalities, poor running terrain, poor running surface, and the presence of poorly rehabilitated/conditioned previous injuries can all predispose the runner to stress fractures. Cook et al. (18) believed that only 22.4% of all stress fractures were associated with training errors and that the affected area was equally distributed throughout the body. These findings, however, contrast greatly with several other reports.

McBryde (44) reported that stress fractures occur mostly in the tibia (34%) but may also occur in the fibula (24%), metatarsals (18%), femur (14%), pelvis (6%), and other bones (4%). Giladi et al. (57) noted decreased medial tibial width and proposed that this was the biomechanical cause of stress fracture. Scully and Besterman (58) documented the response of bony tissue to stress among military recruits. During weeks 1 and 2, increased osteotopic osteoid formation takes place, but tissue strength does not increase. Over weeks 3 and 4, tissue strength gradually increases; however, the rate of strength increase in bony tissue is slower than that for muscle tissue. Scully and Besterman noted that by eliminating jump training during week 3 of recruit conditioning the incidence of stress syndromes decreased from 4.8% to 1.6%. This supports the concept of an adaptive period of bone remodeling, during which its load tolerance improves.

Stress fractures that occur on the tension side of a bone or in regions of poor vascularity have a poor prognosis. This type of stress fracture may occur at the anterior tibial cortex, femoral neck (tension side), proximal fifth metatarsal, and tarsal navicular. Stress fractures generally present a focused pain, in contrast to the rather diffuse pain seen with a MTSS. The single-leg broad jump functional test is usually positive if a stress fracture is present.

Stress fractures of the femoral neck and of the fifth metatarsal (Jones fracture) often require surgical intervention. The most common stress fracture occurs at the medial tibia, with nonsurgical treatment, including the use of an air-stirrup with an anterior tibial pad until focal tenderness ceases (Fig. 34.8). A functional rehabilitation progression, including alternative cardiovascular conditioning and aquatic therapy are implemented within symptom-free limits, and the injured runner is gradually returned to training activities. Low dye taping may be useful when rehabilitating/conditioning the runner who has experienced a Jones fracture.

Heel Pain

Runners often complain of heel pain. The etiology usually involves the plantar fascia. It must be emphasized, however, that central heel syndrome, calcaneal stress fracture, and nerve entrapment also should be considered.

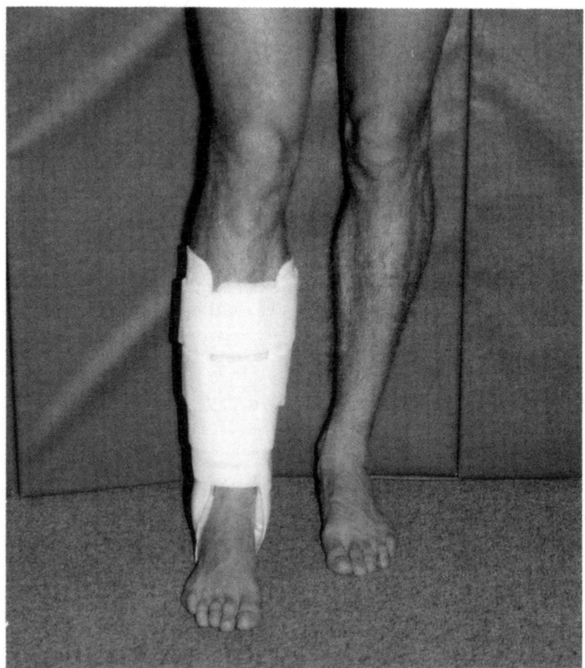

Figure 34.8. Air-stirrup with anterior pad.

Plantar fascitis usually represents a microtraumatic tearing of the medial cord of the plantar fascia, and it has been reported in runners with both cavus and planus feet. Runners with plantar fascitis present decreased static and dynamic range of motion at the knee, ankle, and first toe, in addition to overall decreased lower extremity strength (59). However, it remains unclear whether these deficits arise as a result of plantar fascitis. It should again be emphasized that the entire kinetic chain should be evaluated. Runners with plantar fascitis complain of excruciating heel pain with their first step on arising from bed in the morning. This pain is increased by a generally flexed hip, knee, and plantar flexed ankle sleeping posture. Pain from plantar fascitis is located at the insertion of the medial cord of the plantar fascia on the calcaneus. This is contrasted with central heel syndrome, which presents with central heel pain (Fig. 34.9).

Treatment for plantar fascitis may include NSAIDs, iontophoresis, flexibility exercises for the plantar fascia, and strengthening exercises for the intrinsic muscles of the foot and the muscles of the lower leg. The single most effective treatment for plantar fascitis has been the resting night splint, which the authors have used for many years. This treatment has recently been documented by Wapner and Sharkey (60). D'Ambrosia (61) reported good results with orthotic intervention for runners who pronate excessively, but poor results for runners with cavus feet. This was supported by Gross et al. (62) in their evaluation of 500 long-distance runners.

For central heel pad syndrome, the injection of the injured area with a corticosteroid is not advised because of subsequent fat pad atrophy. If surgical intervention is necessary, no more than 33% of the fascia should be released (63). Approximately 20% of runners

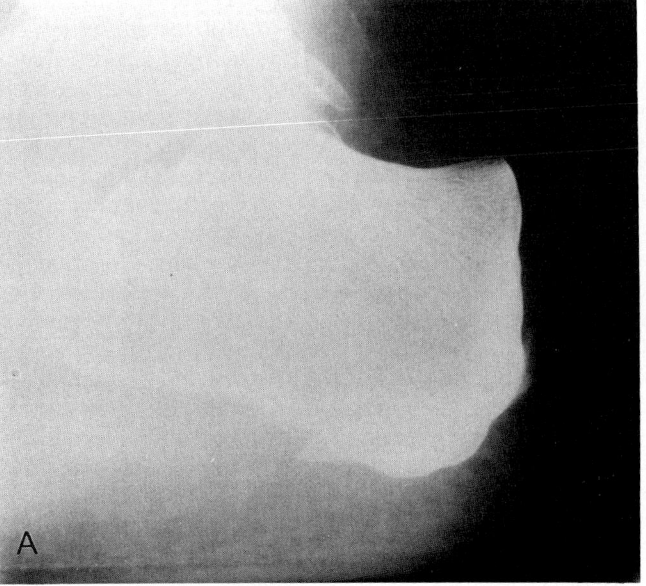

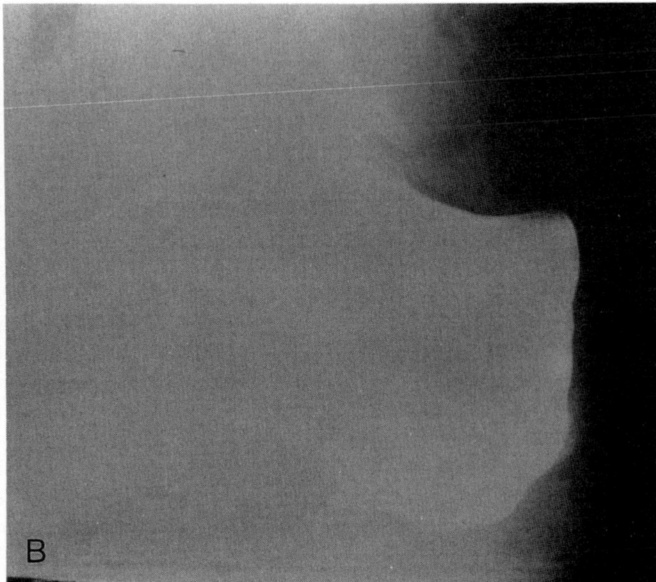

Figure 34.9. Non–weight-bearing (**A**) and weight-bearing (**B**) views of the heel fat pad.

with chronic heel pain may have an underlying nerve entrapment (64).

Functional nerve disorders deserve consideration when the pain presentation is atypical, such as complaints of radiating paresthesia or sudden electric-shock–type sensations. However, this condition may also present persistent toothache-type pain. Close interaction with a skilled electromyographer is necessary to evaluate the signs of functional nerve entrapment. MRI can be useful in exposing edema within the nerve sheath, as noted with posterior tibial nerve entrapment.

Diagnosis

As emphasized by Renstrom and Johnson (13), any overuse running injury should be regarded as a manifestation of kinetic chain dysfunction, and the entire chain must be examined to rule out any asymptomatic injury or dysfunction. Obtaining a pertinent injury history is an important factor in determining present injury etiology.

The comprehensive evaluation of a runner must be a fusion of orthopedic sports medicine, sports physical therapy, biodynamic, and physiologic concepts. The area of biomechanics that studies the relationship between motion and the forces affecting motion is biodynamics. In the next decade, an even greater marriage among biodynamic concepts, and orthopedic sports medicine, and sports physical therapy will occur, as each area recognizes the benefits that can be derived from the others' expertise (65).

Although any structural assessment should include the entire body, the emphasis of the structural assessment of a runner should be on the musculoskeletal system of the lower extremities and back. This assessment should include static and dynamic postural alignment, flexibility, and anthropometry. The data from this assessment provide a basis for determining the effect of body posture on movement; musculature activity; forces, moments, and power; pressure; and metabolic activity.

Static posture should always be evaluated in the frontal and sagittal planes. Deviations in the transverse plane are more difficult to identify but must also be considered. The frontal plane should reveal symmetry of the shoulders, pelvis, hips, knees, and ankles as well as the angle of toeing in or toeing out. Hip anteversion/retroversion, genu varus/valgus, and the magnitude of subtalar pronation also can be appreciated. A low incidence of running injuries is seen with genu varus of <8°; however, an increased incidence is seen when genu varus is >18° (66). Excessive pronation may be physiologic or secondary to tibial varus >10°, functional equinus, talar varus, and forefoot supination (66). Sagittal plane analysis assists in the identification of abnormalities in the truncal posture or carriage of the runner. The segmental relationship of the major joints to a plumb line is well-recognized (67).

Although static alignment provides clues in identifying dysfunction, it must be emphasized that the body is in a constant state of omnidirectional, triplanar motion. Static postural findings may or may not correlate with those noted during the dynamics of walking or running. When an evaluation of each subphase of the gait cycle does not reveal abnormal findings, other means should be used. One interesting concept is to use myriad exaggerated functional activities (68). By using dynamic activities such as excessive knee flexion or "Groucho walking," excessive trunk rotation, increased pelvic translation, and increased stride length, deficiencies in flexibility, strength, and stability may be accentuated. Obscure abnormalities may be further exposed via the technological capabilities of a biomechanics or biodynamics laboratory.

A comprehensive evaluation of the entire lower quadrant is essential; however, attention should be focused primarily on the foot and ankle. Abnormalities in the foot can affect the mechanics of the ankle, knee, hip, and lower back. Neutral subtalar position is of clinical significance because this is considered to be the position of optimal function (69). Neutral subtalar position is identified through palpation of talonavicular congruency. There should be a slight (3° to 4°) varus relationship between the bisection of the distal third of the lower leg and the perpendicular bisection of the calcaneus. The bisection of the calcaneus should be perpendicular to the line of the metatarsals, and the metatarsal heads should be in line with one another. Integrity of the medial longitudinal arch is assessed by the navicular drop test, or Feiss line, which is formed by the tip of the medial malleolus, the navicular tuberosity, and the first metatarsophalangeal joint (70). Normally the navicular tuberosity should be intersected by this line.

Neutral subtalar position is considered to be the norm. The two extremes of this continuum are represented by pes planus and pes cavus. Pes planus, or so-called flatfoot, results in excessive pronation through midstance. Excessively weighted rear-foot valgus and compensatory internal rotation of the tibia often occur in conjunction with hypermobility of the subtalar joint during running. This interaction can predispose the runner to injuries at the medial aspect of the lower extremity. These injuries may include medial tibial stress syndrome; posterior tibial tendinitis; pes anserine tendinitis/bursitis; stress fractures of the tibia, fibula, and tarsal bones; Achilles tendinitis; and plantar fascitis (20, 71, 72). This is contrasted with the cavus, or high-arched foot. The cavus foot presents decreased subtalar motion with resultant decreased mobility of the midfoot and excessively weighted rear-foot varus. The heel of the cavus foot remains in varus at foot strike, the longitudinal arch is maintained, and the foot remains in a locked, rigid posture. Concurrently, the tibia remains in external rotation, resulting in a net increase of stress transference from the ground throughout the midstance phase of running. The reduction of internal tibial rotation increases the stress on the lateral aspect of the foot and lower extremity; therefore, a pattern of lateral injury is seen. These injuries may include iliotibial band syndrome, trochanteric bursitis, stress fracture, Achilles tendinitis, peroneal muscle strain, plantar fascitis, and metatarsalgia (29, 71, 72).

Mobility of the great toe should be assessed with the first ray stabilized. Restriction of the great toe, or hallux limitus, can affect push off and promote the development of early arthritic changes, sesamoiditis, and metatarsalgia (Fig. 34.10). These problems can be treated effectively with the use of a Morton's extension to assist push off and metatarsal pads to unload areas of excessive stress.

Radiologic Evaluation

Only recently has image evaluation played a significant role in the evaluation of overuse injuries. Conventional radiography is obtained to exclude bony pathology; however, 66% of radiographs are initially negative for stress fractures and only 50% ever develop radiographic evidence of stress fractures related to running (73). A stress fracture may become evident when new periosteal formation, endosteal thickening, or a radiolucent line is observed. Occasionally, tomograms may be helpful in delineating a tarsal navicular stress fracture. As with any pathologic bony condition, however, radionucleide imaging is more sensitive than radiography (74).

A triple-phase bone scan may be particularly useful in differentiating soft tissue abnormalities masquerading as stress fracture or vice versa (75). The three phases of a triple-phase bone scan are the angiogram, blood pool, and delayed image phase. Stress fractures are

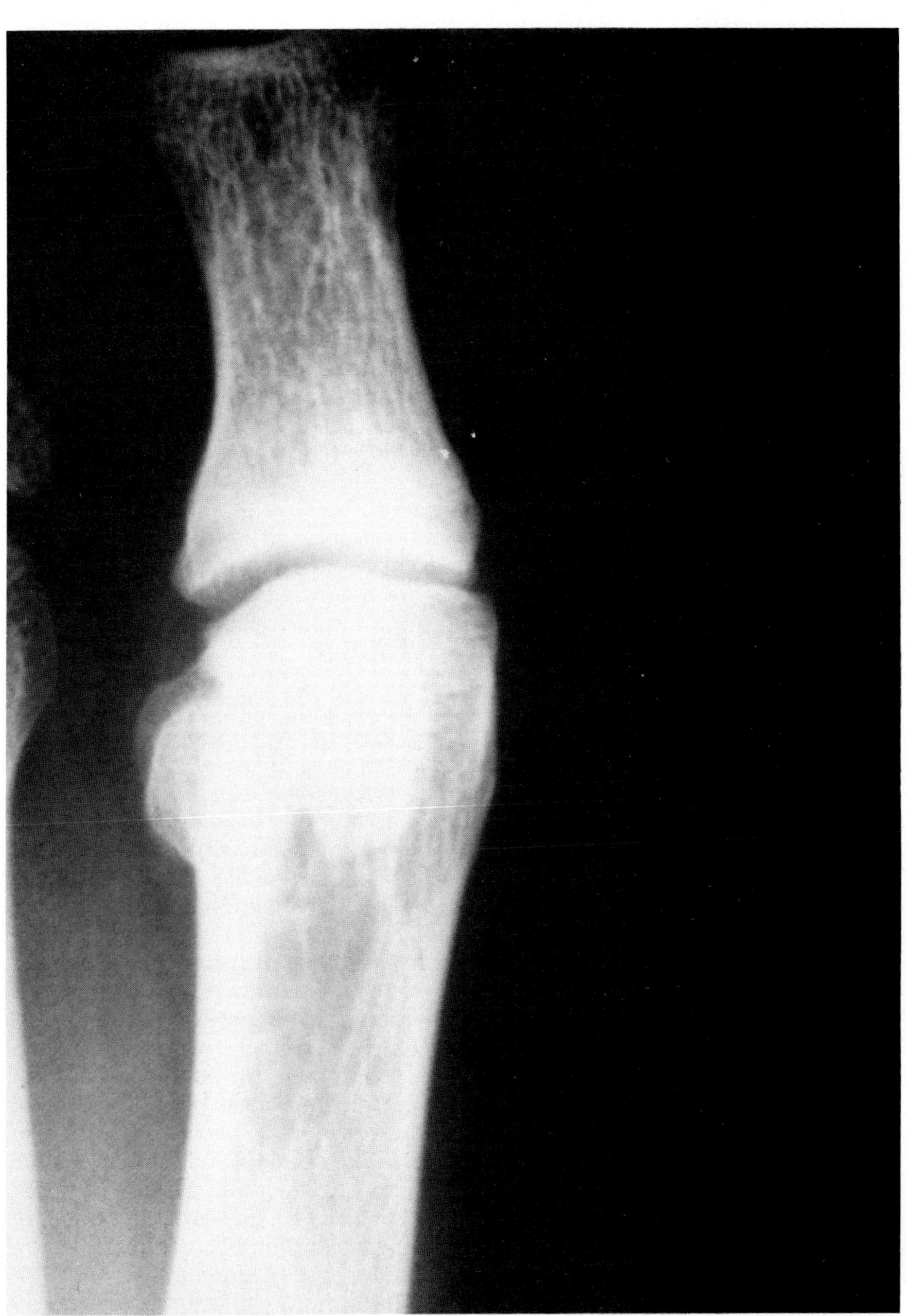

Figure 34.10. Hallux rigidus.

positive for all three phases of the bone scan. In contrast, shin splints are negative for the angiogram and blood pool studies. Plantar fascitis and calcaneal bursitis also present particular patterns that are distinct from calcaneal stress fractures. The use of serial bone scans to evaluate treatment has been proposed with a characteristic progression noted from diffuse uptake early in the stress reaction to sharp fusiform demarcation in advanced stages (76).

The roles of US and computerized tomography (CT) are limited in demonstrating injuries of tendons and muscles, unless complete discontinuity has occurred (77). Standard radiography may be helpful in evaluating accessory ossicle and osteophyte impingement. In addition, a modified zero radiogram is helpful in the evaluation of the heel pad fibrosepta when trying to differentiate central heel syndrome from plantar fascitis.

The role of MRI, although it should be emphasized secondary to clinical evaluation, is adding greatly to the understanding of intrinsic bony and soft tissue pathology. The high intrinsic contrast and spacial resolution of MRI enables a detailed anatomic differentiation of abnormal from normal structures. These capabilities present tremendous potential applications in the sports medicine arena. MRI is particularly useful in providing a detailed assessment of intrinsic abnormalities in tendons, specially at the knee and ankle. However, the use of MRI requires a strong clinical correlation and interaction with a skilled radiologist, because special views may be required. An example of this is modified coronal oblique imaging for cases of suspected posterior tibial tendinitis (78). The role of MRI in the sequential evaluation of stress fractures and soft tissue healing has not yet been clearly defined.

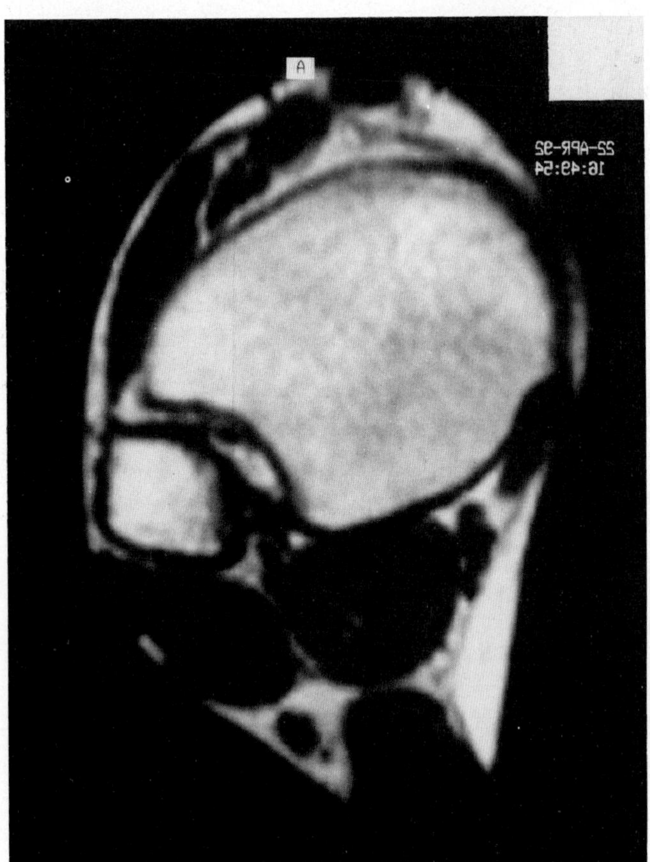

Figure 34.11. MRI view of tibial nerve compression.

MRI also has been useful in the evaluation of entrapment neuropathies. As many as 60% of all entrapment neuropathies occur among the running or jogging population (79). This entity should be considered when atypical, chronic, or recalcitrant pain exists, particularly around the heel and foot. The etiology of this is often dynamic, with the only finding being edema around the nerve, which is not found at the contralateral extremity (Fig. 34.11).

EMG and nerve conduction tests are often unremarkable, unless performed in a dynamic model (79). Therefore, standard EMG and nerve conduction tests that appear to be normal do not preclude a diagnosis of entrapment neuropathy. In conclusion, radiologic and neurologic studies have a role in the evaluation of a runner's injury, however, they are considered secondary to a thorough, and meticulous clinical evaluation.

Soft Tissue Extensibility

Flexibility, hereafter referred to as extensibility, and joint range of motion are often used interchangeably but distinction is warranted. Range of motion refers to the amount of movement about a joint. Extensibility refers to the holistic ability of the soft tissue to elongate through a range of motion (80). Maintenance of adequate range of motion and soft tissue extensibility following injury are critical, because connective tissue may develop scarring, adhesions, and fibrosis. The proliferation of shortened connective tissue can result in the development of a chronic muscle strain cycle.

Soft tissue running injuries are specific to the microtrauma caused by repetitive submaximal loading of musculotendinous structures. The musculotendinous junction is the weakest link of the myotendinous structural unit and is the area in which most strains occur (81). Potential etiologies may include increased collagen content, decreased local extensibility, and the presence of a transitional area of two histologically different tissue types. This is in agreement with the abundance of strains to the gastrocnemius-soleus complex, hip adductors, and hamstring musculotendinous junction observed clinically.

Evaluation of soft tissue extensibility should include all major muscle groups of the lower extremities and lower back. Documentation of initial findings is necessary and periodic comparison may provide motivation to the runner. Gross assessment of the lower back and hips may include the sit and reach (Fig. 34.12) and standing fingertips to floor tests. Specific evaluation of hamstring length can be accomplished by a supine straight leg raise (Fig. 34.13), a 90° hip flexion-knee extension maneuver (Fig. 34.14), or seated-knee extension while maintaining a lordotic posture (Fig. 34.15). Care should be taken to assess lumbopelvic substitutions. Two common tests that assess hip flexor and ili-

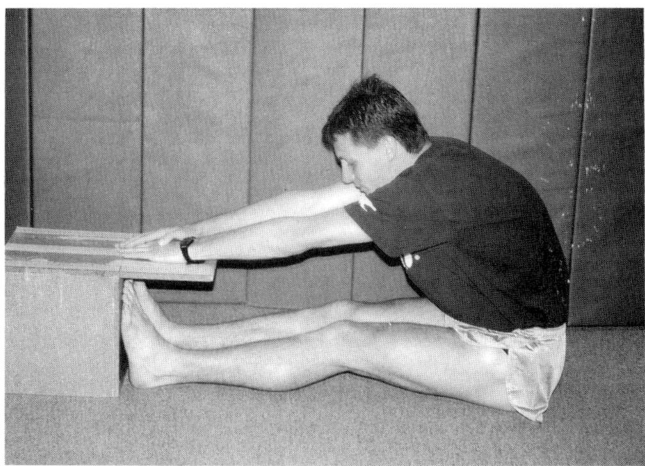

Figure 34.12. Sit and reach test.

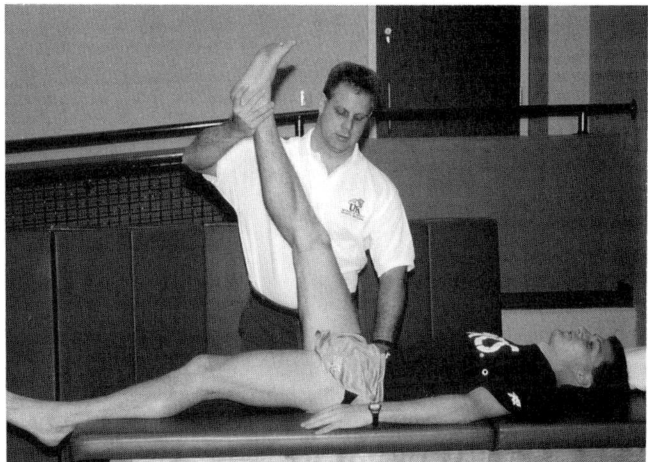

Figure 34.13. Supine straight leg raise test.

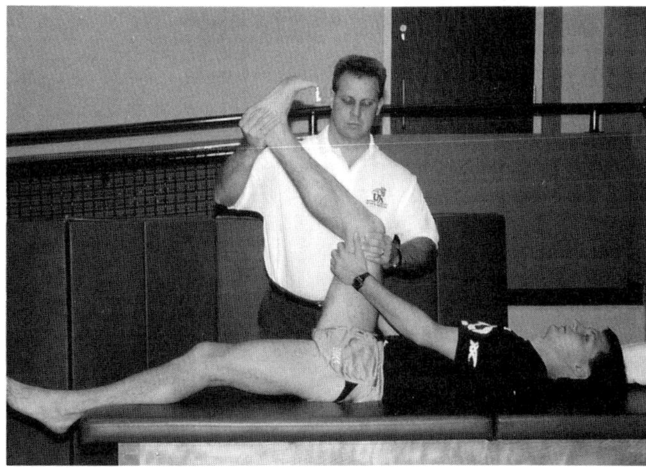

Figure 34.14. The 90° hip flexion–knee extension maneuver.

otibial band extensibility are the Thomas and Ober tests, respectively (Figs. 34.16 and 34.17). The standing hip-drop test is also useful in identifying muscle extensibility and strength imbalances around the hip (82) (Fig.

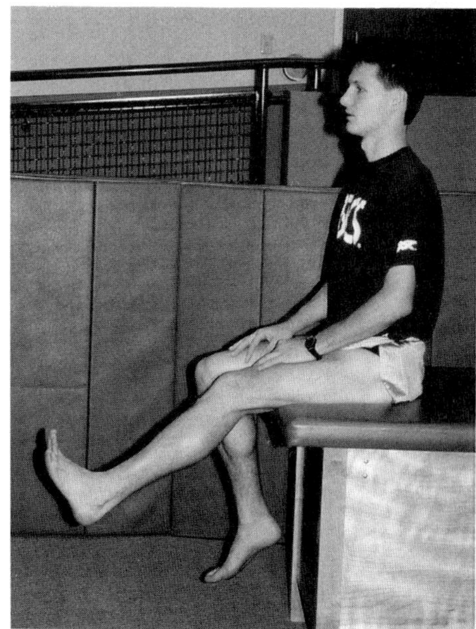

Figure 34.15. Seated-knee extension.

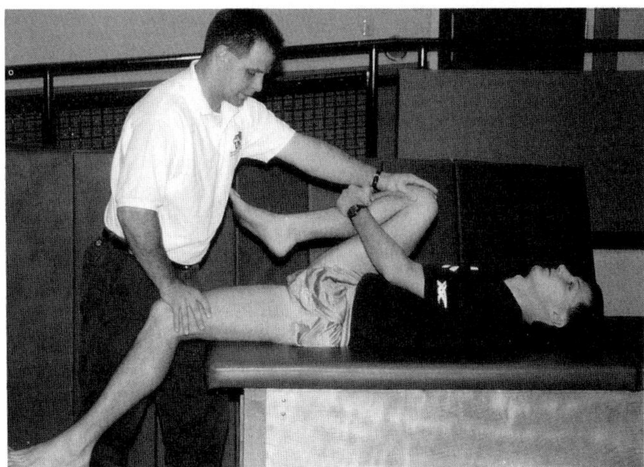

Figure 34.16. Thomas test.

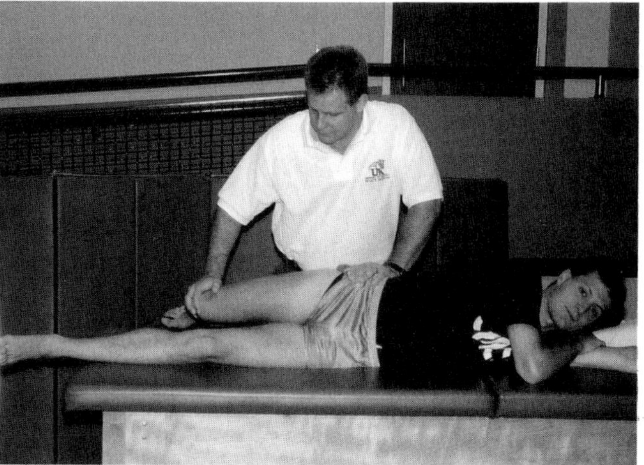

Figure 34.17. Ober test.

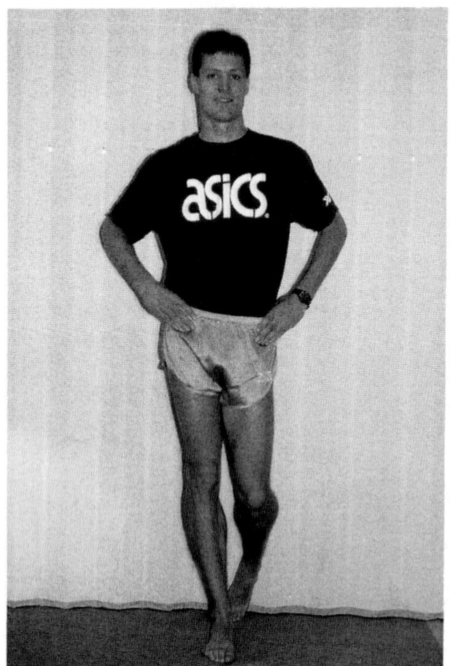

Figure 34.18. Standing hip-drop test.

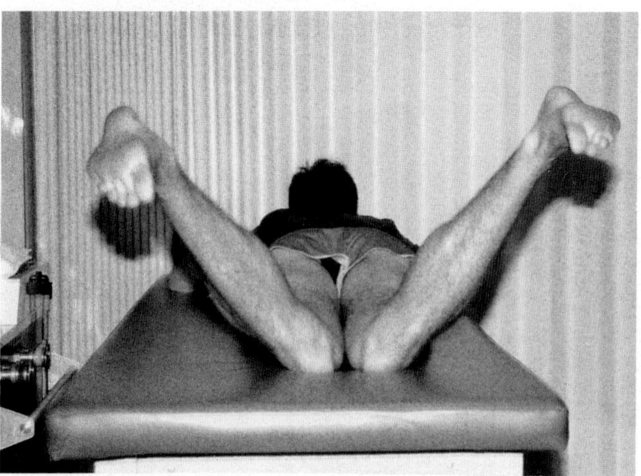

Figure 34.19. Hip rotation assessment.

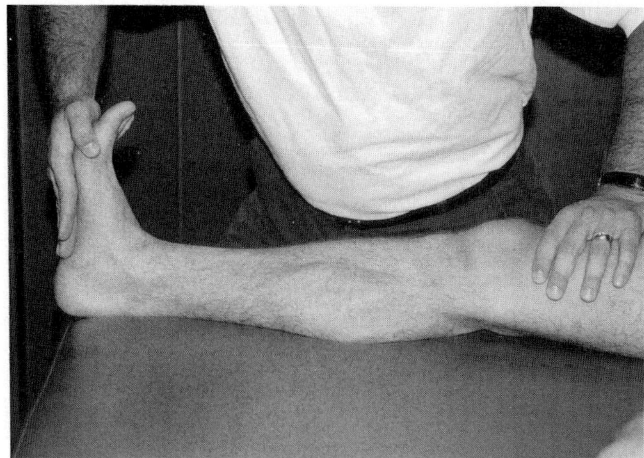

Figure 34.20. Gastrocnemius extensibility assessment.

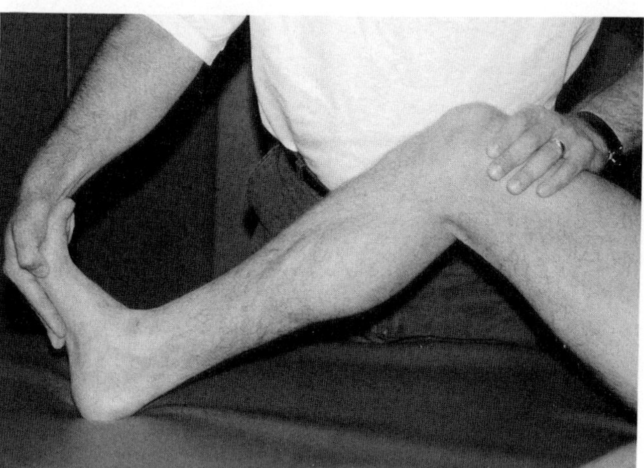

Figure 34.21. Soleus extensibility assessment.

34.18). The hip rotators may be evaluated in a prone position with the knees flexed 90° (Fig. 34.19). Gastrocnemius and soleus extensibility differences can be determined by passively dorsiflexing the ankle with the knee extended and slightly flexed, respectively (Figs. 34.20 and 34.21). Normal ranges of motion have been reported (83).

Innovations in biodynamic analysis are rapidly adding to the understanding of the etiology of running injuries. Those who treat runners should stay current with these innovations and implement them when indicated.

Functional Rehabilitation

Both acute and chronic running injuries should initially be managed with the traditional rest, ice, compression, and elevation (RICE) to diminish pain and inflammation (84). NSAIDs appear to decrease inflammation and promote analgesia while enhancing the return to functional activities and preventing reflex inhibition. Although NSAIDs do not appear to delay the healing process, adverse gastrointestinal affects are common with prolonged use. Because of this, a greater emphasis on local, topical NSAIDs in the form of lotions, ointments, and sprays will likely appear in the near future. The therapeutic effects of US, phonophoresis, iontophoresis, electrical stimulation, and cryotherapy for the treatment of pain and inflammation are well-documented (84, 85). Iontophoresis is superior to US or phonophoresis for treating relatively superficial soft tissue inflammatory conditions, especially when osseous tissues are in the proximity. Several combinations of analgesic and antiinflammatory agents have been suggested, depending on the primary treatment objective (86).

As pain and inflammation are controlled, active mobility and extensibility of the involved tissues should be initiated within symptom-free limits. The exacerbation of any symptom related to the injury site should be interpreted as an indication that the rehabilitation progression is too rapid, the rehabilitation program was poorly designed, something was missed during the initial evaluation, or the runner is noncompliant with the program. Because temperature has been shown to have a profound influence on the viscoelastic properties of connective tissue, a warmup period before the performance of stretching activities is recommended. Although conventional modalities such as hydrotherapy, hot packs, and US may be effective in increasing tissue temperature, a 10- to 15-min session of low- to moderate-intensity stationary cycling or walking is equally effective.

Traditionally, proper stretching is taught as a low-intensity, long-duration, static stretch. The optimal number of repetitions and duration of each stretch remains controversial. One recent study that used an animal model found that 80% of total tissue elongation occurred by the fourth repetition, with the greatest length increase occurring during the initial 12 to 18 sec of each stretch (87). This study supplies valuable information concerning the mechanical properties of the musculotendinous unit, but it does not account for the added difficulty of stretching muscles that act across multiple joints, the components of functional muscle groups that present divergent sites of insertion, or the learning of proper technique.

A recommended stretching routine is three to six repetitions of 15 to 20 sec duration, with total repetitions depending on the functional muscle group being stretched, the ability of the runner to perform the stretch properly, and the amount of warmup before stretch performance. The amount of force during stretching should be subjectively moderate. Static stretching is considered to be safe and can be performed practically anywhere without assistance.

Ballistic stretching attempts to improve extensibility by incorporating gentle bouncing into the stretch. The viscoelastic properties of muscle and the stretch reflex make this technique potentially dangerous if performed by poorly conditioned runners or before warmup.

Dynamic stretching involves moving a joint such as the hip repetitiously through its maximal available range of motion. Because this is considered to be an advanced technique, it should be performed only after subjectively adequate muscle extensibility has been attained through a static stretching program. This method of stretching focuses on the reciprocal action of agonist and antagonist rather than on an isolated muscle group. Dynamic stretching is a useful, but underused rehabilitation tool. It is effective in treating chronic hip adductor, hamstring, and gluteal strains. Examples of this type of stretching include standing hip flexion/extension (Fig. 34.22) and stepping over or under a series of hurdles (Fig. 34.23). Dynamic stretching has the added beneficial component of improving joint/muscle kinesthetic/proprioceptive awareness.

Proprioceptive neuromuscular facilitation (PNF) is a

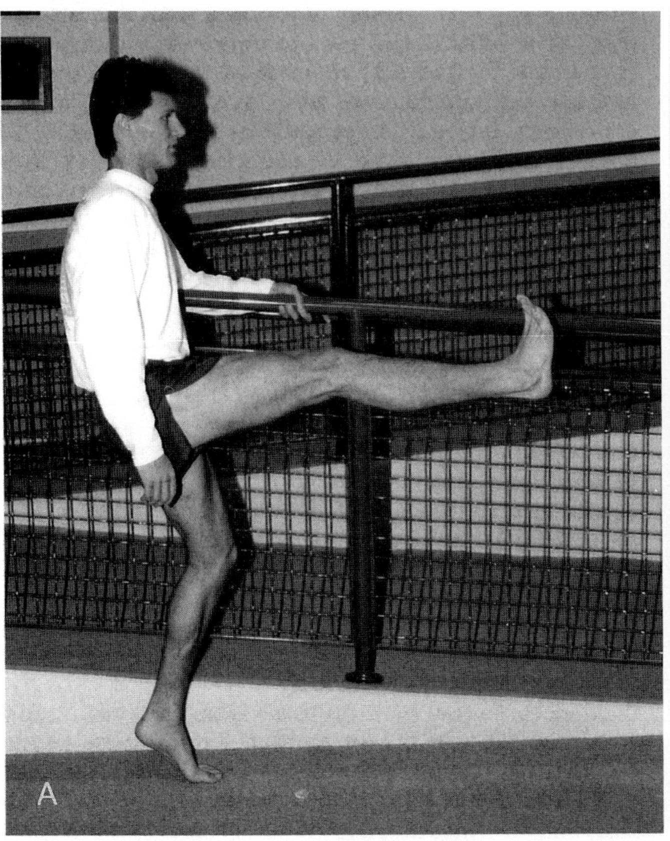

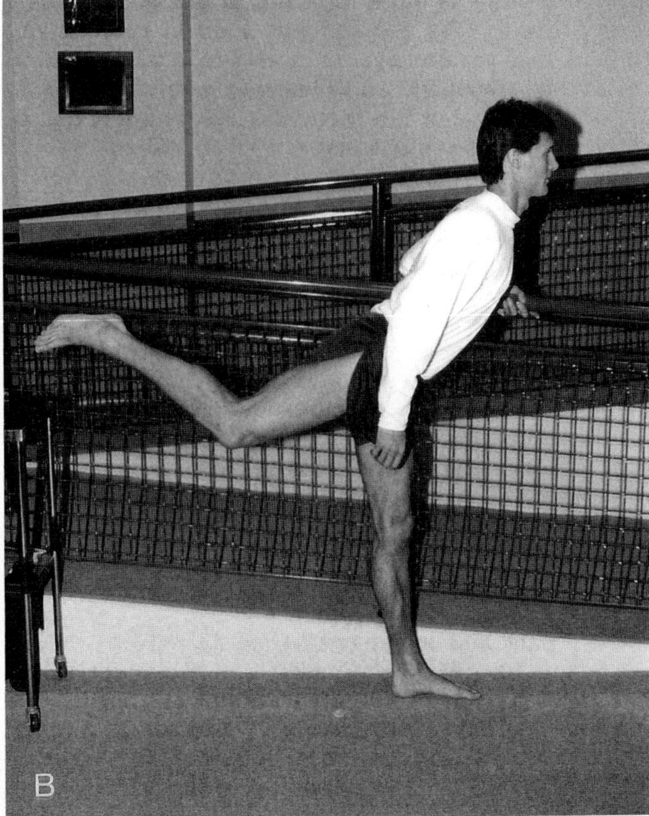

Figure 34.22. Hip flexion (**A**) and extension (**B**) dynamic stretching.

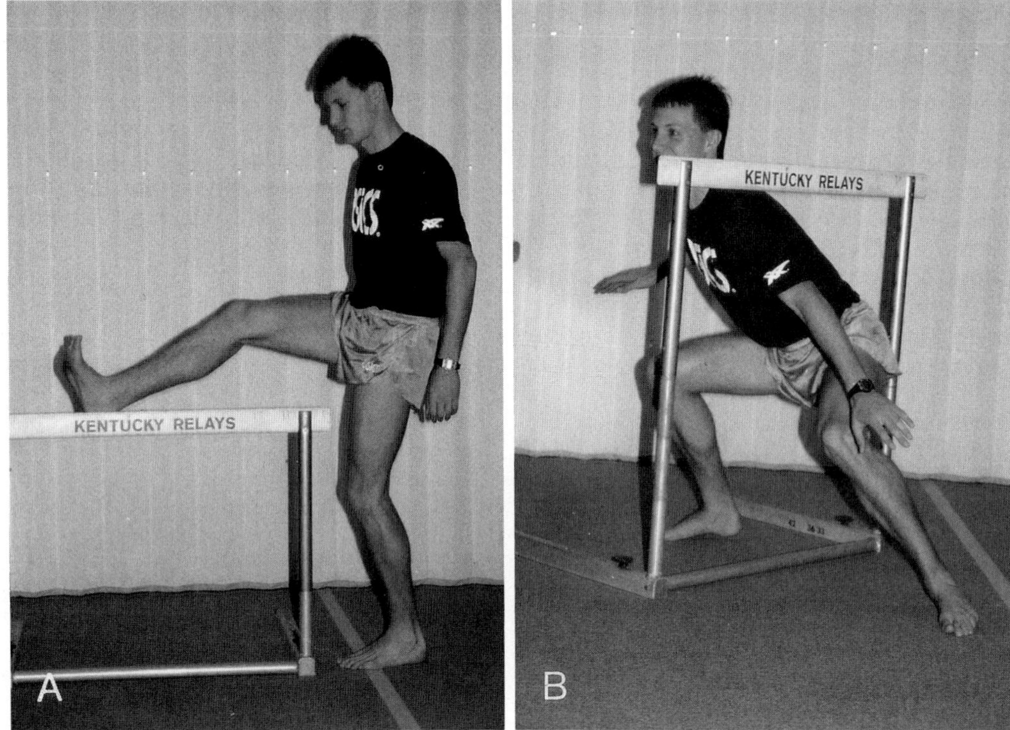

Figure 34.23. Hurdle stepping dynamic stretching involves (**A**) moving over the hurdle in a figure eight motion and (**B**) ducking under the hurdle.

skilled method of promoting neuromuscular activity through a series of quick stretches in functional movement patterns. PNF is frequently used in running rehabilitation programs as a method of manual resistance and also has been shown to improve extensibility (88). The disadvantage of this method of stretching is that it generally requires the assistance of a trained professional.

In addition to pain and inflammation control and the return to improved mobility and extensibility, a cardiovascular maintenance program should be initiated. Immediately, an upper body ergometer may be used. The maintenance of cardiovascular conditioning is an essential component of the total rehabilitation program. As healing progresses, stationary cycling, stepping, rowing, stair climbing, or cross-country skiing devices may be used. Few running injuries require absolute rest from activity. It should be emphasized, however, that it is imperative to minimize reinjury risk factors when planning a rehabilitation and conditioning program. Specific programs should be designed to simulate the demands of the runner's event or training regimen to work effectively the appropriate energy systems.

Once pain and inflammation have resolved, causative factors have been eliminated, and biodynamic limitations such as poor musculotendinous extensibility or a leg length discrepancy have been addressed, a functional rehabilitation plan can be initiated (89). Eccentric muscle action is an important component of this plan when treating the injured runner. The intense eccentric action of the knee extensors during the stance phase of running has been closely associated with the development of tendinitis and muscle injury (81). Running incorporates a rapid role reversal of the knee extensors and the calf musculature from dynamic shock absorbers following impact to propulsive force generators following midstance. The eventual magnitude of these propulsive forces are largely mediated by eccentric muscle action. The specificity principle of rehabilitation suggests that because the lower extremity normally functions through the synergistic action of multiple muscle groups, exercises that enhance this action are desirable. There are instances, however, in which select isolated components (weak links) of the kinetic chain require specific attention, such as isolated exercises for the intrinsic musculature of the feet. A rehabilitation and conditioning program for most runners should emphasize progressive resistance and range of motion squats and multidirectional lunges and stepups. Each movement is performed for approximately two to five sets of 10 to 25 repetitions. Progressive resistance is included with these activities; however, proper technique is obligatory, and each set is terminated at the onset of faulty technique.

Each of the tools previously mentioned as cardiovascular devices may be used to train the anaeorbic capacity of the runner. The performance of multiple anaerobic "bursts" from 10 sec to 2 min in duration help simulate the demands of their event. Intervals of shorter duration are more appropriate for sprinters, whereas longer-duration intervals more effectively train the middle- or long-distance runner. Cross-country skiing machines most effectively train the hip extensors and ankle plantar flexors.

Sliding boards provide total lower extremity rehabilitation with emphasis on the eccentric action of the hip abductors/adductors, whereas the knee extensors/flexors simultaneously act as hip/knee stabilizers. Running against rubber tubing resistance can provide variable resistance for strength and stabilization activities in a variety of functional positions. Each of these activities may be performed for two to five sets of 10 sec to 2 min duration.

The biomechanical ankle platform system (BAPS) (Camp International, Jackson, MI) is an effective rehabilitation tool that can supplement the rehabilitation plan of most running injuries from initial intervention through terminal rehabilitation and conditioning. This device was designed with the triplanar motion of the foot and ankle in mind and is useful for proprioceptive training of this area. This activity is performed for two to three sets of 10 to 30 repetitions. Performing activities such as these while barefoot further strengthens the intrinsic musculature of the foot, thereby improving dynamic impact dampening (90).

Injured runners who rehabilitate in a manner that closely replicates the demands of their event should progress to a running program sooner. No matter how well-designed a rehabilitation or conditioning program is, neglecting structural abnormalities at the lower extremity or lower back will probably result in an unsatisfactory outcome. In particular, a thorough static and dynamic assessment of the feet is encouraged. The emphasis of any rehabilitation program should be on the promotion of a normal ratio between the agonist and antagonist musculature. For example, runners frequently present hamstring dominance, and over time develop a relatively atrophic quadriceps femoris. A proper rehabilitation program should improve this relationship.

Orthotics

Normally, the relationship between the rear foot and fore foot is such that when the rear foot is in a subtalar neutral position, the fore foot is situated transversely to the long axis of the calcaneus. In pathologic conditions, this condition may be altered (12). Orthotics may be used to (*a*) control excess mobility, (*b*) unload a specific region of the foot, (*c*) improve the relationship of the fore foot and rear foot, and (*d*) enhance shock absorption.

When treating the excessively mobile foot of runners who pronate, the physician must determine both the maximal pronation range of motion and the maximum velocity of pronation that occurs during the stance phase. The maximum velocity of pronation can be controlled more effectively by orthotics. Fortunately, this parameter is believed to be of more importance to injury prevention (91). Orthotics have been reported to decrease the rate of pronation by 20% to 70% (91, 92). When treating the relatively hypomobile foot of runners who supinate, the physician may find orthotic intervention that emphasizes shock absorption to be useful. In either condition, posting may be used to improve the fore foot/rear foot relationship.

Runners are generally satisfied with their orthotics, although minor adjustments are often necessary. When orthotics are issued, a dialogue should be maintained to solve problems and evaluate their long-term effectiveness. Further research regarding orthotic and footwear design using recently developed devices such as capacitive pressure distribution platforms that can be inserted into the running shoe is recommended (93).

Return to Running

Returning the injured runner to his or her preinjury level is a complex process. In addition to safely restoring the physiologic and psychological readiness of the runner, care must be taken to avoid reinjury (94). Communication between the runner, coach, and health professionals is vital to prevent training errors. Any return to running program should be goal oriented. By involving the runner in goal planning, the runner's mental outlook will be improved and discouragement caused by the initial absence of competitiveness can be diminished (95). This involvement also increases the likelihood that the runner will have confidence in, and thereby comply with, the program.

Taking these factors into consideration, the concerned personnel can initiate an individualized return to running program that incorporates variable portions of anaerobic and aerobic training based on the specifics of the runner's event. Initially, the following program is recommended: a pace progression from slow to fast, a frequency progression from alternate days to 4 or 5 days/week, and progressive interval training approximately 6 weeks following injury. Before returning to running, the runner should be advised on proper footwear, the avoidance of certain running terrain such as hills, the importance of an adequate warmup, and the importance of compliance with the functional rehabilitation and conditioning program, especially stretching.

Conclusions

As the popularity of running continues to grow, an increased incidence of running injury is likely. Through the implementation of a thorough static and dynamic clinical examination, the use of innovative imaging techniques, and the acquisition of physiologic and biodynamic data, researchers' diagnostic capabilities are greatly enhanced. This information enables the development and optimal use of functional rehabilitation programs, conditioning and coaching strategies, and orthotics. The clinical examination, including a thorough injury history and open communication, will always be the most important component of treating the injured runner.

PART 2

Organization and Administration of Medical Coverage for Road Races

Larry J. Grollman

Frank Shorter's gold medal victory in the Olympic marathon at the Summer Games in Munich in 1972 touched off a running boom in the United States that still continues today. This increase in popularity has led to a change in the types of participants in long-distance road racing. Long-distance road races now attract many novice runners, with a wide disparity in their training, as well as the serious professional and amateur athlete. The increased participation in road racing has made the need for adequate medical support essential.

The percentage of runners who will require medical attention as a result of racing depends largely on environmental conditions and the distance of the run. Injury rates may vary from about 0.1% to 20% of runners treated. The author's experience with the medical coverage of marathon races in Pittsburgh from 1988 to 1992 has included races run in wet bulb globe temperatures ranging from 38° to 84°F (2° to 26°C). Injury rates in Pittsburgh have ranged from 9.6% to 21.8% of runners requiring medical treatment (96).

Proper coordination, training, and supervision of appropriate medical personnel is necessary to provide proper medical care to the runners. The major goals of the medical support should be to (*a*) minimize the potential dangers associated with road racing through the proper organization of medical personnel, equipment, and supplies to manage effectively and efficiently all medical concerns, and (*b*) to promote runner education, prevention of injuries, and proper preparation for participation in the event.

Organizing Committee

The medical support for a road race must include components of both emergency medicine and sports medicine. In reality, preparing for the medical support of thousands of runners is similar to disaster planning. To ensure optimal care, the medical support should be recruited early in the planning of the event. A medical director should be appointed to coordinate and supervise the medical team. A medical doctor (MD) should most likely serve as the medical director for a race. He or she should be knowledgeable in exercise physiology and specific medical concerns of runners.

The medical director must work closely with the race director to coordinate adequately the medical team support. He or she will be responsible for all medical questions that may arise regarding the participants in the race.

Depending on the number of participants and the distance of the race, a medical operations manager or coordinator should be designated by the medical director. The medical operations manager should assist the medical director in securing needed volunteers and provide logistical help in covering the event. The medical operations manager should preferably be an emergency medicine specialist (EMT paramedic), triage nurse, or a sports medicine professional (ATC or PT). He or she should have knowledge in the appropriate personnel as well as the equipment and supplies needed for the race.

A medical organizing committee should be formed for each race event. The committee should consist of the medical director, race director, medical operations manager (if applicable), representatives from the local emergency medical service (EMS) and police force, and a medical communications coordinator. The committee should meet before the event to discuss important issues such as race date and time considerations, recruitment of medical personnel and supplies, runner education programming, and racecourse coordination. A reasonable time limit should be designated for the racecourse (6 hours for a marathon).

The medical organizing committee should carefully consider the time and date for the event. Local weather history should be used to avoid unacceptable levels of environmental extremes. Races should avoid the hottest summer months and the hottest part of the day. The American College of Sports Medicine (97) recommends that "all summer events should be scheduled for the early morning, ideally before 8:00 am, or in the evening after 6:00 pm, to minimize solar radiation." However, caution also should be taken in early fall and late spring races because great variations in local temperatures may occur.

Team Personnel

Medical personnel should include medical doctors (MDs) with an expertise in emergency medicine, sports medicine, orthopedics, or primary care. Nursing personnel (RNs), especially trauma and surgical nurses, are required. Podiatrists (DPMs) should be included to handle foot and ankle concerns. Certified athletic trainers (ATCs) and physical therapists (PTs) who have experience working with injured runners should also serve on the medical team. Massage therapists, primarily those skilled in sports massage, may be included. Additional volunteers serving as recorders for the medical team are useful for race day. The recorders should be responsible for the documentation of all runners' injuries treated at the event as instructed by the members of the medical team.

To secure needed volunteers, members of the medical organizing committee should contact local hospitals and local medical organizations. In addition, mailing lists of various professionals can be obtained from local and state allied health organizations. Recruitment letters can be a successful way to enlist potential volunteers.

Volunteer recruitment forms should include needed demographic information, expertise and experience, and desired location/assignment for the race day. It also may be beneficial to know which volunteers are capable of starting an intravenous injection. Medical volunteers should be questioned on their individual professional liability insurance. Liability insurance that is provided for sanctioned events does not cover medical personnel. Presently, there has been no reported litigation brought on by a competitor regarding the medical care rendered at a road race. However, professional liability should always be considered as an important issue. Each medical volunteer should inform his or her professional liability insurance carrier and/or employer of his or her intent to serve as a medical volunteer at a road race.

All medical volunteers should be clearly instructed that they are under the direction of the medical director. Specific job responsibilities and guidelines should be provided to each medical volunteer before race day. If possible, an orientation program should be provided for the medical volunteers. The program should include aid station reporting and closing times, approximate opening and closing times of the racecourse, overview of the medical support for the race, proper injury management and documentation, and a review of the current Occupational Safety and Health Administration (OSHA) standards of universal precautions for the handling of blood and body fluids (98). All volunteers should be given some type of credential that clearly identifies them as members of the race medical team. In addition, clearly marked medical volunteer T-shirts and hats can be used for easy identification.

The Athletics Congress/USA (TAC)—now called USA Track & Field—has published a manual that provides an overview of medical care for long-distance road races (99). The TAC manual recommends 5 to 10 professional and 5 to 10 nonprofessional volunteers per 1000 runners, depending on the race distance and type of course. Fewer volunteers are recommended for a 10K or out-and-back course. For the Pittsburgh Marathon, which averages 3500 runners, the medical team will number between 800 and 1000 volunteers. These figures include medical personnel and nonmedical (security, dropped-out runner vehicle drivers, and radio operators) personnel.

The level of care provided by the medical team should include instituting basic cardiopulmonary resuscitation (CPR) and advanced life support (ALS), treatment of environmental injuries, first aid treatment for orthopedic and podiatric problems, general medical considerations associated with road racing, and facilities for physically challenged competitors, if appropriate (99).

Communications

A medical communications system should be coordinated by the medical organizing committee. The principal function of the medical communications system is to relay information regarding runners who require immediate medical attention. The communications system also should function to relay necessary information, such as weather conditions, to the medical director. The system can be used to track runners who have received medical attention at an aid station or who are on a dropped-out runner vehicle after dropping out of the race.

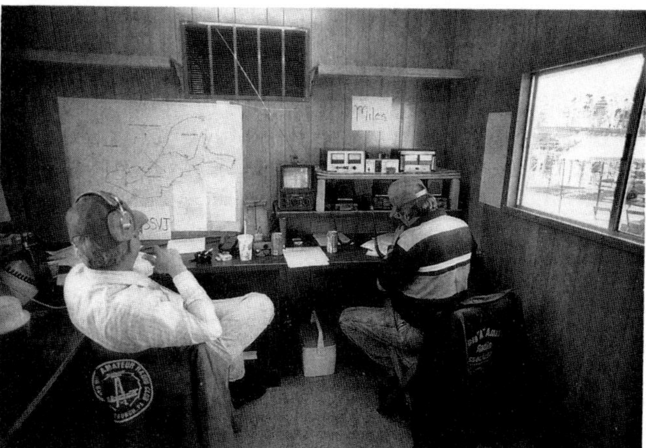

Figure 34.24. Ham radio operators in communications command center at finish line. Courtesy of the University of Pittsburgh Medical Center.

The use of amateur (ham) radio operators or vehicles equipped with citizen band (CB) radios is recommended. The radio operators should be placed every 1 to 2 miles on the racecourse. Ideally, a radio operator should be positioned at the start of the race, at each medical aid station on the racecourse and at the finish line medical area. A radio operator also should be placed in all dropped-out runner vehicles. Cellular phones and long-range pagers can also be used by the members of the medical organizing team on race day to facilitate communications.

The communications system should interface with race operations, local emergency medical services, and the local police force. All communications should be coordinated through a centralized command center, which should logically be located at the finish line (Fig. 34.24). If possible, mobile radio operators should shadow the members of the medical organizing committee so important communications between those parties can be expedited. This will provide the medical communications manager with immediate access to the medical director. Any additional radio operators can serve as medical spotters at various locations on the racecourse.

The medical communications manager should notify all local hospital emergency rooms of the date and time of the race. This will prepare the hospital staffs for any seriously injured runners who may be brought into their facilities. In addition, this will facilitate communication with the emergency room when verifying the status of any injured runners who are treated there.

Aid Stations

Medical aid stations should be located at the start and finish lines for all road races. The finish line medical area should be large enough to accommodate many runners and possibly spectators as well. For a 10K race, there should also be at least two aid stations on the racecourse. Aid stations should be located at least every 2 miles races longer than the 10K. At the Pittsburgh Marathon, aid stations are located every 2 miles for the first 10 miles of the racecourse and then approximately every 1 mile until the finish (Fig. 34.25).

Aid stations should be clearly marked with appropriate signs. The aid station signs should be positioned on posts above eye level so they can easily be viewed by the runners. To assist runners needing medical attention at the aid stations, warning signs that say "aid 100 yards ahead" can be placed on the racecourse (Fig. 34.26).

Noble and Bachman (100) recommend a team of at least three medical personnel consisting of physicians, podiatrists, nurses, or EMTs at each medical aid station per 1000 runners. In addition, each aid station may include an orthopedist and/or podiatrist. At least two physical therapists or athletic trainers should be present at each medical aid station to assist with minor musculoskeletal problems.

The personnel requirements for the Pittsburgh Marathon also take into account the injury data that demonstrates a significant increase in the number of runners treated on the racecourse after mile 15. As a result, the personnel requirements for medical aid stations after mile 15 are approximately twice the number recommended by Noble and Bachman.

The finish line medical area should have one triage officer for races with more than 1000 participants. The finish line medical area should also have a team consisting of at least four to six primary care or emergency room physicians, nurses, or EMTs for every 1000 runners. At least 20 physical therapists and/or athletic trainers should be needed at the finish line medical area.

At the Pittsburgh Marathon, the finish line area consists of a 40 × 100-foot tent that houses three medical areas: acute; general; and sports medicine. Three triage physicians evaluate each runner as he or she enters the medical tent. Upon the results of the evaluation, the runners are moved to the appropriate medical area (Fig. 34.27).

Medical escorts should also be placed in the finish line chutes. The escorts should be medical personnel trained to properly triage the runners (Fig. 34.28). Parallel chutes between the runners' chutes should be planned so the medical escorts are accessible to the runners. Approximately 10 to 15 medical escorts are needed per 1000 runners. To prevent exercise-associated collapse, it is imperative that the escorts encourage runners to continue to move through the chute system. The chutes should be extended far enough so runners will move quickly through and allow for easy access to the finish line medical area. At the Pittsburgh Marathon, the finish line chute area is supervised by an emergency medicine physician and staffed by athletic trainers. Emergency medical personnel with stretchers should be stationed in close proximity to the chute area for downed runners needing assistance.

Nonmedical personnel are also needed at the finish line medical area. Security personnel should be placed at all entrances to the finish line medical area to ensure the privacy of the runners who are treated there. A "Family Reunion/Lost Runner" area should be positioned outside of the finish line medical area. The radio

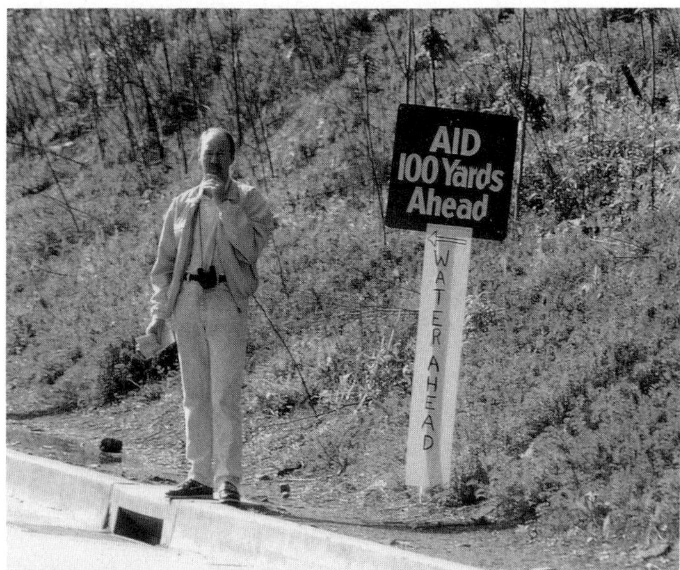

Figure 34.26. Sign to notify runners of upcoming medical aid and fluid stations. Courtesy of the University of Pittsburgh Medical Center.

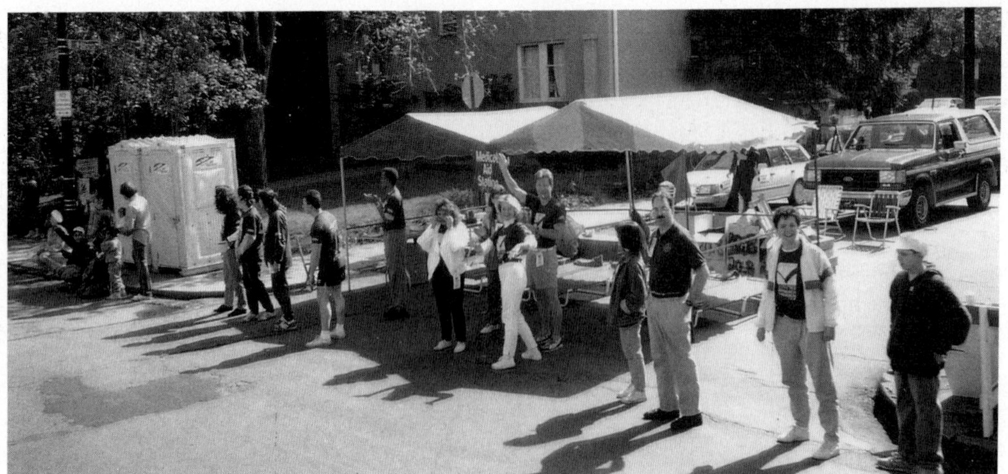
Figure 34.25. Medical aid station on a marathon racecourse. Courtesy of the University of Pittsburgh Medical Center.

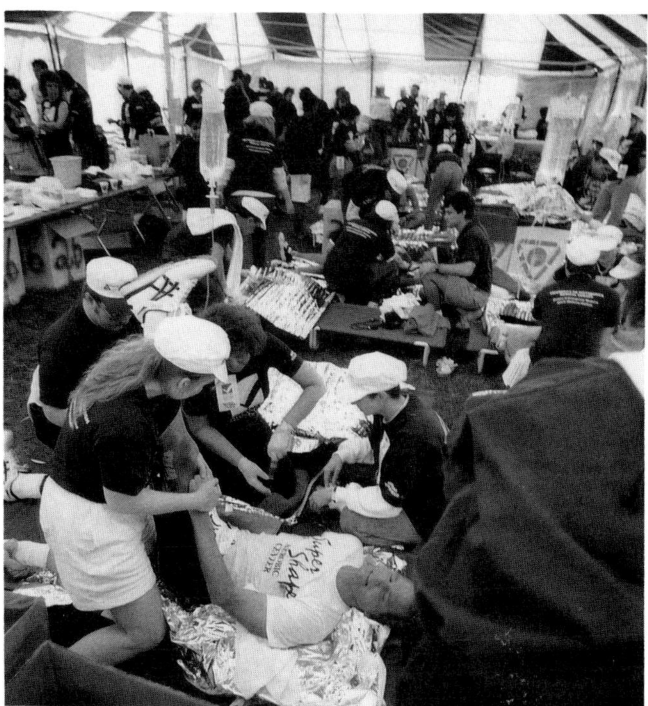

Figure 34.27. Finish line medical area at the Pittsburgh Marathon. Courtesy of the University of Pittsburgh Medical Center.

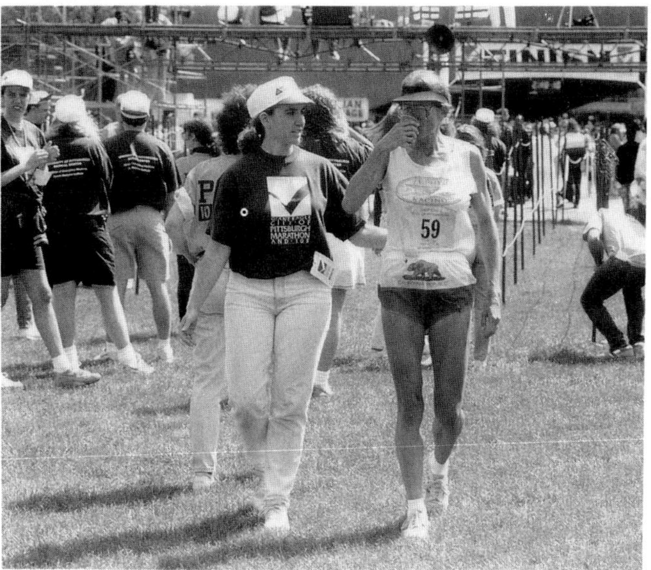

Figure 34.28. Medical personnel escorting runners through finish line chutes. Courtesy of the University of Pittsburgh Medical Center.

operators at the various aid station locations on the course should report periodically to the communications center with the entry number of those participants who were treated at their respective stations. In addition, the operators on the dropped-out runner vehicles should also report periodically on those runners that are being transported on the vehicles. These reports are sent from the communications center to the Lost Runner area. The personnel at the Lost Runner area can provide the status of a runner to a family member or friend who is waiting at the finish line. However, family members are requested to use the services of the Lost Runner area only if they have been waiting longer than 1 hr past the runner's predicted finish time.

Depending on the number of runners, at least two ambulances should be placed at the finish line medical area. There should also be at least two ambulances on the course for every 1000 runners and an additional ambulance for each 1000 runners. For the Pittsburgh Marathon, volunteer ambulance services from the county assist the city's emergency medical services to allow for one ambulance at each medical aid station.

In addition to the emergency vehicles, there should be at least one dropped-out runner vehicle for a 10K race and one vehicle per 1000 runners for a marathon. These vehicles are responsible for transporting runners who have dropped out of the race for nonmedical reasons or for runners who have been treated and released from a medical aid station and will not be returning to the race. One vehicle should serve as a sweep vehicle trailing along the course to pick up runners at the projected time limit per mile (e.g., for a marathon it is 13 to 14 min/mile). A radio operator should be placed in each vehicle so he or she can communicate with the command center.

Equipment and Supplies

The TAC manual suggests equipment and supplies needed per 1000 runners for aid stations and for the finish line medical area (99). As a result of experience with the Pittsburgh Marathon, the author has modified the lists to include intravenous setups at aid stations as well as at the finish line. The modified equipment and supply needs take into account the expected increase in the number of runners treated after the midpoint of the marathon. This list of supplies is presented in Tables 34.2 and 34.3.

Fluid Stations

Adequate fluid stations should be placed throughout the entire racecourse, including the start and finish lines. The TAC guidelines for the starting line are one 8-oz. cup of water per runner for races less than 10 miles and two 8-oz. cups of water for races longer than 10 miles (99). For aid stations, the TAC manual recommends 6 to 8 oz. of water and/or diluted electrolyte replacement drink totaling 1.25 times the number of entrants (99). The finish line area should have at least two 8-oz. cups of water and diluted electrolyte replacement drink per runner. Plans should include having additional fluids and ice available for warmer days.

Appropriate signs should be positioned at each fluid station. The signs should be posted above eye level so they can easily be viewed by the runners. Signs should also be posted before the fluid stations to alert runners of their location. If possible, the runners should be made aware of the brand of electrolyte drink that will be available on race day.

Table 34.2.
The Pittsburgh Marathon Medical Team's Recommended Equipment for All Aid Stations (per 1000 Runners)

Number	Item
4	Cots/stretchers
4	Blankets
10	Mylar (space) blankets
4	Towels
1 set	Weather flags (black, red, yellow, green, and white)
1	Oxygen tanks
1 cooler chest	Ice and zipper-type plastic bags
2	IV setups (normal saline, lactated ringers, D5 1/2 NS, dextrose 50%)
1 container	Blood glucose strips
1	Tourniquet
1	Sharps container
2	Biohazardous wastebags
1	Resuscitation masks
1	Plastic protective eye goggles
10 pair	Rubber gloves
1 bottle	50% Clorox/50% water solution
1 pair	Crutches
2	Stethoscopes
2	BP cuffs
4	Rectal thermometers
4 jars	Petroleum jelly
4 each	Ace bandages (3" and 4")
2 rolls each	Adhesive tape (1" and 1½")
1	Betadine solution
2	Hand cleaner
1 box	Alcohol swabs
20 packets	Antiseptic ointment
1 box each	Tampons/pads
1 box each	Gauze pads (2" × 2" and 4" × 4")
1 box	Band-Aids
10	Tongue depressors
1 pair	Bandage scissors
1 each	Urinals (male and female)
1	Clipboard
20	Injury data cards
30 cups	Water/electrolyte solution (also hot drinks for cold weather)

Table 34.3.
Pittsburgh Marathon Medical Team's Recommended Equipment for Finish Line Medical Area (per 1000 Runners)

Number	Item
10	Cots/stretchers
10	Blankets
200	Mylar (space) blankets
25	Towels
1 set	Weather flags (black, red, yellow, green, and white)
2	Oxygen tanks
4 32 gallon cans	Ice and zipper-type plastic bags
10	IV setups (normal saline, lactated ringers, D5 1/2 NS, dextrose 50%)
2 containers	Blood glucose strips
2	Tourniquets
2	Sharps container
20	Biohazardous wastebags
2	Resuscitation masks
2	Plastic protective eye goggles
50 pair	Rubber gloves
3 bottles	50% Clorox/50% water solution
6 pair	Crutches
6	Stethoscopes
6	BP cuffs
7	Rectal thermometers
4 jars	Petroleum jelly
40 each	Ace bandages (3" and 4")
8 rolls each	Adhesive tape (1" and 1½")
4	Betadine solution
2	Hand cleaner
2 boxes	Alcohol swabs
40 packets	Antiseptic ointment
2 boxes each	Tampons/pads
12 boxes each	Gauze pads (2" × 2" and 4" × 4")
3 boxes	Band-Aids
30	Tongue depressors
5 pair	Bandage scissors
5 each	Urinals (male and female)
5	Clipboard
200	Injury data cards
200 cups each	Water/electrolyte solution (also hot drinks for cold weather)

Environmental Considerations

The ACSM recommends the use of the wet bulb globe temperature (WBGT) for measuring environmental conditions (97). The WBGT measures ambient temperature, humidity, and radiant heat. The following formula is recommended: WBGT = (0.7 Twb) + (0.2 Tg) + (0.1 Tdb), where Twb is temperature, wet bulb thermometer; Tg is temperature, black globe thermometer; and Tdb is temperature, dry bulb thermometer. Instruments to measure WBGT are available commercially. To ensure accuracy, the weather readings should be measured at a location on the racecourse.

The ACSM recommends the use of the color-coded flag system to indicate the risk of environmental stress (97) (Table 34.4). A set of each of the five flags should be included in the supplies and equipment for all aid stations. Weather readings should be taken every 30 min and medical communications should contact all aid stations to indicate the appropriate flag to display. Each aid station should place the appropriate flag at a level easily visible to the runners as they proceed along the course.

Runner Education

Prerace seminars can be extremely useful in educating potential participants, especially the beginning runner. Seminar topics should include medical screening before running a race, guidelines for training, environmental considerations, fluid/electrolyte replacement, and the prevention and management of common running injuries. A seminar on the day before the race should include a overview of the racecourse and the medical support available, final race preparations, expected weather conditions, and techniques to recover quickly from the race.

Medical information can be supplied to the runners in their prerace packets. For the Pittsburgh Marathon, runners receive a medical information brochure that details tips on what they should do from the night before the race through the days following the race. In

Table 34.4.
ACSM Color-Coded Flag System

Color	Meaning	Comments
Black	Extreme risk	WBGT > 82°F (28°C); race has been canceled or modified if conditions exceed this level at starting time
Red	High risk	WBGT from 73° to 82°F (23° to 28°C); all runners should be aware that heat injury is possible and any person particularly sensitive to heat or humidity should probably not run; all runners should slow their pace
Yellow	Moderate risk	WBGT from 65° to 73°F (18° to 23°C); air temperature, probably humidity, and almost certainly radiant heat at the beginning of the race will increase during the course of the race if conducted in the morning or early afternoon; runners sensitive to the heat should slow their pace
Green	Low risk	WBGT from 50° to 65°F (10° to 18°C); no current weather restrictions
White	Risk of hypothermia	WBGT <50°F (10°C); hypothermia may occur, especially in slow runners in long races, and in wet and windy conditions

addition, the participants are asked to provide demographic information and their medical histories. This information will be printed on the back of the entry numbers that are pinned to the runners' shirts on race day.

At least 15 min before and immediately before the start, the medical director should make prerace announcements by loud speaker to the runners. The announcements should include the current and expected weather conditions for the race, review the ACSM color-coded flag system, review the locations of the aid and fluid locations, and any other pertinent information.

Conclusions

Providing for the safety of participants in a road race includes a well-coordinated medical team. Proper planning is essential to effective medical support for a road race. The medical organizing team should be prepared for all potential medical problems. Appropriate personnel and equipment are needed to provide the optimal medical support for the event. A thorough medical communication system will assist in the effectiveness and efficiency of the medical support. In addition to the medical support for the race, runners should be educated on proper training methods and injury prevention.

REFERENCES

1. Jacobs SJ, Berson B. Injuries to runners: a study of entrants to a 10,000 meter race. Am J Sports Med 1986;14:2:151–155.
2. Pollack ML, Gettman LR, Milesis LA, Bak MD, Durstine L, Johnson RB. Effects of frequency and duration of training on attrition and incidence of injury. Med Sci Exerc Sports 1977;9:1:31–36.
3. Bovens AMP, Janssen GME, Vermeer HGW, Hoeberigs JH, Janssen MPE, Verstappen PTS. Occurrence of running injuries in adults following a supervised training program. Int J Sports Med 1989;10:S186–S190.
4. Van Galen W, Diederiks J. Sportblessures breed uitgemeten, Uitg. Haarlem: De Vrieseborch, 1990.
5. van Mechelen W. Running injuries. A review of the epidemiological literature. Sports med 1992;14(5):320–335.
6. Cavanagh PR, Lafortune MA. Ground reaction in distance running. J Biomech 1980;13:393–406.
7. Mann RA, Baxter DE, Lutter LD. Running symposium. Foot Ankle 1981;1:190–224.
8. Ounpuu S. The biomechanics of running: a kinematic and kinetic analysis. In: Greene WB, ed. Instr Course Lect 1990;39:305–318.
9. Mann RA, Moran GT, Doughtery SE. Comparative electromyography of the lower extremity in jogging, running and sprinting. Am J Sports Med 1986;14:6:501–510.
10. Arendt-Nielsen L, Sinkjaer T, Nielsen J, et al. Electromyographic and kinematic profiles during different gait velocities and inclines. In: Anderson PA, Hobart DJ, Danoff JV, eds. Electromyographical kinesiology. Amsterdam: The Netherlands: Elsevier Science, 1991:75–78.
11. Perry J. Gait analysis normal and pathological function. Thorofare, NJ: Slack, 1992:381–411.
12. Jones DC. Foot orthoses. In: Heckman JD, ed. Instr Course Lect 1993;42:219–224.
13. Renstrom P, Johnson R. Overuse injuries in sports: a review. Sports Med 1985;2:316–333.
14. McKenzie DC, Clement DB, Taunton JD. Running shoes, orthotics and injuries. Sports Med 1985;2:334–347.
15. Subotnick SI. The biomechanics of running: implications for the prevention of foot injuries. Sports Med 1985;2:144–153.
16. Nigg BM. The influence of the playing surface. In: Nigg BM, ed. Biomechanical aspects of playing surfaces. Zurich: Juris Verlag, 1978:54–64.
17. Luethi SM, Frederick EC, Hawes MR, Nigg BM. Influence of shoe construction on lower extremity kinematics and load during lateral movements in tennis. Int J Sports Biomech 1986;2:156–165.
18. Cook S, Brinker M, Mahlon P. Running shoes: their relation to running injuries. Sports Med 1990;10:1:1–8.
19. Jorgensson U, Ekstrand J. Significance of heel pad confinement for the shock absorption of heel strike. J Sports Med 1988;9:468–473.
20. Clement DB, Taunton JE, Smart GW, McNicol KL. A survey of overuse running injuries. Phys Sports Med 1981;9:5:47–58.
21. Blair SE, Kohl HW, Goodyear NN. Rates and risks for running and exercise injuries: studies in three populations. Res Q Exerc Sport 1987;58:3:221–228.
22. Walter SD, Hart LE, McIntosh JM, Sutton JR. The Ontario cohort study of running related injuries. Arch Int Med 1989;149:2561–2564.
23. Lloyd T, Triantafyllou SJ, Baker ER, et al. Women athletes with menstrual irregularity have increased musculoskeletal injuries. Med Sci Sports Exerc 1986;18:4:374–379.
24. Konradsen L, Hansson EB, Sandergaard L. Long distance running and osteoarthrosis. Am J Sports Med 1990;18:4:379–381.
25. Lane NE, Bloch DA, Jones HH. Long-distance running, bony density, and osteoarthritis. JAMA 1986;255:9:1147–1151.

26. Lane NE, Bloch DA, Wood PD, Fries JF. Aging, long-distance running, and the development of musculoskeletal disability: a controlled study. Am J Med 1987;82:4:772–780.
27. Felson DT, Andersson JJ, Nainvk A, Walker AM, Meenan RF. Obesity and knee osteoarthritis. The Framington study. Intern 1988;109:18–24.
28. Scott SH, Winter DA. Internal forces at chronic running injury sites. Med Sci Sports Exerc 1990;22:3:357–369.
29. Brody DM. Running injuries. Clin Symp 1987;39:4:1–36.
30. James SL, Bates BT, Osternig LR. Injuries to runners. Am J Sports Med 1978;6:2:40–50.
31. Cibulka MT. Rehabilitation of the pelvis, hip and thigh. Clin Sports Med 1989;8:4:777–803.
32. Bolz S, Davies G. Leg length differences and correlations with total leg strength. J Orthop Sports Phys Ther 1984;6:123–129.
33. Steindler A: Kinesiology of the human body under normal and pathological conditions. Springfield, IL: Charles C. Thomas, 1955:58–86.
34. Gray G. Chain reactions: successful strategies for closed chain testing and rehabilitation. Adrian, MI: Wynn Marketing, 1989.
35. Macintyre JG, Taunton JE, Clement DB, et al. Predicting lower-extremity injuries among habitual runners. Arch Int Med 1989;149:2565–2568.
36. Magee DJ. Orthopedic physical assessment. Philadelphia: WB Saunders, 1987.
37. Macintyre JG, Taunton JE, Clement DB, Lloyd-Smith DR, Mckenzie DC, Morrell RW. Running injuries: a clinical study of 4,173 cases. Clin J Sports Med 1991;1:2:81–87.
38. Drez D. Personal communication, 1990.
39. McConnell J. The management of chondromalacia patellae: a long term solution. Aust J Physiol 1986;32:215–223.
40. Perrin DH. Prophylactic and functional knee braces. Paper presented at the 5th Annual Panther Sports Medicine Symposium, Pittsburgh, PA, 1992.
41. Martens M, Libbrecht P, Burssens A. Surgical treatment of the iliotibial band friction syndrome. Am J Sports Med 1989;17:5:651–654.
42. Styf JR, Kormer LM. Microcapillary infusion technique for measurement of intramuscular pressure during exercise. Clin Orthop 1986;207:253–262.
43. Pedowitz RA, Hargens AR, Mubarak SJ et al. Modified criteria for the objective diagnosis of chronic compartment syndrome of the leg. Am J Sports Med 1990;18:35–40.
44. McBryde AM. Stress fractures in runners. In: D'Ambrosia R, Drez D, eds. Prevention and treatment of running injuries. Thorofare, NJ: Slack, 1982:21–42.
45. Amendola A, Rorabeck CH, Vellett D, et al. The use of magnetic resonance imaging in exertional compartment syndromes. Am J Sports Med 1990;18:29–34.
46. D'Ambrosia RD. Surgical release for exertional compartments syndrome: Don't be too hasty [Editorial]. Orthopedics 1989;12:1413.
47. Martens MA, Moeyersoons JP. Acute and recurrent effort-related compartment syndrome in sports. Sports Med 1990;9:1:62–68.
48. Rorabeck CH. Diagnosis and management of compartment syndromes. In: Barr JS, ed. Instr Course Lect 1989;38:466–472.
49. Rorabeck CH, Castle GSP, Hardle R, et al. Compartmental pressure measurements: an experimental investigation using the slit catheter. J Trauma 1981;21:446–449.
50. Detmer DE, Sharpe K, Sufit RL, et al. Chronic compartment syndrome: diagnosis, management and outcome. Am J Sports Med 1985;13:3:162–170.
51. Michael RH, Holder LE. The soleus syndrome: a cause of medial tibial stress (shin splints). Am J Sports Med 1985;13:87–94.
52. D'Ambrosia RD, Zelis RJ, Chuinard RG, et al. Interstitial pressure measurements in the anterior and posterior compartments in athletes with shin splints. Am J Sports Med 1977;5:127–131.
53. Garth WP, Miller ST. Evaluation of claw toe deformity, weakness of the foot intrinsics, and posteromedial shin pain. Am J Sports Med 1989;17:821–827.
54. Allenmark C, Renstrom P, Peterson L, et al. Ten-year follow-up of conservatively treated partial ruptures of the achilles tendon. New Orleans: American Orthopedic Society of Sports Medicine, 1990.
55. Leach RE, Hammond G. Anterior tibial compartment syndrome. J Bone Joint Surg 1967;49A:451–462.
56. Grimston SK, Engsberg JR, Kloiber R, Hanley DA. Bone mass, external loads, and stress fracture in female runners. Int J Sports Biomech 1991;7:3:293–302.
57. Giladi M, Milgrom C, Simkin A, et al. Stress fractures and tibial bone width, a risk factor. J Bone Joint Surg 1987;69B:326–329.
58. Scully TJ, Besterman G. Stress fracture, preventable training injury. Milit Med 1982;147:4:285–287.
59. Kibler WB, Goldberg C, Chandler J. Functional biomechanical deficits in running athletes with plantar fascitis. Am J Sports Med 1991;19:1:66–71.
60. Wapner KL, Sharkey PF. The use of night splints for treatment for calcitrant plantar fasciitis. Foot Ankle 1991;12:3:135–137.
61. D'Ambrosia RD. Orthotic devices in running injuries. Clin Sports Med 1985;4:4:611–618.
62. Gross ML, Davlin LB, Evanski PM. Effectiveness of orthotic shoe inserts in the long-distance runner. Am J Sports Med 1991;19:4:409–412.
63. Lutter LD. Hindfoot problems. In: Heckman JD, ed. Instr Course Lect 1993;42:195–200.
64. Baxter DE. Functional nerve disorders in the athlete's foot, ankle and leg. In: Heckman JD, ed. Instr Course Lect 1993;42:185–194.
65. Cavanagh PR. Biomechanics: a bridge builder among the sport sciences. Med Sci Sports Exerc 1990;22:5:546–557.
66. Ross CF, Schuster RO. A preliminary report in predicting injuries in distance runners. Podiatr Sports Med 1983;73:275–277.
67. Kendall FP, McCreary EK. Muscles: testing and function. 3rd ed. Baltimore: Williams & Wilkins, 1983.
68. Gray G, Tiberio D. Crayons and computers [Seminar Course Notes]. University of Nevada at Las Vegas, Nevada, 1990.
69. Root ML, Orien WP, Weed JN. Clinical biomechanics. Vol. 2: normal and abnormal functions of the foot. Los Angeles, CA: Clinical Biomechanics, 1977.
70. Norkin C, LeVange P. Joint structure and function: a comprehensive analysis. Philadelphia: FA Davis, 1983.
71. James SL, Bates BT, Osternig LR. Injuries to runners. Am J Sports Med 1978;6:2:40–50.
72. Clement DB, Taunton JE, Smart GW. Achilles tendinitis and peritendinitis: etiology and treatment. Am J Sports Med 1984;12:179–184.
73. Norfray JF, et al. Early confirmation of stress fractures in joggers. JAMA 1980;243:1647–1649.
74. Collier BD, et al. Scintigraphic diagnosis of stress induced incomplete fractures of the proximal tibia. J Trauma 1984;24:156–160.
75. Rupani MD. Three phases of radionuclide bone imaging in sports medicine. Radiology 1985;156:187–196.
76. Roub LW, Gumerman LW, Hanley EN Jr, et al. Bone stress: a radionuclide prospective. Radiology 1979;132:431–438.
77. Pope TF. Radiologic evaluation of tendon injuries. Clin Sports Med 1992;11:3:579–599.
78. Ferkel RD, Flannigan BD, Elkins BS. Magnetic resonance imaging of the foot and ankle: correlation of normal anatomy with pathologic conditions. Foot Ankle 1991;11:289–305.
79. Schon LC, Baxter DE. Neuropathies of the foot and ankle in athletes. Clin Sports Med 1990;9:489–509.
80. Middleton K. Range of motion and flexibility. In: Andrews JR, Harrelson GL, eds. Physical rehabilitation of the injured athlete. Philadelphia: WB Saunders, 1991:141–162.
81. Malone TR. Muscle injury and rehabilitation. Baltimore: Williams & Wilkins, 1988.
82. Sahrman SA. Diagnosis and treatment of muscle imbalances and associated regional pain syndrome [Seminar Course Notes]. Washington University, St. Louis, MO, 1990.
83. McPoil TG, Brocato RS. The foot and ankle: biomechanical evaluation and treatment. In: Gould JA, Davies GJ, eds. Orthopaedic and sports physical therapy. St. Louis: CV Mosby, 1985:313–341.
84. Knight KL. Cryotherapy, theory, technique, and physiology. Terre Haute, IN: Chattanooga Corp., 1985.
85. Prentice WE. Therapeutic modalities in sports medicine. St. Louis: Times Mirror/Mosby College, 1986.
86. Glick E, Snyder-Machler L. Iontophoresis. In: Snyder-Machler L,

Robinson AJ, eds. Clinical electrophysiology, electrotherapy, and electrophysiologic testing. Baltimore: Williams & Wilkins, 1989:247–260.

87. Taylor DC, Dalton JD, Seaber AV, Garrett WE. Viscoelastic properties of muscle-tendon units: the biomechanical effects of stretching. Am J Sports Med 1990;18:3:300–309.
88. Wallin D, Ekblon B, Grahn R, et al. Improvement of muscular flexibility. Am J Sports Med 1985;13:262–268.
89. Graham VL, Gehlsen GM, Edwards JA. Electromyographic evaluation of closed and open kinetic chain knee rehabilitation exercises. J Athletic Train 1993;28:1:23–30.
90. Robbins SE, Hanna AM. Running related injury prevention through barefoot adaptations. Med Sci Sports Exerc 1987;19:2:148–156.
91. Smith L, Clarke T, Hamill C, et al. The effect of soft and semirigid orthoses upon rearfoot movement in running. Podiatr Sports Med 1986;76:227–233.
92. Bates BT, James SL, Osternig LR. Foot function during the support phase of running. Running 1978;3:24–29.
93. Nichol K, Hennig EM. Measurement of pressure distribution by means of flexible large surface mat. In: Asmussen E, Jorgensen K, eds. Biomechanics VI-A. Baltimore: University Park Press, 1978:374–380.
94. Freeman WH. Peak when it counts: periodization for American track and field. Los Altos, CA: Tafnews Press, 1989.
95. Anderson MA. Postinjury rehabilitation in the runner. Techniques Orthop 1990;5:3:64–75.
96. Grollman L, Irrgang J, Dearwater S, Fu F, Verdile V. Defining adequate medical coverage of marathon races: injury surveillance at the Pittsburgh Marathon (1988–1992). Paper presented at the 40th annual meeting of the American College of Sports Medicine, Seattle, 1993.
97. American College of Sports Medicine. Position statement: prevention of thermal injuries during distance running. Phys Sportsmed 1984;12:43–51.
98. Occupational Safety and Health Administration. Occupational exposure to bloodborne pathogens. (Brochure No. 3127). Washington, DC: OSHA, 1992.
99. Robertson J. Sports medicine manual for long distance running. Indianapolis: The Athletics Congress/USA, 1986.
100. Noble HB, Bachman D. Medical aspects of distance race planning. Phys Sportsmed 1979;7:78–84.

35 / SCUBA DIVING

Kevin O'Toole

Introduction

The sport of scuba (self-contained underwater breathing apparatus) diving has had phenomenal growth over the last 20 years. It has gone from an activity that was limited to a relatively few physically fit individuals to one that has many millions of participants, many of whom are not in peak condition. In the United States, it is estimated that there are 3 million active divers. The incident rate for injuries is surprisingly low at 0.04%, which places it at the same level as bowling. However, the types of injuries that occur in scuba diving can be serious, even fatal. In 1990, there were 95 recreational scuba diving deaths involving U.S. citizens. This number has been as low as 66 (1988) and as high as 147 (1976). The fatality rate for scuba diving has declined form 8.6 per 100,000 in 1976 to 3.7 per 100,000 in 1990 (1). This decline in death rate in the face of a large increase in the number of divers may very well be the result of rigorous standards for training recreational divers. It is a tribute to the training organizations involved that there are few deaths in a sport that can be extremely dangerous to its participants. This chapter is intended to allow the primary care physician to recognize injuries and illnesses unique to scuba diving and to initiate treatment. It also will guide the practitioner as to when to refer the patient for specialty care.

History of Diving

Scuba diving as an entity is a relatively new activity. Diving, however, goes back many centuries. Breath-hold diving is the earliest form of diving known to humankind. It has been shown to have been practiced around 4500 B.C. These divers were diving for food and for treasures (2). In early times, the divers also were used for military purposes, as they are today. Free diving continues to be a popular method of diving today. Examples include pearl divers and recreational snorkeling.

The next innovation in diving was the diving bell. This allowed for a longer time underwater as there was an air supply for the diver. It is recorded that Alexander the Great descended in a diving bell in 330 B.C. to view the recovery of a ship (2). The continued problem with a diving bell is that it limited the mobility of the diver. Until the 17th century, the diving bell was state of the art in diving.

The development of surface-supplied diving apparatus in the 17th and 18th centuries dramatically increased the mobility and capabilities of divers. Now a diver was free to move about and not have to worry about returning to the diving bell for the next breath of air. This allowed the diver to do a significantly greater amount of work. This hard-hat diving is still used today by the military and in the underwater construction fields.

The development of a self-contained breathing apparatus was the next evolutionary step in diving. From the middle 1800s, various individuals attempted to create such a device. It was not until 1943, when Emile Gagnan and Captain Jacques-Yves Cousteau unveiled their "Aqua Lung," that the development of the modern scuba gear occurred (2). It is because of the work of these two individuals that we have the sport of recreational scuba diving. It was no longer necessary to be tethered to a surface-supplied air source while wearing a heavy and cumbersome diving suit. This opened the door to ordinary citizens being able to enjoy the underwater environment. All of today's scuba gear is a refinement on this initial apparatus.

The Underwater Environment

The world of the scuba diver, if looked at objectively, is an extremely hostile one. The surrounding "atmosphere" is one that cannot support a diver's oxygen needs without special equipment. This atmosphere is continually changing its ambient pressure with every change in the diver's depth. It is this change in pressure that leads to many of the medical problems that develop in divers. A diver cannot see well if he or she is not wearing a mask. Even with a mask, objects are distorted by appearing closer and larger than they truly are. The surrounding water tends to drain the heat from a diver and expose him or her to the risks of hypothermia. The diver can visit this world for only a limited time, as the air supply is finite and because of the risks of decompression sickness. As can be seen, there are many factors that work against a diver. They are not, however, insurmountable, as evidenced by the popularity of the sport. It is important for the diver as well as the attending physician, to understand the physics of the underwater environment. A diver learns this while undergoing training. For the physician, to understand the pathophysiology of diving injuries requires a basic understanding of underwater physics. As will be shown, most of the common and serious injuries unique to scuba diving occur because of the effects of pressure on gases in the body.

Definitions

Several terms will need to be defined to understand the gas laws that will be discussed below. *Pressure* is defined as an amount of force acting on a unit area. In diving, pressure is usually expressed as pounds per square inch (psi). Mathematically, it can be expressed as pressure = force/area, or $p = F/A$.

The amount of pressure that is exerted on a body by the earth's atmosphere is defined as 1 atm. When measured at sea level, it is equal to 14.7 psi. At higher elevations, it will be less. Atmospheric pressure acts in all directions at any specific point equally. For this reason, its effects are usually neutralized. In diving, pressures also are expressed in atmospheres. For example, a pressure of 147 psi is 10 atm (10×14.7 psi).

Hydrostatic pressure is the pressure produced by the weight of fluid acting on a body submerged in the fluid. It is equal in all directions at any particular depth. In sea water, for every 1 foot a diver descends, the hydrostatic pressure increases 0.445 psi. This number is 0.432 psi for fresh water. For sea water, the pressure at 33 feet is equivalent to 1 atm. For fresh water, every 34 feet is the same as 1 atm, or 14.7 psi.

The definition of *absolute pressure* is the sum of the atmospheric and hydrostatic pressures exerted on a submerged body. Its units of measure are pounds per square inch absolute (psia) or atmospheres absolute (ata). The term *ambient pressure* is defined as the pressure surrounding a submerged body (atmospheric + hydrostatic) and is usually stated in absolute pressure terms.

Gauge pressure is defined as the difference between the pressure being measured and the atmospheric pressure. Most gauges used in scuba diving are calibrated to read zero at normal atmospheric pressures. Gauge pressure is what is measured on a diver's depth gauge. To convert gauge pressure to absolute pressure, one needs only to add 14.7 psi to the gauge pressure.

The final pressure that needs to be defined is *partial pressure.* In a mixture of gases, the proportion of the total pressure contributed by a single gas in the mixture is called the partial pressure. This partial pressure is directly proportional to the percentage of the total volume of the mixture that the individual gas occupies. The partial pressure of a gas determines how much of the gas will be dissolved in the tissues and blood. The concentration of gases in tissues plays an important role in the development of specific diving illnesses such as nitrogen narcosis and decompression sickness.

Gases Used in Diving

There are a number of important gases that are encountered in recreational scuba diving. Air, in a compressed form, is the mixture of gases that are used in sport diving. It is composed of 78% nitrogen, 21% oxygen, 0.9% argon, 0.03% carbon dioxide, and a mixture of other rare gases (0.003%).

Oxygen, as is well-known, is essential to life. It is the only gas that is used metabolically by the diver. All other gases in air serve only to dilute the oxygen concentration. In high enough concentrations, oxygen is toxic to the pulmonary and central nervous systems (3). Sport diving does not include the use of oxygen-enriched gas mixtures for this reason.

Nitrogen is the most abundant gas in air. It is an inert gas and does not support life. Nitrogen is involved in a number of the illnesses associated with diving. Its anesthetic effects at high partial pressure is the cause of nitrogen narcosis, also known as the rapture of the deep (4). The formation of nitrogen bubbles in tissues and blood is the cause of decompression sickness, or the bends (5–7). Nitrogen does serve a useful purpose for the sport diver, however. It dilutes the oxygen so that the diver is not at risk for oxygen toxicity, which would develop at higher partial pressures of oxygen.

Carbon dioxide is normally found in minute amounts in air. It normally is not of any concern to the diver. However, if the diver would happen to get a tank of air contaminated with carbon dioxide, the results could be disastrous. Carbon dioxide in high concentrations (>10%) is toxic to humans and can lead to seizures and death (2, 3, 8). Having a reputable supplier of compressed air is the principal way to prevent this potential disaster.

Carbon monoxide is produced by the incomplete combustion of hydrocarbons in internal combustion engines. It is an extremely poisonous substance that must be excluded from the diver's air supply at all costs. The most common cause of carbon monoxide contamination of a diver's air supply is the intake of an air compressor being near an exhaust system of an internal combustion engine (2). Again, prevention of this disorder can be accomplished by obtaining compressed air only from reputable dealers.

Gas Laws

To understand fully how changes in pressure can lead to the common ailments that are seen in scuba diving, it is important to understand some common gas laws. The effects of change in pressure on liquids is negligible. For this reason, most of the body, which is made up of liquids, has no direct effects from the pressure. It is the air-filled body cavities—the middle ears, sinuses, lungs, and gastrointestinal tract—that are most affected by pressure changes. To understand what changes occur and why they occur, it is essential to discuss several gas laws. The behavior of all gases can be explained by three factors: the pressure, volume and temperature of that gas. The interrelationships between these factors has been explained by the gas laws. There are four of these laws that are applicable to the diver: Boyle's law; Charles's law; Dalton's law; and Henry's law.

Boyle's law can be stated as follows: At a constant temperature, the volume of a gas varies inversely with absolute pressure, while the density of a gas varies directly with absolute pressure. For any gas at a constant temperature, Boyle's law can be written as follows:

$$pV = K$$

where p = absolute pressure, V = volume, and K = constant. This law is vital to the scuba diver in that it describes what happens to an air-filled cavity in the body if it cannot be equalized with the ambient pressure. An example would be barotrauma to the middle ear caused by eustachian tube dysfunction.

Charles's law is stated as follows: At a constant pressure, the volume of a gas varies directly with absolute temperature. For any gases at a constant volume, the pressure of a gas varies directly with absolute temperature. This law can be expressed mathematically as follows:

$$pV = RT$$

where p = absolute pressure, V = volume, T = absolute temperature, R = universal constant for all gases. This law comes in to play when dealing with the compressed air tanks that divers use as their air supply. If a tank is left in direct sunlight, it can be seen from the formula above that either the pressure or volume must increase. Because the air tank is rigid, making the volume constant, the pressure in the tank will increase. This can lead to an overpressurization of the tank and possible tank or valve rupture.

The definition of Dalton's law is as follows: The total pressure that is exerted by a mixture of gases is equal to the sum of the partial pressures of each of the gases if it alone were present in the same volume. The mathematical formula for this law is written as:

$$p_{total} = pp_1 + pp_2 + pp_n$$

where p_{total} = total pressure of that gas, pp_1 = partial pressure of gas 1, pp_2 = partial pressure of gas 2, pp_n = partial pressure of other gas. Dalton's law is important when one is discussing contaminated air supplies, nitrogen narcosis, and decompression sickness.

Henry's law deals with the solubility of gases in a liquid. It can be stated as follows: The amount of any given gas that will dissolve in a liquid at a given temperature is a function of the partial pressure of the gas that is in contact with the liquid and the solubility coefficient of the gas in the particular liquid. To put it simply, in a diver, the amount of gas that will dissolve in blood and tissues will increase with increasing depth until the point of tissue saturation takes place. The formula is as follows:

$$VG/VL = \propto p_1$$

where VG = volume of gas dissolved at standard temperature and pressure (STP), VL = volume of the liquid, $\propto$ = Bunson solubility coefficient at specified temperature, p_1 = partial pressure in atmosphere of that gas above the liquid. Henry's law is the basis for the development of decompression sickness and will be explained later in this chapter.

Heat and Heat Transfer

No matter where a person is diving, be it in the tropics or the cold waters of the Great Lakes, heat loss from the diver's body occurs. Because the human body requires a relatively narrow temperature range to function normally, this loss of heat energy can have significant effects on diver performance and health. There are several mechanisms by which a diver loses body heat: radiation, convection, evaporation, and conduction.

Radiation heat loss by the diver is not significant compared with conduction and convection. Radiation heat loss from the body is in the form of infrared waves. The head, neck, and hands, if left exposed, are areas of the body where radiation heat loss can occur in cold water.

Conduction is the transfer of heat energy by direct contact. This is the most significant cause of heat loss in divers. Water conducts heat much better than air, and a diver that is unprotected loses a great deal of heat by direct contact with the water. The purpose of a diver's wet suit is to prevent the conductive heat loss.

Convection is the transmission of heat energy by the movement of currents. In a diver, even sitting perfectly still, little currents are formed by the rising of water heated by conduction and its replacement by cooler water. This leads to the loss of heat by convective currents.

Evaporation of water vapor from the lungs is another method of heat loss in a diver. The compressed air in a scuba tank has essentially no water vapor present. Each time a diver takes a breath, this air enters the lungs where large amounts of water vapor and thus heat are transferred to it. This heat is lost with each exhalation.

All of the above mechanisms can, in the appropriate setting, combine to cause hypothermia in a diver, leading to physical problems.

Diving Equipment

To better understand the diver and the sport, it is important to know what kinds of equipment and tools are required. Divers frequently carry 50, 60, or more pounds of equipment with them on each dive. Each piece of equipment has a specific and important function. Some equipment failures can be life-threatening and some knowledge by the physician of their purpose is helpful in caring for the diver. The minimum amount of equipment a sport diver uses includes the following:

1. Open-circuit scuba
2. Buoyancy compensator (BC)
3. Face mask
4. Weight belt and weights
5. Fins
6. Submersible timer and depth gauge
7. Knife
8. Protective clothing

Each of these essential pieces of equipment will be discussed briefly.

Open-Circuit Scuba

Open-circuit scuba is what makes scuba diving possible. It consists of the compressed air tank(s), a demand regulator, and a backpack to hold the tank(s). The air tanks are constructed from steel or aluminum and are filled to a pressure of 2000 to 3000 psi. Tanks require an internal visual inspection yearly and hydrostatic testing every 5 years as mandated by federal law. The average tank holds approximately 70 cubic feet of air. This is enough air to fill the average-size phone booth.

The scuba regulator is the key to scuba diving. It is a two-stage apparatus that allows the diver to breath air at whatever ambient pressure he or she is at. It is a demand valve so that air is released only when the diver takes a breath. This allows for conservation of an already small air supply. Modern-day scuba regulators are dependable if the diver cares for it properly. Rarely is a diving accident caused by a faulty regulator.

The backpack that holds the tank is usually part of the buoyancy compensator. It consists of one or two straps that hold the tank in place.

Buoyancy Compensator

The buoyancy compensator (BC in diver terminology) has two functions. First it allows the diver to adjust his or her buoyancy underwater while changing depth. The second function is to act as a life preserver in the event of an emergency. The BC is a vest-like device with air bladders within it. The diver is able to inflate the BC using either a low pressure inflator connected to the regulator or by an oral inflation valve. The same inflaton valve is used to allow air to escape. By adding or emptying air, the diver is able to make himself or herself neutrally buoyant and, therefore, stay at a particular depth effortlessly. Inability to master the use of the BC is a common problem among new divers and can lead to serious medical problems. If a diver inflates the vest too vigorously and shoots to the surface, the possibility of the diver suffering an arterial gas embolism is quite real. Proper instruction is the key to the correct use of this piece of equipment.

Face Mask

The main purpose of the face mask is to allow the diver to see in the aquatic environment. An air pocket is required to be present between the eye and the water so the eye can focus correctly. This air pocket is provided by the face mask. There are many different styles of masks and one offers no distinct advantage over another. Divers who require corrective lenses can have them inserted directly into the mask glass. Glasses should not be worn under the mask. Contacts have been used successfully but can be washed out of the eye if the diver's mask becomes flooded.

Weight Belt and Weights

Because most divers are positively buoyant (i.e., they float) when fully equipped, they require the use of weights. The weights are worn on a belt around the waist. It has a quick-release clasp that allows for rapid removal of the weights in case an emergency ascent is required. The amount of weight a diver will need is highly individual with more obese individuals requiring more added weight than an individual of similar body weight but who is more fit. The most common mistake divers make with weights is to overweight themselves, thus making their buoyancy control more difficult and increasing the work of diving. Experimenting with different amounts of weight will eventually lead to the optimum amount for each particular diver.

Swim Fins

The use of fins allows divers to propel themselves with much less effort than if they were swimming barefoot. They allow divers to swim faster and farther with less effort. There are many different styles and sizes on the market. Larger fins will sometimes cause cramping and exhaustion in divers that do not have strong enough legs to use them. As with the amount of weight a diver should use, the selection of a style and size of fin is best done after trying several different ones.

Submersible Timer and Depth Gauge

These are two very important instruments. They are necessary to keep tract of both the length of time the diver has been submerged and to document the deepest depth of the dive. The timer can be a simple water-resistant watch or a timer that automatically turns itself on when the diver enters the water. The depth gauge is usually part of a console that contains a compass and a pressure gauge that keeps tract of the remaining air supply. The information obtained from these instruments are used to calculate when a dive may require decompression stops as well as for future dive planning. As will be shown in later, the length and depth of a dive are important in the development of decompression sickness.

A relatively new piece of equipment that sport divers are using more is the diving computer. This instrument continually monitors the diver's depth and calculates how much longer the diver can stay at that depth. It has become a popular piece of equipment, because it allows divers to stay under longer compared with the standard decompression tables. It remains to be seen if these dive computers are leading to more cases of decompression sickness. One interesting feature of most of these computers is that they keep in their memory a record of the diver's dives. This becomes important if a diver is believed to have decompression sickness. It is then relatively easy to obtain the pertinent information about the depth and duration of the dives that may have led to the problem.

Knife

Most divers will carry one of several styles of knife with them while diving. Contrary to popular belief, the knife is not for defense against marine life. Its main role is to free a diver that has become entangled in fishing line, kelp, and the like. The knife is usually worn in a sheath attached to the leg for easy access.

Protective Clothing

The type of protective clothing worn by the diver is determined by the diving conditions. A dive in the tropics may require nothing more than a bathing suit. In contrast, an ice diving trip will require at the minimum a 0.25-inch neoprene wet suit. Many divers use a dry suit in these conditions. This is an outfit that keeps the diver's body dry by having waterproof zippers and connections at the neck, wrists and ankles. The diver's environment will dictate to him or her what type of protective clothing will be needed for the dive. It is when the protection is inadequate that the potential for hypothermia is present.

Diving-Related Injury Statistics

As stated earlier, diving has a relatively low injury rate compared with other sports. Diving is, however, a potentially dangerous and deadly sport in which participation must not be taken lightly. The Divers Alert Network (DAN) keeps yearly statistics on diving deaths as well as the most serious diving injuries. The organization's hard work and dedication to diving medicine has led to a better understanding of what leads to deaths in scuba diving. DAN has reported that scuba deaths are the result of multiple factors, leading to a final event that is usually drowning. A look at the 1990 data on contributing factors for drowning deaths shows multiple factors (1). Insufficient air, entrapment, cardiovascular medical problems, and alcohol/drugs lead the list. Remaining factors include air embolism, nitrogen narcosis, boat accident, diabetes mellitus, panic state, head injury, carbon monoxide, and seizure disorder. A review of the list shows that a number of these contributing factors are completely preventable. Running out of air should never occur to a properly trained and motivated diver. Alcohol and drugs are under the control of the diver, who has been made known by his or her instructor that diving and drugs do not mix. Careful and conservative divers should be able to lower their risk of death while diving just by following their training procedures.

In addition to tracking diving deaths, DAN also keeps records on serious diving injuries such as arterial gas embolism and decompression sickness. In 1990, DAN received reports of 589 cases of decompression sickness and 118 cases of arterial gas embolism (AGE) (1). Since 1986, the number of cases have increased each year except for 1988. A full report of each year's statistics can be obtained from the DAN organization.

Medical Problems

The type of medical problems that the scuba diver may encounter are quite varied. Any medical problem that affects the general population can affect a diver. There are, however, a number of unique medical conditions that affect divers. Each will be described and the appropriate immediate treatment as well as definitive treatment will be discussed. Also, recommendations on when to obtain specialty consultation will be made.

Nitrogen Narcosis

Nitrogen narcosis may be better known as the rapture of the deep. As the partial pressure of nitrogen increases with increasing depth, the nitrogen begins to have an anesthetic effect (9). Symptoms usually are not observed until a diver exceeds 100 feet, but there is a wide variation among different divers and even among a single person on different dives. Signs and symptoms are similar to those of ethanol intoxication (10, 11). Initial symptoms may include a feeling of excitement and exhilaration. The diver may notice tingling or numbness in the lips and extremities. He or she may become overconfident at this point. Mental activity becomes increasingly slowed as depth increases. The ability to make rapid and potentially life-saving decisions is impaired. In new divers, there may not be euphoria but more of a feeling of terror. This intoxication leaves the diver more susceptible to having an accident while at the same time less capable of responding appropriately. The only treatment for this disorder is to ascend to a shallower depth. Once this is done the effects dissipate rapidly. The diver should not attempt to return to the deeper depth on the same dive that he or she developed nitrogen narcosis. Factors that can contribute to the development of nitrogen narcosis include fatigue, drug and alcohol use, anxiety, cold, and the use of concurrent sedating medications such as antihistamines and sedatives. By eliminating as many of these factors as possible, a diver will decrease the risk of nitrogen narcosis on future dives.

Barotrauma

Barotrauma is a general term used to describe any injury that has been caused by pressure, specifically pressure changes. Any of the air-filled body cavities are susceptible to barotrauma. The trauma occurs when the pressure is unable to be equalized because of air trapping. This is quite common in the middle ear and can be quite deadly in the lungs. Each specific area will be addressed with emphasis placed on prevention of the barotrauma.

Pulmonary Overinflation Syndrome

Pulmonary overinflation syndrome includes several different possible injuries. The one common underlying mechanism of injury is air trapping within the lung. There are two main reasons that this occurs. The first is that the diver holds his or her breath while ascending. The most common reason for this is that the diver has an underwater emergency and must make an emergency ascent. Divers are taught during their training to exhale continually during ascent. Unfortunately, during an emergency, many divers, especially inexperienced ones, will panic and forget to do this extremely important step. During the ascent with a closed glottis, the air within the lungs continues to expand. If the glottis remains closed, the alveoli will rupture, with air entering the pleural space, subcutaneous tissues, or into the pulmonary veins. Depending on where the air goes, the development of the various components of pulmonary overpressurization will occur.

The second cause of air trapping is the result of underlying lung disease. Individuals with asthma, emphysema, or chronic bronchitis can have areas of the lung that are susceptible to air trapping. Also individuals who have had thoracic surgery or spontaneous pneumothorax can have areas of lung that are abnormal and more prone to air trapping. It is for this reason that individuals with the above illnesses are advised not to scuba dive. No matter what the cause of air trapping, any of the individual illnesses of pulmonary overpressurization can occur. Each of these diseases will be discussed in detail.

Arterial gas embolism (AGE) is perhaps the most feared complication of scuba diving, and with good reason. Many diving experts believe that it is the leading cause of scuba diving fatalities. Many of the diving fatalities that are reported as drowning are more than likely deaths due to AGE. Because the diagnosis of AGE requires a very specific autopsy, many of these deaths go undetected and are simply listed as drowning.

The cause of AGE is the entry of air into the arterial system, which then embolizes to the various organs of the body. With alveolar rupture, air enters the pulmonary veins. It is then carried back to the left side of the heart where it then travels to the brain, heart, and other organs. The air bubbles then occlude the vascular supply to these vital organs, leading to organ dysfunction (10). As the ambient pressure decreases further as the diver ascends, the air bubbles will increase in size, further obstructing blood flow.

The onset of symptoms in AGE are usually immediate and occur not more than 10 min from surfacing (1, 10–15). The diver may surface unconscious or in full cardiac arrest. Those that surface in arrest usually cannot be resuscitated, unless they are immediately placed in a recompression chamber. The signs and symptoms of AGE can include any of the following: headache, shock, unconsciousness, weakness, parathesias, ataxia, visual disturbances, nausea and vomiting, chest pain, shortness of breath, bloody sputum, and confusion. Almost any neurologic symptom or sign can occur with AGE, depending on where the air emboli is lodged. Any diver who within 10 min of surfacing develops any of the above should be considered to have an AGE until proven otherwise.

The appropriate treatment for AGE is recompression therapy at the earliest possible time. Initially, the airway must be secured and adequate oxygenation maintained. The patient should be placed on 100% oxygen as soon as possible. The use of a simple face mask is not adequate as 100% oxygen is not obtainable. One needs to use a nonrebreather mask or endotracheal intubation to obtain as close to 100% as possible. An intravenous line should be started and cardiac monitoring initiated. In the past, much was made of placing the patient in the Trendelenburg position with the left side down. The thinking was that this would trap remaining air bubbles in the apex of the heart and thus prevent further embolization. Recent work in dogs has shown this not to be true. There is no trapping of air at the apex of the heart, because the blood flow through the heart is a strong force and will move any air in the heart out into the systemic circulation. Also, the Trendelenburg position can worsen cerebral edema that can develop with central nervous system (CNS) insults from AGE. Another reason not to place the patient in Trendelenburg position is that this can compromise the patient's pulmonary function as a result of the abdominal organs pushing on the diaphragm, thereby decreasing total lung volume. For these reasons, it is advised to lie the patient flat on his or her back (or side, if vomiting and aspiration are a concern).

As stated earlier, recompression is the only definitive treatment for AGE. Arrangements should be made early for recompression therapy. Tests such as computed tomography (CT) and magnetic resonance imaging (MRI) have no place in the acute management of AGE. The diagnosis is clinically made and any delay to recompression therapy to obtain these tests is unwarranted. The success of recompression is directly related to how soon the patient receives the treatment. If there is no hyperbaric chamber at your facility, make arrangements early for transfer to a hospital with a hyperbaric chamber. These arrangements can be facilitated by contacting DAN at Duke University. This organization can help with patient management as well as helping to arrange transfer of the patient to the nearest appropriate hyperbaric chamber. It must be remembered that the earlier the patient receives recompression therapy, the greater the chance that he or she can make a complete recovery.

Prevention of this disease is the best form of therapy. Vigorous training of individuals learning to dive is and should continue to be the mainstay of prevention. Making potential divers aware of this deadly risk and how to avoid it is the key to lowering the numbers of AGE. Also, until it can be proven otherwise, individuals with asthma, emphysema, and chronic bronchitis should be told that their participation in scuba diving is ill-advised and can be life-threatening.

The second type of pulmonary overpressurization accident is that of pneumothorax. The mechanism is the same as in AGE, i.e., rupture of alveoli secondary to air trapping; however, instead of air entering into the pulmonary circulation, it enters into the pleural space. It should be remembered that pneumothorax also may be present in patients with AGE. A diver is not limited to just one of the overpressurization accidents at a time. As the diver ascends farther, the air in the pleural cavity expands. This can lead to collapse of the involved lung and even the development of a tension pneumothorax. This can lead to cardiovascular collapse and death if not treated appropriately.

The signs and symptoms of pneumothorax include shortness of breath which began acutely, dyspnea, pleuritic chest pain, sudden onset of cough, tachycardia, cyanosis, shock, distended neck veins, and decreased breath sounds on the involved side along with increased tympany on the involved side. If the tension pneumothorax is severe, one may notice a shifted trachea away from the involved side. One may notice the patient bending the chest toward the involved side (12, 14–16).

Treatment of pneumothorax begins with the recognition of the problem. A scuba diver who develops shortness of breath or pleuritic chest pain immediately after a dive should have the diagnosis of pneumothorax entertained. The patient should be put on 100% oxygen and an intravenous (i.v.) line placed. If the patient is stable, a chest x-ray should be obtained. If, however, the patient is in extremis, treatment should proceed before an x-ray. Based on the physical exam, a 12-gauge i.v. catheter should be inserted into the involved hemithorax. The location of the catheter should be the second intercostal space in the midclavicular line. If the patient does have a tension pneumothorax, a rush of air should be heard when the catheter is inserted. Leave the catheter in place so that air does not reaccumulate before the insertion of the chest tube. After the chest x-ray in the stable patient and after the catheter decompression in the unstable patient, a chest tube should be inserted into the involved side. This should be connected to an underwater seal and a post–chest tube x-ray obtained to confirm lung reinflation and proper tube placement. Most of these patients will have an uncomplicated course and will require no further treatment other than the chest tube.

A third component of overpressurization accidents is mediastinal emphysema. The cause is the same as the previous two injuries and develops when air enters the mediastinum after tracking along the larger airways. Signs and symptoms include retrosternal chest pain that may be described as pressure or a dull ache. This pain is made worse with deep breathes or coughing. Swallowing also can make the pain worse. Radiation of the pain occurs to the shoulders, back, and neck. There also may be dyspnea, cyanosis, cough, and in severe cases shock (8, 13–15).

This disease by itself is usually not life-threatening. What it does signify is that an overpressurization accident of the lung has occurred and that the possibility of an AGE or pneumothorax exists. Unless AGE is present, the patient does not need hyperbaric treatment. Placing the patient on 100% oxygen may hasten the resolution of the mediastinal emphysema and improve the patient's symptoms.

The last component of overpressurization accidents is subcutaneous emphysema. This results from the movement of air out of the mediastinum to the subcutaneous tissues of the chest and neck. Although patients with this disease may look terrible, this is usually not a serious illness. The patient may notice a fullness in the neck and crepitence with palpation. Because of involvement of the vocal cords, a change in voice may be noted. Some patients also will develop a cough, but shortness of breath is not a component of subcutaneous emphysema alone (8, 13–15).

Again, unless AGE is present as well, recompression therapy is not needed. Placing the patient on 100% oxygen may be helpful. Reassurance of the patient that he or she is not seriously ill is probably the most important intervention the physician can make.

Ear Barotrauma

There is probably not an active scuba diver alive who has not experienced at least once a middle-ear barotrauma, or squeeze. This is the most common barotrauma experienced by divers (11, 17, 18). This disorder is the result of the inability to equalize the pressure between the middle ear and the environment. It is during the first 10 to 15 feet of a dive that the greatest pressure changes occur. It is in this depth range that the problem of middle-ear squeeze is common. The most common cause of this inability to equalize is eustachian tube dysfunction (10), which can be the result of upper respiratory infections, allergic rhinitis, or smoking. Any process that causes edema and mucous production in the eustachian tube will make the individual more susceptible to middle-ear squeeze.

Most middle-ear squeeze will occur on descent, but a minority of cases can occur on ascent (9, 10). The initial symptom will be a sense of fullness in the ear. If the diver continues to descend without equalizing the pressure, pain will develop. The diver will notice a decrease in hearing in the involved ear. This is secondary to the hemorrhage that has occured within and behind the tympanic membrane. Tinnitus and vertigo can also develop with middle-ear squeeze. If the diver continues to descend despite these symptoms, tympanic membrane rupture can occur. This may lead to severe vertigo and vomiting secondary to the caloric stimulation that will occur with the enterance of water into the middle ear (9–11, 17, 18). This can be life-threatening if the diver vomits into the regulator. Another complication of continued descent is that of round or oval window rupture (9–11). If this occurs, either by the squeeze itself or forceful attempts at clearing the ears, severe long-lasting complications may develop, including hearing loss, tinnitus, and vertigo.

Treatment of middle-ear squeeze begins with prevention. Any diver with upper respiratory infections or active seasonal allergies should delay diving until illness has passed. Many divers will refuse this option and request an alternative. Nasal decongestant sprays and oral decongestants have been recommended and may be useful in some divers. Frequent equalization of the ears during descent, e.g., every foot with the modified Valsalva or the Frenzel maneuver, frequently will prevent middle-ear squeeze. Descending in the head-up position also makes equalizing easier and the descent more controlled. Advise the patient that if he or she encounters difficulty clearing, ascend a few feet and try again. If the diver is still unsuccessful, the dive should be aborted and the diver should go to the surface. Yawning or swallowing has also proven useful for some divers in clearing their ears.

If a diver develops an ear squeeze, further diving should be avoided and the ear should be checked by a physician. Otoscopic examination of the ear may reveal an injected tympanic membrane, hemorrhage within or behind the ear drum, or a rupture of the tympanic membrane. If the drum is not ruptured, decongestants, both spray and oral, along with appropriate pain medication should be given. If the ear drum is ruptured, oral antibiotics can be started. Avoid any medications being placed directly into the ear canal. The rupture will usually heal on its own. Have the patient return in several weeks for a recheck of the ear drum rupture. There should be no further diving until the rupture has healed completely. Ear, nose, and throat (ENT) referral should be made if there is a persistent rupture and the patient wishes to dive again.

Any diver who surfaces with significant acute hearing loss, vertigo, tinnitus, or gait disturbance may have suffered a round or oval window rupture (9–11). These patients should be referred immediately to an ENT specialist as this is considered a serious and emergent condition. These patients may require immediate surgery to prevent permanent damage to the inner ear. Absolutely no further diving should be attempted until cleared by the ENT surgeon.

Sinus Barotrauma

Sinus squeeze occurs when the ostia to the sinuses become obstructed and, therefore, do not allow equalization of pressure while descending (9, 11, 13, 18). Causes of the ostia obstruction are the same as in ear squeeze, namely upper respiratory infections and allergies. Individuals with chronic sinus problems are particularly susceptible to this disorder. One also can develop sinus squeeze on ascent. This tends to happen when a sinus polyp acts as a one-way valve and obstructs the ostia. The unequal pressures in the sinuses lead to exudate and hemorrhage within the sinuses. The diver will first notice a full feeling in the forehead, between the eyes or in the upper teeth. The location depends on which sinuses are involved. This fullness can progress into severe pain and actual numbness. With hemorrhage into the sinus, the diver may develop epistaxis as some blood escapes from the sinus.

Treatment of sinus squeeze again begins with prevention. Diving should not be attempted if one has cold or allergy symptoms. If during descent, the fullness or pain develops, the dive should be aborted and the diver should return to the surface. Treatment with nasal decongestant drops and oral decongestants is usually all that is needed. If the diver develops worsening pain or a purulent nasal discharge, secondary sinus infection should be suspected and appropriate antibiotics started. All diving should be avoided until the symptoms have cleared. Referral to an ENT specialist is advisable if the symptoms become prolonged (longer than 2 weeks) or worsen. Most patients will have an uncomplicated course and should be able to return to diving without any long-term sequelae.

Face Mask Squeeze

An interesting but usually benign condition called face mask squeeze develops when the diver fails to equalize the pressure in the mask (14, 16, 18). The diver is able to do this simply by exhaling occasionally into the mask. The soft tissues of the face, especially the eye and surrounding tissues, can be injured. The diver may notice a suction sensation on the face that can then become pain as the pressure difference increases. When the diver surfaces, the face is noted to be edematous within the region covered by the mask. There may be petechiae and subconjunctival hemorrhage as well (14, 16, 18). There have been reports of optic nerve damage and blindness in severe cases, but this is usually a self-limiting disorder. Prevention by occasionally exhaling into the mask is the best course of action. Ice and analgesia can be prescribed for symptomatic relief.

Ear Canal Squeeze

Ear canal squeeze occurs in divers who wear tight-fitting hoods while diving (9, 13, 14, 16). If the hood is tight enough to prevent water from entering the external ear canal, an air cavity develops that cannot equalize pressure. Symptoms include fullness and/or pain over the external ear region, blood or fluid drainage after surfacing, or a ruptured ear drum. The disorder can be prevented by allowing water to enter the ear canal by holding the hood away from the head while underwater. Once water has entered the canal, the hood can remain tight without causing a squeeze. Treatment includes pain medications and, if the ear drum is ruptured, the same treatment as with middle-ear squeeze and rupture of the ear drum.

Dental Barotrauma

Although relatively rare, dental barotrauma, or aerodontalgia, can be quite painful. It develops in teeth that have gas spaces from either carious teeth or improperly filled teeth (14, 16). During descent, these air spaces become filled with blood or surrounding soft tissue, leading to pain. The pain may become so severe that further descent is impossible. Treatment consists of analgesia acutely with dental repair of the involved teeth. Further diving should not be attempted until the patient has been evaluated and treated by a dentist.

Decompression Sickness

Decompression sickness (DCS), also known as the bends or caisson disease, is a disorder that occurs after inadequate decompression after being exposed to increased pressures. It consists of a constellation of signs and symptoms that can occur after a reduction in barometric pressure leads to the formation of bubbles within the tissues and bloodstream of the body (9, 11, 13, 14, 16, 19–21).

During the time a diver is underwater, there is a continual loading of nitrogen gas into the blood and tissues of the body. The amount of nitrogen dissolved depends on a number of factors but the two most important are depth (pressure) and time. The longer and deeper a dive, the more nitrogen that is forced into solution within the body. There are numerous dive tables that have been devised that take this into account and list safe limits. However, these limits are not absolute and numerous instances of decompression sickness have occurred well within these tables. If a diver returns to the surface too quickly or without making the necessary stops, the blood and tissues become supersaturated from the reduction in ambient pressure, and nitrogen comes out of solution in the form of bubbles. It is the nitrogen bubbles that lead to the disorder known as decompression sickness.

Nitrogen bubbles can cause problems by several different mechanisms (9, 11, 13, 19). Intracellular bubbles can physically disrupt cells. Intravascular bubbles lead to obstruction of vessels, which causes tissue ischemia. Extravascular bubbles can cause extrinsic compression and stretching of nerves and blood vessels. Finally, the bubble-blood interface activates the early phases of blood coagulation and causes the release of vasoactive substances.

There are a number of predisposing factors that can lead to the development of decompression sickness (9, 13, 14, 20, 22):

1. *Pushing the dive tables.* This means going out to the extreme limits on the published diving tables. Most of these tables are based on work done by the U.S. Navy. These limits were calculated using fit, young navy divers. The vast majority of recreational scuba divers would not fit into this category of fitness. So a diver, e.g., who stays 60 min at 60 feet is theoretically within the limits of the table but is placing himself or herself at risk for decompression sickness.
2. *Missed decompression stops.* All the major diving training organizations recommend a stop at between 10 and 20 feet for several minutes at the end of a dive. This is believed to give the body time to rid itself of some of the nitrogen load. Many divers do not follow this advise and may be making themselves more susceptible to developing the bends.
3. *Fatigue.* Divers who are not well-rested are more likely to get "bent."
4. *Vigorous physical activity.* Activity both during and immediately after the dive has been shown to be a risk factor.
5. *Hypothermia.* A cold diver is at greater risk for DCS.
6. *Alcohol use before a dive.* Not only is it unwise to drink because of the effects on cognitive functions but it also appears to make the bends more likely.
7. *Obesity.* Adipose tissue has a great affinity for nitrogen.
8. *Age.* All other factors being the same, the older the individual, the more likely he or she is to develop decompression sickness.
9. *Poor physical condition.* Those who are out of shape are more at risk.
10. *Dehydration.* Increasing the blood viscosity by dehydration further complicates DCS.
11. *Tissues with previous injury.* Any area of the body that may have an underlying injury for which the blood supply is decreased is at increased risk for DCS.
12. Flying too soon after diving. It is advisable to wait at least 24 hr after multiple days of diving. The further decrease in barometric pressure on the aircraft may be just enough to cause bubble formation.
13. *Patent foramen ovale.* Recent studies have shown that a large percentage of patients who have had documented DCS also have a probe patent foramen ovale. It is postulated that bubbles that would normally be safely filtered out by the lungs are crossing through the foramen ovale and manifesting as DCS. This may occur during certain maneuvers such as a Valsalva. Further study will be needed before any recommendations can be firmly made regarding diving and a patent foramen ovale (23, 24).

If decompression sickness is being considered as a diagnosis, asking the patient some specific questions about his or her dives can be helpful. The following questions can be useful in helping to determine if decompression sickness is likely to have occurred.

1. Was the diver using compressed air or another gas mixture?
2. Any preceding alcohol or drug use? Evidence for dehydration?
3. Was there an airplane flight less than 24 hr after the last dive?
4. How many dives were done on this dive trip?
5. How many dives were done a day on average?
6. How deep were the dives and how long did they last (bottom time)?
7. Were deep dives done first or last? Doing deep dives later increases the nitrogen loading.
8. Were there any missed safety stops?
9. How soon after the last dive did the symptoms start?

The answers to these questions will allow the diving medicine specialist to determine the patient's risk of having decompression sickness. Ask to see the diver's log book to help you obtain the above information.

Clinically, decompression sickness is arbitrarily divided into type 1 and type 2. These divisions are helpful in determining the severity and treatment of the DCS, but there is overlap. A certain number of the less severe DCS 1 cases will eventually be determined to be DCS 2. It is important to realize this, because the treatment and outcome can be quite different for DCS 2.

Type 1 DCS is also known as pain only DCS (9, 11, 13, 14, 16, 19–21). This group includes musculoskeletal symptoms and symptoms involving the skin or lymphatics. The symptoms usually begin within several hours of the dive, with the vast majority occurring before 24 hr. There are cases, however, that have begun several days after the last dive. Symptoms within this class include musculoskeletal pain, itching, skin marbling, and lymphatic involvement.

The mildest cases of DCS I are those that involve the skin. Rashes and itching are quite common after diving and are usually transient, requiring no specific therapy. Marbling or mottling of the skin is a form of DCS and may require recompression therapy.

Lymphatic involvement of DCS is unusual and manifests as a painless swelling. This is felt to be caused by obstruction of lymphatic flow by the bubbles. There may be pain in the involved lymph nodes in addition to the edema. Recompression therapy alleviates the pain, but the edema may remain for some time after treatment.

In addition to the above symptoms, excessive fatigue and anorexia are included in DCS 1. A diver may have a general feeling of "something isn't right." There may be no specific complaints that the diver has other than fatigue out of proportion to the amount of physical activity performed. A trial of treatment as outlined below for DCS 1 may be warranted in these particular patients.

The most common symptom of DCS 1 is pain, usually localized to a joint. The joints of the arms are affected more than those of the legs. The onset is gradual and early in the course may be missed or ignored by the diver. The pain is described as dull and throbbing deep in the joint and surrounding tissues. The pain may or may not be increased by movement of the affected joint. The pain may be severe enough that the patient may be unable to use the limb. Rest does not relieve the pain. Physical exam of the involved area is usually unremarkable. There is no edema or discoloration. The area is not tender to palpation. By definition, the neurologic exam of the affected extremity will be normal. If there are any neurologic findings, the diagnosis of type 2 DCS must be made. There are no laboratory tests or radiographic procedures that are helpful in making the diagnosis of DCS 1. The diagnosis is made by history and physical exam and a high index of suspicion.

The treatment of DCS 1 should begin with the application of 100% oxygen. This may be all that is needed to resolve the symptoms. Even if symptoms resolve, the patient should be observed for several hours as recurrences can happen after initial resolution. Look for progression to the more serious type 2 DCS. If there is any doubt as to the severity of the DCS, the patient should undergo recompression therapy. Contact DAN for consultation with a diving medicine specialist. This physician will be of assistance in arranging transportation to an appropriate hyperbaric facility.

Type 2 DCS, also known as neurologic bends, is the more severe form of decompression sickness. This class of DCS includes any cases involving the following: respiratory symptoms, shock, or CNS or peripheral nervous system involvement (9, 11, 13, 14, 16, 19–21).

The signs of symptoms of DCS 2 can be quite varied and multiple in nature. The spinal cord is the most commonly involved organ in recreational scuba divers. Signs and symptoms often do not follow typical nerve distributions and may vary and shift early in the course of the disease. Spinal cord DCS may present with paralysis, sensory loss, paresis, loss of sphincter control, and a girdle-like distribution of pain in the trunk.

Cerebral DCS can have any of the following: headache, visual disturbances, dizziness, tunnel vision, confusion, disorientation, concentration difficulties, psychotic features, and loss of consciousness. DCS involving the labyrinthine apparatus presents with nausea, vomiting, vertigo, and nystagmus. It is also called the "staggers."

Pulmonary DCS is relatively rare, occurring in about 2% of DCS cases. It can be deadly if not recognized and treated appropriately. Symptoms include substernal chest pain worsening with inspiration, coughing, and severe shortness of breath.

In all the various cases of DCS 2, symptoms usually begin within several hours of the dive. They can begin several days out, but this is not common. Treatment before arriving at the hospital should involve the application of 100% oxygen as soon as possible. This may reduce or even relieve the symptoms. Because dehydration plays a factor in the development of DCS, rehydration either orally or intravenously can commence in the prehospital setting. Overhydration should be avoided so as not to further complicate the cerebral and/or spinal cord edema that can develop with DCS. Rapid transport to the hospital should be carried out so that early recompression therapy can begin.

In the hospital, arrangements should be made for the rapid recompression of the patient, as this is the only definitive treatment for DCS 2. If there is not a hyperbaric chamber available at your hospital, make arrangements to transfer the patient with the help of DAN. The rationale for the use of hyperbaric oxygen in the treatment of DCS is as follows:

1. It decreases the volume and thus the diameter of the gas bubbles. This will allow the bubble to pass more distally and, it is hoped, allow the return of blood flow to ischemic tissues.
2. It improves the diffusion gradient of the nitrogen out of the bubble, thus causing the rapid absorption of the bubble.
3. It improves oxygen delivery to ischemic tissues by increasing the amount of oxygen dissolved in the blood to superphysiologic levels.

While waiting for the patient to undergo recompression therapy there are several other interventions that can be done. Hydration should be continued with isotonic solutions to maintain a urine output of 1 to 2 cm^3/kg/hr. For any neurologic involvement, steroids have classically been given. They have never been shown to improve outcome in DCS but are still widely used. If it is decided to use them, hydrocortisone, 1 g, or Decadron, 10 to 20 mg, can be given intravenously. Aspirin, 500 to 1000 mg, should be given by mouth for its antiplatelet activity. Lidocaine may be useful for any cardiac arrhythmias, and it has been shown experimentally to improve neurologic outcome. However, its routine use for this purpose cannot be advised until further studies are done.

Remember, there are no diagnostic laboratory or radiographic procedures for DCS. Delaying recompression therapy to obtain a CT or MRI is unjustified. Patients have the best chance for complete recovery when they undergo early recompression therapy. Even a patient several days out from the start of symptoms should be given the benefit of a trial of recompression therapy.

Table 35.1.
Absolute and Relative Contraindications to Recreational Scuba Diving

Pulmonary
- Absolute: asthma, emphysema, chronic bronchitis, pulmonary blebs, history of spontaneous pneumothorax, lung tumors
- Relative: active pulmonary infections, thoracic surgery, traumatic pneumothorax

ENT
- Absolute: perforation of tympanic membrane, middle-ear surgery, vestibular lesions, inability to clear ears, Ménière's disease, chronic otitis, mastoiditis
- Relative: active upper respiratory infection, acute otitis media, otitis externa, sinusitis, allergic rhinitis, nasal or sinus polyps

Cardiovascular
- Absolute: angina, myocardial infarction, Wolff-Parkinson-White, various cardiac arrhythmias, atrial septal defect, ventricular septal defect, coarctation of the aorta, prosthetic heart valves, pacemakers, history of Adams-Stoke attacks

Gastrointestinal
- Absolute: active peptic ulcer disease, Crohn's disease, ulcerative colitis, hepatitis
- Relative: uncorrected inguinal, abdominal wall hernias

Genitourinary
- Absolute: pregnancy

Hematologic
- Absolute: sickle-cell disease

Endocrine
- Absolute: insulin-dependent diabetes mellitus, most patients taking oral hypoglycemic agents
- Relative: diet-controlled diabetes mellitus

Musculoskeletal
- Absolute: muscular dystrophy, active osteonecrotic lesions
- Relative: healing fractures, any preexisting painful disorder

Psychiatric
- Absolute: psychosis, current drug use, alcoholism, claustrophobia, suicidal ideation
- Relative: depression, anxiety states

Neurological
- Absolute: seizure disorders, unexplained syncope, brain tumor, cerebrovascular accident, transient ischemic attack, arteriovenous malformations, intracranial aneurysms
- Relative: migraine headache

The advantages of the treatment far outweigh the possible complications of the therapy. There have been many reports of patients getting excellent results up to a week out from the start of their DCS.

Prevention of Injuries

Scuba diving is an exiting and popular sport. Many millions in the United States alone are enjoying this sport. However, it is a sport that requires a certain level of physical conditioning and health to remain safe. There are numerous situations in the underwater environment in which good physical conditioning will be the difference between a tragedy and a good outcome. Although being an excellent swimmer is not a prerequisite for diving, being in good physical condition without major medical conditions is necessary for safe diving. Table 35.1 shows the medical conditions that are contraindicated for diving. Many of these conditions are placed in the table for theoretical reasons and have not been well-studied. They appear in the table because they could lead to the death or severe disability of the diver. Some would argue that the decision to dive should be left to the individuals themselves. Others would argue that the individual is placing others at risk as well if he or she should become ill. This includes the dive partners and anyone else with the diver. For many of these illnesses, there is no black or white answer. Each decision about diving must be made individually. Referral to a diving medicine specialist can be helpful in instances for which there is some question about contraindication to diving. DAN maintains a list of physicians throughout the country who have this particular expertise. Table 35.1 shows the absolute and relative contraindications to recreational scuba diving, divided by organ system (16, 25–30).

REFERENCES

1. Divers Alert Network. Report on 1990 diving accidents. Durham, NC: Duke University Medical Center, 1992.
2. NOAA. DIving manual. Washington, DC: U.S. Department of Commerce, 1991.
3. Thom SR, Clark, JM. The toxicity of oxygen, carbon monoxide and carbon dioxide. In: Bove AA, Davis JC, eds. Diving medicine. Philadelphia: WB Saunders, 1990:82–94.
4. Bennett PB. Inert gas narcosis and HPNS. In: Bove AA, Davis JC, eds. Diving medicine. Philadelphia: WB Saunders, 1990:69–81.
5. Kindwell EP. A short history of diving and diving medicine. In: Bove AA, Davis JC, eds. Diving medicine. Philadelphia: WB Saunders, 1990:1–8.
6. Sanford JP. Medical aspects of recreational skin diving. Ann Rev Med 1974;25:401–410.
7. Betts J. Sports medicine (2). Common medical problems in sub-aqua sport. Practioner 1981;225(1358):1169–1174.
8. U.S. Navy. Diving manual. Vol. 1. Air. 2nd rev. Washington, DC: Department of the Navy, 1988.
9. Arthur DC, Margulies RA. A short course in diving medicine. Ann Emerg Med. 1987;16:689–701.
10. Kizer KW. Diving medicine. Emerg Med Clin North Am 1984;2(3):513–530.
11. Melamed Y, Shupak A, Bitterman H. Medical problems associated with underwater diving. N Engl J Med 1992:326(1):3–35.
12. Strauss RH. Diving medicine. Am Rev Respir Dis 1979;119(6):1001–1023.

13. Neuman TS. Diving medicine. Clin Sports Med 1987;6(3):647–661.
14. Dickey LS. Diving injuries. J Emerg Med 1984;1(3):249–262.
15. Bradley ME. Pulmonary barotrauma. In: Bove AA, Davis JC, eds. Diving medicine. Philadelphia: WB Saunders, 1990:188–191.
16. Edmonds C, Lowry C, Pennefather J. Diving and subaquatic medicine. 3rd ed. Oxford, UK: Butterworth-Heinemann, 1992.
17. Replogle WH, Sanders SD, Keeton JE, Phillips DM. Scuba diving injuries. Am Fam Phys 1988;37(6):135–142.
18. Juss JH. Medical aspects of skin and scuba diving. J School Health 1972;42(4):238–242.
19. Francis TJR, Dutka AJ, Hollenbeck JM. Pathophysiology of decompression sickness. In: Bove AA, Davis JC, eds. Diving medicine. Philadelphia: WB Saunders, 1990:170–187.
20. Strauss RH. Medical concerns in underwater sports. Pediatr Clin North Am 1982;29(6):1431–1440.
21. Good RF. Diagnosis and treatment of decompression sickness. A general survey. In: Shilling CW, Carlston CB, Mathias RA, eds. The physician's guide to diving medicine. New York: Plenum Press, 1984:283–312.
22. Vann RD. Mechanisms and risks of decompression. In: Bove AA, Davis JC, eds. Diving medicine. Philadelphia: WB Saunders, 1990:29–49.
23. Moon RE, Camporesi EM, Kisslo JA. Patent foramen ovale and decompression sickness in divers. Lancet 1989;51(1):513–514.
24. Wilmshurst PT, Byrne JC, Webb-Peploe MM. Relation between interartrial shunts and decompression sickness in divers. 1989;2(8675):1302–1306.
25. Anonymous. Appendix 2. In: Bove AA, Davis JC, eds. Diving medicine. Philadelphia: WB Saunders, 1990:314.
26. Linaweaver, PG. Physical and psychological examination for diving. In: Shilling CW, Carlston CB, Mathias RA, eds. The physician's guide to diving medicine. New York; Plenum Press, 1984:489–520.
27. Millington JT. Physical standards for scuba divers. J Am Board Fam Pract 1988;1(3):194–200.
28. Dembert ML. Physical examination of scuba divers. Am Fam Phys 1979;20(2):91–93.
29. Becker GD, Parell GJ. Medical examination of the sport scuba diver. Otolaryngol Head Neck Surg 1983;91(3):246–250.
30. Dembert ML, Keith JF III. Evaluating the potential pediatric scuba diver. Am J Dis Child 1986;140(11):1135–1141.

36 / SOCCER

John H. Lohnes, William E. Garrett, Jr., and Raymond R. Monto

Introduction

Soccer is the world's most popular team sport. Soccer's governing body the Federation International de Football Association (FIFA) reported 60 million registered players in 1984 and estimated there were an additional 60 million unregistered players worldwide (1). In the United States soccer receives less attention as a spectator sport, nevertheless soccer has become the third most popular team sport among children under age 18 in terms of participation, with more than 1.4 million players registered with the U.S. Youth Soccer Association (2).

The incidence of injuries sustained in a soccer game is similar to that observed in sports such as lacrosse and hockey (3). However, because of the rules of play and the mechanisms for advancing the ball, soccer generates its own unique injury patterns and medical problems. The advent of indoor soccer and the growth of women's soccer in the last two decades have added new concerns. This chapter describes the physical demands of soccer; reviews the epidemiology of soccer injuries; and discusses the mechanisms, pathology, and treatment of common soccer-related injuries and medical disorders.

The Game of Soccer

Modern soccer involves two teams of 11 players opposing each other on a field of approximately 75 m wide by 110 m long. The game is played in two 45-min periods with a 15 min halftime. Youth soccer matches may vary in length, depending on the age level. International rules allow only two substitutions during the course of a match, although unlimited substitution is allowed in U.S. interscholastic and intercollegiate soccer.

Field players are allowed to advance the ball with any portion of their bodies except their arms or hands, although the ball is thrown in to restart play when the ball goes out of bounds on the sidelines. Goal keepers may use their arms or hands, but only within the designated "penalty area" about the goal. The ball may be advanced by heading (striking with the head), passing (kicking the ball to another player using any portion of the foot), or dribbling (running while controlling the ball with the feet). The ball also may be controlled with the chest or thighs.

Soccer is a moderate-contact sport where the basic rules are few and open to interpretation by the referee. This can lead to rough play and increased exposure to injury. Recent trends in the style of play have been away from strict position orientation and tactics to the concept of total soccer by which all 11 players are involved with every phase of attack and defense.

Biomechanics of Soccer

Kicking

The ball may be struck with any portion of the foot. The medial and lateral sides of the foot are generally used for making short, accurate passes. However, the instep kick is the primary method for advancing the ball powerfully over a long distance.

The standard soccer ball weighs 400 to 450 g and is made of molded plastic or stitched plastic-coated leather. The plastic prevents the excess weight due to water saturation that plagued previous versions. The standard size 5 ball has a circumference of 68.5 to 71 cm and should be inflated to a pressure of between 8.5 and 15.6 psi. A strong instep kick can accelerate a soccer ball to speeds in excess of 120 km/hr (4). The typical instep soccer kick consists of three main phases: approach; ball strike; and follow-through. Biomechanical analyses of the soccer kick by Gainor et al. (5) have demonstrated that the usual instep kick generates a varus torque on the proximal tibia greater than 200 N-m during approach and ball strike. This is followed by an equally large valgus torque on the tibia during follow-through. There are even higher amounts of extension torque on the proximal tibia during approach, ball strike (280 N-m), and follow-through (230 N-m). By comparison, the standard North American football toe kick exerts similar extension-flexion torque on the knee but does not exhibit varus-valgus torque.

The majority of this torque is generated by the hip flexors that act concentrically with the knee extensors as agonists during the kicking motion (Fig. 36. 1). In addition to the dramatic forces on the thigh and abdominal musculature during a kick, the soccer player's knee joint must withstand large translational and rotational stresses. This may help to explain the frequent occurrence of knee injuries during unchallenged kicks.

The maximum kinetic energy generated by a soccer kick has been estimated at 2000 N-m (5). This force is of sufficient magnitude to fracture a femur. Because only 15% of this kinetic energy is actually transferred to the ball, the remaining amount must be absorbed by the kicking leg. The majority of this force is dissipated by the hamstrings as they fire eccentrically to decelerate the kicking leg during follow-through. Because of this, the leg is quite vulnerable to injury during this stage of the kick. Any incidental contact with the ground or the leg of a defender creates additional impact loads and retards force dissipation in a leg already functioning at the limits of force toleration. This can lead to fracture or, more often, ligamentous disruption.

Because of these high energies, the kicking leg can itself become a dangerous projectile during follow-through. The hazard to the player challenging the kicker is increased because the transferred force cannot be efficiently dissipated.

Heading

One of the unique facets of soccer is the use of the head to advance the ball. A soccer player heads the ball an average of six times during a match (6). Given the large impact energies that are generated at ball contact, the skull, cervical spine, and neck musculature are subjected to high stresses. Several recent biomechanical studies have documented the extent of these stresses and their potential for acute and chronic injury.

Schneider and Zernicke (7) used a dynamic head-neck model to study the biomechanics of the interaction. In a series of studies they compared frontal and lateral head

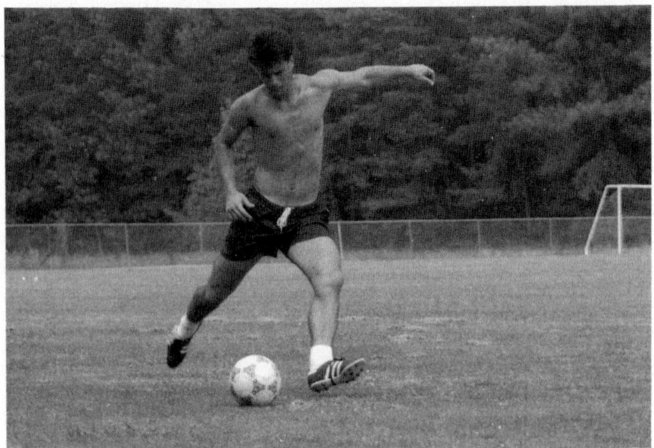

Figure 36.1. The long soccer volley just before ball strike, demonstrating forceful contraction of hip flexors and abdominal musculature.

impacts in adults and children, using various mass ratio/impact velocity combinations. By comparing measurements of linear and angular acceleration velocities with standard industrial head injury tolerance criteria, the relative risks of head trauma were obtained.

They concluded that the injury risk from angular head accelerations is greater than that from linear head accelerations. Lateral head impacts have greater angular accelerations than linear accelerations compared with frontal impacts and are considered more dangerous. This is because the moment of inertia of the head for rotations about the sagittal axis is less than for those about the coronal axis. Linear accelerations are also higher during frontal impacts because of increased axial mobility of the head. The study concluded that at the low mass ratios present when children use a standard soccer ball (size 5), angular accelerations exceeded head injury tolerance levels for frontal impact at ball velocities faster than 9 m/sec and for lateral impacts faster than 7.5 m/sec. These represent relatively slow ball speeds for a soccer match. Linear accelerations were better tolerated, but still eclipsed safe levels at ball speeds greater than 21 m/sec.

For the higher mass ratios in the range commonly seen in adult soccer, angular accelerations were found to result in significant injury risk for frontal impacts at velocities more than 19.5 m/sec and for lateral impacts above 13 m/sec. Unlike the lower mass ratio data found in children, linear accelerations were found to be within safe levels for frontal and lateral impacts at all ball velocities. Based on these data, it is recommended that mass ratios be maximized by using smaller, lighter balls in youth soccer and prohibiting the use of adult-size balls by children under age 12. Hazardous lateral head impacts should also be minimized by emphasizing proper heading techniques. These conclusions were echoed in a mathematical study by Townend (8) that documented a linear relationship between impact force and ball mass. Impact forces were also higher when lighter (i.e., younger) players headed balls of equal size.

Townend calculated the impulsive force absorbed by the head at ball impact to vary between 669 and 689 N. Other experimental measurements at ball velocities of 18 m/sec have found peak impact forces of 851 N for molded soccer balls and 912 N for stitched balls (9). Despite this higher force profile, stitched balls may be safer, because they take nearly 28% longer to reach their maximal force at impact than do molded balls. This increased rise time allows more time for force dissipation by the head and neck.

Although the impact forces during soccer heading may be an order of magnitude lower than the 6300 N that a heavyweight boxer can deliver with a punch to the head, there is a growing body of evidence to suggest that they may still lie in the hazardous range. The average duration of ball impact in soccer heading is 13 to 18 msec (7, 10). Impact forces of only 670 to 1100 N can cause zygoma fractures in cadavers (7). In contrast, the forehead requires much higher impact forces (1700 to 4000 N) for fracture production, again emphasizing the importance of proper heading techniques to avoid injury. Burslem and Lees (10) have demonstrated that, unlike unskilled players, skilled players decelerate their heads to produce head-neck-torso rigidity at ball impact. This lowers the risk of injury by decreasing rotational accelerations of the head at contact and thus minimizing the magnitude of the impact force. With the rigidity afforded by good techniques, these impact forces also are dissipated through a longer kinetic chain. Because the impact forces involved in soccer heading normally lie at the upper limits of safety, significant injury can result from any combination of poor techniques, accidental contact, or ball-to-head weight mismatch.

The incidence of head and neck injuries and clinical evidence of the long-term effects of repetitive soccer heading will be discussed later in this chapter.

Physiology and Conditioning

Soccer requires frequent bursts of high-intensity anaerobic activity within longer periods of aerobic exercise. Rapid changes in speed and/or direction, fast reaction time, and a high level of psychomotor coordination and agility are all key requirements of the sport. Time-motion analyses of soccer players have found that the typical adult competitive field player covers approximately 10 km during a match (11). This distance is covered by a combination of jogging (40%), walking (25%), cruising (15%), sprinting (10%), and backing (10%) (12). Midfielders typically cover 10% greater distance on average than forwards and defenders. Interestingly, the average length of time an individual player actually has possession of the ball during a match is no more than 2 min (13).

The physical demands of a soccer match can be extreme. Aerobic metabolism is frequently stressed to 80% or more of maximum, heart rate may increase to 150/min and venous lactate levels reach up to 12 mmol/liter (14). Muscle glycogen stores have been found to be completely diminished in top-level players following a game, with corresponding decreases in speed and distances traveled as the match progresses. In hot weather, up to 5 kg of fluid loss has been observed (15).

Despite the intense physical demands of a match, the physiologic training effects of soccer tend to be midway between those of a pure endurance sport such as distance running and an anaerobic sporting such as sprinting. $\dot{V}_{O_2}$ max measurements of soccer players have been found to range widely between 50 and 70 ml/kg/min, depending on player position, level of play, and type of training (14). Increased heart size, decreased resting heart rate, and increased forced expiratory volume and flow have been observed as training effects of soccer (16). Muscle fiber number and size, muscle capillary density, and muscular power have also been found to be increased in soccer players compared with nonathletes of the same age (17). The small-sided version of soccer (four or five players to a side) tends to result in a greater physiologic work rate than the normal game and may be a useful training method for improving overall fitness levels (18).

Unlike some other sports, body size and mass are less important determiners of success in soccer than they are in certain other team sports such as American football or basketball. However, several researchers have observed that postadolescent and adult soccer players tend toward mesomorphy or mesoectomorphy (19, 20). The trend toward leaner, taller, and heavier players has been observed in many other sports and may simply be reflective of the general trends in the population (21). It is unlikely that somatotype is an important predictor of individual soccer skill or of team success.

When compared with other athletes, both male and female soccer players tend to fall in the midranges of various measures of fitness, including aerobic endurance, anaerobic power, and strength (12, 22–24). This reflects the hybrid physical demands of the sport. As with other sports, the level of fitness increases with the level of play, with national team and professional players exhibiting the highest fitness levels (23, 25, 26). Differences in fitness levels between different player positions have been observed, with midfielders tending to exhibit greater levels of strength and endurance than other players (27, 28).

Various physical tests to measure soccer fitness have been devised, but no single test has been found to be an accurate predictor of soccer success. Other less easily measured factors such as psychomotor coordination and agility, tactical skill, and even personality type are equally important determiners of soccer ability. Thus conditioning for soccer players consists ideally of a mixture of endurance, strength, and technical skill training plus instruction in tactical strategies.

Nutrition and Fluid Needs

In a typical 90-min soccer match, a field player may use up to 90% of muscle glycogen reserves during a strenuous match or practice (15, 29). Because of the frequency of training and competition during a typical season, soccer players need to pay close attention to the timing, quality, and quantity of carbohydrate consumption.

A competitive adult soccer player will require about 8 g of carbohydrate per kilogram of body weight (3 to 4 g/lb). Carbohydrate loading as practiced by endurance athletes is probably not particularly helpful for soccer players before a match under most circumstances and may be impractical given the frequency of games. However a diet consisting of about 60% complex carbohydrates should be maintained through the competitive season. The pregame meal should be eaten 3 to 4 hr before competition to allow adequate time for gastric emptying. Meat and fried foods should be avoided and liquids encouraged.

When a series of matches are to be played within a short span of time, as in tournament competition, particular attention should be paid to replenishing glycogen reserves. It may take up to 48 hr to replenish muscle glycogen after exhaustive exercise. However, studies indicate that muscle is most avid for glycogen during the first 4 hr after competition; therefore, carbohydrate consumption should be particularly encouraged during this time. The use of glucose polymer drinks has been shown to aid glycogen replacement. In limited quantities they may also be useful immediately pregame and perhaps at halftime. However, because these drinks may also slow fluid absorption they are not recommended for use during games in hot weather, but reserved for immediate postgame consumption.

Endurance training can influence the rate of muscle glycogen depletion by sparing glycogen in favor of fatty acids as a source of energy. Endurance training will be of particular benefit to midfielders who tend to run greater distances during a match.

Soccer players, like most competitive athletes, require between 1 and 1.5 g of protein per kilogram of body weight. Most people typically consume more than this amount daily and so protein supplements are unnecessary, particularly because excess protein is not stored in the body. Likewise, vitamin and mineral supplements are usually unnecessary if the player is consuming a well-balanced diet.

Plenty of plain, cool water should be consumed during matches and heavy practice sessions. During extreme conditions of heat and humidity a player may lose 2 to 3 kg of fluid. To avoid dehydration and heat exhaustion a player should drink 150 ml every 15 min. Weighing before and after exercise can help gauge the amount of fluid lost, with each pound of body weight being equivalent to about 2 cups of water.

Elias et al. (30) established guidelines for tournament play in severe heat conditions based on experience with a large youth soccer tournament. In an effort to avoid morbidity caused by dehydration and heat exhaustion, modification in game timing and structure were recommended based on the wet bulb globe temperature (WBGT), which accounts for both relative humidity and ambient temperature. For WBGT greater than 82°F (28°C), they suggested the following modifications to the game: unrestricted substitutions; shorter game time; fluid breaks during play; quarter breaks; and rescheduling to a later or earlier time of day.

Epidemiology

Given the popularity of the sport, it is surprising that there have been few well-controlled, long-term prospective studies of soccer injuries. Most of the reports describing the incidence of various injuries have been limited in either time or scope or have been retrospective in nature. The results of 20 recent studies published in English are summarized in Tables 36.1 to 36.3.

Three studies (40, 43, 47) reported injuries sustained in large youth tournaments occurring over a span of several days. Although the populations were large and the conditions well-controlled, the definition of injuries was quite variable. The incidences of injuries reported in these studies were higher than those observed in the other studies, possibly because medical care was provided on site, making it more likely that participants would seek medical attention for an injury.

Four studies (34, 39, 44, 45) retrospectively examined soccer injuries gleaned from among emergency room or clinic visits or from insurance reports. Again, al-

Table 36.1.
Epidemiological Studies of Soccer Injuries

Year	Country	Age	Sex	Population Size	Total Injuries	Injury Rate (per 1000 hr)	Reference
1983	United States	Professionals	M	56	142	—	31
1988	United States	6–17	M	681	109	7.3	32
			F	458	107	10.6	
1986	France	10–35	M	123,175	6,153	1.7	33
1986	United States	—	M/F	—	111	—	34
1983	Sweden	17–38	M	180	256	—	35
1991	Sweden	16–28	F	41	78	—	36
1986	United States	8–16	M/F	455 (outdoor)	46	—	37
				587 (indoor)	74	—	
1992	Denmark	5–54	M/F	—	715	—	38
1990	UK	10–45	M	—	200	—	39
1986	Norway	12–18	M/F	14,800	411	11.7 total 17.6 female 8.9 male	40
1978	United States	—	M	15	60	—	41
1991	United States	17–22	M	—	1,221	7.78	3
					595	7.95	
1989	Denmark	16+	M	123	109	14.3 (game)	42
1978	Norway	—	M/F	25,000	1,534	23 (male) 44 (female)	43
1981	United States	14–18	M/F	10,634	436	—	44
1987	Saudi Arabia	11–20	M	—	542	—	45
1980	Finland	10–58	M	—	1,989	—	46
			F	—	83	—	
1985	Denmark	9–19	M/F	6,600	343	19	47
1980	United States	7–18	M/F	1,272	34	0.51 males 1.1 females	48
1990	Denmark	10–18	M	152	62	5.6	49

though the population sizes were fairly large, there is considerable reporting bias inherent in such studies and it is impossible to determine injury incidence or prevalence.

Most of the remaining studies reviewed reported injuries sustained by one or several teams during a league or club season. The ages and numbers of participants, the level of competition, and the methods of injury reporting were quite variable in these studies, nevertheless some general trends regarding injury patterns were consistent.

One of the best controlled of these studies was by Ekstrand et al. (35, 50–54) in Sweden. They observed 180 Swedish Division I professional players between 1979 and 1981 and prospectively examined injury patterns and the effects of various training methods and protective measures on injury incidence. Although the study involved a relatively small number of players, the ob-

Table 36.2.
Locations of Soccer Injuries (Percent of Total)

Head	Upper Extremity	Trunk	Pelvis	Lower Extremity	Thigh	Knee	Leg	Ankle	Foot	Reference
7	8	—	20	—	—	18	29	—	—	31
7	5	3	3	71	8	13	16	19	10	32
12	13	[7	]	61	—	—	—	—	—	33
—	2	—	—	—	—	59	—	9	—	34
—	—	—	13	—	14	20	29	—	12	35
—	—	—	6	—	15	23	9	26	9	36
22	6	—	8	63	—	—	—	—	—	37
8	20	—	15	58	—	—	—	—	—	
2	27	—	—	57	—	—	—	33	—	39
17	14	[7.5	]	61	—	—	—	—	—	40
—	—	—	—	—	—	—	—	—	—	41
9	7	5	6		17	18	7	21	9.5	3
7	7	6	4		18	17	9	22	10	
—	—	—	—	84	22 (includes groin)	18				42
10	15	7	—	68	12	14	13	16	13	43
9	26	—	4	58	—	12	—	—	—	44
—	—	—	—	59	—	—	—	—	—	45
14	12	9	—	64	—	—	—	—	—	46
9	16	7	—	68	—	—	—	—	—	
5	—	[4	]	81	—	—	—	[44	]	47
15	17	—	—	65	—	12	—	41	—	48
4	—	—	—	—	24	19	—	27	19	49

Table 36.3.
Types of Soccer Injuries (Percent of Total)

Contusion	Abrasion	Sprain	Strain	Fracture	Dislocation	"Itis"	Concussion	Reference
16	—	61	15	22	4.5	28		31
35	—	19	28	—	—	—	—	32
21	8	40.5	4	17	—	—	—	33
20	—	29	18	4	2	23	—	35
15	—	33	10	—	—	24	—	36
8	—	16	11	1	—	—	—	37
14	—	30	17	6	—	—	—	
25	5	[46	]	18	2	—	—	38
22	6	33	—	29	2	—	—	39
47	18	22	—	6	—	—	—	40
8	3	35	47	2	5	—	—	41
21	2	27	24	6	2	3	4	3
12	1	27	28	5.5	2.5	4.5	3	
9	—	49	21	6	—	16	—	42
36	39	[20	]	3.5	—	—	—	43
31	7	[38	]	19	2	—	1	44
[23	]	26	—	29	5	—	—	45
42	—	[45	]	[11	]	—	—	46 (males & females)
33	20	—	—	4	—	—	—	47
38	—	35	9	9	—	—	—	48
—	—	49	21	6	—	16	—	49

servations were made in a well-designed, prospective manner with consistent follow-up and reporting methods. The authors also did a retrospective follow-up of these same players in 1988.

The only large ongoing study of soccer league injuries in the United States is being carried out by the National Collegiate Athletic Association (NCAA). The NCAA Injury Surveillance System has been collecting injury statistics on various college sports since 1982. Men's and women's soccer have been included annually since the 1986–1987 season, making it possible to view injury trends over several years. A total of 105 men's teams (601 players) and 61 women's teams (361 players) contributed to this project in 1991–1992, representing Division I, II, and III schools from throughout the country. Injury incidences have tended to remain fairly constant through the seasons examined and will likely become more accurate as the number of participating schools increases. Currently, these data are probably the most reliable figures available for adult soccer injuries in the United States (3).

The reporting system employed by the NCAA is the most commonly accepted method of injury reporting used today. Injury incidence is reported per 1000 hours of "athlete exposure" (AE) rather than as a percentage of total numbers injured. This more accurately reflects the risk of injury. A reportable injury is defined as one that causes the loss of at least 1 day of participation. A number of authors have examined the incidence of specific types of injuries in soccer. Their results are discussed in further detail below. Most of these involved retrospective analyses.

It is impossible to compare directly the results of the various epidemiological studies reviewed in Table 36.1 because of differences in population size and demographics, levels of play and the definition and reporting of injuries. However some general trends can be observed in all studies.

The incidence and severity of injuries increases with increasing age, level of play, and frequency of competition.

Injuries in youth players, especially under the age of 12, are uncommon and typically do not result in significant lost playing time.

For reasons not yet explained, girls appear to be twice as likely as boys to be injured in the younger age groups. This difference is not present in adult players.

Center forwards and midfielders have the highest injury rates, although goalkeepers are the most likely to sustain upper extremity injuries.

Injuries to the lower extremities account for between 50% and 66% of all injuries.

Contusions, ligament sprains (especially ankle sprains), and muscle strains account for 75% of all injuries.

Serious, permanently disabling injuries are, fortunately, rare, accounting for less than 0.1% of injuries at all levels.

Incidence, Treatment, and Prevention

Head and Neck

Acute Injuries

Injuries to the head, face, and neck account for between 5% and 15% of all injuries. Typically, these injuries are minor lacerations, abrasions, or contusions. Skull fractures, concussions, and cervical spine trauma occur infrequently despite the absence of protective headgear and the sometimes large forces sustained by heading the soccer ball. In the NCAA the incidence of concussions was only 0.03/1000 AE.

Sane and Ylipaavalniemi (55) reported on dental injuries sustained in soccer. They reviewed 8640 soccer injuries occurring in players ages 8 to 47 and found 6.4% affected the teeth, alveolar processes, or lower or middle third of the facial skeleton. Only 4.3% of the injuries occurred in players under age 15. These findings are similar to those seen by Nysether (56). Both authors recommended the use of protective mouthpieces or dental guards.

Burke et al. (57) reviewed 12 soccerball-induced eye injuries in youth players (ages 6 to 21). Hyphema and retinal edema were present in all injuries. Vitreous and retinal hemorrhage, corneal abrasion, traumatic iritis, and retinal tear also were observed, although in no case was there any permanent impairment. Similar findings were reported by Orlando (58).

There is some controversy regarding the benefits of protective headgear—helmets, eye protectors, and dental guards—in soccer, especially for children. Serious eye injuries are very rare in soccer and it may be argued that the use of eye protectors actually increases the risk of facial lacerations and contusions. Dental guards, however, can reduce dental injuries and are especially recommended for goal keepers and for players with orthodontic devices, caps, or other dentalwork. The risk of dental injuries for other field players is relatively low and mandatory use of protective mouth guards may be unwarranted. Nevertheless, their use should be encouraged.

The most important preventive measure for avoiding acute head and neck injuries from the ball is to establish proper heading techniques, using the head actively to counteract the force of the oncoming ball with the forehead rather than passively absorbing the shock with the top of the head. As mentioned earlier, the use of smaller balls for youth players also can significantly reduce the risks inherent in heading the ball.

As in all sports, any injured player who loses consciousness should be sent to a medical facility for further evaluation and observation, regardless of his or her symptoms on regaining consciousness. Likewise, any player who complains of neck pain, radicular pain, numbness, tingling, or weakness in the extremities following acute injury should be assumed to have a cervical spine fracture until proven otherwise. These players should be immobilized on the field and transferred to a medical facility for radiographs and evaluation.

Chronic Effects of Heading

The possible chronic effects of repetitive soccer heading have been a subject of some controversy. Reports of cerebral atrophy and brain wave abnormalities have been reported as well as accelerated degenerative changes of the cervical and lumbar spine. Tysvaer et al. (59, 60) have done a series of studies to investigate the neurologic effects of heading. One study of 69 Division I Norwegian players (mean age 25) demonstrated a higher incidence of EEG disturbances in soccer players compared with a control group. A total of 54% and a history of significant head injury while playing soccer and 55% complained of intermittent headaches associated with playing. Another 4 players had had concussions, and 12% gave a history of protracted symptoms related to their head injuries. Although only one of these players had an abnormal neurologic clinical exam, 35% displayed abnormal EEG tracings compared with only 13% in the control group. Abnormal EEGs were seen with more frequency in the younger players: 44% of the 15- to 24-year-olds compared with 26% of the 24- to 34-year-olds. Aross (61) found similar EEG changes.

Sortland and Tysvaer (62) performed computerized tomography (CT) scans of the brains of 33 former elite soccer players with an average age of 49 and compared them with normal standards of cerebral architecture. They found that 27% had central cerebral atrophy with widening of the lateral ventricles. Cortical atrophy was seen in 18%, and 6% had a septum pelucidum cyst. Only 1.5% of normal adults have these type of cysts. Large cysts of the septum pelucidum are classically seen in boxers who have sustained repeated subconcussive blows to the head.

In an attempt to provide clinical correlation for these findings, Tysvaer et al. (60) performed an extensive battery of psychological tests on these former players. Of 37 players examined, 81% exhibited mild to severe deficits in psychologic tests of attention, concentration, memory, and judgment. These results were attributed to neuronal damage caused by repeated minor head trauma.

One study examined the possible chronic effects of heading on the cervical spine. Sortland et al. (62) performed radiologic and clinical examinations on a group of 43 former Norwegian national soccer team players and compared the results with age-matched controls. A total of 21% of the former players had chronic neck pain or stiffness, and 58% had decreased range of neck motion. Five of these players (8%) had evidence of healed compression fractures of the lateral masses, and the majority demonstrated accelerated degenerative arthrosis at all cervical levels compared with the control group.

Further studies will be needed to determine the significance of these findings and to make possible recommendations for prevention. However, players with a history of protracted headaches, nausea, dizziness, visual field disturbances, neck pain, or radicular upper extremity symptoms after heading should be restricted from heading. These players should be further evaluated for subtle brain or cervical spine pathology with EEG, CT, or magnetic resonance imaging (MRI) scans, and/or cervical spine radiographs.

Upper Extremities

Although injuries to the upper extremities (shoulder, elbow, arm, and hand) are commonly encountered in soccer, they seldom result in extensive lost playing time for most field players and will not be discussed in detail here. More detailed descriptions of the evaluation and treatment of upper extremity injuries can be found elsewhere in this text.

Upper extremity injuries account for between 5% and 15% of all soccer injuries and are far more common in goalkeepers than in field players. In the NCAA, the incidences of injuries to the upper extremities (shoulder, arm, and hand) were 0.53/1000 AE for men and 0.47/1000 AE for women (3).

Curtin and Kay (63) reviewed 52 soccer-related hand injuries. Approximately 33% occurred in goalkeepers, mainly the result of contact with the ball. Other players usually injured the hand through contact with the ground or another player. Phalangeal fractures were most common—17 out of 47—and usually involved the dominant hand. For goalkeepers, finger injuries are typically sustained by catching the ball on the end of the finger, with fractures to the distal or middle phalanges or the interphalangeal joints. Forearm fractures

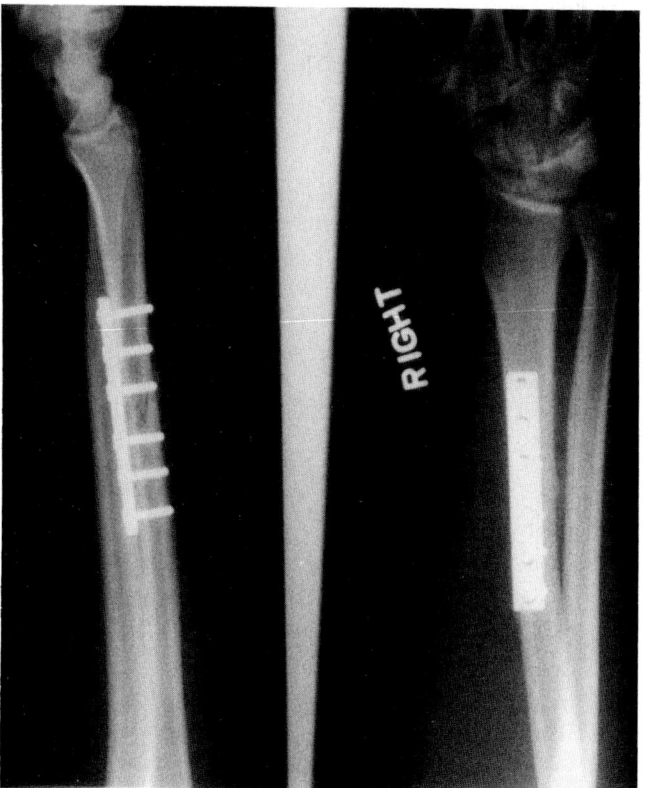

Figure 36.2. Humerus fracture in goalkeeper.

and wrist fractures or sprains may also occur as the goalkeeper attempts to stop the oncoming shot (Fig. 36.2). Despite the advent of padded gloves there has been little change in the incidence of hand injuries in goalkeepers (63).

Shoulder acromioclavicular separations are not infrequent in field players. They are caused by falls on the shoulder or outstretched arm.

Back, Trunk, and Pelvis

Injuries above the waist to the back or thorax are uncommon in soccer. Injuries below the waist to the pelvis, hips, and groin are slightly more common, but combined injuries to the back, thorax, abdomen, pelvis, and groin generally account for less than 10% of all injuries resulting in lost playing time. In the NCAA in 1991–1992, the incidence of back and thorax injuries was 0.41/1000 AE in men and 0.34/1000 AE in women (3).

Complaints of lower-back pain are most often the result of muscle strains or ligament sprains and usually respond well to conservative management. However, persistent or recurrent back pain or radicular symptoms should warrant a further diagnostic evaluation. Congenital spondylolisthesis is not an uncommon source of lumbar pain in young soccer players and is often aggravated by playing on hard or artificial surfaces. Spondylolysis or fractures of the pars interarticularis may also occur in goalkeepers because of the repetitive lumbar hyperextension required in diving saves. Degenerative disc disease and disc herniation are much less common, but both are known to occur at a younger age in the athlete than in the general population.

Groin injuries are perhaps the most common of injuries to the lower trunk, pelvis, and/or upper leg in soccer, although the actual incidence of these injuries is difficult to determine, because the true location of the injury may be obscure and the injury is recorded differently in different epidemiological studies.

The incidence of groin, pelvis, and hip injuries was 0.49/1000 AE in men and 0.42/1000 AE in women in the NCAA (3). Various European studies have reported incidences ranging from 0.5% to 28% (64). Martens et al. (65) in Belgium treated 109 athletes with either adductor tendinitis and/or rectus abdominus tendopathy; of these, 95 (87%) were soccer players. The iliopsoas is also a frequently injured muscle in soccer players (66).

Chronic groin pain (Athletic Pubalgia)

Chronic groin pain, or pubalgia, is often encountered in soccer players and is likely caused by the biomechanics of forceful kicking in which abdominal muscles and hip flexors and adductors are repetitively stressed. Other possible sources of groin pain such as inguinal hernias, osteitis pubis, and prostatitis should first be ruled out. Careful muscle group testing should identify affected muscle groups (67).

A condition quite common in soccer players involves pain related to a defect or weakness in the abdominal wall musculature near the inguinal ligament (68, 69). The external oblique forms an opening through which the spermatic cord runs, forming a roof for the cord proximal to its exit point. The internal oblique begins lateral to the cord and traverses proximally, with a few fibers looping back down behind the cord to attach onto the inguinal ligament along the pectineal eminence. These fibers conjoin with the transversalis tendon and often are quite weak and indeed there may be no contribution of the internal oblique to this conjoined tendon. Repetitive overloading at this site causes recurrent inflammation and groin pain.

The onset is typically insidious, presenting as progressive pain while running and often lasting several hours or days afterward. It is aggravated by activity and relieved by rest but usually returns quickly even after prolonged periods of rest. The pain is usually localized to the inguinal area but frequently radiates posteriorly to the ischium and/or superiorly to the lower abdomen and may be difficult for the player to clearly localize. There may be point tenderness but rarely is an actual hernia or defect palpable. Active flexion and rotation of the torso (e.g., performing a sit-up) usually reproduces sharp pain as the internal oblique muscle is contracted. Diagnostic studies such as radiographs, bone scans, CT, and MRI are frequently negative.

Van Vlierberghe (70) demonstrated that poor lower-back, hip, and knee flexibility and weakness of the abdominal or adductor muscle groups are correlated with groin injuries. Adductor injuries usually respond well to progressive eccentric strength training. Strengthening the internal oblique musculature is more difficult but can be effectively accomplished by lying supine with the arms flat on the floor. The hips and knees are then held in a flexed position and the abdominal muscles are used to lift the buttocks off the floor. The oblique muscles can be further strengthened by pulling the pelvis laterally to either side.

Unfortunately, conservative treatment is often unsuccessful in relieving symptoms in many players. In a study by Martens et al. (71) 70% of the patients treated conservatively did not improve and eventually underwent surgical procedures. Surgical treatment for this type of chronic groin pain involves suturing the transversus abdominus aponeurotic arch to the lacunar-inguinal ligament and reinforcing the conjoined tendon near its insertion along the pectineal eminence in a modified Bassini-type herniorraphy. The results of this procedure are quite successful in relieving pain recalcitrant to conservative measures (68).

Lower Extremities

Lower extremity injuries account for approximately 60% or more of all soccer injuries. Contusions to the lower extremities, muscle strains of the thigh (adductors, hamstrings, and quadriceps), and ankle sprains are the most common acute injuries. Stress fractures and a variety of overuse injuries involving the leg, ankle, and foot in adult soccer are overuse injuries frequently encountered by soccer players.

The location of lower extremity injuries in the NCAA data for 1991–1992 is shown in Table 36.4. These num-

Table 36.4.
Frequency of Injuries to the Lower Extremities in the NCAA Men's and Women's Soccer for the 1991–1992 Season

	Total	Thigh	Knee	ACL	Leg	Ankle	Foot
Men	5.94	1.39	1.48	.13	.54	1.75	.78
Women	6.02	1.45	1.35	.26	.71	1.76	.75

bers have remained fairly constant over the past 6 years of that study.

Contusions

Contusions to the thigh and calf are common but rarely result in much lost playing time. The use of shinguards greatly reduces the frequency of leg contusions and is now required in many leagues. Deep muscle contusions, however, can be quite disabling and may lead to complications such as acute muscle compartment syndrome or myositis ossificans.

Acute Compartment Syndrome. A compartment syndrome is the result of increased pressure within an enclosed fascial space, causing local tissue hypoxia with secondary ischemic muscle and nerve damage. Acute compartment syndrome occurs when local capillary flow is compromised following blunt trauma or fracture when local tissue pressure reaches within 40 mm Hg of the mean arterial pressure. As intracompartmental pressures continue to rise, progressively more severe neuromuscular damage ensues. The duration of compromise is particularly critical. At 30 min tissue compromise is fully reversible. Although capillary damage occurs at 3 hr, full clinical recovery occurs after 4 hr of elevated compartment pressures. After 6 hr, tissue damage is only partially reversible and recovery is incomplete. Delay of 8 hr or more leads to permanent cell death and a poor prognosis for functional recovery. As pressures increase, less time is available for diagnosis and effective surgical relief.

Diagnosis of acute compartment syndrome relies on clinical suspicion and invasive documentation of intracompartmental pressures with wick catheter measurements. Pain is usually the primary symptom and is aggravated by passive motion of the joints adjacent to the involved compartment. Any player with persistent pain and swelling in the calf after sustaining a direct blow should be monitored closely for the next several hours. The presence of pulses can be misleading, because local intracompartmental tissue pressures do not usually exceed arterial blood pressure in even the most severe cases. Numbness and paraesthesias, however, are a disturbing sign of local tissue compromise and possible compartment syndrome. The presence of an open wound does not exclude a concomitant diagnosis of acute compartment syndrome.

Acute compartment syndrome is a surgical emergency. Documentation with Wick catheter measurements of all four compartments (anterior, lateral, posterior, and deep posterior) of the lower leg should be made both before and after surgical release. The limb should *not* be elevated, because this only serves to aggravate the condition by decreasing the local arteriovenous pressure gradient. Ice should also be avoided because of its capillary constrictive effects, which could exacerbate local tissue ischemia.

Myositis Ossificans. Myositis ossificans is another possible complication of deep muscle contusions, especially to the anterior thigh. As Walton and Rothwell (72) suggest, the development of myositis ossificans following blunt trauma may be caused by inefficient force transfer in the deeper muscle layers. Clinical examination reveals a tender, erythematous, firm mass in a previously traumatized muscle group. Radiographs demonstrate a fluffy opacity with increased peripheral density. Histologic studies are frequently misleading and can imply a tumor. For this reason, biopsy of a suspected myositis ossificans lesion should be discouraged.

Treatment of a deep thigh contusion is symptomatic at first with rest, ice, and nonsteroidal antiinflammatory drugs (NSAIDs). Massage should definitely be avoided. Some authors have recommended immobilizing the knee in flexion for the first 24 hr to tamponade the bleeding and avoid the development of a hematoma. Later, passive range-of-motion and whirlpool will help to maintain mobility, although crutches may be required for several days.

Players who do develop myositis ossificans can generally be treated conservatively with antiinflammatory medications. Surgical removal can be difficult and should be reserved only for symptomatic patients with lesions at least 6 months old. This allows the zone of injury to mature and decreases the chance of recurrence (74). Players who develop recurrent or multiple myositis ossificans lesions should have their blood clotting status evaluated with a coagulation profile.

Chronic Compartment Syndrome

Chronic exertional compartment syndrome is frequently seen in soccer players and represents a real diagnostic and therapeutic challenge for the physician. The usual location of chronic exertional compartment syndrome is the anterior compartment of the leg, although it can involve the lateral or deep posterior compartments as well (74). The differential diagnosis includes tibial stress fracture, venous thrombosis, local nerve compressions, and periostitis. In the older player, intermittent claudication should also be considered. Frequently the condition is perceived as shin splints with pain increasing with the intensity of exercise and improving with rest.

Muscle bulk increases up to 20% during exercise and this may contribute to a transient elevation in intracompartmental pressure. As the pressure rises, the bloodflow to muscle during the relaxation phase decreases, resulting in a cramping leg pain. The symptoms are frequently bilateral and sometimes are accompanied by swelling or numbness extending to the dorsum of the foot.

Some key diagnostic clues in the history are that the symptoms tend to resolve quickly, usually within 1 hr after stopping exercise, and are not present with normal daily activities. Furthermore, players with a chronic compartment syndrome cannot play through the pain. This is unusual for the soccer player who is accustomed to frequent lower extremity injuries and typically has some chronic leg or foot complaint.

Diagnosis of chronic compartment syndrome can be confirmed with Wick catheter measurements of preexercise and postexercise intracompartmental pressures. Resting pressures may be slightly higher than normal subjects but frequently are not greater than 15 mm Hg. However, postexercise pressures that remain greater than 15 mm Hg for more than 15 min are considered abnormal.

Chronic compartment syndrome may be treated effectively with elective surgical release of the involved muscle compartment. This may be accomplished on an outpatient basis through small incisions. Total rehabilitation varies from 6 to 12 weeks, with deep compartment involvement leading to a longer recovery period.

Muscle Strain Injuries

Although frequently overlooked as minor injuries, muscle strains can nevertheless become chronic, recurrent, and refractory to therapy. Strains of the hamstrings, adductors, and quadriceps are extremely common in soccer players and result in extended periods of limited or lost playing time. Recent advances in the understanding of the basic pathology and healing of muscle strains has helped in both the treatment and prevention of these troublesome injuries.

Pathophysiology and Healing. Muscle strains typically occur in eccentrically loaded muscles which span two joints (e.g., quadriceps, hamstrings, and gastrocnemius). A high percentage of strain injuries occur in type II muscle fibers, with the tear occurring at the muscle-tendon junction. The syncytial nature of muscle fibers is thought to ensure fiber viability even though the terminal portions of the fibers are disrupted (75). The cellular response following strain injury follows a characteristic sequence. Hemorrhage occurs initially around the ruptured fiber ends followed by fiber necrosis and inflammation during the first 24 hr (Fig. 36.3). By 48 hr after injury there is a proliferation of inflammatory cells and fibroblastic activity at the myotendinous junction with complete breakdown of muscle fibers. After 7 days hemorrhage, edema and inflammation are seen to resolve and muscle regeneration becomes evident with fibrosis and myotube formation (76).

The treatment of grade I and II muscle strain injuries should be accomplished with the above pathophysiology in mind as well as the anatomy and kinematics of the particular muscle involved. Ice, compression, and elevation during the first 24 hr will help to limit bleeding and edema. NSAIDs have been shown to be effective in controlling the pain associated with the inflammatory response, but it remains unclear whether they significantly alter the course of healing (1).

Immobilization of muscle strains is generally not recommended, because it results in muscle atrophy, diminished ability to produce force, and shortening of the muscle-tendon unit. Gentle, passive range of motion should be started soon after strain injury followed by active motion and strengthening as tolerated.

Occasionally complete rupture (grade III) muscle tears do occur and may require surgical repair. However even some grade III tears result in no functional disability because other muscles in the group hypertrophy and compensate. Complete rupture of the rectus femoris is a common example of this in soccer players (Fig. 36.4).

Prevention. Warmup and stretching have been assumed to prevent or limit the severity of muscle strain injuries and are routine in most training programs. However, the amount and type of warmup and

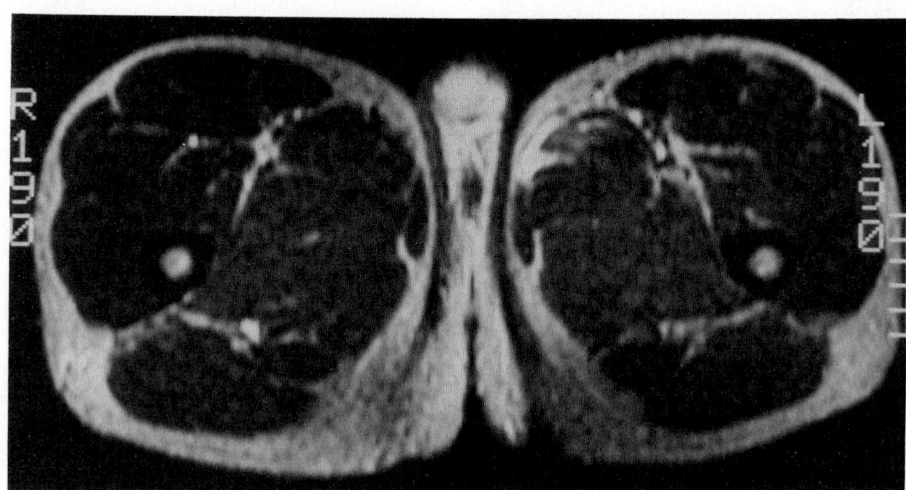

Figure 36.3. MRI scan demonstrating increased signal (edema and hemorrhage) in the left adductor longus following strain injury in 25-year-old professional soccer player.

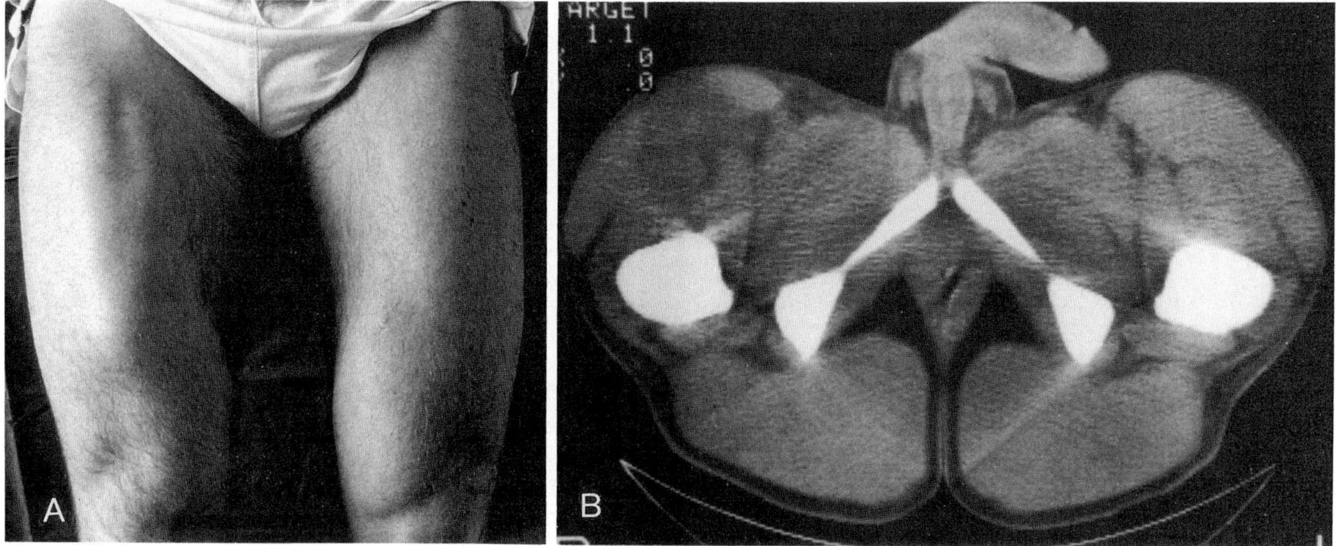

Figure 36.4. **(A)** Clinical appearance and **(B)** CT scan of a rectus femoris rupture.

stretching varies widely. Experimental studies in animal models have demonstrated that activated (contracted) muscle can absorb more energy before tearing than unactivated muscle (77). Likewise, warming of the muscle also increases the load required for failure.

Passive stretching does decrease the stress on a muscle at a given length due to the viscoelastic properties of the muscle fibers (78). In experimental studies only three or four repetitions of a stretch are required to improve muscle elasticity and decrease the risk of strain injury.

Knee Injuries

Acute Knee Injuries. Knee injuries in soccer are less frequent than may be expected but are of great concern because they result in substantial disability, lost playing time, and even the end of a career. Engstrom et al. (79) investigated the incidence and effects of serious knee injuries in a group of 64 elite professional male players. Of these, 12 players sustained major knee injuries that resulted in 80 to 348 days of missed playing time. Of these, 7 of the injuries were to the ACL and/or MCL. The authors concluded that of all the injuries observed in the course of their study, knee injuries accounted for the most time lost.

Meniscal tears and ligament injuries in soccer typically result from pivoting or sudden deceleration stresses rather than from direct contact as in American football or rugby. Articular cartilage or osteochondral injuries are also not infrequent and may result from the hyperextension loading of the strong shot or kick. Such lesions typically occur in the femoral condyle and should be strongly suspected when a persistent effusion develops in the absence of discrete point tenderness or instability (Fig. 36.5). An MRI scan can be extremely helpful in confirming this diagnosis. Osseous or osteochondral injuries should always be suspected in association with ACL or MCL tears. Isolated posterior cruciate ligament tears can occur if the player is struck directly against the anterior tibia as the femur and upper body continue forward.

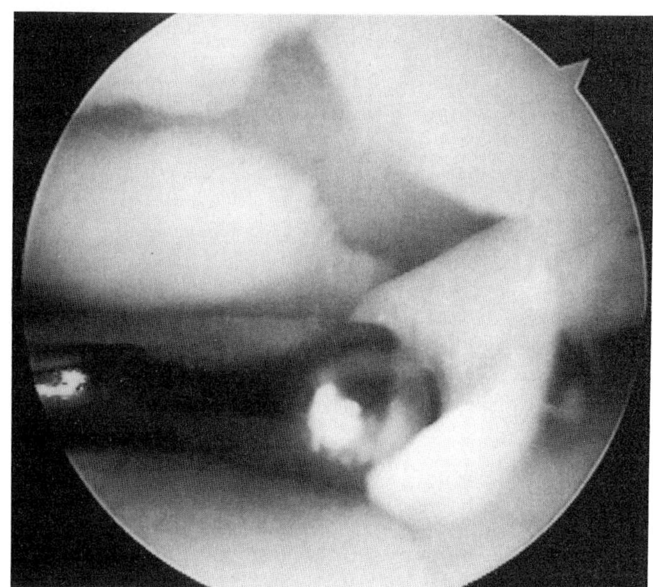

Figure 36.5. Articular cartilage defect of medial femoral condyle in 27-year-old female soccer player.

Tears of the anterior cruciate ligament are generally the most disabling of knee injuries for the soccer player and accounted for the majority of time lost due to knee injuries in most of the studies reviewed. Few soccer players are able to remain competitive with an ACL-deficient knee, despite strengthening and bracing, and surgical reconstruction should be recommended for all patients who wish to continue the sport. The pathophysiology, natural history, and surgical treatment of ACL tears are discussed elsewhere in this volume.

Overuse Syndromes of the Knee. Iliotibial band friction syndrome, popliteus tendonitis, patellar tendonitis (jumper's knee), pes anserine bursitis, and irritation of synovial plicae are common overuse syndromes observed about the knee in soccer players. Iliotibial friction syndrome (or ITB bursitis) presents as lateral knee pain that progressively worsens during running after a pain-free start (71). A tight iliotibial band over the lateral femoral condyle can result in an inflamed bursa with heavy training. Players with varus knees and an oversupinated gait may be more prone to this condition. The treatment is generally conservative with ITB stretching, NSAIDs, and occasional cortisone injection in the bursa. However, chronic cases in elite players may require surgery. Surgery involves excision of the inflamed bursa and excision of a posteriorly based triangular portion of the iliotibial tract at the level of the lateral femoral condyle.

Patellar tendonitis results from cyclic overloading of the extensor mechanism during jumping and kicking. Pain and tenderness is localized to the patellar tendon and can become chronic if not treated early with rest, NSAIDs, and eccentric quadriceps strengthening exercises. Chronic tendonitis may result in a thickened tendon with focal degenerative areas. Steroid injections should be avoided for this reason. Chronic, severe cases may respond well to surgical excision of the nodular degenerative areas.

The chronic effects of playing soccer on the knee was investigated by Chantraine (80). He found that radiological signs of knee osteoarthritis in veteran soccer players increase with age at a much greater percentage than in a random population of the same age. Of the 81 players examined (ages 40 to 74), 56% of the knees had radiologic signs of osteoarthritis. A total of 26% knees had had prior meniscectomies and all of these showed degenerative changes. The author concluded that in the remainder, soccer playing alone had contributed to the degenerative joint changes observed. However, only 30% of the knees with radiologic changes were clinically symptomatic.

Tibia Fractures

Direct kicks to the anterior leg are quite common in soccer and may result in tibia fractures (Figs. 36.6 and 36.7). Fortunately, the use of shin guards can significantly reduce the incidence of these injuries, and shin guards are now mandatory in most youth leagues and many collegiate and adult leagues as well. Experimental studies by Van Laack (81) have shown that shin guards decrease the magnitude of these forces by increasing the amount of contact time. The best results were seen when forces were less than 3000 N. Although the force reduction due to shin guards is substantial enough to prevent some tibial fractures, they were most effective at decreasing the amount of soft tissue damage sustained at impact. Shin guards also decrease the magnitude of the contact forces by dissipating them over a larger area.

Despite the protection afforded by shin guards, it is clear that the forces generated by a direct kick to the tibia can still be sufficient to cause fractures and a fracture should be strongly suspected if an injured player is unable to bear weight due to pain in the shin. Suspected tibia fractures should be referred acutely for radiographs and further treatment by an orthopedist.

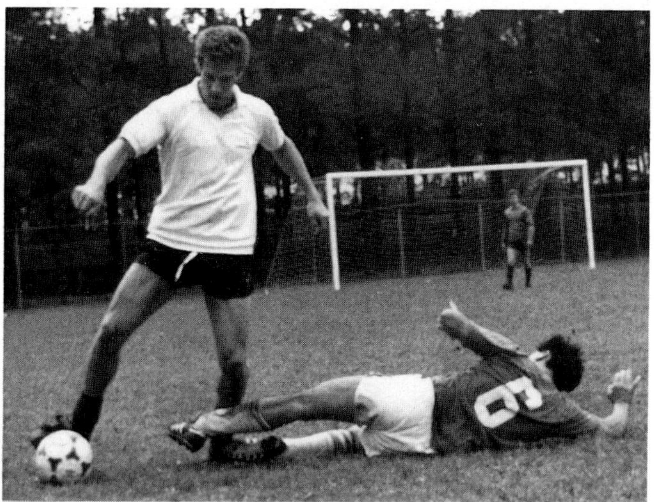

Figure 36.6. Mechanism of injury for tibial fracture.

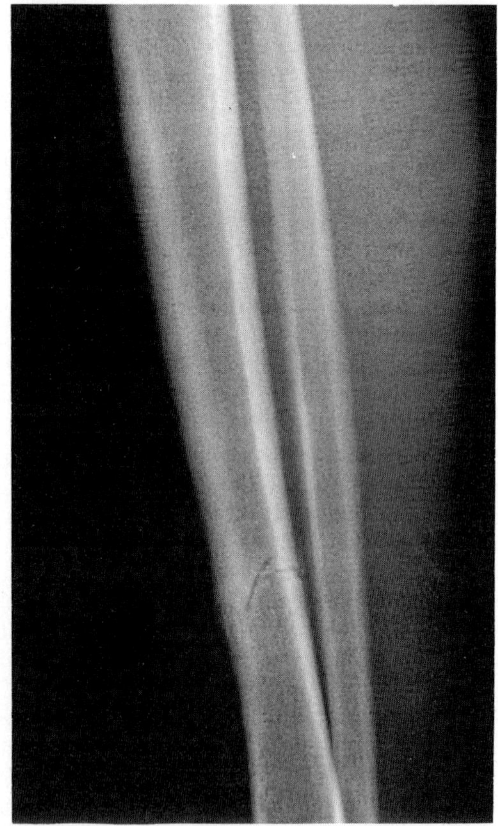

Figure 36.7. Nondisplaced midshaft tibial fracture.

Nondisplaced midshaft tibia fractures may not require casting if the bone is stable and may often be treated successfully with a removable brace and crutches. The advantages to maintaining mobility and muscular strength during the healing phase are obvious for the active player. Comminuted and/or displaced tibial shaft fractures are preferably treated by unreamed intramedullary rodding. This method of fixation offers minimal surgical exposure and early functional return to sport. Its disadvantages are that it does not allow for postoperative adjustments in alignment and at least temporarily disrupts local intramedullary blood flow to the fracture site. Fractures in the proximal and distal shaft can be difficult to stabilize with an intramedullary rod and a circular external fixation device such as the Ilizarov and Monticelli-Spinelli systems can provide an excellent treatment alternative.

Jacchia et al. (82) reviewed 4683 tibia fractures seen at an orthopedic clinic in Florence, Italy, from 1962 to 1988. Of these, 126 (2.7%) were in soccer players. They observed that the development of internal fixation devices and more recently the Ilizarov apparatus significantly reduced the long- and short-term disabilities these fractures cause for soccer players.

Stress fractures of the tibial shaft may become a recurrent problem for some players. Custom-molded orthoses to correct excessive varus or valgus deformities and to increase shock absorption will limit recurrent tibial stress fractures. However, chronic or recurrent tibial stress fractures may progress to complete fractures and require immobilization or even surgical fixation.

Ankle Injuries

Ankle Sprains. Ankle sprains are certainly the most common injuries accounting for lost playing time at all age levels and levels of competition in soccer. In the NCAA, ankle sprains have been the most frequent specific injury reported in each of the six seasons of observation (3). Ekstrand and Tropp (83) found the incidence of ankle sprains in male adult players to vary between 1.7 and 2.0 per 1000 hours of exposure. Between 17% and 20% of all injuries were ankle sprains. They also found a 50% chance of reinjury in players with histories of previous ankle sprains. An observed decrease in the flexibility of soccer players' ankles may contribute to recurrent sprains (84).

As in other sports, the typical ankle injury involves an inversion/plantar flexion stress with injury to the lateral ligaments. In severe injuries with an audible pop and significant pain, swelling, or bleeding, a fracture should always be suspected and radiographs obtained.

A "high" sprain involving an eversion/external rotation stress may tear the anterior-inferior tibiofibular ligament (AITFL), the posterior-inferior tibiofibular ligament (PITL), the inferior transverse ligament, and/or the syndesmotic (interosseus) ligament—the strongest of the group. This sprain is distinguished from the inversion/plantar flexion injury by tenderness along the lateral aspect of the distal tibia. These sprains typically involve much longer recovery times.

The basic tenets of ice, elevation, and compression apply acutely to most ankle sprains and a splint and crutches may be required for several days. However, the trend has been away from strict immobilization, even following severe sprains, and toward allowing the patient to begin weight bearing as tolerated and early range of motion. It is not unusual for a player to experience persistent pain and swelling for many months following a severe ankle sprain, and it is important that rehabilitation continues during this time. As pain and swelling subsides, progressive strengthening and proprioceptive exercises are particularly important components of the rehabilitation process for soccer players, because ball control depends heavily on ankle and foot coordination.

Ekstrand and Gillquist (35) have demonstrated that the incidence of ankle sprains can be significantly reduced through proper preventive measures and rehabilitation following injury. Prophylactic taping is expensive and time-consuming and has not been shown to reduce the incidence of sprains in a previously uninjured player. However, for players with a history of repeated ankle sprains and residual joint laxity, taping or bracing can be effective. Soccer players will typically not tolerate extensive restrictions on their ability to plantarflex the ankle, because this is crucial to controlling, passing, and shooting the ball. Therefore, taping or bracing should emphasize limiting inversion primarily. Players with chronic, recurrent ankle sprains and extreme instability should be referred for possible surgical reconstruction of the lateral ligaments.

Peroneal Tendon Subluxation or Dislocation. Subluxation or dislocation of the peroneal tendon can be one cause of chronic lateral ankle pain. It can occur with forceful ankle plantar flexion and inversion as the peroneal tendon sheath is torn (85). This allows the peroneus brevis to dislocate anteriorly to the lateral malleolus. Despite being the most common tendon dislocation in the foot and ankle, it is still frequently mistaken for a lateral ankle sprain. A split in the tendon also can occur and result in recurrent episodes of peroneal subluxation. A good test to detect these "snapping" peroneal tendons is to have the player roll his or her foot in circles. Another test to elicit subluxation is to perform resisted eversion and dorsiflexion of the ankle.

Radiographs are usually normal but may reveal a small wafer of bone in the event of a severe sheath or peroneus brevis avulsion. Acute cases can be treated with 3 weeks of immobilization but chronic cases require surgical debridement and reconstruction of the tendon sheath (85).

Ankle Fractures. Although ankle fractures are not the career-threatening injuries they once were, their frequency and severity make them problematic for soccer players. Because precise anatomic restoration is necessary to maximize function and minimize osteoarthritis, surgery is usually recommended for competitive players. The biomechanical tolerances of the ankle are so demanding that even a malalignment of 2 mm can lead to disability. Accurate classification of the fracture based on the mechanism of injury and the radiographic appearance will help to guide surgical treatment. The Lauge-Hansen system and the AO system of classifying ankle fractures are the two most commonly used.

Achilles Tendonopathy and Rupture. The ankle is unique in that all of its tendons cross at least two joints. It is, therefore, particularly susceptible to overuse syndromes. These problems can be exacerbated by poor anatomic alignment, surface conditions, or footwear. Conditions can range from mild inflammation and microscopic breakdown to partial or complete tendon rupture. A recent article by Kaanus and Jozsa (86) disclosed preexistent degenerative changes in 97% of Achilles tendons that sustained spontaneous rupture. Changes included tendolipomatoses and calcifying tendinopathy. Despite this, spontaneous rupture occurs in 66% of cases without prodromal symptoms.

In Achilles tendonosis, players present with complaints of calf or heel pain that will often track diffusely along the heel cord. It is worsened during kicking or passive ankle plantar flexion. Overuse leads to microscopic disorganization of the tendon's collagenous bundles. It should be distinguished on physical exam from discrete tendon tears or bursitis. Inspection may disclose diffuse swelling, erythema, and tenderness. Thompson's "squeeze" test of the calf will be negative. Hind-foot varus is sometimes an associated finding.

Radiographic exam is usually negative, but occasional Hagland's exostoses are seen at the calcaneal insertion of the heel cord. MRI scanning or ultrasound also can help differentiate tendonosis from partial tendon rupture.

Treatment should begin with a temporary heel lift, NSAIDs, and a gentle stretching program. Failing this, local excision of the microscopic nests of interstitial degeneration with their central necrotic cores can be performed. Steroid injection in and around the Achilles tendon is to be avoided, because this is a relatively avascular area and the risk of heel cord rupture is increased.

Propagation of local tissue necrosis can result in eventual partial or complete attritional rupture of the tendon. Chronic partial Achilles tendon ruptures do poorly, with approximately 75% unable to return to strenuous activities (87). Chronic partial tears should be explored and repaired early for best results (88).

Acute partial and complete ruptures of the Achilles tendon are seen in the older soccer player and can sometimes be missed. Diagnosis is confirmed by clinical evidence of a positive Thompson's squeeze test of the calf. A palpable defect in the tendon's contour is not always evident. Active plantar flexion of the foot can be misleading because of intact posterior tibial tendon function.

Open surgical repair of Achilles tendon ruptures in soccer players offers the most reliable and predictable results. Closed treatment of these lesions has a recurrence rate nearly twice that of surgical repair (89–91).

Ankle Impingement Syndromes. Impingement syndromes of the foot and ankle are extremely common in soccer players but remain a diagnostic and therapeutic challenge to the clinician. First described by Morris (92) in 1943, and later termed "footballer's ankle" by McMurray (93) in 1950, tibiotalar osteophytes are frequently observed on routine ankle radiographs of soccer players (Fig. 36.8). Monto et al. (94) noted tibiotalar spur formation in 60% of young elite male soccer players; posterior osteophytes were noted in 12%. Similar high incidences also were described by Massada (95). Although the young player may initially be asymptomatic, continued anterior and posterior tibiotalar capsular traction and impingement over a career may lead to chronic ankle pain (Fig. 36.9). In its most severe form, surgical resection of calcified capsular tissue may be necessary if a trial of conservative treatment is unsuccessful.

The os trigonum syndrome is primarily seen in soccer players, ballet dancers, and javelin throwers (96). It presents as vague posterior ankle pain worsened by kicking or passive ankle dorsiflexion. Retrocalcaneal tenderness is noted on physical exam and the differential diagnosis includes Achilles tendonitis, retrocalcaneal bursitis, flexor hallucis peritendonosis, and local stress fractures.

Radiographic evidence of an os trigonum is neces-

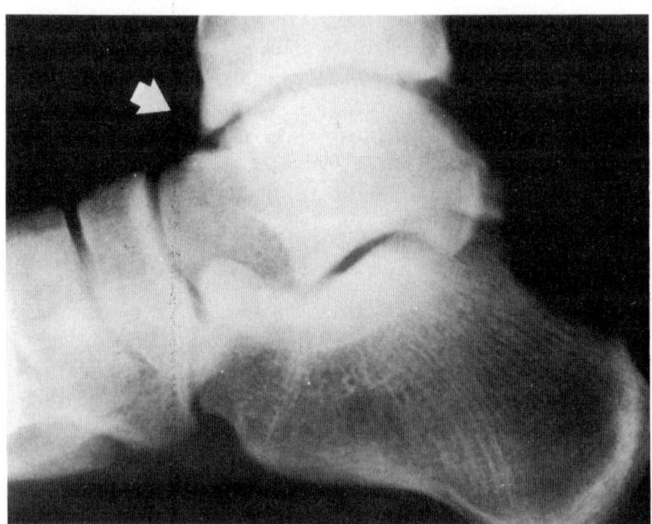

Figure 36.8. Anterior ankle tibial osteophyte *(arrow)*.

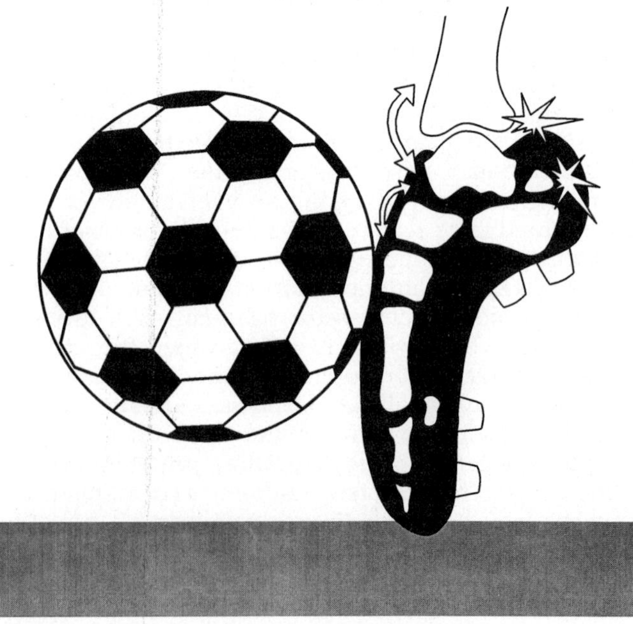

Figure 36.9. Mechanism of anterior traction and posterior impingement of the ankle during the soccer kick.

sary for the diagnosis but not specific for it. Ossa trigona represents a persistent osseous remnant of the posterior calcaneal synchondrosis that normally fuses by age 11. They are found in up to 7% of the general population but were present in 32% of the soccer players reviewed by Monto et al. (94). The incidence is so high that it probably represents a developmental adaptation to the stresses of soccer rather than being congenital in nature. Chronic posterior impingement of the talocalcaneal joint during instep kicking may result in failure of the synchondrosis to ossify or lead to a stress fracture of the posterior talar process.

Symptomatic ossa trigona should be treated conservatively with rest, ice, and short-course NSAIDs. Persistent discomfort may require surgical resection of the bony fragments and inspection of the flexor hallucis longus tendon to rule out peritendonosis or synovitis (96).

Other Tendonitis about the Ankle. Peroneal tendinitis is frequently encountered in soccer players and presents as diffuse lateral retromalleolar pain. It is usually associated with slight heel valgus or tibial varus. Routine radiographs will occasionally disclose calcifications in the region of the peroneal tendon sheath but are often negative. Acute cases can be treated successfully with a lateral heel wedge insert and a brief course of NSAIDs. In refractory or chronic cases, surgical exploration and debridement of degenerative tissue should be considered before an attritional rupture or partial split occurs (86). MRI may be useful in localizing such degenerative changes in the tendon and facilitate surgical planning.

Posterior tibial tendonitis is more common in soccer than other sports because the foot is repetitively forced into hyperpronation during the kick. Symptoms include arch and medial retromalleolar pain. The differential diagnosis includes medial ankle sprain, accessory navicular syndrome, flexor hallucis longus tendonitis, and tarsal tunnel syndrome. Initial treatment should include a medial heel wedge insert and NSAIDs. As in peroneal tendonitis, MRI scanning may disclose discrete areas of degeneration within the tendon. Treatment in these situations should be aggressive because of the potential for tendon disruption. Inability to perform a routine single-legged heel rise on the involved side should raise suspicion of an attritional rupture (so-called acquired flat foot).

Tendonitis of the flexor hallucis longus (FHL) tendon can also present as medial retromalleolar ankle pain. It can be seen alone or in combination with posterior ankle impingement syndromes (96). It results from repetitive hyperplantar flexion of the ankle during kicking. The FHL tendon is particularly vulnerable to irritation because of its passage through a fibroosseous canal, extending from the posterior talus to the sustentaculum tali, and its pully-like mechanism of action. Once established, FHL tendonitis is difficult to treat in soccer players because the flexibility of the toe box and the low-cut design of the shoe accentuate the normal excursion of the FHL tendon. Irritation and thickening of the FHL tendon causes it to catch within its fibroosseous canal and begins a cycle of spiraling inflammation and eventual degenerative damage.

A local injection of 1% lidocaine should eliminate pain with forced plantarflexion and will confirm the diagnosis. This test should help differentiate FHL tendonitis from retrocalcaneal bursitis—another common problem in soccer players, which results from the ankle rubbing against the stiff heel counter of the shoe. Early treatment of FHL tendonitis should include early restrictive taping of the ankle and first metatarsophalangeal joint. If this fails, immobilization may be required. In refractory cases, local debridement may safely be performed through a medial retromalleolar approach with isolation of the neurovascular bundle.

Foot Injuries

Midfoot Sprains. Tarsometatarsal junction injury can occur when the foot is hyperextended and overloaded during a tackle. Repetitive microtrauma and macrotrauma in the midfoot probably accounts for the unexpectedly high incidence of osteophytes in this region seen on plain radiographs of soccer players (94). Acute tarsometatarsal dislocation (Lisfranc injury) is rare in soccer players, but chronic stresses can lead to indolent chronic midfoot pain secondary to ligamentous attrition. The presence of dorsal osteophytes in this zone on radiographs may be adaptive rather than pathologic, so plain films are only diagnostic if subtle evidence of dissociation is seen with bilateral comparative weight-bearing studies.

Plantar Fasciitis. The plantar fascia spans from its origin on the calcaneal tubercle to its insertions at the bases of the proximal phalanges. During phalangeal dorsiflexion at push-off, the plantar fascia tightens by a windlass action and the longitudinal arch is elevated. Repetitive microtrauma during bursts of sprinting can lead to significant damage to the plantar fascia in soccer players and cause arch or heel pain. Microscopic tears at the medial calcaneal origin of the plantar fascia are most commonly seen.

Symptoms are aggravated by the flexible toe box of soccer shoes, which allow excessive dorsiflexion and exaggerate the windlass effect on the plantar fascia. Heel or plantar arch pain can be reproduced in the affected player by passively dorsiflexing the phalanges of the involved foot. Radiographs will sometimes demonstrate a calcaneal traction spur secondary to chronic inflammation. Additional clinical findings of mild foot cavus, pes planus, or Achilles tendon contracture may be present.

Primary treatment should consist of arch supports to unload the tension on the plantar fascia with weight bearing. Progressive stretching of the heel cord is also sometimes helpful. Oral antiinflammatory medications and ice can also afford some relief. Heel cups and cushions are rarely effective. Almost all cases resolve eventually with conservative management and steroid injections and surgery is rarely necessary.

Fifth Metatarsal Fractures. Acute fractures of the fifth metatarsal occur primarily in two forms: diaphyseal and avulsion. Diaphyseal fractures are similar to

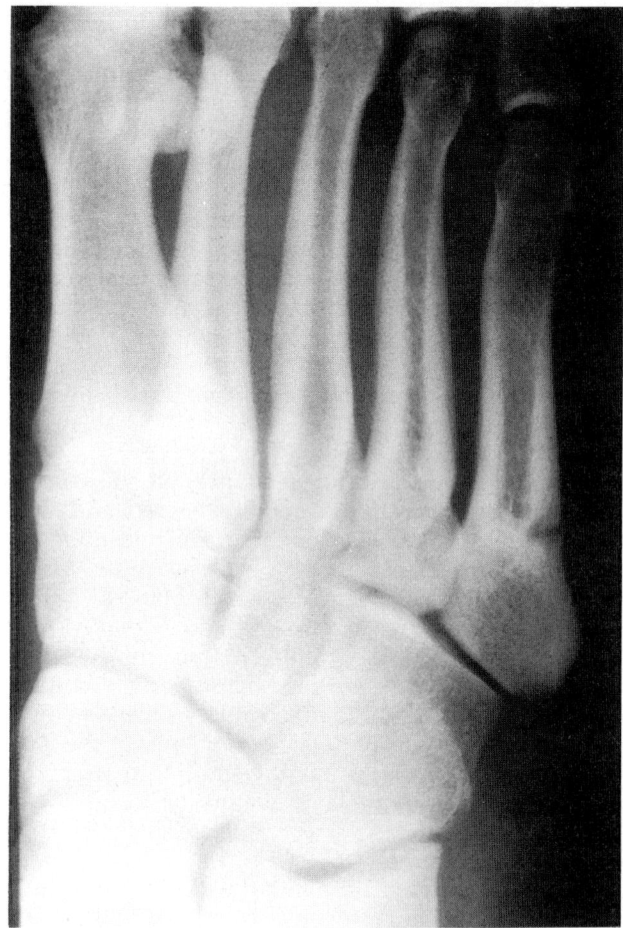

Figure 36.10. Fracture of base of fifth metatarsal.

the classic description of "dancer's fractures" provided by Sir Robert Jones in 1902. It results from forced foot inversion with the heel elevated—a common position for soccer players during tackling. The strong ligamentous attachments between the fifth metatarsal base and the cuboid and fourth metatarsal result in fracture of the diaphysis before dislocation (Fig. 36.10). This fracture is difficult to treat conservatively in the competitive soccer player and may require intramedullary screw fixation for good clinical results.

Avulsion fracture of the base of the fifth metatarsal was once thought to be due to the pull of the peroneous brevis muscle, but is now more correctly acknowledged to be a result of the tough fascial attachments of the plantar aponeurosis and abductor digiti minimi. It may be treated effectively with a short-leg walking cast and rarely results in long-term disability.

Sesamoiditis and Sesamoid Fractures. Pathology of the complex sesamoid-metatarsal-phalangeal joint of the great toe is extremely common among soccer players. Monto et al. (94) noted 47% incidence of partite or fragmented tibial (medial) sesamoids and 19% partite or fragmented fibular (lateral) sesamoids. These figures far exceed the normal incidence of congenitally partite sesamoids in the general population (97). The incidence is so high that it is likely that these too are adaptive changes to the stresses of soccer on the fore foot. Repetitive microtrauma during loading cycles at the halluceal sesamoids during soccer may lead to stress fractures or avascular necrosis from local ischemic insult. Fracture through a previous synchondrosis of a congenitally partite sesamoid also can occur and will cause pain.

There are several reasons why these osseous changes in the sesamoids persist in soccer players. The sesamoids are under constant tensile loading cycles because they are buried in the substance of the flexor hallucis brevis tendon. Because of this, they tend to fracture transversely and have a high nonunion rate. The presence of a metal stud or cleat directly beneath the halluceal metatarsal-phalangeal joint on nearly all soccer shoes may aggravate the problem by increasing local stresses during push off. This may lead to an increase in local ischemia and subsequent avascular necrosis with fragmentation. The diagnosis of sesamoid fracture or fragmentation can be confirmed by comparing clinical findings of localized point tenderness over the sesamoid with an increase in pain on passive dorsiflexion of the toe. Axial radiographs are useful and a bone scan or MRI may provide further diagnostic help (Fig. 36.11). It is difficult to distinguish a discrete sesamoid fracture from sesamoiditis of a congenitally partite sesamoid. Local lidocaine injection can provide pain relief in either case. In the absence of a discrete partite sesamoid with a positive bone scan, the diagnosis of sesamoiditis is more secure.

In either case, treatment is symptomatic with initial rest, ice, and NSAIDs. A custom-molded foot orthosis, incorporating a support proximal to the first metatarsal head can be extremely effective in relieving pain. Cast immobilization may be necessary in both sesamoiditis and stress fractures. If pain becomes refractory, surgical removal of the involved sesamoid has been recommended (98). However complete removal of a sesamoid may result in an imbalanced "cock-up" toe deformity and is not suggested. Return to soccer should be possible even if surgical removal of the fragmented

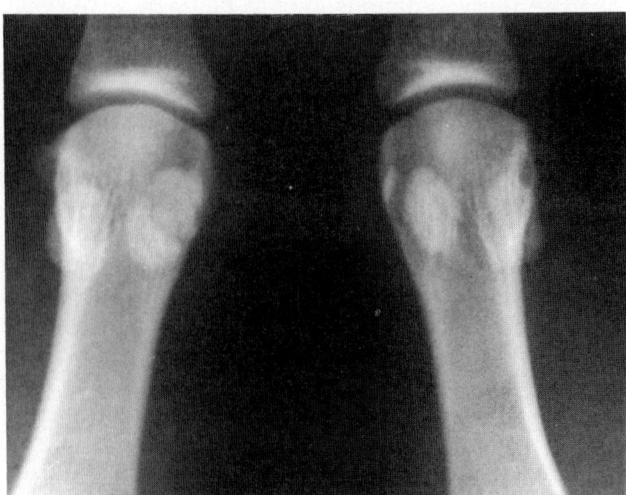

Figure 36.11. Medial sesamoid fracture.

sesamoid is necessary. More typically, the vast majority remain as painless (or tolerably painful) nonunions and require no specific treatment.

Digital Fractures. Contusions to the toes are so common in soccer players that digital, or phalangeal, fractures may go unrecognized. Monto et al. (94) found that 34% of the feet of their group of elite players had previously undiagnosed phalangeal fractures and osteophytes. Osseous damage can easily result from direct trauma during ball strike because of the soft, supple nature of the soccer shoe's toe box. Discrete tenderness of the involved phalanx should alert the physician of a possible fracture and plain radiographs should be obtained. Nondisplaced phalangeal shaft fractures and those that involve less than 30% of the articular surface may be treated conservatively with buddy taping and toe box shoe reinforcement. Displaced fractures require closed reduction, and more severe fractures (i.e., associated with joint subluxation) may necessitate open reduction and internal fixation for a good result. Because of the nature of the sport, toe fractures in soccer players should be treated with the same aggressiveness and expertise that finger fractures would be given in the general athletic population. Protective metallic shoe inserts may be used during the rehabilitation process to hasten healing and return to effective play.

Stress Fractures. Stress fractures of the foot and ankle in soccer are most typically seen in elite or professional players with heavy daily training and game schedules. Stress fractures in the fore foot usually involve the second and third metatarsals, perhaps due to their decreased motion in relation to the midfoot, which results in less contact force distribution and increased local stresses during running. This situation is aggravated by local muscular fatigue and the poor cushioning and support of most soccer shoes. These fractures are usually diaphyseal, whereas stress fractures of the first metatarsal involve the base, because of load transfer to an area with increased cancellus bone content. Stress fractures of the fourth and fifth metatarsals are less common but do occur (99).

Physical exam discloses fusiform swelling, localized tenderness, and pain on passive motion of the involved ray. Radiographs will exhibit a periosteal reaction in diaphysial stress fractures, but can be negative. Basilar stress fractures of the first metatarsal instead display a pattern of basilar sclerosis that may be easily missed. In a case in which clinical suspicion is high in a player with persistent discomfort but negative radiographs, bone scan can be diagnostic (Fig. 36.12). Although a bone scan is the sensitive means of diagnosing stress fractures, it is less specific than other methods such as CT scan. The role of MRI scanning remains unclear, because it may confuse the diagnosis by disclosing subclinical metabolic changes in the bone (99, 100).

Stress fractures of the metatarsals are often already in the healing phase at the time of their diagnosis. Treatment consists of relative rest, i.e., avoidance of pain-producing activity. Immobilization is rarely necessary. Players can be returned to sport earlier when fitted with a custom-molded rigid orthosis. Refractory cases or those involving the fifth metatarsal diaphysis may require casting or surgical fixation.

In contrast to metatarsal stress fractures, stress fractures of the calcaneus, talus, navicular, or malleoli can be quite difficult to diagnose and treat effectively. Players frequently complain of diffuse ankle and midfoot

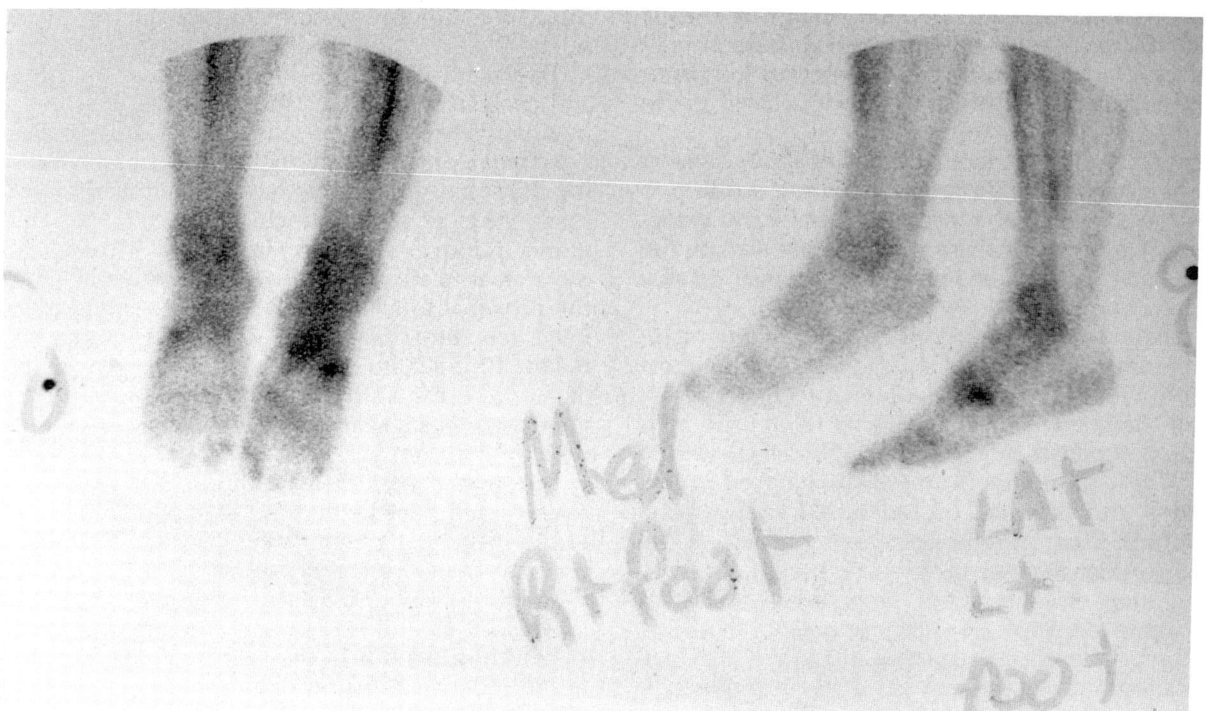

Figure 36.12. Bone scan of 23-year-old soccer player, demonstrating stress fractures of the fifth metatarsal.

pain during running and shooting that is hard to localize. Tarsal-navicular stress fractures are frequently occult on plain radiographs because of routine underpenetration (101). Fatigue fractures in this region are located in the central third of the navicular and are linear in orientation. They tend to begin as incomplete fractures dorsally and propagate to complete fractures if left untreated. Bone scan, plain tomography, and/or CT scanning will confirm the diagnosis.

Initial treatment should include 6 to 8 weeks of cast immobilization. Radiographic evidence of a nonunion does not necessarily preclude a good clinical result, but persistent symptoms may necessitate eventual bone grafting and internal fixation.

Calcaneal stress fractures are infrequent but remain part of the differential diagnosis of heel pain in the soccer player. Symptoms can lead to its delayed diagnosis and confusion with plantar fasciitis, retrocalcaneal bursitis, os trigonum syndrome, and Achilles peritendonosis, which are all common problems in soccer players. Because the calcaneus is primarily composed of cancellus bone, stress fractures appear as dense sclerotic lines on plain radiographs oriented parallel to the line of pull of the Achilles tendon. The diagnosis can be confirmed by bone scan, plain lateral tomography, or CT scanning.

Stress fractures of the talus, cuboid, or cuneiforms are uncommon. However, the possibility of avascular necrosis of the dome of the talus should be considered in complaints of persistent ankle pain.

Malleolar stress fractures can occur in soccer players complaining of persistent pain, especially in the setting of recurrent ankle sprains. Plain radiographs should be inspected carefully for subtle fracture lines oriented perpendicularly to the plafond. Because they are potentially unstable fractures, internal fixation of medial malleolar fractures should be performed. Lateral malleolar stress fractures have a lower potential for nonunion and can be effectively treated with closed methods.

In general, persistent foot and ankle pain in a soccer player should lead to a thorough diagnostic workup to rule out the presence of a stress fracture. Early recognition and treatment of these injuries may obviate the need for later surgical management because of displacement or nonunion.

Turf-Toe. Turf-toe is an injury to the plantar capsule of the metatarsophalangeal (MTP) joint of the great toe. It was first described in American football players following the introduction of artificial turf in the mid-1960s (102). A partial tear of the plantar capsule of the hallucal MTP joint occurs from repetitive forced hyperdorsiflexion and overload caused by flexibility of the standard turf shoe and the increased traction of the surface. Capsular damage in this zone is aggravated by increased shear stresses across the halluceal MTP joint during cutting and push off. Microruptures in the flexor hallucis brevis muscle and collateral ligaments also may be associated and sesamoidal fractures or fragmentations can be seen with this painful condition.

The diagnosis is made by clinical findings of a tender, swollen halluceal MTP joint with increased tenderness on passive dorsiflexion. Initial treatment should include rest, ice, a brief course of NSAIDs, and protective taping to limit MTP dorsiflexion. More severe cases may warrant the use of orthoses or a wooden healing shoe until symptoms resolve. Surgery is only beneficial in cases for which dorsal subluxation of the joint is present or severe osteoarthrosis necessitates arthrodesis of the joint.

Reverse Turf-Toe (Soccer Toe). First described in ballet dancers, reverse turf-toe condition refers to acute and chronic capsular damage to the dorsal aspect of the halluceal MTP joint (103). It results from repetitive forced hyperplantar flexion of the joint, especially during instep ball strike because of the supple nature of the shoe toe box.

The diagnosis is confirmed by physical exam, with swelling and tenderness of the halluceal MTP joint. Pain is exacerbated by passive plantarflexion of the joint. This condition is somewhat less refractory in soccer than turf-toe and generally responds well to conservative treatment with taping to prevent MTP dorsiflexion. Orthoses are rarely needed. However, chronic involvement can lead to hallux rigidus.

Hallux Rigidis. Hallus rigidus represents posttraumatic arthrosis of the hallucal MTP joint secondary to previous fracture, osteochondritis, avascular necrosis, turf-toe, or soccer toe. Dorsal osteophytes form at the halluceal MTP joint, with subsequent pain and stiffness while cutting or pushing off.

Diagnosis is made by the presence of a chronically stiff and tender halluceal MTP joint with a painful, decreased range of motion. Radiographs generally demonstrate evidence of dorsal ostephytic impingement. A diagnostic intraarticular injection with 1% lidocaine provides temporary pain relief and aids in the diagnosis.

Treatment options include the usual rest, NSAIDs, and protective taping or shoe orthosis. However these treatments are often unsatisfactory, and more aggressive therapy is generally required. Intraarticular steroid injection is unpredictable but can help early in the disease. Surgical options include chilectomy, which requires removal of approximately 30% of the dorsal metatarsal head; a dorsally based wedge osteotomy of the proximal phalanx; MTP arthrodesis; and metatarsal head resection. Halluceal MTP arthrodesis is recommended for advanced disease in soccer players because of the need for a strong push off during running. Still, younger players with less severe disease may do well with an osteotomy.

Subungual Hematomas of the Toes. Most soccer players will sustain numerous subungual hematomas of the toes during their career. These injuries generally occur to the great toe as the result of a direct crush by the foot of another player or from the shear stresses of sudden stops and starts as the toe impacts against the close-fitting toe box of the soccer cleat. For many players the toenail becomes dystrophic as the result of repeated damage to the nailbed. Although seldom a serious problem, it can become so troublesome that some professional players have been known to have the toenail of their great toe permanently removed just to prevent its recurrence.

An acute subungual hematoma can be quite painful and the initial treatment should involve releasing the pressure of the blood collected beneath the nail. This can be accomplished with a special drill designed specifically for this purpose; a more convenient technique involves heating the end of a paper clip wire and burning a hole through the nail.

Generally, the nail should be left intact even if it is detached from the nailbed. It should be taped in place if necessary to protect the nailbed as the new nail grows out.

Special Concerns

Indoor Soccer

Indoor soccer is played with only five players on a side on an artificial turf the size of an ice hockey rink. The goal is smaller and the ball may be played off the side walls. It tends to be a much quicker game with more sudden stops and starts and changes in direction. Hoff and Martin (37) found the incidence of injuries in indoor youth soccer to be 4.5 times higher than that observed in outdoor soccer. However, the reporting methods were quite variable and based on survey responses rather than a prospective analysis; therefore, the numbers may be imprecise. Differences in field size and surface, game speed, officiating, and player numbers were all possible causes cited for the increased incidence of injury observed in the indoor game. Another study from Germany found no greater incidence of injuries among adults in the indoor game except for a slightly greater percentage of muscle-tendon injuries (104).

Artificial Surfaces

Ekstrand and Nigg (105) reviewed surface-related injuries in soccer and found that most authors reported no significant increases in injury frequencies on artificial turf. They believed that players who alternate frequently between grass and artificial surface may be at higher risk for injury and thought that a period of adaptation and the use of proper shoe wear would reduce the risk. As more and more facilities adopt artificial turf because of its ease of maintainance, there will be more opportunities to observe any possible differences in injury patterns.

Women's Soccer

The number of women playing soccer has increased rapidly in the past two decades. In a survey conducted by the Soccer Industry Council of America, 38% of females surveyed reported having played soccer at least once during 1989. Most of these (79%) were under age 18. It was estimated that 5.8 million women and girls in the United States participate in soccer at some level.

As mentioned previously, girls under age 12 seem about twice as likely to be injured as boys in soccer. The reasons for this are obscure and have been variously ascribed to differences in physical development, psychomotor coordination, and behavioral patterns. The common practice of mixing boys and girls on the same team at young ages may also be a contributer.

At collegiate and adult levels, overall injury rates for men and women appear to be comparable, but few studies of elite female players have been done. Engstrom et al. (36) reported a significantly higher injury incidence in a study of 41 elite female players in Sweden. The overall incidence of injury was 12/1000 AE with a rate of 24/1000 AE for games and 7/1000 AE for practices. This compared with an overall injury incidence of 5/1000 AE for men at the same level. Engstrom et al. noted that the mean training time for the female players was half that of the males and posited this may have been a factor in the higher injury rate among the women. In the NCAA, where training times are similar for men and women, the overall injury incidence for women was 7.96/1000 AE compared with 7.66/1000 AE for men (3).

In both of these series women were observed to have a greater incidence of knee injuries than their male counterparts. Engstrom et al. found that 23% of all injuries involved the knee, with 17% of players sustaining major injuries involving ligament or meniscus tears. NCAA statistics reveal the incidence of ACL injuries among women to be twice as high as that occurring in the men. This finding mirrors that for other pivoting sports such as basketball. The reason for the high incidence of knee injuries in female soccer players, particularly injuries to the ACL, is unknown. Differences in strength, flexibility, knee anatomy and biomechanics, personality types, and playing styles have all been suggested but no studies have actually examined any of these factors in detail.

Moller-Nielsen and Hammer (106) found a significantly higher incidence of injuries in women during the premenstrual and menstrual period compared with other times of the menstrual cycle. This was attributed to both the physiologic and psychological symptoms that occur during this time such as increased irritability and breast and abdominal pain and cramping.

The physical training and nutritional requirements of female soccer players do not differ significantly from those of men. Douglas (107) examined the hematologic status of 30 collegiate women soccer players through a competitive season and found no evidence that strenuous physical training caused iron-deficiency anemia. However, coaches, trainers, and clinicians should be alert for what has been called the "female athlete triad": amenorrhea, osteoporosis, and disordered eating. Exercise-induced oligomenorrhea or amenorrhea (less than three menstrual periods per year) results from a complex combination of nutritional deficiency, hypoestrogenemia, low body weight, stress, and increased training intensity (especially when premenarchal). Eating disorders such as bulimia and anorexia nervosa and the abuse of diuretics, laxatives, and diet pills has been found in a disturbingly high percentage of competitive female college athletes (108). The combination of these two disorders may result in bone demineralization or osteoporosis and resultant stress fractures of the lower extremities. Female players with unusual weight loss or suspected eating disorders should be referred for nutritional and/or psychiatric counseling.

Youth Soccer

The U.S. Youth Soccer Association registered 1,405,186 players in 1987–1988. This represented more than a 10-fold increase over the 1974–1975 season. The Soccer Industry Council of America estimated 12,009,000 participants under age 18 in the United States. Soccer currently ranks third (after basketball and volleyball) in team sport participation in children under age 18. Under age 12, soccer ranks second. Approximately 46% of all soccer players in the United States are in the 6- to 11-year-old age group.

Injury patterns are different in children and may involve problems not common in adult players. Children are less likely to sustain serious injuries. Contusions and abrasions are the most common injuries and most of these do not result in lost playing time. Most studies of youth soccer have found a slightly higher incidence of upper extremity injuries compared with adult levels. This may be the result of more frequent falls, illegal ball contact, decreased technical expertise, and greater fragility of upper extremity epiphyses.

In the lower extremities, epiphyseal and avulsion fractures, slipped capital femoral epiphysis, and subcapital compression fractures should always be considered when evaluating children's soccer injuries. Apophysitis of the iliac crest, tibial tuberosity (Osgood-Schlatter disease), calcaneus (Sever disease), fifth metatarsal should be suspected in youth players presenting with chronic focal pain at these sites.

The effects of soccer training programs on prepubescent children have been examined. Berg et al. (109) found no significant changes in cardiorespiratory fitness, peak knee torque, or flexibility in a group of 11-year-old boys following a 12-week soccer conditioning program. Mosher et al. (110), however, did find significant increases in aerobic fitness in this same age group following a similar 12-week training program. Although slight gains in aerobic capacity can be achieved through endurance training, the emphasis in youth soccer is probably better aimed at developing basic individual skills and concepts of team play.

REFERENCES

1. Abramson SB. Nonsteroidal anti-inflammatory drugs: mechanisms of action and therapeutic considerations. In Leadbetter WB, Buckwalter JA, Gordon SL, eds. Sports induced inflammation. Park Ridge, IL: American Academy of Orthopedic Surgeons, 1990:421–430.
2. Soccer Industry Council of America. National soccer participation survey. North Palm Beach, FL: America Sports Data, 1988.
3. National Collegiate Athletic Association. Injury surveillance system: Men's and women's soccer injury/exposure summaries, 1986–87 to 1991–92. Overland Park, KS: NCAA, 1992.
4. Keller D, Henneman MC, Alegria J. Fussball: der elfmeter. Leistungsport 1979;9:394–398.
5. Gainor BJ, Piotrowski G, Puhl JJ, Allen WC. The kick: biomechanics and collision injury. Am J Sports Med 1978:6:185–193.
6. Fields KB. Head injuries in soccer. Phys Sportsmed 1989;17(1):69.
7. Schneider K, Zernicke RF. Computer simulation of head impact: estimation of head injury risk during soccer heading. Int J Sport Biomech 1988;4(4):358–371.
8. Townend MS. Is heading the ball a dangerous activity? In: Reilly T, Lees A, Davids K, et al., eds. Science and football: proceedings of the First World Congress of Science and Football. London: E&FN Spon Ltd, 1987:237–242.
9. Levendusky TA, Amstrong CW, Eck JS, Jeziorowski J, Kugler L. Impact characteristics of two types of soccer balls. In: Reilly T, Lees A, Davids K, et al., eds. Science and football. Proceedings of the First World Congress of Science and Football. London, E&FN Spon, Ltd.
10. Burslem I, Lees A. Quantification of impact accelerations of the head during the heading of a football. In: Reilly T, Lees A, Davids K, et al., eds. Science and football: proceedings of the First World Congress of Science and Football. London: E&FN Spon Ltd., 1987:243–248.
11. Reilly T, Thomas V. A motion analysis of work-rate in different positional roles in professional football match-play. J Hum Move Stud 1976;2:87–97.
12. Kirkendall DT. The applied sport science of soccer. Phys Sportsmed 1985;13(4):53–59.
13. Mayhew SR, Wenger HA. Time-motion analysis of professional soccer. J Hum Move 1989;11(1):49–52.
14. Ekblom B. Applied physiology of soccer. Sports Med 1986;3:50–60.
15. Shephard RJ, Leatt P. Carbohydrate and fluid needs of the soccer player. Sports Med 1987;4:164–176.
16. Dibner R. The footballer's heart and its adaptation to physical exercise (Communications to the Second World Congress on Science and Football. J Sports Sci 1992;10:141.
17. Kuzon W, Rosenblatt J, Huebel C, Leatt P, Plyley M, McKee N, Jacobs I. Skeletal muscle fiber type, fiber size, and capillary supply in elite soccer players. Int J. Sports Med 1990;11:99–102.
18. Miles A, MacLaren D, Reilly T, Yamanaka K. An analysis of physiological strain in four-a-side women's soccer (Communications to the Second World Congress on Science and Football). J Sports Sci 1992;10:142.
19. Viviani F, Casagrande G. Somatotype in a group of adolescent soccer players (Communications to the Second World Congress on Science and Football). J Sports Sci 1992;10:158.
20. Garganta J, Maia J, Pinto J: Somatotype, body composition and physical performance capacity of elite young soccer players (Communications to the Second World Congress on Science and Football). J Sports Sci 1992;10:157.
21. Agre JC, Baxter TL. Musculoskeletal profile of male collegiate soccer players. Arch Phys Med Rehab 1987;68:147–150.
22. Tumilty D, Darby S. Physiological characteristics of Australian female soccer players (Communications to the Second World Congress on Science and Football). J Sports Sci 1992;10:145.
23. Davis JA, Brewer J. Physiological characteristics of an international female soccer squad (Communications to the Second World Congress on Science and Football). J Sports Sci 1992;10:142.
24. Rhodes EC, Mosher RE. Aerobic and anaerobic characteristics of elite female university soccer players (Communications to the Second World Congress on Science and Football). J Sports Sci 1992;10:143.
25. Comas ES, Gioarolla RA, Pereira MHN, Matsudo VKR. A comparison of the physical fitness of football players at different levels (Communications to the Second World Congress on Science and Football). J Sports Sci 1992;10:142.
26. Brewer J, Davis JA: A physiological comparison of English professional and semi-professional soccer players (Communications to the Second World Congress on Science and Football). J Sports Sci 1992;10:146.
27. Parente C, Montagnani S, DeNicola A, Tajana GF. Anthropometric and morphological characteristics of soccer players according to positional role (Communications to the Second World Congress on Science and Football). J Sports Sci 1992;10:155.
28. Matkovic BR, Jankovic S, Heimer S. Physiological profile of top soccer players (Communications to the Second World Congress on Science and Football). J Sports Sci 1992;10:152.
29. Jacobs I, Westlin N, Rasmusson M, Houghton B. Muscle glyco-

gen and diet in elite soccer players. Eur J Appl Physiol 1982;48:297–302.

30. Elias S, Roberts W, Thorson D: Team sports in hot weather. Guidelines for modifying youth soccer. Phy Sportsmed 1991;19(5):67.
31. Albert M. Descriptive three year data study of outdoor and indoor professional soccer injuries. Athletic Train 1983;18:218–220.
32. Backous DD, Friedl KE, Smith NJ, Parr TJ, Carpine WD, Jr. Soccer injuries and their relation to physical maturity. Am J Dis Child 1988;142(8):839–842.
33. Berger-Vachon C, Gabard G, Moyen B. Soccer accidents in the French Rhone-Alpes Soccer Association. Sports Med 1986;3(1):69–77.
34. DeHaven KE, Lintner DM. Athletic injuries: comparison by age, sport, and gender. Amer J Sports Med 1986;14(3):218–224.
35. Ekstrand J, Gillquist J: Soccer injuries and their mechanisms: a prospective study. Med Sci Sports Exerc 1983;15(3):267–270.
36. Engstrom B, Johansson C, Tornkvist H: Soccer injuries among elite female players. Am J Sports Med 1991;19(4):372–374.
37. Hoff GL, Martin TA. Outdoor and indoor soccer: injuries among youth players. Am J Sports Med 1986;14(3):231–233.
38. Hoy K, Lindblad BE, Terkelsen CJ, Helleland HE, Terkelsen CJ. European soccer injuries: a prospective epidemiologic and socioeconomic study. Am J Sports Med 1992;20(3):318–322.
39. Hunt M, Fulford S. Amateur soccer: injuries in relation to field position. Br J Sports Med 1990;24(4):265.
40. Maehlum S, Dahl E, Daljord OA. Frequency of injuries in a youth soccer tournament. Phys Sportsmed 1986;14(7):73–79.
41. McMaster WC, Walter M. Injuries in soccer. Am J Sports Med 1978;6(6):354–357.
42. Nielsen AB, Yde J. Epidemiology and traumatology of injuries in soccer. Am J Sports Med 1989;17(6):803–807.
43. Nilsson S, Roaas A. Soccer injuries in adolescents. Am J Sports Med 1978;6(6):358–361.
44. Pritchett J. Cost of high school soccer injuries. Am J Sports Med 1981;9(1):64–66.
45. Sadat-Ali M, Sankaran-Kutty M. Soccer injuries in Saudi Arabia. Am J Sports Med 1987;15(5):500–502.
46. Sandelin J, Santavirta S, Kiviluoto O: Acute soccer injuries in Finland in 1980. Br J Sports Med 1980;19(1):30–33.
47. Schmidt-Olsen S, Bunemann L, Lade V, Brassoe J. Soccer injuries of youth. Br J Sports Med 1985;19:161–164.
48. Sullivan J, Gross R, Grana W, Garcia-Moral C: Evaluation of injuries in youth soccer. Am J Sports Med 1980;8(5):325–327.
49. Yde J, Nielsen AB. Sports injuries in adolescents' ball games: soccer, handball and basketball. Br J Sports Med 1990;24(1):51–54.
50. Ekstrand J, Gillquist J, Liljedahl S: Prevention of soccer injuries. Amer J Sports Med 1983;11(3):116–120.
51. Ekstrand J, Roos H, Tropp H. Normal course of events amongst Swedish soccer players: an 8-year follow-up study. Br J Sports Med 1990;24(2):117–119.
52. Ekstrand J, Gillquist J. The frequency of muscle tightness and injuries in soccer players. Am J Sports Med 1982;10(2):75–78.
53. Ekstrand J, Gillquist J, Moller M, Oberg B, Liljedahl S. Incidence of soccer injuries and their relation to training and team success. Am J Sports Med 1983;11(2):63–67.
54. Ekstrand J, Gillquist J. The avoidability of soccer injuries. Int J Sports Med 1983;4:124–128.
55. Sane J, Ylipaavalniemi P. Maxillofacial and dental soccer injuries in Finland. Br J Oral Maxillofac Surg 1987;25:383–390.
56. Nysether S. Dental injuries among Norwegian soccer players. Community Dent Oral Epidemiol 1987;15(3):141–143.
57. Burke MJ, Sanitato JJ, Vinger PF, Raymond LA, Kulwin DR. Soccerball-induced eye injuries. JAMA 1983;249:2682–2685.
58. Orlando RG. Soccer-related eye injuries in children and adolescents. Phys Sportsmed 1988;16(11):103–106.
59. Tysvaer AT, Storli OV. Soccer injuries to the brain: A neurologic and electroencephalographic study of active football players. Am J Sports Med 1989;17(4):573–578.
60. Tysvaer AT, Storli OV, Bachen NI. Soccer injuries to the brain: a neurologic and electroencephalographic study of former players. Am J Sports Med 1991;19(1):56–60.
61. Aross R, Ohler K, Barolin GS. Cerebral trauma due to heading: computerized EEG analysis in football players. Z EEG EMG 1983;14:209–212.
62. Sortland O, Tysvaer AT. Brain damage in former association football players: an evaluation by cerebral computed tomography. Neuroradiology 1989;31(1):44–48.
63. Curtin J, Kay N. Hand injuries due to soccer. Hand 1976;8(1):93–95.
64. Smodlaka V. Groin pain in soccer players. Phys Sportsmed 1980;8(8):57–61.
65. Martens MA, Hansen L, Mulier JC: Adductor tendinitis and musculus abdominis tendopathy. Am J Sports Med 1987;15(3):353–356.
66. Mozes M, Papa M, Horoszowski H, Adar R. Iliopsoas injury in soccer players. Br J Sports Med 1985;19(3):168–170.
67. Ekberg O, Persson NH, Abrahamsson PA, Westlin NE, Lilja B. Longstanding groin pain in athletes: a multidisciplinary approach. Sports Med 1988;6(1):56–61.
68. Taylor D, Meyers W, Moylan J, Lohnes J, Bassett F, Garrett W. Abdominal musculature abnormalities as a cause of groin pain in athletes. Am J Sports Med 1991;19(3):239–242.
69. Volpi P, Melegati G: La pubalgia del calciatore: aspetti eziopatogenetici e classificativi. Ital J Sports Trauma 1986;8(4):271–274.
70. Van Vlierberghe L. Adductor and rectus abdominis injuries among soccer players (Communications to the Second World Congress on Science and Football). J Sports Sci 1992;10:187.
71. Martens MA, Lilbrecht P, Burssens A: Surgical treatment of the iliotibial band friction syndrome. Am J Sports Med 1989;17:651–654.
72. Walton M, Rothwell AG. Reactions of thigh tissues of sheep to blunt trauma. Clin Orthop 1983;176:273–281.
73. Antao NA. Myositis of the hip in a professional soccer player. Amer J Sports Med 1988;16(1):82–83.
74. Leach RE, Corbett M. Anterior tibial compartment syndrome in soccer players. Amer J Sports Med 1979;7:258–259.
75. Garrett WE. Muscle strain injuries; clinical and basic aspects. Med Sci Sports Exerc 1990;22(4):436–443.
76. Nikolaou P, MacDonald B, Glisson R, Seaber A, Garrett W. Biomechanical and histological evaluation of muscle after controlled strain injury. Am J Sports Med 1987;15(1):9–14.
77. Safran M, Garrett W, Sieber A, Glisson R, Ribbeck B. The role of warm-up in injury prevention. Am J Sports Med 1988;16(2):123–129.
78. Taylor D, Dalton J, Seaber A, Garrett W. Viscoelastic properties of muscle-tendon units. Am J Sports Med 1990;18(3):300–309.
79. Engstrom B, Forssblad M, Johansson C, Tornkvist H: Does a major knee injury definitely sideline an elite soccer player? Am J Sports Med 1990;18(1):101–105.
80. Chantraine A. Knee joint in soccer players: osteoarthritis and axis deviation. Med Sci Sports Exerc 1985;17(6):434–439.
81. Van Laack W. Experimental studies of the effectiveness of various shinguards in association football [Abstract]. Z Orthop 1985;123:951–956.
82. Jaccia GE, Gatti U, Pavolini B, Acanfora A. Leg fractures of football players today. In: Santilli G, ed. Sports medicine applied to football, proceedings of the conference. Rome: MGA, 1990:244–254.
83. Ekstrand J, Tropp H. The incidence of ankle sprains in soccer. Foot Ankle 1990;11(1):41–44.
84. Hattori K, Ohta S. Ankle joint flexibility in college soccer players. J Hum Ergol (Tokyo) 1986;15(1):85–89.
85. Arrowsmith SR, Fleming LL, Allman FL: Traumatic dislocations of the peroneal tendons. Am J Sports Med 1983;11:142–146.
86. Kaanus P, Jozsa L. Histopathological changes preceding spontaneous rupture of a tendon. J Bone Joint Surg 1991;73A(10):1507–1525.
87. Allemark C, Renstrom P, Peterson L and Irstam L. Ten year follow-up of conservatively treated partial ruptures of the Achilles tendon. Paper Presented at the American Academy of Orthopedic Surgeons, New Orleans, February 1990.
88. Nelen G, Martens M, Burssens A. Surgical treatment of chronic Achilles tendonitis. Am J Sports Med 1991;17:754–759.
89. Bradley JP, Tibone JE. Percutaneous and open surgical repairs of Achilles tendon ruptures: a comparative study. Am J Sports Med 1990;18(2):188–195.

90. Mann RA, Holmes GB, Seale KS, Collins DN: Chronic rupture of the Achilles tendon: a new technique of repair. J Bone Joint Surg 1991;73A:214–218.
91. Ma GWC, Griffith TG. Percutaneous repair of acute closed ruptured Achilles tendon: a new technique. Clin Orthop 1977;128:247–255.
92. Morris LH. Athlete's ankle. J Bone Joint Surg 1943;25:220.
93. McMurray TP. Footballer's ankle. J Bone Joint Surg 1950;32B(1):68–69.
94. Monto RR, Lohnes J, Mandelbaum B, Garrett WE. Radiographic abnormalities in the foot and ankle of soccer players. Med Sci Sports Exerc., in press.
95. Massada JL. Ankle overuse injuries in soccer players. J Sports Med Physical Fit 1991;31(3):447–451.
96. Wredemark T, Carlstedt CA, Bauer H, Tonu S. Os trigonum syndrome: a clinical entity in ballet dancers. Foot Ankle 1991;11(6):404–406.
97. Jahss MH. The sesamoids of the hallux. Clin Orthop 1981;157:88–96.
98. Richardson EG. Injuries to the hallical sesamoids in the athlete. Foot Ankle 1987;7(4):229–244.
99. Santi M, Sartosis DJ, Resnick D. Diagnostic imaging of tarsal and metatarsal stress fractures: Part I. Orthop Rev 1989;18(2):178–185.
100. Santi M, Sartosis DJ, Resnick D. Diagnostic imaging of tarsal and metatarsal stress fractures: Part II. Orthop Rev 1989;18(3):205–310.
101. Pavlov H, Torg JS, Freiberger RH. Tarsal navicular stress fractures radiographic evaluation. Radiology 1983;148:641–645.
102. Bowers KD, Martin RB: Turf-toe: a shoe-surface related football injury. Med Sci Sports Exerc 1976;8:81–83.
103. Sammarco GJ, Millar EH. Forefoot conditions in dancers: II. Foot Ankle 1982;3:93–98.
104. Raschka C, Glaser H, Schimmel B, Henke T, de Marees H. Epidemiological characteristics of soccer injuries and proposed programmes for their prevention in Schleswig-Holstein (Communications to the Second World Congress on Science and Football). J Sports Sci 1992;10:189.
105. Ekstrand J, Nigg BM. Surface-related injuries in soccer. Sports Med 1989;8(1):56–62.
106. Moller-Nielsen J, Hammer M. Women's soccer injuries in relation to the menstrual cycle and oral contraceptive use. Med Sci Sports Exerc 1989;21(2):126–129.
107. Douglas P. Effect of a season of competition and training on hematological status of women field hockey and soccer players. J Sports Med Physical Fit 1989;29(2):179–183.
108. Agostini R. Women's fitness and medical disorders. Paper presented at the American Orthopedic Society for Sports Medicine, San Diego, July 6–9, 1992.
109. Berg KE, LaVoie JC, Latin RW. Physiological training effects of playing youth soccer. Med Sci Sports Exerc. 1985;17(6):656–660.
110. Mosher RE, Rhodes EC, Wenger HA, Filsinger B. Interval training: the effects of a 12-week programme on elite, prepubertal male soccer players. J Sports Med 1985;25(1–2):5–9.

37 / SURFING

David A. Stone

In the 200 years since Captain Cook landed in Hawaii, surfing has grown from a pleasure sport to a significant industry for both amateurs and professionals. There may be no sport comparable with that of riding across the face of a moving wave on a specialized board or on one's own body. One has an exhilarating experience that is indescribable. However, whether body surfing or board surfing, there exists a real risk of potentially serious injury and even death, especially for the novice. In this chapter both board and body surfing will be discussed, based primarily on the experience and information derived from the beaches of the island of Oahu in the Hawaiian Islands. A brief history of surfing as well as the incidence and types of injuries and the mechanisms and preventive measures will be discussed.

Historical and Sociologic Background of Surfing

The first form of surfing was probably "belly board" riding. This probably consisted of a small, thin (0.25 to 0.5 inch) board 3 to 4 feet long. It is likely that riding these small belly boards in the prone position was enjoyed by people in various areas of the world, dating back for many centuries. For example, it is known that it was popular in west Africa, where surfing apparently never advanced beyond the belly board stage.

For hundreds of years the Hawaiians rode their heavy koa wood surfboards on waves unseen by foreigners until Captain Cook first landed in the islands. By the early 1900s, surfing had reached California. The legendary Hawaiian Duke Kahanamoku, who represented the United States in the 1912 Olympics and broke the 100-m world swimming record, is credited with popularizing surfing throughout the world.

During the 20th century rapid changes were made in surfboard design. The first breakthrough was the hollow board introduced in 1926 (1). By the 1930s, the boards, although still long (up to 12 feet), were made lighter by combining balsa wood and redwood into a laminated whole or by using plywood shells surrounding a hollow center interrupted by struts, much like airplane wing construction. In the late 1940s and into the 1950s, South American balsa wood was the most popular material for surfboards (2). Also, the fin or "skeg" was introduced to stabilize newer models. Subsequently, in the 1950s board makers coated the soft absorbent balsa wood with Fiberglas to provide a strong, hard outer shell. The balsa and Fiberglas surfboards revolutionized surfing, for although the boards were still relatively long (9 to 12 feet), they were light enough (20 to 30 pounds) so that for the first time one really had control over the waves. It was during this period (1950s) that the giant waves of Makaha Beach on the west coast of Oahu and Sunset Beach and Waimea Bay on the north shore of Oahu were ridden and in a sense, conquered. Waves 25 to 30 feet high were ridden and have been ridden since, but it seems that waves of that size may well be the limit of what can be ridden not only because of limits of the human body's ability to withstand the force of being hit by such a mass of water and the limits of the ability to hold one's breath while being held under water but also because waves of this size bring fear into the hearts of even the bravest surfer, so that attempting to ride waves of even greater height borders on suicide.

In the late 1950s and 1960s, the creation of a light synthetic foam surfboard opened the doors to the present-day surfing age. The balsa interior was replaced with a polyurethane foam, a bubble-filled plastic. With the new foam and Fiberglas boards, one could achieve extreme light weight (<10 pounds), which when combined with short length 6- to 7-foot boards) allowed control over the waves that was previously not possible. The surfboard became a short appendage of the body that could be placed almost anywhere on the wave that the mind willed it to be, rather than a long, heavy plank that had to be forced to respond. The emphasis on riding huge waves seemed to wane in the late 1970s and into the 1980s. The short, lightweight boards and the advent of the leash in the late 1960s (Fig. 37.1), which essentially eliminated swimming after lost boards (much as ski bindings keep skiers and skis together), attracted untold numbers of new surfers, and with the help of

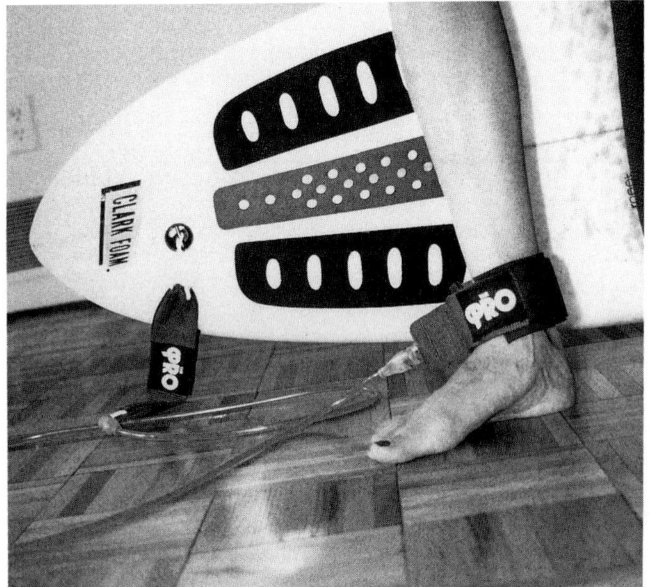

Figure 37.1. The leash prevents a surfer from being hit by another surfer's loose board.

television and international affluence, the sport became a worldwide phenomenon. Surf that had been impossible to ride with longer boards was ridden: The Banzai Pipeline in Hawaii, with perhaps the most dangerous waves of all, was mastered by first a handful and then seemingly countless highly skilled surfers, who with their short boards could drop straight down the face of the waves and make their turn at the bottom—something that had been impossible with longer, heavier boards. The Pipeline, however, differed from big wave sites formerly attempted in one respect: The waves broke in *shallow* water and with tremendous force. Injuries increased—dislocations, fractures, severe lacerations, and deaths occurred as boards rained down on unprotected bodies, and the bodies slammed into the coral sea floor.

By the late 1970s, it became evident that crowding (Fig. 37.2); lack of established rules; and the tendency of surfing to attract people who prefer to live a spontaneous life without coaches, teams, scheduled contests, or time limits had resulted in a sport that has become somewhat more dangerous than the surfing practiced by the ancient Hawaiians hundreds of years ago.

Characteristics of Waves

To understand the mechanisms of surfing injuries it may be pertinent to review briefly the characteristics of

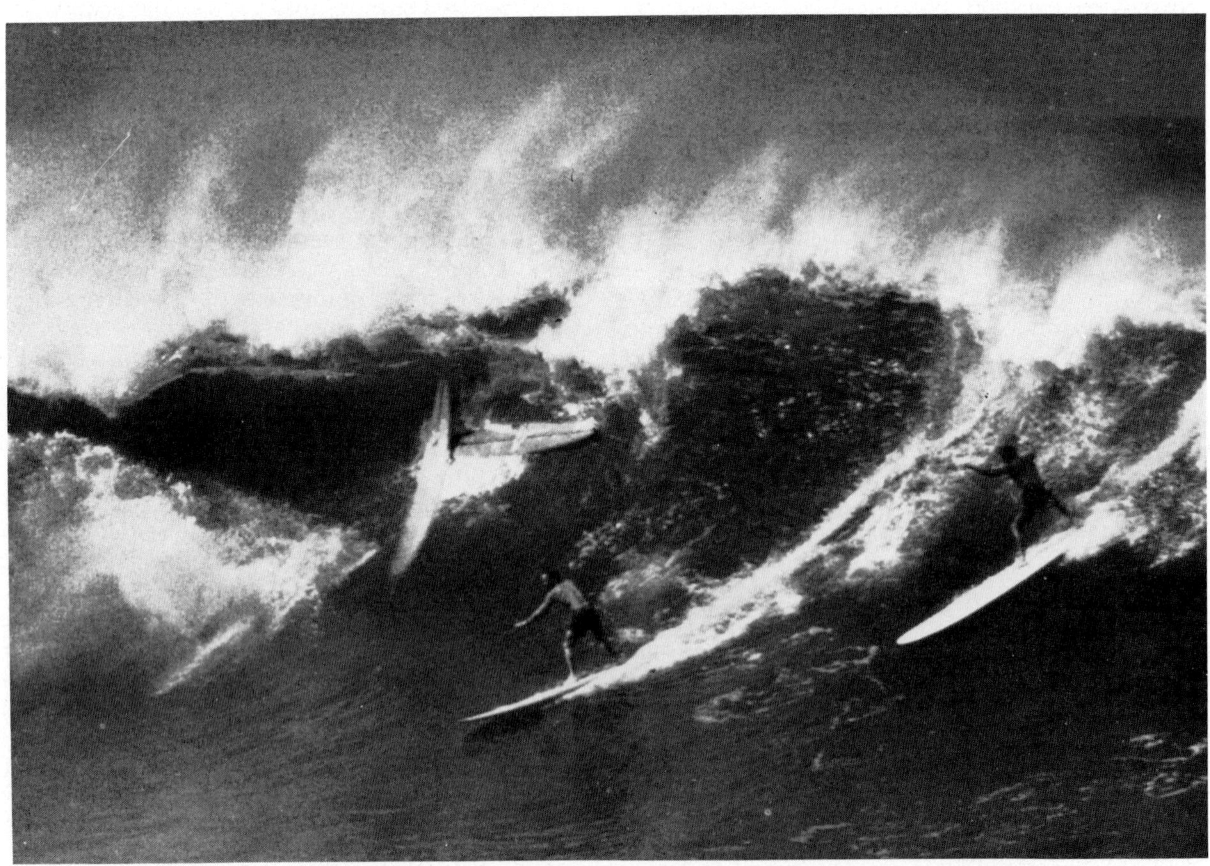

Figure 37.2. Overcrowding in the presence of loose surfboards is a substantial danger in large surf.

a wave, i.e., how waves are formed and where they originate (3). Waves may be created by earthquakes, landslides, passage of the moon, and changes in the atmospheric pressure, but for our purposes, it is the wind that generates the huge waves that hit the north shore of the Hawaiian Islands. These "wind waves" are transmitted throughout all of the shores in the Pacific and are manifested in storms such as the one that devastated the California coast in January 1983. These same waves created huge waves on the north shore of Hawaii. The storm's (or low pressure system's) wind velocity, duration, and direction are important factors in the creation of a wave or waves. When the initial influence of the wind dissipates, the waves blend into smooth, long swells. The swells can travel thousands of miles across oceans, losing little energy. The energy has been transferred from the wind to the ocean, and the resulting waves are pure energy. The water particle that is whipped by a North Pacific storm, of course, never reaches the Hawaiian shore. This is analogous to the energy transferred to the undulations of a whip or the creation of a wave that travels the length of a rope, when it is jerked.

The next phase is understanding how the ocean swell breaks. The wave breaks when it meets the resistance of the ocean bottom. The contour of the ocean bottom is a main determinant in causing a wave to break in a certain way. The winter swells from the north hit the Hawaiian beaches with a tremendous force because, unlike the U.S. mainland or Australia, there is no continental shelf to dissipate the energy. In Australia, for example, the continental shelf extends several miles out, and its slow rising bottom allows the wave to break with less force. In Hawaii, the offshore reef is the first obstacle that the swell encounters after thousands of miles, and the waves are generally much more powerful, faster, and larger than any in the world.

The moving energy in a swell is transferred into moving water in the form of a wave. The open ocean swell is slowed down by the resistance of the rising ocean bottom as the swell approaches shore. The top of the swell is pushed upward, and the swell appears to jump in size. The bottom continues to slow the swell down and push it upward. The swell becomes a steep wall of water with a face (the moving wall) and a crest (top). When the top of the swell (white foam) falls down the face of the swell, the wave turns into a moving wall of water. When conditions are favorably smooth, a tube is actually formed by the moving concave vertical wall and the water of the crest pitching forward. The surfer on the surfboard slices down on the face of the wave, right into the tube, and glides out of the tube and out of the area where all of the water is going to fall at the last moment.

Each surfing area or beach has unique characteristics or wave forms, which are determined by the contour of the ocean bottom and the type of swell that is breaking. In fact, this is so characteristic that often a surfboard is tailor made to the waves of a particular area, and good surfers have two or more boards, each made for a specific spot or beach.

Body Surfing

Body surfing is one of the msot challenging and stimulating individual sports currently enjoyed by many. The Hawaiian Islands (mainly Oahu), southern California, and Australia top the areas where this sport is popular. It may be thought of as a one-on-one competition: the surfer versus the wave, one's body lying on and within a curving wall of rapidly moving water.

The body surfer need only wear a swimsuit and use one necessary accessory, a pair of fins or flippers (occasionally a single fin). The body surfer must be a strong swimmer, as he or she may be carried out beyond the surfline. Foot fins help speed and endurance as well as one's ability to cover longer distances if necessary. *The initial cost is low, but the cost of injury can be horrendous—permanent paralysis secondary to spinal cord injury or death caused by drowning.*

Body-surfing beaches are numerous in Oahu and are named, numbering at least 17. Perhaps the most famous areas are Makapuu, Sandy Beach, Point Panic, Pounders, Waimea Bay, Pipeline, Makaha, and Bellows. Some might even be considered infamous.

In addition to "the wave" and subsequent waves, the body surfer must contend with the ocean bottom (packed sand, coral, and rocks); other surfers (both body and board surfers); and other objects in the water such as surfboards (with their points, tails, and fins), air mattresses, Boogie boards, canoes, kayaks, and catamarans. Some of these are directly dangerous on contact, while others can be distracting or physically upsetting, causing the body surfer to lose control, which could be dangerous.

Knowledgeable body surfers first study the surf from the beach. They then enter the water, put on their fins, tread water (or stand in water about chest deep), and face out to sea, watching each wave as it approaches. When a surfer believes he or she is in a correct position and capable of riding the oncoming wave (usually 2 to 6 feet high) and has analyzed the direction of the break of the wave (left to right, right to left, or straight ahead), he or she then decides whether to "take it" or not. If the surfer decides not to take the wave, he or she dives under and through the base of the wave and comes up on the other side in front of the next wave. It may be necessary to do this several times in a row, thus requiring stamina and good breath-holding abilities. If the surfer decides to take the wave, he or she turns and faces the shore; and when the nearly breaking wave is several feet behind the surfer, he or she begins to swim rapidly with several short, strong strokes and kicks to gain momentum so that as the wave catches the surfer, he or she can ride it. Once caught by the wave, the surfer should be in front of the wave with the upper body, with the remainder of the body encased in the mass of moving water. The surfer extends an arm straight in the direction of the angled body (right arm extended when going to the right on a left to right breaking wave) and rides the wave. It may crash in just a few feet (typical for Sandy Beach) or roll for several yards (10 to 30 would be ideal) and even tube such that the surfer exits far down the tube from where he or she entered, having been completely surrounded by a tunnel of moving water for several ecstatic moments.

Once the ride is almost over, the surfer must safely terminate it before the wave crashes. The proper and safest way is to "curl under" (cut out, kick out) and come out behind the wave, heading out to sea to face the next one. This end of the ride is the most dangerous part, and it is here that even the experienced body surfer can become injured. It is the timing of this critical move that has cost lives as a result of head injury with loss of consciousness, spinal cord injury with paralysis, and drowning. It is here that the now head/neck-flexed surfer can be driven head first into the beach bottom, sustaining a neck injury. The surfer may escape with only a cervical vertebral body compression fracture or perhaps only a spinous process fracture, or he or she may sustain a fracture-dislocation with resultant, usually immediate, spinal cord injury. The experienced body surfer may also be injured by collision with other surfers (body or board) or objects, but the most serious remains a collision with the ocean bottom.

The inexperienced surfer (in Hawaii often the pale tourist or the newly arrived military person) may be injured by just entering unfamiliar waters. If the newcomer should choose to run and dive into the surf, he or she may hit the head, usually the vertex, on the sand or coral bottom, on a projecting hidden rock, or on the head of an oncoming body surfer. The surfer may walk into the water because he or she sees many others in the surf (often 100 or more at Sandy or Makapuu on a Saturday or Sunday), but standing only knee or waist deep, the surfer may be almost immediately pounded downward or thrown backward by a huge wall of water that crashes violently to the ocean bottom. Concussion; near drowning; fractured cervical, thoracic, or lumbar vertebrae; arm/shoulder dislocations; hip dislocations; lacerations; and severe sand abrasions can occur.

If surfing at a lifeguarded beach, there is a good chance of rescue, resuscitation, stabilization, and expeditious transfer to an acute care hospital, all too familiar with the receipt and care of such an injured surfer. Not all body-surfing beaches have lifeguards.

Body surfing can now include riding on an air-filled beach mattress, Boogie board (a soft, light, preformed Styrofoam board about 3 feet long), and short, thin, hard plywood boards. These add a new risk for the rider, because they are frequently ridden directly into shore and can cause an over-the-falls–type of injury, with the rider being thrown forward by his or her own momentum as the wave stops abruptly and crashes down. The surfer may land with neck flexed into the water ahead of the wave (now only inches to perhaps 1 foot deep) or in a head-neck extended position, each causing its own particular type of cervical spine injury.

Most body surfing is done at sand-bottomed beaches, with or without coral, but one challenging area (no beach) is Point Panic. Here, the waves eventually crash on boulders on a projection of land, but the requirement is to ride the wave and then curl out before the final crash! Championship contests are actually scheduled at Point Panic, and winners are determined by style, number of rides, and innovation. Several surfers have ridden a wave too long.

No swimmer or surfer should be in the water alone, and the beginner or novice body surfer must have respect for all waves. Prevention of injury is the only way to enjoy body surfing. One should surf only at a lifeguarded sand beach, be an accomplished swimmer, and choose waves that break slowly and smoothly and are not too high (1 to 2 feet as seen from the front).

Beach areas that allow board surfing, boat launching and landing, and sail-boarding should be avoided. There are beaches that are restricted in use for the appropriate water sport. When a red flag is posted at a guarded beach, the surf is considered dangerous even for the expert!

Sharks, needle fish, sea urchins, sting rays, blow fish, and Portuguese men-of-war have caused injuries to the body surfer, the latter being the most common. Coral cuts and deep sand abrasions also need medical attention. The most devastating of the injuries remains the spinal column injury, usually cervical, often resulting in permanent quadriparesis or quadriplegia.

Epidemiology of Surfing Injuries

Since the first edition of this text several studies of surfing injuries have been reported and case reports have described new injuries. Much of the early data on surfing injuries came from hospital emergency rooms near surfing beaches (4, 5) or from studies of unusual injuries (6). These studies indicated that most surfing injuries were musculoskeletal but did not provide detail; instead, they emphasized nonmusculoskeletal injuries that required hospitalization, usually caused by surfers being hit by a board or losing control of the board and being thrown against coral, rocks, or the beach. Allen et al. (4) a surveyed 36 surfing injuries that occurred from 1969 to 1975 in Hawaii and required hospitalization. A total of 34% of the injuries were craniospinal, almost 50% caused by trauma from a surfboard and the remainder caused by being thrown into the sand by a wave in shallow water. Most of the latter group were body surfers, and this group appears particularly vulnerable to this type of injury. The musculoskeletal injuries included one anterior cruciate ligament (ACL) tear, one tibia-fibula fracture, one fracture of the radius, an acromioclavicular (AC) joint sprain, and a forearm hematoma. There also were three eye injuries, including a globe injury that required enucleation; three maxillofacial injuries, including a compound fracture of the maxilla; a ruptured spleen; three renal contusions; and three ruptures of the tympanic membrane. Mentioned as a mechanism of injury, but not seen in this study, was trauma caused by the surfboard skeg, the stabilizing tail fin that became standard equipment during that time (Fig. 37.3).

Chang and McDanal (5) also reviewed the medical records of patients admitted to the hospital for body-surfing injuries in Hawaii between 1973 and 1977. They found similar mechanisms of injury, in particular trauma

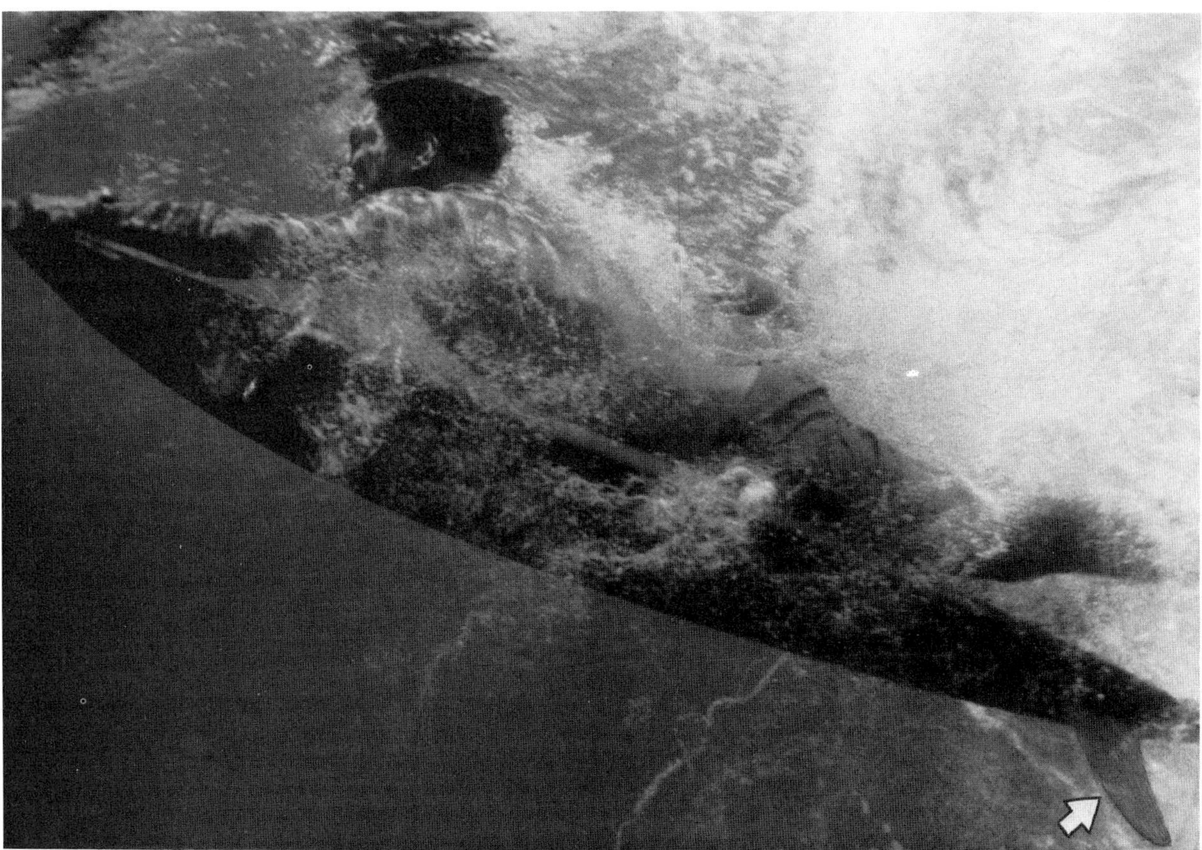

Figure 37.3. Surfboard skeg *(arrow)* was initially a significant source of injury.

caused by loose boards for board surfers and shallow beaches for body surfers. Almost 20% of all injuries were musculoskeletal, including four lower-extremity fractures, four knee ligament injuries, two AC sprains, and a shoulder dislocation. Kennedy et al. (7) studied surfing injuries from emergency rooms near surfing beaches between 1966 and 1969 and again from 1974 to 1975. They also noted that the majority of injuries involved the head and neck and that cuts and bruises predominated. The mechanisms of injury were similar to those in the other studies, most having been caused by loose surfboards or shallow beaches. Both the incidence and mechanism of injury changed little from the first part of the survey to the second, despite the increasing popularity of leg ropes to prevent surfers from losing their boards.

In a second study of injuries in Australia, Kennedy and Vanderfield (8) found that the sides of the board were most responsible for injury, not the nose or skeg as was previously thought. In the mid-1970s, changes in surfboard design emphasized speed and maneuverability, resulting in a shorter, lighter board, thereby decreasing injury potential. Later, soft, durable neoprene rubber was molded onto the nose and tail of boards to further reduce the risk of injury (9) (Fig. 37.4). This, combined with the use of leg ropes in the mid- to late 1970s, reduced the risk of hitting another surfer with a loose board, provided a flotation device, and obviated the need to retrieve lost boards from rocky foreshores with its attendant risk of serious injury. However, detractors cited several disadvantages of leg ropes: greater risk of injuring the surfer attached to the board, greater risk of ankle injury from poorly constructed rope systems, the likelihood that poor swimmers might make use of surfboards as a swimming aid and risk drown-

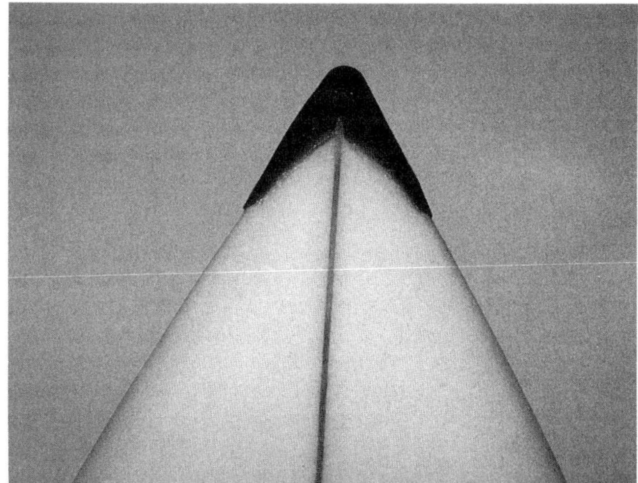

Figure 37.4. A soft neoprene tip on the surfboard reduces risk of trauma from loose boards.

ing if the rope broke, greater probability that surfers would venture too close to rocky or restricted areas (increasing the risk to swimmers) (10). Leg ropes were modified in the latter 1970s from a rope placed through the skeg and tied around the surfer's ankle to rubber tubing and nylon cord attached to the ankle with a Velcro closure and anchored to the surfboard. This adjustment placed less force on the ankle (11).

Investigators also attempted to determine the incidence of injury. Allen et al. (4) estimated this to be 1 injury per 17,500 surfer days with a general downward trend in the data as boards got shorter and lighter. Kennedy et al. (7) estimated the injury rate to be about 1%, indicating that the risk of serious injury to a surfer was low.

The limitations of these early studies were noted by Lowdon et al. (12) who used a questionnaire to obtain injury data from 346 surfboard riders (328 men and 18 women). A total of 33% of the respondents had not sustained an injury; 32% surfed only 2 days/week, but the average was 2.7 days/week, 4 hr/day. The total number of injuries was 337, and a rate of 3.5 moderate to severe injuries per 1000 surfing days was calculated. The most common injuries that required medical attention were lacerations (41%). Approximately 24% of these were on the head and 17%, on the extremities. Injuries to the head an face were most often the result of contact with the surfer's own board; body lacerations were most often caused by contact with the skeg. Lacerations of the lower leg and foot were frequently the result of surfing over shallow reefs.

Soft tissue injuries (i.e., sprains and strains) and fractures were the next most common injuries (35% and 15%, respectively). This group primarily consisted of injuries to the lower back, neck, and shoulder, which represented 16% of all surfing injuries. The isometric hyperextension of the trunk during paddling and the sudden maneuvers during surfing were the causes of the back and neck pain. Four stress fractures of the lumbar spine also occurred, all caused by rotation/hyperextension. Overuse syndromes of the shoulder, similar to those in swimmers, also were noted. The cause was thought to be related to the recovery phase range-of-motion requirements of the shoulder when paddling on small surfboards, which sit lower in the water and require increased motion.

In the study by Lowdon et al. (12) eardrum perforations represented 6% of the total injuries. These occurred more frequently in large surf than did other injuries, and the most common mechanisms were compression on hitting the water, submerging after a wipeout, or rolling under a large wave while paddling out.

Lowdon et al. (13) used questionnaires and interviews to investigate injuries to international competitive surfboard riders. Mean practice time was 3.7 h/day, 5.2 days/week. A total of 187 injuries were reported, an average of 1.1 injuries per surfer per year. Although this is more than double the rate for recreational surfers, the figures are comparable when based on injuries per 1000 surfing days (4.0 versus 3.5), owing to the increased practice time of the professionals. Lacerations were again the most common injury, accounting for 45% of the total. The majority occurred on the head, especially the top and side of the scalp, the chin, and the lips. The surfer's own board was responsible for most of these injuries. A total of 34% were recoil injuries from the elasticized rope attachment. Sprains and strains were second (37%), which the authors believed reflected data collection methods as well as the effect of lighter more maneuverable boards. The back, shoulder, and knee were most commonly affected. In general, recreational surfers and international competitors had many of the same injuries and injury mechanisms.

Renneker (14) reviewed the overall medical aspects of surfing, noting a high incidence of eye problems unrelated to trauma, in particular pinguecula and pterygium, occasional conjunctivitis, and ocular sunburn. Skin problems, especially those related to sun exposure, were common. A skin injury that has been the source of some confusion to the medical community is "surfer's nodules" (15). These are movable, nontender, subcutaneous masses of angiofibroblastic tissue, most often on the knee and usually are caused by the surfer paddling out in a kneeling position. Treatment consists of changing this position, although steroid injections are also effective (6). At one time, nodules developed in about 80% of surfers but are now much less common. Skin ulcers are also common in surfers and are often the result of incidental abrasions or lacerations that progress to ulcers from long days in the ocean. The ulcers often grow *Staphylococcus aureus* or *S. pyogenes albus*, although no systemic symptoms or local lymphangitis was noted. Topical treatment is generally effective, though chronic ulcers often required surgical intervention (6).

Among the idiosyncratic problems for surfers is surfer's ear, the presence of exostosis in the external ear canal. Originally described by Seftel (16), this was considered a compensatory response to irritation of the canal by water and wind. Umeda et al. (17) reviewed the progression of this condition and recommended that surfers wear ear plugs to prevent it. Recommended treatment is similar to that for external otitis media, although severe cases may require surgery to remove exostoses.

A variety of injuries to the shoulder and neck occur when a board surfer or body surfer falls with an arm either hyperabducted or extended (Fig. 37.5). Bailey (18) described a first rib fracture in a board surfer who hyperextended his arm while performing a layback maneuver. Kahn et al. (19) described four cases of luxatio erecta from body surfing, all caused by a wave breaking on the hyperabducted arm. Sage (20) reported a recurrent inferior dislocation of the clavicle in a surfboard rider who caught his arm on the board as he fell. The mechanism was thought to be abduction and distraction.

Prevention of Surfing Injuries

As equipment has changed, some surfing injuries also have changed. Early studies demonstrated a significant

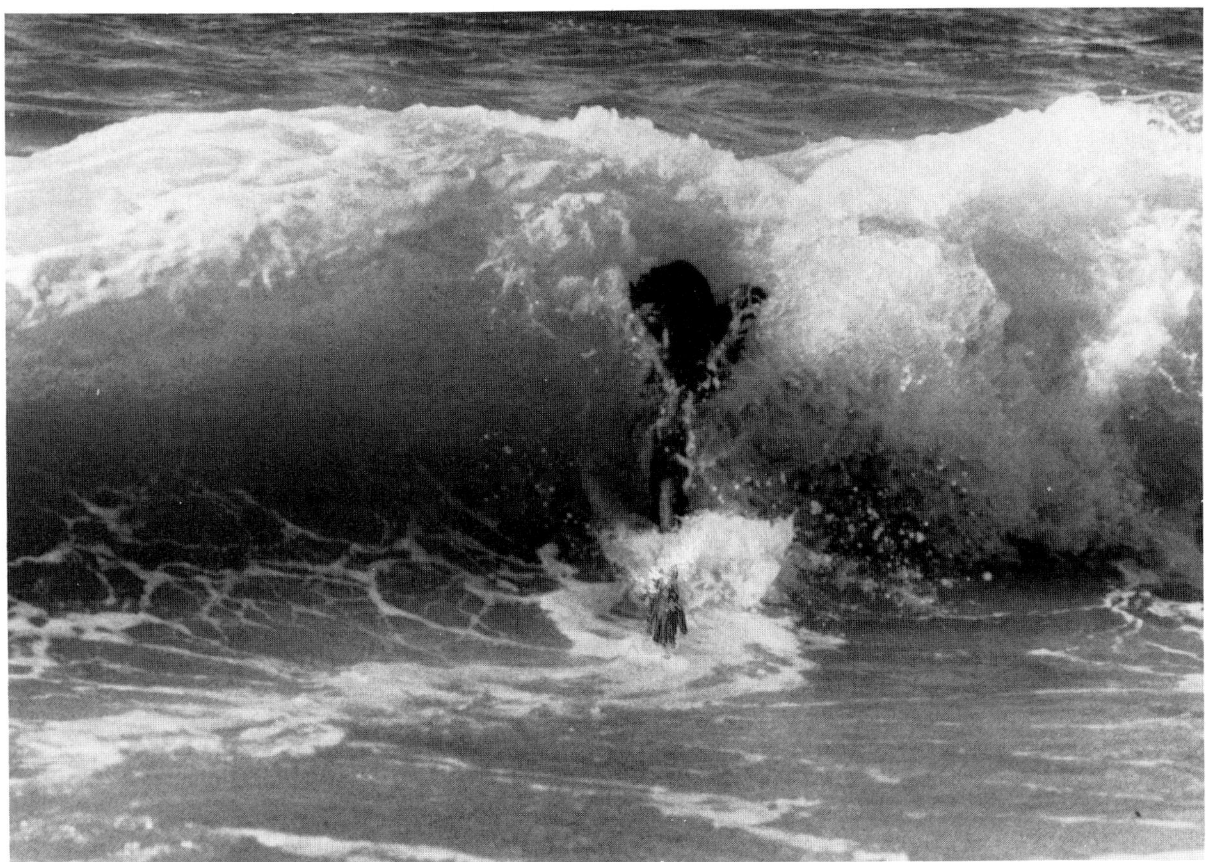

Figure 37.5. The hyperadducted or extended position of the arm as the surfer wave breaks produces a variety of injuries.

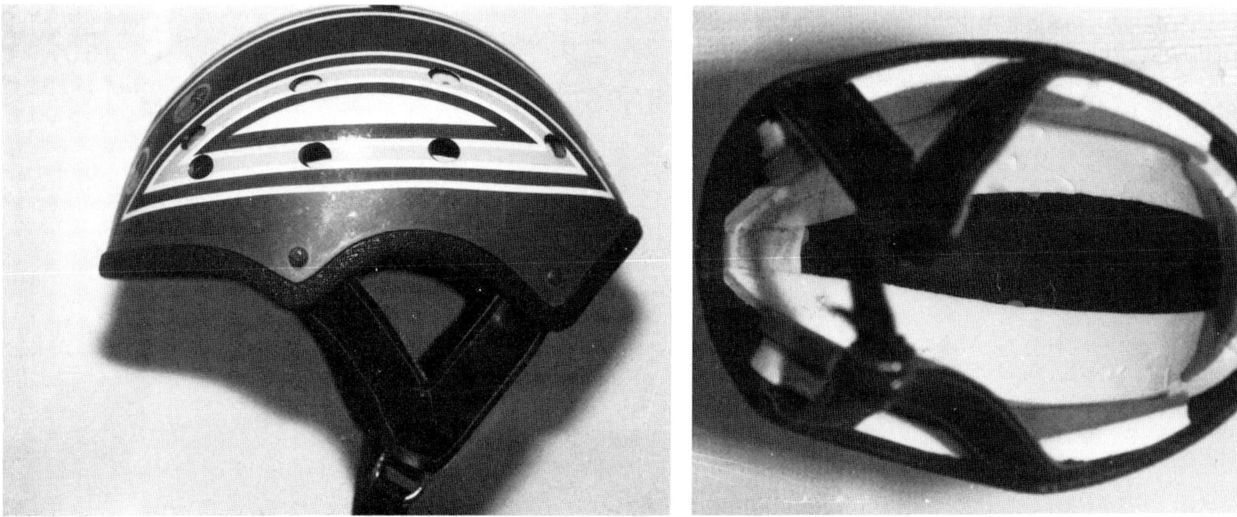

Figure 37.6. One type of surfer's head protection.

risk of being hit with another surfer's board, whereas later studies, undertaken after changes in equipment, have shown increased risk of being injured by the surfboard rider's own surfboard. Injuries to body surfers still involve being hit by the surf or thrown into the sand. As noted by Allen et al. (4) general injury prevention for surfboard riders involves the following recommendations:

1. Study the surf, the bottom, the tides, and traffic.
2. Surf with a companion.
3. Avoid the path of oncoming surfers when paddling

out. If a collision is unavoidable, abandon your board and go deep; stay under longer than is believed necessary.

4. If you fall, try to land behind the board and dive into the fall. Always cover your head and come to the surface with a hand extended to ensure that nothing on the surface is coming down on you.
5. Try to fall on your buttocks or feet first.

For body surfers, recommendations include

1. Avoid areas with surfers, crowds, reefs, and rip currents.
2. Surf where the wave breaks in deeper water and avoid shorebreaks.
3. Arch your body with the head back when riding down the wave, and when exiting a wave, roll to one side and pivot around one shoulder. Never try to somersault.

Lowdon (12) noted the importance of stretching and warming up before board surfing and recommended performing them routinely. Strengthening of neck paraspinal musculature also may reduce the risk of cervical spine injury. The use of a helmet to reduce trauma also has been recommended (Fig. 37.6).

Finally, there is a strong association between drowning and alcohol consumption (21). Anyone entering an ocean under the influence of alcohol is clearly putting himself or herself at great risk.

Acknowledgment

Acknowledgment is made to RM Taniguchi, J. Blattau, WM Hammon who contributed to the previous edition; Surfing. In: RC Schneider, JC Kennedy, ML Plant, eds. Sports Injuries—Mechanisms, Prevention, and Treatment. Baltimore: Williams & Wilkins, 1985.

REFERENCES

1. Wilson G. Surfing in Hawaii [pamphlet]. Honolulu: World Wide Distributors, Ltd.
2. Hemmings F. Surfing. Hawaii's gift to the world of sports. Osaka, Japan: Zokeisha, 1977.
3. Bascom W. Waves and beaches. The dynamics of the ocean surface. New York: Doubleday, 1964.
4. Allen RJ, Eiseman B, Strackly CJ, Orloff BJ. Surfing injuries at Waikiki. JAMA 1977;237:668–670.
5. Chang LA, McDanal CE. Boardsurfing and body surfing injuries requiring hospitalization in Honolulu. Hawaii Med J 1980;39:117.
6. Erickson JG, Gemmingen GR. Surfer's nodules and other complications of surfboarding. JAMA 1967;201:134–136.
7. Kennedy M, Vanderfield G, Huntley R. Surfcraft injuries. Aust J Sports Med 1975;3:53–54.
8. Kennedy MC, Vanderfield GK. Medical aspects of surfcraft usage. Med J Aust 1976;2:707–709.
9. Ryan M. Making your surf board safer. The Surfer 1983;23:26.
10. Department of Culture, Sport and Recreation. Surfboard and leg rope report. New South Wales Sport and Recreation Service, New South Wales, Australia, 1975.
11. Barry SW, Kleinig BJ, Brophy T. Surfing injuries. Aust J Sports Med 1982;14:49–51.
12. Lowdon BJ, Pateman NA, Pitman AJ. Surfboard riding injuries. Med J Aust 1983;2:613–616.
13. Lowdon BJ, Pitman AJ, Pateman NA, Ross K. Injuries to international competitive surfboard riders. J Sports Med 1987;27:57–63.
14. Renneker M. Medical aspects of surfing. Phys Sportsmed 1987;15:96–105.
15. Burdick CO. Surfer's knots [Letter to the Editor]. JAMA 1981;245:823.
16. Seftel DM. Ear canal hyperostosis—surfer's ear. Arch Otolaryngol 1977;103:58–60.
17. Umeda Y, Nakajima M, Yoshioka H. Surfer's ear in Japan. Laryngoscope 1989;99:639–641.
18. Bailey P. Surfer's rib: isolated first rib fracture secondary to indirect trauma. Ann Emerg Med 1985;14:246–349.
19. Kahn ML, Bade HA, Stein I. Body surfing as a cause of luxatio erecta: a report of four cases. Orthop Rev 1987;16:729–733.
20. Sage J. Recurrent inferior dislocation of the clavicle at the acromioclavicular joint: a case report. Am J Sports Med 1985;10:145–146.
21. Mackie I. Alcohol and aquatic disasters. Med J Aust 1978;1:652–653.

38 / SWIMMING

Peter J. Fowler

Swimming

The similar, repetitive movements performed by the competitive swimmer over years of training are associated with a variety of characteristic injuries. These primarily affect the shoulder but they also can involve the lower limb and back. As in all sports, the competitive swimmer's ultimate goal is maximum performance. This goal is shared by all those involved in the athlete's care and development, and, as training programs are organized and implemented, prevention of injuries must be a primary focus. With a basic knowledge of the mechanical details of the sport and an understanding of the related anatomical and biomechanical considerations, physicians and coaches can evaluate the swimmer's performance on an ongoing basis and effectively contribute to his or her progress.

Swimming Strokes

The front crawl, the backstroke, the breaststroke, and the butterfly are the four competitive swimming strokes that are swum in various distances alone or in combination. While it is not the mandate of this chapter to extensively review these strokes, a description of the main components of each will provide a basis for understanding the pathophysiological entities common in competitive swimmers (Table 38.1).

There are four phases common to all strokes: the reach, catch, pull, and recovery (Table 38.2). The main power of propulsion (75%) is provided by arm action during the pull phase in all strokes except the breaststroke, which is unique in both upper and lower extremity motion. In front crawl, backstroke, and butterfly, the motion of the arm through the water starts with hand entry and proceeds with continual adduction and internal rotation of the glenohumeral joint. In the out-of-water phase, the arm is in abduction and internal rotation, so that it is again positioned for hand entry and repetition of the cycle.

Shoulder Injuries

Anatomic Features

As the most mobile joint in the human body, the shoulder has little bony support. The stability that allows the arm to function with power and precision is the result of the interaction of the shoulder capsule, the surrounding ligaments, the rotator cuff muscles, and the pectoralis major and serratus anterior muscles. The rotator cuff muscles, which are supraspinatus, infraspinatus, teres minor, and subscapularis (Fig. 38.1), work in a force couple combination with the deltoid and the long head of the biceps to contain the humeral head in the glenoid fossa. The long head of the biceps is important in stabilizing the humeral head and is active in forward flexion, a function that should not be overlooked in shoulder mechanics. The scapular muscles—the serratus anterior, the rhomboids, and the trapezius—work constantly in swimming arm action. If they fatigue, a downward tilt of the scapula may occur that in turn alters the mechanics of the glenohumeral joint and may contribute to the onset of impingement.

Tendinitis—Swimmer's Shoulder

Because there is a lack of understanding of many of its causes (Fig. 38.2), shoulder pain has become synonymous with the term "impingement." Consequently, inappropriate treatment may be selected for some patients. The term "impingement" should be reserved specifically for those cases where rotator cuff pathology is associated with actual mechanical abutment of the rotator cuff. Rotator cuff tendinitis, which describes existing pathological changes, is a more appropriate term for pain resulting from inflammation of the rotator cuff. The diagnostic challenge lies in determining the exact cause of rotator cuff tendinitis in individual patients.

The term "swimmer's shoulder" was first used by Kennedy and Hawkins in 1974; it refers to tendinitis of

Table 38.1.
Main Components of the Competitive Swimming Strokes

Front Crawl—The fastest, most frequently used practice stroke	Butterfly—Part of competition since 1952	Backstroke	Breaststroke—Oldest swimming stroke
Hand enters water, palm faces downward 12 inches in front of shoulder, reaches ahead until arm is fully flexed Pull phase initiated by sculling motion Torso is rolled about its longitudinal axis; arm is positioned deeper in water S-shaped curving pull, palm facing backward produced under torso Recovery of one arm simultaneous with pull phase of other arm Using body roll, arm is released from water and swept into entry position Arm action continuous; 2 to 6 vigorous flutter kicks per arm cycle	Arms and legs enter water and move simultaneously during pull and recovery phases A dolphin motion with body relieves stress on shoulder Legs perform dolphin kick (a flutter kick with legs moving together)	Arm entry straight with shoulder in fully elevated position Using body roll arm pulls in S-shaped pattern to side Legs perform flutter kick	Arms move together in pull and recovery phases Arms do not pull below waistline *Whip Kick* Begins with legs extended, feet plantarflexed Recovery begins with flexion at hips and knees Recovery ends with foot dorsiflexed and tibia in external rotation Angle between trunk and thigh—120° Knee extends, foot pushes outward and backward Dorsiflexed foot engages water with sole Hip extensors drive thigh toward water surface Extension continues at hip and knees while legs are brought together Knee almost extended and feet a few inches apart Finishes with foot in plantar flexion

Table 38.2.
Components of the Four Phases of the Competitive Swimming Strokes

Reach	Arm reaches forward to enter water Synonymous with term *entry*
Catch	Similar for all competitive strokes Elbow flexes 100° Shoulder extends, horizontally abducts and medially rotates
Pull	Varies slightly with each stroke Swimmer sculls or pushes water The propulsion phase Except in breaststroke, arm action starts at maximum elevation and ends in extension
Recovery	Out-of-the-water phase (except in breaststroke) Arm returns to start pull again

the supraspinatus and/or biceps tendon (1). This was staged chronologically by Neer and Welsh. In Stage I, there is edema and haemorrhage which occurs in athletes under 25 years. In Stage II, fibrosis and tendinitis are seen in those between 25 and 40. In Stage III, there is the formation of osteophytes and the occurrence of partial or complete tendon rupture, in those over 40 (2). In the competitive athlete however, these stages are not age specific. In 1974 Hawkins and Kennedy reported 3% incidence of "swimmer's shoulder" (1). The 50% occurrence more recently reported may be the result of an increase in the intensity of training schedules combined with such anatomical features as acromial shape and shoulder joint laxity along with biomechanical factors such as overwork, impingement, hypovascularity, and stroke mechanics.

Causal Factors

Training

In today's training programs, a swimmer of national caliber typically practices in the water in 2-hr sessions twice a day for a minimum of 5 days a week. A normal range is 4000 to 8000 m during each practice session. This time in the water serves to improve both conditioning and technique. Also part of the routine is dryland training to build strength and endurance. With these rigorous schedules, training sessions must be planned, monitored, and modified on an ongoing basis to prevent and reduce the incidence of swimmer's shoulder. Often, the sports medicine physician becomes involved only after an injury has occurred. Ideally, collaborative efforts involving coaching personnel and the physician will result in the establishment of training programs that are successful in the prevention of injuries and that do not compromise performance.

Overwork

As the least stable joint, the shoulder is the most vulnerable to injury in the overhead position. To keep up with the continuous, repeated demands made by swimming, the muscles of the rotator cuff may be required to work excessively to contain and stabilize the humeral head. With the cuff fatigue that results from

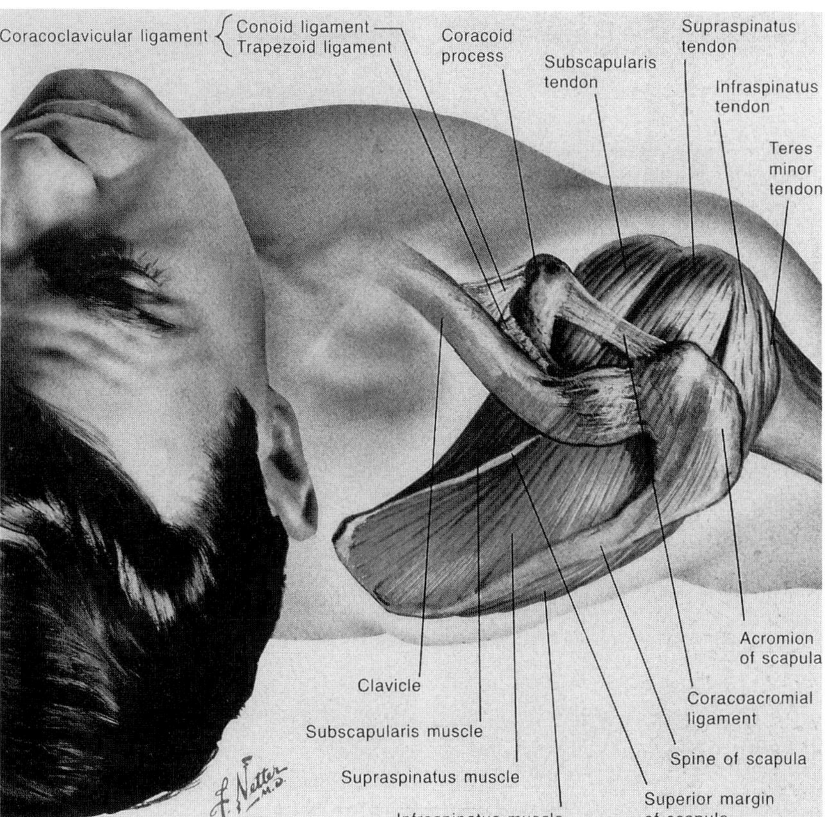

Figure 38.1. Shoulder and acromioclavicular joint from above. (Netter FH. The CIBA Collection of Medical Illustrations. In, Anatomy, Physiology and Metabolic Disorders, Vol 8, part 1, pp 33.)

Supraspinatus ■ inserts on uppermost facet of greater tuberosity ■ active during arm abduction ■ fulcrum for deltoid during abduction ■ helps resist upward displacement of humeral head during other arm actions
Subscapularis ■ primary external rotator ■ resists anterior or inferior displacement of humeral head in glenoid ■ stabilizes humeral head
Infraspinatus ■ external rotator ■ extends humerus in horizontal plane ■ works with supraspinatus and subscapularis to depress humeral head
Teres Minor ■ external rotator

this work, superior migration of the humeral head may occur, and, with this migration, an increase in subacromial loading, which, in turn, may be a factor that triggers the onset of tendinitis.

Hypovascularity

The functional relationship between arm position and blood supply to the supraspinatus and the biceps tendon was studied by Rathbun and Macnab (3). In adduction and neutral rotation, the tendons are stretched tightly over the head of the humerus, compromising their blood supply. Circulation is restored in abduction as the vessels fill. This repeated hypovascularity, known as a "wringing out" mechanism, occurs in the area of the tendon most vulnerable to impingement and, by compounding the potential for damage by repetitive stress, may contribute to early degenerative changes.

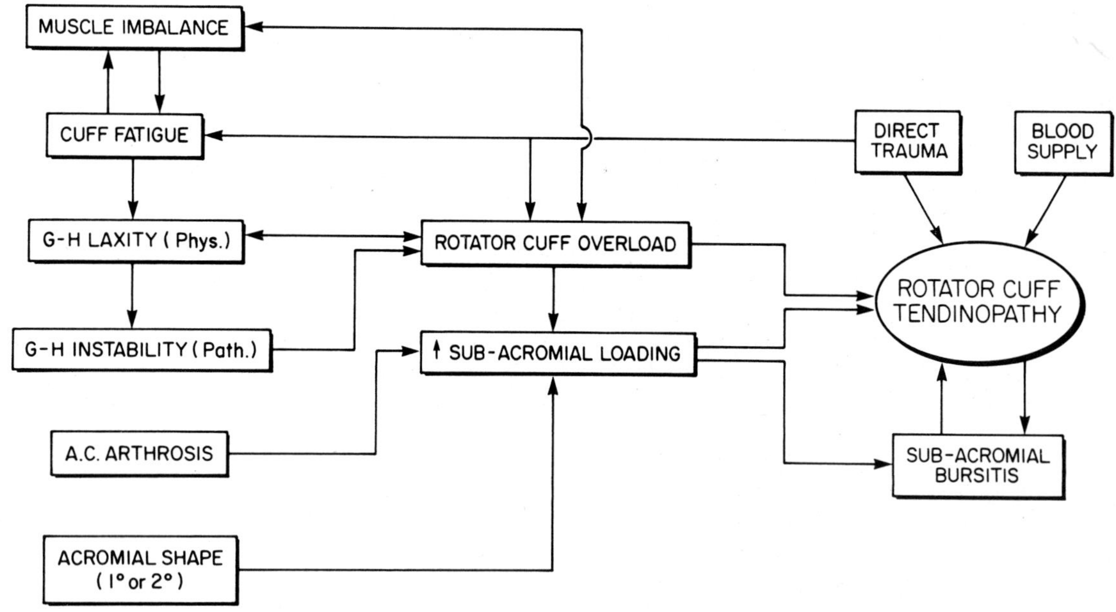

Figure 38.2. This algorithm outlines the many pathological entities that can culminate in rotator cuff tendinitis.

Impingement—Soft Tissue Factors

The supraspinatus and biceps tendons that insert on or across the humerus directly below the coracoacromial arch (formed by the coracoid process, the coracoacromial ligament, and the anterior acromion) are particularly susceptible to impingement. When the arm is in abduction with forward flexion and internal rotation (a position assumed in the catch phase of all competitive strokes), the humeral head moves under the arch and the tendons may be repeatedly impinged here. A mechanical irritation and inflammatory response, which further compromise the space under the coracoacromial arch, may result. An untreated inflammatory process can go on to include the subacromial bursa and the acromioclavicular ligament as well.

Impingement—Osseous Factors

Three acromial shapes have been identified by Bigliani et al.: type I, flat; type II, curved; and type III, hooked (4). Of these, a type III acromion may be an anatomical factor in refractory tendinitis that does not respond to treatment. Because of the already decreased dimensions of the acromial arch, a competitive swimmer with a hooked (type III) acromion may be predisposed to impingement. Consequently, a tendinitis which is resistant to treatment may easily develop. Ogata and Uhthoff have suggested that pathologic changes within the rotator cuff substance may be the result of a primary tendinopathy, and that the acromial changes observed occur as a secondary phenomenon (5). In addition, they suggest that the changes seen within the rotator cuff occur initially on the humeral surface of the tendon near the enthesis, as opposed to the bursal side, where one would expect to see lesions that are a result of mechanical impingement from the acromion. Theories such as this have precipitated a rethinking of shoulder pathology and its underlying causes.

Increased Laxity

Increased laxity may be a contributing factor in the athlete with resistant tendinitis. A loose or lax shoulder in the competitive swimmer may cause the rotator cuff muscles to work hard just to contain the humeral head. These fatiguing muscles are further stressed by the rigors of training. A significant observation of the association between rotator cuff tendinitis and shoulder laxity has been made by Fowler and Webster (6). They assessed 188 competitive swimmers between the ages of 13 and 26 for positive signs of tendinitis and for posterior, inferior, and anterior instability or increased laxity. Fifty recreational athletes without shoulder pain were used as a control group. A formal history was taken of each subject and episodes of shoulder pain were recorded. The "apprehension test" was used to test *anterior instability.* Any sign of pain or anxiety was recorded as a positive response. *Inferior stability* was assessed using the sulcus sign. The "load and shift" test conducted in both the sitting (Fig. 38.3) and supine (Fig. 38.4) positions was used to evaluate posterior laxity. The excursion of the humeral head relative to the posterior glenoid fossa was used as the index for *posterior laxity.* As in many normal asymptomatic individuals, the proximal humerus can be translated posteriorly a distance of to 50% of the glenoid width; any movement greater than this was classified as excessive posterior laxity.

Fifty percent of the swimmers had a history of shoulder pain. Some degree of posterior laxity was present in one or both shoulders in approximately 55% of the swimmers and in 52% of the control group, sug-

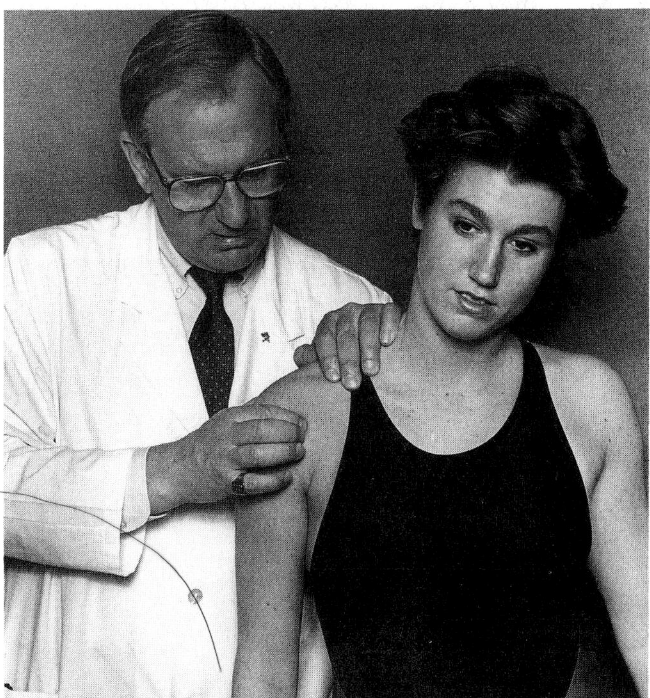

Figure 38.3. A clinical test for posterior laxity. The abducted position imitates arm position in a variety of activities.

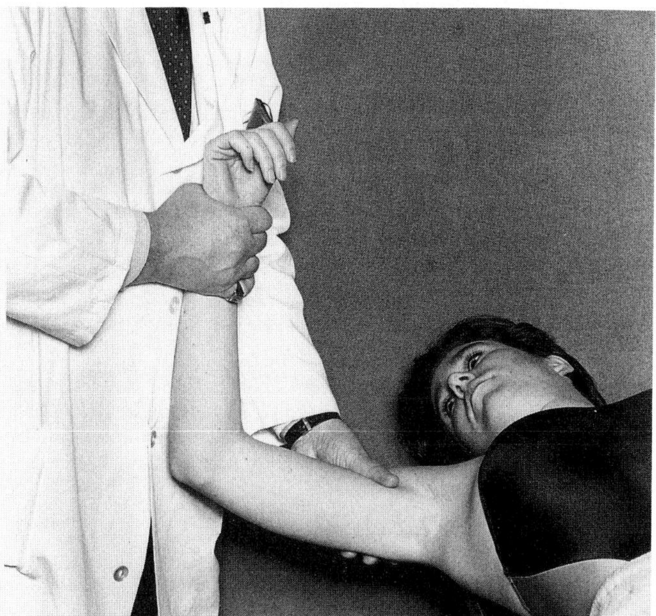

Figure 38.4. A second posterior laxity test. Make sure that the patient maintains the correct position and take care when grasping the humeral head as this area may be tender.

gesting that swimming does not predispose an athlete to increased posterior laxity. A history of tendinitis and increased posterior laxity was present in 25% of the swimmers. In these, tendinitis was always present in the lax shoulder, suggesting a relationship between tendinitis and posterior laxity.

Shoulder Strength Imbalance

Manual testing performed on these same swimmers demonstrated external rotator weakness in one or both shoulders in 40 individuals, with 33 having both weakness and a history of tendinitis in the same shoulder. Based on these findings, a second study was conducted to measure rotation strength about the shoulder (7). A Cybex II Dynamometer was used to test 119 swimmers and 51 controls (participants in activities not requiring arm rotation strength primarily). Internal and external rotation strengths were measured in three arm positions: neutral, 90° abduction, and 90° flexion. There was a significant difference in the rotation torque ratio between swimmers and controls in the neutral and 90° abduction positions (Table 38.3). This was attributed to the greater strength of the internal rotators in swimmers. Because the pull-through phase, which involves adduction and internal rotation at the glenohumeral joint, is the "power" portion of the stroke, most swimmers selectively train their internal rotators to improve power and speed. The resulting imbalance between the internal and external rotators about the shoulder may be a contributing factor in the onset of rotator cuff tendinitis. It is reasonable to assume that a strong muscle will resist stress better than an unconditioned one. There was no significant difference in external rotation strength between the two groups.

Impingement Positions in Swimming Strokes

Positions in swimming strokes during which pain is experienced seem to be associated with the biomechanical factors contributing to tendinitis. This relationship was recognized in a 1981 survey by Webster, which reported that 48.4% of 155 age-group swimmers had an incidence of past or present shoulder pain (8). The front crawl was the main practice stroke used by 99% of this group. Table 38.4 outlines the occurrences of pain during specific phases of the front crawl. During the entry

Table 38.3.
Rotation Strength Ratios About the Shoulder: A Comparison of Competitive Swimmers and a Control Group of Athletes

Position	Swimmers	Controls
Neutral	53.7% (SD = 17%)	65% (SD = 15%)
90° Abduction	62.1% (SD = 14%)	78.2% (SD = 17%)
90° Flexion	Right 46% (SD = 18.4%) Left 42% (SD = 19.7%)	52% (SD = 17%)

Table 38.4.
Pain During Front Crawl Arm Cycle

Position	Percentage
Entry/first half of pull phase	44.7
End of pull	14.3
Recovery	23.2
Throughout cycle	17.8

phase and the beginning of the pull phase (Fig. 38.5), the shoulder is in forward flexion, abduction, and internal rotation, so that the head of the humerus is forced toward the anterior acromion in such a way that the coracoacromial ligament along with the supraspinatus and biceps tendons may be impinged. In the recovery phase, lateral impingement may occur (Fig. 38.6). Here the shoulder is in abduction and internal rotation, so that the head of the humerus comes up against the lateral border of the acromion. When the shoulder leads the arm through recovery, there is less potential for lateral impingement. The "wringing out" mechanism occurs during the end of the pull phase when the arm is in adduction and internal rotation (Fig. 38.7).

Clinical Evaluation of Swimmers for Tendinitis

A thorough history is most important in this assessment. The athlete's pain is characterized in terms of onset, duration, location, quality, and relationship to a specific activity. A systematic physical examination includes inspection, palpation, assessment of range of motion with associated pain, crepitus stability, and motor strength. Tenderness elicited with palpation of the supraspinatus tendon medial to its insertion on the greater tuberosity is indicative of tendinitis. In addition, tenderness over the bicipital groove suggests involvement of the long head of biceps. The "painful arc" syndrome that causes pain with active abduction between 60° and 100° is a classic sign of supraspinatus tendinitis. Biceps tendinitis can be symptomatic of refractory supraspinatus tendinitis. The straight arm raise with the forearm supinated and the examiner resisting forward shoulder flexion can duplicate symptoms of biceps tendinitis.

Impingement Test

There are various tests in which, by placing the shoulder in an impingement-aggravated position, clinical pain is reproduced. An appropriate test for swimmers is one in which the shoulder is flexed forward

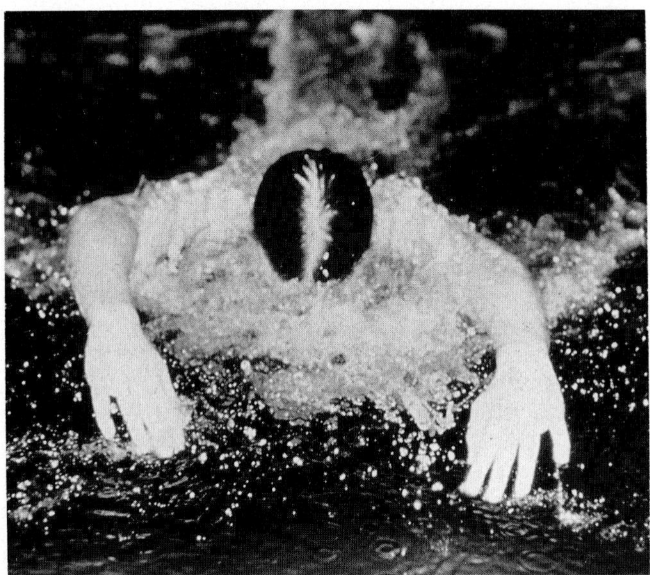

Figure 38.5. The reach or entry portion is similar in all strokes. Here it is shown during the butterfly.

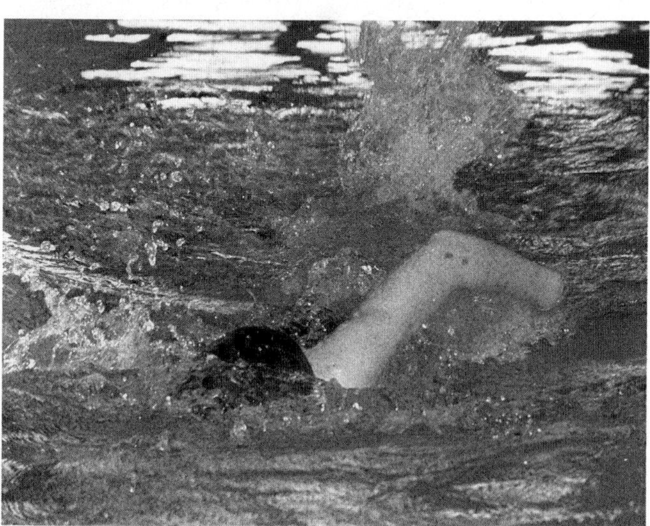

Figure 38.6. The recovery phase of the freestyle stroke. In this position, the amount of subacromial loading is in part determined by the amount of internal rotation of the humerus and the degree of abduction of the arm. The torso should be turned to recover the arm from the water.

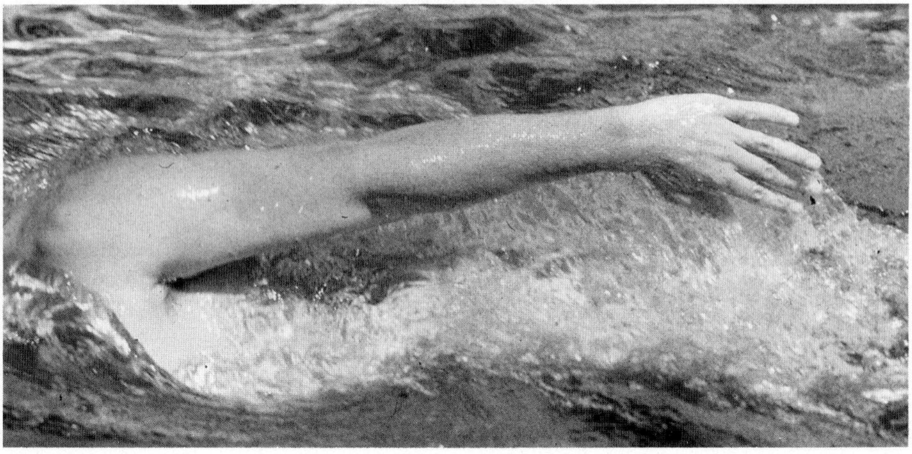

Figure 38.7. The "wringing out" mechanism occurs during the end of the pull phase which is similar for all strokes except the breaststroke.

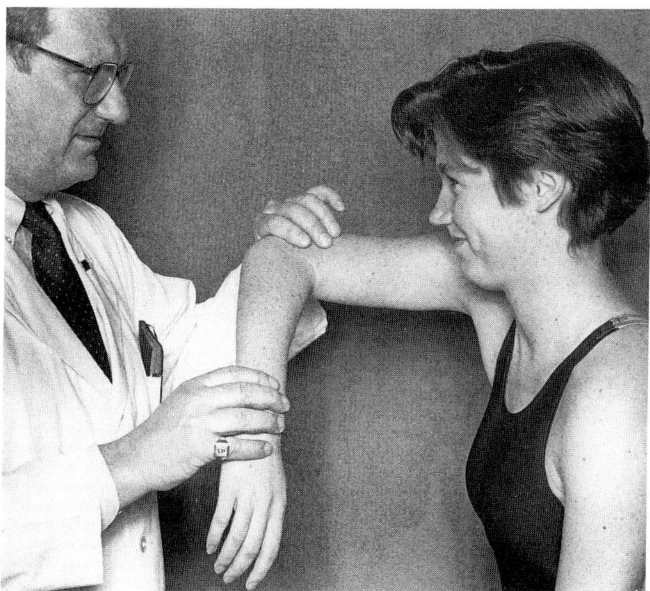

Figure 38.8. A clinical test for impingement. Here the tendons are impinged under the coraco-acromial arch. Since minimal pressure will cause pain, care must be taken when using this test.

90°, the elbow is flexed 90°, and the arm is internally rotated by the examiner (Fig. 38.8). This maneuver pushes the head of the humerus against the coracoacromial ligament, aggravating the inflamed tendon and reproducing pain. In a second test described by Neer, the arm is placed in a forward-flexed position and further stressed by the examiner (Fig. 38.9). This drives the humerus against the anteroinferior border of the acromion.

Muscle Weakness

Internal rotation force, applied by the examiner with the patient's arm in adduction and external rotation and with the elbow flexed 90° (Fig. 38.10), will determine the presence of muscle weakness. Gross weakness will be conspicuous. Pain may accompany this test.

Generalized Laxity

Increased laxity or frank instability may contribute to the progression of tendinitis or may be the total cause of the pain. Fowler and Jobe have described tests in which the humeral head is levered anteriorly in the abducted, externally rotated position. In the presence of anterior glenohumeral instability, this maneuver will exacerbate the athlete's discomfort (Fig. 38.11*A*). Disappearance of the pain with reduction of the humeral head in the glenoid fossa (positive relocation test) (Fig. 38.11*B*) is highly suggestive of a anterior glenohumeral instability that may be the primary underlying pathological process. Other tests, such as Speed's test and Yergason's test, are useful in ruling out bicipital tendinitis.

Posterior Translation

Movement of the humeral head by 50% of the glenoid width is considered normal. Even though movement in excess of 50% is not necessarily abnormal, this amount of movement would increase the work load of the rotator cuff, thereby influencing shoulder mechanics. To assess posterior translation, the patient is su-

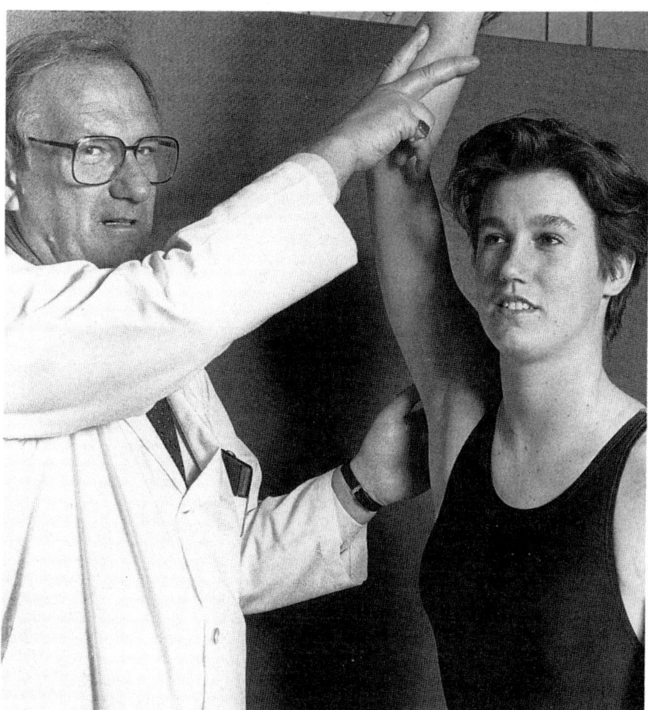

Figure 38.9. Here, pressure is applied to the fully flexed humerus. Pain may be reproduced if already inflamed tendons are impinged against the anterior acromion.

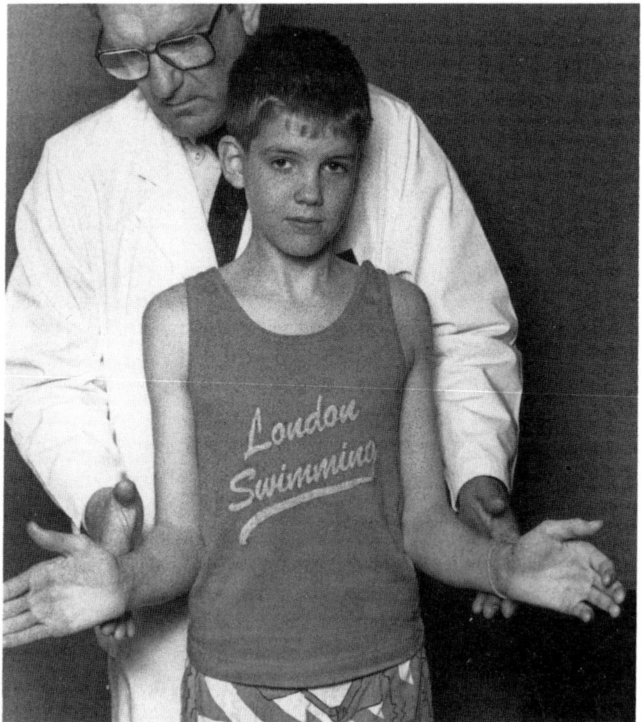

Figure 38.10. This manual test determines the gross external rotation muscle strength.

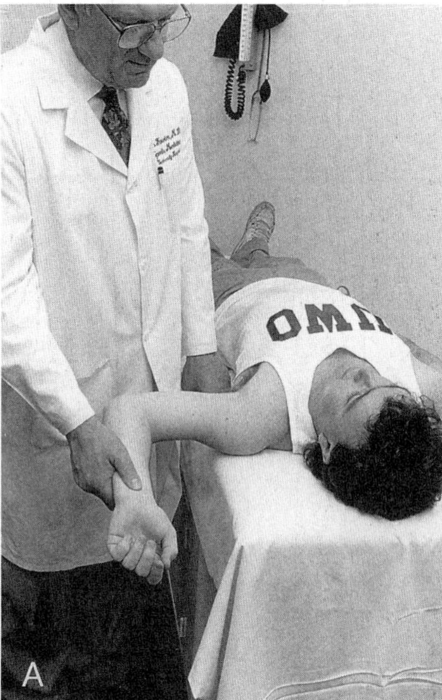

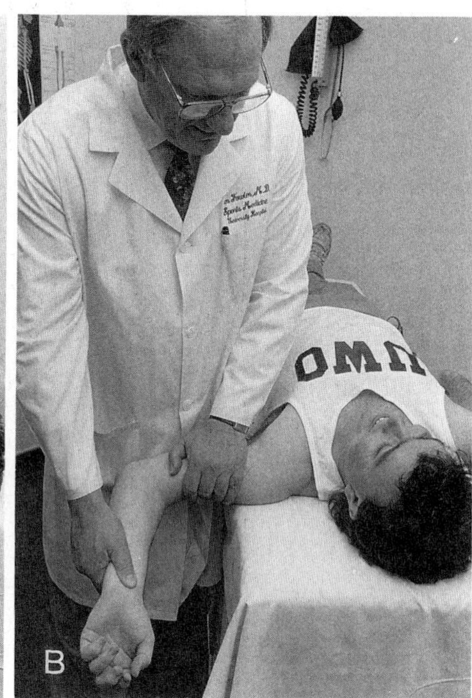

Figure 38.11. A. The arm is abducted and externally rotated, and the humeral head is levered anteriorly. In the presence of anterior glenohumeral instability the athlete will experience apprehension and/or discomfort. **B.** Reduction of the humeral head in the glenoid fossa will relieve the symptoms.

pine and the examiner holds the arm in 90° of abduction, applying posterior pressure to the upper humerus (see Fig. 38.4). If the shoulder is unstable, the application of an axial load may reproduce the symptoms the patient experiences during swimming. In a second test for posterior laxity, the patient sits while the examiner stabilizes the shoulder girdle with one hand and applies posterior pressure with other (see Fig. 38.3).

As tendinitis progresses, generalized pain about the shoulder is often present at night or at rest. The athlete avoids painful positions and those that aggravate the symptoms. To minimize pain during swimming, subtle changes in stroke mechanics may develop. A gradual loss of shoulder range of motion and muscle weakness may occur over time, and supraspinatus and infraspinatus wasting may become apparent. In the mature athlete, this may be an indication of degeneration of the rotator cuff tendon or a partial tear. These conditions are seldom seen in age-group swimmers, and in fact, are rare in athletes under 25 years.

Prevention of Tendinitis

Table 38.5 summarizes a basic preventative program. There are four principles, *balanced muscle strengthening, flexibility, technique modification,* and *avoidance of overwork,* which are fundamental to a preventative program. These can be readily incorporated into a training schedule as it begins; any subsequent adjustments to the regimen should be made with these four principles in mind.

Balanced Muscle Strengthening

As previously mentioned, in competitive swimming, both pool and dry-land training emphasize strengthening the internal rotators and extensors important in propulsion. There is little emphasis on strengthening the antagonists, yet they play a significant role in "containment of the shoulder." This can result in an alteration in the balance of muscle strength between internal and external rotation that contributes to tendinitis. Awareness of an imbalance and early correction plays an important part in prevention. An exercise program that includes strengthening the external rotators as well as the biceps and scapular muscles will help avert this imbalance. These exercises are simple to perform and require a minimum of readily available equipment, such as surgical tubing, pulleys, dental dam, and free weights

Table 38.5.
Prevention of Swimmer's Shoulder

Training Regimen	Gradually increase distance Gradually increase severity Place most vigorous sets at the beginning Proper warm-up and warm-down Warm-up after kicking sets
Strengthening	Include external rotators in dry-land sessions External rotator strengthening more than 3 times per week Include exercises for the muscles surrounding the scapula No pain involved
Stretching	Under 15 years, single stretching Over 15 years, pairs stretching Passive or PNF stretching only No ballistic stretching No pain involved
Stroke Mechanics	Proper mechanics particularly during fatigue situations Proper body roll

(Fig. 38.12*A* and *B*). They are isotonic and eccentric to improve power and control in both prime mover and antagonist muscle functions. In addition, they are performed in neutral, 90° of abduction, and 90° of flexion to reproduce arm positions in the actual sport. Biceps strengthening exercise should incorporate its functions as elbow flexor and forearm supinator and should be performed in several positions of shoulder range of motion as well. When doing weight training, painful subacromial loading positions should be avoided. Note that paddles can produce increased leverage that may overload the rotator cuff muscles and should be used cautiously.

Flexibility

In 1985, Griep conducted a study that determined that regardless of sex or stroke most frequently used, those swimmers with restricted flexibility were more likely to develop tendinitis than those who enhanced their flexibility with a stretching program (9). Stretching should be included in the daily training warm-up routine. Pairs stretching is appropriate for swimmers over 15-years-of-age, since this age group should be sufficiently mature to understand that overstretching soft tissues can cause irritation to the rotator cuff tendons and must be avoided. (Fig. 38.13). Younger swimmers should stretch individually as illustrated in Figure 38.14.

The stretching techniques employed by pairs are either passive stretches or proprioceptive neuromuscular fasciculation (PNF). In the passive, the partner very slowly and gently stretches the swimmer to the pain-free limit. The partner maintains that position while the swimmer contracts against the resistance provided. These stretches are repeated a variable number of times.

Technique Modification

Poor technique not only slows swimmers down but also can be a cause of injury. Again, prevention of overwork and fatigue of the rotator cuff should be foremost in a coach's mind as training programs are planned and the athlete's progress is monitored. Ongoing stroke analysis and recognition of breakdown in stroke mechanics should be part of a routine process that will help the swimmer adjust technique and limit impingement stress. Of particular importance is the analysis of stroke mechanics during fatigue. Lateral shoulder impingement can be a result of insufficient body roll in freestyle or backstroke. A high elbow position during the recovery phase of the freestyle stroke must be achieved by body roll. Attempting to force the elbow into a higher position with muscle activity rather than sufficient body roll can induce subacromial impingement.

Overreach with excessive internal rotation during the catch phase of all swimming strokes may cause undue subacromial loading and excessive activity for the cuff muscles to contain the humeral head. Excessive internal rotation may intensify the "wringing out" phenomenon. Changes to body roll, reach, and the degree of shoulder rotation reduce the frequency and the length of time that the shoulder is in a precarious position.

Evidence as to the effect of breathing patterns on the incidence of tendinitis is contradictory (8). Breathing to

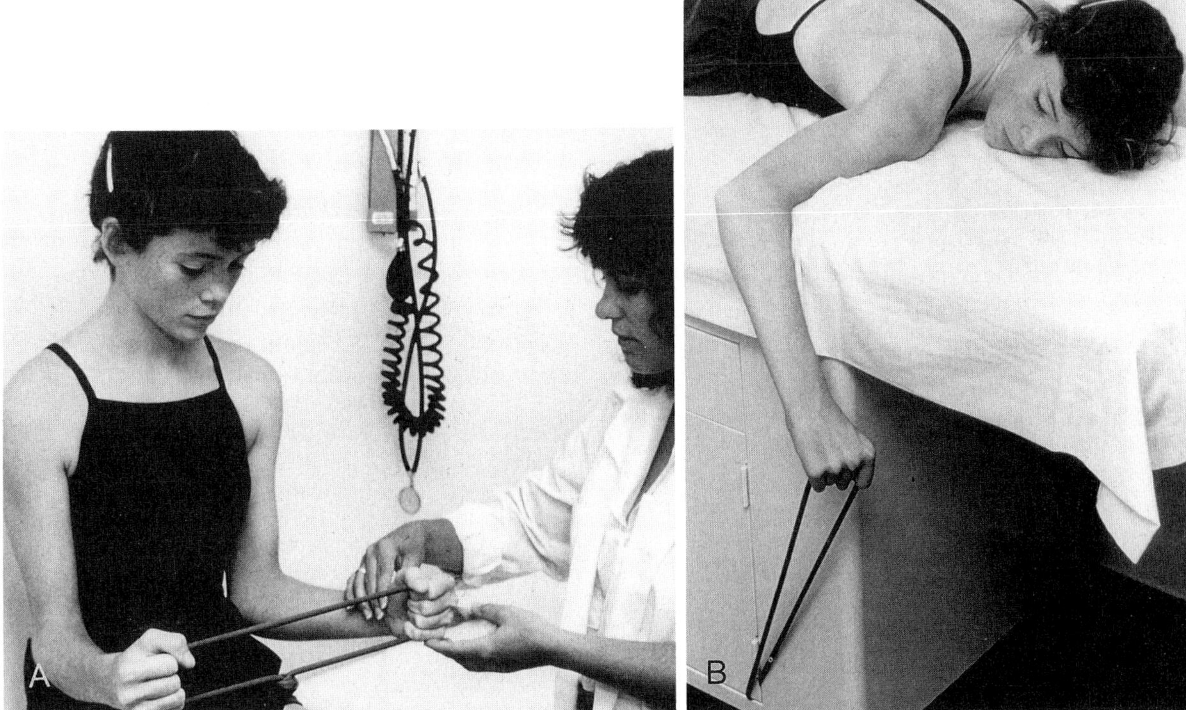

Figure 38.12. A. Strengthening external rotators in neutral. **B.** Strengthening external rotators in 90° abduction.

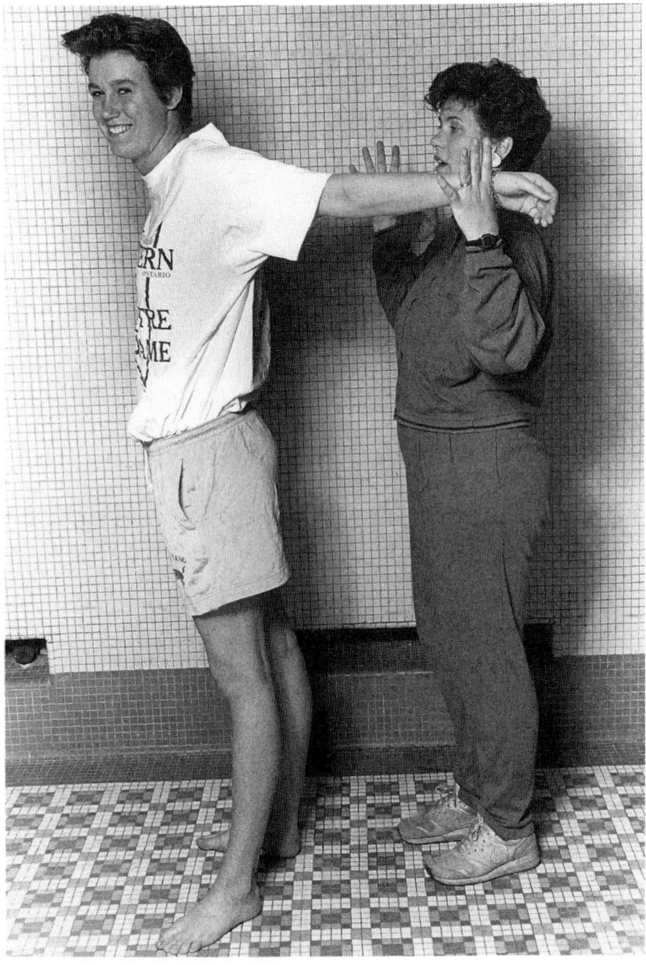

Figure 38.13. Pairs stretching requires a knowledge of proper technique and potential pitfalls.

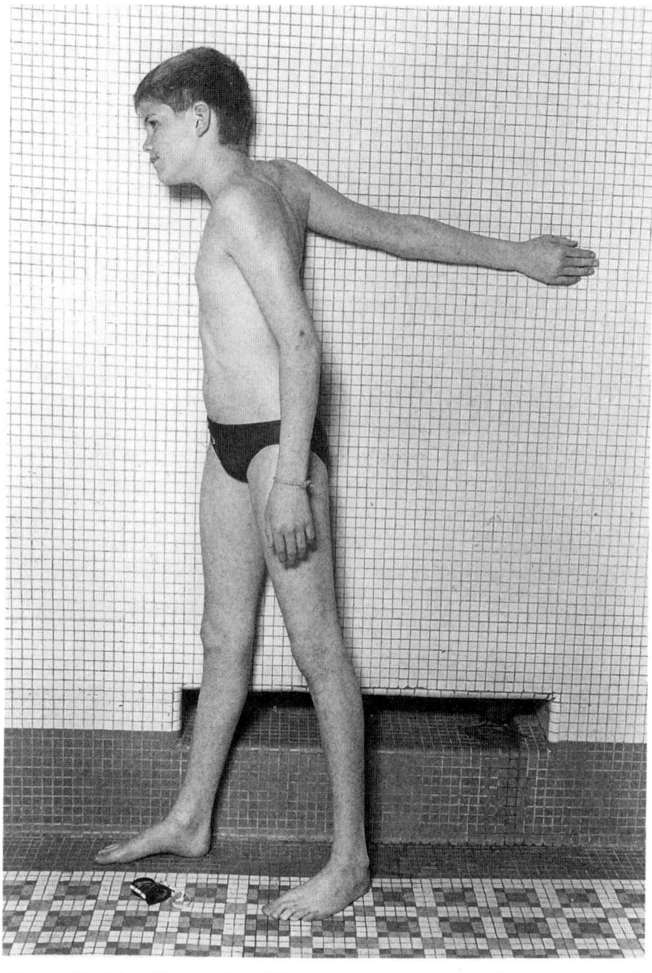

Figure 38.14. Single stretching can accommodate the sarne muscle groups as pairs stretching.

alternate sides keeps the swimmer from leaning constantly on the same shoulder.

Avoidance of Overwork

The demands on the swimmer should be increased gradually. Rigorous training sets before the athlete is ready or "extra hard" practices at the beginning of training regimen can trigger the onset of tendinitis. Training sessions should be designed so that the difficult portion of the workout is completed early in the practice when the swimmer is rested. The workouts should be organized with a focus on providing the swimmer with relative rest to structures at risk. For example, after the difficult work has been completed, the practice can continue with emphasis on stroke drills, alternating stroke and leg work, and start and turn techniques. Minimizing the potential for injury is dependent on proper instruction which will teach the swimmer to guard against fatigue and to be aware of the value of good stroke mechanics.

Treatment of Tendinitis (Table 38.6)

Classification of Tendinitis

Tendinitis is classified in three grades according to the categories for jumper's knee described by Blazina (10).

Grade I—Pain is experienced after the activity.
Grade II—There is pain during and after the sport, but it is not disabling.
Grade III—Disabling pain is present during and after activity.
Grade IV—Pain continues to be experienced in the activities of daily living after the cessation of swimming (11).

Grade I. Conservative management of a grade I tendinitis includes: increases in both warm-up and warm-down times, particular attention to prepractice stretching, icing, correction of external rotation weakness, decrease in work load, and temporary elimina-

Table 38.6.
Treatment of Rotator Cuff Tendinopathy

Treatment of Rotator Cuff Tendinopathy	Rehabilitation Program	
It is important to identify and treat the primary process in order to initiate sensible treatment. 1. REST from aggravation (not complete rest) 2. ALTER mechanics if indicated 3. ANTIINFLAMMATORY medication for a short course 4. ICE—#1 modality, used before and after workouts and therapy 5. PHYSIOTHERAPY modalities—ultrasound, laser, electrical stimulation, friction massage 6. RESTORE motion, strength, power, endurance, stability (individual attention to each depending on deficit) 7. STEROIDS? occasionally in subacromial bursa, repetitive injections may cause further problems 8. FUNCTIONAL sport specific exercises 9. SURGICAL TREATMENT Instability surgery if indicated Decompression surgery *only after 9–18 months of failed conservative Rx* Open or arthroscopic decompression—indications objectives in rehab are same: bursal excision may be sufficient if chronically inflamed and thickened: EUA and explore cuff for tears	Pain/tenderness	Mobilizations (grade I + II), transverse frictions, modalities (ice, US, laser, interferential, TNS)
	Rom/stiffness	ROM (pure and combined AROM movements), mobilizations grade IV + V, stretches—later used as prestrengthening warm-up
	Muscle imbalance	Strengthening—always performed in pain free ROM once shoulder is only mildly irritable Emphasis should be placed on internal/external rotator strength balance, high ratio is important to achieve
		Isometric
		Work all muscle groups, various ranges, maximal contractions—6 reps, 5 sec hold, 3 x per day *Once isometric work causes minimal treatment soreness, progress to isokinetic training.* Isokinetic strength evaluation at slow—60°/sec and fast—240°/sec speeds determines shoulder ratio Training commences in the least irritating position—neutral; progresses to 90° as comfort allows Concentrates on external rotation Tolerance must develop gradually
		Isokinetic
		3 times per week neutral position 240°/sec: 1 × 20 and 2 × 6 reps. 180°/sec: 1 × 15 and 2 × 6 reps. 120°/sec: 2 × 10 and 2 × 6 reps

tion of painful strokes. It is important that practice strokes be painfree. Stretching to increase blood flow, restore range of motion, and decrease potential for impingement should involve all structures about the shoulder, including the anterior ones. These are followed by a prolonged, slow-paced, warm-up in the pool using painfree strokes. Additional arm warm-ups are done after kicking sets. The training session is concluded with a warm-down period in the pool. Icing the shoulder for a maximum of 15 minutes after practice will reduce pain and inflammation. This is conveniently and effectively accomplished using ice cups. Strengthening the external rotators is important in controlling the glenohumeral joint and increasing muscle work efficiency. Strengthening is begun by working the external rotators in adduction and progressing to varying degrees of abduction. If symptoms are caused by one stroke only, that stroke should be discontinued until the symptoms subside when it can be gradually reintroduced. Faulty mechanics must be corrected.

Grade II. Management of grade II tendinitis incudes the activities described above as well as relative rest, physiotherapy, and medication. Relative rest means using strokes that do not cause pain and emphasizing leg work. Kick boards place the shoulder in pain-provoking positions and should not be used. Running and cycling can augment the limited swimming workouts. Antiinflammatory medication along with these measures will help provide symptomatic relief. Physiotherapy is indicated at this stage with treatment based on the therapist's evaluation, an evaluation that includes an assessment to determine the intensity and duration of pain, range limitations, and strength loss in arm and shoulder girdle muscles. Modalities such as ultrasound, interferential (current therapy) and transcutaneous nerve stimulation (TENS) are included in the therapy. Passive immobilization techniques and range of motion exercises are used to treat loss of range. Appropriate strengthening programs are organized to correct muscle strength imbalance or weakness. Exercises are isometric, isotonic, or isokinetic depending on the nature and presentation of the pain, joint range, and weakness. Free weights or surgical tubing can be used effectively in treatment programs as well. It is important that the exercises do not reproduce pain. If pain is felt in certain positions, the exercises should be done around these positions. Exercise that is painful throughout range should be discontinued or decreased in its repetition or resistance to a level that is painfree. A successful treatment program will allow the swimmer gradually to return to a full training schedule. However, therapy should not be discontinued until the preinjury activity level is attained.

A steroid injection into the subacromial space should only be considered if there is no response to treatment and if impingement-aggravated tests still elicit pain. In situations where injection is warranted, the swimmer's load should be decreased following the treatment with a return to previous levels taking place over a 4- to 6-week period. Steroid injections should not be used routinely.

Grade III. If the tendinitis progresses to grade III, becoming refractory in spite of the measures outlined above, the athlete is faced with options that include change of sport or surgical intervention. Most young swimmers choose the former and, in most instances, this is to be encouraged. If the possibility of a career at the national or international level exists, the athlete should be encouraged to weigh carefully the implications of both alternatives and should be assisted in this process by the coach and physician. Surgery, as outlined below, should be planned only if the swimmer clearly understands that the postoperative period demands a serious personal commitment to a rehabilitation program and that the success of the procedure is contingent upon cooperation and compliance with this program. Included in this regimen is a progressive exercise program to restore range of motion and balanced muscle strength. Return to the pool should begin with slow swimming that progresses to interval training and guided stroke modification.

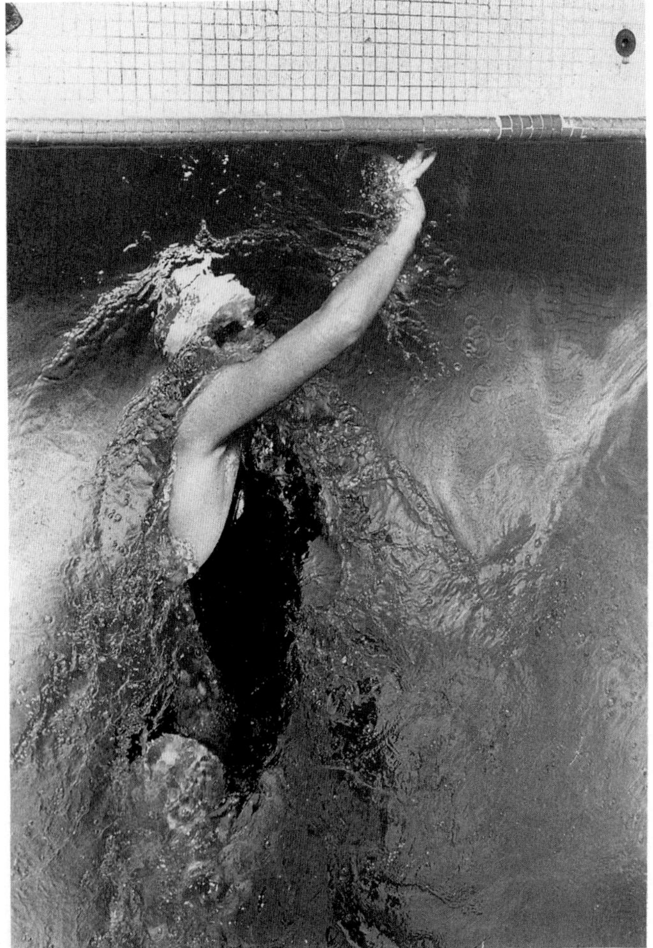

Figure 38.15. Modified backstroke turn. This avoids the provocative position. Turning more than 90° before touching the wall will result in disqualification.

Grade IV. Grade IV tendinitis is most often seen in the mature athlete and may indicate a torn rotator cuff. Imaging techniques such as athrography, ultrasonography, and magnetic resonance imaging may be used to confirm the clinical diagnosis. Lesions such as partial thickness tears and thickened subacromial bursa can be identified by arthroscopy of the shoulder joint and subacromial space. While not a frequent cause of pain in the younger swimmer, anterior and posterior superior quadrant labral tears can cause pain in the swimmer, but can be treated successfully with arthroscopic excision (12). Bursectomy alone followed by appropriate rehabilitation can provide relief in the younger swimmer, but a more radical decompression, which includes resection of the anteroinferior acromion and a portion of the coracoacromial ligament, is usually recommended. However, return to preinjury level of participation is unlikely and this should be explicitly understood by the athlete prior to surgery. Postoperatively, range of motion is often low; muscle strength, endurance, and power deteriorate—particularly in the abductors and external rotators. Physiotherapy that rehabilitates all the muscle groups about the shoulder girdle plays a significant postoperative role.

Shoulder Instability

Anterior Instability: Prevention and Treatment

Anterior instability is not often the cause of pain in competitive swimmers, and usually it is secondary to a traumatic incident in another sport. Compared to throwing activities, the arm is seldom in the provocative position during swimming strokes—with the exception of the conventional backstroke turn where the arm is levered anteriorly.

Primary conservative treatment of anterior instability is stroke modification and balancing-strengthening exercises. The traditional turn in the backstroke, which reproduces the symptoms of shoulder dislocation, can be modified by having the swimmer reach across the body to touch the pool wall and performing a somersault to come out of the turn (Fig. 38.15).

If symptoms do not subside, examination under anesthesia and/or arthroscopy will assist in diagnosing intraarticular lesions such as a Bankart or Hill-Sachs. An anterior stabilizing procedure can provide relief, and athletes can return to preinjury levels if their motion and strength are regained.

Posterior/Multidirectional Instability: Prevention and Treatment

Swimmers with frank posterior instability may have pain from dislocating their shoulders during the swimming stroke cycle. The at-risk position of forward flexion and internal rotation occurs in all strokes. Pain in swimmers with congenital or acquired multidirectional instability must be differentiated from that experienced by those suffering from painful tendinitis who have concomitant increased laxity.

In swimmers with prolonged periods of instability, persistence with a nonoperative program is recommended. In most cases, stroke modification, correction of strength deficits, as well as modification of training programs to minimize the magnitude and incidence of abnormal motion can be successful. Surgical intervention such as an inferior capsular shift, a "reefing procedure" to the posterior cuff and capsule, and a glenoid osteotomy should be considered only when all nonoperative treatments have been exhausted. These procedures, while providing symptomatic relief from pain for daily activities and for recreational participation in swimming and other sports, will, because of restricted motion, terminate a highly competitive swimming career (13, 14).

Knee

In a study of 2496 swimmers, Kennedy and Hawkins found that 90% of 261 individuals with orthopaedic complaints had shoulder, calf, or foot problems (15). Eighty-five calf and foot problems were divided almost evenly among the four competitive swimming strokes. All 70 knee problems were caused by the whip kick during the breaststroke (Table 38.1). The whip kick is considered the superior breaststroke kick in terms of speed and propulsion. However, it subjects the knee to unnatural motion, and, because of the intensity and number of repetitions performed, even proper execution does not protect the breaststroker from knee injury (15). Knee pain in the swimmer is usually caused by:

1. Medial collateral ligament (MCL) stress syndrome;
2. Patellofemoral syndrome;
3. Medial synovitis with or without a pathological medial synovial shelf.

Medial collateral stress syndrome, a common cause of pain in the elite breaststroker, affects the superficial fibers of the MCL that arise from the adductor tubercle of the femur and extend downward and forward to their insertion 4–5 cm distal to the knee joint on the anteromedial surface of the tibia. In a study of the pathomechanics of this problem by Kennedy et al. (16), it was found that tension on these fibers increased as the knee moved from flexion to extension, increased further with a valgus stress, and increased dramatically when external rotation forces were applied to the knee. Point tenderness along the course of the ligament is suggestive of medial collateral stress syndrome. Tenderness is often located at the origin of the MCL at the adductor tubercle and also where the superficial fibers cross the upper tibial margin. Pain may be reproduced when a valgus external force is applied to the knee flexed at 20° to 30°.

Patellofemoral syndrome is an abnormal alignment of the lower extremity as well as hypermobility or frank instability of the patellofemoral joint, which may be associated with patella alta. Palpation of the patellar facets or femoral condyles will elicit tenderness. Carrying out a patellar compression test or laterally deviating the patella may reproduce the symptoms. That more severe patellofemoral syndromes occur in club swimmers may be due to the improper execution of the kick. However, those with inherent instability of the patellofemoral articulations may be precluded from reaching elite levels of breaststroke swimming by the forces generated by the whip kick.

Medial synovitis was confirmed by Keskinen et al. (17) at arthroscopy in 7 out of 9 breaststrokers with knee pain. This synovitis was attributed to a combination of high angular velocities and excessive outward rotation. In a review of 36 breaststrokers with knee pain, Rovere and Nichols (18) found a significant relationship between frequency of knee pain, increased age, increased years in competition, increased training distance, and decreased warm-up distance. They also found that the medial aspect was the most common site of knee pain. Of the subjects examined, 47% had a tender, thickened medial plica (the fold of synovium, often described as the medial shelf). This implicated *medial synovial plica syndrome.* Both the extension phase of the breaststroke kick and plica palpation produce similar pain. During repeated knee flexion and extension, the fold or plica snaps across the medial femoral condyle producing friction that results in pain and inflammation of the plica (18). This synovitis may be the same type noted by Keskinen. Diagnosis is made by eliciting local tenderness and palpating the thickened synovium as it crosses the medial femoral condyle.

Since a multifactorial etiology may be present in many knee problems in swimmers, pathologies such as chronic ligamentous instability, torn medial meniscus (although uncommon in the stable knee), and osteochondritis dissecans must be ruled out as causes of pain.

Prevention of Injury and Treatment

As with other overstress syndromes, prevention is the ideal. An adequate warm-up period is an important first step. A minimum of 1000 to 1500 yards of warm-up prior to beginning hard breaststroke training along with gradual increases in training distances is recommended by Rovere and Nichols (18). Altering training programs so that breaststroke swimmers devote much of their workout time to other strokes and at least 2 months per year of total rest from swimming for elite breaststrokers are suggestions made by Kennedy and Hawkins (15).

Once pain occurs, early diagnosis and identification of the cause are both important. A knowledgeable coach will identify mechanical reasons, such as a faulty whip kick technique, which is known to be a correctable cause of knee pain (19). Communication among coach, physician, therapist, and swimmer is essential. Knee pain in the elite breaststroker is often more easily controlled than severe shoulder pain experienced by swimmers. But anatomical factors such as significant patellofemoral or ligament instability may be incompatible with the stress inherent in the whip kick. Therefore, a prolonged treatment program in such athletes may be doomed to failure. Again, this must be discussed with realistic and honest attitude among the swimmer, coach, and physician.

Therapeutic measures depend on the diagnosis; they include antiinflammatory medication for inflammation of the medial collateral ligament or medial synovial plica; ice and ultrasound may be used to control acute symptoms. For athletes with patellofemoral pain it is important to teach strengthening exercises to overcome muscle deficiencies. A stretching program for lower extremity musculature must be taught as well, and kept up. In addition, the swimmer with knee pain can continue training by swimming other strokes or breaststroke with the arms only. Steroid injections should play only a minor role. When they are used, injections should be directed into the inflamed pathological synovial tissue and not intraarticularly. Rovere and Nichols have noted the effectiveness of such injections in treating inflamed medial synovial plica (18). Once the acute phase of the injury has been handled, ongoing prevention and treatment should continue. The reintroduction of the breaststroke should be gradual and closely monitored to prevent recurrence.

Foot and Ankle

The extensor tendons of the ankle and foot are firmly bound over the dorsum of the ankle by the extensor retinaculum (Fig. 38.16). Tendinitis of these tendons, which are enclosed in sheaths and susceptible to irritation, is the most common cause of pain, regardless of the stroke performed. The foot and ankle are carried into extreme plantar flexion and then back to neutral in both the flutter and dolphin kicks. This repetitive work causes inflammation and edema, which are not well tolerated under the tight retinaculum. In most instances, the diagnosis is obvious since crepitus is both felt and heard when the foot is passively brought from plantar flexion to dorsiflexion. Again, prevention should be stressed with stretching of the extensor tendons routinely carried out prior to practices. Helpful local therapy modalities include ice and ultrasound. Wrapping of the foot and ankle and antiinflammatory medication are often beneficial as well. Swimming can generally be continued with less kicking or no kicking; return to normal kicking should be achieved in a graduated program (11, 20).

Elbow

Stress syndromes about the elbow are caused by the arm pull in the butterfly and breaststroke, and less frequently in the freestyle. The "elbow up" pull, in which the elbow is bent and held higher than the hand throughout the first part of the pull, is used by most competitive swimmers (19). This position allows the swimmer to push the water backward at the most efficient angle with a maximum backward thrust of the hand. The elbow then bends about 100° as the arm is pulled under the body with the upper arm is medially rotated and the forearm pronated. The butterfly stroke is very dependent on this arm pull, and the mechanics are similar to those of the freestyle. The early component of the breaststroke is also comparable to the butterfly and freestyle strokes. In a high elbow position,

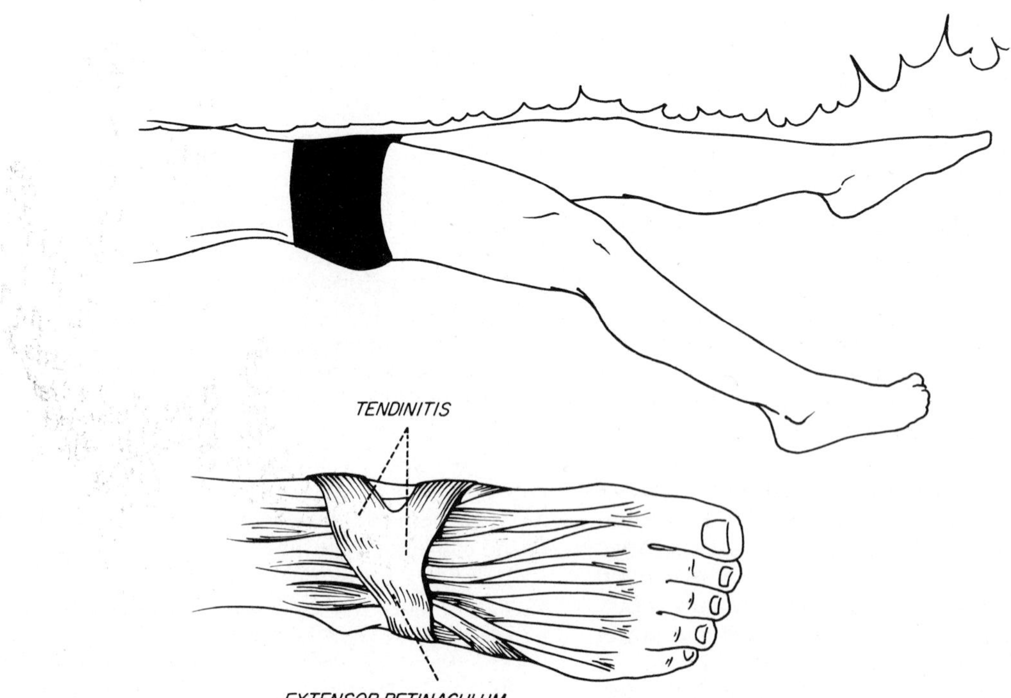

Figure 38.16. *Top.* This overuse syndrome is seen in the flutter kick of both freestyle and backstroke. *Bottom.* Note extreme plantar flexion of the ankle and foot. The tendons become irritated beneath the extensor retinaculum.

the swimmer has the sensation of reaching "over a barrel" (19). Lateral epicondylitis referred to as "tennis elbow" and described by Nirschl and Petrone can ensue (21, 22). With this disorder, the extensor carpi radialis brevis and extensor communis aponeurosis at the lateral epicondyle of the humerus become inflamed. The overwhelming moments of force along with repetition result in a combination of extrinsic overload and excessive muscle contraction. These appear to be the prime etiological factors. "Dropping" the elbow, which results in a less efficient angle and hence requires more force of the common extensor muscles, is recognized as a frequent fault in the swimmer's stroke pattern.

Lateral epicondylitis in the swimmer is treated by application of ice, the discerning use of antiinflammatory medication, and physical therapy modalities such as ultrasound to relieve acute and chronic inflammation. Forearm extensor power, flexibility, and endurance are increased by applying eccentric loads. Stroke alteration may decrease the moments of force placed on the elbow; in most cases, stroke alteration is essential for management over the long term. Steroid injection to the localized area is appropriate in resistant cases. Because there is evidence of collagen disorganization and weakening associated with such injections for up to a 6 week period (23), such injections should be used cautiously, judiciously, and infrequently.

In refractory cases, surgical treatment may include exposure and excision of the degenerative lesion as described by Nirschl (22). This must be followed by a slow and methodical return to training.

Back

Arm action in the breaststroke undergoes frequent change (20). From the glide position with extended arms, many breaststroke swimmers now pull with earlier elbow flexion and arm abduction. This prolongs the "elbow up" position and propels the torso above the water, which aggravates the already lordotic attitude of the lower back. This stress may cause a variety of low back problems including stress fractures of the pars interarticularis or even frank spondylolisthesis. More often however, accentuation of a mildly symptomatic spondylolisthesis or a mechanical low back pain from posterior facet irritation occurs, limiting the competitive breaststroker's training. These back complaints can also occur with the butterfly stroke where inefficient and improper mechanics are often the cause. The main complaint is often back pain with some radiation into the buttocks. Hamstring tightness may direct the physician toward a diagnosis of spondylolisthesis. Positive findings often include a step deformity at the spine of L5 that can be palpated and an abnormal gait with a backward pelvic tilt. The diagnosis is confirmed radiographically. In the presence of normal x-rays, a bone scan will help to diagnose a pars stress fracture. A stress fracture of recent origin requires first and foremost a prolonged period of rest. Spondylolisthesis is treated symptomatically depending on the severity of the complaints. The return to training must be carefully planned and monitored with hamstring stretching and abdominal strengthening playing a particularly important role in the ongoing treatment. If the low back pain is mechanical, a similar program will help. Prolonged treatment that includes other modalities such as transcutaneous nerve stimulations or repeated mobilizations to the affected area may be required in more resistant cases. A steroid injection into the inflamed facet may be necessary for relief as well.

The term "adolescent swimmer's back" was coined by Wilson and Lindseth (24) when they described three adolescent swimmers with backache aggravated by swimming the butterfly stroke. These patients were all diagnosed with Scheuermann's kyphosis. The authors did not determine whether vertebral abnormalities were caused by the forceful contraction of the chest and abdominal musculature or whether these were aggravating factors. Two of three experienced dramatic relief by stopping the butterfly stroke. Patients such as these should be encouraged to continue with their swimming program but to limit their swimming to the backstroke and freestyle.

REFERENCES

1. Kennedy JC, Hawkins RJ. Swimmer's shoulder. Phys Sports Med 1974;2(4):35.
2. Neer CS, Welsh RP. The shoulder in sports. Orthop Clin N Am 1977;8:585.
3. Rathbun JB, McNab I. The microvascular pattern of the rotator cuff. J Bone Joint Surg 1970;52(B):540–553.
4. Bigliani NU, Morrison DS, April EW. The morphology of the acromion and its relationship to rotator cuff tears. Orthop Trans 1986;10(2):216.
5. Ogata S, Uhtoff HK. Acromial enthesopathy and rotator cuff tear. Clin Orthop 1990;254:39–48.
6. Fowler PJ, Webster MS. Shoulder pain in highly competitive swimmers Orthop Trans 1983;7(1):170.
7. Fowler PJ. Shoulder injuries in the mature athlete. In: Grana WA, ed. Advances in sports medicine and fitness. Chicago: Year Book Medical Publishers Inc, 1988:225–238.
8. Webster MS, Bishop P Fowler PJ. Swimmer's shoulder. Undergraduate thesis. Waterloo, Ontario: University of Waterloo, 1981.
9. Griep JF. Swimmers shoulder: The influence of flexibility and weight training. Orthop Trans 1986;10(2):216.
10. Blazina ME. Jumper's knee. Orthop Clin N Am 1980;4(3):65.
11. Kennedy, JC, Craig A, Schneider RC. Sports injuries: Mechanics, prevention, and treatment. Baltimore: Williams & Wilkins, 1985.
12. McMaster WC. Anterior glenoid labrum damage: A painful lesion in swimmers. Am J Sports Med 1986;14(5):383.
13. Fowler, PJ. Evaluation, treatment and prevention of upper extremity injuries in swimmers. In: Nicholas J, Hershman EB, eds. Upper extremity in sports medicine. New York: C.W.Mosby, 1990:891–902.
14. Fowler, PJ, Webster-Bogaert MS. Swimming. In: Reider B, ed. Sports medicine—The school-age athlete. Philadelphia: W.B. Saunders, 1991:429–446.
15. Kennedy JC, Hawkins RJ. Breastroker's knee. Phys Sports Med 1974;2:33.
16. Kennedy, JC, Hawkins RJ, Krissoff WB. Orthopaedic manifestations of swimming. Am J Sports Med 1978;6:309.
17. Keskinen K, Eriksson E, Komi P. Breast stroke swimmer's knee. Am J Sports Med 1980;8(4):228.
18. Rovere G, Nichols AW. Frequency, associated factors and treatment of breaststroker's knee in competitive swimmers. Am J Sports Med, 1985;13(2):164.
19. Counsilman JE. The science of swimming. New Jersey: Prentice-Hall Inc, 1968.

20. Fowler PJ, Regan WD. Swimming injuries of the knee, foot and ankle, elbow and back. Clin Sports Med 1986;5(1):139.
21. Nirschl RP. Tennis elbow. Orthop Clin N Am, 1979;4:787.
22. Nirschl RP, Petrone FS. Tennis elbow. J Bone Joint Surg (AM) 1979;61:832–839.
23. Kennedy, JC, Willis RB. The effects of local steroid injections on tendons. A biomechanical and microscopic correlative study. Am J Sports Med 1976;4:11.
24. Wilson FD, Linseth RE. The adolescent swimmer's back. Am J Sports Med 1982;10:174–176.

39 / TRACK AND FIELD

Jerome V. Ciullo and Jeffrey D. Shapiro

Introduction

Track and field events afford the athlete the opportunity to demonstrate his or her capability in the most basic forms of physical prowess. Running, throwing, and jumping skills are individually emphasized as compared to other sports in which such skills are used in various combinations and for various goals. These events enjoy a rich heritage, tracing their origins to ancient times, as documented in records of the ancient Olympic games.

The Greeks stressed athletics for two reasons. First, their religious beliefs revolved around the "whole man" concept, where integration and development of body, mind, and soul was necessary in order to achieve one's potential. Secondly, athletic competition supplied physically fit soldiers (1). Running and jumping events prepared the soldier for offensive and defensive maneuvers. Throwing sports, such as javelin and discus, emphasized both strength and accuracy and closely paralleled activities of war (2).

The events comprising modern track and field competition fall into two groups, those that have basic explosive power requirements and those that emphasize endurance. Track and field events result in sport-specific injury patterns. To date, no thorough epidemiology studies comparing track versus field injuries have been reported. An epidemiologic analysis of sports injuries at the 1985 Junior Olympics reported that 35% of track participants required medical treatment related to their performance (3).

Analysis of Olympic track and field competitors over the past 100 years has shown that the age at which peak performance is achieved has remained remarkably consistent (4). For both men and women, the age of peak performance increases with the length of the foot race, with women generally achieving peak performance at younger ages. In the 100 meter dash, the mean age of gold medal winners in the last 100 years is 22.85 years for men, and 21.42 years for women. This contrasts with longer distance events. For men, the average age of 10,000 meter winners was 27.53 years. In field events, the mean age for male long jump champions was 23.05 years compared to 24.44 years for women. High jump gold medalists averaged 23.15 years for men, and 22.75 years for women, and shot put gold medalists averaged 24.00 years for men, and 26.11 years for women.

Track athletes with abnormal gait patterns and posture have an increased incidence of stress injuries with performance. A simple preparticipation screen includes assessment of flexibility of all major joints, responsiveness of primary postural muscles, posture, balance, and gait. In addition to a thorough cardiorespiratory evaluation, this basic motor screen is valuable in predicting which athletes are more susceptible to stress injuries.

Exogenous Factors

Running Shoes and Orthotics

There is no single ideal running shoe. Athletes must find a shoe that is comfortable and suits their style of running. Runners compete in spikes, but such shoes are not suitable for either distance or early season training where "flats" or commercial running shoes demonstrate superior shock-absorbing capacity. Some shoes are cut narrow, while others are cut wide; the sole may be curved or straight.

The toe of a running shoe is usually box-shaped and provides enough clearance for slight toe motion. This motion is imperative to prevent blisters, calluses, corns, cracked nails, and hematoma under the nail itself. The runner's foot bends at the ball; therefore, this is the place the shoe should also bend. If it is not flexible for the forefoot, the athlete is forced to "run over" the shoe, which causes a muscular imbalance and stress, so that Achilles tendinitis, shin splints, or strains can occur. If shoes are too stiff, scoring the undersurface at the forefoot with a knife will increase flexibility. The entire sole of the shoe must be well padded, but not too soft. Padding can reduce the incidence of bone bruising of the heel, calcaneal fat pad contusion, midfoot sprains, and spurring at the ball of the foot. The midfoot should be supported with a slight wedge. In addition, the external stripes or "lazy S" pattern of the outside of the shoe also serves to brace and stabilize the foot. The back of the shoe must not irritate the back of the heel. A wider or so-called "wheelbarrow" heel may be of some benefit in distance running where repetitive shock is distributed. Similarly, heel height can decrease strain on the Achilles tendon by slight elevation. Again, this is a matter of preference, since some well-trained athletes are used to walking normally in countersunk or negative heels and may in fact find a lower heel more comfortable.

Inserts or orthotics may be an occasional tool in treating an injury such as posterior tibialis strain. They have not been documented in injury prevention. With excess pronation of the foot, the lower leg compensation may result in a diffuse pain along the patella, which on occasion responds to orthotics.

Hard orthotics are occasionally helpful to recreational athletes, but competitive athletes find them difficult to wear. The musculotendinous unit takes a long time to adapt, and if orthotics are used they must be adapted to also. Runners find soft orthotics more comfortable. Distance runners may need two pairs of orthotics, the first, a hard pair for distance training, and a second softer pair for competition.

In a large series of long distance runners who had used orthotic shoe inserts for symptomatic relief of lower extremity complaints, it was found that these devices are most effective in the treatment of symptoms arising from biomechanical abnormalities such as excessive pronation or leg length discrepancies (5). Other diagnoses in which orthotics were utilized included excessive pronation, leg length discrepancy, patellofemoral disorders, plantar fasciitis, Achilles tendinitis, and shin splints. The results of treatment with the orthotic shoe inserts were independent of the diagnosis or the runner's level of participation.

In a longitudinal, double blind study, the effects of sock fiber composition on the frequency and size of blistering events in long distance runners were examined (6). It was found that socks composed of 100% acrylic fiber were associated with fewer and smaller blisters when directly compared to socks composed of 100% cotton fiber.

Blood Doping

Some Scandinavian and European distance runners have used a method of storing 1 to 2 units of their own blood 2 to 8 weeks prior to their event, and retransfusing it just prior to competition. The added blood volume is thought to allow increased performance by increasing oxygen transfer capability and increasing cardiac contractility (stroke volume) for distribution of the blood. This may be effective in acclimatizing to higher altitude where the air is thinner, thus avoiding the need to train and adapt at that altitude. Otherwise, advantageous effects in training and competition at similar altitudes, are highly controversial.

Diet

Athletes may try to alter their performance by dietary intake. Carbohydrate loading has become popular for the endurance-type athlete, but not for the sprinter or thrower. This is largely due to the muscle fiber type used in specific events. Sprinters and throwers concentrate on development of type II or "fast twitch" fibers. These bulky-type, muscled individuals have fibers that are activated specifically for short bursts. In contrast, endurance runners have developed their "slow twitch," type I, dark, or endurance-type fibers. These are lean muscles that respond to endurance training by increasing capillary supply to deliver oxygen and mitochondrial content to resynthesize adenosine triphosphate (ATP) and are therefore well suited for postural and endurance activity.

In contrast, the fast twitch fibers used in strength events like weight lifting, shot putting, and discus throwing do not respond as well to training in producing mitochondria or increasing capillary supply. Therefore, they have a relatively low capacity to resynthesize ATP through oxidative phosphorylation, and they fatigue quickly.

Muscles store glycogen to use as fuel in endurance-type activity. When not enough oxygen is available to convert this fuel into energy, the fuel is only partially metabolized, and lactic acid is the result. Lactic acid within the muscles or exhaustion of stored fuel quickly causes fatigue. The distance runner will call this "hitting the wall." In the well-trained athlete, this occurs after 1½ to 2 hrs of prolonged activity. In order to avoid this calorie depletion, some athletes have utilized a system called carbohydrate loading.

A well-trained athlete utilizes carbohydrate loading following an exhaustive training period where muscle glycogen is depleted. This is followed by a 3-day period in which carbohydrate intake is kept extremely low. Three days prior to the competitive event, a high carbohydrate diet is initiated. The depleted muscles soak up carbohydrates like a sponge and become supersaturated with glycogen. It is estimated that an untrained individual has approximately 13 g of glycogen per kilogram of muscle, and with training, this can increase to 32 g. After carbohydrate loading in a trained individual, storage can increase up to 35 to 40 g.

Many athletes avoid carbohydrate loading because it is considered to be a major shift from their routine diet. Periods of carbohydrate avoidance are met by the body with burning fat, and the end result is ketosis. This chemical shift can lead to irritability and an electrolyte imbalance resulting in irregularity of the heart beat. Since 3 g of water are stored with each gram of glycogen, a "loaded" distance runner may gain 3 to 5 lbs of weight, leading to a feeling of tightness and heaviness.

Drugs

Drugs have been utilized by athletes and warriors for more than 3000 years to protect them from evil, increase power, and improve performance. Among the agents that have been found in athletic drug use are:

mushrooms, caffeine, alcohol, nitroglycerin, ether, strychnine, cocaine, opium, camphor, ephedrine, glycerine, gelatin, iron, oxygen, aspartic acid, amphetamines, tranquilizers, vitamins, steroids, and red blood cells. Polypharmacy, or the abuse of multiple drugs at the same time, is not uncommon, particularly by the strength event athletes. Vitamins are among the most overused drugs.

The use of multiple vitamins is overrated. A young healthy adult, athletic or otherwise, has no need for vitamins or supplements if a normal diet is eaten. Many vitamins are quickly eliminated from the body after ingestion. Nevertheless, some fat-soluble vitamins like A, D, E, and K are stored within the body and have the potential to achieve toxic proportions.

In strength events, B-complex vitamins are utilized to augment a positive nitrogen balance. They are thought useful in increasing the heme component of both hemoglobin and myoglobin and thus to increase utilization and transfer of oxygen needed for metabolism. Only a small portion of ingested B-complex vitamins are absorbed by the body, and the rest are excreted. Their actual need or value is controversial.

Vitamin C compounds may be of more benefit in the athlete. As collagen turns over in the process of remodeling and adapting to increased stress and in the healing phase encountered with the microtrauma of training, ascorbic acid or vitamin C is a necessary cofactor in sulphur cross-linking and strengthening of the collagen fibrils. Therefore, vitamin C may be useful in coping with the stress of vigorous athletic training. Nevertheless, only approximately 500 mg of vitamin C can be absorbed daily, and megadoses have the potential to lead to crystalline deposits in the kidneys. Ascorbic acid also acts as a cofactor to increase the absorption of B-complex vitamins by the gastric mucosa.

Many athletes involved in strength field sports feel that protein supplements are essential to establish the positive nitrogen balance needed to obtain maximal benefit from anabolic steroids and training. Nevertheless, with megadoses of protein, uric acid levels within the blood increase and microdamage of the kidneys and joints may be the result. Protein is not normally utilized in athletic performance, since the body usually burns protein only in starvation.

The use of anabolic steroids remains controversial. Physicians and the general public tend to view these drugs as dehumanizing, possibly allowing an unfair advantage to the athletes using them, and definitely tainting the spirit of fair play. A report on doping from the health organization of the League of Nations in 1939 was the first official statement to suggest that the use of male sex hormones could theoretically enhance athlete performance (7). The official ban on and testing for anabolic steroids by the International Olympic Committee have reinforced in the athlete's mind that such drugs can indeed enhance performance, and that, in not using drugs, they would be operating at a definite disadvantage. The use of these drugs and possible advantages were discussed at the university level and even down to the junior high level in the early 1970s. The medical community banded together to condemn anabolic steroids (8). Physicians cited known side effects of steroid use such as renal disease, testicular atrophy, and adrenal suppression known to have occurred in diseased individuals. At the same time, they implied that these same side effects could be expected in a healthy athlete. They also cited poorly designed clinical studies in which untrained individuals were utilized, or in which anabolic steroid dosage was very small, in order to demonstrate that use of these drugs was not only dangerous, but ineffective. To tell young athletes that such drugs were of no advantage, and, in fact, had side effects such as decreasing libido has cost the sports medicine community much of its credibility; many track and field athletes have gone elsewhere with their sports-related problems because of this. Track and field athletes have indeed demonstrated enhanced performance despite warnings of adverse side effects. Most notably, Ben Johnson of Canada won the 100 meter dash in the 1988 Olympics but was subsequently disqualified for steroid use. The basic science of steroids is discussed in Chapter 9 on Drugs and Sports.

Caffeine is now considered to be one of the most abused drugs in high performance athletes. Normally, muscles are dependent on stored glycogen. Caffeine from tablets, coffee, or cola drinks will release fats from tissue into the blood stream, making them available to muscle. The muscles then burn these fats in preference to stored glycogen and therefore are able to work longer and to avoid fatigue. Three hundred milligrams of caffeine, or about the amount found in two cups of coffee, have been found to be enough to produce this effect in the trained athletes (9). In fact, any amount above this level can lead to caffeine overdose or fine muscle tremors that decrease athletic performance.

Field Conditions

Important to track and field construction is accessibility of dressing quarters for the athletes and proximity to parking spaces for the spectators. Nevertheless, the surface itself is most important to athletes. Athletes have invested so much time and energy in the training process that they deserve a safe and proper surface on which to compete. Although proper methods of track construction are suggested in the literature, certain errors that can affect performance must be emphasized (2).

Running tracks are essentially oval in shape, with the inner oval length measured at ¼ mile, 440 yards, or 400 meters. Adequate drainage is essential so that the runners need not run in mud. Curving can also help in this drainage effect. A water supply may be needed to sprinkle the surface to make it soft enough for competition, as well as to provide a drinking water supply. Most high schools utilize a cinder-type surface on the track. Clay is commonly used because of cost, but, if utilized, must be watered regularly; otherwise, it will seal and actually prevent seepage of water. If the clay-cinder track is allowed to dry, it becomes brittle and actually flakes under the impact of running shoes.

It is a common error to use 3- to 5-ton street maintenance rollers when leveling cinders. These are used as a matter of convenience, since such equipment is readily available. Nevertheless, this can decrease the resiliency and shock absorption qualities of the track; a ½-ton roller should be utilized instead.

The alternative to frequent maintenance is the all-weather track. The most popular synthetic track is the one popularized in the 1968 Mexico City and the 1972 Munich Olympic Games. With such a surface in conjunction with a good drainage system, little, if any, maintenance is necessary, and lanes and start and finish lines can be permanently marked. Energy storage within the muscles and subsequent muscle contraction have all been found to be enhanced on this synthetic polyurethane surface. With proper engineering, shock to the musculotendinous unit can be minimized, while energy storage and subsequent release are maximized.

Unfortunately, two medical conditions have developed because of these surfaces. The synthetic turf syndrome has been described as painful aching in the ankle joint, thigh musculature, tibia, and patella and has been found in athletes who compete on these synthetic surfaces. It has been suggested that it is related to shock vibrations in these synthetic surfaces that is not found with conventional cinder tracks. Vibration, damping, and elasticity of the track surface as well as ground contact time and step length can be altered by variance of the track stiffness. These need to be adjusted for the individual events to be performed on these surfaces. Rebound variation must be in synchrony with reciprocating eccentric and concentric contraction for energy absorption and release to be maximized. Otherwise, energy handled out of phase will lead to tissue stress and injury.

The second problem encountered with these synthetic polyurethane tracks is abrasion. Synthetic granules, when embedded within the skin surface, lead to a long-lasting weeping reaction. Abrasions encountered with contact with synthetic surfaces must be treated aggressively, that is, with scrubbing and antibiotic solutions, in order to avoid a potentially long-lasting and annoying problem.

In the jumping events, rubberized synthetic surfaces can be used for approach ramps and aprons. In the long jump, triple jump, and pole vault, many schools have limited the width of the approach strip to two feet rather than the standard four feet in order to save money. A misstep from this narrow strip can lead to ankle sprains, twisting of the knee, ligament injuries, or falls and associated contusions. Therefore, the temptation to use narrower approach strips as cost-containing measures should be avoided for the sake of the athlete. Otherwise, the same drainage and building materials can be used for the runways and aprons as is used for track construction itself. The same measures used in maintenance of the track must be carried out in maintenance of the runways. The athlete himself must police the runway prior to utilization to make sure that no holes or obstacles are evident that will cause injury or decrease performance. Takeoff boards at the end of the runway for the broad jump and hop, skip, and jump may need frequent replacement, due to contact with spikes and internal breakdown related to utilization.

The landing pits used for jumping events should extend from a point 10 feet in front of the takeoff board for 20 or more feet beyond. They should be filled with builder's sand and be kept slightly moist. They should be turned daily in order to decrease jarring encountered at the time of contact. At least 12 to 18 inches of builders' sand or foam is necessary to lessen the shock.

The pole vault is a very specific activity, necessitating runways in both sides of the pit to help compensate for wind conditions. Sawdust or sand must be available to place in the planting box to lessen the shock of pole planting if the athlete feels it is necessary. Standards used in the pole vault and high jump should be well machined and weighted to fall away from the individual at contact to avoid athletic injury. The landing pits should be made of foam rubber and should be properly constructed to extend around the planting box, or slightly under the high jump bar, since the athletes frequently do not clear the bar and fall directly downward; therefore, they must be shielded from injury. The crossbar utilized in both pole vault and high jump should be made of fiber glass. Although the metal crossbars may be cheaper, they can cause more injury if the athlete falls on them. The weight circles for discus and hammer must consider the athlete's action of pivoting on the feet so that the texture of the surface and the shoes utilized correspond. It is imperative that the surface be as smooth as possible because of the pivoting so that ankle sprains and stress on the knees can be minimized. The ramp for the javelin throw should be constructed in a manner similar to those of the long jump and pole vault.

Stretching and Weight Training

Slow, steady stretching is common prior to track and field activity. Such eccentric warm-up increases circulation by wasted heat. Contractility is thus increased by enzymatic induction. This effect lasts for up to ½ hr following a single stretch, which can be a significant factor during competition. Stretching after muscular activity, such as a light jog following athletic performance, will help clear metabolites, so that stiffness leading to fatigue will not be a problem in future performance. Stretching following athletic activity also helps overcome biologic creep, viscoelastic contraction of myofibrils and collagen, increasing the limits of flexion and extension somewhat; if muscular hypertrophy develops in proportion to increased range of motion, more effective storage and utilization of contractile energy may be possible. There is a danger of overstretching, however, and it is important to realize that the musculotendinous unit performs optimally at a basal length that is a product of muscle hypertrophy, elasticity, and flexibility.

Weight training is particularly beneficial in increasing myofibril hypertrophy and capillary ingrowth, both of which can increase contractility and decrease fatigue. Nevertheless, if fibers are cold, weakened by previous injury, undernourished, overstretched, or fatigued, chronic strain or tendinitis may develop. Repetitive microtrauma may lead to a major disruption or rupture.

Stretching must become routine to prevent overload of the musculotendinous unit related to training excess or error. Before a race, athletes must warm up to increase efficiency of muscles and thereby reduce the incidence of strain. This also decreases the mental fatigue that leads to strain or sprain injury. Proper warm-up can significantly decrease and even eliminate the initial period utilized to attain the "second wind" level of performance. Middle and long distance runners need more time than sprinters to warm up circulation-dependent type I endurance fibers. A period of easy running and light flexibility exercises working up a slight perspiration followed by a short series of warm-up sprints and easy jogging, striding, and rest before race time can be carried out, followed by a five-minute period of rest to get breathing back to normal. After completing the distance event, athletes must continue to jog for a lap or two in order to encourage circulation and help clear metabolic waste products from muscle so that fatigue and stiffness do not set in during the next few days. Going through a light job and stretching routine the day following competition helps to work out tightness and encourage circulation.

Running Events

Sprints

Sprints are defined as events in which the contestant runs at full speed over the entire distance.

Forward human locomotion is measured within a gait cycle. A normal walking cycle is measured from heel strike to heel strike of the same foot. In sprinting, this changes to analysis from toe strike to toe strike. Motion has been analyzed in terms of a stance or support phase where the foot strikes the ground, attains some support, and then takes off. This is followed by a swing, or recover phase, where there is follow-through, forward swing, and foot descent. In walking, one foot is always on the ground. As speed of gait increases, the stance phase is eliminated when neither lower extremity is in contact with the supporting surface. As the speed of gait increases, the need for forward propulsion and acceleration leads to increased ground reaction force (10).

Sprinters reach top running speed quickly and do this by maximizing initial acceleration. It had been noted that by keeping the center of gravity low, leaning forward, and pushing off with a strong quadriceps, acceleration could be achieved quickly. Sprinters soon learned that kicking holes in the track could be utilized to some advantage in pushing off. Such practices, nevertheless, left the track in poor condition, so that in 1927 removable and adjustable starting blocks were allowed.

Sprinters are said to be born rather than developed (11). A sprinter has a short reflex time and a quick reaction time. Sprinters need a full range of motion for all extremities since they start from a low position to mobilize the body's center of gravity, then move slowly to a more upright position. Initial acceleration necessitates generation of power. This generation of power starts with preloading the muscles by lowering in the starting blocks, and it is aided and amplified by synchronization of upper and lower extremity motion. The hands are thus held tight to generate lower extremity push-off (Fig. 39.1). Sprinters do not burst out of the block, but learn to run out of the blocks. By clinching the fists and swinging the arms strongly, sprinters are able to amplify crossed-extensor reciprocal eccentric and concentric energy utilization.

The starting blocks must be reset for each athlete. Although the setting is somewhat dependent on the athlete's size, flexibility, muscle strength, and stride length are all important factors that necessitate that each athlete find his or her own ideal setting. The sprinter must be quite flexible and capable of reciprocal flexion and extension of the extremities to maximize musculotendinous performance. When the reciprocal pumping action of the arms and legs do not work together, strained muscles are the result. This is either due to overstretch or muscular imbalance overloading antagonistic muscles in the eccentric phase (12).

Because of the need to maintain forward propulsion while the center of gravity is forward of the planted foot and because sprinting is a process of pushing with that extended leg, quadriceps strength is emphasized. In weight work, an emphasis must be made to maintain hamstring strength at approximately 80% of that of quadriceps strength to maintain proper balance. The hamstrings and posterior tibialis muscles must be stretched and strengthened to help prevent injury. In eccentric contraction, the reverse extended leg at the time of the start is capable of generating a tremendous hamstring response. If the muscle is not flexible, or has

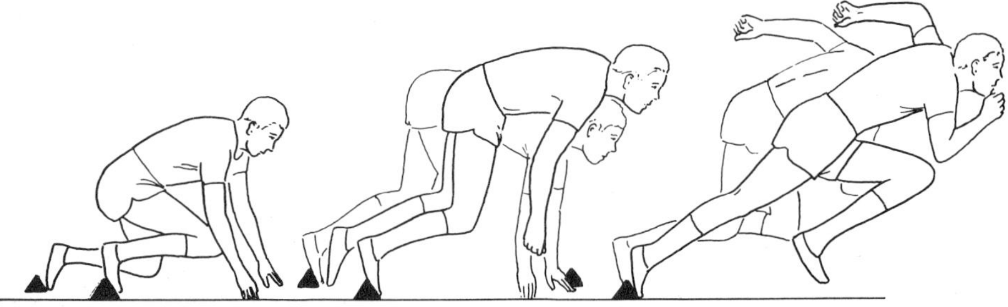

Figure 39.1. Block start. A crouched position is utilized in the start to generate the most effective power by raising the center of gravity slowly. Here efficient utilization of energy, preloaded by lowering oneself into the blocks is maximized.

not been warmed up, a hamstring "pull" or strain results, and, in fact, this is the most common injury in sprinters.

It is important in the evaluation of hamstring injuries to examine the entire musculotendinous complex unit. Avulsion injuries can occur from the ischial tuberosity. These are most often treated nonoperatively, but in cases of considerable displacement, operative treatment can be considered in elite athletes. More commonly, however, these injuries occur within the substance of the muscle belly or at the musculotendinous junction. Stretching and strengthening can help this problem. It is important that the coach allow adequate time for adaptation and rest of the hamstrings. Avoiding block drills too early in the season or on two subsequent days during the season are helpful preventative techniques.

The rehabilitation of hamstring injuries consists of a gradually increasing program of mobilization, strengthening, and increased activity. These injuries frequently heal slowly and can often recur, following premature return to competition. Therefore, return to sport should only be allowed when full muscle strength, endurance, and flexibility have been regained.

Because the sprinter runs on his toes, he is prone to injury of the posterior tibialis, flexor digitorum longus, and flexor hallucis longus musculotendinous units. Most of these injuries consist of tendinitis and can be treated with orthotics, ice, rest, and antiinflammatory medication. Rupture of the posterior tibialis tendon is diagnosed by tenderness at the bony insertion, as well as by loss of the longitudinal arch medially. In addition, when viewed from behind, the patient exhibits the "too many toes" sign where more toes are seen, laterally on the affected side as compared to the unaffected side. Complete tendon ruptures are treated surgically. Stretching is of great importance in avoiding symptoms of tendinitis.

Since greater contact force is generated at higher speed, and since sprinters run on their toes, Achilles tendinitis, or inflammation of the common tendon of the gastrocnemius and soleus muscles, is a frequent problem. Localization of the area of maximal tenderness is usually approximately 2 cm proximal to the insertion of the Achilles tendon on the calcaneus. Nodularity, palpable within the tendon, is indicative of partial tendon injury with subsequent mucinous degeneration of tendon substance. Achilles tendinitis is treated conservatively with stretching, antiinflammatory medication, and heel lifts. Surgery is only performed in recalcitrant cases. Achilles tendon rupture is most commonly seen between the ages of 30 to 40 years. Best results are obtained with surgical approximation of torn tendon ends in elite athletes. Symptoms of Achilles tendonitis are worsened when the sole of the shoe is so rigid that athletes are made to run over it, decreasing their push-off ability and contact time of the ball of the foot. Rigid orthotics may also accentuate the problem. Calf muscle strengthening and heel cord stretching are the keystones of prevention of Achilles tendinitis.

The gastrocsoleus muscle group must be kept strong to allow running on the sprinter's toes. Otherwise, the heel may drop back too far and the stretch placed on the sole of the foot can lead to plantar fasciitis and/or a secondary heel spur. In contrast, running on the toes without proper flexibility can also lead to metatarsalgia. Plantar fasciitis and metatarsalgia are difficult problems to treat; they are best avoided by maintaining proper flexibility and shock-absorbing muscle tone of all groups of lower extremity musculature.

Quadriceps contracture, tight hamstrings, weak vastus medialis, high riding patella, or excess pronation of the foot can lead to a lateral patellar compression syndrome, leading to chondromalacia or roughening of the weight-bearing surface of the underside of the patella. Such roughening increases the coefficient of friction, which will lead to further articular damage, shedding of articular fragments, synovitis and associated effusion of the knee, and early arthritis. Such problems are minimized or avoided by stretching and strengthening the vastus medialis obliquus. Extension exercises are performed in the final 30° of terminal extension to isolate this musculature. Occasionally, because of anatomic variation, a surgical release of the lateral patella retinaculum may be necessary to correct extensor mechanism malalignment.

Stress fractures are usually a product of training error. Fibular and tibial fractures are characteristic of the sprinter and are seen early in the season when the musculotendinous unit has not perfected its shock-absorbing properties, and again late in the season from simple overuse. Highly concentrated muscle force acting across a specific bone because of demands imposed by particular repetitive tasks enhance the loading that occurs merely from direct weight bearing on the affected part (13). Once localized tenderness is elicited on physical examination, x-ray evaluation is mandatory. Stress fractures, however, may take 10 to 14 days to be demonstrable radiographically; they can be diagnosed earlier with technetium scintigraphy. Treatment is by immobilization with weight bearing, depending on the individual fracture. Such complaints can be minimized by avoiding the use of spikes too early in the season and initiating training on soft surfaces, allowing gradual adaptation to occur.

The ankle is most secure due to talar dome configuration in a dorsiflexed position. Thus, the athlete is subject to ankle sprain with a misstep or by turning a plantar flexed ankle on a wet surface. It is, therefore, the athlete's responsibility to inspect the entire lane for wet spots, holes, or debris prior to an event. Since the longer sprinting events must incorporate curves, it may mean that utilizing one of the outside lanes may be safer than an uneven or poorly drained inner lane.

Ankle injuries most commonly occur on uneven surfaces and as the sprinter turns. Although ligamentous sprains are by far the most commonly occurring injuries, chondral and osteochondral lesions of the talar dome, and less commonly of the tibial plafond, can occur. These injuries present in a clinically similar manner to ligamentous injuries, but fail to progress in their healing and rehabilitation. Diagnosis is rarely made by plain x-rays, but can be seen more accurately with computerized axial tomography and magnetic resonance imaging. Treatment is dependent on the size and location of the lesion. Loose or unstable chondral or osteochondral fragments are best excised arthroscopically.

Stress injuries have also been described in the posterior aspect of the talus. These injuries can involve either the os trigonum just posterior to the talus, or the posterior process of the talus. These injuries, if recalcitrant to conservative treatment, are best diagnosed with technetium scintigraphy. Although most injuries to the os trigonum heal after a period of immobilization, recalcitrant cases may require local injection of corticosteroids. Rarely, these injuries require surgical excision of the symptomatic ossicle.

It is customary to run events around the track in a counterclockwise fashion. This causes supinating forces on the left foot and pronating forces on the right foot, leading to torquing and potential incoordination (Fig. 39.2). The pronated outer right foot flattens, and the leg externally rotates to increase the ability to push off and further accelerate around the curve. Torque on the right knee leads to medial symptoms. Voshell's bursa, between the superficial and deep portions of the medial collateral ligament, may become inflamed at the medial collateral ligament just below the joint line. With the internal rotation of the lower leg induced by forced pronation, the outer leg sustains stress in the posterior lateral aspect, which can lead to symptoms of popliteal tendinitis. Point tenderness along the course of the popliteus, particularly posteriorly at the musculotendinous junction or at its femoral insertion just anterior to the fibular collateral ligament, will help make the diagnosis.

The inner left leg being forced into heel supination with corresponding arch elevation and external rotation of the lower leg places stress on the medial hamstrings, which are involved in acceleration around the curve. A strain of the medial collateral ligament is commonly confused with a medial meniscal tear, and in spite of joint tenderness at the joint line, lack of effusion within the joint may be used to lead to proper diagnosis. The above three conditions are best minimized by maximizing the shock-absorbing properties of the musculotendinous unit by strengthening and stretching in an effort to avoid injury.

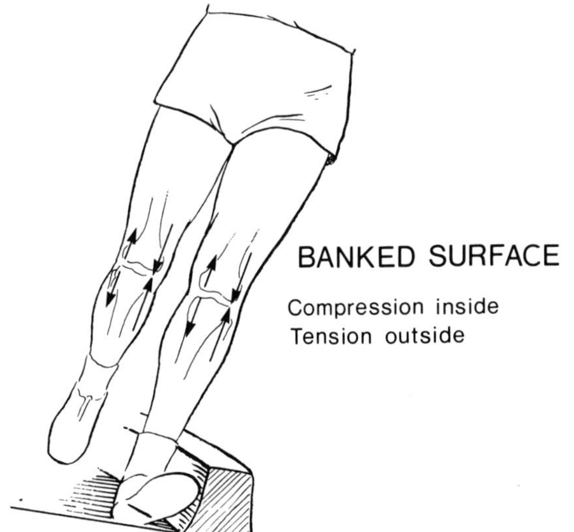

Figure 39.2. The muscular stresses and counter stresses are shown as the runner takes the curve.

The shorter length and increased banking of indoor surfaces can lead to iliotibial band friction syndrome near the lateral knee or hip in athletes with tight structures. It is mandatory to undergo vigorous iliotibial band stretching exercises, particularly if such conditions are anticipated. In running curves indoors, the athlete retains a slight lean to the inside when facing into the turn. The outside arm swings across the body, and the pelvis rotates to potentiate momentum. The athlete should run as close to the inside lane as possible; because of this, short-legged athletes may have an advantage in indoor competition. Since a great deal of energy is expended to maintain angular velocity, the athlete attempts to increase acceleration about the curve to accelerate out of it. In doing so, tremendous torque is generated through the knees and hips.

Although Olympic class outdoor running tracks have an overall lap length of 400 m, turn radii are not specified, thus giving rise to an assortment of tracks with varying aspect ratios. The maximal speed attainable while running on a finite radius turn is considerably less than that running along a straight line. The value of speed reduction to the runner depends on the effective radius of the turn and the runner's top speed. This is secondary to an increase in the foot contact time necessary to maintain constant vertical impulse to compensate for the vectorial decrease of available vertical force as the individual's heel turns over into the turn. The increased foot contact time causes a corresponding decrease in the ballistic air time. As a result, there is a discrepancy in the maximal speed attainable when running different lengths on an oval track. In fact, the outer lanes in a conventional oval race track have a speed advantage over the inner most lanes. This discrepancy is greatest when one considers tracks with tight turns, as is the case with many indoor facilities (14).

Relays

A relay race is an event in which, originally, two and now four runners run a specified distance, each relieving the previous runner at designated points within fixed zones. The first runner is allowed to start from blocks, and all subsequent runners start in an upright position, passing a baton within a 22 m passing zone, although 10 m in front of the passing zone are allowed to build up momentum for the pass. Initially, the relief runner would start his or her leg of the relay after touching the hand of the oncoming contestant. This presented a problem in judging whether such hand contact had actually taken place, so the baton was introduced, bringing an additional hazard to the relay. An attempt is made to exchange the baton with full arm extension by both runners while at maximum speed. There is a right-to-left to right-to-left hand sequence of exchange among the four runners, which must be well practiced. The curve runner holds the baton in the right hand and the straight-away runner holds it in the left. An underhand pass technique is utilized in the sprint; the outgoing runner extends an open hand downward into which the incoming partner slips the baton, a procedure necessitating much practice. The baton missing the open hand can jam into the outgoing runners hip, can lead to contusion or laceration, or result in a misstep or dropping baton.

The runner must establish beforehand which side of the lane to come in on, and on which side of the lane the next runner is to exit. Crossover passing, such as right hand to right hand, must be avoided, since there is a significant risk of running over the partner's feet or heels leading to a spiking injury, sprain, or contusion to the ankle or the calf area.

In the distance relay, the incoming runner will undoubtedly be fatigued, and, therefore, it is necessary for the outgoing runner to look backward and follow the baton visually during the exchange. Unlike the blind pass utilized in the sprint, this must be a visual pass and must be well practiced to avoid the crossover stepping or misstepping that can lead to knee or ankle injury. The baton must be exchanged within the prescribed distance, and, without proper practice, the lead runner may be forced to decelerate to obtain the baton; and this may lead to a torquing anterior cruciate ligament injury.

Baton exchange introduces the factor of hand trauma. Lacerations and jammed fingers are an occasional occurrence. Dislocated phalanges must not be taken lightly, since fracture or collateral ligament damage may be associated. X-ray evaluation is therefore mandatory with these injuries. Ulnar collateral ligament sprain of the thumb can be related to poor passing technique. Obviously these injuries can be minimized by synchronized baton exchange, which can only be accomplished through practice. Walking and jogging through the exchange is mandatory prior to attempting it at full speed.

Hurdles

Although hurdling is erroneously considered a jumping event by spectators, in fact, it is a sprinting event in which the participant must clear obstacles at various heights and because these are sprinting events, the distance is limited to about 440 yards.

As a sprint event, participants utilize blocks and stay within their lanes. Although hurdlers are used to attaining some height to clear obstacles, they must avoid rising up too quickly in their start so that they can both cut down in time and avoid strain to the low back, which can result in either paraspinous muscle spasm or fracture along the transverse process. To avoid rising too quickly as well as to maintain correct body lean, hurdlers must look toward the ground at least until their fifth stride, by which time they have elevated their centers of mass sufficiently to accommodate the first hurdle. Hurdlers approach each obstacle with maximum speed so that they run over the hurdle and do not jump over it. This is important since they decelerate in the jumping process and can only obtain speed by running on the ground.

Hurdlers must drive the knee of the leading leg forward to obtain sufficient spring with the push-off foot to clear the hurdle. The moment they become airborne, they lean forward in order to get the leading leg back on the ground as soon as possible so that they can continue their sprint. If they lean forward too quickly, they will run into the hurdle, and by waiting too long, the center of gravity will land behind the leading leg and they will fall backward. In this way, they drive up with the knee, straighten the leg, and as they are just above the hurdle, they snap their leg down over it. Beginners may want to throw their foot up rather than drive up with the knee. In doing so, they will throw their center of gravity backward and will have a difficult time clearing the hurdle (Fig. 39.3).

Hurdlers keep their arms out in front of the body when accommodating the hurdle. This not only cen-

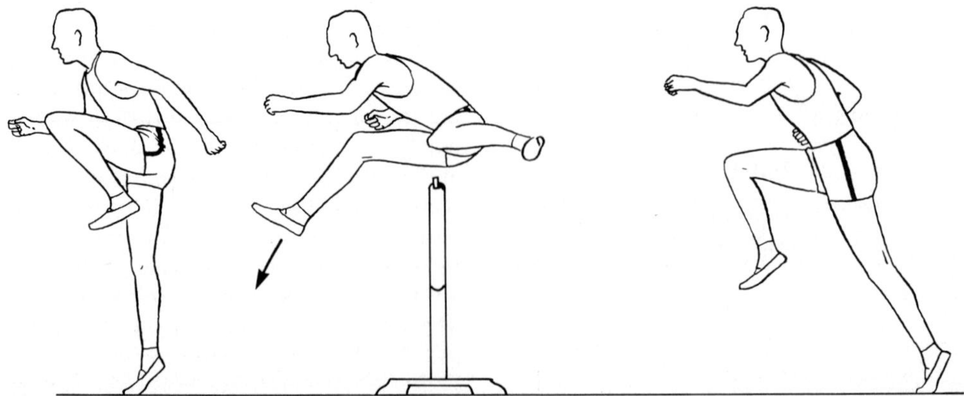

Figure 39.3. Hurdling technique. As the back leg pushes, the leading leg quickly extends helping the back leg to reciprocally flex in order to clear the bar. The front leg then dips over the bar to make ground contact quickly, sine acceleration is only gained on the ground. The center of gravity also remains in a nearly perfect straight line, thus aiding in acceleration.

tralizes the center of gravity, but allows enough clearance to raise the trailing leg so that it can avoid contact with the hurdle. The trailing leg must be brought up into a flexed position and should not be whipped around, because this can lead to an imbalance that is accommodated by straightening the arms out to the side. This slows forward momentum so that the trailing leg or the ankle are at risk of contacting the top of the hurdle.

Hurdlers must lean forward as they come off the hurdle so that the center of gravity is forward, allowing them to sprint toward the next hurdle. They must also know how to clear a hurdle with either leg. Although they may have an ideal number of strides between each hurdle, as the race progresses they may fatigue; the adaptation is a shorter stride length with more strides between each hurdle. If they do not know how to clear the hurdle with either foot, they may have to slow their pace to add an increased stride in order to utilize a favored leg. To do so, they must decelerate. This not only lessens the chance of winning the race, it also can lead to an anterior cruciate ligament sprain in the knee.

As the lead leg snaps down towards the ground, hurdlers must land on the balls of their feet. If they come down too flat footed or on a heel, they will suffer a heel bruise, which is usually one of two entities. The most common is fat pad contusion, where the intracalcaneal fat pad sustains an element of hemorrhage. Clinically, there is point tenderness under the heel. The spongy bone of the calcaneous may also be subject to a micro or stress fracture that may take weeks before it can be demonstrated on standard x-ray. A bone scan may be helpful in delineating the problem sooner, but it is best to avoid the problem with proper technique, because heel injuries commonly take months to clear up.

With the amount of stretch needed to clear the hurdle in both the lead leg and the trail leg, hamstring strain or frank muscle rupture, groin pull, and pelvic avulsion fracture have historically been extremely common. Because of this, hurdlers have religiously done stretching exercises, including the traditional hurdler's stretch, so that in fact the number of such injuries are probably less common than actually found in sprinters. The importance of stretching for the prevention of strain cannot be overemphasized. Nor can emphasis on proper coaching technique, since a misstep can lead to ligament sprain, muscle strain, or repetitive contusion and myositis ossificans.

Hurdlers must make sure that their lane is clear of foreign objects or obstructions, and that the hurdles are square within it. When running, their eyes must be kept forward at all times; if they look back either to see where opponents are, or in response to the sound of an opponent hitting an obstacle, they shorten their stride, decrease their momentum, and interfere with their technique enough that they are at risk of injury.

If hurdlers work hard on one day, they will need a recovery day of gentle stretching and healing. Warm-up takes at least half an hour a day and begins with jogging half a mile or jumping rope. In the off-season, they may be involved with indoor track, but if not, they work on endurance. Since there are so many factors in hurdling techniques, the coach must not confuse the athletes with too many variables at once and must refrain from trying to change technique on the day of the event. This day is for competition, not for training. The technique of lining up a number of hurdles and having athletes run over them in one direction and run back in an opposite direction is extremely dangerous. A hurdle is designed to tip over forwards, and athletes risk broken legs or other injury by running over it from the wrong direction.

Hurdling technique is not easy to learn. Training must start on grass to decrease the number of abrasions and injuries. Soft top hurdles and sponge rubber protectors of the heel, ankle, and knee of the takeoff leg, as well as the knee of the trailing leg, are mandatory in training and should only be eliminated as the athlete gains proficiency. Heel cups are needed throughout the training season to help prevent heel bruising. The old style hurdling shoe had a stiff counter with six spikes in the front and two in the back. This encouraged athletes to land on their heels or flatfootedly, and heel bruising and plantar fasciitis were common. The newer hurdling shoes have spikes in the front and none on the heel; in fact, they have a higher back to encourage athletes to land on their toes and the shoes provide cushioning if they inadvertently land on their heel as they fatigue.

Another injury, which is common in hurdlers, is medial synovial plica syndrome. With repetitive contusions on the medial aspect of the knee of the trailing leg, a synovial plica may become fibrotic. With subsequent sprinting and hurdling techniques, the irritation of the plica rubbing across the medial femoral condyle may become quite severe. Although icing, quadriceps and hamstring stretching and strengthening, or a patella brace are somewhat effective in treatment, arthroscopic resection of the plica may become necessary.

Middle Distance

Standard middle distances today are a half mile, or 880 yards, with an 800 meter equivalent, and a 1 mile event with a 1500 meter equivalent. The half milers are the swing runners, that is, some may be asked to run in the longer distance sprints such as the 440 meter, while others may be asked to run in the 1 or 2 mile events if the need arises. This places a particular burden on the middle distance runner, and therefore some must train as sprint half milers, and others as endurance half milers. Ideal middle distance runners should have the speed of sprinters and the endurance of distance runners. They should have good balance of both type I and type II fibers, and should work hard at interval training to build up both endurance and speed.

The stride of middle distance runners is shorter than that of sprinters, and longer than that of distance runners. They make contact with the surface with the balls

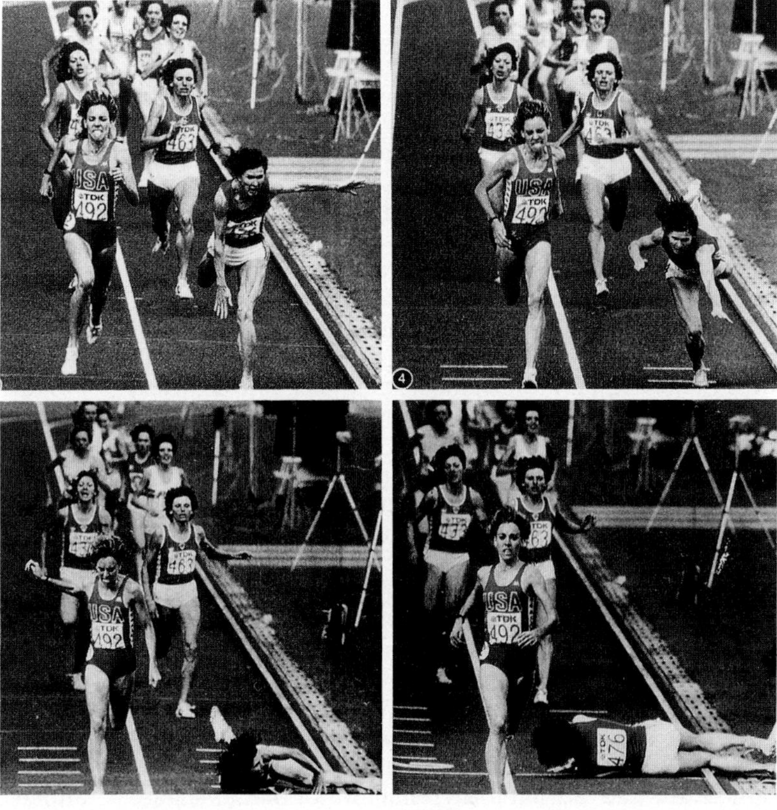

Figure 39.4. Middle distance spring. **(A)** The leading runner on the inside is barely ahead of her outside competitor. She swings her left arm forward, reaching for the tape. **(B)** This maneuver breaks her stride as she lunges forward. **(C)** With a burst of speed, the outer competitor hits the tape as the inner runner hits the track and **(D)** Rolls across the finish line in a frustrated second place finish. (Steve Powell. Sports Illustrated, August 22, 1983:16–17.)

of their feet and roll back onto their heels. As they become more fatigued, they run more flatfooted. Without a proper forward lean, they will land on their heels and may develop heel bruises or calcaneal stress fractures. Like sprinters who accommodate by turning a counterclockwise rotation around the track, they are subject to supinating forces in the left lower extremity and pronating forces in the right. Too much of a body lean around the curves adds torque and increases risk of injury. Sprinter-middle distance runners are therefore subject to the same injuries as sprinters, while endurance-middle distance runners are subject to the type of injury that is discussed with distance runners.

Lead runners have a definite advantage in that they set the pace for the race. In order to avoid injuries, runners must learn to run on the outside shoulder of the runner in front, in an attempt to avoid being boxed in. If boxed in, runners can sustain a strain injury by a misstep associated with being knocked off the track; they can sustain a sprain or a spike injury in an attempt to change position from the cluster. The sprinter distance runner often has a close finish similar to that of the sprinter (Fig. 39.4).

In the off-season, middle distance runners train as distance runners, and as they get into the season, training varies according to their anticipated swing position. In the off-season, they participated in cross-country for stamina and endurance. This is also the time for experiments with running form, such as degree of trunk lean or length of running stride. Athletes must be careful not to mimic the stride length of a teammate, since this stride may not be ideal for them (15). Too long a stride will overstress musculotendinous units and too short a stride will overtax endurance level, leading to fatigue, stiffness, and strain.

Distance, Marathon, and Cross-Country

Long distance events consist of 2 miles (3000 meter equivalent), 3 miles (5000 meter equivalent), 6 miles (10,000 meter equivalent), and a 3000 meter steeplechase. Cross-country courses vary from approximately 3 mile (5 K), 4 mile, or 6 mile (10 K) mile lengths for a sport where approximately 7 team participants work together in order to enable their top five members to score lower than opponents. Marathoning is an individual event covering 26 miles, or 385 yards. Cross-country is considered off-season training for the distance runner, while marathoning and the triathlon are considered the ultimate individual tests of endurance. Technique does not vary much with the different distance events.

In distance running, the trunk angle is straighter. It is inclined from 5° to 9°, depending on stride length and state of fatigue, as compared to 15° in a middle distance runner, and 25° in the sprinter. Sprinting depends on type II fiber, speed, and strength; while distance running depends on type I myofibril and associated capillary hypertrophy for stamina. Distance runners must be able to estimate pace so that they can speed up at the proper time in the race and fall back to a normal pace when appropriate. They can only develop this ability with practice, and they tend to practice mainly at race pace. They must learn to train without straining, because in overuse, their biologic substances break down faster than they adapt. While the sprinter is typically injured by overstressing the musculotendinous unit in an attempt to accelerate, the distance runner typically injures the musculotendinous unit merely by overuse in training.

Distance runners must run relaxed and with a specific cadence in order to develop an efficient stride. This even cadence is the key to success. Distance runners use short strides, low knee lifts, and relaxed arm action. They merely swing their arms and do not pump them. They land on the balls of their feet, drop to their heels, and push off with their toes. They need full flexion and extension of the joints of the lower extremities and have a slight forward body lean. If their stride is too long, if their foot lands in front of the center of gravity, they decelerate and constantly work against themselves; patellar tendinitis and cruciate sprain can result. Ideally, foot plant should always be underneath the center of gravity so that toeing off will produce propulsion.

In changing pace, runners place strain on their well-tuned and conditioned biologic mechanism. Sudden acceleration will increase the energy storage within eccentrically contracting muscle, leading to strain injury. Once fatigue sets in, runners may become unbalanced or attempt to change stride length and also stress the musculotendinous unit. Increasing stride length increases strain during eccentric contraction; decreasing stride length decreases optimal utilization of the energy storage system so that fatigue sets in, and again injury may be the consequence (15).

It is important to train and not to strain, because the body can take only so much pounding; if an athlete is faltering, it is the coach's responsibility to slow down training somewhat. In this way, training programs for distance runners are highly individualized. They should run long runs at less than race pace, distances shorter than the race distance at the race pace, and even shorter distances at faster than race pace. Interval training and work on hills is particularly valuable in developing cardiovascular fitness.

Marathoning is the ultimate in distance training and is often used as an off-season test for endurance in the distance runner. Here again, it is important to run an even pace. This becomes immediately apparent to the well-trained athlete who at the finish of the marathon may feel that he could run much farther at the same pace, but not really much faster over the marathon distance. Runners usually need 6 to 12 months of training to achieve marathon conditioning. This is achieved by mixing long runs of 12 to 20 miles with multiple light runs. They may break up training to two periods daily to decrease lactic acid buildup, fatigue, and the effects of repetitive stress, in order to minimize the chance of injury.

The steeplechase is a particularly difficult 3000 meter event, consisting of 7 laps over 4 fixed hurdles, 3-feet-high, and 1 water jump, with 35 barriers in all. Two different techniques are utilized to accommodate the barriers. The athlete can either hurdle over the barriers or step over them. The standard hurdling technique must be used in attempts to hurdle the barrier. Again, heel bruising and calcaneal stress fractures are common, particularly after fatigue sets in. If athletes land behind their center of gravity, they may fall backward, suffering either a head contusion from contact with the stationary hurdle or a decelerating knee ligament injury. Some runners prefer to "run the barriers," that is, to step over them, opposed to hurdling them. This increases risk of loss of balance or contact deceleration; energy dissipation may result in ankle, knee, or leg injury. The water jump is 12 feet in length on the other side of a barrier. It is impossible to clear with a hurdle, so here stepping over the barrier is the preferred method. Unlike hurdling, in this technique, the lead leg does not become the contact leg. In fact, after contact is made on top of the hurdle, the opposite leg swings forward in a pendulum-like action in an attempt to generate horizontal momentum to clear the water. There is much strain and torque placed on ligaments and joints in this event. Athletes should not compete on a course like this more than once a month. Here athletes concentrate both on endurance training and hurdling techniques. Without adequate ability in both, they are certainly at risk of injury.

Important equipment in endurance training is the running shoe with its padding to absorb the shock of repetitive contact. It also has a heel lift to enhance some forward lean as well as supports at the midfoot to give some strength and to aid the midfoot in locking into position; it also has some flexibility at the ball to allow pushoff. The wheelbarrow heel and doughnut or waffle iron bottom seems to distribute stress well and decrease stress reactions. If the shoe is not broken in slowly or fits improperly, blisters or subcutaneous bursitis ("pump bump") are known to occur. Most distance-related injuries are due to training error, commonly due to overtraining. In overtraining, athletes fatigue; in an effort to accelerate themselves further, they run flat-footed, which leads to increased pronation of the heel.

The ideal running uniform is loose fitting and comfortable. It allows adequate ventilation. It should not bind or prevent free easy movement. Nipple abrasion can be prevented by a thin coat of petroleum jelly and an adhesive strip bandage covering in those particularly susceptible. Thigh chaffing is a particular problem in endurance training, and many athletes will wear a shorter pair of pants over a slightly longer pair to absorb friction; others utilize a commercially available polypropylene long leg girdle. A thin layer of petroleum jelly or talcum powder helps to diminish symptoms while healing and training progress.

Distance training is monotonous and is rarely done around a track. Sometime during the season athletes may demonstrate loss of appetite, worry, excessive fatigue, sleepiness, weight loss, change in attitude towards an event, or illness. These are signs of staleness. Athletes may feel as if they have reached a plateau and are not improving. They will begin to perform at a level much lower than their ability. The psychological and physical fatigue associated with this condition leads to injury if the coach is unable to find the origin of the problem and remove the athlete from it. It is most likely due to the athlete's having settled into a certain pattern of training. Changing this pattern can increase the athlete's feeling of well-being and performance. Varying the method of practice is preventative. Stress-related injuries may occur from overtraining as the body fails from repetitive abuse. Training programs must allow for gradual increases in applied load to biologic tissues.

Endurance runners are subject to what they call second wind. They start off at a slow pace, gradually building up speed while increasing respiratory rate, but eventually reach a point where, when stride is shortened slightly, they run comfortably and breathe easily. At this point, athletes have achieved their second wind, which means that the musculotendinous units have finally warmed up, falling into a cadence or pattern of efficient reciprocal eccentric preloading and concentric contraction. Over time, with proper training and avoidance of injury, this pace will quicken. Occasionally, the novice will develop a pain in the side and label this a second wind. This is a different phenomenon resulting from fatigue of the diaphragm muscles or venous congestion of the spleen and liver circulatory system that becomes active in mobilizing glycogen for endurance work. This is usually a sign of lack of training or of an attempt to perform above the athlete's level of training; decreasing the pace allows circulation to catch up to metabolic demand.

Endurance training is not usually done around a track, since this would become very boring and the surface is usually too hard for continuous training. Therefore, golf courses, cross-country courses, school yards, or local roadways become the training environment. The surface should be relatively even to avoid sprains and strains. Running through the woods may be cooler during summer training and provide a soft surface, but trails must be policed well so that obstacles do not lead to misstep, tripping, or injury. Hills must be avoided since the pronation and corresponding internal leg rotation needed to accelerate uphill leads to knee torque, which may develop symptoms of lateral pain related to stretching of the iliotibial band or lateral patellofemoral compression, or medial pain related to a symptomatic plica or strain of the semimembranosus. Meniscal problems rarely result from track and field activities, but with preexisting injury, symptoms may be accentuated with running hills.

Repetitive downhill running also presents a hazard. Although an increase in stride length with the assistance of gravity can increase speed, acceleration is limited by the need for balance. In deceleration to gain control, runners keep the center of gravity behind the landing foot which slaps down in a plantar-flexed position, they tighten calf muscles and eccentrically contract the extensor mechanism. This leads to corresponding stretch in the posterior aspect of the knee, the musculotendinous junction of calf muscles, the Achilles tendon, and the extensor mechanism itself (16). Extensor mechanism complaints are due to "jamming on the brakes," that is, driving the patella into the femoral trochlear groove while the quadriceps tightens in an effort to decelerate downhill. Lateral retinacular pain and popliteal tenosynovitis frequently result. Medial retinacular pain is occasionally seen. Lateral quadriceps tendon pain occurs, as does chondromalacia and tenderness along either the origin or insertion of the patella tendon. Foot slap associated with downhill running may also aggravate symptoms of plantar fasciitis. The treatment of these conditions consists of decrease and avoidance of inciting factors and temporary change in the contact stress points to help heal damage that has occurred on a microscopic level. This can be done with taping, bracing, or banding to decrease relative tension on the tendons. Stretching of the iliotibial tract and hip abductors is beneficial in prevention of iliotibial friction syndrome (17).

Hyperpronation of the foot in running downhill may lead to popliteal tendinitis due to torque placed in the posterior lateral aspect of the knee. This is similar to the torque the leg sustained while running on a banked track or the banked surface of the gutter of a typical paved street. Posterior pain of the popliteal muscle or tenderness in the popliteal tendon just anterior to the fibular collateral ligament on the femur will make the diagnosis. Alleviating the training error is the solution to the problem.

A word of caution must be given to distance training in an urban environment. First of all, carbon monoxide from exhaust fumes may permanently bind to hemoglobin to decrease oxygen-carrying capacity and relative performance. Overuse problems in training in such an environment are perhaps the more clinically relevant problems. The athlete should attempt to train on a soft grass surface prior to turning to the streets. If a smooth dirt surface such as the shoulder of a road or a maintenance road along a viaduct is available, this should be the next phase, followed by running along an asphalt surface. Running on concrete should be avoided if at all possible, but frequently avoidance is impossible. Training on paved roads may introduce other training errors.

If the runner always runs either with traffic or facing traffic (in some areas this is mandated by local law), one leg becomes the "up leg," while the other becomes the "down leg." This is because most roads are designed with drainage in mind and not the runner. There is a crown at the top and a bank on either side. Running along this bank means that the down leg, or lower leg, does most of the work; that is, it must extend and push off to help the runner run over the upper leg, which is used more or less for balance. The lower foot supinates, and the leg externally rotates, causing stress along the medial joint posteriorly, which can produce semimembranosus strain, medial retinacular stretch, medial collateral ligament strain, medial plateau fractures, and accentuation of preexisting medial meniscal problems. More common is the exacerbation of preexisting lateral meniscal problems. Suprapatellar lateral knee pain in distance runners may be due to a thickened fibrotic suprapatellar plica. Failure to respond to nonoperative management is an indication for arthroscopic resection of this tissue. Occasionally, other symptoms such as lateral retinacular pain may result.

Because of inclement weather, many northern high schools encourage indoor training prior to the beginning of track season. The cement floors of the schools may have fewer shock-absorbing properties than the pavement in the neighborhood streets. The fact that these athletes are relatively unconditioned means that they have decreased shock-absorbing ability of the musculotendinous unit and lack osseous hypertrophy; stress will lead to breakdown. This, in turn, can lead to shin splints (18), a sign of training error. Pain in the shin may be related to overuse or stress of the muscles within the extensor or flexor groups, stress fracture, or induced ischemia within muscular compartments leading to compartment syndrome. Physical examination of the patient with shin splints demonstrates diffuse tenderness along the posteromedial cortex of the tibia along the tibialis posterior muscle. When the tenderness is localized to one particular area on the tibia, consideration is given to possible stress fracture. These can be differentiated with x-rays and bone scanning. Stressing the musculotendinous unit by maintaining stress across the ankle, toe, or foot will increase pain related to a tear within that unit. If weight bearing or longitudinal compression accentuates the constant pain, a stress fracture is suspected. Fatigue fractures occur if the system is continually overloaded. They can occur on more than one level (Fig. 39.5*A–C*) and may not be visualized by standard x-rays until the healing process is established (19). Such reactions can occur on any level in the novice, but, in the well-trained individual, common posterior medial tibial cortical stress fracture is characteristically tender 13 cm above the medial malleolus at the posterior medial margin of the tibia (Fig. 39.6).

Early in the season, as rapid remodeling of bone and tendon collagen turnover occurs in adaptation to increased work load, these structures are found to be particularly at risk. Abuse or overuse may supersede within the adaptation process, leading to stress fracture or strain while in this weakened state. Later in the season as the adaptation has progressed, abuse from overtraining will still lead to breakdown when adequate recovery time is not allowed. Athletes must have enough common sense to discuss their injuries with their trainer and coach so that treatment can begin quickly and loss of performance can be minimized. To play "hurt" is to risk further injury (Fig. 39.7). In distance running, common stress fractures include distal fibula, proximal and distal tibial shaft, second and third metatarsal shaft, and femoral neck and shaft. Although most of these injuries will heal with time, displacement of a fracture, particularly of the femoral neck, can be a devastating injury.

Muscle units within the lower leg are isolated in

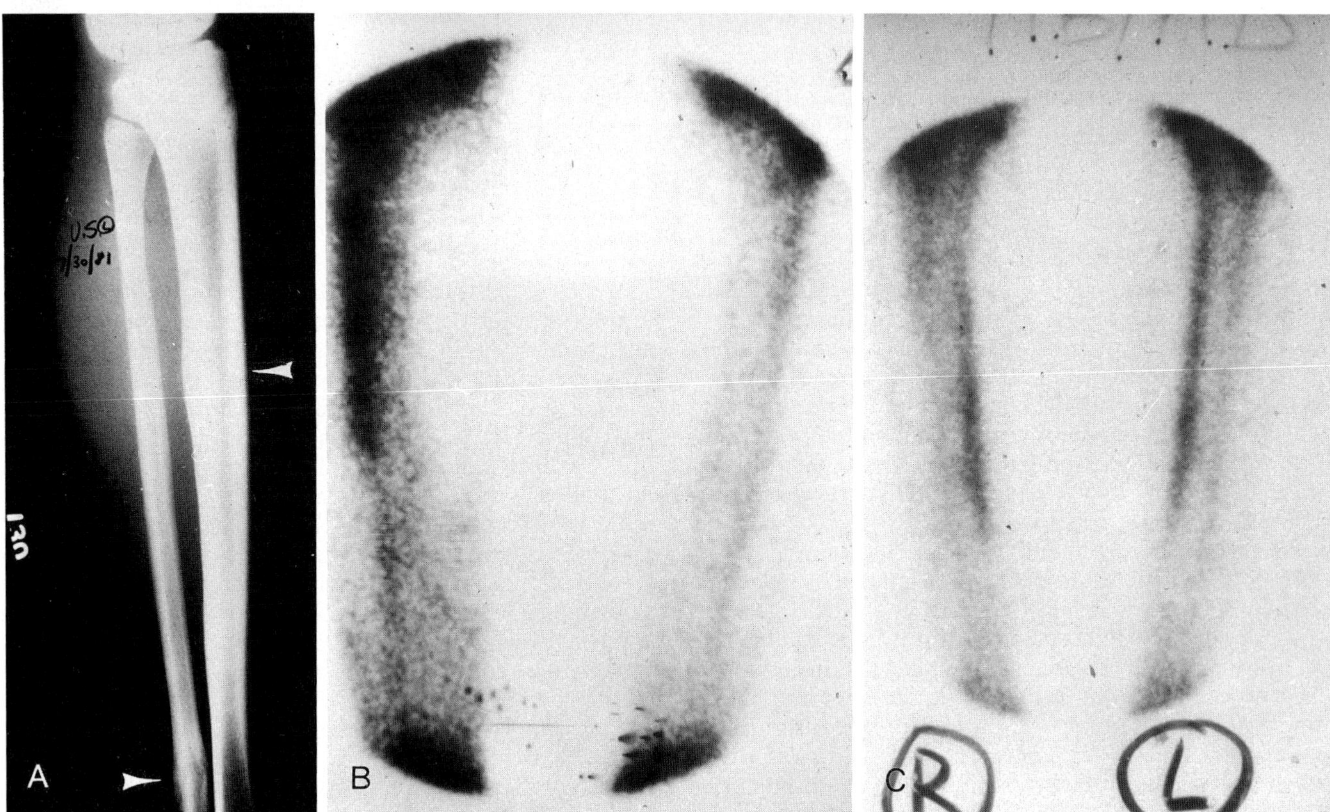

Figure 39.5. Stress fracture. Stress reaction to overtraining or abuse may actually lead to breakdown of bone. **(A)** The microfracture process may not be obvious at first, but eventually will show a periosteal reaction as seen on the posterior cortex of the tibial midshaft. **(B)** The runner may learn to train with pain, so that multiple stress reactions may develop. **(C)** Early in the process, occasionally a fracture cannot be identified, and a bone scan is useful where an unsuspected stress fracture was found in the opposite tibia.

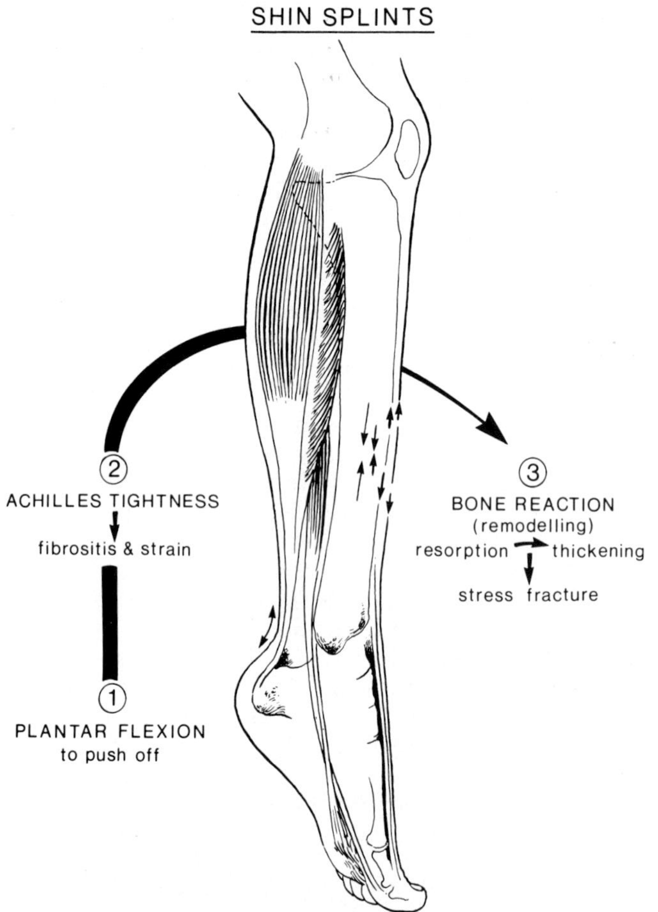

Figure 39.6. Shin splints. Repetitive microtrauma and overuse in running will lead to soft tissue and even bony breakdown, a process commonly called "shin splints." Muscle overpull can lead to periostitis, strain, or trabecular breakdown. The area approximately 13 cm proximal to the tip of the medial malleolus along the posterior tibial cortex appears to be maximally at risk.

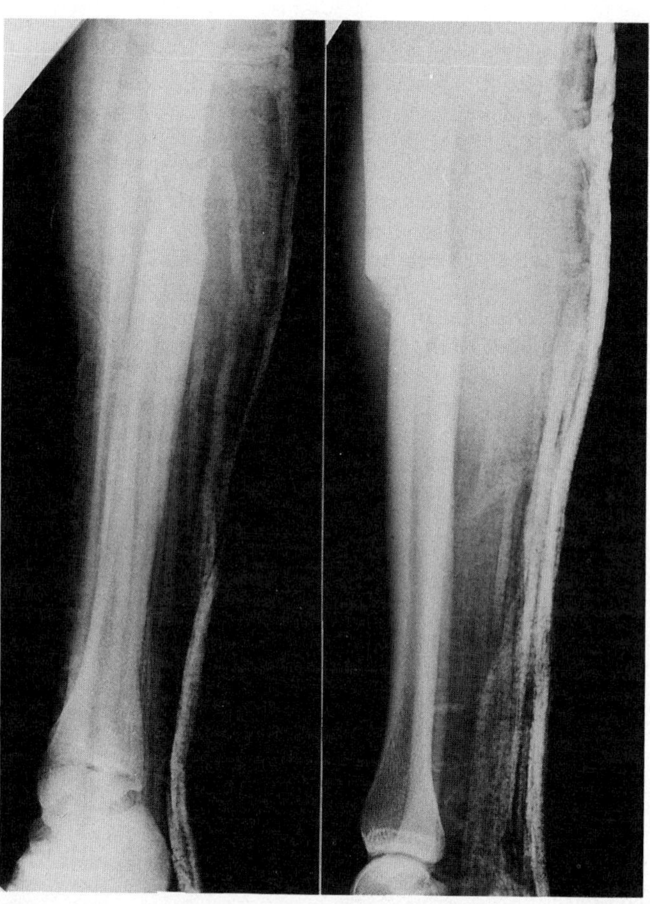

Figure 39.7. "Playing hurt." This 14-year-old female runner had developed pain in the proximal tibia running indoors in gym shoes in preseason practice. She was encouraged to run through her pain. At midseason, in initiating her sprint to the one mile finish, she felt something snap in the area of her previous pain. Although rare, displacement through a stress fracture can occur and emphasized that playing while hurt, the athlete invites further and more significant injury.

closed compartments defined by location within fascial envelopes. With hemorrhage and edema due to contusion or strain, circulation to the muscles and nerves within a compartment may be compromised. Strenuous exercise can initiate compartment syndrome by swelling associated with metabolic waste product buildup. Muscle swelling due to restricted venous or lymphatic outflow may be related to either acute swelling of the muscle due to overuse, or to a transient swelling related to congenital fascial thickening. Most often, findings are transient and related to muscular exertion; symptoms disappear when the inciting activity is stopped only to reappear during a subsequent period of exercise. An acute compartment syndrome may develop primarily or as the result of transient ischemia. Immediate fasciotomy is mandatory to prevent muscle ischemic necrosis. With numbness and pain related to activity, prophylactic fasciotomy is often the treatment of choice in the athlete who wishes to remain active. Although such complications are rare, the physician dealing with track and field athletes must be aware of the potential problems.

Serial biopsies taken from marathon runners at different intervals after competition have shown ultrastructural changes in skeletal muscle (20). In biopsies obtained 1 to 2 days after an event, findings have included focal fiber injury and repair, intra- and extracellular edema with endothelial injury, myofibrillar lysis, dilation and disruption of the T tubular system, and focal mitochondrial degeneration without inflammatory infiltrate. The mitochondrial and myofibrillar damage showed progressive repair by 3 to 4 weeks. At 8 to 12 weeks, biopsies have demonstrated central nuclei and satellite cells characteristic of the regenerative response. Veteran runners have also been noted to have intracellular collagen deposition suggestive of a fibrotic response to repetitive injury.

Back pain is rare in experienced distance runners. If they are executing technique properly by slight forward body lean and placing center of gravity just above the planting foot, locomotion becomes relatively effortless. If, however, they attempt to stand too upright, the center of gravity is shifted behind the planting foot, and they must make an effort to bound over it; the center of gravity moves up and down. In effect, the energy stored in eccentric preloading is wasted in production of a vertical vector of propulsion rather than an efficient horizontal vector. Energy utilized to propel the body upright over a planted foot will produce a bounding type gait in which the head bobs up and down. This leads to quick fatigue and symptoms of stress manifested by heel pain from landing on the heel, plantar fasciitis from rolling over the flatly planted foot, or in back pain developed from the jarring effect of repetitive falling due to inefficient vertical lifting.

Although the generation of heat within the musculotendinous unit is beneficial and increases contractility and pliability of muscle in distance running, it may also have adverse effects. Heat cramping, heat fatigue, and heat stroke are a continuum of maladies discussed in Chapter 4. Acute renal failure is a multifactorial event that is rarely seen in marathon runners (21). The condition is secondary to the combined effects of rhabdomyolysis, dehydration, hypotension, nonsteroidal antiinflammatory drugs, and hyperuricemia. Prevention is by correcting potential dehydration and by minimizing the use of nonsteroidal antiinflammatory drugs.

The maintenance of adequate serum electrolyte concentrations is essential in long distance running (22). In a study of ultramarathon runners racing in a 100 mile race, it was found that with ingestion of sufficient quantities of carbohydrate electrolyte solution, normal metabolic parameters can be maintained. These runners each ingested up to 22.4 liters of fluid during the race.

Stretching must become routine to prevent overload of the musculotendinous unit that is related to training excess or error. Before a race, athletes must warm up to increase efficiency of muscles and thereby reduce the incidence of strain. This also decreases the mental fatigue that leads to strain or sprain injury. Proper warm-up can significantly decrease and even eliminate the initial period used to attain the "second wind" level of performance. Middle and long-distance runners need longer than sprinters to warm up circulation-dependent type I endurance fibers. A period of easy running and light flexibility exercises working up a slight perspiration followed by a short series of warm-up sprints and easy jogging, striding, and rest before race time can be carried out, followed by a 5-min period of rest to get breathing back to normal. After completing the distance event, athletes must continue to jog for a lap or two in order to encourage circulation and help clear metabolic waste products from muscle, so that fatigue does not set in during the next few days. Going through a light jog and stretching routine the day following competition helps to work out tightness and encourage circulation.

Race Walking

Race walking has recently gained public attention and is included in many track and field distance events. The event is often criticized because it "looks funny." This is a walking event; there is no airborne phase as there is in running. The rules clearly state that there must be unbroken contact with the ground and that the advancing foot of the walker must contact the ground before the rear foot leaves the ground. During the period of each step while the foot is on the ground, the leg must be straightened and not bent at the knee for at least one moment (Fig. 39.8)

In order to ambulate with an erect posture and no forward lean, the strain against eccentrically loaded muscle is severe, so that stretching of upper and lower extremities becomes mandatory (23). Rigid orthoses are definitely contraindicated, since athletes would lose stride in vaulting over them. The forefoot of the shoe must be extremely flexible in this event. The upper body is used to amplify lower body motion; most race walkers race with clenched fists. Therefore, race walkers demonstrate the qualities of upper extremity amplification and increased stride length similar to a sprinter, but without forward lean or an airborne phase. To centralize the center of gravity in forward momentum, new, accentuated motions are introduced to allow a narrow-

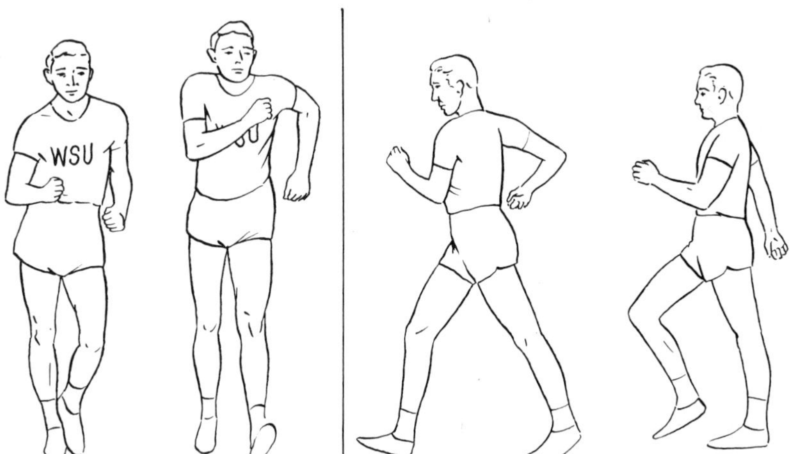

Figure 39.8. Race walking. Proper form necessitated by the rules of race walking place tremendous strain on every muscle of the body. Since the advancing foot must contact the ground before the rear foot leaves the ground, strain in eccentric loading is common. Proper strength training and flexibility and adherence to form is necessary here as in every event to prevent injury.

ing of stride width. This is done by a small burst of hip adductor muscle activity at the end of the swing phase.

Increased ankle dorsiflexion is needed because of lack of an airborne phase, so that pretibial muscles may not overwork and develop symptoms of shin splints. Since erect position due to lack of forward lean is associated with increased trunk rotation, erector spinii and paraspinous muscle strain is extremely common. If the competitor is not flexible, increased stride length will lead to posterior knee pain, heel cord strain, and extensor mechanism complaints. Hyperextension forces of the knee during race walking will put stress on the posterior structures of the knee so that popliteal symptoms commonly occur, which can be prevented by hamstring strengthening and quadriceps stretching. Heel cord strain can be avoided by Achilles stretching exercises; but if strain does develop, heel lifts may aid in limiting symptoms. With increased trunk rotation, strain of the external oblique, transverse abdominus, and rectus abdominus muscles commonly occur. Strain of the abdominal muscles may lead to pain radiating down the inguinal canal, which is particularly bothersome and best avoided. An aggressive program of rotational, abdominal, and paraspinous muscle-stretching and strengthening exercises must be utilized by athletes participating in this sport.

Jumping Events

Long Jump

The running broad jump, or long jump, is one of the five original events of the ancient Olympic games. It was reintroduced in American track and field when the New York Athletic Club was founded in 1868. The Amateur Athletic Union adapted it as a standard event in 1876, and it was adopted for high school use at the University of Pennsylvania High School Relays in 1895. It was formalized as a university level event at the University of Chicago in 1901.

The long jump can be considered to be divided into four consecutive parts: approach, takeoff, flight, and landing. The approach occurs from the moment the athlete starts walking or running toward the board until, but not including, the instant the takeoff foot strikes the ground for the last time prior to takeoff. The second phase is the takeoff, which consists of touch down until the instant at which the takeoff foot breaks contact with the ground. Third is the flight, which is from the instant of take off until the instant the athlete first makes contact with the sand in the landing pit. And lastly, the landing, which occurs from the instant of landing until the athlete's center of gravity passes forward of the feet or comes to rest. Available data suggest that elite long jumpers attain approach speeds of 95% to 99% of their maximum sprinting speed prior to take off.

In the approach, a runoff is used that varies from 120 to 150 feet in college, or less in high school. The object of the approach is to develop maximal speed. There is a short period of half speed, a short period of three-quarter speed, and a long period to adjust to full speed. The jumper sets checkmarks at the side of the runway to signal change of cadence. At the end of the run, eccentrically stored potential energy is released as kinetic energy in production of forward momentum. The number of strides needed to attain full speed comfortably will vary for each competitor. The fewer strides a jumper takes, the easier to keep the checkmarks accurate.

The takeoff distance for the fourth-to-last stride, the landing distance for the last stride, and the height for the center of gravity at takeoff into the jump are significantly correlated with the distance of the jump (24). These three position variables are significantly related to the distance of the jump through their relationships with the velocity of the approach and through the vertical velocity of the center of gravity at takeoff into the jump.

If jumpers miss the mark, they must learn to run over the board and into the pit. They must not suddenly decelerate; to do so risks eccentrically loaded muscle strain or knee or ankle ligament injury. The heel hits the board first and goes through a standard heel, ball, toe motion for takeoff. The opposite knee is driven forward into flexion to drive the center of gravity forward and to amplify the push of the extended takeoff leg. As the center of gravity moves forward, clenched hands, which have been moving in a normal sprinting fashion, drive forward and upward to maintain balance. In the flight or airborne phase, jumpers must maintain balance and must also position the body for an effective landing; some long jumpers attempt to walk in air, while others tuck their knees. In either case, motion must be timed so that landing can occur with both knees partially bent so they can eccentrically absorb contact energy to be used in the forward spring and to prevent falling backward (Fig. 39.9*A*). Falling backwards onto extended hands can result in injuries to the shoulder. This reverse extension combined with contraction of the biceps muscle can result in injury to the superior aspect of the glenohumeral joint, resulting in the so-called SLAP lesion. This is an avulsion of the biceps insertion at the superior labrum in an anterior-to-posterior direction. Nonoperative management consisting of nonsteroidal antiinflammatory medications and physical therapy that emphasize rotator cuff strengthening is stressed initially. Failure to respond to nonoperative management is an indication for operative intervention. These lesions can be debrided or repaired arthroscopically, or may require open surgical superior mechanism reconstruction.

In the early phase of training, hard jumping must be avoided. Throughout training, the pit must be either turned daily if made of builders' sand, or kept dry if the foam rubber-type practice pit is used. Improper acceleration, that is, reaching maximal stride either too early or too late, will lead to strain injury. Inaccurate placement of checkmarks leads to uneven strides, which leads to strain of eccentrically loaded muscles. Contacting the board with the knee too straight settles the center of gravity too far posterior, and induced deceleration detracts from an effective jump or causes knee

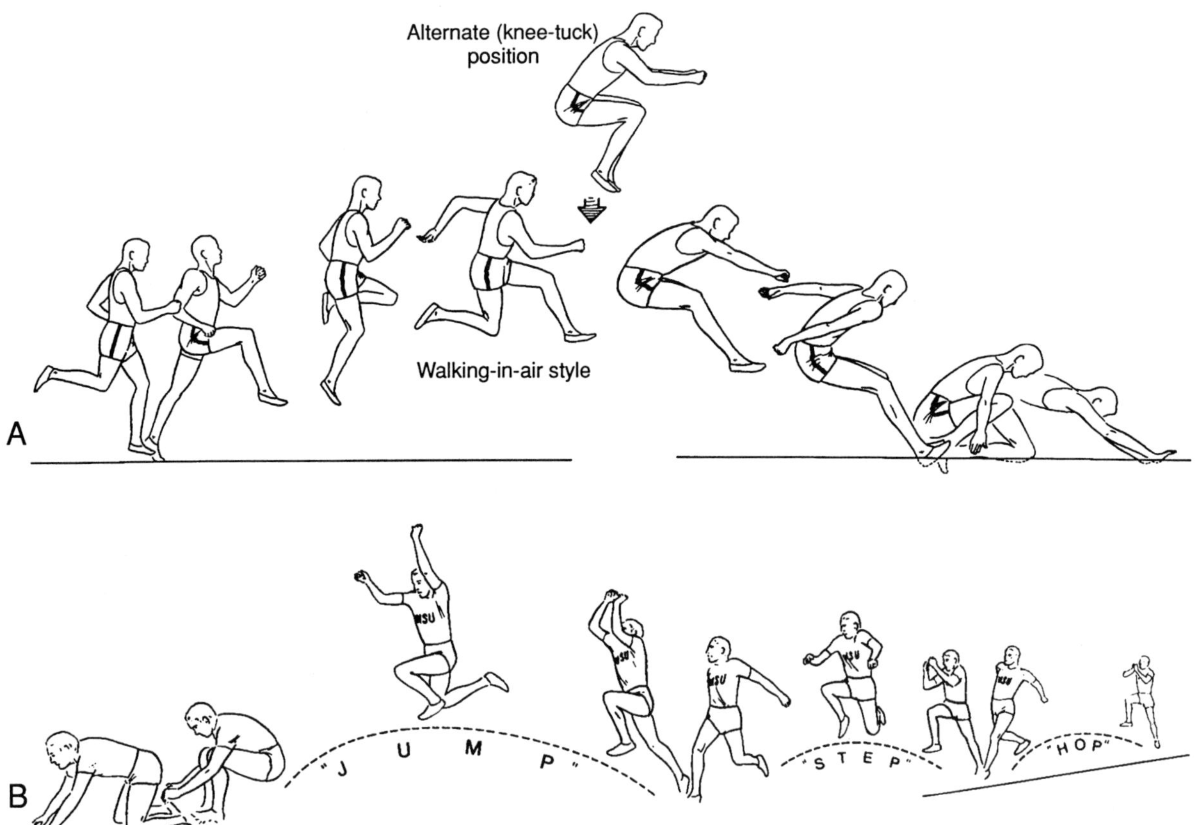

Figure 39.9. Long jump. **(A)** As the planting foot makes contact with the board, this leg extends, propelling the jumper forward. He may either attempt to walk through the air, amplifying crossed-extensor reflex patterns, or may merely tuck his knees in preparation for landing. It is this presetting of muscles that allows the jumper to eccentrically absorb energy at landing for forward propulsion. **(B)** Triple jump. The biologic basis of the triple jump is progressive increase of height and distance made by effective storage of kinetic and contact energy with amplification through reflex integration. The takeoff foot lands in the step. Both feet make contact in the jump. Amplification of energy storage is provided by arm motion, and presetting of muscles allows eccentric energy storage at impact to help propel the body forward.

sprain. Arm action must parallel leg action; when the left knee comes forward, the right arm must also come forward, as it does in sprinting and walking. Any attempt to circumvent the body's natural motion can lead to injury. It is the responsibility of the athlete and the coach to examine the takeoff board. If it is loose, uneven, or excessively worn, its use invites injury.

Triple Jump

The triple jump utilizes the same runway as the long jump. With the "hop," athletes land on the same foot that had been placed on the takeoff board (Fig. 39.9*B*). They then enter the step phase in which they take off on the foot from which they had landed to land on the opposite foot to jump. Essentially, this is a normal long jumping action in which the athletes develop further forward momentum.

Triple jumpers must concentrate on technique in order to maximize forward momentum. A misstep will decrease distance and risk injury. If they concentrate too much on height, they lose distance. Pretensing the hopping leg allows storage of eccentric energy from the landing impact for use in the next "step." Although the heel comes down first on the landing leg, there is a quick roll, so that landing is essentially flatfooted. If it is not, calcaneal fat pad bruising and stress fracture will result; or the braking motion caused by the center of gravity being behind the planted foot may cause a knee ligament injury through deceleration. To absorb the shock of impact, the landing foot is pulled back quickly and preset; otherwise hamstring, quadriceps, or gastrocnemius strain commonly results. After planting the foot, it is important to drive the opposite knee up in order to develop forward momentum through crossed-extensor amplification. In evaluation of lower extremity muscle strain involving the hamstrings, quadriceps, or gastrocnemius, the examiner must delineate the areas of maximal tenderness. Occasionally, the examiner can feel bunched-up areas of muscle within the muscle bellies that are indicative of actual muscle pull. It is important to examine the entire length of the muscle to rule out bony avulsion injuries from the pelvis. With simple muscle strains occurring in the substance of the muscle belly or near the musculotendinous junction, treatment is focused on retaining strength and mobility prior to return to sport.

In the second jump, or the "step," athletes again preset their lower extremity and swing both arms behind the body so that at impact they can swing them forward to drive the body's center of gravity forward in the "jump." Driving the upper extremities forward and backward can cause a rhomboid, pectoralis, levator scapulae, or serratus anterior strain, particularly if athletes are off balance. Flexibility and strength help reduce the incidence of strain injury.

In the third phase of the "jump," athletes must make an effort to attain maximal height and distance, and do so by throwing their hips forward; without proper flexibility and strength, gluteus or paraspinous muscle strain will result (16). Since horizontal speed is diminished greatly, proper technique is necessary to maximize use of energy stored within muscle; foot contact must be perfect, and double arm swing utilization must potentiate energy on pushoff. Ending the "jump," the athlete lands in a near sitting position (Fig. 39.9*B*).

Many characteristics of the kinematic of the triple jump have been found to correlate highly with total jump distance (25). The horizontal position of the center of gravity of the body in relation to the support foot at takeoff correlates highly with the total distance of the jump, as does the distance of the hop phase. The vertical velocity into the hop and step phases correlates highly with the respective distance of each phase and there is an inverse correlation between the maximum height of the center of gravity during flight phase of the step and the total distance.

For optimal distance, the triple jumper must gain great run-up velocity and exert forces during each supporting phase which are 3.6 to 4.4 times the body weight, resulting in a force vector angle of about 101° at each takeoff.

The greatest potential for injury is related to the landing phase. The foot lands in plantar flexion and inversion so that internal rotation injury of the ankle is common; lateral sprain and actual tibial/fibular fractures may be seen. Off-balanced landing in ankle dorsiflexion encourages medial ankle sprain and calcaneal fracture. When evaluating foot and ankle injuries occurring during the landing of the triple jump or the long jump, the examiner must clearly define the areas of maximal tenderness and swelling. If actual bony tenderness over the medial or lateral malleoli or over the calcaneus is found, the examiner must be suspicious of possible fracture and obtain appropriate x-rays. More commonly, however, ligamentous injury occurs in the area of maximal tenderness and coincides with that of the anterior talofibular and calcaneofibular ligaments. Less commonly, deltoid ligament injuries can occur medially. Since the landing is so important in these jumping events, the rehabilitation of these ankle sprains must concentrate on retaining muscle strength and full range of motion of the ankle without pain. Taping is used as necessary. Knee ligament injury and meniscal injury may occur due to compressive and rotatory forces sustained by the knee in an unbalanced impact. If there is not enough spring in the runway contact board, or, if the athlete tends to decelerate at impact with the board, "jumper's knee" patellar tendinitis or peroneal subluxation can develop as discussed in the next section.

High Jump

The running high jump was introduced as an athletic event in one of the ancient Olympiads. It was introduced into American track and field in 1868 with the founding of the New York Athletic Club, and was recognized by the amateur athletic union in 1876.

The original technique consisted of a running start with a "scissors kick" used to clear the bar (Fig. 39.10*A*), and was then modified as an eastern style (Fig. 39.10*B*). In the early 1900s, the western form developed on the Pacific coast. These forms are no longer used on a collegiate level, since they are rarely effective above 6½ feet. They are still used at the high school level.

Fosbury introduced what has been labeled the "Fosbury flop" in the 1968 Olympic Games. This has become the most popular form in attaining height greater than 7 feet. Like the original technique called the scissors jump, takeoff is from the outside foot, but then turns into a back dive over the bar (Fig. 39.10*E*). The jumper is able to obtain full speed on the approach and can convert this momentum into vertical lift. The J-pattern approach is utilized, using a straight line for the first five steps, converting to a semicircular path, maximizing lift with the effects of acceleration in pulling out of centrifugal force. Such an approach is extremely hard on the ankles and leads to frequent ankle sprains. Softer landing pits made the flop a feasible technique by limiting the danger of spinal trauma associated with landing on one's neck and back.

In the 1940s, the "straddle form" developed (Fig. 39.10*D*). Still used today, it is sometimes called the "modified western" or "belly roll". Clearance of the crossbar is made by straddling the bar while facing down. The approach is very similar to the western form (Fig. 39.10*C*), The last stride is lengthened and the rock-up on the toe is from a flatfooted or heel-ball landing of the takeoff foot. The jumper strikes the ground hard with the takeoff foot to obtain a rebound. The opposite leg is swung high towards the bar, not fully straightened and continues to move while slightly bent. Both arms are thrown upwards with emphasis on the arm contralateral to the upswing leg. The center of gravity is over the plant leg, which fully extends at the knee in pushoff. In rocking up on the toe and swinging the opposite leg, the jumper leaves the ground. The lead leg swings over the bar, and the chief concern becomes getting the previous plant leg over the bar without touching. This is often accomplished with a sharp kick in the air, which must be precisely timed. The twisting motion involved leads to a high incidence of abdominal and back strains.

In straddle, western, and belly roll forms, sand or foam pits necessitate falling on both arms and at least one leg, and broken bones in both upper and lower extremities were common. Practice of indoor gymnasium mat falling techniques has been useful in preventing injuries, since rolling at the time of impact was found to reduce the jar and minimize danger of injury. Introduction of foam pits enhanced safety and decreased overall numbers of injury.

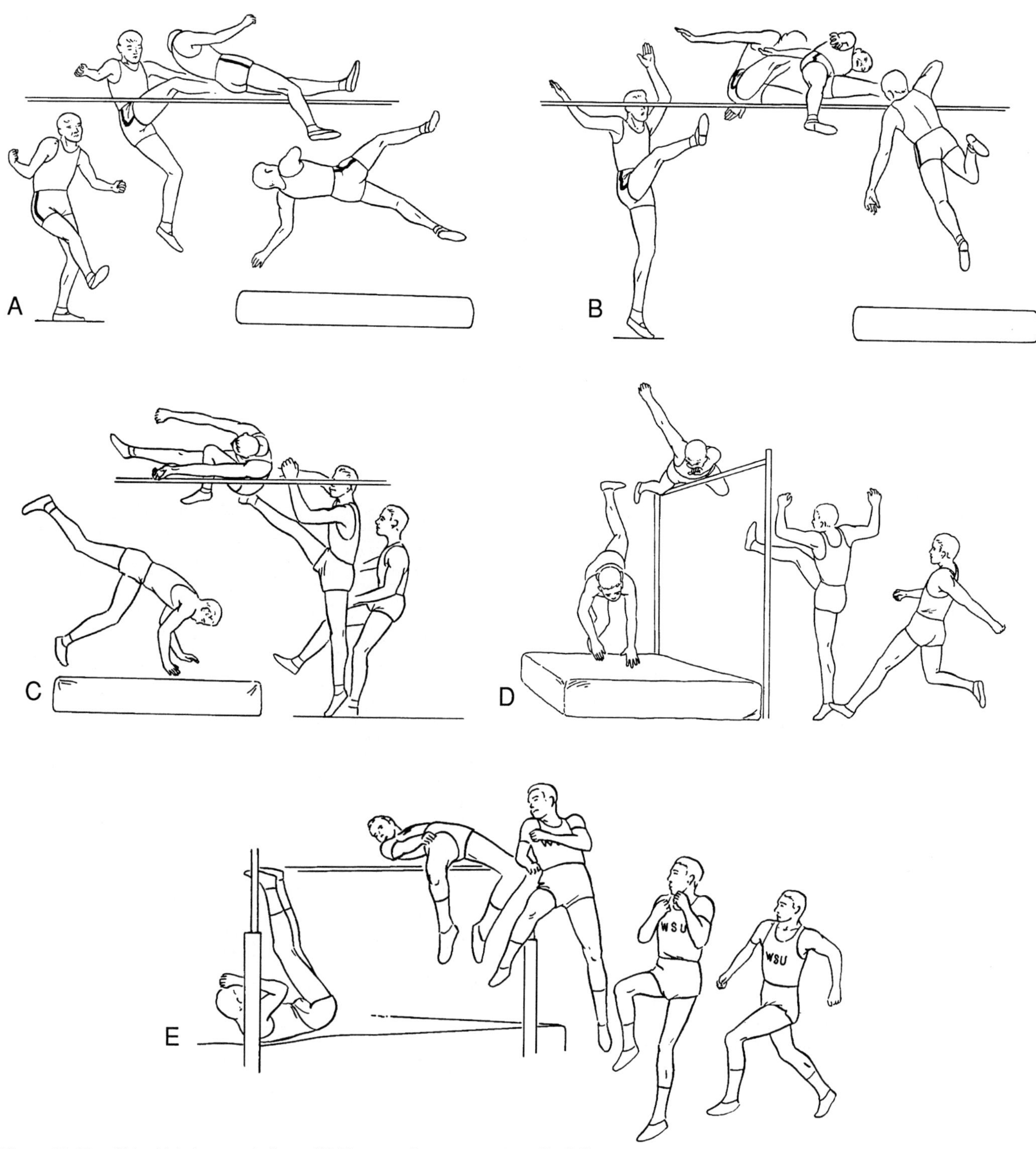

Figure 39.10. Older high jump technique. **(A)** The outer leg was used to propel the body over the bar with the scissors technique and **(B)** eastern technique. **(C)** In the western technique, the inner leg was used in high school where groin, hamstring, and paraspinous muscle flexibility must be emphasized to prevent injury. **(D)** Straddle technique. **(E)** Newer high jump technique. In the Fosbury flop form the jumper crosses on his back. Paraspinous strain and vertebral fracture plague this technique.

Proper foot plant is mandatory; otherwise, the jumper loses control and, in attempting to clear the bar, will strain muscles in the abdomen or lower back.

Because of acceleration of the horizontal approach and translation into vertical lift, braking action is required in conversion of linear motion. Braking is accomplished through quadriceps muscle tension, and extensor mechanism problems may result. These may range from quadriceps tendon superior, medial or lateral strain, chondromalacia of the patella, and patellar tendinitis. Actual rupture of the patellar tendon is more common here than in any other event. Patella tendinitis, or "jumper's knee," is the most common pathologic entity known in high jumpers. The jumper complains of sharp anterior knee pain, which, on physical examination, is found localized to the insertion of the patellar tendon at the inferior pole of the patella (26). In evaluation of the extensor mechanism of the knee, the examiner must palpate for areas of maximal tenderness and carefully feel for any defects either in the quadriceps tendon insertion at the superior pole of the patella or at the patellar tendon origin at the inferior pole. Both quadriceps and patellar tendon ruptures are treated surgically. More commonly, however, these extensor mechanism injuries are tendinitis at both the quadriceps and the patellar tendon insertions on the patella, as well as irritation of the chondral surface of the patella. There may be intrapatellar fat pad hypertrophy and occasionally intraarticular effusion related to associated chondromalacia of the patella. Symptoms may be reproduced by resisted knee flexion and weighted squatting exercises. The pathologic origin of the jumper's knee consists of microscopic disruption of the insertional fibers of the patella tendon at the inferior pole of the patella. Prevention of this condition is accomplished by keeping the quadriceps and hamstring muscles strong and flexible so that their shock-absorbing properties are maximized. This is only useful in conjunction with execution of proper technique. Symptoms range from pain following activity, to pain with and following activity, and, finally, to pain interfering with performance. Icing, antiinflammatory medication, stretching, and patella tendon bracing or strapping may be useful in limiting progression of the disease.

Improper landing technique can result in acute or chronic traumatic injuries to the cervical spine (27). In such cases, repetitive flexion injuries can cause late instability and neurologic damage. They are often not seen on routine lateral radiographs. The presence of slight anterior subluxation, simple compression fractures, or subtle kyphotic angulation at one cervical level should alert the physician to this diagnosis. Flexion/extension views are useful to demonstrate this instability.

In spite of fewer severe injuries due to softer landing areas, the flop technique has introduced more significant injuries. With fatigue and inflexibility, energy utilized in the vaulting technique commonly leads to paraspinous muscle spasm or transverse process fracture. Since jumpers vault over the bar and land on their backs, it is important that they know proper landing technique. Both arms should shoot out and drive into the mat at contact in order to soften the contact of the back and to help limit vertebral compression fractures of the cervical, thoracic, and lumbar spine. Nevertheless, such injury will occur (Fig. 39.11). A backboard and sandbags must be available in high jump and pole vaulting areas because of the potential severity of spine injury.

Energy transfer following foot plant for both eccentric loading and subsequent contracture leave the hamstring and low back muscles particularly at risk. Strains are common, and their incidence can only be reduced with adequate warm-up and stretching. Approach, planting, energy transfer, torquing over the bar, and landing are all difficult techniques, and only one aspect can be coached at a time. Asking the athlete to concentrate on multiple points will lead to confusion. Practice of difficult techniques requires repetition to make such technique habit. The "straddle" form is often used in the lower qualifying heights and the "flop" technique in higher jumps. This conserves energy and lessens the chance of severe injury. Hamstring stretching is mandatory for the first form, while landing technique must be well rehearsed in the second.

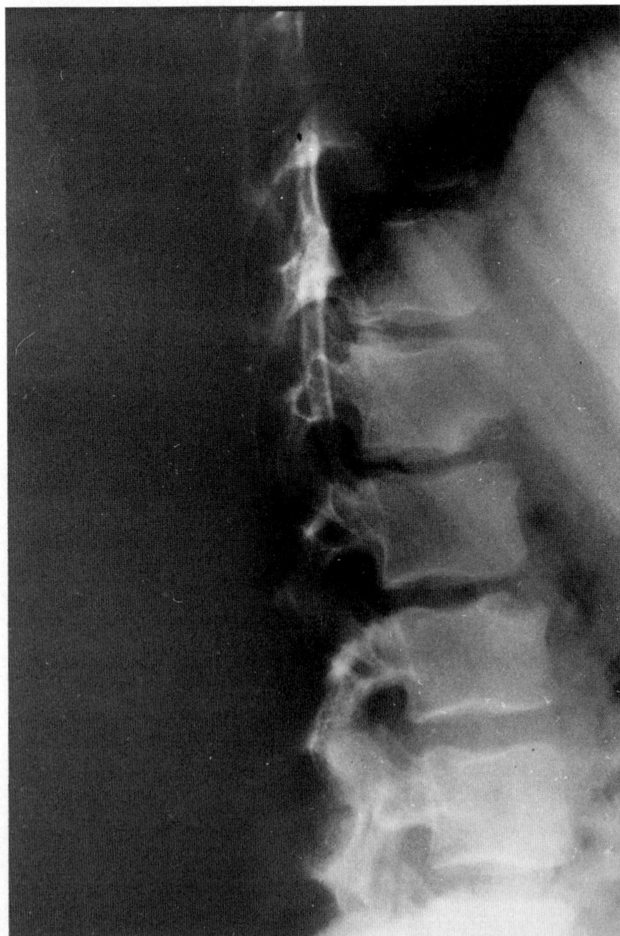

Figure 39.11. Vertebral injury. With the modern techniques incorporating a back landing in the high jump and pole vault vertebral injury is more common, and proper landing technique must be emphasized. Here, a 20-year-old college high jumper who utilizes the "flop" style is found with wedge and compression fractures as well as Schmorl's nodes during evaluation for his back pain (arrow).

Pole Vault

Pole vaulting has prehistoric origins. Ancient man found that by adding the lift of a pole to a running broad jump, barriers such as small streams and gullies could be crossed. Slowly, the concept of competition for height evolved, and, in that form, it was introduced in America in 1877. Vaulters from Northern Britain soon became the early champions, but they were pole climbers and not vaulters (28).

A pole vaulter is essentially a sprinter with a pole. The fiber glass pole, introduced in 1960, allows speed comparable to that of a sprinter. There are four traditional means of pole carrying; high point carry, elevating the tip approximately 45°; intermediate carry, elevating the tip 25°; horizontal carry, with the pole parallel to the ground; and a low point carry, with the tip below horizontal. An effective plant of the pole tip is the most important technique the vaulter must master. If a vaulter misses a plant, the pole tip may lodge in the substance of the foam pit, and sudden jarring will lead to shoulder subluxation or A/C joint sprain. An attempt to decelerate rapidly at the end of a long sprint on the gripping surface of modern synthetic runways while accommodating a heavy pole may lead to anterior cruciate ligament disruption. The vaulter must be taught to slowly decelerate and let the pole slide through his hand if he misses his marks.

The classic technique in the pole vault consisted of an approach of less than full speed, moving the hands closer together, planting the pole, stomping the dominant leg (which is the opposite of the dominant arm due to the crossed-extensor reflex), and propelling one's self upward making one's body parallel to the bar to maximally utilize centrifugal force, turning the body, using the scissors kick to clear the bar, and giving attention to landing to avoid fracture, strain, or sprain (Fig. 39.12*A*). This technique was utilized effectively with a metal pole due to pole stiffness. The same technique will lead to imbalance and injury if used with a fiber glass pole. Unfortunately, many high schools still use metal poles for monetary reasons, and if athletes try to remain competitive, they are most likely to find it impossible to switch techniques if proper equipment become available.

Fiber glass poles are slightly longer than metal poles, being up to 18 feet. The pole tip is held above head level, at about a 15° to 20° angle with a grip wider than shoulder width; both factors allow use of slightly heavier poles. Vaulters are taught that they are sprinters with poles; they are to approach the pit at full speed. Because of this they must have practiced effective plant-

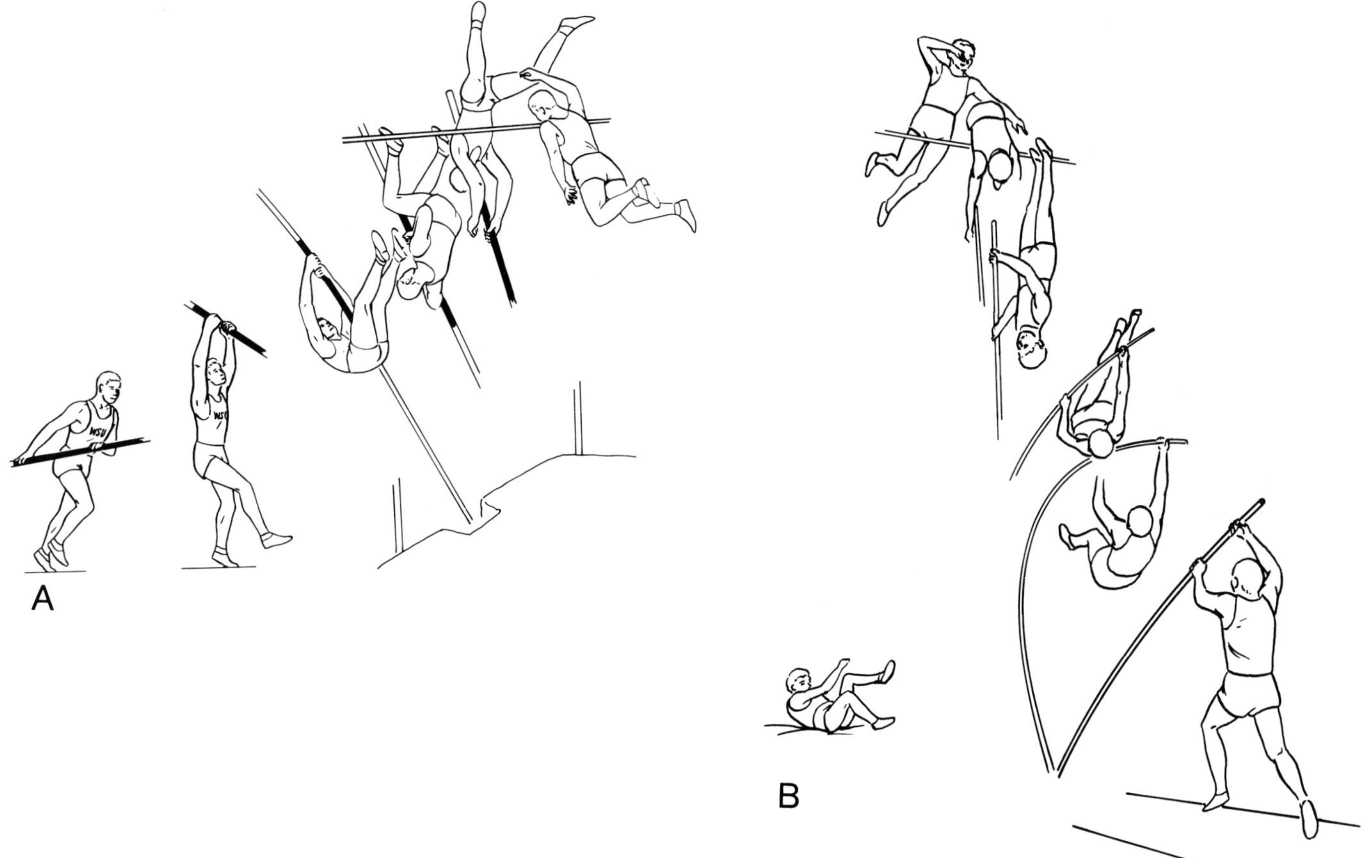

Figure 39.12. Pole vault form. **(A)** With the metal pole, the vaulter must maximize forward momentum in order to propel himself over the bar; thus, he must run through his approach. **(B)** With the fiber glass pole, approach speed can be increased since energy is stored within the pole, which helps catapult the vaulter over the bar; he jackknifes to clear the bar and lands on his back.

ing techniques and an even stride; otherwise, they tend to plant the pole late and decelerate momentum. In the new technique, at the last stride, the pole is held over the head, arms are separated, and with a circular motion, the pole will be planted down into the box. The top hand pulls down while the bottom hand pushes up, making use of their separated positions to store further energy in the pole, effectively using it as a bow and arrow. As the feet continue propelling forward, the pole bends backward, largely encouraged by the separated hand position; the energy of the sprint approach is transferred to the fiber glass pole until rebound release catapults the vaulter over the bar. When the pole is directly vertical, vaulters are thrust upward so they are effectively allowed to do a gymnastic handstand to clear a standard, which is, in fact, higher than the pole they utilize. Abdominal and hip muscles then come into play to help the athletes jackknife over the crossbar and continue the fall to land on their backs. Faulty technique will lead to abdominal, hip, or paraspinous muscle strain, cervical sprain, vertebral and/or skull fracture, or spinal cord injury (Fig. 39.12*B*).

Knowledge and mastery of technique is mandatory in this event. If vaulters have not achieved sufficient speed, the pole will not advance to a full vertical position, and they will fall backward into the box or runway. If they fail to store energy by bending the pole at takeoff, the pole will advance past the standard, and they may even be thrown past the padded pit area. If the plant is not correct, they may be thrown off to the side and into a standard where a laceration or a contusion injury is common.

Vaulters must practice planting technique for 5 or 6 weeks prior to attempting a vault. Their checkmark adjustment and stride length must be accurate, because stepping beyond the ideal takeoff point will lead to shoulder subluxation, and falling short of the ideal takeoff point will lead to decreased momentum so that they will fall back on the runway. They must be taught to run through their plant by relaxing their grip on the pole if they miss their marks. If not, supraspinatus sprain, shoulder subluxation, acromioclavicular (AC) joint sprain, or anterior cruciate ligament disruption will commonly occur.

Examination of the injured shoulder from pole vaulting initially focuses on areas of maximal tenderness. AC joint injury will result in tenderness both over the acromioclavicular joint and, often, just cephalad to the coracoid in the area of the coracoclavicular ligaments, which are also often injured. X-ray examination is mandatory to evaluate AC joint injuries and possible fractures of the distal clavicle. Rotator cuff injuries are best diagnosed by weakness of the supraspinatus in isolation. This is tested by having the patient extend the arms in front of the body, slightly to the outside of straight forward position, with the thumbs pointing down. The examiner then attempts to push downward on the outstretched hands. If pain and weakness are elicited, a supraspinatus strain is likely. Anterior shoulder subluxation is best diagnosed by a positive apprehension sign. This is elicited with the arm abducted, and in external rotation at the shoulder. The athlete notes pain and symptoms of feeling as if the shoulder will pop out of joint. Treatment of these injuries is injury specific. AC joint injuries are most commonly treated nonoperatively. This, however, depends on the degree and severity of ligamentous injury. Full thickness rotator cuff tears are quite uncommon in the younger athletic age group, and most supraspinatus strains will recover with time and rehabilitation, thus avoiding surgical intervention. Shoulder subluxation, if recurrent, may require surgical treatment.

Pole vaulters must have proper flexibility to arch their backs in crossing the bar while keeping their arms down. This facilitates pushing the pole backward with the thumb and prevents them from throwing the arms up in the air, which would force the chest and body into the bar and cause imbalance, thus leading to cervical, paraspinous, abdominal, hip, quadriceps, and gastric strain. They must concentrate on landing as soon as they clear the bar so that they can land relaxed near the middle of the foam pit. The proper technique is to tuck up one's knees while clearing the bar and rolling back for landing. On landing upon the back, the jumper should slap the mat firmly with the arms at a 45° angle to the body to help dissipate energy and decrease the chance of spinous injury.

Throwing Events

Shot Put

Putting a 14-pound stone with rounded edges was a game recorded in Ireland and Scotland as early as 632 B.C. When a 16-pound iron ball was utilized with the modern reintroduction of this event by the Amateur Athletic Union in 1876, the rules were essentially the same. A 7-foot circular platform was utilized in St. Louis in the 1904 Olympics. The metal sphere now utilized is 16 pounds in college, AAU, and Olympic competition, 12 pounds in high school, and 8 pounds for grade school. The spheres are made of iron, bronze, or brass with a lead center. Shot putting is a power event; the missile is pushed rather than thrown.

The restrictions of the 7-foot circle have necessitated developing techniques effective in producing momentum within a small distance. In the 1950s, the long-used straight explosive style was replaced with a low-set rotational style in which the center of gravity started low, from a backward-facing position at the back of the circle, and would rise with rotation along a straight line to gain momentum for release at the front of the circle. Emphasis on weight training helped develop explosiveness for crossed-extensor amplification at release of the shot. In the mid-1970s, the Russians introduced a discus style spin that greatly increased the momentum produced within the limits of the circle and will perhaps be the new dominant form.

Speed must be controlled in order to keep the athlete's balance and rigid attention to form, and practice is the only means to effectively increase speed without injury. Rotational motion in the newer techniques produces tremendous torque. To prevent strain injury, flexibility is necessary. The elbow and throwing shoulder remain behind the shot and hips to produce an effective final push. The newest techniques of spinning in the arc of the discus thrower, consisting of 540° of rotation, is difficult while attempting to accommodate a 16-pound iron weight. In this technique, the weight is kept behind the center of gravity to increase centrifugal force in rotation, producing the effect of an extra burst of energy similar to the effective utilization of the sprinter's blocks (Fig. 39.13).

Warm-up must not be too vigorous, since four quick preliminary trials are necessary prior to qualification for semifinal or final events. However, shot-putters must warm up quickly to maximize quick type II myofibril bursting activity. They must stretch and bend all muscle groups involved in the event, particularly concentrating on the leg, back, and shoulders. The optimal release angle is about 41°, so athletes practice this with a rubberized or indoor shot against set positions on a wall to get the feeling for proper angle. Sprinting, jogging, and agility drills are important in developing speed and coordination. Torquing techniques are particularly hard on the knees, back, and shoulders, so that in midseason, the shot-putter rarely throws the shot in practice more than six repetitions twice a week.

Injury is commonly due to error in technique. Due to torque, generation of momentum, paraspinous muscles spasm at any point along the spine can occur. In combination with hip thrust in the final push, gluteus strain or hip capsular strain will occur if athletes are slightly off-balance. External oblique or transverse abdominus sprain is also common. Athletes commonly plant their nondominant foot under the toe bar at the end of the movement to stop momentum, gain balance, and avoid fouling. This is an extremely dangerous technique, which must be avoided, since continuation of momentum leading to internal rotation on the planted lower leg easily causes anterior cruciate ligament disruption, such that future pivoting on this leg for performance of athletic technique may become impossible.

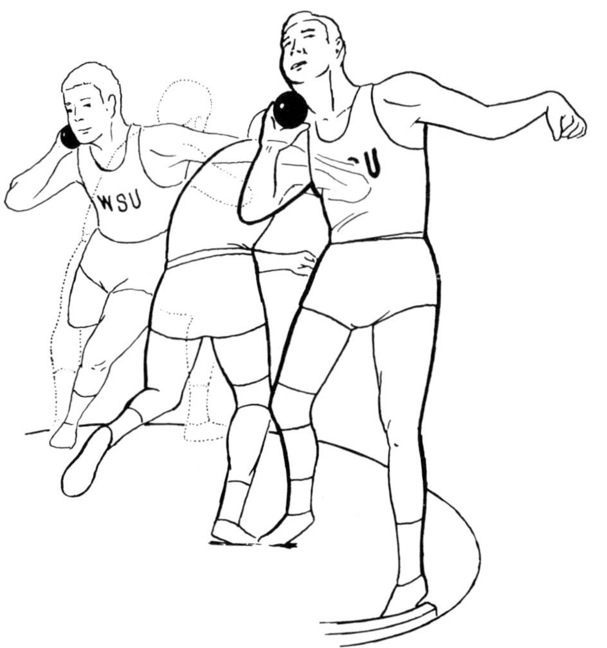

Figure 39.13. Shot put. A whirling discus style has recently been introduced in competition and may eventually prove to be more effective.

The shot is released with a final push resulting from stored energy produced through a complex technique. With the elbow and shot held behind the center of gravity and propelled forward, the push must be straight. If there is slight imbalance, the weight and the push against a shot on the extended fingertips commonly produce lateral epicondylitis, or inflammation of the tendinous origin of the extensor muscles in the forearm. The diagnosis of shot-put tennis elbow is made by finding tenderness with palpation over the lateral epicondyle and pain on resisted wrist extension. The lesion has been found to be consistently located within the origin of the extensor carpi radialis brevis. Epicondylitis is treated with nonsteroidal antiinflammatory medications in mild cases, local cortisone injection or iontophoreses in moderate cases, and cortisone injection with concomitant deep friction massage in recalcitrant cases. Upon cessation of pain, therapeutic exercises are beneficial to strengthen the musculature prior to the resumption of throwing. Surgery is done after exhausting all nonoperative management. Although a tennis elbow strap may help decrease symptoms, pain in the final push will decrease competitive performance. Strict adherence to technique is implicated in injury prevention. Athletes may benefit from wall and standard fingertip push-ups to help coordinate balance and must also choose a shot that feels balanced to hold.

Early in the season, athletes propel the shot forward from the hand. As the season progresses and they gain balance, they both hold and propel the shot from the fingertips. Early in the season, wrist sprain is extremely common and may be prevented by wrist strengthening exercises, avoidance of hyperextension in technique, and taping. Athletes must not progress to fingertip pushoff too early; otherwise, volar plate sprain, collateral ligament sprain, or interosseous and lumbrical muscle strain may commonly occur. Performance of proper technique is only possible through proper progression and attention to form. Athletes must not attempt complex advanced maneuvers until they have been coached properly and are well prepared.

Hammer Throw

Hammer throwing originated in Ireland about 500 B.C. In the 1860s, throwing a 16 pound shot on an oak handle from behind the line was introduced into American collegiate sports. After 1880, a 7-foot throwing circle was utilized. With the introduction of the circle, two circular winds within it preceded delivery of the hammer. With development of technique specific to the sport, three turns were introduced in the 1900s. Offsetting the center of balance to traverse a straight line and develop momentum demands exacting technique, so that technique rather than speed is emphasized. In maximizing centrifugal force, the hammer actually leads the athlete, and by pivoting on one's toes, quick turn and maximal acceleration become possible.

Hammer throwers keep their bodies crossed. This means that the hips are locked into position ahead of the shoulders, which are also locked into position. He generates torque through an almost seated position. In the mid-1960s, the Europeans perfected techniques capable of generating four turns within the 7-foot circle.

Hammer throwers must be quick, well coordinated, and have extremely strong legs and backs. They must be flexible. Rather than worry about rotational speed, technique must be perfect so that extended arms and perfect positioning of the center of gravity will help propel the 16 pound shot forward at the end of the chain.

Throwers learn to lead the hammer and not drag it. The idea is to transfer the energy from powerful leg muscles and the back through the hips, shoulders, and arms ahead of the hammer. In order to keep the hammer in a solid position, throwers must be flexible and strong. They must not allow the hammer to get ahead of them, or the tremendous torque generated will lead to subluxation of the shoulder.

The technique of throwing demands smooth flowing continuous action, such that each turn is faster than the previous one. There are no pauses between different turns, so athletes learn to turn on their toes, and momentum progressively increases. Although athletes must remain in the circle, the hammer does not need to do so; there is, however, no ideal starting position for the hammer.

Athletes start by facing the back of the circle with knees flexed 30°. They start low, generating momentum forward and upward progressively with a smooth lifting motion. As they generate torque, they sit back on their hips, extend their arms and shoulders fully, thus increasing the radius of leverage and achieving a mechanical advantage. Since acceleration can only progress with both feet on the ground, they learn to turn quickly on the ball of the foot. They must emphasize keeping the outer leg close to the body against centrifugal force to prevent imbalance. The back must be locked into position. Without the proper flexibility, paraspinous muscle strain and associated transverse process fracture is extremely common. In sitting back with the arms extended, leverage is increased, utilizing the pelvis to balance the pull of the hammer. Hip capsular sprain, pubic symphysitis, or iliotibial tract friction syndrome commonly occur with slight misstep. To keep control of the hammer, athletes must strive for quick tight turns, attempting to keep the hammer wire-tight through the entire motion. Extreme strength and polished technique are needed.

The speed of the hammer increases progressively with every turn. The hips always lead the shoulders in order to control centrifugal force. Counterbalance of the hips is accomplished by leaning opposite to the direction of the hammer. The torque generated by such training not only stresses the back muscles, but places extreme strain on abdominal muscles, so that the abdominal oblique, transversalis, and rectus muscles can be strained with slight imbalance (Fig. 39.14).

The arms must be kept locked and extended in an X-position behind the pivoting hips. If this position is not maintained, torque on the elbows will lead to medial or lateral epicondylitis. To prevent this, the swing must first be practiced without a hammer. The swing must be even because disruption of rhythm will lead to jerky motion of the hammer, and strains of the hips, back, shoulder, and neck commonly result. Effort must be made to sustain upward and progressive drive, gradually elevating the center of gravity in production of momentum; otherwise, a last minute backward lean to produce elevation will lead to rhomboid, levator scapulae, or a rotator cuff musculotendinous strain. In elevating too quickly at the end of this technique, lateral collateral ligament strain is common.

Athletes must take special care of their equipment and pay strict attention to their competitive area. They must watch out for frayed wires, which may break and cause a fall backward if the weight is released during a turn. The hammer head must revolve freely on its spindle, and if it does not, it should be stored vertically on a hook to prevent the wire from kinking, which leads to wire failure.

Athletes may want to wear a leather glove or tape their fingers to increase grip and decrease friction. They must make sure that the surface is even to help prevent incidence of sprain injury. It is sometimes best to practice with two hammers so that energy can be conserved and not wasted in retrieval. Most importantly, they must pay attention to other athletes on the field to make sure that no one is subject to injury when the hammer is thrown.

Discus

In Homer's epic poetry, the discus was mentioned as an athletic event occurring as early as 1300 B.C. The discus was one of the original five events in the Pentathlon when instituted in 708 B.C. The Greek discus was heavier than the present discus and was thrown from a pedestal, which severely limited background momentum.

The modern discus weighs 2 kg. It has a diameter of at least 21.9 cm. The high school discus is scaled down to 3 pounds, 9 ounces. For practice purposes, the discus may be made of rubber, significantly decreasing contact injury. Standard running or track shoes may be used, but many athletes remove most spikes, particularly in the left shoe, in order to allow pivoting. Small rubberized spikes may be useful on the new synthetic surfaces. The most frequent injury in discus throwing is blistering or laceration of the fingers. Physical examination of deep finger lacerations concentrates on possible injuries to digital nerves and arteries, as well as to flexor tendons. Isolated distal interphalangeal joint flexion is tested to rule out flexor digitorum profundus injury. Tendon lacerations are treated surgically. More commonly, however, lacerations involve only the skin and subcutaneous tissues, which can be treated with

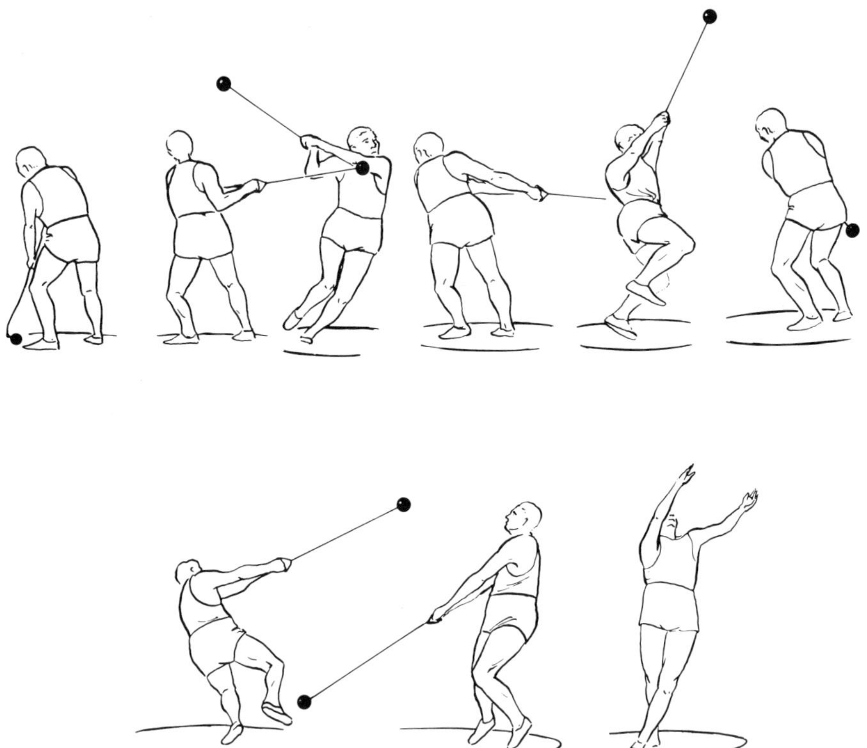

Figure 39.14. Hammer throw. This event is all technique in that the center of gravity and leverage must be perfectly balanced in order to generate momentum and energy. Using abdominal and back muscles to lock the upper body in position over the lower body, energy is stored and amplified by reciprocating crossed-extensor reflex during rotation.

thorough irrigation and primary wound closure. Small spurs that develop on the metallic surface of the discus must be filled immediately, and the use of a compound such as tincture of benzoin or resins are allowed to secure grip, particularly in wet weather.

In the original technique, while standing in a fixed position on a pedestal, the athlete was merely allowed to swing back and forth repetitively to develop momentum (Fig. 39.15*A*). With the institution of a 2.5 m throwing circle in 1910, the momentum of the early swing was potentiated by allowing generation of momentum in a one-and-a-half turn pattern (Fig. 39.15*B*). In the 1930s, a hop was incorporated within the style of one-and-three-quarters turn, which added considerable momentum. The addition of weight training, anabolic steroids, and strict attention to technique have significantly increased the distances generated since the 1950s.

Preliminary swings are utilized to establish proper balance, reassurance, and generation of momentum. From this point, momentum can be either amplified by the crossed-extensor mechanism in rotation, or increased by incorporation of a jump. Athletes must be well tuned to their technique; otherwise, too much speed works against them. They become unbalanced and commonly suffer knee injuries, ankle sprains, shoulder strains, or subluxation. If the knee is not bent enough during rotation, athletes lose considerable drive. Conversely, if the knee is bent too much, the arm does its work prematurely, so that the discus will be hurled before maximum generation of energy (Fig. 39.15*C*).

The feet must be kept close to the body in an effort to consciously counteract centrifugal force. Only while the feet are in contact with the ground can acceleration develop. In the initial swing, throwers are able to preload energy, much like the sprinters lowering into the blocks. The lower body generates energy, and the upper body acts as a sling. The upper body is held rigidly through the back in order to maximize the sling effect because torquing strain to the lumbar, thoracic, and cervical spine muscles is extremely common. If the arm lags too far behind the pivoting motion of the lower extremities, sprain of the anterior capsule of the shoulder, subluxation of the shoulder, or strain to the trapezius or scapular muscles may develop. Athletes start in a crouched position and slowly raise the center of gravity during rotation in order to generate a power snap at the wrist. Wrist sprain is common as is de Quervain's tenosynovitis, when wrist snap is overemphasized. Pain over the first dorsal compartment of the wrist and pain on resisted extension of the thumb are the hallmarks of de Quervain's tenosynovitis. Treatment of mild cases includes nonsteroidal antiinflammatory medications, local cortisone injections, and splinting. In recalcitrant cases, surgical release of the stenotic tunnel in the first dorsal compartment provides excellent relief of symptoms.

Blistering injury is common, and aids to increase

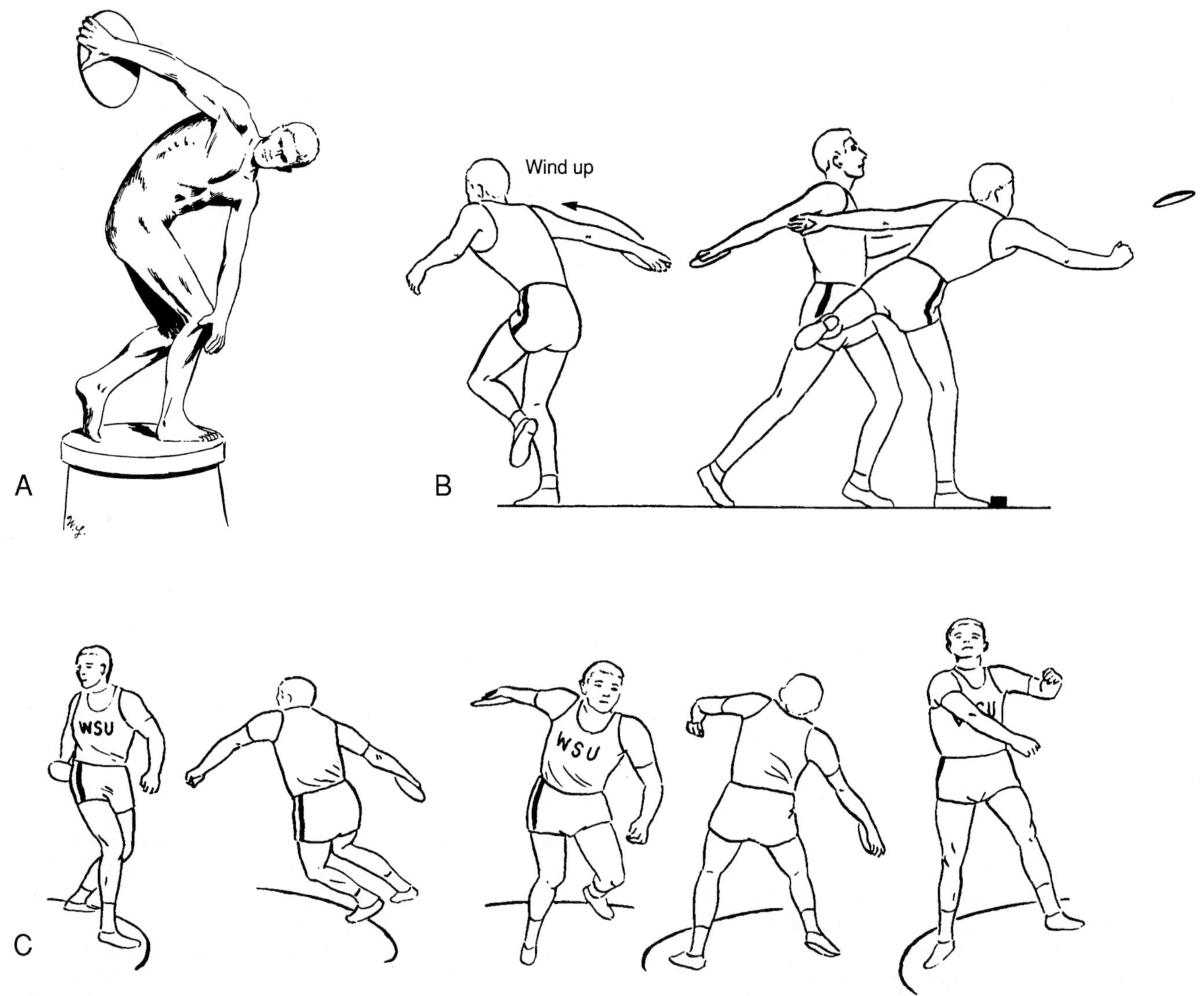

Figure 39.15. Discus. **(A)** Originally, the discus was thrown from a pedestal. **(B)** Additional momentum was gained with the institution of a throwing circle which allowed a pivot rotation energy amplification process. **(C)** A linear rotation pattern, shown above, has since developed which further amplifies momentum.

surface friction are necessary. Holding the discus in the initial swing may also present a problem. If the discus is held in a position too horizontal to the ground, tension is placed on the pectoralis major and conjoined tendons so that strain of these muscles may occur. To eliminate strain, a more perpendicular holding technique is utilized, which, in fact, allows the athlete to turn more in the windup. Unfortunately, changing the plane of the discus from perpendicular to horizontal is not easy and may lead to shoulder, wrist, or elbow strain.

In practice, a strapped discus may be useful in that multiple consecutive turns can be allowed with minimal risk while developing a sense of balance. Balance is also obtained by keeping the knees and trunk bent so that the hips travel through a wider arc in order to develop greater momentum. The center of gravity must be kept ahead of the feet so that the upper body and hips lead into the turn. Nevertheless, the discus throw is a continuous movement. Haltering technique will place tension on ankles, hips, knees, back, and shoulders, and strains will result. Athletes must police the throwing circle for debris that could lead to an ankle sprain. They must follow through on their technique at the completion of the throw so that sudden deceleration will not result in a knee ligament sprain.

Javelin

The javelin was the first field event in the first ancient Olympic Games. It originally consisted of a spear made of wood with a metal point. It also had a qualification of having the foremost point no greater than 110 cm from the center of gravity, or less than 90 cm. A central whip cord near the center of gravity was mandatory, being 16 cm in length. Initially, the overall length of the shaft was not less than 260 cm, and the weight was not less than 800 g. As the modern aerodynamic javelin developed in the 1950s, a fixed size was finally established in 1955; it now weighs less than two lbs.

A system has recently been developed to measure initial conditions in the javelin throw rapidly enough to be used by the thrower for feedback in performance improvement (29). This is achieved with digital high speed video recording with subsequent graphic presentation to the thrower of release conditions and a simulation of the subsequent flight, together with optimal conditions and flight for javelin release. This system allows instant feedback to javelin throwers and is expected to provide greater control and consistency of throwing variables by javelin throwers.

High speed cinematography has demonstrated that in order to attain maximal throwing distance, the javelin thrower should achieve positive acceleration during the running approach, effective thrusting with the right leg on the penultimate stride, and carry the javelin during the last strides at an optimal angle for release between 32° and 36° (30).

Athletes utilize full acceleration and a sudden stop in order to generate tremendous force in throwing the javelin. They hold the javelin above their heads, with the elbow forming about a 90° angle in their approach. As they generate speed, the throwing arm begins to extend with the hand slightly lower than the shoulder and the palm turned out. The cross-over step is used where the body is kept well in front of the javelin to maximize forward momentum, while developing a strong delivery position. The shoulders are kept in line with the direction of the throw. As the arm extends, the body rotates, and the javelin is pulled quickly over the body near the ear. The head leans to the opposite side as the javelin is brought through the center of gravity. The arm must remain flexible to maximize "whip" in the throw. As the javelin is thrown over the contralateral hip and planted foot, the abdominal muscles are activated to pull the chest around and maximize power. The knee ipsilateral to the throwing arm is brought through flexed and high so that it can quickly follow through and block forward momentum just short of the scratch line. This action should square off the body in the direction of the throw so that a sidearm throw, which generates supraspinatus and teres minor shoulder strain, is less likely to occur.

The elbow must lead the hand in the throw. If the arm is too extended, torque is generated through the elbow. Medial epicondylitis at the elbow is the most common javelin injury and can be prevented by flexibility and proper technique. Physical examination of this injury demonstrates tenderness over the medial epicondyle and common flexor wad at the elbow, and pain elicited on resisted palmar flexion of the wrist. Treatment includes nonsteroidal antiinflammatory medication, epicondylitis straps, and, if symptoms continue, local cortisone injection or iontophoresis. Surgery is performed only in recalcitrant cases.

There are two popular styles in approach, a smooth, fast Finnish style, (Fig. 39.16*A*) and a more hopping American style (Fig. 39.16*B*). In the Finnish style, cross-

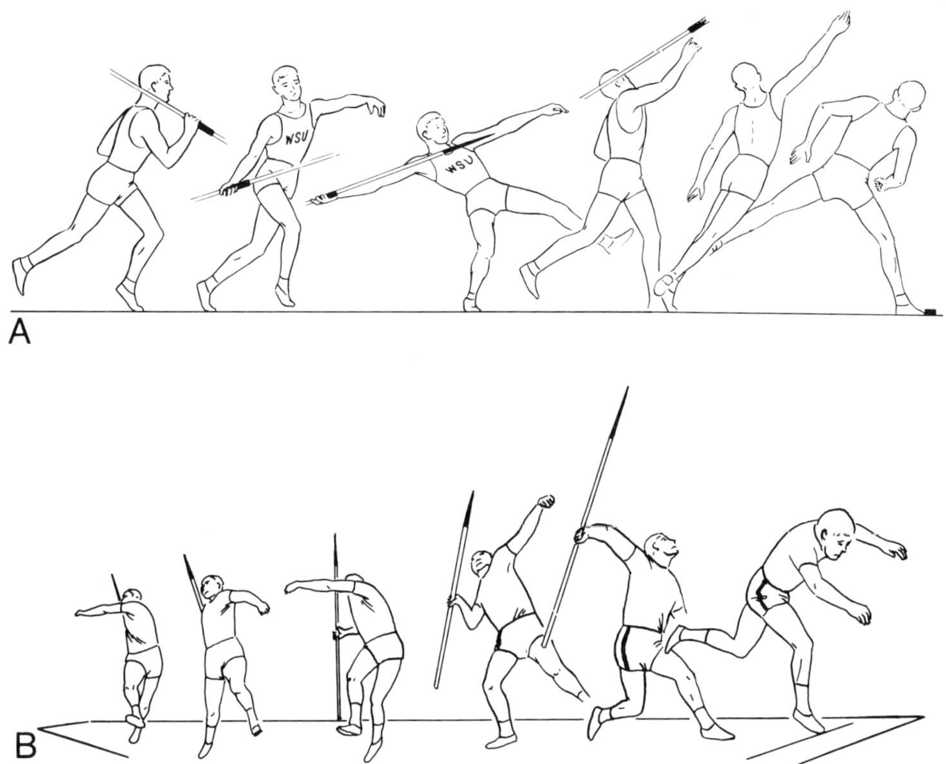

Figure 39.16. Javelin. **(A)** Low cross-stepping Finnish style utilizes abdominal muscles in the throw. **(B)** The American approach utilizes a high cross-step style and a throw in which the shoulders are perpendicular to the direction of throw; this can lead to shoulder impingement and elbow medial capsular injury.

stepping is low, and a front facing position is generated in the throw by strong abdominal muscles. The throw is made over a rigid and fully extended contralaterally planted foot. While approaching the final steps, a series of rapid cross-over steps are utilized, turning the feet slightly to the side of the throwing arm and obtaining a strong throwing position. This hinged-type approach allows progressive and steady acceleration.

American athletes, used to throwing a baseball from center field, have developed a cross-step style of throw. In this cross-over step, the shoulders are in line with the direction of the throw, and the head and feet are turned approximately 45° to the throwing side while the upper body is turned 90°. This style is less energy efficient than the Finnish style and leads to more shoulder injuries because of the torque generated to the upper extremity.

The speed of the approach is related to the athlete's mastery of technique. Too quick an approach will not allow coordination of arm and leg motions so that misstep and related injury occur. If the approach is too slow, power generation is significantly decreased. Nevertheless, the speed of approach is optimally related to the style used.

The angle of release of the javelin is optimal at 35°. In elevating the tip of the spear while producing acceleration, tremendous stress is placed upon the acromioclavicular joint. If technique is not properly executed or if there has been some prior injury to the shoulder or elbow joint, stress to the AC joint is increased, and a sprain of its capsule or disc is common.

Throwing motion must be well rehearsed. It occurs in four stages, and, most important in preparing for the throw, there appears to be a sequential activation pattern of muscular activity. The deltoid fibers fire first, followed by supraspinatus, infraspinatus, teres minor, and finally culminating with subscapularis activity (31). If a throw is not made near the center of gravity, an imbalance will occur and strain to any of these muscles can develop, depending on which phase of activity is stressed. With imbalance of the rotator cuff muscles, scapular strain or subscapular bursitis can occur. Any sporadic motion in the throw may lead to a glenoid labrum tear. Without proper warm-up, a strain of back muscles and triceps is extremely common in the javelin thrower because of torque on these muscles. Insufficient warm-up also leads to impingement and elbow injury.

The most common shoulder injury in javelin throwers is impingement (32). Chronic impingement syndrome of the shoulder from repetitive javelin throwing results in the development of bursitis and supraspinatus tendonitis. Impingement syndrome is described in detail in Chapter 50. Treatment focuses on avoiding this provocative maneuver, strengthening the rotator cuff musculature to enhance depression of the humeral head, and antiinflammatory medications. Nonsteroidal antiinflammatory medications are most commonly used. Cortisone injections are utilized in more severe cases. Continuance of rotator cuff irritation with the development of bursitis and tendonitis can eventually lead to full-thickness rotator cuff tearing. This is diagnosed by loss of strength with pain on resistive maneuvers of the supraspinatus. Full-thickness rotator cuff tears are treated surgically. The bursa is also swollen initially and later becomes fibrotic, in either case, interfering with its normal gliding and lubricating function (33). Maintaining cuff strength, elbow and shoulder flexibility, and utilizing proper technique will decrease incidence of this injury.

Stress fractures involving the olecranon have been reported in javelin throwers (34). These are due to a forceful avulsion force applied by the triceps during the throwing mechanism. These fractures have been treated operatively and nonoperatively. There is, however, a high risk of delayed union and nonunion with this injury, and some authors recommend open reduction and internal fixation of these fractures.

Fingertip lacerations are common because of abrasion against the normal rotation of the grip cord at release. Such injury is minimized by limiting the number of practice throws so that fatigue does not set in. Fatigue-accentuated erratic motions result in injury. In sudden deceleration at the end of the run, athletes must strive for control. In attempting to decelerate momentum while turning inward on a planted and slightly flexed knee, anterior cruciate ligament sprain can occur.

Conclusions

Effective track and field techniques is seen to be dependent on proper form. Each facet of form must be individually emphasized and individually developed to maximize efficiency. Performance hinges on practice and perseverance. Without attention to detail, injury is common.

Proper form maximizes efficiency of energy utilization. Through technique, utilization of the body's own energy-amplifying system can be maximized. Crossed-extensor amplification of energy stored in eccentric contraction becomes the basis of competitive performance. Maximal efficiency is only possible by keeping the musculotendinous unit healthy. Injuries heal with scarring, and scar tissue lacks contractility and energy storage potential. Therefore, to maximize performance, injury must be minimized.

In speed technique, injury is commonly related to avulsion or disruption of cold or fatigued fibers. Injury in track and field is more commonly due to training error. Breakdown of tissue related to repetitive microtrauma leads to a decrease of performance ability, but can be minimized by proper training technique. To train while injured invites further injury.

The musculotendinous unit is particularly at risk in athletic performance. Individual fibrils, if fatigued or cold, will become brittle and easily break down. Keeping fibers warm by stretch and warm-up prior to activity will decrease incidence of breakdown. Strength and flexibility further maximize performance and proper technique while decreasing incidence of injury.

The athlete, coach, trainer, and physician must work together to treat the injury early and aggressively to minimize sequelae. Training errors must be identified early and eliminated if possible. The use of proper equipment and maintenance of that equipment is necessary to help avoid injury, as is policing the area where athletic competition occurs to prevent misstep, strain, and sprain injury. Training must be approached gradually and seriously to avoid injury and to maximize performance.

REFERENCES

1. Gardiner EN. Greek Athletic Sports and Festivals. London: Macmillan, 1910.
2. Bresnahan GT, Tuttle WW. Track and Field Athletics, ed. 2. St. Louis; CV Mosby Company, 1947.
3. Martin RK, Yesalis CE, Foster D. Sports Injuries at the 1985 Junior Olympics, and Epidemiologic Analysis. Am J Sports Med 1987;15(6):603–608.
4. Schultz R, Curnow C. Peak performance and age among superathletes: track and field, swimming, baseball, tennis, and golf. J Gerontology 1988;43(5):113–120.
5. Gross ML, Davlin LB, Evanski PM. Effectiveness of orthotic shoe inserts in the long-distance runner. Am J Sports Med 1991;19(4):409–412.
6. Harring KM, Richie DH Jr. Friction blisters and sock fiber composition. A double-blind study. J Am Pod Med Assoc 1990;80(2):63–71.
7. Boje O: Doping. Bulletin of the Health Organization of the League of Nations. New York: League of Nations, 1939:439.
8. Casner SW, Early RG, Carlson BR. Anabolic steroid effects on body composition in normal young men. J Sports Med Phys Fitness 1971;11:98.
9. Costill DL, Dalsky GP, Fink WJ. Effects of caffeine ingestion on metabolism and exercise performance. Med Sci Sports 1978;10:155.
10. Mann RV. A kinetic analysis of sprinting. Med Sci Sports Exerc 1981;13:325.
11. Bush J, Weiskopf DC. Dynamic Track and Field. Boston: Allyn and Beacon, 1978.
12. Diullo JV, Zarins B. Biomechanics of the musculotendinous unit: Relation to athletic performance and injury. Clin Sports Med 1983;2:71.
13. Stinitski CL, McMaster JH, Scranton PE. On the nature of stress fractures. Am J Sports Med 1978;6(6):391–396.
14. Greene PR. Running on flat turns: Experiments, theory, and applications. J Biomech Eng 1985;107:96–103.
15. Cavagna GA, Thys H, Zamboni A. The sources of external work in level walking and running. J Physiol (Lond) 1976;262–639.
16. Marey EJ, Demeny G. Locomotion humaine: Mecanisma du saut. C R Acad Sci (Paris) 1885;101:489.
17. Sutker AN, Jackson DW, Pagliano JW. Iliotibial band syndrome in distance runners. Phys Sports Med 1981;9:69.
18. Jackson DW: Shinsplints. An update. Phys Sports Med 1978;6:51.
19. Jackson DW, Strizak AM. Stress fractures in runners excluding the foot. In: Mark RP, ed. Symposium on the Foot and Leg in Running Sports. St. Louis: CV Mosby, 1982:109.
20. Warhol MJ, Siegel AJ, Evans WJ, et al. Skeletal muscle injury and repair in marathon runners after competition. Am J Path 1985;118(2):331–339.
21. Seedat YK, Aboo N, Naicker S, et al. Acute renal failure in the "Comrades Marathon" runners. Renal Failure 1989–1990:11(4):209–212.
22. Newmark SR, Poppo FR, Adams G. Fluid and electrolyte replacement in the ultramarathon runner. Am J Sports Med 1991;19(4):389–391.
23. Murray MP, Guten GN, Mollinger LA, et al. Kinematic and electromyographic patterns of Olympic race walkers. Am J Sports Med 1983;11:68.
24. Hay JG, Nohara H. Techniques used by elite long-jumpers in preparation for takeoff. J Biomech 1990;23(3):229–239.
25. Fukashiro S, Miyashita M. An estimation of the velocities of three take-off phases in eighteen meter triple jump. Med Sci Sports Exerc 1983;15(4):309–312.
26. Blazina ME, Kerlan RK, Jobe FW. Jumper's knee. Orthop Ctn North Am 1973;4:655.
27. Paley D, Gillespie R. Chronic repetitive unrecognized flexion injury of the cervical spine (high jumper's neck). Am J Sports Med 1986;14(1):92–95.
28. Ganslen RV. Evolution of modern vaulting. Athlet J 1971;51:102.
29. Hubbard M, Alaways LW. Rapid and accurate estimation of release conditions in the javelin throw. J Biomech 1989;22(6–7):583–595.
30. Kunz H, Kaufmann DA. Cinematographical analysis of javelin throwing techniques of decathletes. Br J Sports Med 1983;17(3):200–204.
31. Jobe FW. Overuse of Throwing Arm and Shoulder. Presented at the 49th Annual Meeting of the AAOS, Anaheim, CA, 1982.
32. Jackson DW. Chronic rotator cuff impingement in the throwing athlete. Am J Sports Med 1976;4:231.
33. Ciullo JV, Guise ER. Coracoacromial arch impingement: clinical presentation, radiographic findings, histological evidence and therapy. Orthop Trans 1981;5:494.
34. Hulkko A, Orave S, Nikula P. Stress fractures of the olecranon in javelin throwers. Int J Sports Med 1986;7(4):210–213.

40 / TRIATHLON

Mary L. O'Toole and T. David Sisk

The triathlon is an endurance competition made up of three events done sequentially with little or no rest between race segments. By definition of the International Triathlon Union (ITU), the world governing body for the sport of triathlon, the sport consists of an open water swim, a bicycle race on roads, and a run on roads (1). Race distances vary, and finish times range from approximately 30 min to several days (Table 40.1). Although the ironman distance race is perhaps the most well-known, races of Olympic distance or shorter are by far the most popular, representing 97% of racing opportunities.

In 1991, approximately 2 million individuals entered at least 1 of the 5000 triathlon competitions held worldwide (2). Diversity of training is undoubtedly a principal reason for the popularity of the triathlon. The athlete must train concurrently in three activities to be successful. Another attraction of the triathlon is the development of a more balanced degree of fitness than that offered by a single sport. Many individuals believe that with such variable training, chance for injury will be minimized without sacrificing overall fitness levels. This chapter examines the medical considerations for participation in triathlon training and competition. The medical and physiologic consequences of multisport training and racing are examined for the primary care physician. Unique aspects of the triathlon will be considered.

Characterization of Triathletes

Physical

Physically, triathletes are a diverse group (3). Contrary to the mental picture of a superfit Spartan, the average triathlete is quite ordinary. The average age of triathletes who have participated in research studies is 32 years old. Those volunteering for research are usually somewhat older than average, so it can reasonably be expected that the average age of triathletes is slightly younger than 30. Ages of those competing range from the mid-teens to older than 70. Average height for the men is 5 feet 11 inches and average weight is 160 lb. Women average 5 feet, 6 inches and 128 lb. Percent body fat is probably the most striking characteristic of triathletes. For men, percent body fat has been reported to range between 5% and 15% (mean = 9.8%), and for women, from 7% to 21% (mean = 15.7%). Although an average is, to a certain extent, a good descriptor, triathletes come in all sizes and shapes. Physique is not a limiting factor to triathlon participation.

Physiologic

Aerobic Capacity

Triathletes have been characterized by measures of aerobic power and anaerobic threshold. A major difference between triathletes and other athletes, however, is that these fitness criteria have been measured in each of the three sports making up the triathlon. Triathletes of varying abilities have been tested with the expected result that their physiologic measures are clearly above those expected in the nonexercising population. Mean $\dot{V}_{O_2max}$ values for treadmill running have been reported to range from 52.4 to 72 ml/kg/min for men and from 58.7 to 65.9 ml/kg/min for women (3). Among triathletes, maximal aerobic power is quite variable, with surprisingly low values and extremely high values being reported. Mean $\dot{V}_{O_2max}$ values during cycling are approximately 3% to 6% lower than those achieved during running. These differences are considerably less than the 9% to 11% that has been reported in single-sport athletes (4). Tethered swimming $\dot{V}_{O_2max}$ values also are closer to treadmill values (9% to 11% less) than those previously reported for athletes doing only run training (13% to 18% less) (5). Maximal aerobic power is only slightly less for triathletes when compared with values reported for comparable single-sport athletes.

Table 40.1.
Standard Distances for Triathlon, in Kilometers (Adopted by ITU, 1991)

Event	Swim	Cycle	Run
Youth or sprint	0.75	20	5
Olympic	1.5	40	10
Long course	2–4	50–180	15–42

Anaerobic Threshold

Both ventilatory and lactate breakpoints have been used as measures of anaerobic threshold in triathletes (6). These thresholds varied between 65% and 85% of $\dot{V}_{O_2max}$. Anaerobic thresholds during cycling were generally at a higher percent of $\dot{V}_{O_2max}$ than were the running thresholds. It is interesting to note that thresholds can vary considerably among sports in any given athlete (7). Because training intensities are often based on thresholds, this becomes an important consideration for the athlete who wants to avoid injury. Economy of motion, particularly running after cycling, also is an important consideration in avoiding injury. Triathletes have been variously reported to have no change in efficiency or decreased efficiency when running after cycling (8).

Training Practices

Distance and Pace

The physiologic demands of different length triathlon competitions are different and, therefore, require slightly different training practices. Table 40.2 presents average training practices of those training for an Olympic distance race. Minimums and maximums vary greatly as does the amount of time spent doing interval or hill workouts. On average, 44% of the swim training was in the form of interval workouts, and 22% of bike and run training was done either with intervals or on hills. The average Olympic distance triathletes trained 4 days per week in each sport. Many augmented their practice with weight training on 2 days per week. The average time commitment for training was 12.25 hr per week or about 1.75 hr per day. Training for shorter races involves lower training distances and more anaerobic or sprint work; training for longer races involves more distance and fewer intervals.

Cross-Training

Technically, as defined in the classic experiments (9), cross-training means deriving benefits in the performance of one activity through training done in another activity. However, the term *cross-training* is commonly used by triathletes and others to mean concurrent training in several activities. The important cross-training issues for a triathlete are optimizing performance and minimizing the chance of injury. For optimal triathlon performance, both central (mainly cardiovascular) and peripheral (mainly musculoskeletal) training adaptations are necessary. The central adaptations result from nonspecific endurance training as long as the load on the heart is adequate (9). Because the musculoskeletal effects of training are specific to the training mode, the triathletes must swim, bike, and run in amounts appropriate to the anticipated competitive distances. The commonly held belief that the cross-training of triathlon participants will result in very few overuse injuries does not appear to be justified by available studies. In addition, the question of relative risk of injury by run training immediately after cycling training compared with separating training periods has not been addressed in well-controlled studies.

Table 40.2.
Average Weekly Training Practices

Aspect	Swim	Cycle	Run
Distance	8.4 km	180 km	48 km
Pace	19 min/km	31 km/hr	4 min 42 sec/km

Training-Related Medical Considerations

Injuries

Many athletes and medical personnel believe that training in multisport activities reduces the chance of training injury because activities are alternated. This has not been borne out in training-injury studies. During training, triathletes have been reported to have a high incidence of injury. Williams et al. (10) reported that 51% of the triathletes surveyed had sustained training injuries. Ireland and Micheli (11) reported that 64% of triathletes they studied had training injuries, whereas Levy et al. (12, 13) reported an injury rate greater than 90%. Triathletes in these surveys were a mixed population, training for events of varying lengths. In a sample of athletes training specifically for the Hawaii Ironman Triathlon, O'Toole et al. (14) reported that 91% sustained at least one training-related injury during the previous year. The most common pattern (72%) was for athletes to sustain multiple injuries (average 2.9 injuries per athlete). The severity of the injuries varied from nuisance to significant. The majority (80% to 90%) of the injuries are overuse syndromes, with the balance being from traumatic events (3, 11, 14, 15). Injury rates were similar in men and women (15, 16). Amid these high injury reports is an encouraging statistic from Williams et al. (10) who report that 68% of the triathletes believed that previously incurred injuries improved during their involvement with triathlon training.

Average training time lost because of injury was 3 weeks (11). However, time lost ranged from 0 to 9 months. Approximately 25% of the injured triathletes studied by Ireland and Micheli (11) reported not changing their training because of the injury. Of those studied by Williams et al. (10), the opposite appeared to be true. Only 20% of that sample indicated that the injuries were severe enough to stop training or withdraw from a race. Not surprisingly, 51% of the worst injuries recurred within a 1-year period (11). It would appear that getting triathletes to allow injuries to heal thoroughly before returning to full training is the largest challenge facing the physician.

Anatomic Location

The lower extremity is involved 85% of the time, with the knee the most commonly involved anatomical site (11, 15, 17). Twenty-two to 32% of the injuries were in or around the knee joint. The foot and ankle were involved 14% to 21% of the time (10, 11, 17). Other anatomical sites mentioned were lower back, 10% to 17%; hamstring 8%; shoulder, 7%; groin, 7%; hip, neck, and Achilles tendon, <5%. In the group of ultraendurance triathletes, the most common injury was to the back, with 72% reporting either lower-back injuries or sciatica. A total of 63% reported having a knee/thigh injury, and 61% reported foot/ankle injury. The most common pattern (34%) was for athletes to have injuries affecting all three of these areas simultaneously (14).

Type of Injury

In the group studied by Ireland and Micheli (11), tendinitis was the most frequent injury (17%), with muscle strains, perhaps related, closely following (16%). Massimino et al. (17) reported muscle strain in 31%, with tendinitis and inflammatory pain each representing 15% of the injuries. Contusions, shin splints, stress fractures, and chondromalacia patella each accounted for approximately 5% of the injuries. Also seen, but occurring in less than 5% of the athletes were iliotibial band syndrome, sciatica, meniscal tear, fracture, abrasion, and plantar fasciitis (11). Bursitis and joint inflammation also were reported to occur during training (15, 16).

Relation to Training

Somewhat surprisingly, none of the studies was able to discern a direct relationship between training practices and incidence of injury. However, Ireland and Micheli (11) noted that athletes who sustained three or more injuries tended to train longer distances in all three disciplines. Because triathletes train concurrently in swimming, biking, and running and because the onset of overuse injury is often insidious, tying an injury to a particular incident or even sport is difficult. However, when the injured athlete was asked to identify the culprit sport, running accounted for 53% to 71%; cycling, 17% to 50%; swimming, 7% to 11%; and combined sports, 5% of the injuries (10, 11, 15, 16). The most common sites of injury associated with the component sports were swimming, the shoulder; cycling, the lower back; and running, the knee (10). According to triathlete perceptions, the majority of injuries (54%) resulted from an increase in training mileage, rather than from actual mileage.

Prevention of Injuries

Prevention of triathlon training injuries should not be different from that of other sports. The hallmark of prevention is gradual progression. The unique aspect of triathlon training, however, is that a triathlete must consider each of the component activities (swim, cycle, run) as separate entities and develop a gradual training program for each. Ability as well as capacity for improvement will likely differ based on athletic background as well as on current status. A rule of thumb that has been suggested for training progression is that no aspect of training should increase by more than 10% at a time. That is, if distance is increased, pace should be kept the same or increased only slightly to keep within the overall 10% limit. Although 10% is an arbitrary value that has not been subjected to scientific appraisal, it appears to be a useful measure. The triathlete should consider not only the increment within a given activity but also the cumulative effect. For example, it probably would be acceptable to increase swim and run training concurrently, but it would probably not be acceptable to increase run and bike training concurrently. There are no studies addressing this important issue or offering scientifically based guidelines.

Treatment of Injuries

Similarly, treatment of triathlon injuries is not different from that of comparable injuries from other sports. The triathlete may have an advantage during injury rehabilitation because he or she can continue to train with musculature not involved in the injury, thereby preserving the central training effects. The most frequently seen injuries in triathletes are tendinitis, muscle strain, patellofemoral syndrome, low-back pain, and stress fractures. The following methods have been found to be effective in the treatment of these common triathlon training injuries.

Tendinitis

The runner suffering from chronic tendinitis poses a major therapeutic dilemma even for the most accomplished practitioner. It is particularly common in athletes ostensively because of the intense functional stresses that the tendon is subjected to in running. The course of tendinitis may be acute or self-resolving, or it may become chronic, resulting in progressive disability with weakening of the tendon. Successful treatment of tendinitis must be preceded by an understanding of the pathogenesis of the process. The cause is usually considered to be mechanical overloading of the musculotendinous unit. Repetitive loading on a tendon that results in microtears has been likened to stress fractures in bone. These microscopic changes evoke an inflammatory healing response, or tendinitis. Excessive tightness or lack or sufficient flexibility in a muscle tendon unit increases the loading effects. Many investigators believe that most tendinitis and tendon ruptures are secondary to eccentric overloading of the system, meaning the muscle tendon unit is lengthening as the muscle contracts.

Treatment of tendinitis involves rest, drugs, physical modalities, rehabilitative exercises, and occasionally surgery. Rest may mean anything from briefly stopping any pain-causing activities to complete cessation or concentration on another phase of training, e.g., swimming rather than running, if that does not produce pain. The concept of limited rest means that the inflamed tendon is used but is protected from stresses that may inflame it further. The use of measures such as strengthening and stretching, designed to correct the underlying cause of the tendinitis, is also appropriate.

Nonsteroidal antiinflammatory drugs (NSAIDs) are usually prescribed but should be carefully monitored by a physician as to the duration needed, potential side effects and so forth. Occasionally, a corticosteroid injection may be appropriate. These must be carefully and sparingly used. Corticosteroids have been shown to decrease the tensile strength of tendon and must never be injected into the tendon itself. If used, it must be placed into the tendon sheath or the adjacent bursa. Injection of a tendon subjected to high tensile loads (e.g., patella, Achilles, or rotator cuff) invites rupture. Physical therapy modalities such as ice, ultrasound, iontophoresis, and so forth may be used. Surgery is unquestionably necessary if tendon rupture results, but its use in other cases of chronic tendinitis is less predictable (e.g., release of constricting tendon sheaths). Once the athlete's pain has resolved, rehabilitating the strength and flexibility of the muscle tendon unit is critical to prevent recurrence. The exercise program should combine stretching and eccentric strengthening exercises, because most of the physiologic changes in the muscle tendon unit have been the result of eccentric overloading. The most common types of tendinitis seen in the triathlete are Achilles, patellar, iliotibial band, popliteus, and posterior tibial.

Achilles Tendinitis. Achilles tendinitis is a painful inflammatory reaction involving the Achilles tendon or its paratenon. This is an especially common type of tendinitis in the triathlete. In the acute case of Achilles tendinitis only the surrounding paratenon and not the tendon itself may be involved. In chronic Achilles tendinitis, a nodule may develop within the tendon that consists of microtears of the tendon with mucinous degeneration and scar tissue formation. The runner often experiences a burning type of pain early in the run that becomes less severe during the run and then worsens after the run. The pain also may appear when the patient gets out of bed in the morning but gradually subsides during the day. Physical examination reveals tenderness about 4 to 5 cm proximal to the insertion of the Achilles tendon into the calcaneous or anywhere along the tendon. In severe cases, crepitation and swelling may result. Conservative therapy is appropriate for acute Achilles tendinitis. Generally, running must cease for a period of time. Ice massage and stretching several times a day is helpful. The use of NSAIDs can be prescribed. The injection of corticosteroids into and around the Achilles tendons are contraindicated because of the risk of tendon rupture. Once the patient's symptoms subside, a program of gentle exercises to stretch the Achilles tendon and to strengthen the anterior compartment (dorsiflexors) should be undertaken. The addition of a heel wedge of approximately 0.5 inch into the running shoe may relieve some of the tensile forces on the Achilles tendon as the athlete resumes training. If pronation is excessive, then an orthotic device may be used to correct the underlying malalignment. Rupture of the tendon secondary to chronic tendinitis generally requires a surgical repair and occasionally, in chronic Achilles tendinitis, a tenolysis and excision of any scar tissue or intratendinous mucinous degeneration may be appropriate.

Patellar Tendinitis. Patellar tendinitis is an inflammatory reaction at the attachment of the patellar tendon into the inferior pole of the patella. Although it is not as common in triathletes as in sprinters and jumping athletes, nonetheless it should be considered in the differential diagnosis of pain about the knee. The hallmark of the diagnosis is exquisite tenderness to palpation at the inferior pole of the patella. Often associated with patellar tendinitis is tightness or lack of flexibility of the opposite hamstring muscle group. This is treated similar to other types of tendinitis with antiinflammatory medications, rest, ice massage, and stretching exercises.

Iliotibial Tract Friction Syndrome. The iliotibial tract is the thickened portion of the fascia lata that passes down the lateral aspect of the thigh and inserts into Gerdy's tubercle. The friction caused by the iliotibial tract rubbing the lateral femoral condyle during running may induce an inflammatory response. The resulting lateral knee pain is felt above the joint with the diagnosis being made by localized tenderness to palpation over the lateral femoral condyle and epicondylar area. It's often been associated with patients with genu varum or with hyperpronation of the feet. Also, the use of badly worn running shoes with worn lateral soles may precipitate this condition. The patient's iliotibial tract may be excessively tight when stretched. Treatment involves the use of ice massage, NSAIDs, stretching of the iliotibial tract and occasionally a corticosteroid injection about the site of maximum tenderness. Surgery is rarely indicated; however, in a few chronic cases, tenotomy of the tract and excision of the underlying bursa may relieve symptoms.

Popliteus Tendinitis. Popliteus tendinitis is an inflammatory reaction involving the popliteus tendon near its insertion on the lateral femoral condyle. It has often been directly related to hyperpronation of the feet and specifically downhill running. The popliteus acts as a check rein to prevent the femur from displacing forward on the tibial plateau during midstance; downhill running, therefore, puts excessive stress on this structure. Running on a banked surface increases pronation; concomitant internal tibial rotation applies traction to the attachment of the popliteus tendon to the lateral femoral epicondyle. There is usually point tenderness to palpation over the attachment of the popliteus just anterior to the fibular collateral ligament. It is managed in a similar way to that described for the iliotibial tract.

Posterior Tibial Tendinitis. Often referred to as shin splint syndrome; posterior tibial tendinitis causes pain along the posterior medial aspect of the distal two-thirds of the tibia shaft. It must be differentiated from tibial stress fractures. Often patients with posterior tibial tendinitis have excessive pronation that results in repeated traction on the posterior tibial tendon at its attachment along the posterior medial aspect of the tibia and interosseous membrane. As previously mentioned, it must be differentiated from tibial stress fractures, and bone scans may be needed to differentiate the two. The treatment is always conservative as described for the other types of tendinitis, and it is especially important to support the longitudinal arch to prevent the hyperpronation that is common in these patients. The use of an orthotic or medial heel wedge to prevent the hyperpronation is usually required.

Muscle Strain

Muscle strains are common in the serious triathlete and usually involve the hamstrings, quadriceps, adductors of the hip, and medial gastrocnemius. Most muscle strains in the conditioned triathlete develop slowly and are often directly related to a sudden change in distance, intensity of training, or change in the terrain on which they are training. Inadequate warmups and stretching of these muscles are frequent predisposing factors. Acute muscle strains are more common in sprinters than in the long-distance runners.

Muscle strains are clinically classified as to severity, depending on the muscle fiber injury, into mild, moderate, and severe grades. Acute rupture of the muscle, while extremely unusual in triathletes, may require surgical repair. Most muscle strains, however, can be treated by conservative measures. Reduction of physical activities, ice application, and compressive support are appropriate acute treatment modalities. The early use of NSAIDs may reduce dramatically the inflammatory response associated with strains, but the athlete should resume his or her training slowly and gradually. Compressive sleeves for the calf or thigh may be useful to control early swelling and later to give support as activities are resumed. As the healing process proceeds, it is important to add stretching to the treatment regimes so contracture does not occur that makes reinjury more likely.

Patellofemoral Syndrome

One of the more common problems in the triathlete is a tracking abnormality of the patella, commonly referred to as patellofemoral stress syndrome. During normal knee flexion and extension, the patella tracks or glides up and down in the grove between the femoral condyles, maintained by the bony anatomy and the muscle and ligamentous balance about the medial and lateral aspect of the patella. In patellofemoral stress syndrome, normal tracking of the patella is disrupted, and often a lateral tracking occurs. This may consist of actual recurrent subluxations or simply a compression between the lateral patellar facet and the lateral femoral grove. Certain anatomic and biomechanical factors contribute to this dysfunction: tightness of the vastus lateralis muscle, the iliotibial tract, and lateral retinaculum; weakness of the vastus medialis; and an increased Q-angle or patellar alta. The patient usually describes the pain as an aching or soreness around the anterior aspect of the knee, and there is usually tenderness to palpation of the medial facet of the patella. The patient's symptoms are usually aggravated by prolonged sitting, stair climbing, or hill running. If the lateral tracking is severe where subluxation intermittently occurs, the patient will often have a positive anxiety or apprehension sign as the patella is manually pushed in a lateral direction. Usually, compression downward on the patella as the patient contracts the quadriceps reproduces the pain. The tangential view of the patellofemoral joint may reveal an increase in the femoral sulcus angle but on occasions is completely normal. Management involves rest, curtailment of activities that place the patella under compressive loading (such as kneeling, stair climbing, or prolonged sitting), and the use of ice massage and hamstring stretching exercises. Once the patient's pain has improved, resistive exercises for the quadriceps should be carried out, either in a short arc technique or isometric exercises. Isokinetic or isotonic exercises through a full range of motion generally exacerbate the patient's condition. Often the tracking problem of the patella can be modified by the use of an orthotic device in the shoe that changes the stress distribution on the lower leg by blocking excessive pronation and internal tibial rotation. Some patients benefit by the use of certain types of knee supports or knee braces that alter the patella tracking movement. NSAIDs are commonly appropriate. Intraarticular injection of corticosteroids have no place in management of this syndrome, and surgery will rarely return the runner to competitive levels of running.

Lower-Back Pain

Back pain in runners is usually the result of a preexisting anatomical abnormality in the lower lumbar spine or to a degenerative condition in the middle-aged or older athlete. Pain is often exacerbated by a change in training techniques, such as increasing the mileage or by hill running. Younger triathletes who develop significant lower-back pain should be studied by x-rays and bone scans to rule out stress fractures in the lumbar spine or developmental spondylolysis or spondylolisthesis. Often excessive tightness in the hamstring muscle group is associated with these conditions. Routine radiographs in the middle-aged and older athlete may show degenerative disc disease and hypertrophic osteoarthritis, with the impact loading transfer from the lower extremities through the pelvis and into the lower spine being responsible for the back discomfort.

Stress Fracture

Stress fractures occur most often when a poorly conditioned athlete tries to increase mileage or speed too rapidly, overwhelming the ability of the bone to withstand the repetitive stresses. Triathletes preparing for a race by rapidly increasing their mileage or speed are also at risk. Stress fractures may occur in the lumbar vertebra body, the pars intraarticularis, sacroiliac joints, symphysis pubis (unilateral or bilateral), iliac crest, femoral neck and shaft, fibula, lateral malleolus, and metatarsals. Ongoing pain and tenderness directly over the bone and a recent increase in mileage strongly suggest the presence of a stress fracture. Often stress fractures are not visible on radiographs for 3 to 6 weeks after the onset of symptoms; therefore, bone scans are most useful in the early diagnosis. Because bone scans may remain positive for 14 to 24 months after injury, they are useful as a diagnostic tool but not for follow-up. As with all stress fractures, running must stop and an alternative training program prescribed. Healing time for these injuries is variable, and certain ones involving the femoral neck or the tibial shaft may require eventual surgical fixation.

Other Medical Care

Primary care physicians responsible for treating various medical illnesses of triathletes should be aware that antidoping regulations that conform to current International Olympic Committee (IOC) guidelines are in effect for all competitors (1). Classes of substances that are banned include stimulants, narcotics, anabolic steroids, β blockers, diuretics, peptide hormones, and analogues. Blood doping as well as pharmacologic, chemical, and physical manipulation of the urine are banned. In addition, the following classes of substances are subject to certain restrictions: alcohol; marijuana; local anesthetics; and corticosteroids. Because athletes may be subject to out-of-competition testing, medications should be prescribed with care. A banned substance is still banned even when prescribed by a licensed physician for legitimate medical purposes. There are other medications that are not banned that can be prescribed to treat all known medical problems. The U.S. Olympic Committee (USOC) has a drug education hotline (800-233-0393) to assist physicians and athletes in complying with the sometimes complicated IOC antidoping regulations. The USOC also has made available a pamphlet that explains in detail their drug education program.

Race-Day Medical Considerations

Medical Coverage

Because competitiveness is part of human nature, a triathlon race usually places more severe physiologic stress on participants than does triathlon training. Triathlon competitors may exceed exercise intensities appropriate for their training level, ignore adverse environmental conditions, and forget to carry out well-planned strategies for fluid and nutrient replacement. Therefore, the first important consideration in making triathlon participation safe is education of the athletes. Competitors should be reminded that each is ultimately responsible for his or her own health and safety. Exercising good judgment along with common sense will not only keep them out of the medical tent but allow them to perform optimally for their level of conditioning and under the conditions of a particular race. Because many race-day medical problems are in some way related to the state of hydration, the emphasis on planning and carrying out an appropriate fluid replacement strategy cannot be overemphasized (18).

Athlete Education

Athletes should be educated through prerace mailings and at the prerace meeting (18). In addition, small symposia can be organized to coincide with race registration—when many athletes are looking for some way to fill the time while waiting for the race. The prerace mailings should include information about conditions to be encountered during that particular race that may have an impact on athlete safety. For example, environmental conditions, such as expected air and water temperature, winds, terrain, etc. should be included. Included in the mailings should also be a worksheet for athletes to complete during training to assess fluid needs and to help them plan appropriate replacement strategies (Appendix 40.A). Also included should be a short, but pertinent, medical history form to be returned prerace so that an alert sheet with the information listed under the contestant's race number and name can be provided to race-day medical personnel (19). It is helpful to have information about allergies, medications, preexisting injuries (such as heat injury), and any other specific medical problem that needs to be brought to the attention of the medical staff. The medical director or representative should be at the prerace meeting to speak briefly to reinforce the information competitors have received in the mailings, answer medical- or safety-related questions, and make athletes aware of location and means of access to race medical facilities. If a registration day minisymposium is desired, the U.S. Medical Triathlon Association (USMTA) can be of invaluable assistance (Appendix 40.B). In addition to providing an extensive, medically oriented triathlon bibliography, the USMTA has a list of well-informed speakers to call on in any particular area of the United States.

Medical Care Guidelines

A physician unfamiliar with triathlon racing, yet responsible for organizing medical care at a triathlon has a number of excellent resources available. The International Triathlon Union (ITU) has a medical committee responsible for establishing standards for the safety and care of triathlon competitors. This committee has developed medical guidelines "based upon the experiences of caring for tens of thousands of competitors in multi-sport/endurance events throughout the world." These guidelines, available from the ITU medical director (Appendix 40.B), can be used as a starting point for developing coverage appropriate for any local situation. TriFed, USA (the U.S. national governing body for triathlon) follows the ITU guidelines and has regional medical directors available for consultation concerning medical coverage of local races (Appendix 40.B).

Expected Medical Problems

Race Length

The frequency and severity of medical problems, excluding trauma, are strongly related to race length. Hiller et al. (18) have reported needs for medical care at three of the most common racing distances. Olympic distance races take from 2 to 4 hr to complete; long-distance races, 4 to 8 hrs; and ironman race times vary between 8 and 17 hr. Based on information from 6245 participants in races of these distances, Hiller et al. (18) make the following recommendations for race-day preparation. In Olympic distance races, a minimum of

2% of participants can be expected to require medical care. Under severe environmental conditions, particularly a combination of high ambient temperatures and humidity, the medical team should be prepared to treat up to 10% of the starters. The most common medical problems seen during this distance triathlon are heat exhaustion (29%), skeletal muscle cramps (29%), trauma or orthopedic complaint (18%), and gastrointestinal problems (12%). During a long-distance triathlon, at least 10% of starters can be expected to present themselves to the medical staff. The majority of these (66%) were reported to be minor complaints requiring less than 5 min of attention. The remainder included heat exhaustion, skeletal muscle cramps, dehydration, hypothermia, gastrointestinal complaints, and trauma/orthopedic complaints. During the Hawaii Ironman Triathlon, an ultradistance race, up to 31% of participants have required medical treatment (20). Dehydration is the most common medical problem in ultraendurance races (approximately 50%).

Race Segment

Type and severity of medical problems encountered in triathlons vary not only with race distances but also with the segment (swim, bike, or run) of the race.

Swim. The swim, although having the greatest potential for a catastrophic event, drowning, usually has the lowest injury rate. Critical to swim safety is a course appropriately manned by lifeguards and spotters in boats. When this is established, Laird (21) reports that the swim leg accounts for only 3% of all race-day medical treatment at the Hawaii Ironman. Similarly, Novak (22) reports that only a small medical staff is needed for the swim. Common medical problems encountered during the swim include psychological as well as physical problems. Anxiety attacks may occur in those unfamiliar with mass starts or open-water swimming. In most cases, reassurance by medical personnel or lifeguards will allow the athlete to continue. Training under expected race conditions is the best preventive measure. Eye irritations may occur because of leaky goggles or irritating defogging solutions. Usually, readjustment of goggles will allow the athlete to continue. If conjunctivitis or corneal abrasions result, medical examination is necessary to treat the eye injury and to judge whether there is sufficient reason for disqualifying the athlete. Treatment should include irrigation, antibiotic ointment, and perhaps patching. Properly fitting goggles should prevent most eye problems. Sea sickness with nausea and vomiting has been reported to occur in rough oceans. Most cases are self-limiting and do not prevent continuation. Particular attention must be paid to fluid and electrolyte replacement in any vomiting athlete, or later dehydration is likely. Athletes with motion sickness predispositions should consider premedication, but only after extensive use during training. Blunt trauma may also occur during mass swim starts. Medical staff members should be aware that potentially serious injuries, although uncommon, can occur. Rib fracture, abdominal injury, and head injury are all possible. Proper seeding of athletes' starting places will help to eliminate this (19).

Hypothermia may be seen in some athletes during the swim and is related to water temperature, length of the swim, and percent body fat of the triathlete. When water temperature is less than 70°F, rectal temperature of swimmers has been reported to decrease (23). Therefore, a lean triathlete swimming a long race (>1.5 km) in cold water is a prime candidate for hypothermia (24). Because mental disorientation often marks thermoregulatory injury, trained spotters should be available to pull symptomatic (uncontrolled shivering, severe cramping, loss of coordination, and disorientation) swimmers form the water (25). Various methods have been used to rewarm hypothermic athletes. Novak (22) reports that hot tubs supervised by a physician and nurses are useful in this regard. When an immersed athlete looks and feels better (clinical judgment), is mentally alert, exhibits good walking balance, and has reasonable standing blood pressure, he or she is allowed to continue. Others prefer to treat hypothermic athletes with blankets, warm drinks, and shelter. The best preventive measures are accurate assessment of water temperature (18 inches beneath the surface at the deepest part) and recommending wet suits be used in very cold water. Other less common medical problems may arise during the swim, such as lacerations from land or water bottom debris and stings from jelly fish or sea urchins.

Bike. The bike portion of the race has been reported to account for 10% of medical visits and the bike-run transition to account for an additional 7% (21). Cycling injuries include trauma of varying severity from falls, sunburn, muscle cramps, hypoglycemia, and sometimes dehydration. Traumatic injuries from bike falls may include serious conditions, such as fractures, usually of the arms, collarbone, or ribs. They may occasionally include head injuries, such as lacerations, or closed-head trauma. More frequently, spills result in abrasions (road rash) that do not force the competitor to drop out. Traumatic injuries should be triaged on site and then evaluated by an orthopedic surgeon for determination of appropriate care. Lacerations and road rash should be thoroughly cleaned and dressed. Head injuries should be thoroughly evaluated. If there is suspicion of significant head injury, the athlete should be disqualified and monitored closely. The best prevention against these injuries is strict adherence to ITU race guidelines. These require that a hard-shell helmet be worn by all competitors during the bike leg and that adequate space be kept between bikers (no drafting rule). Equally important is course layout, surface, and traffic control.

Besides traumatic injury, bikers may be susceptible to severe sunburn, muscle cramps, hypoglycemia, and dehydration. Sunburn and prevention of sunburn should be treated with sun block. Sun block should be easily available to the athletes at transition areas and at aid stations. Muscle cramps are another frequently seen problem, which may or may not be associated with serum electrolyte abnormalities (26, 27) but are often associated with dehydration. Proper conditioning, appropriate fluid replacement, and period shifting of bike position may help prevent skeletal muscle cramps. Hypoglycemia is known to cyclists as "bonking." Classic signs include headache, weakness, dizziness, and diaphoresis. Most hypoglycemia in triathletes is mild and can be managed with oral fluid and sugar (19). Proper nutritional replacement during the bike portion of a long-distance or ultradistance triathlon will prevent this condition. Occasionally, a triathlete will require i.v. fluids to correct either unrelenting muscle cramps or hypoglycemia. The i.v. fluid of choice is D5:NS (18). Unless absolutely necessary, i.v. fluid intervention should be avoided during the race, because in most races, it is grounds for automatic disqualification.

Run. Approximately 15% of medical visits at the Hawaii Ironman occur during the run (21). The majority (65%) of medical visits, however, occur after the athletes have completed the race. Medical problems seen during the run and after completing the race are similar. Common complaints are dehydration, exhaustion, hyperthermia, hyponatremia, skeletal muscle cramps, blisters, diarrhea, and vomiting (18, 19, 24, 26). In triathlon races longer than 4 hr, dehydration is a common problem and is frequently compounded by hyponatremia (18, 28, 29).

The combination of dehydration and hyponatremia is easily understood, considering that during exercise in the heat, evaporation of sweat is the major avenue of heat dissipation. Sweat rate is predominately determined by exercise intensity and total sweat loss by total energy expenditure. Triathletes can easily sweat 1.5 liters per hour (15, 27, 29, 30). Well-trained athletes have sweat sodium concentrations of approximately 1 g/liter. Therefore, it is easy to see that the cumulative effects of these losses throughout a triathlon can be significant. The problem is compounded by the fact that it is much more difficult to replace fluid and electrolyte losses while running than while biking (29, 30).

Diarrhea and vomiting sometimes exacerbate the fluid and electrolyte problems. Both of these problems are most likely associated with gut ischemia secondary to exercise intensity and dehydration. Cramps and exhaustion are likewise related to state of hydration. Prevention of these fluid and electrolyte problems is clearly preferable to treatment. Measuring fluid losses during training will give the athlete an estimate of the amount of fluid he or she needs to consume to remain hydrated. Hiller et al. (18) recommend that 1 g of salt per hour should be consumed if races are longer than 4 hr to avoid hyponatremia. Treatment is based on restoring fluids, electrolytes, and energy. Some physicians prefer replacement through oral fluids and food. Some, however, find i.v. fluids to be more efficacious to restore volumes quickly and avoid the problems associated with nausea and vomiting (21, 31). The recommended i.v. fluid is D5:NS.

Elevated temperatures and hyperthermia also are potential medical problems, particularly during the run. An athlete who exceeds his or her intensity limits or becomes progressively dehydrated is at risk for hyperthermia. Triathletes with rectal temperatures in excess of 106°F should be treated for hyperthermia. This condition has been successfully treated by applying ice over the large blood vessels, particularly in the axillae and groin (31).

Race-day medical problems are reasonably predictable during a triathlon. Education of the triathlete—including appropriate training; heat acclimatization; and fluid, electrolyte, and nutrient replacement—is the key to safe participation. Injuries and medical problems invariably occur in athletes who exceed their limits, regardless of ability level. Conveying this information to the athlete and getting each to assume responsibility for his or her own safety and well-being are the first and most important tasks of the medical personnel. Secondarily, the medical staff is responsible for organizing and giving medical care to those racers who need help. Proper setup of facilities and equipment as well as training of medical personnel in the problems to be anticipated should allow triathlon races to accomplish their goal—safe, healthy fun for all participants.

REFERENCES

1. Technical Committee, International Triathlon Union. International Triathlon Union manual, 1991. West Vancouver, B.C.: Author, 1991.
2. International Triathlon Union. Personal communication, 1991.
3. O'Toole ML, Douglas PS, Hiller WDB. Applied physiology of a triathlon. Sports Med 1989;8(4):201–225.
4. Pechar GS, McArdle WD, Katch FI, Magel JR, DeLuca J. Specificity of cardiorespiratory adaptation to bicycle and treadmill training. J Appl Physiol 1974;36(6):753–756.
5. McArdle WD, Magel JR, Delio DJ, Toner M, Chase JM. Specificity of run training on VO_2 max and heart rate changes during running and swimming. Med Sci Sports 1978;10(1):16–20.
6. O'Toole ML, Douglas PS, Hiller WDB. Lactate, oxygen uptake, and cycling performance in triathletes. Int J Sports Med 1989;10(6):413–418.
7. Town GP. Science of triathlon training and competition. Champaign, IL: Human Kinetics, 1985.
8. Boone T, Kreider RB. Bicycle exercise before running: effect on performance. Ann Sports Med 1986;3:25–29.
9. Clausen JP, Klausen K, Rasmussen B, Trap-Jensen J. Central and peripheral circulatory changes after training of the arms or legs. Am J Physiol 1973;225(3):675–682.
10. Williams MM, Hawley JA, Black R, Freke M, Simms K. Injuries amongst competitive triathletes. N Z J Sports Med 1988;16(1):2–6.
11. Ireland ML, Micheli LJ. Triathletes: biographic data, training, and injury patterns. Ann Sports Med 1987;3(2):117–120.
12. Levy CM, Kolin E, Berson BL. Cross training: risk or benefit? An evaluation of injuries in four athlete populations. Sports Med Clin Forum 1986;3(1):1–8.
13. Levy CM, Kolin E, Berson BL. The effect of cross training on injury incidence, duration and severity (Part 2). Sports Med Clin Forum 1986;3(2):1–8.
14. O'Toole ML, Hiller WDB, Smith RA, Sisk TD. Overuse injuries in ultraendurance triathletes. Am J Sports Med 1989;17(4):514–518.
15. O'Toole ML, Massimino FA, Hiller WDB, Laird RH. Medical considerations in triathletes: the 1984 Hawaii Ironman Triathlon. Ann Sports Med 1987;3(2):121–123.
16. O'Toole ML, Hiller WDB, Massimino FA, Laird RH. Medical considerations in triathletes: a preliminary report from the Hawaii Ironman, 1984. N Z J Sports Med 1985;13:35–37.
17. Massimino FA, Armstrong MA, O'Toole ML, Hiller WDB, Laird RH. Common triathlon injuries: special considerations for multisport training. Ann Sports Med 1988;4:82–86.

18. Hiller WDB, O'Toole ML, Fortess EE, Laird RH, Imbert PC, Sisk TD. Medical and physiological considerations in triathlons. Am J Sports Med 1987;15(2):164–167.
19. Laird RH. Triathlon. In: Schneider RC, Kennedy JC, Plant ML, eds. Sports injuries—mechanisms, prevention and treatment. Baltimore: Williams & Wilkins, 1985:354–367.
20. Laird RH. Personal communication, 1991.
21. Laird RH. Medical complications during the Ironman Triathlon World Championship, 1981–1986. In: Laird RH, ed. Report of the Ross symposium on medical coverage of endurance athletic events. Columbus, OH: Ross Laboratories, 1988:83–88.
22. Novak D. Ironman Canada Triathlon Championship: medical coverage of an ultradistance event. In: Laird RH, ed. Report of the Ross symposium on medical coverage of endurance athletic events. Columbus, OH: Ross Laboratories, 1988:69–73.
23. Galbo H, Houston ME, Christenson NJ, et al. The effect of water temperature on the hormonal response to prolonged swimming. Acta Physiol Scand 1979;105:326–337.
24. Willix RD. Medical coverage for middle-distance triathlons. Ann Sports Med 1987;3(2):111–112.
25. Ivy JL. Recommendations and suggestions for the prevention of injury during endurance athletic events. In: Laird RH, ed. Report of the Ross symposium on medical coverage of endurance athletic events. Columbus, OH: Ross Laboratories, 1988:43–49.
26. Hiller WDB. The United States Triathlon Series: Medical considerations. In: Laird RH, ed. Report of the Ross symposium on medical coverage of endurance athletic events. Columbus, OH: Ross Laboratories, 1988:80–82.
27. Costill DL, Miller JM. Nutrition for endurance sport: carbohydrate and fluid balance. Int J Sports Med 1980;1:2–14.
28. Hiller WDB, O'Toole ML, Laird RH. Letter to the editor. JAMA 1986;256:213
29. O'Toole ML. Prevention and treatment of electrolyte abnormalities. In: Laird RH, ed. Report of the Ross symposium on medical coverage of endurance athletic events. Columbus, OH: Ross Laboratories, 1988:93–98.
30. O'Toole ML, Hiller WDB, Douglas PS, Pisarello JB, Mullen JL. Cardiovascular responses to prolonged cycling and running. Ann Sports Med 1987;3(2):124–130.
31. Laird RH. Medical complications during the Ironman Triathlon World Championships: 1981–1984, Ann Sports Med 1987;3(2):113–116.

APPENDICES

CHAPTER 40/APPENDIX A

Triathlete Fluid Balance Worksheet

SWIM	
Preswim, nude, dry weight	________lb
1-hr swim	
Postswim, nude, dry weight	________lb
Preweight – postweight	________lb[a]
BIKE	
Prebike, nude, dry weight	________lb
1-hr bike	
Postbike, nude, dry weight	________lb
Preweight – postweight	________lb
Add the number of pint bottles drunk	________bottles
Amount of bike fluid loss	________
Add swim loss	________
Total Fluid Needs on Bike	________bottles
RUN	
Prerun, nude, dry weight	________lb
1-hr run	
Postrun, nude, dry weight	________lb
Preweight – postweight	________lb
Add the number of pint bottles drunk	________
Amount of run fluid loss	________bottles
Add swim loss	________
Add bike loss	________
Total Fluid Needs for Run	________bottles

[a] This is the amount of fluid you are behind when you finish a 1-hr swim. Calculations can be adjusted for parts of an hour.

CHAPTER 40/APPENDIX B

Medical Resources for Triathlon

ITU Medical Committee
W. Douglas B. Hiller, M.D., Chairman
1224 Luna Place
Honolulu, HI 96833
phone: 808-484-2042
fax: 808-487-8324

David L. Jackson, M.D.
President USMTA
Department of Rehabilitation Medicine
140 Chambers Medical Plaza
820 South Limestone
Lexington, KY 40536-0226
phone: 606-257-4888
fax: 606-233-6132

TriFed USA, Medical Committee
Thomas K. Miller, M.D., Chairman
4064 Postal Drive SW
Roanoke, VA 24018
phone: 703-776-0256
fax: 703-772-7891

USMTA
P.O. Box 20926
Roanoke, VA 24018
phone: 800-25-USMTA

41 / VOLLEYBALL

E. Lee Rice and Kenneth L. Anderson III

Volleyball is a limited contact sport that is played at all levels of skill and on multiple surfaces, which accounts for a large variety of injuries that result from jumping, diving, and hitting the ball repetitively. At the recreational level, there is a tendency toward acute injuries because practice is limited compared with the time spent in competition. In contrast, overuse injuries are more common at the collegiate and world-class levels as a result of the many hours of practice of specific skills. These overuse injuries are most common in the shoulder, knee, lower back, and foot. The surfaces that volleyball is played on include sand, wood and synthetic floors, concrete, and grass.

Volleyball is composed of a number of techniques that include blocking, passing, setting, hitting or spiking, diving or digging, and serving. Blocking involves extending the arms at the net with the fingers spread (Fig. 41.1). Passing is how the defensive player fields the opposing player's serve (Fig. 41.2) and is accomplished by bumping the ball up with the forearms while the elbows are extended. Setting involves hitting the ball with the fingertips with the wrists radial deviated and hyperextended. Hitting or spiking the ball is done at the maximum height of a vertical jump (Fig. 41.3) and involves hyperextending the back, followed by rotating the body into the ball. The player tries to hit down on the ball, "killing" it so that it cannot be returned. The ball is hit at speeds of up to 80 mph at the advanced levels. Diving is a defensive maneuver to save the ball (Fig. 41.4) and is done with the player's body extended. Players often wear pads on their elbows and knees to soften the impact of these dives. Serves are used to put the ball into play by either hitting it hard or floating it. Acute injuries occur most often close to the net as a result of blocking or hitting. Front-row players do blocking and hitting, while a designated player is the setter for these players. Back-row players are defensive players that do more diving for balls and digging and passing.

At the upper skill levels problems related to traveling to competitions must be taken into account. These include proper immunizations, acclimatization to weather, time differences, and health standards in other countries. Players must ensure adequate fluid intake when traveling to prevent dehydration. They also must be aware of precautions needed to prevent intestinal infections from parasites and bacteria.

The authors studied injuries of the men's US National Volleyball Team from 1981 to 1991. Figure 41.5 shows the incidence of injuries to various joints. The total number of injuries seen was 222, which does not include visits for medical problems other than musculoskeletal injuries. This survey also does not include minor injuries treated during practices or games or injuries sustained while traveling, which were not seen by the authors. Because the authors' clinic is a primary care clinic, acute injuries that were seen first by the team orthopedists also are not reflected. The number of these were few, but may be the reason for the low incidence of internal derangements of the knee. Most of the shoulder injuries were due to impingement. This and patellar tendonitis were the two largest categories of injuries, reflecting the common nature of overuse injuries in these elite volleyball players.

Training Methods

Modern volleyball training techniques have advanced tremendously in the decade. Volleyball requires a well-rounded combination of aerobic fitness, flexibility, strength, power, and agility. In addition, sport-specific skills such as passing, setting, hitting, digging, and blocking must be mastered. Players also must be trained to make rapid mental decisions and to maintain superb psychological concentration and focus during matches. A comprehensive training program involves a variety of methods designed to provide both general conditioning of the athlete and enhanced sport-specific skills that address each of the above needs.

Although volleyball is not a pure aerobic sport, cardiovascular conditioning is of supreme importance, and elite volleyball players are among the most aerobically fit athletes of any team sport. Most coaches prefer many

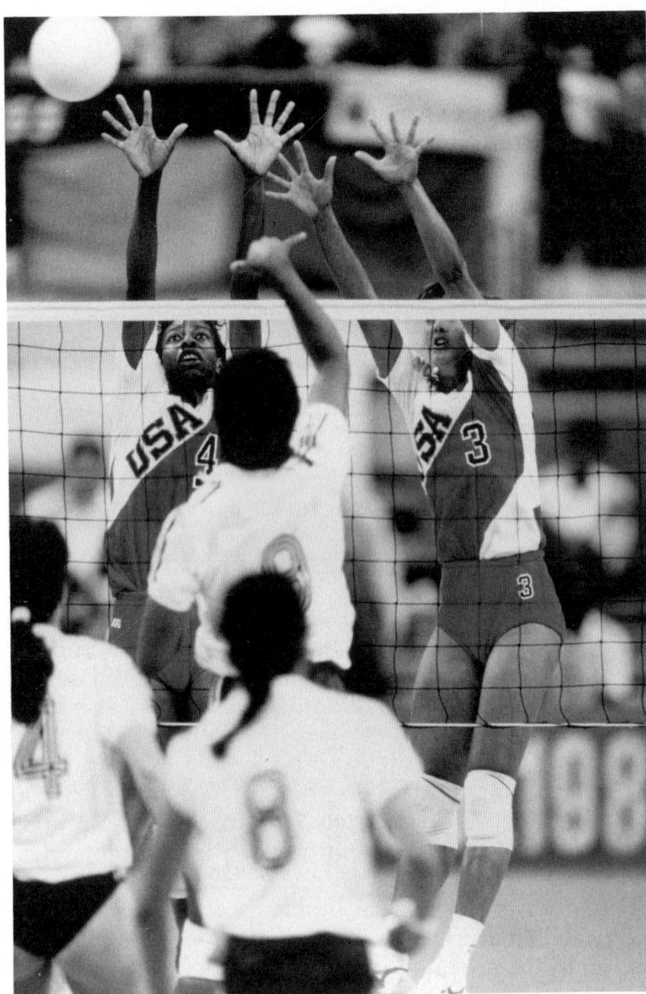

Figure 41.1. Front-row players block the ball for Team USA.

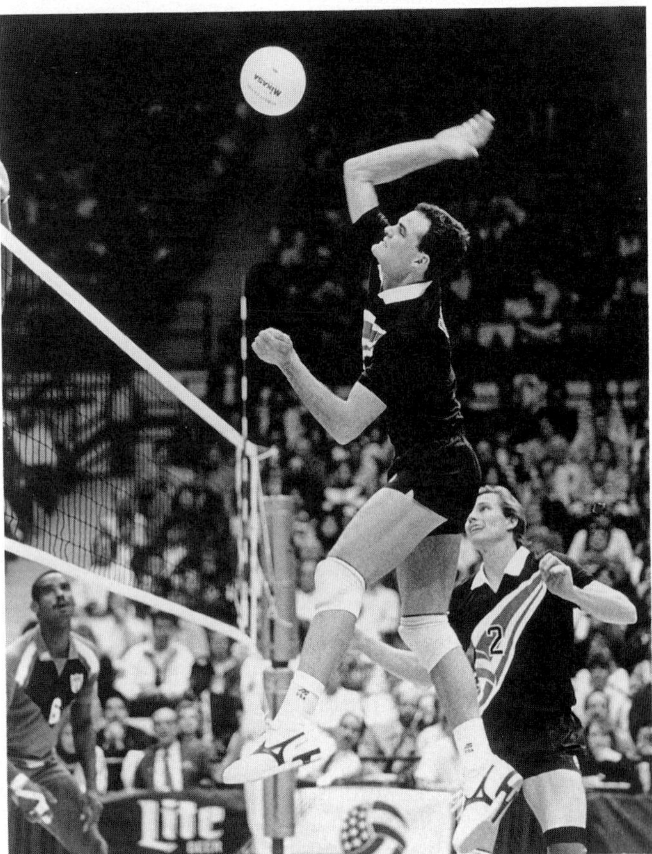

Figure 41.3. Hitting or spiking involves a powerful swing with the player at maximum height during the jump.

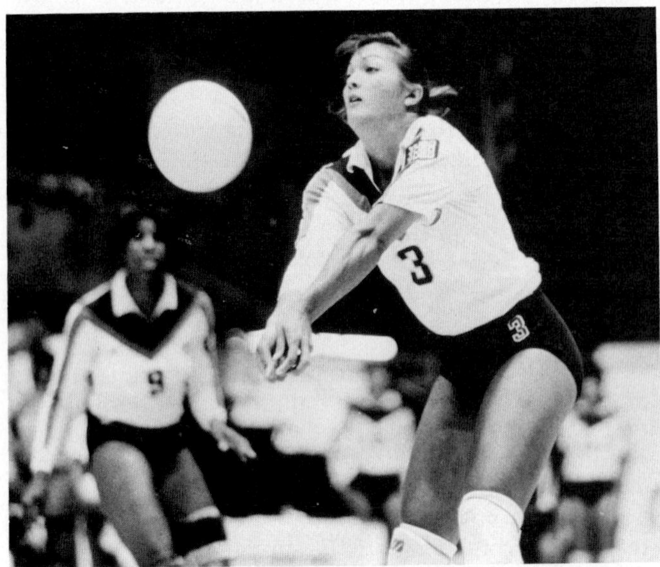

Figure 41.2. A player makes a pass after fielding a serve.

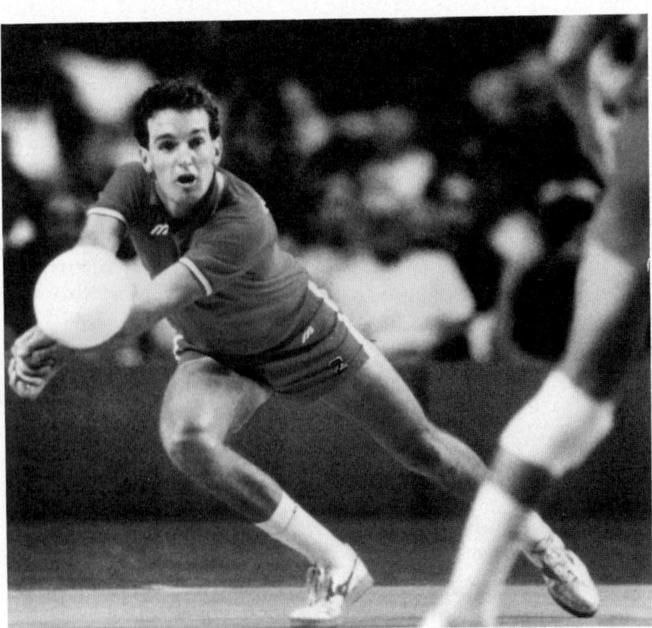

Figure 41.4. A player dives to save the ball.

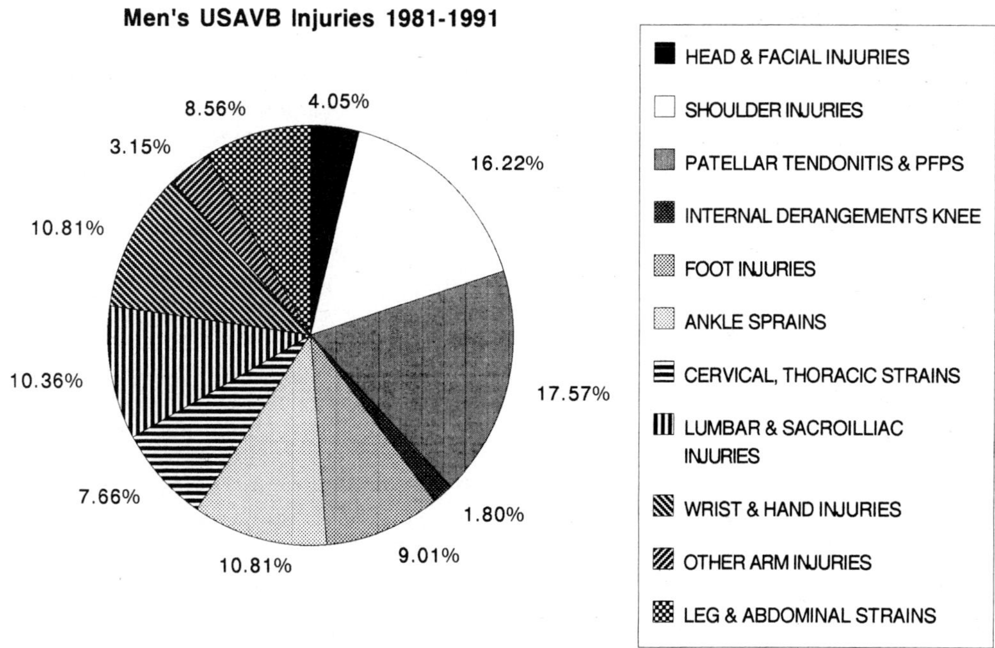

Figure 41.5. Incidence of injuries to various joints.

repetitions to simulate the type of activity required during matches, rather than endurance training involving prolonged continuous activity. Although jogging and biking are often used to improve fitness levels, an emphasis is placed on repetition of drills, involving explosive power, quickness, and agility.

Flexibility is of paramount importance in volleyball, both to improve performance and to prevent injury. Daily stretching is accomplished at the start of practice, with an emphasis on slow, static stretching through the pain-free range of motion of all major joints. Ballistic or bouncing types of movements should be avoided during stretching, because they can cause muscle shortening or even injury. Proprioceptive neuromuscular facilitation (PNF) patterns involving functional rotational movements against light resistance are extremely beneficial. Selected stretching exercises also are recommended after practice to prevent shortening of heavily used muscle groups.

Strength training is usually done two to three times per week. Before the season begins, a base of strength is established, using relatively heavy resistance for all major muscle groups. As the season approaches, the level of resistance is often diminished. The workouts emphasize more repetition and quicker, more powerful movements to satisfy sport-specific needs.

Power is then developed through repetitions of explosive motions. This is especially important for the arms and shoulders to improve hitting skills. It also is important for the legs to maximize vertical jumping ability, an integral part of hitting and blocking.

Plyometric training has recently become a common means of jump training. This involves explosive repetitions of jumping against resistance. The resistance may simply be gravity or it may be provided by elastic bands attached to the player's waist to augment the gravitational force, pulling the athlete back to the ground. Plyometric training in the United States was initially begun for the U.S. national teams, using the "Russian jump box." This is a platform with an adjustable elevation. Players perform drills jumping from the floor to the platform and back as rapidly as possible for a timed period. As ability improves, the elevation of the platform is increased. Elastic bands can be added from the floor to the player's waist to make the resistance even greater. This often provides dramatic improvement in the vertical leap and helps to train lower extremity proprioception, which is necessary for balance and agility. This exercise is reasonably sport specific, because it closely approximates the lower extremity motions necessary for repetitive hitting and blocking during competition.

Unfortunately, plyometric training increases the frequency of patellofemoral syndrome and patellar tendonitis. These problems can be minimized by slowly increasing the intensity and frequency of the exercises over time to allow for proper adaptation of the musculoskeletal structures that are involved. In addition, cushioning the floor surface and wearing proper training shoes will help to minimize these injuries. Athletes who are predisposed to these problems or who develop symptoms of overuse may need to avoid or reduce plyometric training.

Agility drills and exercises designed to improve hand-eye coordination are also essential for a well-rounded training program. These are most helpful if they simulate sport-specific skills and can be efficiently used as part of a team's warmup exercises. Court drills involving game-like conditions, including scrimmages, are essential to allow the athlete and team to integrate all of the previous training techniques into the game itself.

It is invaluable for the team physician to be aware of

the variety and scope of training techniques involved in this sport. All training needs to be evaluated and monitored on an ongoing basis for its appropriateness for any given athlete. Because volleyball by nature involves specific motions, overuse injuries are extremely common. Therefore, adjusting and individualizing training regimens on a continual basis is necessary for prevention and treatment of the injuries inherent in this sport.

Foot and Ankle Injuries

Foot and ankle injuries are quite common in volleyball players. Foot and ankle injuries accounted for almost 20% of the total injuries seen in the US National Volleyball Team. Several other studies also found ankle injuries to be the most frequent type of injury (1–5). Most ankle sprains occur while landing during hitting or blocking at the net. Because of the high number of ankle injuries, prophylactic taping or bracing is recommended for volleyball players.

Inversion ankle sprains are the most common type and result from an inversion force being placed on the supinated ankle during landing. This force usually results in injury to the lateral ankle structures. The first structure that is injured is the anterior talofibular ligament, followed by the calcaneofibular ligament and rarely the posterior talofibular ligament. In one common classification system ankle sprains are graded I, II, and III, with III being rupture of all three ligaments and I being an isolated rupture of the anterior talofibular ligament.

Players with an inversion sprain will complain of pain and swelling over the lateral aspect of the ankle. Examination of the injured ankle should include range of motion, appearance, strength testing, neurovascular status of the foot, radiographs to rule out fractures, and evaluation of the integrity of the ligaments, including the deltoid ligament. Palpation should be performed over the lateral and medial malleoli. Palpation of the proximal fibula also should be carried out to rule out the possibility of a Masionneuve fracture, which involves a tear of the interosseous ligament and fibular fracture. Integrity of the ligaments may be evaluated by an anterior-posterior drawer and inversion-eversion stress.

The anterior drawer is performed by placing one hand on the anterior distal tibia and the other hand on the posterior calcaneus. The calcaneus is then brought forward while the tibia is held in place. Laxity is then assessed by the amount of translation that is present. The talar tilt is performed by placing inversion-eversion stress on the calcaneus while the distal tibia is held in place. Both of these tests may be done with radiographs to measure the laxity more accurately. A talar tilt of greater than 15° on radiography is indicative of a disruption of the anterior talofibular ligament and the calcaneo fibular ligament.

The initial treatment of all ankle injuries includes ice, compression, and elevation. Full weight bearing should not be allowed until the patient can ambulate comfortably without a limp. Third-degree sprains require immobilization for a minimum of 2 to 3 weeks in a cast boot or cast. Surgery may be indicated, depending on a number of factors including the laxity at that time. Third-degree sprains should probably be referred for orthopedic evaluation. First- and second-degree ankle sprains should be treated in a brace such as an aircast to prevent inversion while allowing plantar flexion and dorsiflexion. Range of motion exercises and progressive resistance exercises may be started early through the pain-free range of motion. The patient may be returned to weight bearing as it is tolerated.

Balance exercises, including the use of tilt boards, are helpful to reeducate the proprioceptors in the ankle. Strengthening should be progressed until the strength returns to the same level as the contralateral ankle. Return to activity should be gradual as range of motion is restored and pain eliminated. The first activities allowed are modified-impact exercises such as biking and pool running. This is followed by light jogging, which is advanced to sprints. The final phase involves the addition of cutting and jumping maneuvers.

Whereas casting even first- and second-degree sprains used to be commonplace, complete immobilization is now primarily used for third-degree ligamentous injuries. Although immobilization does allow for excellent tissue repair, the resultant joint stiffness, muscular atrophy, and loss of proprioceptive function can delay total recovery time and even increase the risk of reinjury during rehabilitative process. Immobilization also has been shown to affect articular cartilage adversely.

The benefits of immobilization can be achieved by the use of braces, which provide medial and lateral joint compression and minimize eversion-inversion motion while allowing plantar flexion and dorsiflexion. This enhances stability on weight bearing, allows early range of motion without stressing the injured ligaments, and minimizes both muscular atrophy and loss of proprioceptive function. Pneumatic braces are preferred, although many lace-up braces also provide excellent support.

There are several instances in which casting is appropriate. In the immediate postinjury phase, when rest, ice, compression, elevation, and minimal or no weight bearing are employed, casting may provide excellent pain relief. Removable cast boots are preferred in this situation, so that they can be removed for intermittent cold therapy, treatment with modalities, and early motion through the pain-free range.

Another indication for casting is when the athlete is either unable or unwilling to limit weight-bearing activity that would delay the healing process. Here, the cast is used essentially to protect the athlete from himself or herself. In this situation, the risks of complete immobilization are outweighed by the benefits of greater protection of the joint.

A considerable amount of controversy still exists regarding appropriate indications for surgery. Most third-degree sprains respond well to conservative management, including an initial period of immobilization followed by continued mechanical support and aggressive therapy. However, it is prudent to refer third-degree sprains for orthopedic evaluation. There are some third-degree injuries that will not satisfactorily heal without surgical intervention, including a completely disrupted ligament that has lodged in a position where it mechanically disrupts function or is not in approximation to its normal attachment site. Surgery is necessary to restore normal anatomical position. A magnetic resonance imaging (MRI) scan may be helpful in evaluating which third-degree sprains fall into this category. Another surgical indication is for an athlete with recurrent ankle sprains who is functionally unstable and has failed a trial of conservative treatments, including comprehensive physical therapy. This athlete is unlikely to regain normal stability and function without surgical reconstruction.

Even if conservative treatment is employed, most athletes with third-degree sprains appreciate receiving an orthopedic evaluation and opinion so that they are fully informed concerning the benefits, risks, and potential outcomes of both types of treatment. With increasing frequency, it is the athlete who ultimately makes the decision regarding conservative versus surgical treatment. The orthopedist and primary care physician should work as a team to provide the athlete with all the facts so that he or she can make the most appropriate decision for his or her own situation.

Finally, orthopedic referral is appropriate when any ankle injury is not progressing as anticipated and the primary physician feels uncomfortable with the clinical course of progress, the exact diagnosis, or the next step in the treatment regimen. In these situations, the primary physician will seldom err in seeking an orthopedic opinion and may save both himself or herself and the athlete considerable liability.

Subluxation of the peroneal tendons is an injury that may be first diagnosed an an ankle sprain. This injury usually results from forced supination that ruptures the peroneal retinaculum. The patient will have tenderness and swelling in the region of the peroneal tendons. Computed tomography (CT) or MRI may aid in making the diagnosis. Surgical repair is often required, and injuries left untreated may result in tenosynovitis and chronic subluxation.

Another entity involving the peroneal tendons is tendonitis resulting from forced dorsiflexion in inversion. The patient will usually complain of pain on the lateral aspect of the heel. Tenderness directly over the tendons and increased pain with plantar flexion in inversion are signs of peroneal tendonitis. Conservative treatment involves the use of antiinflammatory medications, ice, stretching of the tendons, and reduction of activities such as jumping. Correction of an ankle that is in varus with orthotics also may help to alleviate the problem. It these measures are not successful, an injection of cortisone around the tendon sheath may relieve symptoms. Care must be taken not to inject the tendon or it may be weakened and rupture.

Achilles tendonitis is another common problem that generally results from overuse. The patient will present with pain and swelling in the retrocalcaneal region. Palpation will reveal thickening along the tendon and crepitus may accompany this thickening. Retrocalcaneal bursitis may be the cause for local tenderness and can usually be diagnosed by compressing this bursa, which lies between the calcaneus and the Achilles tendon, to elicit pain. Dorsiflexion of the feet should be observed to evaluate tightness of the calf muscles. Patients are treated by decreasing jumping, ice, antiinflammatory medication, stretching of the Achilles tendon and its muscles, and the use of ultrasound. A small lift under the heel may reduce stretch on the tendon when symptomatic. Progressive-resistance exercises are added through the pain-free range of motion. This begins with slow, controlled motion and advances to more powerful, high-velocity motions as symptoms and strength allow. As the patient's symptoms decrease and the dorsiflexion increases, he or she may be returned to explosive activity.

Chronic Achilles tendonitis or gastrocnemius tightness may result in a tear of the Achilles tendon and possibly complete rupture. There will be marked swelling and a defect may be palpated on exam. Complete rupture can usually be diagnosed with the patient prone, using the Thompson test. The calf is squeezed while the foot is observed. Movement of the foot indicates some intact tendon, whereas absence of movement indicates a complete rupture. The decision to treat complete ruptures in a long leg cast for 2 to 3 weeks or with surgical repair must be based on the individual patient and the experience of the treating physician. Orthopedic consultation is highly recommended.

Another less common problem seen in volleyball players involves compartment syndromes in the lower legs. Symptoms of compartment syndrome include localized pain and swelling accompanied by parasthesias. These symptoms are exacerbated with certain activities and resolve relatively quickly with rest. The cause of the patients' symptoms is thought to be the result of pressure caused by increased fluid in a closed space. The location of the symptoms vary with the compartment that is involved. Anterior compartment involvement gives a feeling of fullness in the anterior compartment and dorsum of the foot. Posterior compartment syndrome causes discomfort along the posteromedial border of the tibia and medial aspect of the foot. Compartment pressures measured before, during, and after exercise may be diagnostic. Treatment of the exercise-induced compartment syndromes includes avoidance of the offending activity, treatment of biomechanical foot abnormalities with orthotics, stretching programs, ultrasound, ice, nonsteroidal antiinflammatory drugs (NSAIDs), and ultimately fasciotomy, if the other measures fail.

Stress fractures of the tibia and more commonly metatarsals are additional lower extremity problems seen in volleyball players. Symptoms include localized pain and swelling. Initial radiographs may reveal cortical thickening in the painful region or may be negative. Bone scans may be used to confirm a diagnosis, but patients may be treated based on clinical symptoms, alone. Repeat radiographs after 2 weeks also will show signs of the stress fracture, including callous formation or a fracture line.

Initial treatment involves ice, antiinflammatories, and relative rest. This means avoidance of the impact activity that caused the fracture but not complete rest of the extremity. Immobilization is rarely needed to treat these fractures. As the pain resolves, the player may be returned to activities with decreased impact such as pool running or running on a trampoline. Once the time of these activities has been increased without pain, the player may resume full activity for short time periods (15 to 30 min). Activity time is increased gradually. Players with these injuries should be evaluated for biomechanical faults and the possible need for changes in footwear or the use of orthotics to prevent recurrent injury.

Sesamoiditis involves inflammation of the sesamoid structures under the metatarsal phalangeal joint of the great toes. This problem is caused by the repetitive trauma of jumping and landing. Patients will complain of pain under the great toe. A biomechanical exam should be performed to identify and correct any abnormal forces through the area, such as a plantar-flexed first ray. If biomechanical abnormalities are present, orthotics may relieve the added stress to the region. Radiographs should be taken to rule out stress fractures in this region. Treatment is aimed at reducing inflammation with ice and antiinflammatory medications. Loading activities such as jumping and running should be reduced, and padding may be added under the foot to distribute the forces away from the sesamoids. Stretching of the flexor tendons and friction massage will also aid in reducing inflammation. Occasionally, local steroid injection or even excision of the involved sesamoid bone may be necessary.

Plantar fascitis may present with symptoms of heel or arch pain. Physical exam will reveal tenderness along the medial arch or at the insertion of the plantar fascia on the calcaneus. Radiographs may show a traction spur on the anterior calcaneus, which is a sign of increased tension in that area. Treatment of biomechanical problems, such as hyperpronation, may help to relieve symptoms. Treatment also should include stretching of the plantar fascia and Achilles tendon, ice, and antiinflammatory medications. Occasionally, steroid injection at the calcaneal attachment may be helpful in reducing inflammation, but care must be taken to reduce stress on the region, or rupture could occur as a result of weakening of the fascia. Dorsiflexion splints are not routinely used to treat plantar fascitis.

Knee Injuries

A study of volleyball injuries referred to a sports medicine clinic revealed that 59% of injuries were knee injuries (4). The more severe knee injuries were mostly associated with jumping and twisting on landing (Fig. 41.6). Exams of acute knee injuries immediately after injury are usually more accurate and useful than exams done after swelling occurs.

One of the most common problems seen in volleyball players is patellar tendonitis. Inflammation is caused by repetitive jumping and landing during training and play. Chronic patellar tendonitis can infrequently lead to rupture of the patellar tendon, requiring surgical repair. Symptoms of patellar tendonitis are localized pain and swelling in the area of inflammation that is aggravated by activity. Radiographs of the affected knee may show spurring on the distal patella, which is evidence of chronic traction on the insertion of the infrapatellar tendon.

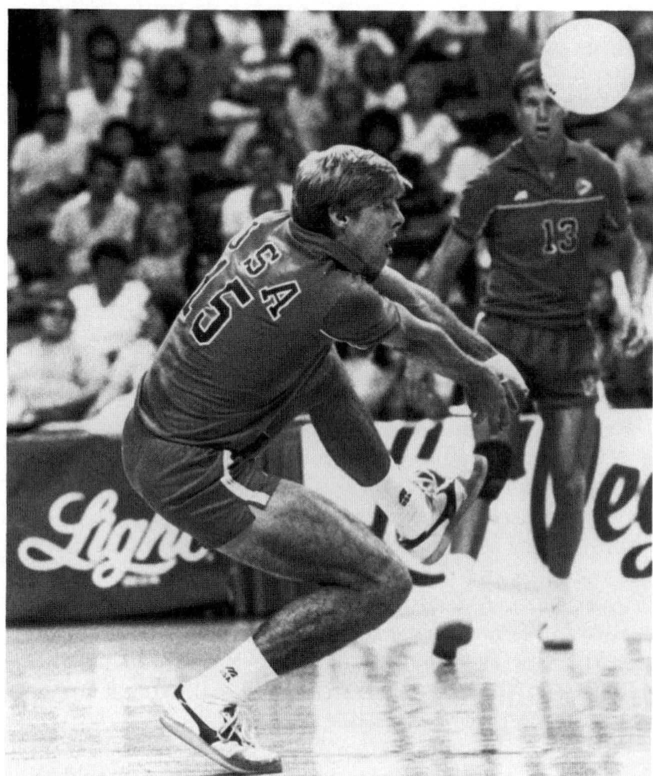

Figure 41.6. Acute injuries frequently occur when landing in unbalanced positions that are accompanied with twisting motions.

Treatment of patellar tendonitis includes decreasing jumping activities, ice, and antiinflammatories. Physical therapy, which includes ultrasound, stretching of the quadriceps, and strengthening, should be instituted with a gradual return to activity as the inflammation subsides. These should be rhythmical activities, such as bike riding (with limited tension on the wheels of a stationary bike or riding on a flat surface), swimming, or running on a trampoline. The last activities added are explosive ones such as jumping repetitively. Patellar tendon straps may help distribute the force across the patellar tendon and provide relief for many players.

Intractable patellar tendon pain that does not resolve with conservative treatment should be referred to an orthopedist for possible surgical debridement. An MRI scan may be helpful in determining the best candidates for the surgery. Focal areas of inflammation and degenerative changes, especially at the distal patellar pole, are indications that debridement may be successful.

Patellofemoral syndrome is another common entity affecting volleyball players. This problem usually results from malalignment difficulties that lead to irritation of the articular cartilage of the patella and/or the patellar groove of the femur. Symptoms of this syndrome include aching of the knee, especially anteriorly; pain with going up and down steps or hills; stiffness after sitting for periods of time, and occasional mild swelling in the patellar region. Evaluation should include a good biomechanical exam while the patient is standing, measurement of the Q-angle, and observing if there is hyperpronation of the feet.

The Q-angle is a measurement of the alignment of the femur on the tibia. The more valgus knee has greater stress placed on the patella, pulling it laterally. The Q-angle is the intersection of two lines at the midpatella. The first line is from the anterior-superior illiac spine to the center of the patella. The second line is drawn from the tibial tubercle to the midpatella. The intersection of these lines is considered normal if it is 10° to 15° in males and 18° to 20° in females. Females have a larger Q-angle because of a wider pelvis, which causes a more valgus alignment.

The knee exam will show some signs of patellar irritation such as tenderness of the surface under the patella with palpation (usually laterally) or crepitus with range of motion. Observation of patellar tracking throughout the range of motion will also reveal any bowstringing laterally, possibly indicating a tight lateral retinaculum. Pain with compression of the patella while the patient extends his or her knee is an extremely sensitive test, but is usually reserved for the subtle cases because of the discomfort that it causes to the patient.

Radiographs may be helpful, especially the sunrise view that shows patellar position in the femoral groove. Lateral riding patellae are indicative of individuals at risk for this problem.

Treatment is directed at reducing inflammation with antiinflammatories and ice and correcting the malalignment problems. Malalignment corrections include strengthening of the vastus medialis muscle and using orthotics if indicated for hyperpronation. The vastus medialis strengthening is done with straight-leg raising, terminal extension, and isometric contraction exercises. Patellar mobilization during physical therapy and stretching of the quadriceps muscle also are effective treatments of this entity. Patellar-stabilizing braces are often helpful as well. If conservative measures do not correct the problem, a surgical release of the lateral retinaculum may be indicated, which may be done arthroscopically.

Acute knee injuries range from mild sprains to significant internal derangements, including torn anterior cruciate ligaments (ACL) and torn menisci. Significant sprains of collateral ligaments (grade II or III) should be placed in a brace that allows controlled extension and flexion, but prohibits varus and valgus motions, and a gradual return to motion is useful in the initial treatment of these injuries. Large effusions should be aspirated for the patient's comfort and to facilitate relaxation for a better exam. The aspirate can provide useful information for the diagnosis, including whether the aspirate is blood or serous fluid, which differentiates between inflammation and an acute tear. If the aspirate contains blood it should be examined for fat, which can be seen as shiny floating cells on the surface of the fluid after it has been placed in a basin. Fat in the aspirate is an indication of a fracture that may not have been seen on initial x-ray, such as a tibial plateau compression fracture. After aspiration, a compression pad should be applied to help reduce the return of an effusion.

A positive McMurray test may be indicative of a meniscal injury. A McMurray test is performed by placing the knee into flexion and rotating the leg in internal and external rotation. As the knee is extended a reproduceable click or pain elicited over the joint line indicates a positive test. The Appley test may also be used to evaluate an acutely injured knee. This test is performed with patient in the prone position. The knee is flexed and pressure is applied downward on the foot as the leg is internally and externally rotated. Joint line pain elicited with this test is an indication of a meniscal injury.

If a meniscal injury is suspected an MRI study or arthroscopy can confirm the diagnosis. The MRI is only necessary if a decision needs to be made about whether the player should be returned to activity or taken to surgery. If the exam clearly indicates a meniscal tear, an MRI is not needed. A study of athletes returning to competition after a menisectomy revealed poor results with volleyball players of international class (6). These results were worse than those for football players and wrestlers. It was thought that this was because of the repetitive jumping that is required for the sport of volleyball.

Patients who feel or hear a "pop" in their knee and then develop an effusion immediately after an injury should be considered to have an anterior cruciate injury until exam proves otherwise. The cruciate may be evaluated with anterior and posterior drawer tests and the Lachman test. Precise measurement of laxity may be done with an arthrometer. Instability may be evaluated by performing a pivot shift test. This test is performed by placing gentle internal rotation on the tibia and valgus stress on the knee, while the knee is flexed 10° to 15°. As the knee is flexed further, a positive test will have a reduction of the subluxation of the tibia that can be felt and seen by the examiner. Good relaxation of the patient's hamstring is essential to perform this test. It is important to assess whether there are accompanying meniscal injuries if the anterior cruciate ligament is disrupted, because meniscal injuries will usually require surgery.

A torn anterior cruciate ligament can be treated conservatively with a derotation brace or by an ACL reconstruction. If the patient wants to limit his or her activities to sports that do not require cutting and jumping, the derotation brace may provide enough stability to allow that athlete to safely compete. If the player wants to return to sports that require a high demand on the knee, such as volleyball, he or she may require the reconstruction to all stability that cannot be achieved in a brace. The advantages of the brace are, obviously, a decreased expense, no surgery, and a shorter rehabilitation period.

A rehabilitation program should be started soon after the injury occurs, and the patient should be on crutches and in a brace that allows flexion without varus or valgus motion. Early range of motion exercises with passive range of motion are crucial to a quicker rehabilitation and full recovery. Isometric quadricep and hamstring strengthening exercises are also recommended. As pain and swelling decrease and active range of motion and strength are regained, the patient may be allowed to bear weight. After the patient's strength has returned, decisions may be made whether a derotation brace is adequate to control stability or if reconstruction is needed. After reconstruction, the patient should wear a derotational brace for high-demand activities, thus the patient may try out the brace before final determination is made concerning the need for surgery.

Hip Injuries

Hip injuries are infrequently seen in volleyball unless the player lands directly on the hip from a dive or fall. Fractures may occur through this mechanism, but more commonly a greater trochanter bursitis may develop. This bursitis may be treated with ice, antiinflammatories, and physical therapy that uses modalities such as phonophoresis and friction massage. Occasionally, a corticosteroid may be injected into the bursa to further reduce inflammation and pain.

Lumbar Spine Injuries

The lumbar spine is placed in extension and rotation when a volleyball is spiked. This leads to strains in the lumbar spine and to sacroiliac joint problems caused by the stresses placed on these joints, especially when landing. All lower-back injuries should be thoroughly examined including x-rays and a neurologic exam. X-rays should include oblique projections to rule out spondylolysis or spondylolisthesis. The neurologic exam should include evaluations of strength, sensation, and deep tendon reflexes. Spinal and extremity range of motion should also be evaluated. hamstring flexibility also must be evaluated and treated with stretching if the hamstrings are tight.

Stresses on the sacroiliac joints can lead to localized dysfunction. Because these joints are the largest articular joints in the body, decreased function can lead to severe pain and discomfort, as well as muscle spasm. Pain is usually felt in the region of the posterior-superior iliac spine (PSIS) and radiates into the buttock. The standing flexion test can be performed to evaluate sacroiliac joint function. The examiner's thumbs are placed on the PSIS and observed as the patient bends forward. If one thumb moves asymmetrically forward, it can indicate dysfunction at that sacroiliac joint. Pain in the sacroiliac joint may also indicate ankylosing spondylitis, which can be seen as narrowing and sclerosis of the sacroiliac joints on x-ray. Sacroiliac dysfunction may also present with groin pain.

The hip flexors should be evaluated to assess their flexibility using the Thomas test. This test involves the patient lying supine with his or her knees at the edge of the table. As the hip is flexed by having the patient pull the knee toward the chest, the contralateral leg is observed. If the thigh comes off the table, the hip flexors are tight. This may add to the patient's back problems because of limited motion. If tightness is observed, a program of stretching for the hip flexors should be instituted.

Treatment of sacroiliac injuries includes cryotherapy, antiinflammatories, and physical therapy. Manipulative therapy also is very useful in the treatment of this injury and other lumbosacral strains. Physical therapy may use transcutaneous electrical nerve stimulation (TENS), ultrasound, and pelvic stabilization exercises to prevent reoccurrence. Stretching of the paravertebral muscles and piriformis should be part of the initial and continuing treatment. The patient also should work on strengthening the abdominal musculature and back muscles with exercises such as abdominal crunches and lumbar extension exercises. These last exercises are done in the prone position with the arms extended. The patient then lifts various extremities off of the floor or table while holding his or her spine in extension. As the patient's strength and range of motion return to normal and he or she becomes pain free, the athlete may gradually be returned to activity. The patient may be returned to partial impact activities such as running in a pool, on a trampoline, or on sand. Explosive running and jumping should be the last activities added before the patient is returned to play.

Spondylolysis is a defect of the pars interarticularis. It is theorized that it may be congenital or may be caused by microtrauma. There is a familial tendency to develop these pars defects. Spondylolysis may lead to spondylolisthesis or subluxation of the spine. Spondylolisthesis of 25% or less (grade I) may treated symptomatically with avoidance of activities that cause pain, such as hyperextension. Strengthening and flexibility exercises should be encouraged to prevent problems. Patients with spondylolysis of greater than grade I should probably be referred to alternative sports that involve less stress on the back than volleyball, but these should be handled on a case-by-case basis.

Care must also be taken during examination of the volleyball player with low-back injuries that the neurologic exam is normal. Repetitive trauma to the supporting structures can lead to herniation of the intervertebral discs. Suspicions of a herniated disc may be confirmed with an MRI study (Fig. 41.7). Neurologic deficits may be evaluated and followed with electromyelograms (EMGs).

Conservative treatment of herniated discs includes limited activities, antiinflammatories, muscle relaxants, extension exercises, and traction and other physical therapy modalities. Treatment may include a medical exercise program that teaches functional stabilization of the spine and postural awareness with daily activities.

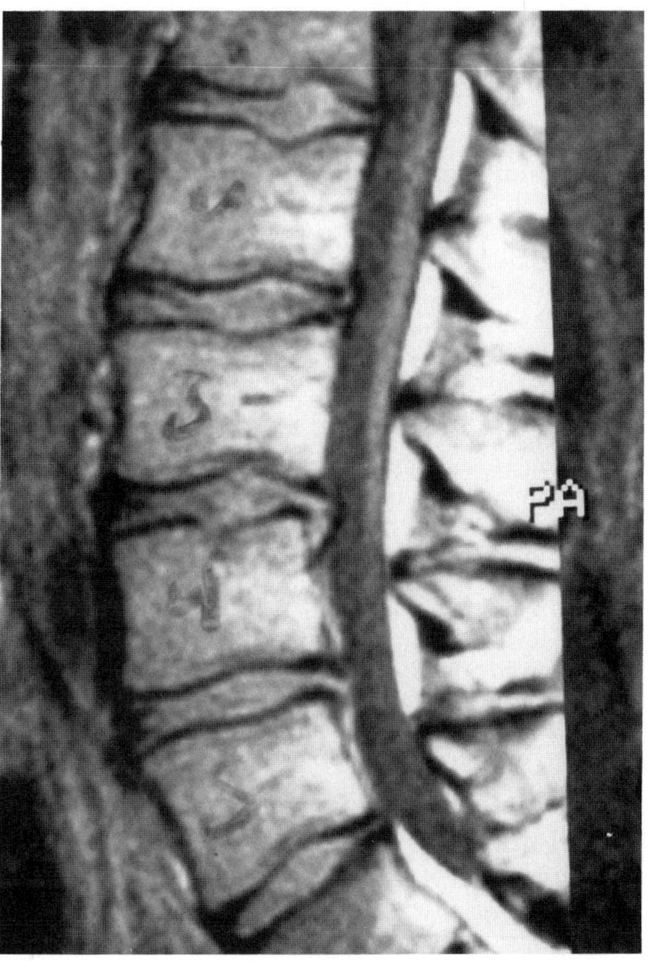

Figure 41.7. Herniated disc at L3-L4 as seen on MRI.

After 8 to 12 weeks, the activity level is gradually advanced to regular activities. Strengthening may include the use of modalities designed to isolate the back muscles such as cybex and med-x, which are forms of dynamic exercise with computer monitoring. Increasing pain or neurologic symptoms as well as failure of conservative therapy may lead to a neurosurgical or orthopedic referral for possible surgical intervention.

Thoracic strains are encountered less frequently than lumbosacral problems, but are seen in conjunction with shoulder problems or as separate entities. These may be treated in a similar manner to lumbar strains and nearly always respond well to conservative management. Regular stretching of the midthoracic and shoulder regions and slow, graduated warmups are extremely important for the player with a thoracic strain.

Shoulder Injuries

Shoulder injuries are seen almost universally in serious volleyball players sometime during their participation. The injuries range from impingement problems and rotator cuff strains to rotator cuff tears and occasionally subluxations or dislocations. One condition that appears to be limited to volleyball players is infraspinatus atrophy secondary to suprascapular nerve injury.

Rotator cuff tears can occur with blocking or diving injuries. The arm is forced into flexion and this force is transmitted through the cuff. The rotator cuff muscles may be previously compromised as a result of chronic strains or impingement problems. This weakness may result in a tear, as this increased force is applied to the muscles. Clinical evidence of a rotator cuff tear is exhibited by significant weakness on external rotation or abduction with or without pain. MRI and diagnostic arthroscopy are used to confirm the diagnosis. A full-thickness rotator cuff tear in an athlete requires surgical repair followed by rehabilitation, as described below for impingement problems. Small partial-thickness tears may heal with conservative management and rest.

Impingement syndrome is usually caused by overuse of the shoulder from repeated hitting of the ball. Some players are predisposed as a result of acromial anatomy, which includes breaking of the anterior aspect of the inferior surface. This "parrot breaking" impinges on the supraspinatus during abduction and rotation of the glenohumeral joint. Impingement also can be initiated by a fall, compressing the joint and causing a subacromial bursitis. Complaints are usually diffuse pain in the shoulder with abduction or overhead activities. Classic complaints include inability to sleep because of shoulder pain at night and acute pain with shoulder rotation or abduction greater than 90°. Impingement is caused by the pinching of the long head of the biceps and supraspinatus tendons as they pass through the subacromial space. In addition to these structures, the large subacromial bursa swells with inflammation.

Physical exam will reveal pain with abduction of the arm or forward flexion greater than 90°. These motions may be limited because of this pain or tightening of the capsule from disuse. The patient may have tenderness at the greater tuberosity where the supraspinatus inserts or in the bicepital groove over the long head of the biceps. The impingement test involves internal rotation of the shoulder while the arm is held at 90° flexion. This forces the greater tuberosity against the inferior acromion and causes pain as the subacromial structures are impinged. Weakness of the infraspinatus is evaluated by locking the elbow at the patient's side and externally rotating the shoulder against resistance. Supraspinatus strength is evaluated by abducting the arm against resistance while held at 90° abduction and 45° forward flexion with the elbow straight and the thumb pointed down. If the patient has profound weakness, the possibility of a rotator cuff tear must be evaluated as discussed above. Radiographs may reveal calcifications in the tendons as a result of chronic problems and also may show narrowing of the subacromial space with acromial spurring. Impingement may also be evaluated by MRI to show the degree of impingement and to rule out a rotator cuff tear or tear of the glenoid labrum.

Management of impingement syndrome includes cryotherapy, antiinflammatories, physical therapy, and reduction of overhead activity and hitting. Physical therapy is aimed at reducing inflammation while maintaining or improving range of motion. Once inflammation has been reduced and pain-free range of motion has been restored, strengthening exercises are begun. These are initially aimed at strengthening the rotator cuff muscles by internally and externally rotating against resistive bands or using very light weights in rotation as well as flexion and extension up to 90°. The supraspinatus may be strengthened with progressive resistance in the same motion as described above for testing the muscle. If the pain continues as conservative therapy progresses, a corticosteroid injection in the subacromial space may reduce inflammation and improve the patient's exercise tolerance.

Failure of conservative therapy is an indication for a subacromial decompression if the athlete wishes to continue to pursue playing volleyball or other activities that cause the impingement. This may be done as an open procedure or through the arthoscope. During this procedure the subacromial bursa is removed and the coracoacromial ligament excised. The inferior surface of the acromion is shaved, especially anteriorly if a spur is present. At the time of the decompression, the rotator cuff should be evaluated for tears. These may be repaired at this time if found during the procedure. Rehabilitation after decompression is similar to what has been described above for the impingement syndrome.

Dislocations of the shoulder are usually anterior dislocations that are caused by the arm being forced into external rotation and extension. The patient will experience pain immediately and a deformity of the shoulder will be noted on exam. Neurovascular status should be assessed distally and radiographic evaluation should be done to rule out fractures.

Initial reduction at the time of injury may be attempted with the patient in the prone or supine position by various methods that all include traction on the arm to counter the traction caused by muscle spasm. Reduction should be done with appropriate analgesia if not done immediately after the injury. Decisions regarding the reduction of the dislocation before taking x-rays should be made by the attending physician based on his or her previous experience with these injuries. After the reduction has been accomplished, the arm should be held in a shoulder immobilizer for at least 3 weeks before gentle range of motion is begun.

Because of the high reoccurrence rate of dislocations, studies are currently evaluating the benefits of surgical repair of the capsule after the first episode of dislocation. Some players may experience chronic subluxations without actual dislocation. These players will feel their shoulder slide in and out of joint. Exam will reveal laxity of the joint capsule and tenderness of the anterior capsule. The patient will also exhibit a positive apprehension test. This test is done by externally rotating the shoulder while the arm is abducted at 90°. A positive test will give the patient the sensation that his or her shoulder is dislocating. Radiographs may show a Bankhart lesion on the inferior glenoid or a Hill-Sachs lesion on the humeral head. If strengthening and modification of activities do not prevent subluxation, surgical tightening of the capsule may be indicated. Posterior dislocations are extremely rare but must be considered with acute shoulder injuries.

The condition of infraspinatus atrophy without pain in athletes has been seen almost exclusively in the dominant shoulder of volleyball players. Atrophy of the infraspinatus is accompanied by weakness on external rotation. This entity is thought to be the result of injury of the suprascapular nerve. Theories for this injury include stretch on the nerve and direct trauma to the nerve when hitting as well as a possible compartment syndrome. It is believed that the injury occurs mainly from serving instead of spiking, because of the tension on the infraspinatus during deceleration. One theory is that follow-through straight down puts more strain on the infraspinatus during deceleration.

Treatment is aimed at encouraging the player to follow-through across his or her body. It also has been postulated that hitting the ball with the arm fully extended rotates the scapula out of the way and puts less stretch on the nerve. There are ongoing studies at this time to test these theories and determine the prevalence of this problem in collegiate players. Because there is no pain involved, it is difficult to convince athletes to rest to alleviate the nerve trauma. Some releases on the suprascapular nerve have been tried surgically without good success. Reduction in play is not always successful at reversing this atrophy.

Wrist Injuries

Most wrist injuries are caused by diving for balls or setting. Injuries sustained by diving are frequently the result of falling on an outstretched hand. X-rays should be taken to rule out any fractures. Tenderness in the anatomic snuffbox is a sign of a possible navicular fracture and should be treated as such even if initial x-rays are negative. This treatment involves a short arm thumb spica splint or cast. The wrist should be reexamined in 10 to 14 days. If the snuffbox is still tender, repeat x-rays should be performed. Resorption at the fracture site by macrophages will make a fracture prominent by that time.

If the patient is nontender, range of motion exercises may be instituted and followed by strengthening. The patient may return to play with a wrist splint after the pain has diminished. Return to practice is first started with gentle bumping and setting. As the patient progresses he or she is allowed to return to hitting and finally blocking.

Hyperextension and radial deviation of the wrist during setting may also lead to overuse injuries. These may be treated with antiinflammatories, ice, and avoidance of hyperextension. This may be prevented by wearing custom splints, such as an orthoplast splint or taping. Strengthening of the wrist flexors will also help prevent hyperextension.

Hand and Finger Injuries

In several studies of volleyball injuries, hand and finger injuries were some of the most common problems. Most of these injuries occurred during blocking

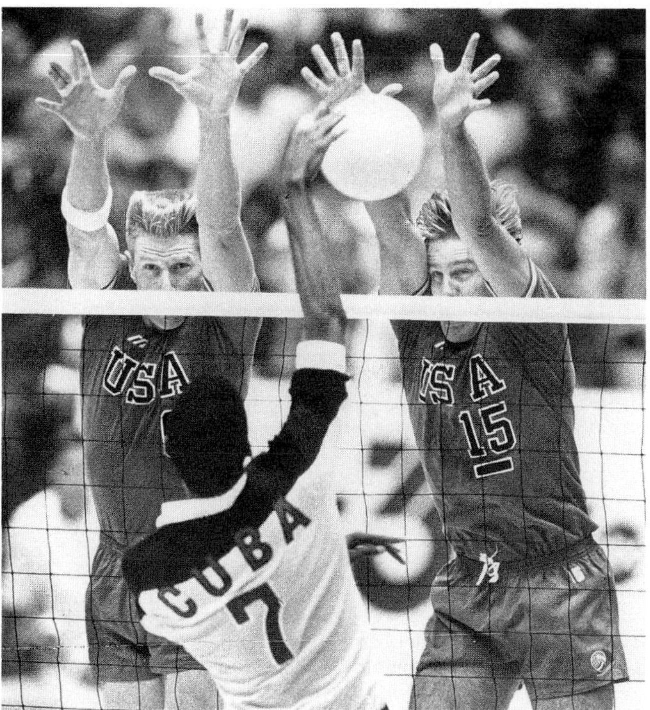

Figure 41.8. Blocking may lead to finger injuries because of the spread fingers.

(Fig. 41.8). This may be because of the technique of spreading the fingers when blocking. These injuries usually are interphalangeal joint sprains and dislocations. Initial treatment includes splinting and ice as well as neurovascular assessment. Finger injuries should be evaluated with x-rays to rule our fracture (Fig. 41.9). Fractures involving greater than 30% of the articular surface may require some form of internal fixation. Stability of the collateral ligaments of the injured joint should be evaluated by stress applied to the joint.

Sprained fingers should be splinted and may be buddy taped to the next finger to allow play. Hitting and blocking with the injured hand should be limited during practice. Dislocations usually occur when the finger is hyperextended. Dislocations may be safely relocated at the time of injury but should have x-rays to evaluate a possible avulsion fracture.

Another injury that occurs is avulsion of the extensor tendon at the distal interphalangeal joint. This usually results from being hit on the distal tip of the finger with a volleyball. This injury is also known as a mallet finger. The joint should be splinted in extension for 6 weeks to allow the tendon to heal. After 6 weeks, the joint should be splinted at night for another 6 weeks.

Fractures of the hand usually occur from diving for balls. There fractures should be evaluated and treated appropriately for the specific fracture. Custom braces may be used to allow the athlete quicker return to play (Fig. 41.10). The length of time that the fracture should be immobilized in a cast before splinting for return to play is determined by the type of fracture, but is usually 2 to 4 weeks.

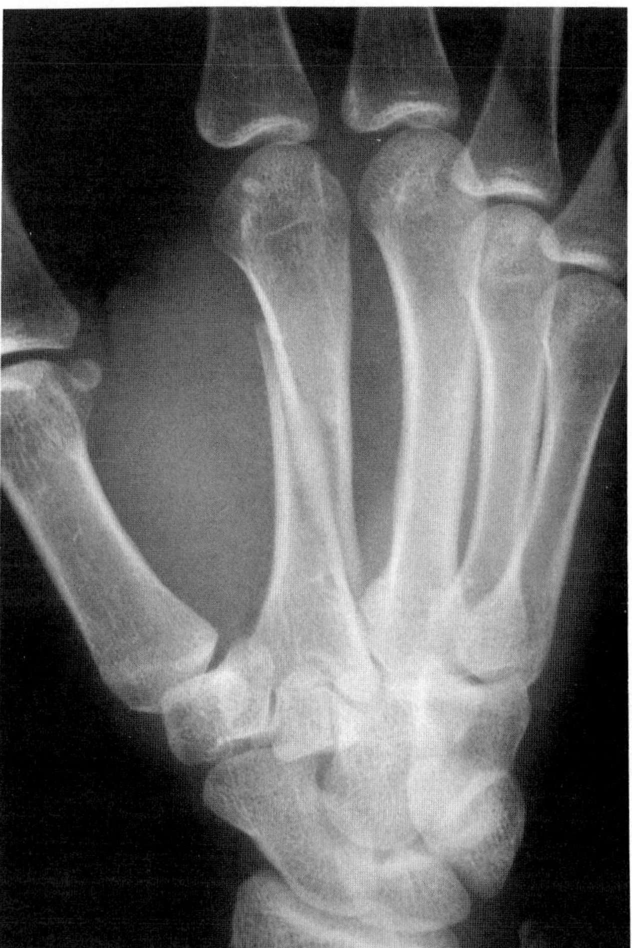

Figure 41.9. Fracture of the second metacarpal.

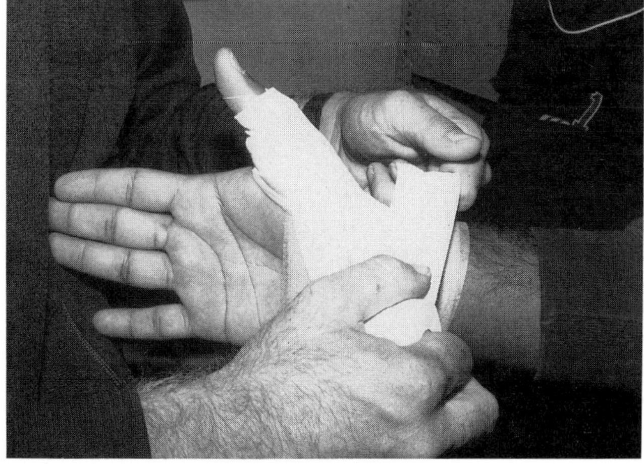

Figure 41.10. Bracing or taping may allow players with hand injuries to return to play earlier.

Head Injuries

Head injuries are rare in volleyball. The ones that occur are usually a result of diving for a ball or a collision between players. The usual injuries are lacerations, especially above the eyebrows or under the chin.

These lacerations should be cleansed and sutured as needed. X-rays should be taken if fractures are suspected. A neurologic exam should be performed to evaluate for a possible concussion.

Any alteration in consciousness or amnesia indicates that a concussion has occurred. The player should be removed from competition and held from activity until all signs of brain dysfunction, including headaches, dizziness, clouded thinking, and blurred vision, have resolved. If the player can then perform aerobic exercise without the return of symptoms, he or she may be allowed to return to full practice and competition. The length of time that a player is held from practice depends on the severity of the concussion and the number of previous head injuries.

REFERENCES

1. Shafle MD, Requa RK, Patton WL, Garrick JG. Injuries in the 1987 national amateur volleyball tournament. Am J Sports Med 1990;18(6):624–631.
2. Hell H, Schonle C. Ursachen und Prophylaxe typischer volleyballvertezungen. Z Orthop 1985;123:72–75.
3. Gangitano R, Pulvirenti A, Ardito S. Lesioni traumatiche da pallavolo: rillevi clinico-statistici. Ital J Sports Trauma 1981;3(1):31–34.
4. Gerberich SG, Luhman S, Finke C, et al. Analysis of severe injuries associated with volleyball activities. Phys Sportsmed 1987;15(8):75–79.
5. Moraldo M, Kirchner HG, Duessen GA. Das Volleyballspiel aus orthopaedischer Sicht. Dtsch Sportmed 1981;11:286–290.
6. Hoshikawa Y, Kurosawa H, Fukubayashi, et al. The prognosis of menisectomy in athletes. The simple meniscus lesions without ligamentous instabilities. Am J Sports Med 1983;11(1):8–13.

SUGGESTED READINGS

Backx FJ, Beijer HJ, Bol E, Erich WB. Injuries in high-risk persons and high-risk sports. A longitudinal study of 1818 school children. Am J Sports Med 1991;19(2):124–130.

Biedert R, Kentsch A. Arthroscopic revision of the subacromial space in impingement syndrome. Unfallchirurg 1989;92(10):500–504.

Bobbert MF. Drop jumping as a training method for jumping ability. Sports Med 1990;9(1):7–22.

Cooney WP. Sports injuries to the upper extremity. How to recognize and deal with some common problems. Postgrad Med 1984;76(4):45–50.

Distefano S. Neuropathy due to entrapment of the long thoracic nerve. A case report. Ital J Orthop Trauma 1989;15(2):259–262.

Dittel KK, Weller S. Isolated acute ruptures of fibular ligaments of the ankle joint in volleyball games. Unfallheilkunde 1980;83(5):219–225.

Duddy RK, Duggan RJ, Visser HJ, et al. Diagnosis, treatment, and rehabilitation of injuries to the lower leg and foot. Clin Sports Med 1989;8(4):861–876.

Ferretti A. Epidemiology of jumper's knee. Sports Med 1986;3(4):289–295.

Ferretti A, Cerullo G, Russo G. Suprascapular neuropathy in volleyball players. J Bone Joint Surg 1987;69(2):260–263.

Ferretti A, Ippolito E, Mariani P, Puddu G. Jumper's knee. Am J Sports Med 1983;11(2):58–62.

Ferretti A, Papandrea P, Conteduca F. Knee injuries in volleyball. Sports Med 1990;10(2):132–138.

Green TA, Hillman SK. Comparison of support provided by a semirigid orthosis and adhesive ankle taping before, during, and after exercise. Am J Sports Med 1990;18(5):498–506.

Holzgrraefe M, Klingelhofer J, Eggert S, Benecke R. Chronic neuropathy of the suprascapular nerve in high performance athletes. Nervenarzt 1988;59(9):545–548.

Israeli A, Engel J, Ganel A. Possible fatigue fracture of the pisiform bone in volleyball players. Int J Sports Med 1982;3(1):56–57.

Jerosch J, Castro WH, Sons UH. Secondary impingement syndrome in athletes. Sportverletz Sportschaden 1990;4(4):180–185.

Kujala UM, Kvist M, Osterman K. Knee injuries in athletes. Review of exertion injuries and retrospective study of outpatient sports clinic material. Sports Med 1986;3(6):447–460.

Lanese RR, Strauss RH, Leizman DJ, Rotondi AM. Injury and disability in matched men's and women's intercollegiate sports. Am J Public Health 1990;80(12):1459–1462.

Lund PM. Marathon volleyball: changes after 61 hours play. Br J Sports Med 1985;19(4):228–229.

Melzer C, Wirth CJ. Complete rotator cuff lesions in athletes. Sportverletz Sportschaden 1989;3(2):81–87.

Novak J, Hlavacek V. Disorders of the upper and lower extremities in members of top junior volleyball teams. Acta Chir Orthop Traumatol Cech 1987;54(5):444–448.

Schmidt-Olsen S. Jorgensen U. The pattern of injuries in Danish championship volleyball. Ugeskr Laeger 1987;149(7):473–474.

Whiteside JA, Fleagle SB, Kalenak A. Fractures and refractures in intercollegiate athletes. An eleven year experience. Am J Sports Med 1981;9(6):369–377.

Williams JM, Tonymon R, Wadsworth WA. Relationship of life stress to injury in intercollegiate volleyball. J Hum Stress 1986;12(1):38–43.

Yde J, Nielsen AB. Epidemiological and traumatological analysis of injuries in a Danish volleyball club. Ugeskr Laeger 1988;150(17):1022–1023.

42 / WATER SKIING

Noëlle Grace, Ross Outerbridge, John F. Pepper, and Wally Sokolowski

Water Skiing

Water skiing enjoys worldwide popularity. Figures suggest that at least 17 million Americans participate in the sport annually. Water skiing was derived from aquaplaning. One historical review credits an 18-year-old, Ralph Samuelson, with the first real water skiing venture (1). In 1922, he set out across Lake Pepin in Minnesota on a pair of barrel slats, towed by a 24-horsepower launch. The sport has evolved since then with improvements in powerboats and skis and is now widely enjoyed as an individual recreational sport. Tournaments at local, national, and international levels are held worldwide, with no major distinctions between the professional and amateur athlete. Waterfront shows often include water skiing exhibitions in the form of show skiing. In evaluating the sport for its potential hazards, one has to look at all its components—from the equipment (including specialized skis and bindings, towboats, and towlines) to the human factors (skier, driver, observer)—that contribute to misadventures. Water skiing may be done in fresh or salt water. Thus, it is subject to varying temperatures, conditions, and hazards. There are two classes of waterskiers; the recreational skier who generally has no formal technical instruction on either driving or skiing safety and the competitor who has detailed knowledge of the sport, its challenges and risks. The competitor usually prepares physically and has individually adapted equipment. The water skier as competitor is much more apt to be disciplined and careful.

In reviewing the medical literature, it is more commonly the recreational skier who is involved in a sensational accident that involves boating or propeller mishaps. Competitive waterskiers participate in any of a variety of events (Table 42.1), each having its own specific equipment and some inherent risks. News reports detail stories of the unusual water skiing injuries, leaving the false impression that the sport can be exceptionally hazardous. A recent report by Kistler (2), for the American Water Ski Association, which used statistics obtained from the United States Coast Guard, disagrees with this view. From 1977 to 1981, there were 3754 boats involved in water skiing accidents in the United States, resulting in 2269 injuries requiring more than first aid. There were 222 fatalities, an estimated fatality rate of 1:32,000 waterskiers. The U.S. Coast Guard summary (whose focus is primarily on the boating aspects of these mishaps) suggests that the single most important factor in these accidents was the towboat driver, whose carelessness or inexperience led to about 33% of the fatalities and significant injuries (Table 42.2).

Interestingly, current competitive water skiing has a remarkable safety record. There has never been, for example, a fatality in the American Water Ski Association tournaments. However, 61 injuries were reported in 1981 from 303 United States tournaments. These injuries were mainly minor cuts, sprains, bruises, torn ligaments, or pulled muscles. Approximately 75% of the reported injuries occurred in the jumping events, 18% in slalom, and 7% in trick riding. Since 1970, there has been a water ski injury report survey in Canada. In 1982, there were 32 sanctioned tournaments involving almost 1,200 skiers, and only one sprained ankle was reported. Although there are still no good epidemiological studies, in the past 4 years from 1987 to 1991 only 3 significant injuries have been reported at Canadian tournaments. In 1970, the Canadian Water Ski Association (WSA) published the first safety manual (3), which became one of the references for the International Water Ski Federation (IWSF) according to a personal communication from R.C. Schneider. The International Water Ski Federation and its national and local subsidiaries have an organized structure for tournament safety. This includes the appraisal of the site from the standpoint of the audience and the skiers, safe water retrieval of injured skiers, first aid, transport and hospital liaison, as well as specific guidelines for equipment.

Types of Injuries

Water ski injuries can be grouped into various categories and discussed under mechanisms, prevention, and treatment (1, 4) (Table 42.3). Many early injuries were the impetus for the presently established rules and regulations in competitive events. The injury categories include skier injuries, which is the authors' major focus here, and the towboat-related accidents where diversion of the driver may have contributed to the mishap (Table 42.3).

"Normal Falls"

All water skiers fall—and they may twist or impact a ski or the water. The impact may be hard if contacted at speed. The usual consequence of this "normal fall" in the recreational skier with or without contacting the ski, are contusions, torn ligaments, occasional dislocations, and sprains. Knees and ankles are the most common sites of injury. The skis of the novice tend to be forced apart, and with the abduction forces, there can be straining and tearing of ligaments around these joints. No study on the breakdown of these ligament injuries has been undertaken. Fractures do occur, but rarely. Although these injuries are often mild, there are sometimes more serious problems. In a personal communication, R.C. Schneider reports of a patient who sustained a thrombosis of an internal carotid artery (Fig. 42.1). When the patient fell forward, his ski struck him on the neck (Fig. 42.2*A*). The more frequent pattern of injury involves the inexperienced recreational skier without body preparation, experience, or protective gear, who is much more likely to sustain stress injuries and to suffer towline entanglements and douche injuries. In competitive skiing, however, the jumper may sustain bruised heels from landing too far back; the trick skier may sprain ankles or worse from a late binding or boat release. Hand calluses can be torn in quick maneuvers. Talus fractures have occurred in a slalom skier. Common injuries seen by event physicians include muscle sprains/strains, disfiguring and painful soft tissue hand injuries, punctured ear drums, costochondral joint separation, ankle injuries, knee ligament strains and hamstring pulls. (See Specific Competitive Water Skiing Injuries below.)

Collisions with Solid Objects

Recreational water skiers at times do not see obstacles or they attempt grandstanding in landings on docks, rafts, diving boards, or the shore. Any misjudgment of speed or angle can result in a direct collision of considerable force. Poor lighting, due to bad weather or the dull light of dusk, aggravates this risk. If the skier and/or driver are in unfamiliar water, they may also not recognize hazardous shoals, reefs, or pylons (Fig. 42.2*B*).

Table 42.1.

	Tournament	
A	Classical	Slalom Trick Jumping
B	Barefoot Competition	Slalom Trick Jumping
C	Speed Skiing	
D	Show Skiing	Jumping Ballet Barefoot Kite Flying Clowning

Table 42.3.

Skiers	Water Ski Boats
1. "Normal Falls" 2. Trick Ski-Delayed Release 3. Stress Injuries 4. Unique Injuries e.g. Collisions with Solid Objects (Hazards) Douche Injuries Towline Entanglements	1. Towboat/Boat Collisions 2. Propeller/Skier (3. Occupant Mishaps)

Table 42.2.
Water Skiing Accidents (Accumulated from Available Literature and Case Reports)

Types of Water Skiing Accidents (% are approximate)	Boat ↕ Another Boat	Solid Objects ↔ (Skier)	Floating Object	← Overboard Passengers	← Propeller Injuries
Injuries (%)	23	12	4	?	?
Fatalities (%)	15	21	5	17	13

	Specific Fault			
	Total ←	Speeding ←	Other Boats ←	Equipment
Injuries (%)	41	7	6	3
Fatalities (%)	24[a]	?	11	3

[a] Half of these drowned.

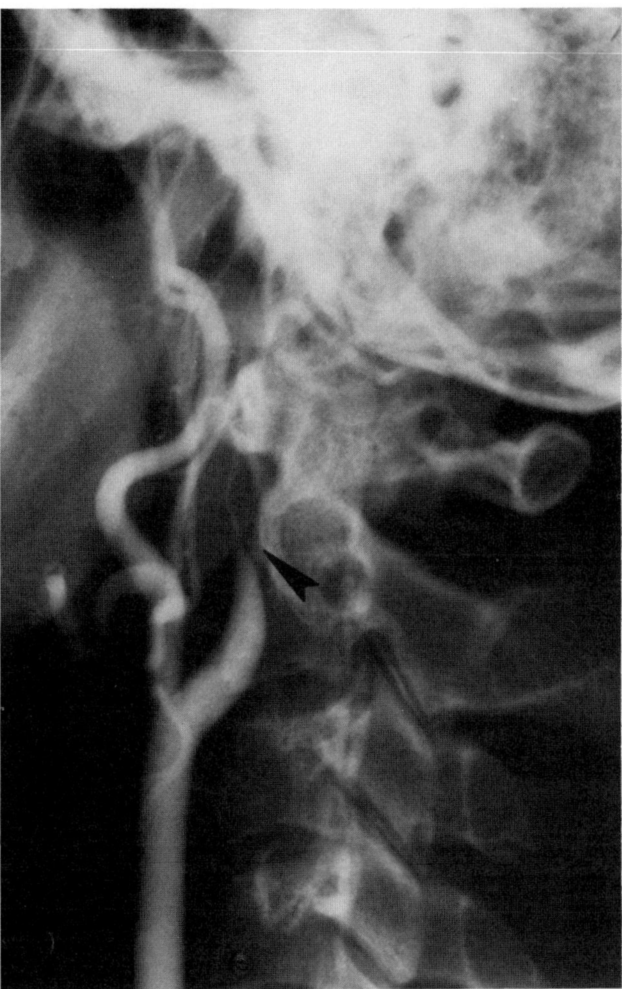

Figure 42.1. Left carotid arteriogram shows the oblique smooth shearing pattern *(arrowhead)* suggestive of a tear of the intima of the thrombosed internal carotid artery.

The authors have seen a teenager sustain a ruptured spleen after colliding with a protruding diving board. A similar accident resulted in the death of a young girl in Ontario, when the severity of her injury went unrecognized and she exsanguinated. The competitive jumping event, the most spectacular of water skiing tournament events, was associated early with some severe injuries of this type. In order to achieve maximum speed, the competitive skier approaches the ramp from the opposite side of the wake (Fig. 42.3) at an acute angle. Misjudging the angle for this double wake crossing, especially in rough water, has led to the deaths of at least three top level competitive skiers, who have either hit the side of the ramp or fallen while sliding up the ramp (Fig. 42.4), sustaining lethal head and neck injuries. Paterson (4) reported a 25-year-old male who hit a submerged sandbank, sustaining a dislocation of C5-C6, and became an instant quadriplegic. R.C. Schneider (personal communication) reported a similar injury that caused neck hyperextension and "hangman's fracture" (95) (Fig. 42.5). These cases are tragic, but with the introduction of mandatory use of personal flotation devices, they have become a present day rarity. Although the early disasters were devastating, a recent national tournament in which hundreds of jumps were taken, had only 3 significant injuries, one of which was an aggravation of a previous costochondral separation. A whiplash and a medial collateral ligament injury to a knee occurred in the same tournament.

Entanglement in Towlines

Experienced skiers and divers are well aware of the necessity for untangling and clearly visualizing the towrope before takeoff (Fig. 42.6*A*). The skier must signal preparedness for takeoff either verbally or by appropriate signal (Table 42.2). Nonetheless, Banta (6) reported that an experienced ski instructor, in attempting an "on the beach start," allowed her left leg to become entangled in the rope (Fig. 42.6*B*). The boat's pilot, an experienced boat driver, (and the ski instructor's husband), stopped the boat immediately, but she was pulled forward, her foot locked in the ski, which resulted in a dislocation fracture of her ankle.

Trick skiing "toehold turns" require the water skier to have one foot anchored into the towrope handle's special grip attachment (Fig. 42.7), while the body pivots back and forth. R.M. Brock (personal communication, 1982) reported an experienced skier who sustained a ruptured posterior cruciate ligament while performing these "toehold turns". As the trick or figure events involve more and more complicated maneuvers over towropes and toehold grips for turns, even the very experienced skier is at some risk. Although toehold grips are designed to allow release of the falling skier's foot, there is a release mechanism now situated in the towboat. Minor injuries involving the towropes themselves can cause rope burn and abrasions which can be treated locally.

Boat Collisions

Boat accidents with other boats occur much as motor vehicle collisions do. There is little or no marine traffic control in most areas, and no safe driver's permit or certificate is necessary before someone can drive a boat. The fact that one of the boats involved in a collision is towing a water skier affects the forward attention of the driver. The U.S. Coast Guard suggested that collisions involving towboats account for 23% of the injuries and 15% of the fatalities associated with water skiing. The law in most countries now requires that an observer be present in the towboat to provide a communication liaison between the driver and skier, thus freeing the driver from watching the skier and ensuring adequate attention forward.

Propeller Injuries

Some of the most devastating injuries are the result of a collision between a boat motor and downed waterskier. The tissue destruction can be massive, with resultant loss of limbs and lives. Propeller injuries usually resemble a sequence of deep transverse incisions as the blades rotate and move along the victim's body

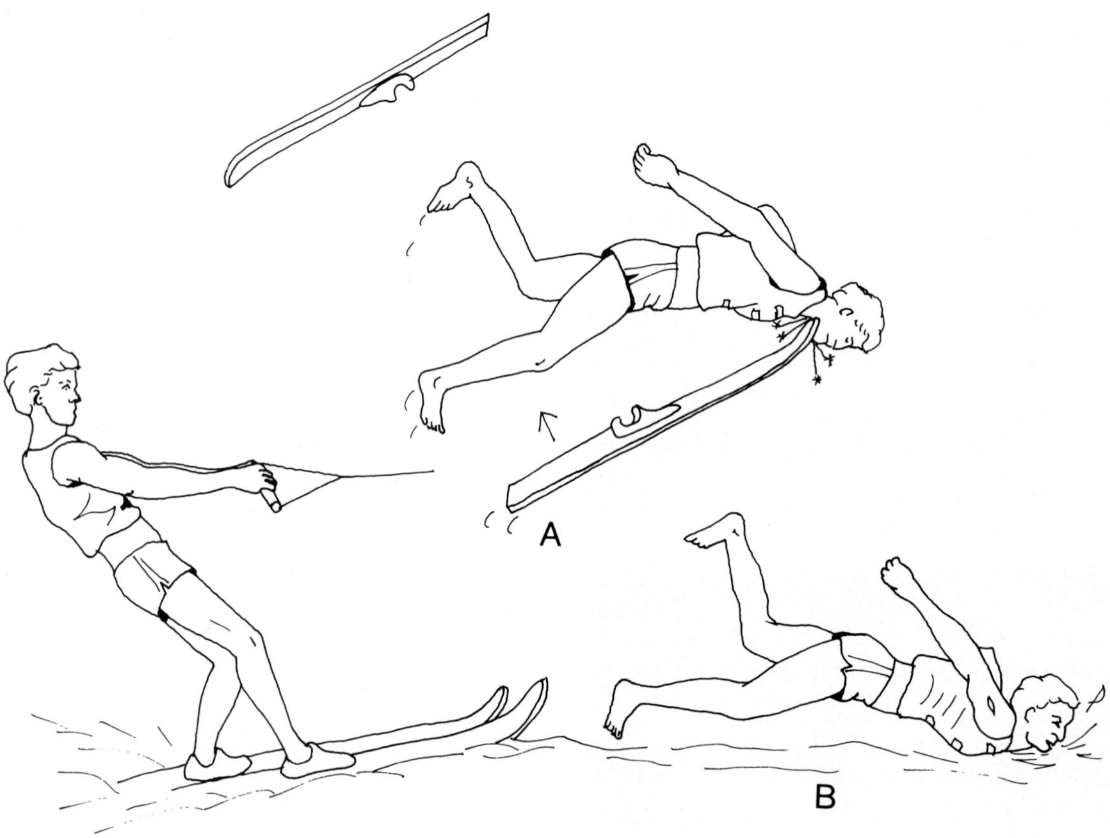

Figure 42.2. Two mechanisms of injury during falls are demonstrated. **(A)** The sharp point of the ski may strike the neck causing the carotid occlusion (see Fig. 42.1). **(B)** The abrupt halt by striking shallow water may cause a fall forward striking the chin on the ground with a forcible hyperextension fracture of the cervical spine (see Fig. 42.5B).

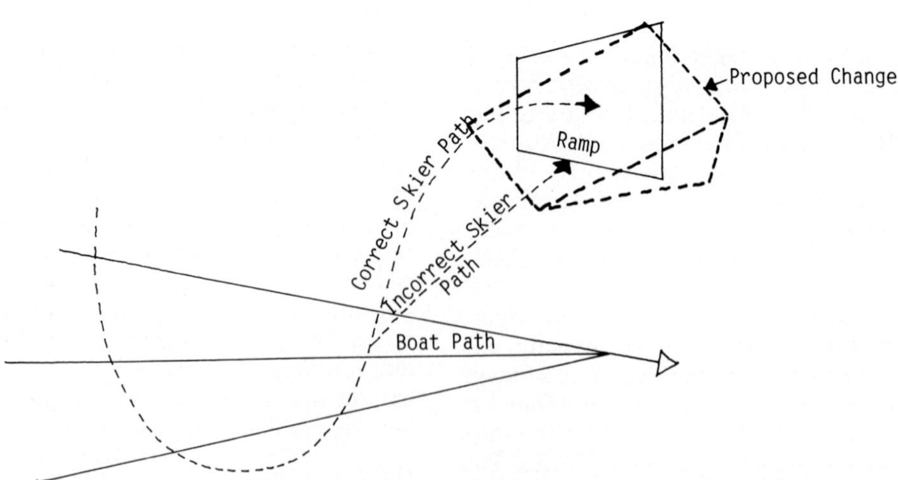

Figure 42.3. In the jump approach, the skier must come from opposite the ramp and cut across the double wake at an acute angle in order to achieve maximum speed at the ramp.

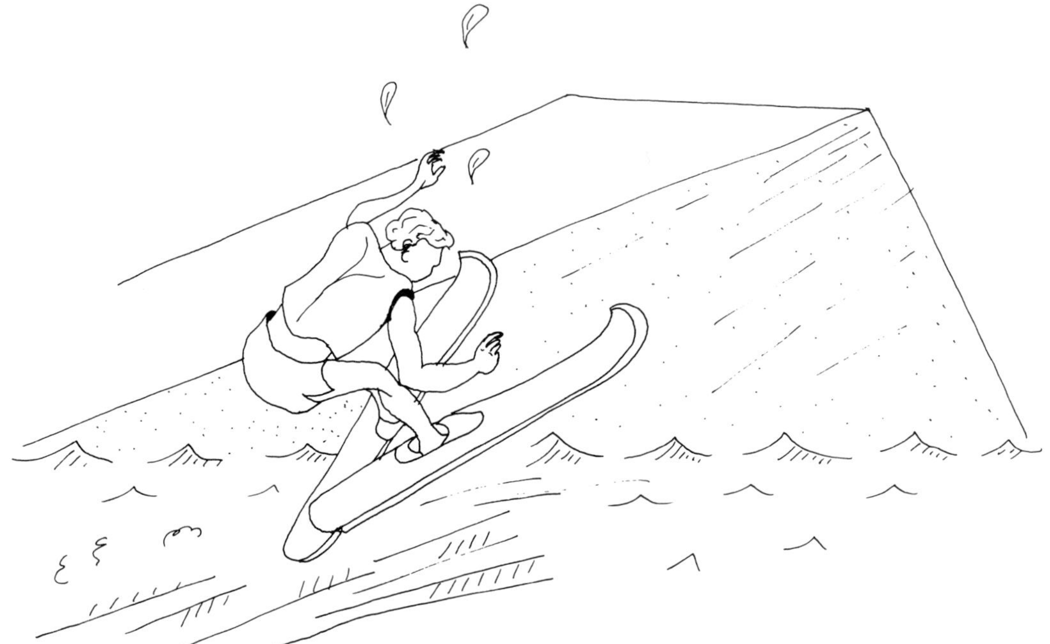

Figure 42.4. The skier misjudged his speed and position on approaching the ramp, sustaining a fatal head and neck injury.

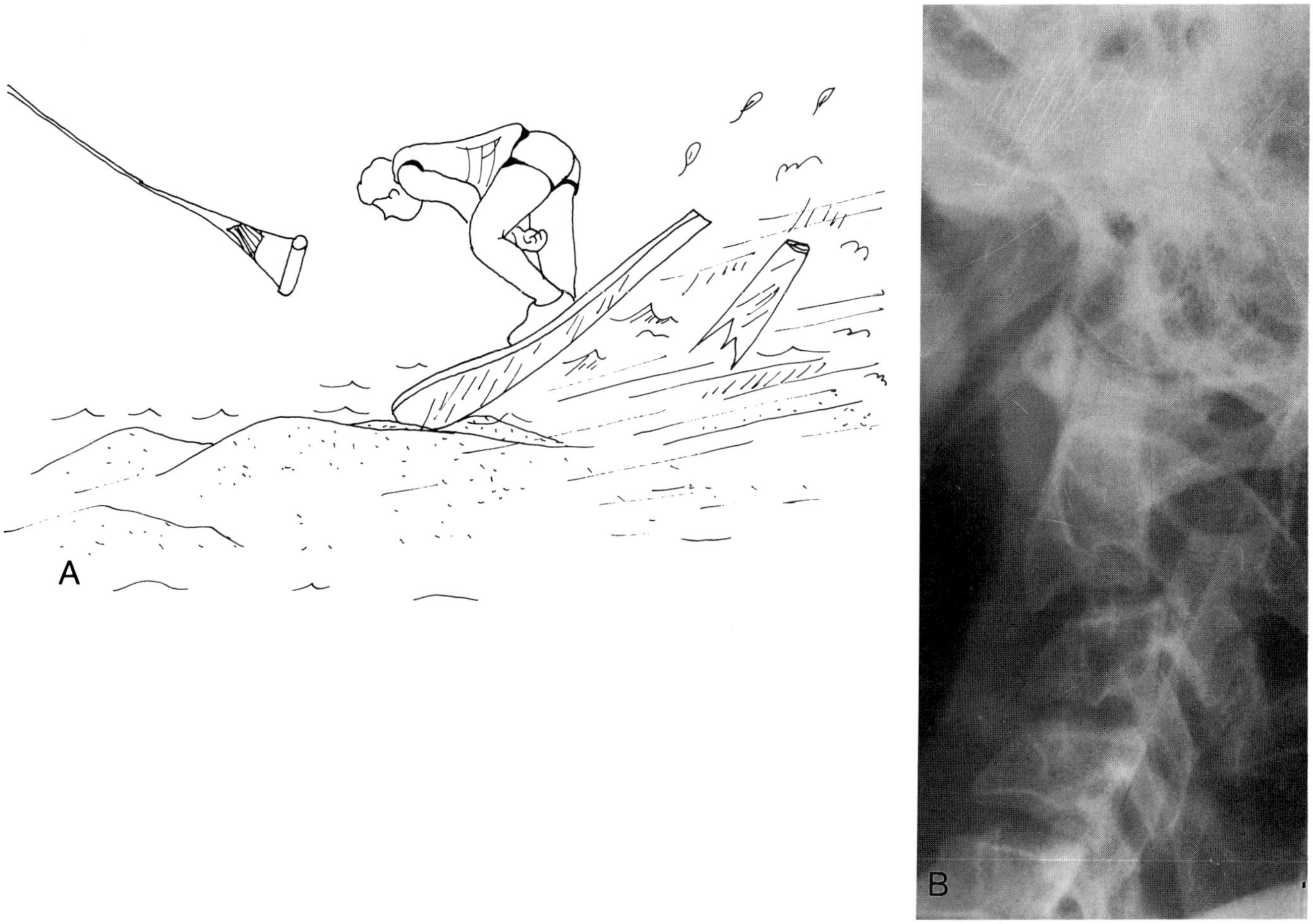

A

B

Figure 42.5. Here the competitor struck the shore **(A),** causing him to be hurled forward so that he sustained a cervical injury **(B)** with a typical "hangman's fracture" and severe quadriplegia.

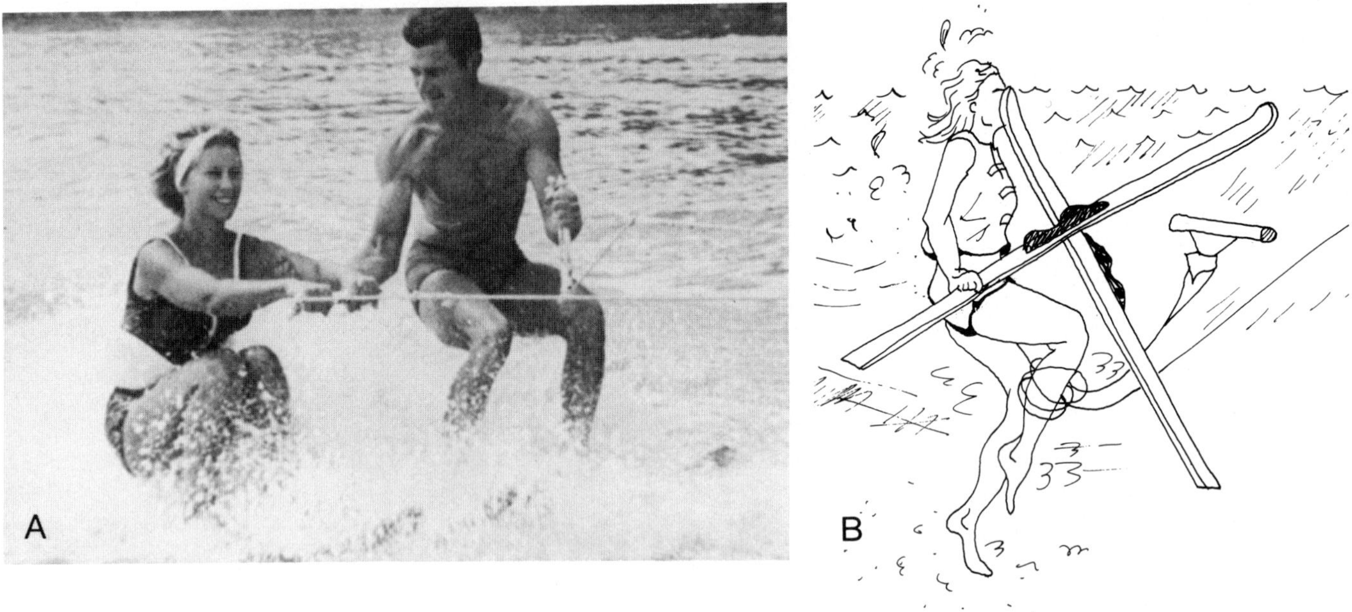

Figure 42.6. This experienced pair have their towropes carefully separated **(A).** Entanglement of the right leg by the towrope **(B)** resulted in a fracture dislocation of the skier's right ankle.

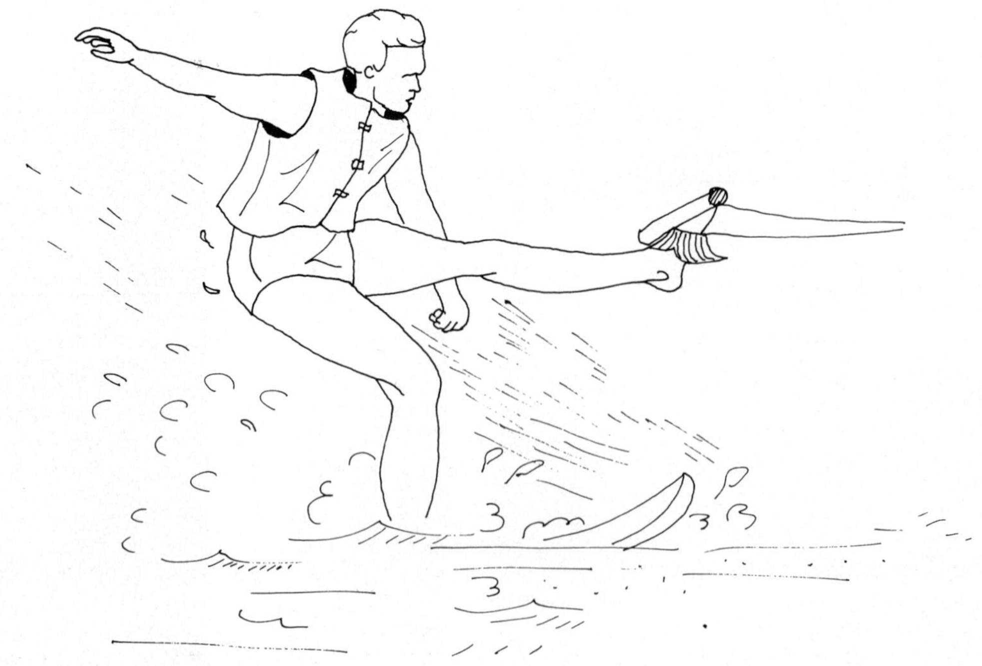

Figure 42.7. Pictured here is the "toe hold grip" for special turns. The trick release is now situated in the boat to prevent dragging a downed skier.

(Fig. 42.8). In addition to massive soft tissue injuries and fractures, these may be complicated by subsequent gross infection, despite vigorous debridement, drainage, and antibiotic coverage. Patterson and Sweeney (7) reported several Australian cases: one, a surfboard rider who was run over by a towboat; another, an 11-year-old swimmer who had not been seen by the water ski boat driver; and the third, run over after falling from a ski. Banta (6) reported three cases; two girls attempting to dive beneath an oncoming water ski towboat sustained massive buttock lacerations and fractures. A 31-year-old female skier was submerged at a boat's stern when it suddenly backed up over her, resulting in amputation of her left leg and thigh.

Boat Occupant Injuries

Boat passengers riding astride the bow or stern or on gunwales are always at risk of falling overboard if the boat turns sharply. May and Piliero (8) recently reported three cases of injury to the water skier observer or "seer" (who was in the boat specifically to provide liaison between skier and driver). As the boat encountered a heavy wake at high speed, a situation not anticipated by the observer who was intent on his job, he (although seated forward in the boat in the front seat) was tossed overboard. The driver then reflexly turned the boat away from the fallen passenger, driving the propeller over him (Fig. 42.9). All three cases sustained severe facial and upper limb wounds associated with fractures. This unusual but repeated experience underlines the importance of following the basic rules of boat safety. The driver should communicate the possibility of sudden changes of direction to his observer, so that extra precautions can be taken. Restraining but nonrestrictive arm grips or seat attachments may minimize the risk of being thrown overboard.

Douche and Enema Injuries

Douche injuries are the result of the forceful entry of a stream of water under high pressure into any of the body orifices. This occurs particularly when the beginner is being dragged through the water in a crouched

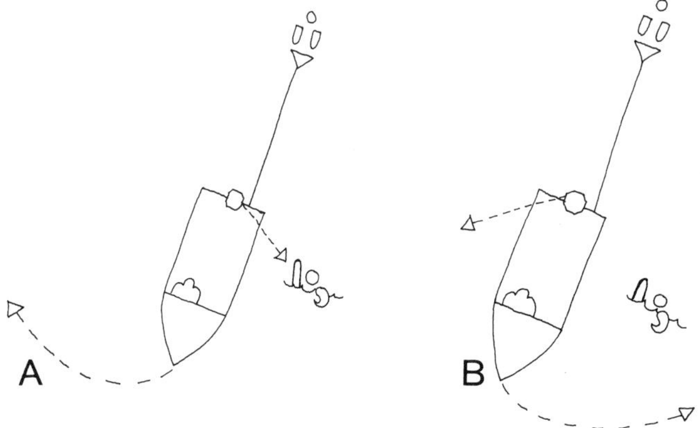

Figure 42.9. **(A)** Pictured here is the incorrect method of turning the boat where an apparent sudden thrust away from the fallen passenger in fact forces the stern and propeller over him. **(B)** The correct method for the boat driver to avoid a fallen passenger is demonstrated here.

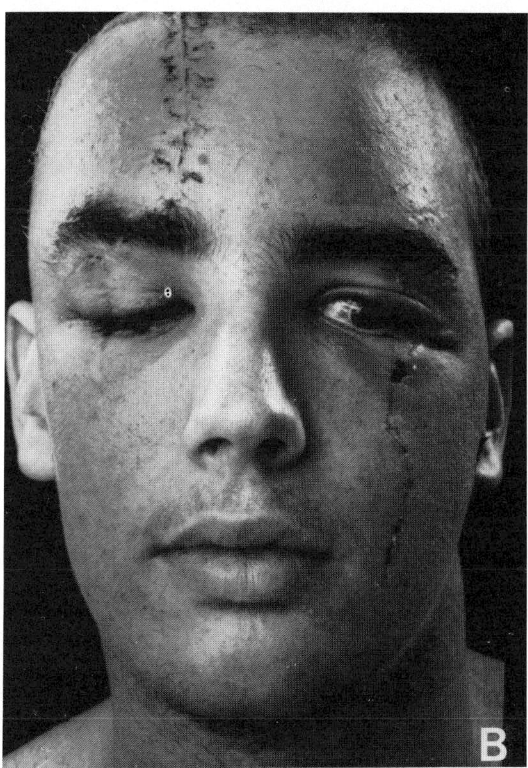

Figure 42.8. **(A)** The bilateral compound fracture from the propeller blade through the right frontal sinus and the left orbit is shown. **(B)** The laceration through the right frontal region damaged the right levator muscle, and there was injury to the left globe.

position, banging the buttocks repeatedly and with increasing speed and force in the water (Fig. 42.10). In the jumping events the measure of slack towrope allowed as the skier is landing may cause the skier to squat at high speeds. In its minor form, the resultant enema, as reported rather facetiously by Kaiser et al. (9), is a rather unpleasant, yet urgent problem, leaving no major sequela. However, extensive rectal lacerations as a result of this mechanism have been reported by Ramey (7) (Fig. 42.11) and others (10).

High pressure vaginal douches can be just as serious. Gray (11) reported a 36-year-old female who sustained a 13 cm vaginal laceration from the posterior wall of the cervix to the vaginal vault that resulted in shock from blood loss and necessitated transfusion and a complicated intraoperative repair. Tweedale (12) reported a similar case, with resultant rupture of a cystocele. Pfanner (13) and McCarthy (14) have reported cases of tuboovarian abscesses after douches sustained in this way, with resultant infertility. Morton (15) has reported miscarriages. Kizer (16) reported a 34-year-old male who was dragged a distance along the surface of the water, receiving considerable amounts of high pressure water into the nose and mouth with subsequent otitis media and sinusitis.

Competition ski jumpers, who squat on landing, are

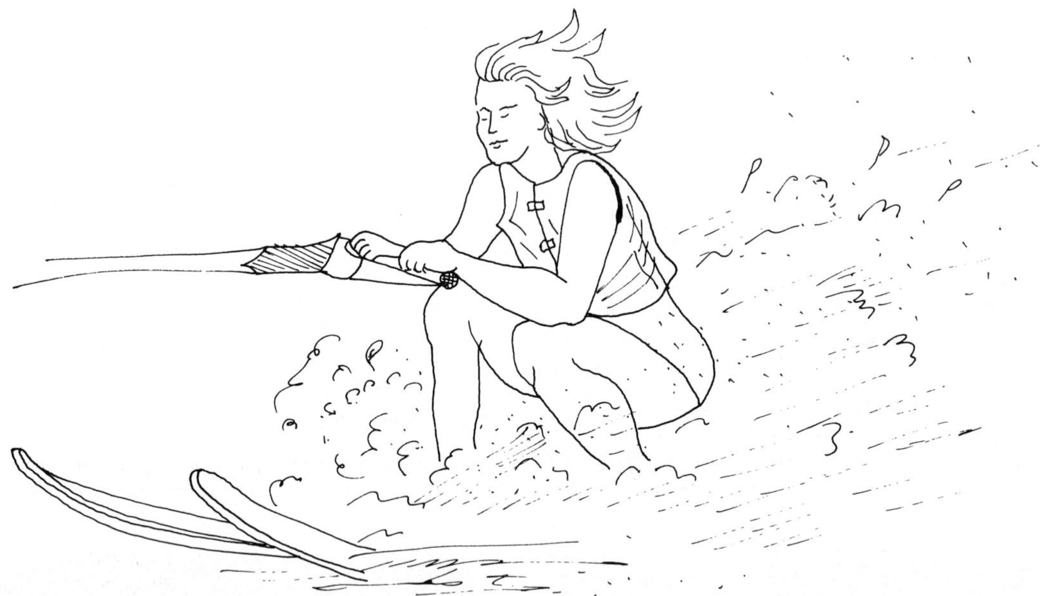

Figure 42.10. In a crouched position with the buttocks banging the water at increasing speeds, there is a risk of injury to the external and internal genitalia. A vaginal douche injury is quite often sustained during takeoff or during loss of balance.

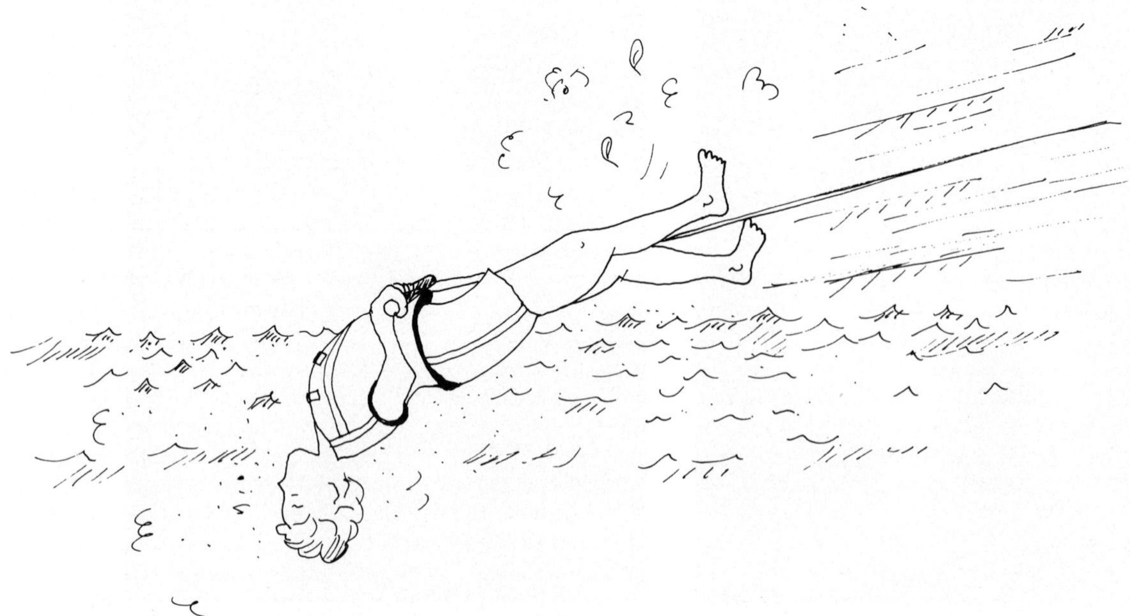

Figure 42.11. With an underwater start the barefoot skier is at risk of a rectal douche.

required to wear reinforced neoprene pants or similar protective gear. Pregnant or potentially fertile women should be aware of the risks of water skiing in regular bathing suits and wear protective equipment. Complaints of rectal and vaginal bleeding after this type of injury must be considered potentially serious. Barefoot skiers are using leg straps and double or triple layers of neoprene over the buttocks.

Miscellaneous

There are unusual and unpredictable types of mishaps. Sometimes these are the consequence of sudden electrical storms or other weather changes. In some areas of Australia, for example, the fallen water skier is vulnerable to shark attacks in ocean skiing (17). Related water sports such as kite flying and barefoot skiing have their own risks. The kite flyer can fall from considerable heights and the barefoot skier must travel at much greater speeds than the average skier, i.e., 40 miles/hr. The water surface becomes very hard in these falls.

Specific Competitive Water Skiing Injuries

Mechanisms and Treatment

Bruised Heels. This injury occurs as a result of landing a jump with the body weight over the heels instead of the toes. Often associated with the injury is inadequate padding in the jump ski binding. Trick skiers, in learning the wake back flip, may land on the opposite wake, not beyond it, with resultant stressful impact and bruising on the rear heel.

The usual signs of bruising, such as swelling and discoloration, may be missing in these cases, with tenderness existing over the sides of the heel, not on the plantar surface; this is probably secondary to the rupture of some heel pad septae.

The injury may be prevented by learning and using appropriate techniques for jumping and wake tricks and by proper padding of ski bindings. Appropriate icing and rest will improve symptoms, which may, however, drag on for a whole season if the vigorous skiing is continued.

Costochondral Separation. This injury may occur as the result of a skipping injury at rapid speed—the skier's chest colliding with the wake as the ski slides out toward the boat.

These separations most commonly involve rib #7, 8 and 9, just inferior to the sternum. Symptomatic treatment and rest over some weeks may suffice, but associated pneumothorax or hemoperitoneum from liver or spleen rupture must be ruled out.

Punctured Ear Drum. If a ski edge is caught with a forceful sideways fall in trick skiing or jumping the blow may produce enough local pressure to rupture an ear drum. Competitive skiers often choose to continue in events despite this injury while using ear plugs and bathing caps.

Otitis Externa. This condition may be a recurrent problem in competitive skiers and requires constant attention.

Hand Callouses. Callouses are often seen early in the season; they are exacerbated by switching from cold to warm water environments. Most commonly they occur on the palmar aspect of the metacarpal phalangeal joints and the distal palmar crease. Neoprene glove liners may be used in the early season to prevent them and to protect the hands.

Muscle Tears and Sprains. These occur most often in the proximal adductor muscle group, associated with toe hold tricks (18). These movements are risky because of the pull, slack, and "catch" after the trick is landed.

Another common area of injury is the flexor and pronator muscle group in the forearm—especially, the pronator teres.

Back Pain. The effect of waterski jumping on the vertebral column on young skiers was questioned without conclusion by Horne (19). Slaloming however, may be responsible for back extension strain with thoracic spine rotation observable when the skier is returning to the wake after a turn. This mechanism may explain back symptoms in water skiers. The elite group have demonstrated higher than average upper and lower back strength. Certainly back symptoms in Canadian National Team members decreased after a specific strengthening program was introduced.

Contributing Factors in Water Skiing Injuries—An Analysis

Many of the changes in water skiing equipment and techniques have been the direct reaction to specific injury types. Laws now regulate boat equipment, traffic, the requirement of an observer, flotation devices, reinforced clothing, etc. for water skiing tournaments. Many factors are involved in accidents. These can be classified into those related to people, equipment, and weather and water conditions.

Human Factors

There are three individuals involved in the water skiing team: the skier, the boat driver, and an observer, each with his or her own responsibilities. Various human traits determine the character makeup of each of these participants, and these traits can be factors in the causes of injuries. For example, personalities vary from introvert to extrovert, confident to insecure. The handling of responsibility for one's own safety and the safety of others may be profoundly affected by these different personality traits. Skill, both natural and acquired, alters risk factors and how potential mishaps are handled. Experienced drivers and skiers have already acquired some facility in avoiding catastrophes, but drugs and alcohol cloud judgment and dull responses for all participants at all levels of experience. Fatigue may slow both reflexes and judgement and lengthen reaction time. Personal physical handicaps (e.g., vision, hearing, and neurological impairments) must always be taken into consideration in planning water skiing expeditions. A specific set of recognized communication hand signals (Fig 42.12), especially noting the skier's "I'm O.K."

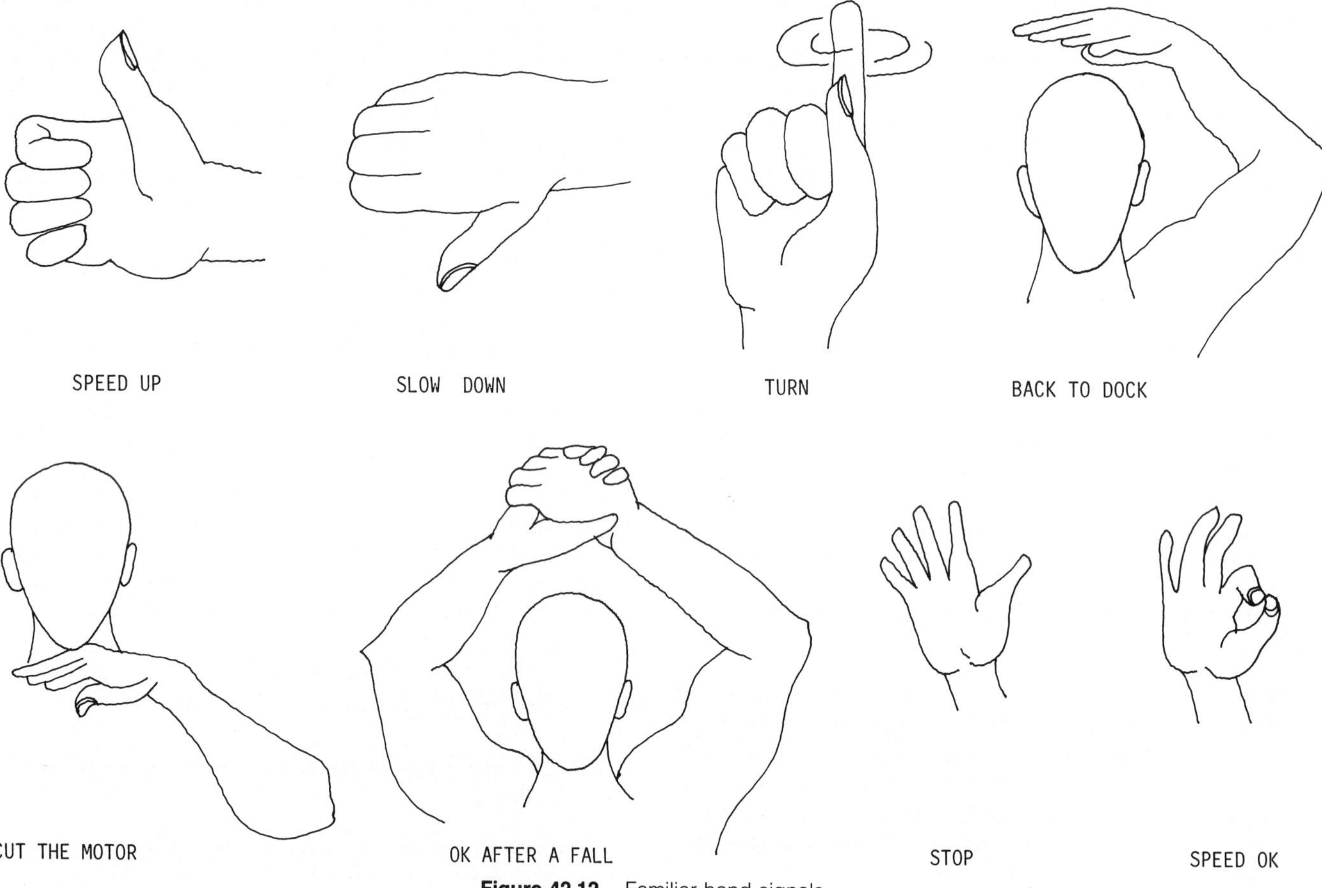

Figure 42.12. Familiar hand signals.

overhead clasp, must be known and discussed before skiing.

Skier. A water skier should be at least a comfortable swimmer, able to swim 50 m and stay afloat, i.e., treading water for a minimum of 5 min. He should be familiar with skiing areas and hand signals. He should be responsible for his own equipment, including an approved flotation device. Even the most accomplished swimmer who sustains a major head injury or loses consciousness while skiing is at risk without a life jacket. Pregnant women should probably avoid water skiing because of the risk of induced abortion from the hydrostatic pressure douches. Beginners and jumpers should wear protective pants (11).

Driver. Driving safety takes priority over skier enjoyment (20). The driver must take his responsibility seriously and should familiarize himself with both "good driving" skills and the skiing area before setting off. He should pay particular attention to the "starts." They should be gradual for water takeoffs and should have sudden acceleration just before the line is taut for dry takeoffs. The towrope must be disentangled and clearly seen between the skis. The skier should give a clear visual or verbal signal, e.g., "hit it," before the boat accelerates. The towboat should clear the dock or shore by 100 ft. for safe skier landing. Speeds must be adjusted according to the skier's skill and needs. Techniques for bringing the towline safely and quickly to the fallen skier must be learned (Fig. 42.13). Sharp, unbalanced turns must be avoided. It is the driver's responsibility to confirm the stability and safety of the towboat, doing so by insisting on an observer and on a minimum number of passengers to avoid weighing down the boat, thus decreasing its maneuverability.

Observer. In most countries and in some local communities, it is a legal requirement that there be an individual seated in the towboat, whose sole responsibility is to provide a liaison between the driver and the skier. He or she must advise the driver of the skier's position, signals, and falls and must provide information about boat traffic approaching from the stern. The observer must be familiar with the hand signals (Fig. 42.12). These signals have been developed as a technique for improving both safety and enjoyment by accurately conveying messages. Because observers can fall overboard and they may be called upon to help retrieve an injured skier, they should be capable swimmers and wear a life jacket.

Equipment (21, 22, 23)

Skis. These are designed differently for the different events (e.g., deep keels for slalom skis), but, in general, they must have simple mechanical bindings that are free of sharp and protruding surfaces, such as screws

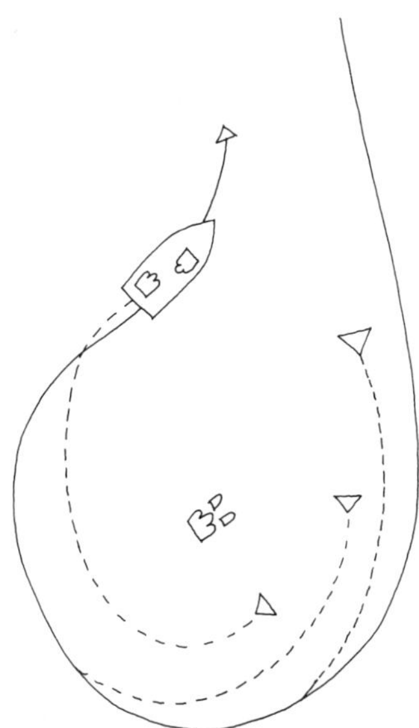

Figure 42.13. The "keyhole method" of skier retrieval is a most important maneuver. The boat passes the fallen skier on the side of the drive so that the rescuer may sideslip into position and provide aid. Care is taken not to turn abruptly away from the skier in order to avoid throwing the motor into the fallen athlete (see Fig. 42.9).

and bolts. Fittings must be easily adjustable, but secure. Although most injuries resulting from collisions with skis are minor, such collisions can sometimes be avoided if a fall is directed backward. Competitive skiers want their body weight centered over the skis and thus have nonadjustable bindings. Even "high wraps" should release during a fall.

Towropes, Handles and Pylons. These connections must be sturdy with strong construction. They must float and be free of knots, irregularities, and hardware. The rope must resist tremendous pressures, and the CWSA rule book specifies 12-strand, braided polypropylene that has minimal stretch.

The pylon must be mounted free of the motor so that the skier's pull is centrally located. This is particularly important for powerful slaloming skiers whose pull at the stern can completely redirect the boat.

Power Boats. The towing craft must be strong enough and yet maneuverable enough to provide a safe ride. The minimal suggested length is 14 feet, although 16 to 18 feet is preferable. Inboard or outboard craft should have at least 30 horsepower, i.e., capable of 20 to 30 mph. Cornering is safer if the beam is at least 60 to 70 inches. A steering wheel is mandatory. Basic safe boating accessories, including life jackets and fire extinguishers are imperative. Optional equipment includes windshields, speedometers, rearview mirrors, stern swim grids and/or boarding ladders.

Flotation Devices. Belt type flotation devices are easily dislodged and they are outdated. The jacket type is mandatory. Some of the early jackets were blamed for neck injuries because they forced the neck into hyperextension or flexion. There are several makes of approved, noninflatable life jackets, which do not impede ease of movement.

Jumps—Ramps and Helmets

Accidents involving competitive jumpers have resulted in a move by the IWSF to change the direction in which the ramp is anchored in the jumping course. The debate still continues, but, if the change is introduced, the jumper will presumably have less chance of misjudging his cut. Since 1975, helmets have also been compulsory for the jumping event in Canadian Water Ski Association sanctioned tournaments (3).

Water Hazards

Major visibility problems must be avoided on the water. Ideally, water skiing should be done on a calm, sunny, warm day in familiar water.

Light. It is both recommended and legislated that no water skiing should be done at night or even in twilight because of the difficulty of identifying water hazards that are not clearly marked, e.g., rafts.

Weather. Severe squalls, steady rain, or fog reduce visibility and increase the risks of collisions with water hazards or with other water sport enthusiasts.

Wind. Especially on large bodies of water, turbulent water markedly increases fatigue factors and sudden balance changes in skiers. If there are waves with white caps, the general rule is, don't ski.

Cold. Hypothermia becomes a risk after prolonged exposure to cold water. Wet suits should be used when conditions indicate.

Depth. A minimal depth of 5 to 6 feet of obstacle-free water is required for safe skiing.

Ski Area

A water skiing course should have a width of at least 200 feet (150 feet for tricks) and should be several thousand feet in length. A long straight run gives the skier a good opportunity to cross the wake and take advantage of the ride.

Traffic

Marinas, swimming, fishing, and sailing areas are generally out of bounds as areas for heavy ski traffic. Timing the use of the water space or using directional traffic controls can help congestion problems.

Obstacles

The area, if not already well known, must be surveyed by the team before starting skiing, so that water depth, docks, rocks, and other potential hazards can be identified. A skier should generally avoid landing on docks or on land and should not attempt to spray members of the audience. Strict attention should be paid to warning buoys.

Miscellaneous

There are special moments in the ski cycle that are most often associated with falls and other problems. These include the takeoff and landing. The skier's position outside on turns and on the bank of turning is important. Turning in on a skier will give tremendous slack rope and a sudden jerk on the arms. Approaching a fallen and possibly injured skier must be done in careful haste, always approaching him or her on the driver's side and cutting the throttle when close to the skier (Fig. 42.13). Even a propeller in neutral can turn enough to cause serious injury. All ropes must be exactly the same length during the multiple skier events. During these events ropes can intertwine, resulting in what can be potentially hazardous endeavors. Takeoff must be synchronized as well. Other skiers should drop as near as possible to an injured skier, but this should be done with extreme caution, since misjudging the drop can further endanger the already injured skier.

Safety

Tournament Level

Safety is a major priority of the International Water Ski Federation, which takes great pride and interest in very specific and controlled safety regulation. Many of the principles of this routine are adaptable to recreational water skiing even without the backup of a first aid station. The technical rules governing tournament procedures are available from the International Water Ski Federation (23).

A Tournament Safety Director is responsible for equipment, facility safety, and tournament operation, according to the safety principles already discussed. A medical advisor should be in attendance and these two individuals are responsible for skier supervision. Two fully equipped safety boats with experienced personnel must be on site in appropriately designated positions. The local governing body must be notified in order to receive permission to hold the tournament. Nontournament boat traffic must be controlled. Submerged hazards, such as rocks or pilings, should be clearly marked. Takeoff and landing areas must be assigned, clearly marked, and free of any sharp protrusions.

Prevention of Water Skiing Injury

1. The skier should be physically fit before water skiing with well-prepared limb muscles.
2. Ski time should gradually increase until the skier is fully fit for long sessions in order to minimize fatigue factors.
3. The hands should be protected with gloves, and they should be conditioned with dry-land practice to minimize blisters, and callouses.
4. Appropriate wetsuits should be worn for protection when conditions merit it.
5. Appropriate dress also should be worn between outings to maintain body heat.
6. Muscles should be warmed up and stretched before skiing; stretching should be repeated afterwards.
7. The skier should prepare mentally before competitive skiing, e.g., by visualizing the program.
8. A skier should train with competent drivers and observers and be knowledgeable in the operation of trick releases in competition.
9. Both the driver and observer should wear hats on sunny days and remain alert. Their roles should rotate often.
10. No skiing should be undertaken in hazardous conditions, such as high winds, large waves, sun glare, blinding rain, darkness, or dusk.
11. The site should be well known to the participants before water skiing.
12. An injury should preclude skiing unless a medical doctor or other health professional has given permission.
13. Courtesy and caution should be maintained toward other craft and the audience.
14. Water skiing should *never* be done under the influence of alcohol or drugs; no one who has been drinking should be allowed to control the towboat.

Note: Fitness for water skiing should include:

1. Endurance aerobics.
2. Specific strengthening exercise programs for hip adductors, full range hamstrings, and quadriceps muscles—with a view to minimizing stress on knee ligaments (e.g., anterior cruciate tears are common).
3. Stretching before and after ski runs is imperative.
4. Complicated trick maneuvers may require work on flexibility.

Specific Management of Injury Types

In water skiing, as with most sports, the occasional unprepared athlete will experience minor muscle aches in arms and legs, even after a short ski tour. With a graduated strengthening program or daily practice, these symptoms diminish. Calluses and blisters often develop in the hands, as discussed earlier. Minor bruises and abrasions usually require no more than the usual first aid, but occasionally, a major soft tissue injury, e.g., in the thigh or breast, will lead to fat necrosis and ultimate skin dimpling.

Added to the usual risks of injury sustained during high speed water skiing collisions, there is a need to treat the injured in the water and to get the skier out of the water without aggravation of the injury. The most important learned signal is the skier's "I'm O.K." shown by two hands clasped over the head. But even this signal can be done semipurposefully by a dazed or injured skier whose prime concern is to reassure others; therefore, this signal from a downed water skier should be evaluated carefully.

The Unconscious Skier

As with the medical evaluation of any unconscious patient, the unconscious skier must have an adequate airway. If the victim is not breathing, artificial respiration must be started, even in the water. Flotation devices keep the skier afloat, but the neck must be kept slightly extended. This position must be held manually or with a collar. The unconscious skier should never be passively hoisted into a boat but should be pulled to shore with head and neck under control where he or she can be floated or lifted on a stretcher or backboard to safety. A skier with vague responses to basic questions may well have a concussion. Any skier with a possible major head injury must be removed from the area and must not be allowed to continue skiing.

Bleeding

Most bleeding can be stopped with direct firm and constant pressure over the site. A bandage can be applied over the area, even if immersed. Water washes away blood clots and may prolong the bleeding. Any rectal or vaginal bleeding must be evaluated quickly and thoroughly, hence the advantage of having good medical facilities at hand. Major lacerations must be repaired at a hospital, where blood can be given to potentially shocked patients.

Suspected Fractures

A suspected fracture should be splinted in the water, preferably with available splints or, alternatively, by taping the injured leg snugly to the opposite leg. An injured arm can be anchored to the chest or supported in a sling. Boat cushions or jump jackets can be used for emergency purposes.

Hypothermia

Wet, shivering, preshock patients may be hypothermic as well. They should be dried and wrapped in blankets after retrieval from the water. Rapid and careful transportation of such victims to shore facilities is mandatory.

Summary

Although water skiing is a most exciting and, ultimately, safe sport, it does have some hazards. The age group participating is generally young and adventurous. Regulations pertaining to the safe conduct of towboats, etc. have evolved as a response to specific injuries. Added to the usual hazards of falls in any sport are the powerful motor boats, various marine obstacles, and the fact that the injured must be rescued from the water. Water ski tournament safety is well controlled, but major safety problems still exist with the recreational group where there is less care taken for safety precautions.

Acknowledgment

Illustrations drawn by Sophie Bodnarchuk-Zaworski

REFERENCES

1. Grace N. Water skiing hazards, nature and prevention. Phys Sports Med 1971;2:655.
2. Kistler B. How safe is water skiing? In: The Water Skier. Winterhaven, FL. American Water Water Ski Association, 1983.
3. Horne, J. The Canadian Water Ski Association Safety Manual. Oakville, Ontario, Publication of the Canadian Water Ski Association, 1973.
4. Paterson DC. Water-skiing injuries. Practitioner 1971;206:655.
5. Schneider RC, Livingston KE, Cave AJE, et al. "Hangman's fracture" of the cervical spine. J Neurosurg 1965;22:141.
6. Banta JV. Epidemiology of waterskiing injuries. West J Med 1979;130:493.
7. Paterson DC., Sweeney JG. Power-Boat injuries to swimmers. Med J Aust 1964;1:320.
8. May JW, Piliero C. The water skier seer syndrome. N Engl J Med 1979;300:865.
9. Kaiser RE, Armenia D, Baron R, Amenia D. Waterskier's enema. N Engl J Med 1980;302:1264.
10. Ramey JR. Intrarectal tear with bleeding from water skiing accident. J Fla Med Assoc 1974;61:162.
11. Gray HH. A risk of waterskiing for women. West J Med 1982;136:169.
12. Tweedale PG. Gynecological hazards of water-skiing. Can Med Assoc J 1973;108:20.
13. Pfanner D. Salpingitis and water skiing. Med J Aust 1964;1:320.
14. McCarthy GF. Hazards of water-skiing. Med J Aust 1969;1:481.
15. Morton DC. Gynaeocological complications of water-skiing. Med J Aust 1970;1:1256.
16. Kizer KW. Medical hazards of the water skiing douche. Ann Emerg Med 1980:9:268.
17. Radford AJ, Baggoley C, Crompton O, et al. Waterskiing injury. Australian Family Physician 1987;16(11):1661–1663.
18. Blazier RB, Morawa LG. Complete rupture of the hamstring origin from a water skiing injury, Am J Sports Med 1990;18(4):435–437.
19. Horne J, Cockshott WP, Shannon HS. Spinal column damage from water ski jumping. Skeletal Radiol 1987;16:612–616.
20. Ostberg JJ. Safer Boat Driving for Water Skiing. Winterhaven, FL. American Water Ski Association.
21. Davis MW, Reichle M, Kistler B. The ABC's of water skiing. Publication of the U.S. Department of Transport and the U.S. Coast Guard.
22. McDonald SH. Safety in Water Skiing. Winterhaven, FL. American Water Ski Association
23. World Water Ski Union. Technical Rules. Winterhaven, FL. The World Water Ski Union, Pub, 1980.

43 / WRESTLING

Mark C. Mysnyk and George A. Snook

Introduction

Wrestling is one of the oldest competitive sports and is practiced in one form or another in all countries. The Olympics and other international competitions involve one of two styles of wrestling. Freestyle is directly descended from ancient forms of wrestling as depicted in Greek and Egyptian art. Greco-Roman wrestling is a more modern form developed in Europe in the late 19th century. Both styles emphasize takedowns and pinning, with little mat wrestling. Greco-Roman differs from freestyle in that no holds can be applied to an opponent below the waist and the legs cannot be used to trip or hold the opponent.

High school and American collegiate wrestling is called folkstyle and was developed from the British Lancashire style. It is similar to freestyle, except the scoring varies slightly and there is relatively less time spent on takedowns and more on mat wrestling. It is popular in the United States, with more than 270,000 high school participants. Its popularity is based in part on the fact that multiple weight classes allow competitors of all sizes to participate.

Incidence of Injury

Unfortunately, wrestling is associated with a high injury rate. Most injury surveillance studies rank wrestling second only to football (1, 2). Depending on how injuries are defined, the injury rate in high school is between 23% and 75% (2–4), whereas in college more than 50% of participants will sustain an injury severe enough to see a trainer or physician (5–7). The number of injuries in collegiate wrestling is even more impressive, though, when expressed as the total number of injuries per wrestler: the rate is an average of 0.7 to 2.4 injuries per wrestler (5–7).

The anatomic area of greatest concern is the knee. It accounts for the most injuries, the most serious injuries, the most surgeries, and the most long-term problems (5–8). Injuries to the shoulder and head/neck (the specific rank order between these two varies in different studies) are also relatively frequent. In addition, although many studies do not include skin disorders in their list of injuries, those that do clearly indicate that skin infections are a major area of concern (5, 6).

More injuries occur in practice than competition, but this is because tremendously more time is spent in practice than in matches. In one report of the injury rate per exposure time, wrestlers were at a 40 times greater risk of sustaining an injury in matches than in practice (7). Takedowns are the highest risk activity (and even more specifically, most injuries occur to the wrestler being taken down); the bottom position on the mat is the next riskiest position, and the top position on the mat is the safest.

Mechanism of Injury

Direct Blows

Direct contact with the mat or the opponent can cause injury. The rules do not allow slams, and at least in high school and collegiate competition, most of the dangerous throws and moves have been made illegal. However, a typically safe move can become dangerous if not done properly or if partially countered, such as demonstrated in Figure 43.1. Direct blows to the head, resulting in compression or stretch injuries to the neck (or brachial plexus), or to the shoulder, resulting in acromioclavicular sprains, are the most frequent injuries from throws. Another way neck injuries occur is with hyperextension. This can occur as a wrestler's head hits his opponent's thigh as he is penetrating for a takedown (Fig. 43.2).

The knee frequently hits the mat during a shot or takedown attempt (Fig. 43.3). Prepatellar bursitis can result from either a single blow or repetitive trauma, resulting in either a bloody or serous effusion.

The most frequent injury caused by contact with the opponent is a nosebleed. Broken noses are much less frequent. Concussions and facial lacerations result from direct head-to-head collisions, such as when both wrestlers attempt a takedown at the same time. Also rela-

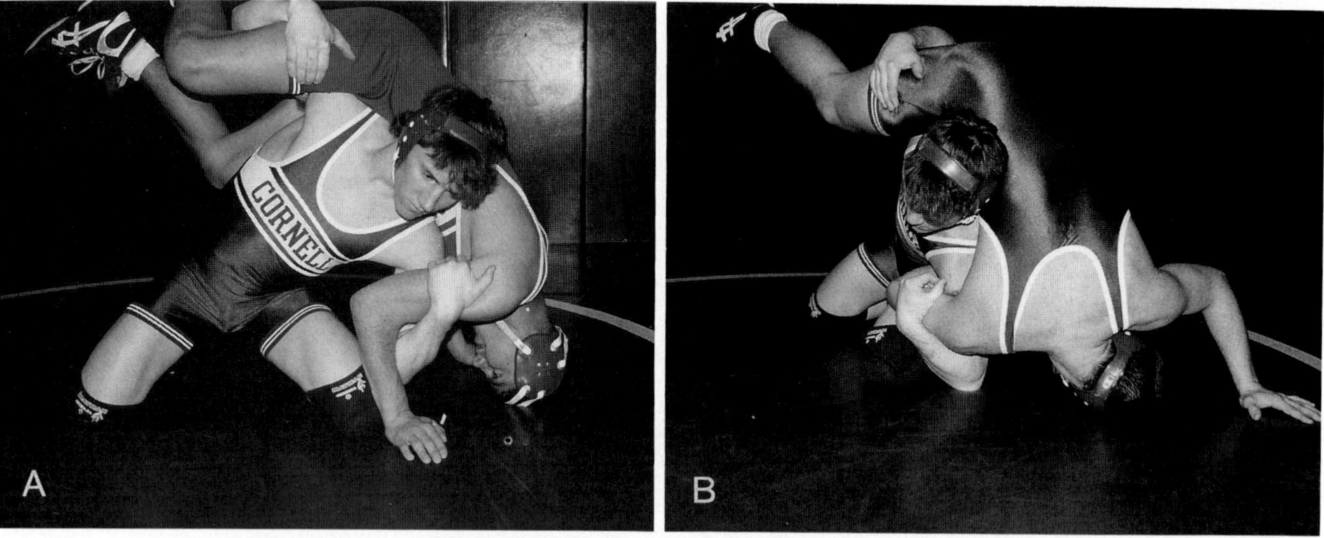

Figure 43.1. The fireman's carry. **A,** There is a direct blow to the top of the head, resulting in a possible compression injury. **B,** The same move is shown, causing a possible brachial plexus stretch injury.

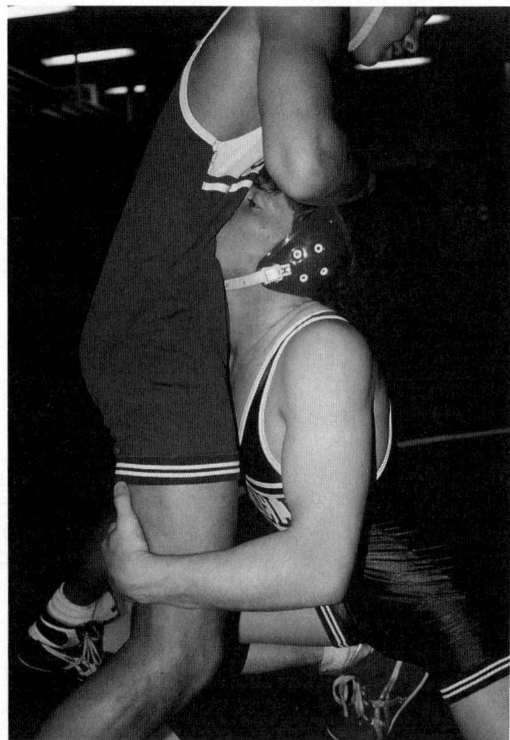

Figure 43.2. A cervical spine hyperextension injury can occur as the wrestler "shoots" or penetrates during a takedown attempt.

tively frequent are auricular hematomas, or cauliflower ear (Fig. 43.4). This is technically a subperichondrial hematoma, and whereas it represents a permanent scar in our culture, it is a source of pride for European and Asian wrestlers who rarely use head gear.

Friction injuries

Friction injuries probably account for most of the infections seen in wrestlers. Herpes simplex, which in wrestlers has been colorfully labeled "herpes gladiatorum" (Fig. 43.5), can spread through an entire team. It has not been well-documented how it is transferred from one wrestler to another, but the primary mechanism is likely direct contact with an infected wrestler, which would explain why most cases are on the face. A possible additional method of transfer is via the wrestling mat. One report sited a 18.8% prevalence and a 7.6% incidence in college wrestlers and a 2.6% incidence in high school wrestlers (9). As with any herpes infection, once an individual is infected, he always harbors the virus, and recurrences can follow emotional or physical stress.

Another common skin infection is impetigo, which is usually caused by *Staphylococcus aureus,* but may be *Streptococcus.* One other infection endemic to wrestlers is septic prepatellar bursitis. Some cases are believed to be blood borne from a distant infected source, but most result from direct penetration of the offending organism, even though a break in the skin is rarely detected. *Staphylococcus aureus* is again the most frequent organism (10).

Twisting and Indirect Force

A common injury mechanism, especially for knee injuries, is twisting and indirect force. Figure 43.6 shows a common mechanism during a takedown, resulting in valgus stress to the knee. Forces such as these result in muscle pulls, ligament sprains, and meniscal tears. The ankle, shoulder, and fingers are all susceptible. Although in other sports and in the general population, medial meniscal tears are approximately four to five times more frequent than lateral tears (11) (when the meniscal tear is not associated with a cruciate ligament injury), in wrestlers, the two are approximately equal. This is probably a result of the twisting forces involved in the sport.

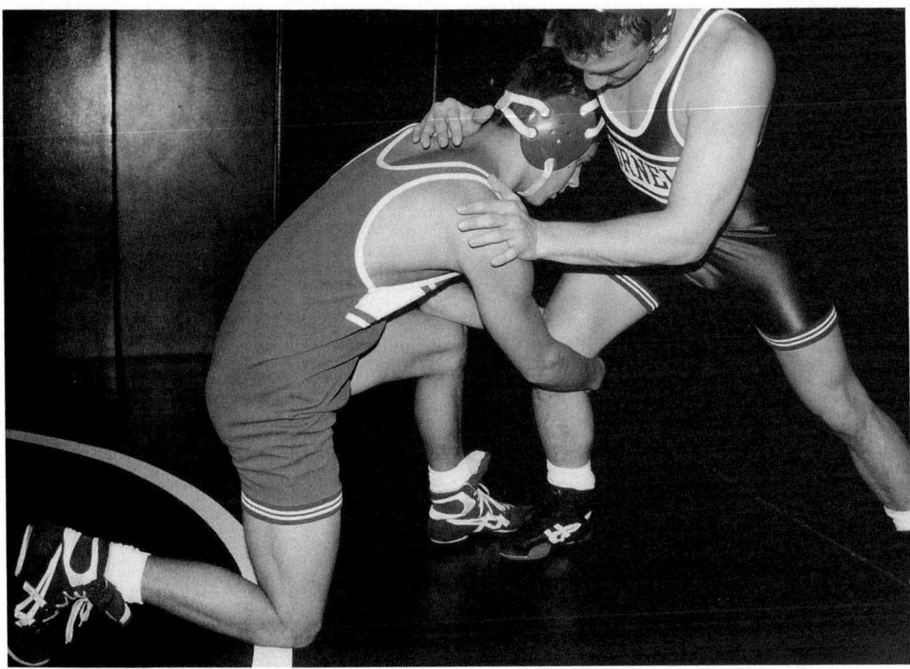

Figure 43.3. The knee is subject to repeated blows. In this case, the attacking wrestler's right knee has hit the mat as he performs a routine single-leg takedown attempt.

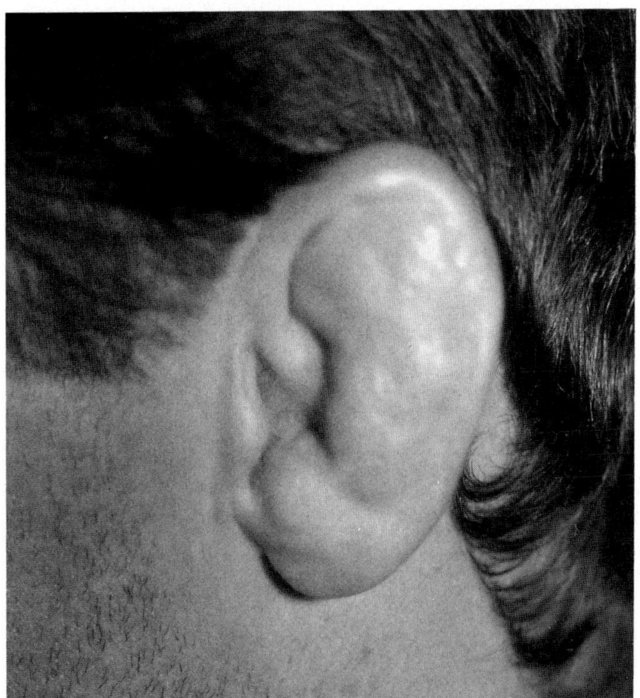

Figure 43.4. Chronic cauliflower ear. This can be prevented if acute episodes are treated properly.

Unknown

In part because of the intensity of the sport and probably also the result of accumulated multiple, and relatively mild stresses, the wrestler will frequently not be able to identify exactly when he got hurt. This is especially true of meniscal tears, which may insidiously start to ache or else lock for the first time following trivial stress. In a worker's compensation case, a similar history may create some question as to the seriousness of the problem, but when dealing with wrestlers, the treating physician should be aware that a significant injury may be present.

Prevention of Injuries

The most important factor in the prevention of wrestling injuries is the coach. The techniques the wrestlers use reflect the coach's teaching, and the athletes' attitude toward the sport reflect the coach's philosophy. He or she is in complete charge of the wrestling room, and absolute discipline is essential. Personal hygiene, proper care of the mats, and ensuring that the wrestlers wear their headgear at all times is the coach's responsibility.

Proper equipment is a necessary part of injury prevention. High school and collegiate rules require the use of headgear in matches, but it is up to the coaches to make sure they are used in practice. Although auricular hematomas can occur even when a wrestler is using his headgear, it happens infrequently, and headgear should be worn at all times. Unfortunately, headgear is illegal in international competition, and although allowed in American freestyle and Greco-Roman competitions, it must be removed if the opponent requests it. These rules should be changed. Once a hematoma occurs, it may help to build up the circumference of the headgear with plastizote to provide further protection (12) (Fig. 43.7).

Mouth guards are not mandatory, but their use should be encouraged. They should be mandatory for wrestlers with braces (for both their own and their op-

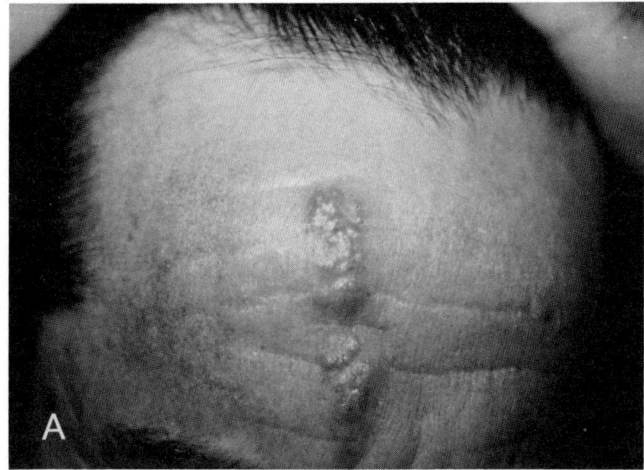

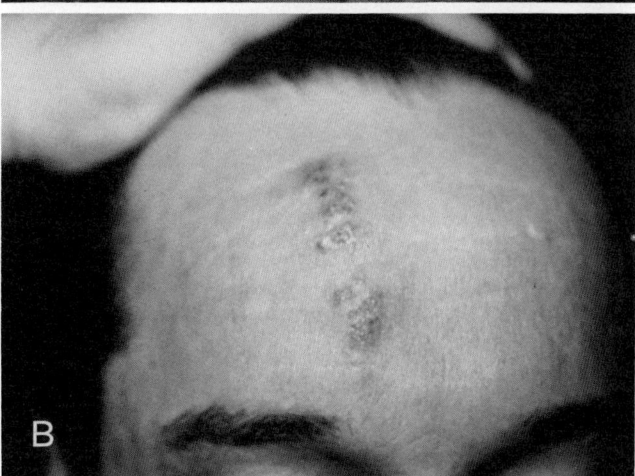

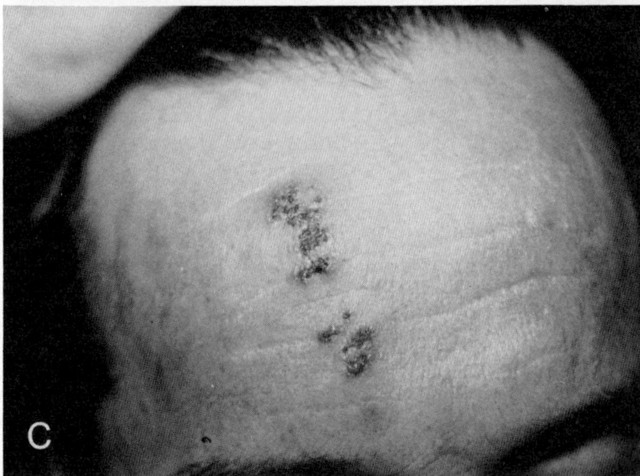

Figure 43.5. Various stages of herpes gladiatorum on a wrestler's forehead. A vesiculopapular rash is seen in **A,** whereas **B** and **C** show the progression to the crusted lesions.

ponents' protection). Likewise, while all wrestlers do not need knee pads, they likely decrease the risk of developing prepatellar bursitis. Especially in a wrestler who is recovering from or has "fully" recovered from an episode of bursitis, the bursa is likely thickened and more prone to recurrence. These wrestlers should wear a knee pad at all times.

Wrestling mats must be of proper resiliency to cushion falls. Because they lose resiliency with time, they should be periodically reconditioned (or if in bad enough shape, replaced). If a school is fortunate enough to have two mats, they should be placed one on top of the other in the practice room to provide extra protection (rather than rolling one of them up and storing it). A wrestling room must be of proper size to accommodate many wrestling pairs. It has been estimated that 50 square feet per participant is the minimum space needed to conduct practices and minimize the collisions (and, therefore, injuries) between pairs of wrestlers (13).

Because in any sport fatigue is an added factor that increases the risk of injury, conditioning is important in the prevention of injuries. It has been reported that the injury rate is highest early in the season, and this is believed to be caused in part by inadequate conditioning (7). If wrestlers want both to maximize their wrestling performance and to decrease the risk of injuries, they need to begin a cardiovascular conditioning program at least 6 weeks before the start of the season (year round is better). Both endurance and strengthening exercises are important, but the former is more critical for injury prevention and success on the mat. Neck conditioning and strengthening exercises are especially important and should be part of the off-season, preseason, and in-season conditioning program.

A final component of prevention, especially as concerns reinjury, is compliance. Wrestlers as a group are notoriously noncompliant (7), and this definitely increases the risk of reinjury. Anything that can be done to increase compliance is obviously important. As an example, if a knee absolutely needs to be immobilized, a cast may be necessary rather than a removable immobilizer. Second, the wrestler, his parents, and the coach should be carefully advised of the nature of the injury and the treatment plan. The treating physician cannot assume that the wrestler is relaying all the details to his parents and coach.

Even if these precautions are followed, though, many wrestlers will still be noncompliant. One wrestler the authors treated was placed in a cylinder cast following excision of a recurrent prepatellar bursitis, and the day after his hospital discharge, he ran 3 miles with the cast on!

Knowing that most wrestlers are compulsive and will seek out some physical activity, it is best to prescribe specifically a safe activity rather than telling the athlete to do nothing. For example, if he has an upper extremity injury, let him continue to run, ride an exercise bicycle, lift weights with his legs, etc. Although it varies for each specific injury, a general ranking of lower to higher risk activities, which can be used to return injured wrestlers gradually back to full participation is listed in Table 43.1.

Finally, a physician should be present at all wrestling matches. This may have no effect in preventing injuries, but as in any sport, proper initial treatment may prevent minor injuries from becoming more severe, and severe injuries from becoming catastrophic.

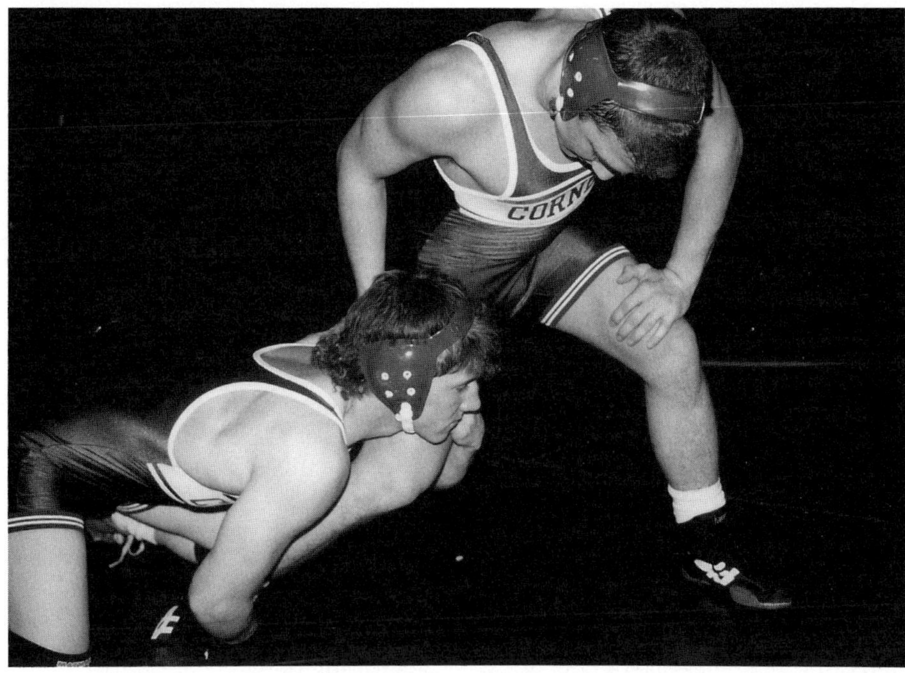

Figure 43.6. As the offensive wrestler is driving into his opponent, significant valgus stress to the knee can result.

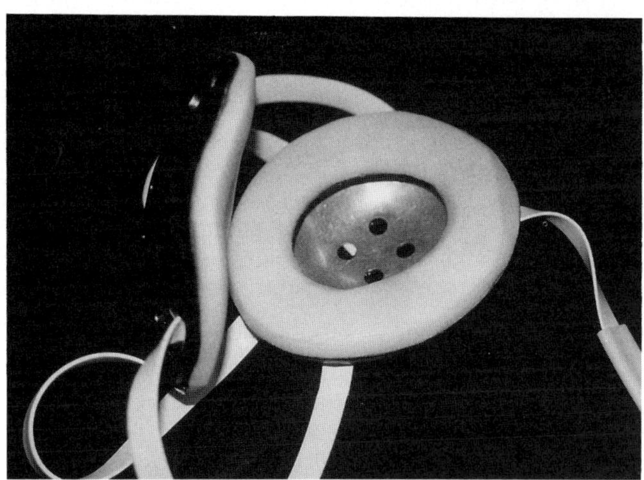

Figure 43.7. This headgear was modified by adding a piece of plastizote to the circumferential cushion to provide additional protection for a wrestler recovering from a cauliflower ear.

Table 43.1.
A General Rank of the Injury Risk of Wrestling Activities That May Be Used to Guide a Recovering Wrestler Back to Full Competition

1. Conditioning
2. Drilling
3. Down (mat) scrimmaging
4. Scrimmaging takedowns
5. Interscholastic competition

In addition, the physician can aid the referee and/or coach in deciding whether an injured wrestler can safely continue or not.

Treatment of Injury

First Aid and Emergency

Collegiate rules allow a competitor 90 sec of injury time. This is accumulative time for both treatment and recovery of injuries. High school competitors are allowed 2 min. The exceptions to this are nosebleeds or other bleeding injuries in which no injury time is counted. The rules also state that in cases of unconsciousness or serious injury to the head, neck, or spinal column, the contestant is not allowed to continue without the approval of a physician. In cases such as these, when the referee questions the ability of the competitor to continue, the examination does not need to be hurried, because if the injury time runs out, an official time-out can be declared to allow completion of the examination (once an official time-out is in effect, an examination only, not any treatment, can be done). If a wrestler is unable to continue because of an injury, the opponent is awarded the bout by default unless the injury occurred by an illegal move, in which case the injured athlete is awarded the decision by default (14).

Nosebleeds are one of the most frequent injuries during matches. Bleeding may be marked, but nearly all cases can be stopped by laying the wrestler down and plugging the nostril with cotton.

Lacerations require pressure to stop the bleeding, followed by butterfly or steristrip closure of the wound and further protection with an elastic wrap. Once the match is completed, if the laceration is severe enough it should be sutured and protected with a sterile dressing, and the wrestler should be allowed to continue competition.

A wrestler frequently can continue to wrestle with finger sprains by simply buddy taping the injured digit to the adjacent one. If an actual fracture is present, treatment must be individualized. Some phalangeal and metacarpal fractures are unstable and need extended cast immobilization or even surgery. Others (especially some metacarpal fractures) are stable, and the treatment just needs to be symptomatic. However, the rules do not allow any bandages, dressing, or casts of any materials that "do not allow normal movement of the joint" (14).

Probably the most demanding injury to evaluate at mat side is the cervical injury. While most cervical injuries are strains, the wrestler must be questioned and examined concerning any radicular symptoms. This can be caused by either a stretch injury of the brachial plexus or compression of a nerve root. If a wrestler suffers only transient radicular pain or burning into one or both arms, but it resolves completely within 1 to 2 min and there is no neurologic deficit (no weakness or sensory or reflex deficit), then the wrestler may return to competition immediately. Also, if there was never any neurologic symptoms but only neck pain and stiffness, the wrestler may continue to wrestle if his neck motion is functional (not necessarily completely normal, but nearly so). In contrast, if any weakness or neurologic deficit remains, a wrestler should not be allowed to continue. Competition may resume when the neurologic symptoms and deficits resolve, and neck strength and motion are normal. The physician should not be intimidated by the injury time clock and rushed into a hasty decision when evaluating a potentially serious injury. As explained above, if evaluation is being made as to the appropriateness of completing the match, an official time-out should be called and enough time for adequate evaluation given (but no treatment can be given during this time).

Subacute

As previously mentioned, the knee accounts for most injuries. Fortunately, the majority of knee injuries are minor, but as is well-known, a knee effusion should alert the treating physician that there may be a serious intraarticular injury. Injuries to the anterior cruciate ligament are much less frequent in wrestlers than other athletes, and in a wrestler, an effusion will usually indicate a meniscal tear (although tears frequently present without an effusion). Sprains of the collateral ligaments are the most frequent knee injury. The wrestler with a first-degree sprain can return as soon as pain allows him to. There may possibly be no time loss, or at most a couple of days. If there is a second- or third-degree sprain, the knee needs to be immobilized initially. At 1 to 2 weeks, range-of-motion, strengthening, and biking exercises can begin, but immobilization should be continued when not exercising. Return to actual wrestling will be variable, but in general should follow the progression of activities as outlined in Table 43.1.

Because prepatellar bursitis is quite frequent in wrestlers, it is important to consider this when evaluating a swollen knee. One simply needs to determine if the swelling is superficial to the patella and/or patellar tendon or deep to them. As prepatellar bursitis frequently recurs in wrestlers, aggressive initial treatment is essential to decrease morbidity and time loss.

An important component of this aggressive but appropriate treatment is aspiration of every acute case of bursitis. Although prepatellar bursitis is usually not painful (and if the wrestler absolutely must wrestle he usually can), it is important to rule out infection and to get the acute episode under control. If only a few milliliters of fluid is present, the wrestler can usually return to practice the next day (with a good knee pad in place). If more than 20 ml is present, the knee should be wrapped, immobilized, and examined (and reaspirated if necessary) daily until the bursitis has resolved. If the wrestler returns too soon and the bursa is traumatized again, the bursal wall can become thickened and recurrences may occur following minimal trauma (chronic bursitis). Although surgery is rarely required for prepatellar bursitis in the general population, it is often necessary in wrestlers if chronic bursitis is established. This is nonemergent, though, and can usually wait until the off-season.

Besides optimizing the chances of an acute traumatic bursitis resolving, a second reason for aspirating all cases of bursitis is to rule out infection. Unlike septic arthritis, septic bursitis is commonly missed clinically—it was unsuspected in more than 50% of the cases in one report (10)—because the wrestler is usually afebrile; has little, if any, pain; and no or minimal erythema, or warmth. The aspirate must be sent for cultures, as the appearance of the fluid and Gram's stain are normal in more than 50% of cases and the white blood cell count is rarely over 30,000 (10).

If diagnosed early, oral antibiotics and frequent aspirations (daily or every other day) may control the infection. If unresponsive, parenteral antibiotics and bursotomy (making a 1- to 1.5-cm incision on the medial or lateral aspect of the bursa, inserting a sterile hemostat to break up any adhesions or loculations, and then wicking the wound) is indicated. If it does not respond to this, surgery (bursectomy) is indicated.

Osgood-Schlatter disease is not caused by wrestling, but because the sport does require its participants to be on their knees, wrestling may aggrevate the condition. If the pain is tolerable, no treatment is necessary. If it becomes more severe, the initial treatment is the use of knee pads and trying to adjust practice and/or techniques so not as much time is spent on the knees. If it does not respond to this, then the wrestler needs to refrain from wrestling until the pain is tolerable.

The most frequent shoulder injury physicians will see is an acromioclavicular (AC) sprain. Treatment for a first-degree AC sprain (no displacement) is symptomatic. Although the injury is caused by a fall on the shoulder, surprising relief can usually be achieved with a doughnut-type pad of firm foam rubber or felt taped over the joint. If there is a step-off (a second- or third-degree sprain), the wrestler will need to be off at least a couple of weeks and not return to scrimmage until he has normal range of motion and at least 90% of his strength.

Numerous treatments have been suggested for auricular hematomas. The traditional treatment is aspiration with an 18-gauge needle and application of a cotton dressing soaked in collodion (15). Even if the wrestler wears headgear, though, it is difficult for him to get back to practice because the dressing frequently falls off. If it is going to be effective, the wrestler probably has to be held out at least a few days. Variations include incorporating a swimmer's nose clip within the collodion (16); substituting felt (white wool) or Webril for the cotton (17); using a plaster (18) or silicone mold (19); suturing buttons (20), or cotton bolsters (dental rolls) in place (21); incising the hematoma and leaving a Penrose (22) or continuous vacuum drain in (23); and allowing open drainage with excision of the fibroneocartilage (24).

When evaluating the alternatives, the following must be considered: effectiveness, invasiveness, cost, complications, and return to wrestling. Given these factors, aspirating (or incising if necessary to totally drain the hematoma) and securing anterior and posterior cotton bolsters with through-and-through suture (21) is probably the best choice. It can be done in the office, allows immediate return to wrestling, and is highly effective. There is a risk of infection; therefore, 4 to 7 days of prophylactic oral antibiotics and a daily application of antibiotic ointment on the suture line should be used. The bolsters are left in place 14 days.

Although not typically considered an injury, herpes simplex (herpes gladiatorum) has become a significant problem in wrestling. Outbreaks of herpes gladiatorum have affected entire teams, resulting in some meets being forfeited. Therefore, as mentioned earlier, wrestlers with herpes must be isolated—they should not resume practice until the lesions have reached the crusted stage (see Fig. 43.5*c*). The lesions will always eventually resolve spontaneously, but a 7-day course of oral acyclovir, 200 mg five times a day, can help speed the process, especially if started within 2 days of the onset of symptoms. Because herpes of any type cannot be cured, in those wrestlers prone to recurrences, a prophylactic dose of acyclovir (200 mg t.i.d.) should be considered for the entire season. In this dose, it is felt to be safe if used no more than 12 months.

Weight Loss and Making Weight

What has generated the most medical interest in wrestling is not the relatively high injury but the health implications of the process of "making weight." In an attempt to reach a lower weight class and, at least theoretically, gain an advantage, wrestlers lose weight through a combination of caloric restriction (dieting), exercise, and short-term dehydration. The dehydration may be from exercise alone, exercise with rubber sweats on, or use of a sauna (the latter two are legal in college but illegal in high school, although still used by some). The use of diuretics, laxitives, and self-induced vomiting have been reported but are not thought to be problematic (25).

Not all wrestlers lose weight to compete, but a large percentage of them do. Reported weight losses from preseason to competitive weight class, which involve both dieting and short-term dehydration, average 7.5% (26) and 7.3% (27) for college wrestlers and 5.7% (26) for high school wrestlers. Weekly weight losses (which in most cases is short-term dehydration) average 3.1% in high school wrestlers and 4.4% in college wrestlers (26). Or, expressed as the amount lost, 49% of high school wrestlers lost 1.4 to 2.3 kg and 23% lost between 2.7 and 4.5 kg weekly. In college wrestlers, 44% reported losing 2.7 to 4.5 kg and 41% stated that they lost 5 to 9.1 kg weekly (25).

For dual meets, college wrestlers typically have at least 5 hr between weigh-ins and competition, and for tournaments, they usually weigh in the night before competition giving them at least 16 hr in which they can eat and rehydrate. Most high school wrestlers weigh in the morning of a match and then have several hours to eat and rehydrate before wrestling that night. They repeat the same process for each competition, and this may be done 20 or more times a season.

Whether of practical use or not (as will be discussed later), attempts are being made to dictate the minimum weight each wrestler can go down to by measuring his fat percentage. The majority of these proposals agree that because of inaccuracies in the estimates physicians should have the final say of whether an athlete can wrestle at a weight lower than what is calculated for him (28–30). To be qualified to make an accurate assessment of what weight class a wrestler should wrestle, the consulting physician needs to be aware of the medical and performance concerns surrounding weight cutting.

In 1967, the American Medical Association's committee on medical aspects of sports came out with a physician stand on weight control in wrestling. In that they quoted their previous "unqualified objection, on both ethical and physiologic grounds, to indefensible practices of 'making weight' " (31). In 1976, the American College of Sports Medicine issued a similar condemnation of weight cutting, stating that it hurt performance and caused numerous adverse physiologic responses (32). Neither organization has issued an updated opinion, which is unfortunate, because not only could they not have possibly included the research that has been reported since that time but also they either overlooked or misinterpreted much of the literature available at that time. Neither statement can be considered an objective, current appraisal, indicating that physicians now dealing with the issue must examine the literature themselves and arrive at their own conclusions. What follows is a review of the issues concerning weight cutting in wrestlers.

Table 43.2.
Concerns of Weight Cutting in Wrestlers

Possible health risks
Cardiovascular or heart disturbances
Heat illness
Impaired renal function
Hypertension
Retarded growth
Decreased metabolic rate
Decreased testosterone levels
Eating disorders
Performance factors
Strength
Endurance
Work capacity

Pros and Cons

Table 43.2 includes a list of the pros and cons of weight-cutting. It can be seen that the only possible "pro" is a competitive advantage, while the "cons" can be divided into possible health risks and performance concerns. Each one of these will be dealt with separately.

Cardiovascular or Heart Disturbances

When wrestlers undergo short-term dehydration, they do not fully rehydrate if they have ≤5 hr between weigh-ins and competition, thus they compete in a dehydrated state (33–37). If dehydration is significant, it can cause a decrease in plasma volume, which in turn decreases stroke volume (38, 39). Following short-term weight losses (primarily through dehydration) of 1% to 11.8%, several studies showed no significant change in exercise heart rates (40–43). Other studies have shown an increased submaximal exercise heart rate following a dehydration weight loss that is reversible after a short period of rehydration. Following weight losses of 3.8% to 6.8%, initial exercise heart rates were increased, but after a partial rehydration period lasting 1 to 5 hr, exercise heart rates were restored to normal (44–47). The first of these studies concluded that ad libitum fluid replacement following a 48-hr weight-loss regimine (as typically practiced by wrestlers) "can effectively restore cardiovascular dynamics within one hour" (44). However, others have demonstrated a persistently increased exercise heart rate (39, 48). The consensus, though, seems to be that short-term dehydration of less than 5% poses no significant load on the heart and no adverse effect on performance.

Heat Illness

Although the decreased plasma volume poses no significant cardiac risk, it can impair sweat production (38), theoretically predisposing the athlete to heat illness. There are four disorders commonly referred to as heat illness: heat cramps, heat syncope, heat exhaustion, and heat stroke. The last of these can go on to death. They are potential risk for any athlete or any individual who works on a hot day or in a hot environment and sweats. Although there are no known reported cases of wrestling-related heat stroke deaths, there were 54 deaths in football players between 1964 and 1983 (49). This is not to say that wrestlers are not at risk, but relatively speaking it does not appear to be a significant problem.

Impaired Renal Function

Blood and urine chemistries of high school and college wrestlers at weigh-ins revealed changes consistent with dehydration (27, 33). It has been speculated that this dehydration can cause acute renal ischemia and perhaps produce renal problems in middle-aged wrestlers (50).

It is well-documented that exercise alone is associated with proteinuria, decreased renal blood flow, decreased glomerular filtration rate, decreased urinary water excretion, changes in electrolyte excretion, hemoglobinuria, and myoglobinuria (51, 52). These changes are associated with any form of exercise and are related to the intensity of exercise and can be exacerbated by dehydration. Wrestling certainly combines intense exercise and dehydration, and therefore, all of these changes can occur in wrestlers. However, all of them are acute changes that are reversible and cause no known long-term problems.

To evaluate for possible long-term effects of wrestling on renal function, the renal function of 320 former wrestlers was compared with 220 controls who had never wrestled. All subjects were between the ages of 30 and 84. Blood samples were used to estimate creatine clearance, and urine specimens were used to calculate a urine protein:urine creatinine ratio as an estimate of proteinuria. It was concluded that in that study population "the reported acute changes in renal function associated with exercise and accentuated by dehydration have no long-term adverse effects on renal function" (26).

Hypertension

There is no evidence that wrestlers, as a group, are hypertensive (50), but it has been suggested that renal damage could cause hypertension later in life (33). As just explained, there is no evidence of any long-term renal damage in former wrestlers. In addition, as part of that same study (26), the blood pressure of all subjects was recorded. There were no significant differences between the wrestlers and controls.

Growth

Because wrestlers typically diet in addition to dehydrating to make weight, it is feared that the process may impede normal growth and development (32). There are anecdotal reports of individuals who wrestled being several inches shorter than their nonwrestling brothers (53), and Tipton (54) has stated that his studies "crude and limited as they are—imply that a reduction in growth will result from chronic weight-cutting." No evidence, however, was presented to support this hypothesis.

It would take a longitudinal study of the growth curves of individuals and controls before they began wrestling and continued until they reached skeletal maturity to determine if wrestling has an effect on height. However, there is evidence to suggest that it does *not*. In adolescents, it has been shown that chronic caloric deficiency can retard normal growth (55–57). Whether the deficiency is corrected (55, 56) or not (57), though, skeletal growth and maturation can be slowed and the growth spurt delayed, but the growth period is prolonged and normal adult height is eventually achieved. It seems that because there is this much resiliency to growth, despite several years of uncorrected caloric deficiency, no adverse effects would be expected in wrestlers who, at worst, have repeated short-term episodes of caloric deficiency interspersed with normal eating during a 3- to 4-month season.

Supporting this is a study that compared the heights of skeletally mature former wrestlers with controls who never wrestled. Both their absolute heights and their heights relative to their fathers' were compared. While former wrestlers were shorter than nonwrestlers, there was *no* correlation between the amount of weight lost during their wrestling careers and their heights relative to their fathers'. It was concluded that wrestlers are not short because they wrestled, but that they became wrestlers because they are short, i.e., there is a selection phenomena (58).

Decreased Metabolic Rate

A group of wrestlers classified as "weight cyclers" (those that lost greater than 4.5 kg at least 10 times a season) was found to have lower resting metabolic rates than a group classified as noncyclers (those who lost less than 1.4 kg weekly). It was concluded that weight cycling produced a lower resting metabolic rate and that in adult life this could cause weight-control problems (59). In contrast to this study, a longitudinal study was done that evaluated the resting metabolic rate in preseason, midseason and postseason. It was shown that the resting metabolic rate did decrease during the season, but that the postseason value was similar to the preseason value. It was concluded that weight cycling did not produce a lasting decreased resting metabolic rate (60).

Testosterone Levels

It has been demonstrated that in wrestlers testosterone levels decreased in midseason and that serum testosterone levels were correlated with low body fat. The levels returned to normal, though, postseason (61). This effect is not unique to wrestling but occurs with any form of intense exercise and is not felt to be of any major significance (62).

Eating Disorders

If a wrestler diets and exercises to make weight an average of two times per week for 3 months (the season is 4 months), is overconcerned about his weight (which could be expected at each weigh-in), and then eats a large amount after making weight, he has met a liberal interpretation of four of the five *DSM*-III-R criteria for bulemia. If during the weigh-in meal, either because of extreme thirst, hunger, or whatever, he feels a lack of control, he has met all five criteria. Although this is not bulemia, an evaluation of college wrestlers suggested that wrestlers may be at risk for the development of sports-induced eating disorders, but no definite abnormalities were found (63). As is clear from the previous discussion of the *DSM*-III-R criteria, it was emphasized that "caution must be invoked in interpreting the results of these questionnaires as measuring symptoms of psychopathy associated with eating."

Performance

There are both proponents and opponents of weight-cutting when performance is discussed. The theoretical reason for losing weight, the experimental findings, and the epidemiologic findings will each be examined.

Theoretical

The theoretical reason for losing weight is to gain a competitive edge in physical size and strength. As an example, imagine two wrestlers of equal ability, both at 14% body fat 2 months before the season begins. One weighs 130 pounds and decides he is not going to lose any weight and will wrestle at 130. The other weighs 151 pounds and begins his diet 2 months before the season starts to lose fat weight and get down to 137 pounds at 5% body fat (Table 43.3). The night before the match he dehydrates 5% of his weight to get down to 130 pounds and, therefore, weighs in at the same weight as the other individual. If they wrestled right as they came off the scales, they would weigh the same, but the wrestler who lost more weight would have a larger body frame and would likely be stronger (the theoretical argument against this is that the weight-cutting process weakens and fatigues the wrestler). In addition, as already mentioned, wrestlers usually have at least 5 hr and sometimes as much as 24 hr to eat and drink before competition. The wrestler who lost no weight and is at his baseline would likely gain no weight in that precompetition period; however, it is not uncommon for wrestlers who have lost a lot of weight to gain 5 to 10 pounds in that period. Because many high school weight classes are separated by just 5 pounds, at the time the two wrestlers get on the mat to face each other, the one could have a one, or even two, weight class advantage.

Experimental Findings

Many experimental studies have been done to assess the effects of weight loss (through various combinations of exercise, dehydration, and caloric restriction) on strength, endurance, exercise heart rate, cardiovascular conditioning ($\dot{V}_{O_2max}$), and work capacity. There are conflicting results found in the literature, largely because of differences in experimental design. It is known that there may be different physiologic affects whether the weight is lost by use of diuretics, sauna, or exercise (64). The environment the tests are conducted in (comfortable, hot-wet, or hot-dry) (38, 65),

Table 43.3.
Ideal Body Weight Determination[a]

Lean Mass	+1%	+2%	+3%	+4%	+5%	+6%	+7%	+8%	+9%	+10%	+11%	+12%	+13%	+14%	+15%
130.72	132	133	135	136	137	139	140	141	142	144	145	146	148	151	153
							Dehydration Tables								
−1%	131	132	132	135	136	138	139	140	141	143	144	145	147	148	149
−2%	129	130	130	133	134	136	137	138	139	141	142	143	145	146	147
−3%	128	129	129	132	133	135	136	137	138	140	141	142	144	145	146
−4%	127	128	128	131	132	133	134	135	136	138	139	140	142	143	144
−5%	125	126	126	129	130	132	133	134	135	137	138	139	141	142	143
−6%	124	125	125	128	129	131	132	133	133	135	136	137	139	140	141
−7%	123	124	124	126	127	129	130	131	132	134	135	136	138	139	140
−8%	121	122	122	125	126	128	129	130	131	132	133	134	136	137	138
−9%	120	121	121	124	125	126	127	128	129	131	132	133	135	136	137
−10%	119	120	120	122	123	125	126	127	128	130	131	131	133	134	135

[a] Current weight, 151 pounds; lean body mass, 130.7 pounds; body fat, 14%.

the subjects' diet (high or low carbohydrate) (66, 67), whether the subjects are heat acclimatized or not (less increased heart rate following dehydration with heat acclimization (36, 68), the conditioning of the subjects (39, 69), whether recovery time and/or rehydration are allowed or not (45, 46, 70, 71), and the time frame for the weight loss can all affect the results.

One final factor that can drastically affect performance in experiments or actual wrestling competition following weight loss is the psychological response to that weight loss. This can vary dramatically with individuals. Because it is impossible to control for this effect, it must also be considered when looking at and comparing the results of the studies. Given these variables, a brief review of the literature follows.

Exercise Heart Rate. As was discussed earlier, although there may be some exceptions, the majority of the research indicates that exercise heart rate, cardiac output, and other hemodynamic variables are back to normal following a 5-hr rehydration period (even if all of the lost fluid is not replaced) (47). Because wrestlers typically have a minimum of 5 hr to rehydrate, there is probably no detrimental effect on any of these variables.

Maximum Oxygen Uptake. There are at least four studies showing no significant decrease in maximum oxygen uptake following a short-term weight loss (39, 42, 67, 72), although one of these did show a "trend" (42).

Strength. From Table 43.4 it can be seen that the majority of studies show no decrease in strength with a weight loss of 8% or even more. Those few studies showing a negative effect on strength demonstrated it in only a minority of the muscles tested.

Endurance and Work Capacity. It has been suggested that weight cutting may impair performance by various means: exercise depleting the glycogen stores; increased muscle temperatures; or dehydration causing a decreased plasma volume and electrolyte shifts (76). The effects of these are hard to separate experimentally, and in addition, there is a psychological effect of weight loss mentioned above. It is not surprising, then, that the experimental effects of weight loss on muscular endurance and work capacity are quite variable.

Table 43.4.
Effect of Weight Loss on Strength

Effect	Reference	Percent Weight Loss	Comment
Increase			
	48	2.25 kg	No percentage was given
No change			
	39	3.6–4	
	43	3.6–4.9	
	36	5	
	72	3.7–9.5	
	41	2.1–11.8	
	40	7.1	
	67	8	
Decrease			
	73	3.1	Significant decrease in one of five muscle groups tested
	74	8	Decrease in only the lowest of three speeds tested
	75	4.9	Decrease in 2 of 16 tests

No effect on endurance was shown in two studies with weight losses of 3.7% to 9.5% (72) and 5% (36). An evaluation of subjects tested in euhydrated, dehydrated, and partially rehydrated states concluded that "both isotonic and isometric endurance . . . decreased significantly" (77). However, an analysis of the data showed that of the four muscle groups tested, two of these groups were not significantly affected isometrically or isotonically by dehydration, and in the rehydrated state (which would parallel a wrestling situation), three of the muscle groups tested isometrically were increased over the euhydrated levels. Another study showed a 10% decrease in work capacity and 12% decrease in run time to exhaustion, but the subjects were tested with no food or water in the 12 to 16 hr before testing, which is not realistic for wrestlers (75).

Three experiments compared euhydrated and dehydrated work performance with no rehydration allowed. In a 6-min arm-crank test, wrestlers who lost approximately 6.2% of their weight over 4 days by a low-carbohydrate diet and restriction, exercise, and dehydration demonstrated a 7.9% decrease in total work. With the same weight loss but on a high-carbohydrate diet, the decrease was significantly less than on a low-carbohydrate diet, and some wrestlers actually improved their performance (66). Following a 3.6% to 4% weight loss in nonwrestlers with "marked differences in fitness," work time was significantly decreased on a bicycle ergometer. The well-trained subjects showed a smaller decreased work time than those in poorer shape (39). In contrast, following a 5% dehydration weight loss, wrestlers showed no significant decrease in average or peak power or in work time on a bicycle ergometer anaerobic test. In fact the wrestlers' total and peak power per kilogram of weight increased with the weight loss, suggesting a benefit of weight cutting (78).

In a situation similar to what a college wrestler would experience, four studies used present or former wrestlers and had them lose 5% (70, 71), 3.7% to 9.5%)72), and 8% (74), respectively, of their weight, and then allowed them to eat and rehydrate over 3 to 5 hr as they would for a match. In two of these, a decreased performance was demonstrated when the subjects were tested within 1 hr of making weight, but all four studies showed a return to normal after 5 hr. One of these studies included muscle biopsies to assess glycogen levels (74). During the 96 hr of weight reduction, muscle glycogen levels decreased 46% and recovered only 14% in the 3-hr rehydration period. Despite this, neither performance, strength, or $\dot{V}_{O_2max}$ were significantly decreased.

In summary, as would be expected, some physiologic changes do occur with weight losses of 3% to 12%. There is no universal effect on all muscle groups. In addition, significant recovery occurs when 5 hr of rehydration (which correlates with the minimum time wrestlers usually have) is allowed before testing. In addition, it appears that if the subjects are regularly consuming a high-carbohydrate diet and are well-conditioned, the changes that do occur will be less. While there may be exceptions, if at least a 5-hr rehydration period is possible, significant detrimental effects on exercise heart rate, $\dot{V}_{O_2max}$, muscle strength, endurance, and performance are unlikely following short-term weight losses of 5% or even more.

Epidemiologic Findings

Table 43.5 shows the fat percentages of various wrestlers. Heavyweights, who do not have to lose any weight, naturally have the highest fat percentage, and in general, the lowest weight classes have the smallest fat percentage. It can be seen that most successful wrestlers are less than 7% body fat, and some even less than 5%. It could be argued that these same individuals would have been as, or even more, successful at a higher fat percentage. However, as can be seen in Table 43.6, in three studies comparing the fat percentages or skinfold totals with the success of the wrestlers, the more successful wrestlers were leaner.

In summary, a reduction to 5% body fat and a short-term dehydration of up to 5% has not been shown to have detrimental effects on health or performance. *Within the parameters discussed,* there is in fact theoretical, experimental, and epidemiologic evidence that performance may be enhanced.

What Weight Class?

Most current recommendations condemn any dehydration and suggest 7% as being the minimum fat percent (85). This does not make sense in light of the above findings that most successful wrestlers are less than 7% or even 5% body fat and that up to a 5% dehydration does not significantly affect performance values, especially if a short rehydration period is allowed.

Because individual wrestlers almost certainly react differently both physiologically and psychologically to dieting and dehydration, there is probably no one ideal

Table 43.5.
Documented Fat Percentages of Wrestlers

Subjects	Range (%)	Average (%)	Comment	Reference
High school wrestlers	4.2–18.3	6.9	Range for lower 12 weight classes was 4.2–6.5%; the average was 5.0%	79
Top four place winners at various high school tournaments	4.4–15.5	6.9	Between the 101- and 170-pound weight classes, range was 4.8–6.7%; the average was 5.8%	80
State finalists	<3–>10	7.3	Approximately 33% were <5%	81
Elite junior wrestlers		7.2±2.4	Not down to competitive weight when measured; therefore, actual values likely lower	82
Junior world team		7.3±0.6	Range for lower 12 weight class was 4.2–6.5%; the average was 5.0%	83
NCAA qualifiers		4.0±0.5		84

Table 43.6.
Studies Comparing Fat Percentage of Skinfold Totals with Levels of Success

Reference	Summary
81	Of NCAA qualifiers, the fat percent of All-Americans was 3.7; of those not placing but winning at least one match, 3.9; and those not winning any matches, 4.2. The most successful wrestlers lost the most weight and were generally the leanest.
28	Skinfold totals were 33% lower in high school finalists than in "average" high school wrestlers.
82	Skinfold totals in state place winners were 34% lower than in non–place winners.

fat percentage that can be applied to every wrestler. Except for the heaviest weight classes, 5% to 7% body fat can be used as a guide, but some wrestlers can more effectively compete at a lower and some at a higher fat percent.

Another reason why everyone should not be encouraged to conform to one "ideal" fat percentage is that the methods used to determine fat percentage are not accurate enough. Hydrostatic weighing (densitometry), anthropometry (either with skinfolds or body dimensions), and bioelectrical impedance analysis (BIA) have been used to estimate fat percentage. Although the prediction of mean values for a large population is relatively good, prediction of individual body fat percentages is not (79), and "it is clear that, regardless of the methods used, determination of minimal wrestling weights is a process which is inherently subject to relatively broad margins of error" (86). Underwater weighing is considered the gold standard, but the calculated fat percentage is accurate only within ±2% to 4% (87). Skinfolds have been used most frequently for wrestlers, because of convenience and cost. The various equations, however, have a 3% to 9% margin of error (88). Even the best skinfold equations have only a 67% confidence level that spans at least 4.88 kg (10.75 pounds) (29). This standard deviation covers more than two high school wrestling weight classes, and in one of three cases the error will be even greater.

While some gifted individuals can wrestle successfully at any of two or three weight classes, there are many more examples of wrestlers who could win, and win safely, a state or NCAA title at one weight class, but not even place at two or even one weight class above that. With the inaccuracies of minimal weight predictions, they should not be used as more than a rough guide to the proper weight class.

What should determine the proper weight class? Performance. Wrestlers, parents, and coaches should be educated on proper weight cutting and nutrition, and then the three parties together should decide on the proper weight class based on performance. This is performance not just on the mat but also in school and at home. If a wrestler is so preoccupied with making weight that family relations are strained or school work suffers, he is either cutting too much weight or losing it incorrectly. If the wrestler is not performing well on the mat and seems to be getting tired near the end of the match, he could be cutting too much weight, be cutting it wrong, be eating incorrectly, be out of shape, or not be getting enough sleep. There are many possible explanations for poor performance besides cutting too much weight, and each must be examined.

It is important that a wrestler not mistake water loss for fat loss. For the 151-pound wrestler with 14% body fat discussed above, Table 43.3 shows how he could get down to 130 pounds by reducing to 5% body fat and then undergoing a short-term 5% dehydration. As outlined above, these would be safe parameters. It would not be prudent, though, for the wrestler to reduce only to 144 pounds (10% body fat) by dieting and then dehydrate 10%. Although this would get him to his target weight, he would have done so by excessive dehydration, which would likely affect his performance. Conversely, if a wrestler seems to be getting beat because he is getting outmuscled, and if the fat percentage estimate indicates he has fat to lose, it can be suggested that he try a lower weight class. No wrestler should ever be forced to go down to a lower weight, though, because that can be the quickest way to make the wrestler lost interest in the sport.

Safe Weight-Cutting Guidelines

There are few absolutes concerning proper weight cutting, but one is that not everyone needs to cut weight. The target figure for most weight classes, as noted, is 5% to 7% body fat. Heavy weights and the upper weights may have much more body fat. Successful wrestlers may be found above and below this range, and it must be remembered that even with the gold standard of underwater weighing, a wrestler told that he has 10% body fat may actually have 8% to 12% body fat, and with skinfold determinations, the range is even larger.

Another absolute concerning proper weight-cutting is that there's no place for diuretics, laxitives, or self-induced vomiting. If a wrestler is going to lost weight, he should start his diet early (1 or more months before the season starts) and plan to lose 1 to 2 pounds per week. More rapid weight loss from dieting could result in loss of lean muscle mass rather than fat. A 1-pound loss is a 3500-calorie deficit; therefore, either input has to be decreased and/or output has to be increased. As a ballpark figure, running 1 mile takes approximately 125 calories and an intense 30-min workout uses 500 calories. The wrestler should consume a minimum of 1500 to 2000 calories a day both preseason and in season. The goal is to lose the fat weight by the start of the competitive season. If he so desires (not everyone needs to), the wrestler can safely dehydrate up to 5% short term (less than 48 hr) to make weight. Dehydration longer than this could interfere with concentration in school or the conditioning and technical aspects of wrestling practice.

The wrestler should regularly consume a balanced

diet of 50% to 60% carbohydrates, 25% to 30% fats, and 10% to 20% proteins. If athletes are regularly consuming a balanced diet with enough calories, they do not require a vitamin supplement. However, in the case of wrestlers, a supplement is a good idea. A simple multivitamin should suffice (there is no need for expensive supplements). Commonsense dieting tips include counting calories (available in food content and calorie books), eliminating junk food and fluid-retaining (salty) foods, consuming low- or no-calorie fluid, substituting white for red meat, and avoiding frying in food preparation.

Because a hard workout and an overnight fast can deplete muscle and liver glycogen stores, wrestlers should ideally have their weight under good enough control so that they can have a good meal high in carbohydrates the night before a match. It is at that time that they should change to fluids with calories. Wrestlers "drift," or lose 0.5 to 2 pounds overnight, and each wrestler should know precisely how much he drifts and take this into account when he plans how much he can eat or drink the night before. If a workout is needed the day of the match, it should be a light one to avoid further glycogen depletion.

The precompetition meal is best consumed 5 or more hr before competition. It should be very high in carbohydrates, because fats slow absorption and excessive protein may worsen dehydration owing to obligatory water excretion with excess nitrogen (89). If less than 2 hr are allowed between weigh-in and competition, a liquid meal should be consumed.

Regardless of the time interval, fluid replacement should begin immediately after the weigh-in. A 6% to 10% carbohydrate drink should be consumed—it is absorbed as fast as water and in addition supplies needed carbohydrates and calories (90). Caffeine should be avoided, as it may have a diuretic effect and, therefore, promote water loss.

During a tournament, athletes may wrestle several times in one day. Thus they should replenish fluids and carbohydrates throughout the day. Although convenient for coaches, the entire team should not wait for a break between matches to go eat. The lighter weight class will finish (and subsequently start) at least 2 hr before the heavyweights and should, therefore, begin to eat and drink soon after they finish their last match of the session to allow as much time possible for rehydration and glycogen replenishment.

Conclusions

Wrestlers as a group pose a definite challenge to their treating physicians. Their sport is arguably the most intense and physically demanding and carries with it a relatively high injury rate. As a group, they are noncompliant. Finally, weight cutting, a process inherent to wrestling, carries with it complex health and performance issues that physicians are expected to be knowledgeable about. To treat wrestlers optimally, the attending physician should be abreast of the principles discussed in this chapter.

References

1. Garrick JG, Requa R. Injuries in high school sports. Pediatrics 1978;61:465–469.
2. National Athletic Trainers' Association. Facts on sports-related injuries in high school wrestling. Greenville, NC: NATA, June 1988.
3. Requa R, Garrick JG. Injuries in interscholastic wrestling. Phys Sportsmed 1981;94:44–51.
4. Estwanik JJ, Rovere GD. Wrestling injuries in North Carolina high schools. Phys Sportsmed 1983;11(1):100–108.
5. Roy SP. Intercollegiate wrestling injuries. Phys Sportsmed 1979;7(11):83–91.
6. Snook GA. Injuries in intercollegiate wrestling: a five-year study. Am J Sports Med 1982;10:142–144.
7. Wroble RR, Msynyk MC, Foster DJ, Albright JP. Patterns of knee injuries in wrestling: a six-year study. Am J Sports Med 1986;14:55–66.
8. Mysnyk MC, Albright JP. Relative risk and long-term impact of injuries from amateur football and wrestling competition. Paper presented at the Sports Medicine Symposium, University of Iowa, Iowa City, May 20, 1988.
9. Becker TM, Kodsi R, Barley P, Lee F, Levandowski R, Nahmias AJ. Grappling with herpes: herpes gladiatorum. Am J Sports Med 1988;16:655–669.
10. Mysnyk MC, Wroble RR, Foster DT, Albright JP. Prepatellar bursitis in wrestlers. Am J Sports Med 1986;14:46–54.
11. Baker BE, Peckham AC, Papparo F, Sanborn JC. Review of meniscal injury and associated sports. Am J Sports Med 1985;13:1–4.
12. Hoegh J. Personal communication. 1991.
13. Rasch PJ, Kroll W. What research tells the coach about wrestling. Washington DC: American Association for Health, Physical Education and Recreation, 1964.
14. National Collegiate Athletic Association. 1993. NCAA wrestling rules and interpretations, rule 7d., p. 50. Overland Park, KS: NCAA August 1993.
15. Stateville OH, Janda CA, Pandya NJ. Treating the injured ear to prevent cauliflower ear. Plast Reconst Surg 1969;44:310–312.
16. Grosse SJ, Lynch JM. Treating auricular hematoma. Success with a swimmer's nose clip. Phys Sportsmed 1991;19(10):99–102.
17. Gernon WH. The care and management of acute hematoma of the external ear. Laryngoscope 1980;90:881–885.
18. Escat M. Simplified treatment of hematoma of the ear. Otorhinolaryngol Int 1946;30:181–182.
19. Bingham BJG, Chevretton EB. Silicone ear splints in the management of acute haematoma auris. J Laryngol Otol 1987;101:889–891.
20. Talaat M, Azab S, Kamel T. Treatment of auricular hematoma using a button technique. ORL. J Otorhinolaryngol Relat Spec 1985;47(4):186–188.
21. Schuller DE, Dankle SD, Strauss RH. A technique to treat wrestlers' auricular hematoma without interrupting training or competition. Arch Otolaryngol Head Neck Surg 1989;115:202–206.
22. Koopmann CF, Coulthard SW. Management of hematomas of the auricle. Laryngoscope 1979;89:1172–1174.
23. Eliacher I, Golz A, Joachims HZ, et al. Continuous portable vacuum drainage of auricular hematomas. Am J Otolaryngol 1983;4:141–143.
24. Griffen CS. The wrestler's ear (acute auricular hematoma). Arch Otolaryngol 1985;111:161–164.
25. Steen SN, Brownell KD. Patterns of weight loss and regain in wrestlers: has the tradition changed? Med Sci Sports 1990;22(6):762–768.
26. Mysnyk MC, Freeman RM, Albright JP, Yesalis CE. Renal function and blood pressure in former wrestlers. Paper presented at the Sports Medicine Symposium, University of Iowa, Iowa City, May 20, 1988.
27. Zambraski EJ, Foster DT, Gross PM, Tipton CM. Iowa wrestling study: weight loss and urinary profiles of college wrestlers. Med Sci Sports 1976;8(2):105–108.
28. Tcheng T, Tipton C. Iowa wrestling study: anthropometric measurements and the prediction of a "minimal" body weight for high school wrestlers. Med Sci Sports 1973;5(1):1–10.

29. Thorland WG, Tipton CM, Lohman TG, et al. Midwest wrestling study: prediction of minimal weight for high school wrestlers. Med Sci Sports 1991;23(9):1102–1110.
30. Oppliger RA, Tipton CM. Iowa wrestling study: cross validation of the Tcheng-Tipton minimal weight prediction formulas for high school wrestlers. Med Sci Sports 1988;20(3):310–316.
31. Committee on Medical Aspects of Sports. Wrestling and weight control. JAMA 1967;201(7):131–133.
32. American College of Sports Medicine. Position stand on weight loss in wrestlers. Med Sci Sports 1976;8(2):11–13.
33. Zambraski EJ, Tipton CM, Jordon HR, Palmer WK, Tcheng TK. Iowa wrestling study: urinary profiles. Med Sci Sports 1974;6(2):129–132.
34. Zambraski EJ, Tipton CM, Tcheng TK, Jordan HR, Vailas AC, Callahan AK. Iowa wrestling study: changes in the urinary profiles of wrestlers prior to and after competition. Med Sci Sports 1975;7(3):217–220.
35. Herbert WT, Ribisl PM. Effects of dehydration upon physical working capacity of wrestlers under competitive conditions. Res Q 1972;43(4):416–422.
36. Serfass RC, Stall GA, Alexander JF. The effects of rapid weight loss and attempted rehydration on strength and endurance of the hand gripping muscles in college wrestlers. Res Q 1984;55(1):46–52.
37. Vaccaro P, Zauner CW, Cade JR. Changes in body weight, hematocrit and plasma protein concentration due to dehydration and rehydration in wrestlers. J Sports Med 1976;16:45–53.
38. Sawka MN, Toner MM, Francesconi RP, Pandolf KB. Hypohydration and exercise: effects of heat acclimation, gender, and environment. J Appl Physiol 1983;55(4):1147–1153.
39. Saltin B. Aerobic and anaerobic work capacity after dehydration. J Appl Physiol 1964;19:1114–1118.
40. Singer RN, Weiss SA. Effects of weight reduction on selected anthropometric, physical and performance measures of wrestlers. Res Q 1968;39(2):361–369.
41. Oehlert WH, Jordan HR, Lauer RM. Metabolic effects of training practices on high school wrestlers. J Iowa Med Soc 1973;63(11):531–534.
42. Bock W, Fox EL, Bowers R. The effects of acute dehydrations upon cardio-respiratory endurance. J Sports Med Physical Fit 1967;7:62–72.
43. Tuttle WW. The effect of weight loss by dehydration and the withholding of food on the physiologic responses of wrestlers. Res Q 1943;14:158–166.
44. Allen TE, Smith DP, Miller DK. Hemodynamic response to submaximal exercise after dehydration and rehydration in high school wrestlers. Med Sci Sports 1977;9(3):159–163.
45. Costell DL, Sparks KE. Rapid fluid replacement following thermal dehydration. J Appl Physiol 1973;34(3):299–303.
46. Palmer WK. Selected physiological responses of normal young men following dehydration and rehydration. Res Q 1968;39(4): 1054–1059.
47. Sproles CB, Smith DP, Byrd RJ, Allen TE. Circulatory responses to submaximal exercise after dehydration and rehydration. J Sports Med 1976;16:98–105.
48. Ahlman K, Karvonen MJ. Weight reduction by sweating in wrestlers and its effect on physical fitness. J Sports Med Physical Fit 1961;1:58–62.
49. Murphy RJ. Heat illness in the athlete. Am J Sports Med 1984;12(4):258–261.
50. Tipton CM. Consequences of rapid weight loss. In: Haskell W, Scola J, Whittam J, eds. Nutrition and athletic performance. Palo Alto, CA: Bull, 1982:176–197.
51. Poortmans JR. Exercise and renal function. Sports Med 1984;1:125–153.
52. Castenfors J, Mossfeldt F, Piscator M. Effect of prolonged heavy exercise on renal function and urinary protein excretion. Acta Physiol Scand 1967;70:194–206.
53. Hanson NC. Wrestling with "making weight." Phys Sportsmed 1978;6(4):107–110.
54. Anonymous. Weight reduction in wrestling [Round Table]. Phys Sportmed 1981;9:79–93.
55. Davis DR, Aply J, Fell G, Grimaloli C. Diet and retarded growth. Br Med J 1978;1:539–542.
56. Pugliese MT, Lifshitz T, Grad G, Fort P, Marks-Katz M. Fear of obesity. A cause of short stature and delayed puberty. N Engl J Med 1983;309(9):513–518.
57. Dreizen S, Spirakis CN, Stone RE. A comparison of skeletal growth and maturation in under-nourished and well-nourished girls before and after menarche. J Pediatr 1967;70(2):256–263.
58. Mysnyk MC, Albright JP, Yesalis CE. The effect of wrestling and weight loss during adolescence on final height. Paper presented at the Sports Medicine Symposium, University of Iowa, Iowa City, May 20, 1988.
59. Steen SN, Oppliger RA, Brownell KD. Metabolic effects of repeated weight loss and regain in adolescent wrestlers. JAMA 1988;260(1):47–50.
60. Melby CL, Schmidt WP, Corrigan D. Resting metabolic rate in weight-cycling collegiate wrestlers compared with physically active, noncycling control subjects. Am J Clin Nutr 1990;52:409–414.
61. Strauss RH, Lanese RR, Matarkey WB. Weight loss in amateur wrestlers and its effect on serum testosterone levels. JAMA 1985;254(23):3337–3338.
62. Cumming DC, Wheeler GD, McCall EM. The effects of exercise on reproductive function in men. Sports Med 1989;7:1–17.
63. Enns MP, Drewnowski A, Grinker JA. Body composition, body size estimation, and attitudes towards eating in male college athletes. Psychosom Med 1987;49(1):56–64.
64. Caldwell JE, Ahonen E, Nousialnen U. Differential effects of sauna, diuretic, and exercise-induced hypohydration. J Appl Physiol 1984;57(4):1018–1023.
65. Craig FN, Cummings EG. Dehydration and muscular work. J Appl Physiol 1966;21:670–674.
66. Horswill CA, Hucker, RC, Scott JR, Costill DL, Gould D. Weight loss, dietary carbohydrate modifications, and high intensity, physical performance. Med Sci Sports 1990;22(4):470–476.
67. Widerman PM, Hagan RD. Body weight loss in a wrestlers preparing for competition: a case report. Med Sci Sports 1982;14(6):413–418.
68. Nadel ER, Pandolf, KB, Roberts MF, Stolwijk AJ. Mechanisms of thermal acclimation to exercise and heat. J Appl Physiol 1974;37(4):515–520.
69. Buskirk ER, Iampietro PF, Bass DE. Work performance after dehydration: effects of physical conditioning and heat acclimation. J Appl Physiol 1958;12(2):189–194.
70. Klinzing JE, Karpowicz W. The effects of rapid weight loss and rehydration on a wrestling performance test. J Sports Med 1986;26:149–156.
71. Ribisl PM, Herbert WG. Effects of rapid weight reduction and subsequent rehydration upon the physical working capacity of wrestlers. Res Q 1970;41:536–541.
72. Kelly JM, Gorney BA, Kalm KK. The effects of a collegiate wrestling season on body composition, cardiovascular fitness, and muscular strength and endurance. Med Sci Sports 1978;10(2):119–124.
73. Bosco JS, Terjung RL, Greenleaf JE. Effects of progressive hypohydration on maximal isometric muscular strength. J Sports Med 1968;8:81–86.
74. Houston ME, Marrin DA, Green HJ, Thomson JA. The effect of rapid weight loss on physiological functions in wrestlers. Phys Sports Med 1981;9(11):73–78.
75. Webster S, Rutt R, Weltman A. Physiological effects of a weight loss regimen practiced by college wrestlers. Med Sci Sports 1990;22(2):229–234.
76. Nielsen B, Kubica R. Bonnesen A, Rasmussen IB, Stoklusa J, Wilk B. Physical work capacity after dehydration and hyperthemia. Scand J Sports Sci 1982;3(1):2–10.
77. Torranin G, Smith DP, Burd RJ. The effect of acute thermal dehydration and rapid rehydration on isometric and isotonic endurance. J Sports Med 1979;19:1–9.
78. Jacobs I. The effect of thermal dehydration on performance of the Wingate anaerobic test. Int J Sports Med 1980;1:21–24.
79. Katch FI, Michael ED. Body composition of high school wrestlers according to age and wrestling weight category. Med Sci Sports 1971;3(4):190–194.
80. Hassler P. Wrestling weight class procedural guidelines. Wrestling USA 1989;(Nov. 15):6–10.

81. Oppliger RA, Tipton CM. Weight prediction equation tested and available. Iowa med 1985;75(10):449–453.
82. Horswell CA, Scott J, Galer P, Park SH. Physiological profile of elite junior wrestlers. Res Q Exerc Sport 1988;59(3):257–261.
83. Silva JM, Shultz BB, Haslam RW, Murray D. A psycho-physiological assessment of elite wrestlers. Res Q 1981;52(3):348–358.
84. Stine G, Ratliff R, Shierman G, Grana W. Physical profile of the wrestlers at the 1977 NCAA championships. Phys Sportsmed 1979;7(11):98–105.
85. Tipton CM. Commentary: physicians should advise wrestlers about weight loss. Phys Sportsmed 1987;15(1):160–164.
86. Thorland WG, Johnson GO, Asar W, Housh TJ. Estimation of minimal wrestling weight using measures of body build and composition. Int J Sports Med 1987;8:365–370.
87. Lohman TG. Body composition methodology in sports medicine. Phys Sportsmed 1982;10(12):47–57.
88. Lohman TG. Skinfolds and body density and their relation to body fatness: a review. Hum Biol 1981;53(2):181–225.
89. Kris-Etherton PM. Nutrition and athletic performance. Contemp Nutr 1989;14(9):366–368.
90. Murray R. The effects of consuming carbohydrate-electrolyte beverages on gastric emptying and fluid absorption during and following exercise. Sports Med 1987;4:322–351.

SECTION

THREE

MANAGEMENT AND TREATMENT OF SYSTEMIC AND REGIONAL INJURIES

44 / SOFT TISSUE ATHLETIC INJURY

Wayne B. Leadbetter

Introduction

Soft tissue athletic injuries are the most challenging and controversial problems encountered in sports medicine. As the most frequent disability associated with athletic competition and recreational athletics, injury to the dense connective tissue of ligament, tendon, and associated muscle are as difficult to qualify as to quantify. Representing the largest tissue component of the body, these "connecting tissues" include a diverse histologic family including not only muscle, tendon, and ligament, but also joint capsule, fascia, meniscus, articular cartilage, synovium, intervertebral disc and adipose tissue. While sports differ in risk because of the quantitative differences in stresses to different anatomic areas, soft tissue injuries still make up the majority of complaints in all sports at all levels of competition. It is estimated that 30% to 50% of all sports injuries are caused by soft tissue overuse (1). While many of these complaints create symptoms of inflammation, a variety of tissue responses may take place when a sports injury occurs. Some of these responses are predictable but others are unanticipated. The predictability of wound healing and repair forms the basis of present day therapy, but those who treat the injured athlete soon become aware of the vast number of variables that defeat textbook application of such logic to any single case. In addition, there is growing evidence for basic pathohistologic and pathophysiologic differences between the acute and chronic (overuse) forms of soft tissue sports injury (2, 3, 4).

The goal of sports medicine therapy is to minimize the adverse effect of traumatic inflammatory responses while promoting tissue repair, thereby expediting a safe return to performance. To do so, the sports medicine clinician must be familiar with human tissue biological capabilities and limitations. This chapter provides an overview of the basic cell and molecular events in wound healing, the initiation and medication of inflammation, repair and degeneration, and the sources of sports-induced athletic pain. Seen within the greater context of cell matrix adaptation and tissue maintenance, additional attention is called to the role of transition as an important injury cofactor. The specific injury response and management are discussed of the most commonly injured soft tissues—muscle, tendon and ligament. Several hypothetical models will be offered to assist in the understanding of these clinically observed patterns of sports injury.

Epidemiology of Sports Induced Soft Tissue Injuries

The epidemiology of sports-induced soft tissue injuries has been analyzed with respect to sites of injury, gender, age, choice of sport, and level of participation.

The sites of injury vary according to the sport. Garrick and Requa pointed out that most sports injuries involve the lower extremities, reflecting the strenuous running, jumping, and cutting maneuvers common to the most popular sports (5). As many as 90% of sports injuries are sustained by the hip, thigh, knee, leg, ankle, and foot. These injuries run the gamut from contusions to sprains and strains. Shoulder and upper extremity complaints predominate for the overhead athlete in racquet, throwing, and swimming sports. DeHaven and Lintner (6) found that 48.1% of baseball injuries involve the shoulder and upper extremity and that 57% of world class swimmers have experienced shoulder pain. Ligament sprains, the most common injuries to joints in general and to the knee in particular, account for 25% to 40% of all knee injuries in most studies. Whitman, et al. (7) in a review of 1280 urban sports medicine patients, with an average age of 30.2 years, found the most frequently injured areas to be the knee, with 45.5%; the ankle, 9.8%; and the shoulder, 7.7%. Of these injuries, 53.9% involved soft tissue.

Gender studies point to a difference in the severity and types of injury in male and female athletes. Chandy and Grana, (8) in a three-year study of seven paired sports in 130 Oklahoma secondary schools involving 24,485 boys and 18,289 girls, found a significant difference in rate of injury only in basketball, in which the girls had significantly more injuries and more severe injuries. Overall, the girls had more sprains and dislocations whereas the boys had more strains and fractures. There was a significant variance in the sites of injuries—boys had significantly more shoulder complaints and girls had more knee injuries. DeHaven and Lintner (6) found patellofemoral pain to be more prevalent in women (19.6% of women versus 7.4% of men). Sprains and strains occurred in 33.4% of men and in 28.7% of women. They also confirmed the higher rate of knee injuries among injured female athletes (20.7% versus 8.5%). In a study of 4 Seattle high schools, Garrick and Requa (5) found the average injury rate for all athletes in ten sports was 5.2%. The rate for girls was 3.5% and the adjusted rate (excluding football and wrestling) for boys was 3%. Again, although the injury rate for all girls' sports was lower, a higher percentage of the girls' injuries required a loss of 5 days or more (52% of girls versus 44% of boys). These studies point to a difference in the severity and types of injuries in male and female athletes, but they do not resolve such variables as level of conditioning, performance technique, anatomic predisposition, or coaching. These studies have not resolved the effect of such variables as level of conditioning, performance technique, anatomic predisposition and coaching.

Age is associated with a changing spectrum of sports soft tissue injury. Of all children participating in sports programs in the United States, 3% to 11% are injured (9). In a survey of Irish school children between the ages of 10 and 18 years, the overall incidence of injury was found to be 2.94 injuries per 100 children per calendar year. More than half of these were sprains, strains, and contusions (10). The rare occurrences of tendinitis or inflammatory changes at the musculotendinous junction in children have been attributed to the transfer of forces to the tendon apophysis. Hoffman and Lyman, (11) assessing sideline injuries in high school football, found that contusions (26.6%), sprains (21.6%), and strains (8.6%) accounted for 56.8% of all injuries. The knee (14.4%), the lower leg (13.7%), and the ankle (11.5%) were the most common sites of injury.

With aging, the injury spectrum shifts towards degenerative processes and gravation of previously acquired injury. Comparatively speaking, the Master athlete may actually have a higher rate of injury. Keller et al. (12) found 15 to 30 times as many soccer injuries in senior and professional athletes as in youths. Hip and thigh injuries were also more common in senior and professional athletes. Notable exceptions were the knee and ligament sprains that accounted for one third of the soccer injuries regardless of age. Contusions were more often significant in youths. These differences can be accounted for in part by the intensity of the game. Menard and Stanish (13) note that "The Masters athlete is often the victim of two sets of injuries: those that are incurred in their youth and those that result from their current training regimen." Inflammatory problems such as tendinitis or bursitis gradually increase in importance. Grossman and Nicholas (14) have called attention to the changing pattern of knee injuries with age. Chondromalacia patellae, patellar tendon rupture and degenerative arthritis are common knee injuries in aging athletes.

Both collision and endurance sports are characterized by the predominance of soft tissue injury. DeHaven and Lintner (6) found 12 times as many injuries in football as in the next sport, basketball. Football accounted for 63.9% of all injuries as well as 60% of all the knee injuries, which were primarily internal derangement and medial collateral ligament injuries. Total injury rate among high school football players range from 25% to 65% depending upon the definition of injury and the method of data collection. Rates of significant injury range from 15% to 18%. Sprains and strains were the most common injuries. Requa and Garrick (5) found wrestling second only to football in knee injuries requiring surgery. Rovere et al. (15) studied soft tissue inflammation in theatrical dance students. Hip tendinitis produced a 6.9 day average loss of participation. For ankle sprains, the average loss was 2.1 days. Soccer caused 2 to 5 times fewer injuries in young athletes than American football. Sprains, strains, contusions and tendinitis dominate the injury patterns. In a collision-prone recreational sport such as downhill skiing, soft tissue injury still predominates. In an analysis of 2596 skiing injuries, Johnson and Pope (16) found that soft tissue injuries accounted for 53.4% of the total. The five most frequent diagnoses were knee sprains (20.9%), thumb sprains (10.2%), leg contusions (8.7%), lacerations (7.8%), and ankle sprains (5.8%).

Endurance sports include jogging, running, swimming, cycling, rowing and race-walking. The incidence of running injuries range from 46.6% to an estimated 70% over the past decade (17, 18, 19). Inflammatory disorders of soft tissue accounted for 5 of the 6 most common problems in the series of James, et al. (17). Musculotendinous injuries predominate in track and field. Knee pain, representing a broad spectrum of overuse soft tissue complaints, occurs in 23% to 40% of all runners (20). While Clement et al. (21) have noted a decrease in the prevalence of Achilles peritendinitis from 11% of all injuries, as reported by James et al. (17) to

6%, possibly due to changes in training and shoe wear, historically, Achilles tendinitis has been a difficult lesion for runners. Welsh and Clodman (22) reported in 1980 that 16% of those affected had abandoned running while 54% still participated despite discomfort. The prevalence of injury in running is directly proportional to the load exposure. Mann (23) has calculated that the ground-reaction force at midstance in running is equal to 2 to 3 times body weight. A 70-kg runner at 1175 steps per mile, absorbs at least 220 tons of force per mile. Swimming is another endurance sport characterized by excessive cumulative load. Competitive swimmers swim 8000 to 20,000 yards per day, 5 to 7 days per week. This distance is equivalent of running up to 45 miles daily. It is estimated that during a 10-month swimming season, a male swimmer performs 400,000 strokes and a female swimmer performs 660,000 strokes (24). Shoulder pain secondary to glenohumeral instability, secondary subacromial tendon impingement, muscle fatigue, and tendinosis are typical causes of "swimmers shoulder" (24). Incorrect mechanics in the whip kick and breast stroke has been given as a primary cause of soft tissue overuse in the medial aspect of the knee, and even inflammation of extensor tendons of the dorsum of the foot has been reported in swimmers (25).

Regardless of the level of play, the factors that contribute to soft tissue injure are frequency, intensity, and duration. Keller et al. (12), in a study of soccer injuries, concluded that professionals sustain a higher rate of injury because of the greater intensity of play. Leach's (26) description of the major league baseball pitcher's typical throwing rotation is another example of the different levels of intensity within sports between amateurs and professionals. A major league baseball pitcher usually pitches every 4 days and throws 110 to 130 pitches in the course of a regular game. The next day his arm is so sore that it is difficult to raise. The second day is characterized by recovery and easy throwing, and the third day by a normal workout. The pitcher returns to starting on either the fourth or fifth day. An injury analysis of the Olympic games from 1968 to 1972 reveals that sprains, strains, and contusions were the most common soft tissue injuries treated, accounting for 61% to 96% of soft tissue problems (27).

Spectrum of Soft Tissue Sports Injury—Term Definition

Sports-induced soft tissue injuries are characterized by a spectrum of interrelated cell matrix responses or by the processes of inflammation, repair, and degeneration (2–4). It is helpful to define these terms in order to more fully understand the observed clinical problems.

Trauma implies an injury from a mechanical force that is applied external to the involved tissue, causing structural stress or strain that results in a cellular or tissue response. *Load* is a measure of external mechanical force. *Use* implies the accumulation of load over time; that is, a rate. Such repetition is seen in endurance sports in the form of cyclic loading and overuse. The effect of load on tissue is described by the terms "strain" and "stress." Strain is the deformation of a structure in response to external load, whereas stress is its internal resistance to such deformation (Fig. 44.1). Sports trauma may be thought of as the mechanism by which injury occurs.

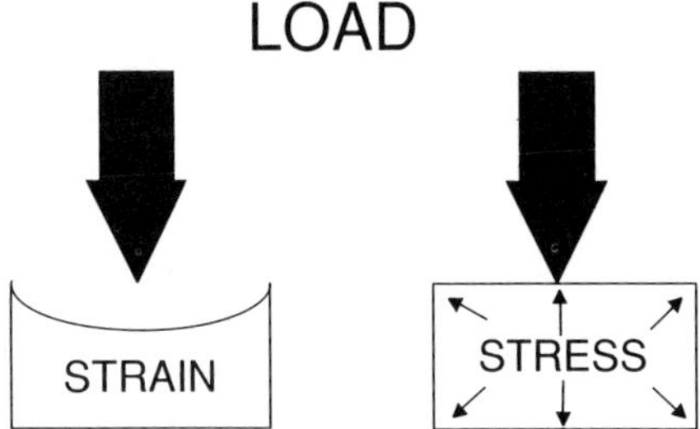

Figure 44.1 Strain—Stress: Strain represents a tissue deformation; stress is the internal tissue resistance to deformation. Both may affect cell matrix biology.

Sports injury (from the Latin *injure*—to make unjust, not right) is the loss of cells or extracellular matrix resulting from sports-induced trauma (28). As in other wounds, an athletic wound is a disruption of normal anatomic structure and function. All wounds result from pathologic processes beginning internal or external to the involved part (29). *Acute wounds* are characterized by generating an orderly and timely reparative process that results in the sustained restoration of anatomical and functional integrity. *Chronic wounds* have failed to proceed through an orderly and timely process to produce anatomical and functional integrity or have proceeded through the repair process without establishing a sustained anatomical and functional result. Injuries are also divided into acute and chronic types, according to rate of onset and the mechanism of the injury. Chronic injury often represents a failure of cell matrix adaptation to load exposure (29).

The mechanism of injury has much to do with the subsequent pathohistologic pattern. "Overuse" and "overload" may not be synonymous terms, because injury can result from excessive and rapid change in use without significant change in resistance—hence, the origin of the term "cumulative trauma disorder," or, as the author prefers, "cumulative cell-matrix adaptive response." Synovial structures, such as the tendon sheath as well as peritenon structures are prone to this form of stress response (2). Injuries can further be divided into acute and chronic patterns according to rate of onset. *Acute* injuries are typified by a sudden crisis followed by a fairly predictable, although often lengthy, resolution. Acute disruptions of structures accompanied by bleeding provide the best model for adherence to the classic acute phase inflammatory reaction seen in other forms of human postnatal wounding. In the tendon, an acute injury often consists of midsubstance ruptures occurring either through aberrant tissue or as the result of high strain rates (30, 31). *Chroinc* injury is characterized by slow, insidious onset, implying an antecedent subthreshold spectrum of structural damage. Eventually this leads to a crisis episode that is often heralded by pain and/or signs of inflammation. Chronic injury may last months or even years and is distinguished by a persistence of symptoms without resolution. Synovitis, bursitis, paratenonitis, and tendinitis are typical of such complaints. It is now known that perturbation of in vivo or in vitro cell populations induces the release of chemical mediators and initiates cascades of inflammatory products (42, 43, 44). How these events lead to further change in matrix integrity of connective tissue is only now becoming understood. Furthermore, it is not clear whether microdamage due to tensile overload and formed element separation with tissue fatigue is the initiating event or whether some overwhelming of the cell metabolism occurs first with resulting loss of the cell to maintain tissue integrity through increasing its synthesis. It is likely that both processes may occur under different circumstances. There appears to be some overlap between acute and chronic injuries, with the bridging stage at 4 to 6 weeks termed the "subacute stage" of injury. Another perspective on the acute versus chronic process would define a chronic injury as an acute injury occurring in association with some impairment to healing (Hunt TK, personal communication). In the athlete, there are both intrinsic and extrinsic factors that can impair recovery (32).

It is difficult to define sports injury clinically. From the athlete's point of view, an athletic injury is any painful problem that prevents or hampers usual sports performance. Furthermore, athletic soft tissue injury complaints are often defined solely by the amount of pain or the inability to perform. Attention has been directed to the inadequacy of this definition of injury and the importance of determining the exact anatomic extent in occurrence of tissue injury (33). Epidemiologic research uses such variables as duration of disability, need for medical attention, and degree of structural tissue damage to define injury (33). Proper therapy often depends on defining the exact anatomic extent and occurrence of tissue injury (33, 39). Classic signs of inflammation after injury are *not* always present or identifiable as a reliable guide. This is typical of deeply located muscle injury. A complaint is not so much identified with a specific structure as within an anatomic area. It is a "painful shoulder," not a painful biceps tendon; It is a "painful knee," not a painful patella tendon. And although the immediate onus on the examiner is to be competent and accurate in making the physical diagnosis, the elicitation of pain does not necessarily shed light on the exact pathology or mechanism of injury. For instance, tendon injury relating to occult joint instability or dynamic tendon stress overload, as may be present with the hyperpronating foot, may be revealed only by further dynamic analysis. Of all the clinical signs, it is loss of function (functio laesa) that provides the necessity for treatment of soft tissue injury, indeed for all sports injury.

Rovere's (15) attempt to define tendinitis in a study of theatrical dance students exemplifies this difficulty. He defined tendinitis as "a syndrome of pain and tenderness localized over a tendon, usually aggravated by activities that bring the particular muscle tendon unit into play, usually against resistance. . . . The syndrome is inclusive of tenosynovitis and tenovaginitis as well as actual inflammation of the tendon substance itself."

Sports-induced inflammation (from the Latin *inflammare,* to set on fire) is a localized tissue response initiated by injury or destruction of vascularized tissues exposed to excessive mechanical load or use (2, 4, 34). It is a time-dependent evolving process characterized by vascular, chemical, and cellular events leading to tissue repair, regeneration, or scar formation. Clinically observed pathways of sports-induced soft-tissue inflammation include spontaneous resolution, fibroproductive healing, regeneration, or chronic inflammatory response (4) (Fig. 44.2). Not all sports injuries produce a classic inflammatory pattern of response, nor are all tissues capable of generating such a response (4, 28, 41, 55). The four cardinal signs of acute inflammation were defined by Celsus (AD 14–37) in the often quoted phrase: "rubor et tumor cum alore et dolore" (redness and swelling with heat and pain) (Table 44.1). It is important to note that this was likely a description of an empyema and fistula of the chest (35). Based upon such historic tradition, pain has assumed a disproportionate importance in the definition of inflammation, such that any painful structure is immediately presumed inflamed. It has taken the advent of more accurate noninvasive assessment such as magnetic resonance imaging and the accumulation of surgical biopsy evidence to correct what may be an improper clinical emphasis. As will be further discussed, the source of connective tissue pain is now known to be multifactorial (36).

Repair of soft-tissue injury has been defined as replacement of damaged or lost cells and extracellular matrices with new cells and matrices (28). Regeneration is a form of repair that produces new tissue that is structurally and functionally identical to normal tissue (28, 54, 58, 61). Repair by scar is the postnatal mammalian response to injury, unlike the fetal wound, which is capable of healing without exuberant scar formation (72). Acutely injured tissues such as tendon or ligament repair by scar deposition that never exactly replicates the histologic or biomechanical properties of the original structures (28, 40). Regeneration is often seen as the ideal wound healing response; whereas, depending on the athlete's demands, the response in soft tissue healing may result in either an adequate or an inadequate response.

Table 44.1.
Recognition of the "Cardinal Signs" of Inflammation

Heat	*Calor*—Metabolic radiant energy
Redness	*Rubor*—Increased vascularity (angiogenesis) and blood flow
Swelling	*Tumor*—Extracellular edema and matrix changes
Pain	*Dolor*—Stimulation of afferent nerve endings by noxious mediators
Loss of function	*Functio laesa*—Decreased performance caused by direct damage or inhibiting pain, edema

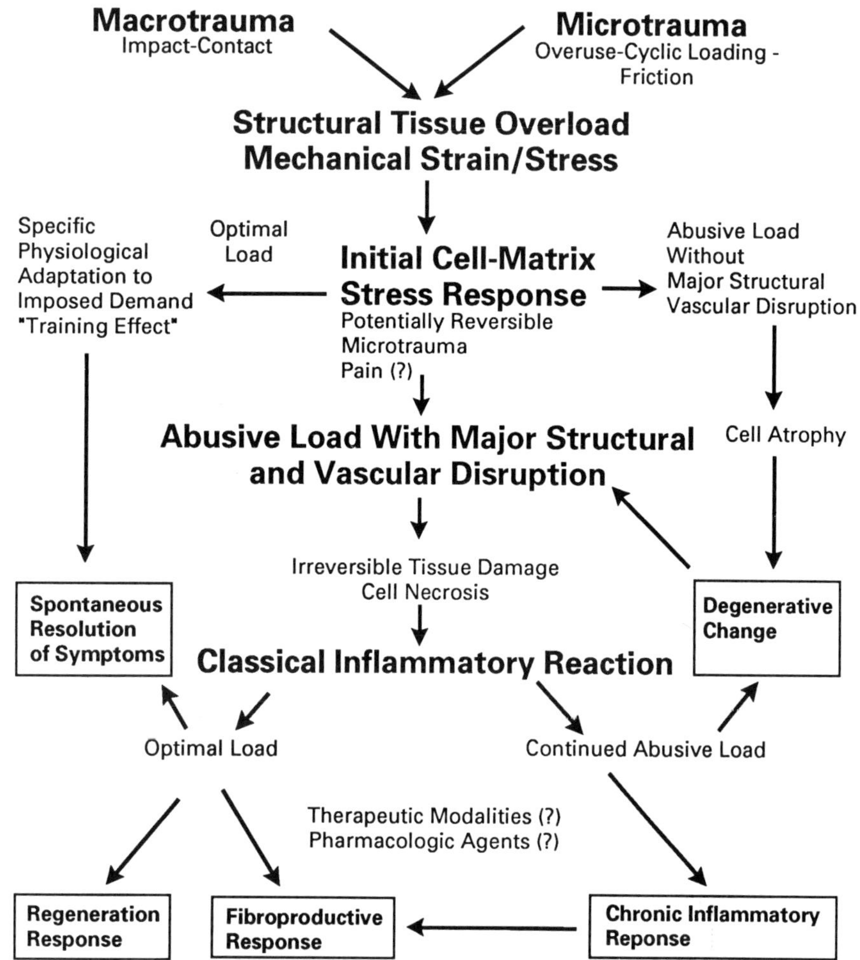

Figure 44.2 Schema of the theoretical pathways of sports-induced inflammatory response. Reprinted by permission from Leadbetter WB. An introduction to sports-induced inflammation. In: Leadbetter WB, Buckwalter JA, Gordon SL, eds. Sports-induced inflammation: Clinical and basic science concepts. Park Ridge, IL: American Academy of Orthopaedic Surgeons, 1990;2.

Healing is a complex dynamic process that results in the restoration of anatomic continuity as a result of an orderly biological repair process (29). Qualities of wound healing have been defined as ideal, acceptable, minimal, and failed (Table 44.2). An ideally healed wound is one that has returned to normal anatomic structure, function, and appearance. An acceptably healed wound is characterized by restoration of sustained function and anatomic continuity (29). A minimally healed wound is characterized by the restoration of anatomic continuity but without a sustained functional result; hence, the wound may recur. In failed wound healing no anatomic restoration or sustained function is achieved. In the treatment of soft tissue injury, ideal wound healing is rarely, if ever, obtained, while acceptably healed wounds are common. It is the challenge of the treating clinician to avoid returning the athlete to play with a minimally healed condition.

Degeneration describes a change in tissue from a higher to a lower or less functionally active form (4). Such weakened structures are then more vulnerable to sudden dynamic overload or cyclic overloading leading to mechanical fatigue and failure. A prominent source of degeneration is cell atrophy, which is the decrease in the size and/or function of a cell in response to a presence (or lack of) an environmental signal (38). Such down-regulation involves decreased protein synthesis and a decrease in such activities as energy production, replication, storage, and contractility. In sports injury, immobilization is a prominent cause of cell atrophy in connective tissues (28). Additional causes include decreased nutrition, diminished endocrine hormonal influence, persistent inflammation, aging, and denervation (4). Reversal of the degenerative process is not a typical feature in degenerative conditions beyond an undefined cell-matrix limit. Ultimately, degeneration represents a profound imbalance in cell-matrix homeostasis (Fig. 44.3).

Table 44.2.
Adequacy of Wound Healing

Ideal	Normal anatomic structural continuity, function, and appearance
Acceptable	Restoration of sustained anatomic continuity and function
Minimal	Restoration of anatomic continuity without sustained function
Failed	No restoration of anatomic continuity or function

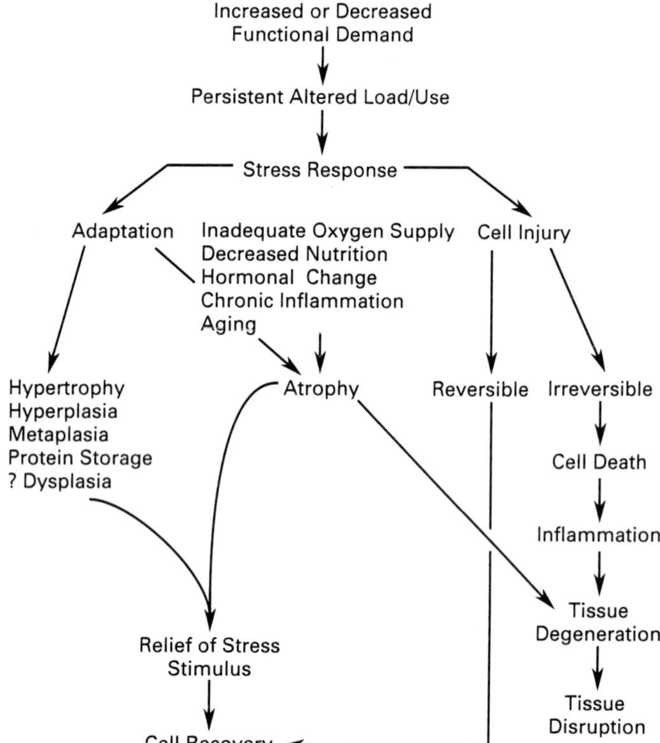

Figure 44.3 Cell matrix response to change in functional level. In this model, tendinosis results from a failed cell matrix adaptation to excessive changes in load use. Such failure is modified by both intrinsic and extrinsic factors. It is likely that all connective tissues demonstrate some type of change in response to functional level. Reprinted by permission from Leadbetter WB. An introduction to sports-induced inflammation. In: Leadbetter WB, Buckwalter JA, Gordon SL, eds. Sports-induced inflammation: Clinical and basic science concepts. Park Ridge, IL: American Academy of Orthopaedic Surgeons, 1990;2.

Necrosis is that structural change occurring in cells subsequent to their death in a living organism (45, 46, 47). This is a focal process resulting both from the presence of extracellular enzymes and from the release within the cell of self degrading lysosomal hydrolytic enzymes in response to the rising acid pH of a hypoxic or anoxic metabolism, a process known as autolysis (47). The process of this enzymatic degradation of cell membrane, lipids, and intracellular organelles, along with the breakdown of tissue macromolecules, provide the prime stimulus for the mobilization of inflammatory cells from blood and nonnecrotic tissues surrounding an area of necrotic injury (38, 45). As Robbins and Cotrane (46) have noted, "Necrotic cells are dead cells, but dead cells are not necessarily necrotic." This refers to the fact that cell necrosis, by definition, cannot occur suddenly; hence, viable cells that are placed in a tissue fixative, such as formalin, do not demonstrate necrosis but do undergo cell death. Furthermore, while initiation of inflammation does not require necrosis (e.g., immune response), necrosis always stimulates inflammation if there is adequate tissue vascularity (38). The severity of sports injury depends upon the extent of cell necrosis.

The pathology of cell injury represents a spectrum of stress responses to the altered environment from the undetectable and totally reversible to the terminally irreversible event of cell death (47, 48). A critical point beyond which cell metabolic function cannot be revived is referred to as "the point of no return" (48). This point remains ill-defined since the exact critical functions which must be compromised before cell death ensues remain controversial. Cell injury or death can be initiated by such factors as ischemia, postischemic reperfusion, inflammation, chemical toxicity, or ionizing radiation (38). The hypovascularized, dense connective tissues of the athlete are vulnerable or irreversible cell damage both during tissue deformation and use (2). Mitochondria are extremely sensitive to this ischemic stress. Mitochondrial swelling with the collapse of the cytochrome oxidase and electron transport enzyme systems results in the release of intracellular calcium stores. Increased intracellular calcium ion is a prominent signal mechanism for increased phospholipase and calcium dependent protease enzyme activity (48). Phospholipid degeneration with a loss of cell membrane integrity resulting from lipid peroxidation is another common pathway of cell injury and is one of the theoretical pathways for all of aging (38). Under such conditions as postischemic reprofusion or inflammation, unstable molecular species resulting from the incomplete reduction of oxygen (O_2 to H_2O) may result. A free radical is any molecule that has an odd number of electrons. These oxy-radicals can react either as electron receptors (i.e., an oxidant) or an electron donor (i.e., a reductant). Free radicals are extremely reactive, chemically unstable, therefore, short-lived, and usually occur in low concentrations (38). They may chemically attack the phospholipid structure of cell membranes by the process of lipid peroxidation, forming unstable lipid peroxide radicals that break down into smaller molecules, leading eventually to the dissolution of the cell wall. Phagocytic cells, such as the neutrophil, generate high volumes of oxygen-free radicals during inflammatory and repair process (49) (Fig. 44.4). This accounts in part for additional tissue injury that becomes the focus of acute athletic treatment. While acute cell injury and cell death always stimulate inflammation (38); in theory, under conditions of microtraumatic sports injury, such factors as tissue hypoxia and cell matrix deformation may alter cell metabolic activity possibly increasing harmful metabolic products, such as free radicals, thus leading to lipid peroxidation. Such theory may provide an explanation for observed degenerative pathology (2, 38, 69).

Chronic inflammation involves the replacement of leukocytes by macrophages, plasma cells, and lymphocytes in a highly vascularized and innervated loose connective-tissue milieu at the site of injury (38). Although findings of chronic inflammation are typical in sites such as the lateral epicondylar lesions of the elbow (50), such responses are not found in all chronic sport injuries (51, 52). The mechanism that converts an acute inflammation to a chronic inflammatory process is not known; continued abusive load and irritation may stimulate the local release of cytokines, resulting in both autocrine (cell self-stimulation) and paracrine (stimula-

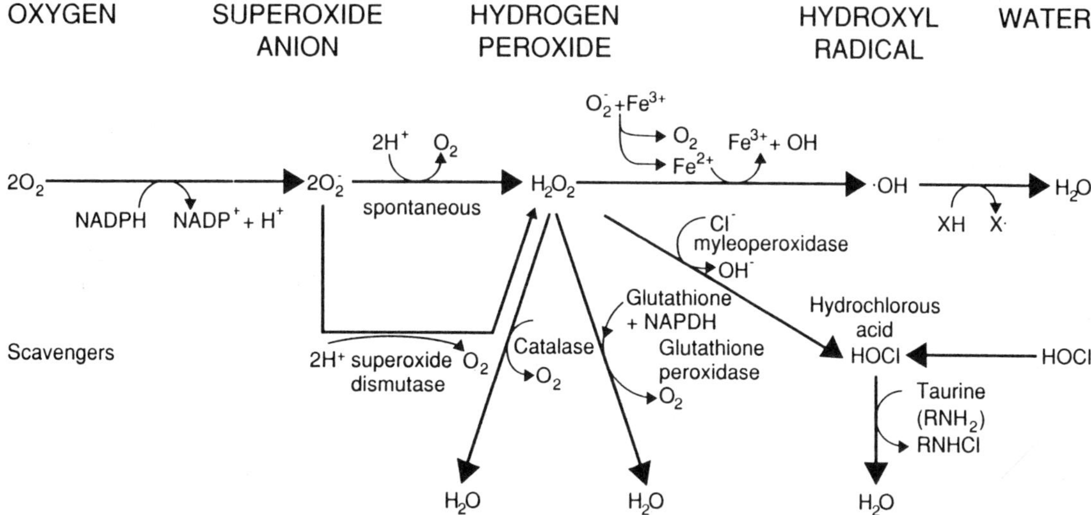

Figure 44.4 Pathway for the production of various activated oxygen species. Reprinted by permission from Wahl SM, Wahl LM. Inflammation. In: Cohen JK, Diegelmann RF, Lindblad WY, eds. Wound Healing. Philadelphia: WB Saunders, 1992;40.

tion of adjacent cells) modulation of further cell activity (42, 53, 54).

Thus, Inflammation, degeneration, and repair form a functional spectrum of cell matrix responses. The predominance of any one response depends on the type of injury, the homeostatic balance of the tissue, and the timing of the observation.

Composition and Function of Injured Tissues

The individual cell holds the key to the regulation of the body's trauma response. Sports medicine therapy is increasingly challenged to understand and anticipate these cellular responses in predicting the recovery from injury or justifying the value of any therapeutic measure. In this context, the clinician must "think like a cell" and come to appreciate that the body's cellular response to sports trauma takes place in the context of a changing biochemical environment, constantly influenced by such factors as oxygen tension, nutrition, genetic endowment, and aging, and modified by physical forces that initiate communication to and between cells. One of the most important results of the integration of these variables is the maintenance of structural integrity during use and of tissue renewal after injury.

Connective tissues are composed of two basic elements: cells and extracellular matrix (41). However, there is great variation in the relative composition and structural characteristics of these two elements in normal connective tissue. Reparative response in connective tissue is essentially a cellular event, the success of which hinges on the ability of a tissue to increase its rate of DNA and macromolecular synthesis (55). Once considered an inert amorphous ground substance, the matrix is now known to be a vital, responsive, biochemical saline jell that contains many important types of macromolecules including collagen, proteoglycans, hyaluronic acid, elastin, and fibronectin (4, 55). There is growing evidence that the matrix may be the modulating medium that prompts cells to change their patterns of protein synthesis in response to load or use. For example, cartilage cells remain in a differentiated state only so long as they are in contact with type II collagen and cartilage specific proteoglycans in the surrounding matrix (55, 56). In muscle injury, the removal of muscle fiber cytoplasm may provide a stimulatory role for myogenesis and repair (64). After forced muscle lengthening of the rat soleus, Fritz and Stauber found an interdependence between myofibers and extracellular matrix proteoglycans (70). This implies both scaffolding functions by matrix components to guide myogenesis and myofiber orientations as well as activation and inhibition effects on cellular repair (70).

Cellular Elements of Connective Tissue

The embryonic mesenchymal cell is the ancestor of most of the indigenous cells of adult dense connective tissues including the fibroblast, tenocyte, and myoblast, or muscle satellite cell (57). These cells make up the resident cell populations of the respective connective tissues. The macrophage and mast cells, which originate from bone marrow stem cells and migrate to their connective tissue site, as well as in situ endothelial cells can be arbitrarily classified as additional resident cells. The immigrant cell population in connective tissue consists mainly of inflammatory cells such as the monocyte (tissue macrophage), neutrophil, lymphocyte, plasma cell, and additional endothelial cells present as a result of chemotaxis and wound repair activation. If an injury results in sufficient damage to create a wound gap or tissue necrosis, new cells must be supplied to reconstruct connective tissue fabric (58, 61). After injury, such new cells are derived from one of three sources: migration of cell populations, replication of resident cells, or the modulation of cells present at the injury site (55). Added variables in sports trauma healing are the differing capacities of resident cell populations to modulate their reparative behavior and of new cells to access the injury site. In most cases, this access is directly the result of adequate vascular supply. Avascular tissue will not heal in vivo (54, 58). The resident cell populations are primarily responsible for tissue matrix maintenance, remodeling, and adaptive change (55, 57).

Fibroblast is a term used to refer to cells with differing functions but similar morphologies (59, 60, 61). The fibroblast is a spindle-shaped cell characterized by tapering eosinophilic cytoplasmic extensions as seen in conventional histologic section. It is the workhorse of most connective tissue injury repair (57). This cell possesses a well-developed, rough endoplasmic reticulum on which the precursor polypeptdes of collagen, elastin, and proteoglycans and glycoproteins are synthesized (57). Not only do tendon fibroblasts have functions and properties different from those of skeletal muscle or liver fibroblast, but the fibroblast within the same tendon also demonstrates different potentiality (43, 62). For instance, the epitenocyte functions as a modified fibroblast with aggressive capability to repair tendon laceration or crush damage. However, the tendon endotenocyte appears to have more limited potential to increase its reparative function (43, 62). The term fibroblast is best understood to be a generic cell phenotype that may refer to connective tissue cells, stem cells, phagocytic cells (histiocytes), protein secreting cells (fibrocytes), and contractile cells (myofibroblasts) (61). In the mature animals, fibroblasts continue to synthesize and maintain elements of connective tissue matrix (e.g. collagens, fibronectin, fibroglycans and other proteins) the matrix is constantly being turned over and being remodeled by fibroblasts and the degraded enzymes that they secrete (e.g., collagenases, proteoglycanases, glycosaminoglycanases, and other proteases (60). By light microscopy, inactive fibroblasts in granulation tissue are oval and show indistinct cytoplasm with an elongated nucleus. Cells with this appearance include at last three functionally distinct mesenchymal cell types: 1) stem cells of connective tissues; 2) cells with FC receptors and phagocytic capabilities (histocytes); and 3) fibrocytes (60). Fibrocytes are those connective tissues cells differentiated by electron microscopy, appearing within days at the site of wound repair. They exhibit active synthesis of extracellular matrix components such as collagens, fibronectins and proteoglycans. Fibroblasts in vivo adhere to and grow in a complex extracellular matrix that is difficult to reliably produce in vitro. The cellular processes or pseudopodia of fibroblasts are attached to substraits at sites known as adhesion-plaques, which are characterized by the presence of increased actin filaments and by the presence of a specific actin-binding protein called vinculin (60). Fibroblasts are capable of considerable modulation in response to lymphokines, monokines, and cytokines; these provide chemotactic signals for direct migration of fibroblasts from neighboring connective tissue to the site of injury as well as for proliferation or mitogenic response (65). This mitogenic response consists of two phases. The first phase is termed "competence;" it occurs in early G1 phase at the cell cycle rendering this cell competent to replicate its DNA, but it does not result in DNA synthesis or the S phase. The second phase, termed "progression," results in DNA synthesis and occurs only in competent fibroblasts. This scheme of cell activation and modulation is typical of cellular reparative cascades in all connective tissues (61). Myofibroblasts are characterized by an abundance of contractile elements (actin-myosin filaments) in the peripheral cytoplasm, a concentration of synthetic organelles (rough endoplasmic reticulum and golgi apparatus) in the perinuclear region, and an indented nucleus (61). These modified fibroblasts are thought to be responsible for wound contraction and are prominent in the wound site in 3 to 10 days after injury (38, 61).

Myoblast is the proper term for a myogenic cell that is withdrawn from the cell cycle, implying a nonproliferating, highly differentiated condition (64). A highly specialized member of the connective tissue family, skeletal muscle cells may derive from embryonic mesoderm. Skeletal muscle cells are permanent cells with no proliferative capacity; the reparative cell in muscle is the satellite tissue cell (61, 64). The muscle satellite cell is a mononucleated cell that lies between a muscle fiber and its surrounding basal lamina. Satellite cells may represent myoblasts that do not fuse into multinucleated muscle fibers during embryonic myogenesis (64). Muscle is formed from the cooperative interplay between cells of two unique and separate developmental lineages, one associated with the formation of individual muscle cells and the other accounting for connective tissue "packaging" of individual muscles (64). This mesenchymal cell lineage provides capacity through differentiation to form bone and cartilage after trauma, as exemplified in myositis ossificans as well as scar (61, 78). Myogenic cells injury response is ultimately related to the innervation pattern and the connective tissue millieu (64, 65). In the face of necrotic muscle degeneration with cell death in vivo, spindle-shaped reserve myogenic cells, with macrophage mediation, are capable of proliferation and limited regeneration (64). More commonly, muscles are prone to form scar after macrotrauma (61, 66, 65, 40).

Endothelial cells are resident within the vascular structures of connective tissue and they also represent a cell population capable of dramatic migration and tissue immigration during the process of angiogenesis in wound repair (38, 61, 54). Entothelial cells are capable of a wide variety of metabolic responses to specific stimuli including immigration, proliferation, and differentiation (54). At the onset of posttraumatic inflammation, stimulation of endothelial cells by vasoactive mediators initiates a complex series of biochemical events, causing cell contraction, loss of tight junctions, and gap formation with extravasation of intravascular fluids (38). Endothelial cells can be induced by cytokines secreted by activated macrophages and lymphocytes to express a distinct set of glycoproteins that promote inflammatory cell adherence and localization to sites of inflammation (38, 40). Interleukin-1 and tumor necrosis factor stimulate the adhesive capacity of endothelial cells for monocytes, a factor critical to the recruitment of circulating cells to sites of tissue injury. Under ischemic conditions, endothelial cells are a source of xanthine oxide and may generate oxygen-free radicals (38, 40).

The immigrant cell populations are primarily involved with connective tissue inflammation, injury repair, and healing. Included in this group are the tissue macrophage or histiocyte, neutrophil, lymphocyte, plasma cell, mast cell, and platelet.

Tissue macrophages function as the "starships" of wound healing and are pluripotential cells capable of generating almost any known mediator (34, 54). These cells are intimately responsible for matrix degradation, remodelling, and regulation (54). Primarily derived from circulating monocytes and, to a lesser degree, from proliferation of local macrophages, the activated macrophage becomes the dominant wound phagocyte upon decline of the neutrophil population, regulating lymphocytic responses to antigen, and cueing the proliferation and functionality of fibroblast, muscle, and endothelial cells (61). While it is possible for wound healing to progress without neutrophils, in the macrophage-depleted animal, there is a marked delay not only in tissue debridement but also in fibroblast proliferation and wound fibrosis (54). The macrophage and fibroblast probably function interchangeably at times in repair (61). Activated macrophages differentiate into multinucleated giant cells and long-lived tissue macrophages, which together with lymphocytes and plasma cells are the hallmark of chronic inflammation (38, 61, 49).

Polymorphonuclear leukocytes (PMN) are highly specialized phagocytic cells capable of both chemotactic response to protein ligands (any molecule capable of interacting with a cell receptor) as well as activation by vasodilating agents such as serotonin histamine, bradykinens, arachidonic acid metabolities, kalkrein and plasminogen activator, the factors involved in coagulation and fibrinolysis, platelet derived growth factor (PDGF); and platelet factor 4 (49, 68). The activated, neutrophil releases lysosomal enzymes metalloenzymes (collagenase, gelatinase) and displays marked activation of NADPH (nicotinamide adenine dinucleotide) oxidase system in the cell membrane. This so-called "respiratory burst" represents a dramatic increase in oxygen consumption with the generation of various activated oxygen-free radical species, including superoxide, anion (O_2), hydrogen peroxide, (H_2O_2) and hypochlorous acid (HOCL) (49, 69) (see Fig. 44.4). These potent products of oxidation are not only bactericidal but are toxic to the neutrophil as well as to the surrounding cells and tissues. Endogenous and exogenous antioxidants, so-called molecular scavengers (e.g., vitamin E; glutathione, superoxide dismutase enzyme) under ordinary conditions provide normal cells with protection from free radical injury (69). Together with the release of other catabolic enzymes oxygen-free radicals contribute to the initiation of a zone of secondary injury (69, 66). During the inflammatory process, there is a balance between tissue injury and host defense that depends in part on the total number of neutrophils. This "neutrophil" load is proportional to neutrophil influx and disposal (54). Reducing the disability of iatrogenic neutrophil injury and the secondary edema and pain after injury is a prime therapeutic target of sports medicine (2, 69). Reactive oxygen metabolites and lysosomal enzymes are synergistic in producing tissue injury. Proteins and glycosaminoglycans exposed to oxidant are rendered more susceptible to degradation by proteases and acid hydrolases respectively (38). Polymorphonuclear leukocytes, although characteristic of acute inflammation, may also be observed at sites of chronic inflammation, demonstrating the continuum of morphologic features between the acute and chronic inflammatory responses.

The *lymphocyte* is a primary cellular component of chronic inflammation and is represented by two subtypes. The first is the "B" lymphocyte, referring to its bursal or bone marrow derivation, is the only cell capable of producing antibodies hence it is characterized by a prominent rough endoplasmic reticulum. This cell often differentiates into a specialized from called the plasma cell. The second is the "T" lymphoctye derived from the thymus, which makes up the cytotoxic lymphocytic population (38, 40, 67). In response to antigenic stimulation, a subset of T-cells, the helper cells, secrete protein hormones called cytokines whose function is to promote the proliferation and differentiation of the T-cells, as well as other cells including B-cells and macrophages (67). Cytolytic T-cells are a second subset of T-cells that lyse cells producing foreign proteins; in addition, they participate in allograft rejection (67). Natural killer cells, also called large granular lymphocytes, are circulating cells derived mainly from the spleen (67). They attack tissue cells and have been implicated in chronic muscle injury (65, 70, 71, 79). Lymphocytes and derived plasma cells are important in both humeral and cell-mediated immune responses (38, 49).

The tissue *mast* cell as well as the related circulating basophil play an important role in the regulation of posttraumatic vascular permeability and smooth muscle tone as well as allergic hypersensitivity reactions (38, 68). Characterized by electron-dense storage granules, this cell is the primary source of histamine, acid mucopolysaccharides (including heparin), and chemotactic mediators for neutrophils and eosinophils (68). By releasing arachidonic metabolites including slow reacting substances of anaphylaxis (SRS-As), which includes leukotriene-C4 (LTC4), leukotriene-D4 (LTD4) and leukotriene-E4 (LTE4) and platelet activating factor (PAF), these cells contribute to increased vascular permeability and edema in the acute phase reaction of inflammation and repair (68). Mast cells enhance the effect of xanthine oxidase and oxygen radical production (69). Mast cells also appear prominently in the early phases of eccentric muscle injury response (70, 71) and delayed onset muscle soreness (80).

The *platelet* is a "cell" without a nucleus. One of the earliest effects of soft tissue injury is the release of granule constituents from activated platelets on the site of vascular disruption. Platelets possess three distinct granules: dense granules rich in serotonin, histamine,

CA_{++}, and adenosine diphosphate (ADP); alpha granules containing fibrinogen, coagulation proteins, platelet-derived growth factor (PDGF), transforming growth factor beta (TGF-beta), and other peptides and proteins, and thirdly, lysosomes containing acid hydrolases (38). Degranulation is associated with the release of serotonin and histamine inducing changes in vascular permeability. In addition, thromboxane A2 is produced to aid further platelet aggregation. Platelets are a major source for growth factors including PDGF, insulin-like growth factor 1 (IGF-1), and, particularly, TGF-beta, all three of which have profound paracrine effects on macrophages and tissue mesenchymal cells (72, 68, 73).

Extracellular Matrix Components

Cell regulation, including migration, differentiation, proliferation, and synthesis, is now recognized to be an important function of cellular interaction with the extracellular matrix components (41, 56). It is the matrix that best defines the structural nature of soft tissue. Matrix components found to have influence on inflammatory reactions and associated tissue repair processes modulate cell activity by direct continuous effect as well as through the byproducts of degradation at sites of tissue injury. For instance, type I collagen in alpha I, alpha II and alpha I CB5 peptides as well as types II, III and IV collagen are able to induce platelet aggregation in vitro (78). Collagen degradation products have been recognized as chemotactic agents for circulating monocytes and connective tissue fibroblasts at sites of injury and inflammation in vivo, based on observations of bacterial degradated collagens on blood monocytes and dermal fibroblasts (79). The collagens form a family of stiff helical and soluble macromolecules providing the scaffold for tensile strength in dense, regular connective tissue (41). Of the dry weight of the ligament and tendon, 70% to 90% is collagen (41). A function of the fibroblast collagen synthesis begins inside the cell and leads to the secretion of a three-peptide chain procollagen molecule. Enzymatic cleavage of the low molecular weight and of the procollagen molecule produces the tropocollagen form that self-assembles extracellularly into the collagen fibral (fibrillogenesis) (Fig. 44.5). Of the types of collagen, type II collagen is the principal collagen of articular cartilage. Types I and III are important in dense musculoskeletal tissues and will be further discussed.

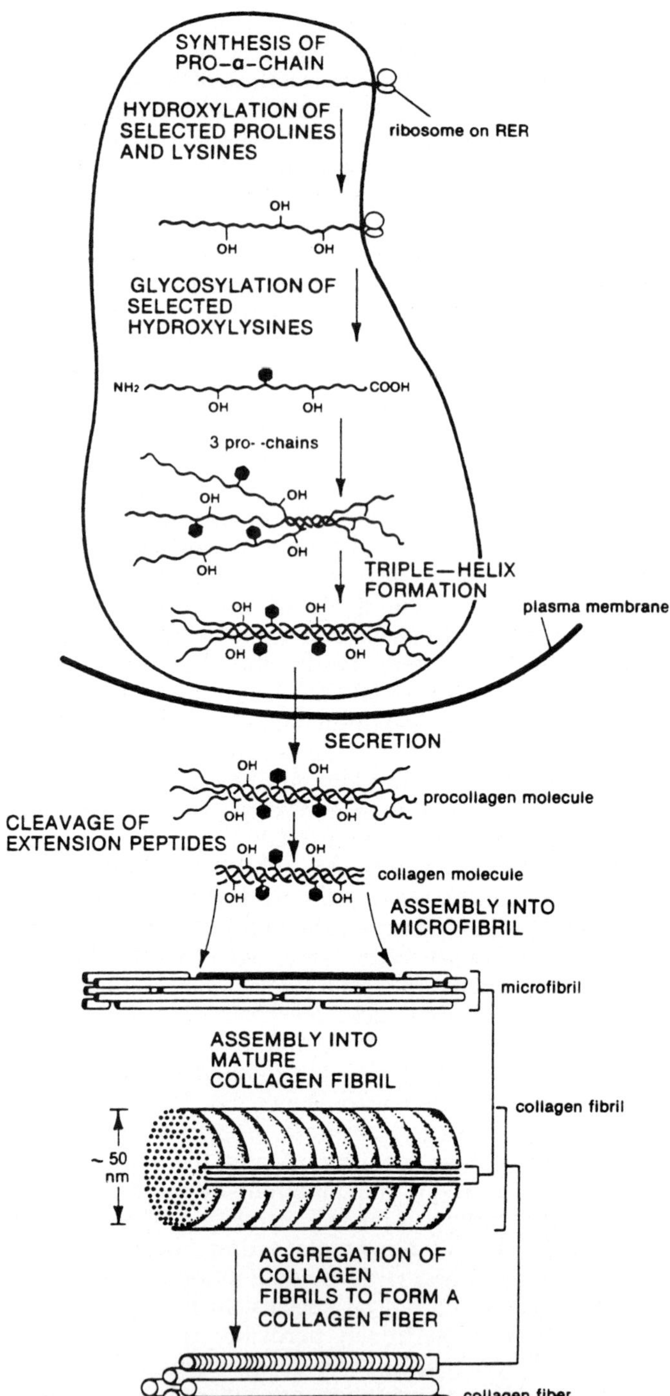

Figure 44.5 Collagen biosynthesis: Intracellular events and secretion. Reprinted by permission from Gamble JG. The musculoskeletal system—physiological basics. New York: Raven Press, 1988;63.

Type I collagen, the normal fabric of tendon, ligament, muscle, as well as bone, derives its strength from two or three covalent intramolecular bonds, or cross-linkings, found in each collagen molecule (41). This cross-linking is tissue-specific with strong trivalent bonding associated with high tensile demands, such as that found in Achilles tendon or anterior cruciate ligament (81). Under increasing load, these cross-links give way, leading to fibril failure and eventual tendon rupture. Failure begins at 8% to 10% strain (change in length/length) (76).

Type III collagen has smaller fibrils and fewer cross-links, and during repair, increased quantities of type III collagen are often deposited, resulting in long-term structural weakening and delayed recovery (81). This initial inadequacy of repair is partially compensated by an increased volume of matrix deposition and collagen synthesis (27). In time, type III collagen is gradually replaced by type I collagen, but this takes several years (41, 81).

Proteoglycans, the other principal group of matrix molecules, possess great waterbinding capacity (41).

Proteoglycans vary in composition according to tissue type and change composition with age (13, 82). The proteoglycan aggregate of connective tissues consists of a glycose aminoglycan side chain attached to a core protein, linked to a hyaluronic acid backbone. These molecular aggregates possess enormous molecular domain and act as electrostatic sponges to provide viscoelastic properties to such soft tissues as tendon, ligament, and cartilage (28) (Fig. 44.6). Hyaluronic acid (HA) is a constituent of the wound extracellular matrix that appears in the early phases of healing to interact with fibrin creating a matrix that facilitates inflammatory, reparative cell migration. The presence of hyaluronic acid appears to affect cell aggregations and chemotaxis during the inflammatory response (54). Subsequent degradation products derived from both fibrin and HA serve as important regulatory molecules to control cellular functions involved in the inflammatory process as well as wound angiogenesis (54, 72). With respect to the effects of the role of extracellular matrix macromolecules in the regulation of connective tissue metabolism, there are several excellent reviews (54, 56, 77, 82).

Fibronectins are noncollagenous glycoproteins with the ability to promote attachment, spreading, and proliferation fibroblasts and phagocytosis by cells (particularly of the endothelial system) thus facilitating repair of damaged connective tissue (61).

Integrins are a group of cell surface proteins containing two polypeptide chains, alpha and beta. These molecules span the extracellular intramembranous and intracellular compartments. As such, they may play an important role in cell matrix communication (61). Interaction of the integrins with the subplasmalemmal protein talin, itself connected to cytoplasmic filaments, results in intra- and extracellular information exchange. Integrins are extracellular matrix binding proteins with specific cell surface receptors. These heterodymic, small molecular-weight polypeptides (MW 140,000) provide a mechanism for cell regulation of tissue adaptation due to mechanical load and use (83), along with cytoskeletal deformation (83, 84).

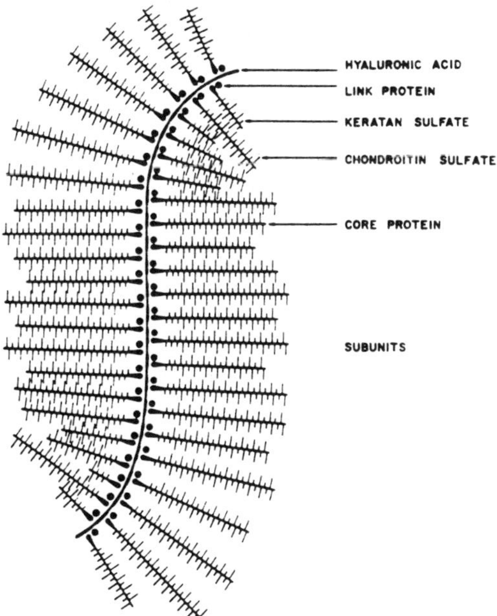

Figure 44.6 Molecular structure of a typical proteoglycan aggregate (courtesy of Dr. Lawrence Rosenberg) Reprinted by permission from Salter RB. Continuous passive motion—CPM—A biological concept for healing and regenerations of articular cartilage, ligaments, and tendons from origination to research to clinical applications. Baltimore, Williams & Wilkins, 1993.

Seven Basic Mechanisms of Sports Injury

There are seven basic mechanisms by which the athlete may sustain injury:

1. contact or impact;
2. dynamic overload;
3. overuse;
4. structural vulnerability;
5. inflexibility;
6. muscle imbalance;
7. growth (Table 44.3).

These mechanisms may occur singularly, as in acute tissue damage resulting from contact or collision, but, more commonly, these mechanisms are seen to occur in combinations, especially in the endurance athlete. Contact is the most obvious source of acute macrotraumatic injury. It generally results in a classic inflammatory wound repair reaction initiated by the onset of a bleeding hematoma and clot formation (2, 66). Direct muscle contusions and severe ligament sprains with possible traumatic joint dislocations are typical examples of soft tissue contact injury. The corollary of contact is impact. This often underrated mechanism of injury is exemplified by the cumulative microtrauma experienced by tissues exposed to repetitive load (23). For example, the ground reactive force at midstance in running is 250% to 300% of body weight. A 70 kg runner at 1175 steps per mile absorbs at least 220 tons of force per mile! (1). While contact may produce more notorious injuries, it is the cumulative damage of impact that produces the more common spectrum of overuse injuries. *Dynamic overload* describes that tissue failure resulting from sudden intolerable strain deformation. An acute tendon rupture or intramuscular strain is often the result of dynamic overloading during jumping, sprinting, or kicking. Tendons are particularly at risk during the eccentric loading that may occur when landing. Overuse or overload represents failed cumulative cell-matrix adaptive responses as seen in the context of the repetitive use of an anatomic part. Of the 30% to 50% of all sports injuries related to overuse, it

Table 44.3.
Seven Basic Mechanisms of Sports Injury

1. Contact
2. Impact
3. Overuse
4. Dynamic overload
5. Inflexibility
6. Structural vulnerability
7. Rapid growth

is estimated that 70% are caused by training errors (1). In the presence of other mechanisms, overuse often is the lighted fuse prior to the occurrence of an injury crisis. Structural vulnerability may contribute to fatigue and eventual tissue failure secondary to focal overload and excessive strain or stress. Hyperpronation of the foot during running, pathologic laxity of a ligamentous support of a joint, or malalignment such as seen with excessive persistent femoral anteversion in the lower extremity constitute structural vulnerabilities capable of contributing to the onset of injury during sports play (21). Inflexibility and muscle imbalance are interrelated mechanisms relating primarily to muscle conditioning and usage. Repetitive patterns of muscle use during athletic activity promote muscular imbalances and resultant joint inflexibility. Muscular fatigue often underlies the promotion of muscular imbalance (85). A fatigued muscle is more prone to strain (87, 86). Joint inflexibility may lead to biases in articular contact, thereby initiating a cycle of degeneration. By definition, growth is a mechanism seen in the growing or child athlete. So-called "overgrowth syndrome" along with "growing pains" are terms emphasizing the muscular imbalances and flexibilities coincident with changing skeletal proportions during maturation (88) that create potential dynamic overload of soft tissue structures. Acquired inflexibilities and muscular imbalance during periods of growth may often persist for inordinate periods of time and even into adulthood in the absence of appropriate rehabilitation and conditioning.

It is important to recognize these common mechanisms of sports injury in order to prescribe useful modifications in behavior, conditioning, rehabilitation, or structural support. In the absence of such intervention, a sports clinician is often left with the alternative of treating the symptoms of tissue injury and inflammation without ever stemming the contributing cause. Such an approach will inevitably lead to persistence of the pain-injury cycle and represents the typical failure of nonsports medicine oriented care.

Tissue Response to Physical Injury

All sports-related connective tissue injury response occurs in the context of two interrelated categories: macrotraumatic—acute tissue destruction, and microtraumatic—chronic abusive load or use.

Acute Macrotraumatic Tissue Response

Acute tissue loss or damage may result from sudden compression, laceration, extreme tensile load, or shear. The moment of tissue injury is defined by the onset of vascular disruption and the initiation of the clotting mechanism with platelet activation. A cascade of overlapping process that has been described as "predictable" then follows: inflammation, cell replication, angiogenesis, matrix deposition, collagen protein formation, contraction (e.g. remodeling), and, in the case of exposed wounds, epithelialization. These highly interdependent events are summarized in Table 44.4 and Fig. 44.7 as Phase One, Phase Two, and Phase Three of the acute injury tissue response. With respect to time, there is great disparity between the phases. While Phase One subsides in a few days, Phase Three may extend indefinitely. Severe muscle strains, spontaneous Achilles tendon ruptures or surgical wounds typically generate this type of response (Fig. 44.8). In fact, this represents an ideal sequence of events that is in fact influenced not only by the type of insult but also such factors as age, vascularity, nutrition, genetics, hormonal changes, innervation and activity level. The literature contains many excellent and exhaustive reviews of the vascular,

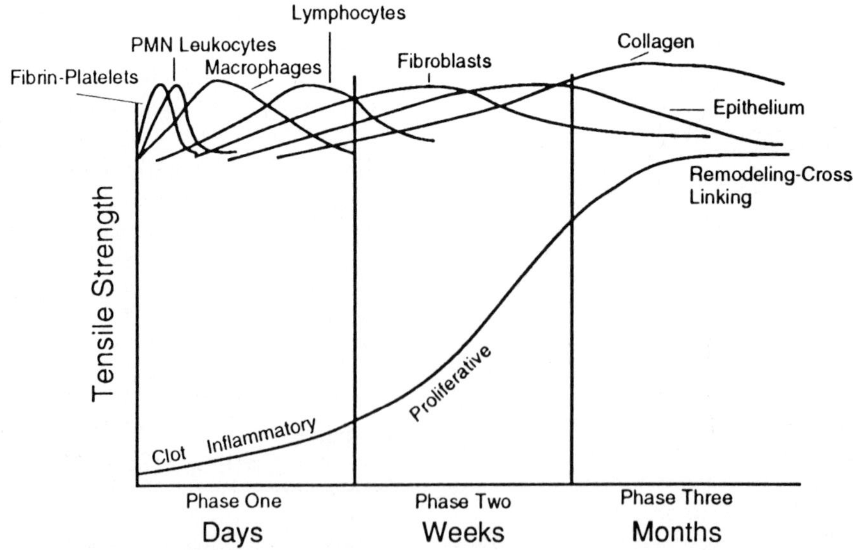

Figure 44.7 Ideal wound healing model. Originally derived from the study of skin lacerations, a variety of factors may distort the actual healing sequence in the tendon. Although this diagram is an accurate portrayal of cell matrix wound healing events, note that the temporal relationship of the various phases is such that the duration of phase one is measured in hours or a few days, but phase three may extend indefinitely. Normal tendon is not regenerated, however. PMN = polymorphonuclear cell. Adapted with permission from Gamble JG. The musculoskeletal system: Physiological basics. In: Hunter-Griffin L, ed. Athletic training and sports medicine. New York, Raven Press, 1988;105.

Table 44.4.
Phases of Acute Injury Tissue Response

Phase	Result
Phase One	
Acute vascular—inflammatory	
Bleeding Coagulation Inflammation	Hemostasis Wound debridement
Phase Two	
Repair—Regeneration	
Cell proliferation Angiogenesis Matrix synthesis	Tissue Reconstruction
Phase Three	
Maturation	
Remodeling Epithelialization	Functional Restoration

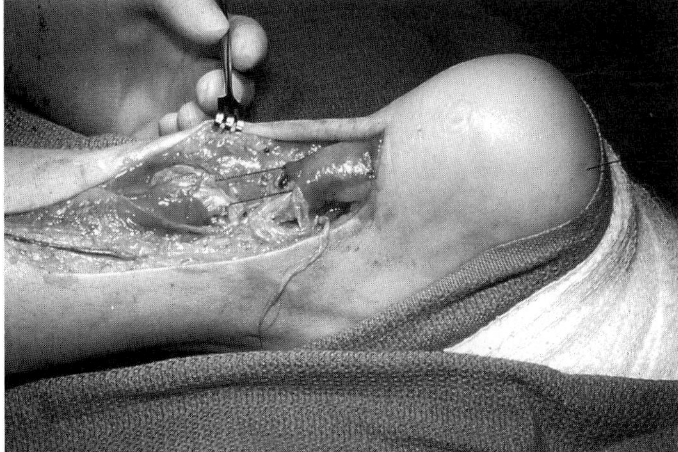

Figure 44.8 Achilles tendon rupture: Hemorrhage, clot, and tissue disruption provide a strong stimulus for an acute injury response.

cellular, and biochemical events in this process (2, 28, 49, 54, 58, 61, 66, 68, 77, 89). What follows is a pertinent summary of some of this literature on the acute connective tissue injury response and its three phases.

Phase One: Acute Vascular-Inflammatory Response

After wounding, the first reparative "cells" to appear in most vascularized wounds are platelets, which are a prominent source of cell mediators such as platelet-derived growth factor (PDGF), platelet factor IV, insulin-like growth factor I (IGF-I), transforming growth factor beta (TGF Beta I and Beta II) and an uncharacterized chemotractant to endothelial cells (72). Activation of the coagulation cascade and formation of a fibrin clot containing fibronectin with crosslinking to collagen, and hyaluronic acid (HA) is vital to facilitate reparative cell activity (54). Also known as the reaction phase, this first phase is characterized by inflammatory cell mobilization aided by an acute vascular response that begins within moments of injury and lasts for a few minutes to several days. Alterations in the anatomy and function of microvasculature are among the earliest responses to injury. An acute vasoconstriction lasts a few minutes and is followed by vasodilatation, primarily of precapillary arterioles that bring increased blood flow to the injured area, causing swelling. Blood from the disrupted vessels collects locally; with cellular debris and early necrotic tissue, it then forms a hematoma. The extent of the initial hematoma in the area of devitalized tissue defines the zone of primary injury (66). A humoral response is nearly coincident with the neurovascular events and centers on the activation of Hagman factor (clotting factor 12) in the plasma, resulting in four subsystems of mediator production that have the following functions:

1. The coagulation systems reduce blood loss by local clot formation, a process activatated in part by collagen exposed in the walls of damaged blood vessels.
2. Fibrinolysis discourages widespread blood clotting by fibrin degradation.
3. Kallikrein produces the strong vasodilator bradykinin, which increases capillary permeability and edema.
4. Complement activation produces anaphylatoxin that activates chemotaxis—the attractant of inflammatory cells in the activation of phagocytosis in wound debridgement (89).

Stimulated by the complement system, mass cells and basophils release histamine. Platelets, in addition to providing clot formation, are primary 'sources of serotonin. Histamine and serotonin work to increase vascular permeability (68).

Fibronectins are a class of noncartilaginous glycoproteins that act as adhesive molecules, integrating the extracellular matrix (61). Hyaluronic acid, a high molecular weight matrix glycosaminoglycan, interacts with fibronectin to create a scaffold for cell migration; later, its degradation by neutrophil hyaluronidases to a smaller molecular form stimulates the angiogenesis that will support fibroblast activity (54). There are three major consequences of the inflammatory phase: first, some initial wound strength is provided by the crosslinking of fibronectin and collagen; second, damaged tissue from the initial trauma is removed, and third, endothelial cells and fibroblasts are recruited and stimulated to divide (72). During this phase, release of complement activates polymorphonuclear cell migration into the extravascular space providing for the removal of cellular debris and initiating chemotaxis of additional inflammatory cells, including the tissue macrophage. Granules within leukocytes release hydrolytic enzymes that hydrolyze cell membrane phospholipids and result in the production of arachidonic acid metabolites, cytokines, proteases, and oxidants (68). The resulting arachidonic acid cascade is an enzymatically driven sequence leading to the marked increased production of prostaglandins, thromboxanes, leukotrienes, eicosanoids and slow reacting substance of anaphylaxis (SRS-A) (68) (Fig. 44.9). Collectively, these polypeptide proteins activate further inflammatory cellular behavior. For this reason, they are the targets of modern day anti-inflammatory drug therapy. The intense chemical activity and exudation of this phase produce the initial clinical signs of inflammation, edema and hypoxia and create the zone of secondary injury (66). (Fig. 44.10) This cascade is the primary chemical event producing the cardinal signs of inflammation. Initiating in minutes, this phase lasts for essentially as long as the body requires and is the ignition for subsequent repair. Assuming no coincident infection or repetitive disturbance to the wound, this usually is a matter of 3 to 5 days (72).

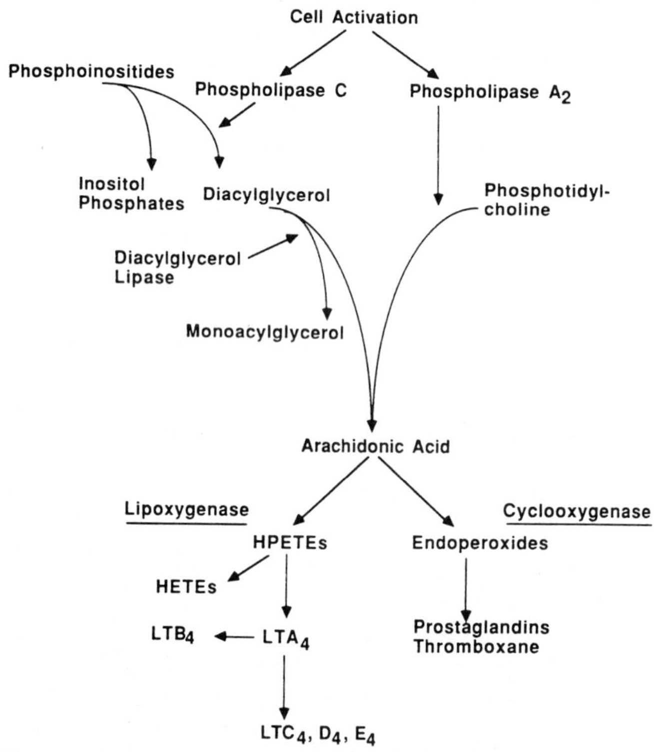

Figure 44.9 Generation of arachidonic acid metabolites. HETEs = hydroxyeicosatetraenoic acids; HPETEs = hydroperoxyeicosatetraenoic acid compounds; LT = leukotriene. Reprinted with permission from Fantone JC. Basic concepts in inflammation. In: Leadbetter WB, Buckwalter JA, Gordon SL, eds. Sports-induced inflammation: Clinical and basic science concepts. Park Ridge, IL: American Academy of Orthopaedic Surgeons, 1990.

Phase Two: Repair–Regeneration

Beginning at 48 hours and lasting up to 6 to 8 weeks, this phase is characterized by the presence of the tissue macrophage, formally a circulating monocyte. This pluripotential cell is essentially capable of directing the complete sequence of events in this proliferative phase (54, 72). The macrophage is characteristically mobile, capable of releasing a wide menu of growth factors, chemotractants, and proteolytic enzymes when appropriate or necessary for the activation of fibroblasts and wound repair. The reparative connective tissue cell, in this phase, is the modified fibroblast, chondroblast, or myofibroblast. This cell is the source of collagen production, protein mediators of repair, and matrix proteoglycans. The fibroblast cell populations of dense connective tissue are typically classified as stable cells, meaning that less than 1.5% are mitotically active at any one time (61). The cells have a characteristic low respiratory quotient and a low rate of collagen turnover (90, 91). Found normally within a dense linear-oriented collagenous matrix, these cells take on a distinct activated behavior and a fibroproductive phenotypic expression that can be further altered by deformation or changes in cell shape. Initially, in acute wounding, type III collagen in a woven pattern is rapidly deposited (30). (Type III collagen is characterized by a small fibril that is deficient in crosslinking.) The remainder of the repair process is characterized by a shift to the deposition of type I collagen that continues for an indeterminate period in the final maturation phase (2). The

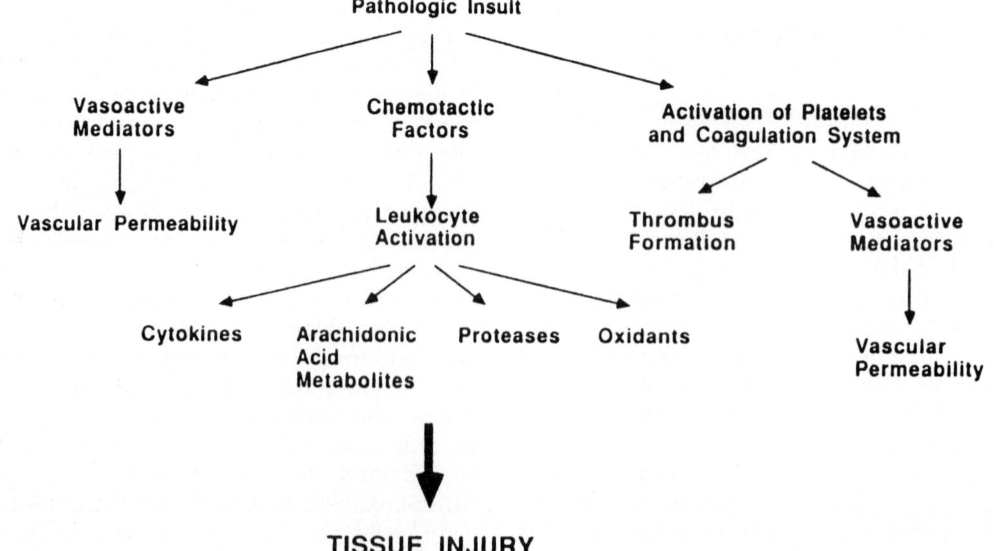

Figure 44.10 Mediators of the inflammatory response. Reprinted with permission from Fantone JC: Basic concepts in inflammation. In: Leadbetter WB, Buckwalter JA, Gordon SL, eds. Sports-induced inflammation: Clinical and basic science concepts. Park Ridge, IL: American Academy of Orthopaedic Surgeons, 1990.

critical driving force in this stage of the wounding response is a relative hypoxia in the wound microenvironment and rising lactate levels contributed in part by the release of large amounts of lactate by the tissue macrophage (72). At the same time, a process of vascular proliferation and ingrowth (angiogenesis) occurs; tiny blood vessels grow and anastomose with each other to form a new capillary bed. Granulation tissue is the visible evidence of this process (54). Various growth factors that promote this activity are prevalent in the wound (54, 61, 68).

Phase Three: The Remodeling-Maturation Phase

This phase is characterized by a trend toward decreased cellularity and an accompanying decrease in synthetic activity, increased organization of extracellular matrix, and a more normal biochemical profile (94). Collagen maturation and functional linear realignment are usually seen by 2 months after injury in ligament and tendon (28, 93). In the lacerated flexor tendon, by approximately 4 months after injury, there appears to be complete maturation of the repair site and the fibroblasts revert to quiescent tenocytes. However, final biomechanical properties can be reduced by as much as 30% despite this remodeling effort (62). The endpoint at which remodeling ceases in soft tissue injury response has not been determined (92, 62). Biochemical differences in collagen type and arrangement, water content, DNA content, and glycosaminoglycan content persist indefinitely, and the material properties of these scars never equal those of the intact tissue (30, 93).

Clinically, it should be appreciated that the human inflammatory repair response to acute injury is not so much purposeful as it is simply an example of the way things work. What factors initiate healing, control its rate, and eventually signal its completeness are not fully understood (58). Whatever relative benefit there may be in the expediency with which initial healing takes place must be balanced against the costs of early loss of function, due primarily to inflammatory pain, and late functional deficit, due to scar. If the "purpose" of inflammation is healing (80), then the body's "good intentions" pave the way to pain and performance loss. While the system works well enough for survival, for the injured athlete with an urgent competitive goal, well enough is seldom soon enough. A summary of these events is presented in Fig. 44.11.

Chronic Microtraumatic Injury Response

Microtraumatic soft tissue injury, as typically occurs in tendons is distinguished by the observation that degenerative changes are a prominent histologic feature, especially in cases of spontaneous tendon rupture (2, 51, 52). This degenerative tendinopathy is thought to be the result of a hypoxic degenerative process involving both tenocyte and matrix components. Inflamma-

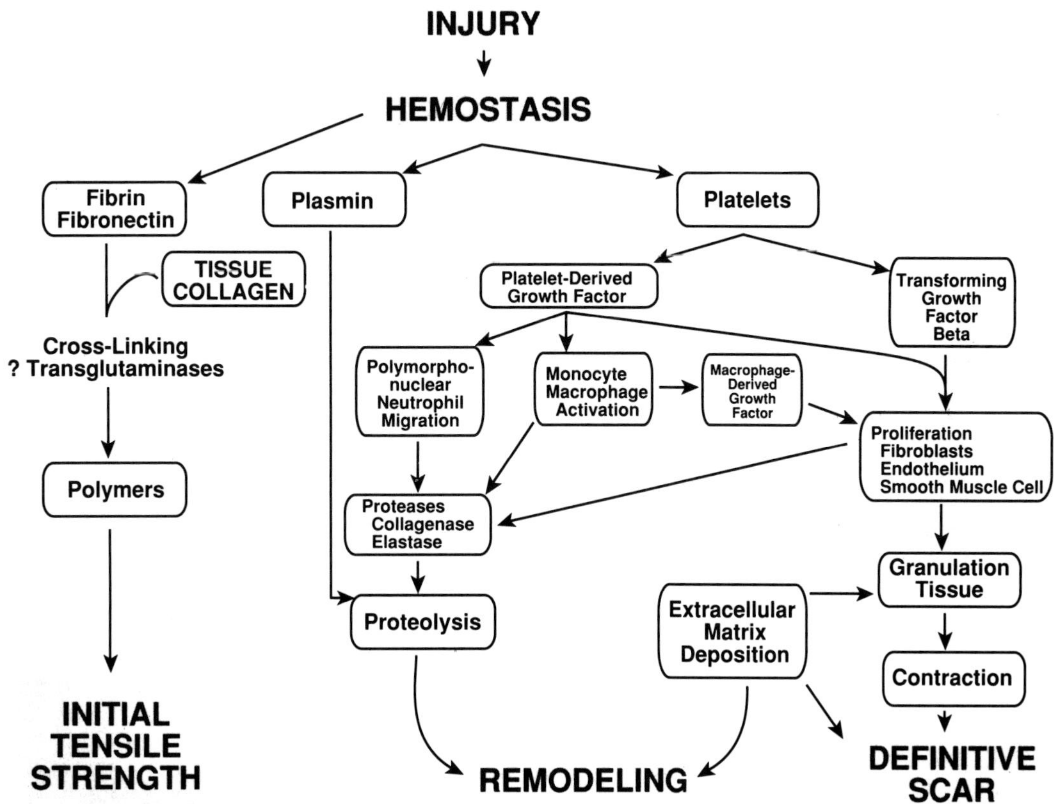

Figure 44.11 Summary of events in macrotraumatic wound response. Reprinted with permission from Martinez-Hernandez A. Basic concepts in wound healing. In: Leadbetter WB, Buckwalter JA, Gordon SL, eds. Sports-induced inflammation: Clinical and basic science concepts. Park Ridge, IL: American Academy of Orthopaedic Surgeons, 1990;78.

tory cell infiltration and an orderly, phased wound repair as seen in macrotrauma seem to be absent or aborted in microtrauma. Much of the histologic evidence for degenerative tendinopathy has been derived from the treatment of spontaneous Achilles tendon rupture. Kannus et al. (51), in a recently published study of the histopathologic changes preceding spontaneous rupture of tendon in 891 patients (397 Achilles tendons, 302 biceps brachii tendons, 40 extensor pollices longus tendons, 82 quadriceps tendons and patella ligaments, and 70 other tendons) found that 97% were affected with prior pathologic change. The mean patient age was 49 years. Of interest was the finding of similar pathologic changes in 34% of the otherwise asymptomatic control population. The microtraumatic response to load and use is best understood within the context of a failed adaptation to physical load and use (2). The histologic picture includes a range from synovial inflammation to tissue degeneration. Leadbetter has reported similar findings in the adult athlete with overuse tendon injury requiring surgical treatment prior to rupture (2, 3). Specimens included Achilles tendon, posterior tibial tendon, digital flexor finger flexor tendon, lateral elbow extensor, medial elbow flexor, patella tendon, and triceps tendon. All specimens displayed varying degrees of the following:

1. Tenocyte hyperplasia;
2. Blastlike change in morphology from normal resting tenocyte appearance;
3. Prominent small vessel ingrowth with accompanying mesenchymal cells;
4. Paravascular collections of histiocytic or macrophagelike cells;
5. Endothelial hyperplasia and microvascular thrombosis;
6. Collagen fiber disorganization with mixed reparation and degenerative change;
7. Microtears in collagen fiber separations (Fig. 44.12, 13).

Statistically, these findings have a strong correlation with aging and with sedentary tissue disuse (94). In theory, epigenetic factors compromise connective tissue cell adaptability to the point where tissue homeostasis and maintenance fails (2). Evidence based upon other models of sublethal cell stress response, such as in cardiac ischemia suggests that fluxes in intracellular calcium ion concentration may play an important role in the signaling of synthesis behavior and be associated with tissue degeneration (47, 95) (Fig. 44.14). The generation of oxygen-free radical species, either as a result of the inflammatory process or hypoxic stress response, leading to cell lipid membrane peroxidation and cell death, is another prominent theoretical model for the observed pathobiology in microtraumatic soft tissue injury (69).

The synovial sheath and peritenon are also involved in microtraumatic injury, especially as a result of friction with excitation of the synovial cells. The synovial A cell, in particular, is an immunologically competent cell with potential for pronounced cytokine production

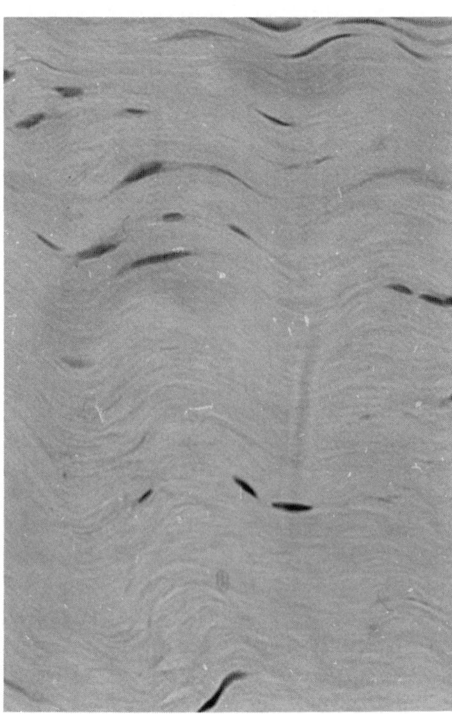

Figure 44.12 Normal tendon: Note relative hypocellularity regular collagen fiber orientations with subtle crimp pattern.

(98) Kvist et al. studied 16 athletes presenting with peritenonitis (96). Increased enzyme activities were mainly found in the fibroblast, inflammatory cells, and vascular walls in the peritenon. The results indicate that marked metabolic changes occur with an increased catabolism, lowered pH, and decreased oxygenation of the inflamed areas. Typical findings included fibroexudation with deposition to fibronectin and fibrinogen, proliferation of blood vessels, and, in some cases, marked endothelial hyperplasia with obliteration of microarterials (96, 97). Growth factors have been substantiated to modulate this process. Badalamente et al. in studying the biopsied tissues of typical cumulative trauma disorders (including trigger-finger de Quervain's disease and carpal tunnel syndrome), identified fibrocartilaginous metaplasia in the trigger-finger and de Quervain's condition, but not synovitis (44). A chondroid metaplasia response appeared to be present. Leadbetter found both chondroid metaplasia in the pulley A1 tissue as well as synovitis in the tenosynovium (3). In carpal tunnel syndrome, a proliferation of the type B synovial cell in the tendon sheath has been found (44). Almekinders et al. have demonstrated an in vitro capacity of the human tendon tenofibroblast to produce inflammatory mediators, including prostaglandin E2 and Leukotriene (LTB 4), in response to repetitive motion (42).

In flat tendons, such as the extensor carpi radialis brevis of the lateral elbow, there are findings of intratendinous degeneration with dull, immature, edematous and gross appearance as well as paratendinous granulation tissue (3, 50) (Fig. 44.15). This tissue has essentially the same appearance as chronic granulation tissue seen in various tendon sites throughout the body

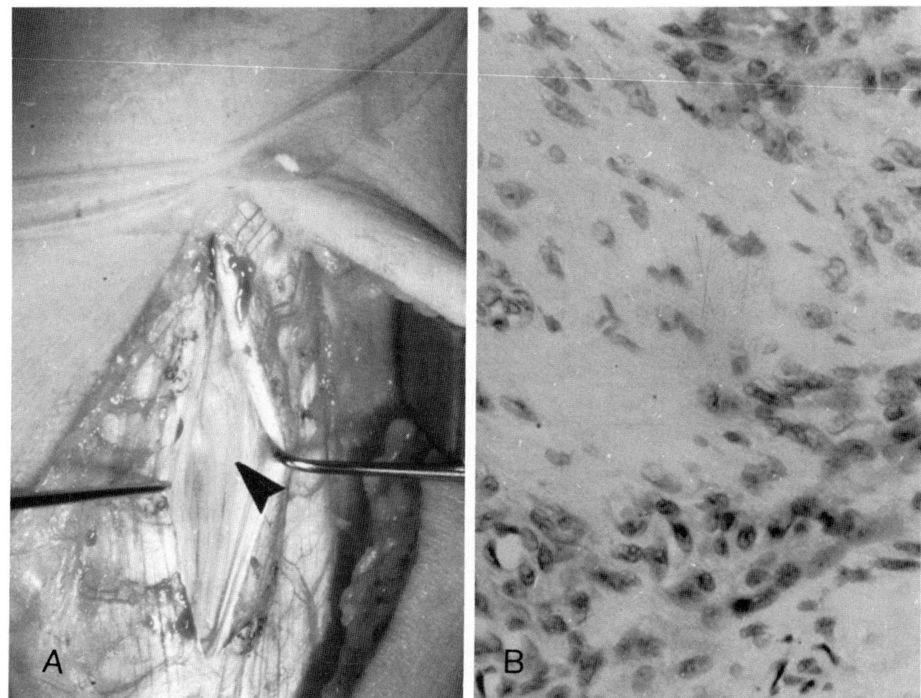

Figure 44.13 **(A)** Tendinosis: Gross appearance of lesion in patella tendon; note dull abnormal intratendinous degeneration *(arrow)* **(B)** Tendinosis *(microscopic):* Chronic inflammatory granulation tissue characterized by abortive scar repair, scattered macrophage-like inflammatory cells and fibroblasts rich in cell mediators and increased microvasculature with accompanying nociceptor innervations (hematoxylineosin).

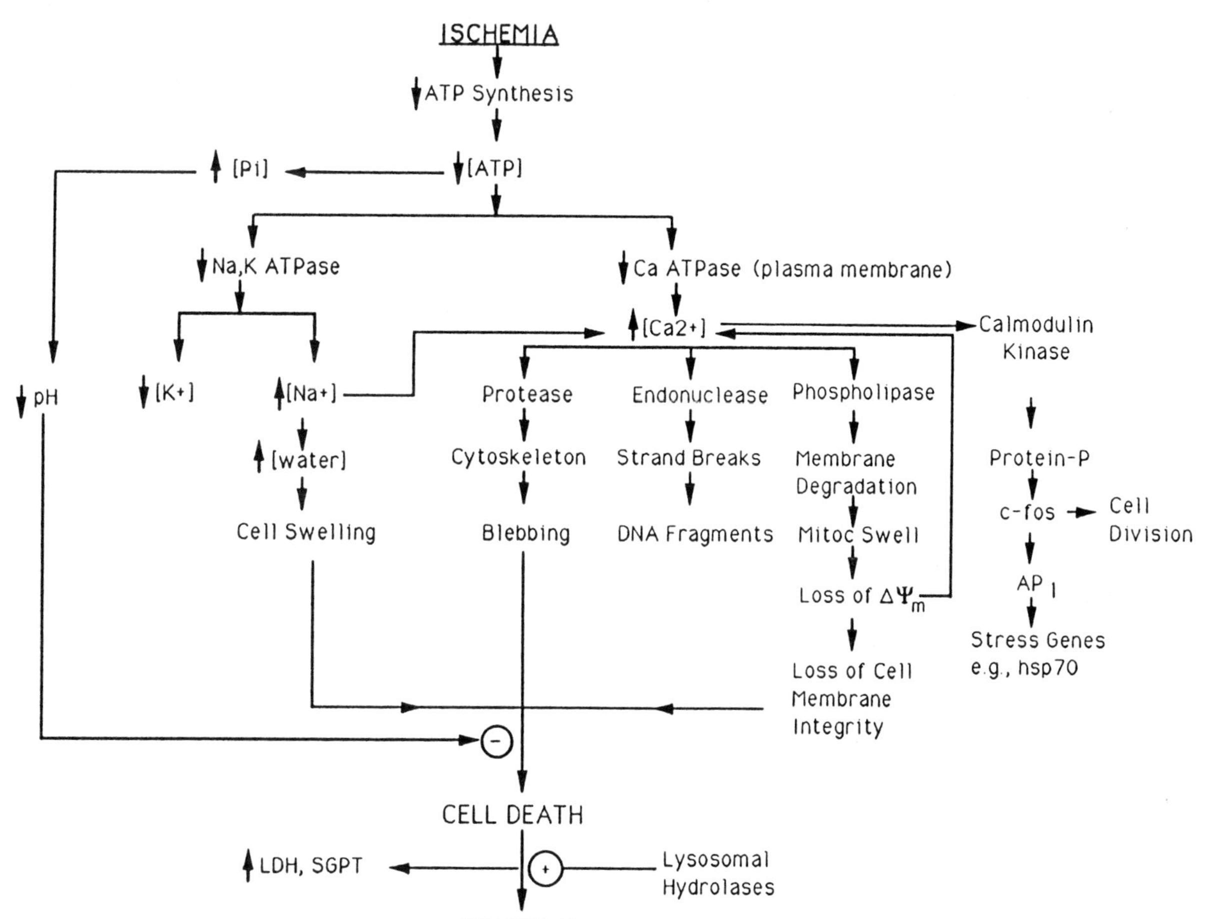

Figure 44.14 Hypothetical scheme for the relationships between ion deregulation and the progression of cell injury resulting from ischemia. Decreased ATP production leads to cessation of Ca 2^{+} and Na^{+}/K^{+}-ATPases accompanied by increases in cytosolic H^{+}, Na^{+}, and Ca^{2+}. The increased Ca^{2+} is detrimental, particularly through activation of proteases, endonucleases and phospholipases. Reprinted with permission from Trump BF, Berrezesky IK, Smith MW, et al. The role of ionized cytosolic calcium (Ca^{2+}) in injury and recovery from anoxia and ischemia. Md Med J 1992;41(6):505–508.

in response to microtraumatic injury. It characteristically has many small fibrosensory nerves, and presumably, a high concentration of nociceptor stimulating substances. The term "angiofibroblastic hyperplasia" (50) coined to describe these findings does not merit recognition as a distinct pathologic entity.

The electron microscopic appearance of microtraumatic injury response is typified in tendons by degenerative findings as reflected in alterations in the size and shape of mitochondria, as well as alterations in the nuclei of the internal fibroblast or tenocyte. Intracytoplasmic or mitochondrial calcification may be seen. Dystrophic calcium pyrophosphate salts precipitate in degenerative connective tissues as a result of mitochondrial injury. The resulting calcification is deposited in the collagen matrix as chalky appearing hydroxyapatite crystals, the "tombstones" of tendon injury (Fig. 44.16*A*, *B*). Cytoplasmic vacuoles, lipid deposition, and cell necrosis changes are thought to result from relative tissue hypoxia (2) (Fig. 44.17). However, similar changes have been documented in reparative cells, after tendon laceration, presumably as a result of the hypoxic wound microenvironment (62). Changes in the collagen fibers at sites of microtrauma in tendons include longitudinal splitting, disintegration, angulation with a unique bent fiber appearance (knicking) and abnormal variation in fiber diameter (52).

The above observations reinforce the concept of chronic injury being that pattern observed when acute injury repair response is impaired.

Acute Versus Chronic Clinical Injury Profile

In addition to the histopathologic pattern of injury and repair, Leadbetter has distinguished acute and chronic injuries according to their clinical injury "profiles" (2). The acute injury profile is characterized by a defined time of onset with the trauma episode generally observed as a sudden catastrophic occurrence, such as a collision or contact injury, or in the case of a tendon, a spontaneous midsubstance disruption. At the moment of injury, pain is likely to be severe. This is

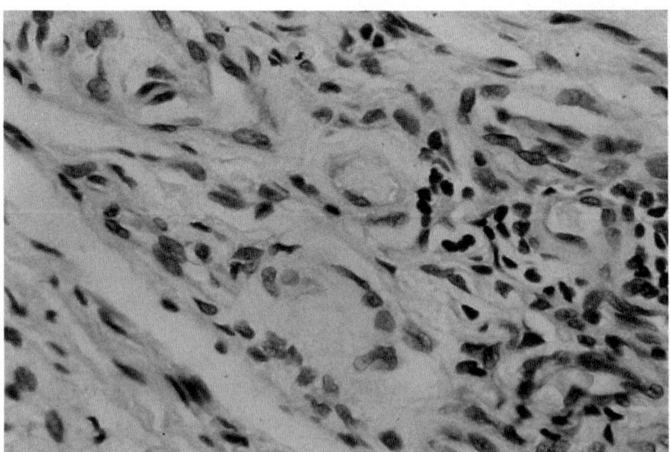

Figure 44.15 Chronic inflammatory granulation tissue characterized by abortive scar repair, scattered macrophage-like inflammatory cells, fibroblasts and neovasculature (hematoxylin-eosin).

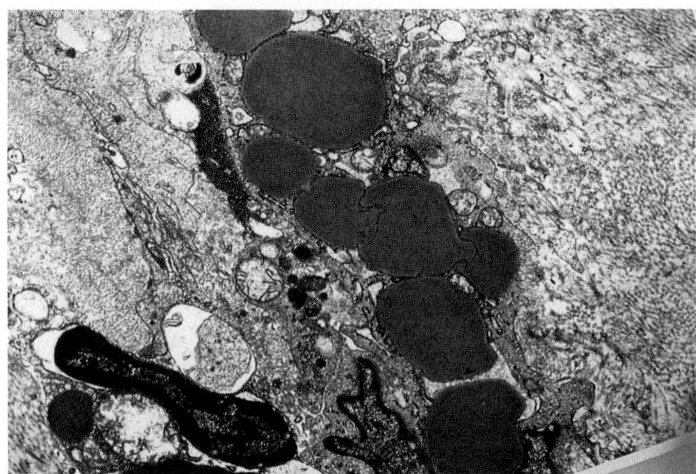

Figure 44.17 Tendinosis: Electron microscopic appearance. Note lipid vascularization, swollen mitochondria and disorganized cell organelles implying hypoxic stress response.

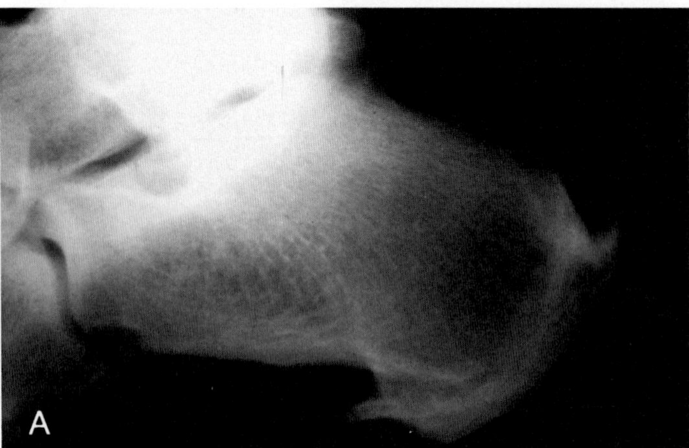

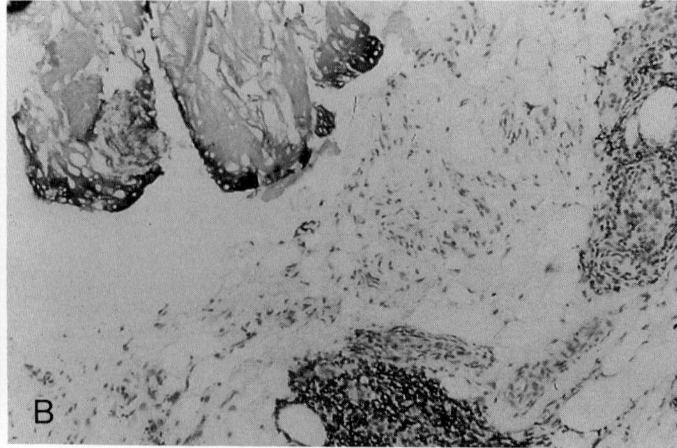

Figure 44.16 **(A)** Typical intratendinous dystrophic calcification of Achilles tendon and calcaneal plantar fascia spur. Occurring at sites of degeneration, these reactions are the "tombstones" of tendon injury. **(B)** Intratendinous calcification with prominent surrounding inflammatory response (hematoxylin-eosin).

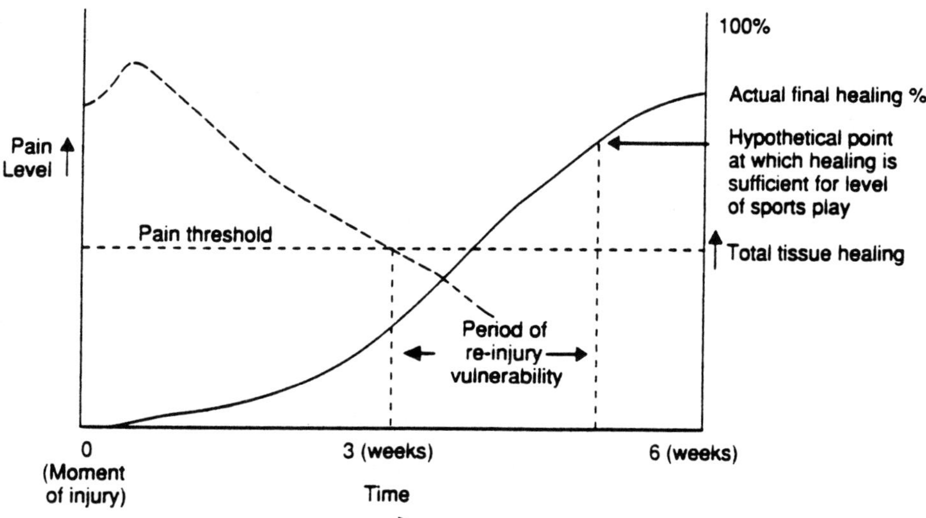

Figure 44.18 Hypothetical profile of acute macrotraumatic tissue injury. This profile is typical of an acute partial tendon strain or the pattern of healing in other acutely injured connective tissues such as a lateral-collateral ligament sprain in the ankle. Curved dashed line = pain; curved solid line = tissue healing. Reprinted with permission from Leadbetter WB. Cell-matrix response in tendon injury. Clin Sports Med, 1992;11(3)553–557.

typically followed by a period of gradually decreasing pain as inflammation is treated intensively. Pain eventually falls below an arbitrary threshold at which time the patient will feel well. When pain is no longer inhibiting, the athlete will request a return to activity; however, when the biologic curve of wound healing is plotted versus the subjective pain response over time, a potential period of reinjury vulnerability appears. The duration of this period of vulnerability is proportional to the original severity of the structural damage, the rate of healing of the given individual, which is likely to be slower with age, the nature of the target tissue that is injured, and, lastly, the expected demand or load exposure upon return to sports. The period of vulnerability after an acute injury would in theory be lengthened by any raising of the arbitrary pain threshold of the athlete or by any rapid removal of the subjective pain (for example, with aggressive antiinflammatory treatment or analgesic treatment). It would be lengthened by the adverse effects of any inappropriate immobilization, but it would be shortened by functional rehabilitation or protective bracing that would either expedite fibrogenesis or decrease tensile load on a tendon. Because research has suggested that an injured connective tissue may attain only 70% to 80% of original structural and biomechanical integrity after as much as 12 months, the period of vulnerability in these injuries can be lengthy, implying the need for protected activity despite the absence of pain, and an ongoing rehabilitation program to recruit muscular support (Fig. 44.18).

Chronic soft-tissue injuries differ from acute injuries in several important ways. The moment of injury, in the athlete's perception, may be a moment of noxious pain. This often occurs after overexertion such as a long-distance run or intense throwing, resulting in pain becoming insidiously inhibiting over a period, or explosively disabling hours or days after the event. Muscle, tendon, and synovial structures typically evidence this type of stress response to sports activity. The examiner's inquiry about the preinjury training patterns and cumulative load exposures is critical to understanding why this type of tissue response has been triggered. For instance, a careful history in a marathon distance runner might reveal that an inadequate amount of time was spent in prerace preparation and that several weeks of mild, but not inhibiting, pain symptoms had been generated by abusive training before the actual moment of injury. This is the transitional injury pattern. In theory, subclinical injury and dysfunction, e.g., microtrauma, precede the moment of conscious injury. The implication is that damage has been accumulating for a long time before the first opportunity for medical treatment. This is distinct from acute injury, in which the onset of injury and initial treatment often closely coincide. The accumulation of repetitive scar adhesions, degenerative change, and adverse effects in chronic microtrauma imply that a recovery will be slower. Again, a period of vulnerability to reinjury results, which is increased when conventional antiinflammatory measures and pain reduction are applied without regard for the lack of adequate structural integrity. In chronic inflammatory injury, it is the history that provides a proper recommendation and adjustment of activity (Fig. 44.19).

Adaptation Versus Injury

Adaptation may be defined as the process by which an advantageous change is achieved in the function or the constitution of an organ or tissue to meet new conditions (99). A maladaptation is a disadvantageous change in an organ or tissue. In pathology, examples of cell adaptation include cell hypertrophy, hyperplasia, metaplasia, protein or lipid storage, dysplasias, increased DNA synthesis, and even changes in cell re-

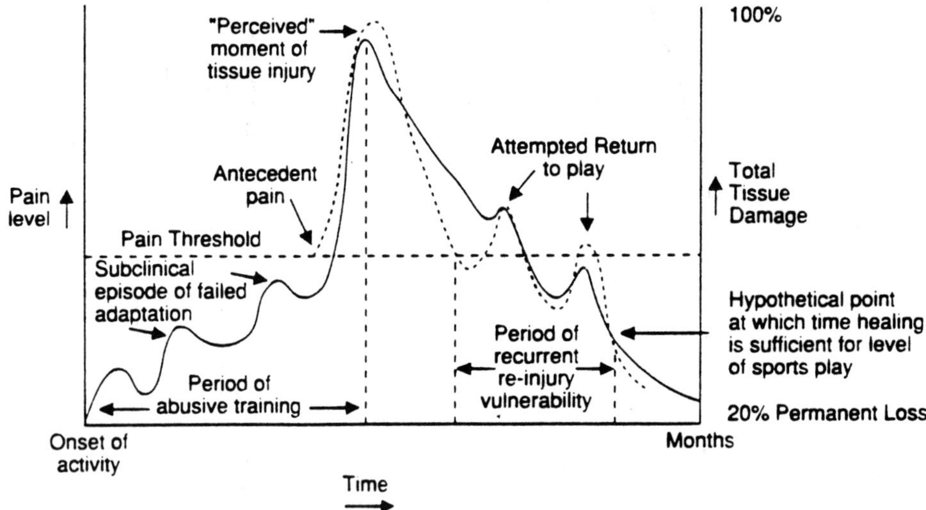

Figure 44.19 Profile of chronic microtraumatic soft-tissue injury. This profile is typical of overuse tendon injury. Solid line = percentage of tissue damage. Reprinted with permission from Leadbetter WB: Cell matrix response in tendon injury. Clin Sports Med, 1992;11(3)533–557.

ceptor properties (38). Such adaptations may prove disadvantageous to the athlete.

The process by which connective tissues renew their cell populations and their matrix contents is known as morphostasis (61). The continual turnover of collagen in dense connective tissue is an example of such tissue maintenance (81). Although difficult to quantify, collagen turnover is most rapid in bone and relatively slower in connective tissue and articular cartilage (81). Mediators are protein hormone messengers (i.e., cytokines or growth factors) that represent the most prevalent and universal method of cell-to-cell and cell-to-matrix regulation throughout the body (56, 100). There are several subcategories of cytokines; these include monokines, so named for their derivation from mononuclear phagocytes; lymphokines, produced by activated T-lymphocytes; colony simulating factors, produced by both lymphocytes and mononuclear phagocytes; interleukins, principally synthesized by leukocytes; and growth factors such as transforming growth factor beta, platelet derived growth factor (PDGF); fibroblast growth factor (FGF); and epidermal growth factor (EGF), produced from a variety of sources including platelets, fibroblasts, and tissue macrophages (101, 102). Such biological response modifiers are not limited to cell synthesized protein molecules. For example, the degradations of products of such structures as cell wall lipoproteins (e.g., prostaglandins) or traumatically induced fragments of proteoglycan molecules (e.g., from muscle or cartilage) act as potent cell stimuli in tissue trauma responses. All of the molecules interact like letters of the alphabet to create words, sentences, and whole messages. Taken out of context, the meaning of any one is often lost. After injury or during exercise-induced adaptations, it is the relative concentrations and the time of appearance of these messengers that often dictate the final tissue response (100, 101, 102). Furthermore, many of these molecules are a normal requirement for tissue or organ functions. For example, prostaglandin E_2 is normally an important factor inhibiting gastric hyperactivity. Likewise, proper hepatic, uterine, and renal functions depend on the presence of prostaglandins; hence, oversuppression of prostaglandin synthesis by nonsteroidal antiinflammatory medication has both advantages (e.g., decreased inflammation) and risks (e.g., peptic ulceration, renal failure). Taken as a whole, mediators influence virtually all tissue cell activity in the body including cell recruitment, migration, differentiation, proliferation and protein synthesis, afterload, use or injury.

Castor (56) has noted that "connective tissue cells function as a community of diverse interacting cell types exerting a high degree of mutual local control over neighboring cells. In perturbed states, as in injury, those metabolic phenomenon with survival value stand out in their major thrust as repair. Metabolic functions of cells during the repair process are genetically programmed activities largely regulated by autacoid mediators (cell self-stimulation), feedback control mechanism, and environmental factors converging on the cell to yield an appropriate metabolic response."

While there may not exist a dominant central control mechanism at the tissue level for such metabolic activity as previously mentioned, the variations in load and use would appear to play a dominant role in the clinically observed maintenance adaptation in injury responses in sports injured tissues (28). Cells may be seen as the transducers of load in this process (84). Cells respond to load by changing shape or composition, protein synthesis, growth rate, mitochondrial density, and collagen turnover rate (84). Extremes of overload or immobilization increase their synthesis of matrix degradation enzymes, a condition clinically known as tissue breakdown. In theory, a physiologic "window of stress" response defines a synthetic homeostatic and degradative cell behavior for any of a given athlete's tissue (2, 28, 31, 93) (Fig. 44.20). The effect of load on tissues is described by strain and stress. Research suggests that

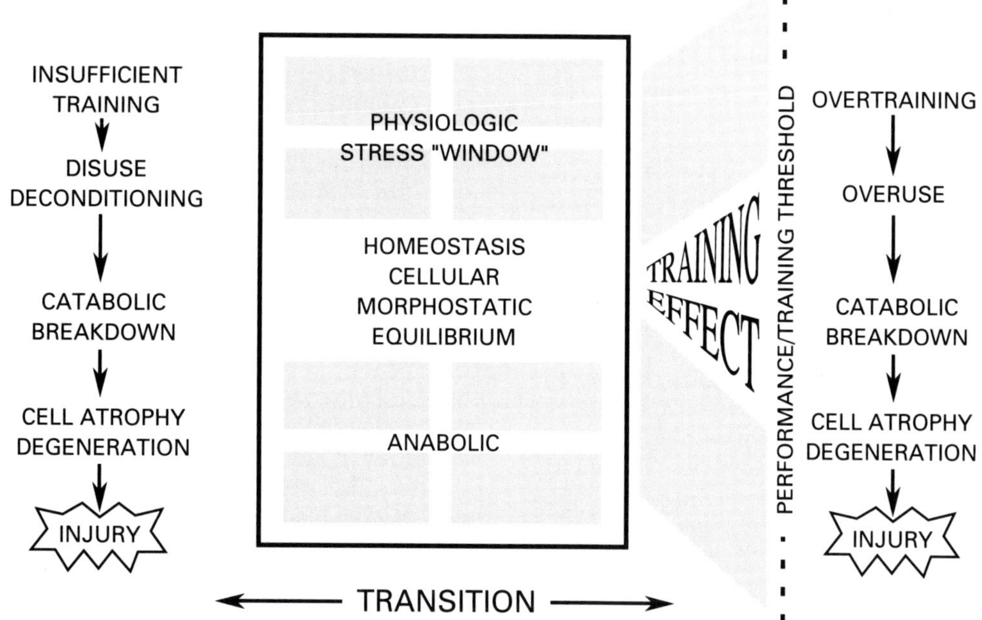

Figure 44.20 Principle of transition: the more rapid the transition, the greater the risk. Reprinted with permission from Leadbetter WB: The physiology of tissue repair. In: Athletic training and sports medicine, 2nd ed. Park Ridge, IL: American Academy of Orthopaedic Surgeons, 1991;96.

both strain and stress may promote cellular or matrix biological responses (28).

For example, tendon structures are subject not only to tensile load but also to high compressive forces (28, 93). Such compression occurs extrinsically at sites of pulleys and bony prominences; intrinsic compression is the result of a cyclic torque load seen secondary to pronation of the foot in the Achilles tendon, in the anterior cruciate ligament during the rotatory movement of the knee, and in the rotator cuff during torque about the shoulder (2). An accumulation of large molecular weight proteoglycans has been demonstrated in regions of human posterior tibial tendon posterior to the medial malleolus, implying a synthetic stress response as a physiologic adaptation to compressive forces (103). Similar findings were noted in the anterior cruciate ligament tissue, as well as the bovine flexor tendons, where fibrocartilaginous matrix metaplasia is a common finding. Woo, in analyzing the mechanical properties of tendon ligaments, has theorized an ideal homeostatic level of stress and strain duration to maintain mechanical properties and tendon mass (28). The cells, collagen, and matrix in tensile and pressure zones of different tendons may differ. Whether these effects are mediated by cytoskeletal deformation or are due to such factors as local piezoelectic effects of matrix on cells is unknown (84). Based upon such observations, a theoretical model has been suggested for Wolf's law of soft tissue (30) (Fig. 44.21).

Epigenetic and Genetic Effects on Soft Tissue Healing

There are both epigenetic and genetic influences upon connective tissue healing. Epigenetic factors are defined as those factors that can influence the phenotypic expression (i.e., protein production) of the cell without altering the genome. Vascularity, hormonal influence, and rest may exert epigenetic influence on tissue injury healing. Genetic factors are intrinsic to the individual but may be variably expressed. In theory, such poorly understood phenomenon as the "quality" of collagen synthesis, the rate of healing, the propensity to inflame after injury and the rate of recovery are to some degree under genetic control. Aging may be considered to have both an epigenetic and genetic role in injury response.

Aging

Aging is best characterized by a failure to maintain homeostasis under conditions of physiologic stress. The salient characteristic of aging is not so much a decrease in basal functional capacity as it is a reduced ability to adapt to environmental stress (38). The aging process is universal, decremental, progressive, and intrinsic to the athlete's tissue (13). Generally, tissue aging parallels overall trends in cellular senescence (59).

There is evidence to suggest that the tendon collagen fiber possesses all of the crosslinkages it will ever have shortly after its synthesis (13). During maturation, reducible crosslinkages gradually stabilize. This results in a less compliant collagen fiber subject to shear-stress injury. Aging results in a significant decrease in tendon and ligament glycosaminoglycan concentration (30). There are extensive data on the aging of cells in vitro (105). Collagen synthesis has long been thought to decrease with age; however, this decrease is not an intrinsic incapability since collagen synthesis can be stimulated in the presence of ascorbic acid (77). Generally, aging results in changes in the matrix integrity and in the rate of wound healing, although aging does not prevent adequate *clinical* wound healing, which can be stimulated by physical training. There are documented morphologic, immunologic, and biochemical aging changes (106). With aging, collagen fibers increase in diameter, vary more in thickness, and there may be an overall increase in insoluble collagen (13). These morphologic changes correspond to biochemical changes that include a decrease in proteoglycans and a decrease in water content. Parallel changes in elastic fibers also occur (106). With age, adaptation requires a longer interval of rest and recovery (38). This is presumably related to the documented down-regulation in the cellular biology of the older athlete. Injured tendons display biochemical and morphologic tissue changes (2, 28, 30, 90). In comparing an area of tendon degeneration, in a 25-year-old adult with spontaneous Achilles tendon rupture with that of a normal 24-year-old, Ippolito noted that, in the area of tendinosis, there was a 34% loss of collagen and an increase in proteoglycans of more than 100% with a significant increase in water and glycoprotein content (107). Similar histologic evidence of this type of tissue response in the very young athlete has not been documented.

Vascularity

Vascularity has long been thought to play a prominent role in tendon degeneration, especially in the supraspinatus portion of the rotator cuff, in the Achilles tendon, and at sites of extrinsic bone pressure (108). Since the injection studies of Rathbun and McNab, a watershed area in the distal supraspinatus tendon has been offered for an explanation of the etiology of rotator cuff degeneration (109). However, there is evidence that the vascularity in the critical zone of the supraspinatus tendon is actually hypervascular secondary to a low-grade inflammatory incitation with neovascularization after mechanical irritation (110). Brooks et al. likewise came to the conclusion that no significant difference existed between the vascularity of the impinged supraspinatus portion and other portions of the rotator cuff. It was concluded that factors other than vascularity were important in the pathogenesis of supraspinatus tendon rupture (11). These assertions tend to shed a different light on the theory of hypoxic intratendinous degeneration and the etiology of tendinosis. Focal load influences on cell matrix metabolism may play as great a role as any proposed diminished vascularity Wilson and Goodship have measured a core temperature increase of 5° to 9°C secondary to hysteresis energy losses in the equine superficial digital flexor tendon during exercise. This radiant energy equals 10% of the lost elastic energy on unloading and it is theorized to be potentially cytotoxic (112). There seems to be a preponderance of support for a diminished microvascular debt in the central core of a round tendon such as the distal third of the Achilles tendon (113). Further research is needed to resolve this question.

Hormonal Influence

Hormonal Influence on tendon biology primarily relates to estrogen and to insulin. It has been suggested that diminished estrogen levels, premature menopause, or premenopausal hystectomy may be associated with incidence of tendinosis in women; no other data are available to support this contention (114). In addition, diabetics are known to heal with some difficulty (115).

Rest

Rest has long been clinically recognized to aid the patient with a soft tissue injury. Yet the beneficial role of rest in the therapeutic intervention of the inflammation repair process remains empirical and undefined. Although it may be said that rest does not heal (39); theoretically, cell reparative efforts may catch up in the face of rest. The effects of rest are probably multifactorial and may include improved vascularity in the tendon at rest or they may represent an improved morphostatic balance between matrix degradation and production. Different forms of rest include total abstinence, protected activity, or altered activity (32). Such classifications imply an attempt to control both cell matrix load signal and the recovery from cell loading. There is evidence that repetitive motion and variation of frequency (i.e., cycles) may create a positive reparative signal postinjury (62). Absolute rest or abstinence does not de facto increase the athlete's potential to tolerate renewed load during participation (2, 32, 39). Modified load rehabilitative prescription has been shown to be important to any successful return to sports performance (76, 116).

Genetic Influences

Genetic Influences are implicated in the modulation of soft tissue cell matrix response based primarily on clinical observations. The mesenchymal syndrome may be a genetically determined cause of failed healing (114). Tendinosis appears in multiple sites in approximately 15% of such patients and in sites not necessarily subjected to obvious overuse (114). An association among lateral epicondyle extensor carpi radialis brevis tendinosis, rotator cuff degeneration, carpal tunnel syndrome, cervical and lumbar disk degeneration, plantar fasciosis, de Quervain's syndrome, and trigger-finger tendinosis has been observed (2, 50). Blood type O has been statistically related to tendon rupture (117). It is interesting that Achilles tendon rupture in children is uncommon and has been encountered only in children whose parents have themselves experienced tendon rupture (118). Young adult herniated disk syndrome is often seen in the presence of a familial history (author's personal observation). An underlying collagen diathesis can be theorized. The clinical significance of the mesenchymal theory is in the early recognition of the patient who presents with frequent tendon complaints disproportionate to the level of activity. In addition to ruling out systemic disease, these patients are unusually vulnerable and must be counseled about proper participation and moderation in their activity.

Structural Variability

Structural variability in connective tissues may explain alterations in response to injury and adaptive capability that are observed both in the animal model and clinically (28). Recent work by Lyon et al. has called attention to the inherent differences between the medial collateral ligament and the anterior cruciate ligament structures that would superficially appear similar but, biologically, behave differently with respect to healing (119). These differences include alterations in basic crimp pattern, a more cartiloid and plumper cellular appearance to the fibroblast in the anterior cruciate ligament, a more spindleshaped linear cellular phenotype of the fibroblast in the medial collateral ligament as well as differences in the cytoplasmic processes between these two structures (119). Chandrasekharam et al., in characterizing the intrinsic properties of the anterior cruciate ligament and the medial collateral ligament cells, revealed in an in vivo cell culture study, a slower rate of proliferation of anterior cruciate ligament (ACL) cells than medial collateral ligament (MCL) cells, a spread-out phenotypical appearance of the ACL cells versus the elongated appearance of MCL cells, relatively more stress fibers and higher actin content in ACL cells, implying possible earlier senescence, a greater tendency towards confluence in cell culture of the MCL cell—all implying a lowered proliferation and migration potential for ACL cells in comparison with MCL cells (120). The authors concluded that these factors may contribute to the differential healing potentials of these ligaments seen in vivo (120). The observed difference in ligaments and tendons in their structure and biochemistry is likely due to different mechanical demands and local nutritional supply (28). Furthermore, ligaments are nonuniform structures. For instance, differences have been found in the thickness, collagen content, hexosomene, and percentage of total water in different areas of the same rabbit medial collateral ligament (121). In the past, ligaments and tendons have been thought to be structurally distinct, with ligaments composed of densely packed collagen bundles arranged in less linear orientation than are tendons (122). However, recent cadaver studies of the rotator cuff tendons have revealed a complex interwoven multilayered orientation combining microscopic features of both ligament and tendon (123). These characteristics impact directly on the potential evolution of injury as well as the location of initial degenerative lesions in such injured tissues. Muscle structure also displays great variability. There are fusiform, parallel, unipennate, bipennate, and multipennate muscle forms. Because of the larger number of their parallel fibers, pennate muscles are more powerful, whereas fusiform muscles allow for greater range of motion (124). Muscles and ligaments display differing failure patterns. Muscles injure primarily at the myotendinous junction or at bony attachment sites (124, 64), while ligaments vary in failure pattern from osseous detachment to intrasubstance disruption, depending on strain rate (31). Thus, it is clear that all connective tissues are not the same. Not only do dissimilar structures possess different biomechanical and biological properties, but similar structures also differ. It is likely that no two ligaments are the same, and that any one ligament may vary from day-to-day and even site-to-site within its structure.

Based on such findings, it is necessary to temper generalizations regarding the adequacy and predictability of connective tissue healing response, unless the wounding mechanism, the biological nature of the involved tissue, and the environmental conditions are carefully defined.

The factors contributing to potential failed healing response in soft tissues are both intrinsic and extrinsic (32) as shown in Table 44.5.

The Principle of Transition

The *principle of transition* states that *sports injury is most likely to occur when the athlete experiences any change in mode or use of the involved part* (4). Transitional injury is rate dependent. Sudden ill-timed activity changes are more injurious. Whether in training or during injury recovery, the result is an undesired breakdown response that may outstrip tissue morphostatic efforts by imposing overload or overuse demands on the cell matrix environment. There is growing evidence for a cellular disuse transitional response, as well as an overuse breakdown response (125). The factors that correlated with the incidence of jumper's knee were hard playing surfaces and an increased frequency of training sessions (126). A relationship between complete rupture of the Achilles tendon and a sedentary lifestyle has been

Table 44.5.
Factors Leading to Failed Soft Tissue Healing

Intrinsic
- Vascular vulnerability
- Limited cell function potential
- Limited cellularity
- Aging
- Genetic predisposition (mesenchymal syndrome, structural variability, ?)
- Degeneration
- Hormonal
- Other (autoimmunity, ?)

Extrinsic
- Overt
  - Incorrect diagnosis
  - Continued self-abuse
  - Improper training (overstimulus or inadequate stimulus)
  - Improper technique
  - Improper equipment
  - Inappropriate treatment
  - Inadequate treatment
  - Harsh environment
- Covert
  - Joint instability
  - Extrinsic pressure
  - Biomechanical fault

noted; although the issue is not specifically addressed in the report, it is likely that many of these injuries occurred in the transition from inactivity to activity (94). A study on Achilles tendinitis and peritendinitis, identified a training error as the primary etiologic factor in more than 75% of all cases (21). Of these, the majority represented a sudden increase in mileage. Too rapid a return to activity was also noted as a prime cause of reinjury (21). Ilizarov, in an attempt to determine the influence of rate and frequency of osseous distraction on cellular behavior, was able to identify a window of tolerable distraction rate of 1 mm per day with as many as 60 incremental lengthenings, thereby creating a gradual transition stress response. He found the rate effects proportional to the growth of the fascial fibroblast and capillary ingrowth (127). Examples of transitional risks include any attempt to increase performance level, any change in position played, improper training, changes in equipment, environmental changes such as a new surface or different training altitude, alterations in frequency, in intensity, and in duration of training, attempts to master new techniques, return to sport too soon after injury, and even body growth itself. Transition theory correlates with current recommendations on periodization in athletic training (128, 129) (Fig. 44.20).

Injury Response Patterns in Specific Tissues

Muscle Injury

A strain is an injury to the musculotendinous unit. Muscle injuries are classified as

1. acute muscular strains and avulsions;
2. contusions;
3. exercise induced muscle injury or delayed onset muscle soreness syndrome (DOMS), (4, 125, 130).

Muscle injuries can be caused by strain or by direct blow (Fig. 44.22). Muscle strain may be generated passive overstretching as well as sudden voluntary eccentric or concentric contracture (124) (Fig. 44.23). Such sudden overloads define the dynamic overload mechanism of injury (18). Fatigue contributes to the risk of injury by decreasing the load-to-failure capacity and absorption of energy to failure of muscle (87). Muscle tissue is well vascularized and capable of generating both acute phase inflammatory responses as a result of disruption of its ultrastructures as well as displaying a variety of metabolic disturbances in muscle homeostasis (64, 80, 84, 132, 134).

Forced lengthening of muscles has been noted by

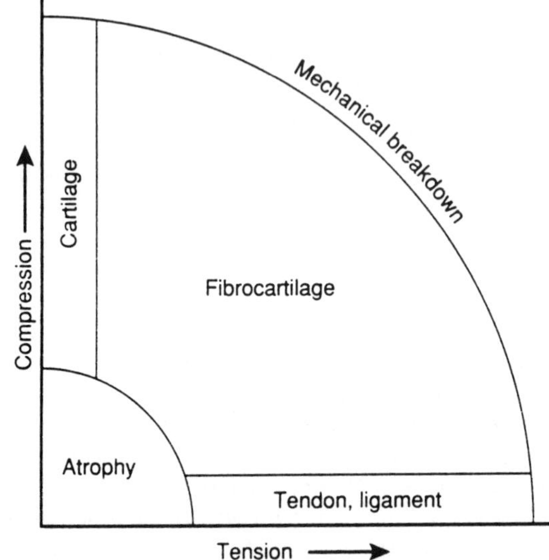

Figure 44.21 Theoretical schema for Wolf's law of soft tissue. Reprinted with permission from Amadio PC. Tendon and ligament. In: Cohen IK, Diegelmann RF, Lindblad WJ, eds. Wound healing: Biochemical and clinical aspects. Philadelphia: WB Saunders, 1992;388.

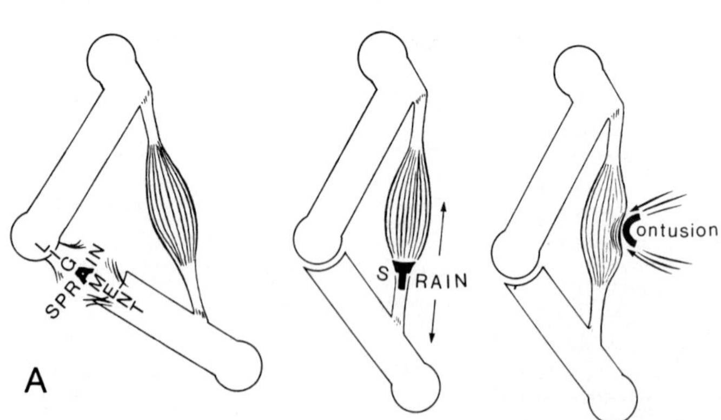

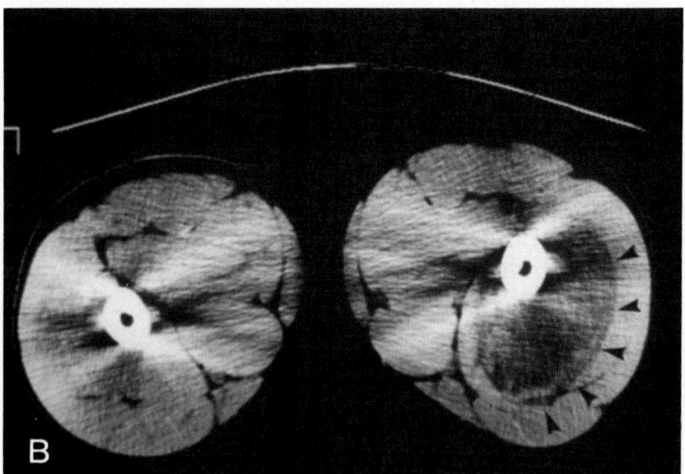

Figure 44.22 **(A)** Mechanism of muscle and ligament injury: The *sprains* are tension injuries while the *contusion* results from compression **(B)** CT Scan of severe intramuscular hematoma, right quadriceps *(arrows)* occurring after direct blow; self treated with immediate application of heat; markedly increased compartment pressure led to emergency fasciotomy of thigh. Reprinted with permission from Ciullo JV, Jackson DW. Track and field. In: Schneider RC, Kennedy JC, Plant ML, eds. Sports injuries—mechanisms, prevention and treatment. Baltimore: Williams & Wilkins, 1985;214.

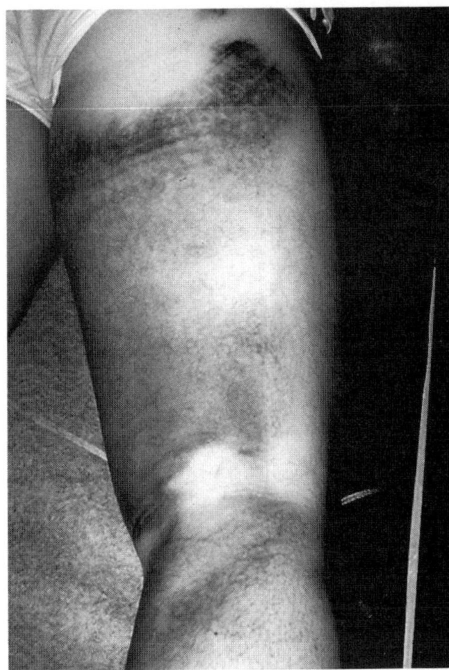

Figure 44.23 Severe hamstring muscle strain. Note pronounced hemorrhage and swelling 72 hours after injury.

Stauber et al. to induce both cellular infiltrative response in muscle tissue as well as alterations in proteoglycan in the surrounding matrix (70, 71). Tissue macrophages and mast cells predominated in the early phase followed by a second wave of lymphoid cells, thought to be cytotoxic and capable of producing both pain and continued elevation of serum enzymes with possible continued muscle damage by cell-mediated response not related directly to initial mechanical damage. There was a prominent degradation in heparan sulfate proteoglycan in the surrounding myofiber matrix. Heparan sulphate proteoglycan is thought to be involved in the regulation of myofibroblast proliferation (70).

The severity of muscle strains is categorized similar to that of ligament injury: first degree, or mild strains, are defined by minimal structural damage, minimal hemorrhage, and early resolution; second degree, or moderate muscle strain, is defined as a partial tear most often at the myotendinous junction accompanied by pain, significant hemorrhage, inflammatory pain, and functional loss; third degree, or severe strain, is accompanied by obvious hemorrhage, swelling, and, often, complete and palpable muscle tissue disruption. As with all soft tissue injury, the inherent difficulty with such a classification is distinguishing moderate from severe muscle strain. Clinical errors, both of undertreatment as well as overtreatment, may result.

Although muscle cells are permanent cells and have no proliferative capacity, reserve cells that lie in the basement membrane of the muscle fiber are able to proliferate and differentiate, forming new skeletal muscle. Thus, the regeneration of muscle fibers in even complete muscle tears is theoretically possible (64). However, when muscle tissue is completely disrupted, it is more common for scar tissue to form (131). Scar tissue prevents the muscle from regenerating and creates adhesions that restrict contractile and adjacent joint function. Initially, injured muscle can lose up to 30% to 50% of its strength (64, 131), primarily due to inflammatory pain (131). Nikolaou et al. have shown that recovery of strength begins as soon as 48 hours postinjury, but that there is significant permanent loss of contractile ability (10% to 20%) (64, 131). What causes this residual weakness is not fully known, but possible causes include intra- or intermuscular restrictive adhesions, change in resting length, as well as coincident or innervation injury.

Delayed onset muscle soreness (DOMS), appears 12 to 48 hours after exercise sessions and represents the clinical syndrome of exertional muscle injury response. DOMS is characterized by tenderness on palpation, by increased muscle stiffness and by direction in range of motion (80, 136). While the exact mechanism remains unresolved, there is considerable evidence for both inflammatory and metabolic dysfunction secondary to muscle damage (80). In support of the inflammatory model, Smith has noted the following similarities between DOMS and classic acute inflammatory response:

1. Pain, swelling, and loss of function are observed;
2. Cellular infiltrates are noted, particularly macrophages;
3. Fibroblasts have been seen in association with both events;
4. Increased lysosomal activity occurs during both events;
5. The progression and the size of the lesion occur in both instances in about 48 hours;
6. Increased levels of Interleukin 1 and acute phase proteins occur in both events;
7. Signs of healing are observed at approximately 72 hours (80).

Structural abnormalities following eccentric exercise have been identified:

1. Primary and secondary sarcolemmal disruption;
2, Swelling or disruption of the sarcotubular system;
3. Distortion of the myofibrils contractile elements;
4. Cytoskeletal damage;
5. Extracellular myofiber matrix abnormalities (133, 135).

Exertional rhabdomyolysis has been associated with elevated plasma levels of intramuscular proteins such as creatinine kinase (CK), lactic dehydrogenase (LDH) and myoglobin (134). The cytokine Interleukin 2 (IL-1) has been called the "endogenous pyrogen" and has been shown to stimulate muscle proteolysis in vitro. Inter-Leukin 1 in vivo is a prominent stimulator of prostaglandin E2 (PGE2), which is known to increase muscle lysosome function (134). As in other sublethal cell stress responses (48) (Fig. 44.14), intracellular CA^{2+} ion levels that may evolve from structural damage to the sarcolemmal especially during eccentric muscular actions (133, 134). This initial calcium overload phase of intracellular accumulation then may precipitate an autolytic phase where proteases and phospholipases increase in activity resulting in myofibrillar and membrane degradation. A regenerative or repair phase would then follow (133, 134).

A muscle contusion results from an external force sufficient to cause muscle damage (Fig. 44.22). Contusions may be graded in severity by restriction in range of motion of the subtended joints. A mild contusion causes a loss of less than one-third of the normal range of motion of the adjacent joint, whereas severe contusions cause limitations to less than one-third of normal excursion. Contusions result in vascular disruption, producing two types of injury: intermuscular hematoma—a hemorrhage occurring along large intermuscular septa or fascial sheaths, or intramuscular hematoma—a hemorrhage occurring within muscle substance. Intermuscular hematomas are more likely to disperse and be reflected by distal ecchymosis and diffusion of degradating blood components, whereas intramuscular hematomas are more difficult to resolve and are associated with scar contraction or myositis ossificans (130). In severe cases, rapid bleeding may cause acute compartment syndrome and require urgent surgical fasciotomy (Fig. 44.22*B*). In the case of contusions of the quadriceps muscles, the Jackson-Feagin classification has proven useful in assessing prognosis and rate of recovery (137). These contusions were classified as mild (localized tenderness, greater than 90° range of motion, normal gait, and the ability to do a knee bend); moderate (swollen and tender muscle mass, less than 90° range of motion, antalgic gait, and inability to climb stairs or arise from a chair without pain); or severe (marked tenderness and swelling, less than 45° range of motion, severe limp requiring crutches for ambulation and pain on the ipsilateral knee) (137, 138). Myositis ossificans developed in 13 of 18 patients with grade II or III contusions, but in none of the 47 athletes with grade I contusions (137).

Myositis ossificans traumatica is a condition of heterotopic ossification response usually confined to a single muscle or muscle group, and occurring in the vast majority of cases after a prior episode of trauma, whether single or repetitive (137) (Fig. 44.24). The pathologic course is that of a benign self-limiting process characterized by both dystrophic calcification (e.g., calcium phosphate precipitation in damaged tissue) and bone formation in areas of preexisting hematoma, and injured tissue as a result of severe contusion, strain, or repeated trauma (139). Clinically, myositis ossificans can be a source of considerable and lengthy disability to the athlete due to inflammatory pain and contracture (64, 78, 124). Parosteal and intramuscular locations are more common than periosteal, which is sometimes helpful in the radiologic differentiation of this lesion from osteosarcoma (138). The most common clinical findings are a soft tissue mass with restriction of joint motion (Fig. 44.25). In myositis ossificans patients, the pain and the size of the mass decrease as the lesion matures, whereas, in osteosarcoma patients, the mass as well as the pain are known to increase as time progresses (138). The quadriceps, femoris and biceps brachii are most often involved, reflecting their exposure to direct trauma. While the exact mechanism of onset remains unknown, experimental evidence suggests that extensive cell necrosis stimulates connective tissue cell metaplasia (78,

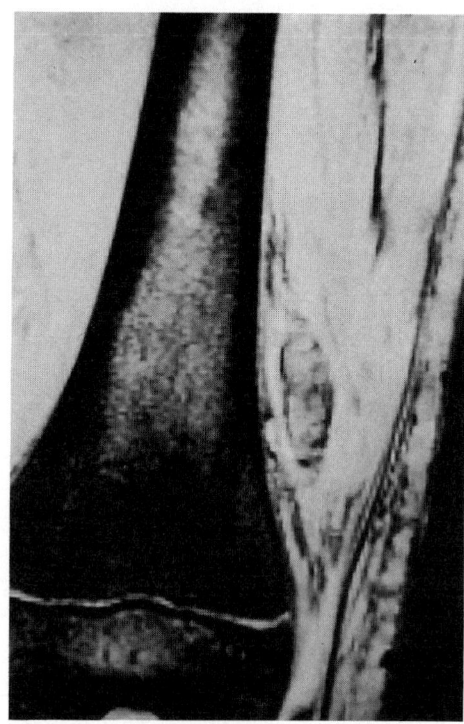

Figure 44.24 Myositis ossificans (MRI vastus lateralis). Note parosteal location and peripheral calcification pattern.

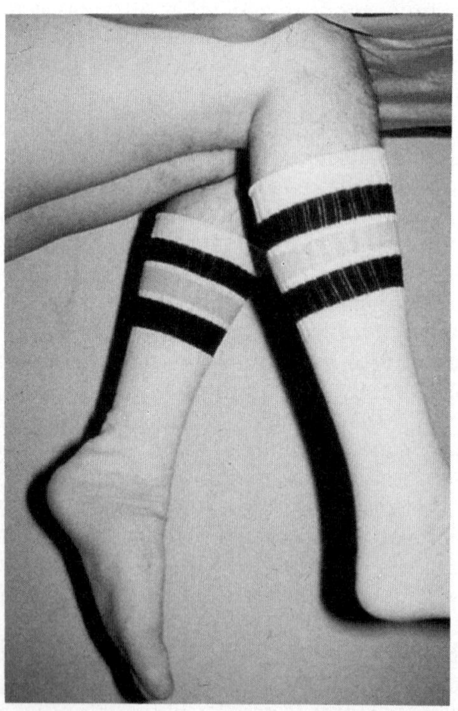

Figure 44.25 Quadriceps contracture secondary to myositis ossificans after contusion injury. Prone examination often best demonstrates loss of knee flexion by eliminating compensating hip flexion.

64). The pathologic process of ossification begins with the initial injury to muscle and connective tissue associated with muscle fiber disruption and hemorrhage. The pathophysiologic sequence may be muscle trauma, inflammation, cellular proliferation, concentration of growth factors, induction of bone forming cells, and, finally, ossification. Nonsteroidal antiinflammatory medications (NSAID's) have been known and have been shown to prevent heterotopic ossification implying that prostaglandins may play a role in the inflammatory generation of myositis ossificans (139). Increased exercise, stress, and younger age have been thought to be associated with heterotopic bone deposition (138). Myositis ossificans is most common in the second and third decades of life. The reason for this is not known, but contributing factors are thought to include high activity level, coupled with rapid growth resulting in increasing muscle length, and larger muscle volume (138). The onset of myositis ossificans has been related to the severity of contusion. Jackson and Feagin found 72% of athletes afflicted by moderate or severe contusions developed heterotopic ossification (141). Reinjury of a contused quadriceps was associated with 100% subsequent development of myositis ossificans. A presentation of pain, a palpable mass, and associated flexion contracture after muscle injury strongly suggest the possibility of early myositis ossificans (138, 141). The clinician may note localized warmth and local tenderness. Radiologic evidence of intramuscular calcification generally is delayed in appearance for 6 to 8 weeks after onset with gradual evolution to mature bone over a period of subsequent months (78, 141, 138). The most important differential diagnosis of myositis ossificans is malignancy, i.e., osteosarcoma. There are some helpful differentiating characteristics between these characteristics. Myositis is characterized by a pattern of decreasing pain and size of the mass over time, a diaphyseal location, a lack of associated bone destruction, the presence of a radiolucent line of separation of the lesion from the adjacent diaphyseal bone, characteristic zones of radiodense mature bone at the periphery of the lesion with a more lucent center correlating with the known histologic zonal maturation pattern of this lesion. This is in contradistinction to tumors, which tend to develop more dense calcification centrally (138) (Fig. 44.25). It should be noted that none of these radiologic features is without exception; recent attention has been called to the wide variety of appearances on all imaging modalities, especially MRI, which can be correlated with different stages of lesion maturation (140). Patients with osteosarcoma have a history of trauma in the involved limb 40% of the time (138). Serial plain radiologic observation is mandatory in all cases and usually suffices to resolve the diagnosis. Surgical biopsy is discouraged due to the confusing callus-like pseudomalignant histology of benign myositis ossificans, the propensity for local recurrence of the lesion, and the tendency for spontaneous resorption (78, 139). In rare cases, surgical removal of a symptomatic lesion is indicated for persistent pain—usually no sooner than a year or more after onset.

Myofascial pain syndrome is a painful musculoskeletal response that can follow muscle trauma. Myofascial trigger-points are small chord-like or nodular sites that are associated with local muscle spasms and are acutely painful (142). Fibrositis is a diffuse multiple site complaint that is not associated with muscle spasm or weakness and that most often affects women between the ages of 30 and 60. It is not caused by trauma and is associated with emotional disturbances (143). One of its symptoms is generalized muscle soreness and deep tenderness to palpation. Orsen has provided an excellent review of myofascial pain (144). Both myofascial pain syndrome and fibrositis have been theorized to have possible neurogenic origin at the central or spinal cord level. Neither condition is known to be inflammatory.

Tendon Injury

Because of their prevalence in sports, injuries to tendons and tendon insertions have received considerable attention. There are many types of tendon and fascial injuries. Enthesopathy is an injury in which tendon fibers are either microtorn or inflamed at their bony insertion (99); it is a term more often reserved for rheumatologic conditions. The tendinosis lesion is an initially asymptomatic tendon degeneration caused either by aging or by cumulative microtrauma without histologic evidence of acute inflammation (2, 52, 90) (Fig. 44.26). Paratenonitis is an inflammation of the tendon sheath and is heralded by pain, swelling, and occasionally, local crepitus (2) (Fig. 44.27*A*, *B*).

In tendinitis, there is injury to the tendon tissue proper, and if partial or complete tearing is involved, there will be capillary damage, vascular injury, and in-

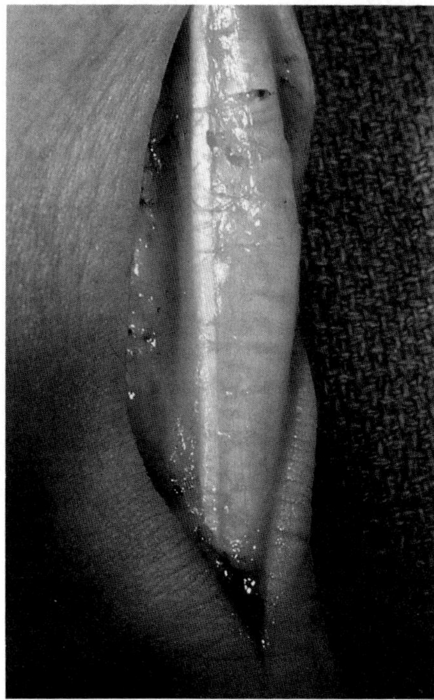

Figure 44.26 Gross appearance of Achilles tendinosis lesion. Note fusiform tendon swelling and hyperemic tenovagium with incidental intact plantar's tendon.

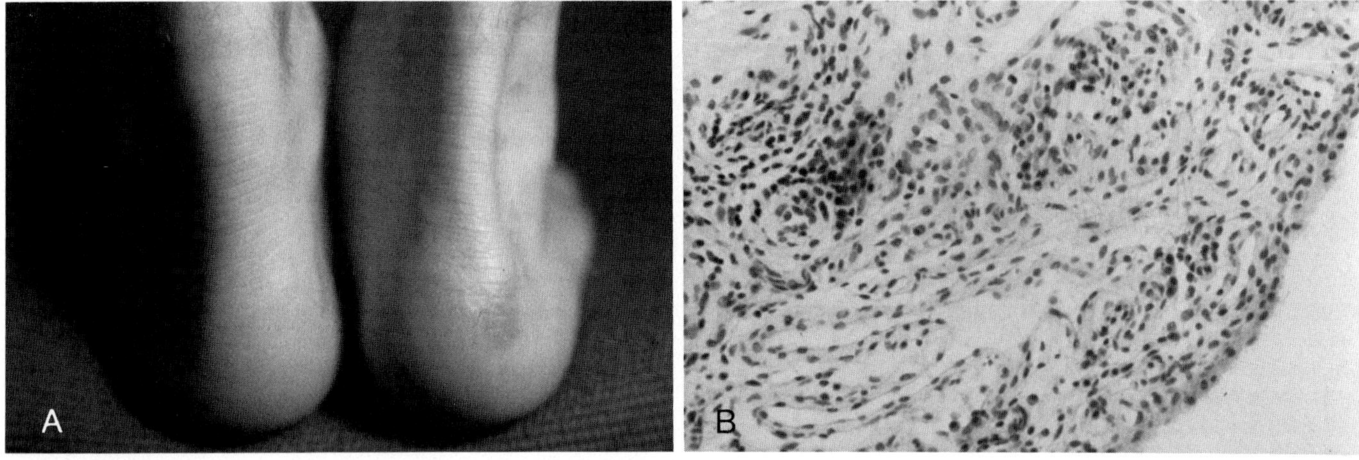

Figure 44.27 **(A)** Typical appearance Achilles paratenonitis. **(B)** Paratenonitis—microscopic appearance. Note prominent inflammatory cells with synovial hyperplasia.

tratendinous inflammation. Depending on the specific tendon, complete tendon tears will require surgical repair (e.g., long head of the biceps, Achilles, pectoralis major, extrinsic tendons of the hand, patella tendon). Normal tendon has a tensile strength that measures 45 to 98 N/mm but at 8% to 10% strain tendon begins to fail (76). The stage at which this failure causes pain and the mechanism involved in healing of this type of injury are matters of conjecture. it is not clear whether inflammation precedes degeneration or if inflammation is incited by gradual mechanical failure. Available evidence from surgical biopsy suggests that inflammation follows tendon tears. The pathology of microtraumatic tendon injury has been extensively discussed in the previous section on physical injury response. The current classification of tendon injury emphasizes the distinction between peritenon or synovial inflammation versus direct involvement of the tendon substance, reflecting the variable stress responses of tendon structure (Table 44.6).

Ligament Injury

A sprain is an injury to a ligament. The nomenclature of ligament injury varies in different schemes (Table 44.7). Healing of sprained ligament tissue is analogous to healing in other vascularized tissues. Disruption of ligament is followed by hematoma and soft tissue inflammatory repair. Full recovery may take more than a year and ultimately tensile strength can be reduced by 30% to 50% (93). This seems to be the result of the differing quality of scar and matrix in healing ligament (93, 28). A corresponding increase in the amount of ligament scar helps to counteract mechanical weakness, but other biomechanical properties such as bending stiffness are not improved (93). Hence, once ligaments are damaged, "normal" ligament tissue is not restored (31, 93). Cell structure, rates of maturation and metabolic activity may differ from ligament to ligament (119, 93). Tendons and ligaments share the structural property of crimp, a regular wavy undulation of cells and matrix that is seen under a microscope (76). This crimp acts as a buffer or shock absorber that allows the ligament to avoid damage during elongation. Under load, the crimp pattern slowly straightens out. Collagen fibers straighten completely at about 4% elongation (93). Beyond this limit, tropocollagen molecular stress occurs. Ligaments display viscoelastic behavior (e.g., a nonlinear deformation with respect to load). This biomechanical characteristic is both rate and history dependent. Therefore, the more rapid a ligament is loaded, the more strain resistance develops. This observation underlines the importance of slow static stretching of both tendon and ligament. A previously deformed ligament remembers "being stretched" by responding slightly differently to each stretch in a series and being able to return to prestretch lengths (93). The mechanism for this response is thought to reside at the molecular level of the matrix and has the additional adaptive advantage of adjusting joint loads under a variety of loading conditions while preventing failure (130). A failure to adapt results in injury.

Synovial Injury

The synovial membrane is a thin layer of cells loosely classified as a specialized form of connective tissue. Synovitis is a frequently associated complaint of tendon and ligament sports-induced injury and therefore deserves some special consideration.

Synovial cells consist of three basic types: synovial type A macrophage-like cells make up 20% to 30% of the synovial lining. The majority of the remaining 70% to 80% of normal synovial lining cells have fibroblast (type B cell) characteristics, including prominent, rough endoplasmic reticulum associated with collagen and scar production. Type AB cells have also been described that represent a combination of characteristics. Synovium functions to regulate the peritendinous environment much as it does the articular cartilage environment in joints (146). Synovial type A cells are active in phagocytosis and the degradation of particular matter from

Table 44.6.
Terminology of Tendon Injury[a]

New	Old	Definition	Histologic Findings	Clinical Signs and Symptoms
Paratenonitis	Tenosynovitis Tenovaginitis Peritendinitis	An inflammation of only the paratenon, either lined by synovium or not	Inflammatory cells in paratenon or peritendinous areolar tissue	Cardinal inflammatory signs: swelling, pain, crepitation, local tenderness, warmth, dysfunction
Paratenonitis with tendinosis	Tendinitis	Paratenon inflammation associated with intratendinosis degeneration	Same as I, with loss of tendon collagen fiber disorientation, scattered vascular ingrowth but no prominent intratendinous inflammation	Same as I, with often palpable tendon nodule, swelling, and inflammatory signs
Tendinosis	Tendinitis	Intratendinous degeneration due to atrophy (aging, microtrauma, vascular compromise, etc.)	Noninflammatory intratendinous collagen degeneration with fiber disorientation, hypocellularity, scattered vascular ingrowth, occasional local necrosis or calcification	Often palpable tendon nodule that can be *asymptomatic,* but may also be point tender. Swelling of tendon sheath is absent
Tendinitis	Tendon strain or tear	Symptomatic degeneration of the tendon with vascular disruption and inflammatory repair response	Three recognized subgroups: each displays variable histology from purely inflammation with acute hemorrhage and tear, to inflammation superimposed upon pre-existing degeneration, to calcification and tendinosis changes in chronic conditions. In chronic stage there may be: 1. Interstitial microinjury 2. Central tendon necrosis 3. Frank partial rupture 4. Acute complete rupture	Symptoms are inflammatory and proportional to vascular disruption, hematoma, or atrophy-related cell necrosis. Symptom duration defines each subgroup: A. Acute (less than 2 weeks) B. Subacute (4–6 weeks) C. Chronic (over 6 weeks)

[a]Adapted from Clancy WG: Tendon trauma and overuse injuries. *In:* Leadbetter WB, Buckwalter JA, Gordon SL, eds. Sports-Induced Inflammation. Park Ridge, IL: American Academy of Orthopaedic Surgeons, 1990; and from Puddu G, Ippolito E, Postacchini P. A classification of Achilles tendon disease. Am J Sports Med 1976; 4:145–150.

Table 44.7.
Schemes for Assessing Ligament Injury

Grade	Severity	Degree	Structural Involvement	Exam	Performance Deficit
1	Mild	1°	Negligible	No visible injury Locally tender, only joint stable	Minimal to a few days
2*	Moderate	2°	Partial	Visible swelling, Marked tenderness +/− stability	Up to 6 weeks (may be modified by protective bracing)
3	Severe	3°	Complete	Gross swelling, Marked tenderness, Antalgic posture Unstable	Indefinite, minimum of 6–8 weeks

*In present schemes for clinical classification of soft tissue injury, it is the intermediate qualities of trauma that form a "gray zone" in clinical decision making.

the cavities they surround, and they demonstrate pronounced immunologic and inflammatory potential. Synoviocytes produce a variety of cytokines including interleukin-I (IL-I), fibroblast growth factor, (FGF), transforming growth factor beta (TGF-B), Beta II microglobulin, amaloyd A, and other unidentified factors (145). Such cytokines are intensely inflammatory and may incite stenosing fibrosynovial response. Bursitis and tenosynovitis are accurate descriptions of the underlying histopathology (Fig. 44.28). Vascular endothelial cells in the synovium maintain nutrition and also participate in inflammatory reactions to trauma. Afferent neurons in the synovium and in the joint capsule contain substance P, a neuropeptide that is a primary source of pain after injury (147). Both connective tissue fibroblasts and macrophages would appear to assume the structure and function of synovial lining cells under conditions as yet to be precisely defined. A special synovial cell has been identified to interdigitate with the immune T lymphocytes, a cell known to mediate chronic inflammatory processes (145). The synovial membrane contains freely available unsaturated phospholipids, a ready source of prostaglandin and prostacyclin production through the arachidonic acid cascade. When in excess, both molecules are potent pain stimulators. Synovial lining cells have been noted to bind antigen antibody complex, present antigen to T lymphocytes, produce cytokines that promote the activation and proliferation of T lymphocytes, and respond to signals from mononuclear cells (145). Explosive swelling such as is seen in the olecranon bursa of the dart thrower or the prepatellar bursa of the wrestler or the marked peritendinous reactions brought on by overuse seem to be triggered by conditions of use as well as frictional shear. It is theorized that wear fragments of matrix molecules may promote this inflammation (148). The type A cell is a secretor of hyaluronic acid that serves as a synovial lubricating factor to counteract frictional irritation (145). Trauma to a bursa or joint with vascular injury and bleeding (hemobursa) rapidly triggers an inflammatory process mediated by the prevalent source of cytokines found in platelets as well as in synovial cells. Lysosomal enzymes released into the bursal or peritenon space may damage exposed tendon surfaces with loss of matrix proteoglycans (146). Medication such as corticosteroid injection or NSAID's reduce synovial inflammation through the direct suppression of the arachidonic acid cascade. (Fig. 44.28)

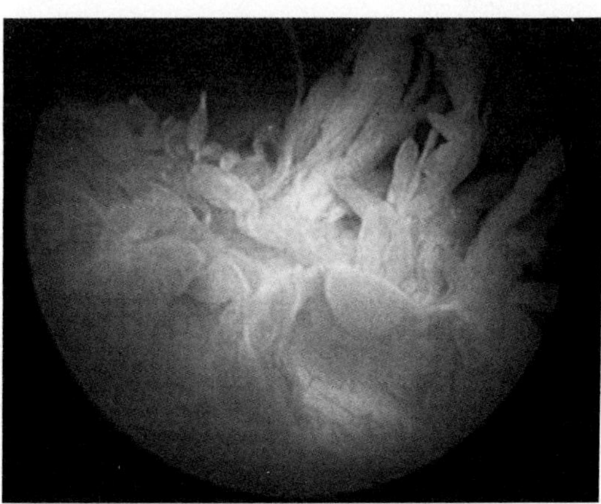

Figure 44.28 Arthroscopic view of synovitis of the knee. The highly vascularized hypertrophic appearance typifies the inflammatory pathology as seen in tenosynovium or bursa.

Sources of Pain in Soft Tissue Injury

The sources of soft tissue pain are multifactorial and include both inflammatory and biomechanical sources (36) (Fig. 44.29). Synovial sites are capable of secreting a wide variety of inflammatory mediators, in particular IL-1 and PGE-2, and provide a ready source of nociceptor stimulation in synovial lined joints, bursa, and peritenon. The internal tendon fibroblast is capable of producing inflammatory mediator proteins under repetitive stress (42). Elongation of a tendon or ligament beyond its elastic limit may trigger nociceptors as well as myotendinous reflexes (149). Direct injury to small connective tissue nerves may be a source of retinacular pain in the knee (150). Substance P is a peptide neurostimulating substance found in high concentrations at sites of soft tissue pain and inflammation (147, 36) (Fig. 44.30).

There would appear to be a distinction between the pathobiology of pain due to inflammation and that due to degeneration. Pain due to inflammation evolves when excessive loading results in immediate tissue damage and necrosis, producing the onset of an acute inflam-

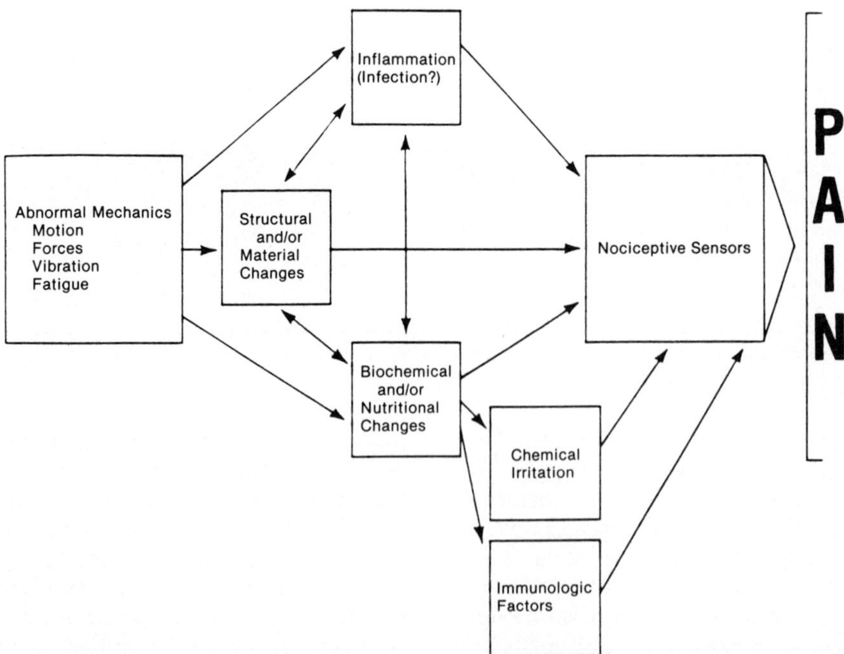

Figure 44.29 Possible mechanisms of musculoskeletal pain. Reprinted with permission from White AA III. The 1980 symposium and beyond. In: Frymoyer JW, Gordon SW, eds. New perspectives in low back pain. Park Ridge, IL: American Academy of Orthopaedic Surgeons, 1989;3–17.

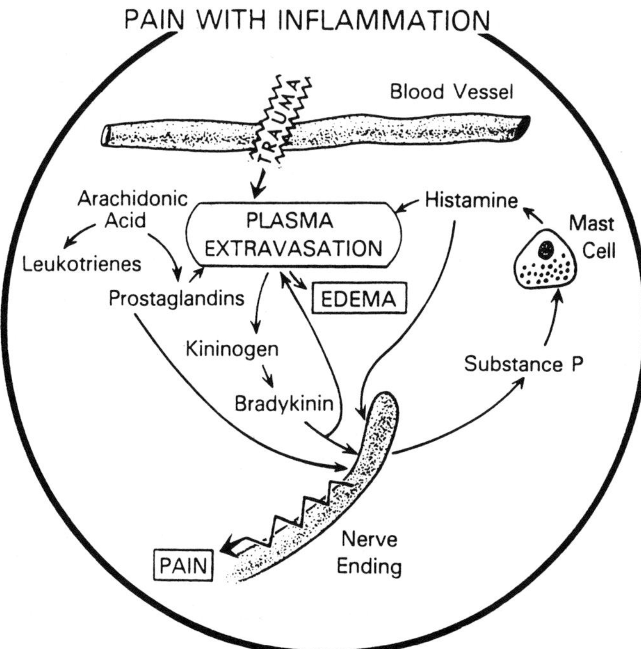

Figure 44.30 Schema of the positive-feedback relationship that develops during the course of inflammation secondary to sports-related injuries. Reproduced with permission from Hargreaves KM, Troullos ES, Dionne RA. Pharmacologic rationale for the treatment of acute pain. Dent Clin North Am 1987;31:675–694.

matory cascade as seen in typical macrotrauma with resulting chemical nociceptor stimulation. Degenerative pain may evolve when excessive cyclic microloading results in matrix molecular alterations, loss of tissue strength, resultant increased strain deformation with loading, and subsequent stimulation of pain mechanoceptors.

Systems for grading the severity of sports-induced soft tissue inflammation and the progress of healing are used to recognize the severity of injury, to judge its resolution, and to make recommendations on level of activity and return to competition (152). Such staging concepts for sports trauma, which have been applied to both acute and chronic injuries, attempt to describe subjective or qualitative symptoms or behaviors in quantitative terms. An early example, the traditional American Medical Association classification of ligament injury, set up three grades: grade 1, mild stretching; grade 2, partial tear; and grade 3, severe complete tear. These grading systems are based on these assumptions

1. There is a measurable response to soft tissue injury;
2. The duration and subjective appreciation of severity and type of pain correlate directly with the degree of tissue injury;
3. A given level of pain correlates with a specific quality of tissue pathology (152).

The scheme for identifying ligament injury severity in the prototypical example is shown in Table 44.7.

Although these assumptions have been substantiated in selected cases, they usually cannot be scientifically documented by such parameters as histologic biopsy. Therefore, in the individual athlete there are exceptions to the arbitrary application of these grading systems. In the traditional scheme of defining three grades of injury, the grade 2 injury is the "gray zone", for it often shares signs and symptoms of both lesser and higher grades of injury. The resolution of this question is no small point. The clinician is at liberty to allow return to play with fairly minimal concern for the grade 1 injury, aside from preventing recurrence and identifying initial contributing causes. Grade 1 injuries, by definition, produce only localized pain and tenderness without any significant disability or lengthy interruption of play and may resolve fairly spontaneously. With experience, the clinician will not find it difficult to identify the grade 3 injury because soft tissue signs and symptoms are pronounced and the disability is prohibitively severe. The distinguishing features between grade 2 and grade 3 injuries are often best determined by stress assessment of the injured part. Palpable loss of muscle continuity or a stress x-ray which reveals instability of a joint defines a grade 3 injury. Grade 3 injuries require prohibition from play. Grade 2 injuries remain the challenge in both diagnosis and recommended intervention. It is often possible, with additional brace and support protection, to allow limited participation in athletic competition. For example, if an athlete presents with a swollen lateral ligament injury of the ankle and stress x-rays of the ankle mortise reveal a stable mortise, intensive treatment of the acute phase inflammation followed by dynamic ankle support with a playing brace or taping, may allow for an earlier return to competition without prohibitive risk.

The decision on when to allow athletic competition after soft tissue athletic injury is not only determined by the initial assessment of the grade or severity of injury, but also by the progression or trend in the recovery from that injury. In this respect, grading systems have been useful in allowing a consistent albeit subjective way of quantifying and qualifying the healing progress of the athlete. The clinician can often improve upon the grading concept by having the athlete create a log, noting the level of activity and including such variables as frequency, intensity, and duration, along with recording the symptom severity, whether pain or a physical manifestation such as swelling, using a scale of 1 to 10. This can be surprisingly helpful in revealing what levels of activity and what forms of activity precipitate or what patterns of rest facilitate recovery.

These staging systems do not accurately distinguish between the symptom of pain and the real presence of inflammation. To the degree that there are multiple pathways for the origin of pain, as well as modifications of its appreciation at the cerebral level, attention is again called to possible mechanically and biochemically mediated effects on cell and matrix (36). A cautionary word must be mentioned regarding the symptom of night pain. While it is not uncommon for the patient with a chronic tendon injury such as to the rotator cuff, pain that awakens the patient at night may be the harbinger of a more serious coincident lesion, notably neoplasms. So-called sports tumors often pre-

Table 44.8.
Clinical Grading of Sports-Induced Soft Tissue Inflammations

Grade	Subjective Pain Pattern	Physical Signs	Tissue Damage	Healing Potential	Relevant Therapeutic Measures	
I	Pain after activity only. Duration of symptoms less than two weeks. Spontaneous relief within 24 hours.	Nonlocalized pain.	Micro Injury	Potential spontaneous resolution	Proper warmup and conditioning. Avoidance of abrupt transition in activity level.	Training, coaching and self-help measures often effective.
II	Pain during and after activity, but no significant functional disability. Duration of symptoms greater than two weeks, less than 6 weeks.	Localized pain. Minimal or no other signs of inflammation.			Analysis of technique and efficiency. Decrease transitional abuse and improve training.	
III	Pain during and after sport lasting for several days despite rest with rapid return upon activity. Significant functional disability. Duration of pain greater than 6 weeks. Night pain may occur.	Intense point tenderness with prominent inflammation (edema, effusion, erythema, crepitus, etc.).	Macro Injury	Permanent scar and residual tissue damage more likely	Medical assessment of structural vulnerability (e.g. flat feet, inflexibility, muscle weakness, etc.). Protected activity (e.g., bracing). Modification or substitution of different sports exercise to avoid excessive load on injured part.	Medical diagnosis and opinion valuable.
IV	Continuous pain with sport and daily activity. Total inability to train or complete. Night pain common.	Grade III symptoms plus tissue breakdown, atrophy, etc. Impending or actual tissue failure.			Surgical treatment often indicated to stimulate fibrous scar and repair or create structural alteration such as releases or decompression, potential permanent withdrawal from activity (e.g., deg. joint disease).	

Adapted from Leadbetter WB, Buckwalter JA, Gordon SL, eds. *Sports-induced inflammation: Clinical and basic science concepts.* Park Ridge, IL: American Academy of Orthopaedic Surgeons, 1990.

sent with night pain; the clinician should be alert to reassess his or her diagnosis and to repeat, if necessary, appropriate imaging in the face of this persistent symptom (153). A summary grading scheme is shown in Table 44.8.

Therapeutic Management of Soft Tissue Sports Injury

The therapeutic management of soft tissue athletic injury requires first establishing an accurate diagnosis; second, understanding the mechanism contributing to the injury; and thirdly, providing an intervention that ensures the most benefit for the least risk to the athlete. Ultimately, successful management is the sum of diagnosis, treatment, and preventative rehabilitation. Depending upon the type of injury, treatment decisions may be readily apparent or arrived at only through a trial of therapy. The traditional approach has been to view athletic soft tissue injuries as either acute or chronic. This oversimplification often breaks down because previous or recurrent acute injuries may contribute to an evolving chronic pattern. The following discussion will emphasize the principles and rationale underlying current sports medicine diagnostic and therapeutic practice.

General Principles

The key steps in the management of soft tissue athletic injury have been defined as follows (154):

1. To establish an accurate and complete diagnosis of all the anatomic and functional deficits resulting from the injury.
2. To minimize the deleterious local effects of the acute injury.
3. To allow anatomic healing of the injury.
4. To maintain other components of athletic fitness.
5. To regain previous athletic function.

Both acute and chronic injury may lead to functions and inflammatory symptoms (Fig. 44.31). The first objective in acute injury treatment is to control hemorrhage and initial excessive inflammatory pain (acute phase response effects) and to limit subsequent necrosis and tissue edema (zone of secondary injury). These principles are summarized in the mnemonic RICE'M: *R*est, *I*ce, *C*ompression, *E*levation and *M*obilization (Figs. 44.32, 33).

The initial objective in the treatment of chronic overuse injury is to recognize the problem in the greater context of inadequate or abusive training. This shift in

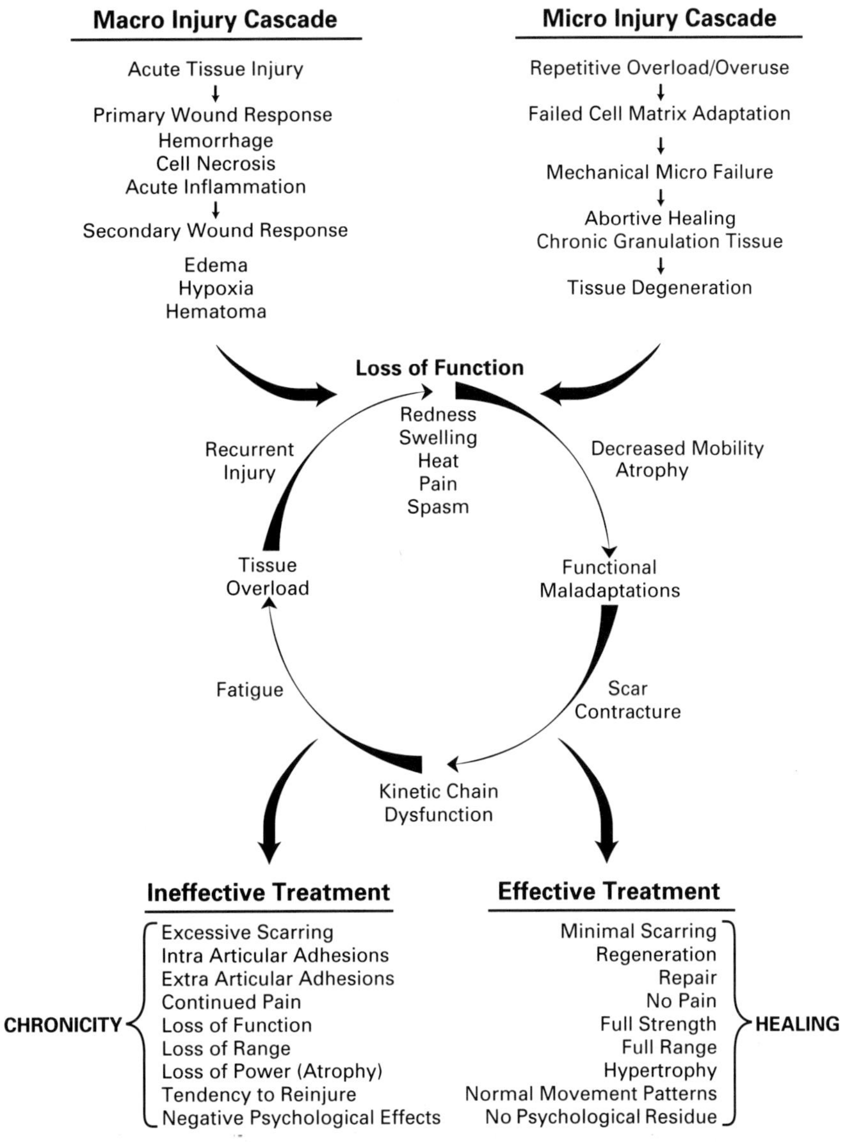

Figure 44.31 Injury-pain cycle. The promotion of healing and performance depends upon accurate diagnosis of excessive inflammatory response and adequate rehabilitation.

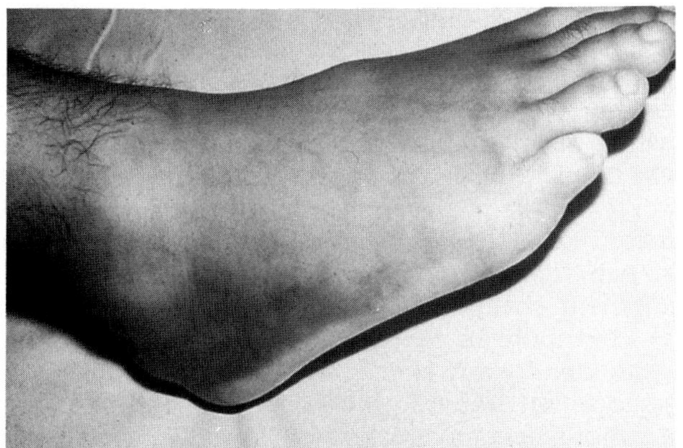

Figure 44.32 Severe acute ankle sprain. Hemorrhage and edema contribute to the zone of secondary injury. Note the "antalgic posture" with early Achilles contracture and plantar flexion of foot and ankle. Immobilization and splinting in positions of function are essential early treatment.

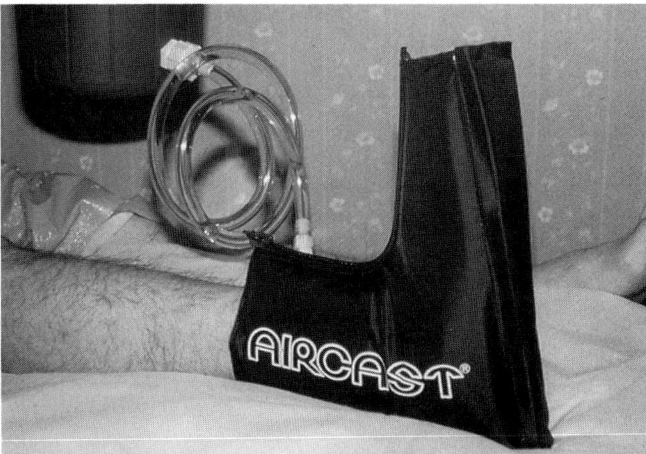

Figure 44.33 Ankle Sprain: Cryotherapy. Immediate controlled compression and cooling is expedited by a cryocuff.

emphasis is summarized in the mnemonic REST'M: Rest and Rehabilitation, Education, Support of the injured part, Training and technique, Modification of activity, Modalities and Medication (32).

Regardless of the type of injury, first, do no harm. In prescribing treatment, it is wise to remember that every treatment has its cost as well as proposed benefit. A NSAID drug may add cost and side-effect risks without significant improvement in soft tissue healing. Improper or lengthy immobilization that results in atrophy or contracture can delay functional recovery despite immediate pain relief. No cure should be worse than the problem it addresses. While acute injuries are often accompanied by obvious physical findings, the diagnosis of most overuse injuries requires familiarity with a good history, physical examination techniques, and proper radiographic imaging (39). Plain x-rays may reveal unsuspected arthritis, tumors, or stress reaction and they should always be done. With the exception of dystrophic calcification, plain radiographs may only confirm negative findings in true soft tissue injury; however, the triphase technetium bone scan, the MRI, and ultrasound scan have proven useful in the identification of persistent, chronic structural soft tissue injury (156) (Figure 44.34). The focus of the therapeutic program may vary, depending on the soft tissue structure involved. The primary consequence of muscle injuries is loss of strength, mobility, and potentially adverse cosmetic effect (e.g, rupture of the pectoralis major muscle in a body builder). Tendon injuries result in persistent pain and loss of movement. The disability of ligament injuries is instability. Diagnosis and treatment should proceed on a need-to-know basis, which is established by the nature of the structure injured, the competitive level of the athlete, and the specific sport. Establishing what the athlete can do, what he cannot do, and what he wishes to do helps to determine the extent of the diagnostic evaluation. The clinician must "know the sport" with respect to the techniques and dosing demands of musculoskeletal load and use if a successful sports-specific solution is to be prescribed. When encountering the injured athlete, be prepared to *L*isten, *L*ook, and then *L*ocate the problem.

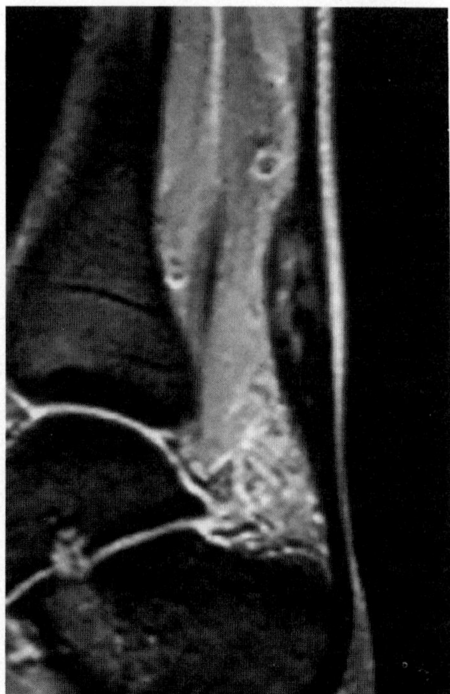

Figure 44.34 Achilles Tendinosis (Typical MRI appearance). Note bright intratendinous signal implying matrix degeneration or injury.

Basic Elements of Diagnosis

History and Physical

It is helpful to establish a consistent mental approach in the diagnosis of athletic soft tissue injury. Keeping in mind the seven basic mechanisms of injury can be useful, since, by a process of elimination, the examiner will single out the most likely contributing causes to the athlete's pain. The differentiation of acute from chronic injuries is made easier by simply asking the athlete, "Did this problem begin by your hurting it or did it begin hurting you?" It is the absence of a contact or single sudden injury that often defines the overuse mechanism. Basic fact-finding should include asking when the injury began, what the exact activity was at the time of injury, what the athlete felt at the time he or she became "injured," and whether there was a previous injury. If a previous injury did occur, it is mandatory to spend time defining exactly what occurred at that time. Oftentimes, the injured athlete glosses over such occurrences, not recognizing a causal relationship with the current complaint. A statement such as, "I twisted my knee two years ago skiing" may reveal the onset of an incompletely evaluated ligamentous instability; stating that there was a prior fracture of an ankle requiring cast immobilization may provide the clue for a persistent atrophy or proprioceptive deficit. Such disabilities may exist for years without the benefit of diagnosis or complete rehabilitation. The pattern of pain may be helpful. A history of immediate disability after injury or the loss of ability to play sports from an injury is a more ominous symptom implying significant structural damage. Any persistent dysfunction such as a limp requires full evaluation.

While the history is helpful to the acute injury assessment (e.g., the acknowledgement of a "pop" on twisting of knee that implies an anterior cruciate ligament injury), the history is invaluable in assessing the chronic complaint. Overuse injury is a diagnosis by deduction. Questions of training load, athletic technique, rest patterns, competitive schedule, playing position, equipment changes, nutrition and hydration patterns may contribute to that diagnosis. The history should seek to identify any change or transition in athletic performance that would imply a legacy of abusive overuse (i.e., improper training) and new adaptive demand. This can be best summarized by the Rule of Too's—too often, too hard, too soon, too much, too little, too late, etc. (32). Work exposures also contribute to adaptive demands. The weekend tennis player who happens to carry a briefcase or perform extensive labor with the

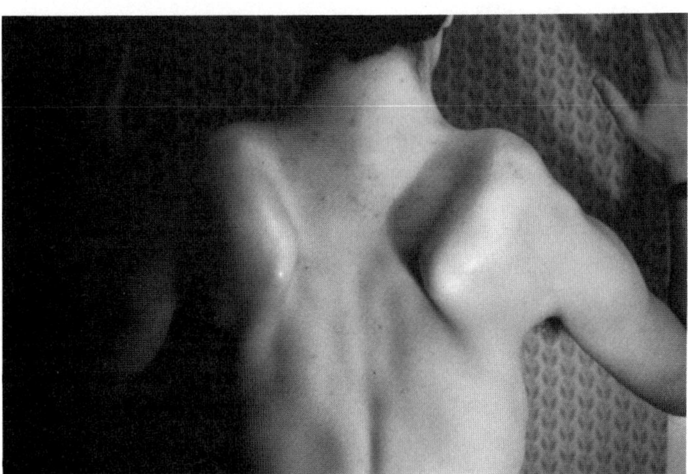

Figure 44.35 Severe scapular winging associated with scapulo-facial-humeral dystrophy. Patient presented de novo with complaint of weakness.

affected arm during the week may accumulate more adverse effects than would be apparent from his or her sports participation alone. If a fitness jogger with a painful Achilles tendon must, in addition to jogging, repeatedly climb stairs or use a ladder while working, improvement from conventional treatment may be frustrated. The onset of pain immediately upon activity implies a structural deficit; pain that is absent at onset and increases during the activity implies an underlying mechanical deficiency with fatigue or chronic inflammation. In the face of a subsequent benign physical exam with no initial traumatic episode by history, the examiner may often be confronting an overuse injury. However, the examiner should beware of spontaneous afflictions producing synovial inflammation, a mass, unrelenting pain, or prominent limb dysfunction. Neoplasms, systemic or rheumatologic disease, and primary muscle disease may present as athletic injury (Fig. 44.35). A brief medical history should disclose allergies and drug intolerances, important coincident illness such as a history of peptic ulcer, as well as current list of medications. It is important to know what previous therapeutic measures were prescribed, whether there was proper compliance by the athlete, and the relative effect. Has the problem improved, stayed the same or become worse, and what contributes to these trends. Pain diagrams and analog scales have been useful in aiding in such description.

Physical Examination

The physical examination of athletic soft tissue injury requires familiarity with a variety of evocative tests and maneuvers. Competence with these techniques allows the examiner to more accurately differentiate specific structural injuries in the same anatomic area. For example, differentiation of chondromalacia patella versus patella tendinitis, the dysfunction of the scapula stabilizing muscles versus glenohumeral instability, the presence of an attenuation of the posterior tibial tendon versus a flexor hallucis longus tendinitis hinges on the examiner's familiarity with both anatomy and examination technique. In this respect, the physical assessment of athletic soft tissue injury is a lifelong learning experience. Specific methods for physical assessment are further described throughout this text.

The examiner should strive to develop a precise and organized approach. Remember to compare and to first examine the uninjured limb; this will help to reduce the athlete's anxiety and will establish the range of normal individual variation. Since most chronic injuries do not occur as an isolated event, but represent a failure in a complex kinetic chain (39, 85), the physical examination provides an opportunity to identify intrinsic alignment abnormalities and soft tissue (musculous, tendinous and ligamentous) insufficiencies (39, 85). The overhead athlete complaining of shoulder pain may require assessment of more proximal scapular stabilizing musculature or even lumbar pathomechanics; a runner with a knee complaint may clearly demonstrate persistent femoral anteversion with increased torque upon the patellofemoral joint or excessive pronation as structural vulnerabilities that can be supported and palliated by an orthotic. While the physical examination provides ample opportunity for static assessment, dynamic contributions to athletic soft tissue injury are often overlooked. Whenever possible, provide the athlete with the opportunity to imitate the sports motion during which pain is experienced. Examples of such techniques include providing a racquet in the clinic, a ball for making short tosses, a treadmill or even larger space for sprint or jogging, or a simple stair-step to assess patellofemoral confidence.

Specific Treatment Alternatives

The treatment of athletic soft tissue injury may target both the cellular as well as the functional level of the injured athlete. The former is an attempt to influence the resolution of inflammation, whereas the latter represents an effort to increase the rate of repair and repel cummulative adverse injury effects on various body tissues and systems. Changing the inflammatory repair process in connective tissues implies controlling a cellular and/or matrix tissue response (2).

In clinical medicine, such attempts are common and involve the prescription of a modifier. Potential modifiers include antiinflammatory medications (which may be oral, injectable, or topical) and physical techniques such as thermotherapy, cryotherapy, electrical field induction, ultrasound, and rehabilitative exercise. At the cellular level, modifiers are intended to reduce extracellular edema, improve oxygenation, improve bloodflow, correct pH imbalance, and generally improve the cell matrix environment. At the tissue level, such modifiers are intended to decrease pain, reduce immobilization effects, improve neuromuscular coordination, avoid adhesions and adjacent joint stiffness, and decrease pain, thereby allowing compliance with a rehabilitation protocol. Such modifiers are intended to decrease pain, reduce immobilization effects, improve neuromuscular coordination, avoid adhesions and adjacent joint stiffness, and decrease pain, thereby allowing compliance with a rehabilitation protocol.

The effectiveness of these interventions depends in large part on where in the spectrum of tissue injury between inflammation-dominant and degenerative-tissue-dominant conditions the particular athletic injury lies (Fig. 44.36). At the onset, it should be emphasized that with the exception of therapeutic rehabilitation, significant promotion of healing has been poorly documented for all other forms of intervention. Use of these other forms remains largely adjunctive to the normal, time-dependent healing process of the body. Whatever the treatment program selected, it must adhere to the following principles:

1. Protection of the early phases of tissue healing, while "normalizing" as much as possible all remaining limb function.
2. Avoidance of excessive immobilization.
3. Restoration of total limb function by emphasizing the timely application of therapeutic and rehabilitation techniques.
4. Retraining and establishment of appropriate criterion for return to play.
5. Elimination of faulty or abusive technique (1, 39, 85, 154, 157, 158).

Medical Modifiers

Nonsteroidal Antiinflammatory Drugs (NSAIDs)

NSAIDs block the cyclooxygenase enzyme breakdown of arachidonic acid to prostaglandins and derivatives (38). The toxicity of nonsteroidal antiinflammatory drugs is related to their capacity to inhibit normal prostaglandin function in such organs as the liver, lining of the stomach, and kidney (158). Since the initiation of the arachidonic acids cascade is a critical step in igniting the further steps in acute injury repair, NSAIDs could seriously inhibit injury repair. Unlike the derivatives, NSAIDs have not been shown to significantly slow the normal healing process, a reflection of their more selective site of action in the arachidonic acid metabolism (Fig. 44.37). Paradoxically, the suppression of prostaglandin synthesis by NSAIDs has been shown to unmask other mediators, such as, in particular, leukotrienes and thrombaxins, (Fig. 44.9), and, in a complex fashion, to result in potentially increased damage from inflammation (160, 157). The effectiveness of NSAIDs in the treatment of acute and chronic soft tissue injury remains controversial. Using a prophylactic dosage with ibuprofen, either prophylactically or 24 hours after onset of eccentric exercise of the knee, Hasson et al. found

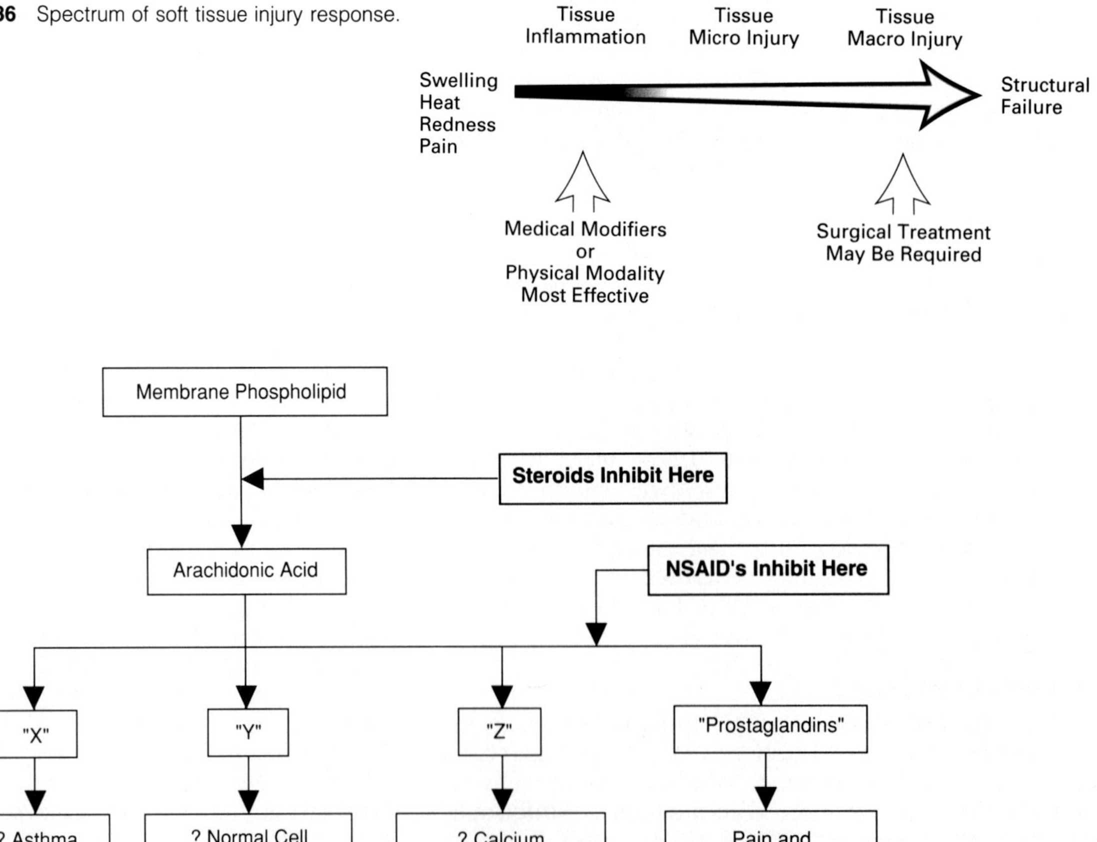

Figure 44.36 Spectrum of soft tissue injury response.

Figure 44.37 Scheme for arachidonic acid metabolism showing how the sites of action of corticosteroids differ from those of nonsteroidal antiinflammatory drugs. Because corticosteroids suppress other pathways in addition to pain and inflammation, their potential side effects are greater. (From Goodwin, JS. Mechanism of Action of Corticosteroids. In: Mediguide to inflammatory Diseases. New York: Lawrence Delacorte Pub, 1987;6:1)

improvement in perceived muscle soreness, knee extensor torque decline, less decline in vastus lateralis EMG magnitude (161). The group of patients treated prophylactically displayed between 40% and 50% less muscle soreness and significant less decline in isometric, concentric, and eccentric torque at 24 hours. There was no difference in treated and untreated groups with respect to measured muscle damage as determined by creatinine kinase (CPK) levels. The effect of piroxicam on the healing of an experimental injury to the medial collateral ligament in the rat demonstrated increased early strength in the treated ligament when dosage was administered for short periods of time after injury, but did not improve the ultimate strength when healing was complete (162). Other experimental evidence suggests a delay in muscle regeneration after strain injury treated with piroxicam (163). Weiler, in an exhaustive review of the literature, could find only 11 studies that were double blinded, randomized and placebo controlled for the efficacy of NSAIDs in sports related injury (160). Of these, 8 reported positive results and 3 reported negative results. It was also noted that topical applications of NSAIDs seemed to fare better than placebos when treating acute injury without subjecting the athlete to the myriad of adverse events associated with oral administration of NSAIDs. Weiler further concluded that despite such benefits seen in the treated patients as slightly more rapid healing and decreased inflammation, the use of NSAIDs could neither be condemned or strongly recommended at present (160). In general, about half the patients who receive NSAIDs will have an adverse event associated with the use of these medications, and 1% to 2% of these reactions may be serious (160). The toxic effects of aspirin may be enhanced when a nonaspirin, nonsteroidal or corticosteroid is used in conjunction (159). The risks of NSAIDs may be minimized by prescribing short-term (7 to 10 day dosage in acute injury) and by careful monitoring in the chronically treated patient.

Corticosteroids

Corticosteroids may be administered either orally or by injection. Oral corticosteroids have generally been avoided in the treatment of sports-related injury. Claims that short-burst, low-dose prednisone, in the form of a Dose-pak, may be helpful for neuritis, paratenonitis, and bursal inflammation remain empirical but in the author's experience, appear helpful. By contrast, corticosteroid injection therapy continues to be widely employed, although the mechanism of its alleged therapeutic effect has not been documented in the human. In the animal model, corticosteroid tendon injection has resulted in early collagen disarray and degenerative effects followed over a period of weeks by a trend of reparative healing (164). The functional significance of these improvements is not known. Likewise, spontaneous tendon rupture occurring after corticosteroid injection remains a controversial phenomenon. The argument centers on whether tendon degeneration precedes the injection effect, thus the tendon rupture being inevitable or whether repeated tendon injection damage directly precipitates a spontaneous rupture (164). Alternatively, corticosteroid injection anabolic effects may further potentiate sports-induced cell matrix failure. To date, efforts to resolve these questions have been frustrated by the lack of adequate animal models. Bachman et al. have described a rabbit model for chronic Achilles paratenonitis with tendinosis (165). However, the consistency and reproducibility of such a model has not been validated; therefore, either normal tendons have been injected, or inflammatory injury has been artificially induced by acute wounding (164). In addition, such animals may not react to these substances in the same way as humans (166). Because there remains controversy regarding the suppression of collagen synthesis during the repair phases of healing, current clinical practice avoids injecting steroid preparations directly into tendons. The best indication for steroid injection remains a localized inflammatory site such as a synovial cavity, bursa or tendon synovial sheath (164). Side effects observed after corticosteroid injection can problematic and the athlete should be warned of the risk of local skin depigmentation (Fig. 44.38*A*, *B*), subcutaneous atrophy with hypersensitivity, spontaneous tendon rupture, and the potential for chemical irritation from intratendinous or intrabursal precipitate (164). A common adverse systemic effect of local injection in the diabetic is sudden transient elevation of serum glucose levels. The author has documented serum rises of 300–400 mg/ml in a 24-hr period. While usually controllable, this effect could cause clinical symptoms. Patients should be appropriately cautioned as to their diabetic control. Factors contributing to lack of response to injection therapy may be either athlete-related (e.g., persistent overuse, faulty technique, or evidence of advanced tissue trauma) or physician related (e.g., improper diagnosis, inadequate injection technique) (164). It is the author's impression that there is indeed a "tissue responder" that seems uniquely predisposed to inflammatory reaction in the face of soft tissue sports microtrauma and whose inflammatory cycle can be mollified by the proper timing of corticosteroid injection. Since surgical options are often considered after a trial of nonoperative care that includes injection, corticosteroid injection should not be the first treatment alternative nor should it be the last used in aiding the athlete. Efforts should be made to dispel the false sense of security in the athlete that symptomatic relief following steroid injection may produce that may lead to self abuse and more serious reinjury. Sports participation after injection adjacent to a major tendon should be delayed a minimum of 3 weeks (164, 39). Recommendations for injection of acute muscular strain or ligamentous sprain injury to reduce the acute inflammatory phase after injury have not been substantiated by controlled study. Guidelines for the appropriate clinical use of corticosteroid injection have been defined (Table 44.9).

Anabolic Steroids

Anabolic steroids have gained attention as possible modifiers of healing and repair because of the observed increases in strength and muscle size that anabolic ste-

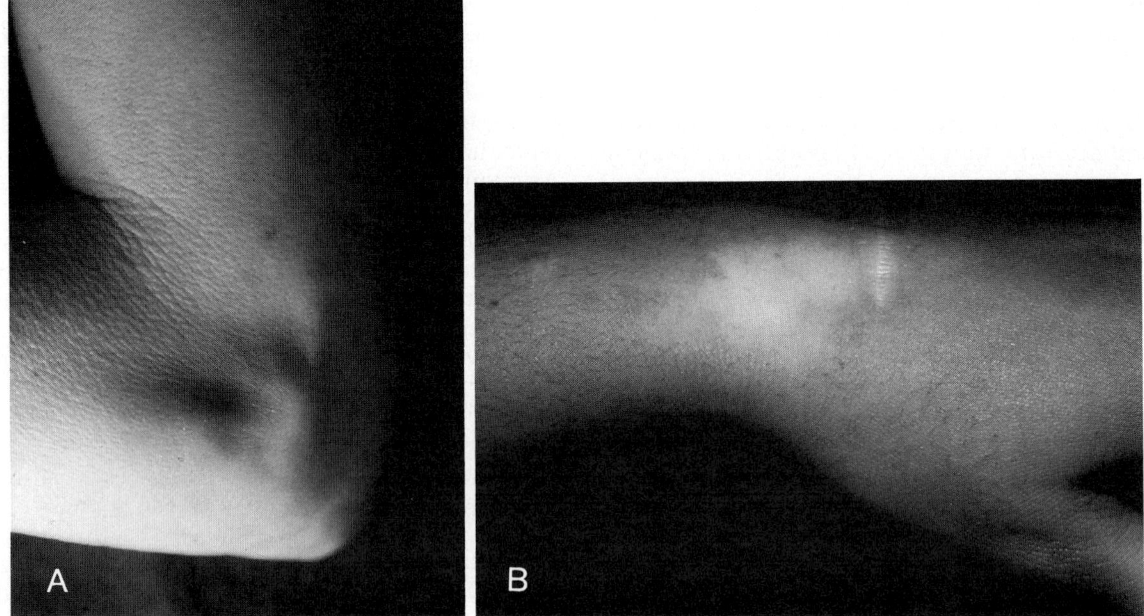

Figure 44.38 **(A)** Complications of steroid injection. Subcutaneous atrophy most often seen at the elbow epicondyle. Note loss of subcutaneous fat; skin becomes hypersensitive. **(B)** Complications of steroid injection. Cutaneous depigmentation after wrist paratendinous injection.

Table 44.9.
Use and Abuse of Corticosteroid Injection[a]

Proper use
Six-week preinjection trial of rest, adjusted level of play, and conditioning
Discrete, palpable site of complaint (avoid tendon)
Peritendinous or inflammatory target tissue
Limit of three injections, spaced weeks apart, given only if first led to demonstrated improvement
Rest (protection) for 2 to 6 weeks after injection
Avoidance of contributing mechanical cause (e.g., equipment, conditioning)
Improper use
Acute trauma
Intratendinous injection
Infection
Multiple injections (>3)
Injection immediately before competition
Frequent intraarticular injections

[a]Adapted with permission from Leadbetter WB, Buckwalter JA, Gordon SL, eds. Sports-Induced inflammation: Clinical and basic science concepts. Park Ridge, IL: American Academy of Orthopaedic Surgeons, 1990.

roid regimens produce in the intensively strength-training athlete (167, 168). Irrespective of the documented adverse side effects of anabolic steroids, (which include an increased risk of coronary artery disease, impaired glucose tolerance, dysfunction of the liver, hepatic cancer, reproductive alterations, psychological changes, and premature epiphyseal closure), anabolic steroids have documented catabolic as well as anabolic effects on connective soft tissue (167). Miles et al. found that, in the rat, anabolic steroid treatment produced a stiffer tendon that absorbed less energy to failure. Alterations in the size of collagen fibrils was noted on electron microscopy (169). In a study of anabolic steroid effect on collagen synthesis in rat skeletal muscle and tendon, a transient decrease was noted in collagen biosynthesis, implying another underlying rationale for spontaneous rupture (170). The mechanism and physiologic effect of anabolic steroids in resolution of soft tissue inflammation and repair remain at present unsubstantiated (168).

Dimethol Sulfoxide (DMSO)

DMSO is a commercial, chemical byproduct of the wood pulp industry; it is a powerful solvent and a medium for other chemical reactions (171). It lowers the freezing point of biological fluids, a quality useful in cryopreservation of animal and human tissues and cells. Since the early 1960s, DMSO has gained notoriety, especially among athletes as a black market therapy for the treatment of injury. Claims of reduction in pain, swelling, and more rapid return to sports play led to a series of clinical studies. Percy and Carson reported on the use of DMSO in tennis elbow and rotator cuff tendinitis. No therapeutic effect could be demonstrated (172). In a study of DMSO effects on mice Achilles tendon, decreasing mean separation force of up to 20% after a 7 day treatment was found (171). Myrer et al. applied DMSO topically to traumatized muscle in adult male rats and found significantly fewer healing cells were present in the experimental group than in the control during the early period of inflammation. This was construed to imply that some antiinflammatory effect might be rendered. However, no improved healing response was noted during the course of the experiment (173). Complications of DMSO use have included local rash, burn, blisters, itchiness, hives, scaling, dryness of the skin, foul breath, and potential teratogenic effects (171).

The role of DMSO in the treatment of athletic injury remains unsubstantiated and is not recommended.

Antioxidants

Antioxidants are chemical scavenger molecules that buffer excessive production of oxygen-free radicals, themselves by-products of oxidative damage and exercise induced lipid peroxidation of cell membranes (69, 174). Antioxidants are normally present in the body to help reduce the activity of these radical induced reactions. As previously mentioned, such reactions commonly occur due to the lysosomal activity of neutrophils in the acute phase response after injury. Oxidative distress is also a by-product of intensive exercise (175). Normal tissue sources of antioxidant defense include the enzyme superoxide dismutase, catalase, glutathione peroxidase, and the antioxidant vitamins (69). Vitamin E (α-tocopherol) and Vitamin C (ascorbate) are powerful antioxidants implicated in the treatment of cancer, aging, arthritis, as well as exercise-induced oxidative stress (174). In athletics, the role of vitamin E has been studied in a number of endurance sports. There is conflicting evidence of improved performance (174, 176). Since evidence of muscle damage following exercise has been widely reported, the question arises whether lipid peroxidation is a cause or a consequence of tissue damage. While oral antioxidant therapy is relatively safe, a significant effect on tissue repair and injury recovery has not been demonstrated.

Physical Modalities

Physical modalities are frequently prescribed to promote healing and recovery after injury (177, 157, 158, 130). There is much claimed and much more unknown about these various physical techniques, their indications, efficacy, and potential to modify the inflammation repair cycle, yet it is safe to say that the role of physical modalities remains largely experiential and theoretical.

Cryotherapy

Cryotherapy remains a mainstay in the physical treatment of sports injury (177). External application of cold has been demonstrated to result in decreased regional blood flow, decreased and more rapid resolution of edema, decreased local hemorrhage, and improved analgesia (157, 177). A primary goal of cryotherapy is to reduce the zone of secondary injury in acute macrotrauma (177) (Fig. 44.39). Ice therapy has the additional advantages of being adaptable, available, cheap, and relatively safe. However, there have been reports regarding cryogenic superficial nerve injury as well as the risk of frostbite from inappropriate application (178). The risk of such injury can be diminished by limiting ice application to 20 minutes or less, avoiding excessive compression, and protecting the underlying skin from direct contact (178). Cryotherapy has been attempted synergistically with other modalities. In a study combining transcutaneous electrical nerve stimulation and cold application, a significant decrease in perceived pain, an increase in elbow range of motion but no significant improvements in muscle strength has been shown (179). In the author's experience, cooling is used after acute injury until signs of swelling and hemorrhage have completely abated. This may take many days.

Thermotherapy

Thermotherapy (heat application) produces physiologic effects as a result of vasodilatation, increased nutrition, and increased enzymatic activity (180). There is evidence that collagen synthesis increases with the application of exogenous heat (157, 56). Tissue extensibility and metabolism are enhanced and muscle spasm decreased (157, 180). Thermotherapy is usually applied in the range of 102° to 110° fahrenheit (130). The amount of permanent elongation resulting from a given amount of stretching will increase in a thermal environment of 103° fahrenheit or greater. At 104° fahrenheit and above there is a thermal transition in the microstructure of collagen that significantly enhances the viscoelasticity of collagen tissues allowing for greater deformation without excessive strain. This observed phenomenon is thought to be due to changes in molecular creep and increased viscoelastic properties (130). Structural weakening produced by loading varies inversely with temperature. In addition, tissues that are stretched under heated conditions and then allowed to cool while under tension, maintain a greater proportion of their plastic deformation than structures not allowed to cool in an unloaded state. The mechanisms for these observations remain controversial but it is presumed that an alteration occurs in the collagenous microstructure (130). These observations provide a rationale for application of therapeutic modalities in the treatment of connective soft tissue injury. Guidelines for the safe application of heat after injury remain argumentative. While some would apply heat to aid in the resolution of inflammation and employ ultrasound or diathermy in an effort to encourage the resolution of a thigh contusion (130), other opinions oppose any use of heat under these conditions (158). The premature use of heat after acute injury runs the risk of encouraging intracompartmental hemorrhage (Fig. 44.39). In the author's opinion, heat application is reserved for chronic conditions and to warm up indolent tissue damage prior to rehabilitative exercise.

Therapeutic Ultrasound

Therapeutic ultrasound is another energy source resulting in the heating of deep tissues. Conflicting reports exist as to its effectiveness. Pulsed ultrasound would appear more therapeutically effective (181). Various studies have suggested that wound healing is improved by ultrasound application, for example, in venous stasis ulcers or in an animal wound model (181). Such studies suffer from a lack of direct application to the athlete in that the form of wounding, the environmental stress, and the biological system vary from sports medicine experience. In a study of acute wound healing of rat Achilles tendon, Frieder et al. found a thera-

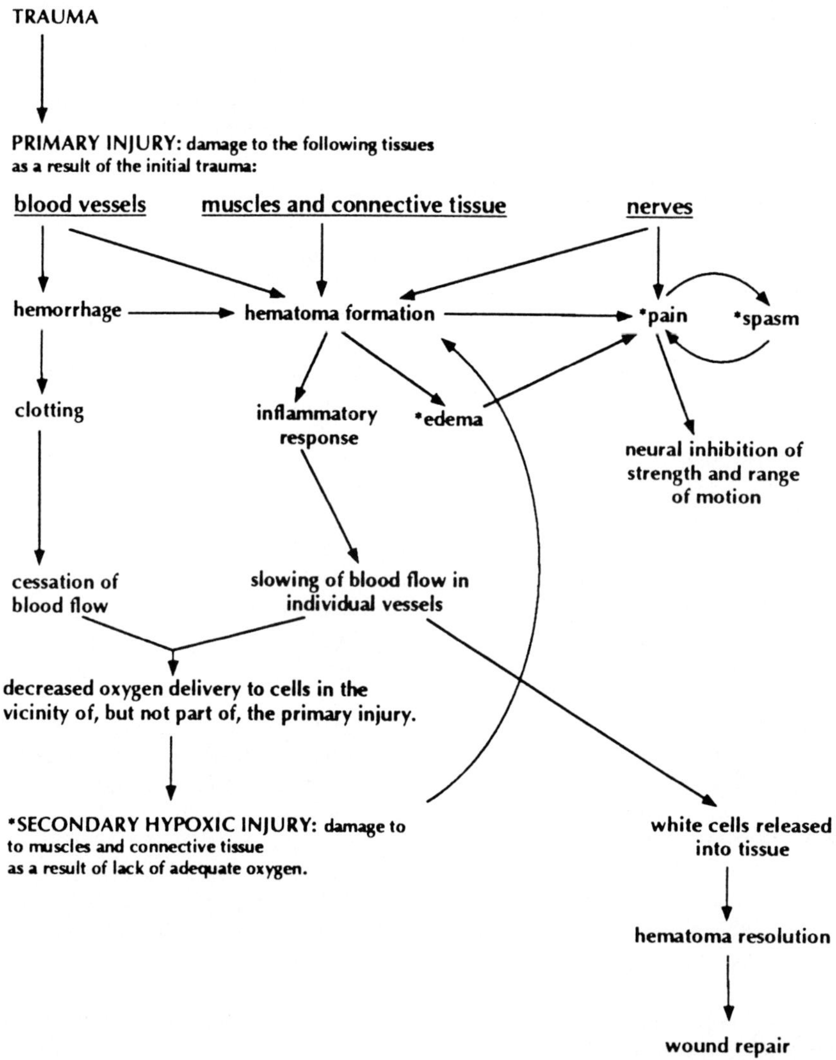

Figure 44.39 Summary of the response of the inflammatory system to acute trauma. The phases that respond to intervention by cold applications to the injury site are labeled with asterisks. Reproduced with permission from Knight KL. Cryotherapy: Theory, technique, and physiology. Chattanooga, TN: Chattanooga Corp, 1985.

peutic effect only after 9 treatments over a 3 week period (182). However, in a similar study, collagen synthesis was increased 5 days postinjury with evidence of increased collagen synthesis (183). Diathermy is a high frequency current, short-duration impulse form of electromagnetic radiation, which is used as another vehicle for delivering heat to an injury area; its general physiologic actions are unknown (181).

High Voltage Pulse Galvanic Stimulation (HVPGS)

High voltage pulse galvanic stimulation is currently advocated for both acute and chronic athletic soft tissue injury treatment. HVPGS is an electrical stimulation unit with an output of more than 100 to 150 V and a pulsatile monophasic wave form, often twin peaked, from 5 to 100 micro s in duration (184). The short pulse and the high voltage dramatically reduce skin resistance to current flow, thus allowing potentially unlimited depth of penetration. HVPGS applications include temporary relaxation of muscle spasm, preventing or retarding disuse atrophy, increasing local blood circulation, reeducating muscles atrophied from disuse, and in the biofeedback control of trigger point pain. Alterations in ion, free amino acid, and protein flow (cataphoresis) by this imposed electrical current are thought to account for observed therapeutic effects (184). Used in conjunction with cryotherapy, high voltage galvanic stimulation may reduce edema by reducing microvascular permeability to plasma proteins (184).

There is still much to be learned regarding the ultimate cell matrix effects, dosage, timing, and synergistic or additive effects of modalities. In a comparative study of ice massage, ultrasound, iontophoresis (transcutaneous electrically driven corticosteroid application) and phonophoresis (corticosteroid applied transcutaneously in conjunction with continuous ultrasound) for shin splint syndrome, Smith et al. found no treatment modality superior to another, yet all were clearly superior to a control treatment program (185). The controversies underlying modality use in athletic injury were underlined in an exhaustive review by LaBelle et al. regarding the lack of scientific evidence for the treatment of epicondylitis of the elbow (186). Of 185 articles published since 1966, only 18 were randomized, controlled studies. The remaining papers were reviewed with respect to therapy used: ultrasound, iontophoresis, oral NSAIDs, and steroid injection. It was noted that these studies were characterized by: 1) poor methological design, 2) prominent placebo effect, 3) small sample size, and 4) the finding that significant improvements from baseline were found in all studies, confirming either that all treatments had a therapeutic effect or that the condition improved spontaneously with time. The authors concluded that there was not enough scientific evidence to favor any particular treatment for acute lateral epicondylitis (186).

In a review of the effective use of physical modalities, Polikoff has stated (and we agree), "When using physical therapy modalities, it is important to avoid implanting the thought of permanent disability and invalidism. The patient should be encouraged to go through an orderly program and encouraged to progress. As soon as possible the patient should be discontinued from attendance at specific sessions with a therapist since this may perpetuate modality dependency. There is no objection to placing the patient on a home program reinforcing responsibility for self help, and emphasizing that the patient is in a mending state rather than in a continued state of physical disability" (187).

Rehabilitative Therapeutic Exercise

Rehabilitative therapeutic exercise has the strongest rationale for use in the treatment of sports induced soft tissue athletic injury (39, 85, 84, 130, 154, 157, 188). Cellular and biomechanical responses to exercise documented in tendon, ligament, and muscle include changes in collagen turnover rate; changes in collagen cross linking at the intramolecular and intermolecular level; alteration in tissue water and electrolyte content; and changes in the arrangement, number and thickness of collagen fibrils (158, 28). Both tissue stress and strain may play a role in modifying changes in cell matrix synthesis (28). Exercise counteracts the hazards of prolonged immobilization after injury (189, 190) (Table 44.10). Goals of a rehabilitative prescription include:

1. the prevention of further contractural loss of motion and tissue atrophy;
2. promotion of resolution of the acute phase response to injury;
3. promotion of the reparative phase of collagen synthesis;
4. reclamation of performance attributes such as strength, endurance, power, agility, speed, range of motion, and sports-specific technique (27, 34, 39, 154, 158).

It is important to emphasize what the athlete can do, as well as his limitations during recovery. Beyond physiologic limits, rest and antiinflammatories do not heal (39). A rest program allows for decreased sensitivity, early initiation of healing, and decreased pain disability, but only rehabilitation will restore performance ability. In addition to rehabilitation of the injury site, a total body fitness program emphasizing aerobic conditioning as well as maintenance of general body performance reduces the risk of reinjury on return to sport (154). O'Connor et al. has identified the advantages of such a program:

1. increasing regional perfusion through central and peripheral aerobics,
2. providing neurologic stimulus to the injured tissue through neurophysiologic synergy and overflow,
3. minimizing weakness of adjacent uninjured tissue (decreases or eliminates destructive domino effect in the kinetic chain),
4. minimizing negative psychological effects, and
5. controlling unwanted fat and accumulated weight (39).

Surgical Indications in Soft Tissue Injury

Surgery may be indicated in both acute and chronic forms of athletic injury. It is less appropriate to speak

Table 44.10.
Adverse Effects of Immobilization[a]

Muscle	Ligament	Joint
Decrease in muscle fiber size Decrease in mitochondria size and number Decrease in total muscle weight Increase in muscle contraction time Decrease in muscle tension produced Decrease in resting length of glycogen and ATP More rapid decrease in the ATP level with exercise Increase in lactate concentration with exercise Decrease in protein synthesis	Significant decrease in linear stress, maximum stress and stiffness Decrease in ligament fibril cross-sectional area, resulting in a reduction in fibril size and density Decrease in synthesis and degradation of collagen Haphazard arrangement of new collagen fibers Reduction in load and energy-absorbing capabilities of the bone-ligament complex Decrease in the GAG level Increase in osteoclastic activity at the bone-ligament junction, causing an increase in bone resorption in that area	Reduction in water and GAG content, decreasing the extracellular matrix Reduction in extracellular matrix associated with decrease in lubrication between fiber cross links Reduction in collagen mass Increase in collagen turnover, degradation, and synthesis rate Increase in abnormal collagen fiber cross links Reduction of hyaluronic acid

[a] Adapted from Andrews JR, Harrelson GL. Physical rehabilitation of the injured athlete. Philadelphia: WB Saunders, 1991.

of "conservative" versus "aggressive" alternatives than to consider all treatment in terms of nonoperative and operative solutions. In the case of a severe rotator cuff tear, an acute rupture of the tendon Achilles, or a patellar tendon or biceps tendon disruption, timely surgical intervention may be appropriate and, indeed, conservative. In general, grade III injuries of both ligament and tendon often require surgical repair, the notable exception being ankle sprains and medial collateral ligament injuries of the knee. Because of the technical difficulty of suturing muscle tissue and the extensive scar reaction, direct repair of muscle tissue disruption is not commonly advocated. Repair attempts are usually superceded by protection followed by aggressive rehabilitation of the remaining intact fibers.

The surgical treatment of overuse injury is only indicated after failure to respond to a rigorous nonoperative program. Thus, the athlete must qualify for surgery. Lack of compliance and inadequate rehabilitation most often lead to inappropriate surgery and a poor result. An analysis of currently recommended surgical procedures in chronic overuse tendon injury reveals a variety of surgical goals:

1. To alter the tissue structure and restore strength by inducing reparative scar;
2. To remove a nidus of offending adherent scar (e.g., chronic granulation tissue, degenerative tendon, hypertrophic synovium, calcific deposit);
3. To encourage revascularization of tendon tissue;
4. To relieve extrinsic pressure, either bony or soft tissue;
5. To relieve tensile overload,
6. To discover and repair gross interstitial tendon rupture,
7. To repair or augment injure tendon structure (e.g., transverse grafts) (32). See Figure 44.40 and Table 44.11.

Indications for such soft tissue surgery include: 1) a failed monitored rehabilitative program of at least 3 to 6 months duration, 2) altered quality of life, 3) persistent pain with or without activities or sports play, 4) night pain (grade IV), 5) objective signs of radiologically confirmed lesion (plain x-ray, arthrogram, MRI, sonogram, bone scan) and 6) persistent weakness, atrophy, and dysfunction (39, 32). The perioperative considerations and preoperative management of chronic overuse injury is depicted in Figure 44.41.

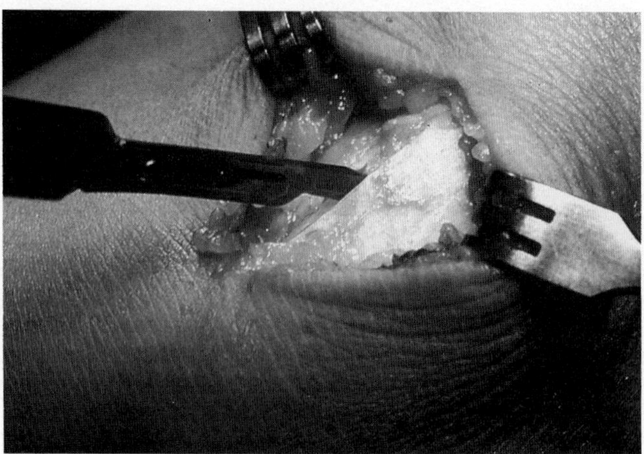

Figure 44.40 Typical surgical technique in tendinosis of patella tendon. Excision of degenerated tissue or calcific deposit is formed by reparative scar response.

Surgical treatment of tendinitis and chronic overuse injuries induces a change in the tendon cell matrix environment by promoting a renewed wound repair cycle and by removal of aberrant tissue (32). However, the end result will not be regenerated tendon or ligament or muscle, but remodeled connective tissue and scar repair, which is indeed different. With so many variables surrounding the postoperative management, including extended rest, immobilization, and rehabilitation, it has been emphasized that the factors responsible for clinical improvement postoperatively are not well established.

Insidious onset, the inherent nonoperative nature, and the lack of opportunity for tissue assessment postoperatively have slowed surgical insight. The primary reason to employ operative treatment in athletic soft

Table 44.11.
Common Surgical Techniques in the Treatment of Overuse Tendon Injury

Technique	Typical Application
Intratendinous or paratendinous excision	Persistent ossicle in Osgood-Schlatter's disease Rotator cuff calcific tendinosis Debridement chronic granulation tissue (e.g., lateral elbow epicondyle, subacromial space) Retrocalcaneal bursectomy Excision of accessory tarsal navicular
Decompression	Subacromial impingement syndrome Haglund's syndrome De Quervain's tenovaginitis Trigger finger release Achilles paratenonitis (fibrosheath inflammation)
Synovectomy-bursectomy	Subacromial impingement Retrocalcaneal bursectomy Tenovaginitis
Longitudinal internal tenotomy (linear tendon incision)	Achilles tendinosis Patella tendinosis Elbow extensor or flexor origin injury
Tensile "release"	Plantar fasciitis (fasciosis)
Repair	Rotator cuff Elbow extensor or flexor origin injury Achilles tendon interstitial tear
Drilling or scarification of bone tendon attachment	Elbow extensor or flexor origin injury Patella bone (Sinding-Larsen-Johansson)
Tendon transfer	Posterior tibial tendinosis with attenuation

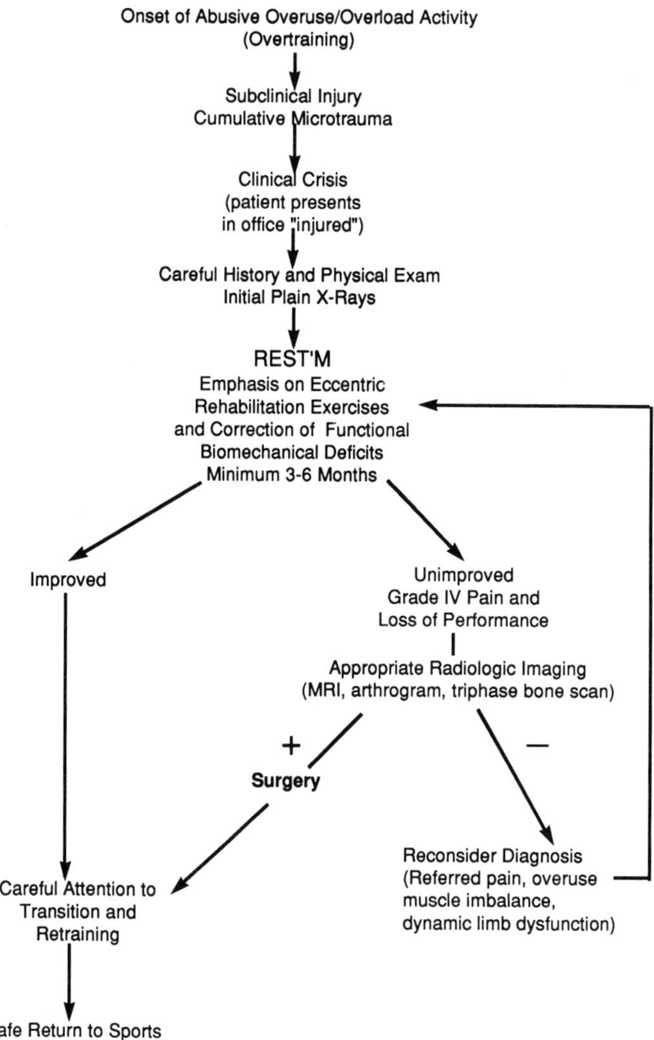

Figure 44.41 Algorithm for the treatment of overuse tendon injury. Surgical treatment is only one alternative in an extensive therapeutic plan.

tissue injury remains the empiric observation that improvement can be achieved in selective cases; the main argument against surgical treatment remains the fact that the improperly selected patient may do poorly and that the majority of chronic overuse complaints do not require such intervention for improvement (32). While a well-timed surgical incision may be a powerful stimulus to initiate the local tissue release of biological cell mediators for repair, the factors that contributed to the chronicity of the injury may not be altered (e.g., genetic predisposition, aging, biomechanical deficiencies, etc.). It is simplistic to claim that "bad scar" is replaced by "good scar" as a result of surgical intervention. More often, structurally inadequate or excessively inflamed tissue is replaced by an initially immature and disorganized collagen fabric that may evolve into adequate tissue but not normal tissue. Placed under the repetitive demands of sports performance, such tissue may be very sensitive to transitional stress and of vulnerable durability.

Returning the Athlete to Sports Participation

Guidelines for return to activity should be provided to the athlete to allow a safe progressive return to competition. Blazina and associates first developed the phasing concept of overuse injury with their description of "jumper's knee syndrome" or patella tendinitis (191). Since that initial description, guidelines have come into common usage (18, 34, 39, 76, 154, 152, 158, 188). These are summarized in Table 44.8. In counseling return to activity, it is the progression in the pattern of pain that dictates success. Participation is usually prohibited if the athlete has any daily activity pain. Pain should be assessed as to intensity, duration, and length of recovery time needed after activity. Keeping a log may help the athlete to quantify the subjective experience. With respect to physical findings, local swelling, tenderness, and loss of motion should be monitored. In managing the athlete, it is important to point out that the rate of tissue healing is roughly proportional to the visible resolution of hematoma or the progressive healing of the cutaneous postoperative scar. In addition, objective standards of strength, endurance, power, agility, speed, and range of motion must be assessed. Such testing should not rely merely on manual judgments, but on mechanical measurement, in order to provide a comparative record of performance. While sports drills may begin at around 80% strength and endurance levels, unrestricted play is not allowed until 90% or better comparative functional return. The well-equipped sports medicine rehabilitative center will provide some methodology for such testing to be carried out. Functional testing, such as jumping, sprinting, carioca drills, and sports-imitative skill exercises, provide another opportunity to observe and counsel the athlete on readiness for competition. A pattern of increasing pain or physical findings such as swelling or warmth should be viewed with caution and should initiate readjustment of the training schedule. The variables affecting athletic performance after injury are the same as those of all fitness attainment, namely, frequency, intensity, and duration. It is appropriate to initiate an alternating day participation program and to allow increases in intensity only after frequency and duration of exercise are significantly improved. A typical example of a progressive return to sports program is Brody's plan for a return to running activity after injury (192) (Table 44.12).

Ultimately, the athlete should not be allowed full athletic competition until after all clinical symptoms and biomechanical deficits have resolved and are no longer causing subclinical maladaptations (154).

Finally, attention must be given to faulty technique and abusive play that often has initiated the current injury. The sports medicine clinician is obligated to educate the patient about the potential risks of inappropriate training and to make suggestions regarding improved equipment as well as technique. It is often appropriate to prescribe professional teaching and fitness training for the highly competitive athlete. In grade I and II soft tissue injuries as well as in the return to

Table 44.12.
Return to Running After Injury[a]

The runner must be free of pain and tenderness, with normal daily activities before resuming his or her training program. (On a scale of 0 to 10, on which 0 is normal and 10 is the worst, the runner is asked to rate his or her pain with normal activities; the rating must be at 0).

(A) If 0: Run every other day for two weeks, then a maximum of 5 days a week for the next four weeks. If the previous level was 4 to 6 miles per session, begin with one mile. (If previous level per session was less than 4, begin with 0.5 mile per session). If no pain with running, follow the following weekly mileage schedule:

1	0	1	0	1	0	2	
0	2	0	2	0	3	0	
3	2	0	3	3	0	4	
3	0	4	4	0	5	4	
0	5	5	0	6	5	0	etc.

(B) If you have short intervals of pain with running:
- A. No running for 2 weeks.
- B. 10 minute total workout, alternating 4 minute run and 1 minute walk. If no pain, add 5 minutes every 3 days, working up to 30 minutes, then progress to the next step. If you experience pain, cut back 5 minutes and work up.
- C. 15 minutes total workout, alternating 4½ minute run and ½ minute walk. If no pain, add 5 minutes every 3 days, working up to 30 minutes, then progress to next step. If you experience pain, cut back 5 minutes and work up.
- D. Run steadily for 15 minutes, adding 5 minutes every 3 days. If you experience pain, cut back 5 minutes and work up.

(C) If you have pain after running:
- A. Cut your workout by 50% and progress by adding 10% a week.
- B. If you cut your workout 50% and still have pain, cut it by 50% again and progress by adding 10% a week.

(D) Running routine

moist heat (5 minutes) → stretch → run as prescribed → ice massage (10 minutes)

At night: moist heat (20 minutes) → stretch
weight lift
back exercises

[a]Adapted with permission from Brody DM. Techniques in the evaluation and treatment of the injured runner. Orthop Clin North Am 1982; 13:541–558.

sports phase, performance may be empowered by a variety of supportive devices. These include taping, neoprene sleeves, force-sparing braces and constraining functional braces. In the case of the ankle and elbow, such braces have been shown to be of value in improving performance, possibly through subtle neuromuscular feedback (193). Potential adverse effects and impairments of limb function have also been identified, emphasizing the importance of comprehensive rehabilitation and patient education (194).

Conclusions

Athletic soft tissue injury presents an intriguing problem to the sports medicine clinician. As Bowerman (195) has aptly stated, "It is the circumstances of the injury, the risk taking involved, and the continued exposure to risk, that produce interesting characteristics of the injury in sport." In this respect, the clinical predictability of soft tissue healing in sports-induced trauma must always be qualified by the imposed demand. All connective tissues are not the same. Intrinsic differences in the biologic nature of connective tissues have yet to be fully understood in their impact on the quality of healing. There are basic differences in the acute trauma response and overuse trauma tissue response, both of which are processes that are time and cell matrix dependent. Transition plays an important role in the determination of these processes. The success of treatment often depends on its timing and the relative balance of inflammation and degeneration that is present at the site of injury. What distinguishes the "fast healer" from the "slow healer" remains obscure. Reliance on rest and on medical and physical modalities should not be a substitute for a comprehensive therapeutic program. Physical rehabilitation remains a singularly important solution to sports-induced inflammation, scar, or degeneration, and the resultant biomechanical dysfunction. Hippocrates (196) noted that "Healing is a matter of time but is sometimes also a matter of opportunity." In this age, when sports medicine has been an art, earnestly seeking its science, the modern sports medicine clinician must be increasingly aware of the biological events and reparative capabilities of human tissues. For while the art of sports medicine may be extended through experience, the future therapeutic opportunities of sports medicine will only be extended by its scientific basis.

REFERENCES

1. Herring SA, Nilson KL. Introduction to overuse injuries. Clin Sports Med 1987;6:225–239.
2. Leadbetter WB. Cell-matrix response in tendon injury. Clin Sports Med 1992;11(3)533–577.
3. Leadbetter, WB. Histopathologic characteristics of overuse tendon injury in sports. Presented at Keystone Symposia on Molecular and Cellular Biology (wound repair), Keystone CO, April 1–7; American Academy of Orthopaedic Surgery, 59th Annual Meeting, Washington, DC, 1992.
4. Leadbetter WB. An introduction to sports-induced inflammation. In: Leadbetter WB, Buckwalter JA, Gordon SL, eds. Sports-induced inflammation: Clinical and basic science concepts. Park Ridge, IL: American Academy of Orthopaedic Surgeons, 1990: 3–23.
5. Garrick JG, Requa RK. The epidemiology of foot and ankle injuries in sports. Clin Sports Med. 1988;7:29–36.
6. DeHaven KE, Lintner DM. Athletic injuries: Comparison by age, sport and gender. Am J Sports Med 1986;14:218–224.
7. Witman PA, Melvin M, Nicholas JA. Common problems seen in a metropolitan sports injury clinic. Phys Sportsmed 1981;9:105–110.

8. Chandy DA, Grana WA. Secondary school athletic injury in boys and girls: A three-year comparison. Phys Sportsmed 1985;13:106–111.
9. Goldberg B. Injury patterns in youth sports. Phys Sportsmed 1989;17:175–184.
10. Watson AW. Sports injuries during one academic year in 6799 Irish school children. Am J Sports Med 1984;12:65–71.
11. Hoffman MD, Lyman KA. Medical needs at high school football games in Milwaukee. J Orthop Sports Phys Ther 1988;10:167–171.
12. Keller CS, Noyes FR, Buncher CR. The medical aspects of soccer injury epidemiology. Am J Sports Med 1987;15:230–237.
13. Menard D, Stanish WD. The aging athlete. Am J Sports Med 1989;17:187–196.
14. Grossman RB, Nicholas JA. Common disorders in the knee. Orthop Clin North Am 1977;8:619–640.
15. Rovere GD, Webb LX, Gristina AG, et al. Musculoskeletal injuries in theatrical dance students. Am J Sports Med 1983:11:195–198.
16. Johnson RJ, Pope MH. Safety in skiing. In: Scott WN, Nisonson B, Nicholas JA, eds. Principles of Sports Medicine. Baltimore: Williams & Wilkins, 1984;367–374.
17. James SL, Bates BT, Osternig LR. Injuries to runners. Am J Sports Med 1978;6:40–50.
18. Leadbetter WB: Getting ahead of running injury. Emerg Med June 15, 1979;27–39.
19. Jacobs SJ, Berson BL. Injuries to runners: A study of entrants to a 10,000 meter race. Am J Sports Med 1986;14:151–155.
20. Newell SG, Bramwell ST. Overuse injuries to the knee in runners. Phys Sports Med 1984;12:80–92.
21. Clement DB, Taunton JE, Smart GW, et al. A survey of overuse running injuries. Phys Sportsmed 1981;9:47–58.
22. Welsh RP, Clodman J. Clinical survey of Achilles tendinitis in athletes. Can Med Assoc J 1980;122:193–195.
23. Mann RA. Biomechanics of running. In: Mack RP, ed. American Academy of Orthopaedic Surgeons Symposium on the Foot and Leg in Running Sports, St. Louis: CV Mosby, 1982;1–29.
24. Richardson AB, Jobe FW, Collins HR. The shoulder in competitive swimming. Am J Sports Med 1980;8:159–163.
25. Johnson JE, Sim FH, Scott SG. Musculoskeletal injuries in competitive swimmers. Mayo Clin Proc 1987;62:289–304.
26. Leach R. Tennis serving compared with baseball pitching. In: Zarins B, Andrews JR, Carson WG. Injuries to the Throwing Arm. Philadelphia: WB Saunders, 1985;308.
27. Zarins B, Ciullo JV. Acute muscle and tendon injuries in athletes. Clin Sports Med 1983;2:167–182.
28. Woo SL-Y, Buckwalter JA, eds. Injury and Repair of the Musculoskeletal Soft Tissues. Park Ridge, IL: American Academy of Orthopaedic Surgeons, 1988.
29. Lazarus GS, Cooper DM, Knighton DR, et al., eds. Definitions and guidelines for assessment of wounds and evaluation of healing in Scars and Stripes, The Newsletter of the Wound Healing Society, 1992;2:(3):7–14.
30. Amadio PC: Tendon and ligament. In: Cohen IK, Diegelmann RF, Lindblad WJ, eds. Wound Healing: Biochemical and Clinical Aspects. Philadelphia: WB Saunders, 1992:384.
31. Butler DL, Groodes ES, Noyes FR, et al. Biomechanics of ligaments and tendons. In: Hutton RS, ed. Exercise and sports sciences reviews. Washington, DC: Franklin Institute Press, 1978:125–181.
32. Leadbetter WB, Mooar PA, Lane GJ, et al. The surgical treatment of tendinitis. Clin Sports Med 1992;11:No(4):679–712.
33. Noyes FR, Lindenfeld TN, Marshall MT. What determines an athletic injury (definition?) Who determines an injury (occurrence)? Am J Sports Med 1988;16(suppl 1):S65–S66.
34. Leadbetter WB. Physiology of tissue repair. In: Athletic training and sports medicine. 2nd ed Park Ridge, IL: American Academy of Orthopaedic Surgeons, 1991:96.
35. Majno G. The healing hand: Man and wound in the ancient world. Cambridge, MA: Harvard University Press, 1975:29, 102, 165, 373.
36. Hargreaves KM: Mechanisms of pain sensation resulting from inflammation. In: Leadbetter WB, Buckwalter JA, Gordon SL, eds. Sports-Induced Inflammation: Clinical and basic science concepts. Park Ridge, IL: American Academy of Orthopaedic Surgeons, 1990:383.
37. Weiss JA, Woo Sl-Y, Obland KJ, et al. Evaluation of a new injury model to study medial collateral ligament healing: Primary repair versus inoperative treatment. Orthop Res 1991;9:516–528.
38. Rubin E, Farber JL, eds. Pathology. Philadelphia: JB Lippincott, 1988:4.
39. O'Connor FG, Sobel JR, Nirschl RP: Five-step treatment for overuse injuries. Phys Sports Med 1992;20:(10):128–142.
40. Gallin JI, Goldstein IM, Snyderman R, eds. Inflammation: Basic principles and clinical correlates. New York: Raven Press, 1988.
41. Gamble JG: The musculoskeletal system, physiological basics. New York: Raven Press, 1988.
42. Almekinders LC, Banes AJ, Ballinger CA: Inflammatory response of fibroblasts to repetitive motion. Trans Ortho Res Soc 1992;17: 678.
43. Banes AJ, Donlon K, Lind GW, et al. Cell populations of tendon: A simplified method for isolation of synovial cells and internal fibroblasts. Confirmation of origin and biologic properties. J Orthop Res 1988;6:83–94.
44. Badalmente MA, Sampson SP, Dowd A, et al. The cellular pathobiology of cumulative trauma disorders/entrapment syndromes: Trigger finger, De Quervain's disease and carpal tunnel syndrome. Trans Ortho Res Soc 1992;17:677.
45. Grisham JW, Nopanitaya W. Cellular basis of disease, in Anderson's pathology, 9th ed. St. Louis: CV Mosby, 1990.
46. Robbins SL, Cotran RS. Pathologic basis of disease, 2nd ed. Philadelphia; WB Saunders, 1979.
47. Scarpelli DG, Iamnaconne PM. Cell injury and errors of metabolism. In: Kissane J, ed. Anderson's pathology. Vol 1, 9th ed, St. Louis: CV Mosby, 1990.
48. Scarpelli DG, Trump BF. Cell Injury. Universities, Bethesda, Md: Associated for Research and Education in Pathology, Inc., 1971.
49. Wahl SM, Wahl LM. Inflammation: In: Cohen JK, Diegelmann RF, Lindblad WY, eds. wound healing. Philadelphia: WB Saunders, 1992:40.
50. Nirschl RP, Pettrone FA. Tennis elbow. The surgical treatment of lateral epicondylitis. J Bone Joint Surg 1979;61A:832–839.
51. Kannus P, Jozsa L. Histopathological changes preceding spontaneous rupture of a tendon. J Bone Joint Surg 1991;73A:10, 1507–1525.
52. Puddu G, Ippolito I, Postacchini F: A classification of achilles tendon disease. Am J Sports Med 1976;4(4) July/August.
53. Bailey AJ, Bazin S, Delaunay A: Changes in the nature of the collagen during development and resorption of granulation tissue. Biochem Biophys Acta 1973;328:383–390.
54. Clark RAF, Henson PM, eds. The molecular and cellular biology of wound repair. New York: Plenum Press, 1988.
55. Mankin HJ. The response of articular cartilage to mechanical injury. J Bone Joint Surg 1982;64-A:460–466.
56. Castor CW. Regulation of connective tissue metabolism. In: McCarty DJ, ed. Arthritis and allied conditions: A textbook of rheumatology. 11th ed. Philadelphia: Lea & Febiger, 1989:256–272.
57. Goldberg B, Rabinovitch M. Connective tissue. In: Weiss L, ed. Cell and tissue biology—A textbook of histology. 6th ed. Baltimore: Urban and Schwarzenberg, 1988:157.
58. Hunt TK, Dunphy JE, eds. Fundamentals of wound management. New York: Appleton-Century-Crofts, 1979.
59. Stanulis-Praeger BM. Cellular senescence revisited: A review, mechanisms of aging and development 1987;38:1–48.
60. Postlethwaite AE, Kang AH. Fibroblasts. In: Gallen JI, Goldstein IM, Snyderman R, eds. Inflammation: Basic principles and clinical correlates. Raven Press, 1988:577.
61. Martinez-Hernandez A. Repair, degeneration, and fibrosis. In: Rubin E, Faber JL, eds. Pathology. Philadelphia: JB Lippincott, 1988:68–95.
62. Gelberman R. Goldberg V, An KN, et al. Tendon. in Woo SL-Y, Buckwalter JA eds. Injury and repair of the musculoskeletal soft tissues. Park Ridge, IL: American Academy of Orthopaedic Surgeons, 1988:5.
63. Postlethwaite AE. Failed healing responses in connective tissue and a comparison of medical conditions: In: Leadbetter WB, Buckwalter JA, Gordon SL, eds. Sports induced inflammation:

Clinical and basic science concepts. Park Ridge, IL: The American Academy of Orthopaedic Surgeons, 1990.
64. Caplan A, Carlson B, Faulkner J, Fischman D, et al. Skeletal Muscle. In: Woo SL-Y, Buckwalter JA, eds. Injury and Repair of the Musculoskeletal Soft Tissues. Park Ridge, IL: American Academy of Orthopaedic Surgeons, 1988.
65. Stauber WT. Repair models and specific tissue responses in muscle injury. In: Leadbetter WB, Buckwalter JA, Gordon SL, eds. Sports-induced inflammation: Clinical and basic science concepts. Park Ridge, IL: The American Academy of Orthopaedic Surgeons, 1990:205.
66. Arnheim DD. Modern principles of athletic training. St. Louis: Times Mirror/Mosby, 1989:230.
67. Abbas AK, Lichtman AH, Pober JS. Cellular molecular immunology. Philadelphia: WB Saunders, 1991.
68. Fantone JC. Basic concepts in inflammation. In: Leadbetter WB, Buckwalter JA, Gordon SL, eds. Sports-induced inflammation: Clinical and basic science concepts. Park Ridge, IL: The American Academy of Orthopaedic Surgeons, 1990:25.
69. Ward PA, Till GO, Johnson KJ. Oxygen derived free radicals and inflammation. In: Sports-Induced Inflammation: Clinical and basic science concepts. American Academy of Orthopaedic Surgeons, 1990:315–325.
70. Fritz VK, Stauber WT. Characterization of muscles injured by forced lengthening, II proteoglycans. Med Sci Sports Exerc, 1988;20(4)354–361.
71. Stauber WT, Fritz VK, Vogelback DW, et al. Characterization of muscles injured by forced lengthening, I. Cellular infiltrates. Med Sci Sports Exerc 1988;20(4)345–353.
72. Jennings RW, Hunt TK. Overview of post-natal wound healing. In: Adzick NS, Longaker MT, eds. Fetal Wound Healing. New York: Elsevier, 1922:25.
73. Wilder RL, Lafyatis R, Remmers EF. Platelet-derived growth factor and transforming growth factor beta: Wound healing and repair. In: Leadbetter WB, Buckwalter JA, Gordon SL, eds. Sports-induced inflammation clinical and basic science concepts. Park Ridge, IL: The American Academy of Orthopaedic Surgeons, 1990:301.
74. Beachey EH, Chiang TM, Kang AH. Collagen—platelet interaction Connect Tissue Res 1979;8:1–21.
75. Postlethwaite, AE. Cell-cell interaction in collagen biosynthesis and fibroblast migration. In: Weissman G, ed. Allowances in Inflammation Research. New York: Raven Press, 1983:27–55.
76. Curwin S, Stanish W. Tendinitis: Its etiology and treatment. Lexington, MA: Collamore Press, 1984.
77. Adzick NS, Longaker MT. Fetal wound healing. New York; Elsevier, 1992.
78. Estwanik JJ, McAlister JA. Contusions and the formation of myositis ossificans. Phys Sportsmed 1990;18(4)53–64.
79. Clarkson PM. Exercise-induced muscle damage—Animal and human models. J Am Coll Sports Med 1992;24,(5)510–511.
80. Smith LL. Acute inflammation: The underlying mechanism in delayed onset muscle soreness. Med Sci Sports Exerc 1991;23(5):542–554.
81. Eyre DR. The collagens of musculoskeletal soft tissues. In: Leadbetter WB, Buckwalter JA, Gordon SL, eds. Sports induced inflammation: Clinical and basic science concepts. Park Ridge, IL: American Academy of Orthopaedic Surgeons, 1990:161.
82. Rosenberg L, Choi HU, Neame PJ, et al. Proteoglycans of soft connective tissues. In: Leadbetter WB, Buckwalter JA, Gordon SL, eds. Sports-Induced Inflammation: Clinical and basic science concepts. Park Ridge, IL: American Academy of Orthopaedic Surgeons, 1990.
83. Heidemann SR. A new twist on integrins and the cytoskeleton. Science 1993;260:1080–1081.
84. Frank CB, Hart DA. Cellular response to loading. In: Leadbetter WB, Buckwalter JA, Gordon SL, eds. Sports-induced inflammation: Clinical and basic science concepts. Park Ridge, IL: American Academy of Orthopaedic Surgeons, 1990:555.
85. Kibler WB, Chandler TJ, Stracener ES. Musculoskeletal adaptations and injury due to overtraining. In: Holloszy JO, ed. Exerc sports sci rev 1992;20:99.
86. Garrett WE, Lehnes J. Cellular and matrix response in mechanized injury at the myotendinous junction. In: Leadbetter WB, Buckwalter JA, Gordon Sl, eds. Sports-Induced Inflammation: Clinical and basic science concepts. Park Ridge, IL: American Academy of Orthopaedic Surgeons, 1990.
87. Chow GH, LeCroy CM, Seaber AV, et al. The effect of fatigue in muscle strain injury. Trans Orthop Res Soc 1990;15:148.
88. Micheli LJ, Fehlandt AF. Overuse injuries to tendons and apophyses in children and adolescents. Clin Sports Med 1992;11:713–726.
89. van der Meulen JC. Present state of knowledge on processes of healing in collagen structures. Int J Sports Med 1982;3(suppl 1):4–8.
90. Clancy WG. Tendon trauma and overuse injuries. In: Leadbetter WB, Buckwalter JA, Gordon SL, eds. Sports-Induced Inflammation: Clinical and basic science concepts. Park Ridge, IL: American Academy of Orthopaedic Surgeons, 1990:609.
91. Gerber G, Gerberg G, Altman KI. Studies on the metabolism of tissue proteins: I. Turnover of collagen labeled with poline-U-C14 in young rats. J Biol Chem 1960;235:3653.
92. Laurent TC. Structure, function and turnover of the extracellular matrix. Adv Microcirc 1987;13:15–34.
93. Frank C, Amiel D, et al. Normal ligament properties and ligament healing. Clin Orthop 1985;(196)15–25.
94. Jozsa L, Kvist M. Balind BJ, et al. The role of recreational sport activity in Achilles tendon rupture. A clinical, pathoanatomical and sociologic study of 292 cases. Am J Sports Med 1989;17:338.
95. Trump BE, Berezesky IK, Smith MW, et al. The role of ionized cytosolic calcium (CA_2) in injury and recovery from anoxia and ischemia. Md Med J 1992;41:505–508.
96. Kvist M, Jozsa L, Jarvinen MJ, et al. Chronic Achilles' paratenonitis in athletes: A histological and histochemical study. Pathology 1987;19:1–11.
97. Kvist MH, Lehto MUK, Jozsa L, et al. Chronic Achilles' paratendinitis. Am J Sports Med 1988;16:616–623.
98. Fox RI, Lotz M, Carson DA. Structure and functions of synoviocytes in arthritis and allied conditions. In: McCarty DJ, ed. A textbook of rheumatology. 11th ed. Philadelphia: Lea and Febiger, 1989:273–287.
99. Stedman's Medical Dictionary, 25th ed. Baltimore: Williams & Wilkins, 1990.
100. Moelleken BRW. Growth Factors in Wound Healing. In: Esterhai JL, Gristina AG, Poss R, eds. Musculoskeletal Infection. Park Ridge, IL: American Academy of Orthopaedic Surgeons, 1992:311.
101. Fong Y, Moldawer LL, Shires GT, et al. The biologic characteristics of cytokines and their implication. In surgical injury. Surgery, gynecol obstet 1990;170(4):363–378.
102. Goldring MB, Goldring SR. Skeletal Tissue Response to Cytokines. 1990;258:254–277.
103. Vogel KG. Proteoglycans accumulate in a region of human tibialis posterior tendon subjected to compressive force in vitro and in ligaments. Trans Combined Meeting Orthop Res Soc USA, Japan and Canada, October 21–23, 1991, p. 58.
104. Koob TJ, Vogel KG, Thurmond FA. Compression loading in vitro regulates proteoglycan synthesis by fibrocartilage in tendon. Trans Orthop Res Soc 1991;16:49.
105. Hayflick L. Cell aging. Ann Rev Gerontol Geriatr 1980;1:26–67.
106. Ippolito E, Natali PG, Postacchini F, et al. Morphological, immunological, and biochemical study of rabbit Achilles tendon at various ages. J Bone Joint Surg 1980;62A:583–598.
107. Ippolito E, Postacchini F, Riccardi-Pollini PT. Biomechanical variations in the matrix of human tendons in relation to age and pathological conditions. Ital J Orthop Traumatol 1975;1:133–139.
108. Uhthoff HK, Sarkar K. Classification and definition of tendinopathies. Clin Sports Med 1991;10:707–720.
109. Rathbun JB, McNab I. The microvascular pattern of the rotator cuff. J Bone Joint Surg 1970;52B:540–553.
110. Chansky HA, Iannotti JP. The vascularity of the rotator cuff. Clin Sports Med 1991;10:807–822.
111. Brooks CH, Revell WJ, Heatley FW. A quantitative histological study of the vascularity of the rotator cuff tendon. J Bone Joint Surg 1992;74B:151–153.
112. Wilson AM, Goodship AE. Hysteresis energy losses in the equine superficial digital flexor tendon during exercise produce a local temperature sufficient to damage fibroblasts in vitro. Trans Orthop Res Soc 1992;17:769.

113. Schatzker J, Branemark PI. Intravital observation on the microvascular anatomy and microcirculation of the tendon. Acta Orthop Scand 1969;126(suppl):1–23.
114. Nirschl RP. Mesenchymal syndrome. Va Med Monthly 1969;96:659–662.
115. Madden JW, Arem AJ. Wound healing: Biologic and clinical features. In: Sabiston DC ed. Textbook of surgery, 14th ed. Philadelphia: WB Saunders, 1991:167.
116. Teitz CC. Overuse injuries. In: Teitz CC ed. Scientific foundation of sports medicine. Toronto: BC Decker, 1989:299.
117. Jozsa L, Balint JB, Kannus P, et al. Distribution of blood groups in patients with tendon rupture. J Bone Joint Surg 1989;71B:272.
118. Singer KM, Jones DC: Soft tissue conditions of the ankle and foot. In: Nicholas JA, Hershman EB, eds. The lower extremity and spine in sports medicine. St. Louis: CV Mosby, 1986:148.
119. Lyon RM, Akeson WH, Amiel D, et al. Ultrastructural differences between the cells of the medial collateral and the anterior cruciate ligaments, Cl Ortho and Rel Res 1991;272:279–280.
120. Chandrasekharam NN, Amiel D, Green MH, et al. Characterization of the intrinsic properties of the anterior cruciate and medial collateral ligament cells: An in vitro cell culture study. J Orthop Res 1992;10:465–475.
121. Frank C, McDonald D, Lielser RL, et al. Biochemical heterogeneity within the maturing rabbit medial collateral ligament. Clin Orthop 1988;236:279–285.
122. Warwick R, Williams PL. Gray's anatomy. 36th ed, Edinburgh: Churchill Livingston, 1980.
123. Clark JM, Harryman DT. Tendons, ligaments, and capsule of the rotator cuff—Gross and microscopic anatomy, J Bone Joint Surg 1992;74-A:713–25.
124. Garrett WE. Muscle strain injuries: Clinical and basic aspects. Med Sci Sports Exerc 1990;22:436–443.
125. Harper J, Amiel D, Harper E. Changes in collagenase and inhibitor in ligaments and tendon during early development of stress deprivation. Trans Orthop Res Soc 1991;16:114.
126. Colosimo AJ, Bassett III, FH. Jumper's knee: Diagnosis and treatment. Orthop Rev 1990;19:139–149.
127. Illizarov GA. The tension-stress effect on the genesis and growth of tissues: II. The influence of the rate and frequency of distraction. Clin Orthop Rel Res 1989;239:263–285.
128. Periodization—Part I. National Strength and Conditioning Association Journal. 1993;15(1)57–67.
129. Periodization—Part II. National Strength and Conditioning Association Journal. 1993;15(1)69–76.
130. Reid DC. Sports injury assessment and rehabilitation. New York: Churchill-Livingston, 1992.
131. Nikolaou PK, Macdonald BL, Glisson RR. Biomechanical and histological evaluation of muscle after controlled strain injury. Am J Sports Med 1987;15:9–14.
132. Russell B, Dix DJ, Haller DL, et al. Repair of injured skeletal muscle: A molecular approach. Medicine and Science in Sports and Exercise, 1992;24(2)189–196.
133. Armstrong RB. Initial events in exercise-induced muscular injury. Med Sci Sports Exerc 1990;22(4)429–435.
134. Evans WJ. Exercise-induced skeletal muscle damage. Phys Sports Med 1987;15(1)89–100.
135. Waterman-Storer CM. The cytoskeleton of skeletal muscle: Is it affected by exercise? A brief review. Med Sci Sports Exerc 1991;23(11)1240–1249.
136. Armstrong RB. Mechanisms of exercise-induced delayed onset muscular soreness: A brief review. Med Sci Sports Exerc 1984;16(6)529–538.
137. Jackson P, Feagin J. Quadriceps contusions in young athletes. J Bone Joint Surg 1973;55:95–105.
138. Cushner FD, Morwessel RM. Myositis ossificans traumatica. Orthop Rev 1992;21(11)1319–1326.
139. Finnerman GAM, Shapiro MS. Sports induced soft tissue calcification. In: Leadbetter WB, Buckwalter JA, Gordon SL, eds. Sports-induced inflammation: Clinical and basic science concepts. Park Ridge, IL: American Academy of Orthopaedic Surgeons, 1990:257–275.
140. Mono JOV, Pope TL, Ward WO, et al. Magnetic resonance imaging of myositis ossificans. J South Med J 1993;2(2):67–76.
141. Hughston J, Whatley G, Stone M. Myositis ossificans traumatica, South Med J. 1962;55:1167–1170.
142. Travell JG, Simons DG. Myofascial pain and dysfunction: The trigger point manual. Baltimore: Williams and Wilkins, 1983.
143. Smyth HA. Nonarticular rheumatism and psychogenic musculoskeletal syndromes. In: McCarty OJ, ed. arthritis and allied conditions. 11th ed. Philadelphia: Lea and Febiger, 1989:1241–1254.
144. Rosen WB. Myofascial pain: The great mimicker and pretender of other diseases in the performing arts: 88, Md Med J 1993;42(3):261–266.
145. Fox RJ, Lotz M, Carson DA. Structure and functions of synoviocytes. In: McCarty OJ, ed. Nonarticular rheumatism and psychogenic musculoskeletal syndromes in arthritis and allied conditions. 11th ed. Philadelphia: Lea and Febiger, Chapt. 15, 1989;273–287.
146. Evans CH. Response of synovium to mechanical injury. In: Finerman GAM, Noyes FR, eds. biology and biomechanics of the traumatized synovial joint: The knee as a model. Rosemont, IL: American Academy Orthopaedic Surgeons 1992;17–26.
147. Deleted in proof.
148. Rodesky MW, Fu FH. Indications of synovial inflammation by matrix molecules, implant particles and chemical agents. In: Leadbetter WB, Buckwalter JA, Gordon SL, eds. Sports-induced inflammation: Clinical and basic science concepts. Park Ridge, IL: American Academy of Orthopaedic Surgeons, 1990:357–381.
149. Biedert RM, Stauffer E, Freiderich NK. Occurrence of free nerve endings in the soft tissue of the knee joint. Am J Sports Med 1993;20(4):430–433.
150. Fulkerson JP, Hunderford DS. Disorder of the patellofemoral joint. 2nd ed. Baltimore: Williams & Wilkins, 1990.
151. Gronblad M, Korkala O, Konttinen YT, et al. Immuno reactive neuropeptides in nerves in ligamentous tissue—An experimental neuroimmunohistochemical study. Clin Ortho Rel Res 1991;265:291–296.
152. Leadbetter WB. Clinical staging concept in sports trauma. In: Leadbetter WB, Buckwalter JA, Gordon SL, eds. Sports-induced inflammation: Clinical and basic science concepts. Park Ridge, IL: American Academy of Orthopaedic Surgeons, 1990;587–596.
153. Torg JS, Schneider R. Sports medicine tumors. Presented at the annual meeting American Academy of Orthopaedic Surgeons, San Francisco, CA, February 20, 1993.
154. Kibler WB. Concepts in exercise rehabiliation of athletic injury. In: Leadbetter WB, Buckwalter JA, Gordon SL, eds. Sports-induced inflammation: Clinical and basic science concepts. Park Ridge, IL: American Academy of Orthopaedic Surgeons, 1990;759–769.
155. Fry HJH. The treatment of overuse injury syndrome. Md Med J 1993;42(3):277–282.
156. Baker BE, Levinsohn ME. Radiologic diagnosis of pain in one athlete. Clin Sports Med 1987;6:4.
157. Andrews JR, Harrelson GL. Physical Rehabilitation of the Injured Athlete. Philadelphia: WB Saunders, 1991.
158. Roy S, Irvin R. Sports medicine prevention, evaluations, management and rehabilitation. Englewood Cliffs, NJ: Prentice Hall, 1983.
159. Amadio Jr, P, Cummings DM, Amadio P. Nonsteroidal antiinflammatory drugs: Tailoring therapy to achieve results and avoid toxicity. Postgrad Med 1993;93,(4)73–97.
160. Weiler JM. Medical modifiers of sports injury: The use of nonsteroidal anti-inflammatory drugs (NSAID's) (n sports soft tissue injury in tendinitis I: Basic concepts. Clin Sports Med 1992;11(3)625–644.
161. Hasson SC, Daniels JC, Divine JG, et al. Effect of ibuprofen use on muscle soreness, damage and performance: A preliminary investigation. Med Sci Sports Exerc 1993;(1)9–17.
162. Dahners LE, Gilbert JA, Lester GE, et al. The effect of nonsteroidal antiinflammatory drug on the healing of ligaments. Am J Sports Med 1988;16(6)641–646.
163. Almekinders LC, Gilbert JA. Healing of experimental muscle strains and the effects of nonsteroidal antiinflammatory medication. Am J Sports Med 1986;14(4)303–308.
164. Leadbetter WB. Corticosteroid injection therapy. In: Leadbetter WB, Buckwalter JA, Gordon SL, eds. Sports-induced inflam-

mation: Clinical and basic science concepts. Park Ridge, IL: American Academy of Orthopaedic Surgeons, 1990;527–545.

165. Backman C, Boquist L, Friden J, et al. Chronic Achilles paratenonitis with tendinosis: An experimental model in the rabbit. J Orthop Res. 1990;8:541–547.
166. Bowen DL, Fauci AS. Adrenal corticosteroids. In: Gallin JT, Goldstein IM, Snyderman R, eds. Inflammation—Basic principles and clinical correlates. New York: Raven Press, 1988;877–895.
167. Haupt HA, Rovere GD. Anabolic steroids: A review of the literature. Am J Sports Med 1984;12:469–484.
168. Haupt HA. Anabolic steroids as modifiers of sports-induced inflammation. In: Leadbetter WB, Buckwalter JA, Gordon SL, eds. Sports-induced inflammation: Clinical and basic science concepts. Park Ridge, IL: American Academy of Orthopaedic Surgeons, 1990;449–454.
169. Miles JW, Grana WA, Egle D, et al. the effect of anabolic steroids in the biomechanical and histologic properties of rat tendon. J Bone Joint Surg 1992;74-A:411–422.
170. Karpakka JA, Pesda MK, Takala TE. The effects of anabolic steroids on collagen synthesis in rat skeletal muscle and tendon—a preliminary report. Am J Sports Med 1992;20(3):262–266.
171. Percy EC. Dimethyl sulfoxide: Its role as an anti-inflammatory agent in athletic injuries. In: Leadbetter WB, Buckwalter JA, Gordon SL, eds. Sports-induced inflammation: Clinical and basic science concepts. Park Ridge, IL: American Academy of Orthopaedic Surgeons, 1990;443–447.
172. Percy EC, Carson JO. The use of DMSO in tennis elbow and rotator cuff tendinitis: A double blind study. Med Sci Sports Exerc 1981;13:215–219.
173. Myrer JW, Heckman R, Francis RS. Topically applied dimethyl sulfoxide—its effects on inflammation and healing of a contusion. Am J Sports Med 1986;14:165–169.
174. Packer L. Protective role of vitamin E in biological systems. Am J Clin Nutr 1991;53:1050S–1055S.
175. Alessio HM. Exercise-induced oxidative stress. Med Sci Sports Exerc 1993;25(2)218–224.
176. Goldfarb AH. Antioxidants: role of supplementation to prevent exercise-induced oxidative stress. Med Sci Sports Exerc 1993;25(2)232–236.
177. Knight KL. Cryotherapy: theory, technique and physiology. Chattanooga, TN: Chattanooga Corp, 1985.
178. Bassett FH, Kirkpatrick JS, Engelhardt DL, et al. Cryotherapy-induced nerve injury. Am J Sports Med 1992;20(5):516–518.
179. Denegar CR, Perrin DH. Effect of transcutaneous electrical nerve stimulation, cold, and a combination treatment on pain, decreased range of motion and strengthening associated with delayed onset muscle soreness. J Athletic Train 1992;27(3):200–206.
180. Prentice WE. Therapeutic modalities in sports medicine. St. Louis: Times-Mirror/Mosby, 1986.
181. Gieck JH, Saliba E. Therapeutic ultrasound: Influence on inflammation and healing. In: Leadbetter WB, Buckwalter JA, Gordon SL, eds. Sports-induced inflammation: Clinical and basic science concepts. Park Ridge, IL: American Academy of Orthopaedic Surgeons 1990;479–492.
182. Frieder S, Weisberg J, Fleming B, et al. A pilot study: The therapeutic effect of ultrasound following partial rupture of Achilles tendons in male rats. J Ortho Sports Phys Ther 1988;10(2):39–46.
183. Jackson BA, Schwane JA, Starcher BC. Effect of ultrasound therapy on the repair of Achilles tendon injuries in rats. Med Sci Sports Exerc 1991;23(2):171–176.
184. Quillen WS, Mohr TM, Reed BV: High voltage pulsed galvanic stimulation as a modifier of sports induced inflammation. In: Leadbetter WB, Buckwalter JA, Gordon SL, eds. Sport-induced inflammation: Clinical and basic science concepts. Park Ridge, IL: American Academy of Orthopaedic Surgeons 1990;493–498.
185. Smith W, Winn F, Parette R. Comparative study using four modalities in shin splint treatments. J Orthop Sports Phys Ther 1986;8(2):77–80.
186. LaBelle H, Gilbert R, Joncas J, et al. Lack of scientific evidence for the treatment of lateral epicondylitis of the elbow. J Bone Joint Surg 1992;74-B,646–651.
187. Policoff LD. Effective use of physical modalities. Ortho Clin N America 1982;13(3):579–586.
188. Stanish WD, Curwin S, Rabinovitch M. Tendinitis. The analysis and treatment for running. Clin Sports Med 1985;4:593–609.
189. Akeson WH, Amiel D, Abel MF, et al. Effects of immobilization on joints. Clin Orthop 1987;219:28–37.
190. Salter RB. Continuous passive motion—CPM—A biological concept for healing and regenerations of articular cartilage, ligaments, and tendons from origination to research to clinical applications. Baltimore: Williams & Wilkins, 1993.
191. Blazina ME, Kerlan RK, Jobe FW, et al. Jumper's knee. Orthop Clin North Am 1973;(4)665–678.
192. Brody DM. Techniques in the evaluation and treatment of the injured runner. Orthop Clin North Am 1982;13:541–558.
193. Groppel JL, Nirschl RP. A mechanical and electromyographical analysis of the effects of various counterforce braces on the tennis player. Am J Sports Med 1986;14(3):195–200.
194. Ott J, Clancy WG. Function knee braces, A review. Orthopaedics, 1993;16(2):171–176.
195. Bowerman JW. Radiology and injury in sport. New York: Appleton-Century Crofts, 1977.
196. Hippocrates. Writings on the articulations. In: Hutchin RM, ed. Great Books of the Western World. Chicago: Encyclopedia Britannica, 1952;(10)91–121.

45 / DIAGNOSIS AND TREATMENT OF DERMATOLOGIC PROBLEMS IN ATHLETES[a]

Wilma Fowler Bergfeld and Dirk M. Elston

Introduction

Skin problems are common among athletes and may be debilitating. Some skin problems are also unique to athletes; some, indeed, are unique to a particular sport. The majority of dermatologic disorders observed in the youthful and in mature athlete are secondary to physical and chemical agents, climatic conditions, infections, infestations, and exacerbations of preexisting cutaneous disorders. Most of these cutaneous disorders represent common dermatologic entities, which are exacerbated by environmental climatic conditions. The more common and interesting disorders will be elaborated in this presentation with discussion of the accepted therapies (1–6).

In sports medicine, a frequently asked question is: What are the disqualifying dermatologic disorders in a contact or individual sport? In answer, a general statement is that all infectious disorders and infestations temporarily disqualify the athlete until these have been treated. More specific recommendations are discussed later in this chapter.

Mechanical and Physical Injury

Physical agents account for a significant number of the athlete's cutaneous injuries. The majority of these injuries are minor, although frequently painful, and avoidable. Sudden frictional forces directed to the skin are the primary factor producing petechiae, hemorrhage, or blisters, especially on acral areas.

Most physical injuries sustained during sports affect deeper tissues, the associated skin injury being only incidental. Friction blisters represent a mechanical injury in which only the skin is affected. Friction blisters are common in athletes and may produce significant disability. Blisters primarily occur on weight-bearing surfaces and are especially noted on the feet and hands of athletes such as runners, basketball, football, soccer, or volleyball players (Fig. 45.1) (1). Blisters occur secondary to frictional force on the skin. The effect of friction is exaggerated by increased humidity and heat. Common sites of involvement are joints, tips of fingers and toes, the heel of the foot and under calluses. Prevention of blisters can be achieved by hardening the skin with 10% tannic acid soaks, wearing two pairs of powdered socks to decrease frictional force on the foot, and wearing appropriate well-fitted hand and foot gear. The treatment of blisters consists of draining them with a sterile needle and covering the blisters with occlusive pressure dressings, such as adhesive tape (7). Some synthetic wound dressings may also be helpful in the management of extensive friction blisters. DuoDerm, a synthetic hydrocolloid dressing, is a self-adhesive dressing, which may serve as a physical barrier to infection and further trauma. Thin-film, adhesive polyurethane dressings, such as Op-Site, have also been used. It is necessary to exercise caution when removing these dressings because they have been known to strip the new epithelium from a healing wound. Vigilon, a gel-type dressing, may be refrigerated and applied to a cutaneous injury as a cool compress and dressing in one. Treatment of friction blisters may include the use of antibiotics to prevent secondary infection. The topical antibiotic mupirocin (Bactroban) may be especially useful. It offers effective coverage against *Staphylococcus aureus*.

Another lesion produced by frictional forces is the black heel, which represents palmar or plantar petechiae at the site of injury and is most commonly observed in athletes involved in running sports, and in weight lifters. The therapy of this disorder includes skin lubrication and tincture of time. Prophylaxis may require a change of foot gear.

[a] The views and opinions expressed in this chapter are those of the authors and not to be construed as official or reflecting those of the United States Army or the Department of Defense.

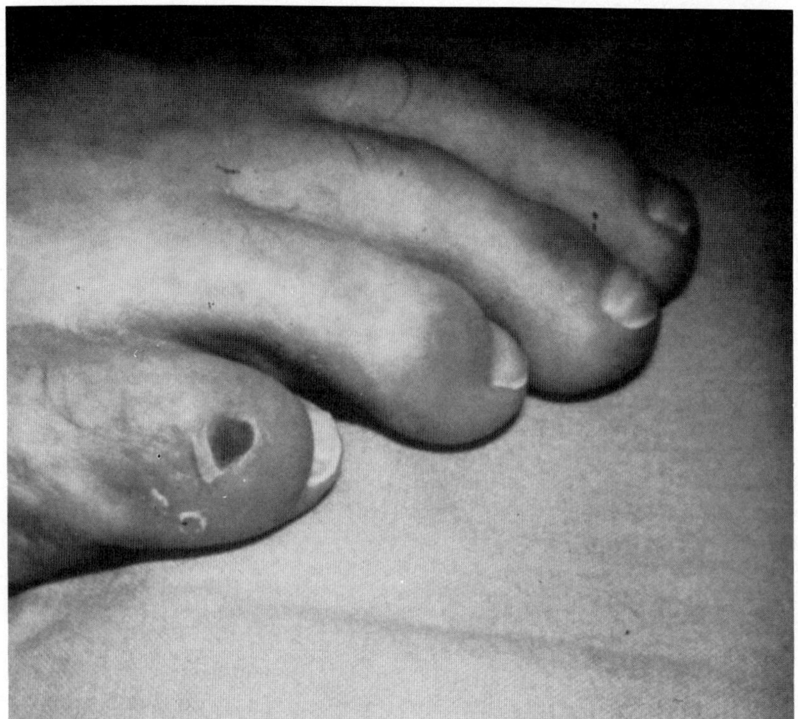

Figure 45.1. Friction blisters are seen in areas of pressure and rubbing and are exaggerated by increased humidity and heat.

The tennis toe represents a painful splinter hemorrhage beneath the nailplate primarily of the great toe (1). Injury is incurred by the nail abruptly hitting the top of the shoe. The treatment is basically preventive and includes properly fitting shoes and appropriate padding of the distal toe.

Subungual hematomas are painful hemorrhages, which are also produced by sudden blunt external force to the nailplate (1). The toenail is the most common site involved. Treatment consists of incisional drainage of the painful hemorrhage, which is usually accomplished by hot wire puncture of the nailplate.

Stria distensae (stretch lines or bands) represent the sequela of extensive stretching of the skin with fragmentation of elastic supporting fibers. Common sites of involvement are the sites of greatest tension or stretch, such as the shoulders, back, and thighs as seen in weight lifters, gymnasts, and runners. Weight gain can also induce striae over similarly stretched areas of skin. Essentially, there is no treatment once striae have occurred. Hydration and lubrication of skin are helpful in preventing striae; however, prevention is best accomplished by avoidance of overstretching the skin.

Calluses are ubiquitous among athletes and are observed over bony prominences where there is increased pressure (Figs. 45.2 and 45.3). Formation of calluses represents a protective response of the skin to increased pressure or rubbing. In certain sports, calluses may be advantageous to the sporting event, such as on the hands of gymnasts or archers or on the feet of runners, basketball players, or football players. If calluses are painful, reducing the size is indicated and can be accomplished by hydration and subsequent paring with a shearing implement or pumice stone. Cushioned small pads are especially helpful on the feet to reduce pain on specific pressure sites.

Abrasions are superficial erosions or ulcerations that commonly occur over joints or at the site of a shearing force directed to the skin. Abrasions are observed in all athletes but are more prone to occur in football players and soccer players who perform on Astroturf (Fig. 45.4) or in those who run on cinder tracks. Abrasions have even occurred under poorly fitting gear, such as the football helmet. The preferred treatment is preventive, i.e., by wearing appropriate protective clothing and hand and foot gear. Once an abrasion has occurred, the treatment of choice is debridement and cleansing with frequent applications of an antimicrobial agent. If the abrasion becomes secondarily infected, systemic antibiotics are indicated, such as cephradine 500 mg BID for 2 weeks.

Climatic Injuries

Urticaria can be induced by a variety of etiological agents, including such physical agents as cold, heat, exercise, and ultraviolet light. Urticaria induced by physical agents presents as localized, pruritic, transient swellings of the skin or mucous membranes (Fig 45.5). The etiological causes are determined by clinical history. Specific tests include exercise to produce increased core body temperature, which induces cholinergic urticaria; the ice cube test for cold urticaria; and phototesting for solar urticaria. Specific laboratory tests might include eosinophil counts, sedimentation rate, serum levels of C4, C2, or both, and quantitative C1

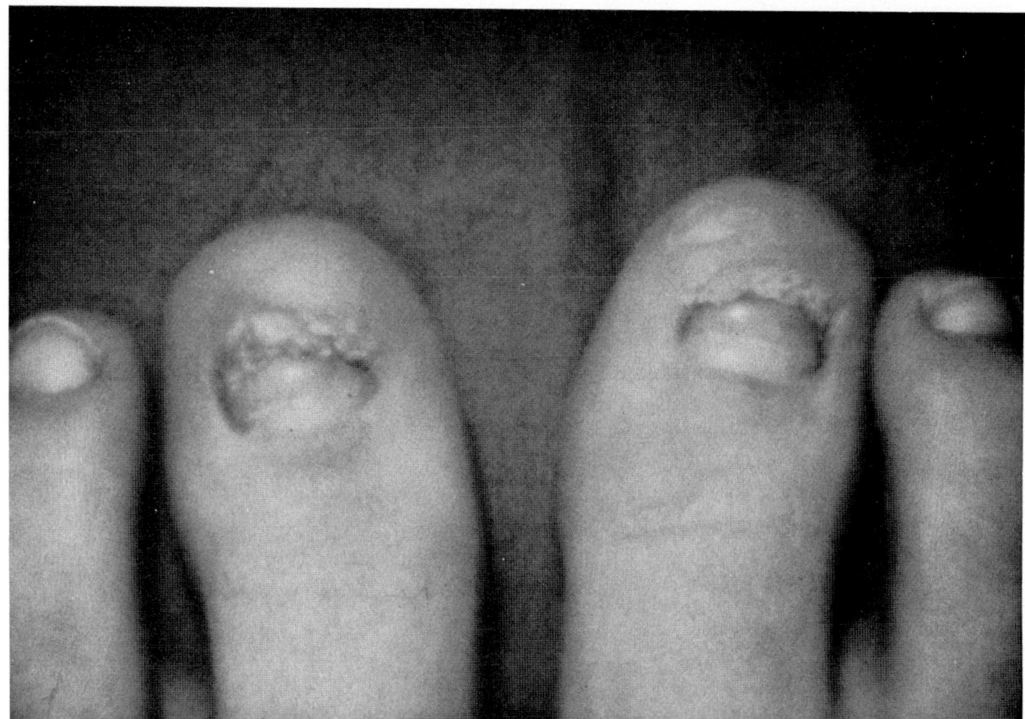

Figure 45.2. Dystrophic nails. Unusual nail formation and loss of nails can be seen with chronic pressure and secondary to frictional forces, such as in ballet dancers and figure skaters.

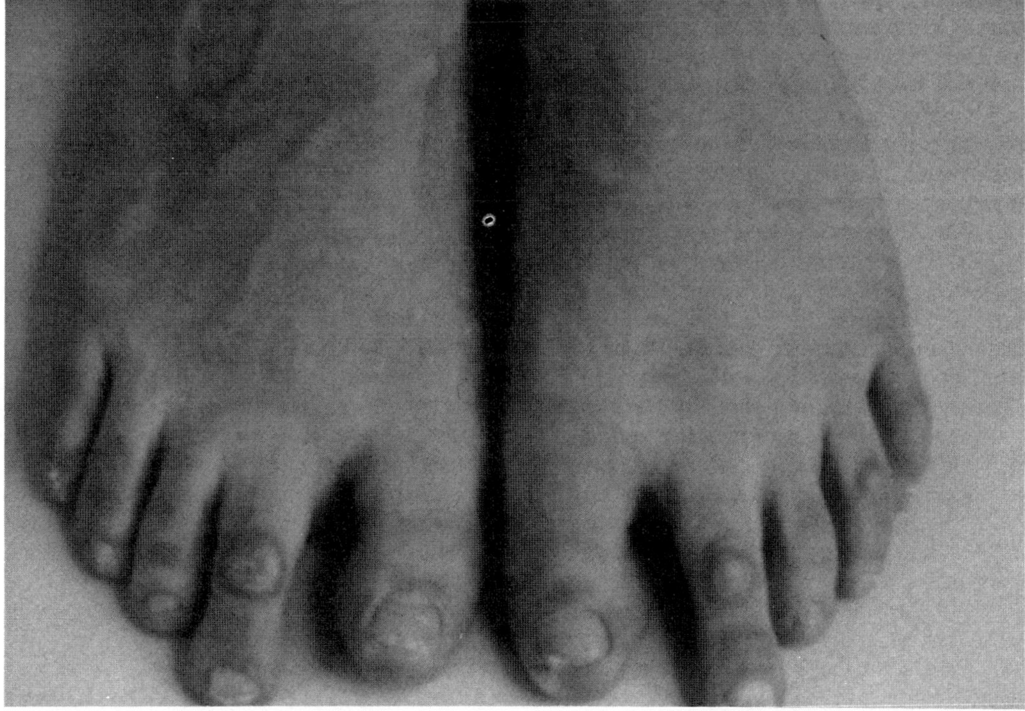

Figure 45.3. Dystrophic nails and calluses. In such sports as ballet and figure skating where both pressure and movement are involved, nail dystrophy as well as callus formation is frequently observed.

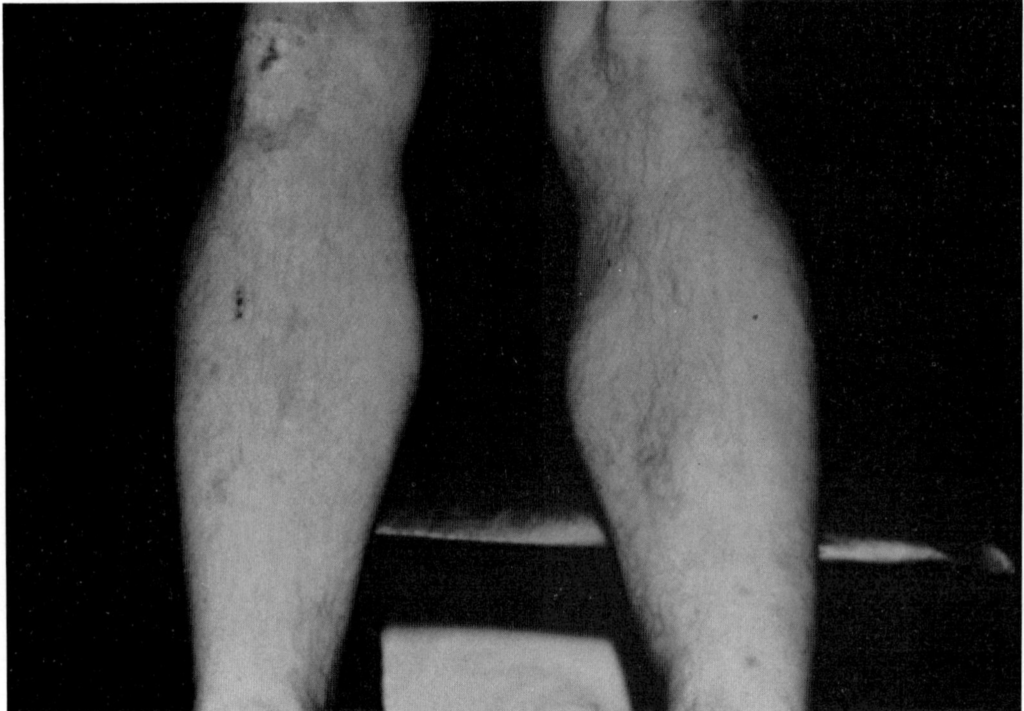

Figure 45.4. Astroturf burns are superficial abrasions or erosions that are secondary to a frictional force on the skin surface.

esterase. These complement tests would define hereditary angioneurotic edema (8, 9).

Treatment of urticaria is best accomplished by elimination of the causative agent. Immediate treatment is directed at reducing skin pruritus and discomfort. Drugs that are commonly used include antihistamines, such as hydroxyzine (Atarax), given in doses of 10 to 50 mg every 4 to 6 hours. Other antihistamines include chlorpheniramine maleate (Chlor-Trimeton) given in doses of 4 to 8 mg every 4 to 8 hours or diphenhydramine hydrochloride (Benadryl) given in doses of 50 to 100 mg every 4 to 6 hours. In addition, epinephrine given as a subcutaneous injection will give the most rapid relief of transient urticaria. Epinephrine is injected as an aqueous USP 1:1,000. The usual dose is 0.3 cc given subcutaneously. The dose should be repeated in 10–15 minutes if necessary.

Antihistamines are given until relief of urticaria or pruritus is obtained and sustained. Treatment periods may range from 1 week to several months (10).

Miliaria, or prickly heat, is often seen in the athlete who is participating in an environment with increased heat and humidity (Fig 45.6). Miliaria refers to a group of cutaneous disorders in which rupture of the sweat duct produces visible raised papules and anhidrosis. Three types of miliaria are recognized: miliaria crystallina in which the sweat duct is occluded within the horny layer of the epidermis; miliaria rubra (prickly heat), which follows obstruction of the duct within the epidermis; and miliaria profunda, a less common variety, resulting from obstruction of the sweat duct deep to the dermal-epidermal junction. Miliaria crystallina presents as the sudden onset of hundreds of small crystal-like, superficial vesicles on the skin surface. The vesicles are generally asymptomatic. Miliaria rubra presents as hundreds of small, itchy, red papules. Often, the patient believes that the lesions represent hundreds of insect bites.

Miliaria is commonly observed in football players who practice during the summer months. Miliaria rubra may occasionally become pustular, especially when they are secondarily infected. The deeper lesions of miliaria profunda are white papular or pustular lesions of 4 to 6 mm in size that clinically are not pruritic. All three types of miliaria can be seen as manifestations of the heat-stress syndromes and are interpreted as cutaneous signs of these syndromes. Compensatory facial hyperhidrosis is a common clinical marker in athletes with extensive miliaria rubra or profunda. There are no laboratory findings or diagnostic tests that are prognostically important. Diagnosis can be made by clinical observation and skin biopsy.

Treatment is mainly aimed at the prevention of miliaria by controlling the humidity and heat of the skin. When miliaria is present, application of topical drying agents and mild topical corticosteroids is helpful. Avoidance of extreme heat and humidity is essential to allow for recovery of the sweat duct occlusion.

Another unusual heat-induced cutaneous disorder is erythema ab igne (11). This is a nonpainful pigmentary change of the skin induced by extreme heat. Clinically, it appears as a reticulated erythema with ultimate hyperpigmentation at the site of heat application. In athletes, this can be seen at the site of hot packs or heating pads and occasionally at the site of electrostimulation. The clinical presentation is diagnostic, and biopsy is

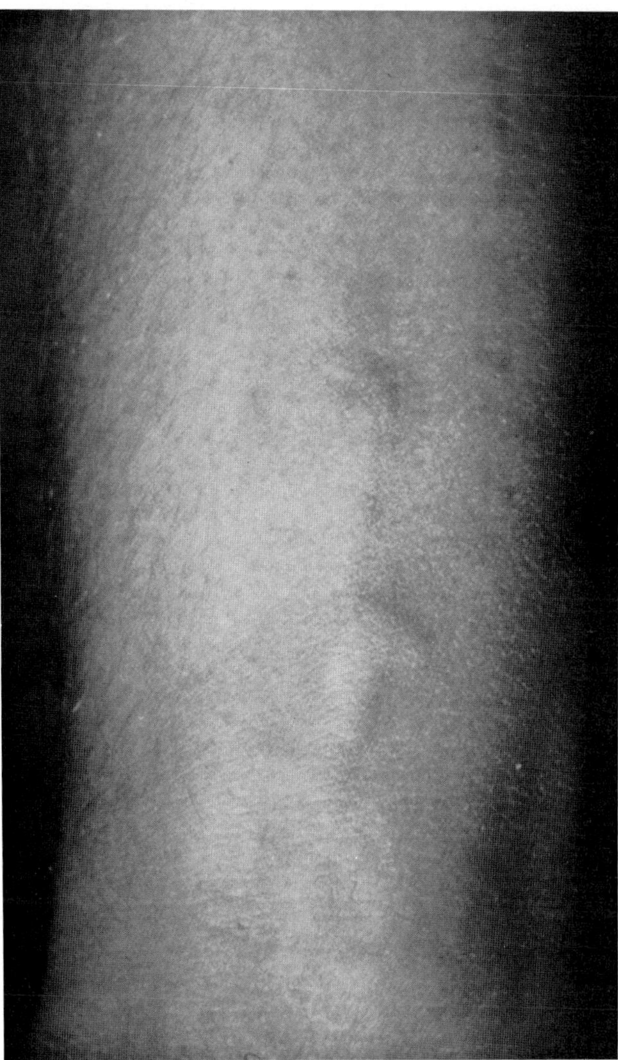

Figure 45.5. Cold urticaria. Urticaria can be induced by physical agents, such as cold, heat, exercise, and ultraviolet light.

unnecessary. Treatment is preventive. Once the pigment tattoo is present, only tincture of time will lighten the skin. Bleaching agents are not helpful.

Sunburns represent a phototoxic reaction of the skin from ultraviolet light. Clinically, sunburn presents as an intense erythema with or without blistering at the site of sun exposure (Fig 45.7). Historically, sunburn reactions have been classified as first degree burns, consisting of mild erythema; second degree burns, consisting of erythema and blister formation; and third degree burns, consisting of erythema, blistering, and ulceration.

The second and third degree burns may induce pigmentary changes as well as superficial scars (12). The ultraviolet light capable of producing a sunburn reaction is the short ultraviolet light ranging from 290 to 320 nm. This ultraviolet light meets the surface of the earth at its greatest intensity between the hours of 10 AM and 3 PM in the northern hemisphere. Factors that influence the intensity of ultraviolet light include cloud coverage and humidity, both of which reduce the short ultraviolet light's penetration to the earth's surface but do not alter the long ultraviolet light. The short ultraviolet light is known to induce skin cancers, whereas the long ultraviolet light alters the collagen and may induce premature aging, wrinkling, and hyper- and hypopigmentation. The long ultraviolet light also has limited capability of inducing sunburn and ultimately tanning; however, it has a greater destructive effect on the dermal collagen. The athlete's response to ultraviolet light is dependent primarily on his or her skin type, time of day and duration of exposure, protective clothing, and the use of sunscreens. Light-colored skin, will need the greatest sun protective agents. Phototoxic reactions to oral drugs such as tetracycline and sulfa resemble sunburns, but are caused by long wave UV light.

Acute sunburn can act as a triggering mechanism for a variety of sun-related disorders, such as herpes sim-

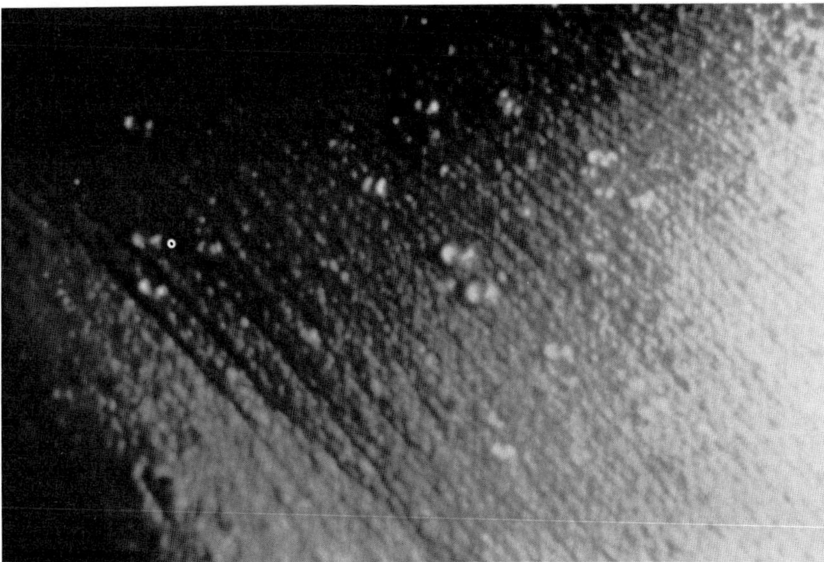

Figure 45.6. Miliaria, or prickly heat, is often seen in athletes who are participating in environments with increased heat and humidity.

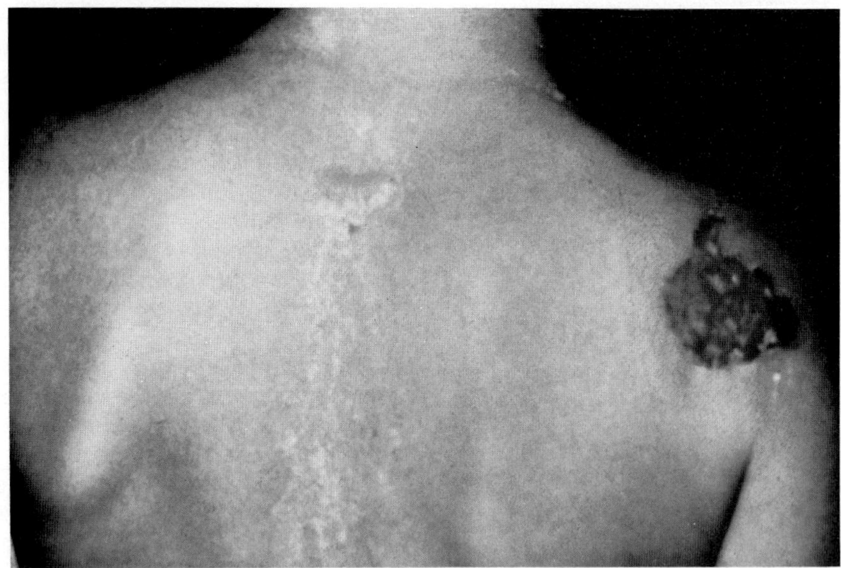

Figure 45.7. Sunburn presents as an intense erythema with or without blisters at the site of sun exposure.

plex, lupus erythematosus, porphyria cutanea tarda, solar urticaria, polymorphous light eruption, vitiligo, telangiectasia, premature aging of the skin, and sunstroke (13).

The treatment of sunburn is directed toward reducing the skin's inflammation and heat. Cool water compresses are effective in reducing skin heat. Topical corticosteroid creams and antiinflammatory agents offer minimal improvement when used 2 to 3 times a day. Oral antiinflammatory medications include aspirin 600 mg 2 times a day, indomethacin (Indocin) 25 mg 3 times a day, and/or oral short courses of corticosteroids. Preventive treatments are multiple and diverse and include protective clothing, topical sunscreens, and careful, short sun exposure to promote tanning rather than sunburn. Aspirin, taken in therapeutic doses 1 to 2 hours prior to sun exposure, will reduce redness. Pretanning has been useful in very sun-sensitive individuals.

Exposure to a hot, humid environment may lead to maceration and intertrigo. Macerated skin is prone to injury. Maceration softens the protective stratum corneum and predisposes to blistering of the skin. Socks should be changed frequently to avoid maceration. Intertrigo results from an overgrowth of bacteria and yeast in intertriginous areas. Lesions of intertrigo are characteristically bright red, moist, and tender. Treatment of intertrigo includes the use of topical antiinflammatory and antiinfective agents. Topical corticosteroids and antifungal preparations may be useful. Broad spectrum antiinfective agents such as phenol and resorcinol are commonly combined in formulas such as Castellani's paint. These agents are generally effective, and they avoid the use of topical corticosteroid agents or creams, which may worsen maceration. Zinc oxide ointment may also be helpful, especially in acutely inflamed lesions, which may be irritated by phenol or resorcinol preparations.

Chemical Injuries

Contact dermatitis in the athlete is secondary to either a cutaneous irritation or allergy. Contact dermatitis appears as an acute or chronic dermatitis at the site of contact of the specific chemical or physical agent. Contact irritant dermatitis is a nonallergic reaction of the skin resulting from exposure to irritating or caustic agents that produce skin damage, ulceration, and ultimately pain. Increased sweating may induce eczematous dermatitis changes on the hockey player's hands (Fig 45.8).

Athletes commonly engage in outdoor activities, which, in North America, is a certain formula for acquiring poison ivy. Rhus—poison ivy, oak, and sumac—is the most common cause of allergic contact dermatitis in North America. Nickel, a ubiquitous metal found in clasps, buckles, and whistles is also a common cause of contact dermatitis in athletes. Rubber compounds found in athletic shoes are a common cause of athletic shoe dermatitis (Fig 45.9) (14, 15). Athletic shoe dermatitis is common and may be debilitating. Patch testing to determine the offending allergen is essential in managing these patients. Once the allergen is identified, athletic shoes free of the offending chemical may be substituted.

Topical medications, which have been used specifically to treat skin disorders, have induced allergic contact dermatitis. Some of these agents include benzocaine, nitrofurazone (Furacin), topical antihistamine preparations, ammoniated mercury, neomycin, penicillin, sulfonamides, tincture of benzoin, and paraminobenzoic acids.

The appearance of both irritant and allergic dermatitis can be either dry, thickened skin or an acute eczematous dermatitis, which commonly produces symptoms of itching or pain.

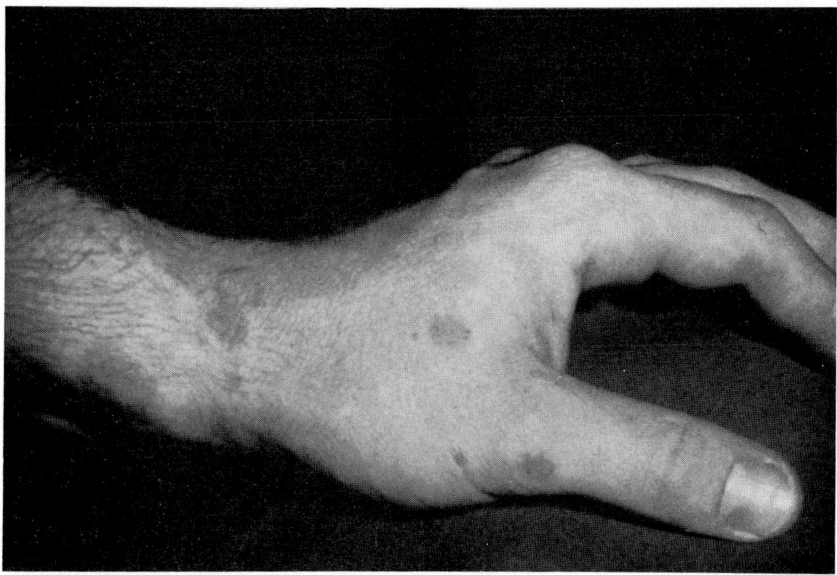

Figure 45.8. Contact irritant. Nummular eczema is observed in hockey players beneath their protective gloves. This is secondary to overhydration of the hand.

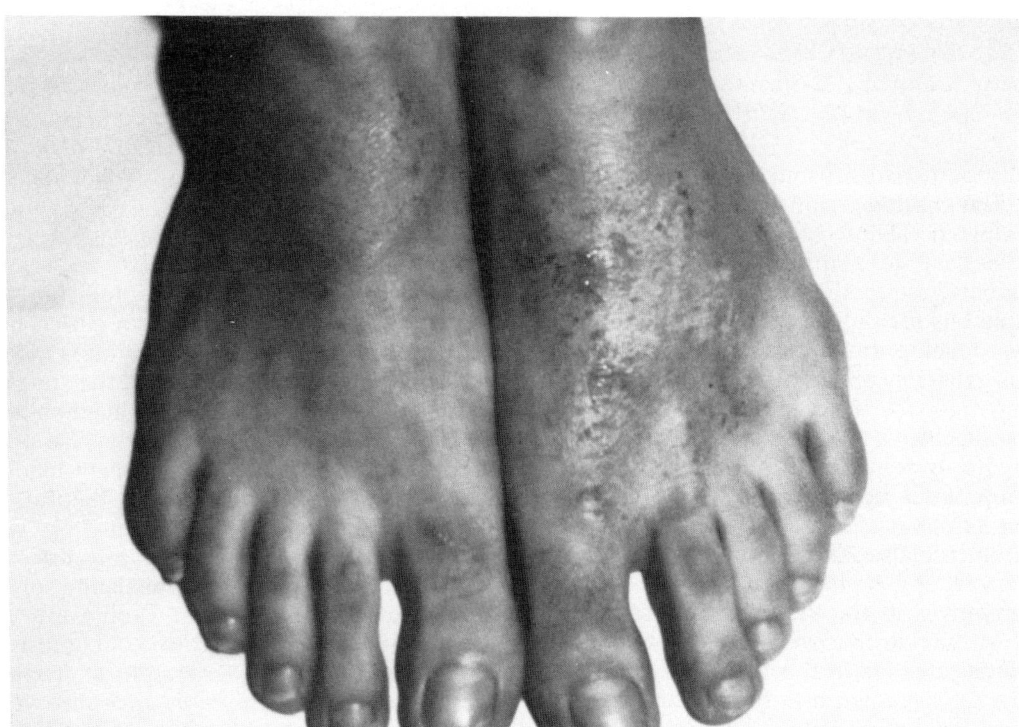

Figure 45.9. Contact allergic dermatitis is due to five major allergens, which include rubber compounds and chromates. Shoe allergic dermatitis is common in basketball players.

The therapy for contact dermatitis is based upon avoidance of the contactant responsible for the skin reaction. The eczematous reactions should be treated with cool compresses or soaks and topical corticosteroid preparations. Systemic antihistamines and aspirin will reduce pruritus. Limited courses of oral corticosteroids may be indicated for a severe dermatitis. The disqualification of an athlete is totally dependent upon the degree of skin involvement and the severity of the cutaneous symptoms and signs.

Infections

Bacterial Infection

Bacterial infections in the athlete may take many forms; however, the most common bacterial infections are impetigo, folliculitis, and furunculosis.

Impetigo is a common disorder seen in athletes, especially those participating in swimming and wrestling (Fig 45.10) (16). Impetigo is caused by the beta-hemolytic streptococci and *Staphylococcus aureus*. Impetigo

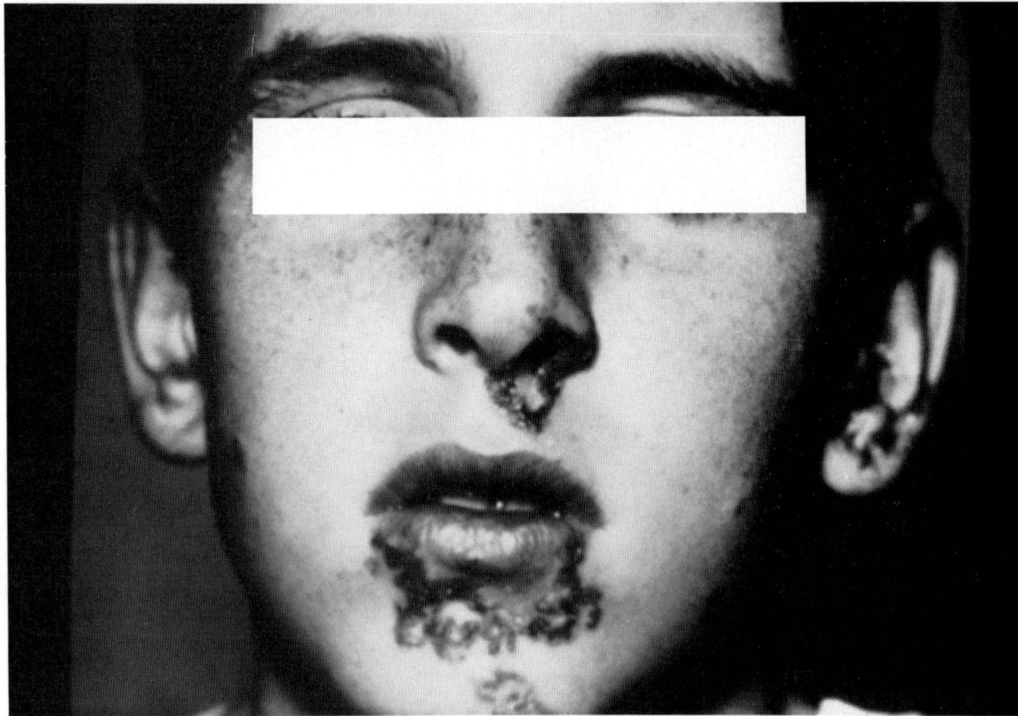

Figure 45.10. Impetigo is a common disorder seen in athletes, especially those participating in swimming and wrestling and is caused by B-hemolytic streptococcal or *Staphylococcus aureus* phase II organisms.

appears clinically as honey-crusted lesions, pustules, and/or blisters. The crusted lesions frequently are secondary to a streptococcal infection, while the blisters formed are secondary to staphylococcal organisms. Younger individuals frequently present with a single blister or multiple blisters on normal skin, while older individuals may develop small vesicular lesions with serosanguineous crust on an erythematous base. The diagnosis of impetigo is suspected clinically and confirmed by bacterial cultures (17). The treatment consists of both topical and systemic medications. The topical treatments include local debridement with soap and water, astringent lotions or alcohol solutions for drying, and topical antimicrobials. Antibiotics are frequently indicated and consist of a cephalosporin, erythromycin or penicillin derivatives in the therapeutic doses for 7 to 10 days (18). Mupirocin (Bactroban) is a new topical antibiotic, which is effective in the treatment of impetigo. The use of a topical agent may be desirable in athletes because this avoids the nausea and diarrhea that may be associated with oral antibiotics.

Athletes with active lesions of impetigo are contagious. They should not participate in contact sports of any kind until all crusts, pustules, and blisters have resolved.

Pseudofolliculitis is a disorder in bearded men, especially those with coarse, curly beards (Fig 45.11). Pseudofolliculitis is primarily a foreign-body reaction to ingrown hairs. Acute lesions are commonly pustular and may suggest an infectious disorder to the attending physician. Secondary infection, especially with *Staphylococcus aureus,* may occur. Gram stain and culture will help to differentiate pustular foreign-body reaction from true infection. Chronic, nonpustular, pseudofolliculitis is not an infectious disorder. The presence of nonpustular lesions should not bar an athlete from competition.

The primary lesion of pseudofolliculitis is an inflammatory papule within which is a curled hair that reenters the skin surface. The condition is most common in black males. Growing a beard is the simplest and most effective treatment for pseudofolliculitis. For those who do not wish to grow a beard, the use of chemical depilatories or specially designed razor blades which prevent overly close shaving can be helpful. Topical corticosteroids will reduce the inflammatory response.

Furunculosis is a bacterial infection secondary to staphylococcal organisms consisting of tender, red, perifollicular swellings that evolve into fluctuant abscesses (18, 16). The diagnosis is confirmed by clinical presentation and bacteria culture. Topical treatment consists of warm compresses and benzoyl peroxide, 5% to 10%, applied 2 to 3 times a day. In addition, oral antibiotics effective against *Staphylococcus aureus* should be given for 10 to 14 days. A semisynthetic penicillin or cephalosporin would be appropriate. If the treatment is initiated early it is not necessary to incise and drain these lesions. Athletes with furunculosis should be disqualified from contact or swimming sports.

Diphtheroid skin infections present as erythrasma or pitted keratolysis. Erythrasma appears predominantly in the intertriginous areas of the body and frequently mimics a tinea infection, such as tinea cruris or pedis. However, this condition is caused by the bacterial diphtheroid, *Cornebacterium minutissimum* (19). Clinically, the infections are erythematous with a fine scale

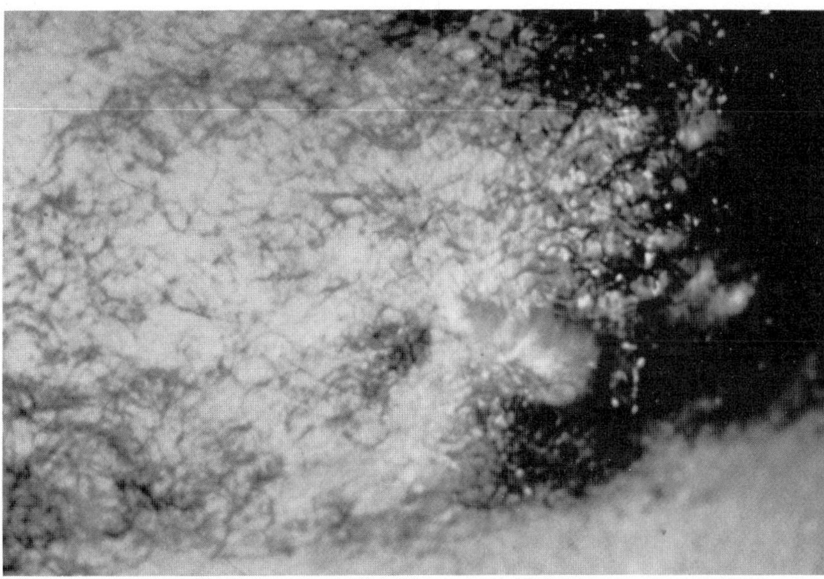

Figure 45.11. Pseudofolliculitis is a common disorder of bearded men, especially those with coarse curly beards, and induces an acneiform-like eruption.

and are well demarcated at their peripheral borders. Potassium hydroxide examination of the scale is negative for fungus. Wood's light examination (black light) reveals a characteristic coral-red fluorescence. Treatment of choice consists of topical debriding agents, topical germicidal agents applied 2 to 3 times a day, and oral antibiotics, such as erythromycin 1 g/day for 7 to 10 days (20).

Pitted keratolysis is also a bacterial infection precipitated by occlusive footwear, exertion, and/or essential hyperhydrosis. Clinically, the palmar or plantar aspects are involved and appear to have dirty peppered pits, especially on weight-bearing areas. The treatment of choice is to decrease localized moisture, which can be accomplished by changing footgear and socks frequently and applying topical drying agents such as aluminum chloride solutions. Oral erythromycin, in the same dosage as for erythrasma, is helpful in reducing the pitted lesions. These pitted keratolyses are most frequently observed in basketball and tennis players.

Fungal Infections

Superficial fungal infections are the most common dermatologic infectious disorders in the athlete. These organisms invade and are nourished by the keratin layer of the skin and hair follicles. With their invasion, cutaneous inflammation may be observed. A vesicular inflammatory dermatitis that accompanies a tinea infection is the hallmark of hypersensitivity to the invading organism. The causative organisms include the genera *Trichophyton, Microsporum, Epidermophyton,* and *Candida.* The clinical presentation of the cutaneous tinea infection is dependent on the site involved. Fungal infections of the hair and scalp are called tinea capitis and tinea barbae. These infections are characterized by patchy hair loss and frequent broken hair fibers. *Trichophyton tonsurans* is a common scalp tinea infection that induces a noninflammatory alopecia. The inflammatory type of alopecia is secondary to tinea organisms primarily belonging to species of *Microsporum.*

Tinea corporis (of the body) of the nonhairbearing skin is characterized by circinate patches with mild cutaneous inflammation with an advancing scaly border. The most common causative organism is *Trichophyton rubrum.* Tinea cruris (of the groin) presents as a scaly, slightly erythematous patch with discrete borders that spares the scrotum (Fig 45.12). The two most common causative organisms are *T. rubrum* and *Trichophyton mentagrophytes.* Tinea pedis (of the feet) presents usually as a dry, scaly, erythematous patchy or vesicular dermatitis and occasionally has a moist erythematous intertrigo. When hands and feet are involved, nail infection (onychomycosis) is common (21).

Candida infections are generally beefy red with superficial erosions and peripheral folliculitis. Candida infections are most commonly observed in intertriginous areas and may involve the perineum and scrotal skin.

Diagnosis of fungal disease is suspected clinically and is confirmed by potassium hydroxide examination of skin scrapings, vesicle tops, or hair shafts and by a fungal culture (22).

The topical treatment of choice involves the use of imidazole products (Micatin, Mycelex, and Lotrimin creams and solutions) applied twice a day for at least 1 month (23, 24). These chemicals are active agents against cutaneous dermatophytes, *Candida,* and tinea versicolor infections. For eroded areas of skin, vital dyes may lend a drying effect. Oral griseofulvin is effective only in dermatophytosis and is ineffective in *Candida* infections. The usual dose of ultramicrosize griseofulvin is 250 mg/B.I.D for at least 1 month or the equivalent. The period required for treatment of onychomycosis is 6 to 12 months due to the extended growth periods of the nailplates.

Tinea versicolor is a mild, occasionally pruritic, chronic

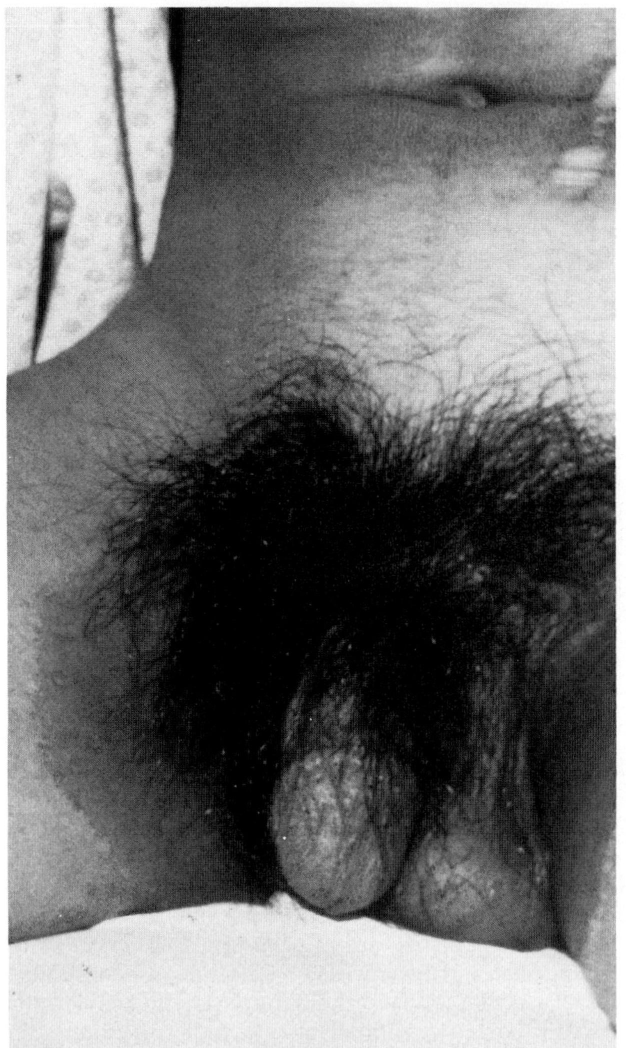

Figure 45.12. Tinea cruris. Tinea infections in the athlete are the most common infection and frequently involve the intertriginous areas of the skin. Tinea cruris is common secondary to dermatophytes or *Candida* organisms.

superficial fungal infection caused by malassezia *furfur*, a dimorphic fungus. Clinically, it is characterized by salmon-pink macules with fine scaling that principally affects the trunk and extremities. Afflicted areas fail to pigment with ultraviolet light exposure and ultimately are paler in color than normal skin. When this color difference is noted, the patient frequently seeks therapy. Diagnosis of tinea versicolor is made by clinical presentation and confirmed by potassium hydroxide examination of skin scrapings. Treatment consists primarily of topical treatment with selenium sulfide 2.5% (Selsun) applied to the skin surface for 6 to 12 hours and rinsed off and then reapplied 1 week later (25). Other antifungal agents may also be used, but, because of the large surface areas to be treated, selenium sulfide is preferred because it is less expensive than other antifungal agents. Oral ketoconazole (Nizoral) is effective in the treatment of tinea versicolor. Nizoral taken orally in a 400 mg dose will result in peak blood levels approximately 1 hour after ingestion. At this time, the athlete is to engage in vigorous exercise that causes the medication to be transferred via sweat to the skin surface. The sweat must be allowed to dry on the skin surface for 1 hour after exercise. This regimen is highly effective; however, it must be emphasized that ketoconazole may result in hepatic toxicity. In general, topical agents such as selenium sulfide are safer.

Viral Infections

Herpes gladiatorum is a cutaneous infection of wrestlers caused by the herpes simplex virus. Large outbreaks of Herpes gladiatorum have been described. Any athlete involved in a contact or swimming sport should be barred from competition until herpetic lesions have healed.

Herpes simplex infections are caused by Herpes simplex virus types I and II. (26–30). Herpetic infections are extremely contagious and are clinically characterized by three states: primary infection, latent phase, and recurrent infection. Primary infections are generally severe and localized and are associated with intense erythema, swelling, vesiculation, and pain. Primary and recurrent lesions have in common the erythema, localized tenderness, or pain that precedes the vesicle formation. Malaise, fever, and a local neuralgia may occur. After the presentation of painful erythema, small 1- to 2-cm vesicles appear on the erythematous base (Fig. 45.13). In later stages, these vesicles ulcerate and may become impetiginized. The usual duration of a herpes simplex infection is 10 to 14 days. These lesions are self-limited and generally resolve without therapy. However, therapy may be employed to alleviate pain and to promote early healing.

Diagnosis is primarily made by clinical inspection and a Tzanck or Papanicolaou smear of the vesicle or vesicle base. The smear demonstrates multinucleated epithelial cells with intranuclear herpetic inclusions. Other more elaborate diagnostic tests include viral tissue culture and neutralizing antibody titers of acute and convalescent sera. The type I and type II infections can be distinguished from one another in viral culture. Type I infections are more commonly associated with extragenital lesions and type II, with genital lesions.

The treatment of herpes simplex infection has been directed at reducing symptoms and hastening healing. The oral antiviral agent acyclovir (Zovirax) is highly effective in the treatment of herpes simplex infections. Long-term suppressive doses may be used to reduce the frequency of recurrence. An alternative method of treatment is to provide the patient with a prescription for a 5-day supply of acyclovir taken in 200 mg doses 5 times daily while awake. The patient will begin the medication at the first sign of a tingling prodrome of herpetic infection. Refills should be given on the prescription so that the patient will always have a supply of medication to begin, on his or her own, at the first sign of prodromal symptoms.

Other medicines employed have included topical agents such as hydrogen peroxide, povidone-iodine (Betadine), chlorhexidine gluconate (Hibiclens), iodoquinol hydrocortisone (Vytone cream), and low po-

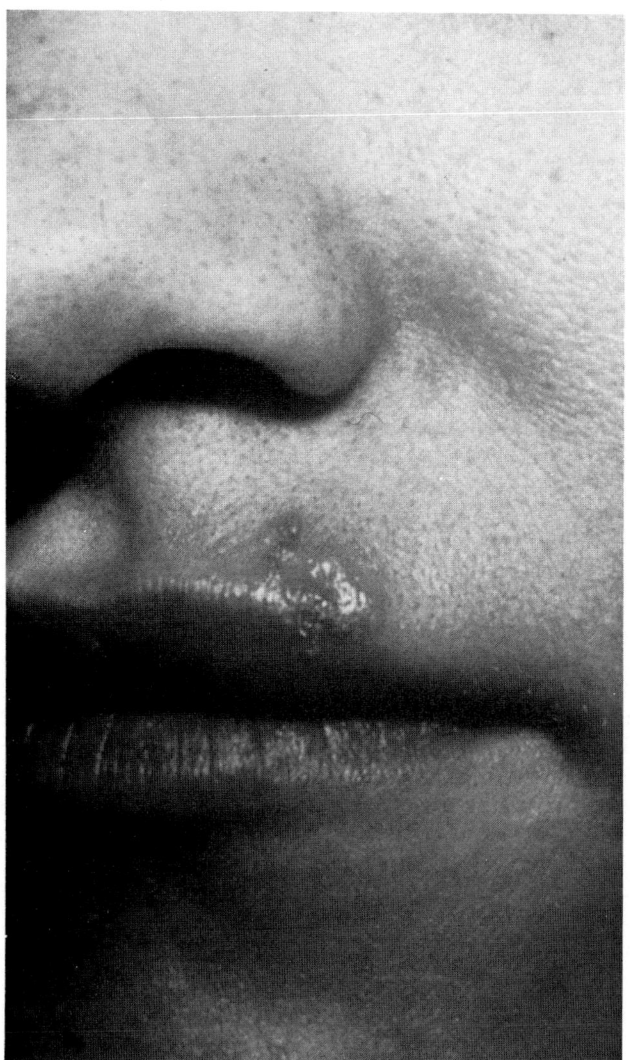

Figure 45.13. Herpes simplex. Various infections are secondary to the herpes simplex type I or type II viruses, which are highly contagious and are disqualifying infections.

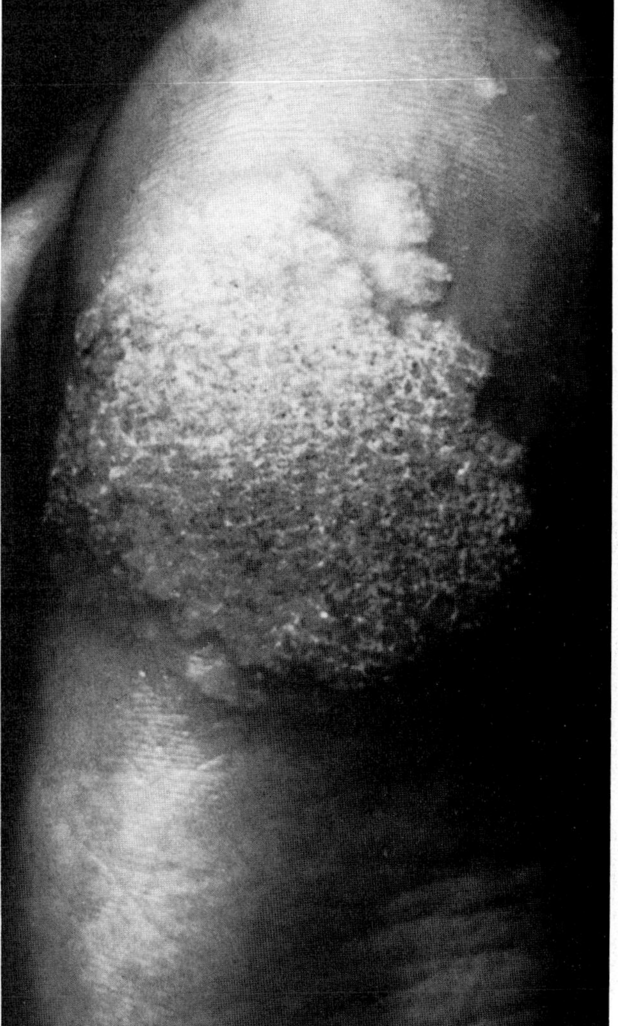

Figure 45.14. Plantar warts are secondary to the papule virus infection of the skin and have an incubation period of 6 months.

tency corticosteroid creams. Antiinflammatory agents are most helpful in the early erythematous stage or in the late crusted stage. They are minimally effective during the blistering or vesicular stage. Oral L-lysine, 1 g/day ad infinitum, has been used, but definitive proof of its efficacy is lacking. Parenteral antiviral agents are not indicated unless the patient has a life-threatening disseminated infection (31, 32).

Warts

Warts are benign viral epithelial tumors that are induced by strains of human papilloma virus. Clinical lesions occur in the skin and mucous membranes and range from 1 mm to large fungating tumors (Fig 45.14). Characteristically, lesions are well circumscribed, firm, and elevated with a verrucous surface. When present on pressure sites such as the feet, lesions become endophytic and may resemble a callus or corn (Fig 45.15). The average incubation period for the wart virus, from contact to development, is approximately 6 months (33). The most acceptable therapies represent tissue-destructive techniques, such as chemical cautery with caustic acids, cryotherapy, liquid nitrogen, and electrodesiccation (2, 34). These forms of therapy should be avoided during the athletic season since they disable the athlete and thus reduce his or her performance. Treatment with topical salicylic acid preparations may be used during the competitive season. These treatments can be palliative, reducing the bulk of a wart which is causing pain and interfering with function. Prolonged treatment with salicylic acid compounds can result in complete resolution of a wart. Sometimes, it is best simply to palliate the wart until after the competitive season because attempts at complete ablation of the wart may result in an ulcer or an erosion that may interfere with competitive athletics. A number of salicylic acid preparations are available, including 40% salicylic acid plasters, and liquid preparations such as Duofilm and Compound W. Excision of warts may be highly effective therapy, but may also result in disability during the competitive sea-

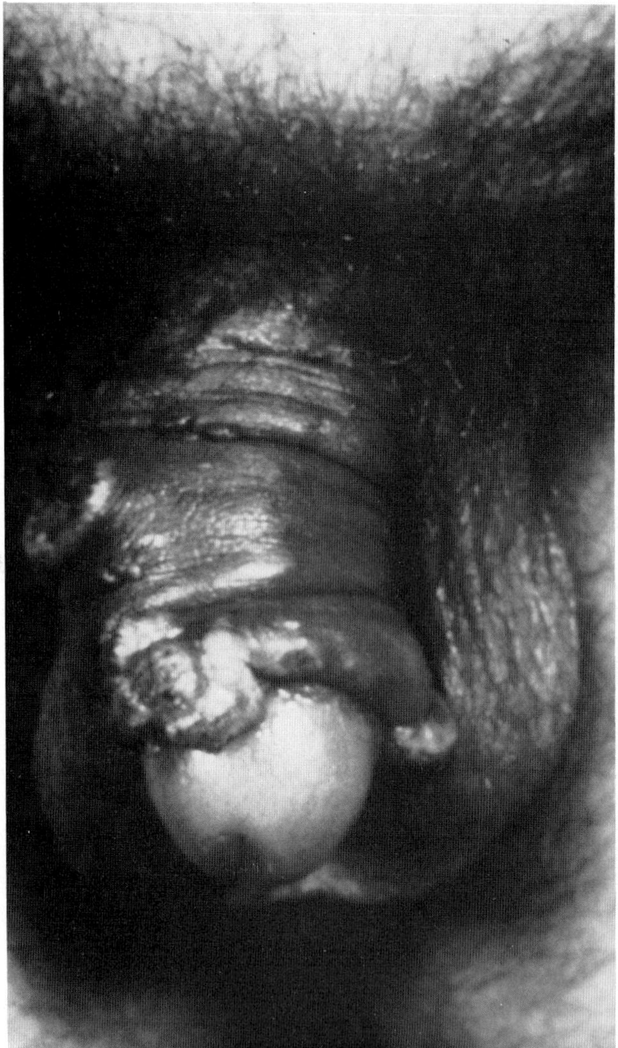

Figure 45.15. Condylomata accuminata is a papilloma virus.

son. Excision of warts on the plantar surface of the foot may occasionally result in a chronically painful scar.

Molluscum Contagiosum

Molluscum contagiosum, another cutaneous viral tumor, is caused by a pox virus. The epithelial tumor can present as a solitary lesion but commonly it appears in multiples and clusters. Clinically, it is characterized as a flesh-colored papule with a central umbilication filled with keratogenous debris and virions. The surrounding skin is essentially noninflamed.

Human Immunodeficiency Virus (HIV) Infections

Unfortunately, HIV infection is no longer uncommon. Questions whether HIV-infected patients should participate in contact sports have already surfaced in the news media. Obviously, active bleeding of an HIV-infected individual poses a risk of contagion. The risk from sweat and saliva is probably minimal and may not be significant. With the present state of knowledge, the authors believe that individual cases should be decided by the sports associations involved, based on expert medical advice. The rights of the HIV-infected athlete must be preserved whenever possible.

Infestations

Scabies

Large groups of people, especially those living in close quarters, are especially susceptible to scabies infestation. Athletes participating in contact sports, especially those with prolonged contact such as wrestling, may be more prone to scabies infestation. Affected individuals usually present with intense pruritus. Web spaces of the fingers areolae, and the glans penis are common sites of involvement (Fig. 45.16). The diagnosis is confirmed by demonstration of an adult mite, eggs, or feces in scrapings from a burrow (Fig. 45.17). In adults, scabies may be transmitted by sexual contact. Physicians are encouraged to examine the patient for signs of other sexually transmitted diseases when the diagnosis of scabies is made.

Permethrin (Elimite), lindane (Kwell), and crotamiton (Eurax) have been used to treat scabies infestation. Of these agents, permethrin appears to be the most active agent. Care must be exercised to treat *all* infected areas, especially web spaces, the umbilicus, and under fingernails. All close physical contacts of an infected patient must be treated. This is critical to prevent further spread of the infestation, especially in group settings such as dormitories.

Lice

The crab louse, *Pthirus pubis,* is mainly transmitted by intimate contact, especially sexual contact (Fig 45.18). Crab lice tend to live on short thick hairs, such as the hairs of the perineum, abdominal wall, legs, axillae, and eyelashes. *P. pubis* is rarely observed in the scalp.

Pediculus capitis, the head louse, commonly affects scalp hairs. Head louse infestation is seldom a sexually transmitted disorder. Pruritus is often the presenting symptom. On close inspection, adult lice or, more commonly, nits are observed on affected hairs. On the scalp, the occipital region and retroauricular regions are the best areas to examine for nits. Treatment of lice may be accomplished with permethrin (Nix), pyrethrins and piperonyl butoxide (RID, A-200), malathion, or lindane (Kwell). Of these agents, permethrin is generally the best tolerated. Nits may be removed with the use of a nit comb. Formic acid preparations (step II) may also be helpful for removing nits. It is essential that individuals with pediculosis be barred from competitive sports until they have been treated and all nits have been removed.

Miscellaneous Disorders

Acne Vulgaris

Acne vulgaris is a common inflammatory disorder observed in adolescent and young athletes (Fig 45.19) (2, 35). The primary lesion is an open or closed comedo resulting from a defect in intrafollicular keratinization and increased sebum production. Secondary inflam-

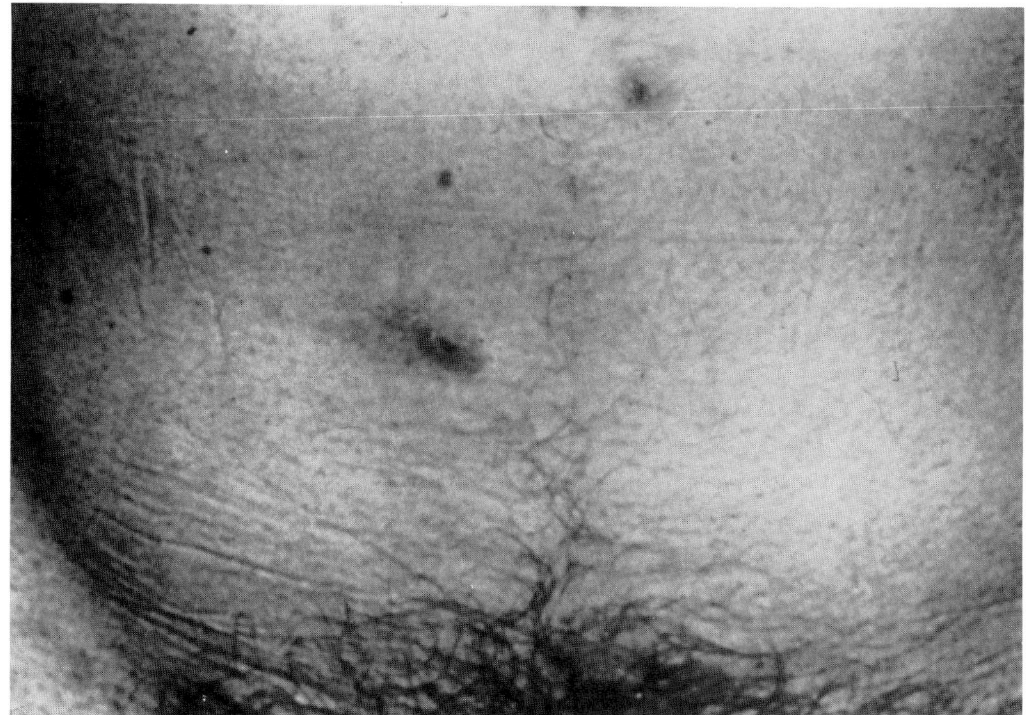

Figure 45.16. Nodular scabies. Human scabies caused by the mite *Sarcoptes scabiei* produces severe pruritus and is highly transmittable.

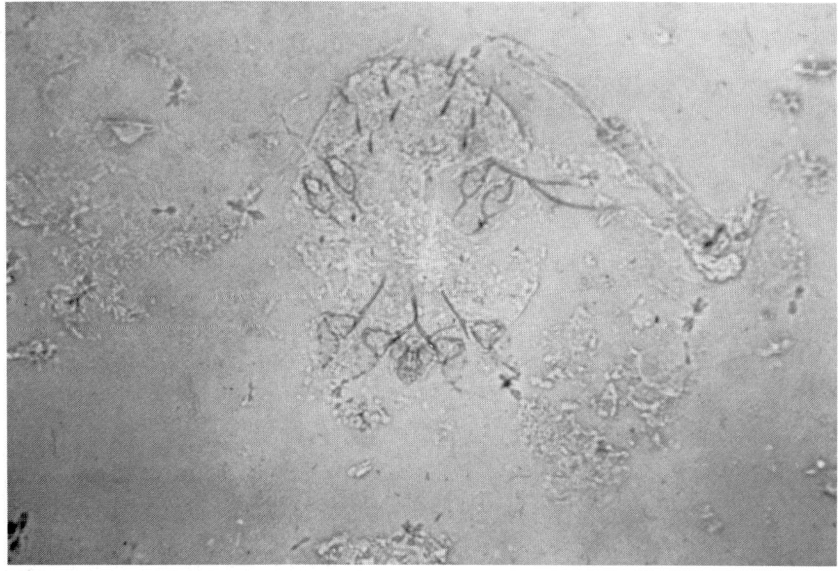

Figure 45.17. Scabetic mite. Skin scrapings from tortuous burrows or nodules demonstrate scabetic mite eggs or feces.

matory lesions, such as papules, pustules, and cysts, are a result of an inflammatory response to sebum, keratin, bacteria, and yeast. These cutaneous lesions are observed at the sites where the sebaceous glands are of greatest density—face, scalp, trunk, and, less commonly, on the extremities. The acne condition can be exacerbated by heat, humidity, mechanical irritation, manipulation, stress, occlusive cosmetics, and certain topical and oral medications.

The treatment of early acne consists of the removal of comedones or the suppression of their formation. Manual extraction of comedones by an experienced person is frequently helpful. The daily use of topical comedolytic agents—especially tretinoin (Retin-A)—is helpful in reducing formation of new comedones. Topical and systemic antibiotics are useful in inflammatory acne because they alter the migration of the inflammatory cells to the acne lesion and reduce the presence of

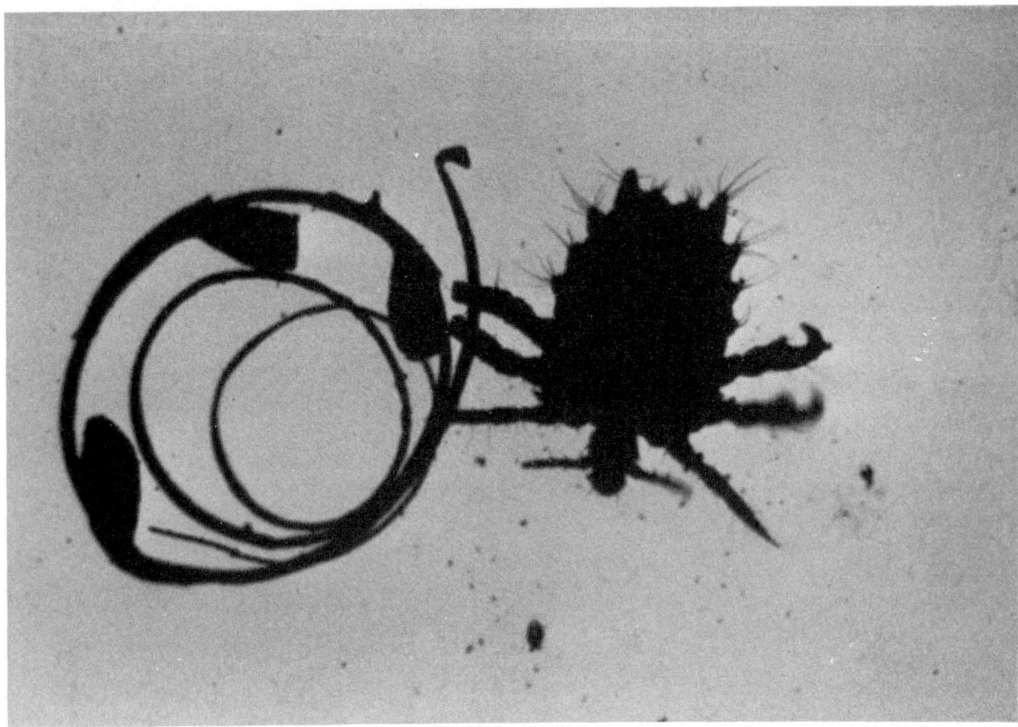

Figure 45.18. The crab louse is one of the most common infestations of athletes.

Figure 45.19. Acne vulgaris is a noninfectious disorder of the hair follicle and sebaceous gland and is worsened by increased heat and humidity.

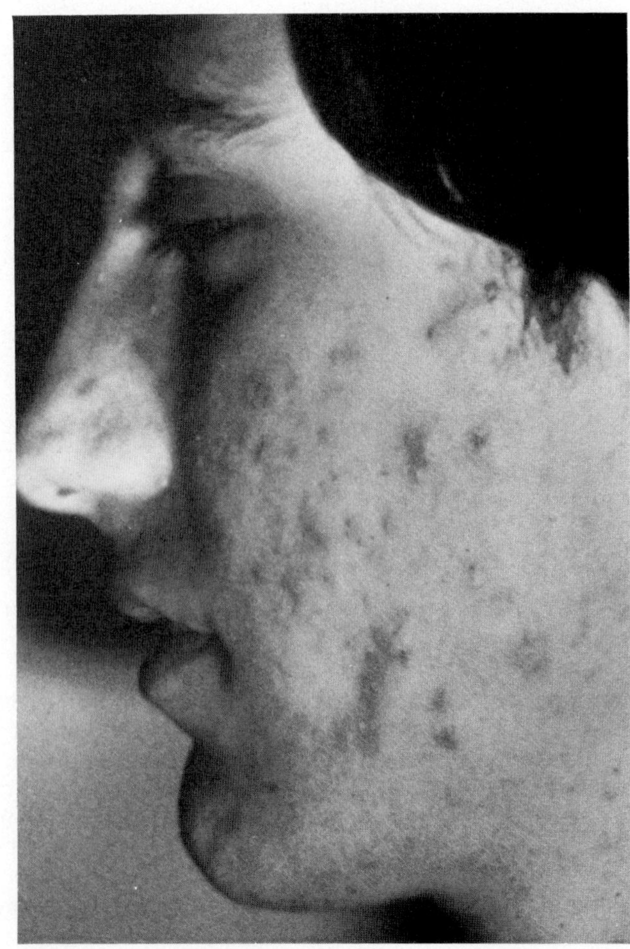

the saprophytic organisms's lipase activity, thereby reducing the formation of short chain fatty acids. Topical antibiotics include tetracycline, erythromycin, and clindamycin in alcoholic suspensions (36). These topical antibiotics are used twice a day and are said to be as effective as 500 mg of parenteral tetracycline. When acne lesions include inflammatory lesions and comedones, treatment may include topical tretinoin (Retin-A Gel or Cream), benzoyl peroxide 5 to 10%, and topical antibiotics. The clearing effect can be appreciated within 4 and 12 weeks. Systemic antibiotics, specifically tetracycline, are most widely used and have a favorable safety profile. Systemic antibiotics are necessary for the management of severe acne vulgaris. Corticosteroids have been used parenterally and as intralesional injections in severe acne patients to reduce the inflammatory papules, pustules, and cysts. This therapy is the last resort and should be used only by experienced physicians. Cyclic estrogen and progesterone therapy in the form of birth control pills can reduce the formation of acneiform lesions in females. Suitable oral contraceptives may include Demulen, Desogen, and Ortho-Cept. The general rule of thumb is that birth control pills should be administered by a gynecologist who will initiate the appropriate safety followups with the patient.

The systemic retinoid 13-*cis*-retinoic acid (Accutane) is a relatively new drug that effectively reduces sebum production and alters abnormal intrafollicular keratinization. Clinical toxicity is related to dosage and includes extreme dryness of skin and mucous membranes, hypertriglyceridemia, liver enzyme abnormalities, and bone and joint pain. The suggested dose is 0.5 to 2 mg/kg/day for a 4-month treatment period. The Food and Drug Administration has recommended Accutane therapy only for severe, recalcitrant cystic acne, and only for the prescribed 4-month treatment period with appropriate rest periods (37). Accutane has been associated with severe birth defects, and is absolutely contraindicated in any female who might become pregnant during or within 1 month after treatment.

Conclusion

This chapter has dealt with the common dermatologic entities seen in the athlete to aid the physician in diagnosis and to outline currently accepted therapies. Skin disorders in athletes are common, and they may interfere with athletic competition. Prompt diagnosis and treatment of these disorders can be of great benefit to the athlete and to his or her athletic performance.

REFERENCES

1. Bart B. Skin problems in athletics (sports medicine, fitness and nutrition corner). Minn Med 1983;66:239.
2. Bergfeld WF. Dermatologic problems in athletes. Symposium on pediatric and adolescent sports medicine. Clin Sports Med 1982;1:419.
3. Freeman MJ, Bergfeld WF. Skin diseases of the football and wrestling participants. Cutis 1977;20:333.
4. Houston SD, Knox JM. Skin problems related to sports and recreational activities. Cutis 1977; 19:487.
5. Muller SA. Dermatologic disorders in athletes. J Ky Med Assoc 1976;74:225.
6. Robinson HM Jr. Skin problems in athletes. Md State Med J 1969;18:81.
7. Seder JI. Treatment of blisters in the running athlete. Arch Podiatr Med Foot Surg 1978;(suppl 29).
8. Akers WA, Naversen DN. Diagnosis of chronic urticaria. Int J Dermatol 1978;17:616.
9. Monroe EW, Jones HE. Urticaria, an updated review. Arch Dermatol 1970;113:80.
10. Speer F, Carrasco LC, Kimura CC. The management of urticaria. Ann Allergy 1978;40:387.
11. Daniels F. Physiologic factors in the skin's reactions to heat and cold. In: Fitzpatrick TB, Eisen AZ, Wolff K, et al., eds. Dermatology in general medicine, 2nd ed. New York: McGraw-Hill 1979;921.
12. Lorincz AL. Physiological and pathological changes in skin from sunburn and sun tan. JAMA 1960;173:1227.
13. Epstein JH. Polymorphous light eruption. Ann Allergy 1966;24:397.
14. Fisher AA. Contact Dermatitis, 3rd ed. Philadelphia: Lea & Febiger, 1986.
15. Pystowsky SD, Allen AM, Smith RW, et al. Allergic contact hypersensitivity to nickel, neomycin, ethylenediamine and benzocaine: relationships between age, sex, history of exposure and reactivity to standard patch tests and use tests in a general population. Arch Dermatol 1979;115:959.
16. Steele RW. Recurrent staphylococcal infection in families. Arch Dermatol 1980;116:189.
17. Leyden JJ, Stewart R, Kligman AM. Experimental infections with group A streptococci in humans. J Invest Dermatol 1980;75:196.
18. Dillon HC Jr. Topical and systemic therapy for pyodermas. Int J Dermatol 1980;19:443.
19. Sarkany I, Taplin D, Blank H. The etiology and treatment of erythrasma. J Invest Dermatol 1961;37:283.
20. Schlappner OLA, Rosenblum GA, Rowden G, et al. Concomitant erythrasma and dermatophytosis of the groin. Br J Dermatol 1979;100:147.
21. Frisk A, Heilborn H, Melen B. Epidermic occurrence of trichophytes among wrestlers. Acta Derm Venereol 1956;46:453.
22. Eaglstein WH, Pariser DM. Office techniques for diagnosing of skin disease. Chicago, Yearbook Medical Publishers, 1978.
23. Borgers M. Mechanism of actions of antifungal drugs, with special reference to the imidazole derivatives. Rev Infect Dis 1980;2:520.
24. Smith EB. New topical agents for dermatophytosis. Cutis 1976;17:54.
25. Catterall MD. Tinea versicolor. In: Maddin S, ed. Current dermatologic therapy. Philadelphia: WB Saunders, 1982;463.
26. Porter PS, Baughman RD. Epidemiology of herpes simplex among wrestlers. JAMA 1965;194:998.
27. Selling B, Kibrick S. An outbreak of herpes simplex among wrestlers (herpes gladiatorum). N Engl J Med 1964;270:979.
28. Shelley WB. Herpetic arthritis associated with disseminate herpes simplex in a wrestler. Br J Dermatol 1980;103:209.
29. Shute P, Jeffries DJ, Maddocks AC. Serum-pox caused by herpes simplex virus. Br Med J 1979;2:1629.
30. Wheeler CE, Cabaniss WH. Epidemic cutaneous herpes simplex in wrestlers (herpes gladiatorum). JAMA 1965;194:145.
31. Jones BR, Coster DJ, Fison PN, et al. Efficacy of acycloguanosine (Wellcome 248U) against herpes simplex corneal ulcers. Lancet 1979;1:243.
32. Spruance SL, Overall JC, Kern ER, et al. The natural history of recurrent herpes simplex labialis: Implications for antiviral therapy. N Engl J Med 1977;297:69.
33. Massing AM, Epstein WL. Natural history of warts: a two year study. Arch Dermatol 1963;87:306.
34. Bender ME, Pass F. Anogenital warts (condylomata acuminata). In: Maddin S, ed. Current dermatologic therapy. Philadelphia: WB Saunders, 1982:483.
35. Farber GA, Burks JW, Hegre AM, et al. Football acne—an acneiform eruption. Cutis 1977;20:356.
36. Thomsen RJ, Stranieri A, Knutson D, et al. Topical clindamycin treatment of acne. Arch Dermatol 1980;116:1031.
37. Peck GL, Olsen TG, Butkus D, et al. Isotretinoin versus placebo in the treatment of cystic acne. J Am Acad Dermatol 1982;6: 735.

46 / SPORTS NEUROLOGY

Lawrence R. Wechsler and Neil A. Busis

Introduction

Sports-related neurologic syndromes are being increasingly recognized and can affect the central or peripheral nervous systems. Some syndromes are directly related to athletic endeavors. Others are common in the general population and occur in nonathletes as well as athletes. Some athletes may have preexisting conditions (e.g., hereditary liability to pressure palsies) that predispose them to specific sports-related neurologic injuries (1). This chapter reviews several topics in sports neurology: headache, seizures, stroke, and peripheral nerve injuries. A monograph on the topic is also available (2).

Headache

Headache is one of most frequent complaints in clinical practice. The most common etiologies include tension or muscle contraction headaches and migraine (Table 46.1). Although muscle injuries occurring during exercise cause head or posterior neck pain, they seldom result in diagnostic confusion. Migraine headaches with or without neurologic accompaniments present a more dramatic picture that alarms both athletes and trainers.

Estimates of migraine prevalence vary from 5% to 30% of the population (3). Common migraine refers to unilateral throbbing headaches accompanied by nausea, vomiting, and photophobia without aura or neurologic accompaniments. Similar headaches preceded by visual disturbances or other neurologic symptoms are called classic migraines. Neurologic accompaniments may occur without headaches or with only minor headache, often raising concerns about cerebrovascular disease or other neurologic conditions. Visual symptoms, including flashing lights, fortification spectra, or wavy lines, are the most common neurologic accompaniments. Numbness or tingling in the face or extremities also occur, but weakness is rare and should prompt a search for other diagnoses. Migrainous visual or sensory disturbances characteristically evolve over 15 to 30 before reaching maximal intensity. This slow buildup or spread is unusual with TIAs or focal seizures and helps identify the process as migraine. Headache usually follows resolution of the neurologic symptoms by minutes to hours.

Posttraumatic Headache

Headaches with characteristics of common or classic migraine may be precipitated by minor head trauma encountered during athletic activities. In some cases, there is a background of similar spontaneous headaches; in others, the headache occurs for the first time during sports. Matthews (4) described headaches following repeated heading maneuvers in soccer players using the term *footballer's migraine.* Neurologic symptoms similar to the aura of classic migraine sometimes preceded the headaches. Repeated head blows in boxing may cause similar headaches. The trauma is usually minor, not resulting in loss of consciousness or significant memory loss. In some cases, headaches recur with repeated injuries in a stereotyped fashion. This type of headache occurs most frequently in children or adolescents but occasionally occurs in adults.

The pathogenesis of headache associated with minor head trauma is uncertain. Vasospasm induced by "jarring" of arteries and spreading depression have been suggested as causes of the neurologic accompaniments associated with posttraumatic migraine (5). Dynamic isotope brain scans within 3 days in eight patients with classic migraine related to head traumas were normal (5). In a few cases, investigations with angiography demonstrated vascular occlusions (6, 7) in cerebral branch vessels suggestive of arterial embolization. This is not a likely mechanism for most cases, because permanent neurologic sequelae would be expected. It is possible individuals with headache or neurologic accompaniments following minor head trauma have a predisposition to migraine. Trauma serves as a triggering mechanism similar to certain foods or stress.

Table 46.1.
Causes of Headache in Athletes

Exertional migraine
Posttraumatic headache
Neck strain with secondary headache
Subarachnoid hemorrhage
Increased intracranial presssure (severe head injury only)

Treatment is problematic because not every head blow precipitates headache. Ergotamine prevented attacks in a soccer player with recurrent headaches (4). Ergots may cause nausea and vomiting and are contraindicated with hepatic or renal dysfunction. Preventive therapy with β-blockers or calcium blockers are indicated only if headaches occur frequently without exercise.

Headache with Exertion

Exertion associated with weight lifting, running, or swimming has been reported to cause headache. Headaches associated with weight lifting begin abruptly and are usually brief (8, 9). An interval of a few minutes to several hours occurred between exertion and onset of headache. Pain recurs with repeated attempts to lift weights, and in some cases, orgasmic migraines or onset with other types of exertion also occurred. Headaches often resolved within 6 months, and full activity levels could resume without further events. Rooke (10) followed patients with exertional headaches and found that 70% became headache free after 10 years. Case reports of exertional headaches were unfortunately often incomplete. Computed tomography (CT) scans of lumbar punctures were not performed to exclude clearly other etiologies for headache. Subarachnoid hemorrhage from a cerebral aneurysm may be preceded by one or several "warning leaks." These are brief severe headaches with abrupt onset, sometimes accompanied by neck stiffness. CT may be negative but lumbar puncture usually reveals blood or xanthochromia. These headaches may resolve within hours, mimicking a migraine. Exertion, particularly activities such as weight lifting, may trigger small leaks and must be distinguished from weight lifter's cephalgia. Following a first such event, a CT and lumbar puncture should be performed if there is a clinical suspicion of a warning leak.

Weight lifters are subject to neck strain, which can also lead to headaches (9). These headaches are typically occipital, although there may be radiation to the frontal region. Headaches have been associated with tight-fitting goggles in swimmers ("goggle migraine") (11). Other athletic activities and equipment also are likely to precipitate migraine in susceptible individuals, and adjustment of an exercise regimen or equipment should be considered when repeated headaches occur.

The mechanism of migraine induced by exercise remains speculative. Hyperventilation and hypocapnia associated with exercise possibly leads to vasoconstriction of the basal cerebral arteries and migrainous auras (12). Vasodilation follows, causing headache by stretching of pain-sensitive fibers in the walls of these vessels (13). Distention of venous sinuses during exercise, particularly straining during weight lifting, has also been proposed (8). As more is learned about the mechanism of migraine, the role of exercise in inducing such headaches will likely be clarified.

Unless headaches occur frequently it is not usually necessary to institute preventive treatment. Indocin prevented headaches in some cases (14), but no large clinical studies have been reported. Other causes of headaches should be considered before concluding that headaches induced by exercise represent migraine. Examination for signs of raised intracranial pressure or focal neurologic signs should be performed. Sinus problems or temporal mandibular joint dysfunction can occasionally mimic migraine. If there is any suspicion of an intracranial process, a CT scan of the head should be obtained. Migraine should be diagnosed when symptoms are typical and all other potential sources of headaches are excluded.

Prognosis

Return to exercise in patients with migraine is limited primarily by the pain induced by specific activity. Once the headaches spontaneously remit or respond to medication, previous levels of exercise can resume. Headaches following minor head injury must be approached more cautiously. Relatively minor head trauma during sports rarely results in rapid development of coma and death caused by cerebral edema (15). A previous recent concussion possibly predisposes to this complication (16). Complete resolution of headache and any postconcussion symptoms such as dizziness, confusion, or headache should be required before returning to sports. If symptoms persist, a CT scan of the head should be performed. Headaches following even minor head injury occasionally signify intracranial hemorrhage or vascular injury such as dissociation of an intracranial or extracranial artery. Examination by an experienced physician is mandatory whenever symptoms become persistent or are out of proportion to the perceived injury.

Seizures

Epilepsy refers to a pattern of recurrent seizures. A single seizure does not necessarily imply a seizure disorder. Most issues in sports concern the safety of individuals with seizure disorders while participating in athletics. Children with seizures are often unnecessarily encouraged not to participate. If seizures are well-controlled and easily identified, most sports can be enjoyed with minimal risk.

Classification

Seizures are divided into partial and generalized seizures (Table 46.2). Partial seizures include focal discharges within the brain, causing localized motor or sensory phenomenon without loss of consciousness. Generalized seizures include grand mal, complex partial or temporal lobe, and petit mal seizures. Loss of consciousness occurs in all generalized seizures. Partial seizures occasionally become secondarily generalized

Table 46.2.
Classification of Seizures

Classification
Partial seizures
Simple partial seizures
Complex partial seizures
Partial seizures with secondary generalization
Generalized seizures
Absence seizures
Myoclonic seizures
Clonic seizures
Tonic seizures
Tonic-clonic seizures
Atonic seizures

(e.g., Jacksonian seizures in which focal motor activity spreads to become a generalized motor seizure).

Grand mal or generalized motor seizures usually begin with a tonic stage with rigidity of all muscles, at times resulting in transient respiratory paralysis and cyanosis. This may be followed by clonic jerking movements of the extremities with return of respirations. Incontinence occurs when motor activity ceases. Consciousness returns initially with confusion and agitation that gradually clears. There is typically amnesia for events during and immediately after the seizure. Muscle aches, headache, tongue soreness and sleepiness frequent sequelae. Seizures are occasionally preceded by an aura consisting of odd smells, sensations, or experiences.

Complex partial seizures also include loss of consciousness but without the generalized motor activity characteristic of grand mal seizures. Lip smacking, repetitive hand movements, or other automatic motor activity are the hallmarks of this seizure type. Again there is amnesia for events during the seizure. Confusion and sleepiness also frequently follow complex partial seizures. Petit mal or absence seizures occur mostly in children and are characterized by brief staring spells with immediate return of full awareness. A sentence may be interrupted by a seizure with continuation of the sentence at the point of interruption when the seizure ends. Several seizure types may occur in a single individual, and a careful history is essential to proper diagnosis and assessment of response to therapy.

Etiology

The most frequent causes of seizures varies with age. Idiopathic seizure disorders usually begin by age 30. Brain tumors, head trauma, and infections predominate between ages 30 and 60. Cerebrovascular disease becomes the most common etiology over age 60. Alcohol or barbiturate withdrawal may cause a single seizure or a series of seizures. Sleep deprivation, stress, or medications can precipitate seizures in susceptible individuals.

Sports and Seizures

Many physicians advise patients with seizures against participation in sports. Transient loss of consciousness may lead to injury, particularly in contact sports such as football or boxing. Sports in which driving is necessary pose an obvious hazard. Exercise decreases absorption of many drugs and reduces hepatic as well as renal clearance (17), potentially altering anticonvulsant levels. No data are available concerning the effects of exercise on the pharmacokinetics of anticonvulsants, thus the clinical significance of these changes is unknown.

Another concern is whether overexertion or injury during sports causes seizures with or without an underlying seizure disorder. Several cases of seizures occurring during strenuous exercise have been reported. Korczyn (18) described 5 patients with seizures during a variety of athletic activities. Seizures recurred later under similar circumstances in some patients and occasionally were unrelated to exertion. A total of 90 other epileptic patients were surveyed, but none suffered seizures during sports, suggesting this is an infrequent phenomenon. Ogunyemi et al. (19) reported 3 patients with seizures related to exertion. EEG recordings while riding a stationary bike demonstrated epileptiform discharges not seen at rest or during hyperventilation (19). In a similar study, Goetze et al. (20) recorded EEG in 30 patients with epilepsy while they performed deep knee bends. Seizure discharges diminished during exercise, in contrast to the previous study, suggesting an increase in seizure threshold during exercise and a decrease in the likelihood of clinical seizure activity. No information regarding the relationship of seizures to physical activity is included for these patients. Animal models also suggest exercise might reduce the probability of seizures. Stress lowers seizure thresholds, possibly by release of endogenous epinephrine (21). Stress factors were associated with seizures in only 37 of 1250 patients surveyed by Friis and Lund (22). The most common factors were sleep deprivation and emotional stress, although overexertion was reported in 16. In most cases there were multiple stressful influences.

Data regarding effects of exercise on seizure threshold are conflicting. Seizure thresholds may increase or decrease in different individuals. Clinical data indicate seizures precipitated by physical activity rarely occur, and it would seem unfair to prohibit all patients with seizures from sports. Accident rates during physical activity are no different for epileptics than nonepileptics (23) and minor head injuries likely to be encountered during sports do not increase the likelihood of seizures in susceptible individuals (24). Epilepsy often accompanies physical and cognitive deficits that preclude most athletic endeavors. Those patients with well-controlled seizures and the ability and desire to engage in sports should be encouraged to participate.

Treatment

Anticonvulsant therapy should be administered whenever recurrent seizures occur. Treatment of a single, unprovoked seizure is controversial. Some physicians advocate observation rather than immediate treatment, because seizures recur in only 20% to 70% of patients (25, 26). The decision to treat can be further complicated by the desire to participate in athletics. Sports predisposing to minor head trauma, such as football, or activities with potential danger should a seizure occur, such as swimming, might favor treatment to avoid the risk of recurrent seizures in those settings. Dilantin or Tegretol is usually the initial choice for anticonvulsant treatment. Both potentially cause sedation or cognitive impairment when given in therapeutic doses. Careful gum hygiene is important when taking Dilantin, because of the possibility of gum hypertrophy, particularly in children. Zarontin is used as a first-line agent to control petit mal seizures. In most cases, a single drug adequately controls seizures, regardless of type. If there is any question that seizures are continuing despite treatment, contact sports, swimming, and other activities in which brief loss of consciousness could lead to injury, should be avoided.

Stroke

Only 3% of strokes occur before the age of 40. The incidence of stroke in the young adult population has been estimated at 25/100,000. Even fewer occur in otherwise healthy individuals engaging in vigorous sports. Atherosclerosis occurs less frequently in this age group, but accounts for 20% of all strokes (27). Embolism, primarily from cardiac sources, and hypercoagulable states cause much of the remainder. Arterial disorders, including vasculitis and dissection, are rare but important etiologies, as specific therapy is required.

Most strokes in young individuals are unrelated to physical activity. Sedentary lifestyle predisposes to stroke, and physical stress has not been identified as a risk factor. Physical activity, however, occasionally triggers a cardiac or vascular process that results in cerebral ischemia. Because these strokes are rare in comparison with more common stroke types, a statistical association would not be identified. Dissection of the major cerebral vessels, cardiac arrhythmias, and paradoxical embolism may be precipitated by vigorous physical activity and should be considered when a stroke occurs in this setting.

Carotid Dissection

Dissection of the cerebral vessels results from blunt trauma to the neck but also occurs with minor or seemingly insignificant trauma. In some cases, no definite injury is identified. Carotid artery dissection has been reported in association with a variety of sports, including jogging (28), football, tennis, basketball, volleyball, skiing, and bowling (29). The extracranial carotid artery becomes compressed against the transverse process of the cervical vertebra with neck extension and rotation, possibly tearing the wall of the vessel (29). Underlying vascular pathology such as fibromuscular dysplasia or cystic medial necrosis predisposes to dissection with minor trauma. Dissection into the adventitia or media creates a false lumen and expands the size of the vessel. Subintimal dissection narrows the true lumen and may lead to carotid occlusion. Although expansion of the artery with compression of adjacent structures causes a variety of symptoms, the most serious consequence of dissection is vascular occlusion. Reduction of perfusion in the ipsilateral hemisphere may lead to stroke when collaterals are inadequate. In addition, thrombus forming at the site of recent occlusion may fragment and result in embolic occlusion in the intracranial vessels. In one population-based study of young adults, dissection accounted for 4% of all strokes (27).

The most common symptoms of carotid dissection include ipsilateral headache or neck pain, Horner's syndrome, visual scintillations, self-audible bruit, and dysgeusia (30). Head pain is typically around the eye or in the temple ipsilateral to the dissection (30). Angiography demonstrates narrowing of the vessel, extending from several centimeters beyond the carotid bifurcation to the base of the skull (31). This contrasts to the typical site of atherosclerotic narrowing within the first 3 cm of the internal carotid artery. The other common site of carotid dissection is in the upper cervical region at the level of C1–C2. Bilateral or multiple dissections occur occasionally and are usually associated with fibromuscular dysplasia (32).

Symptoms of head or neck pain typically follow a sudden twist or extension of the neck. Examination reveals signs of a Horner's syndrome including ptosis and meiosis. The hypoglossal nerve may be compressed causing ipsilateral tongue weakness (33). Amaurosis fugax or sudden stroke often follows the injury by one or several days. Recognition of the early signs of dissection is critical, because institution of appropriate therapy may prevent subsequent stroke. Anticoagulation with heparin is usually administered initially, and Coumadin is given for long-term treatment. Although worsening of dissection with anticoagulation seems plausible, this has not been observed in practice. The optimal duration of treatment for dissection has not been established, but in some cases stenotic vessel recanalizes, eliminating the need for continuing anticoagulation. Surgical intervention to remove occluding thrombus may be considered within the first few hours after dissection, but it is unclear whether the risk of this procedure is warranted and whether outcome is improved when compared with medical management. Athletic activities can be resumed after recanalization of dissection or after an occluded vessel has been allowed sufficient time to ensure organization of intravascular thrombus. If angiography demonstrates evidence of fibromuscular dysplasia or other vascular anomalies predisposing to additional dissections, strenuous sports, particularly those involving sudden head and neck movements, should be avoided.

Vertebral Dissection

Dissection also occurs in the vertebral and basilar arteries. The cervical or intracranial segment of the vertebral artery may be involved. Adventitial dissection in the intracranial segment causes subarachnoid hemorrhage in addition to the typical symptoms of dissection. Pain from vertebral dissection most frequently localizes in the posterior neck or behind the ear. Vertigo, diplopia, and other symptoms of vertebral-basilar ischemia may occur at the onset of dissection or within the next several days. Basilar artery dissection is rare. Pain is usually suboccipital and clinical syndromes correspond to the distribution of ischemia in the basilar artery territory. This often occurs in young individuals and in males more frequently than females (34).

Chiropractic manipulation has been associated with vertebral dissection (35), but other types of neck manipulation may also cause vessel injury. Vertebral dissection has been reported with yoga (36), gymnastics (37), archery (38), and swimming (39). Other sports involving sudden turning of the neck would likely also potentially lead to dissection. Fibromuscular dysplasia or cystic medial necrosis are found in some but not all patients. Sudden neck rotation causes stretching of the vertebral artery and sometimes mechanical injury. The most common site of dissection is between C1 and C2 (40). The mechanism of intracranial vertebral or basilar artery dissection is unknown.

Anticoagulation is usually begun if the vessel is severely stenotic or occluded to prevent extension of thrombus or distal embolization. Subarachnoid hemorrhage must be excluded in cases of intracranial vertebral dissection before initiating anticoagulation.

Cardiac Arrhythmias

In a large stroke data bank study, cardioembolic stroke accounted for approximately 19% of all ischemic strokes (41). Atrial fibrillation is an important risk factor for stroke and 15% of all strokes are associated with atrial fibrillation (42). Stroke occurs with increased frequency in patients with atrial fibrillation regardless of etiology (43). However, young patients with atrial fibrillation and no clinical heart disease may represent a subgroup with low stroke risk (44, 45). Atrial fibrillation is occasionally found in otherwise healthy athletes (46). Whether transient fibrillation in a healthy individual without heart disease explains some cases of cerebral embolization associated with exercise is unknown.

Paradoxical Embolus

Atrial or ventricular septal defects predispose to right-to-left shunts and possible paradoxical emboli causing stroke. Contrast echocardiography in one study demonstrated a potentially patent foramen ovale in 40% of patients with stroke of unclear etiology (47). In addition to a communication between the right and left heart, right heart pressures must be elevated before a paradoxical embolus occurs. There also must be a source of venous thrombus such as deep-vein thrombosis. Pulmonary hypertension or multiple pulmonary emboli increase right heart pressures, but this would not likely occur in an individual well enough to participate in sports. Valsalva acutely raises right heart pressures and may transiently open a potentially patent foramen ovale allowing right-to-left shunting. Exercise or exertion involving Valsalva in predisposed individuals creates circumstances favoring paradoxical embolization and possibly stroke. The frequency of such events is unknown, but in most patients with stroke associated with exercise contrast echocardiography is not performed. This mechanism should be considered and investigated whenever stroke occurs at the time of strenuous physical activity.

Drug Abuse

Substance abuse has become increasingly frequent among athletes. Some agents such as steroids may lead to a hypercoagulable state (48) and predispose to stroke. Amphetamines cause subarachnoid and intracerebral hemorrhages. Angiography and pathologic studies often show evidence of cerebral vasculitis (49). Although some reports emphasized intravenous administration as the major risk for stroke, many cases are associated with oral amphetamines (47). Cocaine has been associated with stroke, although a definite cause-and-effect relationship has not been convincingly established (50). A careful history of drug use should be elicited in any young patient with stroke, including those occurring during sports.

Peripheral Nerve Injuries

Overview

The peripheral nerves of athletes can sustain several types of injury. Trauma can be macroscopic or microscopic, with remodeling of connective tissues near the nerve or direct nerve damage caused by repetitive stresses (51). Pressure, stretch, angulation, and friction all play a role. Nerves can be exposed to brief periods of high pressure or chronically to lower pressures. Nerves and their blood supply can be compressed in tight fibrous or fibroosseous passageways, by anomalous or hypertrophied muscle, soft tissue swelling, scar tissue, tumor, or orthopedic deformity. Stretch can result from anatomic deformity such as occurs in displaced fractures. The nerve axon, myelin sheath, connective tissue sheath, or various combinations of these tissues can be damaged. Nerve injuries can be classified according to the type of anatomical structures that are involved (52, 53).

Neurapraxia is focal demyelination without axonal damage. It is the result of relatively blunt trauma or compression. Demyelination leads to segmental conduction block, which leads to weakness and sensory loss. A lesser degree of demyelination leads to segmental conduction slowing, which is useful diagnostically on neurophysiologic studies but may not be clinically significant. Recovery occurs following remyelination, a process that takes several weeks to a few months.

Axonotmesis is axonal interruption with preservation of the connective tissue sheath around the peripheral nerve. The distal nerve stump undergoes Wallerian degeneration over the first 3 to 5 days after the injury, then the proximal axonal stump attempts to regenerate. Axons can regenerate at a rate of about 1 mm per day or 1 inch per month. The preserved connective tissue sheath acts as a guide for axonal regeneration and reinnervation. However, recovery is not always predictable.

Neurotmesis is interruption of axons and the endoneurial connective tissue sheath. More severe types of neurotmesis are associated with interruption of perineurium or perineurium and epineurium (transection of the nerve trunk). Reanastomosis of the connective tissue sheath is necessary if regeneration is to occur. Traumatic neuromas can form at the proximal stump that can impede further axonal growth and become spontaneously electrically active, causing pain. Aberrant regeneration can occur, causing synkinetic movements.

Peripheral nerves are subdivided into fascicles, each containing many individual axons. In many nerve injuries, different fascicles sustain different degrees of damage to axons and myelin and connective tissue sheathes. Recovery from these mixed nerve injuries is biphasic, with the early phase of recovery caused by remyelination and the later phase, the result of axonal regrowth. Diagnosis of focal sports-related neuropathies depends on an accurate history, physical examination, and often on electromyography (EMG) and nerve conduction studies and imaging procedures.

Injuries to nerve roots, plexuses, and individual nerves or their branches cause specific patterns of motor and sensory alteration, pain, reflex change, and sometimes autonomic dysfunction. Motor and sensory symptoms can be caused by over- or underactivity of motor and sensory axons. These symptoms are termed *positive* and *negative* respectively. Positive motor symptoms are cramps, fasciculations, and other types of abnormal motor activity. Negative motor symptoms are weakness and wasting. Positive sensory symptoms are paresthesias such as pins and needles or tingling feelings, or pain. Tinel's sign refers to the paresthetic feeling elicited by tapping over the site of an injured nerve. Negative sensory symptoms are sensory loss to one or more modalities.

EMG and nerve conduction studies are often of critical importance in diagnosing peripheral nerve injuries in athletes (54). These studies may confirm the clinical diagnosis and determine its pathophysiology, severity, and perhaps its prognosis. At times a neurologic problem different from that initially suspected will be revealed, and at other times, a negative examination will help diagnose a soft tissue injury without neurologic involvement.

There are certain limitations to EMG and nerve conduction studies that must be recognized to interpret the results correctly. These studies can potentially distinguish between nerve injuries caused by segmental demyelination and those caused by axonal interruption, but timing of the studies is crucial. As discussed above, Wallerian degeneration of axons takes at least 3 to 5 days to occur. Denervated muscles first develop fibrillation potentials and positive sharp waves (the EMG hallmarks of denervation) within 10 to 14 days. Thus, after an acute nerve injury, the full range of pathologic findings will generally be present only if the EMG and nerve conduction studies are performed 3 to 5 weeks after the injury. Timing of EMG and nerve conduction studies is less critical in the diagnosis of a chronic process. Only surgical exploration of the nerve can determine the integrity of the connective tissue sheath.

Nerve conduction studies primarily measure the number and conduction velocity of the large-diameter, fastest-conducting sensory and motor fibers. Syndromes in which the symptoms are predominantly the result of positive phenomena (e.g., pain); in which the symptoms are caused by intermittent, reversible impingement of nerve fibers (especially those with mainly sensory involvement); or in which small-diameter fibers are preferentially affected may be associated with normal nerve conduction studies. EMG and nerve conduction studies are most likely to be abnormal in subacute syndromes (3 weeks to 6 months) in which weakness is present.

In neurapractic lesions, the demyelinated segment may be quite short. Focal conduction slowing, an electrodiagnostic hallmark of neurapractic lesions, may not be detected if only long segments of the affected nerve are studied. Sometimes only the "inching technique" in which 1- to 2-cm-long segments of a given nerve are studied serially will reveal the conduction slowing.

Although a majority of focal sports-related nerve injuries involve the shoulder girdle, routine median and ulnar motor and sensory nerve conduction studies do not adequately assess the cervical roots and brachial plexus. Additional, less commonly studied nerves should be assessed if the examination is to be maximally helpful. Furthermore, many of the important shoulder girdle muscles are difficult to study because they overlie one another, and it is difficult to activate them selectively.

The presence of a severe peripheral nerve lesion may mask another, more proximal, one. For example, a patient with a severe brachial plexopathy may also have coexistent cervical radiculopathy that would not necessarily be detectable electrophysiologically.

There are relatively little data on the usefulness of preoperative EMG and nerve conduction studies in predicting prognosis after surgery, and there is often poor correlation between the degree of clinical and electrophysiologic recovery after surgery. In particular, there can be persistence of EMG and nerve conduction abnormalities postoperatively, even when there has been marked clinical improvement. This observation complicates the interpretation of abnormal EMG and nerve conduction studies found in a patient in which surgery, such as carpal tunnel release, did not lead to the expected improvement.

Treatment options for focal neuropathies include both nonsurgical and surgical approaches. In general, conservative nonsurgical measures such as rest, splinting, recognition, and amelioration of provocative factors as well as nonsteroidal antiinflammatory drugs (NSAIDs) are tried first. Local anesthetic or steroid injections can be useful in certain situations. If symptoms and signs persist and are severe, surgical treatment may be indicated. Surgical approaches usually involve decompression of the nerve by removing those anatomic structures thought to be responsible for the entrapment. Sometimes the nerve itself is moved to another location. Because scarring of the nerve trunk itself can cause persistent entrapment, epineurectomy or epineurotomy is sometimes indicated. The utility of extensive internal neurolysis, in which individual nerve fascicles are decompressed, is more controversial.

Well-defined and easily diagnosed disorders such as carpal tunnel syndrome are often treated quite successfully by nonsurgical or surgical approaches, depending on the severity of the lesion. Less well-defined or controversial syndromes, such as resistant tennis elbow, carry a less optimistic prognosis. A detailed discussion of the treatment of each of the focal neuropathies reviewed below is beyond the scope of this chapter.

Excellent reviews of the etiologies, clinical presentation, evaluation, differential diagnosis, and treatment of entrapment neuropathies have been published (55, 56). Much of the material presented below is discussed in greater detail in these publications.

Specific sports-related peripheral nerve injuries are reviewed in the following sections and have also been reviewed recently (2). Much of the data come from individual case reports, several of which are not detailed. Some of the "focal neuropathies" in the sports neurology literature may really represent other entities. For example, some of the reported mononeuropathies about the shoulder girdle may actually be the result of idiopathic brachial plexus neuropathy, a well-described condition in the general population (67).

Cervical Radiculopathy and Brachial Plexopathy

The "stinger" or "burner" is a common syndrome affecting football players (54, 55). After a tackle or similar types of hard jolts in which the ipsilateral shoulder is depressed or the head is deviated back or toward the contralateral shoulder, the player develops stinging or burning pain in the arm, which can radiate from shoulder to hand, and arm weakness. The pain subsides in seconds and the weakness resolves in minutes. Repeated episodes may lead to more prolonged weakness. Usually, the arm weakness is nonsegmental, although if it persists, shoulder abductors and external rotators and forearm flexors are involved. Sensory dysfunction also is not usually dermatomal. Lateral flexion of the neck to the painful side is usually limited and may reproduce the sensory symptoms.

The site of pathology underlying the stinger is not certain. EMG and nerve conduction studies have variable results. Some suggest cervical radiculopathy (58), but others suggest brachial plexopathy (59, 60). Some patients who suffered from the syndrome underwent cervical laminectomy and had scarred C5 and C6 nerve roots at the point where they emerge from the vertebrae (61).

Repeated occurrences may result from chronic instability caused by ligamentous or facet laxity in the cervical spine or fibrosis with edema around the nerve roots. The patient should forego athletic participation until symptoms and signs have resolved. Preventive measures include a cervical collar, possibly raising the shoulder pads, and neck-strengthening exercises.

Acute trauma can cause severe brachial plexopathy in football, bicycle and dirt bike accidents, snow-related sports, equestrian sports, and water-related sports. Some patients may require operative intervention (62). Brachial plexopathy as a late complication of clavicular fracture in a football player has been reported, which was caused by callus formation (63). However, brachial plexopathy coming on acutely, without specific inciting trauma or long after acute trauma, is probably acute brachial plexus neuropathy, as mentioned above (57).

Cervical radiculopathies must be distinguished from brachial plexus injuries. Although there can be differences in history and examination findings in these entities, neuroimaging studies and EMG and nerve conduction studies (64) are often crucial for differentiation.

Specific Nerve Injuries

Spinal Accessory Nerve

The spinal accessory nerve may be injured by local trauma in stick-handling, sports such as hockey and lacrosse, or stretch of the supraclavicular area during exercise (65). Symptoms consist of shoulder aching and difficulty lifting the arm. On examination, there is scapular winging when the arm is abducted to the side and there is weakness of shoulder shrugging or abduction. EMG and nerve conduction studies can confirm the diagnosis and provide prognostic information by quantitating axonal loss and continuity (66). Conservative therapy consist of analgesia and physical therapy. Surgical exploration should be considered for a persistent deficit.

Supraclavicular Nerve

A patient with midclavicular pain and tenderness, with associated sensory loss over the anterior shoulder and under the midportion of the clavicle was found to have entrapment of the supraclavicular nerve as it passed through a canal in the clavicle. Pain was relieved, but numbness persisted (67).

Suprascapular Nerve

There are several potential sites of entrapment for the subscapular nerve, including the suprascapular notch, superior transverse scapular ligament, inferior transverse scapular ligament (68), and the spinoglenoid notch at the lateral border of the spine of the scapula. Repetitive shoulder movements in baseball pitchers (69), fencers (70), weight lifters (71), and volleyball players (72) can injure the nerve. Blows to the suprascapular region or anterior dislocation of the shoulder can also cause the syndrome (73–76). The primary symptom is pain in the posterior-lateral shoulder that can be increased by flexing the shoulder. Shoulder weakness may be noted. Examination reveals weakness or atrophy of the supraspinatus and infraspinatus muscles or just of the infraspinatus muscle. Pain can be reproduced or aggravated by scapular abduction maneuvers or neck rotation toward the asymptomatic shoulder. Tenderness at the site of entrapment may be noted. EMG and nerve conduction studies may differentiate between suprascapular nerve injury, cervical radiculopathy, and brachial plexus palsy. Surgical exploration is indicated for persistent signs and symptoms despite conservative therapy or in cases of acute onset without obvious cause (77).

Long Thoracic Nerve

The long thoracic nerve can be injured by heavy backpacks or in the course of weight training (78), swimming the backstroke (79), tennis, bowling, golf, soccer, hockey, gymnastics (80, 81), and volleyball (82). Many "injuries" may actually be formes frustes of idiopathic brachial plexus neuropathy (57). Symptoms include dull aching shoulder pain and shoulder weakness. Examination reveals a sagging, weak shoulder. With arms extended forward, the scapula will wing. In one series, patients required an average of 9 months before full recovery. Traumatic etiologies are associated with a relatively poor prognosis (83).

Axillary Nerve

Most axillary mononeuropathies are caused by overt trauma such as shoulder dislocation, humeral head fracture, traction injuries, or direct blows to the shoulder (84, 85). Symptoms consist of shoulder weakness. On examination there is deltoid weakness and there may be deltoid atrophy and sensory loss over the lateral shoulder. Conservative treatment includes splinting the shoulder in partial abduction. If there is no significant improvement in 3 months, then the nerve should be explored.

The axillary nerve can be entrapped in the quadrilateral by abnormal fibrous strands or muscle hypertrophy (86) as described in baseball pitchers (87, 88), foot ball players, and a rower. Symptoms include pain in the anterior shoulder, which is worsened by abduction and external rotation of the humerus. Shoulder and upper arm paresthesias may be present. Subclavian arteriography can confirm the diagnosis, demonstrating occlusion of the posterior humeral circumflex artery with the arm in abduction and external rotation. Surgical correction is possible (89).

Musculocutaneous Nerve

The musculocutaneous nerve may be injured by strenuous exercise—in which case the entrapment may be the result of a hypertrophic coracobrachialis muscle (90)—or in contact sports such as football (91), hockey, and rugby. Symptoms consist of elbow flexion weakness. Examination reveals painless weakness of biceps and brachialis muscles and can show sensory loss over the lateral forearm. EMG and nerve conduction studies can confirm the diagnosis and assess axonal continuity. Treatment consists of a sling and physical therapy. Surgery is rarely indicated.

The lateral antebrachial cutaneous nerve, the sensory termination of the musculocutaneous nerve, may be entrapped by the biceps aponeurosis and tendon at the antecubital fossa (92). This injury may be caused by repetitive forceful forearm pronation with the elbow extension, direct trauma, or muscular hypertrophy and has been reported in swimmers, weight lifters, racquetball players, and athletes in throwing sports. Symptoms include pain in the proximal forearm and elbow, worsened with elbow extension or repeated pronation and supination of the forearm, and dysesthesias and numbness over the anterolateral forearm. On examination, there is tenderness over the nerve at the antecubital fossa and sensory loss over the anterolateral forearm. If conservative therapy fails, surgical decompression is indicated.

Radial Nerve

Radial nerve injuries at several levels have been reported in swimming, tennis, golf, weight lifting, and throwing sports (93). Mechanisms include direct trauma or stretch and compression either by the lateral head of the triceps muscle or a fibrous arch coming from this muscle (94, 95).

High radial nerve injuries are defined as those lesions proximal to the bifurcation of the nerve into the posterior interosseous nerve and the sensory branch. In such lesions, triceps function may or may not be affected, depending on the level of injury. There can be pain, paresthesias, and numbness along the superficial radial nerve distribution (dorsal radial area of the hand) and wrist and finger drop. There may be tenderness and a Tinel's sign at the site of entrapment.

Compression of the posterior interosseous nerve is entrapment at the arcade of Frohse. Symptoms are wrist and finger weakness. Pain is not prominent in the classic syndrome. It is noted in only half the cases and is usually brief. On examination, there is prominent finger extensor weakness. Wrist extension may be weak, but only partially so, because innervation to extensor carpi radialis longus and brevis is proximal to the lesion. Tenderness may be present over the nerve in the extensor muscle mass just distal to the elbow.

EMG and nerve conduction studies are useful in confirming these two classic syndromes of radial neuropathy and can quantitate the deficit, assisting management.

The classic symptom of tennis elbow is pain over the lateral epicondyle, although pain in the medial elbow has also been reported. Although one potential source of the pain is the result of muscle or tendon damage (96–98), it is possible that some patients actually have entrapment of the posterior interosseous nerve by the extensor carpi radialis brevis, arcade of Frohse, or the supinator muscle (99, 100). This syndrome is called "resistant tennis elbow" or "radial tunnel syndrome." In these patients, forceful supination or wrist or middle finger extension will produce pain, and there is tenderness over the radial nerve and not the lateral epicondyle. EMG and nerve conduction studies sometimes reveal pathognomonic abnormalities (101). Surgical decompression of the posterior interosseus nerve has led to improvement in a number of patients (102, 103).

The superficial branch of the radial nerve can be entrapped in the distal forearm. Repetitive pronation, supination, and ulnar flexion may produce stretch injury in the nerve, presumably at the site where it exits from under the brachioradialis to assume a subcutaneous position, because it is relatively fixed there. The nerve also can be directly compressed by tight wrist bands or direct trauma. Symptoms include pain and paresthesias over the dorsoradial aspect of the hand. Examination reveals radial distribution sensory loss and a Tinel's sign at the site of entrapment. Pain is worsened with ulnar deviation and flexion of the wrist (104, 105). EMG and nerve conduction studies can confirm the diagnosis and rule out more proximal radial nerve pathology and cervical radiculopathy or brachial plexopathy.

Median Nerve

The median nerve may be entrapped at the ligament of Struthers in distal humerus, the proximal forearm (pronator teres syndrome), midforearm (anterior interosseous syndrome), or wrist (carpal tunnel syndrome) from repetitive upper extremity exertion or direct trauma.

About 5 cm proximal to the medial epicondyle, some patients have a bony spur, a supracondylar process. The ligament of Struthers runs from this spur to the medial epicondyle. Symptoms and signs in this syndrome are poorly defined, but may consist of varying degrees of pain above the elbow, tenderness over the ligament, weakness of pronation, wrist and finger flexion and thumb abduction, and median distribution sensory loss. The diagnosis can be supported by radiographic demonstration of the supracondylar process, although the ligament can be present in some patients without this bony protuberance. Surgical exploration is sometimes indicated.

In the pronator teres syndrome, the median nerve is entrapped within the pronator teres muscle itself by hypertrophy or a fibrous band, in a tight fibrous arch of the flexor digitorum superficialis, or in a thickened lacertus fibrosus (106). This syndrome has been reported in sports requiring forceful repetitive forearm pronation or gripping such as baseball (107, 108), racquet sports, weight lifting, and gymnastics as well as in contact sports, following acute trauma to the proximal forearm. Symptoms include anterior forearm pain on exertion with or without clumsiness, loss of dexterity, hand weakness, and paresthesias. Accentuation of symptoms by forceful forearm pronation or repetitive elbow motion supports the diagnosis. On examination, pain or median-distribution paresthesias may be produced by forcefully compressing the pronator muscle mass. Tinel's sign may be present. Median motor deficits are sometimes present but are variable. Sensory findings are usually poorly defined. Although EMG and nerve conduction studies are rarely abnormal, in some patients the studies clearly demonstrate a median nerve lesion proximal to the wrist. EMG and nerve conduction studies may also rule out other conditions in the differential diagnosis such as carpal tunnel syndrome and cervical radiculopathy. If conservative therapy is unsuccessful, surgical decompression is indicated.

The anterior interosseus nerve can be compressed at the tendinous origins of the deep head of the pronator teres muscle or flexor digitorum superficialis to the long finger or by several types of accessory muscles, tendons, and blood vessels (109). Acute trauma or chronic trauma, with a preexisting anatomical disposition, can cause anterior interosseus entrapment. Settings include weight lifting and activities requiring repetitive elbow flexion and pronation. Symptoms include pain in the proximal forearm or arm, loss of dexterity, and loss of the ability to pinch. On examination there is weakness of flexion of the interphalangeal joint of the thumb (flexor pollicis longus) and distal interphalangeal joint of the index finger (flexor digitorum profundus of the index finger). In addition, there is weakness of forearm pronation when the elbow is flexed (pronator quadratus). There can be tenderness over the pronator muscle mass and increased pain on resisted pronation. Tinel's sign can be present. There is no sensory loss. EMG and nerve conduction studies may show denervation in the involved muscles or prolonged distal motor latency to the pronator quadratus. If a prolonged trial of conservative therapy fails, surgical exploration is indicated.

Median nerve entrapment at the wrist (carpal tunnel syndrome) can occur from bicycling, excessive forceful gripping, excessive throwing of a curve ball (baseball pitchers), performing repetitive wrist flexion-extension movements (various racquet sports) (110), or direct trauma to the volar surface of the wrist (111), including fracture-dislocation and crush injuries. Symptoms include pain and paresthesias in the wrist and hand, which is often worse at night or with use of the hands. The pain can spread all the way to the shoulder in some patients, although the paresthesias are present only in the fingers. Hand clumsiness or weakness can also be noted. On examination, sensory loss can be found in the median-innervated digits (thumb, index, middle, and lateral border of ring finger). There can be weakness of the abductor pollicis brevis muscle and atrophy of the thenar eminence. Tinel's sign or Phalen's sign may be present, although these are sometimes present in the absence of carpal tunnel syndrome.

EMG and nerve conduction studies should confirm the diagnosis of carpal tunnel syndrome in all but a small minority of patients. Conservative treatment consists of immobilization of the wrist with a splint, worn at night, and NSAIDs. Injection of corticosteroids into the carpal tunnel is sometimes helpful. Failure of conservative treatment and a severe median nerve lesion are indications for surgical treatment.

Ulnar Nerve

Ulnar nerve entrapment at the elbow (condylar groove or cubital tunnel) can be caused by repetitive elbow flexion, an inflamed or calcified collateral ligament, loose bodies in the cubital tunnel, osteoarthritis, a severe valgus deformity, an anomalous muscle (112), or hypermobility of the nerve caused by lax or ruptured ligaments (113). There can be inflammation or a constricting band that entraps the nerve at the entrance to the cubital tunnel, the origin of the flexor carpi ulnaris. Entrapment has been reported in baseball pitchers (114–118), weight lifters, and racquetball players and other stick-handling athletes (119).

Symptoms consist of elbow pain, intermittent paresthesias in the fourth and fifth digits, and sensory alteration in the fourth and fifth digits and ulnar border of the hand. A sensory deficit over the medial dorsal aspect of the hand (distribution of the dorsal cutaneous branch of the ulnar nerve) implies that the lesion is proximal to the wrist. Weakness, if present, can range from mild clumsiness to definite weakness associated with intrinsic hand muscle atrophy. On examination, there can be ulnar distribution sensory loss (palmar and dorsal surfaces of medial hand, entire fifth digit, medial half of fourth digit) and weakness of flexor carpi ulnaris, flexor digitorum profundus of fourth and fifth digits, and abductor digiti minimi and first dorsal interosseous weakness); but partial deficits are more common than complete ones, probably because of unequal involvement of the different ulnar fascicles. Tinel's sign or tenderness over the nerve at the elbow may be present. EMG and nerve conduction studies can often confirm the diagnosis, but do not always demonstrate focal slowing or conduction block across the elbow, probably due to the fascicular nature of the injury in many patients.

If definite bone or joint deformities are absent, conservative treatment of ulnar neuropathy at the elbow with splinting and protection of the elbow with a soft pad along with a short course of NSAIDs is tried first. If conservative measures fail, then surgical intervention is indicated. Surgical treatments include decompression of the nerve at the cubital tunnel or anterior transposition of the ulnar nerve. The results of surgical decompression are variable.

Ulnar nerve entrapment at the wrist may result from chronic or repeated trauma; from hamate or pisiform bone fractures; or rarely from ganglia, arthritis, anomalous muscle, lipomas or other tumors, arteriovenous fistulas, aneurysms, or thrombosis of the ulnar artery at or near Guyon's canal (120). Bicyclists ("handlebar palsy") (121, 122), baseball catchers, weight lifters, gymnasts, martial arts practitioners, racquetball players, golfers, video game enthusiasts (123), and a man who did a lot of push-ups on a hard floor (124) have been reported with this injury.

Depending on the site of the lesion, four different syndromes of ulnar nerve entrapment at the wrist have been described. Compression of the nerve just proximal to or within Guyon's canal will cause weakness of all ulnar-innervated hand muscles and sensory loss over the palmar aspect of digit five and the medial aspect of digit four. Entrapment of the proximal-most deep terminal branch will result in pure weakness but no sensory loss. Compression of the deep terminal branch distal to the innervation of the hypothenar eminence results in weakness of ulnar-innervated hand muscles, except those of the hypothenar eminence. Compression of the superficial terminal branch in or just distal to Guyon's canal result in pure sensory loss involving the distal palmar hypothenar area and the palmar aspects of the ulnar-innervated digits. There may be pain and local tenderness and, in cases caused by repetitive trauma, a callus over the base of the palm may be present. Diagnostic tests include x-rays of the wrist with a carpal tunnel view to look for fractures and EMG and nerve conduction studies.

Initially, conservative treatment of ulnar neuropathy at the wrist is recommended. Avoidance of external pressure, the use of protective padding, and NSAID therapy are usually adequate. In cyclists, preventative measures include well-padded gloves and handlebars, correct bicycle frame size and distance from seat to stem, and frequent changing of hand positions on the handlebars (125). If conservative measures fail or if a mass is present at Guyon's canal, surgical exploration at Guyon's canal and distally may be indicated (126).

Digital Nerves in the Upper Extremities

Bowler's thumb is a digital neuropathy of the thumb (127). A cheerleader who did a lot of clapping and cartwheels developed a median palmar digital neuropathy (128). Digital neuropathies have also been described in catchers and batters (129). Symptoms consist of pain over the nerve, and paresthesia and hypesthesia in the distribution of the involved nerve. Tinel's sign may be present, and skin atrophy and callus formation may be present as well. For digital neuropathies, surgical correction may be indicated if conservative measures fail.

Pudendal Nerve

The pudendal nerve may be damaged along with a pelvic fracture from a bicycle or motorcycle fall. Numbness of the shaft of the penis (130) and impotence (131) have been reported from prolonged bicycle riding. The symptoms presumably resulted from compression of the pudendal nerves between bicycle seat and pubic symphysis.

Sciatic Nerve

Sciatic nerve entrapment can occur in the gluteal region around the sciatic notch and gluteal fold or in the thigh (132). The most common cause of sciatic nerve injury is trauma such as fracture-dislocation of the hip or severe traction injury as seen in motorcycle racing accidents. Transient sciatic neuropathy in cyclists has been reported, presumably the result of pressure on the nerve in the perineal area (133) or at the sciatic notch from the bicycle seat (134).

The sciatic nerve may also be injured in the thigh. Complete sciatic nerve laceration caused by a closed femoral shaft fracture in a motorcyclist has been reported (135). Traumatic hematomas of the thigh and myositis ossificans in the biceps femoris muscles (reported in a cricket and soccer player) may also cause sciatic entrapment (136–138).

A complete sciatic nerve lesion results in paralysis of the hamstrings and all muscles below the knee, sensory loss in all areas below the knee except for the medial calf, and an absent ankle jerk reflex. Most sciatic nerve lesions are incomplete, however. The lateral (peroneal) trunk is more vulnerable than the medial (posterior tibial) trunk, so that in some patients with sciatic neuropathy, the clinical findings are similar to those expected for a lesion of the common peroneal nerve at the fibular head (139). EMG and nerve conduction studies, including evaluation of the short head of the biceps femoris (the only muscle innervated by the lateral trunk proximal to the fibular head) can establish the diagnosis. Imaging studies to look for fractures and pelvic masses are also useful.

Compression of the sciatic nerve in the piriformis muscle is a controversial entity (140). No patients reported to have this syndrome had significant neurological deficits, although EMG evidence of sciatic distribution denervation was noted in one. Some authors state that lack of a neurologic deficit is an essential diagnostic criterion. Symptoms have been relieved by surgical exploration and division of the piriformis muscle in some patients (141).

Posterior Cutaneous Nerve

A bicyclist developed a neuropathy of the posterior cutaneous nerve of the thigh (142). Symptoms of this entrapment include paresthesias over the lower buttock and/or posterior thigh.

Femoral Nerve

Femoral neuropathy has been reported in gymnasts (143), judo practitioners, parachute jumpers, dancers performing exercises in which their hips are hyperextended (144), and in athletes doing repeated somersaults. Sudden flexion or extension or stretching of the nerve during hyperextension of the hip for a long period and compression of the nerve under the inguinal ligament may be etiologic factors.

Symptoms and signs of femoral neuropathies include weakness and atrophy of the quadriceps muscle, reduction or absence of the knee jerk reflex, and sensory loss over the anteromedial thigh and along the medial aspect of the lower leg. Little or no sensory loss can be seen in partial nerve lesions. Iliopsoas or thigh adductor weakness rules out pure femoral nerve involvement. Iliopsoas muscle weakness can be seen in an upper lumbar plexopathy or L2–L3 radiculopathy. Thigh adductor weakness can be seen in obturator neuropathy, lumbar plexopathy, or L2–L3 radiculopathy. EMG of the lumbar paraspinal muscles, iliopsoas, thigh adductors, and quadriceps can assist in the differential diagnosis. Imaging studies of the lumbar spine and pelvis (which may reveal a hematoma or mass) are also useful (145).

Conservative treatment includes analgesics and physical therapy. Bracing may be necessary. Surgical exploration may be indicated if the lesion is severe or if laceration of the nerve is suspected.

Saphenous Nerve

Surfers can develop a saphenous neuropathy caused by pressure on the nerve when the medial aspects of knees are pressed against the surfboard (146). Symptoms consist of dysesthesia over the anteromedial aspect of the leg below the knee. Examination revealed sensory loss in the saphenous distribution.

Obturator Nerve

The obturator nerve is most often injured from trauma such as pelvic fractures. Symptoms and signs include weakness of hip adduction, sensory loss, pain and/or paresthesias in the medial thigh, and sometimes groin pain. Quadriceps strength and the knee jerk reflex are normal. In most cases of obturator nerve involvement, a lesion of the femoral nerve also is present. EMG and nerve conduction studies are useful in the diagnosis as are imaging studies of lumbar spine and pelvis. Treatment depends on the cause of the neuropathy.

Lateral Femoral Cutaneous Nerve

Lateral femoral cutaneous nerve entrapment is termed meralgia paresthetica (147). The lateral femoral cutaneous nerve enters the thigh by passing through a tunnel in the lateral attachment of the inguinal ligament to the anterosuperior iliac spine and supplies sensation to the anterolateral aspect of the thigh. Meralgia paresthetica has been reported in weight lifters who wear tight corsets, belts, or trusses (perhaps the result of direct compression of the nerve at its point of exit from the pelvis), in gymnasts (perhaps due to the impact of the thighs on the uneven parallel bars or to repetitive flexion and extension of the hip in rope jumping) (148), and in a jogger. Symptoms and signs include pain, paresthesias, and sensory loss in the anterolateral thigh. A Tinel's sign or tenderness at the anterosuperior iliac spine may be present. Symptoms often increase while standing or walking. EMG and nerve conduction studies are valuable in excluding lumbar radiculopathy, lumbar plexopathy, and femoral neuropathy, but nerve conduction studies of the lateral femoral cutaneous nerve are unreliable in most hands. Conservative treatment consists of analgesics and avoidance of precipitating factors such as certain exercises or tight corsets, belts, or trusses. Nerve blocks or local steroid injections may help. If conservative therapy fails, surgery may be indicated. The nerve can be released at a level of exit from the inguinal ligament. Nerve section carries the risk of producing unpleasant paresthesias due to neuroma formation.

Peroneal Nerve

The peroneal nerve is injured most frequently at the head and neck of the fibula. Acute adduction of the knee joint with rupture of the lateral ligaments, twisting of the ankle or sudden stretching may lead to a severe traction injury of the nerve (149). Peroneal nerve entrapment at the fibular head has been reported in tennis and racquetball players (150), in runners (151, 152), and in a skier who had distal fractures of the tibia and fibula caused by severe ankle inversion injuries (153). An athlete with exertional knee pain had entrapment of the peroneal nerve in the popliteal space by a fibrous band (154). Symptoms and signs include footdrop with weakness or paralysis of the ankle and toe dorsiflexors, and weakness of ankle evertors. Sensory loss involving the anterolateral aspect of the lower leg and dorsum of the foot can be present. Variable patterns of motor and sensory deficit can be seen, depending on the relative involvement of the superficial and deep peroneal branches. Tinel's sign can be present at the fibular head. Persistent pain implies a true entrapment in the fibular tunnel or compression by tumors or cysts. EMG and nerve conduction studies can help confirm the diagnosis and can help rule out lumbar radiculopathy, lumbar plexopathy, and sciatic neuropathy. Imaging studies of the knee can also be useful. Conservative treatment consists of bracing with a plastic orthosis molded to the posterior calf of the foot to provide stability while walking and avoidance of extrinsic pressure at the fibular head (e.g., by avoiding crossing the legs at the knees). Surgical therapy is indicated in patients with persistent pain and progressive motor and sensory loss.

The deep peroneal nerve can be entrapped in runners, soccer players, and skiers. The most common site of entrapment is the anterior tarsal tunnel (inferior extensor retinaculum), although other nearby entrapment sites have been described. Recurrent ankle sprains or trauma may be contributory. Symptoms include pain in the dorsum of the foot with radiation to the first web space, worsened by running. Examination reveals decreased sensation in the first web space, and there may be extensor digitorum brevis weakness and atrophy. Pain can be provoked by dorsi- or plantar-flexion of the foot, depending on the site of entrapment.

Entrapment of the superficial peroneal nerve can occur in runners as well as soccer, hockey, tennis, and racquetball players. The usual point of entrapment is at the exit point from the deep fascia 10.5 to 12.5 cm proximal to the lateral malleolus. About 25% of patients have a history of previous trauma, most commonly an ankle sprain. Injuries to the superficial peroneal nerves may also result from wearing tight ski boots or roller skates (155). Fascial defects with muscle herniation may be present (156). Symptoms include pain over the outer border of the distal calf and dorsum of foot and ankle. There may be sensory loss in the same distribution. The pain is worse with exertion. On examination, there may be point tenderness where the nerve exits the deep fascia. Tinel's sign may be present. Sensory loss can be noted, as can a palpable fascial defect.

Injuries to the deep and superficial peroneal nerves leading to pain and numbness on the dorsolateral foot may result from ankle sprains, blunt trauma, or rupture of the peroneus longus muscle (157).

Posterior Tibial Nerve

An athlete with exertional knee pain had entrapment of the tibial nerve in the popliteal space by fibers of the medial gastrocnemius muscle (154). The distal tibial nerve or its major distal branches can be entrapped at the ankle or foot (158).

The posterior tibial nerve can be entrapped in the tarsal tunnel in runners and other athletes. In some cases there are abnormalities of the fibroosseus tunnel or its contents. Extrinsic pressure can also be involved. Tight golf shoes caused the syndrome in a patient of one of the authors. About 33% of cases are related to trauma. Symptoms consist of burning, sharp pain, and paresthesias that radiate into the sole of the foot. Standing, walking, or running will exacerbate the symptoms. Numbness and nocturnal pain are less common. On examination, there may be a Tinel's sign over the tarsal tunnel. Sensory loss in the medial and/or lateral sole may be noted. Intrinsic foot muscle weakness may be present.

Entrapment of the medial plantar nerve occurs in joggers in the region of the master knot of Henry. Patients often run with excessive pronation of the feet or excessive heel valgus. Arch supports may compress the nerve. Symptoms include pain in the medial aspect of the arch, worsened by running or the use of a new orthosis. On examination, there is tenderness near the navicular tuberosity. Tinel's sign may be present. Decreased sensation on the medial sole may be present after running.

The first branch of the lateral planar nerve can be entrapped (usually in runners) between the deep fascia of the abductor hallucis muscle and the medial caudal margin of the quadratus planae muscle, over the plantar side of the long plantar ligament, or in the osteomuscular canal between the calcaneus and the flexor digitorum brevis. Symptoms consist of chronic heel pain worsened with walking or running. On examination, there is tenderness over the nerve deep to the abductor hallucis muscle. Tinel's sign is sometimes present over the nerve.

Entrapment of the calcaneal nerve branch has been reported in athletes with chronic heel pain that was unrelieved by conservative therapy (159). This neuropathy occurred in long-distance runners and a badminton player.

Therapy for these disorders is primarily conservative. Tight shoes, straps, or taping are to be avoided. Alteration in technique or playing surface, appropriate exercises, antiinflammatory drugs, rest, ice or heat, massage, and injections may be helpful. Surgery may be needed if conservative measures result in no improvement.

Sural Nerve

The sural nerve may be injured by avulsion fracture of the base of the fifth metatarsal bone in runners (160), a tight-fitting ski boot, fibrosis secondary to recurrent ankle sprains, ganglions, and myositis ossificans at the musculotendinous junction of the Achilles tendon. Symptoms include pain and paresthesias in a sural distribution. Examination may reveal tenderness over the nerve, a Tinel's sign, and sensory loss.

Digital Nerves in the Lower Extremities

Measurable differences in vibratory sensation threshold and in lower extremity nerve conduction were found in long-distance runners compared with controls, perhaps because of multiple small injuries to toes and feet (161). However, none of the runners had clinical symptoms or signs of neuropathy.

Interdigital neuromas (Morton's neuroma) are not uncommon in runners (158). Plantar digital nerves are subjected to repetitive microtrauma against the distal edge of the intermetatarsal ligament. Usually, the third web space is involved. Symptoms include plantar or forefoot pain associated with running. Numbness or tingling of affected toes is sometimes present. On examination, there is point tenderness on the plantar aspect between the metatarsal heads at the affected web space.

Supraorbital Nerve

Supraorbital neuropathy has been reported in a swimmer, presumably caused by pressure on the nerve from tight swimming goggles. Symptoms consisted of ipsilateral headaches and supraorbital ridge pain. Tinel's sign was present at the supraorbital notch (162).

Conclusions

Awareness of sports-related neurologic syndromes should lead to more rapid and precise diagnosis and should improve the development and institution of preventative measures.

REFERENCES

1. Pritchett JW. Preexisting musculoskeletal conditions presenting as school sports injuries. J Adolesc Health Care 1989;10:212–216.
2. Jordan BD, Tsairis P, Warren RE. Sports neurology. Rockville, MD: Aspen, 1989.
3. Stewart WF, Lipton RB, Celentano DD, Reed ML. Prevalence of migraine headache in the United States. Relation to age, income, race and other sociodemographic factors. JAMA 1992;267:64–69.
4. Matthews WB. Footballers migraine. Br Med J 1972;2:769–770.
5. Bennett DR, Fuenning SI, Sullivan MA, Weber J. Migraine precipitated by head trauma in athletes. Am J Sports Med 1980;8:202–205.
6. Haas DC, Pineda GS, Lourie H. Juvenile head trauma syndromes and their relationship to migraine. Arch Neurol 1975;32:548–554.
7. Oka H. Kako M, Matsushima M, et al. Traumatic spreading depression syndrome. Review of a particular type of head injury in 27 patients. Brain 1977;100:287–298.
8. Powell B. Weight lifter's cephalgia. Ann Emerg Med 1982;11:449–451.
9. Paulson GW. Weightlifter's headache. Headache 1983;23:193–194.
10. Rooke ED. Benign exertional headache. Med Clin North Am 1968;52:801–808.
11. Pestronk A, Petronk S. Goggle migraine [Letter to the Editor] N Engl J Med 1983;308:226–227.
12. Seelinger DF, Coin GC, Carlow TJ. Effort headache with cerebral infarction. Headache 1975;15:142–145.
13. Dalessio DJ: Mechanism of headache. Med Clin North Am 1978;62:429–442.
14. Diamond S. Prolonged benign exertional headache: its clinical characteristics and response to indomethacin. Headache 1982;22:96–98.
15. Schneider RC. Head and neck injuries in football: mechanisms, treatment and prevention. Baltimore: Williams & Wilkins, 1973.
16. Saunders RL, Harbaugh RE. The second impact in catastrophic contact-sports head trauma. JAMA 1984;252:538–539.
17. Rosenbloom D, Sutton JR. Drugs and exercise. Med Clin North Am 1985;69:177–187.
18. Korczyn AD. Participation of epileptic patients in sports. J Sports Med 1979;19:195–198.
19. Ogunyemi AO, Gomez MR, Klass DW. Seizures induced by exercise. Neurology 1988;38:633–634.
20. Goetze W, Kubicki St, Munter M, Teichmann J. Effect of physical exercise on seizure threshold. Dis Nerv Sys 1967;28:664–667.
21. Swinyard EA, Miyahara JT, Clark LD. The effect of experimentally-induced stress on pentylenetetrazol seizure threshold in mice. Psychopharmacologia 1963;4:343–353.
22. Friis ML, Lund M. Stress convulsions. Arch. Neurol 1974;31:155–159.
23. Aisenson MR. Accidental injuries in epileptic children. Pediatrics 1948;2:85–88.
24. Livingston S, Berman W. Participation of epileptic patient in sports. JAMA 1973;224:236–238.
25. Hauser WA. Should people be treated after a first seizure? Arch Neurol 1986;43:1287–1288.
26. Hart RG, Easton JD. Seizure recurrence after a first, unprovoked seizure. Arch Neurol 1986;43:1289–1290.
27. Hart RG, Miller VT. Cerebral infarction in young adults: practical approach. Stroke 1983;17:110–114.
28. Kelly WF, Roussak J. Stroke while jogging. Br J Sports Med 1980;14:229–230.
29. Hart RG, Easton. Dissections of cervical and cerebral arteries. Neurol Clin 1983;1:155–182.
30. Fisher CM. The headache and pain of spontaneous carotid dissection. Headache 1982;22:60–65.
31. Fisher CM, Ojemann RG, Roberson GH. Spontaneous dissection of cervico-cerebral arteries. Can J Neurol Sci 1978;5:9–19.
32. Ringel SP, Harrison SH, Norenberg MD, et al. Fibromuscular dysplasia: multiple "spontaneous" dissecting aneurysms of the major cervical arteries. Ann Neurol 1977;34:251–252.
33. Goodman JM, Zink WL, Cooper DF. Hemilingual paralysis caused by spontaneous carotid artery dissection. Arch Neurol 1983;40:653–654.
34. Hart RG, Easton JD. Dissections and trauma of cervico-cerebral arteries. In: Barnett HJM, Stein BM, Mohr JP, Yatsu FM, eds. Stroke: pathophysiology, diagnosis and management. New York: Churchill Livingstone, 1986:775–788.
35. Katirji JB, Reinmuth OM, Latchaw RE. Stroke due to vertebral artery injury. Arch Neurol 1985;42:242–248.
36. Hanus SH, Homar TD, Harter DH. Vertebral artery occlusion complicating yoga exercises. Arch Neurol 1977;34:574–575.
37. Nagler W. Vertebral artery obstruction by hyperextension of the neck: report of three cases. Arch Phys Med Rehabil 1973;54:237–240.
38. Sorensen BF: Bow hunter's stroke. Neurosurgery 1978;2:259–261.
39. Tramo MJ, Hainline B, Petito F, Lee B, Caronna J. Vertebral artery injury and cerebellar stroke while swimming: case report. Stroke 1985;16:1039–1042.
40. Barnett HJM. Progress towards stroke prevention: Robert Wartenberg lecture. Neurology 1980;30:1212–1225.
41. Sacco RL, Ellenberg JH. Mohr JP, Tatemichi TK, Price TR, Wolf PA. Infarcts of undetermined cause: the NINCDS stroke data bank. Ann Neurol 1989;25:382–390.
42. Mohr JP, Caplan LR, Melski JW, et al. The Harvard cooperative stroke registry: a prospective registry. Neurology 1978;28:754–762.
43. Sherman DG, Goldman L, Whiting RB, Jurgensen K, Kaste M, Easton JD. Thromboembolism in patient with atrial fibrillation. Arch Neurol 1984;41:708–710.
44. Stroke Prevention in Atrial Fibrillation Study Group Investigators. Preliminary report of the stroke prevention in atrial fibrillation study. N Engl J Med 1990;322:863–868.
45. The Boston Area Anticoagulation Trial for Atrial Fibrillation Investigators. The effect of low-dose warfarin on the risk of stroke in patients with nonrheumatic atrial fibrillation. N Engl J Md 1990;323:1505–1511.
46. Huston TP, Puffer JC, Rodney WM. The athletic heart syndrome. N Engl J Med 1985;313:24–32.
47. Lechat Ph, Mas JL, Lascault G, et al. Prevalence of patent foramen ovale in patients with stroke. N Engl J Med 1988;318:1148–1152.
48. Frankle MA, Eichberg R, Zachariah SB. Anabolic androgenic steroids and a stroke in an athlete: case report. Arch Phys Med Rehabil 1988;69:632–633.
49. Caplan LR, Hier DB, Banks G. Current concepts of cerebrovascular disease—Stroke: stroke and drug abuse. Stroke 1982;13:869–872.
50. Brust JCM. Stroke and substance abuse. In: Barnett HJM, Mohr JP, Stein BM, Yatsu FM, eds. Stroke: New York: Churchill Livingston, 1986:903–920.

51. Cofield RH, Simonet WT. The shoulder in sports. Mayo Clin Proc 1984;59:157–164.
52. Seddon HJ. Three types of nerve injury. Brain 1943;66:237–245.
53. Sunderland S. Nerves and nerve injuries. 2nd ed. New York: Churchill Livingstone, 1978.
54. Wilbourn AJ. Electrodiagnostic testing of neurologic injuries of athletes. Clin Sports Med 1990;9:229–245.
55. Dawson DM, Hallett M, Millender LH. Entrapment neuropathies. 2nd ed. Boston: Little, Brown, 1990.
56. Stewart JD. Compression and entrapment neuropathies. In: Dyck PJ, Thomas PK, Griffin JW, Low PA, Poduslo JF, eds. Peripheral neuropathy. 3rd ed. Philadelphia: WB Saunders, 1993:961–979.
57. Hershman EB, Wilbourn AJ, Bergfeld JA. Acute brachial neuropathy in athletes. Am J Sports Med 1989;17:655–659.
58. Poindexter DP, Johnson EW. Football shoulder and neck injury: a study of the "stinger." Arch Phys Med Rehabil 1984;65:601–602.
59. Robertson WC, Eichman PL, Clancy WG. Upper trunk brachial plexopathy in football players. JAMA 1979;241:1480–1482.
60. DiBenedetto M, Markey K. Electrodiagnostic localization of traumatic upper trunk brachial plexopathy. Arch Phys Med Rehabil 1984;65:15–17.
61. Rockett FX. Observations on the "burner"; traumatic cervical radiculopathy. Clin Orthop 1982;164:18–19.
62. Kline DG, Lusk MD. Management of athletic brachial plexus lesions. In: Schneider RC, Kennedy JC, Plant ML, eds. Sports injuries: mechanisms, prevention, and treatment. Baltimore: William & Wilkins, 1985:724–742.
63. Matz SO, Welliver PS, Welliver DI. Brachial plexus neuropraxia complicating a comminuted clavicle fracture in a college player. Am J Sports Med 1989;17:581–583.
64. Clancy WG, Brand RL, Bergfield JA. Upper trunk brachial plexus injury in contact sports. Am J Sports Med 1977;5:209–216.
65. Logigian EL, McInnes JRM, Berger AR, Busis NA, Lehrich JR, Shahani BT. Stretch-induced spinal accessory nerve palsy. Muscle Nerve 1988;11:146–150.
66. Wright TA. Accessory spinal nerve injury. Clin Orthop 1975;108:15–18.
67. Gelberman RH, Verdeck WN, Brodhead WT. Supraclavicular nerve-entrapment syndrome. J Bone Joint Surg 1975;57A:119.
68. Kaspi A, Yanai J, Pick CG, Mann G. Entrapment of the distal suprascapular nerve. An anatomical study. In Orthop 1988;12:273–275.
69. Ringel SP, Treihaft M, Carry M, Fisher R, Jacobs P. suprascapular neuropathy in pitchers. Am J Sports Med 1990;18:80–86.
70. Aiello I, Serra G, Traina C, Tugnoli V. Entrapment of the suprascapular nerve at the spinoglenoid notch. Ann Neurol 1982;12:314–316.
71. Agre JC, Ash N, Cameron C, House J. Suprascapular neuropathy after intensive progressive exercise: case report. Arch Phys Med Rehabil 1986;68:236–238.
72. Ferretti A, Cerullo G, Russo G. Suprascapular neuropathy in volleyball players. J Bone Joint Surg 1987;69A:260–263.
73. Zotlan JD. Injury to the suprascapular nerve associated with anterior dislocation of the shoulder: cases report and review of the literature. J Trauma 1979;19:203–206.
74. Goodman GE. Unusual nerve injuries in recreational sports. Am J Sports Med 1983;2:224–227.
75. Hashimoto K, Oda K, Kuroda Y, et al. Case of suprascapular nerve palsy manifesting as selected atrophy of the infraspinatus muscle. Clin Neurol 1983;23:970–973.
76. Drez DJ Jr. Suprascapular neuropathy in the differential diagnosis of rotator cuff injuries. Am J Sports Med 1976;4:43–45.
77. Murray JWG. Surgical approach for entrapment neuropathy of the suprascapular nerve. Orthop Rev 1974;3:33–35.
78. Stanish WD, Lamb H. Isolated paralysis of the serratus anterior muscle: a weight training injury: case report. Am J Sports Med 1978;6:385–386.
79. Bateman JF. Nerve injuries about the shoulder in sports. J Bone Joint Surg 1967;49A:785–792.
80. Gregg JR, Labosky D, Harty M, et al. Serratus anterior paralysis in the young athlete. J Bone Joint Surg 1979;61A:825–832.
81. Johnson TH, Kendall HO. Isolated paralysis of the serratus anterior muscle. J Bone Joint Surg 1955;37A:567–574.
82. Distefano S. Neuropathy due to entrapment of the long thoracic nerve. Ital J Orthop Traumatol 1989;15:259–262.
83. Goodman CE, Kernick MM, Blum MV. Long thoracic nerve palsy: a follow-up study. Arch Phys Med Rehabil 1975;56:352–355.
84. Blom S, Dahlback CO. Nerve injuries in dislocations of the shoulder joint and fractures of the neck of the humerus. Acta Chir Scand 1970;136:461–466.
85. Berry H, Bril B. Axillary nerve palsy following blunt trauma to the shoulder region: a clinical and electrophysiological review. J Neurol Neurosurg Psychiatry 1982;45:1027–1032.
86. Cahill BR, Palmer RE. Quadrilateral space syndrome. J Hand Surg 1983;8:65–69.
87. Redler MR, Ruland LJ III, McCue FC III. Quadrilateral space syndrome in a throwing athlete. Am J Sports Med 1986;14:511–513.
88. Cormier PJ, Matalon TAS, Wolin PM. Quadrilateral space syndrome: a rare cause of shoulder pain. Radiology 1988;167:797–798.
89. Petrucci FS, Morelli A, Raimondi PL. Axillary nerve injury: 21 cases treated by nerve graft and neurolysis. J Hand Surg 1982;7:271–278.
90. Braddom RL, Wolfe C. Musculocutaneous nerve injury after heavy exercise. Arch Phys Med Rehabil 1978;59:290–293.
91. Kim SM, Goodrich JA. Isolated proximal musculocutaneous nerve palsy: case report. Arch Phys Med Rehabil 1984;65:735–736.
92. Bassett FH, Nunley JA. Compression of the musculocutaneous nerve at the elbow. J Bone Joint Surg 1982;64A:1050–1052.
93. Posner MA. Compressive neuropathies of the median and radial nerves at the elbow. Clin Sports Med 1990;9:343–363.
94. Lotem M, Fried A, Levy M, et al. Radial palsy following muscular effort: a nerve compression syndrome related to a fibrous arch of the lateral head of the triceps. J Bone Joint Surg 1971;53B:500–506.
95. Mitsunaga MM, Nakano K. High radial nerve pasy following strenuous muscular activity. Clin Orthop 1988;234:39–42.
96. Coonrad RW, Hooper WR. Tennis elbow: its course, natural history, conservative and surgical management. J Bone Joint Surg 1973;55A:1177–1182.
97. Van Rossum J, Buruma OJS, Kamphuisen HAC, Onvlee GJ. Tennis elbow—a radial tunnel syndrome? J Bone Joint Surg 1978;60B:197–198.
98. Nirschl RP. The etiology and treatment of tennis elbow. J Sports Med 1974;2:308–323.
99. Werner CO. Lateral elbow pain and posterior interosseous nerve entrapment. Acta Orthop Scand 1979;174:1–62.
100. Roles NC, Maudsley RH. Radial tunnel syndrome. Resistant tennis elbow as nerve entrapment. J Bone Joint Surg 1972;54B:499–508.
101. Rosen I, Werner CO. Neurophysiological investigation of posterior interosseous nerve entrapment causing lateral elbow pain. Electrophys Clin Neurophysiol 1980;50:125–133.
102. Lister GD, Belsole RB, Kleinert HE. The radial tunnel syndrome. J Hand Surg 1979;4:52–59.
103. Jalovaara P, Lindholm RV. Decompression of the posterior interosseous nerve for tennis elbow. Arch Orthop Trauma Surg 1989;108:243–245.
104. Rettig AC. Neurovascular injuries in the wrists and hands of athletes. Clin Sports Med 1990;9:389–417.
105. Aulicino PL: Neurovascular injuries in the hands of athletes. Hand Clin 1990;6:455–466.
106. Hartz CR, Linscheid RL, Gramse RR, et al. The pronator teres syndrome: compressive neuropathy of the median nerve. J Bone Joint Surg 1981;63A:885–890.
107. Barnes DA, Tullos HS. An analysis of 100 symptomatic baseball players. Am J Sports Med 1987;6:62–67.
108. Khurana RK. Schlagenhauff RE, Zwirecki RJ. The pronator syndrome (A case report and reappraisal). Neurology (India) 1975;23:46–48.
109. Hill NA, Howard FM, Huffer BR. The incomplete anterior interosseous nerve syndrome. J Hand Surg 1985;10:4–16.
110. Layfer LF, Jones JB. Hand paresthesias after racquetball. Ill Med J 1977;152:190–191.
111. Match RM. Laceration of the median nerve from skiing. Am J Sports Med 1978;6:22–25.

112. Hirasawa Y, Sawamura H, Sakakida K. Entrapment neuropathy due to bilateral epitrochleoanconeus muscles: a case report. J Hand Surg 1979;4:181.
113. Childress HM. Recurrent ulnar nerve dislocation at the elbow. J Bone Joint Surg 1956;38A:978–984.
114. Godshall RW, Hansen CA. Traumatic ulnar neuropathy in adolescent baseball pitchers. J Bone Joint Surg 1971;53A:359–361.
115. DelPizzo W, Jobe FW, Norwood L. Ulnar nerve entrapment syndrome in baseball players. Am J Sports Med 1977;5:182–185.
116. Indelicato PA, Jobe FW, Kerlan RK, et al. Correctable elbow lesions in professional baseball players: a review of 25 cases. Am J Sports Med 1979;7:72–75.
117. Hang YS. Tardy ulnar neuritis in a Little League baseball player. Am J Sports Med 1981;9:244–246.
118. Wojtys EM, Smith PA, Hankin FM. A cause of ulnar neuropathy in a baseball pitcher. A case report. Am J Sports Med 1986;14:422–424.
119. McCue FC III. The elbow, wrist and hand. In: Curland D, ed. The injured athlete. Philadelphia: JB Lipincott, 1982:295–329.
120. Kaplan EB, Zeide NS. Aneurysm of the ulnar artery: case report. Bull Hosp Joint Dis 1972;33:197–199.
121. Eckman PB, Perlstein G, Altrocchi PH. Ulnar neuropathy in bicycle riders. Arch Neurol 1975;32:130–131.
122. Noth J, Dietz V, Mauritz KH. Cyclist's palsy. J Neurol Sci 1980;46:111–116.
123. Friedland RP, St. John JN. Video-game palsy: distal ulnar neuropathy in a video-game enthusiast. N Engl J Med 1984;311:58–59.
124. Walker FO, Troost BT. Push-up palmar palsy. JAMA 1988;259:45–46.
125. Mellion MB. Common cycling injuries. Management and prevention. Sports 1991;11:52–70.
126. Adelaar RC, Foster WC, McDowell C. The treatment of cubital tunnel syndrome. J Hand Surg 1984;9:90–95.
127. Dobyns JH, O'Brien ET, Linscheid RL, Farrow GM. Bowler's thumb: diagnosis and treatment. J Bone Joint Surg 1972;54A:751–755.
128. Shields RW, Jacobs IB. Median palmar digital neuropathy in a cheerleader. Arch Phys Med Rehabil 1986;67:824–826.
129. Belsky M, Millender LH. Bowler's thumb in a baseball player. Orthopedics 1980;3:122.
130. Goodson JD. Pudendal neuritis from biking. N Engl J Med 1981;304:365.
131. Solomon S, Cappa KG. Impotence and bicycling. A seldom-reported connection. Postgrad Med 1987;81:99–102.
132. Stewart JD, Angus E, Gendron D. Sciatic neuropathies. Br Med J 1983;287:1108–1109.
133. Gold S. Unicyclist's sciatica—a case report. N Engl J Med 1981;305:231–232.
134. Haig AJ. Pedal pusher's palsy. N Engl J Med 1989;320:63.
135. Spiegel PG Johnston MJ, Harvey JP Jr. Complete sciatic nerve laceration in a closed femoral shaft fracture. J Trauma 1974;14:617–621.
136. Zimmerman JE, Afshar F, Friedman W, et al. Posterior compartment syndrome of the thigh with a sciatic palsy: case report. J Neurosurg 1977;46:369–372.
137. Jones BV, Ward MW. Myositis ossificans in the biceps femoris muscles causing sciatic nerve palsy. J Bone Joint Surg 1980;62B:506–507.
138. Gristina JA, Horelick MG. An uncommon location and complication of myositis ossificans: a case presentation. Contemp Orthop 1981;3:1035–1037.
139. Sunderland S. The relative susceptibility to injury of the medial and lateral popliteal divisions of the sciatic nerve. Br Med J 1953;41:2–4.
140. Pace JB, Nagle D. Piriformis syndrome. West J Med 1976;124:435–439.
141. Solheim LF, Siewers P, Paus B. The piriformis muscle syndrome: sciatic nerve entrapment treated with section of the piriformis muscle. Acta Orthop Scand 1981;52:73–75.
142. Arnoldussen WJ, Korten JJ. Pressure neuropathy of the posterior femoral cutaneous nerve. Clin Neurol Neurosurg 1980;82:57–60.
143. Brozin IH, Martfel J, Goldberg I, Kuritzky A. Traumatic closed femoral neuropathy. J Trauma 1982;22:158–160.
144. Miller EH, Benedict FE. Stretch of the femoral nerve in a dancer. J Bone Joint Surg 1985;67A:315–317.
145. Simeone JF, Robinson F, Rothman SL, et al. Computerized tomographic demonstration of a retroperintoneal hematoma causing femoral neuropathy: report of 2 cases. J Neurosurg 1977;47:946–948.
146. Fabian RH, Norcross KA, Hancock MB. Surfer's neuropathy. N Engl J Med 1987;316:555.
147. Ecker AD, Wolman HW. Meralgia paresthetica: a report of 150 cases. JAMA 1938;110:1650–1652.
148. MacGregor J, Moncur JA: Meralgia paresthetica—a sports lesion in girl gymnasts. Br J Sports Med 1977;1:16–19.
149. White J. The results of traction injuries to the common peroneal nerve. J Bone Joint Surg [Br] 1968;50:346–350.
150. Streib EW. Traction injury of peroneal nerve caused by minor athletic trauma. Arch Neurol 1983;40:62–63.
151. Massey EW, Pleet AB. Neuropathy in joggers. Am J Sports Med 1978;6:209–211.
152. Leach RE, Purnell MB, Saito A. Peroneal nerve entrapment in runners. Am J Sports Med 1989;17:287–291.
153. Nobel W. Peroneal palsy due to hematoma in the common peroneal nerve sheath after distal torsional fractures and inversion ankle sprains. J Bone Joint Surg 1966;48A:1484–1495.
154. Ekelund AL. Bilateral nerve entrapment in the popliteal space. Am J Sports Med 1990;18:108.
155. Dewitt LD, Greenberg HS. Roller disco neuropathy. JAMA 1981;246:836.
156. Garfin S, Mubarak SJ, Owen CA. Exertional antero-lateral compartment syndrome. Case report with fascial defect, muscle herniation, and superficial peroneal-nerve entrapment. J Bone Joint Surg 1977;59A:404–405.
157. Davies JAK. Peroneal compartment syndrome secondary to rupture of the peroneus longus. J Bone Joint Surg 1979;61A:783–784.
158. Schon LC, Baxter DE. Neuropathies of the food and ankle in athletes. Clin Sports Med 1990;9:489–509.
159. Henrickson AS, Westlin NE. Chronic calcaneal pain in athletes: Entrapment of the calcaneal nerve? Am J Sports Med 1984;12:152–154.
160. Gould N, Trevino A. Sural nerve entrapment by avulsion fracture of the base of the fifth metatarsal bone. Foot Ankle 1981;2:153–155.
161. Dyck PJ, Classen SM, Stevens JC, O'Brien PC. Assessment of nerve damage in the feet of long-distance runners. Mayo Clin Proc 1987;62:568–572.
162. Jacobson RI. More "goggle headache": supraorbital neuralgia. N Engl J Med 1983;308:1363.

47 / HEAD INJURIES

Donald W. Marion

Introduction

In the United States, sports and recreational activities cause far fewer head injuries than do motor vehicle accidents, falls, or assaults. Because the brain is so intolerant of trauma, however, head injuries that do occur in sports are often more debilitating to the athlete than injuries involving most other areas of the body. Moreover, rehabilitation of the damaged brain is not nearly as successful as rehabilitation of a damaged limb. Although the treatment of head trauma has made great strides over the past 20 years, those who suffer a severe injury and are rendered comatose for a prolonged period still are unlikely to recover fully from all neurologic or cognitive impairment.

The team sports that most commonly cause head injuries are the contact sports, primarily football, boxing, rugby, and ice hockey. Other sports associated with a high risk are gymnastics, diving, horseback riding, bicycling, and skiing. Fortunately, these activities do not often result in injuries severe enough to cause prolonged coma. "Mild" head injuries are quite common in contact sports, however, and there now is a large amount of data indicating that these injuries can lead to substantial and, at times, incapacitating behavioral and cognitive deficiencies. Persistent dizziness, headaches, inattentiveness, or memory problems can impair an athlete's performance significantly and preclude his or her return to play. In addition, recent studies have found that sustaining one mild head injury increases the vulnerability to future injury (1).

The best treatment for head injury is prevention. The use of protective head gear in most contact sports significantly limits the severity of injury from a cranial impact. Yet protective helmets still are not worn in many situations that pose a significant risk of injury, such as bicycle riding. In some sports, the best preventive measure would be modifications that eliminate particularly dangerous practices such as "high sticking" in ice hockey.

After reviewing the epidemiology of sports-related traumatic brain injury, this chapter will describe the anatomic and physiologic characteristics of the various types of head injury and their treatment and prognosis. Finally, the cognitive sequelae of minor head injury will be discussed as well as return-to-play issues.

Epidemiology

Because most severe head injuries occur between 14 and 30 years of age, they account for more potential years of life lost than do cancer and cardiovascular disease combined. In 1984, an estimated 500,000 hospital admissions or deaths in the United States resulted from traumatic brain injury (2). Between 3% and 10% of these were caused by sports or recreational activities. Of the 43,000 outpatient emergency department visits for head injuries in the state of Pennsylvania in 1988, 13% were caused by a sports-related injury (3). Table 47.1 provides the incidence of head injuries among various sports considered to be particularly hazardous.

Published statistics are not available for minor head injuries, that is, for those that lead to a brief period of confusion but allow the player to return to competition within minutes. Even in those sports causing the highest incidence of head trauma, however, the great majority of injuries are minor and do not require hospitalization. A 10-year survey of football injuries in the U.S. determined that the yearly incidence of severe head injuries causing intracranial hemorrhage was no more than 4/100,000 among college athletes and less than 2/100,000 among high school students (4). The study also found that only 1/100,000 football players in college and half as many in high school died each year of a head injury. During the 1975–1984 seasons, a total of 69 deaths resulted from head injuries in organized football at all levels of play; 87% of these were caused by a subdural hematoma (5).

Minor head injuries are not necessarily innocuous, however. They not only can cause immediate confusion and alterations of consciousness, but also can lead to prolonged headaches, dizziness, memory difficul-

Table 47.1.
Incidence of Head Injuries/Concussions in Selected Series of Several of the Highest Risk Sports[a]

Sport	Incidence (%) Among	
	Population of Participants	Injured Participants
Football, college (54, 55)	34	4.5
Football, high school (1, 56)	19	5
Boxing, adults (57, 58)	5–6[b]	81
Bicycling, college (59)	5	18
Rugby, college (60)	NA	15
Ice hockey, professional (61)	NA	13
Horseback riding, adults (62)	NA	9
Alpine skiing, young adults (63)	NA	4

[a] These statistics include only those athletes who come to medical attention.
[b] Incidence of those knocked unconscious. NA, not available.

ties, and irritability. These symptoms are a part of the postconcussion syndrome and can be so severe that they limit the athlete's ability to function in the sport, at work, or in school. In soccer, a sport in which players frequently use their heads to hit the ball, a recent study revealed that 16.4% of players complained of some constellation of postconcussive symptoms (6).

The risk of head injury from bicycling accidents is low, relative to most other sports. Nonetheless, bicycle riding is an increasingly popular activity that causes an estimated 1300 deaths each year, and the cause of death is attributed to head trauma in 70% to 80% of all bicycling fatalities (7). The estimated chance that a fall from a bicycle will cause a head injury is 50%, and a fall from a bicycle traveling 20 mph can be fatal if the unprotected head strikes a hard object (8).

As the typical age of bicycle riders has increased over the past several years, so has the age of those suffering severe head injuries. In the 1960s, most victims of fatal bicycling accidents were under 15 years of age, whereas in 1985, two-thirds of bicycling fatalities occurred in those older than that. Thompson and colleagues found that the use of an approved bicycle helmet reduced the risk of brain injury by 88% (9). Despite these facts, it is estimated that fewer than 1% of bicycle riders wear an approved helmet.

Helmet use also has been shown to reduce the frequency of head trauma in football and ice hockey (10, 11). In football, the number of head-injury related fatalities that occurred between 1975 and 1984 was dramatically lower than in the previous 10 years (69 vs. 162 deaths) (5). This sharp decline was attributed partially to the first national safety standards for football helmets, which went into effect for college football in 1978 and for high school football in 1980. Unfortunately, few well-designed studies have been conducted to establish the safety factors for these helmets. Nevertheless, most experts agree that the best helmets are those with a hard shell and polystyrene liners (12). Under impact conditions that emulate contact sports, such helmets have proved far superior to the once-popular suspension helmets, which no longer are recommended for use (13). The thickness of the liner, and not the rigidity of the shell, has been correlated most closely with protection from severe head injury. Because impact distorts the liner, causing it to lose some of its thickness, either the helmet or the liner should be replaced after each severe impact.

Changes in the rules of play over the past 20 to 30 years have been another measure designed to reduce the number and severity of head injuries in particularly high-risk sports such as football, ice hockey, and boxing. In 1976, the National Collegiate Athletic Association and the National Federation of State High School Athletic Associations implemented severe penalties for intentionally striking a runner with the crown of a helmet and for "spearing." Such rule changes share the credit with helmet improvements for the reduction in fatal head injuries in this sport. For boxing, most states now impose mandatory suspensions for boxers who suffer even minor head injuries. In ice hockey, however, the current penalty system seems ineffective in reducing head injuries. Pforringer and Smasal reviewed the causes of head injury in 246 ice-hockey players and concluded that 76% were caused by violence that was not a necessary part of the game: 45% from a blow with a hockey stick (high sticking), 20% from a deliberate push, and 11% from a fist fight (14). Less than 20% of the head injuries were caused by mechanisms of injury traditionally associated with hockey, such as checking, sliding into the boards, or being hit by a hockey puck. Thus, more stringent rules appear to be necessary in this sport.

Anatomy and Pathology

The management and prognosis of head injuries are related not only to the severity of the injury, but also to the cause. There are important differences in the treatment required for various types of brain injury and in their neurologic prognoses, depending to a large extent on the mechanism of injury. It is useful to consider a head injury as either a closed or a penetrating wound, because each has certain unique characteristics. Closed head injuries are those in which the entire head undergoes translational or rotational acceleration, and this motion damages the enclosed brain or its covering. In penetrating head injuries, a missile or missile fragments actually pierce the skull and brain. Penetrating injuries are subdivided further into low-velocity and high-velocity injuries, the latter usually being a gunshot wound.

Closed Head Injuries

Most sports-related head injuries result from the rapid acceleration or deceleration of the brain within the skull after a blunt force has been applied to the head. Fortunately, the victim usually is not permanently disabled and may only lose consciousness or experience amnesia briefly after the impact. The incidence of severe injury causing prolonged loss of consciousness or requiring surgical intervention is very low, and sports injuries rank far behind motor vehicle accidents and falls as causes of fatal head injuries.

Mild closed head injuries commonly are referred to as concussions, and, traditionally, this term has excluded anatomic disruption of brain tissue. Rather, there is a transient, physiologic disruption leading to a brief loss of consciousness or amnesia surrounding the traumatic event. However, recent studies have demonstrated that even these "mild" injuries can cause profound long-term behavioral or cognitive deficits that severely limit the victim's ability to perform in sports, in school, or at work (15).

More severe trauma can cause injuries of various types to the soft tissues surrounding the skull, fractures of the skull, blood clots between the skull and the brain, or damage to the brain itself. The types of injuries sustained depend on the mechanism of injury and, in the case of low-velocity injuries, on the location of impact on the skull. Therefore, knowledge of the mechanism and location of the injury can help the physician to anticipate the type and severity of damage that might follow the accident.

Hematomas and focal contusions that produce a mass effect and require immediate surgical intervention are much more common after low-velocity blunt trauma to the head, such as occurs with falls or assaults. In contrast, head injuries caused by motor vehicle accidents are more likely to involve diffuse injury to the brain with brain swelling but often do not cause hematomas or other focal mass lesions requiring surgery. With high-speed motor vehicle accidents in particular, the injury often has a prominent rotational component. Because the cortex of the brain is more dense than the underlying white matter, severe rotational forces cause disproportionate acceleration of these two layers, leading to shear injuries at the gray-white interface. This kind of injury leads to diffuse brain swelling and is often neurologically devastating but usually does not lead to large hematomas that require emergent surgery.

Blunt trauma can cause a contusion, abrasion, or laceration of the scalp. The scalp is composed of five layers: the skin, subcutaneous fibrous tissues, the galea aponeurotica, loose areolar tissue underlying the galea, and the pericranium attached to the outer table of the skull (Fig. 47.1). A blunt injury of the scalp can rupture the small vessels within it, and the blood from these vessels will tend to dissect into the plane of least resistance, the loose areolar tissue under the galea. Thus, a soft, sometimes boggy area of the scalp found after blunt trauma usually represents a subgaleal hematoma. In the frontal scalp regions, blood can dissect this plane down to the periorbital soft tissues and cause periorbital ecchymoses. Patients with large frontal subgaleal hematomas should be forewarned that they can expect to have "black eyes" in several days.

Trauma to the scalp should raise the suspicion of an underlying skull fracture, which should be investigated radiographically. Skull fractures can occur either over the convexity of the skull or through the skull base. Low-velocity blunt trauma is more likely to cause convexity fractures, whereas basilar skull fractures usually are caused by high-velocity acceleration injuries. Blunt trauma to the surface of the head can cause a linear fracture, the edges of which may or may not be separated. Separation of the fracture edges is referred to as "diastasis." When inspecting x-ray films of the skull for the presence of linear skull fractures, confusion often arises as to which linear markings on the film represent fracture lines and which are normal sutures of the skull. The coronal sutures frequently are mistaken for skull fractures. True skull fractures have smooth, sharp edges and not the serrated edges of sutures (Fig. 47.2). Knowledge of the normal location of the major sutures also helps in distinguishing them from fractures. As might be expected, linear skull fractures are most common in the thinnest areas, which includes the squamous portion of the temporal bones (lateral surfaces of the skull).

The single most important feature of a linear skull fracture is its location relative to major venous sinuses

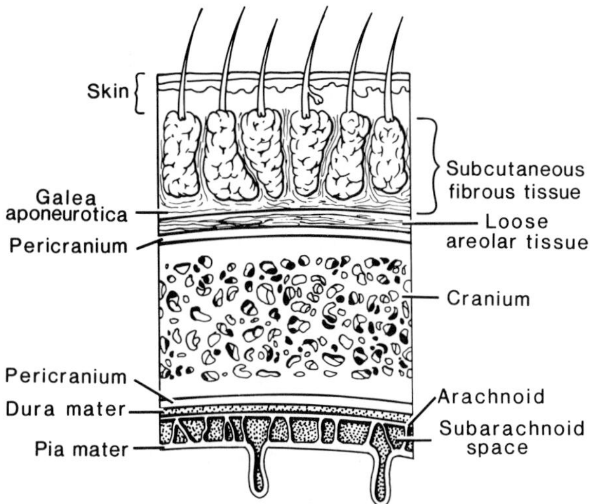

Figure 47.1. Layers of the scalp and meninges.

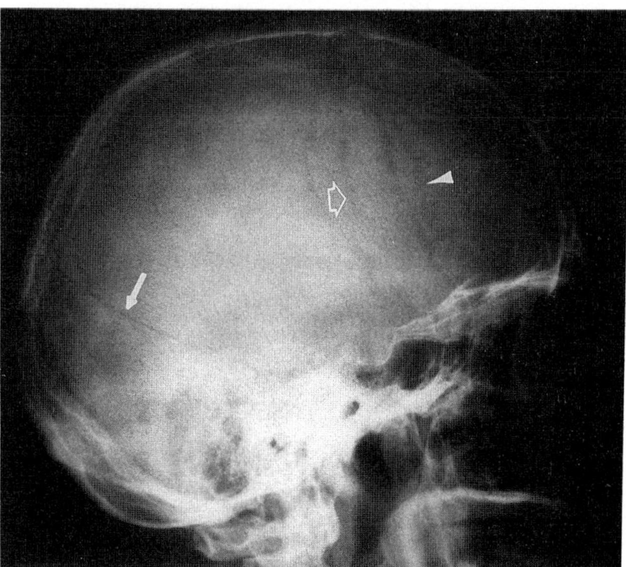

Figure 47.2. Lateral skull radiograph of a linear skull fracture *(solid arrow)*. The sharp edges of the fracture are in contrast to the serrated edges of the coronal suture *(arrowhead)* or the meandering and blurred appearance of normal vascular markings *(open arrow)*.

or arteries that lie adjacent to the inner table of the skull. Convexity fractures that cross the midline at the vertex of the skull or fractures that extend posteriorly and cross the occipital protuberance or nuchal line can disrupt the underlying superior sagittal sinus or transverse sinuses and thus cause an intracranial hemorrhage (Fig. 47.3). Fractures through the temporal bones anterior to the ear can lacerate the middle meningeal artery or one of its branches, causing a massive hemorrhage into the space between the inner table of the skull and the dura mater (epidural hematoma, Fig. 47.4). Linear skull fractures per se usually are not significant problems and rarely require surgical repair, but they do indicate a certain severity of injury. Their presence thus should raise concern about underlying injuries such as intracranial hematomas or cerebral contusions.

Blunt impact to the head also can cause fracture and depression of a skull fragment (depressed skull fracture, Fig. 47.5). If the depressed fragment of bone extends beyond the inner table of the skull, it is likely that the underlying dura has been torn and that the surface of the brain is contused. Depending on the location of the depressed skull fracture, injury to the underlying brain tissue may cause neurologic deficits as well as seizures. The depressed fragment often maintains some continuity with the skull on one side and therefore may maintain some of its blood supply.

"Open" depressed skull fractures can result from severe blunt head injuries, such as when the head is struck by a hockey puck or baseball bat. By definition, an open depressed skull fracture involves a depression of the skull with a laceration of the scalp overlying the depression. An edge of the depressed fragment of skull may lacerate the meninges of the brain and the brain tissue. Thus, risks are present for neurologic dysfunction, depending on the area of the brain that is damaged, and for seizures, because the cerebral cortex has been disrupted. In addition, the scalp laceration opens a direct route from the contaminated scalp and hair to

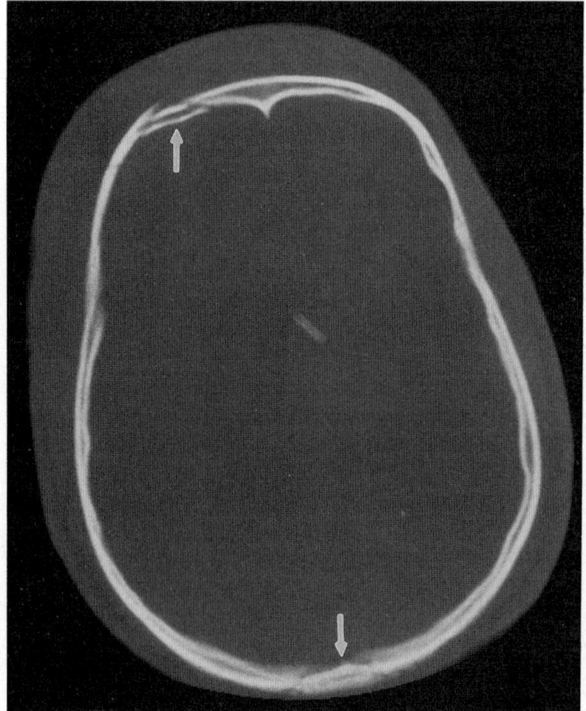

Figure 47.3. Axial CT image of right frontal and occipital comminuted skull fractures. The occipital fracture is particularly ominous because it lies over the superior saggital sinus and may have lacerated it, causing an intracranial hematoma.

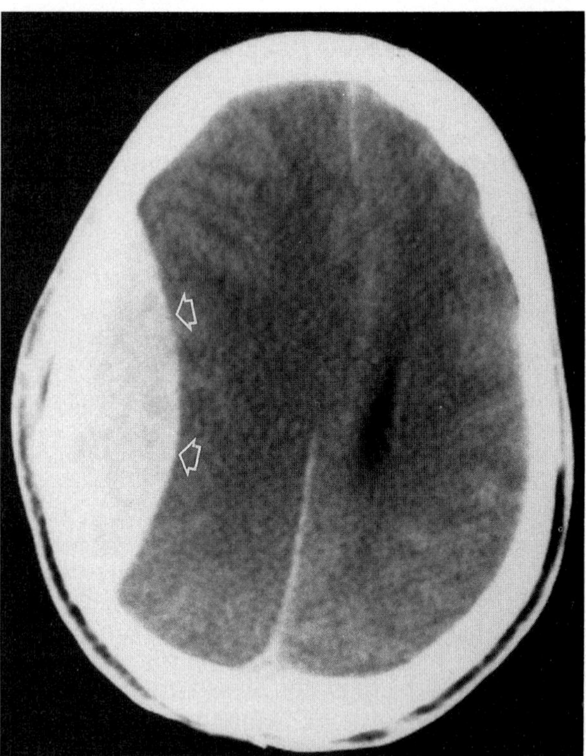

Figure 47.4. Typical appearance of an epidural hematoma on an axial CT image.

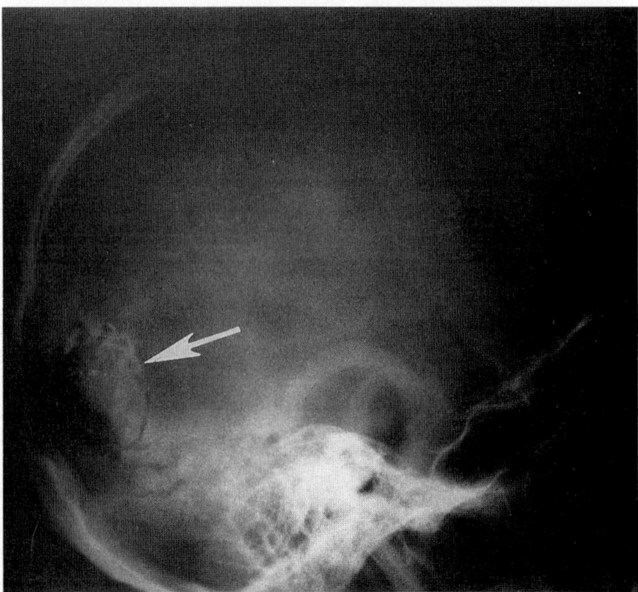

Figure 47.5. A lateral skull radiograph demonstrating a depressed skull fracture.

the depressed bone fragment and cerebrospinal fluid (CSF). As a result, bone-fragment infection, meningitis, or cerebritis can develop. Patients with open, depressed skull fractures therefore require careful observation and antibiotic treatment to help reduce the risk of serious central nervous system (CNS) infections.

Rapid acceleration or deceleration injuries and some forms of blunt impact can cause fractures through the base of the skull. The most common basilar skull fractures are those through the cribriform plates of the anterior cranial fossa. These fractures often are accompanied by laceration of the underlying dura and, if so, result in a CSF communication between the subarachnoid space and the nasal cavities or paranasal sinuses. Because both the nasal cavity and paranasal sinuses normally harbor bacteria, this passage is another potential route of CNS infection. In addition, air can enter the cranial cavity through such a fistula and become trapped, leading to pneumocephalus and producing a mass effect on the brain (tension pneumocephalus). Fractures through the floor of the anterior cranial fossa frequently extend through the orbital rim (Fig. 47.6), rupturing small vessels in the overlying soft tissues or causing bleeding from the bone itself. The resultant bleeding leads to periorbital ecchymoses, commonly called the raccoon's sign; therefore, this sign is a physical indication of a possible basilar skull fracture. Other important signs of a basilar skull fracture are CSF leakage from the nose (CSF rhinorrhea) or profuse bleeding from the nose after blunt head trauma. Fractures through the floor of the anterior cranial fossa also can extend posteriorly and involve the optic canals, damaging the optic nerves. Most anterior basilar skull fractures severe enough to cause CSF rhinorrhea also disrupt the olfactory nerves and cause a loss of the sense of smell.

Basilar skull fractures through the petrous bone are less common than those through the anterior cranial fossa, but they can cause CSF leakage from the ear and a CNS infection. Longitudinal fractures of the petrous bone often continue into the mastoid eminence, and associated bleeding results in ecchymosis over this prominence (Battle's sign). If the fracture extends into the middle ear (Fig. 47.7), bleeding may cause a hemotympanum, and if the tympanic membrane is disrupted, a CSF leak through the external auditory canal can develop (CSF otorrhea). In either case, a conductive hearing loss is common but usually transient. Fractures that traverse the internal auditory canal often damage the seventh and eighth cranial nerves. Consequently, facial paresis and sensorineural hearing loss may develop, and deficits thus caused usually are permanent. All patients suspected of having a posterior basilar skull fracture based on radiographic evidence or on the presence of CSF or on blood leaking from the ear should undergo thorough testing of hearing and facial nerve function.

In short, the real danger from a skull fracture is not the fracture itself, but rather the risk of a CNS infection with open, depressed or basilar skull fractures and, with any skull fracture, the potential for intracranial hemorrhage or cerebral contusion. Contusions or hemorrhage

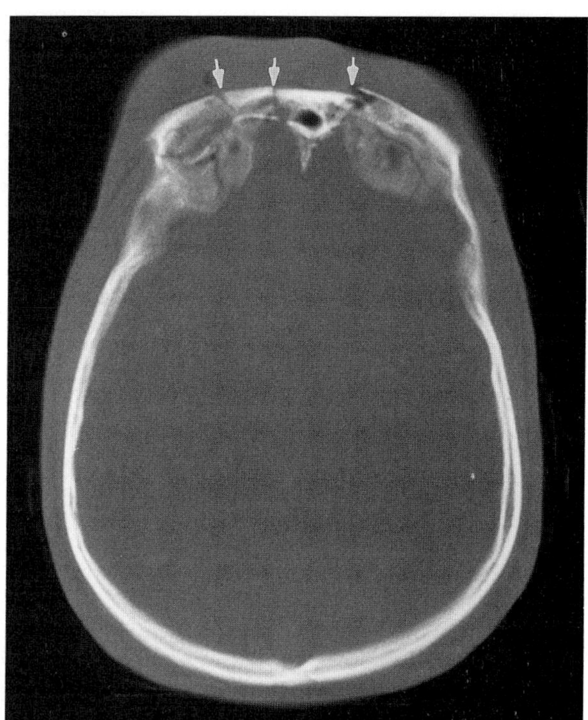

Figure 47.6. Axial CT image showing multiple fractures through the orbital rims, extending into the floor of the anterior fossa.

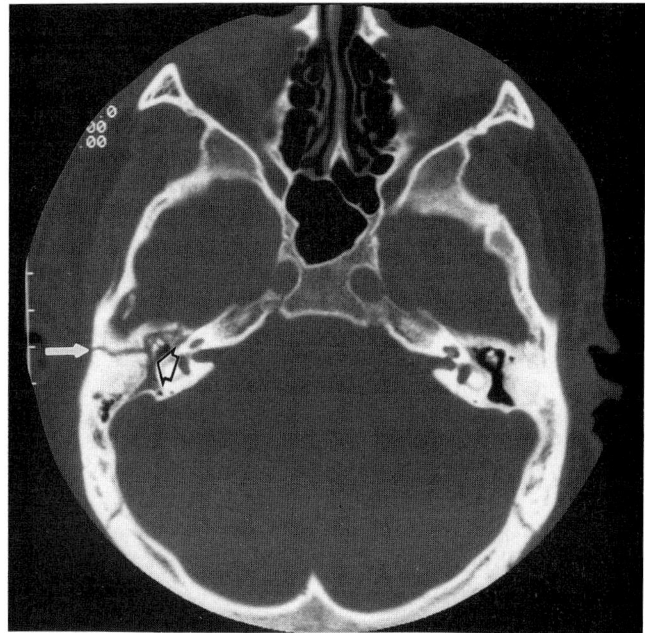

Figure 47.7. A basilar skull fracture involving the petrous bone is seen on this axial CT image *(solid arrow)*. The fracture extends into the middle ear *(open arrow)* and can cause a conductive hearing loss by disrupting the tympanic membrane or the ossicles of the middle ear. The fracture also can cause hemorrhage into the middle ear cavity, which will result in hearing loss.

are not always apparent on the initial CT scan and may take 24 to 48 hours to develop (Fig. 47.8). It has been estimated that intracranial hemorrhage is 20 times more likely to follow a head injury if there is a skull fracture

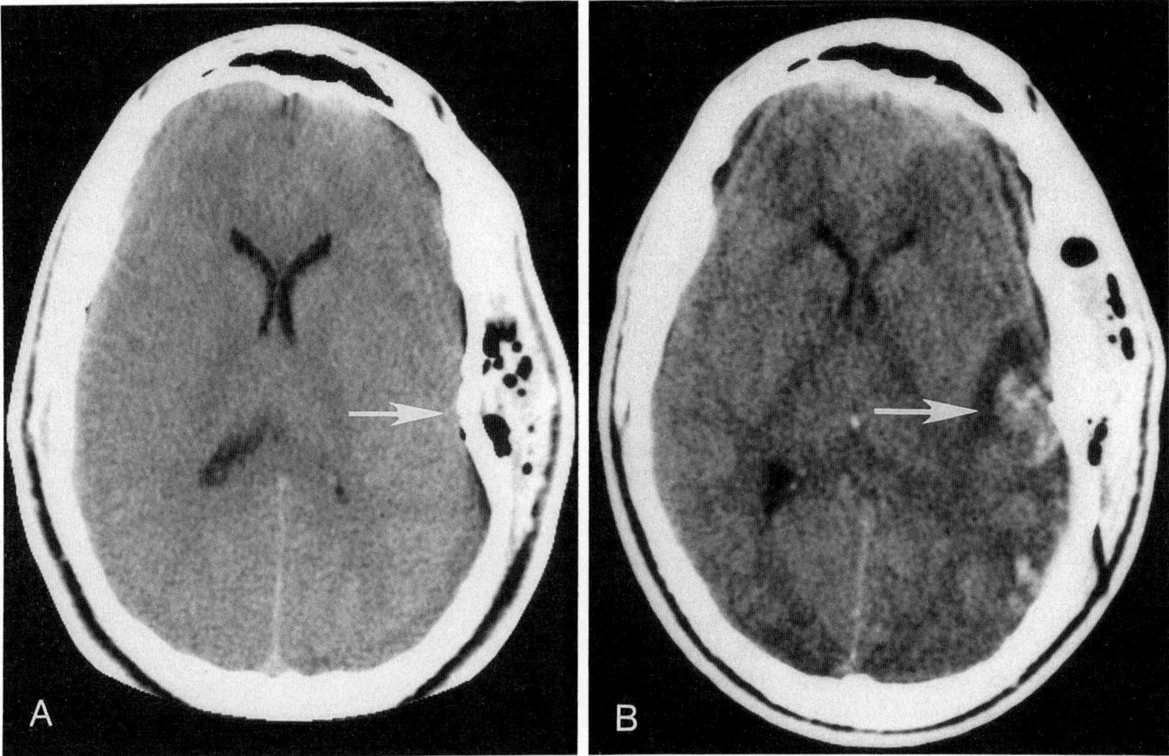

Figure 47.8. Intracranial hemorrhage or cerebral contusions are not always apparent on CT images obtained immediately after the injury. The axial CT images above were obtained from a patient with a left-sided open depressed skull fracture 3 hours **(A)** and 36 hours **(B)** after the injury. Note the appearance of a hemorrhagic contusion underlying the fracture on the later scan.

than if not (16). Chan and associates studied 418 patients, 11 to 15 years old, who were admitted to their hospital with closed head injuries (17). Twenty-six had skull fractures, and an intracranial hematoma developed in 13 of them, even though, at admission, 10 of these 26 patients had a Glasgow Coma Scale (GCS) score of 15 (alert, oriented, following commands). In contrast, no patient without a skull fracture had an intracranial hematoma. Multivariate analysis of the study population showed that skull fracture was the only significant independent risk factor predictive of intracranial hematoma in adolescents.

Posttraumatic hemorrhage inside the skull can occur in several intracranial compartments, which are separated by the membranes covering the brain, or within the brain substance itself. Between the inner table of the skull and the surface of the brain are three membranes and three potential or real spaces: the epidural potential space, dura mater, subdural (potential) space, arachnoid membrane, subarachnoid space, and pia mater (Fig. 47.1). These membranes and spaces are invested with an abundance of arteries and veins. Rapid acceleration or deceleration, blunt trauma, or skull fractures can lacerate or rupture these vessels, causing them to bleed into any of the three spaces.

Intracranial hematomas that develop after a severe head injury are described according to their location, either within these spaces that surround the brain or within the brain or its ventricles. The most common location for posttraumatic intracranial hemorrhage is the subarachnoid space. A subarachnoid hemorrhage usually can be detected on computed tomographic (CT) images of the brain (Fig. 47.9). The most likely cause of subarachnoid hemorrhage is rupture or tearing of bridging vessels in the subarachnoid space. Posttraumatic subarachnoid hemorrhage usually does not cause permanent neurologic morbidity, although recent evidence suggests that there is a risk of vasospasm (18, 19). Bleeding into the subarachnoid space can cause headaches and neck pain in the first few weeks after a head injury.

The most common intracranial hematoma of surgical consequence is the subdural hematoma. These blood clots most often are seen after relatively low-velocity trauma such as that caused by a fall or an assault. They result from the tearing of larger veins on the surface of the brain or laceration of the cortical surface after a blow to the head. Subdural hematomas thus tend to develop slowly and usually do not cause rapid neurologic deterioration. Often, though, they cause a mass effect that shifts the intracranial contents to the opposite side. When the shift seems out of proportion to the size of the subdural hematoma, there may be diffuse swelling of the ipsilateral hemisphere (Fig. 47.10), and the injury may be more complicated than just a clot. In such cases, surgery to evacuate the clot is treacherous, because swollen brain tissue can herniate through the craniotomy site.

Epidural hematomas occur in the potential space between the dura mater and the inner table of the skull.

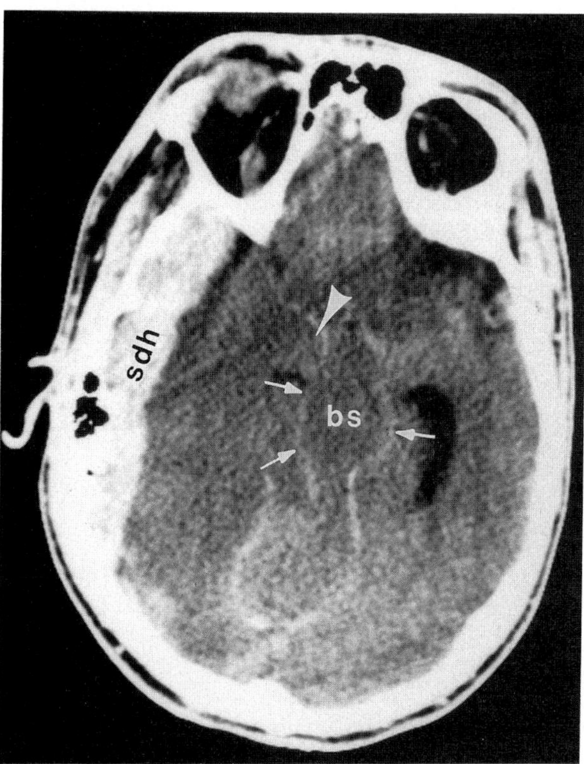

Figure 47.9. Axial CT image demonstrating an acute subdural hematoma (sdh) on the right side, with herniation of the medial temporal lobe into the tentorial notch *(arrowhead)*. The midbrain is outlined by subarachnoid hemorrhage in the perimesencephalic cistern *(arrows)*. bs, brainstem

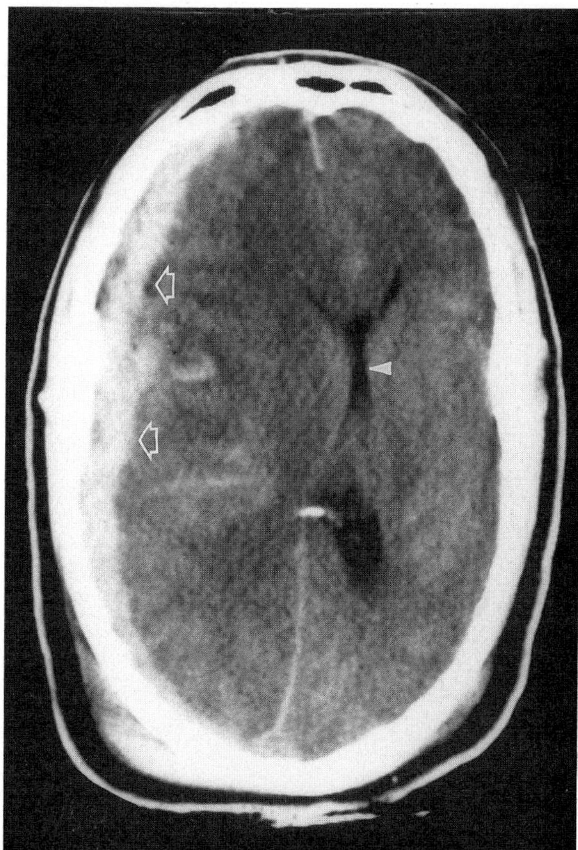

Figure 47.10. Typical appearance of an acute subdural hematoma *(open arrows)* on an axial CT image. The degree of shift of the midline structures *(arrowhead)* is greater than the thickness of the subdural hematoma, suggesting significant parenchymal injury to the hemisphere in addition to the hematoma.

They usually are the result of a tear in the middle meningeal artery caused by a skull fracture in the adjacent temporal bone. In the squamous (lateral) portion of the temporal bone, this artery lies within a groove in the bond (Fig. 47.11). The artery is trapped or tethered at this point, and fractures through the temporal bone easily can tear it, leading to an epidural hematoma. These lesions extend by stripping the dura mater from the inner table of the skull and form clots that have a classic lenticular shape on CT images. Because of their arterial source, epidural hematomas rapidly enlarge and can cause abrupt neurologic deterioration. However, these hematomas rarely cause damage to the underlying brain, and their early evacuation often leads to an excellent recovery.

Severe head trauma can disrupt or contuse the brain parenchyma and vessels within the substance of the brain, leading to intracerebral hematomas or hemorrhagic contusions. The most common sites for these lesions are the anterior portions of the temporal lobes and the inferior portion of the frontal lobes (Fig. 47.12). At these locations, the brain comes in contact with irregular surfaces of the skull (Fig. 47.13) so that rapid shifts of the intracranial contents more easily can cause contusions. However, low-velocity blunt force also can cause focal contusions in other areas of the brain. Depending on the mechanism of the injury, the focal contusion may be adjacent to the point of impact (coup contusion) or contralateral to the point of impact (contrecoup contusion). If the head is in motion before impact with a stationary object, as in a fall, contrecoup damage is usually much more extensive than coup damage. Conversely, if the head is stationary and sustains a severe blow, contrecoup damage is rare and coup damage severe (20).

After very severe injuries, intracerebral hematomas can develop quickly. More often, though, the hematoma will not appear until 12 to 24 hours after the injury, because the source of the hematoma is located in slowly oozing small vessels. Large intracerebral hematomas can cause damage by compressing surrounding tissues or by rupturing into the ventricles of the brain (intraventricular hemorrhage). In most cases, however, posttraumatic intracerebral hematomas are secondary to very severe cerebral contusions, which are the immediate cause of the brain damage.

Intracranial hematomas as well as severe brain swelling can lead to neurologic deterioration by causing a mass effect and shifting of the brain. The intracranial contents are divided into three compartments by two semirigid dural membranes—the falx cerebri and the tentorium cerebelli (Fig. 47.14). The tentorium cerebelli separates the posterior cranial fossa from the

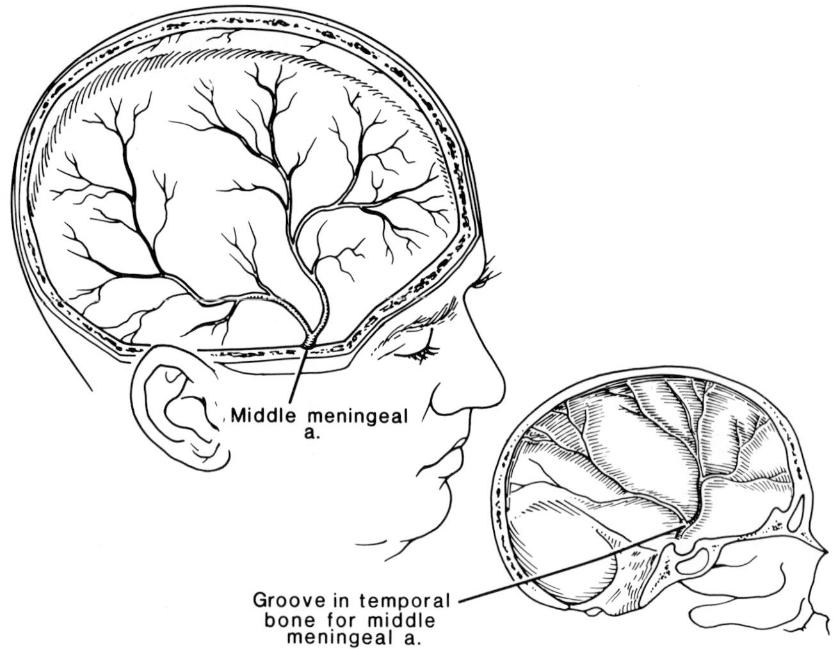

Figure 47.11. The middle meningeal artery is tethered in a groove in the temporal bone and is easily lacerated by fractures through this bone. Hemorrhage from the middle meningeal artery causes an epidural hematoma.

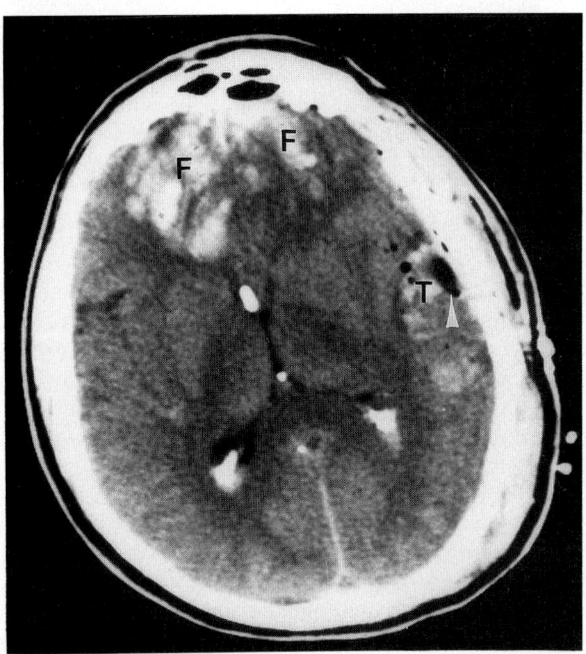

Figure 47.12. Hemorrhagic contusions of the inferior frontal lobes *(F)* and left temporal lobe *(T)* are demonstrated on this axial CT image. The left-sided temporal hemorrhagic contusion also contains air *(arrowhead)*, which was entrained through an overlying scalp laceration, skull fracture, and dural laceration.

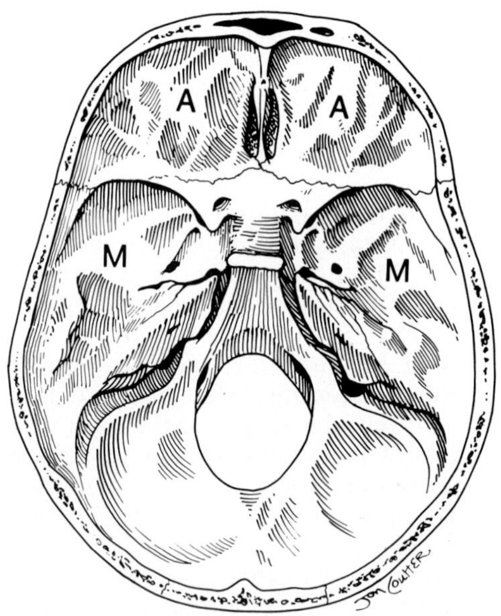

Figure 47.13. The floors of the anterior *(A)* and middle *(M)* cranial fossae are very irregular, and acceleration of the inferior frontal and temporal lobes against these surfaces often causes contusions of these lobes.

middle and anterior fossae. A curvilinear notch, Kernohan's notch, provides an opening between the two compartments, through which the brainstem passes. The midbrain lies within the notch. A second important dividing structure is the falx cerebri, a dural membrane that separates the two hemispheres of the cerebrum. This membrane also is incomplete, and a central opening allows passage of the corpus callosum and the third ventricle. The inferior border of the falx is at the level of the cingulate gyri, which lie just above the corpus callosum.

When a lateral vector of force is produced by a large mass, such as a blood clot or focal brain swelling, there is a potential for herniation of the brain tissue that is adjacent to the openings in these dural partitions. Masses in the temporal or inferior parietal lobe can push the medial temporal lobe (the uncus) into the the tentorial notch (transtentorial herniation, Fig. 47.9). Such herniation can compress the brainstem and cause unconsciousness, because the reticular activating system (responsible for consciousness) is located largely in the midbrain. In addition, transtentorial herniation often causes torsion of the midbrain, from which the third cranial nerve (the oculomotor nerve) emerges, together with its parasympathetic fibers, which provide pupillary constrictor tone. Midbrain torsion can stretch the third cranial nerve, causing a third nerve palsy, manifest by a fixed and dilated pupil. Very severe herniation may affect the third nerve of both sides, whereas moderate herniation affects the nerve only ipsilateral to the herniation. In patients with a head injury, transtentorial herniation most often results from an acute subdural hematoma, but it also can be caused by an epidural hematoma and by intracerebral hematomas or severe brain contusion and swelling in the temporal or parietal lobes. Although less common, diffuse brain swelling involving large portions of both cerebral hemispheres also can cause a rostral-caudal vector of force, leading to transtentorial herniation.

Subfalcine herniation, that is, herniation of the cingulate gyri under the inferior border of the falx cerebri, frequently accompanies acute subdural hematomas or unilateral cerebral swelling. Although the patient usually has no focal neurologic deficit directly attributable to this type of herniation, it can cause compression of the distal branches of the anterior cerebral artery.

Herniation of the cerebellar tonsils into the foramen magnum and compression of the medulla oblongata can result from post-traumatic cerebellar hematomas (Fig. 47.15). Because central control of breathing resides in the medulla oblongata, this type of herniation can cause apnea. Cerebellar tonsillar herniation also can cause lower cranial nerve dysfunction, leading to swallowing and speech difficulties. Severe cerebellar injuries are rare after trauma, however, occurring in less than 5% of patients with severe head injuries.

Penetrating Head Injuries

Penetrating head injuries can be caused by either low-velocity or high-velocity missiles. In most cases, the high-velocity missile is a bullet, and gunshot wounds to the head carry a very high mortality rate. The higher the muzzle velocity of the bullet, the greater the damage to the brain, because the energy imparted to the brain is proportional to the square of the velocity of the bullet. As a high-velocity bullet penetrates the brain, it destroys a cylinder of brain tissue that may be 10 to 20 times the diameter of the bullet (Fig. 47.16). Thus, injuries caused by a high-velocity rifle are much more destructive than those from a relatively low-velocity handgun. The prognosis after a gunshot wound to the head also depends on the trajectory of the bullet. Bullets that traverse the basal ganglia, brainstem, or posterior fossa or that ricochet off the inner table of the skull and traverse the brain several times carry a much higher mortality rate than bullets that penetrate only one lobe or hemisphere of the brain.

Low-velocity penetrating head injuries generally cause much less brain damage and, therefore, are associated with a much better prognosis. These are the kinds of injuries likely to occur in sports such as javelin throw or archery. Although the neurologic sequelae of low-velocity penetrating injuries largely depend on the location of the injury, several other issues also must be considered. Slow penetration of brain tissue by a missile causes direct damage, and the location of the dam-

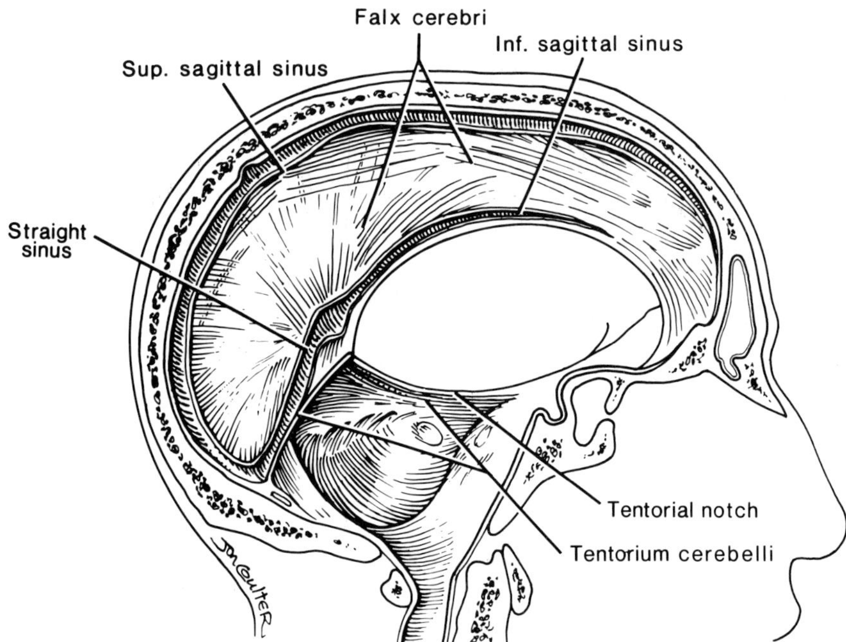

Figure 47.14. Location of the falx cerebri and tentorium cerebelli within the skull.

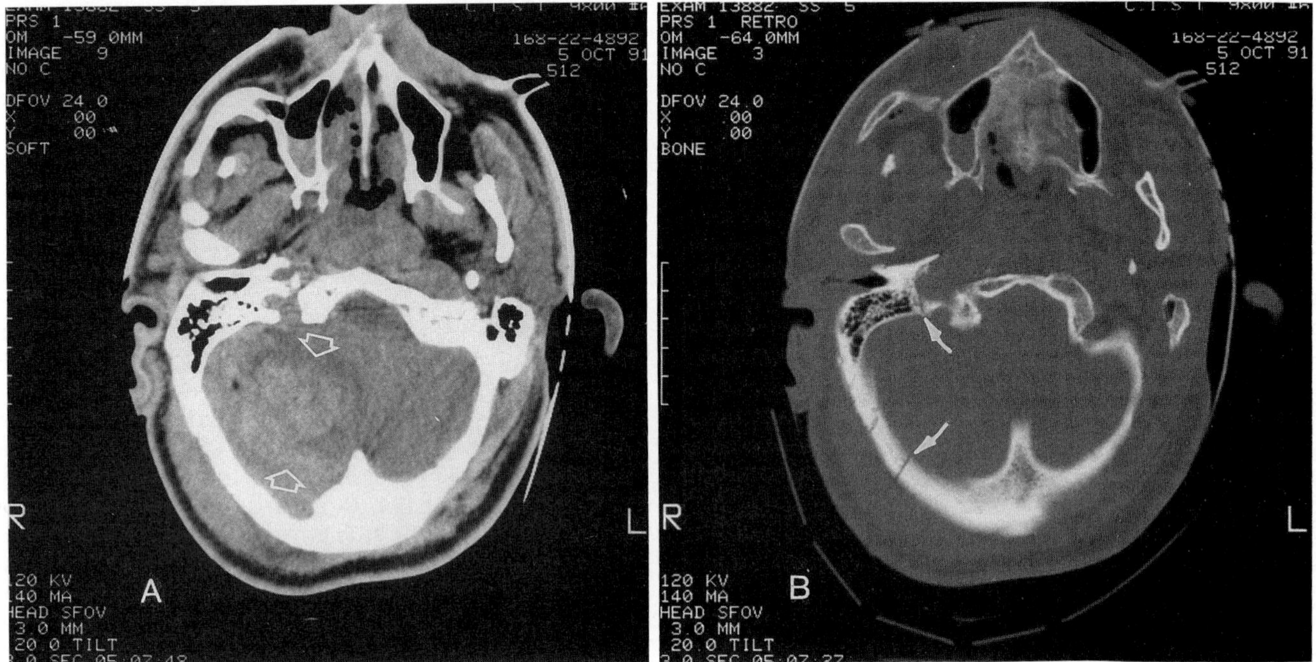

Figure 47.15. A, B. Axial CT images demonstrate a hemorrhagic contusion of the right cerebellar hemisphere **(A)** associated with a fracture through the floor of the posterior fossa on the right side **(B).**

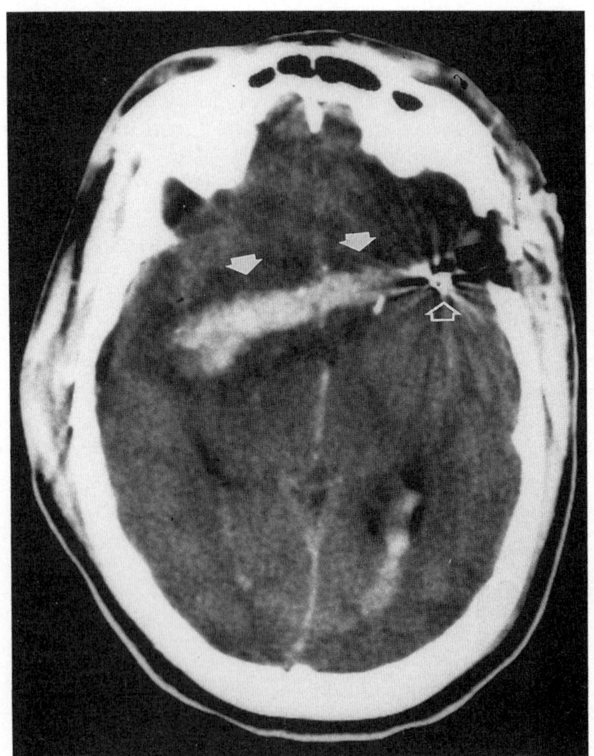

Figure 47.16. Hemorrhagic contusion and edema demarcate the bullet path in this axial CT image *(closed arrows).* A fragment of the bullet is visible in the left temporal lobe *(open arrow).*

aged brain tissue determines what neurologic deficits can be expected. For example, if a missile damages a large portion of the motor cortex on the left side, the patient will have right-sided hemiparesis. Cerebral blood vessels also may be damaged, causing much more devastating injuries. If the injury causes occlusion of a major cerebral artery, the result can be infarction of the brain tissue supplied by that artery (a stroke) and subsequent hemiparesis, aphasia, or both. Rupture of a major vessel can cause development of a life-threatening blood clot (a subdural or intracerebral hematoma) that will require immediate surgical evacuation.

Because the intracranial portion of a missile, such as an arrow or knife, may be acting as a tamponade in a large vessel, a missile usually should not be removed until the patient is in the operating room, where the surgeon can deal with the hemorrhage that might result. An insidious consequence of some penetrating injuries is damage to the wall of an artery that weakens the wall but does not cause an immediate hemorrhage. Weeks or even years later, the pulsatile action of the blood on this weakened area can cause an aneurysm to develop and rupture, leading to a sudden and often fatal intracerebral hemorrhage. Because of the potential for vascular damage and a sudden intracranial hemorrhage, most authorities advocate cerebral angiography as part of the initial evaluation of patients who suffer penetrating head injuries.

Infection and seizures are two other potential complications of penetrating head injuries. Missiles that pierce the skull and outer meninges of the brain carry with them fragments of skin and hair laden with bacteria. For this reason, there is an estimated 10% chance that an infection will develop in the brain or its coverings after a penetrating head injury. Potential infections include cerebritis, cerebral abscess, meningitis, and vasculitis; they usually are caused by typical skin flora (staphylococci streptococci, or Gram-negative rods). High-velocity missile injuries frequently carry skin and fragments of bone from the skull deep into the brain, and infected bone fragments are particularly difficult to treat. However, most such wounds can be treated successfully with early (within 12 hours) debridement of the entrance wound and superficial missile tract in the brain, closure of the dura and scalp, and a 10- to 15-day course of intravenously administered antibiotics. The antibiotic choice should provide both Gram-negative and Gram-positive coverage and good CNS penetration. We advocate using a third-generation cephalosporin and an aminoglycoside.

Most penetrating head injuries pose a risk of seizures. The degree of risk depends on the location of brain penetration (the motor strip and adjacent cortex are most sensitive), the extent of brain injury, and the presence of an infection. Nevertheless, most patients with such injuries should be given anticonvulsants prophylactically, either carbamazepine (Tegretol) or phenytoin (Dilantin), for 6 months. Both drugs have proven equally effective in lowering the risk for posttraumatic seizures (21). Anticonvulsant levels should be monitored once a month to avoid toxicity from high serum levels. Because Tegretol can cause leukopenia, which is usually reversible, weekly white blood cell counts also should be monitored during the first month that a patient takes this drug and once a month thereafter. Dilantin is associated with an elevation of liver enzymes in some patients; therefore, liver function tests should be performed on a similar schedule for patients taking this drug.

The prognosis after a penetrating head injury is related closely to the neurologic status of the patient immediately after the injury and to the velocity of the missile. Among patients who suffer a gunshot wound to the head and are rendered comatose, 80% will die, whereas a good outcome can be expected for more than 80% of those who have a low-velocity missile wound to the head and are conscious after the injury.

Primary Injury Versus Secondary Injury

Trauma to the head causes mechanical deformation of the brain, which can result in various degrees of physiologic and anatomic disruption of brain tissue, depending on the severity of the impact. Disruption of brain tissue that occurs at the time of the impact is called "primary brain injury" and, if severe enough, the patient will die within minutes or hours after the injury. Although the majority of patients who are comatose after head trauma do not have severe primary brain injury, many still succumb within days of weeks after the incident. Often, brain swelling and ischemia develop, followed by brain death.

Brain injury that occurs after the traumatic event is referred to as "secondary brain injury." Whereas severe primary brain injury generally is considered irreversible, secondary brain injury may be treatable and reversible. The existence of secondary brain injury and the potential for effective intervention are supported by several lines of evidence. Povlishock demonstrated that some types of structural brain damage previously thought to be the result of the impact, such as diffuse axonal injury, actually do not appear until 24 to 48 hours after impact and likely are caused by potentially reversible metabolic consequences of secondary brain injury (22). In addition, many patients with a severe head injury have a relatively lucid period prior to neurologic deterioration, suggesting that much of the brain injury does not occur at the time of impact but is the result of later events occurring in the brain.

Local or regional ischemia is the most likely cause of secondary brain injury. Graham and colleagues found ischemic cell changes to be common in patients who died after a severe head injury (23). Moreover, the author and colleagues have documented abnormally low cerebral blood flow in patients during the first 4 to 6 hours after a severe head injury (24), and studies of cerebral oxygen extraction and lactate production indicate that such low blood flow reflects ischemia (25). Ischemic cell damage, at least in part, represents an excitotoxic lesion caused by enhanced release and/or diminished uptake of glutamate or related excitatory amino acids. Normally, glutamate is cleared rapidly from the synapse after its release, but during ischemia, the glutamate concentration at the synapses surrounding the focal ischemic lesion can be increased for sustained periods. The toxic action of this and related excitatory amino acids is caused mainly by enhanced calcium influx into the cell. High intracellular levels of calcium initiate several biochemical reactions that ultimately lead to the production of free radicals. Ionized intracellular calcium is a catalyst for the arachidonic acid cascade and lipid peroxidation and interrupts normal oxidative phosphorylation. The metabolic byproducts of these reactions are free radicals. Free radicals are toxic to cell membranes and cause their disruption (Fig. 47.17). They also may disable autoregulatory mechanisms of the cerebral vessels, leading to vasodilation and cerebral hyperemia. The end result is brain swelling, which can cause increased intracranial pressure, compromised cerebral blood flow, and further brain damage or brain death.

The recent discovery and characterization of these biochemical events, occurring within the first few hours after injury and leading to brain swelling, have provided a number of opportunities for therapeutic intervention. A recent clinical study demonstrated that administering high doses of methylprednisolone, a free radical scavenger, in the first 24 hours after CNS (spinal cord) trauma led to an improved neurologic outcome (26). Ongoing clinical studies are evaluating other

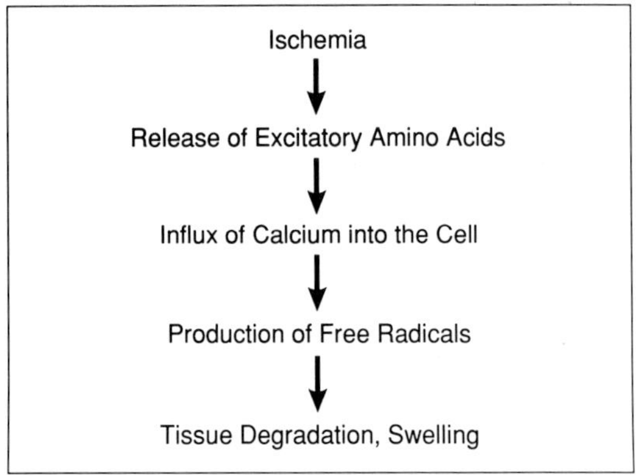

Figure 47.17. The progression of major neurochemical and physiologic events thought to be responsible for secondary brain injury.

free radical scavengers, such as 21-aminosteroids and superoxide dismutase. Clinical investigators also are studying the efficacy of treatment to reduce the extracellular concentration of excitatory amino acids (moderate hypothermia), the blockade of the membrane-bound receptors mediating calcium entry into the cell (MK-801, naloxone), and the blockade of the arachidonic acid cascade with nonsteroidal antiinflammatory agents. Results of this research should be available within the next 2 to 3 years. Rather than any individual measure, however, the optimal treatment for secondary brain injury probably will be some combination of these therapies. It also is anticipated that some types of brain injuries will respond better to one combination and other types to different combinations.

Management

Prehospital Treatment

The initial treatment of patients with head injuries depends largely on the severity of the injury. Nevertheless, several principles apply regardless of the severity. The most important of these is that attention be focused on the entire individual and not just the CNS. In most sports-related head injuries, victims will have only a brief loss of consciousness from which they recover rapidly. Persons who have no neck or back pain and no major injury elsewhere can be allowed to walk. To estimate the duration of pretraumatic and posttraumatic amnesia, injury victims should be asked about the incident with special attention given to their recollection of the events immediately before and immediately after it occurred. They also should be asked several questions to determine the level of their orientation and attention span (e.g., their name, address, the date, and where they are) and short- and long-term memory (e.g., the names of the president and vice-president and a description of a recent event). In addition, calculation abilities are tested by asking the victim to subtract 7 from 100 and to continue subtracting 7 from each subsequent answer. Finally, abstract thinking is tested, for example, by asking what they would do if they were in a crowded theater and smelled smoke. Many of these questions, particularly the serial sevens, provide information about attention span as well as calculation and other abilities.

Responses to these questions also provide a quick estimate of the victim's response time, ability to function independently, and general ability to perform on the playing field. Problems in responding to these questions suggest that the patient may not be able to function well and should not be allowed to return to play until the sensorium has cleared. In many cases, the sensorium clears within 10 to 15 minutes and activity may be resumed.

Those who are unresponsive for longer than 5 minutes have a more severe head injury; their evaluation and treatment must proceed rapidly and systematically. The first priority is to establish and maintain adequate breathing, including intubation if necessary. Intubation of an unresponsive patient with a head injury can be difficult and should be performed only by someone experienced in the necessary technique. The presence of a cervical spine fracture should be presumed; therefore, the patient's neck must not be hyperextended to facilitate intubation.

Blind nasotracheal intubation usually is the safest intubation technique when cervical spine instability is suspected, but orotracheal intubation occasionally can be accomplished without extending the neck. If the first responders are not comfortable with these intubation techniques, the patient with respiratory distress is often best treated by bag-valve-mask ventilatory assistance until more experienced personnel arrive or the patient has been transported to an emergency department. Portable pulse oximetry equipment is becoming widely available and provides immediate information about the adequacy of ventilation.

While emergency resuscitation is underway, the cervical spine should be immobilized by a second person, who applies gentle axial traction to the head. Angular movement of the neck must be avoided in the patient who is comatose or complains of neck pain. If the athlete is wearing a helmet, the helmet should be left in place until arrival at an emergency care facility. A face mask, if present, may need to be removed to provide adequate access to the airway. If this cannot be done without removing the helmet from a patient who is in respiratory distress, the helmet can be removed if one person supports the patient's neck and applies gentle axial traction while another person manually distracts the sides of the helmet and slides it off. Bolt cutters, if available, should be used on the face mask.

The next priority is the patient's blood pressure. Venous access always should be established as soon as possible for obtunded patients, preferably by inserting a large-bore (14- to 16-gauge) catheter in a large arm vein. Measurement of the blood pressure or assessment of skin color and capillary refill will provide vital information. If the patient is hypotensive (systolic blood pressure <90 mm Hg), 500-cc boluses of isotonic saline should be given as rapidly as possible. Pressure dressings are applied to any site of active bleeding. Posttraumatic hypotension never is due to an intracranial hemorrhage and most commonly is caused by intraabdominal hemorrhage.

These basic principles of hemodynamic and pulmonary resuscitation are included in this chapter on head injuries because hypotension and hypoxia occurring immediately after the injury are important causes of permanent brain damage and can undermine any neurosurgical attempts to treat patients with severe head injuries. Because the injured brain is particularly vulnerable to ischemia, permanent neurologic deficits often can be avoided if adequate cerebral perfusion and oxygenation are restored soon after a head injury.

After the airway and blood pressure have been attended to and the spine has been immobilized, the patient's neurologic status is assessed and scored according to the GCS (27, 28). This score can be obtained quickly and provides important information about the patient's neurologic status in a convenient shorthand that can be transmitted to neurosurgeons and emergency medicine physicians at the receiving hospital. The overall GCS score ranges from 3 to 15 and is composed of points assigned as follows: motor response, 1 to 6; verbal response, 1 to 5; and eye-opening response, 1 to 4 (Table 47.2). The highest scores in each category are assigned when a patient can comprehend and respond appropriately to verbal requests; the lowest scores, when there is no response even to painful stimuli. Testing is an active process—the tester must provide verbal stimuli and, if the patient does not respond, must apply painful stimuli in the form of a sternal rub or supraorbital pressure. When there is asymmetry of the right and left eye-opening or of motor scores, the side with the best scores is used for calculating the GCS.

The size and reactivity of the patient's pupils also should be observed. Normally, pupils are 3 to 7 mm in diameter, depending on the ambient light, and they constrict briskly in response to direct light. A pupil that does not respond to light or is larger than 8 mm in diameter may indicate transtentorial herniation of the medial temporal lobes caused by an intracranial blood clot or cerebral contusion. However, 20% of the population normally may appear to have asymmetric pupils, and 5% have measurable differences of 1 to 2 mm (29). Therefore, if the patient is alert and awake, the finding of asymmetric pupils after a minor head injury generally does not indicate significant intracranial injury.

Table 47.2.
Glasgow Coma Scale (27, 28)

	Score
Eye Opening	
Eyes open spontaneously	4
Eyes open to verbal command	3
Eyes open only with painful stimuli	2
No eye opening	1
Verbal Response	
Oriented and converses	5
Disoriented and converses	4
Inappropriate words	3
Incomprehensible sounds	2
No verbal response	1
Motor Response	
Obeys verbal commands	6
Response to painful stimuli (upper extremities):	
Localizes pain	5
Withdraws from pain	4
Flexor posturing	3
Extensor posturing	2
No motor response	1

Total Score = Eye + Verbal + Motor and ranges from 3 to 15 points

If a patient has a GCS score of 9 to 15, the brain injury usually is not severe and is unlikely to require surgery. For those with a GCS score of 8 or less, however, the probability of a surgical intracranial mass lesion is much higher. This group of severely injured patients almost always benefits from early endotracheal intubation. If the patient's neurologic status remains stable, the ventilatory rate should be approximately 12 breaths/minute. Those who deteriorate during transport should receive ventilatory assistance at 20 to 25 breaths/minute to help reduce intracranial pressure. Elevated intracranial pressure, often from a mass lesion such as a hematoma, is a common cause for progressive neurologic deterioration after a head injury, and hyperventilation is a rapid and effective technique for reducing intracranial pressure. However, because ischemia is so common immediately after a head injury, and hyperventilation (>12 breaths/minute) exacerbates cerebral ischemia by causing cerebral vasoconstriction, its use is not recommended for neurologically stable patients.

Patients who have severe head injuries causing prolonged loss of consciousness should be transported as quickly as possible to the emergency department of the nearest trauma center. Trauma centers are those hospitals capable of dealing with all aspects of trauma care and have a surgeon in house at all times. Such hospitals also should have neurosurgical and orthopedic support available within 10 to 15 minutes after the patient arrives. Many states in the U.S. have established mechanisms for systematically evaluating and designating trauma centers, and patients with severe head injuries are best served by rapid transport to such centers. Stopping at a nearby emergency department not equipped to deal with trauma is usually appropriate only if the patient does not have a severe head injury, or if airway or hemodynamic instability persists despite field resuscitation efforts.

Specific indications for transport to a trauma center include either the loss of consciousness or retrograde amnesia lasting more than 5 minutes. Both of these are associated with a significant risk of intracranial hematomas. A victim of a head injury who has any of the following signs or symptoms also should be taken to an emergency room: neck or back pain, disorientation or confusion for longer than 15 minutes; an intense headache, blurred vision or diplopia, a focal neurologic deficit (weakness, numbness), a scalp laceration, or discharge of CSF or blood from the nose or ears. Those who have neck or back pain should be kept immobile during transport. Paramedical personnel should be involved as quickly as possible; such personnel should be skilled in providing intravenous access, administering sedative medications, and intubation. Patients with neck or back pain who are agitated must be sedated to be adequately immobilized. Occasionally, this may require intubation. If protective head gear is present it should be left in place until the patient is evaluated in an emergency department, unless it significantly compromises the airway or causes difficulties in protecting the airway or intubating the patient.

Steriods have not been found to be beneficial for patients with head injuries and are not recommended. Many investigators have reported finding no improvement in the rate of good recovery with the use of steroids (30–32). Although steroids reduced the mortality rate in some studies, careful analysis of those studies suggests that the only additional survivors were patients in a persistent vegetative state who otherwise would have died.

Emergency Department Management

Once the victim of a head injury has arrived at the emergency department, we advocate the Advanced Trauma Life Support protocol for initial assessment and stabilization (33). The primary survey includes airway assessment and stabilization, assessment of breathing with treatment of respiratory distress, and stabilization of the blood pressure. Sources of internal or external hemorrhage are sought and controlled rapidly. The spine remains immobilized until these immediate life-threatening problems have been addressed adequately. The secondary survey involves a more detailed clinical and radiographic assessment of the patient, including a neurologic examination and a CT scan of the head. Once the patient's neurologic status has been evaluated thoroughly, a systemic neuromuscular-paralyzing agent often is given to calm an agitated but seriously injured patient so that good-quality imaging studies can be obtained. When patients with unstable spine fractures are agitated, such medication also can prevent them from seriously injuring themselves. If the CT scan reveals a surgical intracranial mass lesion such as a subdural or epidural hematoma, the patient is taken immediately to the operating room to undergo a craniotomy and evacuation of the mass. Not infrequently, neurosurgeons and general surgeons operate simultaneously on a patient who has serious cranial and abdominal or thoracic injuries.

The need to elevate depressed skull fractures depends somewhat on the severity of the depression. If the depressed bone does not extend beyond the inner table of the skull, there is no evidence that elevation of the fracture reduces the risk of seizures or of a permanent neurologic deficit. If there is an overlying scalp laceration (open depressed skull fracture), recent reports suggest that elevation of the depressed fragment also does not reduce the risk of infection, provided that the scalp wound had been debrided, thoroughly irrigated, and closed (34, 35).

For patients who have severe, open, depressed skull fractures in which bone fragments penetrate the meninges, the brain, or both, operative debridement and elevation of the bone fragments are advocated. However, the purpose of these measures is not to reduce the risk of seizures or neurologic deficits; the risk of these complications is determined by the severity of the underlying brain injury and is not increased by the presence of the depressed bone fragment. Rather, when bone fragments are depressed through the meninges and into the brain, the risk of infection is increased and cannot be adequately prevented with scalp debridement and antibiotics.

In all cases of open depressed skull fractures, the author advocates the prophylactic use of antibiotics (a cephalosporin and an aminoglycoside) for 10 to 15 days and anticonvulsants (carbamazepine or phenytoin) for 6 months.

The next priority is to identify spinal injuries. Anteroposterior and lateral radiographs are obtained of the entire spine if the patient is comatose or of the spinal areas where there is pain in the awake patient. In addition, an open-mouth odontoid view of the cervical spine is obtained. Because the cervical spine is injured in 5% to 10% of all patients who suffer a severe head injury, the obtunded patient must be assumed to have an unstable spine until radiographically disproved. Cervical spine injuries account for 50% of all traumatic spine injuries, and manipulation of an unstable cervical spine quickly can lead to irreversible quadriplegia. Thus, every effort must be made to identify cervical spine fractures as soon as the patient is stable.

Recent evidence supports the following protocol for radiographically clearing the cervical spine (36). Three cervical spine views are obtained: lateral, anteroposterior, and open-mouth odontoid views. The lateral view must reveal the entire cervical spine from the occiput to the upper border of the T-1 vertebra. Axial CT scans are obtained through any areas where the plain films indicate a possible fracture. Patients who have a short neck or large body habitus that precludes obtaining radiographs of the lower cervical spine undergo axial CT scanning of the lower cervical spine instead. If a patient is awake and complains of severe neck pain, but findings on all of the previous radiographs and CT scans are normal, the author also obtains flexion and extension lateral cervical spine radiographs. If no abnormalities are found on these films, the cervical spine can be considered stable. When a patient has a neurologic deficit referable to the cervical spine, and radiographs do not show a dislocation of the vertebrae, further evaluation with magnetic resonance imaging (MRI) or myelography must proceed immediately to exclude the possibility that there is soft tissue compression of the spinal cord. Such soft tissue compression may be caused by a herniated disc or an epidural hematoma, and immediate surgical removal of such lesions may prevent permanent neurologic deficits in patients with incomplete spinal cord injuries.

Intensive Care

Once the life-threatening issues have been addressed and emergent surgery has been completed, patients with severe head injuries should be admitted to an intensive care unit capable of comprehensive physiologic monitoring. The nursing staff should be experienced in identifying subtle signs of neurologic deterioration and should perform a neurologic assessment at least every 30 minutes for the first several days after the injury. The detailed medical treatment of the patient with a severe head injury is outside the scope of this chapter, but its primary goal is to prevent secondary brain injury. Because regional cerebral ischemia is the most likely cause of secondary brain injury, every effort is made to keep the cerebral perfusion pressure above 70 mm Hg. Cerebral perfusion pressure is defined as the difference between mean arterial pressure and intracranial pressure; therefore, it is important to maintain an intracranial pressure below 15 to 20 mm Hg and a mean arterial pressure above 90 mm Hg.

Hyperventilation traditionally has been used to help reduce intracranial pressure, but recent evidence suggests that it often can exacerbate the problem of regional cerebral ischemia. The reduction in the partial pressure of carbon dioxide (P_{CO_2}) caused by hyperventilation results in vasoconstriction and a reduction in cerebral blood flow. If the brain already has critically reduced blood flow, the further reduction in cerebral blood flow caused by hyperventilation could lead to ischemia or infarction. We therefore recommend that hyperventilation not be used prophylactically for patients with severe head injuries, that it be used only when absolutely necessary to control intracranial pressure and, then, only for brief periods.

The injured brain also is very sensitive to hypoxia, hypotension, hyperthermia, and hyperglycemia. Every attempt should be made to maintain an arterial oxygen partial pressure value above 96 mm Hg, a mean arterial pressure above 90 mm Hg, and a core body temperature below 38° C. The author does not use glucose-containing intravenous solutions during the first 24 to 48 hours after injury and maintains the serum glucose level below 200 mg/dL, administering insulin if necessary.

Minor Head Injuries

The most common head injuries encountered in athletic competition are collisions that cause a concussion. These injuries do not cause prolonged loss of consciousness, and the victims usually can function normally soon after the impact. Ommaya and Gennarelli observed that the level of consciousness and the presence and extent of pretraumatic and posttraumatic amnesia were associated with the likelihood of subsequent disability, leading them to describe five grades of concussion (Table 47.3) (37). A grade I concussion is defined as mild, temporary confusion after impact with no loss of consciousness and no amnesia for events before or after the impact. He or she may have a dazed look and some unsteadiness of gait, but all symptoms subside within 5 to 15 minutes after the injury. If the athlete has posttraumatic amnesia in addition to these symptoms, the concussion is considered grade II. A grade III concussion is characterized by all of the symptoms of the lower grades plus retrograde amnesia lasting several minutes or more. Consciousness also may be lost for several seconds or even a few minutes. A grade IV concussion involves the loss of consciousness lasting 5 to 10 minutes, and grade V describes a concussion causing a prolonged loss of consciousness. The higher the grade of the concussion, the greater the likelihood that the victim will not be able to function normally, either in the game or otherwise, for an extended period after the injury. More importantly, those with a grade III and, particularly, a grade IV or V concussion are at increased risk for a surgical intracranial mass lesion.

Table 47.3.
Grades of Concussion

Grade	Amnesia: Posttraumatic	Amnesia: Retrograde	Loss of Consciousness
I	No	No	No
II	Yes	No	No
III	Yes	Yes	No or seconds
IV	Yes	Yes	Yes, 5–10 minutes
V	Yes	Yes	Yes, prolonged

The more severe grades of concussion also carry the greatest likelihood of postconcussion syndrome, although at least one study found no clear relationship between the duration of posttraumatic unconsciousness or amnesia and the onset of postconcussive symptoms (38). Postconcussion syndrome is characterized by a constellation of symptoms that includes headaches, inattentiveness, vertigo, gait unsteadiness, emotional lability, sleep disturbances, intermittent blurring of vision, and irritability. Not all of these symptoms are apparent in every patient, and symptoms may not emerge for several weeks after a minor head injury. They can last for several months or even several years in some instances but are rarely permanent. In a study of 114 adults who suffered minor head injuries, 90% of the victims experienced one or more of the above symptoms after their injury, but the symptoms lasted an average of only 2 weeks (39). This study also suggested that hospitalization may have prolonged the symptoms and did not reduce their incidence or severity. Patients with postconcussion syndrome often are suspected of feigning their symptoms for the purposes of secondary gain, but in most cases, the symptoms do not subside even after compensatory damages have been awarded to the victim (38).

The etiology of postconcussion syndrome is poorly understood. The symptoms are particularly difficult to treat and can be quite disabling, not infrequently precluding the return to school or work. A minority of patients benefit from treatment with tricyclic antidepressants or ⟨β⟩-adrenergic blocking agents. The best approach in particularly severe cases of postconcussion syndrome is to enroll the patient in a multidisciplinary treatment program that includes physiatrists, physical therapists, psychotherapists, and pain specialists. Such programs are usually available through local rehabilitation hospitals.

There is increasing evidence that even minor head injuries can lead to both measurable deterioration of subtle cognitive functioning and electrophysiologic abnormalities. In addition, structural disruption of brain tissue has been detected with MRI performed days or even months after such injuries. In most cases, particularly with the less severe injuries, these abnormalities are reversible. However, after relatively severe injuries, especially those that involve prolonged loss of consciousness, subtle alterations in attention, memory, and the speed of processing information may last for 10 to 20 years and endure long after the level of intelligence has normalized (as measured by conventional psychometric tests such as the Wechsler intelligence scales) (40). One of the most extensive studies of psychological deficits caused by minor head injury was reported by Gronwall and Wrightson in 1974 (41). They studied patients aged 17 to 25 years who had suffered a minor closed-head injury and had had no previous concussion. Compared to age-matched, uninjured control subjects, psychological testing revealed that the trauma victims had a slower rate of information processing and an increased central processing time but were not significantly more distractible. Most patients, especially those with the least severe injuries, recovered normal function after 4 weeks. Subsequent studies have shown that both attentional and information processing deficiencies are common after mild closed-head injuries. Reaction time typically is slowed, an impairment most prominent under complex conditions and during the 1st month after the injury (42). Pretraumatic abilities usually return within 3 months after the injury (43). Long-term recovery from cognitive deficiencies has been most closely correlated with the severity of impairment during the first few days after the injury (44).

A minor head injury, particularly for athletes, increases the risk for sustaining future head injuries. One study of high school football players found a 4-fold risk of head injury among those who had suffered a previous minor head injury (1). Moreover, neuropsychological defects following a second minor head injury have been shown to last longer and to be more severe than those caused by the first (45).

Several recent studies demonstrated abnormalities in cerebral electrical conduction after minor head injuries. Tysvaer and Storli studied 69 soccer players, a group of athletes who often use their head to hit the ball as a routine part of the game. They found a significantly higher incidence of electroencephalographic abnormalities in this group than in age-matched control subjects, the greatest incidence occurring in the youngest players (46). Gorke and Schmidt performed visual-evoked potentials in 50 children who had had minor head injuries. Although none had lost consciousness from the injury, 36% had significantly prolonged latencies, which usually returned to normal within 2 to 3 months (47). Abd al-Hady and coworkers studied brainstem auditory-evoked potentials in 40 adults who had suffered minor head trauma and found high-frequency conductive and sensorineural hearing losses in 20% (48). They also found a significant increase in the absolute wave V latency and in the wave III-V interpeak latency in these patients. Among 15 adults with minor head injuries, Podoshin et al., demonstrated that such abnormalities were usually temporary and that brainstem conduction latencies had returned to normal 2 months after the injury (49). They concluded that the reversibility of the evoked potential abnormalities supported the hypothesis that transient ischemia rather than structural or axonal damage cause the symptomatic abnormalities associated with a minor head injury.

MRI recently has become available at most hospitals and provides much more sensitive imaging capabilities than does CT scanning. Yokota and colleagues compared MRI and CT findings for 134 victims of mild head trauma (initial GCS scores of 13 to 15) (50). Almost half of the patients were studied within 6 hours of their injury, and all within 3 days. Parenchymal lesions of the brain were detected in 34 of the 134 patients with MRI but in only 9 of the patients with CT. Most of the lesions demonstrated by MRI but not by CT were in the cerebral cortex. The significance of such lesions is unclear, however. It has been our experience that for patients with a mild head injury, most of the lesions detected on the acute MRI studies no longer are visible on MRI scans obtained 3 months later. Because MRI is particularly sensitive to edema (51), we suspect that the lesions seen on MRI and not on CT images during the first few days after injury represent very small contusions magnified by the presence of surrounding edema. Any structural or permanent damage is probably minimal in such cases.

Who Can Return to Play?

Familiarity with the characteristics of minor head injuries, as described in the previous section, can help to determine when a player should be allowed to return to the game. We emphasize that the degree of impairment within the first few hours after the injury is one of the best predictors of cognitive function several months later. Impaired cognition primarily is manifest as a slowing of both information processing and reaction time, the latter being particularly severe in complex situations. Thus, it is not surprising that the likelihood of a second injury is increased by returning to the game too soon after a minor head impact. In most cases, congnitive deficits that result from minor head trauma are worst during the 1st month after injury.

Based on these facts and on the recommendations of several experts who have extensive experience in treating college and professional football players with head injuries (52, 53), The following guidelines are suggested for determining when participation in sports can resume (Table 47.4). In general, return to play should not be allowed until the athlete is completely lucid and asymptomatic. Those with a grade I concussion may return to the game within 5 to 15 minutes after they are completely lucid. Head injuries in this grade do not cause a loss of consciousness. If the player has suffered

Table 47.4.
Recommendations for Return to Play

Grade of Concussion	Recommendation for Return to Play
After First Minor Head Injury	
I	Return 5–15 minutes after completely lucid; asymptomatic
II	No return that day
III	No return for 1 week after completely lucid, asymptomatic; detailed neurologic evaluation
IV	No return for 1 month; detailed neurologic evaluation
V	No return for 3 months; detailed neurologic evaluation
After Additional Minor Head Injuries	
I–II	No return for at least 1 week; detailed neurologic evaluation
III	No return for at least 1 month; detailed neurologic evaluation
IV–V	No return for at least 1 year; also consider discontinuing sport

a grade II concussion (demonstrating posttraumatic amnesia), play should be prohibited for the rest of the day, and the team trainer or physician should thoroughly examine the victim before permitting future participation. For a grade III concussion, in which there is retrograde amnesia with or without a brief loss of consciousness, return to play should be delayed for 1 week after the victim becomes completely lucid. In addition, the player should undergo a thorough neurologic evaluation immediately after the injury and again prior to play. Ideally, such an examination includes a CT scan of the head and neuropsychological tests of information processing and reaction times. Without baseline (preinjury) studies, neuropsychological tests can be difficult to interpret, but gross abnormalities can be identified and should preclude return to play until there is improvement. Anyone who has lost consciousness for more than 5 minutes (grade IV or V concussion) should not return to play for 1 to 3 months. In most cases, such persons should be taken immediately to a nearby trauma center for evaluation by a neurosurgeon and for a CT scan of the head. After 1 to 3 months, the resumption of sports activities is advisable only if a full recovery is confirmed as the result of appropriate neurologic testing. Anyone who is allowed to play again after a minor head injury must be watched closely by the coaching staff and trainer and removed from the game if he or she does not appear to be functioning normally.

If the player suffers a second head injury, the author advocates removal from competitive sports for a minimum of 1 week. During that time, a thorough neurologic evaluation should be performed, including neuropsychological testing; participation should be prohibited until the results of these tests are considered within normal limits. Any person who is rendered unconscious for longer than 5 minutes more than once should not be allowed to participate in sports for the remainder of the season and should be counseled on the advisability of returning to the sport in the future.

The author recognizes that these guidelines are relatively conservative and emphasizes that they are meant to aid coaches, trainers, and physicians in developing their own policies. Each victim of head injury must be considered individually, and these recommendations may not apply in specific cases.

Summary

Although sports and recreational activities cause far fewer head injuries than do motor vehicle accidents, those that do occur are often more debilitating than injuries elsewhere in the body. The prevention of head injuries must be a concern of all those involved in sports, including the players, coaching staff, and trainers. It is recommended that, during particularly high-risk sports such as football and boxing, protective head gear should be worn at all times. It is also recommended that authorities in schools, professional athletic organizations, and communities regularly monitor the incidence of head injuries in the various sports, updating rules and regulations as needed. At the present time, these recommendations seem particularly urgent for activities such as bicycle riding and ice hockey.

Preparations should be made in advance of organized athletic competition for rapid evaluation and triage in the event of a head injury. The coach, team trainer, or team physician must be well versed in the principles of advanced trauma life support and immediately available to direct the proper care of the athlete from the moment of injury. In the field, emphasis should be placed on establishing or maintaining hemodynamic and respiratory stability and on immobilizing the cervical spine if the injured party is rendered unconscious or is complaining of neck pain. All victims of head injury who remain unconscious, confused, or disoriented should be taken to the emergency department of the nearest trauma center as soon as possible. The same recommendation applies to those who have persistent headaches, nausea, vomiting, or focal neurologic deficits.

Most sports-related head injuries do not cause prolonged unconsciousness, however. Players who suffer only brief confusion or who are temporarily dazed may be allowed to resume play 10 to 15 minutes after the injury, but only after the coach or team trainer has carefully assessed the mental status of the victim and has determined that he or she is completely alert and oriented in all spheres. Both those supervising and those participating in sports should be aware that the speed of information processing typically is slowed after a minor head injury and that the likelihood of further injury is increased by the first injury. The possibility of posttraumatic symptoms such as prolonged headaches, dizziness, memory loss, or emotional lability also must be considered. However, such symptoms never should be ascribed to posttraumatic syndrome until the victim has had a thorough neurologic evaluation, usually including a CT or MRI scan of the head. Neuropsychological testing may be very helpful in documenting the severity of subtle cognitive deficits caused by a minor head injury. Such testing also can be used to guide the determination of when to allow the victim to return to play. The role of MRI in this regard is not yet clear. Although MRI is more sensitive than CT in detecting small parenchymal brain injuries, as yet there is no documented correlation between these small injuries and subsequent neurologic capabilities.

Acknowledgement

The author gratefully acknowledges the editorial assistance of Helene Marion in the preparation of the manuscript.

REFERENCES

1. Gerberich SG, Priest JD, Boen JR, et al. Concussion incidences and severity in secondary school varsity football players. Am J Public Health 1983;73:1370–1375.
2. Kraus JF. Epidemiology of head injury. In: Cooper PR, ed. Head injury. 2nd ed. Baltimore: Williams & Wilkins, 1987:1–19.
3. Young WW, Gunter MJ. A study of the head injured population in Pennsylvania. Pittsburgh: The Pittsburgh Research Institute, 1991:58–59.
4. Torg JS, Vegso JJ, Sennett B. The national football head and neck injury registry: 14-year report on cervical quadriplegia (1971–1984). Clin Sports Med 1987;6:3439–3443.
5. Mueller FO, Blyth CS. Fatalities from head and cervical spine injuries occurring in tackle football: 40 years' experience. Clin Sports Med 1987;6:185–196.
6. Tysvaer A, Storli O. Association football injuries to the brain. A preliminary report. Br J Sports Med 1981;15:163–166.
7. National Safety Council. Accident facts. Chicago: National Safety Council, 1982:45–91.
8. Greensher J. Non-automotive vehicle injuries in adolescents. Pediatr Ann 1988;17:114–121.
9. Thompson RS, Rivara FP, Thompson DC. A case-control study of the effectiveness of bicycle safety helmets. N Engl J Med 1989;320:1361–1367.
10. Hodgson VR. National operating committee on standards for athletic equipment. Football helmet certification program. Med Sci Sports 1975;7:225–232.
11. Bishop PJ. Impact performance of ice hockey helmets. Safety Res 1978;10:123–129.
12. Bishop PJ, Briard BD. Impact performance of bicycle helmets. Can J Appl Sport Sci 1984;9:94–101.
13. Kersey RD, Rowan L. Injury account during the 1980 NCAA wrestling championships. Am J Sports Med 1983;11:147–151.
14. Pforringer W, Smasal V. Aspects of traumatology in ice hockey. J Sports Sci 1987;5:327–336.
15. Rimel RN, Giordani B, Barth JT, et al. Disability caused by minor head injury. Neurosurgery 1981;9:221–228.
16. Edna TH. Acute traumatic intracranial hematoma and skull fracture. Acta Chir Scand 1983;149:449–451.
17. Chan KH, Mann KS, Yue CP, et al. The significance of skull fracture in acute traumatic intracranial hematomas in adolescents: A prospective study. J Neurosurg 1990;72:189–194.
18. Gomez CR, Backer RJ, Bucholz RD. Transcranial Doppler ultrasound following closed head injury: Vasospasm or vasoparalysis. Surg Neurol 1991;35:30–35.
19. Compton JS, Lee T, Jones NR, Waddell G, et al. A double blind placebo controlled trial of the calcium entry blocking drug, nicardipine, in the treatment of vasospasm following severe head injury. Br J Neurosurg 1990;4:9–15.
20. Yanagida Y, Fujiwara S, Mizoi Y. Differences in the intracranial pressure caused by a "blow" and/or a "fall"—An experimental study using physical models of the head and neck. Forensic Sci Int 1989;41:135–145.
21. Mattson RH, Cramer JA, Collins JF, et al. Comparison of carbamazepine, phenobarbital, phenytoin, and primidone in partial and secondarily generalized tonic-clonic seizures. N Engl J Med 1985;313:145–151.
22. Povlishock JT. Diffuse deafferentation as the major determinant of morbidity and recovery following brain injury [Abstract]. Status report on CNS trauma. VII, 1990.
23. Graham DI, Ford I, Adams JH, et al. Ischaemic brain damage is still common in fatal non-missile head injury. J Neurol Neurosurg Psychiatry 1989;52:346–350.
24. Marion DW, Darby J, Yonas H. Acute regional cerebral blood flow changes caused by severe head injuries. J Neurosurg 1991;74:407–414.
25. Robertson CS, Narayan RK, Gokaslan ZL, et al. Cerebral arteriovenous oxygen difference as an estimate of cerebral blood flow in comatose patients. J Neurosurg 1989;70:222–230.
26. Bracken MB, Shepard MJ, Collins WF, et al. A randomized, controlled trial of methylprednisolone or naloxone in the treatment of acute spinal-cord injury. Results of the Second National Acute Spinal Cord Injury Study. N Engl J Med 1990;322:1405–1411.
27. Teasdale G, Jennett B. Assessment of coma and impaired consciousness: a practical scale. Lancet 1974;2:81–84.
28. Jennett B, Teasdale G, Galbraith S, et al. Severe head injuries in three countries. J Neurol Neurosurg Psychiatry 1977;40:291–298.
29. Jaffe R. Sports medicine emergencies. Prim Care 1986;13:207–215.
30. Giannotta SL, Weiss MH, Apuzzo ML, et al. High dose glucocorticoids in the management of severe head injury. Neurosurgery 1984;15:497–501.
31. Dearden NM, Gibson JS, McDowall DG, et al. Effect of high-dose dexamethasone on outcome from severe head injury. J Neurosurg 1986;64:81–88.
32. Braakman R, Schouten HJA, Dishoeck MB, et al. Megadose steroids in severe head injury: Results of a prospective double-blind clinical trial. J Neurosurg 1983;58:326–330.
33. Committee on Trauma, American College of Surgeons. Advanced trauma life support student manual. Chicago: American College of Surgeons, 1989:1–243.
34. Braakman R. Depressed skull fracture: Data, treatment and follow-up in 225 consecutive cases. J Neurol Neurosurg Psychiatry 1971;34:106–110.
35. Van den Heever HJ, Van der Merwe JJ. Management of depressed skull fractures: Selective conservative management of nonmissile injuries. J Neurosurg 1989;71:186–190.
36. Borock EC, Gabram SGA, Jacobs LM, et al. A prospective analysis of a two-year experience using computed tomography as an adjunct for cervical spine clearance. J Trauma 1991;31:1001–1006.
37. Ommaya AK, Gennarelli TA. Cerebral concussion and traumatic unconsciousness. Correlation of experimental and clinical observations on blunt head injuries. Brain 1974;97:638.
38. Bornstein RA, Miller HB, van Schoor JT. Neuropsychological deficit and emotional disturbance in head-injured patients. J Neurosurg 1989;70:509–513.
39. Lowdon IM, Briggs M, Cockin J. Post-concussional symptoms following minor head injury. Injury 1989;20:193–194.
40. Stuss DT, Stethem LL, Hugenholtz H. et al. Reaction time after head injury: Fatigue, divided and focused attention, and consistency of performance. J Neurol Neurosurg Psychiatry 1989;52:742–748.
41. Gronwall D, Wrightson P. Delayed recovery of intellectual function after minor head injury. Lancet 1974;2:605–609.
42. Hugenholtz H, Stuss DT, Stethem LL, et al. How long does it take to recover from a mild concussion. Neurosurgery 1988;22:853–858.
43. Levin HS, Mattis S, Ruff RM, et al. Neurobehavioral outcome following minor head injury: a three-center study. J Neurosurg 1987;66:234–243.
44. Dikmen S, Reitan RM, Temkin NR. Neuropsychological recovery in head injury. Arch Neurol 1983;40:333–338.
45. Grunwall D, Wrightson P. Cumulative effect of concussion. Lancet 1975;2:995–997.
46. Tysvaer AT, Storli OV. Soccer injuries to the brain. A neurologic and electroencephalographic study of active football players. Am J Sports Med 1989;17:573–578.
47. Gorke W, Schmidt U. Non-target visual event-related potentials in evaluation of children with minor head trauma. Neuropediatrics 1991;22:79–84.
48. Abd al-Hady MR, Shehata O, el-Mously M, et al. Audiological

findings following head trauma. J Laryngol Otol 1990;104:927–936.
49. Podoshin L, Ben-David Y, Fradis M, et al. Brainstem auditory-evoked potential with increased stimulus rate in minor head trauma. J Laryngol Otol 1990;104:191–194.
50. Yokota H, Kurokawa A, Otsuka T, et al. Significance of magnetic resonance imaging in acute head injury. J Trauma 1991;31:351–357.
51. Fumeya H, Ito K, Yamagiwa O, et al. Analysis of MRI and SPECT in patients with acute head injury. Acta Neurochir [Suppl] (Wien) 1990;51:283–285.
52. Wilberger JE Jr, Maroon JC. Head injuries in athletes. Clin Sports Med 1989;8:1–9.
53. Vegso JJ, Lehman RC. Field evaluation and management of head and neck injuries. Clin Sports Med 1987;6:1–15.
54. Albright JP, McAuley E, Martin RK, et al. Head and neck injuries in college football: an eight-year analysis. Am J Sports Med 1985;13:147–152.
55. Canale ST, Cantler ED, Sisk TD, et al. A chronicle of injuries of an American intercollegiate football team. Am J Sports Med 1981;9:384–389.
56. Thompson N, Halpern B, Curl WW, et al. High school football injuries: Evaluation. Am J Sports Med 1987;15:S-97–S-104.
57. JAMA Council on Scientific Affairs. Brain injury in boxing. Chicago: AMA, 1983:252–257.
58. Enzenauer RW, Montrey JS, Enzenauer RJ, et al. Boxing-related injuries in the US Army, 1980 through 1985. JAMA 1989;261:1463–1466.
59. Kruse DL, McBeath AA. Bicycle accidents and injuries. A random survey of a college population. Am J Sports Med 1980;8:342–344.
60. Blignaut JB, Carstens IL, Lombard CJ. Injuries sustained in rugby by wearers and non-wearers of mouthguards. Br J Sports Med 1987;21:5–7.
61. Jorgensen U, Schmidt-Olsen S. The epidemiology of ice hockey injuries. Br J Sports Med 1986;20:7–9.
62. Grossman JA, Kulund DN, Miller CW, et al. Equestrian injuries. Results of a prospective study. JAMA 1978;240:1881–1882.
63. Sahlin Y. Alpine skiing injuries. Br J Sports Med 1989;23:241–244.

48 / TREATMENT OF SPORTS EYE INJURIES

Thomas J. Pashby and Robert C. Pashby

Introduction

The eye accounts for only .002% of the body's surface area and 0.10% of the erect frontal silhouette, yet it is the victim of 1% of sports-related injuries (1, 2).

Injured eyes require immediate assessment and early treatment. Ideally, every eye injury deserves treatment by an ophthalmologist or a medical doctor who is familiar with using the ophthalmoscope and able to interpret the finding of an intraocular examination.

However, the optimum treatment is not always immediately available. Often, the athletic trainer or first aid attendant must deal with the injured player. Therefore, it is extremely important that these people understand the anatomy and physiology of the eye, the means of testing and assessing central and peripheral vision, and the equipment required to examine and treat minor eye injuries.

This chapter presents guidelines to enable trainers and first aid attendants to examine the eye and recognize minor ocular injuries they can handle, injuries that require ophthalmological care, and injuries that demand immediate, on-the-spot treatment before the person is sent for specialist care.

In addition to familiarizing themselves with the present material, athletic trainers and paramedical personnel should be aware of more detailed texts (3) and should avail themselves of management courses that include study of the eye. The need for physicians who practice sports medicine to serve as instructors in such courses is obvious.

Assessing an Eye Injury

Minimum Equipment Needed by Team Physicians and Trainers

Probably the minimum equipment (Fig. 48.1) necessary to perform an eye examination is as follows:

vision card,
penlight,
sterile fluorescein strips,
sterile eye pads,
eye shields,
tape,
sterile cotton-tipped swabs, and
sterile irrigating solution.

Examining the Injured Eye

A routine ocular examination is necessary to determine the seriousness of an eye injury. A penlight is used to obtain an oblique illumination of the eye that may indicate damage to the conjunctiva, cornea, anterior chamber (the area bounded by the cornea and the iris-lens diaphragm), pupil, iris, and lens (Figs. 48.2 and 48.3). This procedure is followed:

1. Inspect the lids and brow for lacerations, bruising, and hematoma.
2. Inspect the conjunctival sac for hemorrhage, laceration, and foreign bodies. Eversion of the upper eyelid often shows a foreign body that can easily be brushed away. Displaced contact lenses are often found by this means.
3. Examine the cornea for any foreign body, abrasions, or lacerations. Abrasions are well outlined by fluorescein dye, which is applied by pulling the lower lid downward and then dipping a sterile fluorescein strip into the pool of tears in the lower fornix.
4. Assess the clarity and depth of the anterior chamber and compare with the other eye.
5. Compare the size, shape, and light reaction of the pupil in the injured eye with the other eye.
6. Compare the iris colors of each eye.
7. Test visual acuity using a reading card or newspaper and compare with the uninjured eye. It is useful to know the patient's vision in each eye with glasses or contact lenses before injury. Vision less than 20/40 should be referred.
8. Test peripheral vision (confrontation perimetry) by having the patient fix on the examiner's nose and, after occluding the other eye, having patient iden-

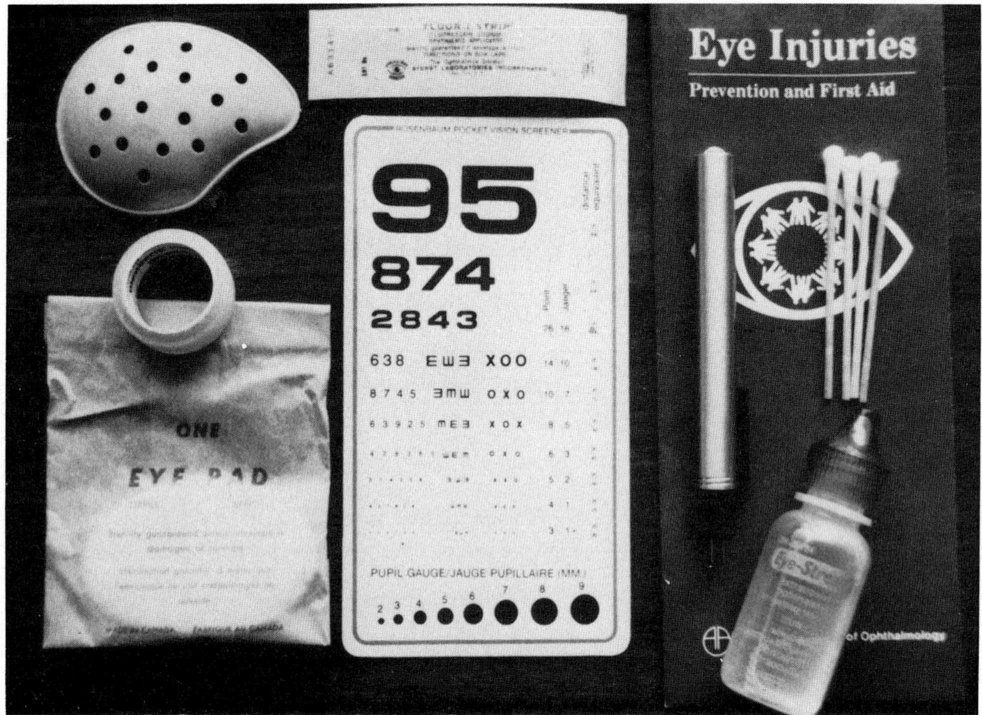

Figure 48.1. This display shows probably the minimal equipment necessary to examine the injured eye in an emergency.

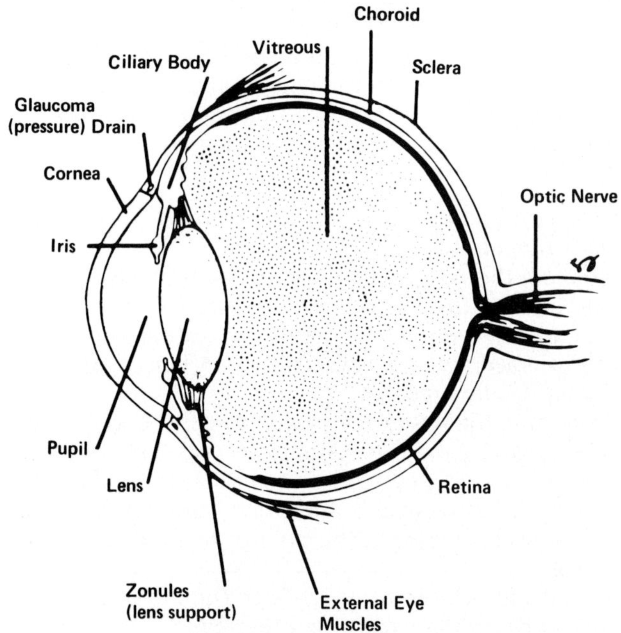

Figure 48.2. The eye is shown in sagittal section.

tify the number of fingers held up in all fields of gaze (Fig. 48.4). A normal minimal visual field extends 85° temporally, 65° downward, 60° nasally, and 45° upward. Any person with a loss of field must be referred for specialist care.

9. Assess ocular movements by asking the patient to look to the right, then upward, then downward, similarly to the left, up and down (the 6 cardinal positions of gaze). With both eyes moving together, there should be no diplopia (double vision) when a light is held in the primary position and the 6 cardinal positions of gaze. Any double vision must be referred for specialist care.
10. Compare the eyes to determine whether the injured eye is sunken, making the palpebral aperture narrower, or proptosed, in which case the aperture would be enlarged. A fracture of the orbital floor results in enophthalmus (a sunken eye), while a retrobular hemorrhage causes proptosis (a pushing forward of the eye).

If a medical doctor is available, an intraocular examination should be performed with an ophthalmoscope to identify damage to the lens, vitreous, and retina.

After the eye examination is completed, a decision must be made regarding management. Always err on the side of caution. If there is any doubt about the seriousness of the injury, make sure the patient is seen by an ophthalmologist as soon as possible.

Forcing the Injured Eye Open

To examine an injured eye, it is necessary to have the eye open. However, the injured person may have an obviously lacerated eyelid or present with pain, lacrimation, and blepharospasm that make opening the eye and its examination difficult. If these symptoms are severe, it is better not to force the lids open, since this could cause further damage. Such patients should have a sterile eye pad applied and be transported to hospital for ophthalmological care.

The reverse is the case with chemical burns (Fig. 48.5), as for example, from lime on the playing field. Such

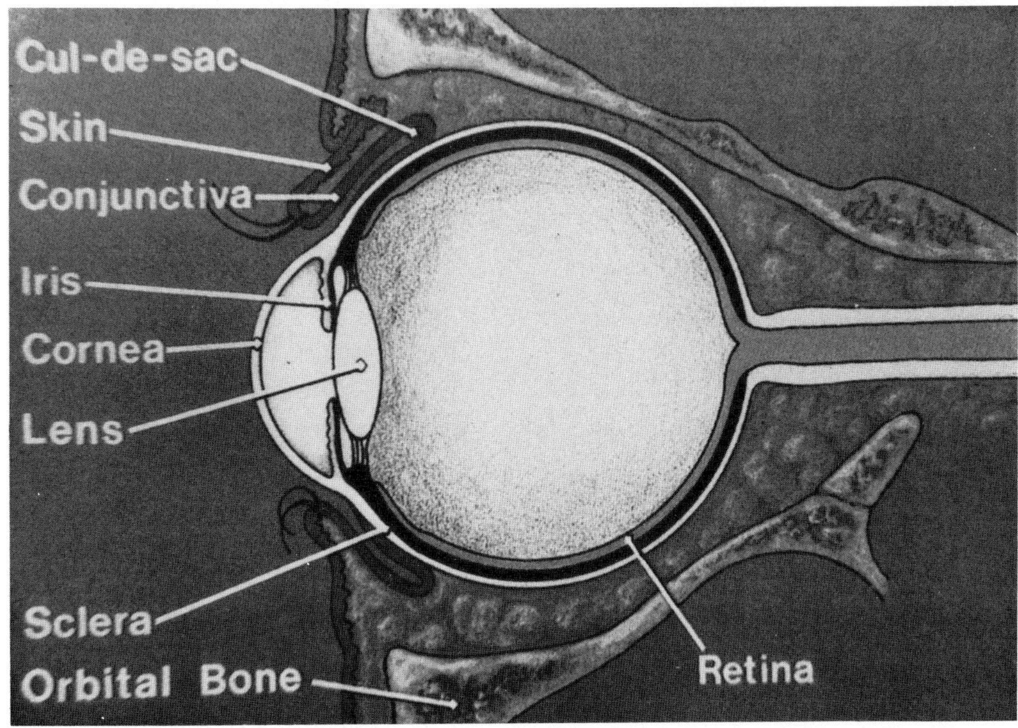

Figure 48.3. This view demonstrates the eye in relationship to its surrounding structures.

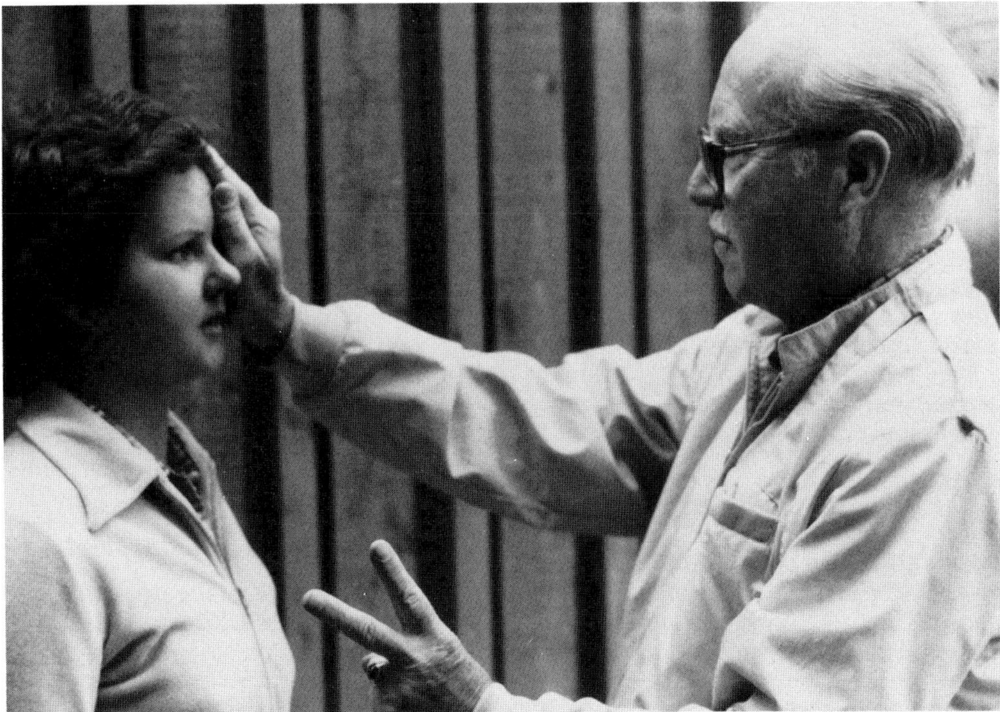

Figure 48.4. Peripheral vision is being tested by confrontation perimetry.

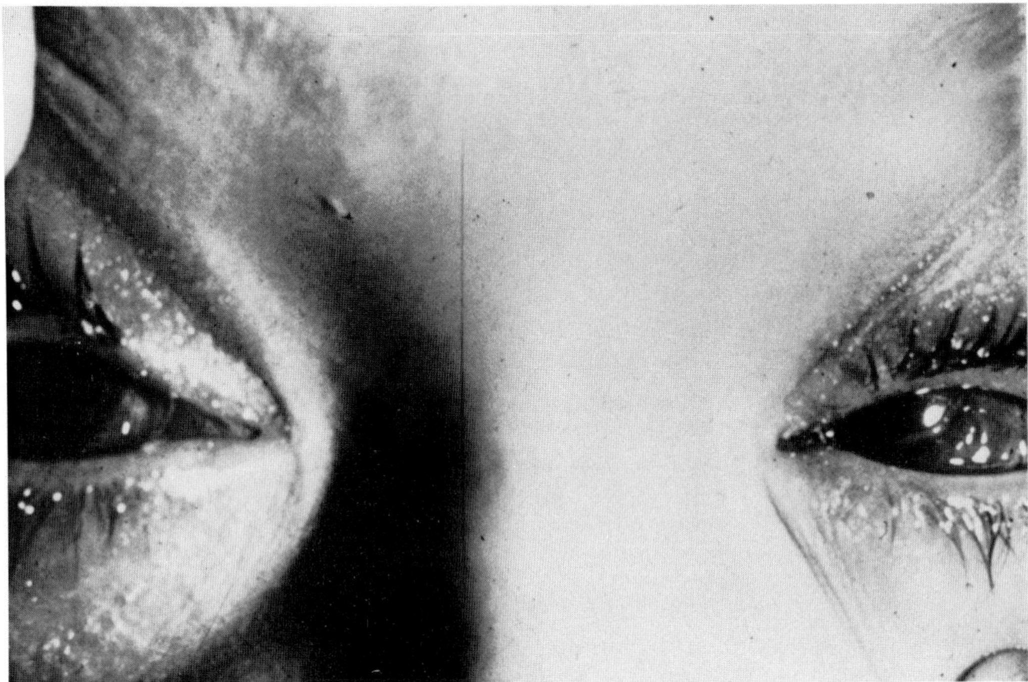

Figure 48.5. Lime burns occasionally result from the chemical contact on the playing field.

injuries demand immediate treatment by forcibly opening the eye, removing any solid particles with a cotton-tipped swab, and irrigating the opened eye with copious amounts of water (at the very minimum a quart and for at least 5 min). If water is not available, soda pop or Gatorade can be used. While this is being done, another person should notify the nearest emergency facility, describing the type of injury and giving the patient's name. The patient must be transported to hospital with the eye uncovered. A chemical burn is an emergency and must be treated at once.

Types of Eye Injuries and Their Management

In personal experience of over 3800 eye injuries associated with sports, (4–7) the incidence of the various types of eye injuries was as follows: soft tissue injuries, 34%; hyphemas, 27%; other intraocular injuries, 23%; corneal injuries, 9%; orbital fractures, 4%; ruptured globes, 3%. Approximately 11% of these injuries rendered the eye legally blind (20/200 or less).

Soft Tissue Injuries

Orbital Hemorrhage

Orbital hemorrhage (black eye) (Fig. 48.6) may occur after blunt trauma to the orbital region. Proptosis of the affected eye, associated with hemorrhage into the lids and beneath the conjunctiva, and restriction of ocular movement may occur. If the hemorrhage is severe, the vascular supply to the optic nerve and retina may be shut off, causing visual loss. It is urgent that ophthalmologic consultation be sought immediately. During transport, an ice pack should be applied and the head kept elevated.

Any soft tissue lid injury should be assessed before extreme swelling ensues which would preclude a proper examination of the globe. Such an examination includes visual acuity and fields; pupillary size, shape, and reaction; iris color; and tests for diplopia. Any foreign body in the eye must be identified and recorded.

Lid Lacerations

Lid lacerations (Fig. 48.7) may be caused by sharp objects, blunt trauma, or objects that catch the lid and actually tear it. Bleeding is controlled by direct pressure, allowing the extent of the laceration to be assessed. Lacerations through the lid margin require meticulous surgical repair for proper cosmetic results and the prevention of subsequent tearing. Lacerations or punctures of the upper or lower lid should be repaired by an ophthalmologist, who will clean the wound thoroughly, explore for foreign material, and make anatomical closure of muscle and skin layers. Lid tissues that may appear to be irreparably jeopardized, with respect to blood supply, should not be discarded but repaired. A sterile eye pad is applied prior to transport to control bleeding and prevent infection.

Lacerations of the Lacrimal Apparatus

Medial lacerations of the upper and/or lower lid usually involve the lacrimal drainage system (Fig. 48.8). The canalicular laceration is best repaired by an ophthalmologist using a microscope. Do not repair the lid laceration but refer the person for canalicular repair immediately.

In case of severe eyelid trauma, the eyelids may become disinserted from their attachments of the medial or lateral orbital margins. Reattachment of the liga-

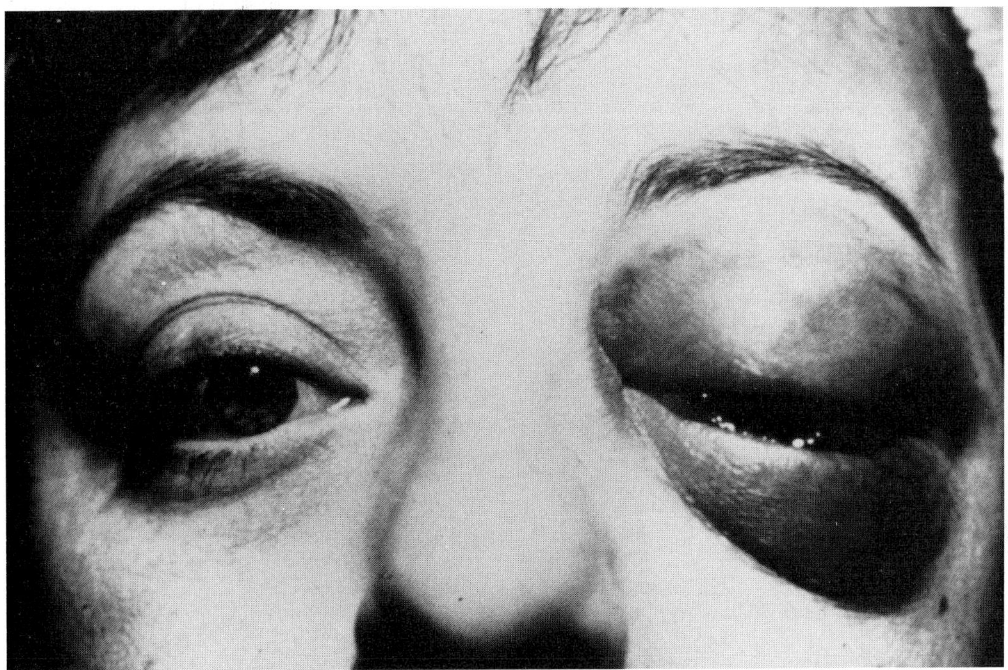

Figure 48.6. The left eye has sustained a contusion and an orbital hemorrhage.

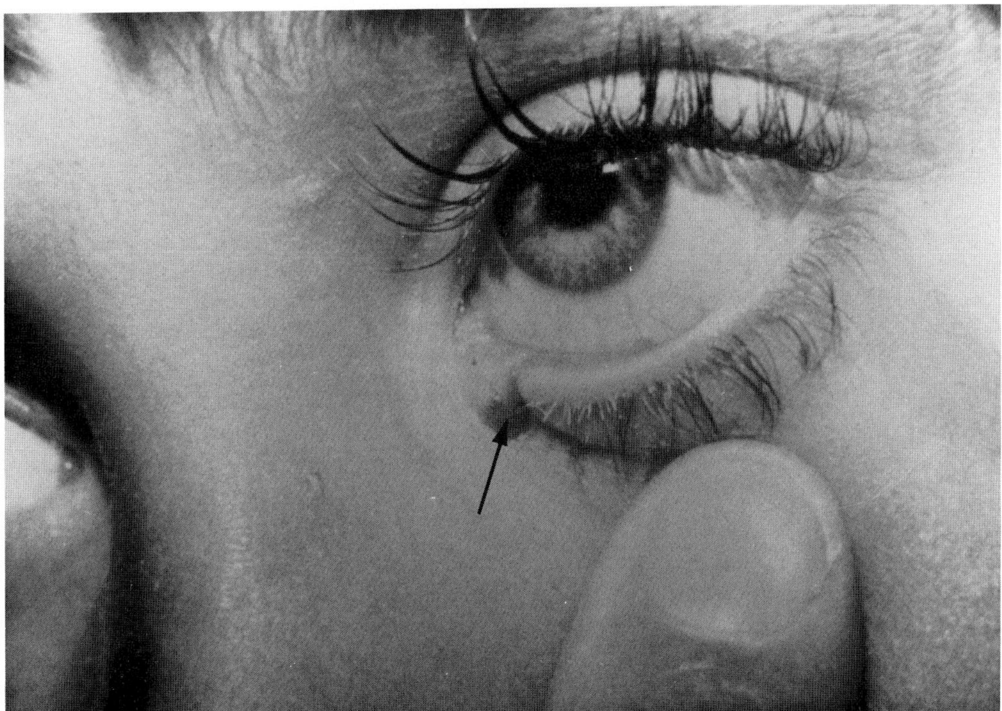

Figure 48.7. Such a lower lid laceration *(arrow)* may occur from a hockey stick blow.

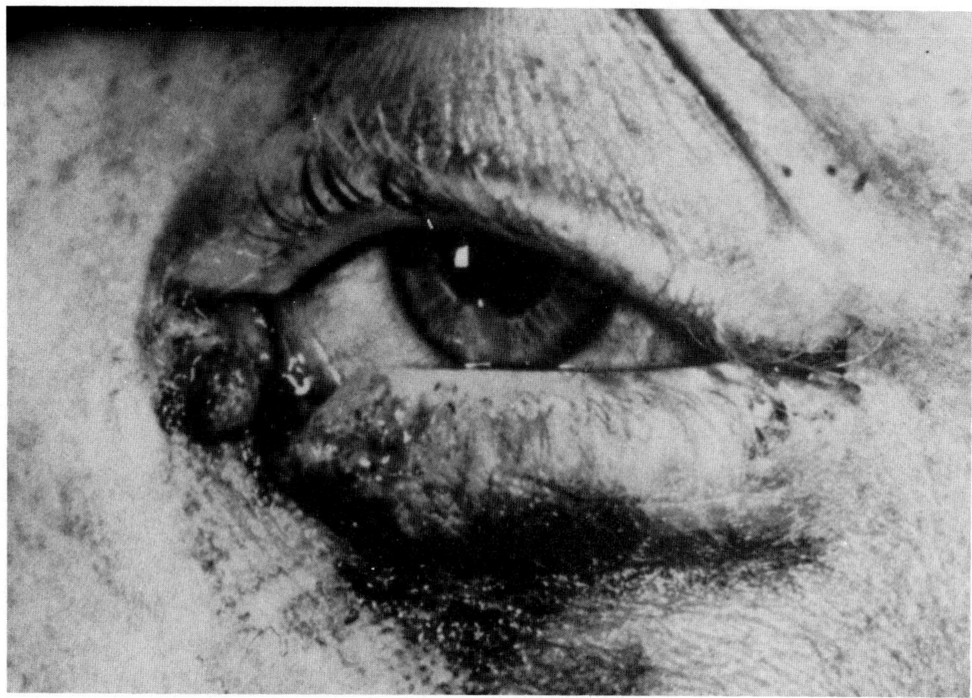

Figure 48.8. The right lower lid laceration involves the lacrimal system.

ments to bone is necessary for good functional and cosmetic results.

With lid lacerations, as with any wound, general considerations must be remembered, namely: control of bleeding with sterile gauze, assessment of globe damage, application of a sterile eye pad, and general tetanus prophylaxis. The importance of examining the globe cannot be stressed enough, and, for this reason, any significant injury in the region of the eye should be assessed by an ophthalmologist. Remember, it is much easier to examine the globe before lid swelling occurs.

A record must be kept of visual acuity, visual fields, the presence or absence of diplopia, and intraocular findings.

Conjunctival Injuries

In minor lacerations of the conjunctiva, suturing is not necessary. A search for and removal of any dirt particles or other foreign material must be carried out. An eye pad is applied for 24 hours, and a follow-up examination is made at that time.

Foreign bodies often lodge just under the margin of the upper eyelid (Fig. 48.9). Eversion of the eyelid will reveal their presence, and removal is usually achieved by wiping with a moist cotton-tipped swab. The first aid attendant should be familiar with the procedure of everting the upper eyelid (Fig. 48.10).

Foreign Bodies in the Eye

Foreign bodies in the eye are a common problem on the playing field. They are commonly lodged under the upper eyelid (Fig. 48.10).

To examine the area, the upper eyelid must be everted by having the patient look down with both eyes open; then, the upper lid lashes are grasped and the lid is pulled away from the eyeball. Counter pressure on the upper lid with a Q-tip will evert the lid. (The lashes are rolled over the cotton-tipped swab.) (Fig. 48.9). The foreign body can often be wiped away with a moist cotton swab. It helps to have inserted a drop or two of local anaesthetic solution into the eye beforehand (Pontocaine or Ophthetic).

After removal, the player can return to play in 15 or 20 min when the anesthetic effect has worn off.

Hyphema

Hyphema is a collection of free blood in the anterior chamber of the eye. It is the most common intraocular injury associated with sports, occurring in 27% of injured eyes in the authors' series. This percentage may seem high; however, all reported injuries required ophthalmological care. The person rendering first aid must be familiar with its appearance.

At the time of injury, a hyphema appears as a haze in the anterior chamber. The iris looks somewhat muddy in color compared to the fellow eye, and the pupil is usually irregular in shape and sluggish in reaction to light. Vision is somewhat blurred. With rest, the blood settles to form a level in the anterior chamber (Fig. 48.11), unless bleeding continues; in this case, blood fills the chamber to create an "eight ball" eye. Most hyphemas clear in a few days, but, in about 15% of cases, a secondary hemorrhage occurs, usually between 2 and 5 days after the initial injury. For this reason all hyphemas demand ophthalmological care. They must be rec-

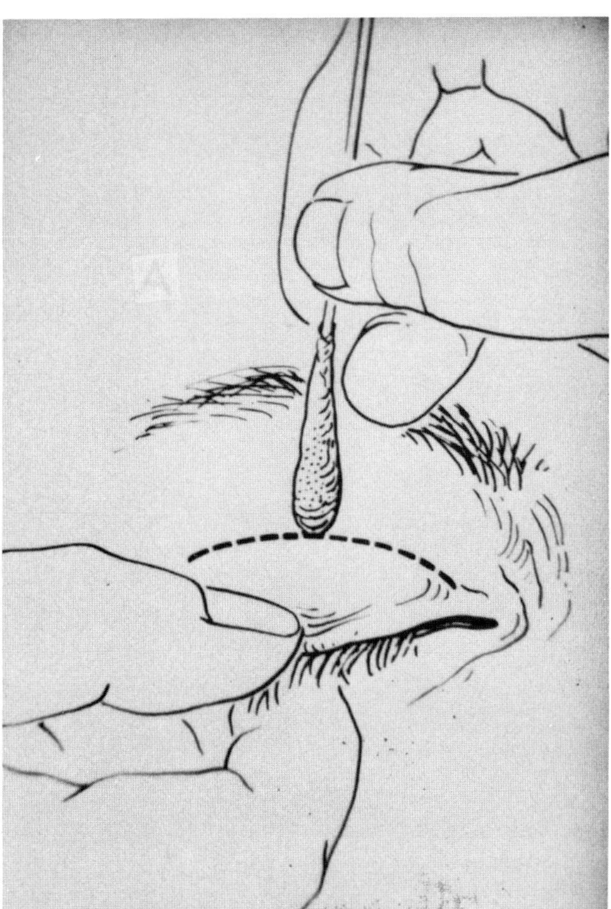

Figure 48.9. The patient is told to look down while the examiner grasps the upper lid lashes pulling them away from the eye while at the same time exerting counter pressure backward with a cotton swab at the upper border of the tarsus. The upper lid is then readily everted.

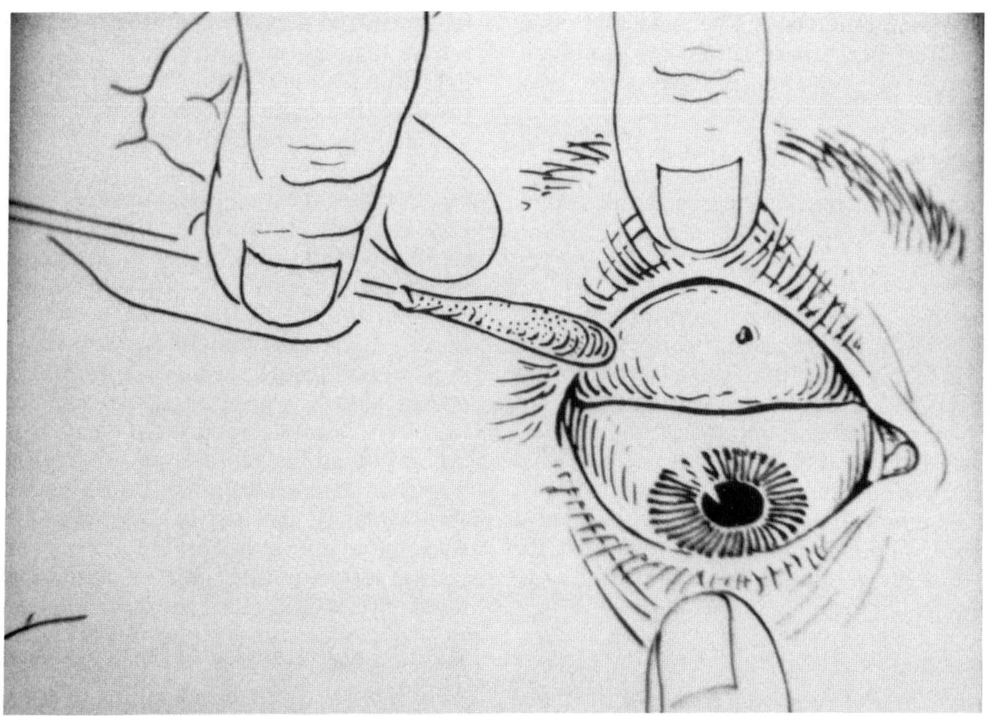

Figure 48.10. Eversion of the upper lid of the right eye has exposed the foreign body.

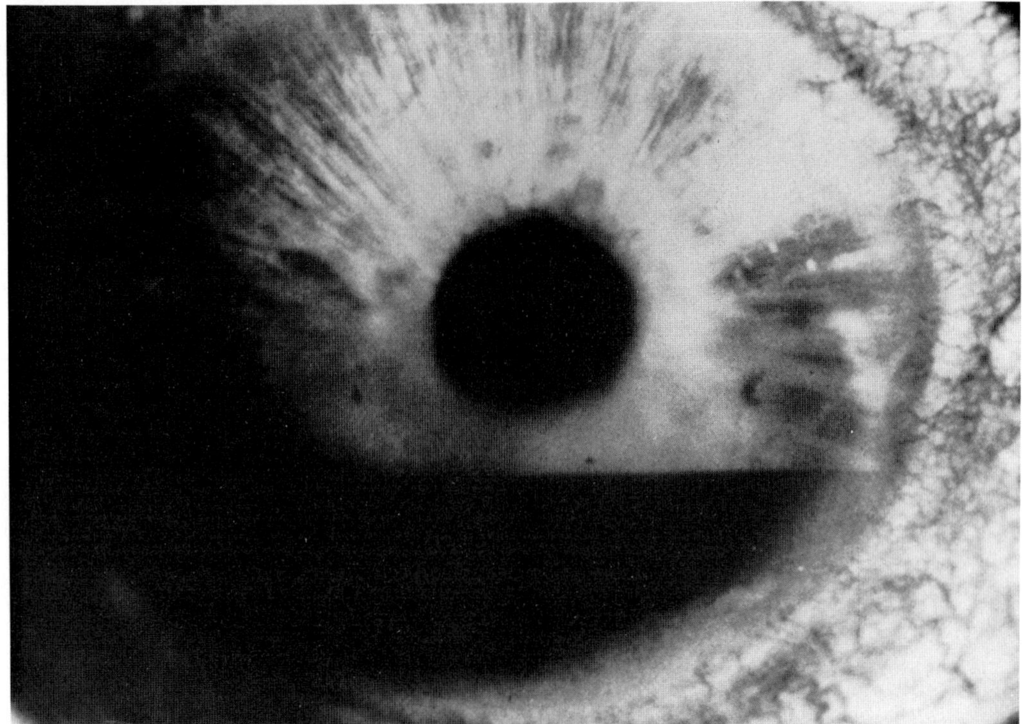

Figure 48.11. This hyphema or blood in the anterior chamber resulted from a contusion to the eye ball.

ognized and must be referred. Treatment, although controversial, entails sedation, usually hospitalization (especially for children), and often bilateral bandaging of the eyes for 5 or 6 days. In most cases, the blood settles down and forms a level in the anterior chamber which absorbs in a matter of 4 or 5 days, depending on the amount.

Secondary glaucoma and blood staining of the cornea are worrisome complications of hyphema that often result in prolonged or permanent disability. Antiglaucoma medical therapy or even surgical intervention may be necessary.

Other Intraocular Injuries

Injuries to the posterior part of the eye are also common, occurring in 23% of the authors' series.

Choroidal Injuries

Choroidal ruptures result when a contrecoup force from a blow by a blunt object to the front of the eye produces a wave of pressure that forces the choroid against the sclera. A split occurs, and, if this split involves the macular area, the visual acuity is markedly reduced in the injured eye (Fig. 48.12).

Choroidal hemorrhages may occur without rupture. Such hemorrhages result in necrosis of the choroid and retina in that area. There is no specific treatment for these injuries, but they should be followed by an ophthalmologist.

Macular Injuries

Macular edema follows severe concussion of the globe with contrecoup force. Central vision is seriously affected. The macular swelling may result in the formation of a macular cyst that may rupture, causing a macular hole and permanent visual impairment (Fig. 48.13). There is no treatment.

Retinal Injuries

Hemorrhages into the retina frequently follow blunt injuries to the eye (Fig. 48.14). They are not incapacitating unless they occur in the macular area. However, retinal tears are not uncommon and may lead to retinal detachment (Fig. 48.15). Detachment may also occur at the ora, the retina's most anterior attachment, resulting in a dialysis of the ora. Early recognition and treatment of the tears and holes will prevent retinal detachment (8). For this reason, eye injuries of even moderate degree deserve ophthalmoscopic examination. Testing of peripheral field may reveal the presence of a retinal detachment.

Detachments of the retina require immediate treatment. If the detachment is allowed to progress, as it most certainly will, to involve the macular area, normal central vision cannot be restored even though the retina is successfully reattached. Any loss of visual acuity accompanied by a loss of field, suggests retinal detachment. Follow-up examination is necessary, and the patient must be warned to report any loss of vision, especially to the side, up, or down. Over one-third of retinal detachments, due to contusion, are sports related. Successful recovery depends on early treatment.

Rupture and Avulsion of the Optic Nerve

A severe, direct blunt injury to the eye may rupture the optic nerve where it enters the eye. One injury,

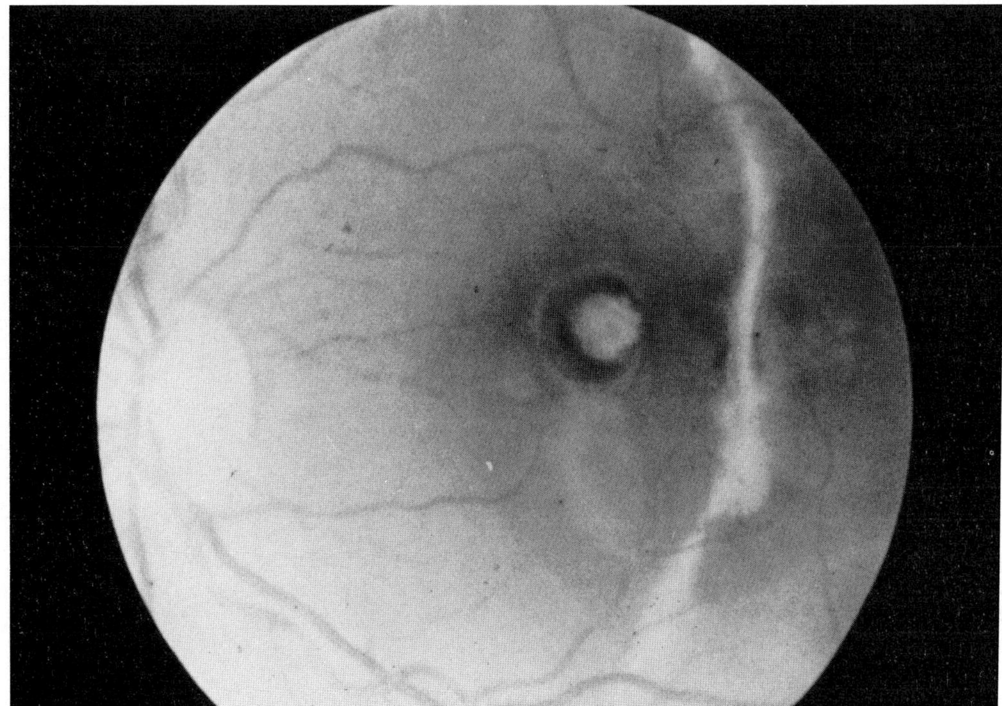

Figure 48.12. This choroidal tear resulted from a blow to the eye such as occurs in racquetball players.

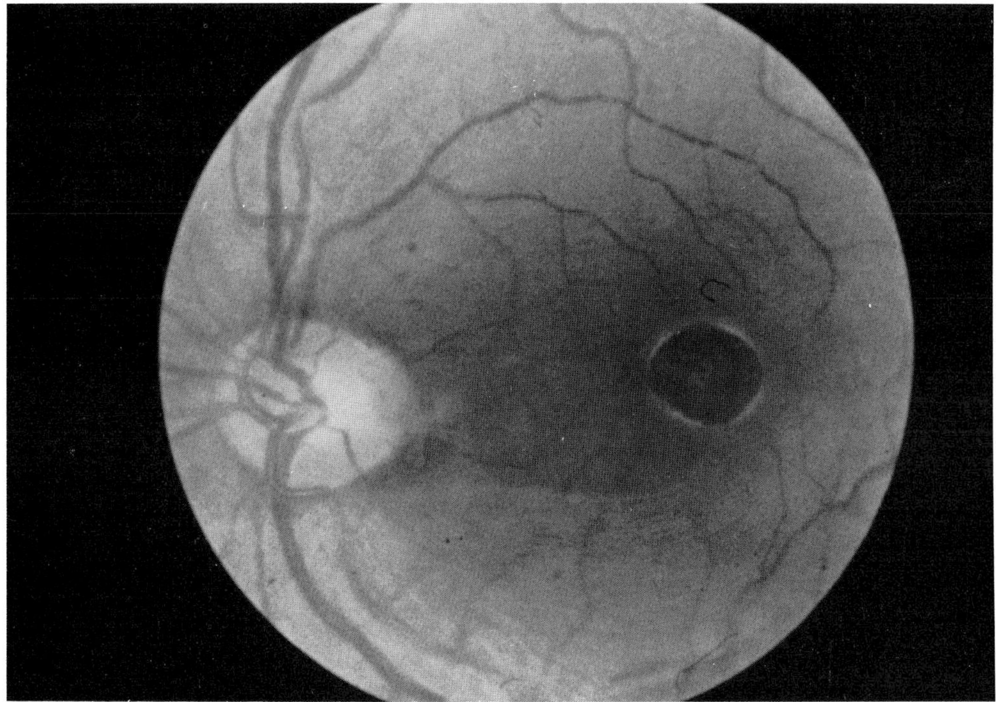

Figure 48.13. Trauma caused this hole in the retina at the site of the macula.

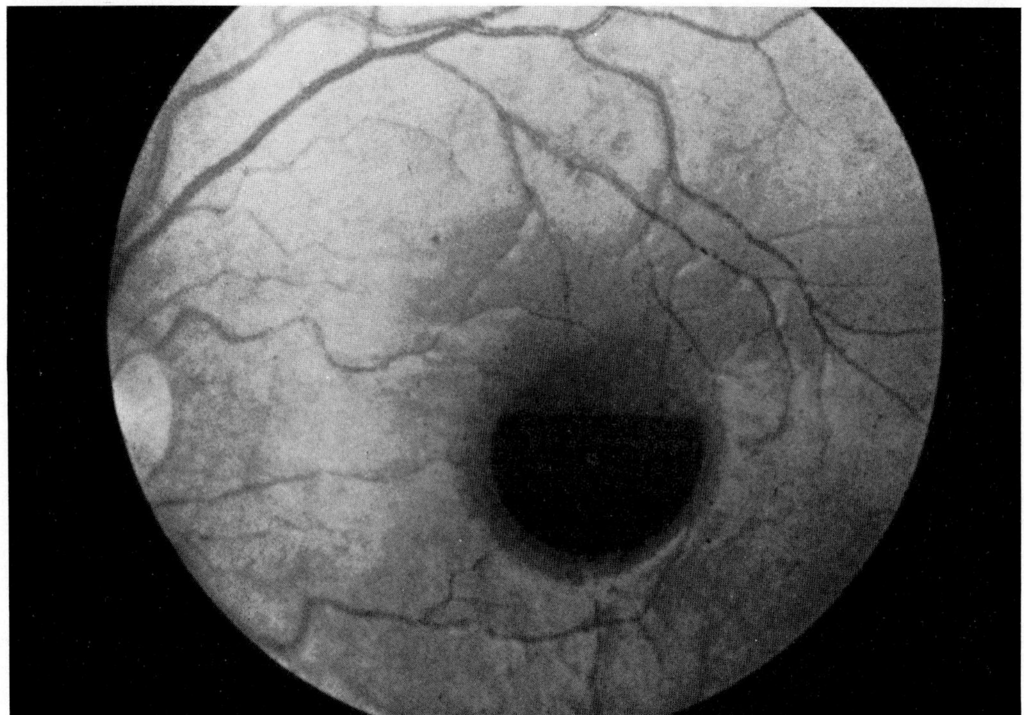

Figure 48.14. Such a retinal hemorrhage may result from a blow to the eye by an opponent's elbow in a basketball game.

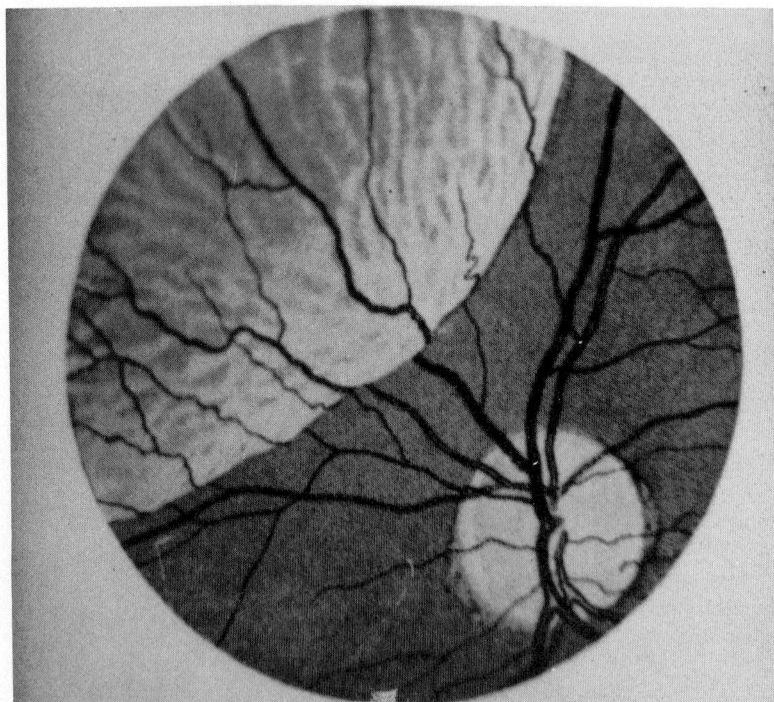

Figure 48.15. This pathologic lesion of retinal detachment is not too uncommon in boxers.

personally seen by the author, resulted in immediate blindness to an eye kicked by a boot. This is an unusual but very sickening injury for which there is no chance of visual recovery.

Corneal Injuries

Corneal injuries cause lacrimation, photophobia, and blepharospasm. There is sudden onset of sharp pain.

Foreign bodies (Fig. 48.16), if superficial, can either be brushed off using a moist, sterile cotton-tipped swab or irrigated off using a sterile irrigating solution. If not easily removed, a sterile eye pad should be applied, and the person taken to the hospital for removal, using the slit lamp and a sterile needle or spud. After removal a firm eye pad is applied for 24 hours, at which time, a follow-up examination is carried out.

Corneal abrasions produce similar symptoms (Fig. 48.17) and can be outlined with fluorescein, which stains the denuded area green. After determining that no other eye problem exists, a sterile eye pad is applied for 24 hours, and then a follow-up examination is conducted.

Corneal lacerations are accompanied by severe pain with tearing, photophobia, and blepharospasm (Fig. 48.18). If the eye can be opened easily, the pupil will be seen to be irregular, the anterior chamber shallow, and the iris adherent to or prolapsed outside the wound (Fig. 48.19). Do not forcibly open the lids because this will cause further damage. Immediate ophthalmologic treatment is necessary. A sterile eye pad and shield should be taped in place (Fig. 48.20) with the patient transported to hospital for repair.

In case of corneal injury or any other ocular injury, a record must be kept of visual acuity, fields of vision, and diplopia (if present) as well as intraocular findings, if possible.

Injuries to the Lens

The lens can be injured by blunt trauma causing concussion that results in cataract formation. This may occur immediately or after a few days, weeks, or even months. In mild cases, the iris, driven forcibly against the anterior lens capsule, leaves a circular mark like that of a rubber stamp on the anterior lens capsule. This is readily seen as the pupil dilates. As a rule, this type of blow does not lead to cataract formation.

More severe blows can cause a rupture of the lens capsule allowing aqueous (the clear fluid in the anterior chamber of the eye) to enter, causing the lens to become cataractous. Localized cataracts may develop after a blow without capsular rupture. Such opacities often take the form of a rosette in the subcapsular areas of the lens (Fig. 48.21).

Blunt injury may cause the lens zonule to rupture so that the lens loses its moorings. If the entire zonule ruptures, the lens becomes dislocated and may disappear into the vitreous or even migrate forward to appear in the anterior chamber. If only part of the zonule ruptures, subluxation occurs, and the lens will shift away from the zone of zonular rupture (Fig. 48.22).

Treatment of cataracts entails removal of the cataractous lens and restoration of visual function using a contact lens. Some professional athletes have continued their careers under these circumstances. Direct injury to the lens, after penetrating wounds of the cor-

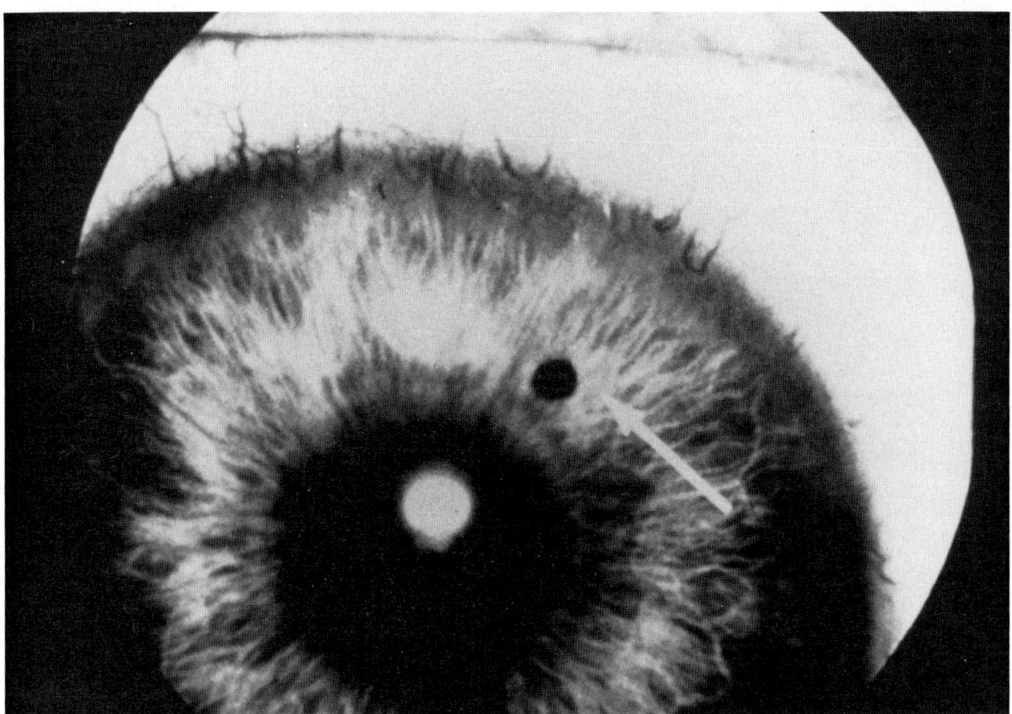

Figure 48.16. While sliding into second base a baseball player occasionally gets a corneal foreign body in his eye.

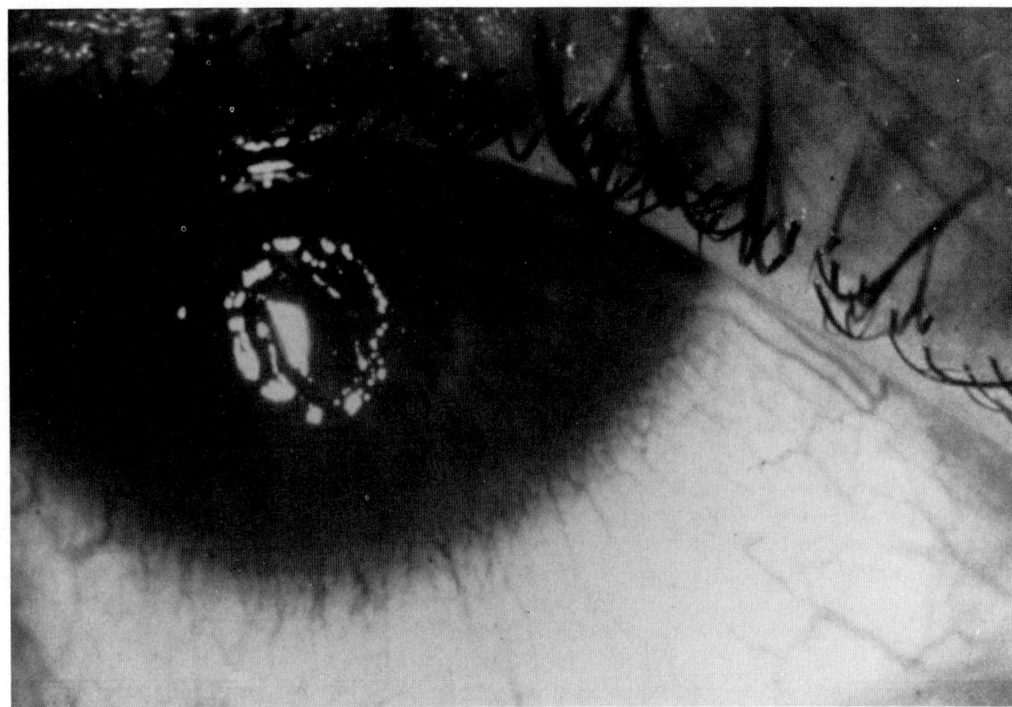

Figure 48.17. Corneal abrasions occur in contact sports as the elbow or padded thighs brush against the player's eye.

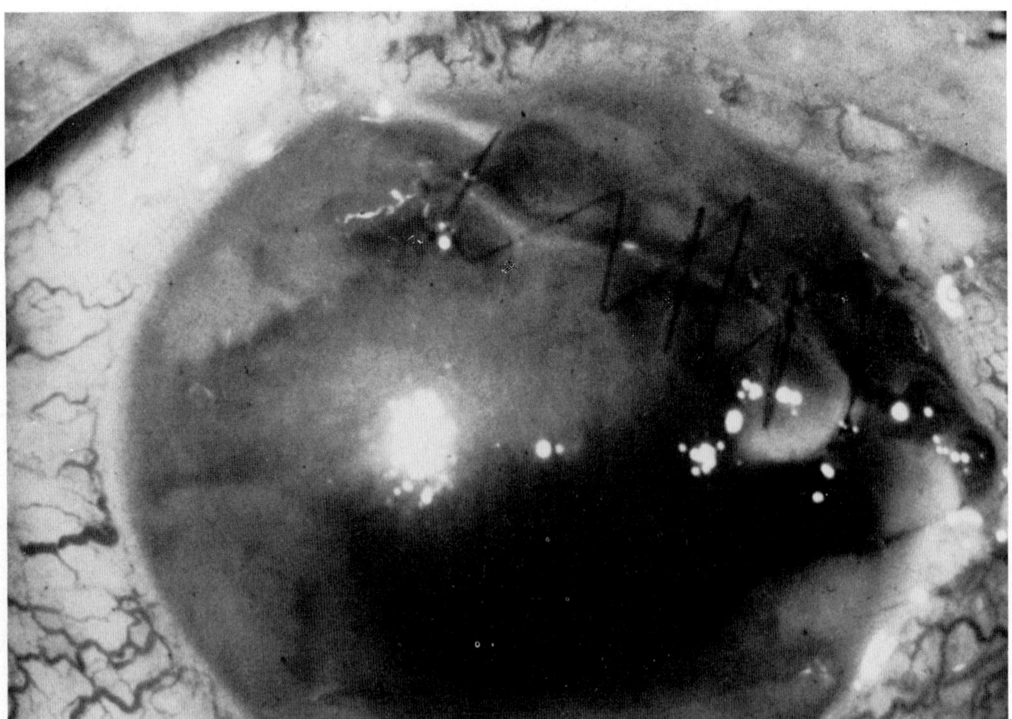

Figure 48.18. A blow to the cornea may cause more than an abrasion with a true tear or laceration of the cornea.

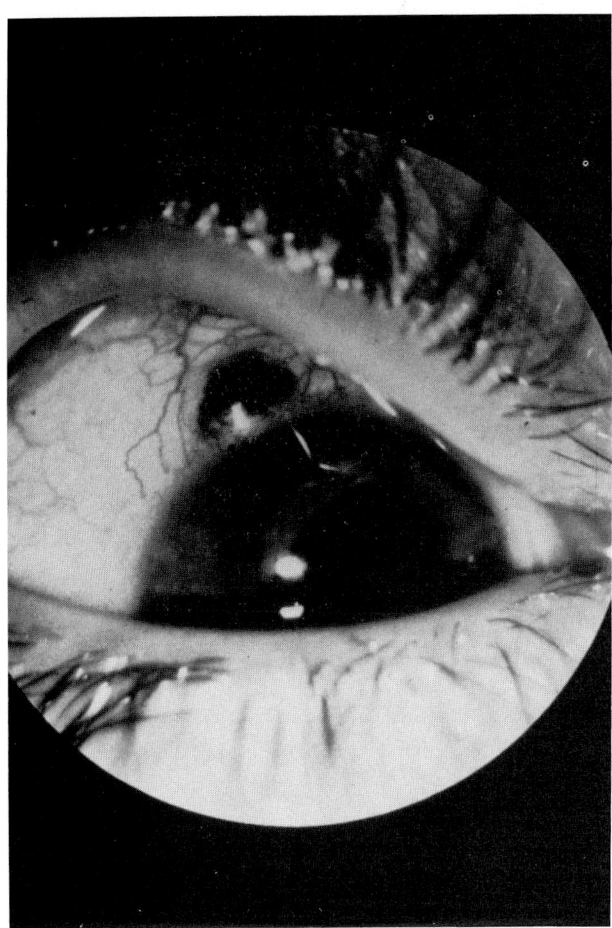

Figure 48.19. With more severe trauma of the eye there may be an iris prolapse.

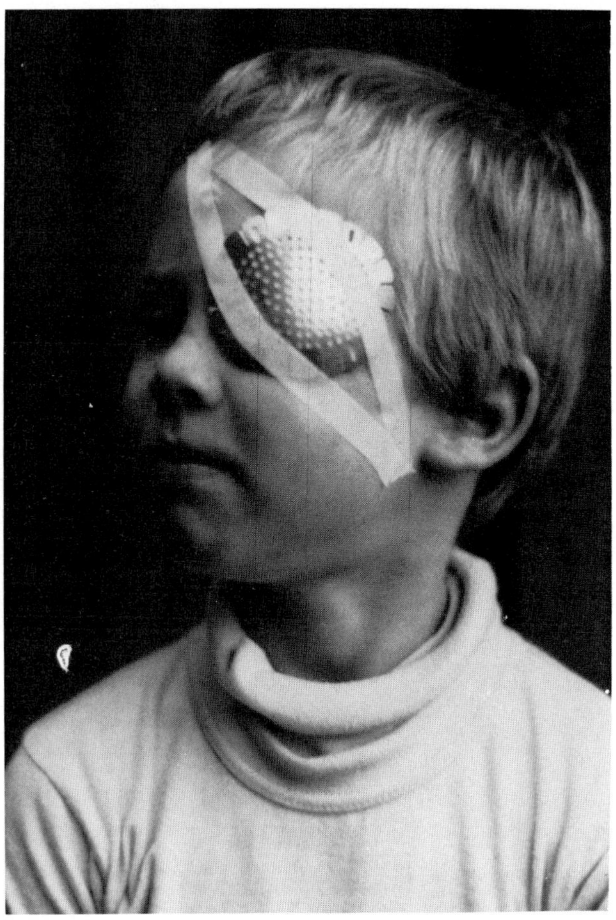

Figure 48.20. After examination and first aid, the eye may be covered with the pad and eye shield in place.

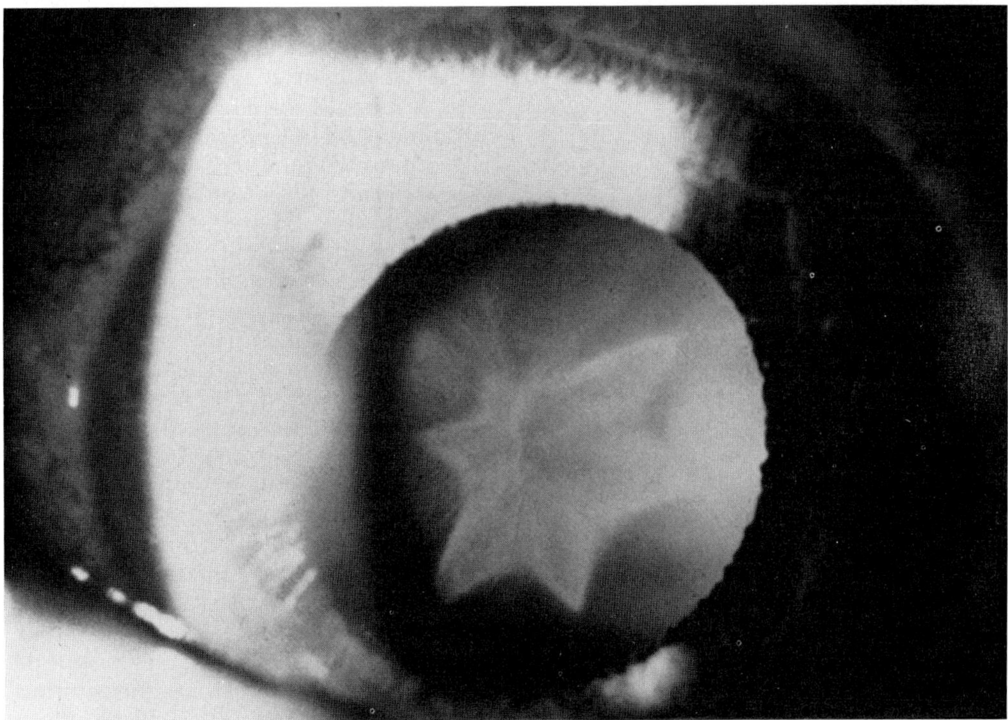

Figure 48.21. A severe blow has caused a localized cataract, resulting in a rosette effect.

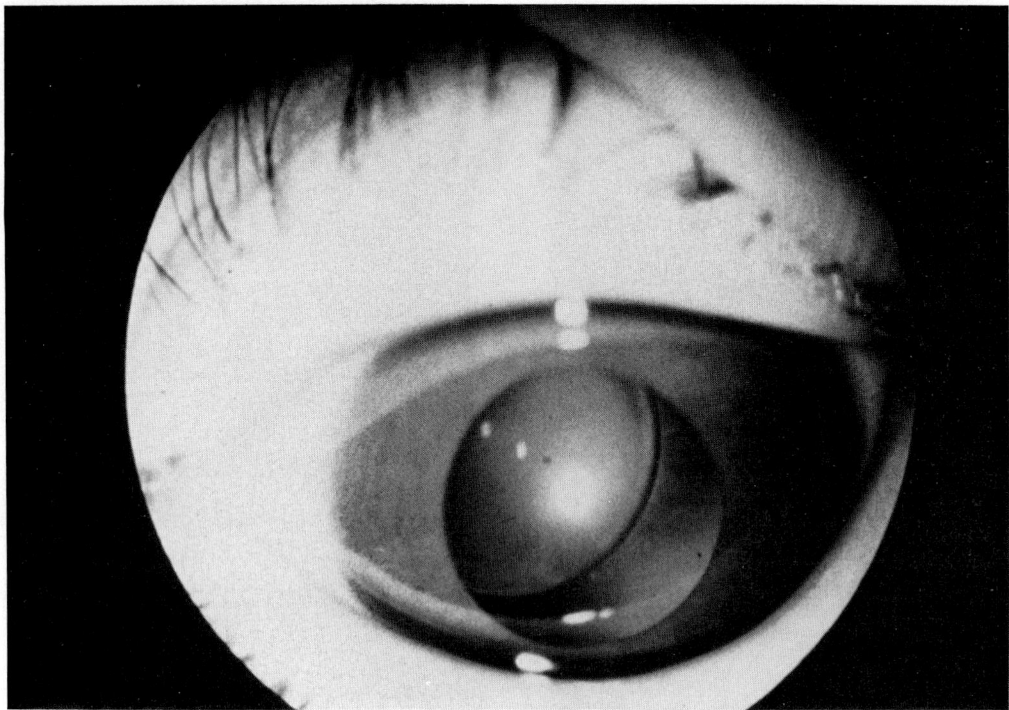

Figure 48.22. This lens has been dislocated by a direct blow to the eye.

nea, is common. The lens material is removed at the time of corneal repair. Injuries to the lens must be recognized by the person rendering first aid and referred for ophthalmological care.

Traumatic Glaucoma

Following blunt injury to the eye, the intraocular pressure may rise and fall, swinging between hypertension and hypotension for a few days, before settling back to normal. In such cases, there is usually no permanent structural damage within the eye. However, blunt injury may damage the anterior chamber angle, resulting in a split of the ciliary body with deepening of the angle and interference with aqueous outflow.

Glaucoma develops in 10% of cases of split angle: it may occur soon after injury or even many years later. Problems of this type should be followed by an ophthalmologist, who can monitor intraocular tensions, because the development of glaucoma is usually insidious, causing damage to the optic nerve without the patient being aware of anything happening.

Any loss of peripheral vision (field loss) resulting from glaucoma cannot be restored. A dislocated lens is another cause of secondary glaucoma; in this case, it is necessary to remove the lens for control of intraocular pressure.

Secondary glaucoma is common with hyphema, especially with secondary hemorrhages. Irrigation of the anterior chamber and removal of the blood clot are indicated. Should the intraocular pressure remain high with blood in the anterior chamber, not only is the optic nerve in danger, but blood staining of the cornea may occur (Fig. 48.23). Even when the intraocular pressure is controlled, the blood staining remains, taking years to absorb.

Orbital Fractures

Orbital fractures are usually sustained by blunt trauma. The most frequent is a fracture of the orbital floor caused by blunt trauma to the eye. This forces the eye back into the orbit, thereby increasing the orbital pressure and causing a "blow out" of the thin, weak orbital floor. One may see limitation of ocular movement, especially on elevation (Fig. 48.24), because of entrapment of the inferior ocular muscles in the fracture. Enophthalmos (Fig. 48.25), due to orbital tissue herniation into the maxillary sinus, is usually evident. Diplopia is also commonly present, being more marked on upward and downward gaze.

Ophthalmologic examination of the globe and investigation of the fracture with x-rays, etc. are mandatory, but not an absolute time emergency. The entrapped muscle can at times be freed by forcibly elevating the eye with forceps after topical anesthesia. Should this not be possible, surgical exploration may be necessary as may the insertion of a Teflon support along the orbital floor to cover the fracture.

Additional orbital fractures may occur in the maxilla or other portions of the orbital rim. These often can be diagnosed by direct palpation and must have appropriate x-ray and clinical evaluation. Fractures of the roof necessitate neurosurgical assessment, with the ophthalmologist in a secondary position.

Fracture into one of the sinuses often leaks air into the orbital cavity, which produces crepitus (a crackling sound) when finger pressure is applied on the swollen

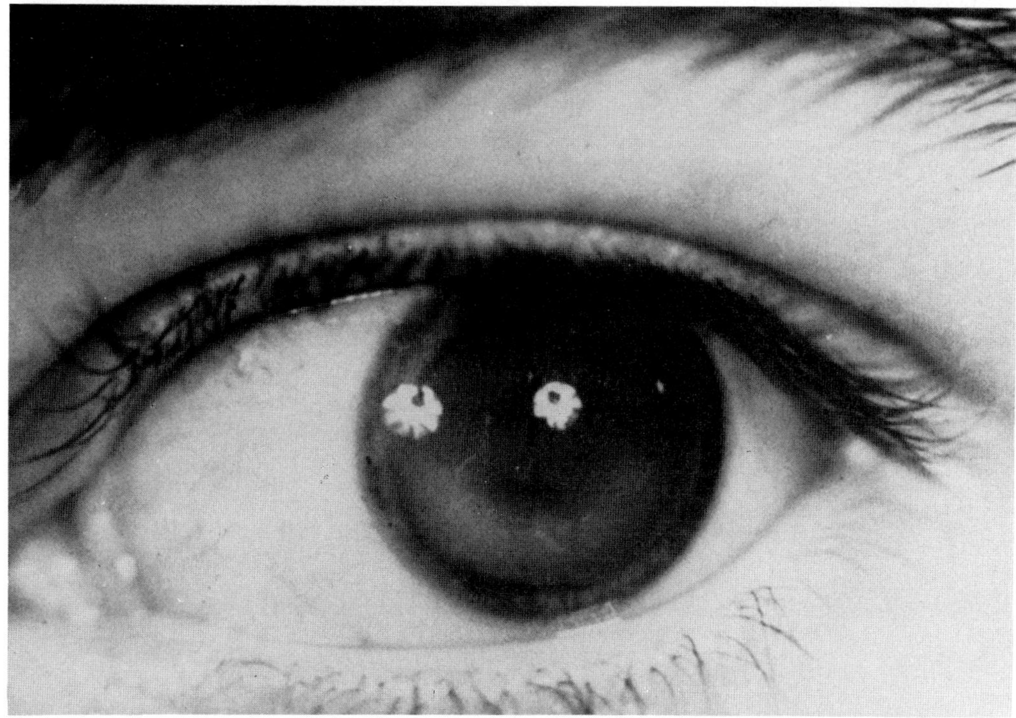

Figure 48.23. Such blood staining of the cornea may be slowly absorbed.

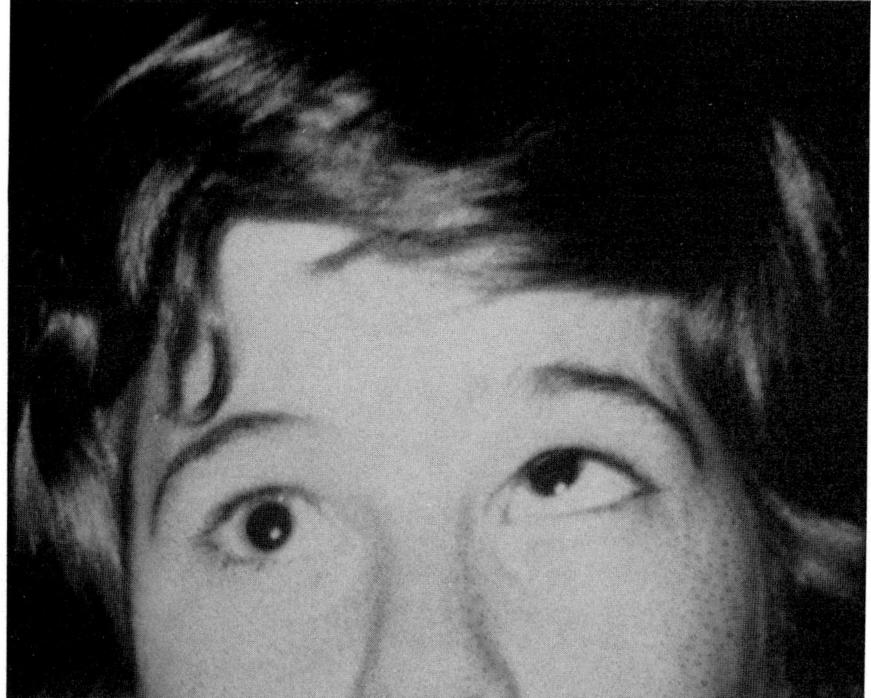

Figure 48.24. A blunt orbital floor trauma resulted in a fracture and left inferior rectus muscle entrapment with double vision.

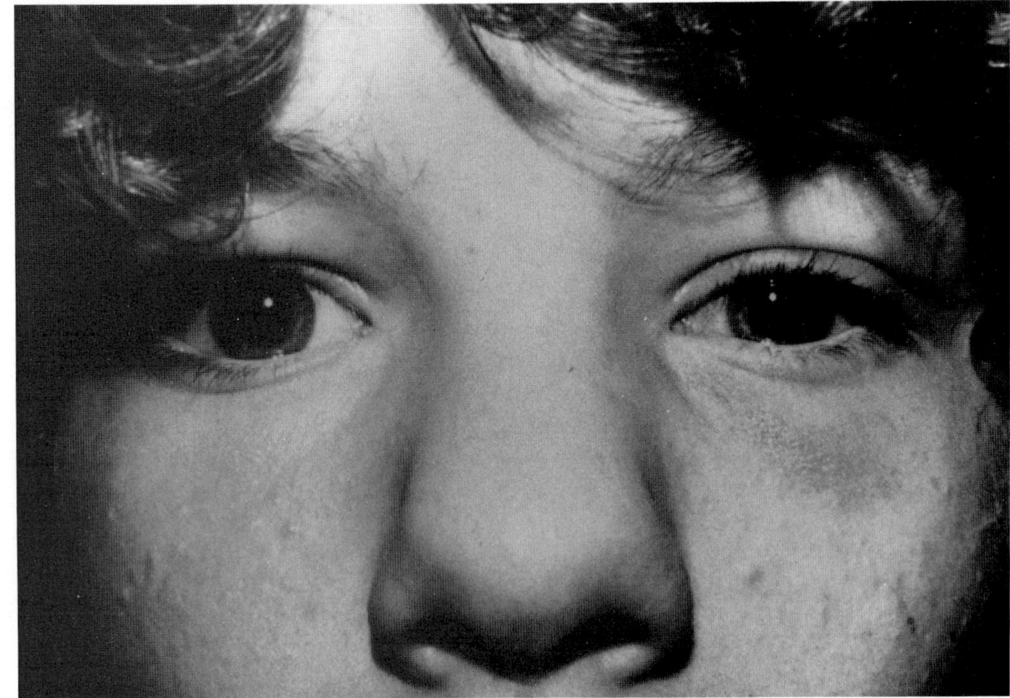

Figure 48.25. Note the narrowing of the left orbital fissure due to escape of orbital contents through the orbital floor fracture into the maxillary sinus.

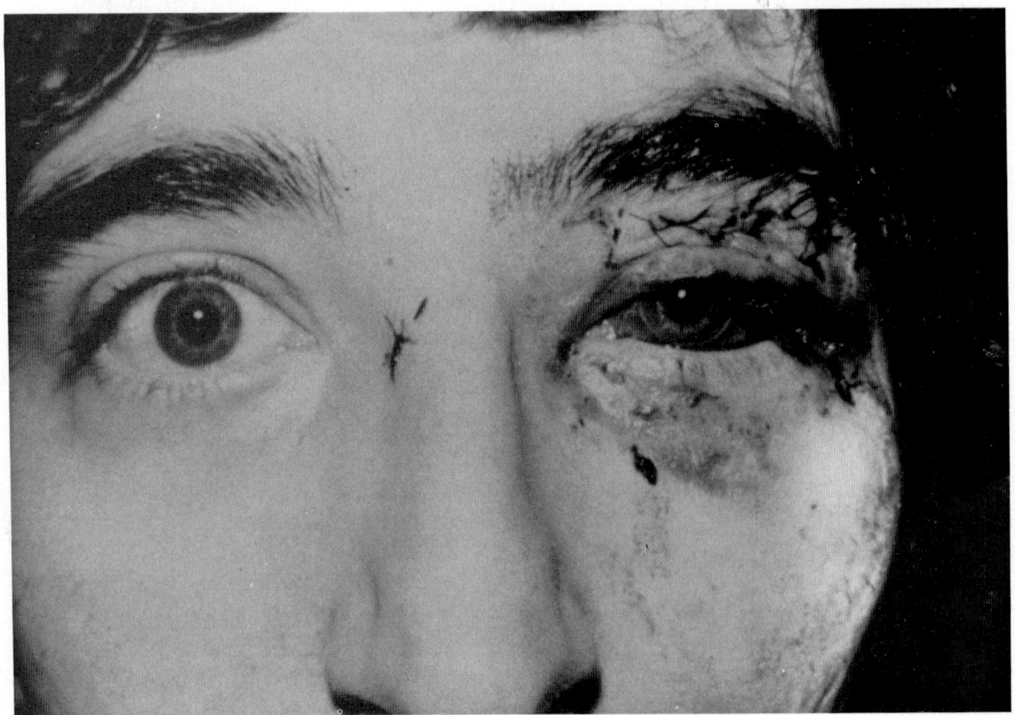

Figure 48.26. There has been resolution of the fracture into one of the sinuses without surgical intervention.

area. The air and fracture are readily demonstrated on x-ray. Resolution without surgical intervention is usual (Fig. 48.26), but prophylactic antibiotic treatment is a good idea.

Ruptured Globe

Ruptured globes (Fig. 48.27) usually result from contact with a hockey stick or puck, a golf ball or club, a ski tip, a squash ball or racquet, a tennis ball, or a baseball. They are usually caused by high-velocity, low-mass missiles. Rupture can also occur when a slower moving, high-mass object, such as a fist or large ball, strikes the eye with a glancing blow. This type of rupture usually occurs near the limbus where the sclera is thinnest. Most of these injuries result in enucleation (9).

A direct blow on the front of the cornea by an object larger than the orbital opening is more likely to produce a blow-out fracture. When ruptured, the globe will appear soft or collapsed and sunken in the orbit. Such an eye must be gently covered with a sterile eye pad and shield, and the patient must be transported directly to the hospital for ophthalmologic repair.

Contact Lenses

In the 1940s, scleral contact lenses were custom-made for a National Hockey League player. These lenses cleared the cornea and rested on the sclera. The corneal cup was filled with a balanced salt solution before insertion. However, this solution tended to cloud during play, and fresh solution was required between periods of the hockey game. These lenses were difficult to make and somewhat uncomfortable.

Late in the decade, hard corneal lenses became available. They were easier to fit and insert, but also more easily displaced after a blow. They might also migrate down into the lower fornix or more commonly up under the upper lid (Fig. 48.28*A*). The displaced lens could either be removed by irrigating with sterile eye solution or lifted off by applying a small suction cup.

A hard contact lens has been known to split in two halves from a blow in a hockey game (Fig. 48.28.*B*) with resultant corneal abrasion, but no permanent visual defect. Both halves were found in the fornix and preserved as a trophy. At times, small foreign bodies could become trapped under these hard contacts, scratching the cornea, causing much pain and preventing continuation of play.

In the 1960s, soft contact lenses became available. They were more comfortable but more fragile and required nightly disinfection and cleaning to prevent bacterial and fungal growth. They did not dislocate easily from the cornea and they sealed out foreign bodies because of their larger size and snugly fitting edge. There was no spectacle blur on switching to regular glasses as had commonly been the case with hard contacts. Soft contacts were usually replaced every 6 to 12 months because of the buildup of tear deposits.

A wide range of soft hydrophilic lens materials became available with higher water content and greater oxygen permeability. The very thin, high water content lenses were approved for extended wear, but experience showed that this regimen led to a substantial increase in ocular infections.

Recently, disposable soft contact lenses have become available and can be recommended. They are available in powers up to 9 diopters of myopia and will compen-

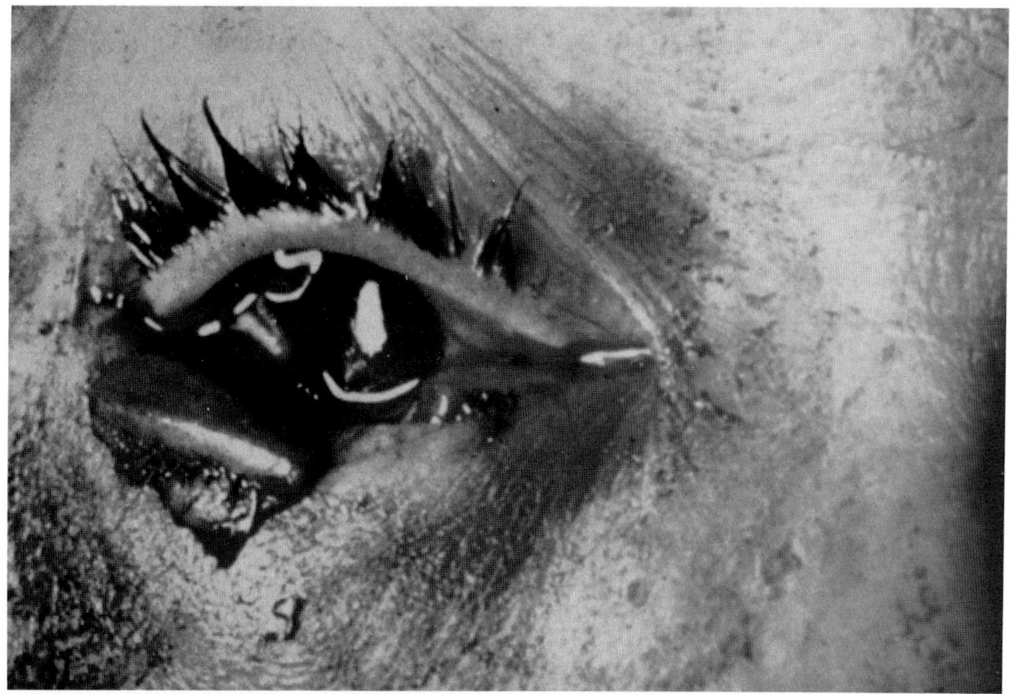

Figure 48.27. A severe glancing or direct blow to this right eye has resulted in a rupture globe.

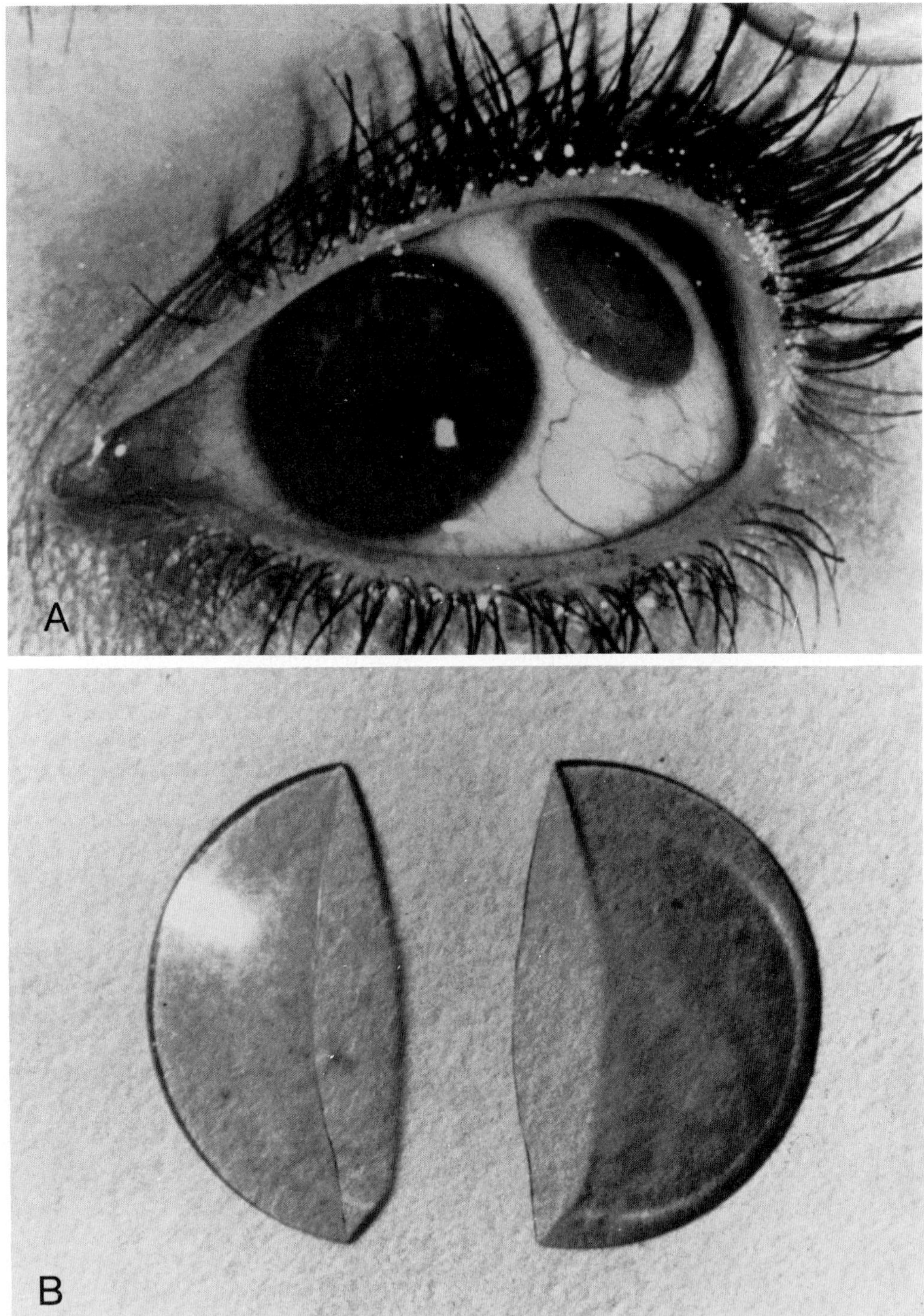

Figure 48.28. A, The contact lens has been displaced upward and laterally by a blow to the eye. **B,** Traumatic hockey injury resulted in this split of the hard contact lens.

sate for up to 2 diopters of astigmatism. The Canadian cost is approximately $12.00 per pair. They are discarded after 1 week of wear. Because of their high water content, they are very comfortable, and because they are discarded after 1 week of wear, there is no problem with protein deposits on the lens. They are easy to insert and remove.

The advantages of contact lenses over regular glasses include improved peripheral field of vision and less tendency to be displaced; in addition, they do not fog. It must be stressed, however, that they provide no protection against injury. Safety glasses or other types of eye protection must be worn where indicated.

Table 48.1.
Commonly Used Eyedrops

1. Antiinfective—Bacitracin	500 units per mL
—Chloramphenicol	0.5%
—Framycetin	0.5%
—Gentamicin	0.3%
—Polymyxin	0.25%
—Tobramycin	0.3%
—Sulfacetamide	10.0% and 30.0%
2. Antiallergic—Naphazoline	0.1%
3. Local anesthetics—Lidocaine	2.0%
—Pontocaine	0.5%

Common Eye Infections

Bacterial and viral infections of the external eyes and lids are frequently contagious and can be passed from one individual to others. Individual wash cloths and towels should be used to prevent spread of the infection. Warm compresses 4 times daily followed by sulfacetamide or broad-spectrum antibiotic drops are needed for 5 to 7 days until the infection clears.

Contact lenses must not be worn while an eye infection is present.

Infections of the Eyelids

Blepharitis is a low-grade chronic infection of the eyelid margins, usually due to *Staphylococcus aureus*. The eyelids are red and often scaly and sticky, particularly on awakening. Scrubbing the eyelid margins with a clean moist face cloth or with baby shampoo-soaked cotton-tipped swabs and then applying an antibiotic ointment at bedtime is indicated.

Hordeolum, styes, are infections in the eyelash follicles causing redness, swelling, and pain. Warm compresses and antibiotic drops are indicated. Staphylococci are the usual cause.

Chalazions occur with a blockage of the meibomian glands of the eyelid, forming a granuloma. Swelling, redness, and pain in the lid proper is the rule. The chalazion may point toward the skin but usually points backward toward the eye causing a foreign body sensation. It is better seen by everting the lid, unless too painful. Warm compresses and antibiotic drops are indicated, plus the addition of systemic antibiotics, if severe or with involvement of the preauricular gland. When persistent, surgical incision and curettage is indicated.

Conjunctivitis

Conjunctivitis of bacterial or viral origin is contagious. The eye is red ("pinkeye"), often photophobic, and sticky discharge is present. Warm compresses 4 times daily, followed by the instillation of antibiotic drops is indicated for 5 to 7 days, or until the infection subsides.

Allergic conjunctivitis causes swelling, redness and itching. Tearing is present but without sticky discharge. Treatment with systemic antihistamine tablets and antiallergy eye drops afford relief. (Table 48.1 lists commonly used eyedrops.)

Table 48.2.[a]
Eye Injuries in Canadian Sports

Sport	Injuries	Blind Eyes
Ice Hockey	1790	275
Racquet Sports	1028	45
Baseball	426	24
Ball Hockey	336	29
Football	170	8
Golf	53	16
Skiing	33	9
Volleyball	27	4
Broomball	25	2
Basketball	37	1
Snowmobiling	11	5
War Games	61	24
Other Sports	139	14
Total	4136	456

[a]Data to July 1, 1993.

Conclusion

In conclusion, it may be noted that eye injuries incurred during sports participation have been recorded over the past 20 years by Canadian ophthalmologists with 4136 sports eye injuries recorded to date (October 1993), including 456 blind eyes (Table 48.2). It is estimated that 90% of these injuries could have been prevented had the participants worn available certified eye protection.

REFERENCES

1. Hornblass A: Eye injuries in the military. Int Ophthalmol Clin 1981;21:121.
2. Vinger PF, ed. Ocular sports injuries. Int Ophthalmol Clin 1981;21:21.
3. Vaughan D, Asbury T. General Ophthalmology. 9th ed. Los Altos, CA: Lange Medical Publications, 1980.
4. Pashby TJ. Eye injuries in Canadian hockey. Phase II. Can Med Assoc J 1977;117:671.
5. Pashby TJ. Eye injuries in Canadian hockey. Phase III: Older players now at most risk. Can Med Assoc J 1979;121:643.
6. Pashby TJ, Bishop PJ, Easterbrook WM. Eye injuries in Canadian racquet sports. Can Fam Physician 1982;28:967.
7. Pashby TJ, Pashby RC, Chisholm LDJ, Crawford JS. Eye injuries in Canadian hockey. Can Med Assoc J 1975;113:663. 674.
8. Antaki S, Labelle P, Dumas J. Retinal detachment following hockey injury. Can Med Assoc J 1977;117:245.
9. Diamond GR, Quinn GE, Pashby TJ, Easterbrook WM. Ophthalmologic injuries. Clin Sports Med 1982;1:469.

49 / CERVICAL SPINE AND SPINAL CORD INJURIES

Robert G. Watkins and William M. Dillin

In many of today's sports, particularly in contact sports, the neck is at risk for injury because of an inability to pad, brace, or protect the cervical spine and allow it to maintain its function. The flexibility and motion of the cervical spine must deliver the head and eyes to the right place at the right time. The function of the spine also includes being a conduit for the central nervous system, with the spinal cord and the cervical nerve roots passing through, making injury to the neck a potentially catastrophic event. The incidence of sports-related injuries to the spinal cord in football has been reported by Clark (1) to be 54% of all spinal cord injuries in school and college athletics. Torg (2) has reported on the findings of the National Football Head and Neck Injury Registry, which was established to document the incidence and nature of severe intracranial and cervical spine injuries resulting from tackle football. The criteria for inclusion in the Registry are injuries that require hospitalization for at least 72 hours, injuries of the neck involving fracture subluxation or dislocation, injuries involving intracranial hemorrhage, or injuries with associated quadraplegia or death. A recent update on the Registry (2) has shown that between 1971 and 1984, there were 1412 cervical spine injuries meeting these criteria. The prevention of cervical spine and spinal cord injuries is of paramount importance. The responsibility for educating athletes in methods to prevent neck injury is most important in those sports in which the risk of trauma to the cervical spine is the highest. Contact sports, such as football, rugby, and wrestling, have been identified as being particularly high-risk activities for cervical trauma (2). The use of the head as an offensive weapon to block and tackle makes football a significant source of cervical injuries. Even noncontact sports, such as diving, water skiing, surfing, water polo, and body surfing, can be responsible for traumatic spinal injuries (3). The prevention of neck injuries in athletes involves the education of players, trainers, and physicians.

Prevention of these injuries must incorporate appropriate rule changes for those sports that are at highest risk. After research by Dr. Joseph Torg (2) and others proved the role of head contact in catastrophic injuries of the head and neck in football players in the mid-1970s, the National Collegiate Athletic Association (NCAA) made rule changes that condemned the use of the head in tackling and effectively outlawed the technique of blocking and tackling known as spearing. These rule changes have been noted to have had significant impact on the instance of traumatic cervical spine and spinal cord injuries in football players from the high school through the collegiate level and up to the professional level (2). Also, modification of protective gear to incorporate newly developed modern materials and equipment into properly fitting shoulder pads and neck pad modifications has added, it is hoped, to the decrease incidence of neck injuries in athletes.

The treatment of the athlete with neck, cervical spine, or spinal cord trauma, remains one of the most medically challenging of all aspects in sports medicine. There have been no "miraculous" medical breakthroughs that have made a significant impact on the catastrophic consequences of a young, active athlete suffering a complete spinal cord injury. Recently, Braacken et al. (4), published their findings of a study of high-dose intravenous corticosteroids administered immediately after spinal cord injury and its effectiveness on the subsequent neurologic outcome of those patients. They showed that a 24-hour course of corticosteroids administered within 6–8 hours after cervical spinal cord injury may be associated with an improved prognosis for cervical nerve root sparing and may lead to the cervical spinal cord injury patient recovering one to two more cervical nerve root levels. However, even this ray of hope in the treatment of spinal cord injury is not enough to allow for complacency in the continual goal of the sports medicine community to decrease further the incidence of cervical spine and spinal cord injuries in athletes.

Football players are at greater risk for cervical injury than are the average adult in the United States. The nature of the game of football requires violent contact between the head and shoulders of a player and the body of his opponent or the hard surface of the playing field. Besides protective equipment and educational techniques to enhance the football player's awareness of the potential for neck injury, several other protective factors can be maximized to decrease the risk of cervical spinal cord injury in these athletes. Neck-strengthening exercises can build muscle bulk and increase the protective capability of the thick sleeve of neck and shoulder muscles that surround the cervical spine. The biomechanical advantage afforded by powerful and bulky neck flexors, extensors, and rotators, as well as massive trapezius and shoulder girdle musculature is evidenced in the modern professional football player. This is particularly true when it is understood that many of the professional football athletes playing today may have narrowed cervical spinal canals secondary to degenerative changes in the cervical discs and cervical facet joints with hypertrophic bony encroachment of the spinal canal. Yet, the incidence of catastrophic cervical spinal cord injuries in professional football players is exceedingly low. By increasing the level of conditioning of the athlete and improvements in balance, coordination, and skill, the natural and acquired protective actions of the cervical musculature and shoulder musculature are increased. The likelihood of fatigue causing a diminution of these protective mechanisms is decreased.

The responsibility for teaching and enforcing proper tackling techniques must fall to the football coaches and referees. Safe tackling techniques must become second nature to the player and must be enforced. Safe blocking and tackling avoid the use of the head in initial contact. Spearing and the use of the head as an offensive weapon increase the risk of cervical spine fractures and quadraplegia. Since the rule changes banning the use of the head as a battering ram, the incidence of quadraplegia in football players has dropped dramatically (2). The biomechanics of cervical spine fracture illustrates that direct head compression, with axial loading and flexion, is a major mechanism of injury fracture or dislocation of the cervical spine in football players. To resist the loading impact, attacking players straighten out their cervical spine to a neutral position. The loading on the crown of the athlete's head plus the velocity of body weight compress the cervical spine. Just as one would buckle a simple soda straw by squeezing the ends between the fingers, the spine buckles in the middle, and produces an axial loading flexion rotation injury. There is an accordion effect of bone and ligamentous failure of the cervical column (2). This is exactly the injury pattern that may occur to the cervical spine when the player uses the head as a battering ram, particularly when that player is fatigued, is wearing inadequate protective equipment, does not have adequate neck strength and muscle bulk, and does not have adequate levels of overall conditioning.

Clinical Anatomy, Signs, and Symptoms

The cervical spinal cord is housed in the neck by the rigid intercollated spinal motion units. Rigid bony protection against direct blows as well as protection against axial loading, flexion, extension, and torsional injuries is afforded by the lamina, spinous processes, facet joints, and vertebral bodies of the cervical spine. However, with axial loading and bending that surpasses the bony element's biomechanical capability and strength, there may be the resultant fracture, dislocations, or both. This failure of the bony elements of the spine may cause injury to the spinal cord or cervical nerve roots. The same may occur when the mechanical limits of the ligamentous and muscular support of the neck are exceeded in traumatic situations.

The spinal cord begins at the cervical medullary junction and extends through the cervical and thoracic spine to terminate caudally at the L1-L2 junction as the conus medullaris. From the conus medullaris, the lumbosacral nerve roots emanate like a horse's tail, the cauda equina. The lumbar and sacral nerve roots exit the spinal cord via the corresponding neural foramina. In the neck, the cervical spinal cord produces the cervical nerve roots, which exit above the named cervical vertebra via the neural foramina. For example, the sixth cervical nerve roots exit the cervical spinal canal via the neural foraminal formed by the fifth cervical vertebra, cephalad, and the sixth cervical vertebra, caudally. This relationship between spinal level and root level has important diagnostic and prognostic implication when an athlete sustains a spinal cord injury. From a surgical viewpoint, the precise anatomic level corresponding to nerve tissue damage is critical in assuring that surgical intervention, if warranted, is performed at the correct level. Prognostically, the potential for functional independence in a quadraplegic patient increases dramatically with each functioning root level below the fourth cervical nerve root. Clinically, the difference between a C5-level quadraplegic and a C7-level quadraplegic is dramatic. In fact, the recovery of a single additional cervical nerve root level in a quadraplegic patient can mean the difference between a completely dependent existence and a completely independent and functional life.

Cervical spine or spinal cord injury has a more favorable prognosis when identification of the injury is made prior to any further movement of the injured patient. An unstable fracture or dislocation without neurologic injury has catastrophic sequelae if improper transportation techniques are utilized, even if performed by well-meaning and concerned individuals. The player with an unstable cervical spine injury may not be aware of the magnitude of the injury because of the minimal amount of pain felt by the player at the time of injury. When in a game situation, it is not unusual for the player to shrug off even the most serious neck injuries as minor because of the minimal symptomatology present on the playing field. However, once identified as a spinal cord injury, the level of cord injury can be quickly assessed by simple pinprick sensation testing along the cervical dermatomes and by manual muscle strength testing. The fifth cervical nerve root supplies sensation to the deltoid region in lateral brachium distally to the elbow. The sixth cervical nerve root supplies the skin sensation to the lateral forearm from the elbow distally to include the thumb and index finger. The seventh cervical nerve root supplies the sensation to the upper extremity and the dermatomal pattern that includes the midpalm as well as the long finger. The eighth cervical nerve root supplies the dermatomal pattern that includes the ulnar border of the forearm as well as the ring and small fingers. The first thoracic nerve root supplies the dermatomal region medially at the elbow and proximally up toward the middle part of the arm. It is not unusual for there to be some overlap of adjacent dermatomes in individuals.

The motor deficits identifiable in cervical spinal cord injury are categorized according to which motor groups are spared. Remember, the third cervical root exits at the level of the second and third cervical disc level. Schneider (5) has summarized the injury levels.

C3-C4 Level

Injury at the C3-C4 level may result in complete paralysis of the trunk and extremities, with a complete loss of all normal unassisted respirations due to a paralysis of the diaphragm as well as of the thoracic musculature. A loss of pain to pinprick, to a point just below the clavicle, including the upper extremities, may be evidenced.

C4-C5 Level

Athletes can only shrug their shoulders, indicating trapezius innervation via the second and third cervical nerve roots to the motor branch of the spinal accessory nerve. The arms, the lower extremities, and trunk will be without movement with the toes pointed outward These patients will have only abdominal breathing. The progression of spinal cord swelling or hemorrhage may occur, particularly if inappropriate immobilization techniques are utilized, even if only one more segment toward the head, may mean the cessation of spontaneous respirations. The motor fibers to the diaphragm via the phrenic nerve, from the C3 and C4 nerve cell bodies exit from the spinal cord with the upper portion of the C5 root. The absence of pain sensation is present to the level of the outer border of the upper extremity between the shoulder and elbow.

C5-C6 Level

At this level, players will be able to bend their arms at the elbows and they will tend to remain flexed in that position unless they fall downward with gravity. Attempted movements of the hands result in hyperextension at the wrists with inability to close the fingers voluntarily. Extension of the arms is markedly impaired. There may be a loss of pain on pinprick over the region of the thumb and index finger of the hand.

C6-C7 Level

With injury at this level, athletes will be able to close their hands very weakly and grasp with the fingers. The arms can be flexed and extended weakly at the elbows. They may be unable to spread the fingers apart strongly because of loss of the intrinsic musculature innervation to the hands. Pinprick sensation will be intact over the thumb and index finger, but will usually be lost over the middle and radial half of the ring finger.

C7-T1 Level and Below

Injuries occurring at the C7-T1 junction and below can result in complete sparing of the muscle function of the upper extremities with only lower extremity paraplegia resulting. Trunk control, including the control of the rectus abdominis, internal and external oblique muscles, and the spinal extensor muscles is, however, affected by the level of the thoracic spinal injury. With a more caudal level of thoracic spinal cord injury, there is an increased ability of the patient to adapt to activities requiring controlled and coordinated trunk musculature activity. Pinprick sensation will be impaired from the dermatomal level corresponding to the level of injury. Fracture dislocations of the thoracic or lumbar spine are much less common in the athlete, in part, because of the benefit of protective equipment, such as shoulder pads covering the area. Also, the thoracic rib cage imparts significant structural support to the thoracic spine. The lumbar spine is more protected than the neck because of the increasing size and strength of the vertebra and of the surrounding trunk musculature.

Schneider has stressed that these are rather simple tests that are far from a complete neurologic examination and are meant only as a quick method of determining the level of neurologic injury in a player that is, for example, laying on the playing field (6). A very high degree of suspicion must be maintained when examining players injured on the field if there are indications that a neck injury has occurred. When there are questionable findings or when the examining coach, trainer, or physician believes that a neck injury has occurred, but the player's complaints include only some vague neck stiffness or neck pain, or when there are minimal objective findings to support concern, these players should be treated as if they have a true injury until this can be proven otherwise.

Much more common than complete or incomplete spinal cord injury are the lesions known as burners and stingers. The characteristic motor and sensory manifestations are thought to be quite common among football players. At least 50% of college players have experienced a burner (7). Cervical nerve root or brachial plexus neuropraxia is considered to be the etiology of stingers and burners. Such lesions are identified by intense burning pain accompanied by numbness, paresthesias, and transient weakness in the arm. The symptoms usually last from a few seconds up to 15 minutes. The symptoms start immediately after head and shoulder contact, usually with the opponent, but sometimes after striking the playing surface. The pain typically involves the entire arm from the fingertips up to the neck and shoulder. Commonly, the last symptoms to resolve are that of the C5 or C6 dermatomal pattern. Players may complain of recurrent stingers and burners throughout the season and in the offseason. Almost always, when the symptoms are recurrent, the same dermatomal pattern is present, the same motor deficit is present, and the same biomechanical mechanism of injury is present in the subsequent episodes. However, it is not unusual for a multiroot pattern to be found. Repeated episodes over a season may result in significant weakness of the deltoid and biceps (8). A residual neurologic deficit may persist for days to months following more severe episodes. Burners are very common in football players. Most teams have a certain number of burners every season.

The mechanism of injury most often seen in professional football players is an off-center axial load that is applied to the head with the head uncontrollably forced both into extension and lateral flexion. This forces the head toward the ipsilateral side of the resultant burner and stinger. Biomechanically, the cord, nerves, and canal will respond in a predictable manner.

Extension of the spine produces a slackening of the cord and spinal nerves; whereas flexion increases nerve tension. Extension decreases the size of the spinal canal and foraminae, and flexion increases the size of the canal and foraminae. With extension and bending of the cervical spine toward the involved shoulder and arm, the neural foramina are abruptly narrowed, allowing for the bony walls of the neural foramina, or for intervertebral disc or osteophytes to pinch the nerve root as it exits the spinal canal.

The mechanism of injury is equivalent to the Spurling's maneuver (9), which is a diagnostic sign that can be elicited in the clinical examination in the office setting of patients with cervical radiculopathy. The Spurling's maneuver consists of extension of the head and lateral bending and rotation of the head and neck toward the painful side. When these maneuvers are performed together, a positive Spurling's sign is identified by pain that is reproduced in the patient's shoulder and arm, identical to the pain that is the patient's presenting clinical complaint. A positive Spurling's test indicates cervical foraminal stenosis due to either soft disc herniation or osteophytes encroachment of the neural foramina. This ipsilateral rotation and axial loading mechanism of injury seen with burners implies that the pathomechanics involve a multilevel root contusion from narrowing the canal and foramina. It may be possible to detect a subtle foraminal narrowing at one or more levels on a contrast CT scan. Other cases may demonstrate a profound central canal and foraminal narrowing. There are certainly cases, however, when complete diagnostic evaluation including magnetic resonance imaging, CT myelography, and electromyelographic (EMG) / nerve conduction studies will fail to reveal the source of pathology.

The other possible mechanism of injury in the production of burners and stingers involves an abrupt stretching of the existing cervical nerve roots or the adjacent brachial plexus. The head is forced away or to the opposite side of the depressed shoulder and symptomatic arm. There is an increased tautness to the brachial plexus with this mechanism. While this mechanism of injury is also associated with transient signs and symptoms, the potential for long-term neurologic deficit is present, as it is with the pinching mechanism previously described.

Two distinct and useful classification systems of burners and stingers have been described by Seddon (9), and Clancy and associates (10). In Seddon's classification system, neurapraxia is the mildest lesion that has identifiable histologic findings and corresponds to demyelonization of the axon sheath without intrinsic axonal disruption. Recovery of neural functioning generally occurs within 3 weeks. Axonotemesis includes disruption of the axon and the myelin sheath with preservation of the fibrous epineurium. The epineurium serves as a conduit for the regenerating axon in axonotemesis. In most healthy adults, the rate of recovery in axonotemesis can be expected to be approximately 1 mm/day with an initial 7-day delay from the time of injury. This expected rate of recovery is measured from the site of injury to the motor endplate to which the nerve supplies motor impulses. Neurotemesis corresponds to complete nerve transaction. In neurotemesis, there is generally no possibility of distal nerve regeneration without surgical repair and reapproximation of the nerve sheath.

Clancy et al. utilized Seddon's classification system for definition of the burner syndrome from brachial plexus injury (10). Grade I injuries had an initial recovery of motor and sensory function generally within several minutes of injury and with a complete recovery noticed by 2 weeks. These injuries correspond to Seddon's definition of neurapraxic lesions. Grade II injuries can result in motor loss to the deltoid, biceps, intraspinalis, and supraspinalis muscles. Weakness can last from weeks to months and corresponds to axonotemesis. Grade III lesions would be quite rare and are more typically seen in trauma patients who have suffered from penetrating injury to the neck or shoulder region from a motor vehicle accident, knife fight, gunshot wound, or shrapnel injury from an explosion. Additionally, falling in this classification of injuries would be the scapulothoracic dissociation injury that is associated with high-energy trauma and results in evaluation and separation of the shoulder girdle from the thorax. Scapulothoracic dissociation is additionally associated with significant trauma to the traversing major blood vessels, neurologic structures, and muscular structures. EMG studies will show abnormalities in type II and type III lesions. Generally, the type I or grade I (neurapraxia) will not show EMG or nerve conduction velocity abnormalities. The long-term EMG findings have been studied in a group of 20 athletes with burners by Bergfeld et al. (11). They selected a group of players with clinical findings of severe neurologic involvement after athletic injuries that caused burners or stingers. In the study by Bergfeld et al. (11), the EMG findings generally localized to the upper trunk of the brachial plexus, as well as cervical nerve root and peripheral nerve root levels. This study demonstrated that the EMG abnormalities lagged behind the motor strength recovery of the individual as the injury resolved. They demonstrated that utilizing the EMG as a criterion for return to play after a burner or stinger is an inaccurate and ineffective prognostic measure. We routinely utilize a precise history of symptoms, a detailed neurologic examination, along with provocative testing such as the Spurling's maneuver to decide on a player's timing for return to play after a burner or a stinger. Certainly, an appropriate diagnostic imaging work-up is included in the evaluation of patients with burners or stingers so that the underlying pathology can be identified. Especially in the older athlete, a severe first-time burner may be the symptom of a cervical disc herniation. Under these circumstances, restricting play until the chance of a disc herniation is eliminated by MRI is a safe procedure.

Examination of the player on the sidelines will usually reveal the mechanism of injury by careful questioning and head range-of-motion testing. Spurling's maneuver will reproduce the symptoms. The shoulder abduction test, in which the hand is placed palm down on the top of the head, may alleviate the symptoms somewhat (7). Davidson et al. (12) have observed a series of patients with cervical myeloradiculopathies due to extradural compressive disease in whom clinical signs included relief of radicular pain with abduction of the shoulder. The mechanism by which shoulder abduction may relieve pain from cervical root impingement at the level of the neural foramen was thought to be due to the shorter distance that the nerve root must traverse and is, thus, under less tension when the shoulder is abducted. The study by Davidson et al. included two patients who had myelographically proven extradural impingement of the cervical root. Of the patients in the study by Davidson et al., 68% noted relief of pain with abduction of the affected shoulder. On the field, players with burners or stingers classically hold themselves with the head forward and flexed posture, and they complain of a stiff neck. The arm is too weak to elevate. Attempts to elicit the Spurling's sign are generally met with pain. Occasionally, head compression will reproduce the symptoms. Persistent neck pain with head compression may be considered a fracture or disc herniation until proven otherwise.

Garfin and associates (13) have studied the question of whether compressive neuropathy of spinal nerve roots is a mechanical or a biologic problem. They believe that, pathophysiologically, nerve root pain production is a complex issue. They have identified clinical data and basic science data that suggest mechanical compression, per se, may not always be the sole cause of radicular pain and dysfunction. Specifically, they have identified that acute compression of a normal cervical nerve usually does not cause pain but rather causes numbness, paresthesias, motor weakness, and related signs and symptoms. They also identified mechanical compression of a normal spinal nerve root, which also seems to induce similar senory and motor impairment without associated pain. However, the compression of inflamed nerve roots and mechanical deformation of inflamed and irritated nerve roots will cause pain. This has been proven in neurophysologic studies in which the experimental response to manipulation of normal vs. irritated nerve roots has been dramatically different indicating that, for consistent reproduction of pain in a nerve root distribution, there is generally an underlying degree of inflammation and nerve root irritation suggestive of repetitive mechanical deformation of the nerve. The sources of inflammation, acute nerve compression, and the symptoms of burner or stinger are difficult to correlate. Animal and in vitro studies may fail to simulate the true clinical situation seen in football players.

Prevention of Burners

The primary preventive rule for burners is wearing properly fitting shoulder pads. Shoulder pads should accomplish four basic functions: *(a)* absorb shock; *(b)* protect the shoulders; *(c)* fit the chest; *(d)* fix the midcervical spine to the trunk. The typical shoulder pad (Fig. 49.1), worn by a professional defensive lineman, is a soft arc, very thin-padded material that has questionable shock-absorbing properties and fits the chest in a semiarc type of configuration. The fixation to the chest is less than ideal and allows sliding of the shoulder pads on the shoulder during contact. In order to fit the chest properly, the pads should be more of an A-frame type with very rigid, long, anterior and posterior panels. The shoulder pads should fit well to the subxiphoid portion of the chest and fit snugly around the chest. A proper shoulder pad should encompass many of the characteristics of proper cervicothoracic orthosis.

Immobilization of the cervical spine in any type of cervical orthosis requires rigid fixation to the chest. All studies evaluating fixation methods that include only the neck, such as a hard or soft cervical collar, demonstrate poor fixation and limitation of cervical spine motion. It is only when the base is extended and fixed firmly to the chest, as in a proper cervicothoracic orthosis, that there is any restriction of cervical spine motion. Although there are limitations on the ability to fix the head to the chest in football players because they must have full range of motion of the cervical spine, it is possible to fix the chest rigidly to the base of the neck, and the shoulder pads should accomplish this.

The majority of neck rolls that are attached to the top of the shoulder pads rotate away from the neck at the moment of contact (Fig. 49.2). This rolling back of the shoulder pads adds to a lack of protection for the cervical spine in resisting compression. This axial compression mechanism of injury is commonly seen in serious neck injuries and plays a big role in burners. As a shoulder pad rolls back, the head coils into the hole in the shoulder pad. There is no protection against head compression in injuries and the extension, compression, and rotation mechanism of the burner. It

Figure 49.1 The typical shoulder pad worn by a professional defensive lineman is a soft arc of very thin padded material that has questionable shock-absorbing properties and fits the chest in a semiarc type of configuration.

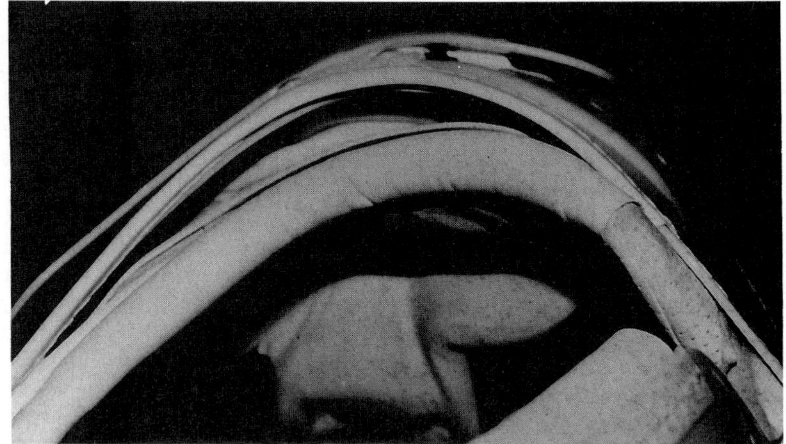

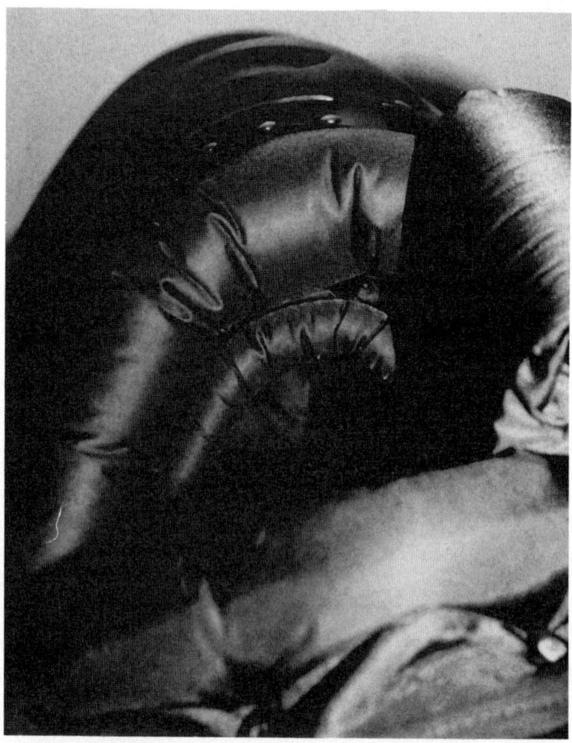

Figure 49.2 A well-constructed shoulder pad.

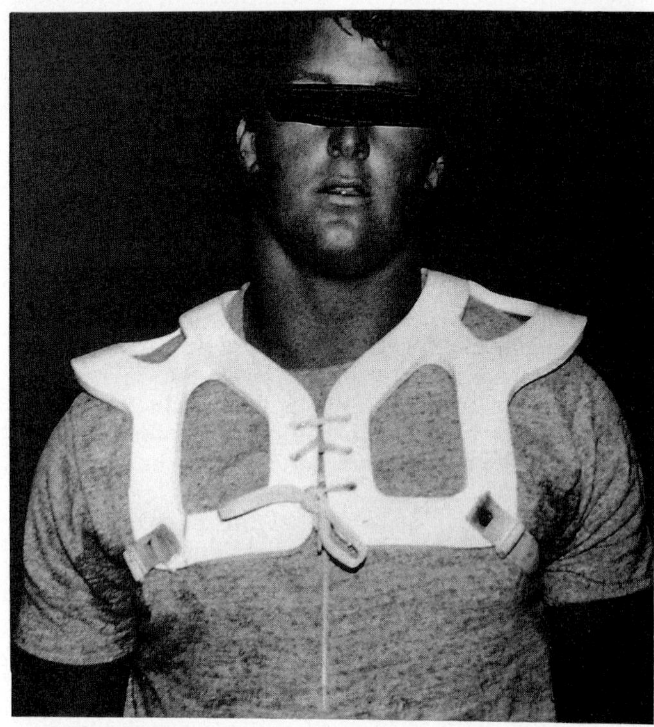

Figure 49.3 Lifters provide additional neck support.

is very difficult to get a collar roll on the back of the shoulder pads that can block extension during contact. One professional veteran used a stiff cervical collar that was tied tightly around his neck posteriorly and attached to the shoulder pads by strings to the laces on the front of the pads. This was an attempt to prevent the failure to block extension seen with collar rolls (Fig. 49.3).

Important characteristics of a proper shoulder pad include a modified A-frame shape to the shoulder pad that fits the chest and prevents shoulder pad roll during contact. Firm circumferential fixation to the chest is important. After fixing the chest, fix the neck to the chest by the fit of the shoulder pad at the base of the neck. Thick, comfortable, stiff pads at the base of the neck are the key. It is this support laterally at the base of the neck that offers fixation to the cervical spine. Some posterior support could be helpful but is very difficult to obtain. Higher, thicker lateral pads inside the shoulder pad that are tighter at the base of the neck can improve fixation of the cervical spine, especially when the pad fits the chest and shoulders well. The lateral pad seen in the Donzis shoulder pad is a good example of a proper pad.

A common method of adapting pads is to add lifters (Fig. 49.4). The lifters provide a pad at the base of the neck that supplements the typical shoulder pad. Often, a combination of lifters, the pre-existing pad, and the neck roll will all add to an improved fit of the pad laterally at the base of the neck. Because most of the rotation in the cervical spine occurs at C1-C2, it is believed that this support should not limit the player's

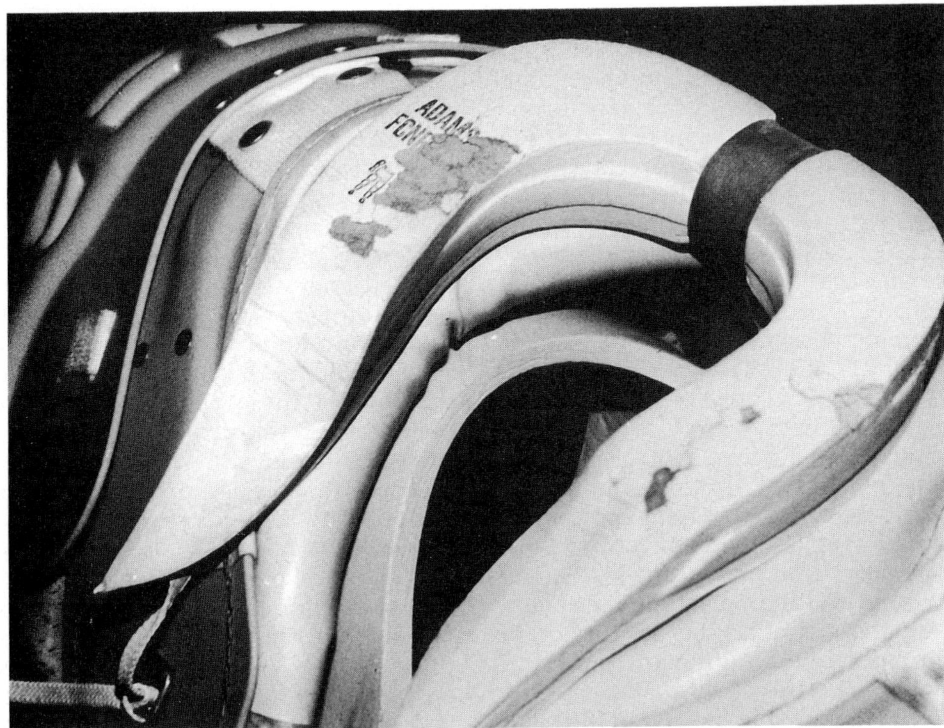

Figure 49.4 This illustration shows shoulder pads after they have been modified.

visibility and should provide some added support in the mid and lower portion of the cervical spine.

Regarding the shock-absorbing capability of the shoulder pad, proper fit to the chest is important in distributing the shock to the shoulders evenly, over the pad and to the thorax. Better resistive padding and better plastics in the outer shell of the pad will absorb shock and allow the use of the shoulder in proper blocking and tackling techniques. Better shoulder protection should allow one to de-emphasize the use of the head as a blocking and tackling instrument.

Treatment of Burners

In addition to prevention, treatment is critically important. Once the symptoms occur, we emphasize the chest-out posturing and thoracic outlet obstruction exercises. Chest-out posturing produces three effects.

1. It opens the intervertebral foramina to its maximum size. Sticking the chest out brings the head back over the body and produces a strengthening or less extension in the cervical spine. Flexion in the cervical spine, while tightening the nerve roots slightly, does increase the size of the intervertebral foramina. Extension closes the foramina and decreases the central canal's diameter.

2. It reduces the effect of the weight of the head. The lever arm effect of the weight of the head on the cervical spine is eliminated as the head is brought back over the body with the chest-out posturing. This is important in relieving neck strain and decreasing the force exerted on the spine by the weight of the head.

3. It opens the thoracic outlet. By changing the alignment of the scalene muscles and the clavicle relative to the neck, the thoracic outlet is opened with a chest-out posturing. A stoop-shoulder, head-forward posture adds to thoracic outlet obstruction and will cause the symptoms of brachial plexus irritation to persist. Many heavily muscled athletes have adopted a round-shoulder, head-forward posture. When they sustain an injury to a nerve root or brachial plexus, symptoms will persist because of an inability to produce proper chest and head alignment. All strengthening of weak muscles owing to a brachial plexus and or nerve root injury should be conducted while emphasizing a chest-out posture.

We frequently use a basic group of preventive and therapeutic exercises designed for neck and shoulder problems. The key to these exercises is emphasizing the chest-out posture. By emphasizing the chest-out posture during upper extremity, shoulder, and neck exercises, proper head and neck alignment is enhanced. A general exercise program could include the shoulder and rotator cuff exercises as well as dorsal glides, midline neck isometrics, shoulder shrugs, arm rolls, and a weight program. The athlete should stick the chest out, and not attempt to hold the shoulders back or forcefully tuck the chin. The chest, abdomen, and buttock muscles should be used. The important factor is the chest-out posture.

Neck strengthening is also important. Neck and radicular pain will cause muscle weakness and dysfunction in the muscles that support the head. The same emphasis that is used on quadraceps strengthening for knee injuries should be used for neck muscles in neck injuries, but it must be done carefully. Resistive neck exercises are begun very slowly so that the compressive load on the cervical spine does not produce pain. Neck isometrics should be done with the head in the midline only, and resisting forces should be applied perpendicularly to the head from every direction. Very slowly, the head can be taken out of the midline after there is no pain whatsoever with strengthening in the midline, but extremes of head flexion, either anteriorly, posteriorly, or laterally against resistance, are seldom indicated for adequate neck strengthening. Our emphasis has been on midline isometric strengthening.

Stretching exercises are critically important to allow for the protective flexibility and range of motion for the cervical spine. Cervical stiffness is produced by nerve, ligament, or disc injury. The reactive stiffness can produce chronic contractures and a loss of range of motion if not corrected. Chronic contractures are a great enemy of a pain-free neck that if a contracture exists, sudden motion at a moment of contact through that restricted range of motion will reproduce the injury and severe pain. Relieve those contractures and restore a protective range of motion with a program of cervical active range of motion exercises. Use motion into the painless areas initially, then slowly move into the painful areas. Extension is usually the most painful, but it cannot be neglected. Dorsal slides and passive neck stretches are important. Remember that chest-out posturing should be used during the exercises. Aggressive stretching and motion exercises should be done with extreme caution, as it is the most common cause of flare-ups in therapy.

Decision-Making in Neck Injuries in Athletes

Decision-making in neck injuries to athletes often centers around whether or not a player is cleared to return to play. It involves a more complex decision centered around what risks are involved in returning to play either on that day or later. The decision that allows a player to resume football play depends upon the diagnosis, prognosis, and risk factors for future injury. Crucial to the decision-making process is a physician who is trained in evaluating, diagnosing, and treating neck injuries, and who also has a thorough understanding of the game. When dealing with football players, it is important that the physician has an understanding of the mechanics involved in football as well as the effects of the stress of the game upon the particular injury that the player has received. For the physician to make a reasonable recommendation for return to play, factors such as the mechanism of the player's injury, any prior history of neck injury, the findings on the initial physical examination of the player immediately after injury, as well as the diagnostic studies that have been obtained must be assessed. Factors to be avoided in this decision-making are contract provisions, disability contracts, the player's desire to play, and the desires of others (girlfriends, wives, coaches, team owners, parents). Everyone, regardless of what is said, is looking to the team physician for medical advice only. The physician should stick closely to the medical facts of the case and provide the same information to all concerned about the known risk factors. To help in our decision-making, we have developed a system for classifying the risk of continued play or return-to-play, based on the radiographic findings after a specific type of neck injury, coupled with the patient's current signs and symptoms, as well as the patient's detailed prior history of neck injury. The history of prior neck injury must include the frequency of occurrence of such incidents as burners, stingers, transient neuropraxia, and neck stiffness, as well as the length of duration of these episodes of neurologic embarrassment or neck injury. The type of treatments that the player has received as well as the player's response to these treatments is important in assessing the readiness of the player for return to play. The classification system that has been developed combines the published clinical and scientific information related to specific neck injuries as well as our experience in diagnosing and treating neck injuries in football players. We utilize radiographic component studies and many other factors in the final outcome of such a decision-making process. We categorize the player's case into risk categories. The risk categories are both the risk of permanent injury and the risk of recurrent symptoms.

On-Field Decisions

Decision-making begins with the player that has been injured in the game and is down on the field. The only diagnostic capabilities will be the physician's history, physical examination, and knowledge of the mechanics of the injury.

The key decision to make is whether to move the player (whether he has a spinal cord injury or not). The first issue is whether a player has radiating arm pain and loss of function, such as paresthesias and weakness, or more global paresthesias and weakness indicative of a transient neuropraxia of the cervical spine cord. Radiating arm pain and neurologic deficit can be indicators of a more serious problem, such as spinal instability, that can lead to a permanent neurologic deficit from further cord or nerve root injury. Additionally, some players may be neurologically intact but may have a stiff, painful neck. Neck stiffness and loss of cervical range of motion may indicate a cervical fracture.

Initial muscle spasm that occurs after a cervical spine injury can mask an underlying unstable cervical spine lesion. The patient's pain perception may be altered by the emotion of the game, as well as by the player's dedication to the coach and the team. A controlled head compression test that produces radicular arm pain or significant neck pain may indicate a cervical fracture. Players with a new pain and residual loss of neck range of motion and neck stiffness should not be allowed to return to play until further diagnostic evaluation is performed. No return to play is suggested in players with a significant neck injury until further diagnostic evaluation has been obtained.

Spinal cord neuropraxia with four-extremity involvement, including, possibly, loss of consciousness, temporary quadraplegia or quadraparesis, or burning dysesthesias of the arms and legs indicates a significant but temporary injury to the spinal cord. Players who have transient neurapraxia of the spinal cord that lasts for less than 10–15 seconds may arise from the playing field and exit the field on their own power. Only when the player is at the sideline is the trainer or team physician made aware of the symptomatology. Examination of these players on the sideline or on the field involves evaluation for motor weakness, sensory deficits, and signs of myelopathy. It is important that all players with the possibility of cervical spine injury and acute neurologic deficit are treated with cervical spine immobilization and appropriate transportation and diagnostic studies.

Transportation and Immobilization

When confronted with an individual on the playing field who complains of symptoms of neck pain or stiffness, or any upper or lower extremity neurologic manifestations, the initial response of the trainer or team physician is to assure prompt and adequate immobilization of the cervical spine and establish an airway. In the acute emergency setting, the helmet should not be removed in a player suspected of cervical spine injury. In a player with neck injury and respiratory compromise, either the mask must be a removable face mask or the availability of large bolt cutters capable of transecting the metallic face mask are mandatory. If the provision of an adequate airway is necessary, then the bolt cutters should be utilized to transect the metal stays attaching the face mask to the helmet. If the player is unconscious and having inadequate respiratory effort, then the airway may be opened by grasping the angle of the mandible with both hands and thrusting the jaw forward. Hyperextension of the head to obtain an open airway is usually not necessary when cervical spine injury is considered a possibility. It is only after cervical spine immobilization has been provided that the individual may be transported to the sidelines, the locker room, or the emergency room. When there is doubt concerning the necessity for neck immobilization and player transportation, the recommendation is to transport players as if they had a spine injury until further evaluation is possible. The precise and safe implementation of cervical spine immobilization and transportation of a player with neck injury require proper instruction of the coach and trainer by the team physician as well as practice in the transportation techniques by those involved in the provision of transportation (Figs. 49.5 and 49.6). The team trainer as well as the fire rescue personnel in attendance at the game must be provided with and comfortable with the application of the standard cervical immobilization collars. The most common collars in use include the Nek-loc, and the Philadelphia collar. When appropriate, these collars can be applied to the player before transportation.

The transport technique should be standardized and

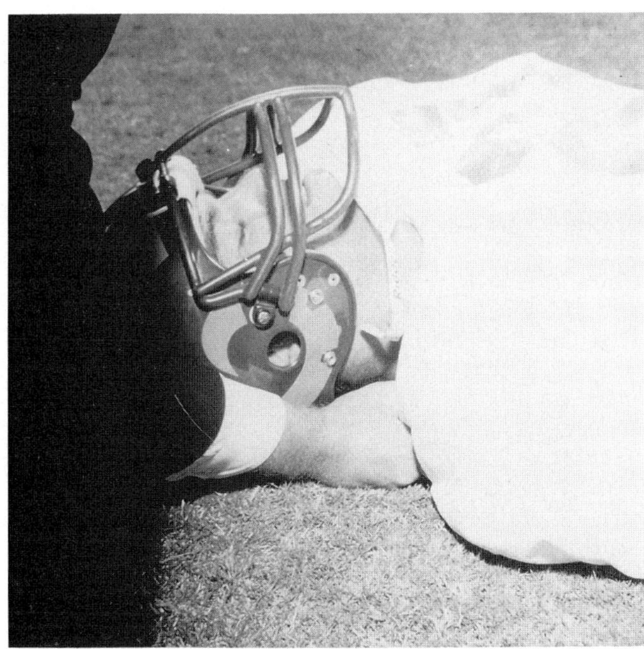

Figure 49.5 Immobilization of the head to the trunk. The person in charge holds the trapezius-clavicle-scapula area with his hands and holds the head between his forearms.

practiced by the trainer, coach, and team physician before the start of the playing season and requires five to six people to move the player safely. Trying to transport the patient with only three people is inappropriate. A frequent error in transport is not having enough people available who know how to transport a player with a potentially unstable cervical spine injury (Fig. 49.7). The most important key to the technique is to have one person controlling the head and shoulders, not just the head. Holding the head only and trying to visually match the head to the body is impossible. This individual is in charge of the timing of transportation. This person should grab the trapezial, clavical, and scapular area with his/her hands while cradling the helmeted head of the player between the forearms. The person in charge should not be responsible for any of the weight of the transfer. The additional members of the transportation team include one individual holding the player's shoulders and upper torso. The third and fourth persons holding the player's trunk and upper thighs on each side of the player. The fifth and sixth members of the turning team are responsible for lifting and turning the legs.

The person holding the head is responsible for announcing each move in the transportation process. At no time should the person in charge hold only the head and not the shoulders. When practicing these maneuvers, try having the person in charge hold only the head in an awake, uninjured volunteer, and proceed through the turning maneuvers. Then ask the awake volunteer how much he felt his neck move during the turning procedure. Generally, a significant amount of neck motion can be felt, thus reinforcing the need for the person in charge to maintain a firm grasp connecting the shoulders to the head, thus assuring adequate immo-

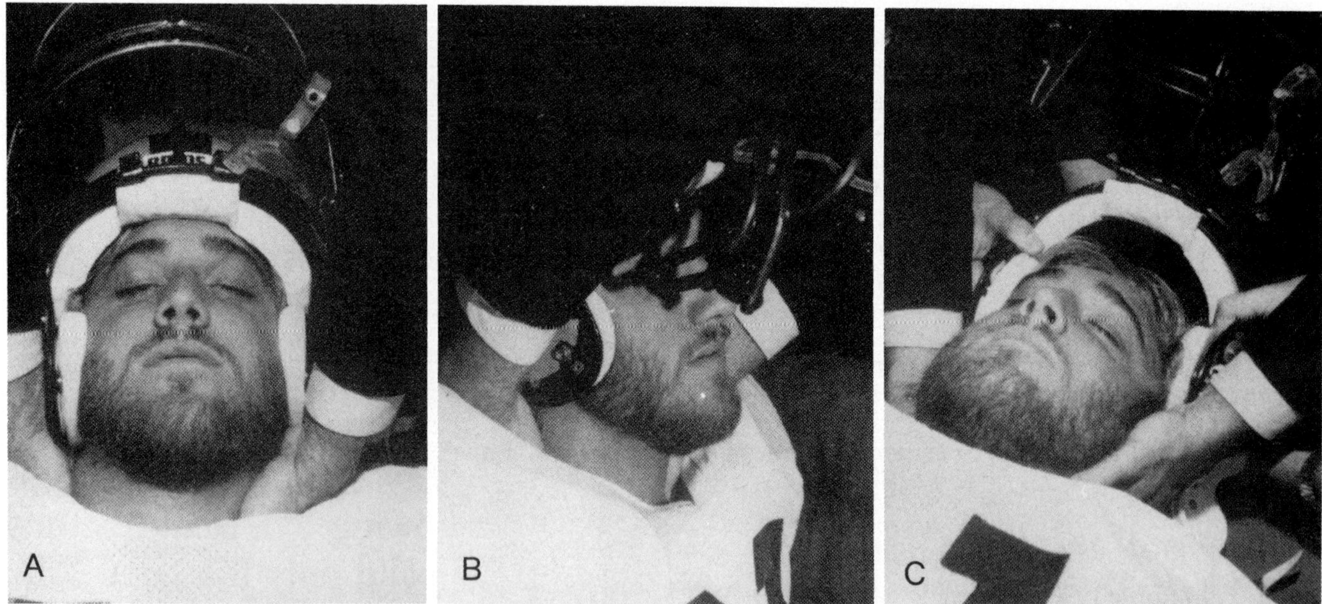

Figure 49.6 *(A)* Hand position for helmet removal. *(B)* Helmet removal, side view. *(C)* Helmet removal, the assistant pulls out on the helmet and slips it off.

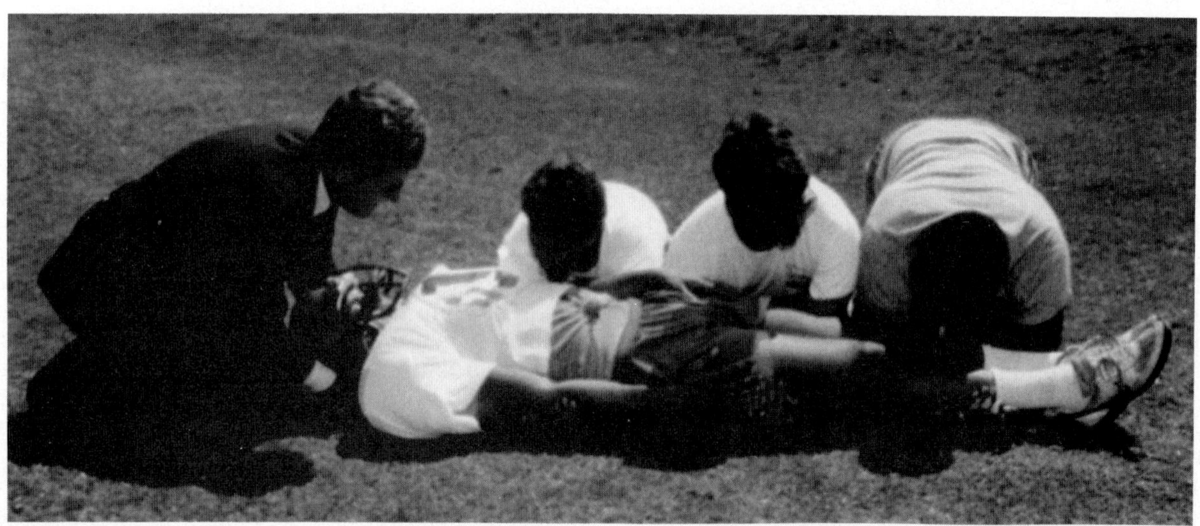

Figure 49.7 The transport technique should be standardized and practiced, and it requires five or six people to safely move the player. This figure illustrates the multiman carry. The "chief" immobilizes the head, neck, and shoulder and calls the signals. Three men on each side of the body (the three on the near side are not pictured) join hands and lift the player on the "chiefs'" command. The spine board is brought underneath the player.

bilization of a potentially unstable cervical spine. It is possible for the person in charge to grasp both the trapezius inside and a shoulder pad outside, but this is not quite as stable as the prior recommended method. Another person may be utilized to squeeze the forearms of the person in charge to the head, thus further increasing the stability of the grasp on the player's shoulders and head. Once all individuals are in place, the team members on each side of the body then join hands in a weaved grip, with the palm placed against the forearm of the individual directly across from them, underneath the player. When the team chief calls the signal, the assistants gently elevate the player off the ground while a rigid backboard is slid directly under the player.

If the player is face down on the field, the chief rotates the player's arms and grasps his head and shoulders in a similar fashion. In this situation, it is mandatory that an assistant grasp the chief's arms and squeeze them together to increase the hold on the player's shoulders and head. Safely turning the prone player to the supine position requires multiple assistants to roll the player over gently while the team chief maintains the alignment of the head with the shoulders during the turn. Once the player is turned, then the standard transportation protocol is utilized (Fig. 49.8).

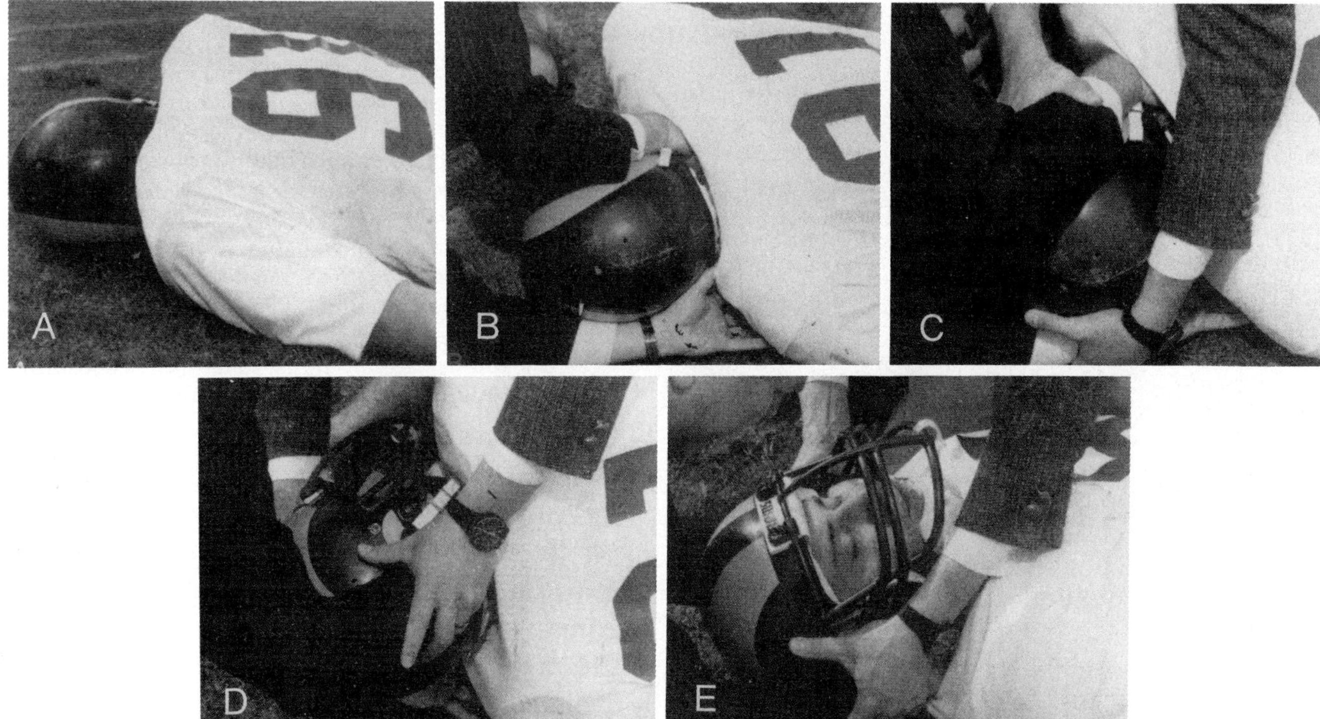

Figure 49.8 *(A)* If the player is face down on the field, *(B)* the chief rotates his arms and grasps the player's head and shoulders in a similar fashion. *(C)* In this situation, it is mandatory that an assistant grasp the chief's arms and squeezes them together to increase the hold on the player's shoulders and head. *(D)* Safely turning the prone player to the supine position requires multiple assistants to gently roll the player over while the team chief maintains the alignment of the head with the shoulders during the turn. *(E)* Once the player is turned, then the standard transportation protocol is utilized.

Once the player is on the backboard, then the player can be safely transported off the field to the appropriate health care facility, while the team chief maintains the grasp on the player's shoulders and head. Once the player is on the backboard, if an appropriate cervical orthosis is available, such as a Philadelphia collar, then the team chief may safely relinquish his hold on the neck at the same time applying the cervical orthosis. If the cervical orthosis cannot be applied because of the helmet or the shoulder pads, then the team chief must maintain his grasp on the individual until transportation to the locker room or emergency room is completed. It may be necessary to utilize a backboard that has built-in neck and head supports or utilize the sandbags taped into place rather than the original grasp of the person in charge.

Locker Room Decisions

Our decision-making process involves evaluating players for return to play who have had either significant, persistent, or severe enough symptomatology to warrant transportation to a medical facility or to a locker room where x-rays are available.

Radiographic Evaluation

Once x-rays are available, it is mandatory to obtain adequate visualization of the cervicothoracic junction at C7-T1 as well as an adequate quality x-ray that can be safely interpreted. Generally, the lateral x-ray is obtained first (Fig. 49.9) and should be interpreted and evaluated before proceeding with the remainder of the radiographic evaluation. Thomas (14) has reported the appropriate sequence of x-rays that should be obtained in the neck-injured player include the anteroposterior projection, the lateral x-ray and the neutral position, the open mouth view of the atlantoaxial articulation, and each oblique position. It is not until the initial sequence of cervical spine films has been reviewed and evaluated for any potential instability, fracture, or dislocation that subsequent flexion-extension x-rays should be considered. If such instability, fracture, or dislocation is identified, then the next appropriate step is to continue cervical spine immobilization and proceed with definitive treatment or further diagnostic studies including CT scan or MRI as indicated by the nature of the lesion. When the basic radiographic evaluation indicates spinal instability, fracture, or dislocation, then the lateral flexion-extension films may be contraindicated and unsafe.

The x-rays should be evaluated for obvious vertebral body fracture or malalignment; also, the anterior retropharyngeal space should be evaluated. At the anterior aspect of the body of C3, there should be no more than 4 mm of space between the posterior pharynx and the anterior vertebral body. Increase in the retropharyngeal space indicates soft tissue swelling and may be indicative of cervical spine injury. The posterior margins of the vertebral bodies and the spinal laminar lines should

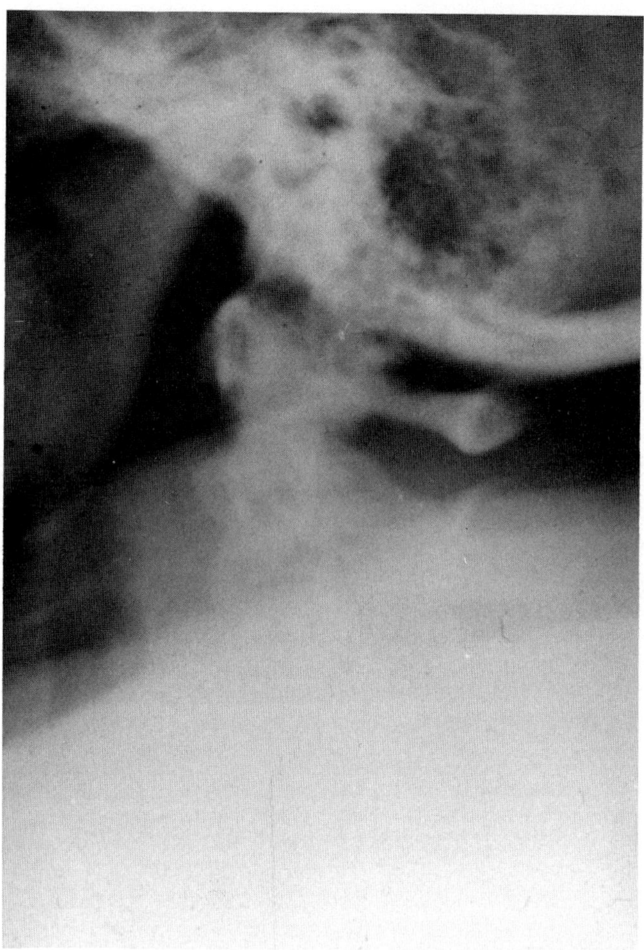

Figure 49.9 A typical lateral x-ray of a football player.

be evaluated for a symmetric and smooth contour. The facet joints should be evaluated for symmetry and congruity. Changes in the rotational position of the spinal column from one motion segment to the next may be indicative of facet subluxation or dislocation. The criteria of White and Panjabi (15), including subluxation of 3.5 mm or more and kyphotic angulation of the injured level that is 11° or greater than an adjacent level, is generally considered as cervical spine instability. These criteria pertain to any lateral cervical spine view including flexion view.

The evaluation of C1 through T1 is imperative and can be facilitated by the use of traction on the player's hand in a downward fashion by an assistant during the radiograph or by the use of the Boger straps. We prefer the Boger straps, which are passive action Velcro straps that are connected to the wrists and passed around the bottoms of the feet. They are tightened with the knees flexed. As the knees are straightened out by pushing down on the knees, the straps tighten and pull the arms down. A sandbag can be placed on the knees in an unconscious patient, thereby maintaining traction on the arms. We have never had a patient in which C7 was not visualized using the Boger straps. Occasionally, traction on an arm with cervical radiculopathy produces too much pain to pull for a long time. If Boger straps are not available, then the "swimmer's view," a special radiographic view obtained by centering the beam on the lateral projection at C7, can be utilized. The patient's arm closest to the source of the radiographic beam is left at the patient's side, while the opposite arm that is adjacent to the radiographic plate is fully abducted over the patient's head. If adequate visualization of the cervicothoracic junction remains a problem after the swimmer's view is obtained, then the next step in radiographic evaluation is a CT scan to include that region. We will not clear a patient's cervical spine film unless the full cervical spine is visualized. Also important on the lateral view is the atlantodens interval. An atlantodens interval of greater than 2–3 mm may be considered indicative of cervical spine instability at the atlantoaxial articulation, particularly if this atlantodens interval markedly increases on flexion films.

One difficult aspect of the radiographic evaluation is to determine if there is an acute injury, an old injury, or an asymptomatic finding. One complicating factor is the presence of a hypermobile segment over a stiff, arthritic segment. Many athletes who do neck strengthening exercises on a regular and consistent basis, especially those starting at a young age, have relative osteoarthritic changes in the lower cervical spine region. The biomechanical stiffness of these levels may produce a relative increase in mobility through a compensatory mechanism at the levels just above these less mobile lower segments. To find an asymptomatic never-injured level that exceeds the White-Punjabi criteria would be rare (15).

The adequate identification of an area of ligamentous instability may be particularly difficult in the acute situations secondary to the associated muscle spasm from the injury.

Compression fracture noted in the lateral film must be interpreted with caution. What may be interpreted as a simple compression fracture may, in fact, include an injury with associated cervical spine instability. A review of 27 patients with cervical compression fractures revealed that six of these injuries were later noted to have associated spine instability (16). When doubt continues as to the stability of a cervical spine injury, such as when there is too much spasm to obtain flexion-extension views, continued immobilization with a cervical orthosis is expected until additional radiographic evaluation in subsequent days with flexion-extension views at that time is obtained. Once a fracture has been identified on plain film or CT scan, it should be classified into the standard classification system utilized today, depending upon the spine level affected and the fracture configuration.

Often important in the radiologic evaluation is the determination of whether a radiographic finding is an acute injury, on old injury, or an asymptomatic degenerative change. Boden et al. (17), have identified the incidence of asymptomatic degenerative changes occurring in the cervical spine in a group of volunteers that underwent MRI of the cervical spine while being asymptomatic for problems related to the neck. They were able to identify a 14–35% incidence of herniated cervical disc, osteophytes, and degenerative disc disease in these completely asymptomatic individuals. They underscored the importance of the clinical correlation among the radiographic findings and the history and physical examination findings and individuals being evaluated for cervical injuries.

Once in a controlled environment, then removing the player's helmet should be accomplished in a safe fashion. First, remove the face mask. The appropriate hand position of the team chief for helmet removal includes having that team chief grasp the base of the occiput and the base of the neck with open palms and fingers. An assistant may first spread the sides of the helmet, then gently slide the helmet in a cephalad direction and off the player while neck control is maintained by the team chief. Absolutely no cervical flexion should be allowed during this maneuver. If the shoulder pads do not allow for adequate cervical spine examination and radiograph, then they should be removed at this time. They should be removed in a similar fashion, while maintaining cervical immobilization and not allowing cervical and head flexion.

When to Do In-depth Studies

The logical answer to this question is "when they are needed to make the diagnosis" or "when the results would change your treatment." As a practical measure, studies are obtained on players with severe, persistent, or reccurring problems. For a stiff, painful neck due to recent injury, a bone scan may identify an acute fracture. MRI and plain CT scans are helpful and a contrast CT scan will help identify disc herniations and fractures. An EMG with nerve conduction study is helpful in distinguishing a peripheral nerve problem from a cervical nerve root problem, but not as helpful in following a case for progression. Liberal use of whatever tests are taken to diagnose the problem properly is the way to proper treatment and prognosis.

Continued Play Decision: Risk Categories

The spinal consultant or the team physician is often called upon, in the preseason, to examine players and evaluate their risk for play during the upcoming season. The team physician must be able to give a clearcut "yes" or "no" answer to the team's management and to the player, himself, or the player's parents. It is often the spinal consultant who is asked to make that decision in players who have had documented neck injury and are thought to be at some risk for further play. As consultants, the radiographic data will be combined with the history and physical examination of the player to develop a risk category into which that particular player can be placed in regard to his chance for permanent damage to the neck, spinal cord injury, permanent nerve root injury with paralysis and pain, or death. Also, risks may be categorized in terms of percentage of chance of recurrence of symptoms that would hinder future play. Very important in this decision is the level of play in which the player participates. In a high school player, of course, the parents' opinion is very important. If there is a suggestion of structural damage and even a minimally increased risk to a high school player, the decision is often for the athlete to discontinue playing football. In professional football, the players themselves need to be advised of the approximate level of risk, so that they may have received an informed consent as to their future play and an appropriate decision can be made by the player and all concerned.

Although no published data can precisely dictate the individual player risk for return to play, a system that incorporates clinical experience in dealing with football players and the published literature related to cervical spine injuries is utilized. A *minimal risk* is the term used to suggest that there is very little increased risk, as compared with playing the game as it is normally done. *Moderate risk* means that there is a reasonably high percentage chance that the patient will have recurrence of symptoms and a reasonable chance that he will run some risk of permanent damage. *Extreme risk* means that the patient runs a very high risk of permanent damage and recurrence of symptoms. It is critical that all factors related to the player's symptomatology, history of injury, radiographic findings, results of any special studies needed, and expectations be included in the ultimate recommendations made to the player in regard to his likelihood of injury if he returns to the sport of football. When considering other sports that involve bodily contact, similar recommendations can be made.

Extreme Risk Category

Fractures of the first cervical vertebra (Jefferson fractures) generally represent an axial loading injury often resulting from head-on collision by the player with the opponent or the ground. The Jefferson fracture is disruption of the ring of the first cervical vertebra and may be identified on the open mouth AP view as eccentric or excessive overhang of the lateral mass of the first cervical vertebra on the second cervical vertebra. CT scan is excellent as precisely identifying the configuration of a C1 fracture. At the level of the atlas, there is considerable room for the spinal cord secondary to the large central spinal canal at that level. As such, neurologic injury secondary to Jefferson fracture is unusual. The mechanism of injury involves axial loading that forces the occipital condyles into the lateral mass of the atlas, resulting in failure of the ring of the atlas, often at the thinner region just medial to the trough that lies at the level of the vertebral artery. Certainly, return to play after a recent Jefferson fracture is contraindicated. It is only after bony healing has occurred and appropriate tests for ligamentous stability can be obtained that a recommendation as to return to play can be made. If the bone completely heals, a full, normal range of motion is present and no residual instability noted on flexion-extension views is present, then return to play is possible. Certainly, if there is any residual instability or if there is residual neck stiffness or discomfort, then the recommendation for return to play would include placing that player in an extreme risk category. Occasionally, C1 ring fractures heal with a fibrous union as evidenced on CT scan and in these players with no re-

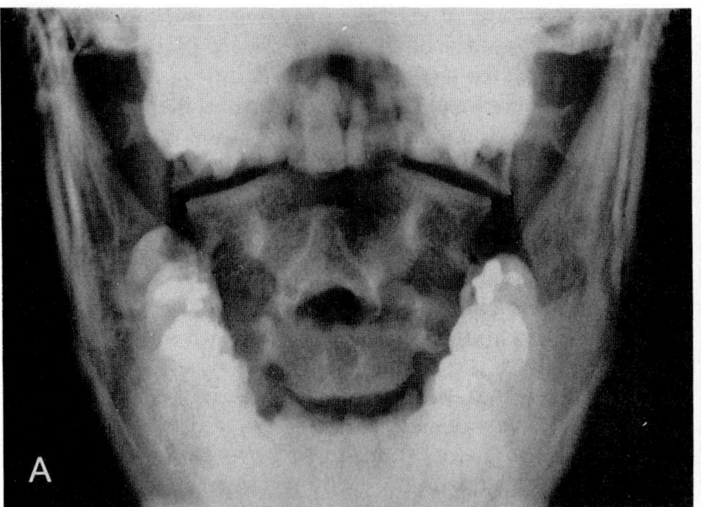

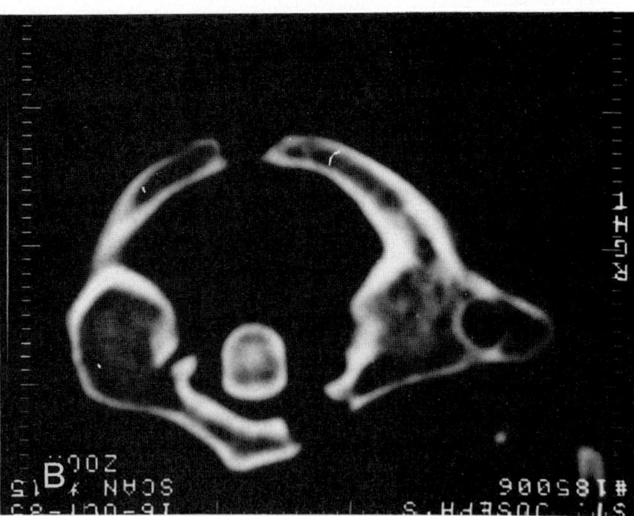

Figure 49.10 *(A)* This flexion fracture resulted from a head-first tackle. The key measurement is the amount of lateral overhang. An amount over 7 mm may indicate a ruptured transverse ligament. *(B)* CT scan shows a fracture with separation.

sidual neck stiffness or pain, then a moderate, significant risk category for return to play would be offered.

Figure 49.10 illustrates a Jefferson-type fracture with 7 mm of overhang resulting from head-on collision; the player is a college senior defensive back. Projected as a first round draft choice in the National Football League, this injury certainly placed the player in a high-risk category.

Transverse ligament ruptures result from high velocity axial loading injuries. Transverse ligament injuries are quite rare and occur in only 3% of all cervical spine injuries (18). The odontoid is held snugly against the back of the atlas by the strong fibers of the transverse ligament. These fibers arise from the lateral masses of the atlas, just behind the origin of the accessory ligament. Rupture of the transverse ligament is identified by abnormal motion between the atlas and the odontoid on the flexion-extension views or by an atlantodens interval greater than 5 mm on the neutral lateral film. Partial tears of the transverse ligament may be identified by an atlantodens interval of 2–5 mm. We have treated a player who had a partial tear of the transverse ligament; he was a starting professional defensive tackle who had suffered a high velocity injury with residual stiffness and pain in his neck. This player was thought to be in an extreme-risk category for futher play. We have also treated a 17-year-old high school football player who presented after a significant neck injury that resulted in upper cervical spine stiffness and pain. He presented with a "V"-shaped atlantodens interval. The diagnosis for this youngster was the partial transverse ligament tear, even though there have been references made to this entity being an incidental finding. Our recommendation to this child and his parents was that he would be at an increased risk of neurologic injury from continued participation in football.

The open-mouth view is utilized to identify odontoid fractures and can be classified according to the system of Anderson and Alonzo (19) into either type I fractures, which include the tip of the odontoid and are thought to be stable fracture configurations. A type II fracture is through the base of the odontoid and is the least stable and most likely to lead to nonunion, and type III odontoid fractures, which involve variable components of the vertebral body of C2, are likely to lead to early union. Odontoid fractures that heal completely, without deformity and with free, unrestricted, pain-free neck motion are considered to place that player at a mild risk of secondary injury from continued play. However, any residual deformity or the suggestion of a fibrous union between the odontoid and the body of C2 is considered a potentially unstable situation and a football player who can be expected to place significant biomechanical stress on that fracture, would place that player in an extreme-risk category.

Fracture of the pedicles of C2 is termed a "hangman's fracture" because of its association with the sudden hyperextension provided by the hangman's noose. Hangman's fractures have been classified according to the system of Effendi (20) and modified by the system proposed by Levine and Edwards (21). Type I injuries are considered stable and are fractures through the pars interarticularis with less than 1–2 mm of displacement at that fracture site. Type II injuries often have some degree of displacement and occur through the isthmus. In these fractures, there may also have been some rebound flexion with associated disruption of the posterior ligamentous structures or the C2-C3 disc resulting in residual angulation and subluxation.

Type IIA fractures have been introduced by Levine and Edwards (21) and include fractures that have less displacement, but more angulation than the type II injury described by Effendi et al (20). These fractures may have been associated with primary flexion force and are particularly prone to increased angulation and displacement when traction is applied. Type III fractures are generally secondary to flexion injury and may be associated with facet capsule disruption between C2 and C3. This allows for fracture through the pars interarticularis. If the hangman's fracture heals completely, with no fibrous union, and there is satisfactory reestablishment of the posterior arch of C2, then this is thought to signal only a mild risk for subsequent injury in that player. However, any suggestion of fibrous union or significant residual deformity after bony union would increase the chance of injury and would be considered an extreme risk category. Often, the soft tissue injury involves both the posterior and middle column and, occasionally, the anterior column as well and is an extreme risk.

The hidden flexion injury of McSweeney can be identified as a subtle subluxation presenting on the flexion view that is actually a total ligamentous disruption. This diagnosis is made on the lateral or flexion film (22). The x-ray findings may include a gapping of the spinous processes, a localized endplate deformity, or a subtle avulsion fracture of the anterior edge of the vertebral body. The findings may be quite subtle and the radiographic findings may take several weeks to become apparent secondary to the residual stiffness and spasm present immediately after the accident. Failure to diagnose this residual ligamentous stability and allowing these players to return to play would be extremely dangerous. This type of residual ligamentous instability certainly places these players at extreme risk. Herkowitz et al. (23) have documented this particular ligamentous and radiographic finding after cervical spine trauma. Delay in the diagnosis and treatment of this injury can also lead to a fixed kyphotic deformity placing the patient or player permanently in the extreme-risk category.

Fractures of the vertebral bodies, C3-C7, can be associated with compression and flexion forces as well as torsional forces that may leave the player with a significant cervical spine instability. Vertebral burst fractures may include significant spinal cord injury and are occasionally associated with facet dislocations that place the player at significant risk for complete neurologic injury. Certainly, there is not always a good correlation between the degree of spinal cord injury and the amount of bony injury or dislocation on the plain films. The prognosis for return to play after vertebral burst fractures, which may or may not have included subluxation or dislocation in the cervical spine, is quite dependent on the neurologic injury and the residual deformity present after complete healing. Certainly, if there is no residual neck pain or stiffness, no residual neurologic deficit, no residual associated cervical instability, and no residual deformity or canal narrowing, then players having suffered cervical spine compression or burst fractures may be allowed to return to play, but still are at some mild risk.

Facet dislocations, bilateral and unilateral, can occur with head compression and flexion-rotation injury. The facet dislocation that reduces completely and heals with no residual deformity or instability, would place that player in a moderate-risk category because of the damage to ligamentous support for that segment. Facet dislocations that heal with any residual deformity or instability would certainly place the player at an extreme risk of further injury.

Moderate-Risk Category

Fractures of the cervical facet or pillar fractures through the lateral mass may present like a facet dislocation because of the frequently seen anterior subluxation of one vertebral body on another. For these fractures the ultimate recommendation as to return to play depends most significantly on any residual deformity that persists after healing has occurred as well as any residual instability or cervical stiffness that is manifested after appropriate treatment has been completed.

Herniated cervical discs are reasonably common in adult football players. Most of the herniated cervical discs that we identify in athletes have a lingering or persistent radiculopathy in those players with a first time severe burner at the professional or college level. Because the incidence of disc bulges and herniations in asymptomatic people and players is significantly high, the finding of a herniated cervical disc in a football player who was completely asymptomatic for signs and symptoms of cervical myelopathy or radiculopathy related to that herniation would not be considered to place that player at an increased risk of injury. However, players who have evidence of radiculopathy are in a moderate-risk category. There is often a great deal of difficulty in determining whether a disc herniation is acute, chronic, hard as in a cervical osteophyte, soft, whether it is a free fragment, or simply a contained disc bulge. It is very important in these players that any radiographic diagnostic imaging abnormalities be closely correlated with the physical findings. It is important that the physical findings match the herniation for an accurate prognosis to be made. The treatment for herniated, extruded cervical discs is an anterior cervical discectomy and fusion. After such treatment, we often place the player in a mild-risk category, secondary to the biomechanical alterations that must necessarily occur above and below the fused cervical motion segment. It is for this reason that, if given the appropriate clinical indications, we might recommend a microscopic cervical foraminotomy for the treatment of monoradiculopathy secondary to foraminal stenosis in an athlete involved in contact sports. For the athlete with significant intermittent radiculopathy, a positive Spurling's hyperextension test, and foraminal stenosis, a posterolateral foraminotomy is a reasonable approach. The technique of this operation is adopted from Robert Warren Williams (24) and includes a minimal resection of the posterior wall of the foramina only until nerve root pulsations are clearly present. A significant facet resection would make return to football contraindicated.

Minor-Risk Category

Undisplaced fractures that heal without any residual deformity indicate a low risk for return to play. Clay-shoveler fractures are avulsion fractures of the tip of the spinous process of C7 caused by strong muscular contractions of the trapezius and shoulder. They present with point tenderness, otherwise negative studies, and dual rigidity. Lateral mass fractures always heal but may have a slight subluxation of one vertebra on another. The degree of risk depends on the degree of subluxation. There is rarely ligamentous damage with this injury. Laminar fractures that heal without deformity are a minor risk condition. Disc herniations that have become asymptomatic over many months or years are not of significance except as to how they have left the central canal narrowed. Foraminal stenosis is important when symptomatic but, because of the high incidence of asymptomatic foraminal stenosis, we would not consider a nerve root to be in danger just because radiographic foraminal stenosis is present.

Congenital Abnormalities

Congenital abnormalities of the cervical spine may or may not place the player at an increased risk for neurologic damage, depending upon the precise morphology of the congenital abnormality present. Os odontoideum, which has been documented in the literature as most likely secondary to a traumatic lesion is a potentially significant unstable situation in which the risk of injury places the player in an extreme-risk category (Fig. 49.11). Not infrequently, os odontoideum will present in the younger player as an asymptomatic and incidental finding and, as such, can be a particularly difficult problem to explain in the otherwise young, healthy, high caliber athlete. Multiple levels of failure of segmentation, as found in the klupophile syndrome, place the adjoining spinal motion units at an increased biomechanical disadvantage secondary to the compensatory increased motion that occurs adjacent to the fused levels. We, in general, would list this constellation of segmentation defects as a moderate to extreme risk that would depend somewhat upon the findings on flexion-extension films as well as on the distribution of the fused segments. Springle's deformity in association with klupophile is not unusual and is an extreme risk. Some examples in the high-risk category:

a. Os odontoideum;
b. Ruptured transverse ligament C1-C2;
c. Occipitocervical dislocation;
d. Odontoid fracture;
e. Total ligamentous disruption of a neuromotor segment of the lower cervical spine;
f. An unstable fracture dislocation;
g. Unstable Jefferson's fracture;
h. Cervical cord anomaly;
i. Acute large central disc herniation.

Examples in the moderate-risk category:

a. Facet fractures;
b. Lateral mass fractures;
c. Nondisplaced healed odontoid fractures;
d. Nondisplaced healed ring of C1 fractures;
e. Acute lateral disc herniations;
f. Cervical radiculopathy due to a foraminal spur.

Examples in the minimal risk category:

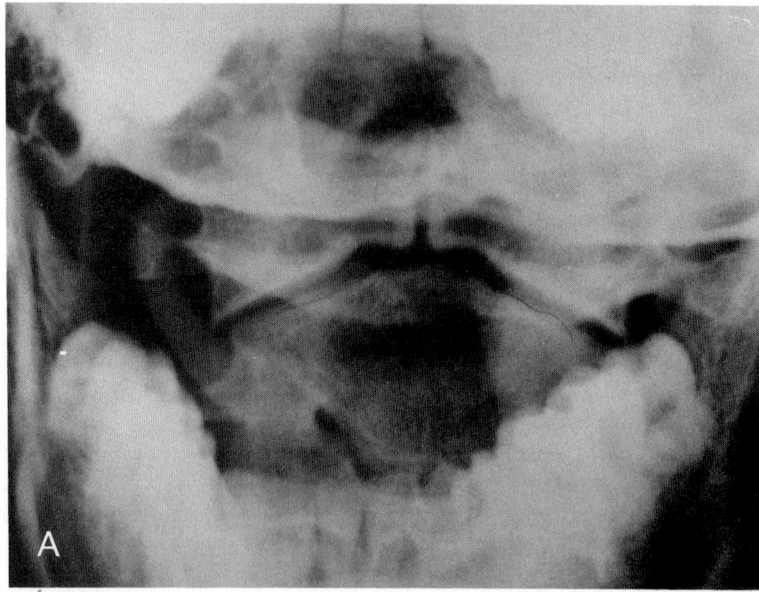

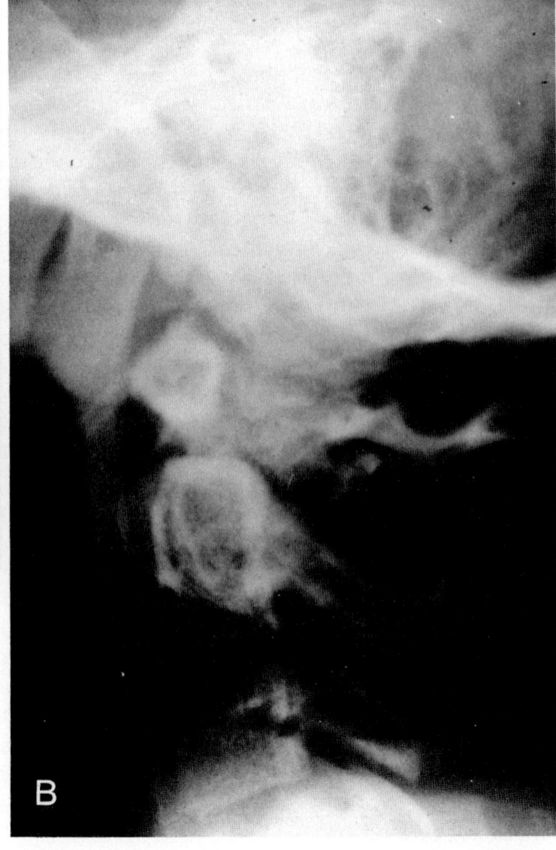

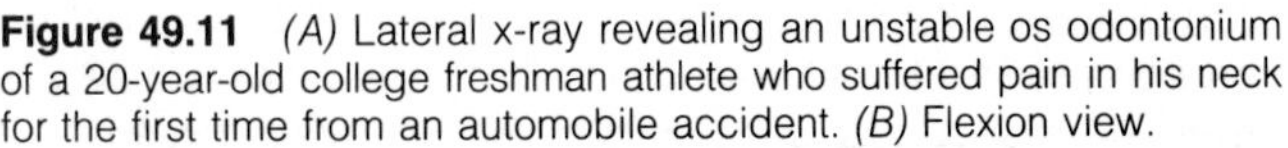

Figure 49.11 *(A)* Lateral x-ray revealing an unstable os odontonium of a 20-year-old college freshman athlete who suffered pain in his neck for the first time from an automobile accident. *(B)* Flexion view.

a. Asymptomatic bone spurs;
b. Certain healed facet fractures;
c. Burners;
d. Stingers;
e. Healed disc herniation;
f. Healed lamina fracture;
g. Fractured tip of the spinous process;
h. Asymptomatic foraminal stenosis.

In conclusion, the decision-making process that each team physician uses when approaching the cervical spine-injured football player must rely on the medical facts and the current medical knowledge. Attention to detail, with structured preplanning and a practiced on-the-field routine are critical to ensuring that no additional damage is done to the injured player after the accident. Counseling the player and other concerned individuals must be uniform and should only include the medical facts. It is important to remember that the team physician's role is only to convey the medical information as well as to instruct and to train the players, coaches, and trainers in techniques that will be useful to prevent player injury and to prevent further injury once a player is down on the field. There are no strict guidelines that have been published that are considered the standard of care. The ultimate recommendation of the team physician must be based on the medical facts as he or she finds them. Familiarity with the game of football or the particular athletic event for which the team physician is covering, and the particular needs and desires for those athletes will help shape a more appropriate decision-making process. An understanding of the relative risk of a spine disorder or a spine injury to an individual player both at the time of injury and for recommending return to play must come from advanced training in sports-related spine injuries or from clinical experience that comes from active participation in the care of athletes on a regular basis.

Rehabilitation of Neck Injuries

Certainly, for the athlete who is expecting to return to contact sports, it is imperative that the individual regains a full, pain-free range of motion of the cervical spine before being allowed to return to the sport. In football, in particular, the interrelationship among the head, neck, and shoulders in the development of a synchronous flow of movement is imperative to minimize the risk of recurrent injury. As such, the rehabilitative protocol must concentrate on strength, bulk, and coordination in the rehabilitation of the spinal flexors, extensors, as well as the shoulder girdle musculature. Once the acute phase of the injury has subsided, and the player is regaining the less painful range of motion of the neck, then progressive isometric strengthening of the neck musculature is begun. As symptoms further diminish, the player is progressively allowed to resume a normal weight training schedule in the attempt to regain any lost muscle strength and to regain the muscle bulk that is necessary to protect the underlying skeletal structures. Posture correction is the key to neck rehabilitation.

We recommend a progressive isometric trunk-strengthening exercise program aimed at placing the neck in a biomechanically sound position with the shoulders, back, and chest in a posturally correct position. This exercise program concentrates on trunk strengthening and trunk mobility. Throughout the program, the patient is instructed in postural modifications that place the patient in a chest-out posture, which effectively normalizes the lumbar lordosis while bringing the shoulders backward and bringing the head and neck back over the shoulders. This is quite similar to the military position of attention and, in that position, the cervical lordosis is normalized while the neural foramina are opened. Athletes involved in the use of the upper extremities require a rigid cylinder of strength in their torso to transfer torque from their legs to their upper extremities. Trunk and leg strength generate the strength of the upper extremity activity while the arms and hands generally provide the fine control. Fatigue in the trunk or legs can reduce the fine control in the upper extremities available for overhead activities such as in racquet sports and throwing sports. When there is loss of the rigid trunk cylinder strength, there is a resultant loss of synchrony between the arms and legs. There is a similar linkage among the legs, trunk, neck, and head in regard to the fine control available for blocking and tackling techniques that must be utilized precisely and reproducibly throughout a game. Loss of synchrony between the arms and legs can cause a resultant loss of coordination between the trunk and neck as well as a loss of precise coordination between the trunk and upper extremities. As the trunk flexors and abdominal musculature weaken due to fatigue, the lumbar lordosis increases and low back pain may result. Asymmetrical, asynchronous upper extremity athletic activities can result in neck pain, neck strain, and cervical spine injury. Interscapular pain can be directly related to bad posture, round shoulder/head forward posture, and asynchronic muscle activity. A weak trunk produces undue arm and shoulder strain because the upper extremity must compensate for the weak trunk, and arm muscles are used for strength instead of fine control. The joints, cervical spine, shoulder, and elbow are not under undue strain. Nowhere is this better demonstrated than in athletes who throw as part of their sport.

Throwers require a rigid cylinder of strength to transfer torque from their legs to their throwing arms. Trunk and leg strength generate the velocity of the throw and the arm provides the fine control strength. Fatigue reduces the control of the pitching motion and ball location. A major factor in ball control is a loss of tone and strength in the trunk caused by trunk muscle fatigue. A loss of the rigid trunk cylinder produces a loss of synchrony between the legs and arms. This causes a change in the pitching motion. As the trunk flexors and abdominal musculature weaken because of fatigue, lumbar lordosis increases and the back arches. The subtle change of a few degrees puts the arm behind in the pitching motion, promoting earlier ball release, and the pitch comes up. Arm strain increases as the trunk musculature fatigues. Attempts to compensate for loss of trunk strength and a "slow arm" increase the use of the arm musculature and predisposes the shoulder to injury.

Attempts to compensate for loss of trunk strength may involve the use of blocking and tackling techniques that are more dangerous, placing the player at an increased risk for cervical spine injury. As such, our trunk conditioning program is aimed at developing power in the torsional strength of the trunk musculature including the trapezius muscles, the spinal erector musculature, the latissimus dorsi, the internal and external obliques as well as the transversus abdominus, the rectus abdominus sheath of muscle, the gluteal musculature as well as the hip flexors, extensors, abductors, adductors, and the thigh musculature. Trunk-strengthening exercises are designed not only to enhance performance, but also to prevent subsequent injury to the back, the neck, and the arms.

We have recognized that attempts to increase the strength of the trunk or neck musculature by exercising the neck and back through a full range of motion may be counterproductive to the ultimate goal of relieving neck and back pain. Rather, we stress an isometric set of exercises that can accomplish adequate trunk and neck strengthening to diminish or relieve symptoms of neck or back pain. However, most important to recognize is that the isometric trunk-strengthening program that we have designed is easily taught to athletes without back or neck pain. When an individual trainer or physician is treating an athlete with neck or back pain after an injury, then the full clinical details of that patient must be incorporated into the development of a rehabilitation and exercise protocol that is designed specifically for that individual and for that individual's injuries. However, we have found that our isometric trunk-conditioning program is effective at preventing back injuries and is useful in many individuals with active neck or back pain. While treatment plans for symptomatic back and neck pain patients as well as patients who have suffered cervical spine spinal cord injury may include similar exercises, each of the treatment plans should be designed to match the examination and the symptoms. Any trunk-strengthening and -conditioning program necessarily faces a biomechanical strain on the spine and can exacerbate any underlying inflammatory or degenerative condition that is symptomatic. Therefore, the implementation of this isometric trunk-strengthening and trunk-conditioning program requires a safe and controlled program that proceeds progressively from less vigorous activity to more vigorous activity as the patient's symptomatology diminishes.

The key to safe strengthening of the back and neck is the ability to maintain the spine in a safe, neutral position during the strengthening exercises. For upper body strengthening, the spine must be well aligned with a chest-out posture. Isometric trunk exercises and upper body exercises that emphasize this chest-out posture also strengthen the supporting structures for the cervical spine and the postural muscles necessary for maintaining proper body alignment; ultimately, these exercises are useful preventive measures for neck pain during athletic activity. In individuals other than football players, we do not recommend specific neck-strengthening exercises except for modest isometric exercises that can be performed manually only. There are certainly exceptions in sports, such as wrestling, rugby, and other contact sports; the individual neck-strengthening exercises must be tailored appropriately.

The establishment of a finely coordinated set of muscles that transfer the torque from the lower extremities up through the trunk, chest, and back musculature to the arms and neck requires a practiced and controlled sequence of exercises aimed at increasing the coordination among these interlinked musculoskeletal elements. Establishing finely coordinated control through a series of exercises that enhance the coordination between these muscle groups is the theory behind this isometric trunk-conditioning program. The key to the trunk stability exercises is learning to maintain and control a neutral, pain-free position of the trunk. Every exercise in this program could be done by any reasonably conditioned athlete with no training whatsoever, but the key is doing the exercises correctly. The program initially starts with the athlete learning to obtain and maintain a neutral, pain-free position for the trunk and being able to hold the trunk muscles including the buttocks, the paraspinus musculature, the abdominal oblique musculature, the rectus abdominus musculature, and the thigh musculature in a tight, rigidly controlled trunk position. One objective of the trunk-stabilization program is to retrain the trunk muscles to fire to protect the spine when the person is using his or her arms and legs. Another objective is for these muscles to work and function in a coordinated fashion during activities in which the individual does not have time consciously to think and activate the trunk musculature in the sequence of firing that is necessary to perform the particular activity. This exercise program retrains trunk muscles through a balancing and coordinating group of exercises. These exercises teach a balanced and coordinated muscle-firing sequence of adequate strength to protect the spine during the sport activity. Ability to do 5000 sit-ups may protect the back while doing the sit-up but not while throwing a football, throwing a baseball, or tackling another player. The key to the exercises is the first step, being able to isolate trunk musculature, provide a tight contraction, and hold the spine in a neutral, pain-free position. The therapist and trainer initially assist the individual in learning where the neutral, pain-free position is and how to use the muscles to maintain that position.

We have found this particular program of exercises helpful in the postoperative recovery of patients after neck and back surgery. After neck surgery, an appropriate period of spinal immobilization with an orthotic device is required. Then, the patient may initiate this series of exercises with the assistance of the physical therapist.

Generally, within 3–6 weeks after neck or back surgery that does not require bony healing or bony fusion to take place, we will initiate our isometric trunk-stabilization program. If the wound is well healed, the patient is able to take part safely in a water rehabilitation program. We will allow patients to enter into a gentle water rehabilitative program at 3 weeks, doing exercises in the swimming pool, with the individual running in the water while using the wet vest. By 6 weeks postoperatively, the patient has been able to advance to dry land exercises that have included progressive walking for aerobic conditioning.

Once well into the healing process, the individual can progress to the Swedish ball exercises, which utilize a large beach ball that is able to support the weight of the individual. A whole host of exercises is then performed on the beach ball, progressing from crunches to wall slides, all the way through full sit-ups, as well as rotational sit-ups and resistive exercises on the ball.

Isoband exercises utilize a flexible rubber stretch band and are useful in all aspects of rehabilitative programs including upper and lower extremity strengthening and, in particular for hip extensor and hip adductor strengthening. Aerobic conditioning includes skipping rope, exercise bicycle, climbers (Versa Climber), ski machines (Nordic Trac) and stair machines (Stairmaster). We have been particularly pleased with water running, which includes the performance of running in place while wearing a flotation-type wet vest. A buoyancy vest or life jacket from a boat can also be useful for these individuals. As the individual progresses in his aerobic conditioning, he or she may even assume the use of old tennis shoes to increase the weight and resistance on the legs and, thus, increase the aerobic capacity. The water running is particularly useful in postoperative lumbar spine patients because the non-weight-bearing activity significantly limits the amount of low back pain present. In fact, it is extremely unusual for even the most severely affected postlaminectomy syndrome patient to be unable to adapt progressively to a water running program. We recommend *Water Workout Recovery Program* (25) as a source of useful techniques for treating patients in the weight-free environment of the swimming pool.

Cervical Stenosis

Cervical spinal stenosis and its associated transient neuropraxia of the cervical spinal cord is a source of great controversy as to recommendations for continued play. Grant (26) first described the clinical entity of cervical spinal cord neuropraxia with transient quadraplegia. Torg describes the clinical picture as an acute transient neurologic episode of cervical cord origin with sensory changes that may be associated with motor paresis involving either both arms, both legs, or all four extremities, following forced hyperextension, hyperflexion, or axial loading of the cervical spine (29). The sensory changes include burning pain, numbness, tingling, or loss of sensation, and motor changes consist of weakness or complete paralysis. Congenital cervical spinal stenosis is associated with a decreased anteroposterior diameter of the cervical spinal canal as measured from the posterior vertebral body to the anterior spinal laminar line on the lateral radiograph. Acquired spinal stenosis is more likely to occur in the professional level football player with multiple levels of degenerative disc disease, multiple levels of osteophyte formation, disc bulging, disc herniation, hypertrophy of ligamentum flavum as well as hypertrophy of the facet joints. This combination of degenerative and hypertrophic changes in the professional football player are not unusual. The absolute minimum sagittal diameter of the cervical spinal canal that can accommodate the spinal cord without cord compression is somewhere between 11 and 13 mm, depending upon the relative diameter of the spinal cord. The classic work of Penning (28) documented that if the sagittal diameter is less than 11 mm in extension, there is a strong suspicion of spinal cord compression. It was Penning who illustrated the "pincer's mechanism," in which the spinal cord is pinched between posterior vertebral osteophytes off of the lip of the vertebral endplate and the posterior lamina. Certainly, this mechanism of injury is commonly responsible for the production of the central cord syndrome in individuals with preexisting degenerative disc disease and osteophyte formation who suffer a hyperextension injury of the head and neck. However, there is ample clinical experience in dealing with professional football players with sagittal cervical spinal canal diameters of less than 11 mm who have no signs or symptoms of spinal cord compression. Therefore, as with all radiographic findings precise clinical correlation of the radiographic findings with the patient history, the patient's physical examination, as well as a basic understanding of the mechanical considerations of the patient's sport must be considered before making a judgment as to the individual player's risk category. Torg has concluded that, on the basis of his data, which involved the evaluation of 32 patients in whom an acute transient neurologic episode resulted from forced hyperextension, hyperflexion, or axial loading of the cervical spine, clearly, those individuals with developmental spinal stenosis are not predisposed to more severe injuries with associated permanent neurologic sequelae. However, he believed that athletes who have developmental spinal stenosis as well as demonstrable cervical spine instability, or acute or chronic intervertebral disc disease should not be allowed further participation in contact sports (27). We believe there are many factors that must be considered prior to making such a determination.

Types of Stenosis

There are three basic types of cervical stenosis:

1. Congenital stenosis—which is typified by the short pedicles and funneling shape to the basic bony structure of the spinal canal, observable on the lateral x-ray
2. Developmental stenosis—which occurs during life and may be the result of thickening of the bone due to increased stress. For example, upper body weight lifters, strengtheners, and people who do upper body- and neck-strengthening exercises produce a larger cervical spine bone, just as they produce larger mus-

cles in the neck and upper extremity and, as a result, the spinal canal may narrow as the bone increases in size.

3. Acquired cervical stenosis—which is due to cervical spondylosis with bone spurs, disc bulges, bulges of ligamentum flavum occurring with disc space narrowing and osteophytes on the facet joints, all contributing to the cervical stenosis. Of course, there may be more than one type of cervical stenosis present in any patient.

Measurement of Cervical Stenosis

There are different techniques for measuring the size of the spinal canal in order to assess the presence and degree of cervical stenosis. Pavlov and Torg (29) described a ratio of the central canal sagittal diameter to the vertebral body sagittal diameter measured on the lateral x-ray in order to remove the x-ray magnification that is always a consideration in direct measurements. The determination of what is a normal Pavlov ratio in certain population groups is still somewhat unclear. A Pavlov ratio of 0.8 or less has been used to indicate cervical stenosis, but the ratio was based on symptoms of transient cord neuropraxia in people with 0.8 or less and a lack of symptoms in people with ratios higher than that and was scientifically correlated to stenosis. In a group of myelopathic and radiculopathic nonfootball patients, Schnebel et al. (30) compared the ratio to CT scan central canal diameters and found the 0.8 ratio to be an extremely sensitive but not specific measurement. Every patient who had 10 mm or less of central canal diameter had a 0.8 ratio or less. The excellent study by Herzog et al. (31) that used CT scans and plain x-rays of football players provided the key factors concerning the Torg ratio. He showed that 78% of the football players with an abnormal Torg ratio had a normal-sized spinal canal. The football players had larger vertebral bodies, therefore distorting the ratio and rendering it useless in identifying players with cervical stenosis. The report also showed that standardized distance lateral x-rays—with calculations done to eliminate magnification—do correctly identify bony spinal stenosis.

The contribution made by Joseph Torg cannot be underestimated. The 20 years of acquiring records concerning injuries to football players provided great insight into the overall problem of cervical paralysis in football players. While many cases show distinct differences and have characteristics of a number of different injuries, it was Torg's impression and understanding that there were no instances of permanent quadraplegia in football players that resulted from disc herniations or spinal stenosis only (2). Certainly there are cases of fracture dislocations that may have had characteristics of stenosis or a disc herniation, but as isolated entities, there are no records of football players having been totally paralyzed with these two entities. The 0.8 ratio should not be used as a screening tool because whether there is a 0.8 ratio or not has no correlation to permanent neurologic deficit. If there is an episode of transient quadraparesis, then there is a 90% chance there will be a ratio of 0.8 or less, but, since the incidence of the transient quadraparesis has been estimated to be 7 in 10,000 ball players, then whether there is a 0.8 ratio or not cannot be statistically correlated with any increased chance of transient neuropraxia or permanent deficit. The Torg ratio is of little value for screening and should not be used for continued play decisions.

Since 17 ± 5 mm is the normal sagittal diameter (32), 10 mm is considered by most to be abnormal stenosis. The contrast CT scan is the definitive technique for measuring central canal diameter. The contrast CT scan allows one to measure not only the central canal diameter, but also a functional central canal diameter. The functional central canal diameter in the sagittal plane can be defined as the amount of canal available for the dural sac and spinal cord. The trefoil-shaped canal or the canal with the small, peaked empty space, exactly in the midline, are canal shapes that do not allow full expansion of the dural sac and cord throughout its central diameter. When measuring the central canal diameter, including a small, peaked area of space that could account for 2 mm of measurement yet will not accommodate the dural sac gives a measurement that is of little consequence to cord function. This is seen also in the lumbar spine where lateral recess stenosis very commonly produces a major compression on the entire sac, leaving an empty dorsal portion of the spinal canal.

Matsuura et al. (33), at Rancho Los Amigos Hospital, found a strong coordination between the shape of the spinal canal and the extent of neurologic injury with fracture/dislocations. They used the ratio of sagittal to transverse diameter and found a strong positive correlation between this ratio and spinal cord injury when compared with controls. While the transverse diameter was inversely proportional and the sagittal diameter was directly proportional to the spinal cord injury, the area of the spinal canal was not. The exact mean ratio varied at different levels but was best correlated at the three most important levels, C4, C5, and C6. The control mean was approximately 0.6 and the spinal cord injury mean was 0.5. In this report, the Torg ratio was stated to be not as powerful a discriminator as the sagittal diameter. Ogino, et al. (34) used the sagittal to transverse "compression" ratio as an indicator of cord damage in myelopathy patients. This study, done on cadaveric specimens, shows a relationship between compression ratio and the degree of cord damage in people with cervical stenosis and myelopathy.

The area of the canal as related to the area of the cord has been found to be important in radiculopathy and myelopathy (35) (Fig. 49.12). Measuring surface area of the dural sac vs. the canal has some difficulties in determining the surface area of canal available for the sac. The lateral portions of the canal and the area of the nerve root sleeves, which will not accommodate much cord expansion, should not be included in the area available for cord expansion.

There are cases with a larger spinal cord or a smaller cord/sac ratio. Measuring exact cord shapes are dependent upon exact radiologic technique. The presence of a large volume of dye circumferentially around the cord

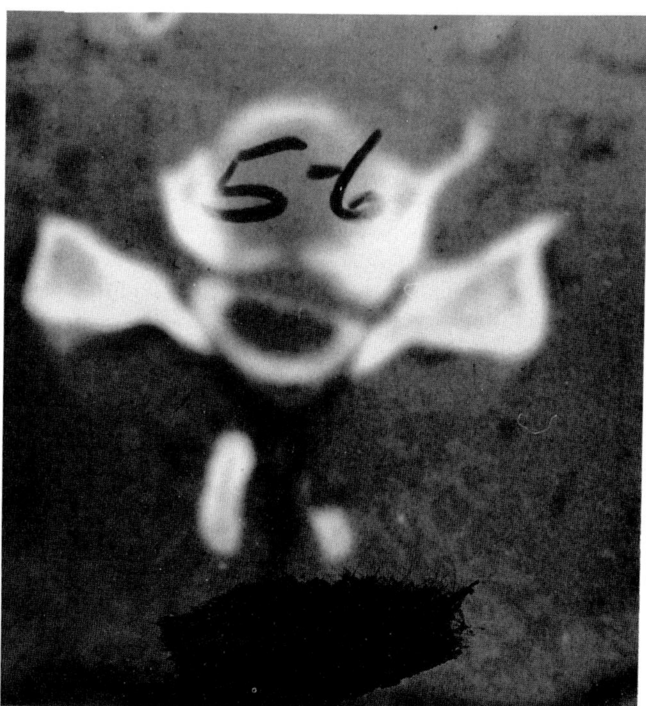

Figure 49.12 X-ray of a professional football player who persisted with a C6 radiculopathy. The symptoms began with a forearm blow to the head. Although no myelopathy was present, there was a significant distortion of the cord and dural sac.

is a good sign and the obliteration of dye volarly can be an important sign of volar compression and, as seen in cases with a poor compression ratio, a flat spinal cord is a bad sign.

The amount of motion in the cervical spine is probably proportional to the risk from stenosis. Dynamic MRI has been used to demonstrate the narrowing of the cervical canal that occurs with extension (36). It is well known that that the cervical spinal canal can narrow up to 2 mm in full extension as compared with the neutral or flexion position. Neurologic tissue in the spine becomes slack and loose in extension, taut in flexion, and the spinal canal narrows in extension and opens in flexion (37). Numerous clinical syndromes are dependent upon these dynamic factors affecting spinal cord and nerve root function in addition to exact central canal measurements and ratios. The biomechanic of the spinal column and neurologic tissue motion must be considered in continued play decisions in cases of cervical stenosis.

Bohlman (38) has pointed out the importance not only of canal diameter but, also, of blood flow to the cord and cervical motion as three important factors in the determination of symptoms of cervical myeloradiculopathy. Exact quantification of vascularity to the cervical cord is difficult clinically, but there are vascular abnormalities and insufficient areas of flow that can certainly predispose an individual patient to neurologic injury.

A fixed kyphotic cervical spine does not respond to axial loading normally and may present a volar cord compression with the cord tethered over volar osteophytes. Batzdorf and Batzdorf (39) showed that patients with a kyphotic cervical spine had more neck pain and responded more poorly to laminectomy for cervical myelopathy than did patients with a lordotic cervical spine.

Factors in Decision-Making in Transient Quadraparesis and Spinal Canal Stenosis

There are numerous decision-making factors in these cases. Among them, severity of the episode, extent of neurologic deficit, severity of the symptoms, age, player position, and neck size. The numerous methods of assessing cervical canal size bear consideration. Regardless of the canal diameter, there is certainly more danger to someone who suffers a greater neurologic injury with the episode. The severity of the episode is important. A person who had symptoms of myelopathy lasting more than 6 months is obviously at greater risk for return of those symptoms than someone who had the episodes for 5 seconds. Each case will be a variation of severity of symptoms, type of neurologic deficit, extent of neurologic deficit, and longevity of the symptoms. The important things are the history and physical examination. One must document very, very carefully exactly what happened through the history and physical examination. The neurologic examination must be immaculate to identify and to quantify the deficit present.

We have found the rating system shown in Table 49.1 to be helpful in assessing the severity of the episode. However, every factor in a case may be considered in its entirety.

Table 49.1
Rating System To Assess Severity[a]

Rating	Extent of Neurologic Deficit
1	Unilateral arm—numbness or dysesthesia, loss of strength
2	Bilateral upper extremity loss of motor and sensory function
3	Hemi arm and leg and trunk loss of motor and sensory function
4	Transitory quadriparesis
5	Transitory quadriplegia
Rating	**Time Ratings**
1	Less than 5 minutes
2	Less than 1 hour
3	Less than 24 hours
4	Less than 1 week
5	Greater than 1 week
Rating of Central Canal Diameter	**Canal Narrowing**
1	Greater than 12 mm
2	Between 10 and 12 mm
3	10 mm
4	10 to 8 mm
5	Less than 8 mm

[a] Any existing neurologic deficit due to a cord neuropraxia should exclude an athlete from play in any case. As a general guideline: less than 4 is a mild episode, 4–7 a moderate episode, and 8–10 is a severe episode. When combined with canal size, the severity of the episode can lead to some guidelines for recurrence.

In terms of the three major risk factors in Table 49.1, adding in the canal diameter rating to the time and extent of deficit scale, we use a general rating of 6 or below as a mild risk factor, 6–10 as a moderate risk and 10–15 as a severe risk category. It must be emphasized, however, that each case is very individualized. For example, a player with a brief episode with a 4-mm canal or 6 months of myelopathy with a 15-mm canal may be precluded from play forever. The rating scale is only a guideline. Clinically, we use the rating scale, extenuating factors such as the level of play and the risk vs. benefit to the patient. The risk vs. benefit ratio is often an unquantifiable factor. An informed consent concerning continued play with cervical stenosis and a prior episode of transient quadraparesis should include an accurate assessment of as many known facts as possible. The incidence of permanent paralysis in professional football is rare. Permanent paralysis in any football player is most related to blocking and tackling techniques. An episode of transient quadraplegia does not necessarily precede an incident of permanent neurologic loss. Cantu (40) reports three cases in which this occurred but did not have such a case in the Registry. Just because one has stenosis does not mean he will smash someone with his head, get a fracture dislocation, and be a permanent quadraplegic. Indeed, it may have no specific relation to such a future incident.

A good example of a consent would be to inform those concerned that there is no direct predisposition between having stenosis and getting the fracture dislocation that typically paralyzes football players. Give advice concerning what we do know about nonfootball players. There are several facts known about cervical stenosis in nonfootball players. The report by Eismont's et al. (41) demonstrates that the greater degree of cervical stenosis with a specific cervical spine injury, the greater the neurologic deficit. Matsuura et al., as stated previously, found that it is not just the central canal diameter but the shape of the canal that is important. The greater the compression ratio, the greater the degree of neurologic deficit with a spine injury. Edwards et al. (42) demonstrated that an individual with a cervical canal stenosis is more likely to require surgery with a cervical disc herniation and less likely to be able to get well nonoperatively (42, 43). Radicular pain is more common in smaller canals (44).

In the Epstein study (45), there were 20 patients of 200 admissions to an acute spinal cord injury unit who had no fracture or dislocation, but had complete neurologic deficit. Among these cases were various diagnoses of cervical spondylosis, congenital stenosis, and others, but the study indicates that permanent neurologic deficit can occur with spinal stenosis (17). The incidence of permanent tetraplegia in spinal column injury has varied from 4–70% of pediatric neck injuries, depending on the sample studied. Others have hypothesized on the etiology of quadraplegia without fracture dislocation to be a combination of injury to microvascular blood supply, longitudinal traction on the cord, acute disc prolapse, and/or compromise of the vertebral spinal arterial system (46–50). A common pathology in these cases is a central cord infarct (51).

As for recurrence of symptoms, multiple episodes do occur but can potentially be prevented through proper equipment, conditioning, and technique.

Other Factors in Any Continued-Play Decision

While every position on the football field is subjected to head trauma, the worst are the impact positions of defensive back and linebacker. Blocking and tackling techniques can rarely be changed at the professional level. If the player is a head-hitter, he usually stays a head-hitter. Education for proper blocking and tackling by using the shoulders, not the head, must be aimed at athletes at younger ages, starting with those in grade school and continuing through college.

What are the chances of recurrent injury once a player has been injured? Albright et al. (52) have offered some excellent insight into this situation. At the high school level, the reinjury rate, after all neck injuries, one-third of which had extremity or neurologic symptoms, was 17.2%. The twice injured players at all levels of play had an 87% chance of future injury or significant history of past injury. After a time-lost injury, the recurrent injury rate was 42%; 62% in the next season; and 67% in future seasons (37). Therefore, the recurrent injury rate is significant regardless of the type of injury received and is higher with the time-lost neck injury.

What can be done to prevent this recurrence? Conditioning can prevent injury. Preconditioned response to predicted head stresses can allow an increased protective muscle reflex response to ward off even relatively unexpected blows (53). Neck strengthening can help protect the player from neck injury (54). Probably the greatest testament to conditioning is the ability of professional football players to deliver or receive high impact blows without injury.

Using the head for contact produces dangerous mechanisms for cervical injury (55). Protective wear is limited to good shoulder pads with a high neck roll that is built up on the lateral neck. The posterior rolls are not as helpful as the side rolls because the shoulder pads are more likely posterior at contact and the neck straight. The spine straightens with slight flexion to deliver the axial loading blow with the top of the head (53). While the mechanism of pure extension has been implicated as a source of serious injury, others believe that it is not a significant source of major cervical injury in football. The lateral pads can help with lateral flexion and rotation toward the painful arm so common in burners and stingers. The majority of stingers and burners are a root injury, not a brachial plexus traction injury, and C6 is the most common root involved. The most effective method of preventing the high risk of recurrent neck injury is to allow total recovery of pain, relief from tenderness, and restoration of a normal range of motion as well as maximum strength before returning to action. Normal clinical muscle function is more important than changes, for example. Good nonoperative cervical care, such as may be used with a herniated cervical disc, can improve symptoms from neck injuries in football players. A mainstay of our exercise rehabilitation program is a chest-out posturing exercise program concentrating on entire trunk strength as well as neck and upper extremity strength.

Responsibility is always a consideration and it is important to emphasize that the doctor who performs the players' physical examinations and clears them to play bears a certain responsibility to the patient. Through proper informed consent, the patient and family are also responsible. The team, as an employer, in any worker's compensation situation, is naturally responsible for the health of its employees as well as for fielding an effective team. Earlier, reference was made to risk vs. benefit to the patient. The benefit of continued play to the patient will be well known to the patient, family, agent, team, and others. The risk to the patient can be very difficult to define as a reality. Proven facts are science and predictions are basically educated guesses. Nevertheless the physician must present the risks to the patient as clearly as possible.

It is hoped that this chapter will provide some guidelines for decision-making in situations where football players have injured their necks and want to return to football. Obviously, there are many factors to consider in a decision that is of great importance to those involved.

REFERENCES

1. Clark KS. The survey of sports related spinal cord injuries in schools and colleges: 1973–1975. J Safety Res, 1977;9:140.
2. Torg JS, Vegso JJ, Sennett B, et al. The National Football Head and Neck Injury Registry. 14 Year report on cervical quadraplegia, 1971–1984. JAMA 1985;254:3439–3443.
3. Burke DC. Spinal cord injuries from water sports. Med J Austral 1972;2:1190.
4. Bracken MB, Shepard MJ, et al. A randomized controlled trial of methylprednisolone or naloxon in the treatment of acute spinal cord injury. N Engl J Med 1990;322:1405–1411.
5. Schneider RC. The treatment of the athlete with neck, cervical spine and spinal cord trauma. In Schneider, Ed. Sports injuries: Mechanisms, prevention and treatment. Baltimore: Williams & Wilkins, Baltimore, 1985.
6. Schneider RC. Serious and fatal neurosurgical football injuries. Clin Neurosurg 1966;12:226.
7. Watkins RG. Neck injuries in football players. Clin Sports Med 1986;5:215–246.
8. Jackson DW, Lohr FP. Cervical spine injuries. Clin Sports Med 1986;5:373–386.
9. Seddon H. Surgical disorders of the peripheral nerves. Edinburgh: Churchill Livingstone, 1972.
10. Clancy W, Brand R, Bergfeld J. Upper trunk brachial plexus injuries in contact sports. Am J Sports Med 1977;5:209.
11. Bergfeld JA, Hershman EB, Wilbourn AJ. Brachial plexus in sports, a five year followup. Orthop Transac, 1988;12:743–744.
12. Davidson RI, Dunn EJ, Metzmaker JN. The shoulder abduction test. Spine 1981;6:441–446.
13. Garfin SR, Rydevik BL, Brown MD. Compressive neuropathy of spinal nerve roots. Spine 1991;16:162–166.
14. Thomas JC. Plain roentgenograms of the spine in the injured athlete. Clin Sports Med 1990;5:353–371.
15. White AA III, Johnson RM, Panjabi MM, et al. Biomechanical analysis of clinical stability in the cervical spine. Clin Orthop Relat Res 1975;109:89–96.
16. Mazur JW, Stauffer ES. Unrecognized spinal instability associated with seemingly simple cervical compression fractures. Spine 1983;8:687–692.
17. Boden SD, et al. Abnormal magnetic resonance scans of the cervical spine in asymptomatic subjects. A prospective investigation. J Bone Joint Surg (Am) 1990;72:1178–1184.
18. Davis D, Bohlman H, Walker AE, et al. The pathologic findings in fatal craniospinal injuries. J Neurosurg 1971;34:603.
19. Anderson LD, D'Alonzo RT. Fractures of the odontoid process of the axis. J Bone Joint Surg 1974;56A:1669.
20. Effendi B, Roy D, Cornish B, et al. Fractures of the rim of the axis. J Bone Joint Surg 1981;63B:319.
21. Levine AM, Edwards CC. The management of traumatic spondylolisthesis of the axis. J Bone Joint Surg 1985;67A:217.
22. Watkins RG. Neck injuries in football players. Clin Sports Med 1986;5:215–246.
23. Herkowitz H, Rothman R. Subacute instability of the cervical spine. Spine 9:May–June, 1984.
24. Williams RW. Microcervical foraminotomy: A surgical alternative for intractable radicular pain. Spine 1983;8:708–716.
25. Watkins RG, Buhler W, Loverock P. Water workout recovery program. Philadelphia: Contemporary Books, 1988.
26. Grant J, Sears W: Spinal injury and computerized tomography; a review of fracture pathology and a new approach to canal decompression. Aust NZ J Surg 56:April 1986.
27. Torg JS. Cervical spinal stenosis with cord neurapraxia in transient quardraplegia. Clin Sports Med 1990;9:279–296.
28. Penning L. Some aspects of plain radiography of the cervical spine in chronic myelopathy. Neurology 1962;12:513–519.
29. Torg JS, Pavlov H. Cervical spinal stenosis with cord neurapraxia and transient quadriplegia. Clin Sports Med 1987;6:115–133.
30. Schnebel B, Kingston S, Watkins RG, et al. Comparison of MRI to contrast CT in the diagnosis of spinal stenosis. Spine 1989;14:3.
31. Herzog RJ, Weins JJ, Dillingham MF, Sontag MJ. Normal cervical spine morphometry and cervical spinal stenosis in asymptomatic professional football players. Plain film radiography, multiplanar computer tomography, and magnetic resonance imaging. Spine 1991;16 (Suppl):178–186.
32. Wilkenson H, Lemay M, Ferris E. Roentgenographic correlations in cervical spondylosis. AJR 1969;105:370.
33. Matsurra P, Waters R, Adkins RH, et al. Comparison of computerized tomography parameters of the cervical spine in normal control subjects and spinal cord injured patients. J Bone Joint Surg 1989;71A:183–188.
34. Ogino K, Tada K, Okada K, et al. Canal diameter, anteroposterior compression ratio and spondolytic myelopathy of the cervical spine. Spine 1983;8:1–15.
35. Chrispin AR, Lees F. The spinal canal in cervical spondylosis. J Neurol Neurosurg Psychiatr 1963;26:166–170.
36. Cervical Spine Research Society Meeting, Key Biscayne, FL, 1988.
37. Brieg A, Turnbull I, Hassler O. Effects of mechanical stresses on the spinal cord in cervical spondylosis. J Neurosurg 1966;25:45.
38. Bohlman H. Cervical spondylosis with moderate to severe myelopathy. Spine 1977;2:151.
39. Batzdorf U, Batzdorf A. Analysis of cervical spine curvature in patients with cervical spondylosis. Neurosurgery 1988;22:5.
40. Cantu RC. Head and spine injuries in the young athlete. Clin Sports Med (US), 1988;7:459–72.
41. Eismont FJ, Clifford S, et al. Cervical sagittal spinal canal size in spine injuries. Spine 1984;9:663–666.
42. Edwards W, La Rocca H. The developmental segmental sagittal diameter of the cervical spinal canal in patients with cervical spondylosis. Spine 1983;8:20.
43. Wolf B, Khulnani M, Malis L. The sagittal diameter of the bony cervical spinal canal and its significance in cervical spondylosis. J Mt Sinai Hosp 1976;23:283.
44. Williams JPR, McKibben B. Cervical spine injury in the rugby union football. Br Med J'1978;2:1747.
45. Epstein J, Carras R, Hyman R, Costa S. Cervical myelopathy caused by developmental stenosis of the spinal canal. J Neurosurg 1972;51:362–367.

46. Burke DC. Traumatic spinal paralysis in children. Paraplegia 1974;11:268–276.
47. Cheshire DJE. The paediatric syndrome of traumatic myelopathy without demonstrable vertebral injury. Paraplegia 1977;15:74–85.
48. Hill SA, Miller CA, et al. Pediatric neck injuries: A clinical study. J Neurosurg 1984;60:700–706.
49. Pang D, Wilberger JE Jr. Spinal cord injury without radiographic abnormalities in children. J Neurosurg 1982;57:114–129.
50. Scher AT. Vertex impact and cervical dislocation in rugby players. S Afr Med J 1981;59:227–228.
51. Ahmann PA, Smith SA, et al: Spinal cord infarction due to minor trauma in children. Neurology 1975;25:301–307.
52. Albright JP, Moses JM, Feldick HG, et al. Non-fatal cervical spine injuries in interscholastic football. JAMA 1976;236:1243–1245.
53. Reid SE, Reid SE Jr. Advances in sports medicine: Prevention of head and neck injuries in football players. Surg Annu 1981;13:251–270.
54. Funk FJ, Wells RE. Injuries of the cervical spine in football. Clin Orthop Relat Res 1975;109:50–58.
55. Bauze RJ. Experimental production of forward dislocations in the human cervical spine. J Bone Joint Surg (Br) 1978;60:239–245.

50 / LUMBAR SPINE INJURIES

Robert G. Watkins and William M. Dillin

Introduction

Low back pain has been a significant factor in many different types of athletic activity. The severity and extent of back pain often determines the actual ability to compete and is a worry to all concerned: athlete; family; coaches; trainers; and those responsible for paying the bills. Essentially, treatment of the athlete with a lumbar spine injury involves an understanding of basic anatomy, biomechanical function of the spine, the diagnosis of conditions affecting the lumbar spine, proper use of diagnostic studies, and a systematized all-inclusive history and physical examination. It is necessary to understand some factors that are important in predisposing the athlete to lumbar spine problems as well as training and therapeutic techniques to prevent lumbar spine problems in athletes. Among the predisposing factors to back pain in athletes are increased trunk length, and stiff lower extremities (1). Spina bifida occulta is found in a high percentage of patients who develop lower lumber spondolytic defects (2). The exact relation of exercise and back pain in athletes compared with the average population does not demonstrate an increased incidence in back pain in athletes participating in organized sports. Fairbank et al. (1) found that back pain was more common in students who avoided sports than those who participated. Fisk et al. (3) found that prolonged sitting was the important factor in the pathogenesis of Scheuermann's disease compared with athletes lifting weights, undergoing compressive stresses, or doing heavy lifting and part-time work. This study of 500 students (17 and 18 years old) showed that 56% of males and 30%of females had some x-ray evidence of changes similar to Scheuermann's disease.

An interesting review (4) found that 80% of back injuries occurred during practice, 6% during competition, and 14% during preseason conditioning. A total of 8% of the men and 6% of the women had injuries; this was of no statistical significance. The nature of the injury was acute for 59% of cases, overuse for 12%, and aggravation of preexisting conditions for 29%.

Anatomy

The vertebral column is a series of linked intervertebral joints. The joint is made up of the intervertebral disc, its two facet joints, concomitant ligaments, vessels, and nerves; it is referred to as a neuromotion segment. A neuromotion segment is considered to be one of the basic units of spinal anatomy and function. The lumbar spine has a lordotic curve and plays an important role in the biomechanics of the lumbar spine. The spine is broken down into two basic columns. The anterior column consists of the disc and vertebral bodies and the accompanying longitudinal ligaments, the anterior longitudinal ligament, and the posterior longitudinal ligament. The posterior column consists of the facet joints, lamina, spinous process, ligamentum flavum, and pars inarticularis. The disc itself may be described as a circular, multilaminated ligament that connects the two vertebrae together. The nucleus pulposus is the central, gelatinous-like portion of the disc; the annulus is the multilayered woven basket with fibers at precise angles to resist torsional and compression forces. The annulus is firmly anchored to the end plate of the vertebrae. The annulus, nucleus, and the accompanying end plates are excellent at resisting compressive forces but do not resist torsional forces well. The orientation of the facet joint is different at every level of the spine. In the lumbar spine, the facet joints are oriented in a transitional plane between the parasagittal orientation in the upper lumbar spine to the more coronal orientation in the lower lumber spine. This parasagittal orientation allows good motion in flexion and extension and less motion in lateral flexion. The parasagittal orientation of the facet joints naturally resist rotation, but fall victim to high torsional forces that overcome the strength of the joint, tearing the annulus and injuring the facet joints. When considering the anatomy of the spine, one must consider the important role of the entire cylinder of the trunk and its supporting muscles. The static ligamentous structures of the spine provide considerable resistance to injury, but this resistance in itself would be insufficient to produce proper spine strength without the additional support provided through the trunk musculature and lumbodorsal fascia. Muscle control of the lumbodorsal fascia allows a much higher resistance to bending and loading stresses. The lumbodorsal fascia and the muscles attaching to it must be considered of equal importance to the more specialized function of the intervertebral disc and facet joints.

Diagnosis

It cannot be emphasized enough that obtaining a proper diagnosis in the athlete presenting with low back pain is crucial. It is the key to initiating an appropriately aggressive diagnostic and therapeutic plan (5, 6). Especially in the adolescent and younger athlete, a high index of suspicion must be maintained to diagnose accurately conditions such as stress fractures and spondolytic defects (7). A great variety of pathologic conditions can be diagnosed on plain x-ray, and their relationship to the athlete and his or her sport can be more specifically addressed (8). The bone scan is a vital part of the diagnostic armamentarium of the physician caring for lumbar spine problems in athletes. An adolescent athlete with significant back pain persisting longer than 3 weeks should have x-rays and a bone scan. Possible conditions ranging from the rarer, osteoid osteoma, infections, and stress fractures of the sacroiliac joint to the more routine spondolytic defects. The incidence of spondolytic defects seen on x-ray is approximately 30% to 38%, and 35% of young athletes presenting with significant lumbar pain have a positive bone scan (7, 9).

In diagnosing the exact etiology of the lumbar spine pain in athletes, age is an important factor. Younger athletes are certainly more likely to have stress fractures and to have congenital predispositions to stress fractures. Diseases that affect growing cartilage (e.g., Scheuermann's disease) are more common in young athletes. In the mature athlete, often the radiological assessment involves distinguishing between age-related, asymptomatic changes and symptomatic recent trauma. Is the L5–S1 disc degeneration symptomatic in a 30-year-old athlete or is it an asymptomatic finding? The diagnostic plan must use an organized system of identifying the most common conditions as well as retain the ability to diagnose the rare conditions such as a herniation of the inferior lumbar space (10) or osteoid osteoma.

One of the most important diagnoses to make in the athlete with back and leg pain is that of peripheral nerve injury and peripheral nerve entrapment. There is a great variety of peripheral nerve problems including generalized peripheral neuropathy, carpal tunnel syndrome, piriformis syndrome, peroneal nerve injury, femoral neuropathy, and interdigital neuroma. The chief reason for getting an electromyogram (EMG) and nerve conduction (NC) study of the lower extremities is to diagnose a peripheral nerve problem. The nerve conduction study combined with a careful physical examination can at least raise the distinct possibility of a peripheral nerve problem and heighten the diagnostician's skepticism concerning small, potentially asymptomatic spinal lesions in the role of the patient's extremity nerve pain.

Spondylolysis and Spondylolisthesis

Age is important in the natural history of spondylolysis and spondylolisthesis. There is a 4.4% incidence at age 6, increasing to 6% by adulthood. It is unusual for children to present with spondylolysis before the age of 5, and it is unusual for young children to present with severe spondylolisthesis (grade 3 or 4). Most symptoms appear in adolescence, but luckily, the risk of progression after adolescence is low, being approximately 15%. Symptoms cannot be correlated with the degree of slip; a high degree of slip may present with deformity and little pain. Many times, it is the pain of an injury that leads to the identification of spondylolisthesis that may not be originating in the spondylolisthetic segment.

Isthmic spondylolisthesis develops as a stress fracture. It is believed that there is a hereditary predisposition to developing such a stress fracture, and there is certainly a genetic predisposition for conditions in which the bone of the pars inarticularis is not sufficient to withstand normal stresses. Furthermore, certain mechanical activities that expose the patient to repeated biomechanical challenge and increase the stress concentrated on the pars interarticularis have a higher incidence of spondylolisthesis. The concept of repeated microtrauma with concentration of these stresses in the pars has become increasingly recognized in adolescent athletes participating in sports such as gymnastics and weight lifting.

The most common site for spondylolysis and spondylolisthesis is L5–S1. The slippage in spondylolisthesis results from the lack of support of the posterior elements produced by the stress fracture of the pars. The spectrum of neurologic involvement runs from rare to more common with higher degree slips. The majority of neurologic deficits are an L5 radiculopathy with an L5–S1 spondylolisthesis. Cauda equina symptoms are more likely in grade 3 or 4 slips. Cauda equina neurologic loss is rare.

The diagnostic and therapeutic plan for spondylolisthesis begins with a high degree of diagnostic suspicion in the adolescent athlete with low back pain. Up to 33% of adolescent athletes presenting with low back pain will have a positive bone scan for a stress fracture. Certainly, a low back pain that is not resolved within 3 weeks should be examined with a bone scan. If the bone scan is positive, the patient should have a computed tomography (CT) scan to see if there is a demonstrable stress fracture or if the bone is hot as a result of an impending fracture. If the bone scan is negative and the patient persists with lumbosacral pain, a magnetic resonance image (MRI) is indicated. A combination of an MRI, bone scan, and CT used in this manner should diagnose most of the significant pathologies in the lumbar spine.

The treatment plan for spondylolisthesis is basically rest or restriction of enough activity to relieve the symptoms. This may vary from simply removing the athlete from the sport until the pain has significantly improved to immobilization in a lumbosacral corset, Boston brace, or thoracolumbar orthosis (TLSO) to bed rest and casting.

In summary, stop the pain through whatever amount of inactivity it takes. The authors routinely brace the patient with a hot scan and restrict his or her activity for a minimum of 3 months. The bone scan is then repeated, and if it is negative, sufficient healing has taken place to allow the athlete to begin a rehabilitation program. If the bone scan is still positive and the athlete is asymptomatic, it can be difficult to decide whether the athlete should begin a rehabilitation program or continue with restricted activity. The authors usually continue restrictions for another 3 months. Unilateral hot bone scans with or without a demonstrated fracture have a reasonably high incidence of healing, and adolescent athletes in general should be treated with the idea in mind of healing the defect. Bilateral stress fractures are less likely to heal, despite comprehensive nonoperative therapy.

If the bone scan is cold and there is a spondylitic defect present, the patient should be treated for mechanical low back pain. This usually involves a progressively vigorous trunk stability rehabilitation program. The authors put no permanent restrictions on athletes with spondylolysis or spondylolisthesis. It should be obvious that patients with grade 3 to 4 spondylolisthesis are less likely to be able to participate in vigorous sports activities without pain and discomfort. They should probably avoid the heavy strength sports such as football and weight lifting.

There is a high incidence of spondylolysis and grade 1 and 2 spondylolisthesis in sports. As a long-term factor, this condition is not considered to be significant in an athlete's ability to play.

Biomechanics

The understanding of the basic biomechanics of the lumbar spine begin with an understanding of the forces and stresses applied to the spine as related to its normal curvatures. Because of its lordotic shape, the spine experiences a vectoral force as a vertical axial loading compressive force perpendicular to the surface of the disc and a compressive force horizontal to the disc. The combination of these two forces produces both tensile stress in the annulus fibrosis and a shear force on the neural arch. The center of gravity of body weight is anterior to the spine. This weight times the distance back to the spine produces a lever-arm effect of the weight of the body. This is resisted by the erector spinae muscles and the lumbodorsal fascia. Abnormal stresses applied to this equation may result in annular tears of the intervertebral discs or stress fractures on the neural arch, because of the excessive resistive force. The most common place for stress fracture, of course, is the pars interarticularis.

The basic mechanism of injury produces a combined vector of force that may be difficult to analyze in a force diagram. The three basic mechanisms of injury to consider are the following:

1. Compression or weight loading to the spine.
2. Torque or rotation, which may result in various shear forces in a more horizontal plane.
3. Tensile stress produced through excessive motion on the spine.

The compressive type of stress is more common in sports that require high body weight and massive strengthening such as football and weight lifting. Torsional stresses occur in sports involving throwing such as javelin, baseball and golf. Motion sports that put tremendous tensile stresses on the spine include gymnastics, ballet, other dance, pole vault, and high jump.

Sprains and strains result from direct blows. In sports like football, there can be muscle contusions; muscle stretches; and tears of fascia, ligaments, and occasionally muscle.

Lumbar fractures can occur from direct blows to the back, with fracture of the spinous process or twisting injuries that avulse the transverse process. A vertebral body end-plate fracture caused by an axial compression load on the disc is a relatively common compressive disc injury. The annulus is likely to be injured in rotation, and the end plate is vulnerable to compression. Flexion rotation fracture dislocations of the cervical and lumbar spine are certainly possible. Axial-loading compression injuries can result from jarring injuries in motor sports or boating. In any sport in which one athlete falls on another, the mechanism is similar to that of the coal-face injury in which a rock falls on the miner while he or she is on all fours. An athlete can suffer an asymmetric loading, rotational injury to the thoracolumbar spine.

The intervertebral disc is injured predominantly through rotation and shear, producing circumferential tears and radial tears. Initially, the layers may actually separate or the inner layers may break. As the inner layers weaken and are torn, there is added stress on the outer layers. This can produce a radial tear of the intervertebral disc. With the outer layers torn, the inner layers of annulus break off, and portions of the nucleus are forced with axial loading to the place of least resistance, the weak area in the annulus. The outer areas of annulus are richly innervated, producing tremendous pain and reflex spasm when the annulus tears. The spasm and pain is mediated through the sinuvertebral nerve, with anastomosis through the spinal nerve to the posterior primary ramus. As the herniated material extrudes and produces pain from the transversing or exiting nerve root itself, the patient may develop sciatica or radiculopathy. Intradiscal infiltration of the granulation tissue adds increased potential for painful sensation in the annulus. The annulus, with time, can heal, although the healing annulus will not retain the same biomechanical function capability as the original intervertebral disc.

Biomechanical functioning of the spinal column and its relationship to the biomechanics of nerve tissue involves several basic concepts:

1. Flexion of the lumbar spine increases the size of the intervertebral canal and the intervertebral foramina (11).
2. Extension decreases the size of the intervertebral canal and the intervertebral foramina (11).
3. Flexion increases dural sac and nerve root tension (12).
4. Extension decreases dural sac and nerve root tension (12).
5. Front flexion, axial loading, flexion, and upright posture increase intradiscal pressure.
6. With flexion, the annulus bulges anteriorly (13).
7. With extension, the annulus bulges posteriorly (13).
8. Nuclear shift in an injured disc is poorly documented, but probably corresponds with annular bulge (11).
9. Rotation and torsion produces annular tears and disc herniations (14).

Conclusion of these facts indicate that motion does have an effect on the nerves and the neuromotion segments of an injured area. For example, if there is a spinal obstructive problem such as spinal stenosis, extension exercises can further compress the neurologic structures and make them worse; or if there is a nerve root tension problem such as disc herniation, then flexion can produce increased tension in an already tense nerve and increase symptoms.

History and Physical Examination

The key to a proper history and physical examination is to have a standardized form that accomplishes the needed specific objectives.

1. *Quantitate the morbidity.* Use a scale value of pain, function, and occupation to understand how sick the patient is. Converse in detail with the patient to hear the inflections and manner of pain description. Detail the time of disability and the time of origin of the pain.
2. *Delineate the psychosocial factors.* Know what psychological effect the pain has had on the patient. Know the social, economic, and legal results of the patient's disability. Understand what can be gained by his or her being sick or well. Derive an understanding of what role these factors are playing in the patient's complaints.
3. *Eliminate the possibility of tumors, infections, and neurologic crisis.* These diseases have a certain urgency that requires immediate attention and a diagnostic therapeutic regimen that is different from disc disease.
4. *Diagnose the clinical syndrome.*
   a. Nonmechanical back and/or leg pain: inflammatory; constant pain; minimally affected by activity; usually worse at night or early morning.
   b. Mechanical back and/or leg pain: made worse by activity and Valsalva; relieved by rest.
   c. Sciatica: predominantly radicular pain; positive stretch signs; with or without neurologic deficit.
   d. Neurogenic claudication: radiating leg pain or calf pain, worse with ambulation; negative stretch signs, worse with spine extension, better with flexion.

Pinpoint the pathophysiology causing the syndrome. Three important determinations are

1. What level? Which neuromotion segment?
2. What nerve?
3. What pathology: what is the exact structure or disease process in that neuromotion segment that is causing the pain?

The history and physical examination together make up the first step in determining the clinical syndrome. Some key factors are the following:

1. The time of day during which the pain is worse.
2. A comparison of pain levels during walking, sitting, and standing.
3. The effects of Valsalva, coughing, and sneezing on pain.
4. The type of injury and duration of the problem.
5. A percentage of back versus leg pain. The authors insist on getting an accurate estimate of the amount of discomfort in back and legs. There must be two numbers that add up to 100%.

The physical examination should address these factors:

1. The presentation of sciatic stretch signs.
2. The neurologic deficit.
3. Back and lower extremity stiffness and loss of range of motion.
4. The exact location of tenderness and radiation of pain or paresthesias.
5. Maneuvers during the examination that reproduce the pain.

The history determines whether it is an axial (back pain) or extremity (leg pain) problem. What is the exact percentage of back versus leg pain? Is the pain made worse by the mechanical activity or is it a constant resting pain? It the pain worsened by maneuvers that increase intradiscal or intraspinal pressure? Is there significant night pain?

Classic radiculopathy causes radicular pain to radiate into a specific dermatomal pattern, with paresis and loss of sensation and reflex. The radicular pattern of the pain and neurologic examination determines the nerve involved. The usual history for radiculopathy caused by a disc herniation is back pain that progresses to predominantly leg pain. It is made worse by increases in intraspinal pressure such as coughing, sneezing, and sitting. Leg pain predominates over back pain and mechanical factors increase the pain. Physical examination shows positive nerve stretch signs. A dermatomal distribution leg pain that is made worse by straight-leg raising, sitting or being supine, leg-straight foot dorsal flexion, neck flexion, jugular compression, and direct palpation of the popliteal nerve or sciatic notch is characteristic of radiculopathy. A source of radicular pain not found in this description is that caused by spinal stenosis. Spinal stenosis usually lacks positive nerve stretch signs but has the characteristic history of neurogenic claudication (i.e., leg and calf pain produced by ambulation). Pain that does not go away immediately after stopping is made worse with spinal extension and is relieved by flexion. The pain progresses from proximal to distal.

The pain drawing is a major help in accomplishing the objectives of the physical examination. Each patient completes the pain drawing using a rating system, which distinguishes organic from psychologic pain fairly well. It also helps localize the symptoms for future reference with pain reproduction studies such as with discography and postoperative evaluations.

The initial history and physical evaluation determines the aggressiveness of the diagnostic and therapeutic regimen. The morbidity rating and the time the patient has had the problem are important parts of the history and physical examination that help determine the aggressiveness and invasiveness of the diagnostic plan. The leg pain versus back pain ratio is an important factor in determining which diagnostic tests are indicated. Leg pain leads to test for nerve function and obstructive pathology in EMG/NC, myelogram, contrast CT scan, and MRI. Back pain evaluation includes at times bone scan, MRI, and discograms. The clinical syndrome should be divided into predominantly mechanical pain, axial pain, and leg pain. An appropriate treatment program can begin, based on the initial evaluation.

Most athletic injuries to the lumbar spine fall under the category of mechanical, axial, back, or leg pain. Within this category a number of different syndromes exist.

1. *Annular tear of the intervertebral disc.* This is usually a loaded compressive rotatory injury to the lumbar spine producing severe, disabling back spasm and pain. The pain is usually worse in flexion with coughing, sneezing, straining, upright posture, sitting, and with any other situations that increase intradiscal pressure. There may be referred leg pain, low back pain with straight-leg raising, and anterior spinal tenderness. Annular tears can be produced with as little as 3° of high-torque rotation (15). Facet joint alignment that protects the disc from rotatory forces may lead to facet joint injuries as the annulus fails in rotation.
2. *Facet joint syndrome.* This more typically occurs in extension with rotation, reproduced with extension rotation during the examination. It may present with a pain on rising from flexion, with a lateral shift in the extension motion. There may be point tenderness in the paraspinous area over the facet joint and associated referred leg pain.
3. *Tears of the lumbodorsal fascia and muscle injuries and contusions.* These present with muscle spasm, stiffness, and many of the characteristics of facet joint syndrome in annular tears.
4. *Sacroiliac joint pain and pain in the posterior superior iliac spine.* The most common referred pain area for pain from the annulus in the intervertebral disc and the neuromotion segment of the spine is across the posterior surface of the ilium, which includes the posterior-superior iliac spine and sacroiliac (SI) joint. Sciatic pain can hurt in the sciatic joint area as well as the sciatic notch and buttocks. While injuries can occur to the sacroiliac joint, the vast majority of syndromes presenting with SI joint pain are thought to be the result of referred pain from a neuromotion segment in the spine.

The most important thing to be done with the physical examination of the athlete is to demonstrate what types of motions reproduce the patient's pain. Where exactly is the tenderness present. What deformity is present in the spine? If there is a lateral shift, in which direction? The chief advantage that physical therapists have in the treatment of the athlete with lumbar spine pain, is the hands-on approach directed specifically to motions and activities that produce and relieve the pain. Local modalities can be directed specifically to localized areas of inflammation and pain. Treatment of referred pain areas through localized treatment in the area of the referred pain plays a major role in the relief of symptoms and return to performance. Therefore, techniques of treatment of referred pain should be understood and used. This may include injections of local anesthetic, cortisone injections, transcutaneous nerve stimulator (TENS) units, ultrasound, and ice.

Another important diagnostic category in these patients is to identify areas of contracture and weakness on the physical examination. The physician and therapist can make the diagnosis by carefully examining the patient for areas of muscle atrophy and loss of range of motion. Sophisticated tests and dynamic EMG function analyses have identified localized areas of weakness in the shoulders of pitchers as well as in the abdominal musculature of baseball pitchers (16). There is a great deal of skill involved in being able to recognize these deficiencies during the physical examination and in designing a rehabilitation program to correct them.

Nonoperative Care

The nonoperative treatment plan begins with several basic rules:

1. Stop the inflammation.
2. Restore strength.
3. Restore flexibility.
4. Restore aerobic conditioning.
5. Return to full function.

Stopping the inflammation in an injured athlete of the spine often requires rest and immobilization. The authors try to limit the rest and immobilization to the minimum. Bed rest produces stiffness and weakness, which cause the pain to persist and are antithetical to the body functions necessary for athletic performance. Every day of rest and immobilization may produce weeks of rehabilitation before the athlete is able to return to performance. As in motion treatment of lower extremity injuries (i.e., fracture bracing and postoperative continuous motion machines), rapid rehabilitation of lumbar injuries in athletes requires effective means of mobilizing the patient. Bed rest longer than 3 to 5 days is not of any benefit in the natural history of the disease.

Rapid mobilization requires strong antiinflammatory medications, including epidural steroids, oral Medrol Dosepak, Indocin SR, other nonsteroidal antiinflammatories, and aspirin. Lots of ice; TENS unit; and mobilization with casts, corsets, and braces can also help. Corsets and braces are used for only limited periods of time, and strengthening techniques are used so that the braces can be removed as soon as possible. Braces in themselves can cause a significant amount of stiffness and weakness. Exact timetables are difficult, because the duration of immobilization should be based on the individual patient's history and physical examination. As a general rule, acute disc herniations are treated with 3 to 5 days of bed rest. Patients work with a physical therapist within 7 days. A corset is worn for no longer than 10 to 14 days. Patients may be given Indocin, occasionally Medrol, and less commonly, epidural injections. The therapist begins with the neutral position, isometric trunk-strengthening program and, depending on the response of the patient, evolves into resistive strengthening, motion, and aerobic conditioning as tolerated.

Part of the key to being able to initial early therapy is understanding, based on the physical examination, what makes the patient symptomatic. Nonoperative care should be the basis of any therapeutic approach to athletes with lumbar spine injuries. With the exception of cauda equina injuries, this should also be true in the athlete with neurologic deficit. The key to effective nonoperative care is to have a well-thought-out, balanced biomechanical approach. Common questions asked are whether to do extension exercises, flexion exercises, or twisting exercises; what type of aerobic exercising should be done; when weight lifting can begin; what role Nautilus beautification exercises have in rehabilitation of the athlete, and what the best type of nonoperative rehabilitation is for the individual athlete's sport.

Everyone is concerned about the risks of increasing or producing a neurologic deficit through nonoperative care. So often, nonoperative care in the face of a neurologic deficit consists of no care. Bed rest is the usual initial stage of treatment for the athlete with a lumbar spine injury and neurologic deficit. It is felt that bed rest best protects the patient from increasing injury to the spine and thus increasing the neurologic deficit. Unfortunately, bed rest also produces profound weakness and loss of biomechanical function, and it actually increases the risk of injury as a result of weakness and stiffness. If the purpose of bed rest is to decrease inflammation, the logical substitute would be aggressive antiinflammatory medication. If the objective of bed rest is to prevent motion, braces and casts can be substituted. If the objective of bed rest is to prevent abnormal motion that could injure the spine, it is with the understanding that certain mechanical functions must take place. Patients get on and off of bed pans; they get up to go to the bathroom. They roll over in bed. They cough, sneeze, and eventually have to walk. It seems logical that if it were possible to design an exercise system that would prevent abnormal motion while restoring strength and flexibility in a biomechanically sound fashion, then the spine would be protected from the abnormal motion that produces injury, and healing would be potentially enhanced. This enhancement takes place through normal biomechanical motion in the injured part by increasing strength and flexibility in the adjacent portions of the body that can absorb the stress potentially directed to the injured part and by preventing the atrophy, weakness, and stiffness caused by inactivity.

Lumbar spine injuries in athletes make up a category that often demands prevention of atrophy and stiffness, and restoration to maximum function as early as possible. It follows that if this restoration can be achieved in athletes, it can function just as effectively in steelworkers, secretaries, weekend athletes, and homemakers. The key to the program obviously lies in safety and effectiveness. If you could summarize an overall basis to the preferred rehabilitation program, it would lie in the concept of neutral position isometric strengthening for the spine. This program is derived from work by Saal, White, and others, including Randolph, Robinson, Brewster, and others at the Kerlan Jobe Orthopedic Clinic.

Trunk Stretching and Strengthening Program

The athlete should be given an exercise program that concentrates on trunk strength and trunk mobility, balance, coordination, and aerobic conditioning. A practical application of the use of trunk strengthening in back treatment, injury prevention, and improved performance is for athletes who must throw.

It certainly appears that the place to begin the rehabilitation program for an injured lumbar spine, with or without neurologic deficit, should be with neutral position isometric strengthening. The basis of the trunk stability program is to have the patient find a neutral, pain-free position, laying supine on the ground with the knees flexed and feet on the ground. This position is about as untraumatic as possible for beginning rehabilitation, and it also forms the basis of an important concept in not only athletic function but activities of daily living for everyone. Muscles are retrained to work to support the spine while the patient is using his or her arms and legs. It is not only theoretically ideal but practically possible. The athlete who learns to control muscles by tight, rigid contraction and to control the spine with the lumbodorsal fascia, gluteus maximus, oblique abdominals, and latissimus dorsi can protect the lumbar spine while improving athletic performance. The power and strength of any throwing athlete comes from the trunk. Lifting weight requires functioning of the lumbodorsal fascia.

Trunk strength also prevents back injuries and is an important treatment method for back pain. While treatment plans for symptomatic back pain patients may include similar exercises, each of the treatment plans should be designed to match the exam and the symptoms. Any trunk strengthening plan puts strain on the spine and can produce back pain as a result of overload. Therefore, such a plan should be conducted in a controlled, progressive manner.

The key to safe strengthening is the ability to maintain the spine in a safe, neutral position during the strengthening exercises. For upper body strengthening, the spine must be well-aligned in a chest-out–chin-tucked posture. Doing isometric trunk exercises and upper body exercises emphasizing this posture will strengthen the support for the cervical spine, strengthen the postural muscles necessary for maintaining proper body alignment, and prevent neck pain caused by athletic activity.

For the lower body, trunk control plays a vital role in the ability to rotate and transfer torque safely. Trunk strengthening exercises such as sit-ups and spine extensions produce strength. Flexibility produces a protective range of motion, but often the key is providing trunk strength and control at the proper moment during the athletic activity. For example, a baseball hitter goes from flexion through rotation to extension. If the hitter's trunk musculature does not maintain rigid control, despite the changes in the axis of alignment, he or she may lose power or get a back injury. Therefore, although the muscles may be strong, if they do not fire in sequence at the proper time, they will not protect the athlete from injury and certainly will not enhance performance. A key to producing a safe range of motion is to begin trunk control in the safe neutral position, establish muscle control in that position, and maintain it through the necessary range of motion to perform the athletic activity.

The authors begin identification of the neutral spine position with the dead-bug exercises (Fig. 50.1). Dead-bug exercises are done supine with the knees flexed and feet on the floor. With the assistance of the trainer or therapist, the athlete pushes the lumbar spine toward the mat until he or she exerts a moderate amount of force on the examiner's hand. This is not an exaggerated, back-flattening, extreme force, but a moderate amount of painless force on the examiner's hand. The athlete is then taught to maintain this same amount of force through abdominal contraction while doing the following:

1. Raising one foot.
2. Raising the other foot.
3. Raising one arm.
4. Raising the other arm.
5. Raising one leg.
6. Raising the other leg.
7. Flexing one leg and extending with the foot.
8. Flexing the other leg and extending with the foot.

These same exercises can be performed with weights on arms or legs.

The next stage for torque-transfer athletes is resistance to rotation; first supine; then sitting; then standing. The athlete maintains the neutral spine control position while resisting rotation of the upper body on the lower body. The player resists the rotational force exerted by the therapist or trainer.

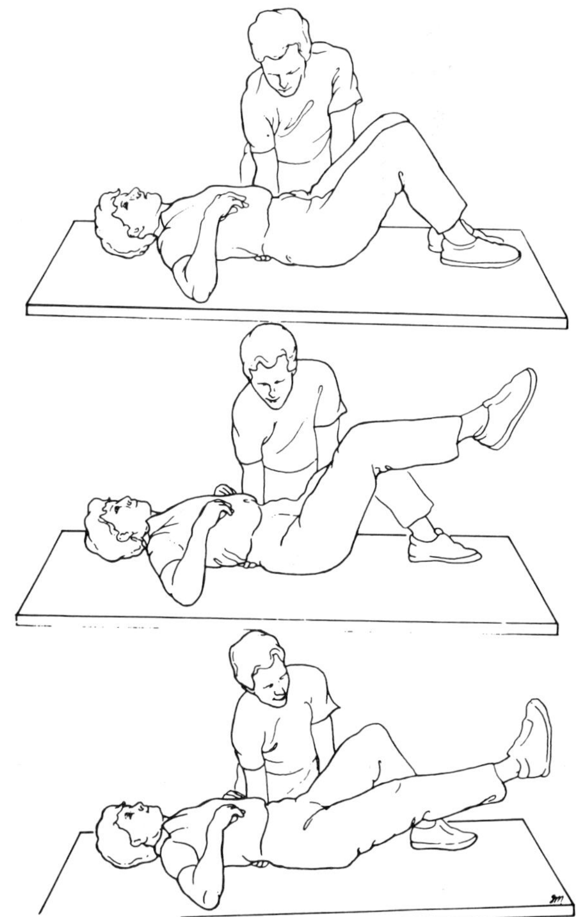

Figure 50.1. Identification of the neutral position begins with the dead-bug exercises.

In the next stage, the player maintains trunk control while actively rotating through a short range of motion against the trainer's resistance. This is done in numerous positions to teach trunk control, regardless of the position of the patient (Fig. 50.2).

Additional benefits can be gained through beach-ball exercises. A 4-foot-diameter base can be used to do partial sit-ups while the athlete maintains control of the ball and keeps the trunk in neutral position. Partial sit-ups and resistive sit-ups are done on the ball (Figs. 50.3 and 50.4).

Lower extremity, trunk, and upper extremity strengthening must be done with concentration on maintaining the controlled neutral trunk position. This control must be taught as a descrete activity and not as part of the athlete's sport. A routine is established for the player: think trunk control; neutral position; and tense contractions. Trunk control is incorporated into throwing or batting. This will ultimately produce a more efficient transfer of torque from the lower to the upper

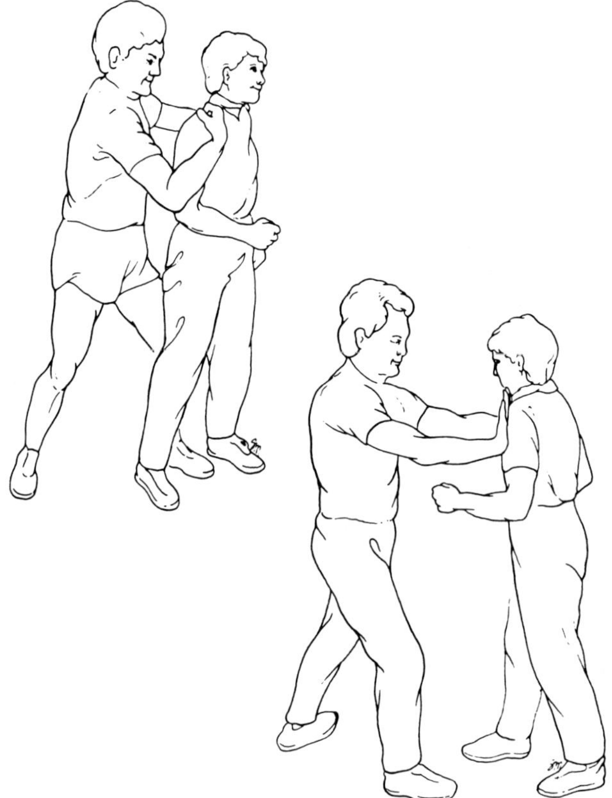

Figure 50.2. The athlete learns trunk control, regardless of his or her position.

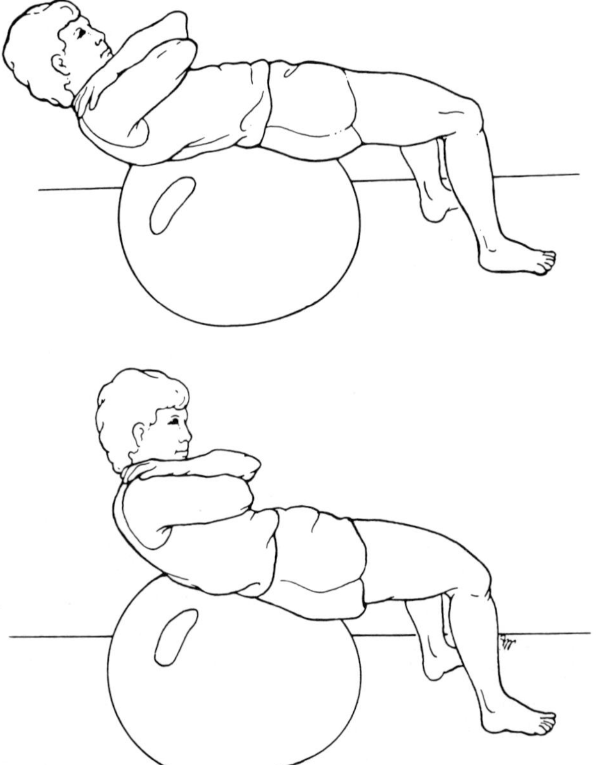

Figure 50.3. The athlete performs partial sit-ups on an exercise ball while maintaining control of the ball and keeping the trunk in the neutral position.

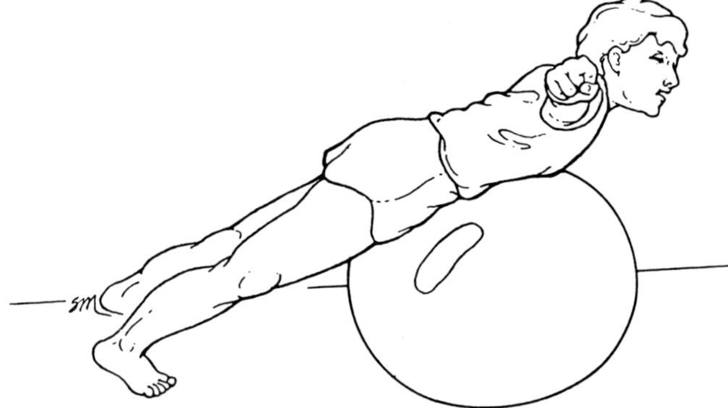

Figure 50.4. The athlete performs extension exercises on an exercise ball while maintaining control of the ball and keeping the trunk in the neutral position.

extremities, e.g., better bat control for a hitter and better endurance and ball control for a pitcher. An additional valuable benefit can be prevention of spine injuries and spinal pain caused by the athletic activity.

After establishing neutral position isometric control of the spine, extremity strengthening can begin. Probably the most important muscles needed to protect the spine itself is the quadriceps. The ability to return to work after a back injury has been directly related to quadriceps strength. Yet quadriceps strengthening should not be done in the standard, sitting, full-knee extension position in a patient with severe lower back pain. The quadriceps strengthening should be done without irritating the lumbar spine mechanical pain. Note that the ability to move a weight from 90° to 0° may not relate as specifically to lumbar spine function as quadriceps strength obtained through functional strengthening.

Functional strengthening is done initially by wall slides: sliding down the wall, holding the position for 10 sec, and moving back up at varying depths of slide. This is begun immediately postoperatively. Throwing a medicine ball in a flexed-knee position is another good exercise. Exercise machines such as a Versa Climber and stationary bicycle are used to strengthen quadriceps function while learning to maintain trunk control during sports-related activity. Gluteal strengthening and hip extensor strengthening are important, but must be done without inadvertently hyperextending the lumbar spine. Exercise bands that provide resistance to hip extension without a lot of spine extension are important as are other techniques that deemphasize spine motion while producing isometric extensor strength. The key to the use of Nautilus machines, which can be important in a safe, protected range of motion for extremity strengthening, is good isometric trunk control in a pain-free neutral position before exercise begins. If trunk control is established first, then a safe, protected range of motion can be performed while a good spinal position is maintained. Therefore, military presses and latissimus dorsi, arm, and leg strengthening with machines can be of benefit while protecting the spine. Spine strength testing machines have been shown to be helpful in predicting return to work. The ability to perform flexion extension exercises or resistance rotational exercises on a machine may not translate to functional spine activity during athletics. The authors have not recommended those machines for treatment of lumbar injuries.

Stretching exercises are an important part of any rehabilitation program. The more flexible the legs, arms, and upper body, the more likely there will be a proportional decrease of motion stress on the injured lumbar spine. If some muscle control is established first, through the strengthening program, then the spine can be held in a stable position while stretching of the extremities takes place. It is important to note that hamstring stretching too often is taken to the extent that abnormal lumbar spine motion is produced. Stretching the leg past the point of pelvic motion only strains the spine and does not increase hamstring looseness. Lumbar spine conditions are frequently irritated because of excessive lumbar motion during hamstring stretching. The spine should be neutralized and held in that neutral stable position when doing hamstring-stretching exercises. Lumbar spine motion is important also, but it is not part of the initial stage of the rehabilitation program. Lumbar spine motion is begun with good muscle control of the spine during the motion exercises. During the initial stage, the most common position is the cat/cow position, on all fours, in which muscle control can be easily maintained.

The stretch exercises are a critical component of the program. Stretching increases the functional range of motion of the trunk and legs. Increasing the functional range of motion decreases the likelihood of lumbar spine injury during the strengthening program and during play.

Most low back injuries occur when the player exceeds the strength of the spine and its range of motion. The stretching program provides a greater area of pain-free and injury-free function. For example, if an athlete who is stiff, having 10° of spine extension and 20° of spine rotation, suddenly reaches for a ball producing 25° of extension and 40° of rotation, he or she may injure the back by tearing the stiff tissue. If the mobility exercises produce a functional range of motion of 40° of extension and 50° of rotation, injury is less likely to occur. This is a protective range of motion.

The authors' chief findings from ball players with back pain are loss of spine extension, loss of rotation (usually more in one direction), poor mechanics in rotation, and weak abdominals. Once the back pain starts, the weakness and contractions increase. Note that the program outlined here is designed for performance enhancement and injury prevention, not the treatment of back pain.

Aerobic Conditioning

There are numerous methods available for aerobic conditioning. The authors often see athletes who prefer a specific technique such as running, but have developed pain and problems directly related to running.

Cross-training is critically important in getting over aerobic exercise-induced injury. The runner with an injured back not only must do the stretching and strengthening rehabilitation program but must learn cross-training for aerobic exercise. Water running, swimming, cycling, Nordic Trac, Versa Climber, and rowing machines can all produce the needed aerobic conditioning outside of the injurious sport. The benefit of a swimming or water running program (17) should be obvious. The total unweighting of the spine in water removes many of the compressive loads and allows good physical activity without the tremendous pounding and straining of running. The Nordic Trac builds tremendous conditioning with strong use of the arms and increasing cardiac output without the pounding of running. The Versa Climber and cycling have several things in common. First, the back can be positioned in a beneficial position for back protection while still getting good aerobic conditioning. Cycling is done slightly bent forward, which, of course, helps the stenotic spine. The Versa Climber is done erect, which removes as much nerve root tension as possible. Both have the same potential hazard in that the pelvis should not tilt laterally during exercise. For the Versa Climber, short steps should be taken to prevent a lot of pelvic tilting with the motion, and in cycling, the legs should not become fully extended, allowing the pelvis to tilt when reaching for the peddles. The athlete should keep the pelvis and spine in a firm, neutral position, using good isometric control during the aerobic conditioning. Running stairs or stair-walking machines produce good leg strength and good hip extensor strength. Rowing machines can injure the back, but if done property—with rigid muscle control of the spine, in a neutral pain-free position—they offer benefits to upper and lower extremity function, quadriceps strengthening, and aerobic conditioning without spine stress. The better aerobic condition the athlete is in, the less likely he or she will sustain injury, including lumbar spine injury. Therefore, aerobic conditioning is an important part of every spine rehabilitation program.

An effective nonoperative treatment program for lumbar spine injuries includes the following elements.

1. *Stop the inflammation.* Antiinflammatory medications are preferred, and Indocin SR is the standard medication. Patients should be advised of potential complications of any antiinflammatory medication. Medrol Dosepak may be used in increasing difficult clinical situations as can epidural cortisone injections.
2. *Restrict activity.* This may vary from 24 to 72 hr of bed rest to immediate immobilization in a lumbosacral corset and restriction of painful activities.
3. *Begin a spine stability rehabilitation program.* Rehabilitation should begin as soon as practically possible: in bed, in the hospital, at 24 hr, or at the first available outpatient appointment in physical therapy.

The following are answers to some of the questions asked earlier.

1. *Do you start flexion or extension exercises?* The answer is you start neither. You start neutral isometric control exercises.

2. *Do you do twisting exercises?* Twisting exercises can be the most injurious exercises in any rehabilitation program, yet torsional rotation is an important part of many sports. The answer lies in producing tight, rigid trunk control that holds the spine during rotational activities, with the motion occurring predominantly in shoulders, hips, and legs. The athletes should be able to produce a parallelism between the shoulders and pelvis during rotation, especially during the contact portion of the rotational sport. A twisting exercise that allows loss of muscle control of the spine during exercise can be injurious and may not be of benefit. Rotational strengthening can be important but must be started with close observation and control. People twist many times in an average day and twisting is a part of many sports. Having a pain-free rotational range of motion is important; therefore, proper, slow, active stretching in rotation is important. Part of the key is to not twist and to learn to rotate with the whole body.
3. *What type of aerobic conditioning should be done?* The type that holds the spine in its most advantageous position and best unweights the spine from injurious compressive loads. Cross-train and use a variety of aerobic conditioning techniques.
4. *When can someone lift weights?* An athlete can lift weights when he or she can do it safely, meaning with tight, rigid trunk control. Athletes can protect their spines while strengthening their extremities and can lift weights when they understand the role of balance, speed, and proper mechanical advantage in weight lifting. The key to functional weight lifting for the athlete is not to lift the weight at the greatest mechanical disadvantage, but to simulate the positioning used in the sport. Isometric trunk control and position protection first, then resistive weight lifting.
5. *What role do weight machine exercises have?* Weight machines can offer distinctly advantageous control situations for resistive weight lifting. All machines that strengthen the extremities require proper spine control first. The authors have not used trunk strengthening machines such as the flexion, extension, or rotation machines in patients with back problems. Questions still linger as to their benefit. The key probably lies in proper use of the equipment and combining the equipment with a functional isometric control-type system, such as the trunk stability rehabilitation program.
6. *What type of nonoperative rehabilitation is best for the individual athlete's sport?* It depends much on the sport and the demands of rotational activity, compressive load, and tensile extremes of range of motion.

Operative Care

The chief indications for surgery in the athlete are the indications for surgery in any patient. The basic principle as in dealing with any patient is still of major importance in the athlete:

1. Sufficient morbidity to warrent surgery.
2. Failure of conservative care.
3. An anatomic lesion that can be corrected with a safe, effective operation.
4. A proper, fully developed postoperative rehabilitation program.

It is not possible to place too much emphasis on a proper postoperative rehabilitation program. To fail to do postoperative spinal rehabilitation would be similar to a failure to do postoperative knee strengthening after reconstruction of the knee or a failure to do postoperative strengthening and range-of-motion exercises after surgery on a shoulder. The patient wants restoration of function. The surgeon should be able to guide the patient through restoration to function. The morbidity of the patient, the amount of pain and loss of function, and the occupation are the critical factors.

Spinal operations to enhance performance rather than relieve disabling pain are a part of managing the care of athletes, a part that requires a great deal of experience not only in spinal surgery but also in dealing with athletes.

There are numerous factors to consider. One must always keep in mind the full longevity of the patient. Young players can lay out a year after a significant spinal surgery and still return to play. Older players are less likely to return to play after a major spinal reconstructive operation.

What the player will be like after his or her career—the condition of the spine at that time—should be of major importance in decision making early on. A principal factor is calculating the risk if the operation is successful. In many sports, after, for example, a spinal fusion or major resection of a supporting structure in a decompression injury, the percentage chance of return may be no greater after the operation than without the operation.

Surgeons must carefully question their advice concerning surgery if they do not have a proper alternative to the surgery and good, effective nonoperative care. Frankly, if all one knows is the surgical technique and if one does not have a proper understanding of and delivery system for a nonoperative care program, then that person should not advise surgery for the athlete. An appropriate team approach among specialists in nonoperative care and specialists in operative care can be worked out so that the decision for surgery is well-founded, but the surgeon must understand and participate in that portion of the decision-making process, i.e., he or she must determine if the patient has had a sufficient nonoperative treatment plan.

The anatomic lesion is critically important. A simply extruded disc herniation, of course, can be amenable to a one-level microscopic lumbar discectomy, but an annular tear of the intervertebral disc with mild nerve root irritation will not be made better by a decompressive laminectomy and usually will be made worse, because of abnormal motion in the injured disc (segmental instability) with a nerve root scarred to the back of the annulus. In spondylolisthesis, the obvious solution may be, as it is in the majority of the patients facing surgery for spondylolisthesis, a spinal fusion. Some athletes can return to their sport after a successful spinal fusion and some may not be able to. Part of the danger is in curing the x-ray and not the patient. Another possibility is curing the patient with a successful operation and leaving the player without a job. As with everyone, an absolute indication for surgery and lumbar disc disease is progressive cauda equina syndrome or progressive neurologic deficit. Strong, relative indications are static and significant neurologic deficit, unrelenting night pain, and major loss of functional capability. Mild relative indications for surgery fall more under the category of performance enhancement and return to play. There will always be patients who could live the way they are but cannot perform the way they are. This is a relative indication for surgery, but it must be a frequent consideration in lumbar spine injuries in athletes.

Individual Sports

The lumbar spine is a highly vulnerable area for injury in a number of different sports. The incidence varies from 27% to 7% to 13% (4, 6, 18). Although the incidence is significant and the time lost may be significant, the most important problems lie in fear of spinal injuries and the necessity of a therapeutic plan. Lumbar pain is a big part of many sports, but an organized diagnostic and therapeutic plan can prevent permanent injury and allow full function and maximum performance.

Gymnastics

With reference to lumbar spine injuries, gymnastics is probably the most commonly mentioned sport. The motions and activities of gymnastics produce tremendous strains on the lumbar spine. The hyperlordotic position used with certain maneuvers (such as the back walkover) exerts tremendous forces on the posterior elements and requires a great deal of flexibility. The amount of lumbar flexion/extension used during flips and vaulting dismounts require a great deal of strength to support the spine during these extremes of flexibility. Female gymnasts have an incidence of spondylolysis of 11% (2). Spondylolysis is a fatigue fracture of the neural arch, and it is felt that the vigorous lumbar motion in hyperextension in gymnastics produces the fatigue fracture. It is also interesting to note that Jackson et al. (2) found spina bifida occulta in 9 of the 11 gymnasts with pars interarticularis defects. It is known that there is a hereditary predisposition to the stress fracture of the spondylolysis, and the findings of occult spina bifida may point out a weakness of the dorsal arch in certain of these gymnasts. But the nature of the sport itself plays a tremendous role in a much higher incidence of spondylolysis and a much higher incidence of back pain in general. Garrick and Requa (19) noted a high incidence of low back pain in female gymnasts and recommended the vigorous trunk strengthening exercises that are used today to prepare gymnasts properly for their sport.

Ballet

Many of the motions used in ballet are similar to those in gymnastics. The classic maneuver that produces back pain problems is the arabesque position. This position requires extension and rotation of the lumbar spine. Performing a proper arabesque maneuver is the key to preventing lumbar strain. Several points have been emphasized: keep the pelvis stable; keep the extension of the spine symetrical over all the levels of the spine; and obtain good extension through the hip joints (20).

Ballet involves the lifting of dancers, especially lifting in awkward positions. The outstretched hand produces tremendous level-arm stresses across the spine of the lifting partner. Off-balance bending and lifting is a hallmark of back problems in industrial workers, and yet ballet, while balanced, is designed often to produce some of the most difficult lifts. The male dancers follow the body weight of their female partners very closely. Spondylolysis and spondylolisthesis play critical roles in dancers and may often produce severe mechanical back dysfunction.

Water Sports

In addition to injuries to the wrist and cervical spine, a lumbar spine in diving is subjected to added strain caused by only rapid flexion/extension changes but the severe back arching after entering the water. While swimming and water exercises are a major part of any back rehabilitation program, certain kicks (such as the butterfly) produce a lot of vigorous flexion/extension of the lumbar spine, especially in young swimmers. The swimmer must have good abdominal tone and strength to protect the back during a vigorous kicking motion. Thoracic pain and round-back deformities in young female breaststrokers can be a problem because of the repeated round-shoulder-type stroke motion.

Pole Vaulting

Pole vaulting is another sport that involves a maximum flexion/extension and muscle contraction during performance. The range of motion of the lumbar spine has been documented with high-speed photography from 40° of extension to 130° of flexion in 0.65 sec. One can imagine the tremendous forces generated across the spine with these functional demands (21).

Weight Lifting

Of the sports that require strength, lifting, and high body weight, the most common is weight lifting. The incidence of low back pain and problems in weight lifters is estimated to be 40% (22). The tremendous forces exerted on the lumbar spine by lifting weights over the head produces extreme lever-arm effects and compressive injury to the spine. Weight lifting is begun with the spine in tight, rigid position of flexion, and the lifter lifts with the legs. Tremendous extension force is produced at the hips and knees, while the spine is kept in a rigidly stable position. Success in this portion of the lift requires the body to generate rigid immobilization of the spine in the power position of slight flexion. To do a forward bent motion with the spine out of this position can be quite dangerous, resulting in large shear forces across the spine. Lifting weights with the spine flexed at 90°, whether they be lighter arm weights or heavier weights across the upper back, generates tremendous lever-arm effect forces. The weight times the distance back to the spine results in shear forces across the lumbar spine, especially if the weight is to be moved from this position. One cannot imagine the muscles that must be strengthened in this dangerous and mechanically disadvantagous position. A dangerous time for weight lifters is the shift from spinal flexion to extension that occurs with lifting the weight over the head as in the clean-and-jerk maneuver or the "snatch." The transition from flexion to extension must be done with rigid, tight muscle control. Inexperienced lifters, especially, will have no muscle control as the spine shifts from flexion to extension. A trained lifter controls that shift with rigid muscle control of the lumbodorsal fascia. The position of holding the weight over the head invariably draws increased lumbar lordosis. These tremendous extension forces of the lumbar spine naturally lead to the possibility of spondylolysis and spondylolisthesis. The incidence of spondylolysis in weight lifters has been estimated at 30%, and the incidence of spondylolisthesis at 37% (23). Many newer training techniques in weight lifting emphasize the role of general body conditioning, flexibility, aerobic conditioning, speed, and cross-training in addition to the ability to lift weight.

Football

Football players lift weights. It is part of the sport. The upper body forces and leg strength necessary to play football for most of the athletes involved in the sport require tremendous strength. Some football players, of course, rely on great agility and jumping ability, throwing ability, and eye-hand coordination, but strength is the backbone of football. Every year, every professional team needs heavier, stronger athletes. The offensive line players, in particular, go through a period of mechanical back pain as training camp begins. It is difficult to prepare an athlete in the off-season for the tremendous, rapid back extension against weight necessary for blocking in the offensive line. Extension jamming of the spine produces facet joint pain, spondylolysis, and spondylolisthesis. It is similar to the weight-lifting position of the weight held over the head, except it must be generated with forward leg motion and off-balance resistance to the weight while trying to carry out specific maneuvers such as blocking a man in a specific directions. Lumbar spine problems in these athletes requires specific training in back strengthening exercises to prevent injury (24, 25).

Safety in weight lifting is an important part of football. To have a promising football player injured in the weight room is not an uncommon occurrence. It has been estimated that more injuries may actually occur in training rather than in competition (26). This can be avoided through proper weight-lifting techniques. In addition to these extension lifting forces, football involves sudden off-balance rotation. This rotation may produce transverse process fractures, torsional disc injuries, and tears in the lumbodorsal fascia. Sudden off-balance twisting is part of the game and may be caused by tremendous loads or in a loose, unloaded position. Football has the added dimension of receiving unexpected, severe blows to the lumbar spine that may produce contusion or fracture. A helmet in the ribs produces rib fractures, and a helmet in the flank can produce renal contusion, retroperitoneal hemorrhage, and transverse process and spinous process fractures. Many aerobatic receivers and runners suffer spondolytic defects for the same reasons as gymnasts and ballet dancers, but the most common incidence of problems is in weight lifting. The role of the strength coach in teaching proper weight-lifting techniques and designing training schedules that prepare the lumbar spine for what is expected with football is important to prevent lumbar spine injuries in football players.

Running

In addition to weight lifting, another sport that produces stiffness is running. Distance runners must cross-train with flexibility to prevent injury. Running involves maintenance of a specific posture with tremendous muscle exertion over a long period of time. Low back pain as well as interscapular and shoulder and neck pain are commonly reported in runners. The vast majority of runners who have mechanical low back pain can be cured with stretching exercises. There also is the natural tendency in runners to develop isolated abdominal weakness. Running does not naturally involve constriction of abdominal and spine-stabilizing musculature. Frequently, there is a significant inbalance between flexors and extensors, not only in the legs but also in the trunk. Intrascapular and back pain results from abnormal posture during running. The key to posture in runners, as in all patients, is good isometric trunk strength that holds the body in an upright-chest-out position. Runners with low back pain should be treated with the following:

1. A vigorous stretching program that stretches the trunk as well as lower extremities. The basis of back pain in runners is stretching exercises.
2. Cross-training and muscle strengthing techniques that strengthen the antagonist muscle such as hip extensors and knee extensors.
3. Abdominal strengthening and isometric trunk stability exercises to enhance abdominal control.
4. Chest-out strengthening exercises, beginning with abdominal strengthening and adding upper body exercises to emphasize the chest-out posture and tight abdominal control.
5. Proper footwear for cushioning and enhancement of foot function.

Rotational and Torsional Sports

Rotational and torsional sports have certain characteristics in common. Baseball, golf, and the javelin all require rotation but have distinctly different demands on the spine. The javelin requires a tremendous amount of force to be generated in going from a hyperextended to a full flexion forward-through position. A javelin is not thrown 200 feet with only the arm. While shoulder and arm injuries are common in javelin throwers, the key is rigid abdominal strength that produces the torque necessary to throw the javelin. Throwing with only the arm will produce injury and in no way will generate any type of distance. Every arm injury in a javelin thrower has to be treated with trunk exercises and trunk strengthening. A rotatory lumbar spine injury in a javelin thrower is a completely debilitating injury that requires tremendous care and correction before returning to the sport.

Golfers notoriously have the highest incidence of back injury of any professional athlete. Callaway and Jobe reviewed injuries of 300 golfers on the 1985–1986 PGA tour. A total of 230 of the golfers experienced an injury, making the incidence 77%. Approximately 44% of all injuries were spine related, and about 42% were lumbosacral (5, 6). Lumbar spine pain in golfers result in torsional stress on the lumbar spine. The key to prevention of lumbar spine pain in golfers is to minimize the torsion stress by absorbing the rotation in the hips, knees, and shoulders and by spreading the rotational stresses on the spine out over the entire spine. Maintaining rigid, tight control through the power portion of the swing is critical. Proper technique in golf begins when addressing the ball. The knee flexion of the address position tenses the abdominal musculature. This abdominal tension is initiation of the trunk control necessary for a properly placed swing. The majority of the emphasis is on maintenance of parallel shoulders and pelvis through most of the swing. This requires rigid abdominal control and rotation between shoulders and hips, and loss of this rigid parallelization of the shoulders and pelvis can generate rotational strain on the lumbar spine. Rotation occurs between the hips and shoulders in the backswing, and the amount of backswing is not as important to the power of the swing as the ability of the golfer to regain tight muscle control as he or she proceeds from maximum backswing down through the power portion of the swing. It is the ability to obtain tight control and parallelism, and to maintain them, that produces the power of the swing and protection for the lumbar spine. The first advice for any recreational golfer with back pain is to cut down the backswing and the follow-through and to concentrate on the power portion of the swing. The golfer should concentrate on tight abdominal control during the power portion and minimize the excesses of rotation with backswing and follow-through. It is important also that the golf swing be symmetrical. The same amount of extension on the backswing as in the follow-through is important. Lateral bending should be avoided, especially in the follow-through. There is a tendency to bend to the left side, an off-balance lateral bending position, thus loading the spine asymmetrically and producing injury. Golf is usually restricted according to the patient's symptoms.

There is no condition of the lumbar spine for which the authors specifically restrict golf. Many people with spondylolisthesis, through superb conditioning and care, can play relatively pain free. Premature, symptomatic degenerative disc disease is common among golfers who play a great deal, especially among professionals who not only play but practice long hours. People can return to golf after decompressive lumbar surgery or spinal fusions. There are significant questions about the effect of a spinal fusion on an adult, professional golfer. The effect on adjacent segments and on overall spine function may not allow any better function. Under these circumstances, a fusion should be a last resort.

Baseball

Torsional problems develop in both baseball pitchers and baseball hitters (7, 8). Hitters are required to initiate a violent lumbar rotation based on instantaneous ocular information, and the role of the lumbar spine in a baseball hitter begins with visualization of the ball. If a hitter is not seeing the ball properly, the mechanics of the swing will be disturbed; the most common is delayed recognition of the ball, producing a rotation with the hips in front of the shoulders, a loss of parallelism of shoulders and hips, and increased torsional strain of the lumbar spine. As step one, the player must see the ball properly and initiate a symmetrical swing. The trunk should move quickly, as a solid unit, through the baseball swing.

Throwers require a rigid cylinder of strength to transfer torque from the legs to the throwing arm (9). Trunk and leg strength generate the velocity of the throw, and the arm provides the fine control strength. Fatigue reduces the control of the pitching motion and ball location. A major factor in ball control is a loss of tone and strength in the trunk caused by trunk muscle fatigue. There is a loss of the rigid trunk cylinder that produces a loss of synchrony between the legs and arms. This causes a change in the pitching motion. As the trunk flexors and abdominal musculature weaken because of fatigue, lumbar lordosis increases and the back arches. The subtle change of a few degrees puts the arm behind in the pitching motion, promoting earlier ball release, and the pitch comes up. Arm strain increases as the trunk musculature fatigues. Attempts to compensate for loss of trunk strength and a slow arm increase the use of the arm musculature and predisposes the shoulder to injury. Developing power in torsion depends on trunk strength, i.e., strengthening abdominal, back, buttock, and thigh muscles. Trunk strengthening exercises are designed not only to enhance performance but also to prevent arm injury. Trunk strength is superseded only by balance and coordination. The firing sequence of trunk muscles in a professional baseball player follows a consistent median pattern. Alteration in that pattern produces an inconsistent,

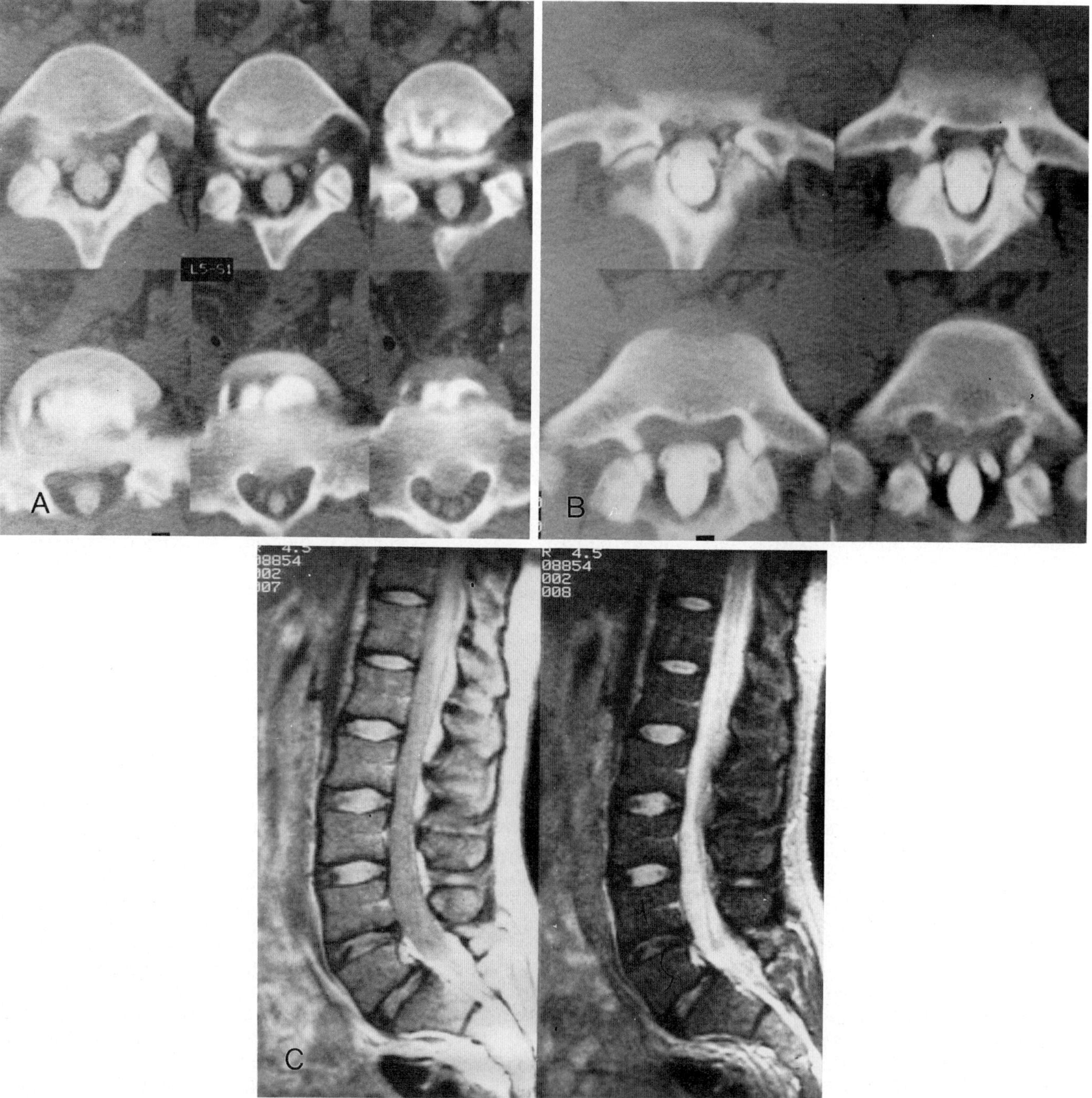

Figure 50.5. A 34-year-old professional golfer with L5–S1 spondylolisthesis and L4–L5 and L5–S1 disc degeneration. Discography reproduced the patient's L5 radiculopathy from the L5–S1 disc. The contrast CT scan demonstrates the close proximity of the bone spur and the caudal facet of the pseudarthrosis, which is in close proximity to the L5 nerve root. A two-level fusion would be the most definitive solution to the problem. A limited decompression may play a role in relief of the radicular symptoms, and a postoperative rehabilitation program may produce sufficient stability to avoid the fusion.

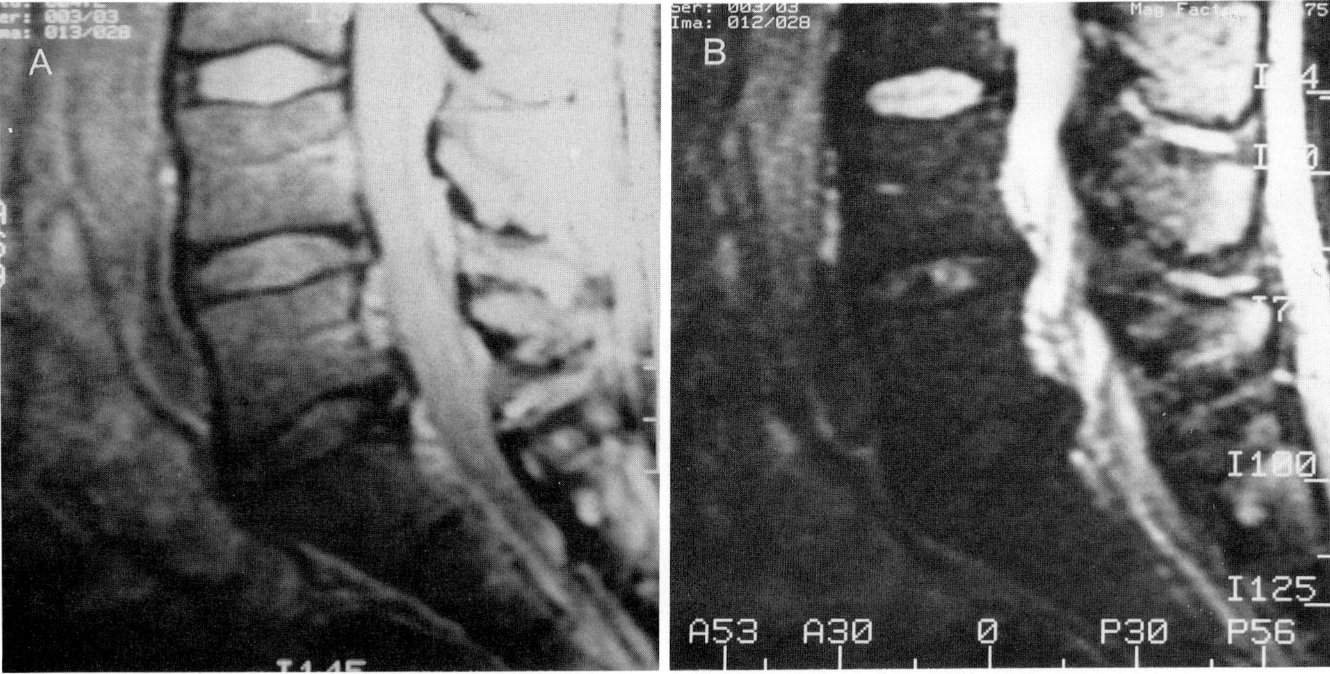

Figure 50.6. This 30-year-old professional golfer has a L5–S1 spondylolisthesis and severe two-level degenerative disc disease with a large pseudodisc at L5–S1. He responded to a trunk stability rehabilitation program. Because he did his exercises, he has been able to perform effectively and remain relatively asymptomatic.

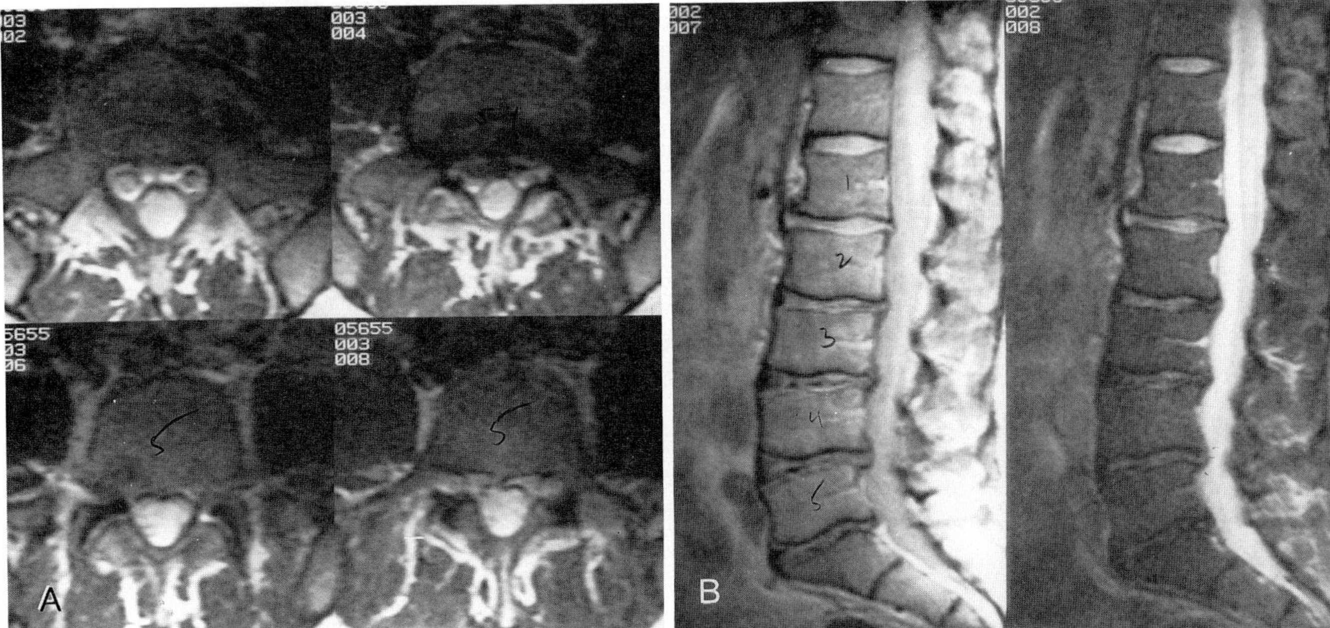

Figure 50.7. The MRI of a 34-year-old starting American League third baseman. This patient suffered multiple episodes of mechanical back dysfunction without significant radicular symptoms.

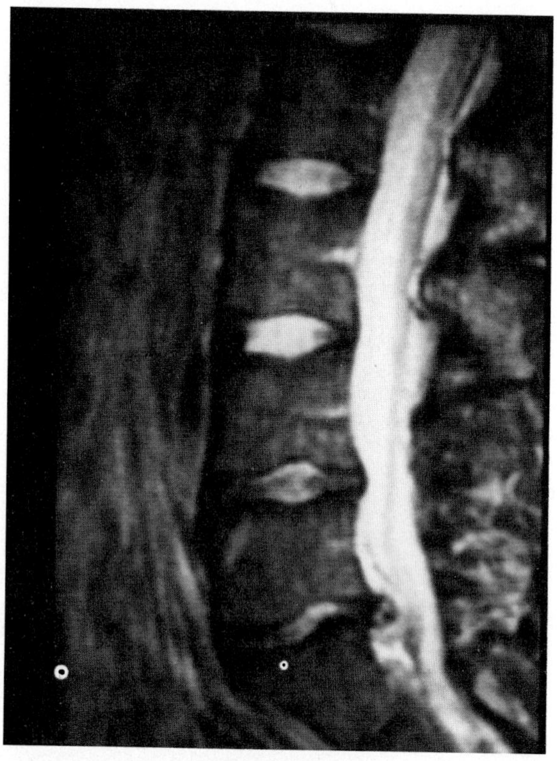

Figure 50.8. This 21-year-old infielder had an L5–S1 radiculopathy. Recommended treatment was a one-level microscopic lumbar discectomy and postoperative rehabilitation. It can be seen that the patient suffers from two-level degenerative disc disease and has significant degenerative changes in the L5–S1 disc space. It is predicted that the patient will need significant postoperative rehabilitation to return effectively to his sport.

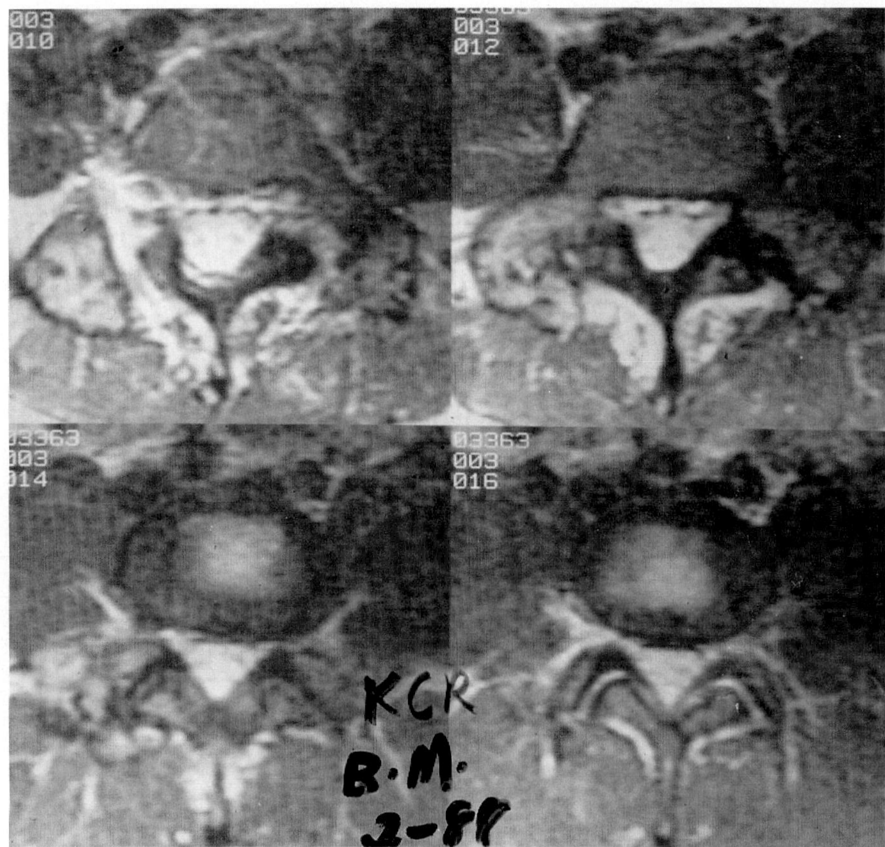

Figure 50.9. This 22-year-old American League baseball pitcher had bilateral spondolytic defects. T2-weighted MRI revealed normal water content. The patient reproduced his pain, and it was blocked by injection of the spondolytic defects. He failed to respond over 1 year of nonoperative rehabilitation and underwent a posterolateral fusion and returned to pitch with minimal lumbar spine symptomatology.

uncoordinated pattern leading to arm strain and back injury (16).

Tennis

Chard and Lachmann (27) examined racquet sport injuries and reported the incidence of injury as follows: squash 59%, tennis 21%; and badminton 20%. A total of 38% of professional tennis players have missed tournaments because of back pain. Trunk strengthening should be a principal part of the tennis player's regimen (28).

Tennis as a sport involves speed, rotation, extremes of flexion, lateral bending, and extension. It involves the power aspects of the overhead serve, the effect of trunk strength on shoulder function, and many of the other aspects mentioned for other sports. The one most important factors in protecting the spine in tennis is to bend the knees. Leg strength, quadracep strength, and the ability to play in a bent-knee–hip-flexed positioned while protecting the back are the keys to prevention of back pain. Proceeding from the back-extended position to the follow-through position in the serve requires strong abdominal control. The strength of the gluteal latissimus dorsi, abdominal obliques, and rectus abdominus controls the lumbodorsal fascia and delivers the power necessary through the legs up into the arm.

Conclusions

In summary, the keys to proper management of lumbar spine problems is athletes include the following.

1. Comprehensive diagnosis
2. Aggressive, effective nonoperative care.
3. Pinpoint operations that do as little damage as possible to normal tissue but correct the pathologic lesion.

REFERENCES

1. Fairbank JC, Pynsent PB, Van Poortvliet JA, et al. Influence of anthropometric factors and joint laxity in the incidence of adolescent back pain. Spine 1984;9:461–464.
2. Jackson DW. Low back pain in young athletes: evaluation of stress reaction and discogenic problems. Am J Sports Med 1979;7:364–366.
3. Fisk JW, Baigent ML, Hill PD. Scheuermann's disease: clinical and radiological survey of 17 and 18 year olds. Am J Sports Med 1984;63:18–30.
4. Keene JS, Albert MJ, Springer SL, et al. Back injuries in college athletes. J Spinal Dis 1986;2:190–195.
5. Keene JS. Low back pain in the athlete from spondylogenic injury during recreation or competition. Postgrad Med 1983;74:209–217.
6. Spencer CW, Jackson DW. Back injuries in the athlete. Clin Sports Med 1983;2:191–215.
7. Micheli LJ. Back injuries gymnastics. Clin Sports Med 1985;4:85–93.
8. Cacayorin ED, Hochhauser L, Petro GR. Lumbar thoracic spine pain in the athlete: radiographic evaluation. Clin Sports Med 1987;6:767–783.
9. Papanicolaou N, Wilkinson RH, Emans JB, et al. Bone scintigraphy and radiography in young athletes with low back pain. AJR Am J Roentgenol 1985;145:1039–1044.
10. Light HG. Hernia of the inferior lumbar space. A cause of back pain. Arch Surg 1983;118:1077–1080.
11. Schnebel BE, Simmons JW, Chowning J, et al. A digitizing technique for the study of movement of intradiscal dye in response to flexion and extension of the lumbar spine. Spine 1988;12:309–312.
12. Schnebel BE, Watkins RG, Willin WH. The role of spinal flexion and extension in changing nerve root compression in disc herniations. Spine 1989;14:835–837.
13. White AA, Panjabi MM. Clinical biomechanics of the spine. Philadelphia: Lippincott, 1978.
14. Farfan HF. Mechanical disorders of the low back. Philadelphia: Lea & Febiger, 1973.
15. Farfan HF. Muscular mechanism of the lumbar spine and the position of power and efficiency. Orthop Clin North Am 1975;6:135–144.
16. Watkins RG, Dennis S, Dillin WH, et al. Dynamic EMG analysis of torque transfer in professional baseball pitchers. Spine 1989;14:404–408.
17. Watkins RG, Buhler B, Loverock P. The water workout recovery program. Chicago: Contemporary, 1988.
18. Sieman RL, Spangler D. The significance of lumbar spondylolysis in college football players. Spine 1981;6:174–179.
19. Garrick JG, Requa RK. Epidemiology of women's gymnastics injuries. Am J Sports Med 1980;8:261–264.
20. Howse AJG. Orthopedist's aid ballet. Clin Orthop Relat Res 1972;89:52–63.
21. Gainor BJ, Hagen RJ, Allen WC. Biomechanics of the spine in the polevaulter as related to spondylolisthesis. Am J Sports Med 1983;11:53–57.
22. Aggrawal ND, Kaur R, Kumar S, et al. A study of changes in weight lifters and other athletes. Br J Sports Med 1979;13:58–61.
23. Kotani PT, Ichikawa MD, Wakabayashi MD, et al. Studies of spondylolisthesis found among weight lifters. Br J Sports Med 1981;9:4–8.
24. Cantu RC. Lumbar spine injuries. In: Cantu RC, ed. The exercising adult. Lexington, MA: Collamore, 1980.
25. Ferguson RJ, McMaster JH, Staniski CL. Low back pain in college football linemen. J Sports Med 1974;2:63–69.
26. Davies JE. The spine in sports injuries, prevention and treatment. Br J Sports Med 1980;14:18–20.
27. Chard MD, Lachman SM. Racquet sports—patterns of injury presenting to a sports injury clinic. Br J Sports Med 1987;21:150–153.
28. Marks MR, Haas SS, Weisel SW. Low back pain in the competitive tennis player. Clin Sports Med 1988;7:277–287.

51 / SHOULDER INJURIES

Michael G. Maday, Christopher D. Harner, and Jon J. P. Warner

Introduction

The shoulder is a frequent site of injury in competitive athletes. Shoulder injuries comprise between 8% and 13% of all athletic injuries (1). These injuries may result from repetitive overhead activities (in swimmers, baseball pitchers, tennis players, and javelin throwers) and direct or indirect trauma (in football and rugby players). Certain shoulder injuries are more specific or typical of certain sports. Table 51.1 lists examples of the incidence of typical injuries seen in specific sports. Furthermore, within a given sport, shoulder injuries become more prevalent among certain participants. For example, in baseball, shoulder injuries are more common among pitchers, and in swimming, shoulder injuries are most common in swimmers who compete in butterfly, freestyle, and backstroke events. In addition to the nature of the sport, shoulder injuries in the athlete depend on the level of overhead activity, level and length of participation, the techniques used, age and conditioning of the athlete, and anatomic considerations specific to the athlete.

An increased understanding of shoulder abnormalities and the existence of newer diagnostic modalities such as magnetic resonance imaging (MRI), shoulder arthroscopy, and ultrasound have led to an increased awareness of problems specific to the shoulder in athletes and to more successful treatments. In this chapter, the more common shoulder problems seen in athletes will be discussed. The emphasis will be on the relevant biomechanics and pathophysiology, and special attention will be given to diagnosis and treatment. The discussion will begin with a section on functional shoulder anatomy and biomechanics. Then physical examination, diagnostic imaging of the shoulder, and specific shoulder injuries and problems will be discussed.

Functional Anatomy and Biomechanics of the Shoulder

Functional Anatomy

An understanding of normal shoulder anatomy is essential to diagnosing and treating shoulder injuries. Normal shoulder motion is actually a combination of motions of four joints: *(a)* the glenohumeral joint; *(b)* the scapulothoracic joint; *(c)* the sternoclavicular joint; and *(d)* the acromioclavicular joint. The glenohumeral joint contributes approximately 120° of the 180° of upward motion of the arm. The remaining 60° is the result of scapulothoracic motion. Virtually all rotation of the upper arm occurs at the glenohumeral joint. The glenohumeral joint is encased by a capsule that, to accommodate a large range of motion of the shoulder, is of necessity loose and redundant. The joint capsule is reinforced by thickenings that form three ligaments: the superior, middle, and inferior glenohumeral ligaments (Fig. 51.1). The superior glenohumeral ligament arises from the glenoid labrum anterior to the biceps tendon and inserts into the humeral neck in the region of the bicipital groove of the lesser tuberosity. The glenoid labrum is a fibrocartilage structure that rings the glenoid cavity and acts as an attachment for the inferior glenohumeral ligament and serves to "deepen" the socket and contain the humeral head as the shoulder moves through a range of motion (12, 13). The superior glenohumeral ligament helps to control inferior translation when the shoulder is adducted and posterior translocation when the shoulder is adducted, flexed, and internally rotated (14). The middle glenohumeral ligament acts as a secondary restraint to inferior translation when the shoulder is in the position of adduction and external rotation (14). The inferior glenohumeral complex is a hammock-like support for the glenohumeral

Table 51.1.
Incidence of Sport-Specific Shoulder Injuries

Sport	Percent Injury	Typical Injuries Seen Involving the Shoulder	References
Baseball	11–57	Acromioclavicular joint injuries, impingement syndrome, rotator cuff tendinitis	2, 3
Wrestling	17	Glenohumeral subluxation, acromioclavicular joint injuries, glenohumeral dislocation	1
Tennis	56	Rotator cuff tendinitis, impingement syndrome	1
Football	8–14	Acromioclavicular joint injuries, glenohumeral dislocations	4
Gymnastics	1–18	Impingement syndrome, biceps tendinitis, glenohumeral instability	5
Swimming	3–50	Impingement syndrome, glenohumeral instability	6, 7
Golf	3–13	Impingement syndrome	8
Basketball	3	Glenohumeral subluxation	9
Skiing	6–9	Glenohumeral dislocation, glenohumeral subluxation, acromioclavicular joint injuries	10
Volleyball	44	Biceps tendinitis, impingement syndrome	11
Javelin throwers	29	Biceps tendinitis, impingement syndrome	11

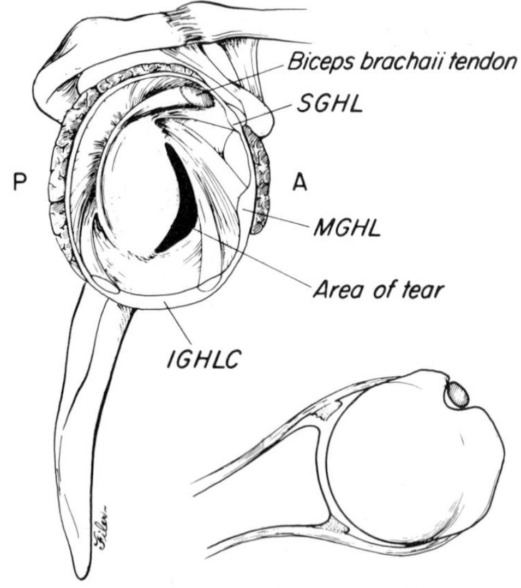

Figure 51.1. Diagram of the Bankart lesion. *SGHL*, superior glenohumeral ligament; *MGHL*, middle glenohumeral ligament; *IGHL*, inferior glenohumeral ligament; *A*, anterior; *P*, posterior.

joint and is a primary restraint to anterior-posterior and inferior translation in the abducted shoulder (15).

The scapula with its glenoid, acromion and coracoid processes rests on the chest wall and is suspended by the levator scapulae muscles, the trapezius, serratus anterior, and the coracoclavicular ligaments. Attached to the coracoid process are the coracoacromial ligaments, the coracoclavicular ligaments (the conoid and the trapezoid ligaments), the pectoralis minor muscle, and the conjoined tendon of the coracobrachialis and the biceps brachii muscle (Fig. 51.2). The coracobrachialis and biceps brachii share a common nerve supply—the musculocutaneous nerve. Although the sternoclavicular joint tilts approximately 40° in all directions, the acromioclavicular joint has limited motion of approximately 20° secondary to the attachments of the coracoclavicular ligaments. Because these four joints move both simultaneously and synchronously, an abnormality in any of these four will have a direct effect on the others.

The primary muscles around the shoulder consist of two layers. The outer layer, the deltoid muscle, and the inner layer consisting of the rotator cuff muscles: the supraspinatus; the infraspinatus; the teres minor; and the subscapularis. The deltoid muscle (axillary nerve) along with the pectoralis major (medial and lateral pectoral nerves) and the latissimus dorsi (thoracodorsal nerve) supply most of the power for shoulder motion. The rotator cuff muscles act primarily to control the humeral head within the glenohumeral cavity. The supraspinatus (suprascapular nerve) originates on the medial three-quarters of the supraspinatus fossa of the scapula and inserts into the greater tuberosity of the humerus. This muscle passes under the coracoacromial ligament and is primarily responsible for initiating shoulder abduction and containing the humeral head in the glenoid during abduction. The teres minor (axillary nerve) and infraspinatus (suprascapular nerve) act as external rotators of the humerus. The teres minor originates on the axillary border of the scapula, while the infraspinatus originates in the medial three-quarters of the scapula in the infraspinatus fossa. Both muscles insert on the greater tuberosity and are supplied by the suprascapular nerve. The subscapularis muscle originates on the medial four-fifths on the anterior surface of the scapula and inserts into the lesser tuberosity of the humerus. This muscle is innervated by the upper and lower subscapular nerves and acts as an internal rotator of the humerus. The long head of the biceps passes through the interval between the subscapularis and supraspinatus.

Biomechanics

Injuries to the shoulder are commonly seen in athletes who are throwers or swimmers. To understand the nature of these injuries, it is necessary to understand the biomechanics of shoulder motion during throwing and swimming. Forces on the shoulder gen-

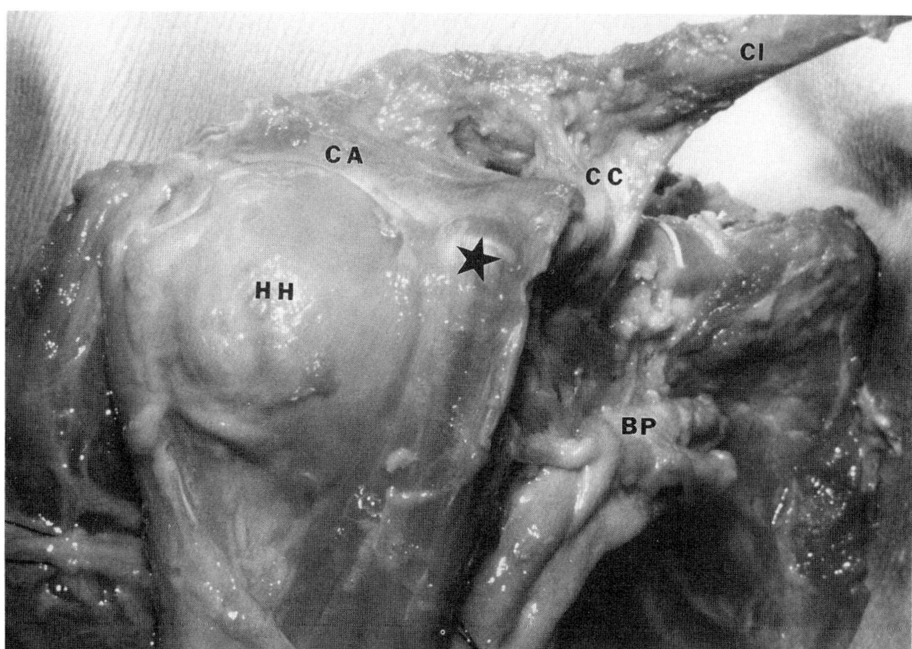

Figure 51.2. Shoulder specimen dissection to show attachments to coracoid process *(star)*. *CI*, clavicle; *HH*, humeral head; *CC*, coracoclavicular ligaments; *CA*, coracoacromial ligament; *BP*, brachial plexus. Pectoralis minor attachment has been removed.

erated during the acceleration and deceleration of throwing are explosive. Although each throwing sport has specific mechanistic patterns, there are similarities between the sports (16). Because of these mechanistic similarities in the patterns of throwing and because most of the current understanding of sport-specific biomechanics comes from examination of pitchers, the discussion of throwing biomechanics is based on the baseball pitch.

The baseball pitch involves five stages (17, 18) and is discussed in detail elsewhere in this book. Pitching involves a coordinated motion of the entire body to generate momentum for the throw. The muscles of the shoulder alone cannot generate the kinetic energy required to throw a baseball at high velocities nor can these muscles alone adequately dissipate the energy once the throw is completed. Injuries can, therefore, occur when the shoulder muscles generate or dissipate energies beyond their capabilities. Studies have shown that professional pitchers are able exclusively to use the subscapularis muscle while the remaining rotator cuff muscles remain silent during the acceleration phase of pitching. Amateur pitchers, on the other hand, tend to use all the rotator cuff muscles as well as the biceps muscle (19). Therefore, overuse injuries may occur often and earlier in those pitchers who use these rotator cuff muscles unnecessarily. Proper throwing mechanics are essential to the prevention of overuse injuries of the shoulder.

The swimming stroke basically consists of a pull-through and a recovery phase (20). During the recovery phase the supraspinatus, infraspinatus, and middle deltoid are primarily active. They function to rotate externally and abduct the arm in preparation for a new pull-through phase. The recovery phase is similar to the cocking phase seen in throwing. It is in this position that subacromial impingement may occur (21). The serratus anterior allows the acromion to rotate clear of the abducting humerus and provides a stable glenoid platform for rotation of the abn, thereby decreasing the risk for impingement or instability. The biceps, as in pitching, functions primarily at the elbow. The latissimus dorsi and pectoralis major are the major propulsive muscles during the swimming stroke, and their actions are similar to the acceleration phase seen in throwing. Therefore, baseball pitching and swimming can be thought of as highly complex, repetitive, coordinated efforts of the muscles about the shoulder. It can then be appreciated that any abnormality in biomechanics or technique will be greatly magnified as the result of the repetitive increased stress during swimming or pitching. These increased stresses can lead to shoulder injury.

Physical Examination of the Shoulder

History

A thorough examination of the athlete's shoulder involves a careful history, a generalized examination, and provocative testing as needed. The history should include present symptoms, a detailed discussion of the nature of the symptoms, and the response to medication and therapy. The history of the present symptoms should include a description of events surrounding the current complaint and a prior history of shoulder problems. The physician should establish whether or not trauma was involved, the mechanism of injury, length of symptoms, and specific symptomatic activities and arm positions. For example, swimmers may complain of shoulder pain only during one type of stroke or baseball pitchers may complain of pain only during a certain portion of their throwing motion. Symptoms may not involve only pain, but the athlete may complain of stiffness, weakness, catching, or a feeling that his or her shoulder is "giving-out." It is also important to inquire about associated neurovascular symptoms in the arm and pain in the neck. The physician should also establish whether or not the athlete has been treated with medication, pain modalities, or formal physical therapy and what response, if any, there has been to treatment. Finally, the physician should determine whether or not the patient has any previous diagnostic studies.

Physical Examination

Following a complete history, a careful physical examination should be performed. The cervical spine should be examined for range of motion and reproduction of symptoms. The arm should also be examined for neurologic or vascular pathology. The shoulder can be thought of as four separate joints: the sternoclavicular; the acromioclavicular; the glenohumeral; and the scapulothoracic joint. A careful examination includes each of these joints and proceeds by inspection, palpation, range of motion testing, strength testing, and provocative tests.

The physical examination begins with the patient seated, relaxed, and both shoulders exposed. Men should be undressed above the waist and women should wear halter tops or have the gown positioned above the breast with the straps tied in back. Both shoulders must be free for comparison. Inspection of the sternoclavicular joint involves looking for prominences, depressions or asymmetry. As will be discussed later, this joint can be involved in sprains, subluxations, dislocations, fractures, or degenerative arthritis. The sternoclavicular joint may be palpated while standing behind the patient. The physician should palpate the medial end of the clavicle and determine if gentle pressure over the articulation elicits pain. Pain without a palpable deformity is consistent with a sprain or arthritis, whereas a palpable deformity is consistent with a subluxation or dislocation. In an anterior subluxation or dislocation, the sternal end will be prominent and may be mobile in the superior-inferior direction. With a posterior dislocation, clavicular depression is palpable. Because a posterior dislocation can be associated with acute neurovascular compromise, the athlete's peripheral pulses and airway must be assessed. Adduction of the arm across the chest compresses the joint and may cause pain in cases of degenerative arthritis or trauma.

Following examination of the sternoclavicular joint, the acromioclavicular joint should be evaluated. The most common disorders of this joint are traumatic ligamentous injury and arthritis. The lateral aspect of the clavicle should be inspected bilaterally for prominence relative to the acromion. The clavicles should be palpated beginning medially and progressing laterally toward the acromioclavicular joint. Tenderness or deformity along the clavicle should be noted. Direct pressure over the acromioclavicular joint will elicit pain in the setting of an acute injury or arthritis.

The glenohumeral joint and its surrounding bony and soft tissue structures allows for a complex balance of mobility and stability. Examination of the glenohumeral joint begins with careful observation. The physician should observe the shoulders from the front and back and look for any asymmetry. This asymmetry may take the form of muscle atrophy or abnormal prominences. The deltoid, infraspinatus, and supraspinatus should be examined for atrophy (Fig. 51.3). The biceps should be inspected for evidence of distal enlargement, which may be consistent with a rupture of the long head. An anterior prominence of the humeral head is suggestive of an anterior dislocation, whereas a posterior dislocation may present as a prominence of the coracoid process. Most important, the symptomatic side must be compared with the asymptomatic side for evidence of subtle atrophy or abnormal prominences.

Following inspection, the bony prominences surrounding the glenohumeral joint are palpated. With the physician standing behind the patient, the coracoid process, acromion, and greater tuberosity of the humerus can be palpated. Anterior and medial to the greater tuberosity lies the bicipital groove, which is bordered medially by the lesser tuberosity and laterally by the greater tuberosity. Inflammation of the biceps or its synovial lining may result in pain with palpation. Deep palpation of the biceps tendon in a normal shoulder can result in considerable discomfort. The spine of the scapula with the surrounding infraspinatus and su-

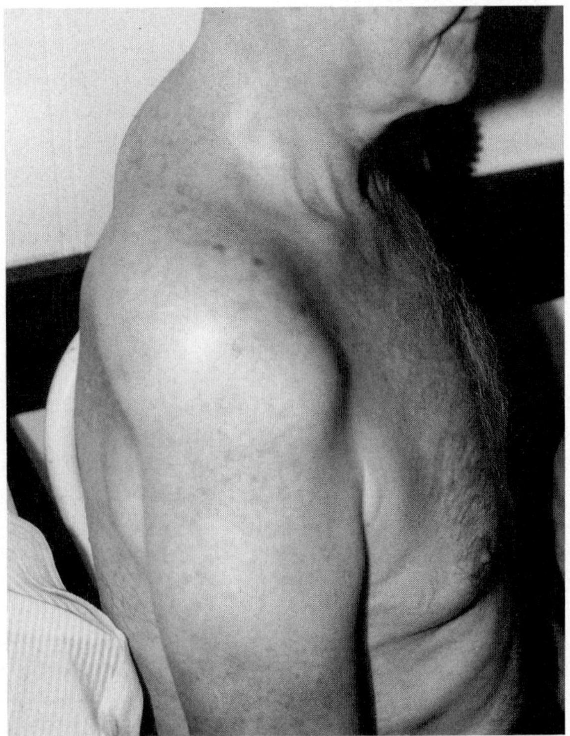

Figure 51.3. Example of infraspinatus wasting secondary to suprascapular nerve entrapment.

praspinatus muscles should also be palpated. A depression at the site of the supraspinatus or infraspinatus can be indicative of a muscle tear or suprascapular nerve injury. Following gentle palpation of the shoulder girdle, the glenohumeral joint should next be evaluated for passive and active motion.

The shoulder has motion in every plane, and to access initial function and to follow progress, both passive and active motion must be documented accurately. Passive and active motion should be measured and recorded separately because active motion can be altered by pain and may be a less accurate assessment of progress. Motion of the opposite shoulder should always be measured and recorded for comparison. The passive motion of forward elevation, internal rotation, external rotation, and rotation in abduction should be measured and recorded. Passive forward elevation is measured with the patient supine. Neer (22) advocates measuring elevation in the scapular plane because there is less tightening of the glenohumeral capsule and thus less restriction of motion than either in the coronal (abduction) or sagittal (flexion) planes. The total elevation is the combination of the scapular and glenohumeral motion (Fig. 51.4). Passive external rotation also is measured with the patient supine, which provides a reference point and eliminates trunk rotation and scapulothoracic contribution. Rotation is remeasured with the arm at the side and the elbow flexed at 90°. In this position, the capsule and glenohumeral ligaments are relaxed. Active internal rotation is measured with the patient sitting and the thumb is brought up the spine by the examiner. The highest level on the spine that the thumb reaches is recorded. It should be noted that this measurement also reflects shoulder extension and elbow flexion, and a stiff elbow will affect this measurement. Scapulothoracic motion and its contribution to total shoulder motion is best determined by viewing the patient from the back. Any asymmetries of motion should be noted and may be seen with such conditions as adhesive capsulitis and winging of the scapula. Internal and external rotation should also be measured and recorded with the arm in 90° of abduction. This position eliminates scapulothoracic motion and tests for pure glenohumeral motion.

Pain, instability, strength, motivation, and passive motion all affect active shoulder motion (22). Active and passive motion should be recorded separately. Total active elevation is measured and recorded by having the sitting patient raise his or her arm against gravity. Active internal and external rotation can also be tested with the patient seated. Any differences recorded between active and passive motion should be noted and investigated. A patient with a nerve injury or a rotator cuff tear, for example, may have full passive motion but lack some degree of active motion.

After passive and active motion of the glenohumeral joint have been evaluated, the shoulder muscle strengths should be measured. The muscles that should be tested include the deltoid, external rotators, internal rotators, supraspinatus, trapezius, biceps, triceps, and serratus anterior. The strengths are graded from 0 to 5. According to the American Shoulder and Elbow Surgeons' examination form (Table 51.2) the strength scale is as follows:

5. Normal—complete range of motion (ROM) against gravity with full resistance.
4. Good—complete ROM against gravity with some resistance.
3. Fair—complete ROM against gravity.

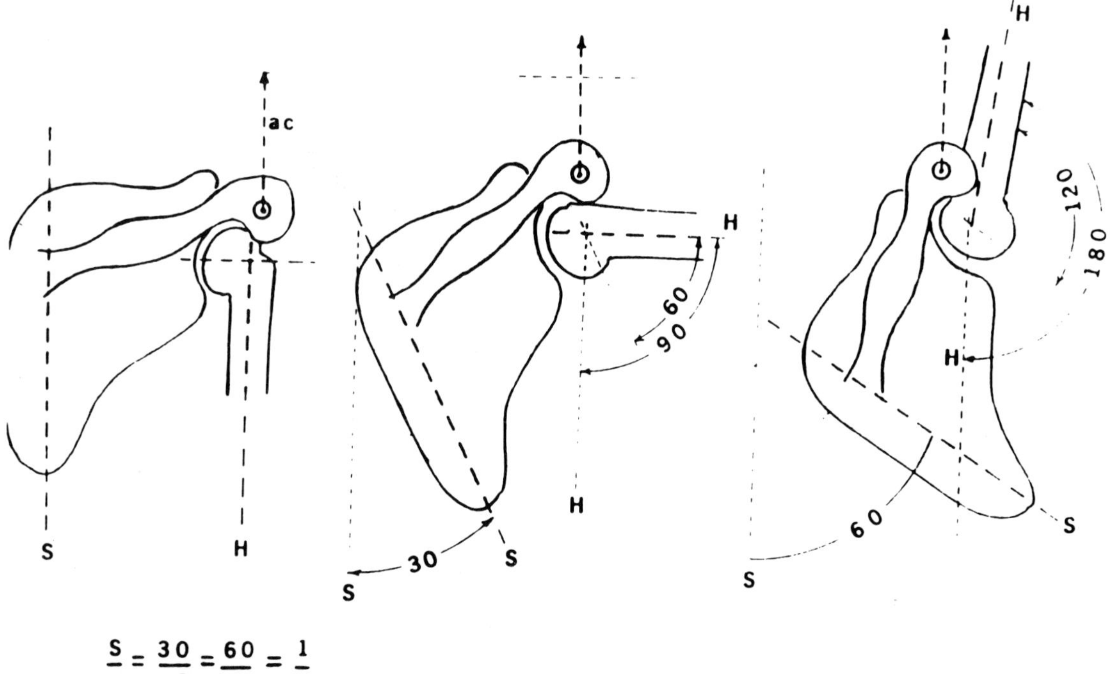

Figure 51.4. Total shoulder abduction is the result of combined glenohumeral-scapulothoracic motion in a ratio of about 2 to 1.

Table 51.2.
The Society of the American Shoulder and Elbow Surgeons Evaluation Form

I. Pain (circle one): (5 = none; 4 = slight; 3 = after unusual activity; 2 = moderate; 1 = marked; 0 = complete disability; and NA = not available)

II. Motion

A. Patient sitting (enter motion or NA if not measured):

1. Active total elevation of arm: ______ degrees
2. Passive internal rotation (circle segment of posterior anatomy reached by thumb; Enter NA if reach restricted by limited elbow flexion):

1 = Less than trochanter	8 = L2	15 = T7
2 = Trochanter	9 = L1	16 = T6
3 = Gluteal	10 = T12	17 = T5
4 = Sacrum	11 = T11	18 = T4
5 = L5	12 = T10	19 = T3
6 = L4	13 = T9	20 = T2
7 = L3	14 = T8	21 = T1

3. Active external rotation with arm at side: ____ degrees.
4. Passive external rotation at 90° abduction: ____ degrees. (Enter "NA" if cannot achieve 90° of abduction)

B. Patient supine:

1. Passive total elevation of arm: ____ degrees.[a]
2. Passive external rotation with arm at side: ____ degrees.

III. Strength (5 = normal; 4 = good; 3 = fair; 2 = poor; 1 = trace; 0 = paralysis, and NA = not available) (enter numbers below):

A. Anterior deltoid ____
B. Middle deltoid ____
C. External rotation ____
D. Internal rotation ____

IV. Stability (5 = normal; 4 = apprehension; 3 = rare subluxation; 2 = recurrent subluxation; 1 = recurrent dislocation; 0 = fixed dislocation; and NA = not available) (enter numbers below):

A. Anterior ____
B. Posterior ____
C. Inferior ____

V. Function (4 = normal; 3 = mild compromise; 2 = difficulty; 1 = with aid; 0 = unable, and NA = not available) (enter numbers below):

A. Use back pocket (if male); fasten bra (if female) ____
B. Perineal care ____
C. Wash apposite axilla ____
D. Eat with utensil ____
E. Comb hair ____
F. Use hand with arm at shoulder level ____
G. Carry 10 to 15 pounds with arm at side ____
H. Dress ____
I. Sleep on affecfed side ____
J. Pulling ____
K. Use hand overhead ____
L. Throwing ____
M. Lifting ____
N. Do usual work ____ (Specify type of work) ____________
O. Do usual sport ____ (Specify sport) ____________

VI. Patient response (circle choice):
(3 = much better; 2 = better; 1 = same; 0 = worse; and NA = not available/applicable)

[a]Total elevation of the arm is measured by viewing the patient from the side and using a goniometer to determine the angle between the arm and the thorax.

2. Poor—complete ROM with gravity eliminated.
1. Trace—Evidence of contractility.
0. Paralysis—no contractility.

The anterior, middle, and posterior divisions of the deltoid can be tested by resistive testing with the arm in slight flexion, abduction, and posterior extension, respectively. The examiner attempts to push the arm into the neutral position while the patient attempts to resist. Most tears or disruptions of the deltoid can be palpated during resisting testing.

The external rotators of the glenohumeral joint (infraspinatus and teres minor) are best tested with the arms at the side and the elbows flexed to 90° (Fig. 51.5*A*). The examiner stands behind or in front of the patient and attempts to push both hands together as the patient resists. Similarly, the internal rotators of the shoulder (subscapularis, pectoralis major, latissimus dorsi, and teres major) can be evaluated (Fig. 51.5*B*). With the arm at the patient's side and the elbow at 90°, the patient is asked to resist an external rotation force placed by the examiner. The pectoralis major and latissimus dorsi can be tested by placing the arm at 30° of abduction and asking the patient to adduct and internally to rotate the arm. The latissimus dorsi can be palpated to assess strength and integrity.

The trapezius is innervated by the spinal accessory nerve and is tested by asking the patient to shrug his or her shoulders while slowly increasing downward resistance. Normally, the other scapular elevators will contribute significantly to the action of the trapezius; therefore, differences between the sides should be noted. The serratus anterior is responsible for scapular protraction and is innervated by the long thoracic nerve. Scapular winging is noted with paralysis of the long thoracic nerve or weakness of the serratus anterior and is evident when the patient does a push-up or pushes against a wall (Fig. 51.6). Winging of the scapula may also be noted in a patient with adhesive capsulitis who tries to compensate for decreased motion at the glenohumeral joint by increasing scapulothoracic motion.

The supraspinatus can be isolated by having the patient hold his or her arms at 90° of abduction, 30° of forward flexion, and internal rotation with the thumbs pointing downward (Fig. 51.7). The patient is then asked to resist the examiner's downward force. Pain or weakness is indicative of supraspinatus pathology. Because the biceps acts as both a flexor and supinator of the elbow, it can be tested by having the patient flex his or her arm against resistance and supinate his or her arm against resistance. The triceps is tested by having the patient extend his or her elbow against resistance.

Provocative Tests

Often the history alone will give the physician enough information to form a presumptive diagnosis. The general physical examination of the shoulder then helps to confirm that diagnosis. With a particular diagnosis in mind, there are a number of provocative tests that the physical can perform to confirm or redefine the diagnosis. These specialized tests should be part of the complete physician examination of the shoulder in any athlete with suspected glenohumeral instability, impingement, rotator cuff tears, and bicipital tendinitis (Table 51.3).

Glenohumeral Instability Tests

Instability of the glenohumeral joint is defined as excessive symptomatic translation of the humeral head on

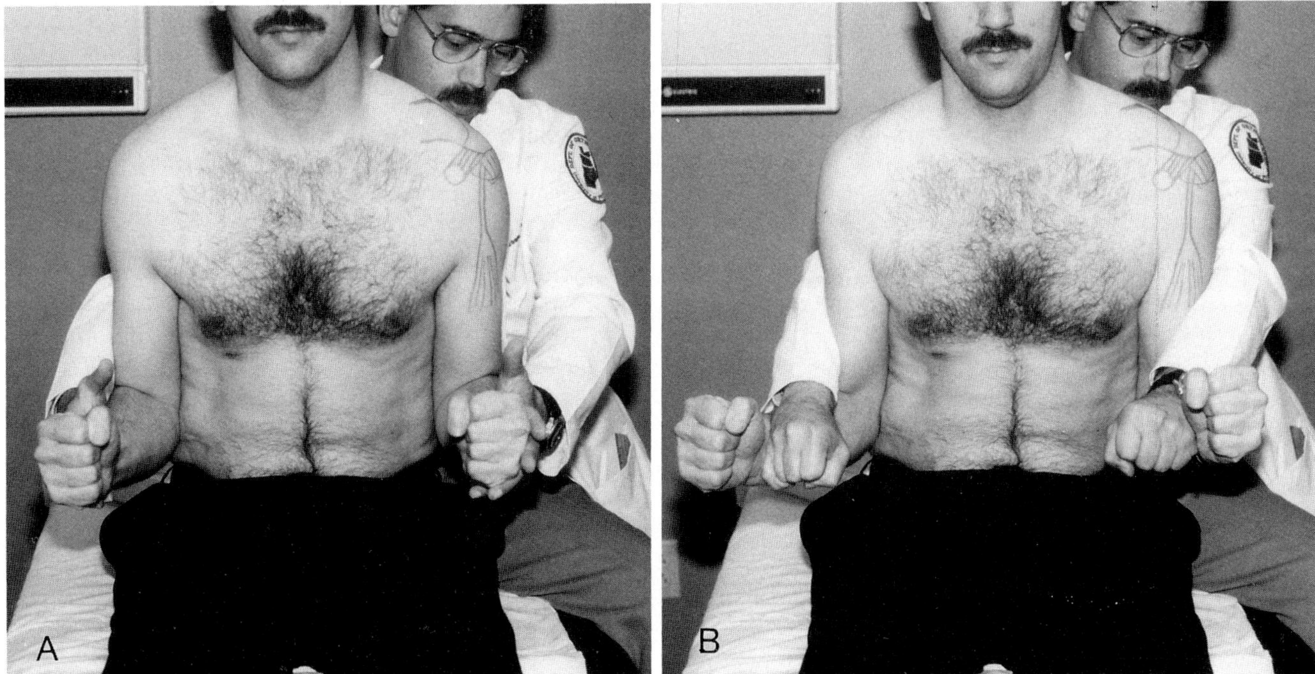

Figure 51.5. A, Manual muscle test of external rotators of the shoulder. **B,** Manual muscle test of internal rotators of the shoulder.

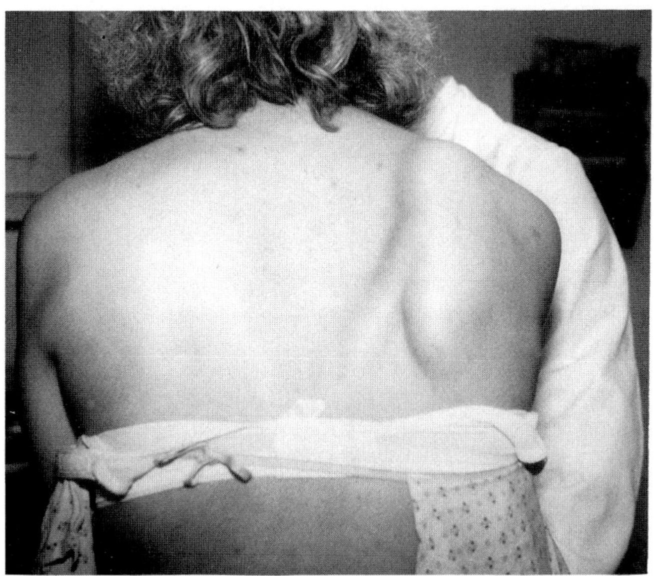

Figure 51.6. Scapular winging due to paralysis of the right long thoracic nerve.

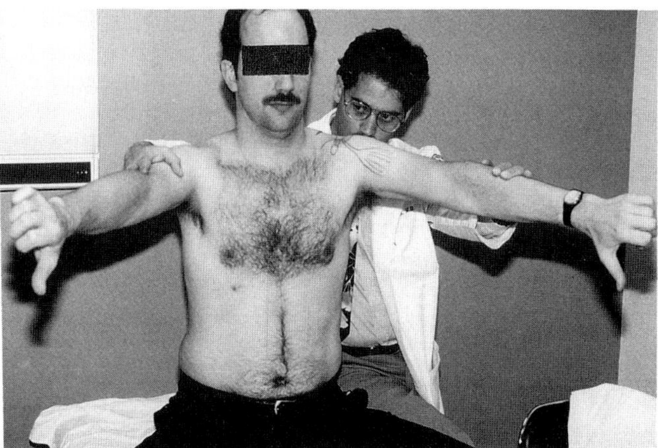

Figure 51.7. The supraspinatus resistance test.

the glenoid during shoulder rotation. Because shoulder instability may be a manifestation of generalized ligamentous laxity, it is necessary to examine the athlete for generalized ligamentous laxity by the criteria described by Steiner (23), Schwartz et al. (24), and Beighton and Horam (25). These criteria include *(a)* abduction of the thumb to touch the forearm with the wrist fully flexed, *(b)* hyperextension of the little finger metacarpophalangeal joint beyond 90°, *(c)* elbow hyperextension beyond 10° and *(d)* knee hyperextension beyond 10°. If three of four of these criteria are satisfied,

Table 51.3.
Provocative Tests and Imaging Studies for Specific Shoulder Disorders

Diagnosis	Provocative Test	Imaging Study
Genohumeral instability	Apprehension Relocation Translation testing Load and shift	Trauma series Stryker-Notch view West Point axillary Arthro-CT scan
Rotator cuff tear	Drop arm Supraspinatus weakness External rotation weakness Lift-off test	Scapular outlet view Caudal tilt view Ultrasound Arthrogram
Impingement	Impingement sign Impingement test	Scapular outlet view Caudal tilt view
Biceps tendinitis	Yerguson's test Speed's test	Fisk view

then the patient is considered to have ligamentous laxity (25). Assessment of increased laxity in the glenohumeral joint is determined by the following tests: *(a)* apprehension; *(b)* relocation; *(c)* glenohumeral translation; and *(d)* sulcus sign. It is important to compare side-to-side differences with all of these tests.

Anterior glenohumeral instability is perhaps best demonstrated by the anterior apprehension sign. In patients who subluxate or dislocate their shoulders anteriorly, the "provocative position" or position in which they feel most fearful that the shoulder will "come out" is that of abduction and external rotation. The apprehension test is performed with the examiner standing behind the sitting position. The examiner palpates the humeral head while gently placing the arm in abduction and external rotation. The test also may be performed in the supine position with the patient's shoulder at the edge of the table. A positive apprehension sign is one in which the patient complains of pain and/or contracts his or her muscles to resist further movement of the arm with the fear that the shoulder may come out if the stress is continued (Fig. 51.8).

If a positive apprehension sign is elicited, then the relocation test as described by Jobe and Bradley (26) can be performed with the patient supine. for the relocation test, the examiner places the arm in abduction and external rotation and places a gentle posteriorly directed force on the humerus with the thenar eminence of the opposite hand (Fig. 51.9). The test is considered positive if pain reduction occurs with this maneuver. The response can be graded as mildly positive, positive, or negative. An abrupt release of the posteriorly directed force may elicit an immediate feeling of pain and/or apprehension. This test is sensitive but not necessarily specific for increased anterior laxity. Because other pathologic conditions, such as superior labrum anterior posterior (SLAP) lesions and biceps tendinitis, may elicit a similar response, additional clinical and imaging studies may be necessary to confirm the diagnosis.

In addition to the anterior apprehension test, a posterior apprehension test should also be performed. The test is performed with the patient seated and the arm held across the chest with the elbow flexed to 90°. As the arm is brought across the chest, a posteriorly directed force is placed on the elbow, which places a posteriorly directed force across the glenohumeral joint. If posterior instability exists, the humeral head will slip posteriorly and the patient will experience pain and/or apprehension. Some authors, however, feel that apprehension related to posterior instability is not a reliable sign and translation of the humeral head in the glenoid socket should be assessed.

In addition to reproducing a symptomatic apprehen-

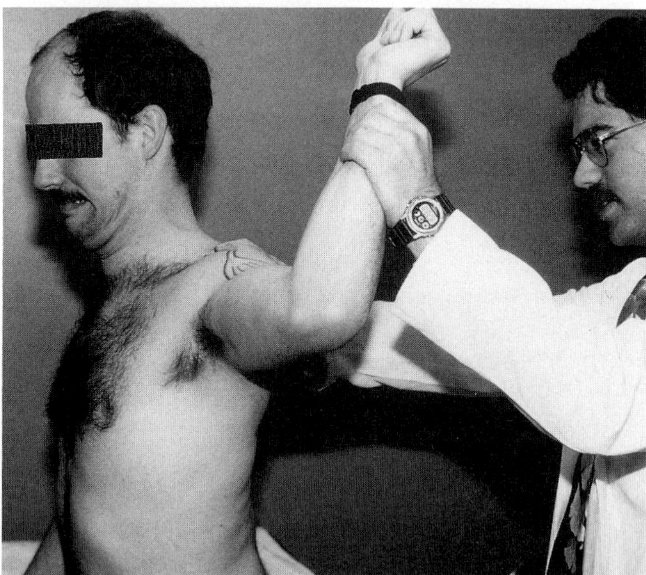

Figure 51.8. The apprehension test for anterior shoulder instability.

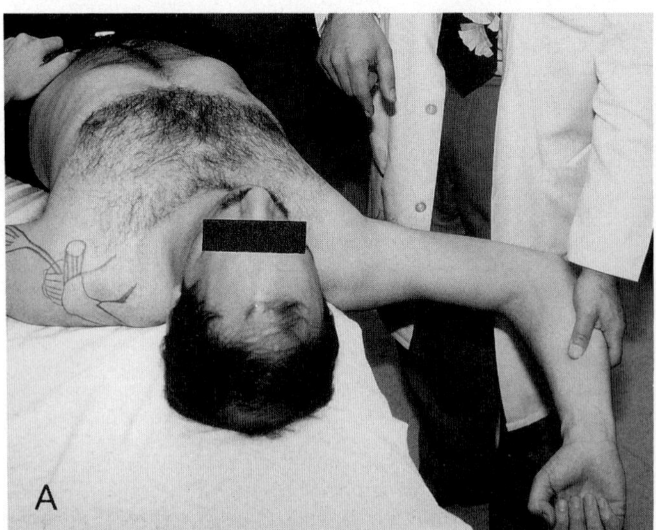

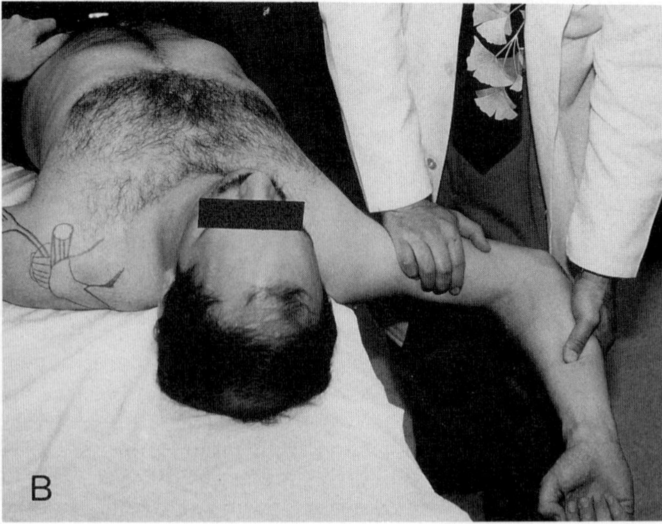

Figure 51.9. A, With patient lying supine, the apprehension test is performed by placing the arm in abduction, external rotation, and extension. **B,** The relocation test is performed by applying posterior pressure to the humerus. A positive test is the reduction of pain and apprehension.

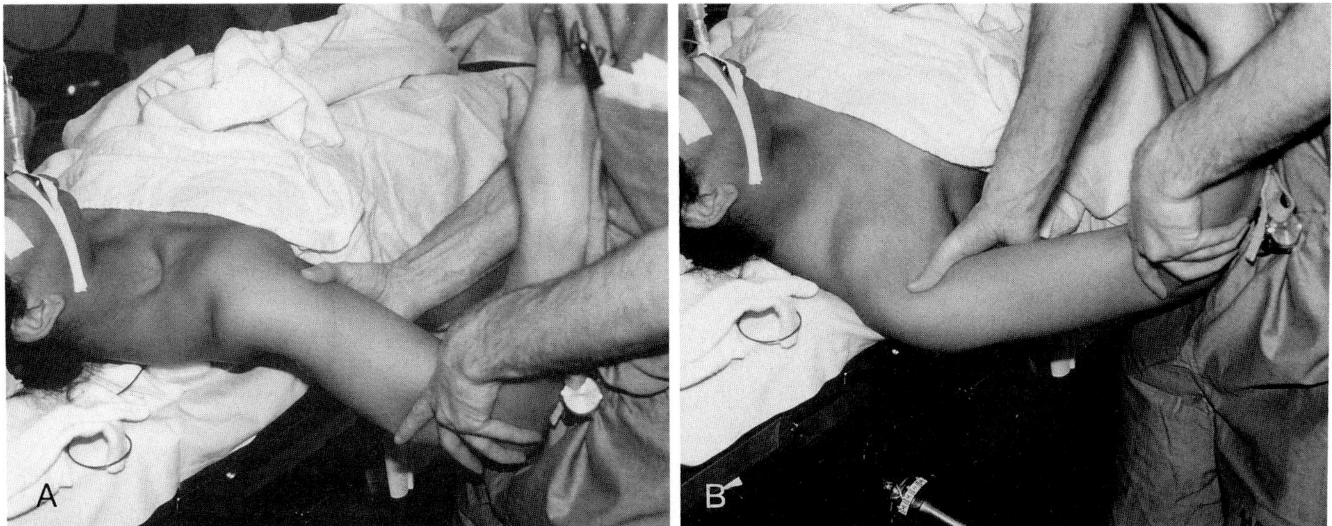

Figure 51.10. A, Anteior drawer demonstrates a complete dislocation (grade III). **B,** Posterior drawer demonstrates complete dislocation (grade III) in a patient with multidirectional instability.

sion or subluxation by stressing the glenohumeral joint, instability may be assessed by documenting the amount of translation possible between the humeral head and glenoid fossa when stressed by the examiner. An assessment of anterior and posterior translation of the humeral head on the glenoid socket is often difficult to appreciate even for the experienced physician. A demonstrable difference in the amount of translation between sides is considered abnormal, and the amount of translation can be graded (27). Grade 0 is normal or no instability. Grade I is translation of up to 50% of the diameter of the humeral head. A feeling that the humeral head is riding over the glenoid rim and spontaneously reducing is considered grade II. In grade III translation, the examiner experiences the feeling that the humeral head rides over the glenoid rim, but remains dislocated upon release (Fig. 51.10). This test is most sensitive when performed with a patient under general anesthesia.

The translation of the humeral head can be demonstrated by the "load-and-shift" test (28) It is first necessary to ensure that the humeral head is reduced with the glenoid fossa and not translated anteriorly, posteriorly, or inferiorly. To ensure this reduction, the humeral head is "loaded" by being grasped and pushed into the glenoid fossa. Once the head is loaded, the examiner applies directional stresses. The athlete is initially seated with the examiner standing behind and to the side. The examiner places one hand on the shoulder and scapula and the other hand grasps the humeral head. The examiner applies anterior and posterior directed forces and notes the amount of translation as above. Next, with the athlete supine, the arm is grasped and positioned in 20° of abduction and forward flexion. With the humeral head loaded, an anteriorly and posteriorly directed force is applied and the degree of translation noted. As noted by Hawkins and Bokor (28), the accuracy of the load-and-shift test depends on the examiner's skill and the ability of the patient to relax. It is often necessary to perform the examination under

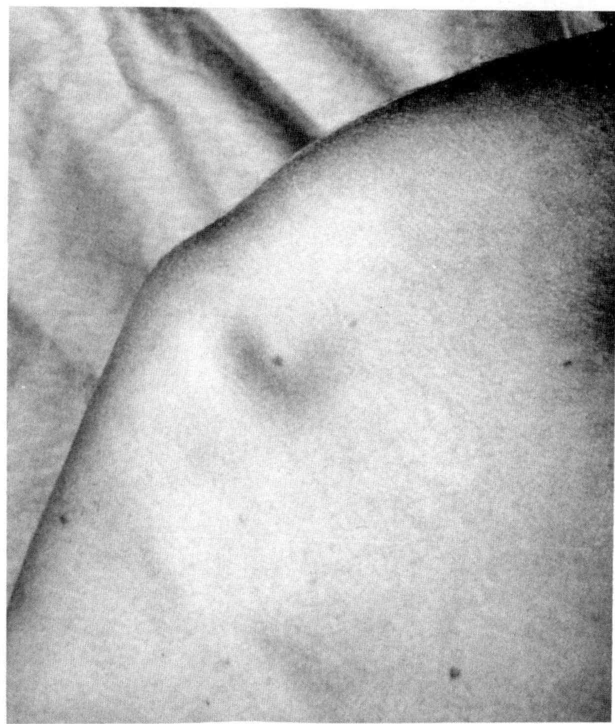

Figure 51.11. The sulcus sign is demonstrated by pulling inferiorly on adducted arm.

anesthesia to maximize the information obtained. Most normal shoulders translate up to a grade II posteriorly and up to a grade I anteriorly (28). Therefore, correlation should always be made with the uninvolved shoulder. Significant inferior glenohumeral instability is the hallmark of multidirectional instability.

The sulcus sign is indicative of inferior instability and is demonstrated by applying an internally directed longitudinal force in line with the humerus. The appearance of a sulcus or depression in the subacromial region as the humeral head translates inferiorly is the sulcus sign (Fig. 51.11). Thus apprehension and translational testing should be performed in all athletes suspected of having glenohumeral instability. The examiner should be able to reproduce the instability pattern (anterior, posterior, inferior, or multidirectional) via a thorough examination.

Rotator Cuff Test

Impingement is defined as encroachment of the rotator cuff on the coracohumeral arch (acromion-coracoacromial ligament) with forward flexion of the humerus (29). Patients with impingement often have palpable crepitation and an arc of pain. As the arm is raised from the side and lowered in various degrees of rotation, the patient may experience pain within an arc of motion. The maximum joint reaction forces and rotator cuff tension occur as the arm passes between 70° and 120°. Pain within this range is consistent with a positive arc of pain. Impingement lesions can be separated from other causes of shoulder pain by the impingement sign and the impingement test (29). The humerus is forward flexed as the scapula is stabilized with the opposite hand so that the greater tuberosity comes directly under the coracoacromial arch (Fig. 51.12). Although this maneuver is sensitive for impingement, it is not specific, because pain may be elicited with other conditions, including frozen shoulder, glenoid labrum pathology, acromioclavicular joint inflammation, and rotator cuff biceps tendinitis. The impingement test is used to exclude these other conditions. With the impingement test, the range of motion of the shoulder is noted before and after the injection of 10 ml 1% lidocaine into the subacromial space (Fig. 51.13). The patient is asked to evaluate subjectively the degree of pain relief by rating from 0 to 10, with a 10 representing

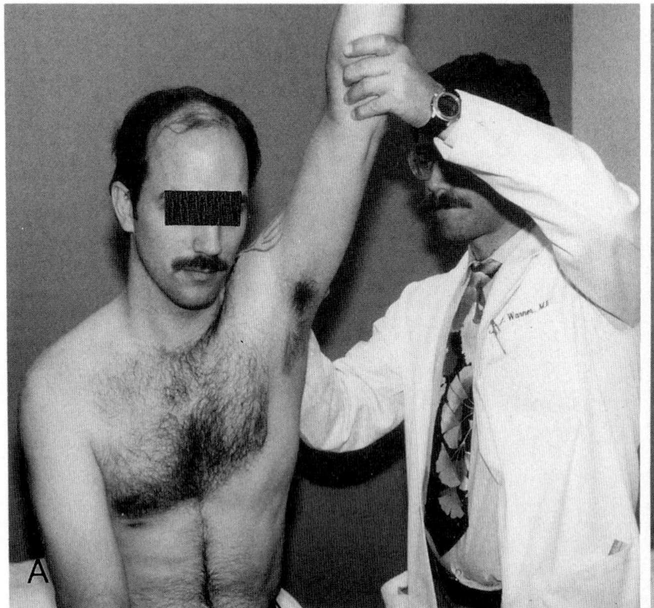

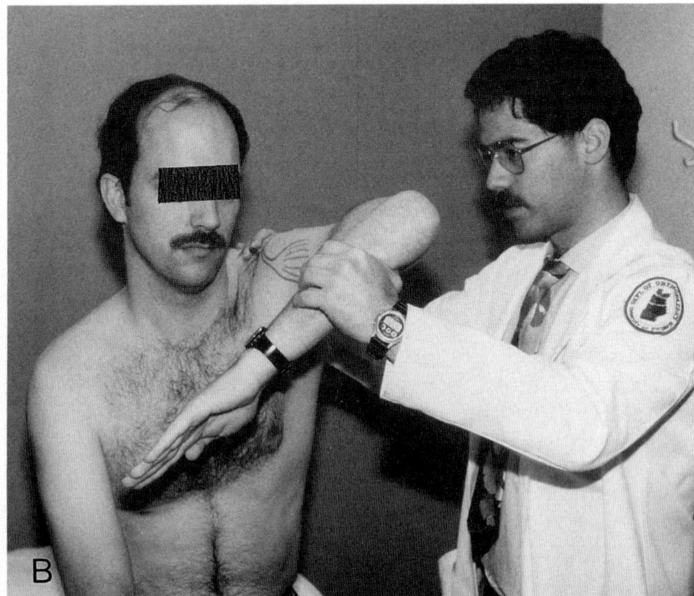

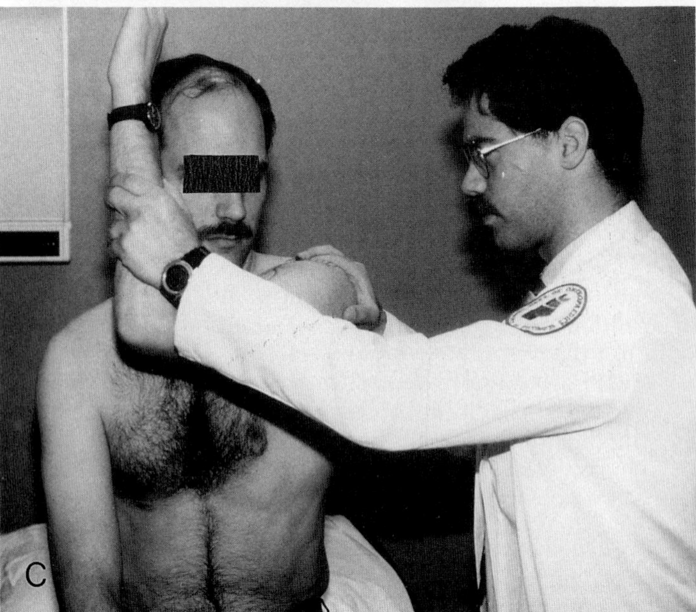

Figure 51.12. A, The impingement sign of Neer. **B,** The modified impingement sign of Hawkins. **C,** Cross-chest adduction elicits pain from acromioclavicular joint pathology.

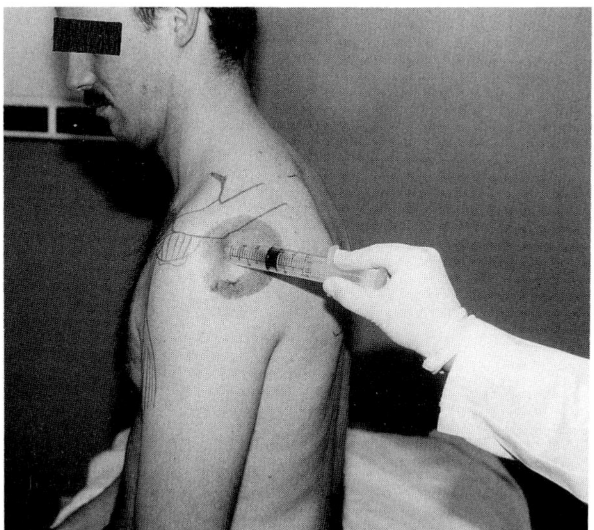

Figure 51.13. The impingement (injection) test.

complete pain relief. If the pain relief is only partial and the acromioclavicular joint is tender, an injection is made into the acromioclavicular joint. If no relief or only mild relief is obtained with an appropriate subacromial injection, another diagnosis must then be entertained.

The physical examination with a possible rotator cuff tear should include the drop arm test (30). With the patient standing, he or she is asked to abduct the arm to 90°. The patient is then asked to lower the arm slowly. If the patient has a large tear of the rotator cuff, he or she may not be able smoothly and slowly to lower the arm to the side.

The strength of the rotator cuff muscles should be tested in athletes suspected of a rotator cuff tear. Manual muscle testing should include external and internal rotation and abduction against resistance. Any weaknesses should be noted and testing should be repeated following subacromial injection. Supraspinatus weakness in athletes with suspected rotator cuff tears may be caused by pain. In this situation, relieving the pain by a subacromial injection can resolve the weakness on manual testing.

In the majority of cases, the rotator cuff tear occurs in the supraspinatus insertion on the greater tuberosity. Although it is difficult to determine the exact size of the rotator cuff tear by physical examination, it is often possible to estimate the size by selective manual muscle testing. A small tear may only show weakness on isolated supraspinatus testing. A larger tear, on the other hand, may extend into the external rotators and become evident on resisted external rotation. Only patients with large or massive rotator cuff tears will have a positive drop arm sign. Rare cases of traumatic isolated subscapularis tears have been noted. In these cases, the patient will demonstrate a positive "lift-off" test. In this test, the patient attempts to lift the dorsum of the hand to his or her lumbosacral spine. A positive test is one in which there is severe weakness; it is indicative of injury to the subscapularis muscle. Resistive internal rotators, on the other hand, will not necessarily be effective because other muscles can substitute for the subscapularis (e.g., pectoralis major).

Biceps Tendinitis

Biceps tendinitis rarely occurs as an isolated entity in the athlete and is usually secondary to impingement. The athlete with biceps tendinitis will complain of anterior shoulder pain that is less intense with rest. The pain of tendinitis may be masked by pain secondary to impingement. Biceps subluxation is exceedingly rare and never occurs without a subscapularis tear. Biceps subluxation can present with a similar pain pattern to bicipital tendinitis, but the athlete may complain of a palpable snap or pop with shoulder motion. The athlete with biceps tendinitis will have point tenderness in the bicipital groove, which can be localized with the patient's arm held in 10° of internal rotation (31). The point of maximal tenderness is located approximately 3 inches below the anterior ridge of the acromion and will move as the arm is rotated. This "tenderness motion" sign is thought to be specific for bicipital tendinitis.

Yerguson's sign (32) for biceps tendinitis is elicited with the elbow flexed and the patient forcibly supinating against resistance. A positive test is one in which pain is referred to the anterior aspect of the shoulder. In Speed's test (33) (Fig. 51.14), with the elbow extended and the forearm supinated, the patient flexes his or her shoulder against resistance. Pain localized to the bicipital groove constitutes a positive test. With de Anguin's test (34), the examiner has his or her finger in the bicipital groove. A positive test occurs when the patient feels pain as the tendon glides beneath the finger.

Radiographic Evaluation of Athletic Shoulder Problems

Once a thorough history and complete physical examination of the shoulder are performed, the physician may then obtain the appropriate adjuvant diagnostic studies. The studies requested depend on the presumptive diagnosis.

Although injuries to the sternoclavicular joint can often be diagnosed clinically, appropriate x-rays should be taken to evaluate fully the injury and rule out associated fractures. The standard AP or PA chest x-ray is often useful to demonstrate asymmetry of the sternoclavicular joint. The 40° cephalic tilt view as described by Neer and Rockwood (35) is easy to obtain and useful in demonstrating anterior or posterior subluxations or dislocations of the sternoclavicular joint. The view is taken with the patient supine, a cassette is placed behind the patient, and the beam is angled 40° from the vertical and aimed at the manubrium. Computed tomography (CT) scans offer the best information for evaluating the sternoclavicular joint. For posterior sternoclavicular dislocations with possible vascular compression, contrast CT studies are valuable. A bone scan

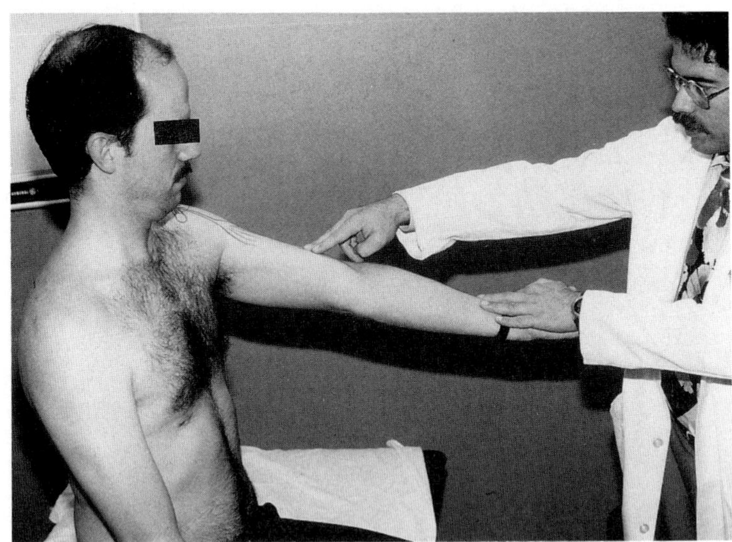

Figure 51.14. Speed's test for biceps tendinitis.

may also be used to detect inflammatory or degenerative changes of the sternoclavicular joint.

Athletic injuries to the acromioclavicular (AC) joint are readily evaluated by radiographs. Because the AC joint is relatively more superficial than the glenohumeral joint, 50% less x-ray voltage is necessary to expose the AC joint than is necessary to expose a typical glenohumeral joint. The best unobstructive view of the distal clavicle and AC joint is the Zanca view (36). This x-ray is obtained with a 10° cephalic tilt. An AP view of the acromioclavicular joints can be taken with the patient sitting or standing. Both shoulders should be imaged on a single cassette to compare the acromioclavicular joint and the coracoacromial distance of the injured versus the uninjured shoulder. If the AP views are not conclusive for a complete acromioclavicular dislocation, but there is clinical suspicion, stress x-rays should be obtained. An AP x-ray of the AC joints is taken with 10 to 20 pounds of weight strapped to the patient's wrists (Fig. 51.15). If these x-rays reveal a less than 25% difference in coracoclavicular distance between the injured and normal shoulder, then a complete separation can be ruled out. The standard axillary view taken with the x-ray beam placed inferior to the axilla and aimed at an x-ray cassette superior to the shoulder with the arm held in 70° to 90° of abduction should be obtained to demonstrate anterior or posterior displacement. The degree of clavicle elevation combined with anterior and posterior displacement determines the severity of the injury and the type of treatment necessary.

Diagnostic imaging of the glenohumeral joint begins with the trauma series. (AP and axillary or scapular lateral) as advocated by several authors (35, 37–40). A more complete series involves the AP and lateral in the scapular plane and the axillary view. The AP view in the scapular plane is obtained with the beam angled 45° to the patient so that the scapula is parallel to the x-ray cassette. With this view, the glenoid appears in profile and can be seen separately from the humeral head. Any

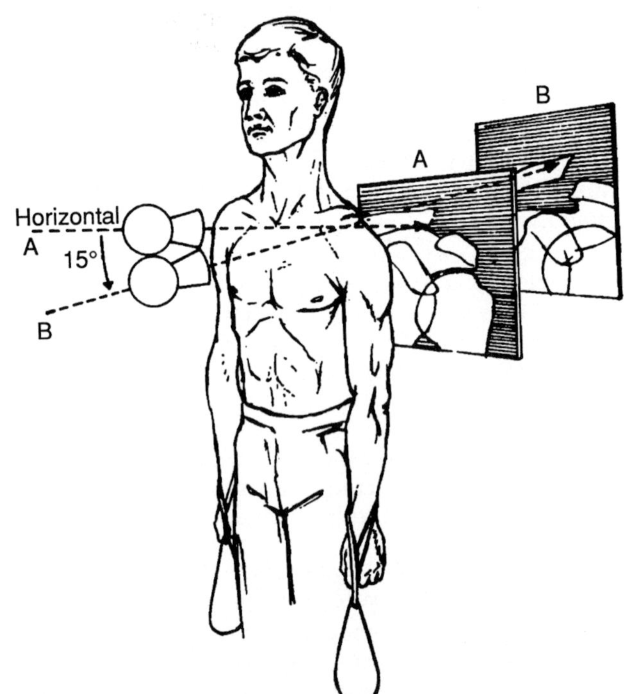

Figure 51.15. Acromioclavicular joint view with weights to rule out AC separation.

overlapping of the glenoid and humeral head is indicative of a glenohumeral dislocation.

The lateral view in the scapular plane is also called the transcapular or Y lateral view (41). This view is a true lateral of the scapula and is helpful in determining the anterior and posterior displacement of the humeral head relative to the glenoid. The axillary lateral, on velpeau lateral view, when combined with the AP and lateral in the scapular plane, maximizes the information available. The axillary view clearly delineates the relationship between the humeral head and the glenoid and allows for identification of dislocations. If because of pain or muscle spasm a true axillary view cannot be obtained, then a Velpeau axillary view should be obtained. This view, described by Bloom and Obata (42), eliminates the need for shoulder abduction. The patient stands or sits at the end of the x-ray table and leans backward over the table. The x-ray beam is aimed directly over the shoulder and passes through the shoulder joint toward the cassette (Fig. 51.16). In addition to the standard trauma series, fracture dislocations involving the glenohumeral joint can be further evaluated by CT scan.

Following the standard trauma series, special radiographic views and imaging techniques are available to assess specific pathology. Anterior shoulder dislocation or subluxation may be accompanied by small fractures of the glenoid or calcified soft tissues of the anterior or anterior-inferior aspect of the glenoid rim. If the fracture is anterior and inferior, it may not be seen on the routine axillary view. In this case, the West Point axillary view will provide more information than the axillary view. The West Point is taken with the patient prone, the x-ray cassette positioned against the superior aspect of the shoulder, and the x-ray beam angled 25° downward and 25° toward the midline (Fig. 51.17). Fractures or calcification about the glenoid rim may also be seen on CT scans or arthro-CT scans.

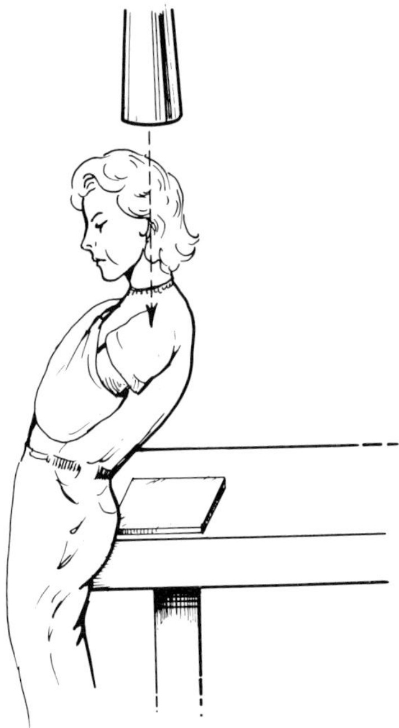

Figure 51.16. The Velpeau axillary view.

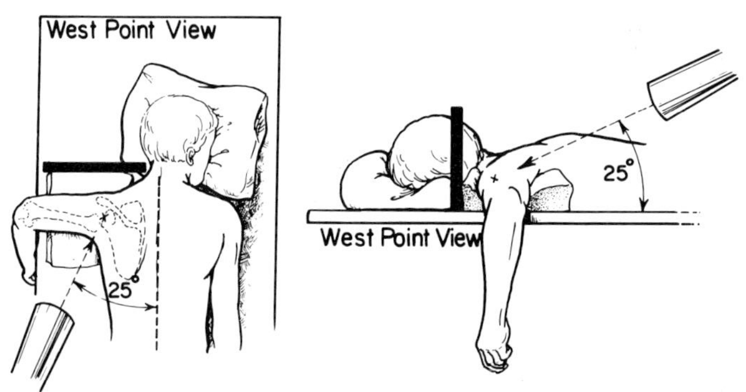

Figure 51.17. The West Point axillary view.

The Hill-Sachs (43) lesion is a compression fracture of the posterolateral humeral head, which is often the result of anterior shoulder dislocations. The Hill-Sachs lesion may occur following a single anterior dislocation or be the result of recurrent anterior dislocations. Because this lesion is on the posteriorlateral aspect of the humeral head, it can often be seen on the anterior-posterior x-ray of the shoulder with the arm held in full internal rotation (Fig. 51.18). Perhaps the best view to see the Hill-Sachs lesion is the Stryker-Notch view (35, 44). For this view, the patient is positioned supine with the x-ray cassette behind the shoulder with the x-ray beam angled toward the shoulder at 10° The patient touches the top of his or her head and holds the arm in approximately 120° of flexion (Fig. 51.19). In this position, the arm is in internal rotation. The presence of the defect on x-ray confirms that the shoulder has been dislocated. A CT scan is also useful in documenting the presence and size of the Hill-Sachs lesion.

Athletes with a history of shoulder dislocations may have soft tissue injury to the shoulder. Bankart (45) described an avulsion of the anterior capsule and glenoid labrum of the glenoid rim (see Fig. 51.1). This lesion is known as the Bankart lesion and is associated with anterior shoulder instability. These lesions can be seen on arthrogram (46), pneumoarthocomputed tomography (47), arthro-CT (48), and MRI.

Posterior shoulder instability is less common than anterior instability. Posterior glenohumeral dislocations are often missed if an inadequate physical examination is performed or inadequate x-rays are obtained. The trauma series should be adequate to reveal a posterior

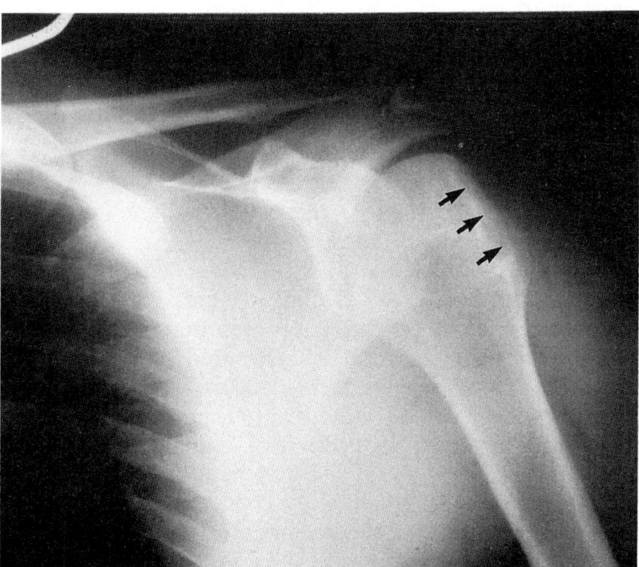

Figure 51.18. Hill-Sachs lesion *(arrows)* is demonstrated on AP view with arm in internal rotation.

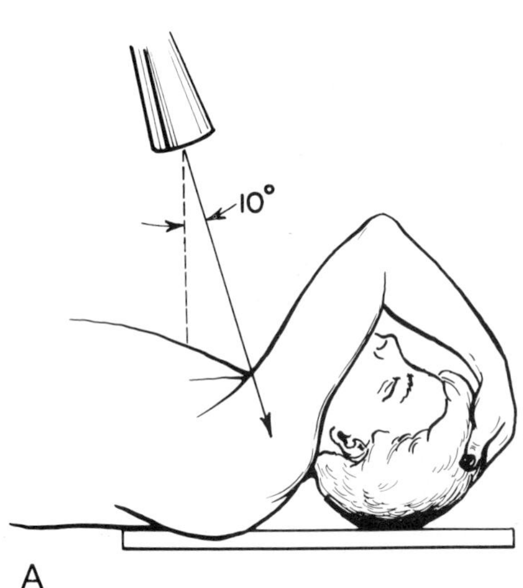

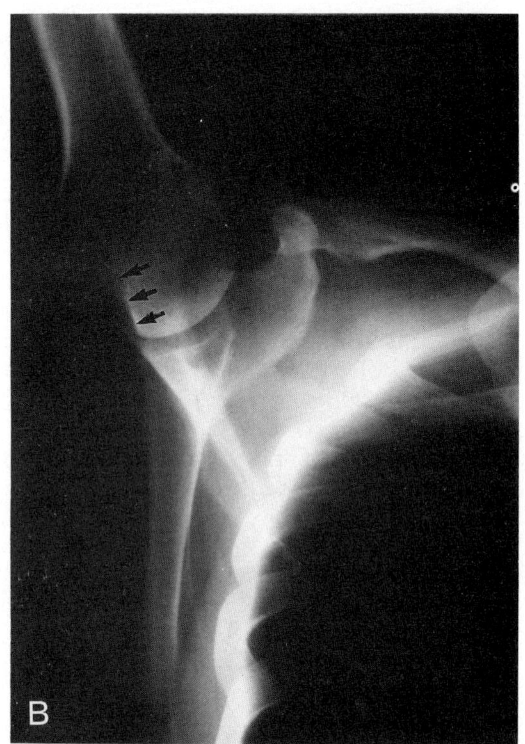

Figure 51.19. A, Positioning of the Stryker-Notch view. **B,** Example of the Hill-Sachs lesion on Stryker-Notch view *(arrows)*.

dislocation. Posterior glenohumeral instability may result in an avulsion of the posterior glenoid labrum known as a reverse Hill-Sachs lesion. This lesion is seen in the anteromedial surface in the humeral head. Axillary x-rays and CT scans are useful for evaluating bony lesions of the posterior glenoid rim.

Radiographic techniques are important in evaluating impingement and rotator cuff pathology. The x-ray evaluation of impingement consists of the standard AP view, a 30° caudal tilt view, and the scapular outlet view. The standard AP view of the shoulder can reveal superior migration of the humeral head under the acromion and narrowing of the acromiohumeral interval. A more sensitive measurement of rotator cuff dysfunction is to take several AP views while the shoulder is abducted and measure the position of the center of the humeral head relative to the equator of the glenoid. Normally, the humeral head remains perfectly centered. In the case of a rotator cuff tear, the humeral head translates superiorly (Fig. 51.20). The 30° caudal view is taken as the standard AP view with the x-ray beam angled with a 30° caudal tilt. This view demonstrates acromial spurring or proliferation of the anterior-inferior acromion that is associated with impingement. The scapular outlet view is taken with the patient positioned for a lateral view in the scapular plane, but the beam is angled 5° to 10° in the caudal direction (Fig. 51.21). Bigliani et al. (49) used this view to identify three types of acromion, which they correlated with the incidence of rotator cuff disease. Although arthrography is considered the gold standard for identification of full-thickness rotator cuff tears, the sensitivity rate of the arthrogram for detecting full-thickness rotator cuff tears is estimated to be between 95% and 100% (40). Because

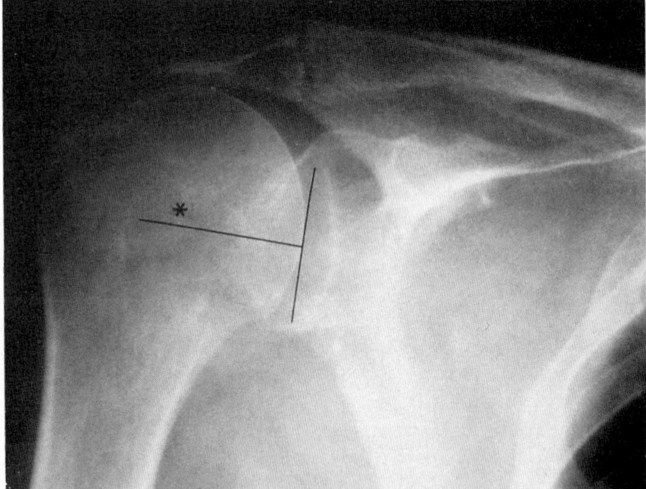

Figure 51.20. The center of the humeral head (*) moves above the equator of the glenoid as this patient with a rotator cuff tear attempts to raise the arm.

of the invasiveness of arthrography, other techniques for evaluating the rotator cuff have been studied. The sensitively of the MRI for diagnosing full-thickness rotator cuff tears is estimated to be between 95% and 97% (50, 51). MRI also is useful in identifying partial-thickness tears and edema within the tendons. Real-time ultrasound also is used in some centers for identification of rotator cuff pathology. The results appear to be user dependent, but an accuracy of between 82% and 100% (50–53) has been reported. Compared with other imaging studies, ultrasound is reported to be safe, rapid, noninvasive, and inexpensive.

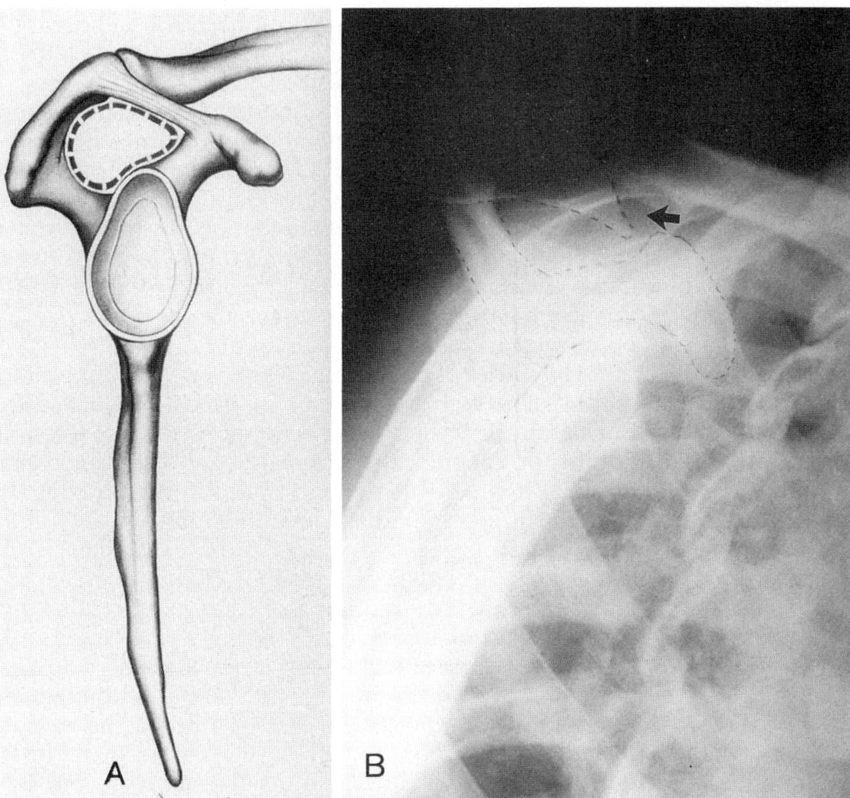

Figure 51.21. A, The supraspinatus outlet is formed by the coracoacromial arch. **B,** Narrowing of the supraspinatus outlet by a larger anterior acromial osteophyte *(arrow)*.

The radiographic evaluation of the athlete with tendinitis or biceps tendon subluxation involves the Fisk (54) view. In this view, the x-ray beam is superior to the shoulder. The beam is angled perpendicular to the bicipital groove. The patient holds the cassette while leaning over the table. Patients with primary bicipital tendinitis may have degenerative changes in the walls of the groove, whereas patients with subluxation may have a relatively shallow groove. Dislocations of the biceps tendons can be seen on arthrogram (55) and biceps tendon lesions can be seen on ultrasound imaging (56) and MRI. Table 51.3 summarizes the provocative tests and imaging studies for glenohumeral instability, rotator cuff tears, impingement, and biceps tendinitis.

Injuries to the Athletic Shoulder

Instability

The glenohumeral joint has an unique anatomic arrangement that balances mobility and stability. This unique balance makes the shoulder susceptible to injury when subject to athletic demands and especially in sports that require throwing or repetitive overhead maneuvers. These sports can stress both the dynamic (rotator cuff) and static stabilizers (ligaments) of the glenohumeral joint beyond their physiologic limits and eventually can lead to the breakdown of these stabilizers. This breakdown can result in glenohumeral instability. In addition to this repetitive, chronic pattern of instability, instability may result from a single episode of stress or trauma. Furthermore, specific pathologic lesions have been implicated as causes of or have been seen in association with glenohumeral instability that includes glenoid labrum detachment (Bankart lesion), excessive capsular laxity, subscapularis insufficiency, posterior lateral humeral head defect (Hill-Sachs lesion), abnormal humeral and glenoid version, rotator cuff tears, and lateral capsular avulsion.

Instability of the glenohumeral joint is defined as symptomatic excessive translation of the humeral head on the glenoid during shoulder rotation. There is a spectrum of instability that represents increasing degrees of injury to the dynamic and static stabilizers of the glenohumeral joint. Subluxation is defined as increased humeral head translation beyond that permitted by normal tissue laxity without complete separation of the articular surfaces. Because normal shoulders have a certain degree of play, clinical subluxation requires increased translation of the humeral head in association with symptoms. These symptoms include pain, a feeling that the shoulder is "loose," or a painful giving way of the shoulder associated with neurologic symptoms. This phenomenon is known as the "dead-arm" syndrome. This translation can occur in the anterior, posterior, or superior-inferior planes.

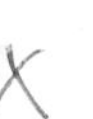

Glenohumeral instability can be categorized into five groups, depending on the mechanism of injury and the direction of instability:

1. Posttraumatic anterior subluxation/dislocation.
2. Posttraumatic posterior subluxation/dislocation.
3. Atraumatic anterior subluxation/dislocation.
4. Atraumatic posterior subluxation/dislocation.
5. Multidirectional subluxation/dislocation.

The stability of the glenohumeral joint is based on the interaction of the static and the dynamic constraints about the shoulder. Although there is some overlap of the anatomic structures in each category, the static constraints primarily include bony anatomy, the glenoid labrum, and the capsular ligaments (superior, middle, and inferior glenohumeral ligaments). The dynamic constraints of the glenohumeral joint are the rotator cuff muscles and the biceps. These muscles function dynamically to contain the humeral head in the glenoid by causing joint compression. They also act synergistically by contracting in a coordinated fashion to steer the humeral head into the glenoid in different arm positions, which leads to tightening of the static capsular ligamentous structures.

A careful history should be obtained from any athlete suspected of having glenohumeral instability. This historical evaluation should attempt to classify the nature and degree of the instability, which will in turn affect the prognosis and treatment. The classification should include the frequency or timing of the occurrences leading to the instability. For example, does the athlete describe an acute presentation of a one-time event, or does he or she describe multiple episodes. The direction of the instability should also be determined. By the description of the arm position when symptoms occur, the direction of the instability (anterior, posterior, or multidirectional) can often be determined. The onset of the instability should be determined. It should be noted whether the instability was traumatic or atraumatic in origin or was the result of overuse. The physician should also ascertain if the subluxation/dislocation is completely involuntary or if there is a voluntary component. Some patients may be able willingly to demonstrate their instability and are considered "voluntary" dislocators. Whereas, patients who demonstrate their instability through arm positioning alone are considered involuntary dislocators. The degree of instability should be noted. It should also be determined whether the shoulder subluxated or completely dislocated and either spontaneously reduced or had to be reduced on the field, in the training room, or in the emergency room. Finally, a history of generalized laxity of other joints should be obtained.

The hallmark of multidirectional instability is a positive sulcus sign on physical examination. Patients with multidirectional instability may give a history of pain and instability with activities such as lifting light objects. Neurologic symptoms such as transitory numbness of the hands or arm are common in patients with inferior instability. It is important to consider the possibility of multidirectional instability in all patients being evaluated for instability, because when standard treatments for recurrent unidirectional instability are applied to patients with multidirectional instability, they often fail. Multidirectional instability can be the result of one or more episodes of significant trauma (football or wrestling), repetitive minor injuries seen in overhead activities, or varying degrees of inherent ligamentous laxity (57, 58).

Despite a careful history and physical examination and in light of inconclusive or negative radiographic studies, approximately 10% of patients with instability remain a diagnostic dilemma. These patients have usually undergone a trial of nonoperative management without success. An examination under anesthesia and diagnostic arthroscopy may be considered for such patients. With the patient free of pain and without muscle guarding, a detailed examination, including translational testing of both shoulders can be performed. Often a surgical decision will be made on the basis of this examination. In other cases, arthrography may be performed to identify and treat labral lesions or identify Hill-Sachs lesions that were not seen on radiographs. The arthroscope can be used to visualize the translation of the humeral head, stretching or attenuation of the capsule, displacement of the inferior glenohumeral ligament complex, impaction fractures of the glenoid rim, loose bodies, and labral damage (59). Evaluation of an unstable shoulder can be a difficult problem. The differential diagnosis of glenohumeral instability must include acromioclavicular joint sprains and subacromial impingement.

These diagnoses will be discussed in detail below. A careful history, a thorough examination, and adequate radiographs should all be used to assess the mechanisms, degree, and direction of the glenohumeral instability, so that the pattern of instability can be put into one of the five categories and a treatment plan can be formulated.

Traumatic anterior dislocations of the glenohumeral joint account for more than 98% of shoulder dislocations (60). Often excessive abduction and external rotation forces will be responsible for levering the humeral head out of the glenoid fossa. Anterior dislocations may also be the result of a direct blow from behind. The anterior capsule stabilizing structures are usually torn with the dislocation. The athlete will complain of acute pain and have a severely decreased range of motion secondary to guarding. Often the diagnosis can be confirmed by the history and physical exam before obtaining x-rays (Fig. 51.22). The physical examination should include a neurovascular examination of the upper extremity with particular attention to the sensory distributions of the axillary and musculocutaneous nerves. The physician may be able to feel the humeral head displace anteriorly. An immediate reduction may be attempted on the playing field. If this reduction is unsuccessful, further attempts can be made in the locker room before muscle spasm has set in. Frequently, the shoulder can be reduced with the Stimson (60) maneuver in which the athlete is placed prone on the examination table with a 10-pound weight hanging from the wrist (Fig. 51.23). A variety of other techniques may be used as well. Any technique used should involve only gentle traction and manipulation to avoid iatrogenic fracture or nerve injury (Fig. 51.24). If reduction cannot be accomplished, then the athlete should be taken to the hospital for x-rays and muscle relaxation medication. If possible, x-rays should be obtained both before reduction, to excluded fracture, and after reduction, to confirm the reduction.

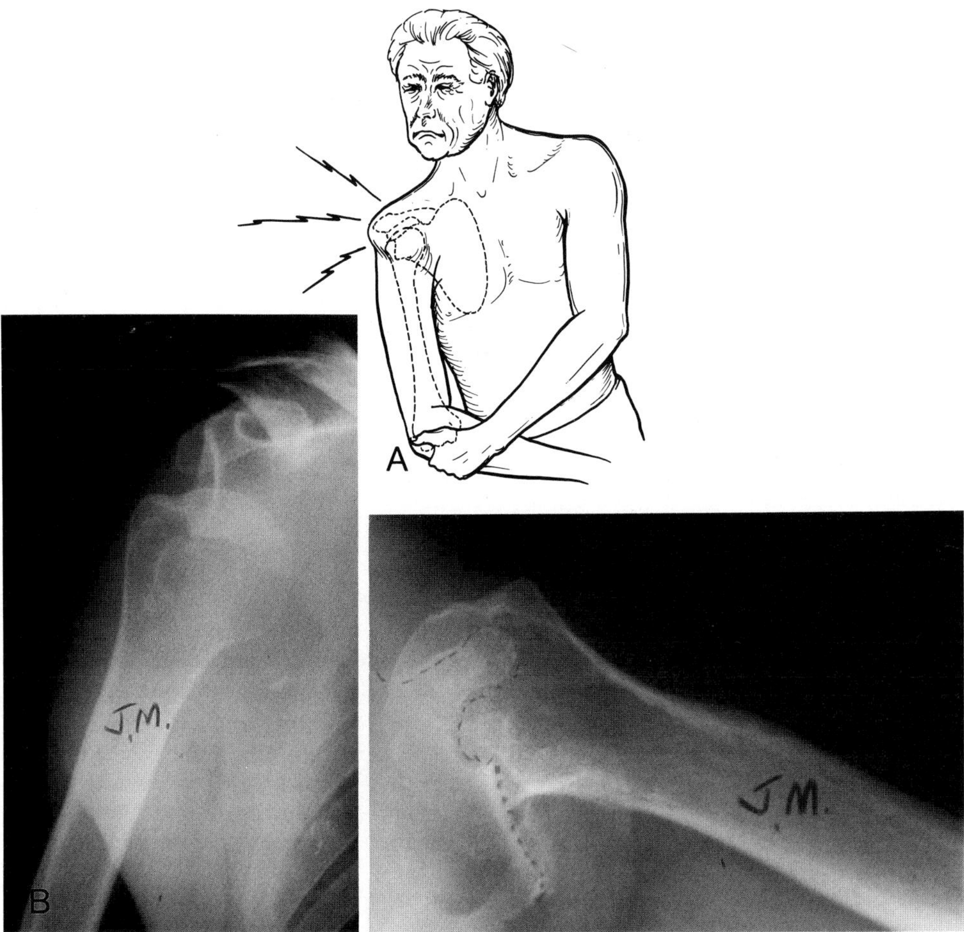

Figure 51.22. **A,** In an anterior glenohumeral dislocation, the arm is held to side and patient leans toward affected side. **B,** Example of a locked anterior (chronic) dislocation as seen on AP and axillary view.

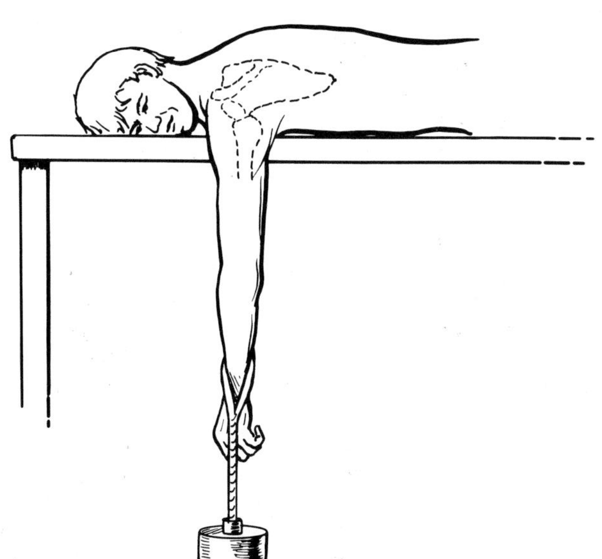

Figure 51.23. Stimson reduction maneuver for anterior dislocation.

A neurovascular examination should be done as soon after reduction as possible. If the athlete has no prior history of shoulder instability following reduction, a sling should be used to immobilize the arm in internal rotation for 6 weeks. (60). Following immbolization, rehabilitation exercises are begun, consisting of shoulder strengthening with emphasis on the internal rotators. In athletes over 40 years old, there is a greater incidence of rotator cuff tears and adhesive capsulitis following traumatic anterior dislocations or subluxations (61). These athletes should, therefore, be immobilized for only 7 to 10 days and then begin range-of-motion and strengthening exercises. The incidence of recurrence depends primarily on the age of the patient at the time of the initial dislocation. In a series by Rowe and Sakellarides (62), it was noted that patients less than 20 years old have a greater than 90% chance of recurrence, whereas patients greater than 40 years old have less than a 25% chance of recurrence. It is extremely important that the shoulder be completely rehabilitated

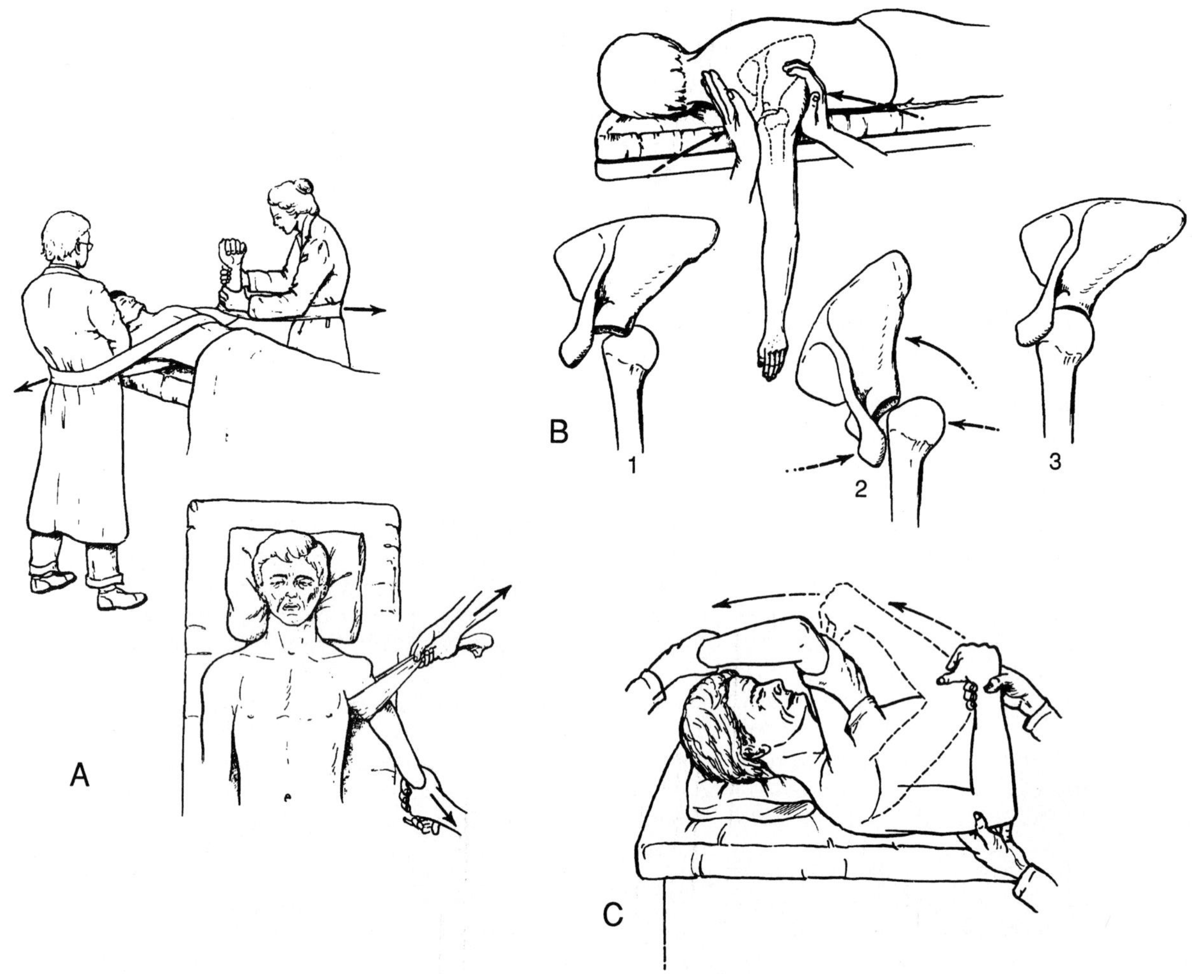

51.24. A, Reduction of anterior glenohumeral dislocation by traction-countertraction method. **B,** Reduction by scapular manipulation method. **C,** Reduction by Rowe's technique of traction and gentle forward flexion.

before returning to athletics. The criteria for returning to sports are based on a full range of motion and full strength.

Posterior traumatic subluxation or dislocation is much less common than anterior subluxation or dislocation. An acute traumatic posterior dislocation is usually the result of a direct blow to the anterior shoulder or the result of direct forces with the arm held in flexion, adduction, and internal rotation. Posterior dislocation can also result from seizures or electrical shock. The patient usually presents with the arm adducted and internally rotated with limitation of external rotation. Most posterior dislocations spontaneously reduce (60). The axillary view is critical in making this diagnosis. As with anterior dislocations, a careful neurovascular assessment is essential. Following reduction, the shoulder should be immobilized in a position of external rotation to allow tightening of the posterior capsule. In the young athlete less than 40 years old, immobilization is continued for 4 to 6 weeks followed by an aggressive physical therapy program that emphasizes strengthening of the external rotators of the shoulder. In athletes older than 40 years old, immobilization should only be 2 to 3 weeks (63). There is little documentation regarding recurrences of posterior dislocations, but as with anterior dislocations, the younger the patient, the higher the recurrence rate.

Athletes, especially those involved in repetitive overhead activities, can experience signs and symptoms of shoulder instability without significant initial trauma. Symptomatic anterior subluxation in throwers is often manifested during the acceleration phase of throwing when the arm is maximally abducted and externally rotated. Swimmers may notice symptoms during the back stroke or during turns. The pain associated with anterior subluxation may be posterior because of the stresses placed on the posterior tissues during anterior humeral head translation. The initial treatment of symptomatic anterior dislocation involves a sling and antiinflammatory medication until acute pain and inflammation subside (60). After the initial pain and swelling has subsided, a vigorous physical therapy program should be initiated with range-of-motion and strengthening exercises for the rotator cuff.

Unlike posterior dislocations, which are rare in athletes, posterior subluxation is relatively common. The athlete usually complains of pain rather than instability. The pain may be either anterior or posterior. The pain generally occurs when the posterior capsule is stressed. This pain occurs most notably with follow-through in pitching, during the pull-through phase in swimming, and during serving motions or backhand in tennis. The initial treatment is similar to that of anterior subluxation with sling and nonsteroidal antiinflammatory drugs (NSAIDs). Physical therapy is then initiated when pain and swelling subside. The goal of therapy is to increase strength of the external rotators of the shoulder.

Multidirectional instability of the shoulder is defined as instability occurring in more than one plane. This may involve the anterior-inferior, posterior-inferior, or instability in all three directions. Multidirectional instability may have atraumatic origins in persons with extensive ligamentous laxity, especially in those athletes who perform repetitive overhead activities, or may be the result of a traumatic insult to the shoulder in a person with generalized ligamentous laxity. The clinical findings depend on the predominant direction of the instability. The patient may have multiple apprehension signs and a positive sulcus sign. As with anterior and posterior instability, the initial treatment is conservative involving NSAIDs and physical therapy.

Physical therapy for patients with instability involves first a stretching program to restore full motion to the shoulder. Once full motion has been achieved, strengthening can begin. The goal of strengthening is to eliminate imbalance in the rotators due to a deficiency caused by the subluxation. With posterior subluxation, the external rotators are often deficient and with anterior subluxation it is the internal rotators that are deficient. Generally, spring exercises or rubber tubing is used to provide resistive strengthening. The athlete may return to activities at a low level during therapy as long as the specific activities that cause symptoms are avoided. The therapy will vary with the age, motivation of the patient, and the degree of damage to the shoulder. Therapy should progress until the patient can return to activities without symptoms.

In traumatic and posttraumatic anterior, posterior, and multidirectional instability of the shoulder, operative intervention should be considered for those athletes who fail at an adequate trial of physical therapy. These athletes are those whose pain and instability preclude adequate functioning of the involved shoulder. Many surgical procedures have been described to address glenohumeral instability. The type of procedure depends on the direction of the instability and the pathology involved. In general, athletes who have surgical treatment for instability may lose some range of motion of the shoulder, especially internal or external rotation. In the athlete who performs repetitive overhead activities, this loss of rotation may result in some diminution of performance in his or her sport.

Rotator Cuff Problems, Impingement, and Biceps Tendinitis

Subacromial impingement is one of the most common causes of shoulder pain in the athlete (64, 65). Impingement is defined as encroachment of the acromion coracoacromial ligament and the acromioclavicular joint on the rotator cuff mechanism that passes beneath them when the glenohumeral joint is moved (see Fig. 51.21A). Recently, a close relationship of impingement to lesions of the rotator cuff, biceps, subacromial bursa, and acromioclavicular joint has been recognized. Impingement lesions can be classified as outlet impingement and nonoutlet impingement.

Outlet impingement is by far the most common type and is defined as narrowing of the supraspinatus outlet (66) (see Fig. 51.21*B*). The impingement occurs against the anterior one-third of the acromion and the acromioclavicular joint. Narrowing of the supraspinatus outlet can be caused by an anterior acromial spur at the attachment site of the coracoacromial ligament. These spurs rarely occur in patients under the age of 40 years (66). The shape of the acromion, the slope of the acromion, and the prominence of the acromioclavicular joint all can result in outlet impingement. The shape of the supraspinatus outlet can be radiographically evaluated by the "outlet view."

Nonoutlet impingement occurs with a normal supraspinatus outlet. Causes of nonoutlet impingement include a prominent greater tuberosity of the humerus, malunion of the greater tuberosity fracture or surgical neck fracture, lesions of the acromion, thickening of the subacromial bursa, loss of humeral head depression, and loss of glenohumeral fulcrum (66). When the deltoid contracts, the humeral head is displaced upward. The rotator cuff and biceps tendon act to prevent the ascent of the humeral head. Loss of the stabilizing function of the rotator cuff causes displacement of the humeral head upward and results in impingement. Loss of these stabilizing factors can occur with rotator cuff tears or tears of the long head of the biceps. An unstable head that subluxates anteriorly due to capsular laxity may displace upward against the acromion. This creates two clinical problems that can coexist: instability and impingement (67, 68). Once the shoulder is sufficiently stabilized either though physical therapy or surgical intervention, the impingement is usually eliminated.

Impingement that is caused by instability of the glenohumeral joint is referred to as secondary impingement (67, 68). Secondary impingement may be the most common type of impingement seen in young athletes. As already noted, overhead activities in the athlete place tremendous stress on the dynamic and static stabilizers of their shoulders. Repetitive stresses result in microtrauma to the glenohumeral ligaments and eventually may lead to attenuation of these structures. Without these stabilizers, an instability pattern can develop that places increasing demands on the rotator cuff. Fatigue of the rotator cuff allows the humeral head to translate anteriorly and results in secondary mechanical impingement of the supraspinatus tendon on the coracohumeral arch. This overlap of impingement and instability was recognized by Jobe et al. (68). They noted that athletes who had shoulder pain and were involved in overhead activities could be divided into four groups based on their history, physical exam, and arthroscopic findings: *(a)* pure impingement; *(b)* instability secondary to anterior ligamentous labral injury with subsequent impingement; *(c)* instability caused by hyperelastic capsular ligaments and tissues with secondary impingement; and *(d)* pure anterior instability.

The first group consists of athletes with pain secondary to pure impingement. The diagnosis of impingement is made by history and physical examination. A patient with impingement will usually have an arc of pain, i.e., when the arm is raised from the side and lowered from overhead at various positions, pain will occur. The arc through which this pain occurs is called the arc of pain. The examiner might also notice crepitus as the front and back edges of the acromion are palpated and the humerus is rotated. These athletes will have a positive impingement test. The impingement sign maneuver, however, may elicit pain in several other conditions as well, including frozen shoulder, glenohumeral instability, anterior acromioclavicular joint arthritis, and calcium deposits in the rotator cuff. Therefore, the impingement induction test is used to exclude these other conditions. In athletes with pure impingement, the joint will be stable on stress testing and will have a normal labrum and normal glenohumeral ligaments arthroscopically. These patients are usually over 35 years of age and should be placed on a 6-month program of strengthening and avoidence of offending activities. Most of the patients have been found to have a tight posterior capsule, which increases superior translation and aggravates impingement. Stretching of the posterior capsule is critical in treating these athletes. If nonoperative treatment fails, surgical treatment usually consists of an open or arthroscopic subacromial decompression with resection of the coracoacromial ligament.

The second group of athletes are those with impingement pain secondary to glenohumeral instability. These patients have pain with the apprehension test, a positive relocation test, and a positive impingement sign. Arthroscopic examination reveals either an anterior labral tear of deficient anterior-inferior glenohumeral ligament. Most of these athletes will improve with strengthening of the rotator cuff or scapular rotators. For those that do not improve with conservative strengthening exercises, operative repair of the capsular labral complex is an alternative. Because these patients have impingement secondary to instability, it is necessary to address their instability. An isolated anterior acromioplasty is unlikely to relieve their symptoms.

The third group of athletes consists of those with impingement pain secondary to instability because of hyperplastic capsular ligaments. Like the patients seen in group 2, these patient will have a positive impingement sign, positive apprehension test, and a positive relocation test. These patients may have generalized ligamentous laxity and an examination under anesthesia reveals laxity of both shoulders with the dominant one being most involved. Arthroscopic findings may include redundancy of the anterior capsule and a lax inferior glenohumeral ligament with an easily manipulated humeral head. Initial treatment involved strengthening of the rotator cuff and scapular rotators. If at the end of 6 months this treatment fails to relieve symptoms, an operative procedure may be necessary.

The fourth group of athletes are those with pure instability without impingement. These patients have a negative impingement sign but have pain with apprehension testing and relief of their pain with relocation. Arthroscopy in these patients may reveal labral damage and possibly a Hill-Sachs lesion. There may also be evidence of a loose anterior capsule and a lax inferior glenohumeral ligament complex. Treatment for this group consists of physical therapy. Again, if physical therapy fails to relieve symptoms, operative capsular reconstruction is indicated.

Impingement of the subacromial space is intimately related to rotator cuff disease. The wear on the humeral side is centered at the supraspinatus tendon. Neer (69) classified three progressive stages of outlet impingement leading to rotator cuff disease. In stage 1, there is edema and hemorrhage secondary to repetitive overhead activities. This lesion is typically seen in patients who are younger than 25 years old and is completely reversible with rest, oral antiinflammatories, and a strengthening program. In stage 2 impingement leading to rotator cuff disease, there is fibrosis and tendinitis from repeated mechanical insults. This type of impingement is usually seen in the 25- to 40-year-old age group. In patients who fail to respond to the nonoperative treatment and whose disability has persisted for more than 6 months, the authors approach is to remove the thickened fibrous subacromial bursa, divide the coracoacromial ligament, and perform an anterior acromioplasty, which is usually possible with an arthroscopic technique. Stage 3 lesions are categorized by complete impingement tears of the rotator cuff. These lesions are rare in patients under 40 years old, although athletes may present at a young age. If full restoration of strength is desired, it is usually necessary to repair the torn tendons in addition to performing an acromioplasty.

In the young athletic patient, on the other hand, rotator cuff tears may result from a breakdown of fibers within the tendons as a result of a repetitive microtrauma. This microtrauma is seen in activities that place unusual stresses on the shoulder and subject the rotator cuff tendons to large compressive and tensile forces and eccentric loading such as pitching. Occasionally cuff disruption in athletes can occur as the result of a single traumatic event such as an anterior shoulder dislocaton. This mechanism is more common in the older athlete, and it is now recommended that any individual older than 40 who has had an anterior dislocation and complains of persistent pain and weakness following closed reduction should be evaluated for a rotator cuff tear (70). While impingement may precede rotator cuff tears, it is more likely in the young athlete that repetitive high loads impinge the rotator cuff tendons during overhead activities and lead to gradual failure. This mechanism may be the cause of rotator cuff tears in competitive throwers. Rotator cuff tendon injures are rarer in swimmers. Rotator cuff inflammation most often results from transient shoulder instability (71, 72). This impingement-type pain does not represent true impingement but rather is the result of repetitive traction and compression of the rotator cuff during subluxation of the glenohumeral joint.

Many of the characteristics of rotator cuff tears seen in the elderly are not present in the young athletic patient. While the young will usually complain primarily of pain during and after activities, the older athlete may complain of weakness as well as pain. The throwing athlete with a rotator cuff tear will complain of a decreased velocity (78). The differential diagnosis of rotator cuff injuries in the throwing athlete includes glenohumeral subluxation, multidirectional instability, and nerve injury. On physical exam, the size of the tear may be determined by the loss of strength. A significant loss of external rotation strength usually indicates a large tear, involving the infraspinatus as well as the supraspinatus tendons.

In general, the treatment of a partial-thickness rotator cuff tear in a young athlete is a rotator cuff–strengthening program. If tendinitis persists but instability is absent, arthroscopic subacromial decompression may relieve pain, but the athlete may not be able to return to his or her previous level of overhead activity (72, 74). Operative repair usually gives excellent pain relief; however, the athlete's functional performance with overhead activities is variable. Following rotator cuff repair and 6 months of rehabilitation, throwing activities are begun gradually over the next several months. Swimmers may begin swimming the breast stroke at approximately 6 months after surgery (74–78).

Biceps Tendinitis and Subluxation

Biceps tendinitis and subluxation are causes of anterior shoulder pain in athletes involved in overhead activities (79, 80). The biceps tendon runs in the bicipital groove between the greater and lesser tuberosities. It is surrounded by a synovial sheath and is stabilized in the groove by the transverse humeral ligament. The biceps tendon functions as a depressor of the humeral head preventing upward migration into the acromion (81).

Biceps tendinitis can be classified as primary or secondary. Secondary biceps tendinitis is by far the more common problem and can result from osteoarthritis, rheumatoid arthritis, or impingement syndrome. The impingement syndrome, as previously noted, may be primary impingement or secondary to instability. With elevation and rotation of the arm, the biceps tendon becomes vulnerable to impingement between the head of the humerus, the acromion, and the coracoacromial ligament. Biceps tendinitis is most commonly seen in athletes who participate in golf, tennis, swimming, and throwing sports. The athlete usually complains of anterior shoulder pain that is less intense with rest. One or more of the previously mentioned provocative tests will be positive. The treatment of biceps tendinitis secondary to impingement closely follows that of impingement alone. If the impingement is caused by underlying glenohumeral instability, then the instability should be addressed (82).

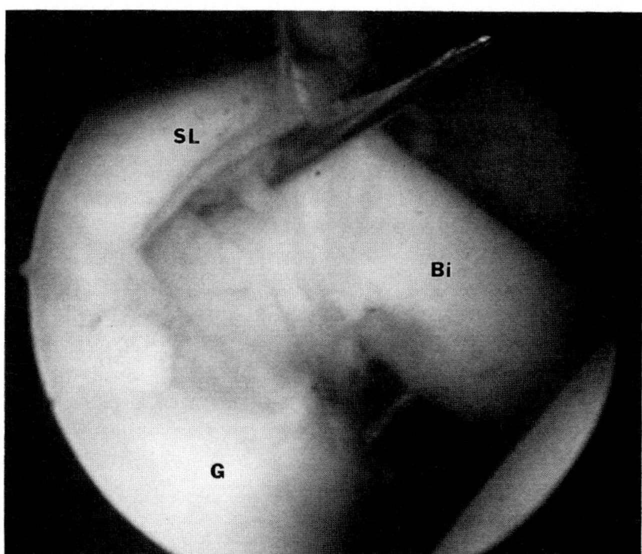

Figure 51.25. Arthroscopic view of a SLAP lesion. *Bi*, biceps; *SL*, superior labrum; *G*, glenoid. The probe is underneath the superior portion of the labral tear.

If the tendinitis is secondary to pure impingement and the athlete does not improve with conservative treatment, then an arthroscopic or open anterior acromioplasty should be considered. If the biceps tendon is extremely frayed in association with stage II impingement, biceps tenodesis may be indicated (83).

Biceps instability is often related to degeneration and associated with a tear of the subscapularis tendon (84). It is rare in the young athlete. Treatment involves repair of the rotator cuff, anterior acromioplasty, and fixation of the biceps tendon (85).

Recently, superior labrum anterior posterior (SLAP) lesions have been addressed (83) (Fig. 51.25). The SLAP lesion is a condition in which there is damage to the superior labrum of the shoulder from anterior to posterior in the area beneath the biceps tendon. These lesions have been associated with partial-thickness tears of the rotator cuff, compression injury to the superior humeral head, and anterior shoulder instability. The lesion of the biceps and labrum may be associated with instability of the glenohumeral joint (83). The most common cause appears to be the result of a compression injury from a fall onto the outstretched arm (83). The clinical examination is consistent with tenderness with resisted biceps motion, as noted by Speed's test. Ultrasound, plain x-rays, arthrogram, CT scans, and MRI are usually inconclusive, and the definitive diagnosis is made by arthroscopy. Based on the clinical symptoms of the patient and the findings at arthroscopy, a decision is made concerning treatment. The treatment options involve debridement or repair of the labrum and repair, resection, or tenodesis of the involved tendon (83).

Injuries to the Acromioclavicular Joint

Problems involving the acromioclavicular joint in athletes can be divided into two categories: acute traumatic injury and chronic pain. Chronic pain is usually the result of repetitive microtrauma such as weight lifting or repetitive overhead activities. The most common mechanism of injury to the acromioclavicular joint is a direct fall or direct blow to the acromion (35). The result of the shoulder being depressed is either a clavicular fracture or a tearing of the acromioclavicular ligaments. The acromioclavicular ligaments are primarily responsible for horizontal stability of the acromioclavicular joint. With progressively more severe trauma, the coracoclavicular ligaments will tear. The coracoclavicular ligaments are primarily responsible for vertical stability (86). In the most severe injuries involving the acromioclavicular joint, the deltoid and trapezius can be torn from their attachments on the outer end of the clavicle. Other less common mechanisms of injury include a fall onto the outstretched hand and an indirect downward force that may result from severe distraction of the abducted arm (35).

The most commonly used classification of acromioclavicular injuries is the six-grade classification (87, 88). This classification system is based on the degree of ligamentous damage and the direction of distal clavicular displacement.

Type I acromioclavicular separations are those in which there is no disruption of the acromioclavicular or coracoclavicular ligaments, but rather there is a stretch of the acromioclavicular ligament. With a type I injury the athlete experiences pain and tenderness on palpation. There is usually minimal displacement of the acromioclavicular joint seen on x-ray.

A type II separation involves disruption of the acromioclavicular ligament, but the coracoclavicular ligaments remain intact, whereas in a type III injury, the coracoacromial ligaments are disrupted as well. In type II and III injuries deformity of the joint is obvious, and there is exquisite tenderness over the joint. On x-ray, the distal clavicle in a type II injury is displaced up approximately one-half the normal superior inferior height of the joint compared with the normal side. In a type III injury, this distance is greater than one-half the normal superior-inferior height (Fig. 51.26). In certain cases, anterior-posterior stress views with 10 to 15 pounds of weight in each hand may be helpful for differentiation of a type II from a type III injury. Rockwood and Young (89) suggested that a 3-mm or 25% increase in the normal coracoclavicular distance of 1.1 to 1.3 cm compared with the other side is diagnostic of a complete disruption of the coracoclavicular ligaments.

In a type IV injury, the distal clavicle is displaced posteriorly and may be buttonholed through the trapezius muscle (Fig. 51.27). A type V injury is similar to a type III injury but more severe with disruption of the deltoid and trapezius attachments to the clavicle (Fig. 51.28). A type VI injury results from abduction forces. The distal clavicle is displaced underneath the acromion or coracoid process and may be associated with a brachial plexus injury (89).

Type I injuries are treated with ice for 24 hr, and then a sling is worn for 4 to 7 days until pain subsides. Once a full range of motion has been achieved and pain has resolved, athletic activity can be resumed. This time usually is 1 week. Type II injuries are treated with ice for 24 hr and in a sling for 1 to 2 weeks, followed by range-of-motion exercises. Athletic participation can usually be resumed in 3 to 4 weeks although throwing may require 6 weeks. There exists controversy concerning the treatment of type III injuries. The patient will usually not be clinically symptomatic following nonoperative treatment, but a cosmetic deformity will be present. Many studies have confirmed the fact that there is no objective or subjective evidence to support the conclusion that operative treatment of type III injuries is better than nonoperative treatments. Therefore, if the athlete accepts this deformity, the authors' treatment consists of a sling, range-of-motion exercises beginning at 1 week, and strengthening begun during the 2nd week. The athlete can usually return to throwing as soon as 4 weeks. Posterior displacement associated with type

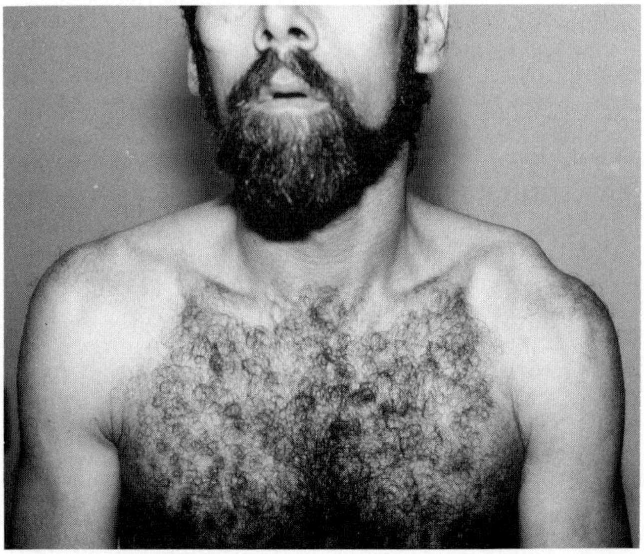

Figure 51.26. Patient with left shoulder type III A-C separation.

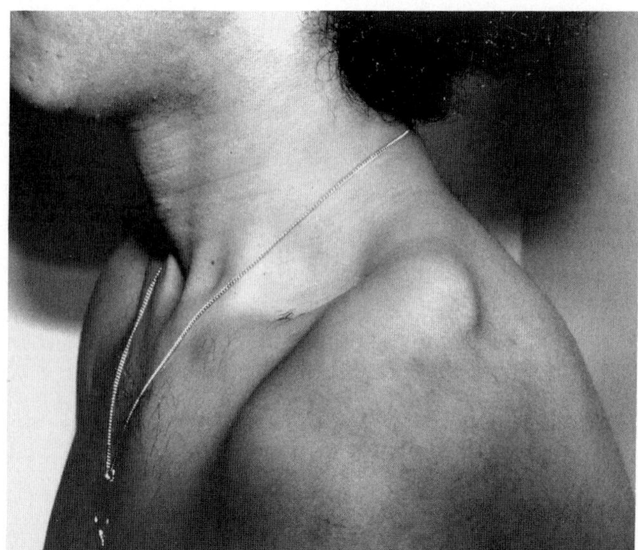

Figure 51.27. Patient with left shoulder type IV A-C separation. Note the posterior displacement.

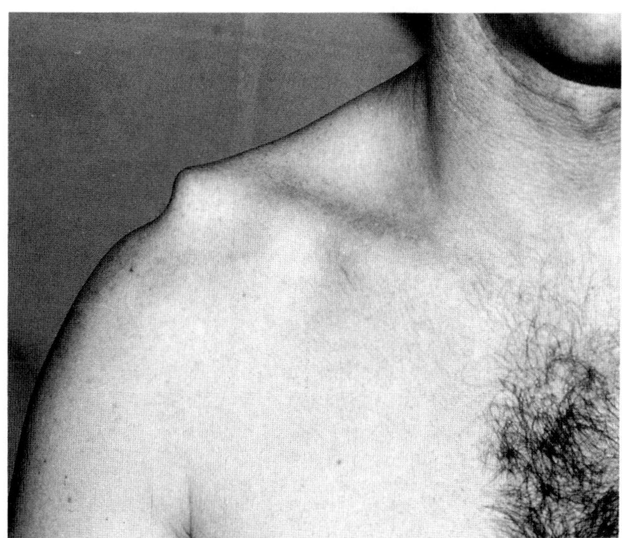

Figure 51.28. Type V A-C separaton. The distal clavicle is subcutaneous.

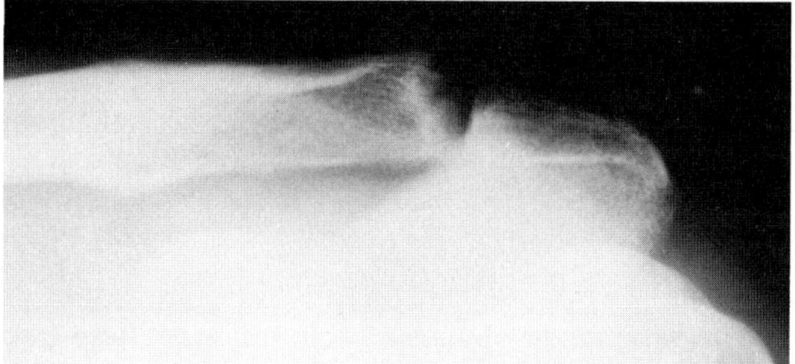

Figure 51.29. Distal clavicle osteolysis.

IV acute injuries is treated by the authors by open reduction and acromioclavicular fixation or ligamentous reconstruction (87, 89). Open reduction also is the treatment of choice for type V and VI injuries (87, 89).

Not all acromioclavicular joint injuries can be attributed to a single, specific injury. When subjected to the repetitive stresses experiences by baseball pitchers or when following a type I and type II dislocation, degenerative changes may occur. These changes may be associated with severe pain. Often there is narrowing of the joint with subchondral cyst and osteophyte formation. Long-term pain relief can be achieved by resection of the distal clavicle, which allows for return to competitive throwing (90).

Osteolysis of the distal clavicle may result from an acute injury or be the result of repeated stress on the shoulder (i.e., weight lifters) (91). Typical symptoms are those of a dull ache, which is exacerbated by overhead activities. A bone scan or AC joint injection may help to confirm the diagnosis (classic x-ray changes include osteoporosis, osteolysis, tapering, or osteophytes of the distal clavicle) (Fig. 51.29). The symptoms are usually self-limited and resolve with reduction of offending activities. If symptoms persist despite conservative treatment, distal clavicular resection is usually curative.

Sternoclavicular Joint

Traumatic dislocation of the sternoclavicular joint is a rare injury, because of the strong surrounding ligamentous structures and the tremendous forces required to dislocate the joint. The sternoclavicular joint may be injured either by direct or indirect trauma. A growing athlete usually sustains an epiphyseal fracture rather than a ligamentous dislocation following trauma. Traumatic injury may be classified in the adult as a mild sprain, if the ligaments remain intact and the joint is stable, and a moderate sprain, if there is anterior-posterior subluxation of the sternoclavicular joint. In the case of the moderate sprain, the ligaments are partially disrupted. A severe sprain is one with complete disruption of the sternoclavicular ligaments. This complete disruption or dislocation may be either anterior or posterior and presents with pain that is increased with arm movement. With an anterior injury, the medial end of the clavicle will be prominent anterior to the sternum. A posterior dislocation is more serious because of the possibility of the distal clavicle causing occlusion or tearing of large vessels as well as dyspnea from tracheal compression. X-rays of the sternoclavicular joint are often difficult to interpret, but occasionally an AP view of the chest will reveal asymmetry of the sternoclavicular joints. As mentioned previously, tomograms or CT scans may be necessary to view the dislocation.

The treatment of those injuries without instability involves only symptomatic treatment using a sling, ice, and gradual return to activities. A subluxation is usually treated with ice for 12 hr and then heat and a well-padded figure-eight clavicular strap. If the strap does not provide pain relief, then the arm is supported by a sling for 7 to 14 days. The athlete gradually increases arm motion until full motion is achieved. Most anterior dislocations are unstable. A reduction is carried out with suitable anesthesia and lateral traction placed on the abducted arm and direct pressure over the medial clavicle. A figure-eight bandage can be used to hold the reduction. Reduction may be lost but does not appear to interfere with normal shoulder function, and operative repair is usually not necessary (92).

If a posterior dislocation is present and there is evidence of compression of the great vessels in the neck or difficulty breathing or swallowing consistent with pressure on the mediastinum, it should be considered a medical emergency. The appropriate cardiothoracic specialist should be contacted, and closed reduction should be performed as soon as possible. Because of the serious complications associated with an unreduced posterior dislocation, an open reduction should be performed if closed reduction fails (92). Symptomatic chronic posterior dislocations of the sternoclavicular joint should be treated with a proximal clavicle resection (92).

Spontaneous recurrent dislocations of the clavicle are rare but may be present in athletes who have repeated stresses on the sternoclavicular joint. These athletes include swimmers and tennis players. These dislocations are usually anterior, and the patient complains of pain and weakness. When symptoms persist, surgery may be indicated to reduce and stabilize the sternoclavicular joint. Osteoarthritis secondary to trauma may develop and result in chronic pain. Chronic pain can usually be relieved by resection of the medial end of the clavicle.

Fractures

Fractures of the proximal humerus in the athlete are rare and the result of considerable trauma. These fractures may also be associated with glenohumeral dislocations. Fractures were classified according to Neer (93) by the number of major segments involved. For a segment to be considered displaced, it must be displaced 1 cm or angulated 45° from its original position. The four segments are the head, neck, greater tuberosity, and lesser tuberosity. A greater tuberosity fracture can be associated with an anterior dislocation of the glenohumeral joint, and a lesser tuberosity fracture is most often seen with a posterior dislocation. These fractures can be seen on the standard anterior-posterior lateral views in the scapular plane and axillary x-ray views. Following glenohumeral reduction, displacement of the fracture fragments requires an open reduction and internal fixation. With secure internal fixation, motion may be started immediately. Nondisplaced proximal humeral fractures may be treated with a sling and swathe until comfortable, and gentle range-of-motion exercises are recommended.

Glenoid fractures in athletes are also rare. Approximately 20% of traumatic shoulder dislocations have an associated glenoid rim fracture (35). These fragments are generally small and best seen on axillary x-rays or CT scans. On the other hand, a large central depression fraction can occur by violent central impact of the head of the humerus. These fractures may render the joint unstable and incongruous and require surgical treatment. Occasionally, osteochondral prominences can be seen at the posterior inferior aspect of the glenoid. These prominences have been seen in baseball pitchers and are attributed to violent triceps contracture during throwing (35).

Fractures of the body and spine of the scapula are rare and are usually associated with direct trauma. These injuries are usually treated by care for the surrounding soft tissues. This care involves ice for 48 hr followed by heat. The patient also is immobilized in a sling until comfortable (35).

Clavicular fractures can result from similar forces as those producing acromioclavicular separations. Approximately 80% of clavicular fractures involve the middle third of the clavicle, 15% involve the distal third, and 5% the proximal third (35). Fractures of the middle third usually can be manipulated into alignment and held in a modified shoulder spica or a sling. Fractures of the inner third that do not involve the joint can be treated with a supportive sling. Fractures of the distal third have been divided into three types (94). Group I, the most common type of distal clavicle fracture, have minimal displacement, intact coracoclavicular ligaments, and require only a sling for treatment, because the tendency for displacement and nonunion is low. In group II (distal clavicle fractures), the coracoclavicular ligaments are detached and are, therefore, unstable. The coracoclavicular ligaments remain with the lateral portion of the clavicle fracture. Because adequate reduction is difficult to maintain, open reduction and internal fixation are advocated for group II fractures of the distal clavicle. Group II fractures can lead to symptomatic arthritic changes in the acromioclavicular joint. These fractures can be subtle and may be misdiagnosed as a grade I AC separation. High-quality x-rays are necessary to detect these injuries. If x-rays are negative and there is a clinical suspicion, a CT scan may be helpful. These injuries are managed conservatively; however, if chronic pain persists, a simple distal clavicular resection will usually be curative (94).

Neurovascular Injuries about the Shoulder

Neurovascular problems in the shoulder of athletes are rare but potentially serious. It is important to include a thorough neurovascular examination in any athlete complaining of shoulder pain. Perhaps the most serious arterial problem recognized in the shoulder of a throwing athlete is an acute axillary artery thrombosis. A recent study concluded that repetitive overhead activities in throwers can cause intermittent compression and intimal contusion of the axillary artery by the humeral head (95). These changes result in a decreased blood flow and increase the likelihood of axillary artery thrombosis. Anterior instability produces more impingement of the artery and increases the potential for thrombosis. The clinical presentation may vary from muscle ache, fatigue, intermittent paresthesia, to loss of pulses, cyanosis, and decreased skin temperature. When the diagnosis is suspected, an arteriogram is usually necessary for confirmation. Acute treatment consists of thrombotic therapy with possible need for long-term anticoagulation.

Neurologic entrapment syndromes include suprascapular nerve entrapment, quadrilateral syndrome, and thoracic outlet syndrome. The suprascapular nerve is a motor nerve origination from the C5-C6 nerve roots and passes to the upper border of the scapula and through the scapular notch. The scapular notch is roofed by the transverse scapular ligament. The nerve innervates the supraspinatus before passing along the neck of the scapular spine, where it then innervates the infraspinatus. The cause of the suprascapular nerve dysfunction may be from entrapment of the nerve as it passes throughout the suprascapular notch, a traction injury in the spinous glenoid area, or vascular compromise to the nerve (96). Because the supraspinatus and infraspinatus are not functioning properly, other problems may occur such as rotator cuff tendinitis and bicipital tendinitis. The athlete with suprascapular nerve entrapment may complain of deep diffuse pain often localized to the posterior lateral aspect of the shoulder, but it may radiate down the arm or into the neck (96). On physical examination, the athlete may have pain with adduction of the extended arm and/or tenderness to pressure over the suprascapular notch. There may also be significant wasting of the infraspinatus alone or in combination with the supraspinatus, depending on the level of entrapment. The diagnosis may be confirmed by electromyographic (EMG) studies. Initial treatment includes rest, flexibility, and a strengthening program (97). Chronic cases may require a surgical release of the nerve.

The quadrilateral space syndrome results from compression of the neurovascular structures that pass through the quadrilateral space. The quadrilateral space is formed laterally by the neck of the humerus, medially by the long head of the biceps, superiorly by the teres minor, and inferiorly by the teres major. The axillary nerve and posterior humeral circumflex vessels pass through this space. These structures can be compressed during throwing when the arm is maximally abducted and externally rotated (98). The athlete may complain of pain or paresthesis with a particularly hard throw or during the accleration phase of throwing (99). The examination of the shoulder may be normal except for tenderness over the quadrilateral space. EMG studies are usually normal and the diagnosis is confirmed by a subclavian arteriogram, which will reveal occlusion of the posterior humeral circumflex artery during humeral abduction and external rotation. Surgical decompression may be necessary for athletes who remain symptomatic.

Thoracic outlet syndrome is a complex of symptoms resulting from neurovascular compression to the arm. The clinical presentation may vary, depending on the structures involved. The athlete may have vague complaints and confusing physical signs (100). The thoracic outlet is defined as the area in which the great vessels leave the chest to enter the arm and the nerves exit the neck to joint them. The brachial plexus courses to the upper extremity through the interscalene interval formed by the anterior scalene muscle anteriorly, the middle scalene posterolaterally, and the anterior surface of the first rib. Direct or indirect injury to the scalene muscles or muscular imbalance of the suspensory muscles of the scapula can result in compression (101). Two other potential sites of compression include the clavicle compression on the first rib with shoulder abduction and in the subacromial region at the insertion of the tendon of the pectoralis minor.

The clinical presentation may vary and include pain in the shoulder and arm paresthesia (usually along the ulnar aspect of the forearm) and weakness of the ulnar-nerve-innervated intrinsics. The periodicity of symptoms and their relationship to the position of the arm and shoulder are crucial in the diagnosis (102). Symptoms of venous occlusion include pain and swelling following activities.

The physical examination should include careful evaluation of the cervical spine and trapezius muscles and intrinsic musculature of the hands. An overhead exercise test is performed by having the patient elevate the arms and flex and extend the fingers. A positive test is one in which cramping and fatigue occurs within 20 sec. Several provocative tests have been described, including Adson's and Wright's maneuvers. In Adson's maneuver, the arm is placed at the side and the

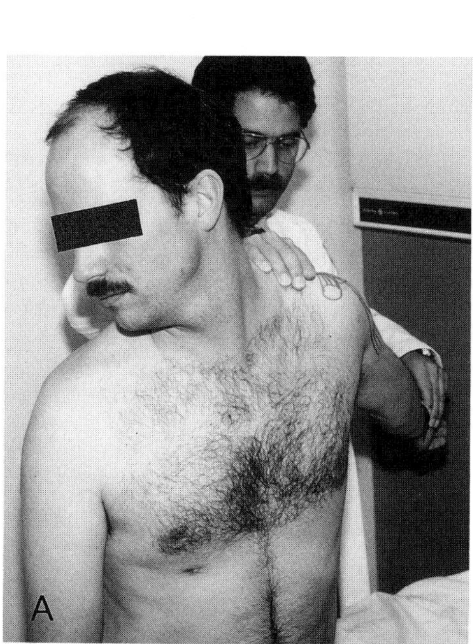

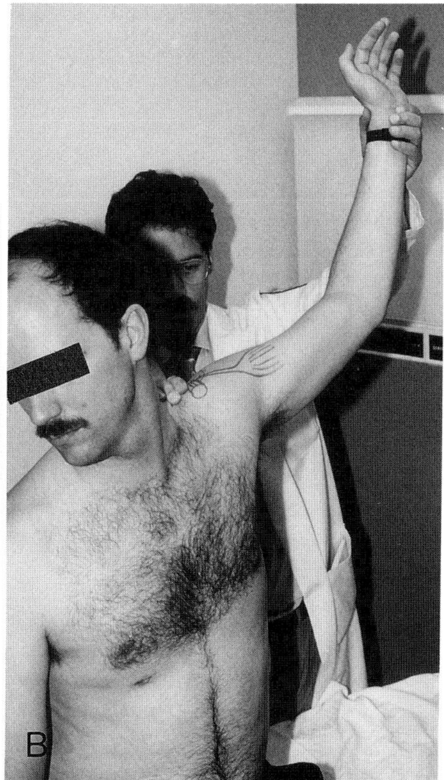

Figure 51.30. **A,** Adson's maneuver for thoracic outlet syndrome. **B,** Wright's maneuver for thoracic outlet syndrome.

neck is rotated to the ipsilateral side and hyperextended while the patient inspires. In Wright's maneuver, the arm is abducted and externally rotated with the neck rotated to the opposite side (Fig. 51.30). The patient then takes a deep breath in order to reproduce symptoms.

X-rays should include the cervical spine and first rib. Nerve conduction studies are useful to rule out more peripheral lesions, such as ulnar neuropathy at the wrist or elbow or carpal tunnel syndrome. Noninvasive vascular studies should be obtained in symptomatic patients. The differential diagnosis includes cervical spine abnormalities, lesions at the lung apex, brachial neuritis, carpal tunnel syndrome, reflex sympathetic dystrophy, and shoulder pathology.

Most athletes respond to conservative therapy, involving heat, ultrasound, massage, oral antiinflammatory agents, and an exercise program. The exercise program should emphasize correction of postural abnormalities and strengthening of the muscles of the neck and shoulder girdle. In those athletes who do not respond to conservative treatment in 2 to 3 months, surgical intervention should be considered (102). Surgical intervention may involve first rib resection or release of the anterior scalene muscles.

REFERENCES

1. Hill JA. Epidemiologic perspective on shoulder injuries. Clin Sport Med. 1983;2(2):24–246.
2. Slager RF. From Little League to big league, the weak spot in the arm. Am J Sports Med 1977;10:37–48.
3. Yocum LA. Reporting athletic injuries. Paper presented at the 81st annual meeting of Major League physicians and trainers, Dec. 6, 1982, Honolulu.
4. Dagiau RF, Dillman CJ, Milner EK. Relationship between exposure time and injury in football. Am J Sports Med 1980;8:257–260.
5. Weiker GG. Club gymnastic. Symposium in gymnastics. Clin Sports Med. 1985;4:39,1985.
6. Kennedy JC, Hawkins RJ: Swimmers shoulder. Phys Sportsmed 1974;2:35–38.
7. Dominquez RH. Shoulder pain in age group swimmers. In: Eriksson B, Furbert B, eds. Swimming medicine. Vol. 4. Baltimore: University Park Press, 1978;105–109.
8. McCarrol JR, Gioe TJ. Professional golfers and the price they pay. Phys Sportsmed 1982;10:64.
9. Henry JH, Lareau B, Neigut D. The injury rate in professional basketball. Am J Sport Med 1982;10:16–18.
10. Carr D, Johnson RJ, Pope MH. Upper extremity injuries in skiing. Am J Sports Med 1981;9:378–383.
11. Yokoe K, Nanjima H, Yamazaki Y, et al. Injuries of the shoulder in volleyball players and javelin throwers. Orthop Trauma Surg 1959;22:351–359.
12. Galinat BJ, Howell SM. The containment mechanism: the primary stabilizer of the glenohumeral joint. Orthop Trans 1988;12:458.
13. Howell SM, Galinat BJ. The glenoid-labral socket: a constrained articular surface Clin Orthop 1989;243:122–125.
14. Warner JP, Deng X, Warren RF, Torzilli PA, O'Brien SJ, Altchek DW. Static capsuloligamentous restraints to superior-inferior translation of the glenohumeral joint. Am J Sport Med 1992;20:625–685.
15. Schwartz RE, O'Brien SJ, Warren RF, Torzilli PA. Capsular restraints to anterior posterior motion of the abducted shoulder: a biomechanical study. Orthop Trans 1988;12:727.
16. Perry J. Anatomy and biomechanics of the shoulder in throwing, swimming, gymnastics, and tennis. Clin sports Med 1983;2:247–270.
17. King JW, et al. Analysis of the pitching arm of the professional baseball pitcher. Clin Orthop 1979;67:16.
18. Pappas AM, Zawacki RM, Sullivan TJ. Biomechanics of baseball pitching. Am J Sports Med 1983;13:223–235.
19. Gowan ID, Job FW, Tibone JE, et al. A comparative electromyographic analysis of the shoulder during pitching. Am J Sports Med 1987;15:586.
20. Richardson AB, Job FW, Collins HR. The shoulder in swimming competition. Am J Sports Med 1980;81:159.
21. Hawkins RJ, Hubeika PE. Impingement syndrome in the athletic shoulder on injuries to the shoulder in the athlete. Clin Sports Med 1983;2:391.
22. Neer CS II. Shoulder reconstruction. Philadelphia: WB Saunders, 1990.
23. Steiner ME. Hypermobility and knee injuries. Phys Sportsmed 1987;15:159–165.
24. Schwartz E, Warren RF, O'Brien SJ, et al. Posterior shoulder instability. Orthop Clin North Am 1987;18:409–419.
25. Beighton PH, Horam FT. Dominant inheritance on familial generalized articular hypermobility. J Bone Joint Surg 1970;52B:145–147.
26. Jobe FW, Bradley JP. Rotator cuff injuries in basketball. Am J Sports Med 1988;6:378–389.
27. Hawkins RJ, Schutte JP, Huckell GH, et al. The assessment of glenohumeral translation sing manual and fluoroscopic techniques. Orthop Trans 1988;12:727–728.
28. Hawkins RJ, Bokor DJ. Clinical evaluation of shoulder problems. In: Rockwood CA, Matsen FA, eds. The shoulder. Philadelphia: WB Saunders, 1990;167–169.
29. Neer CS II. Impingement lesions. Clin Orthop 1983;173:70.
30. Hoppenfeld S. Physical examination of the spine and extremities: New York: Appleton-Century Crofts, 1976.
31. Burkhead WZ. The biceps tendon. In: Rockwood, CA, Matsen FA, eds. The shoulder. Philadelphia: WB Saunders, 1990;791–832.
32. Yerguson RM. Rupture of the biceps. J Bone Joint Surg 1931;13:160.
33. Gilcrest EL, Albi P. Unusual lesions of muscles and tendons of the shoulder girdle and upper arm. Surg Gynecol Obstet 1939;68:903–917.
34. Steindler A. Interpretation of pain in the shoulder. In: WA Larmon, ed. AAOS Instructional Course Lecture. Ann Arbor, MI: JW Edwards, 1958:159.
35. Neer CS II, Rockwood CA. Fractures and dislocations of the shoulder. In: Rockwood CA, Green DP, eds. Fracture. 2nd ed. Philadelphia: JP Lippincott, 1984;675–950.
36. Zanca P. Shoulder pain: involvement of the A-C joint: analysis of 1000 cases. AJR AM J Roentgenol 1971;112(3):493–506.
37. Neer CS II. Displaced proximal humeral fractures. J Bone Joint Surg 1970;52A:1077–1089.
38. McLaughlin H. Posterior dislocation of the shoulder. J Bone Joint Surg 1952;34A:524–590.
39. Neviaser RJ. Radiologic assessment of the shoulder: plane and arthrographic. Orthop Clin North AM 1987;18(3):343–349.
40. Rockwood CA, et al. X-ray evaluation of shoulder problems. In: Rockwood CA, Matsen FA, eds. The shoulder. Philadelphia: WB Saunders, 1990:178–207.
41. Rubin SA, Gray RL, Green WR. The scapular "Y" view—a diagnostic aid in shoulder trauma. Radiology 1974;110:725–726.
42. Bloom MH, Obata WG. Diagnosis of posterior dislocation of the shoulder with use of Velpeau axillary and angle up roentgenographic views. J Bone Joint Surg 1967;49A(5):943–949.
43. Hill HA, Sachs MD. The grooved defect of the humeral head: a frequently unrecognized complication of dislocations of the shoulder joint. Radiology 1940;35:690–700.
44. Hall RH, Isaac F, Booth CR. Dislocations of the shoulder with special reference to accompanying small fractures. J Bone Joint Surg 1959;41A(3):489–497.
45. Bankart ASB. Recurrent or habitual dislocation of the shoulder joint. Br Med J 1923;2:1132–1133.
46. Pappas AM, Goss TP, Kleinman PK. Symptomatic shoulder instability due to lesions of the glenoid labrum. Am J Sports Med 1983;11:279.
47. Matsui K, Ogawa K. Pneumoarthro-computed tomography of the

shoulder joint for anterior and multidirectional instability. In: Post M, Morrey BF, Hawkins RJ, eds. Surgery of the shoulder. St. Louis: CV Mosby, 1990;14–17.
48. Shuman WP, Kilcoyn RF, Matsen FA III, Rogers JV, et al. Double contrast computed tomography of the glenoid labrum. AJR AM J Roentgenol 1983;141:581–584.
49. Bigliani LU, Morrison D, April EW. Morphology of the acromion and its relationship to rotator cuff tears. Orthop Trans 1986;10:228.
50. Craig EV, Fitts HM, Crass JR. Noninvasive imaging of the rotator cuff. In: Post M, Morrey BF, Hawkins RJ, eds. Surgery of the shoulder. St. Louis: CV Mosby, 1990;6–10.
51. Resch H, Furtshegger A, Diterzur N, Glotzer W, Wanitschk P. The value of different screening methods in the diagnosis of shoulder lesions: ultrasonography, arthrography, CT, MR imaging, arthroscopy, bursoscopy. In: Post M, Morrey BF, Hawkins RJ, eds. Surgery of the shoulder. St. Louis: CV Mosby, 1990:22–26.
52. Hodler J, Fretz CJ, Terrier F, Gerber C. Rotator cuff tears: correlation of sonographic and surgical findings. Radiology 1988;169:791–794.
53. Mack LA, Matsen FA, Kilkoyne RF, Dovies PK, et al. Ultrasonic evaluation of the rotator cuff. Radiology 1983;157:205–209.
54. Fisk C. Adaptation of the technique of radiography of the bicipital groove. Radiology Tech 1965;37:47–50.
55. Hawkins RJ, Kennedy JC. Impingement syndrome in athletes. Am J Sports Med 1980;8:151–158.
56. Middleton WD, Reinus WR, Tooty WG, et al. Ultrasonographic evaluation of the rotator cuff and biceps tendon. J Bone Joint Surg 1986;68A(3):440–450.
57. Neer CS II, Foster CR. Inferior capsular shift for involuntary inferior and multidirectional instability of the shoulder. J Bone Joint Surg 1980;62:897–908.
58. Altchek DW, Warren RF, Skyhar MJ, Ortiz G. T-plasty modification of the Bankart procedure for multidirectional instability of the anterior and inferior types. J Bone Joint Surg 1991;73A:105–112.
59. Baker CL. Arthroscopic evaluation of the unstable shoulder. Operat Tech Orthop 1991;1(2):164–170.
60. Neer CS II. Dislocation. In: Shoulder reconstruction. Philadelphia: WB Saunders, 1990:299–309.
61. Hawkins RJ, Bell RH, Hawkins RH, Koppert GJ. Anterior dislocations of the shoulder in the older patient. Clin Orthop 1986;206:192.
62. Rowe CR, Sakellarides HT. Factors related to recurrences of anterior dislocations of the shoulder. Clin Orthop 1961;20:40.
63. Skyhar MJ, Warren FR, Altchek DW. Instability of the shoulder. In: Nicholas JA, Hershman EB, eds, The upper extremity in sport medicine. St. Louis: CV Mosby, 1990:181–220.
64. Hawkins RJ, Kennedy JC. Impingement syndrome in athletes. Am J Sports Med 1980;8:151.
65. Tibone JE, et al. Surgical treatment of tears of the rotator cuff in athletes. J Bone Joint Surg 1986;68A:887.
66. Neer CS II. Cuff tears, biceps lesions and impingement. In: Shoulder reconstruction. Philadelphia: WB Saunders, 1990:41–142.
67. Fu FH, Harner CD, Klein AH. Shoulder impingement syndrome. Clin Orthop 1991;269:162–173.
68. Jobe FW, Tibone JE, Jobe CM, Kvitne RS. The shoulder in sports. In: Rockwood CA, Matsen FA, eds. The shoulder. Philadelphia: WB Saunders, 1990:961–990.
69. Neer CS II. Impingement lesions. Clin Orthop 1983;173:70.
70. Neviaser RJ, Neviaser TJ, Neviaser JS. Concurrent rupture of the rotator cuff and anterior dislocation of the shoulder in the older patient. J Bone Joint Surg 1988;70:1308.
71. Jobe FW, Giangara CE, Glousman RE, Kuitne RS. Anterior capsulolabral reconstruction in throwing athletes. Paper presented at the annual meeting of Shoulder and Elbow Surgeons, Las Vegas, Feb. 12, 1989.
72. Altchek, DW, Skyhar MJ, Warren FR, Wickiewicz TL. Arthroscopic acromioplasty: a prospective analysis of 43 patients. Paper presented at the annual meeting of Shoulder and Elbow Surgeons; Las Vegas, Feb. 12, 1989.
73. Warner JJP, Warren RF. Consideration and management of rotator cuff tears in athletes. Ann Chir Gynaecol 1991;80:160–167.
74. Tibone JE, Elrod B, Jobe FW, et al. Surgical treatment of the tears of the rotator cuff in athletes. J Bone Joint Surg 1986;68:887.
75. Ellman H, Hanker G, Bayer M. Repair of the rotator cuff end-result study of factors influencing reconstruction. J Bone Joint Surg 1986;68:1136.
76. Gore DR, Murray MP, Sepic SB, Gardiner GM. Shoulder muscle-strength and range of motion following surgical repair of full-thickness rotator cuff tears. J Bone Joint Surg 1986;68:266.
77. Hawkins, RJ, Misamore GW, Hubeik PE. Surgery of full thickness rotator cuff tears. J Bone Joint Surg 1985;67:1349.
78. Bigliani, LU, Kimmel J, McCann PD, Wolfe, I. Repair of the rotator cuff in tennis players. Am J Sports Med 1992;20:112.
79. McCue FC III, et al. Throwing injuries to the shoulder. In: Zarins B, Andrew JR, Carson WG, eds. Injuries to the throwing arm. Philadelphia: WB Saunders, 1985:98.
80. O'Donohue D. Subluxating biceps tendon in the athlete. Clin Orthop 1982;164:26.
81. Lucas DB. Biomechanics of the shoulder joint. Arch Surgery 1973;107:425–432.
82. Burkhead WZ. The biceps tendon. In: Rockwood, CA, Matsen FA, eds. The shoulder. Philadelphia: WB Saunders, 1990:827–829.
83. Synder SJ, Wuh HCK. Arthroscopic evaluation and treatment of the rotator cuff and superior labrum anterior posterior lesion. Operat Tech Orthop 1991;1(3):207–220.
84. Gerber C, Krushell RJ. Isolated rupture of the tendon of the subscapularis muscle. J Bone Joint Surg 1991;73B:389.
85. Abbott LC, Snders LB de CM. Acute traumatic dislocation of the tendon of the long head of biceps brachii: report of 6 cases with operative findings. Surgery 1939;6:817–840.
86. Fukuda K, Craig EV, et al. Biomechanical study of the ligamentous system of the acromioclavicular joint. J Bone Joint Surg 1986;68A:434–439.
87. Gerber C, Rockwood CA. Subcoracoid dislocation of the lateral end of the clavicle: a report of three cases. J Bone Joint Surg 1987;69A:924–927.
88. Tossy JD, Mead NC, Sigmond HM. Acromioclavicular separations: useful and practical classification for treatment. Clin Orthop 1963;28:111–119.
89. Rockwood CA, Young CD. Disorders of the acromioclavicular joint. In: Rockwood CA, Matsen FA, eds. The shoulder. Philadelphia: WB Saunders, 1990;413–476.
90. Cook F, Tibone JE. The Mumford procedure in athletes. Am J Sports Med 1988;16(2):97–100.
91. Madsen B. Osteolysis of the acromial end of the clavicle following trauma. Br J Radio 1963;36:822.
92. Rockwood CA. Disorders of the sternoclavicular joint. In: Rockwood CA, Matsen FA, eds. The shoulder. Philadelphia: WB Saunders, 1990:477–525.
93. Neer CS II. Displaced proximal humeral fractures part I: classification and evaluation. J Bone Joint Surg 1970;52A:1077–1089.
94. Neer CS II. Fractures of the distal third of the clavicle. Clin Orthop 1968;58:43.
95. Rohrer MJ, et al. Axillary artery compression and thrombosis in throwing athletes. J Vasc Surg 1990;11:761–769.
96. Post M, Mayer J. Suprascapular nerve entrapment: diagnosis and treatment. Clin Orthop 1987;223:126–136.
97. Pappas AM. Injuries of the shoulder complex and overhand throwing problems. In: Grana WA, Kalenek A, eds. Clinics in sports medicine. 1991:335–360.
98. Redler MR, et al. Quadrilateral space syndrome in the throwing athlete. Am J Sports Med 1986;14:511–513.
99. Gambardella RA, Job FA, Nicholas JA. Diagnosis and treatment of shoulder injuries in throwers. In: Hershman EB, ed. The upper extremity in sports medicine. St. Louis: CV Mosby, 1990:751–766.
100. Strukel RJ, et al. Thoracic outlet syndrome in the throwing athlete. Am J Sports Med 1978;6:35.
101. Capistrant TD. Thoracic outlet syndrome in whiplashing. Ann Surg 1977;185:175–178.
102. Leffert RD. Thoracic outlet syndrome and the shoulder. Clin Sports Med 1983;2(2):439–452.

52 / ELBOW INJURIES

James P. Bradley

Anatomy and Biomechanics

Comprehension of the basic anatomy and biomechanics of the elbow is helpful in both the diagnosis and treatment of athletic elbow maladies. Although a detailed description of the anatomy and biomechanics of the elbow is beyond the scope of this chapter, some salient points are highlighted.

The elbow articulation is one of the most congruous joints in the body and, therefore, is one of the most stable. This characteristic is the result of an almost equal contribution from the soft tissue constraints and the articular surfaces. Static stability is provided by the articular surface and ligamentous and capsular structures, while dynamic stability is provided by the musculotendinous units crossing the elbow. The elbow functions as a hinge or pin-type joint. This has been illuminated by investigations of the joint surface contact area, of the collateral ligaments, and of the importance of the proximal ulna to elbow stability (1, 2). Normal range of motion of the elbow is (*a*) 0° to 150° flexion/extension, (*b*) 80° pronation, and (*c*) 85° supination. Functional testing has shown that for most activities of daily living 30° to 130° flexion/extension and 50° pronation and supination are required (1).

The primary stabilizer of the elbow is the medial collateral ligament complex, which is composed of three distinct bundles: the anterior bundle; the posterior bundle; and the transverse bundle (Fig. 52.1). The anterior and posterior bundles stabilize the elbow to valgus stresses, whereas the transverse bundle adds little to elbow stability. Biomechanically, the medial ligamentous complex tightens as the elbow is flexed as a result of the bony cam effect that is created.

The lateral ligamentous complex is the prime stabilizer to varus stress. Unlike the medial complex, the lateral complex is less discreet and some individual variation is common (3). The radial collateral ligament originates from the base of the lateral epicondyle and inserts on the annular ligament. The annular ligament provides stability by tightening from the pull of the supinator muscle during forearm supination (Fig. 52.2) (1). The lateral ulnohumeral ligament originates from the inferior lateral epicondyle and inserts onto the crista supinators of the ulna. Morrey and An (1) have shown that this ligament plays an important role in elbow stability, particularly after radial head excision. Incompetence of the lateral ulnohumeral ligament can be documented by a "lateral pivot shift" of the proximal ulna on the humerus (4).

The bony articular anatomy is a significant contributor to elbow stability. Theoretically, elbow stability can be considered to be approximately 50% a function of the collateral ligaments and anterior capsule and 50% of a function of the bony articulation, primarily from the ulnohumeral joint (5). An and Morrey (6) showed that with serial excision of the olecranon (25%, 50%, 75%, 100%) that there is a near linear decrease in elbow stability provided by the ulnohumeral joint in both 0° and 90° of flexion. The olecranon and distal humerus (trochlea) are steadfastly seated together during compressive loads by contractions of the brachialis and biceps muscles, thus providing important anteroposterior stability, especially during lifting. Recently, the stabilizing effect of the radial head on the elbow was examined. The radial head does furnish some resistance to varus stress, varying between 15% and 30%, depending on the load configuration and orientation of the joint (7). Studies of force transmission across the elbow have shown that forces across the radial head are greatest in the first 0° to 30° of flexion and decrease with further flexion (2). During valgus stress, the radial head absorbs 30% of the initial load, and the anterior capsule and medial collateral complex share the remaining stress (2). The resistance of the radial head to valgus stress may be more during throwing, but additional information is needed to better understand the role of the radial head during throwing (8).

Varus stress applied during extension shows that the anterior capsule carries 30%, the joint surface 50%, and the radial collateral ligament complex 15% of the applied load (2). In flexion, however, the joint surface

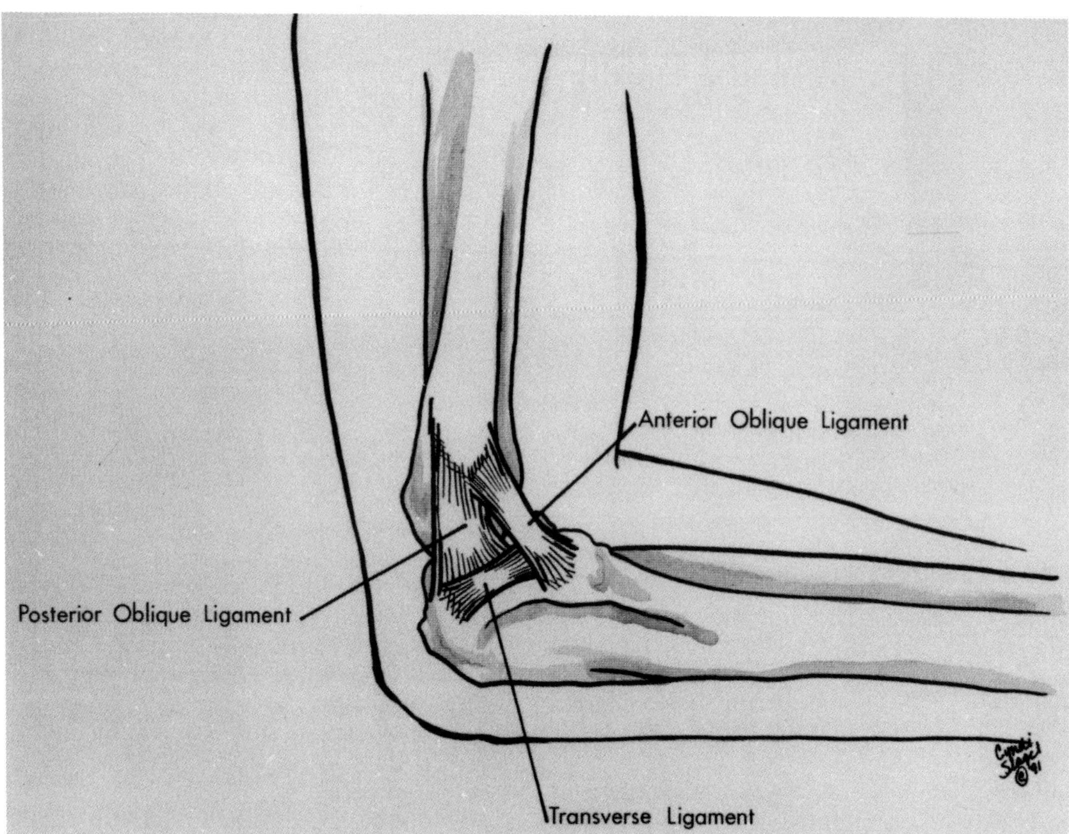

Figure 52.1. Medial collateral ligament complex of the elbow.

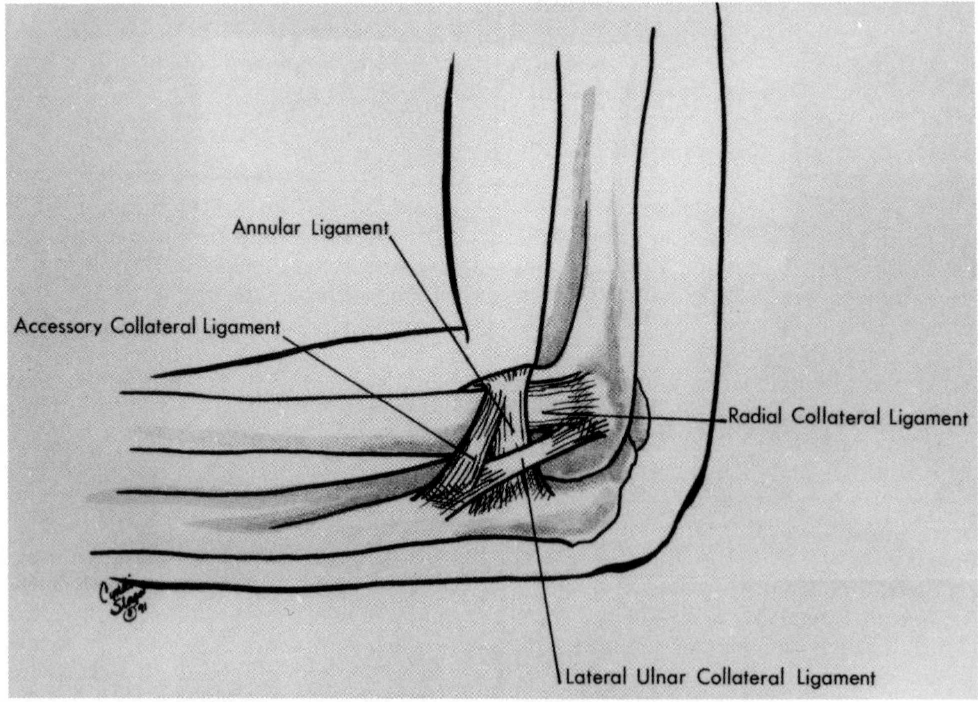

Figure 52.2. Lateral collateral ligament complex of the elbow.

supports 75% of the load, and the radial collateral complex supports only 10% (2).

The amount of force transmitted across the joint varies with specific factors which include (*a*) loading configuration and (*b*) angular orientation of the joint. A magnitude of close to three times body weight has been speculated in certain functions (8, 9). Activities of daily living necessitate approximately 50% of body weight transmitted across the joint, with maximal loads noted at about 90° of flexion (10, 11).

These studies primarily examined the elbow during activities of daily living and isometric lifting, which cannot be extrapolated to the tremendous demands imposed on the elbow during throwing and contact sports. Considering this, it is not surprising that a small deficiency in the elaborate stability and controlling mechanisms of the elbow would have a significant and cumulative effect on elbow function during sports.

Throwing Injuries

Athletes who participate in overhead sports can sustain myriad injuries to the elbow. Chronic stress is initiated by the repetitious high-velocity nature of these activities and often predispose the elbow to overuse syndromes. Many of these overhead activities (e.g., baseball pitch, tennis serve, javelin throw, slap shot in hockey, and football pass) require similar movements: rapid forceful extension of the elbow, frequently accompanied by valgus stress and pronation of the forearm. It is estimated that the range of motion of the elbow exceeds 300° per second during throwing. The forces at the elbow include (*a*) traction of the medial side, (*b*) compression of the lateral side, and (*c*) medial shear posteriorly (Fig. 52.3). The normal valgus angle of the elbow in extension may particularly bias the medial aspect of the elbow to overuse injuries. The velocity, power, and repetitiousness of the throwing motion all contribute to the ensuing microtrauma. Thus overuse injuries are encountered when the body's physiologic ability to heal itself lags behind the incessant microtrauma.

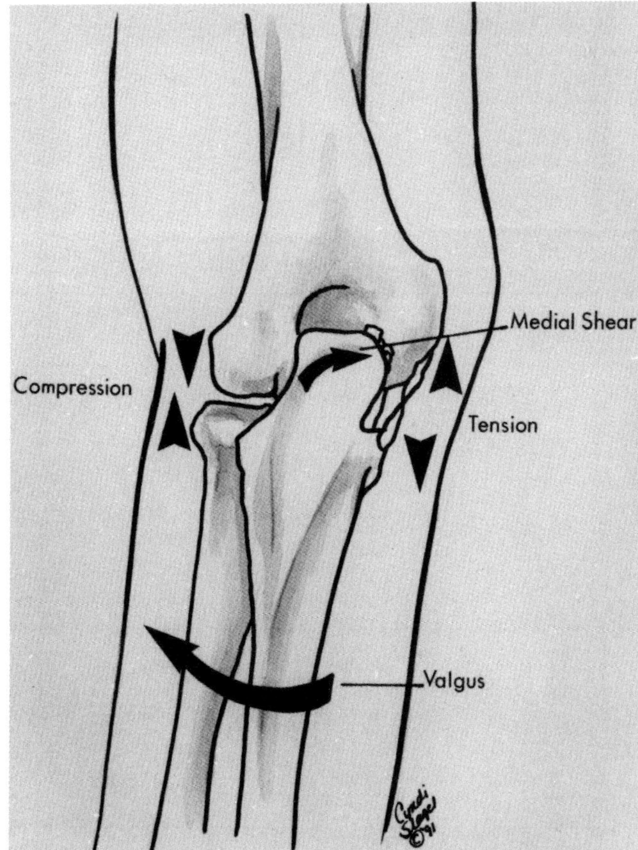

Figure 52.3. Elbow forces during throwing.

Young Athletes

The generic term *Little League elbow* has been commonly used to depict a group of pathologic entities in and about the elbow joint in young, immature throwers. It is important to realize that each of these entities are specific elbow injuries with individual personalities regarding prognosis and treatment. In addition, it is salient to understand that the throwing motion is common to many sports (e.g., the tennis serve, football pass, and javelin throw). The typical pathologies include (*a*) medial epicondylar fragmentation and avulsion (Fig. 52.4), (*b*) delayed or accelerated apophyseal growth of the medial epicondyle, (*c*) delayed closure of the medial epicondylar physis, (*d*) osteochondrosis and osteochondritis of the capitellum (Fig. 52.5), (*e*) deformation and osteochondrosis of the radial head, (*f*) hypertrophy of the ulna, and (*g*) olecranon apophysitis with or without delayed closure of the olecranon apophysis (12–17). Many authors have attributed these abnormalities to be secondary to the biomechanical throwing stresses placed on young, developing elbows (18–23). The classic stresses associated with throwing produce exceptional forces in and about the elbow (24). These include traction, compression, and shear, localized to the medial, lateral, and posterior aspects of the elbow (24). Any or all of these forces may contribute to the alteration of normal osteochondral development of the elbow (25).

Typically, the young athlete will complain of elbow pain while throwing; less common are complaints of fatigue or a decay of performance. Obviously, a timely and accurate diagnosis is the cornerstone to successful treatment of the many permutations of Little League elbow. A fastidious history and physical examination are primary tools in achieving this goal, routine x-rays excluded. The use of special tests such as the arthrogram, computed tomography (CT) and magnetic resonance imaging (MRI) are often necessary, but theirs is a confirmatory role rather than a diagnostic one. Salient factors in the history include age, duration of pain, location of pain, radiation, trauma, nature of onset, mechanism of injury, and past medical history. By simply focusing on these factors, it is often possible to acquire a good working diagnosis.

Physical examination begins with inspection of both elbows. Loss of motion, muscle atrophy or hypertrophy, bony deformity, and elbow asymmetry are ascertained. Palpation follows, focusing on the medial and

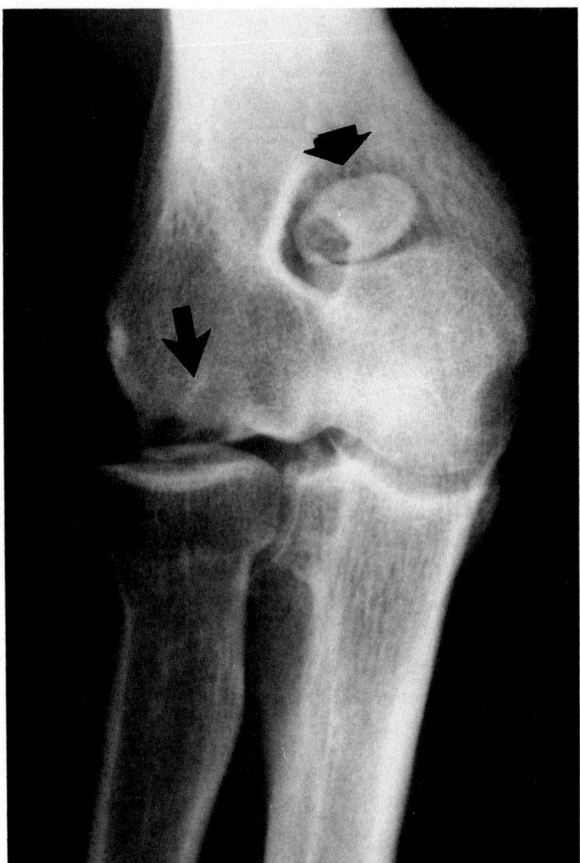

Figure 52.4. Medial epicondylar avulsion (*arrow*).

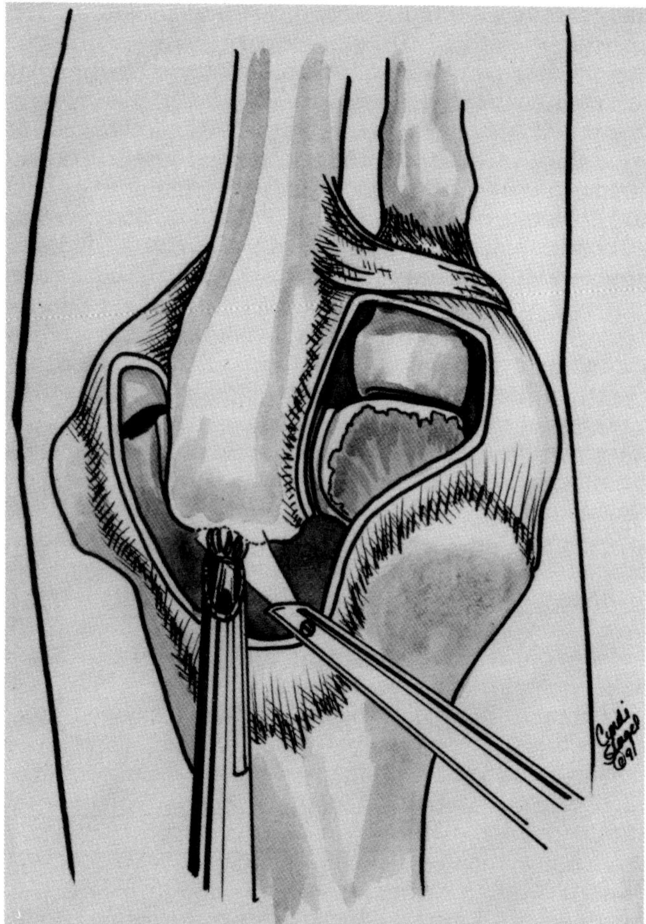

Figure 52.5. Osteochondritis dissecans of the capitellum (*arrows*).

lateral epicondyles, olecranon process, radial head, and collateral ligaments. Palpation of the ulnar nerve in both flexion and extension is helpful in evaluating subluxation. Examination of the olecranon fossa by flexing the elbow and application of pressure in the fossa to delineate between posterolateral and posteromedial pathology are also done. The physician should unlock the olecranon from the fossa (15° to 25° of flexion) and evaluate the medial and lateral ligamentous integrity. Stability testing requires sensitive fingers to detect the subtle differences in laxity noted between elbows. Finally, a complete neurologic and vascular examination of the extremity is performed.

Routine x-rays are essential in the diagnosis of this type of elbow pathology. Standard anteroposterior, lateral, reverse axial, and comparison radiographs are helpful. Stress films may be added in cases of suspected elbow instability. Prevalent medial findings in the immature elbow include enlargement, fragmentation, physeal widening, beaking of the epicondyle, and occasionally avulsion of the medial epicondyle. Lateral pathology classically involves the subchondral bone and manifests as osteochondrosis or osteochondritis dissecans of the capitellum or radial head. This may eventually result in loose bodies and terminally degenerative arthritis. Posterior lesions commonly present with hypertrophy of the ulna, causing chronic impingement of the olecranon tip into the olecranon fossa. Repetitive impingement of the olecranon causes osteophytic enlargement with resultant loose bodies in the fossa. Rarely, stress fractures of the ulna, olecranon apophysis, or delayed fusion of the olecranon apophysis transpires. If the elbow radiograph appears normal, carefully reevaluate the growth plates for irregularity or widening, because this usually is the weakest link in the chain.

Medial Tension Injuries

Most cases of Little League elbow present with medial elbow complaints. The common triad of symptoms include progressive pain, decreased effectiveness, and decreased throwing distance. Usually these are caused by subtle apophysitis or a stress fracture through the medial epicondylar epiphysitis. In most cases, a 4- to 6-week course of abstinence from throwing will result in a cessation of symptoms. Initially, ice and nonsteroidal antiinflammatory drugs (NSAIDs) will help to decrease the acute symptoms. After cessation of symptoms, a strengthening rehabilitation protocol and gradual throwing program is instituted.

Medial Epicondylar Fractures

When application of a more violent valgus stress is applied while throwing, an avulsion fracture of the medial epicondyle may ensue. Acute pain, point tenderness, and a flexion contracture are usually present. X-rays most often only show a minimally displaced epicondylar fragment; however, sometimes significant displacement with or without displacement in the joint is apparent (Fig. 52.6). Treatment depends on the extent of the epicondylar displacement. Although controversy exists on appropriate treatment, the author advocates anatomic surgical reduction in any medial epicondylar fracture demonstrating greater than 2 mm of displacement.

Medial Ligament Ruptures

Medial ligament rupture is uncommon in young throwers, except in the cases of violent trauma (e.g., elbow dislocation). Most cases occur in adult throwers, with years of insidious microtrauma and scarring of the medial collateral complex.

Treatment is generally conservative, which includes initial immobilization followed by functional bracing and, finally, a gradual rehabilitation program of symptomatic control, range of motion, and strengthening. Surgical reconstruction of the medial collateral ligament complex would only be considered in a young athlete who desires to continue in aggressive overhead sports in which prolonged symptomatology has occurred.

Lateral Compression Injuries

Panner's Disease (Osteochondrosis). Panner's disease is described as a disturbance of the growth or ossification centers in children (ages 7 to 12 years) that commences as a degeneration or necrosis of the capitellum and is followed by regeneration and reossification (25). The child presents with dull aching elbow pain that is exacerbated by activity, especially overhead sports. The elbow is swollen, but flexion contractures are uncommon. The differentiation between Panner's disease and osteochondritis dissecans (OCD) must be established. The difference focuses on age and degree of involvement of the capitellar secondary center of ossification. Panner's disease is a focal, localized lesion of the subchondral bone and its overlying articular cartilage (anterior central capitellum) in a young child (7 to 12 years) (26). Osteochondritis dissecans is a focal lesion in the capitellum demarcated by a rarefied zone, with or without loose bodies in an older athlete (13 to 16 years) (27).

Initial treatment should consist of rest, avoidance of throwing, and sometimes splint immobilization until pain and tenderness subsides. X-ray follow-up is recommended until healing is documented. Late deformity and collapse of the articular surface is rare.

Osteochondritis Dissecans. Osteochondritis dissecans presents in an older child (13 to 16 years) complaining of dull lateral elbow pain associated with a flexion contracture and sometimes locking. X-rays exhibit a focal island of subchondral bone demarcated by a rarefied zone, with or without loose bodies (Fig. 52.7).

Treatment is determined by lesion site, size, fixation, and condition of the articular cartilage of the capitellum and radial head. Type 1 lesions are intact with no evi-

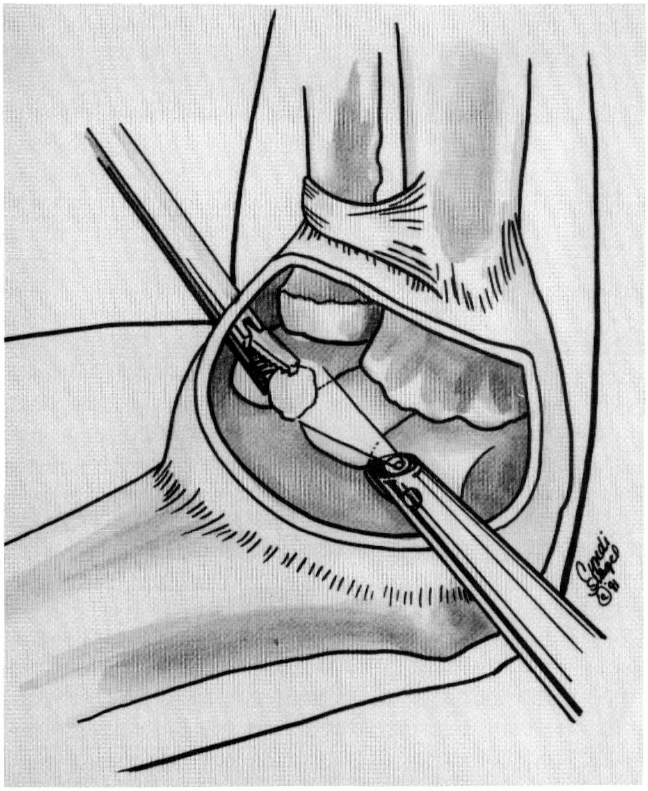

Figure 52.6. Medial epicondylar avulsion with displacement into joint.

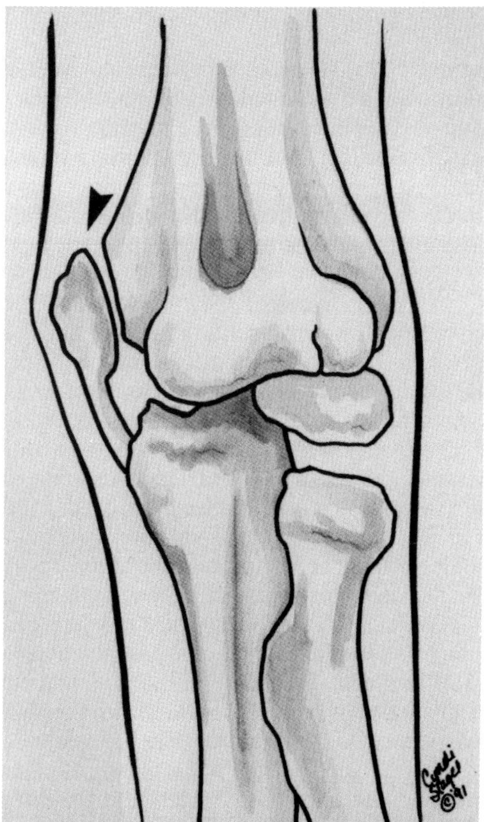

Figure 52.7. Osteochondritis dissecans of the capitellum (*arrow*).

dence of displacement and no articular cartilage fracture. Rest and splinting for 3 to 4 weeks will help with symptomatic control; range-of-motion exercises follow. Protection of the elbow should continue until radiographic evidence of healing is apparent. Type 2 OCD demonstrates fracture or fissure of the articular cartilage and/or partial detachment of the nonvascular fragment. If the fragment is partially detached, an elbow arthroscopy with either in situ pinning (large fragment) or removal and burring of the base of the lesion (small lesion) is recommended. Type 3 lesions are completely detached and lying free in the joint. Usually, the loose fragment is hypertrophied and rounded; the crater is obscured by fibrous tissue and is subsequently much smaller than the loose body. Treatment involves elbow arthroscopy with removal of the loose fragment and curettage of the crater. Late sequelae of OCD include loose bodies, residual deformity of the capitellum, and often residual elbow disability.

Posterior Extension and Shear Injuries

Posterior elbow injuries are uncommon in young athletes. Most posterior injuries of childhood are centered on the secondary ossification center of the olecranon, producing irregular patterns of ossification and secondary pain from repeated stress. Complaints, pathophysiology, and treatment are representative of osteochondrosis (25). During adolescence, the injury pattern progresses to avulsion fractures and/or lack of fusion between the secondary ossification center and the olecranon (25). Loose bodies, osteophytes, and partial avulsions are most common in the young adult population.

Treatment is individualized to the age and the specific condition. Children with osteochondrosis usually respond to rest from pitching in association with range-of-motion, flexibility, and strengthening exercises. Adolescents with persistent pain from lack of fusion may require a bone graft to induce union across the physis; rare avulsion fractures should be stabilized.

Adult Athletes

In the young throwing athlete as well as in the mature thrower, four distinct areas are vulnerable to throwing stresses: (*a*) tension overload of the medial elbow; (*b*) compression overload to the lateral articular surface; (*c*) posterior medial shear forces to the posterior articular surface; and (*d*) extension overload to the lateral restraints (24). In the adult, however, the weakest link is the ligamentous and bony surface as opposed to the physis of the young thrower. Therefore, a separate and distinct group of injury patterns are evident.

In the adult as well as in the young thrower, medial tension injuries are the most common, because of the tremendous valgus stresses applied to the elbow. A significant distraction tension force is applied to the medial restraints during the late cocking and acceleration phases of the throwing cycle. The resultant force presents as tension on the medial epicondylar attachments, including the flexor muscle origin and medial collateral ligaments. Commonly with overuse (microtrauma) or altered throwing mechanics, the weakest link in the medial complex can be injured. In young athletes, the medial epicondylar ossification center is targeted. Conversely, in adult athletes, the medial collateral ligament may become overstretched, resulting in traction spurs at the origin of the flexor wad and ligament complex. Treatment of these injuries varies on the integrity of the medial collateral ligament complex and the resultant stability of the joint. However, for most cases of medial ligament strain and epicondylitis, conservative measures will suppress the acute symptoms. Treatment consists of rest (from pitching), ice, and NSAIDs, followed by strengthening exercises for the forearm flexors and a progressive throwing protocol as the symptoms permit.

If microtrauma and secondary inflammation of the medial ligament complex become chronic, calcification of the ligaments may occur. Biomechanically, this further compromises the ligament complex, which may ultimately fail if the insults are continued. If the conservative regiment noted above fails to correct the problem, excision of the calcified degenerative tissue may be helpful. Careful examination of medial elbow stability should be conducted after removal of the degenerative tissue. If medial elbow stability has been compromised by the removal of the calcified tissue, reconstruction of the medial collateral ligament may be necessary.

Infrequently, chronic microfractures in the fibers of the ligament will cause a complete ligament rupture. The history commonly will include multiple bouts of medial elbow pain during and after pitching that will respond to conservative treatment. Then there is often a single episode of "giving away," which is distinct and isolated and represents the final insult. Pitchers and gymnasts are particularly at risk for this malady (28).

Valgus instability can be diagnosed initally by history, then confirmed clinically by first flexing the elbow (15° to 25°) to unlock the olecranon from its fossa and then applying gentle valgus stress. "Instability" of the joint will allow the medial side of the joint to open; however, this requires sensitive fingers and experience. Radiograph gravity stress tests of the elbow may confirm the diagnosis (Fig. 52.8). MRI has recently been used to isolate the medial collateral complex, detecting both incomplete and complete disruption. Treatment depends on the goals of the patient and the degree of instability. Surgical reconstruction consists of replacing the medial collateral ligament with a substitute ligament, which in most cases is the palmaris longus tendon. Indications for surgical reconstruction include (*a*) acute rupture in throwers; (*b*) significant chronic instability; (*c*) after debridement for calcific tendinitis, if there is insufficient tissue remaining to effect a primary repair in a throwing athlete; and (*d*) multiple episodes of recurring pain (with subtle instability) with throwing after periods of conservative care. Medial collateral ligament reconstruction has been gratifying and will usually allow a return to full throwing activities within an 18-month period.

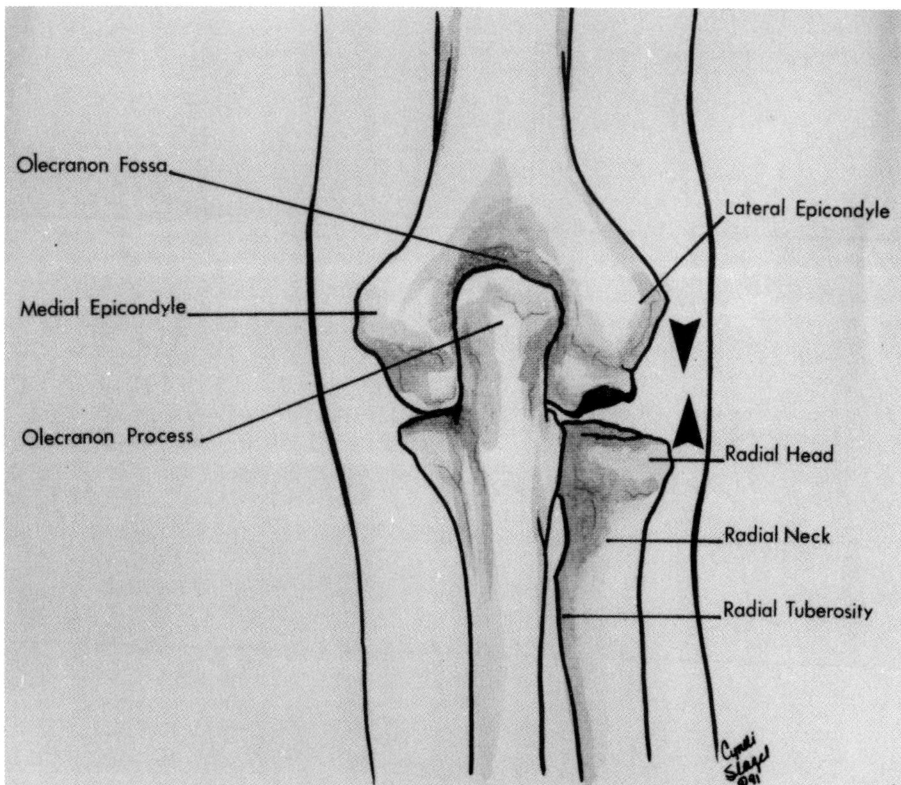

Figure 52.8. Stress x-ray showing rupture of the medial collateral ligament complex with valgus instability (*arrow*).

Posterior articular damage is common in adults and develops in two phases of throwing. A posterior medial shear force develops about the olecranon fossa, amid late cocking. Throughout, follow-through hyperextension of the elbow may be present, thereby placing stress on the olecranon and anterior capsule. These stresses commonly induce three sites of pathology: posterior medial spurs; pure posterior olecranon spurs (triceps tendinitis); and osteophytes in the olecranon fossa (Figs. 52.9 and 52.10). These sites may then contribute to loose body formations in the olecranon fossa (Fig. 52.11).

Initial treatment is conservative with accentuation on symptomatic control. Usually, however, arthroscopic burring of the spurs and removal of loose bodies may become necessary.

Lateral extension overload occurs during the acceleration phase of throwing, when forearm pronation stresses cause a tension force to the lateral ligaments and extensor attachment at the lateral epicondyle. This cascade may consequently induce lateral epicondylitis.

Biceps Tendonitis

Biceps tendonitis occurring at the elbow is uncommon. Hyperextension at follow-through or repetitive forceful pronation-supination activities may cause microtears/tendonitis at the musculotendinous junction or tendon insertion on the radial tuberosity.

Physical examination demonstrates tenderness about the insertion of the biceps at the radial tuberosity. Additional findings include pain with resisted supination

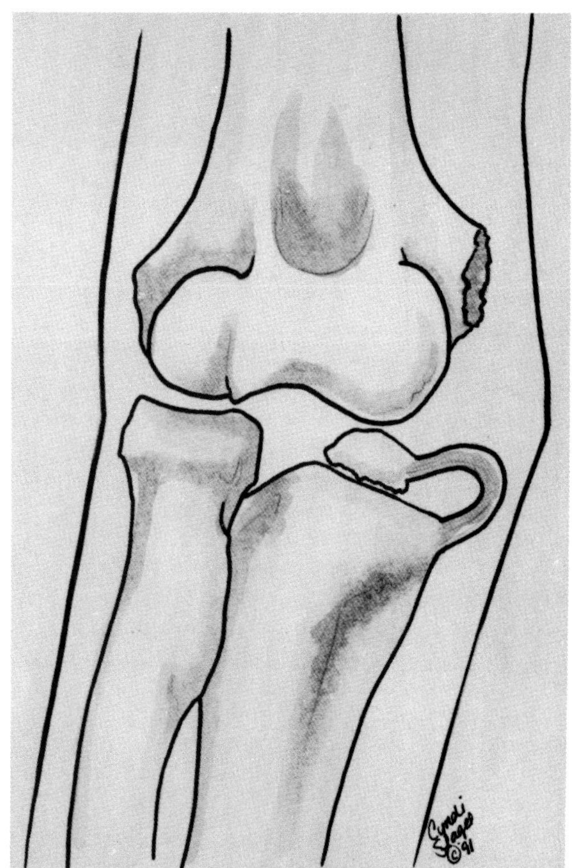

Figure 52.9. X-ray showing posterior medial spur (*arrow*).

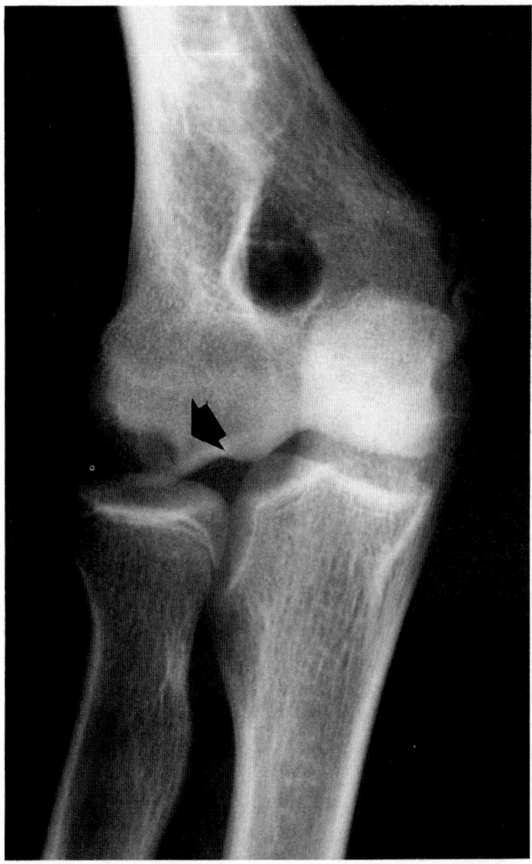

Figure 52.10. X-ray showing fluffy calcification at triceps insertion.

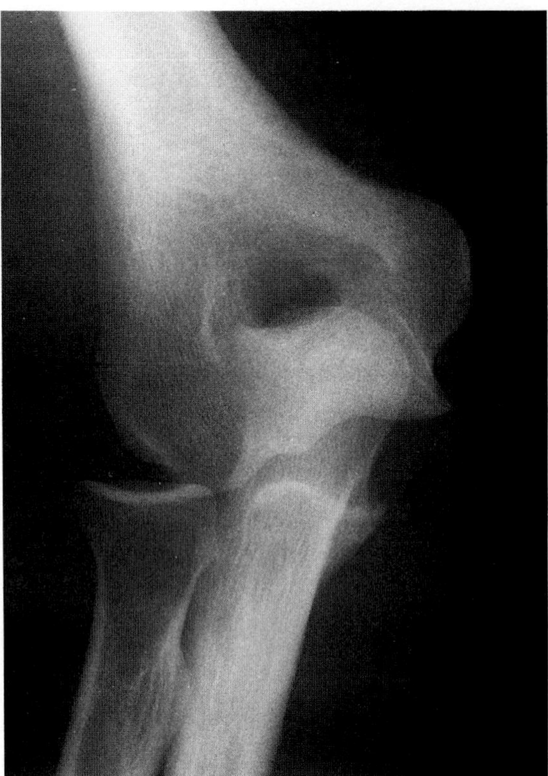

Figure 52.11. X-ray demonstrating a large loose body in the posterior compartment (*large arrow*) and osteochondritis dissecans of the capitellum (*small arrow*).

and weakness in supination secondary to pain. Treatment is conservative, consisting of rest from throwing, NSAIDs, and ultrasound. Once the symptoms have decreased, longitudinal massage of the tendon and submaximal supination strengthening have been helpful. Once painless exercise is apparent, a throwing protocol is instituted. Slow, steady improvement is typical and surgical intervention is rarely warranted.

Ulnar Nerve Injuries

Chronic valgus stresses applied to the medial side of the elbow by the repetitious high-velocity nature of many overhead sports often incite inflammation of the ulnar nerve in the cubital tunnel. Biomechanically, during flexion, the ulnar nerve elongates an average of 4.7 mm and can be pushed over 7 mm medially by the medial head of the triceps (28). Cubital tunnel volume can be reduced by concomitant stretching of the arcuate ligament and bulging of the posterior division of the medial collateral ligament complex (chronic ligament inflammation) (28). Entrapment and/or dislocation of the nerve are conditions seen most often in athletes whose arms repeatedly perform a throwing motion. This population includes baseball players, tennis players, javelin throwers, gymnasts, and football quarterbacks. The chief clinical symptom is pain about the medial elbow, sometimes radiating distally down the ulnar aspect of the forearm into the hand. Numbness and tingling of the ring and little fingers is occasionally present. Additional symptoms include clumsiness, heaviness, and problems with grasp, especially after activities. Painful snapping or popping sensations, while the elbow is rapidly flexing and extending, combined with sharp pains radiating into the forearm and hand, are indicative of recurrent dislocations of the ulnar nerve.

The physical examination will elicit tenderness over the ulnar nerve in the cubital tunnel. Upon palpation, the cubital tunnel may feel thickened or "doughy" and the nerve may be subluxed manually. Tinel's sign may be localized to the cubital tunnel. Neurologic anomalies in the domain innervated by the ulnar nerve, including hypoesthesia, interosseous washing, and dry skin, may be present. Subtle changes in two-point discrimination over the ring and little fingers and loss of fine intrinsic muscle control may be noted periodically.

Treatment of acute cases of ulnar neuritis, in which symptoms are not yet severe and intrinsic atrophy is not present, may respond well to conservative treatment. Rest and ice should be applied along with immobilization with a splint for 2 to 3 weeks. Antiinflammatory medications may also be helpful. Steroid injections into the cubital tunnel is not recommended. In most cases, surgical intervention is not required. If symptoms recur and chronic elbow pain develops following resumption of throwing, then a surgical decompression may be indicated. A transfer of the ulnar nerve deep to the flexor muscles with the brachialis as the floor (submuscular transposition) is the author's preference. This approach will allow inspection of the medial collateral ligament complex and permits reconstruction if necessary. Technical points of the transposition include (*a*) release proximally of the arcade of Struthers, (*b*) resection of a portion of the intermuscular septum where the new course of the nerve lies, (*c*) preservation of the elbow articular branches of the ulnar nerve, and (*d*) preservation of the motor branches to the flexor carpi ulnaris.

Postoperatively, the joint should be splinted in 90° of flexion, leaving the wrist free, for 10 days. The patient should start squeezing a sponge or soft ball as soon as comfort permits. Range-of-motion exercises emphasizing extension should begin at 2 weeks. After full range of motion is attained, a gradual strengthening program of the forearm flexors and extensors is instituted. Care must be taken not to avoid the other major muscle groups of the upper extremity during rehabilitation. At 2 months postoperation, the patient may begin gently to toss a ball, followed by a progressive throwing protocol. Return to full activities is permitted at about 6 months.

Medial Epicondylitis

Chronic valgus stress to the medial aspect of the elbow will cause microtrauma to the medial restraints and subsequent inflammation. Three types of athletes who commonly present with medial epicondylitis are golfers, tennis players, and pitchers. In golfers, the trauma is induced by repeatedly hitting behind the ball (hitting it fat), imparting large amounts of stress to the medial structures. Conversely, it is noted in advanced tennis players who forcibly extend their wrist while striking the ball on overheads and serves. The etiology in pitchers was discussed earlier. Pain and tenderness at the medial epicondyle and positive provocative tests (pain with resisted wrist flexion and pronation) are the hallmarks of the examination. If diffuse medial pain and tenderness and/or neurologic findings are present, then other sources for the pain should be explored (e.g., medial ligament laxity).

Initial treatment consists of ice, rest from sport, phonophoresis, and antiinflammatories. Recalcitrant cases will sometimes need injections of steroids at the site of maximal tenderness. Once the symptoms have abated, a systematic regimen of strengthening exercises are initiated. As strength improves, a counterforce brace is applied and sports are resumed. However, the patient is advised to seek professional advice to improve the biomechanics of the desired sport. If intractable symptoms recur despite conservative measures, surgery is sometimes indicated. The surgery entails release of the flexor origin with excision of granulation tissue, burring the medial epicondyle and reconstruction of the medial musculotendinous unit, thus reinstating a good vascular bed to induce healing. Postoperative care is similar to the rehabilitative regimen of the transposition of the ulnar nerve.

Lateral Epicondylitis

Inflammation of the lateral musculotendinous structures originating at the lateral epicondyle is termed lateral epicondylitis. This entity is much more common in tennis players than in other athletes (e.g., baseball) and is known by the generic term *tennis elbow*. Many authors have investigated this malady and most feel that the primary pathology lies in the extensor carpi radialis brevis. Nirschl (29) has termed the histologic pathology fibroangiomatous hyperplasia provoked by repetitive trauma .

The typical patient is middle-aged (30 to 50 years old) and involved in racquet sports with poor stroke mechanics. Poor mechanics usually center on the backhand, for which the patient will lead with the elbow rather than the body and shoulder. Increased racquet vibration typically initated by off-center hitting (miss hits) that has a direct correlation with poor mechanics is another inciting factor. Both will subsequently place additional stress on the lateral musculotendinous restraints, thereby inciting inflammation and microscopic tears in the tendons.

The athlete will complain of a dull pain localized to the lateral elbow, which comes on after playing tennis for a period of time. Frequently, the pain will be present when turning a door knob, lifting a milk carton, or opening a jar. Night pain is not common but may appear in chronic cases.

Physical examination will elicit discreet tenderness over the lateral epicondyle of the elbow. Provocative tests such as lateral elbow pain with resisted wrist dorsiflexion or supination also are present. Roentgenograms do not classically reveal any abnormalities; however, in chronic long-standing cases, a small calcific deposit over the lateral epicondyle may be present. This calcification is secondary to the chronic repetitive tension forces placed on the common extensor origin.

The initial treatment of acute epicondylitis includes rest from provocative movements, ice, and NSAIDs. Care must be taken to educate the patient that this is an overuse syndrome. If the symptoms are not abated and functionally severe enough, a steroid injection to the lateral epicondyle is sometimes helpful. It is important to realize that repeated steroid injections may lead to tendon compromise and complications. Therefore, only three injections over a 1-year time interval are prudent. After the symptoms abate, a comprehensive rehabilitation program is initiated, emphasizing strength and flexibility of the forearm extensors and flexors. Strengthening is best accomplished by initially starting with a 1-pound dumbbell doing extensions of the forearm with three sets of 10 repetitions per day. The weight is increased in increments of 1 pound per week until the patient can easily lift 8 to 10 pounds. Flexion and flexibility exercises are simultaneously done during the above protocol. The patient is then allowed to start his or her desired racquet sport. The patient is urged to change to a newer composite racquet, use a racquet with a larger head, increase the grip size, and use a string tension between 55 and 60 pounds. Different racquet compositions have different string tensions, e.g., Vortex is 40 to 50 pounds and Prostaff is 55 to 60 pounds. The use of an elbow counterforce brace is also helpful. Most important, the patient should be encouraged to seek professional instruction to eliminate biomechanical errors in stroke production. Typical errors include (*a*) improper weight transfer (hitting off the back foot), (*b*) hitting with the leading elbow during the backhand, and (*c*) excessive pronation of the forearm during the serve or the overhead.

In the 5% to 10% of patients who fail conservative measures over a 6-month period, a surgical approach may be indicated. Although many different surgical techniques have been touted for correcting lateral epicondylitis, the author favors the removal of granulation tissue and reconstruction of the lateral epicondyle. Basically, the common extensor hood is fastidiously elevated, and the underlying granulation tissue is excised. The epicondyle is burred to bleeding bone to create a good vascular bed and the extensor hood is reconstructed, utilizing sutures directly through the lateral epicondyle. Any calcium or spurs that may be present are removed at the time of the reconstruction.

Postoperatively, the patient is started at once on gentle range-of-motion exercises and progressed in the rehabilitation of strength and flexibility as tolerated. Full strength and flexibility are usually attained by 3 months, and resumption of athletic activity, with a counterforce brace, is initiated. High-speed rehabilitation with Cybex II equipment has been helpful in recreating the forces encountered during racquet sports and should be incorporated during the rehabilitation phase.

Posterior Elbow Problems

Problems about the posterior elbow are relatively uncommon compared with the medial and lateral elbow. The triceps musculotendinous unit and the olecranon are overloaded in activities that require repetitive forceful extension of the elbow. These activities include racquet sports, pitching, gymnastics, shot putting, javelin throwing, and weight lifting. It is helpful to divide posterior problems into two groups: triceps musculotendinous strains and bony pathology of the olecranon and its fossa.

Triceps Tendinitis. Inflammation of the triceps insertion at the proximal olecranon is common in athletes who lift inordinate amounts of weight or in explosive field events such as the shot put. The patient will isolate the pain to the tip of the olecranon and will rarely complain of neurologic symptoms. On examination, the maximal tenderness is just superior to the attachment of the triceps on the olecranon, or exactly where the triceps inserts. Provocative tests such as resisted extension of the elbow will increase the pain. Roentgenographic evaluation is usually normal. The pathology is similar to lateral epicondylitis, and the ensuing treatment is the same as most tendinitis conditions. In the acute phase, rest, ice, and NSAIDs are used. Steroid injection of the tendon and/or tendon sheath is not recommended, because of the possibility of rupture of the triceps tendon. Infrequently, the symptoms may become chronic and disabling, at which time surgery may be indicated. Initially, an MRI has been helpful in localizing the specific area of degeneration. The surgical procedure encompasses exploration of the tendon with excision of intratendinous and extratendinous degeneration and granulation tissue. If the degeneration is primarily located at the distal triceps insertion, curettage of the insertion is performed, and if there is significant degeneration, reattachment of the triceps tendon is undertaken. Postoperatively, the rehabilitation is similar to that presented for lateral epicondylitis.

Olecranon Bursitis. The olecranon bursa does not exist in children under 7, and by the age of 10 some form of bursa is present. The size of the bursa is proportional to age and activity of the extremity (30). Olecranon bursitis is an inflammation of the olecranon bursa caused by either a traumatic inflammatory response or by an infectious etiology. The patient will complain of pain and/or tightness of the posterior elbow associated with swelling of the elbow about the olecranon tip. Overuse, direct trauma or bacterial inoculation of the bursa all have been described as the initial inciting event. X-rays denote posterior soft tissue swelling, and sometimes calcification of the triceps insertion on the olecranon is present (Fig. 52.11).

Treatment usually consists of rest, protection and antiinflammatories. If an infectious etiology is suspected, aspiration of the bursa with cultures and Gram strain, followed by the appropriate antibiotics, is necessary. Persistent traumatic symptoms occasionally require aspiration, a steroid injection into the bursa, and rest and immobilization. Chronic insistent bursitis or infectious bursitis requires surgical bursectomy, either by open or arthroscopic means.

Bony Posterior Problems

Bony posterior compartment injuries are common in racquet sports, baseball, and javelin throwing in contrast to triceps musculotendinous injuries. In these sports, the olecranon is repeatedly and forcefully driven into the olecranon fossa. In addition, there is typically a valgus stress that causes the olecranon to abut against the medial wall of the olecranon fossa. These repetitive compressive forces generate bony osteophyte formation on the olecranon and loose body formation. Loose bodies are produced by the olecranon impacting the wall of the olecranon fossa, thus shearing off osteocartilaginous fragments. Occasionally, this repetitive abutment can cause a stress fracture of the olecranon.

The patient usually localizes the pain to the posterior elbow, sometimes with subjective clicking and grating. Infrequently, the elbow may become locked, and the patient will manipulate it until it releases. Examination uncovers tenderness posteriorly along the margins of the olecranon; rarely, loose bodies will be palpated. Crepitus may be noted with range of motion. Full extension is blocked by the osteophytes and/or loose bodies. X-rays show the offending osteophytes, enlargement of the olecranon, and sometimes the loose bodies (Figs. 52.9 and 52.11). CT scans have been helpful in localizing the osteophytes and loose bodies.

Treatment initially depends on the presence of loose bodies. If no loose bodies are discovered, a conservative protocol of rest and nonsteroidal agents will usually control the acute symptoms. This is followed by a

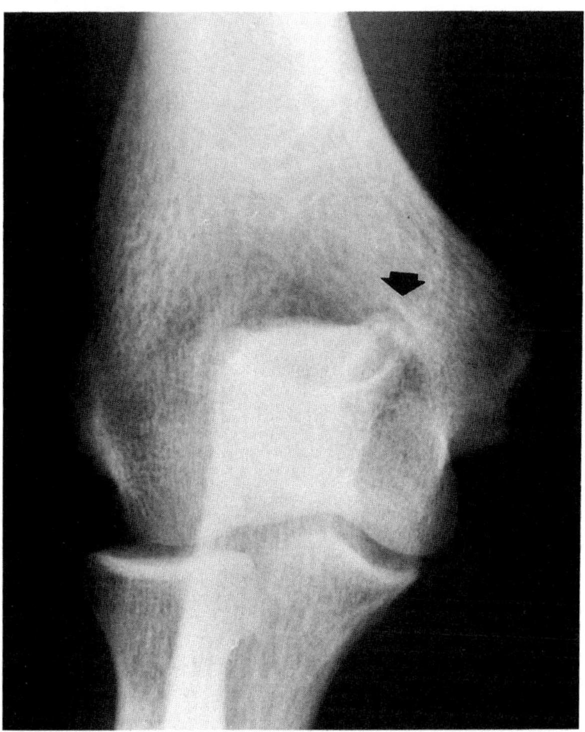

Figure 52.12. Arthroscopic burring of olecranon osteophytes.

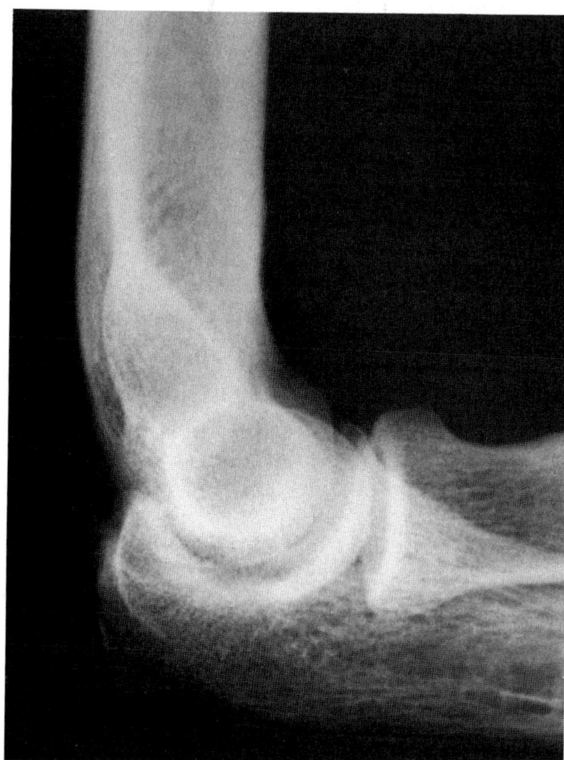

Figure 52.13. Arthroscopic removal of loose bodies.

rehabilitation regiment of strengthening and flexibility exercises. Typically, the athlete will be able to resume activities in 4 to 6 weeks.

However, if loose bodies are present or if symptoms persist, surgical intervention may be advisable. Arthroscopic removal of loose bodies and burring of osteophytes with simultaneous removal of the distal tip of the olecranon has been rewarding (Figs. 52.12. and 52.13). Removal of the olecranon tip allows it to fit into the olecranon fossa better and helps prevent impingement against the wall of the fossa. Because this procedure does not involve cutting any musculotendinous groups, rehabilitation may begin immediately to regain flexibility, especially extension. After 3 weeks, strengthening and a progressive throwing protocol is initiated.

Fractures and Dislocations

Fractures of the Humerus

Sports-related fractures of the humerus can occur from both direct (contact) and indirect (rotational) forces. Tremendous torques are applied to the humerus in the act of throwing, arm wrestling, and shot putting (31, 32). Rotational forces with the forearm used as a lever are common to these sports. Indirect distal humeral fractures generally occur in the unconditioned athlete who lacks the necessary amount of biceps and triceps strength to counterbalance the rotational stresses or in athletes who have intrinsic bone weakness (e.g., tumor).

The patient will complain of a sudden sharp pain with the inability to continue the activity. Physical examination reveals discreet tenderness of the humerus and sometimes obvious deformity distally. X-ray denotes a typical spiral-like fracture, involving the distal end of the humerus. Conversely, pathologic fractures are usually seen in direct continuity with the intrinsic site of bone weakness and may have numerous configurations.

Treatment of distal rotational fractures can be adequately managed with coaptation splints and immobilized until radiographic union is present. Clear evidence of clinical and radiographic union must be noted before a rehabilitation protocol is instituted. This protocol involves progressive range of motions and strengthening of the entire upper extremity. The patient must regain normal range of motions and strength before he or she is permitted to resume sporting activities.

Treatment of a pathologic fracture depends on the cause of the intrinsic bone weakness. Obviously, the treatment of a solitary bone cyst will differ dramatically from a sarcomatous neoplasm of the humerus.

Supracondylar Fractures

Supracondylar fractures are the second most common fracture encountered in a pediatric age group (33). Basically, they are classified into two types: extension and flexion. The extension types are usually produced by extension injuries (i.e., fall onto outstretched hand) in which the distal fragment is pulled proximally and posteriorly by the pull of the triceps (Fig. 52.14). The much less common flexion type is produced from a direct injury to the back of the elbow. Clinically, it is important to distinguish supracondylar fractures from pure

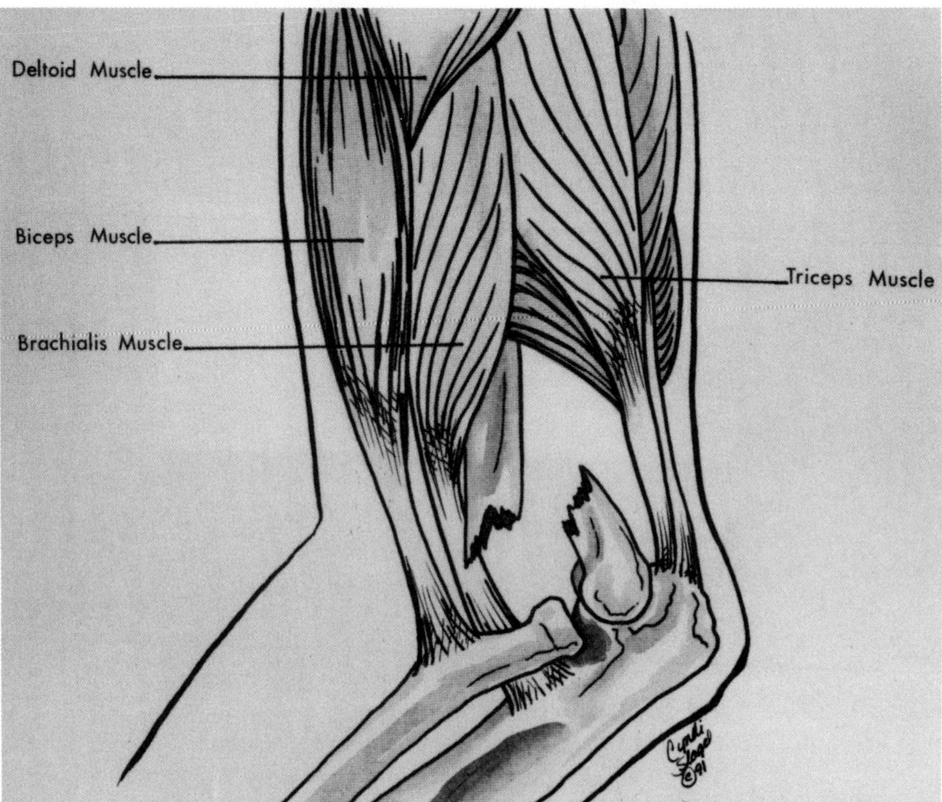

Figure 52.14. Supracondylar humeral fracture (extension type).

elbow dislocations. In supracondylar fractures, the normal triangular anatomic relationship between the medial and lateral epicondyle and the olecranon process does not change, which is not the case in elbow dislocations.

Treatment of displaced supracondylar fractures in the pediatric age group is fraught with potential problems. Treatment is based on the neurovascular status of the distal extremity and the ability to maintain the alignment of the fracture fragments. Generally, gentle closed reduction (using skin traction, gentle manipulation, or skeletal traction through the olecranon) followed by cast immobilization is adequate. However, if the reduction cannot be maintained or if neurovascular compromise is present, percutaneous or open surgical treatment may be indicated.

Dislocation of the Elbow

In children under 10, dislocation of the elbow is the most common dislocation seen, whereas in adults it is seconded only to shoulder dislocations. Most of the dislocations are either posterior or posterolateral. The mechanism of injury is usually a fall onto an outstretched extremity or by direct trauma. The athlete immediately notices pain, disability, and sometimes deformity. Examination reveals a disruption of the normal triangular relationship between the medial and lateral epicondyles and the tip of the olecranon. Because of the possibility of neurovascular compromise in these injuries, a careful examination of the neurologic and vascular status of the extremity is paramount.

Treatment is gentle reduction of the dislocation. The athlete should be removed from the field and in the calm of the locker room, a gentle reduction should be attempted. Smooth, progressive traction is applied with the elbow in 30° of flexion; direct pressure on the olecranon is sometimes helpful. If reduction cannot be accomplished, the athlete should be taken to the hospital for radiographic examination. Once x-rays confirm the displacement, the above maneuver is attempted again; first correct the medial or lateral displacement and then the posterior component. Hyperextension of the elbow should be avoided during this maneuver. If this fails, the athlete should be taken to the operating room for reduction under anesthesia. Immediately postreduction, the neurovascular status should be checked again. Smooth flexion and extension of the elbow should be apparent without catching. Postreduction intraoperative x-rays are mandatory to confirm reduction and to determine if any subtle fractures are present. A posterior splint is applied with the elbow in its most stable position (usually 90° of flexion) for 1 week. The parents are instructed to watch for circulatory or neurologic changes. After 1 week, the patient is fitted for a hinged elbow brace and gentle active flexion and extension range of motions are encouraged under the supervision of a physical therapist. At 3 weeks postreduction, the stability of the reduction will determine the course of therapy or bracing. This protocol of early motion with bracing has been helpful in avoiding flexion contractures of the elbow, initiating early rehabilitation and return to athletics. Persistent instability and redislocations are rare in athletes; however, if apparent, reconstruction of the elbow ligaments may be necessary.

Fractures about the Elbow

Many of the sports-related fractures about the elbow were discussed earlier in this chapter. Because a complete fracture text is beyond the scope of this chapter, this section will focus on sports-related fractures of the radial head and their treatment.

Radial head fractures are common in athletes, especially in the adult population. The typical mechanism of injury is a fall onto an outstretched hand, which transmits force to the elbow. They can also occur concomitantly with elbow dislocations. Fractures of the radial head and neck are associated with injuries of the distal radioulnar joint, interosseous membrane, and nerve injuries. Mason's classification of radial head fractures has proven a helpful guideline for treatment (34). Type 1 fracture is an undisplaced fracture involving less than 25% of the radial head. Type 2 fractures are marginal with displacement, including either angulation, impaction, or depression. Type 3 fractures involve the entire radial head and are comminuted. Type 4 fractures are associated with dislocations of the elbow.

Treatment of type 1 fractures is nonsurgical and includes splint support and early range-of-motion exercises. Multiple options are reliable for Mason type 2 fractures, which include (*a*) splinting and early range of motions, (*b*) open reduction and internal fixation, and (*c*) excision of the radial head. The final outcome for the above treatment methods are about the same. If conservative methods fail, late resection of the radial head is equal to early excision (35). However, to avoid complications of myositis ossificans, it is recommended to wait 3 to 4 weeks before late excision. Open reduction and internal fixation with either Herbert screws or cannulated interfragmentary screws is best achieved when at least 50% of the radial head remains intact to provide stable fixation platform.

Mason type 3 fractures usually require excision of the radial head. In the past, an anconeus approach was popular, but recently a direct lateral approach to spare the lateral ulnohumeral ligament is favored.

A Mason type 4 fracture associated with a elbow dislocation is a complex problem, and controversy exists. If the radial head is comminuted, excision should be contemplated; however, if open reduction and internal fixation is feasible, the radial head should be retained. Because late excision of the radial head has proven gratifying, preservation of the radial head for almost all Mason type 1 and 2 fractures is recommended. Preservation of the radial head for type 3 and 4 fractures is recommended when practical.

It has been helpful to allow early range of motion, when possible, with radial head fractures. Range of motions coupled with a supervised rehabilitation program have aided in decreasing the occurrence of contractures about the elbow. In the author's clinic, these programs must be individualized and supervised to produce the expected results.

Conclusions

The specific emphasis in this chapter has been directed toward common athletic elbow problems and their diagnosis and treatment. The interest in sports has blossomed in recent years, producing a wide spectrum of athletic elbow injuries across a broad age range. It must be recognized that the prevalence and type of injury are determined not only by sport but also by age. Fastidious adherence to a complete history, physical examination, and a high index of suspicion for uncommon disorders is paramount. Understanding the basic elbow anatomy, biomechanics, and common sport-specific pathology will enable the clinician to predict the common lesions and suspect the uncommon problems. The importance of well-supervised and comprehensive rehabilitation protocols cannot be overemphasized and are paramount to the successful return to sport.

REFERENCES

1. Morrey BF, An KN. Functional anatomy of the ligaments of the elbow. Clin Orthop 1985; 201:84–90.
2. Stormont TJ, An KN, Morrey BF. Elbow joint contact study: comparison of techniques. J Biomech 1985;18:329–336.
3. Morrey BF. Anatomy of the elbow joint. In: Morrey BF, ed. The elbow and its disorders. Philadelphia: WB Saunders, 1985:7–42.
4. O'Driscoll DW, Bell DF, Morrey BF. Posterolateral rotatory instability of the elbow. J Bone Joint Surg 1991;73A:440–446.
5. Morrey BF, An KN. Articular and ligamentous contributions to the stability of the elbow joint. Am J Sports Med 1983;11–315–319.
6. An KN, Morrey BF. Biomechanics of the elbow. In: Morrey BF, ed. The elbow and its disorders. Philadelphia: WB Saunders, 1985:43–61.
7. Bradley JP, Perry J, Jobe FW. The biomechanics of the throwing shoulder. Perspec. Orthop Surg 1990;1(2):49–59.
8. Halls AA, Travill A. Transmission of pressures across the elbow joint. Anat Rec 1964;150:243–247.
9. Hui FC, Chao Ey, An KN. Muscle and joint forces at the elbow during isometric lifting [Abstract]. Orthop Trans 1978;2:169.
10. Elkins EC, Leden UM, Wakin KG. Objective recording of the strength of normal muscles. Arch Phys Med 1951;32:639–647.
11. Larson RF. Forearm positioning on maximal elbow flexor force. 1966; 196:99–104.
12. Trias A, Ray RD. Juvenile osteochondritis of the radial head—report of a bilateral case. J Bone Joint Surg 1963;45A:576–582.
13. Tullos HS, Erwin WD, Wouds GW, et al. Unusual lesions of the pitching arm. Clin Orthop 1972;88:169–182.
14. Adams IE. Injury to the throwing arm: a study of traumatic changes in the elbow joints of boy baseball players. Calif Med 1965;102:127–132.
15. Gugenheim JJ, Stanely RF, Wood GW, et al. Little League survey: the Houston study. Am J Sports Med 1976;4:189–199.
16. Larson RL, Singer KM, Bergstrom R, et al. Little League survey: the Eugene study. Am J Sports Med 1976;4:201–209.
17. Hang, YS. Little League elbow: a clinical and biomechanical study. In: Matsui H, Kobayashi K, eds. Biomechanics VIII—A&B: proceedings of the 8th international Congress of Biomechanics, Nagoya, Japan. Champagne, IL: Human Kinetics, 1983:70–85.
18. Brogdon BG, Crow NE. Little Leaguer's elbow. Am J Roentgenol 1960;83:671–675.
19. Brown R, Blazina ME, Kerlan RK. Osteochondritis of the capitellum. Am J Sports Med 1974;2:27–46.
20. King IW, Brelsford AJ, Tullos HS. Epicondylitis and osteochondritis of the professional baseball pitcher's elbow. AAOS Symp Sports Med 1975;75–88.

21. Lipsomb AB. Baseball pitching injuries in growing athletes. Am J Sports Med. 1975;3:25–34.
22. Middleman IC. Shoulder and elbow lesions of baseball players. Am J Surg. 1961;102:677–632.
23. Slager RF. From little League to big league, the weak spot is the arm. Am J Sports Med. 1977;5:37–48.
24. Pappas AW. Elbow problems associated with baseball during childhood and adolescence. Clin Orthop 1986;701:84–90.
25. Bianco AJ. Osteochondritis dissecans. In: Morrey BF, ed. The elbow and its disorders. Philadelphia: WB Saunders, 1985:254–259.
26. Panner HI. A peculiar affection of the capitellum humeri, resembling Calvé-Perthes disease of the hip. Acta Radiol 1929;10:234–242.
27. Bennett JB, Tullos HS. Ligamentous and articular injuries in the athlete. In: Morrey BF, ed. The elbow and its disorders. Philadelphia: WB Saunders, 1985:502–522.
28. Jobe FW, Bradley JP. Ulnar neuritis and ulnar collateral ligament instabilities in overarm throwers. In: Torg JS, ed. Current therapy in sports medicine—2. Toronto: BC Decker 1990:419–424.
29. Nirschl RP. Tennis elbow. Orthop Clin North Am 1973;4:787–792.
30. Chen J, Alk D, Eventov I. Development of the olecranon bursa: an anatomic cadaver study. Acta Orthop Scand 1987;58:408–409.
31. Santavirta S, Kiviluoto O. Transverse fracture of the humerus in a shotputter: a case report. Am J Sports Med 1977;5(3):122–123.
32. Whitaker JH. Arm wrestling fractures-a humerus twist. Am J Sports Med 1977;5(2):67–77.
33. Hanlon CR, Estes WL. Fractures in childhood: a statistical analysis. Am J Surg. 1954;87:312–323.
34. DeLee JC, Green DP, Wilkens KE. Fractures and dislocations of the elbow. In: Rockwood CA, Green DP, eds. Fractures in adults. 2nd ed. Philadelphia: JP Lippincott, 1984;1:559–652.
35. Broberg MA, Morrey BF. Results of delayed excision of the radial head after fracture. J Bone Joint Surg. 1986;68A:669–674.

53 / HAND AND WRIST INJURIES

Dean G. Sotereanos, Jon A. Levy, and James H. Herndon

Introduction

Injuries to the hand and wrist are common at all levels of sport. These injuries can be the consequence of either an isolated traumatic event or repetitive actions that result in an overuse syndrome. For diagnostic purposes, the first important step is a detailed history and physical examination, paying special attention to the reported mechanism of injury. Subsequent evaluation also must include appropriate roentgenograms or studies pertinent to the suspected injury.

Following diagnosis, the proper treatment must be matched with the specific injury. Appropriate measures can range from simple techniques such as splinting to more invasive procedures such as primary surgical repair. Treatment goals should include returning the athlete to his or her previous level of function, preventing permanent disability, and expediting care to enable an early return to the playing field. Although these are similar to treatment goals for the general population, time tends to play a larger role in the care of the injured athlete. Coaches, players, and families often pressure the physician to accelerate the treatment protocol to allow a return to play. This must be kept in mind initially when choosing the treatment and throughout the recovery period.

In this chapter, the mechanisms of injury; diagnostic routines; and treatment plans for the more common fractures, ligamentous injuries, and nerve compression syndromes seen in the hands and wrists of athletes will be discussed.

Wrist Injuries

Distal Radius Injuries

Fractures of the distal radius are sustained by falling onto an outstretched hand with the wrist in extension. The well-known Colles fractures is a typical example (1). Classically, this term describes a distal radius fracture with dorsal displacement and dorsal angulation, resulting in a so-called silver-fork deformity. Other frequently cited eponyms for these injuries include Smith's fracture, which represents volar displacement and volar angulation of the distal radius (2), and Barton's fracture, a dorsal or volar (reverse Barton's) fracture dislocation of the wrist, in which the carpus is translocated with the distal fragment of the radial fracture (3). Unfortunately, these eponyms often are misused.

Clinically, a patient with a distal radius fracture has an edematous, tender wrist with or without deformity. The physical checkup must include a thorough neurovascular examination with special attention paid to median nerve function (4). Also, as with all fractures, the skin over the fracture must be evaluated closely to rule out an open injury.

Initial roentgenograms must include anteroposterior (AP) and lateral views. The radiographic assessment should document whether there is intraarticular fracture extension into the radiocarpal or radioulnar joints. The degree of displacement and angulation should be noted as well. Radiographic parameters describing the anatomy of the normal radius are well-documented. On the lateral radiograph, the distal radius normally has a volar tilt of 11° to 12°. On the AP view, the normal inclination of the radius averages 22° to 23° (5). Radial length can be measured on the AP radiograph, normal being 11 to 12 mm. This distance is measured by comparing the length of two lines perpendicular to the long axis of the radius. One line is drawn at the level of the radial styloid; the second, at the level of the articular surface of the distal radius at its most proximal point (6). AP and lateral tomograms are often quite helpful in assessing the degree of comminution or joint incongruity. By assessing the fracture radiographically, the physician can ascertained the severity of the injury relative to the distortion of normal anatomy.

Frykman (7) developed a classification system of distal radius fractures based on involvement of the radiocarpal joint, the radioulnar joint, and/or the ulnar styloid. Gartland and Werley (8) classified these fractures based on whether they are intraarticular or extraarticular relative to the radiocarpal joint. As with the eponyms, the classification systems are deficient in that they are not used universally and they do not directly correlate with available treatment modalities.

The treatment of distal radius fractures has become increasingly complex over the years. Initial management, however, has not changed. The extremity should be splinted following closed reduction. Then observation is required to rule out neurovascular compromise. Further radiographic evaluation may be performed using tomography. Ideally, definitive treatment is provided within 7 to 10 days after the fracture occurs.

Treatment modalities range from casting to internal fixation, the primary goal being to achieve anatomic reduction with the least-invasive technique. Persistent intraarticular incongruity can result in osteoarthroses; therefore, intraarticular displacements of more than 2 mm must be addressed (6). Similarly, persistent loss of volar tilt can lead to radiocarpal or radioulnar pain, decreased grip strength, and carpal instability (9, 10).

The historic method of closed reduction and casting remains a viable and frequently chosen treatment option. Extraarticular and/or minimally displaced fractures are amenable to this modality. Close observation early in the treatment course is necessary to avoid loss of reduction. Neither the method of immobilization, the choice of short-arm versus long-arm casts, nor the position of the forearm have been shown to have a significant influence on outcome (11, 12), although discretion must be based on the injury. For some fractures, closed reduction will restore the anatomy, but pins or external fixation may be necessary to maintain the reduction.

For intraarticular fractures with extensive comminution, open reduction and internal fixation are frequently necessary to achieve treatment goals. Treatment must be tailored to the particular type of fracture. Internal and external fixation may be used in combination. Bone grafting also may be necessary to provide the requisite structural support to the articular surface.

After the initial treatment, physical therapy should be started while the patient is still immobilized. Such therapy should focus on metacarpophalangeal (MCP), proximal interphalangeal (PIP), and distal interphalangeal (DIP) motion and should aim to prevent further joint stiffness and potential reflex sympathetic dystrophy (13). Once radiographic and clinical union have been achieved, generally within 6 to 8 weeks, gentle range of motion of the forearm and wrist should be instituted. The rate of progression and degree of protection must be individualized to match the patient, his or her sport, and severity of initial injury.

In the pediatric patient with open physes and wrist pain, one must suspect a Salter physeal fracture. Cheerleaders and gymnasts frequently have this type of fracture. Pain directly over the physis upon palpation is indicative of this injury. Roentgenographic findings often are negative. The treatment consists of casting for 3 to 4 weeks. Following cast removal, a series of gentle stretching and strengthening exercises is recommended, with a progression of cheerleading or gymnastic tasks. These are often performed with some type of wrap to limit terminal wrist extension, which prevents early and excessive loading of a fracture site and prevents development of tendinitis in a deconditioned wrist.

Scaphoid Fractures

The scaphoid is the most frequently fractured of the eight carpal bones. Generally, it is injured from axial loading on a dorsiflexed wrist, as occurs in a fall or during contact sports. Scaphoid fractures are seen most often in young male adults and are quite rare in children.

Initial symptoms include radial wrist pain with focal tenderness over the anatomic snuffbox. This may or may not be accompanied by localized edema. Radiographic evaluation must include AP, lateral, and ulnar deviation views of the carpus as well as a posteroanterior (PA) clenched-fist view. Because of carpal mechanics, the clenched fist brings the wrist into dorsiflexion and ulnar deviation, thus providing an excellent view of the scaphoid.

When suspicion is high for a fracture, based on the patient's history and physical examination, treatment should be instituted even if the findings on preliminary radiographs are normal. A thumb spica cast or splint should be applied, and 10 to 14 days later, radiographic evaluation should be repeated. By this time, bone resorption at the fracture site often enables better visualization. The authors also recommend that all patients with a scaphoid fracture undergo AP and lateral tomography to assess displacement and angulation.

Fractures of the scaphoid generally can occur at any of five sites: the tuberosity, the proximal third, the waist, the distal third, or the scaphotrapezial joint (osteochondral fractures) (14). A clinically important difference is that the distal fractures have essentially a 100% union rate, whereas the rate of nonunion and avascular necrosis increase as fractures become more proximal. This is because the blood supply to the scaphoid is composed of a branch of the radial artery, which enters the dorsal ridge distally. This branch provides 70% to 80% of the intraosseous blood supply and supplies essentially the entire proximal pole. An additional 20% to 30% of the blood supply enter volarly at the level of the tuberosity (15).

Our preferred treatment for nondisplaced fractures, regardless of location, is application of a long-arm thumb spica cast for 4 to 6 weeks (16). Then a short-arm thumb spica can be substituted until union is documented by tomography. Many professional and amateur sporting associations do not allow players to participate with rigid immobilization of upper extremity injuries. To facilitate the return to play, athletes with stable scaphoid fractures can practice while wearing Fiberglas or plaster short-arm thumb spica cast. This in turn may be exchanged for a Silastic spica cast for game play. This requires significant time and attention and frequent cast changes. The benefit is that the athlete can return to his or her sport almost immediately.

Displaced fractures, as defined by Cooney et al. (17), are those with a gap wider than 1 mm, a scapholunate angle greater than 60°, or lunocapitate angle greater than 15°. These fractures require a more aggressive approach in an attempt to prevent nonunion or future carpal instability. Open reduction and internal fixation with either a Herbert screw or an AO 3.5-mm screw have proven to be effective for this purpose. On a rare occasion, closed reduction and percutaneous pinning can be used. Early return to play is not advised because of loss of fixation. In fact, postoperative loss of fixation is a significantly greater problem than is angulation of a conservatively treated fracture. Therefore, it is recommended that after internal fixation, play not be resumed until there is evidence of fracture healing.

The treating physician must be wary of an acute injury superimposed on a chronic union. Radiographically, this may manifest as sclerosis of the fracture fragments, cyst formation, and fracture-gap widening. The treatment of nonunions includes corticocancellous bone grafting with or without internal fixation. The modified Russe technique also has proven effective, reportedly achieving union rates of up to 97% (18, 19). The volar approach is preferred to minimize further compromise of the blood supply to the scaphoid.

Rotary Subluxation of the Scaphoid

Hyperextension injuries of the wrist can cause many combinations of ligamentous injuries, fracture dislocations, or both. Mayfield (20) showed experimentally that a spectrum of ligamentous injuries generally begins on the radial aspect of the carpus and propagates toward the ulna. The most common of these injuries results in a scapholunate dissociation, representing a disruption of the scapholunate interosseous ligament and the volar extrinsic ligaments.

Clinically, rotary subluxation of the scaphoid or scapholunate dissociation (used interchangeably) is characterized by tenderness over the snuffbox and point tenderness over the dorsum of the scapholunate joint. A useful diagnostic test is that described by Watson (21): With passive motion of the wrist from ulnar to radial deviation and with volar pressure on the scaphoid tuberosity, the proximal pole of the scaphoid can be displaced from the scaphoid fossa of the radius. This cannot be accomplished on the contralateral (normal) side.

The definitive diagnosis of scapholunate dissociation is made radiographically. On the AP view of the wrist, the scapholunate interval will be wider than its normal 2 mm (22). In addition, the scaphoid generally adopts a palmar flexed orientation. Therefore, the AP view demonstrates foreshortening of the scaphoid and a "cortical ring" sign. On the lateral view, the scapholunate angle is often increased consistent with a dorsal intercalated segmental instability (DISI) pattern (23). In questionable cases, arthrography can be helpful for better documentation.

Treatment options differ depending on whether the injury is acute or chronic. Most of these injuries are discovered late and often are not associated with an isolated traumatic event. Options for early treatment include closed reduction with percutaneous pinning and primary ligamentous open repair.

Although its use is controversial, the authors prefer primary open repair to ensure anatomic reduction and ligamentous healing. When the injury is found relatively late, the clinical picture is often complicated by arthritic changes in the involved carpal bones and radius. Therapeutic choices include ligamentous reconstruction, carpal arthrodesis, and wrist arthrodesis. The authors prefer to perform ligamentous reconstruction, such as dorsal capsulodesis as described by Blatt (24), because it preserves wrist motion, which is sacrificed with arthrodesis. As salvage procedures, limited carpal arthrodesis or wrist arthrodesis remains options.

Ulnar Wrist Pain

Diagnosing the cause of ulnar wrist pain in athletes can be difficult. The history and physical examination must note findings such as clicking, snapping, or clunking of a tendon or bone. The differential diagnosis must include tears of the triangular fibrocartilage complex (TFCC), of the lunotriquetral ligaments, or of both.

Clicking and pain with ulnar deviation of the wrist are typical signs of TFCC tears. The diagnosis can be confirmed only by wrist arthrography, arthroscopy, magnetic resonance imaging (MRI), or some combination. Treatment consists of debridement of the TFCC if the tear is central and repair of the TFCC if peripheral. Debridement can be performed either open or arthroscopically.

Lunotriquetral ligament tears also are characterized by clicking and/or clunking with ulnar circumduction of the wrist. A diagnosis can be attained with lateral radiographs if a volar instability pattern is noted. Often, however, wrist arthroscopy or arthrography is necessary. Treatment consists of ligament repair or intercarpal fusion, depending on the degree of instability and pain.

Carpal Dislocation

High-energy hyperextension wrist injuries can result in massive ligamentous damage to the carpus, thereby leading to true carpal dislocations. Such dislocations represent the extreme of Mayfield's (20) "progressive perilunar instability" spectrum. Because the ligamentous injury theoretically begins on the radial aspect of the carpus and propagates toward the ulna, the result is either a lunate or perilunate dislocation. The latter describes a carpal dislocation in which the lunate remains in the lunate fossa of the radius, and the remainder of the carpus undergoes dorsal or volar dislocation. In the reverse scenario (lunate dislocation) dorsal or volar dislocation of the lunate occurs, while the remainder of the carpus maintains its anatomic position. Dislocation patterns can become more complex because these injuries also can be associated with fractures. On the radial aspect of the carpus, either the scapholunate interosseous ligament is disrupted or the scaphoid fractures. Thus, aside from a perilunate dislocation, one may suffer a transscaphoid perilunate dislocation, which is accompanied by a scaphoid fracture. Classification of these injury patterns is complex (25) but is based on the basic premise that the range of carpal dislocations represents a broad spectrum of injury.

Clinically, the patient has a painful, edematous wrist with marked limitation of motion. Aside from a history of significant trauma, patients often have bruises over their thenar or hypothenar eminence, suggesting hyperextension-type injuries. Median nerve compression symptoms also are common, secondary to local compression and/or the initial injury. Radiographically, carpal dislocations can be obvious or quite subtle. Initial AP, lateral, and oblique views are often adequate for diagnosis. A PA film with ulnar deviation of the wrist is also helpful. If a carpal dislocation is present, the PA view will show one or more of the following: a triangular lunate or elongation of the volar lip of the lunate, loss of congruity between the radiocarpal articulations, loss of carpal height, or overlapping carpal bones (26).

The goal of treatment of these complex injuries is to restore the anatomic alignment of the carpus by closed or open means. One recognized treatment includes closed reduction and splinting. If closed reduction is accomplished, the subsequent radiographs must be examined very closely. Because of the severity of ligamentous damage, they usually show residual ligamentous carpal instability. This instability may include rotary subluxation of the scaphoid or a volar intercalated segmental instability (VISI) or dorsal intercalated segmental instability (DISI) pattern (27). These findings are manifest on the lateral radiograph by abnormalities in the scapholunate angle (normally 30° to 60°), the radiolunate angle (normally 0° to 15°), or the capitolunate angle (normally 0° to 15°). Although closed reduction with percutaneous pinning is an option, open reduction with percutaneous pinning usually is required.

Once anatomic reduction is achieved, prolonged immobilization with casting is necessary for 10 to 12 weeks. During this period, the injury must be observed closely to monitor for loss of reduction. Participation in sports without the protection of a rigid or soft cast is not recommended immediately after closed treatment or open ligamentous repair. The extremity should be immobilized for 6 to 8 weeks to allow ligamentous healing. The use of protective orthotics must be continued during play until full, pain-free motion is possible. Potential sequelae of these injuries include late carpal instability, avascular necrosis of the scaphoid or lunate, and carpal arthrosis.

Hamate Fractures

Fractures of the hook of the hamate bone can occur from a direct blow while falling onto an outstretched palm. However, athletes tend to sustain such injuries while swinging a bat, golf club, or racquet.

Patients with these injuries experience pain when firm pressure is applied over the hook of the hamate. Their grip strength may be mildly decreased as well. Infrequently, patients complain of paresthesias or numbness in the ring or little finger; this is because the fracture is close to the ulnar nerve. On routine AP and lateral roentgenograms, these fractures are difficult to recognize. They are best visualized on either a carpal tunnel view or an oblique view with the forearm supinated 45° and the wrist dorsiflexed. On rare occasion, a computed tomography (CT) scan may be required to better demonstrate the base of the hook or the body of the hamate.

Recent literature has reported a considerably high incidence of nonunion or chronic pain related to these fractures. The pisohamate and transverse carpal ligaments as well as the flexor digiti minimi brevis and the abductor digiti minimi muscles are attached to the hook. Therefore, the fracture site has a high propensity for motion even with cast immobilization. To minimize future disability and to facilitate an early return to athletics, the current recommended treatment is excision of the hook of the hamate. This treatment is recommended for all patients, whether the injury is new or old. Competitive athletes may return to play 4 to 6 weeks after excision (28).

Kienböck's Disease

Avascular necrosis of the lunate bone, or Kienböck's disease, is a clinical entity seen in the general population. The loss of vascularity to this carpal bone has no known cause. Although Kienböck's disease can be related to a traumatic injury such as a carpal dislocation, often no prior injury can be implicated.

Clinical signs and symptoms include a painful, possibly edematous wrist, a loss of grip strength, and localized tenderness. Radiographically, Kienböck's disease includes a spectrum of findings ranging from lunate sclerosis in the early stages to complete carpal collapse and arthrosis later. In the early phase, plain films and MRI are quite useful diagnostically. Kienböck's disease has been associated with an ulnar-minus relationship between the distal radius and the distal ulna, although this is not always present (29). On a PA roentgenogram of the wrist in the neutral position, the relationship between the articular surfaces of the distal radius and the ulna can be assessed. In the normal wrist, the articular surfaces are most often lined up equally; in the ulnar-minus variant, the ulna is shorter than the radius; and in the ulna-plus variant, the reverse is true.

Early recognition of Kienböck's disease is important to prevent carpal collapse and arthrosis. Unfortunately, no treatment option is universally successful in halting progression. The authors currently prefer radial shortening in an effort to equalize the radial and ulnar lengths and theoretically "unload" the lunate (30). If the disease is advanced at the time of diagnosis, options are limited to carpal or radiocarpal arthrodesis as salvage procedures.

Metacarpal Fractures

Metacarpal fractures are among the most common fractures in both the competitive athlete and the general population. These fractures can be classified based on their anatomic location: head, neck, shaft, or base.

The hand with a metacarpal fracture has dorsal swelling, with localized tenderness over the involved metacarpal. If the patient makes a fist, the dorsal prominence of the MCP joint is often decreased or absent. The involved digits must be assessed for rotational malalignment and axial shortening. Shortening can be ascertained with the digits in full extension; rotation, by asking the patient to flex the MCP and PIP joints while extending the DIP joints. With the hand in this position, all digits should point to one imaginary point on the forearm; there should be no digital divergence or overlap. In addition, the nail surfaces should lie roughly in the same plane. Patients who sustain metacarpal fractures by striking a person in the mouth must be examined closely for dorsal skin wounds. Often, a small, superficial puncture represents a large dorsal rent in the extensor hood. These fractures must be treated aggressively as open fractures, because they pose a high risk for joint infection.

For radiographic evaluation, AP and lateral roentgenograms generally surface, though oblique views occasionally are needed. The classic posture of neck and shaft fractures is apex dorsal angulation, which is caused by the deforming force of the interosseus muscles.

Metacarpal fractures involving the joint must be approached in a manner similar to other intraarticular injuries. If the joint surface is substantially displaced, the fracture and joint surface may have to be stabilized with internal fixation.

A metacarpal neck fracture, referred to improperly as a boxer's fracture, typically causes volar angulation. Of importance is the fact that carpometacarpal motion of metacarpals two and three is markedly less than that of metacarpals four and five. Therefore, volar angulation of up to 40° or 50° can be accepted with the fourth and fifth metacarpals, whereas the second and third cannot withstand such severe angulation. After the length and rotation of the metacarpals are assessed, these fractures usually can be treated with closed reduction and splinting. The splint must hold the MCP joints flexed at an angle of 70° to 90° degrees with the PIP and DIP joints in 5° to 10° of flexion. This position keeps the collateral ligaments taut, thereby preventing later joint stiffness. If attempts at closed reduction fail, an open or percutaneous operative method is the next step. Immobilization is necessary for 3 to 4 weeks to achieve clinical union. Range-of-motion exercises can be started before union is confirmed radiographically.

Shaft fractures are plagued by the same potential problems as neck fractures, including shortening, angulation, and rotational deformities. The treatment methods are also similar, beginning with closed reduction and splinting and, if necessary, progressing to open reduction and internal fixation. Spiral or oblique fractures have a significant potential for shortening and rotating, and they often must be treated more aggressively. For the athlete, an orthoplast splint often can be fabricated to allow an early return to play. Use of silicone casting (RTV 11) is effective for skill positions and offers the advantage of easy, on-field adjustment for fine-tuning. However, this option poses the potential for loss of fracture reduction. Open reduction and internal fixation of shaft fractures with AO techniques enables the earliest return to motion and sports for fractures that require stabilization.

Fractures of the metacarpal base generally are stable, but again, rotational deformity is possible. Also, radiography must be adequate to rule out a carpometacarpal dislocation. More important, fractures at the base of the thumb and fifth metacarpal must be distinguished from those of the other rays because of their greater risk for displacement such as in Bennett's and reverse Bennett's fractures.

Axial loads on the metacarpal of the thumb can fracture the first carpometacarpal joint. This often leads to a volar lip fracture with radial and dorsal subluxation of the metacarpal fracture, or a so-called Bennett's fracture. If this is a T- or Y-intraarticular fracture, the eponym *Rolando's fracture* may be applied. These injuries are true fracture dislocations and, therefore, must be treated more aggressively than most Bennett's fractures. The treatment of choice usually is closed reduction and percutaneous pinning, but open reduction remains a viable, sometimes necessary option. Intraarticular fractures of the fifth metacarpal base (reverse Bennett's fracture) can be treated similarly.

In summary, metacarpal fractures are common injuries with relatively straightforward treatment. However, these injuries must be taken seriously, because they can lead to significant deformity and disability. The potential for shortening, rotation, angulation, and joint stiffness is always present throughout the treatment course. Therefore, close observation and serial radiographs are necessary during the initial 3 to 6 weeks (31).

Soft Tissue Injuries

Metacarpophalangeal Joint Dislocations

Dislocations of the MCP joints in the fingers or injuries of their collateral ligaments are relatively uncommon in the athlete. This is because of the inherent ligamentous stability of these joints, which is provided by the soft tissue complex including the volar plate, collateral ligaments, and transverse metacarpal ligaments. Nonetheless, the MCP joint is vulnerable to injury from dorsally directed forces, and therefore, most MCP injuries result from hyperextension.

MCP dislocations can be either dorsal or volar and are further classified as simple or complex (32). A simple dislocation is reducible by a closed method, whereas the complex type is not. With a simple dorsal dislocation, the MCP joint is hyperextended 60° to 90°, and the PIP and DIP joints are slightly flexed. Although reduction usually can be achieved by closed means, excessive traction and/or hyperextension can convert a simple dislocation into a complex one (33). The reduction maneuver includes wrist flexion and gentle MCP hyperextension followed by flexion of the MCP joint, while contact is maintained between the articular surfaces of the metacarpal and proximal phalanx.

With a complex dorsal MCP dislocation, hyperextension of the involved joint is minimal, and the distal joints are slightly flexed. In addition, the volar skin of the MCP is dimpled. Radiographically, the proximal phalanx overlies the metacarpal head, and they are almost parallel. A pathognomonic radiographic sign of a complex dislocation is a sesamoid lying within the joint space (32). Reduction of a complex dislocation is obstructed by the interposition of soft tissue—usually the volar plate. Consequently, open reduction is required and can be accomplished through either a dorsal or volar approach. The authors prefer the dorsal approach.

After open or closed reduction, dorsal MCP dislocations require protective splinting to prevent hyperextension. The preferred method is extension block splinting for 3 to 4 weeks, allowing early motion. When the dislocation is simple, buddy taping to an adjacent digit is acceptable treatment, but protective splinting or taping must be adequate during athletic participation to prevent reinjury.

Volar MCP dislocations are exceedingly rare, but irreducible dislocations have been reported. The affecting structures in such cases may include the dorsal capsule, the volar plate, or the collateral ligaments. Therefore, a dorsal and volar approach to reduction occasionally is required (34).

Collateral ligament injuries or lateral dislocations of the MCP joints of the fingers can result from laterally directed forces. The patient has pain and swelling over the involved ligament, and stressing the affected structure elicits pain and instability. Adequate treatment often can be provided by 3 weeks of splinting with the joint flexed 50° to 90° (35). In rare instances, these injuries are accompanied by avulsion injuries. If a significant portion of the metacarpal is involved, open reduction with internal fixation may be indicated (31).

Injuries of the Metacarpophalangeal Joint of the Thumb

Injuries of the MCP joint of the thumb are seen frequently in skiers, football players, and participants in racquet sports. This condyloid joint provides flexion/extension, adduction/abduction, and a minor degree of rotation. The range of motion is quite varied from one individual to another. Abduction and hyperextension injuries to this joint often completely or partially tear the ulnar collateral ligament. If unrecognized, such lesions can result in chronic pain, instability, and decreased pinch strength.

Clinically, a hyperextension/abduction injury to this MCP joint causes pain and localized edema. Partial and complete tears must be differentiated because their treatments differ. A clinical examination and stress radiographs generally are adequate to make this distinction, and patients often require local anesthesia to undergo an adequate examination. To stress the joint, the metacarpal must be stabilized while abduction stress is applied to the proximal phalanx. This should be performed with the MCP in extension and repeated with the joint flexed 30°. Comparison with the uninjured side is mandatory, because of the wide range of motion in this joint. When there is a complete tear, the joint often can be abducted 45° or more, and no end point can be noted (36). Another indicator is the ability to abduct the joint at least 10° more than the contralateral thumb (37).

Partial ulnar collateral ligament tears can be treated successfully with a short-arm thumb spica cast for 4 to 6 weeks. Although taping or orthoplast bracing can be used instead, complete immobilization is preferable.

Football players may return to play with adequate splinting in 3 to 10 days. Volleyball and basketball players, however, require protective splinting for an entire season because these sports cause frequent loading. Skiers can use gauntlet casts or commercially available gloves with no time lost.

Due to the local anatomy of the ulnar collateral ligament, complete tears do not often fare as well with conservative treatment. There is a propensity for the adductor aponeurosis to become interposed between the torn ends of the ligament, thereby resulting in the so-called Stener's lesion (38). Moreover, a complete tear with adductor interposition cannot be differentiated from one without. Because Stener's lesions have a relatively high incidence, primary surgical repair must be considered for all complete tears of this ligament. Most often, the ligament is torn from the base of the proximal phalanx and, therefore, must be reattached to bone. However, if the tear is midsubstance, primary repair can be performed (Fig. 53.1).

For the patient with chronic game-keeper's thumb, the treatment plan often must be altered. Delayed treatment frequently precludes primary anatomic repair. Thus more extensive reconstructive procedures, including free tendon grafts or tendon transfers, may be necessary. Following early or delayed repair of gamekeeper's thumb, protective splinting is necessary to prevent recurrent abduction stresses on the MCP joint.

Injuries of the radial collateral ligament of the thumb are less common and generally less debilitating because the thumb is subjected to abduction stress more frequently than to adduction stress. The author's favor a diagnostic and therapeutic approach similar to that for injuries of the ulnar collateral ligament.

Dislocations of the MCP joint of the thumb can occur in the volar or dorsal plane, the latter being much more common. Simple dorsal dislocations can be reduced with wrist flexion, interphalangeal joint flexion, and gentle volar pressure on the proximal phalanx. Complex dislocations require open reduction. Generally with a dorsal dislocation, the volar plate is torn, but the collateral ligaments remain intact. For any of these dislocations, postreduction examination is mandatory immediately to assess joint stability. If the joint is unstable, the collateral ligaments must be examined and treated as previously described.

Proximal Interphalangeal Joint Injuries

The PIP joints of the hand have a great deal of inherent bony and ligamentous stability. The volar plate and the radial and ulnar collateral ligaments are the soft tissue constraints that allow the joint to flex and extend while limiting rotation and lateral deviation. The bicondylar nature of the bony architecture forms a hinge joint

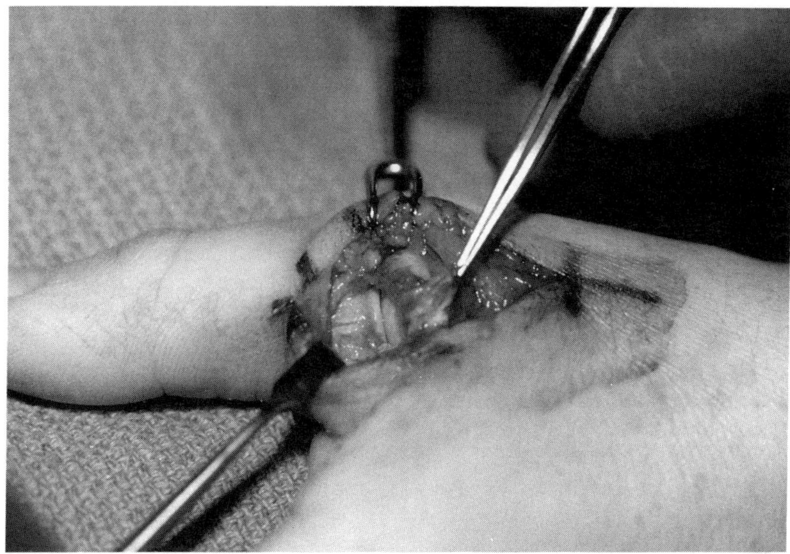

Figure 53.1. In the Stener lesion, the adductor aponeurosis is trapped between the ulnar collateral ligament and its insertion, which prevents healing.

that permits only flexion and extension. The normal range of motion is approximately 0° to 105°, although flexion can be up to 120° in some individuals. The PIP joint is highly susceptible to injury because of the long proximal and distal levers of the proximal and middle phalanges. Unfortunately, this joint also is prone to stiffness after injury. Therefore, PIP injuries should be treated early and aggressively.

Collateral Ligament Tears

Collateral ligaments of the PIP joint usually are injured by laterally directed stresses while the joint is extended (39). Participants in football, wrestling, and baseball are particularly prone to such injuries. Victims generally have edematous, tender PIP joints, and this pain tends to limit motion. The point of maximal tenderness—the volar plate, central slip, or collateral ligaments—must be thoroughly examined because the dislocated PIP joint frequently has been reduced by this time.

An isolated collateral ligament tear should be defined as either partial or complete. Although the symptoms are similar, true lateral instability can be elicited when the tear is complete. Under a digital block, the PIP joint can be stressed medially or laterally. Studies have shown that a deviation of greater than 20° is indicative of a complete tear (40). Stress films can be helpful for confirmation. The examiner must also be certain that the joint has a fully congruous range of motion.

Partial collateral ligament injuries respond nicely to taping to the adjacent digit. This buddy taping limits radial and ulnar deviation while allowing active flexion and extension. It is recommended that the tape be worn for 3 to 4 weeks and that protection with specialized gloves or taping be added for up to 6 weeks during athletic activities.

The treatment of complete collateral ligament ruptures remains controversial. The options are *(a)* initial immobilization of the joint in one of various degrees of flexion followed by buddy taping and *(b)* primary repair (41, 42). The authors prefer to immobilize the PIP in 25° to 30° of flexion for 3 weeks and then tape the injured finger to the adjacent digit for 4 weeks. Primary repair should be considered when the radial collateral ligament of the index finger is injured. The potential loss of motion related to surgery must be weighed against the likelihood of chronic instability. Although chronic instability can be treated with reconstructive procedures, they are technically demanding, and the results vary.

PIP Joint Dislocation

Dislocation of the PIP joint can result from hyperextension, axial loading, or rotational force on the joint. Resultant dislocations are of three types: dorsal, volar, and rotatory. Often these injuries are reduced on the playing field before full evaluation. Reduction on the field with temporary protective taping or splinting may nable an immediate return to play. From a diagnostic standpoint, however, it is desirable to delay reduction until a radiographic evaluation has been completed. Both AP and lateral roentgenograms of the involved digits are crucial to determining the complete extent of the injury. Moreover, postreduction radiographs are necessary to document a congruous reduction without evidence of soft tissue interposition.

Dorsal dislocations (the middle phalanx lies dorsal to the proximal phalanx) are by far the most common dislocations of the PIP joint. These sometimes are accompanied by a volar fracture of the middle phalanx. In such cases, the volar plate usually is torn from its insertion on the middle phalanx. This is often manifested radiographically by a small fleck of bone volar to the middle phalanx. Although the collateral ligaments may be involved, they usually are not disrupted.

The simple dorsal dislocation can be reduced by gentle traction and mild hyperextension of the PIP, followed by gradual flexion of the joint. However, excessive traction can lead to soft tissue interposition or avulsion. Therefore confirming reduction, the authors institute dorsal extension block splinting for 3 weeks. The splint allows PIP flexion but prevents full extension, thus preventing stiffness while preserving stability of the joint. After this brief period of immobilization, active range of motion with buddy taping is encouraged for an additional 4 weeks. The taping serves to prevent hyperextension and subsequent redislocation. If closed reduction is unsuccessful, open reduction (43) is required, followed by a similar postoperative treatment course.

A more complicated situation arises when the dorsal dislocation is associated with a significant intraarticular fracture of the middle phalanx. Often this comprises 25% to 75% of the joint surface. For patients with such injuries, only one attempt at closed reduction is advised. The goal of treatment is to reduce subluxation of the remaining dorsal articular surface. Anatomic reduction of the volar lip fragment is not necessary to achieve a good functional outcome. If congruous reduction can be achieved, a program of dorsal extension block splinting (44) is recommended: Initially, extension is limited to the degree necessary to maintain reduction. Thereafter, at 1- to 2-week intervals, gradually increasing extension is permitted. Throughout the therapeutic course, active range of motion of the PIP is allowed to reduce residual stiffness. In the event that closed reduction cannot be achieved, operative intervention is required. Surgical treatments include open reduction with internal fixation and a volar plate arthroplasty. The volar plate arthroplasty as described by Eaton and Malerich (45) is a good option, whether performed soon after injury or later. This procedure involves excising the volar fragment and advancing the volar plate to fill the defect and maintain PIP reduction.

Volar dislocations of the PIP joint are quite rare. They cannot occur unless the central slip of the extensor tendon is disrupted. This injury may be overlooked if reduction is performed before radiographic evaluation. Unrecognized, it can lead to a posttraumatic boutonnière deformity. Whether a bony or strictly soft tissue injury, the residual boutonnière deformity can be prevented by 4 weeks of splinting with the PIP joint held in extension (46). This should be followed by 4 to 6 weeks of either dynamic extension splinting or buddy taping.

Another rare form of PIP joint dislocation is rotatory subluxation. This results from a rotational injury that causes one of the condyles of the proximal phalanx to herniate through a "buttonhole" formed in the extensor hood (47). The condyle then becomes lodged between the central slip and the lateral band. Often, findings on the lateral radiographs are diagnostic of this injury; a true lateral film of the proximal phalanx that does not provide a true lateral view of the middle phalanx indicates the presence of a rotational deformity. Although closed reduction may be successful, open reduction frequently is necessary. After reduction, a splint is applied until stability is achieved.

Distal Interphalangeal Joint Injuries

DIP Joint Dislocation

Dislocations of the DIP joint are less common than those of the PIP joint. The injury usually occurs from the direct impact of a solid object such as a ball or a helmet. Once again prereduction films are helpful in assessing the degree of injury, but usually, the phalanx is reduced on the playing field by longitudinal traction.

Although some DIP joint dislocations are volar, most are dorsal. In either event, closed reduction usually is successful. Open reduction may be required if soft tissues block reduction or the initial injury is open. Once reduction is accomplished, immobilization of the DIP joint in 10° to 20° of flexion for 2 to 3 weeks usually provides adequate treatment (41).

Fracture dislocations of the DIP joint may be accompanied by avulsion of either the flexor digitorum profundus or the extensor mechanism. These injuries are discussed in the following sections.

Avulsion of the Flexor Digitorum Profundus

Avulsion at the insertion of the flexor digitorum profundus into the base of the distal phalanx most often occurs in the ring finger. This injury occurs when the DIP is forcibly extended while the flexor digitorum profundus is actively contracted. The common scenario is that a tackler grabs an opponent's jersey and feels sudden pain. Unfortunately, the victim's pain and local edema often cause the loss of flexion to go unnoticed. This diagnosis may be difficult to establish, and often, the patient has pain in the palm or the PIP joint rather than the edematous DIP joint. If the patient can comply, limitation of DIP motion and grip weakness can be demonstrated.

As described by Leddy and Packer (48), three types of this injury can occur, distinguished by the level of tendon retraction. In the type I lesion, the tendon retracts into the palm, thereby severing the tendon's blood supply. With type II, the tendon retracts to the level of the PIP joint, and a portion of the blood supply remains intact. Avulsion of a large bony fragment causes the type III lesion. With this type, the tendon's retraction is limited by the A-4 pulley.

In all cases, surgical intervention is required to reconstruct the flexion mechanism of the DIP joint. When the tendon retracts into the palm, reconstruction must be performed within 7 to 10 days. Even after successful reconstruction, the tendon can rupture because of the initial vascular insult. For the patient with a type II lesion, primary repair can be performed up to 3 weeks after the injury, although earlier repair is recommended. If the tendon is avulsed with a large bone fragment, this can be anatomically reduced and secured with a button and pull-out wire.

Of primary importance with these lesions is early recognition. If diagnosed late, they may require reconstructive procedures, including tendon grafting, DIP joint arthrodesis, or excision of the flexor digitorum profundus. Delayed symptoms include decreased grip strength with limited DIP joint flexion, decreased range of motion in the PIP joint, and fullness and pain in the palm.

Injury to the Extensor Tendon of the DIP Joint

Damage of the extensor mechanism of the DIP joint is a prevalent injury among athletes. This injury is sustained either by a hyperflexion force on an already-extended DIP joint or simply a hyperextension injury of the DIP. The latter mechanism often results in a significant intraarticular fracture. The so-called mallet finger (49) refers to extensor tendon rupture from the base of the distal phalanx.

The clinical signs of these injuries are a flexed posture and decreased or absent active extension of the involved DIP joint. If left untreated, a swan-neck deformity can develop. Attempts at DIP extension result in PIP hyperextension and accentuated DIP flexion from the unopposed forces of the flexor digitorum profundus. This deformity may be subtle or absent soon after the injury occurs but becomes more evident later, when the lateral bands subluxate dorsally and the volar plate stretches. A mallet deformity can be caused by attenuation of an intact tendon or complete avulsion from its insertion. On the lateral radiograph, this avulsion may be accompanied by a small fleck of bone. A large bony fragment also can be avulsed with the tendon, resulting in a significant intraarticular fracture. This then leads to volar subluxation of the distal phalanx.

The acute injury can most often be treated adequately with conservative measures—specifically, immobilization of the DIP joint in a neutral position or slight hyperextension. This can be achieved with a variety of splinting techniques, including stack splints, dorsal or volar aluminum splints, and digital casting. By leaving the pulp free, dorsal splints enable tactile sensation and thus may be preferable. The goal of splinting is to allow unresisted extension for 6 to 8 weeks. The patient may remove the splint for hygiene, but the DIP joint must not be permitted to flex throughout the treatment course. Active PIP joint motion is encouraged throughout the recovery period.

If the injury has a significant bony intraarticular component (i.e., 25% to 50%) with or without DIP subluxation, splinting should be attempted, followed by a lateral radiograph. If the joint can be reduced congruously, this injury may be treated similarly to a soft tissue mallet finger. Close follow-up is necessary to monitor joint congruity and fracture reduction. The appropriate treatment for such an injury remains controversial, with many authors recommending open reduction and internal fixation of the fragment (50). Although open treatment remains a viable option, it is often associated with the subsequent loss of DIP joint motion (notably flexion). Therefore, a closed treatment for soft tissue and bony mallet fingers is recommended when such treatment can maintain joint congruity. A splint should be used for 6 to 8 weeks, and for the next 6 weeks, the digit should be protected during athletic activities by taping or splinting. Often the athlete is able to resume play immediately after the previously mentioned splinting techniques are initiated, regardless of whether the chosen treatment is open or closed.

Phalangeal Fractures

Fractures of the proximal, middle, and distal phalanges of the hand are among the most common injuries in athletes. Their treatment can range from splinting to open reduction and internal fixation and must be individualized for each of these fractures. The therapeutic goals are to avoid rotational deformity, angulation deformity, and axial shortening, while maintaining the range of motion of the MCP, PIP, and DIP joints. If a residual deformity persists after treatment, the patient may be left with a significant cosmetic and functional deficit.

As a rule, nondisplaced intraarticular or extraarticular phalangeal fractures can be treated with a short course of splinting followed by gentle, active range-of-motion exercises. Although the radiographic documentation of union may take several months, the more important clinical union of these fractures occurs after 3 to 4 weeks.

Extraarticular fractures of the proximal phalanx generally take on an apex-volar angulation. Transverse fractures often can be reduced by closed methods, but the chosen technique must prevent angular and rotational deformity. An angular malunion of this fracture often markedly decreases the range of motion of the PIP joint. If reduction cannot be maintained by splinting, either longitudinal or transverse K-wire percutaneous fixation (51) is recommended. Spiral fractures are amenable to the use of transverse wires, whereas transverse fractures lend themselves to longitudinal fixation.

An extraarticular fracture in the middle phalanx is less common than in the proximal phalanx. These fractures can have dorsal or volar angulation, depending on the level of the fracture. Again the therapeutic goals are to achieve an anatomic reduction, if possible by a closed method. Extraarticular fractures of the distal phalanx are adequately treated by protective immobilization. However, if the fracture is in the tuft, it may be associated with a nail bed injury. If so, a rather benign-appearing injury may in fact be an open fracture.

Intraarticular fractures of the MCP, PIP, or DIP joint must be assessed relative to joint congruity and stability. Significant displacement may predispose the involved joint to a decreased range of motion and/or posttraumatic arthritis. Condylar fractures of the PIP or DIP joint must be treated aggressively if the joint is displaced. Appropriate fixation methods include the use of percutaneous K-wires or open reduction and internal fixation with small screws (52).

Phalangeal injuries can be debilitating to certain athletes (e.g., basketball or racquet sports players). Football players, on the other hand, often can return to play almost immediately with the use of orthoplast protective splints. Phalangeal fractures usually heal in 3 to 5 weeks, and within 8 to 12 weeks, full motion is often restored.

Nerve Compression Syndromes

Athletes sometime suffer compression neuropathies of the forearm, hand, or wrist, although these account for only a small portion of sports-related hand injuries. Nonetheless, repetitive blunt trauma and/or repetitive motion place the athlete at risk for median, ulnar, radial, and digital nerve compression. Athletic injuries can cause nerve compression syndromes of the upper extremity, but such cases are relatively rare. In all cases, a thorough physical examination, including a neurologic evaluation is necessary to identify the source of site of the disorder.

Carpal Tunnel Syndrome

Defined as compression of the median nerve at the wrist, carpal tunnel syndrome is the most common upper extremity compression neuropathy. Classically, the patient describes paresthesias in the median nerve distribution. The paresthesias usually are transient and nocturnal. Patients with chronic or more advanced cases tend to have thenar atrophy, decreased two-point discrimination, and motor weakness. The Tinels's sign and Phalen's test (53) also are diagnostically helpful. In general, carpal tunnel syndrome is diagnosed on the basis of clinical findings, but electromyography is recommended for further documentation or confirmation. However, it should be remembered that electromyograms can be falsely negative, despite an obvious median nerve compression.

For mild or early cases of carpal tunnel syndrome, conservative treatment is recommended. Nonsteroidals and extension splinting frequently help to alleviate symptoms. Steroid injection (54) also has been shown to be successful, but only in a minority of patients, and it remains controversial. Many patients ultimately require surgical intervention. In cases of failed conservative therapy or advanced disease, including thenar atrophy, surgical carpal tunnel release is advised. The authors currently recommend open surgical release through an incision adequate for visualizing the nerve and its branches; at this time, arthroscopic release of the carpal canal is in the early stage of evolution. Furthermore, open operative treatment is quite reliable and is associated with a low recurrence rate. It should be noted that the patient's full grip strength and activity may not return for 3 to 4 months postoperatively.

Ulnar Nerve Compression

The ulnar nerve can become compressed at the level of the elbow (cubital tunnel) or wrist (Guyon's canal). Athletes subject to repetitive trauma in the hypothenar region, such as bicyclists or racquet-sport players, are at risk for ulnar neuropathy at the wrist. To determine the appropriate treatment, ulnar nerve compression must be characterized by the anatomic lesion. At the level of the wrist, the patient may have a pure sensory, pure motor, or combined lesion. The symptoms can include pain or paresthesia in the ulnar nerve distribution, motor weakness, or a combination of these symptoms. Advanced lesions can cause intrinsic wasting as well as power pinch weakness. Sensory and motor lesions occur when the nerve is compressed proximal to the point where it bifurcates into a deep branch and a superficial branch. If paresthesia is present in the dorsal ulnar sensory distribution, the compression usually is located at the elbow. Clinically, Tinels's sign can be elicited by percussing the cubital tunnel as well as Guyon's canal. Electrodiagnostic studies are also recommended to differentiate between proximal and distal compressive lesions.

Ulnar nerve compression at the wrist also can be caused by a hamate hook fracture (55). Baseball players, golfers, and racquet-sport competitors are susceptible to these fractures. This lesion must be considered when the patient is subject to repetitive trauma in the hypothenar region. A carpal tunnel view roentgenogram is suggested for diagnosis.

Two other ulnar nerve compression syndromes are described in the literature. "Handle-bar palsy" (56) sometimes develops in long-distance cyclists. It results from using the handle bars to support a substantial portion of body weight, thereby causing repetitive trauma to the hypothenar region of the hand. This can often be alleviated by wearing well-padded cycling gloves or by temporary abstinence from cycling. "Racquet player's pisiform" is thought to be caused by compression of the ulnar nerve, resulting from focal synovitis or arthritis of the pisotriquetral joint (57).

For all patients with a compression neuropathy at the wrist, the Allen test is mandatory to rule out a vascular anomaly or lesion, such as an ulnar artery aneurysm or thrombosis, as the source of pain. Early or mild cases of ulnar nerve compression at the wrist (transient symptoms without muscle weakness or atrophy) initially should be treated with rest, nonsteroidals, and protection. For advanced or unresponsive cases, surgical decompression of the nerve in Guyon's canal is recommended. In those patients with ulnar neuropathy accompanied by a hamate fracture, excision of the fragment has been advised (see discussion of carpal fractures).

Cheiralgia Paresthetica

The sensory branch of the radial nerve (58) can become compressed or entrapped where it exits from under the muscle belly of the brachioradialis. Consequently, the patient experiences pain and paresthesia in the radial sensory distribution. This lesion can develop from either a direct contusion or repetitive trauma. Patients with this lesion have a Tinels's sign in the region and often have false-positive findings on a Finkelstein's test. Conservative treatment with splinting, nonsteroidals, and injection frequently helps to alleviate symptoms. In resistant cases, surgical decompression may be required.

Bowler's Thumb

Perineural fibrosis of the ulnar digital nerve of the thumb is caused by the repetitive blunt trauma involved in gripping and releasing a bowling ball and thus has been referred to as "bowler's thumb" (59). The most common symptom is paresthesia in the distribution of the ulnar digital nerve of the thumb; tenderness or hyperesthesia also may occur. Generally, the nerve is enlarged, and thus this disorder may be confused with a cyst. Sensation over the thenar aspect of the thumb may be impaired, and on occasion, a Tinels's sign is noted. The recommended therapy is for this lesion conservative. Redrilling of the bowling ball or adjustment of the grip are often adequate to relieve symptoms. A protective thumb shell may be required for the resistant case.

Conclusions

Sports-related injuries of the hand and wrist are common. These injuries are not unlike those sustained by the general population, but certain sports put an individual at increased risk for specific injuries. The treating physician of the high-level athlete is given the additional burden of choosing the treatment that allows the earliest return to the sport. Treatment regimens can often be accelerated to return the athlete to play if adequate protective splints or casts are used. One must be cautious of not jeopardizing the athlete's long-term career goals by returning to play too soon. This chapter has provided a brief summary of a vast array of injuries and therapeutic options. In all cases, treatment must be individualized to suit the athlete and his or her particular situation.

REFERENCES

1. Colles A. On the fracture of the carpal extremity of the radius. Edinburgh Med Surg J 1814;10:182–186.
2. Smith RW. A treatise on fractures in the vicinity of joints, and certain forms of accidental and congenital dislocations. Dublin: Hodges & Smith, 1854.
3. Barton JR. Views and treatment of an important injury to the wrist. Med Examin 1838;1:365.
4. McCarroll HR Jr. Nerve injuries associated with wrist trauma. Orthop Clin North Am 1984;15:279–287.
5. Gruberg, Suen, Lundstrom. Radiographic measurements of the radio-carpal joint in normal adults. Acta Radiol 1976;17:249–256.
6. Jupiter JB. Fractures of the distal end of the radius. J Bone Joint Surg 1991;73A:461–469.
7. Frykman G. Fracture of the distal radius including sequelae shoulder-hand-finger syndrome, disturbance in the radio-ulnar joint and impairment of nerve function. Acta Orthop Scand Suppl 1967;108:3–153.
8. Gartland JJ Jr, Werley CW. Evaluation of healed Colles' fractures. J Bone Joint Surg 1951;33A:895–907.
9. Fernandez DL. Correction of post-traumatic wrist deformity in adults by osteotomy, bone-grafting and internal fixation. J Bone Joint Surg 1982;64A:1164–1178.
10. Talesnik J, Watson HK. Midcarpal instability caused by malunited fractures of the distal radius. J Hand Surg 1984;9A:350–357.
11. Pool C. Colle's fracture: a prospective study of treatment. J Bone Joint Surg 1973;55B:540–544.
12. Solgaard J, Burger C, Solund K. Displaced distal radius fractures. A comparative study of early results following external fixation, functional bracing in supination or dorsal plaster immobilization. Arch Orthop Treatment Surg 1989;109:34–38.
13. Cooney WP III, Dobyns JH, Linscheid RL. Complications of Colles' fractures. J Bone Joint Surg 1980;62A:613–619.
14. Cooney WP, Dobyns JH, Linscheid RL. Fractures of the scaphoid: a rational approach to management. Clin Orthop 1980;149:90–97.
15. Gelberman RH, Menon J. The vascularity of the scaphoid bone. J Hand Surg 1980;5:508–513.
16. Gellman H, Caputo RJ, Carter U, Aboulataic A, McKay M. Comparison of short and long thumb spica casts for non-displaced fractures of the carpal scaphoid. J Bone Joint Surg 1989;71A:354–357.
17. Cooney WP, Dobyns JH, Linscheid RL. Nonunion of the scaphoid: analysis of the results from bone grafting. J Hand Surg 1980;5:343–354.
18. Russe O. Fracture of the carpal navicular: diagnosis, non-operative treatment and operative treatment. J Bone Joint Surg 1960;42A:759–768.
19. Stark A, Brostrom L, Suantengren G. Scaphoid non-union treated with the Matti-Russe technique: long-term results. Clin Orthop 1987;214:175–180.
20. Mayfield JK. Patterns of injury to carpal ligaments. A spectrum. Clin Orthop 1984;187:36–42.
21. Green DP: The sore wrist without a fracture (AAOS Instructional Course Lecture No. 34). St. Louis: CV Mosby, 1985.
22. Linscheid RL. Scapholunate instabilities (dissociations, subdislocations, dislocations) Ann Chir Main 1984;3:323–330.
23. Linscheid RL, Dobyns JH, Beckenbaugh RD, Cosney WP, Wood MG. Instability patterns of the wrist. J Hand Surg 1983;8:682–686.
24. Blatt G. Capsulodesis in reconstructive hand surgery: dorsal capsulodesis for the unstable scaphoid and volar capsulodesis following excision of the distal ulna. Hand Clin 1987;3:81–102.
25. Green DP, O'Brien ET. Classification and management of carpal dislocations. Clin Orthop 1980;149:55–72.
26. Gilula LA. Carpal injuries: analytic approach and case exercises. AJR Am J Roentgenol 1979;133:503–517.
27. Linscheid RL, Dobyns JH, Beabout JW, Bryan RS. Traumatic instability of the wrist: diagnosis, classification and pathomechanics. J Bone Joint Surg 1972;54A:1612–1632.
28. Stark HH, Chao EK, Zemel NP, Richard JA, Ashworth CR. Fracture of the hook of the hamate. J Bone Joint Surg 1989;71:1202–1207.
29. Gelberman RH, Salamon PB, Jurist JM, Posch JL. Ulnar variance in Kienböck's disease. J Bone Joint Surg 1975;57A:674–676.
30. Almguist EE, Burns JF. Radial shortening for the treatment of Kienböck's disease. A 5 to 10 year follow up. J Hand Surg 1982;7:348–352.
31. Green DP, Rowland SA. Fractures and dislocations in the hand. In: Rockwood CA, Green DP, Buchholz RW, eds. Fractures in adults. Philadelphia: JB Lipincott, 1991:441–562.
32. Green DP, Terry GC. Complex dislocation of the metacarpophalangeal joint. J Bone Joint Surg 1973;55A:1480–1486.
33. McLaughlin, HL. Complex "locked" dislocation of the metacarpophalangeal joints. J Trauma 1965;5:683–688.
34. Moneim MS. Volar dislocation of the metacarpophalangeal joint. Pathologic anatomy and report of two cases. Clin Orthop 1983;176:186–189.
35. Eaton RG. Joint injuries of the hand. Springfield, IL: Charles C Thomas, 1971.
36. Smith RJ. Post-traumatic instability of the metacarpophalangeal joint of the thumb. J Bone Joint Surg 1977;59A:14–21.
37. Bowers WH, Hurst LC. Gamekeeper's thumb. Evaluation by arthrography and stress roentgenography. J Bone Joint Surg 1977;59A:519–524.
38. Stener B. Displacement of ruptured ulnar collateral ligament of the metacarpophalangeal joint of the thumb. A clinical and anatomical study. J Bone Joint Surg 1962;44B:869–879.
39. McCue FC, Honner R, Johnson MC, Gieck JH. Athletic injuries of the proximal interphalangeal joint requiring surgical treatment. J Bone Joint Surg 1970;52A:937–956.

40. Kiefhaber TR, Stern PT, Grood ES. Lateral stability of the proximal interphalangeal joint. J Hand Surg 1986;11A:661–669.
41. Eaton RG, Lutter JW. Joint injuries and their sequelae. Clin Plast Surg 1976;3:85–98.
42. Moberg E. Fractures and ligamentous injuries of the thumb and fingers. Surg Clin North Am 1960;40:297–309.
43. Green SM, Posner MA. Irreducible dorsal dislocations of the proximal interphalangeal joint. J Hand Surg 1985;10A:85–87.
44. McElfresh EC, Dobyns JH, O'Brien ET. Management of fracture-dislocation of the proximal interphalangeal joints by extension-block splinting. J Bone Joint Surg 1972;54A:1705–1711.
45. Eaton RG, Malerich MM. Volar plate arthroplasty of the proximal interphalangeal joint: a review of ten years' experience. J Hand Surg 1980;5:260–268.
46. Peimer CA, Sullivan DJ, Wild DR. Palmar dislocation of the proximal interphalangeal joint. J Hand Surg 1984;9A:39–48.
47. Nevaiser RJ, Wilson JN. Interposition of the extensor tendon resulting in persistent subluxation of the proximal interphalangeal joint of the finger. Clin Orthop 1972;83:118–120.
48. Leddy JP, Packer JW. Avulsion of the profundus tendon insertion in athletes. J Hand Surg 1977;2:66–69.
49. Stark HH, Boyer JH, Wilson JN. Mallet finger. J Bone Joint Surg 1962;44A:1061–1068.
50. Stark HH, Garmor BJ, Ashworth CR, Zemel NP, Rickard JA. Operative treatment of intra-articular fractures of the dorsal aspect of the distal phalanx of digits. J Bone Joint Surg 1987;69A:892–896.
51. Green DP. Non-articular hand fractures. The case for percutaneous pinning. In: Nevalser RJ, ed. Controversies in hand surgery. New York: Churchill Livingstone, 1990:81–89.
52. Heim V, Pfeiffer KM. Small fragment set manual. Technique recommended by the ASIF group. New York: Springer-Verlag, 1982.
53. Phalen GS. The carpal tunnel syndrome: clinical evaluation of 598 hands. Clin Orthop 1972;83:29–40.
54. Gelberman RH, Aronson D, Weisman MH. Carpal tunnel syndrome, results of a prospective trial of steroid injection and splinting. J Bone Joint Surg 1980;62A:1181–1184.
55. Carter PR, Eaton RG, Lottler SW. Ununited fracture of the hook of the hamate. J Bone Joint Surg 1977;59A:583–588.
56. Smail DF. Handlebar palsy. N Engl J Med 1975;292:322.
57. Helal B. Racquet player's pisiform. Hand 1978;10:87–90.
58. Ehrlich W, Dellon AL, MacKinnon SE. Cheiralgia paresthetica (entrapment of the radial sensory nerve). J Hand Surg 1986;11A:196–198.
59. Dobyns JH, O'Brien ET, Linsheid RL, Farow GM. Bowler's thumb: diagnosis and treatment. J Bone Joint Surg 1972;54A:751–755.

54 / KNEE INJURIES

Mark B. Silbey and Freddie H. Fu

Anatomy

The knee is composed of a hinge joint between the femur and tibia and an arthrodial joint between the femur and patella. It is divided into three compartments: medial, between the medial femoral condyle and medial tibial plateau; lateral, between the lateral femoral condyle and lateral tibial plateau; and patellofemoral, between the patella and the femur.

The femoral condyles form the rounded, articulating portion of the distal femur. The medial femoral condyle has a larger anterior-to-posterior diameter and a more symmetric curve than the lateral femoral condyle. The lateral femoral condyle is shorter than the medial femoral condyle and has a larger medial-to-lateral diameter. Between the two condyles is the intercondylar notch, which is contiguous with the anterior surface along which the patella tracks, known as the trochlear groove.

The proximal tibia is composed of the medial and lateral plateaus, the tibial spines, and the articular facet for the head of the fibula and has a 10° posterior slope. The medial plateau is larger and flatter than the lateral plateau, which is concave. The medial and lateral tibial spines arise between the two plateaus.

The patella is a sesamoid bone located within the tendon of the quadriceps femoris muscle. It is divided by a ridge into a larger lateral and smaller medial segment. These are then subdivided into thirds, plus a seventh or odd facet along the medial border. With extreme flexion, only the odd facet is in direct contact with the trochlear groove.

The proximal tibiofibular joint is a diarthrodial joint composed of the head of the fibula and its tibial articulation just distal to the lateral tibial articular surface. It allows for a slight up and down gliding motion and is stabilized by an articular capsule, small anterior and posterior ligaments, and the interosseous membrane.

Joint Capsule

The articular capsule surrounds the knee joint and is lined by a synovial membrane. This membrane extends proximal to the patella beneath the vastus muscles. It extends distally beneath the patellar tendon with the infrapatellar fat pad separating the synovium from the tendon. The synovium is reflected anterior to the cruciate ligaments and inserts on the tibia. The capsule joins with the menisci at their periphery, forming the meniscocapsular junctions. Also, medially and laterally, synovial folds may converge in the joint cavity to form a plica on either side. Posterior to the lateral meniscus, the capsule forms a sac between the meniscus and the popliteus tendon.

Extensor Mechanism

The extensor mechanism is composed of the quadriceps tendon, the patella, and the patellar tendon. The quadriceps tendon is formed by the tendinous distal expanses of the rectus femoris, vastus medialis, and vastus lateralis muscles, inserting on the proximal pole of the patella and forming a retinacular sheath over the patella. The vastus medialis obliquus muscle has its own insertion at the proximal pole. The distal portion of the exensor mechanism is formed by the patellar tendon (ligament), extending from the inferior pole of the patella to its insertion on the tibial tubercle. These structures form the primary extensors of the knee, with the tensor fascia lata performing a secondary role.

Medial Ligamentous Complex

The medial and lateral sides of the knee are each composed of three layers (I, II, and III from superficial to deep) which have been well described (1–3). On the medial side, the outer layer consists of the deep fascia that supports the muscle bellies and neurovascular structures in the popliteal region. It contains the insertion of the sartorious muscle. Separating layers I and II are the tendons of the gracilis and semitendinosus muscles. These tendons insert on the tibia along the sartorius muscle at the pes anserinus (Fig. 54.1).

The medial or tibial collateral ligament extends from the medial epicondyle to the medial aspect of the medial tibial plateau. It is composed of superficial and deep portions. The superficial medial collateral ligament makes up layer II. This structure, along with the tendon sheath of the semimembranous muscle blends with layer III, the capsule of the knee joint, at the posteromedial corner forming the posterior oblique ligament. In addition, the oblique popliteal ligament is formed by fibers of the semimembranous tendon sheath that pass obliquely across the knee to insert on the posterior aspect of the lateral femoral condyle. Also, the patellofemoral ligament is formed by a band of fibers running from the anterior portion of the superficial medial collateral ligament to the lateral patella, deep to the vastus medialis. It helps provide stability to the patellar-tracking mechanism. The deep portion of the medial collateral ligament is formed by a thickening of the capsular fibers of layer III and extends from the femur to the peripheral aspect of the meniscus and tibia. The remainder of the capsule attaches the meniscus to the tibia, forming the meniscotibial or coronary ligament that prevents excessive motion of the meniscus.

Lateral Ligamentous Complex

On the lateral side, the lateral or fibular collateral ligament extends from the posterior aspect of the lateral femoral condyle to the lateral side of the head and styloid process of the fibula. The superficial layer of the lateral side, layer I, is composed of two parts: the iliotibial tract anteriorly and the biceps femoris posteriorly (Fig. 54.2) (1). Just posterior to the biceps tendon is the peroneal nerve. Layer II is formed anteriorly by the retinaculum of the quadriceps tendon. Posteriorly, it is made up of two patellofemoral ligaments, one proximal and one distal. A patellomeniscal ligament is also present. Layer III is the lateral joint capsule. A coronary

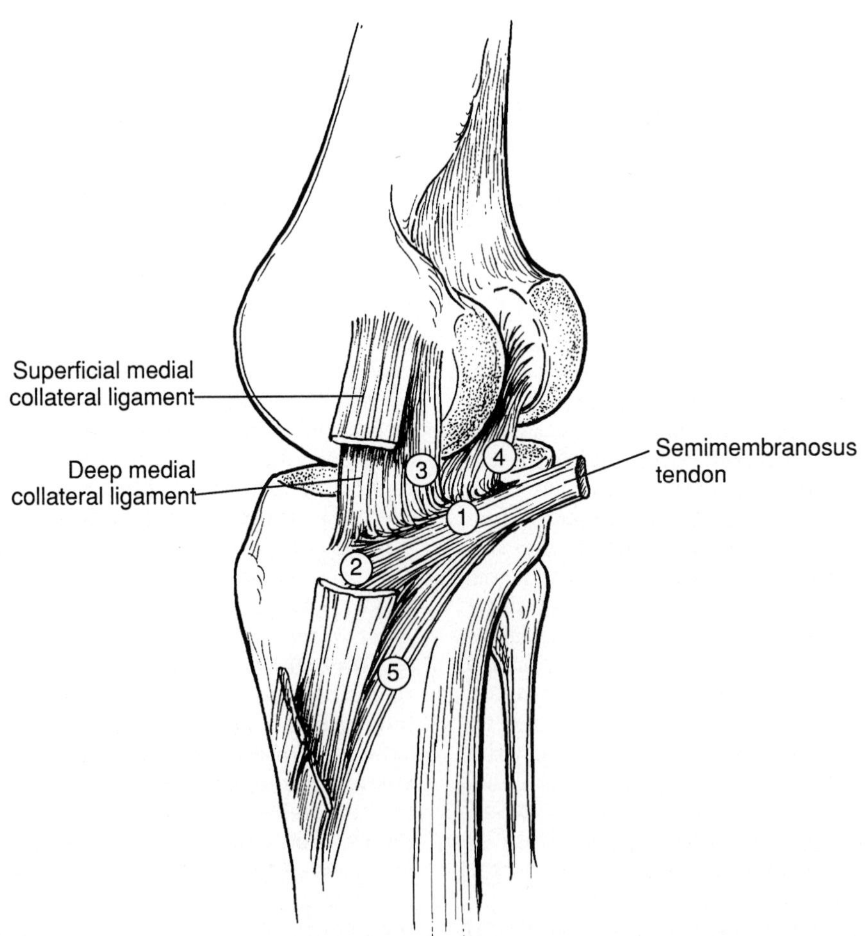

Figure 54.1. The posteromedial corner of the knee. Numbers correspond to the insertions of the semimembranosus tendon and its sheath. From Warren LF, Marshall JL. The supportive structures and layers on the medial side of the knee. An anatomical analysis. J Bone Joint Surg 1979;61:56.

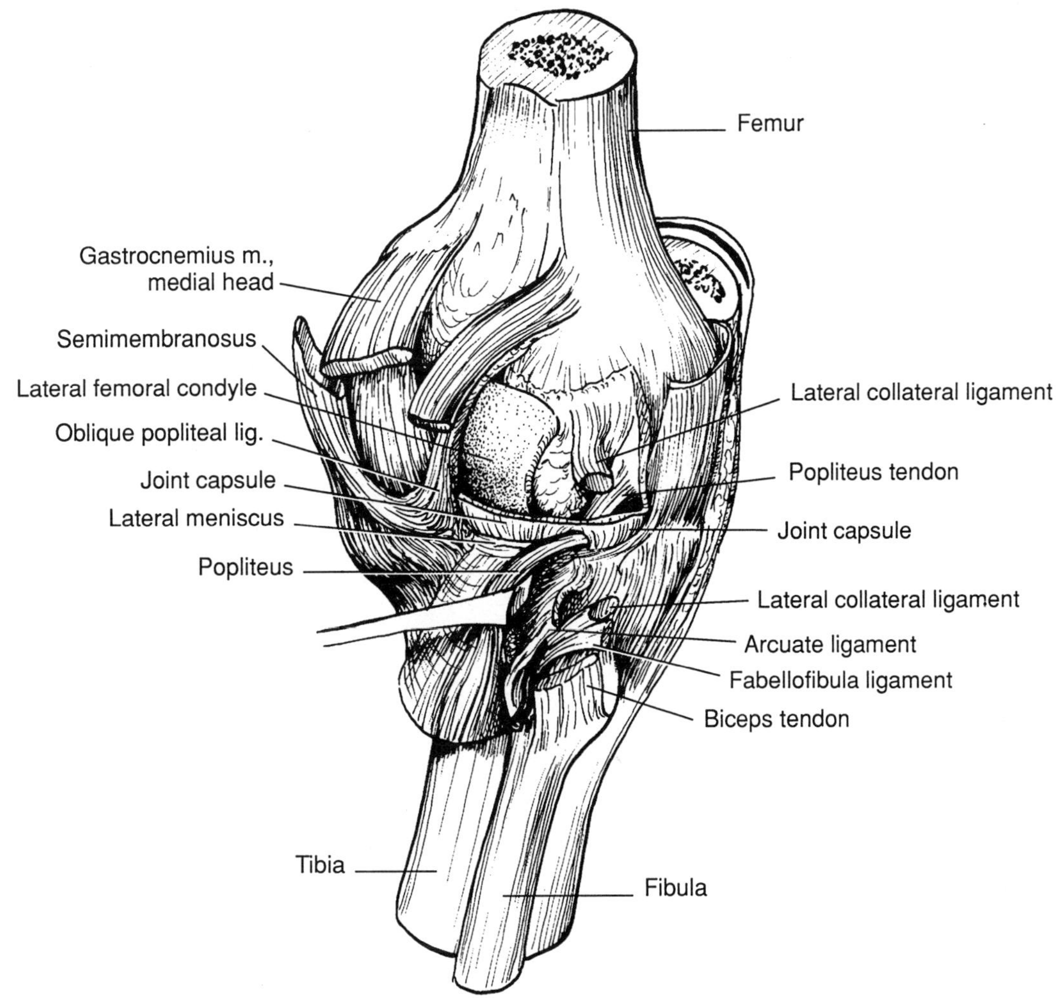

Figure 54.2. The posterolateral corner of the knee. From Seebacher JR, Inglis AE, Marshall JL et al. The structure of the posterolateral aspect of the knee. J Bone Joint Surg 1982;64:536.

ligament extends from capsule to meniscus, just as on the medial side. The popliteus tendon passes through an opening to the coronary ligament, the popliteal hiatus. The capsule divides into two laminae. The superficial lamina encompasses the lateral collateral ligament and forms the patellofibular ligament posteriorly. The deeper lamina forms the arcuate and coronary ligaments. The arcuate and patellofibular ligaments insert on the fibular styloid process and extend proximally to the lateral head of the gastrocnemius muscle. At this point, they merge with the oblique popliteal ligament.

Cruciate Ligaments

The two cruciate ligaments help to check extension, lateral rotation, and motion of the tibia on the femur. The anterior cruciate ligament extends from the posterior aspect of the lateral femoral condyle anteriorly to the tibial eminence and controls anterior motion of the tibia on the femur. The posterior cruciate ligament extends from the lateral aspect of the medial femoral condyle to the posterior aspect of the lateral meniscus and proximal tibia and controls posterior motion of the tibia on the femur (Fig. 54.3). These ligaments are discussed in more detail later in this chapter.

Menisci

The menisci are cartilaginous structures that deepen their respective tibial articular surfaces. The medial meniscus is crescent shaped and attaches to the tibia in front of the anterior cruciate ligament and in the posterior intercondylar fossa. The lateral meniscus is more circular and attaches to the tibia in front of the anterior cruciate ligament and posteriorly behind the tibial eminence but anterior to the medial meniscus. It also is attached to the medial femoral condyle through the anterior and posterior meniscofemoral ligaments, known as the ligament of Humphrey and the ligament of Wrisberg, respectively. The anterior horns of the menisci are interconnected by the transverse ligament (Fig. 54.4).

Popliteal Fossa

Posteriorly, the popliteal fossa is a diamond-shaped space. It is bounded by the biceps femoris muscle laterally and above, the semimembranosus and semiten-

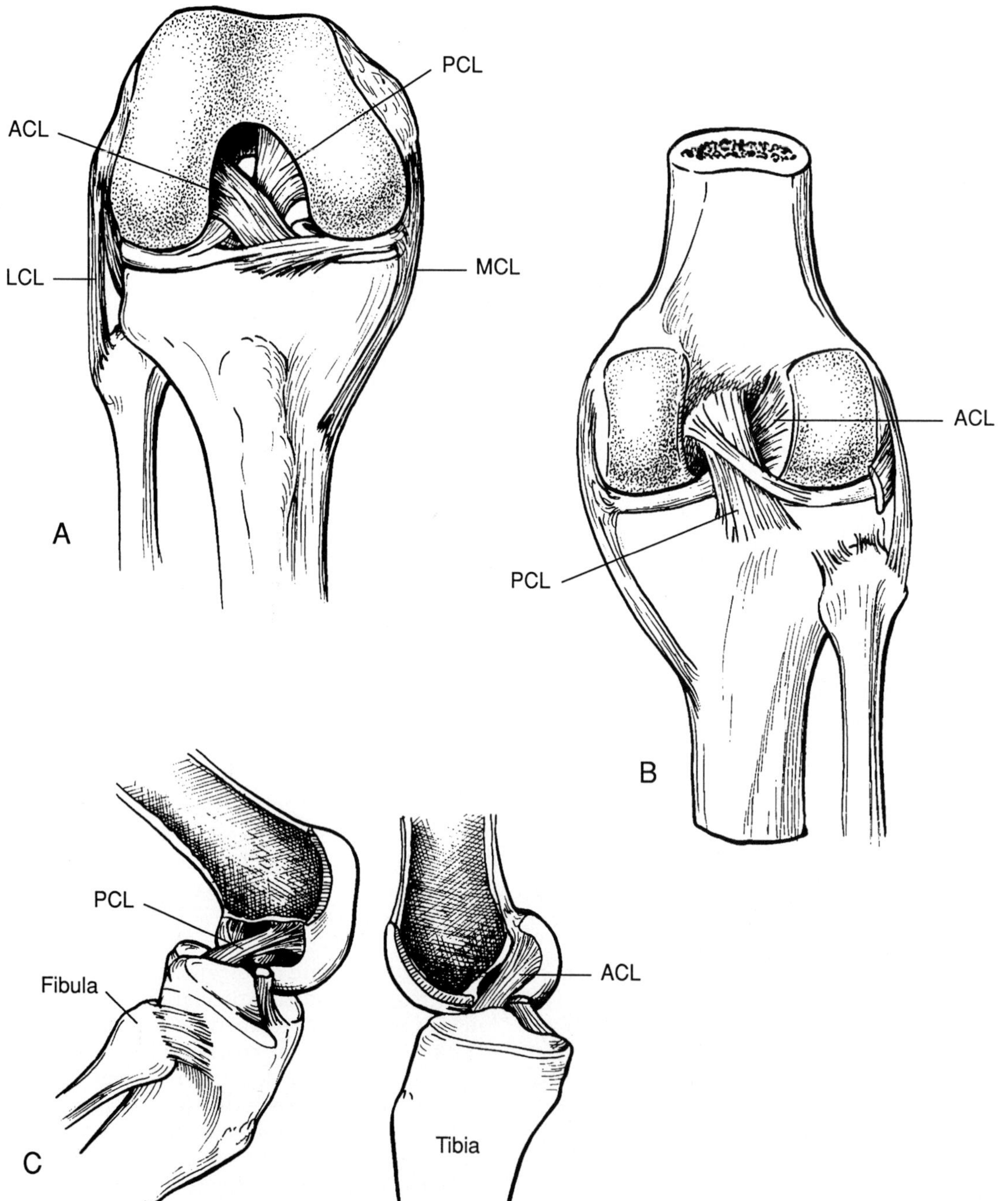

Figure 54.3 **A,** Anterior view of anterior and posterior cruciate ligaments. **B,** Posterior view of anterior and posterior cruciate ligaments. **C,** Lateral views of anterior and posterior cruciate ligaments.

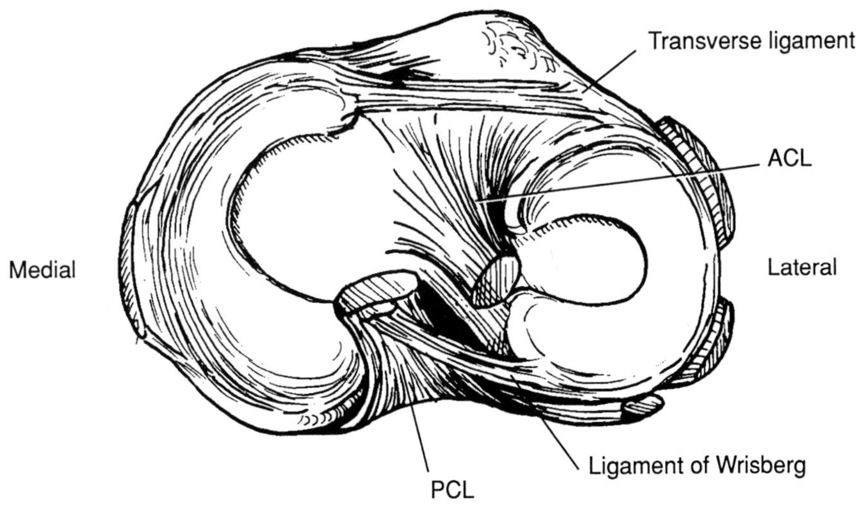

Figure 54.4. Tibial articular surface.

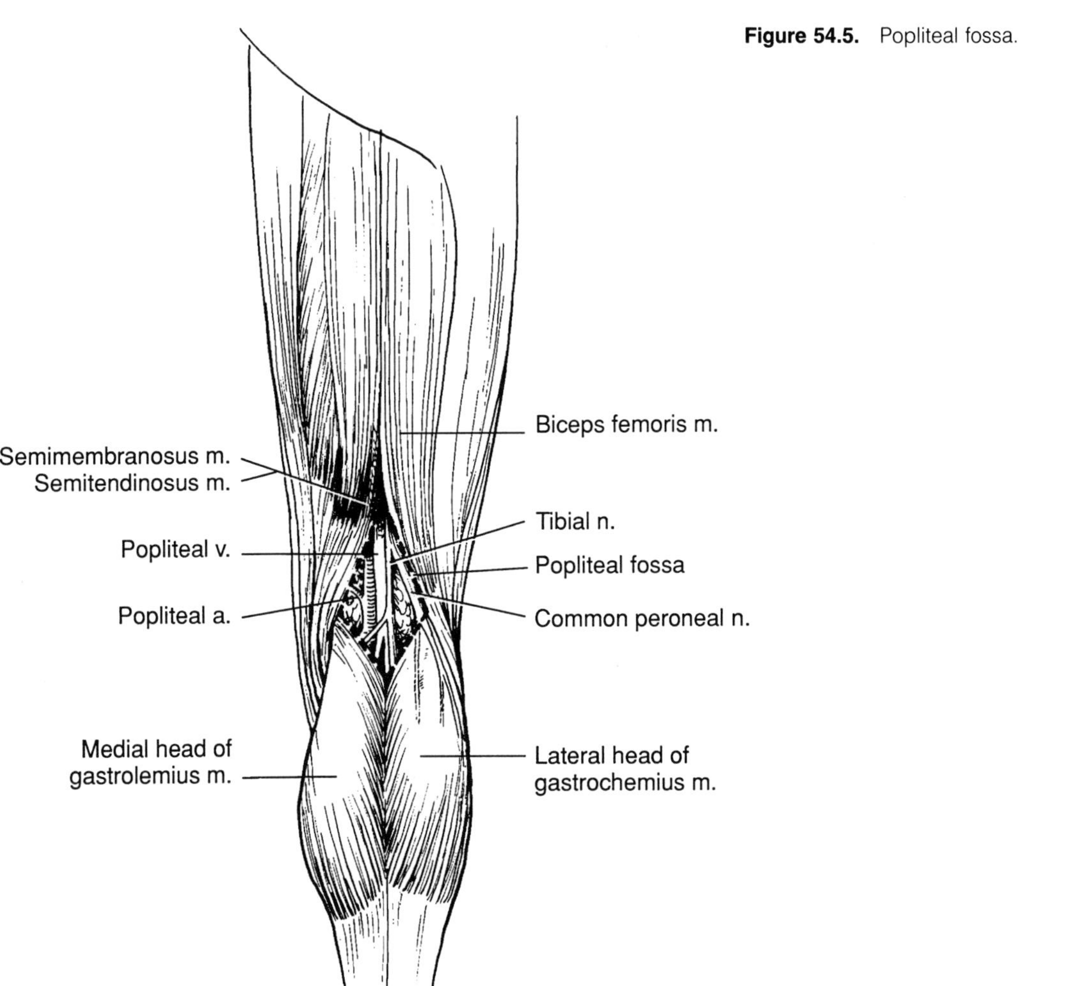

Figure 54.5. Popliteal fossa.

dinosus medially and above, the lateral head of the gastrocnemius muscle laterally and below, and the medial head of the gastrocnemius medially and below. The floor is formed by the femur, oblique popliteal ligament, and popliteus muscle. The popliteal fossa contains the popliteal artery and vein, tibial and common peroneal nerves, the termination of the small saphenous vein, the distal end of the femoral cutaneous nerve, and articular branches of the obturator nerve (Fig. 54.5).

Hamstrings

The semimembranosus and semitendinosus muscles (innervated by the tibial nerve) along with the sartorius and gracilis muscles (innervated by the femoral and obturator nerves, respectively) make up the medial hamstring group. The biceps femoris muscle makes up the lateral hamstring muscle and is composed of a long head (innervated by the tibial nerve) and a short head (innervated by the common peroneal nerve). These act as the flexors of the knee joint along with the popliteus, gastrocnemius, and plantaris muscles. As previously mentioned, the quadriceps femoris muscle (innervated by the femoral nerve), and the tensor fascia lata (innervated by the superior gluteal nerve), are responsible for knee extension. Medial rotation of the knee is achieved by the popliteus, semimembranosus, semitendinosus, sartorius, and gracilis muscles. Lateral rotation is achieved by the action of the biceps femoris.

Neurovasculature

The arterial network about the knee arises from the popliteal artery, which is a continuation of the femoral artery as it emerges from the hiatus of the adductor magnus muscle. The popliteal artery passes into the popliteal fossa, giving off superior medial, lateral and inferior medial, and lateral geniculate branches. The popliteal vein is formed by the anterior and posterior tibial veins at the level of the popliteus muscle insertion on the tibia. It continues proximally to form the femoral vein.

The sciatic nerve divides into tibial and common peroneal branches in the posterior thigh just proximal to the knee. The tibial nerve passes deep to the biceps femoris and then crosses superficially to the vessels to reach the medial side. It then continues distally as the posterior tibial nerve. The common peroneal nerve passes along the deep medial border of the biceps femoris and distally around the fibular neck before dividing into the superficial and deep peroneal nerve branches (4–18).

Biomechanics

An understanding of the fundamental biomechanical principles of knee motion is crucial to the diagnosis and management of sports injuries of the knee. As both a hinge joint and an arthrodial joint, the knee operates with 6° of freedom. There are three planes of translation and three of rotation. Translation occurs in the anterior-posterior plane (5 to 10 mm), the medial-lateral plane (1 to 2 mm), and the compression-distraction plane (2 to 5 mm). Rotation occurs as flexion/extension, varus/valgus, and internal/external. The normal range of extension is from 0° to 15° of hyperextension, and flexion from 130° to 150°. Internal and external rotation range from 20° to 30° with the knee in full extension.

During the first 15° to 20° of flexion, there is a pure rolling motion of the femoral condyles relative to the tibial plateau. By 10° to 15° of flexion on the medial side and 20° on the lateral side, gliding of the femur posteriorly on the tibia begins and becomes progressively more important as flexion continues. Subsequently, the femoral condyles rest on the posterior horns of the menisci (4). In addition to the rolling and gliding motions, during terminal extension, the tibia must externally rotate to accommodate the larger AP diameter of the medial femoral condyle relative to the lateral femoral condyle. This is known as the "screw home mechanism" and is dictated by the asymmetry of the condyles as well as the mechanical alignment of the knee and the integrity of the surrounding capsular and ligamentous structures.

Evaluation of Injuries

The sports medicine history and physical examination are critical to the accurate diagnosis and treatment of injuries. Physical examination will be discussed as it relates to specific injuries. However, a thorough history should be taken as part of the examination and evaluation process. A basic history-taking format is followed, including chief complaint, history of present illness, past medical history, and review of systems. History taking and examination should not be confined to the knee, as spine or hip problems, leg length discrepancy, or other musculoskeletal pathology may result in symptoms referable to the knee. In addition to a basic history, a relevant sports history should include types of sports and level of involvement as well as prior injuries. A history of prior or concomitant injuries may be helpful in assessing compensatory changes in the biomechanics of running, for instance, that may have produced the current knee symptomatology. Similarly, changes in the training regimen may have resulted in an overuse syndrome. The mechanism of injury plays a large role in assessing the location of the pathology. Was the onset of pain sudden or gradual? Was this a repetitive stress situation or was there an acute episode? If the episode was acute, was there a blow to the knee? If so, in what direction was the blow struck? Was there a twisting injury? Was there an audible "pop"? Did the knee swell? Was the swelling gradual or immediate? Does the knee lock or give way? When does the pain occur, while starting to run, after a few miles, or after completing the run? Is there pain going up and/or down stairs (19, 20)?

Disorders of the Extensor Mechanism

Extensor mechanism disorders may result from trauma but are often associated with intrinsic bone or soft tissue abnormalities: Symptoms are related to alterations in patellar tracking in the trochlear groove and/or patellofemoral contact forces (21). The patellofemoral joint is exposed to large forces, as reflected by the fact that the articular cartilage on the posterior aspect of the patella that acts to transmit this force is the thickest cartilage in the human body. The force is expressed as a load transmitted from the extensor mechanism to the trochlea by the patella. This load is directly proportional to the force generated by the quadriceps mechanism and indirectly proportional to the angle of the knee flexion. The patellofemoral joint reaction (contact) force varies from one-half times body weight with level walking to seven times body weight with squatting or jogging (22–26).

The patella also serves to increase the effective power of the quadriceps muscle by increasing the distance of the quadriceps mechanism from the axis of knee motion, thereby increasing the lever arm of the quadriceps mechanism. Patellar tracking is affected by several factors. The quadriceps muscles and, in particular, the vastus medialis obliquus muscle help to maintain the patella within the trochlear groove throughout the full range of knee motion. Similarly, the integrity of the medial and lateral retinaculum and patellofemoral ligaments help to maintain proper tracking. Also, the shape of the patellar and trochlear groove plays a role in patellar tracking. For instance, a flattened lateral femoral condylar ridge may allow for lateral subluxation of the patella. The Q angle is defined as the angle formed by a line drawn from the anterior superior iliac spine to the midpatella and a line drawn from the midpatella to the tibial tubercle (Fig. 54.6). A normal Q angle is up to 10° for males and up to 16° for females (26). The Q angle may be increased by external rotation of the tibia or a laterally positioned tibial tubercle, resulting in abnormal patellar tracking. Similarly, rotational deformities of the hip or foot may alter the biomechanics of patellar tracking. Also, a high-riding patella (patella alta) may be associated with tracking problems, whereas a low-riding patella (patella baja) results in increased patellofemoral joint reaction force and subsequent arthrosis.

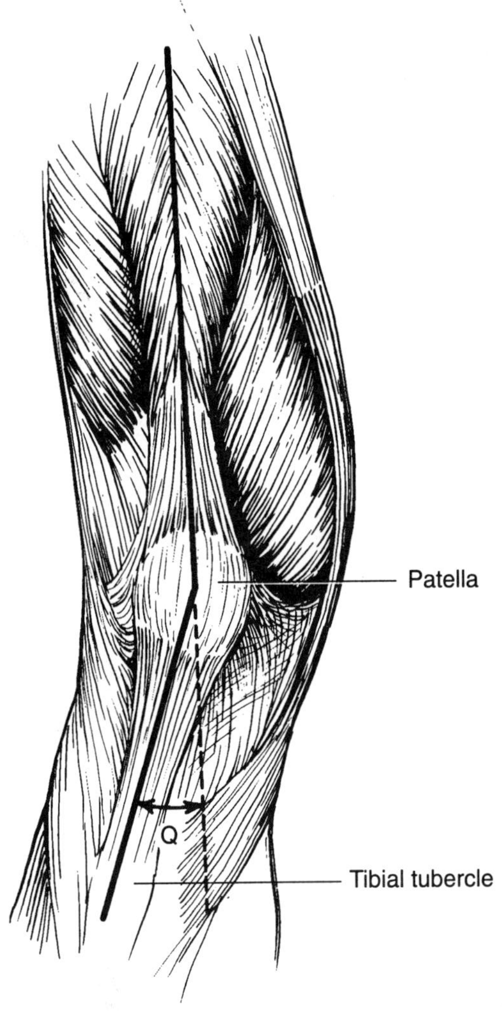

Figure 54.6. Q angle.

Evaluation

Extensor mechanism problems may be attributed to one of three subgroups: (*a*) problems of the patellofemoral articulation; (*b*) problems of the supporting muscles, tendons, ligaments, and retinaculum; and (*c*) problems of mechanical alignment, resulting in altered knee mechanics (27–31).

Physical Examination

Examination of the function and integrity of the extensor mechanism includes evaluation of the entire lower extremity. Initially, the patient's gait pattern is evaluated. Is the gait antalgic? Is there in-toeing or out-toeing that may reflect excessive internal or external tibial torsion or femoral anteversion or retroversion? Next, a standing examination is performed. Is there excessive genu valgum or varum? From the lateral view, is there genu recurvatum or a flexion contracture? This is followed by evaluation of the lower leg and foot alignment. In runners, in particular, it is important to assess the position of the distal tibia relative to the floor. If the angle formed between the distal tibia and the floor deviates laterally to 10°, then excessive subtalar joint pronation must occur to produce a plantigrade foot. This may occur with tibia vara or genu varum and produce peripatellar pain (28).

The knee is next examined with the patient in the sitting position. The legs hang freely with the knees flexed 90°. First, patellofemoral crepitation may be tested by placing the examiner's fingertips on the patella and having the patient actively flex and extend the knee. Crepitation may be graded a 1+, slight "scratching" sensation; 2+, more coarse "sandpaper-like" scratching; 3+, palpable grinding; and 4+, palpable and audible grinding. This must be distinguished from the more discrete synovial "pop" that may be normal and nonpathologic or may represent a symptomatic plica (synovial fold).

Position of the patella may also be evaluated from the sitting position. Normally, the patella rests in the trochlear groove. When the knee is flexed 90°, displacement is easily detected by palpating the position of the patella relative to the femoral condyles. Proximal displacement is referred to as patella alta and distal displacement is referred to as patella baja. In addition, the position of the patella relative to the tibial tubercle is noted. Normally, with the knee flexed 90°, the midline of the patella lines up with the tibial tubercle. Deviation from this axis may contribute to patellar tracking problems. As the patient extends the knee, the patella is noted to migrate proximally 5 to 7 cm. In the case of abnormal lateral tracking, the patella is noted to sweep abruptly laterally as it exits the trochlear groove as the knee reaches full extension.

The patient is next examined in the supine position on the examining table. Initially, the presence or absence of an effusion is assessed. With the knee in the extended position, the distal thigh is cupped in the palm of the examiner's hand and fluid from the suprapatellar pouch is gently milked distally (Fig. 54.7). Using the opposite hand, the examiner then palpates the peripatellar region for any accumulation of fluid. With the knee remaining extended, the medial and lateral retinaculum is then palpated and any tenderness is noted. By gently moving the patella medially and laterally the extent of patellar mobility may be assessed. Patellar gliding may be quantitated by dividing the patella longitudinally into four quadrants and noting the amount of medial and lateral displacement. For example, gliding of the patella medially so that two quandrants are displaced across the medial femoral condyle is denoted 2+ medial glide. Apprehension or guarding of the patient on glide testing reflects a tendency toward patellar subluxation or dislocation (Fig. 54.8). In conjunction, tenderness along the medial retinaculum and/or the medial patellofemoral ligament or patellomeniscal ligament may reflect a recent subluxation or dislocation. This test may more easily be performed with the knee supported in a flexed position at 30°. Also, as the patella is moved medially and laterally, medial and lateral patellar facet tenderness may be assessed by palpation of these regions.

Next, the patient is asked to perform a straight-leg raise by tightening the quadriceps muscle and elevating the leg. An inability to elevate the leg reflects a disruption in the extensor mechanism (quadriceps tendon rupture, patellar tendon rupture, or patellar fracture), and any soft tissue or bony defects should be palpated and noted. Occasionally, a patient will be unable to perform a straight-leg raise because of pain and accompanying effusion from another knee pathology. Under such circumstances, the knee may be aspirated and injected with 10 ml of lidocaine. Such a procedure temporarily alleviates the discomfort and allows for testing of the extensor mechanism. If this is done, the character and amount of the effusion should be noted (yellow, blood-tinged, bloody, and/or cloudy) as well as the presence of any fat droplets, which are indicative of fracture.

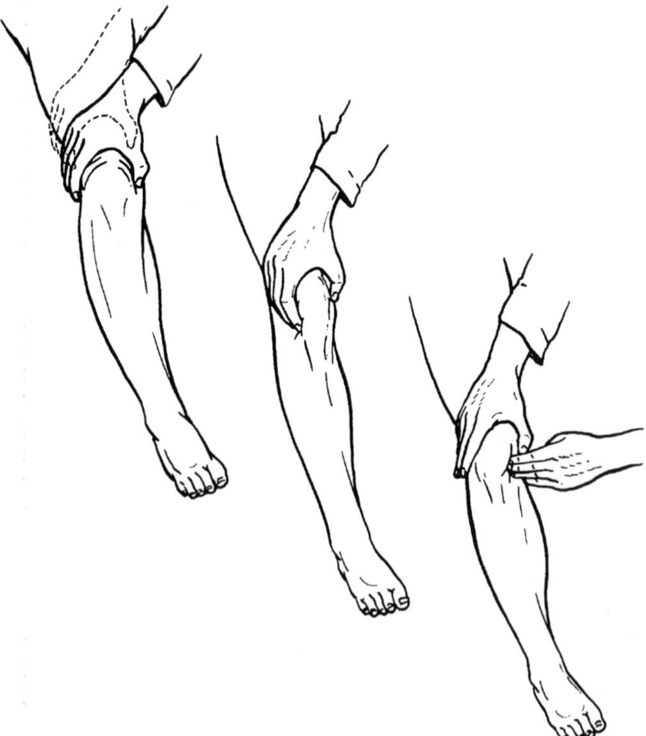

Figure 54.7. Evaluation of a knee effusion.

The functional quality of the quadriceps muscle is assessed by noting the size and tone of the musculature. In particular, the degree of the development of the vastus medialis obliquus muscle is noted. If an effusion is not present, an objective assessment of muscular development may be obtained by measuring the circumference of the distal thigh at a specific point (i.e., 10 cm proximal to the superior pole of the patella). In the case of unilateral involvement, a relative comparison is made to the unaffected limb. The Q angle may be estimated by a line drawn from the anterior superior iliac spine to the center of the patella and a line drawn from this point to the tibial tubercle.

Radiographic Evaluation of the Patellofemoral Joint

A standard knee x-ray series includes AP and lateral weight-bearing views and a tangential view of the patellofemoral joint (Fig. 54.9). The AP and lateral views are useful in determining patella alta and baja. This can be done by a number of methods. Insall and Salvati (32) described a ratio of length of the patellar tendon: greatest diagonal length of the patella, as seen in the lateral view (Fig. 54.10). The average value of the ratio is 1.02. This ratio should not deviate by more than 20°. Therefore, a ratio of 0.80 or less represents patella baja,

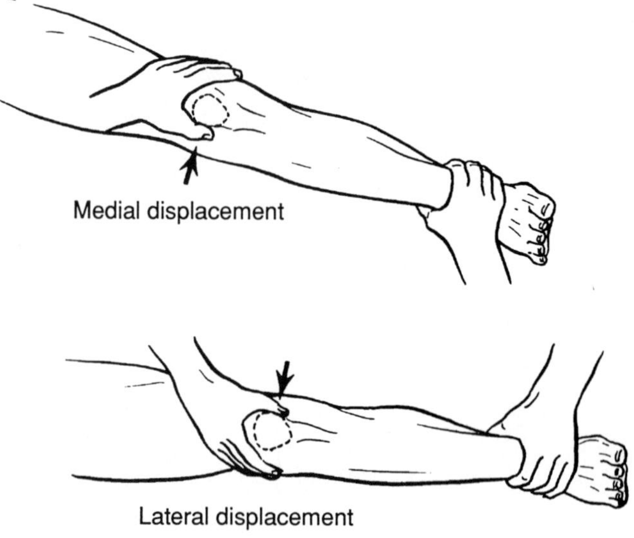

Figure 54.8. Evaluation of patellar mobility.

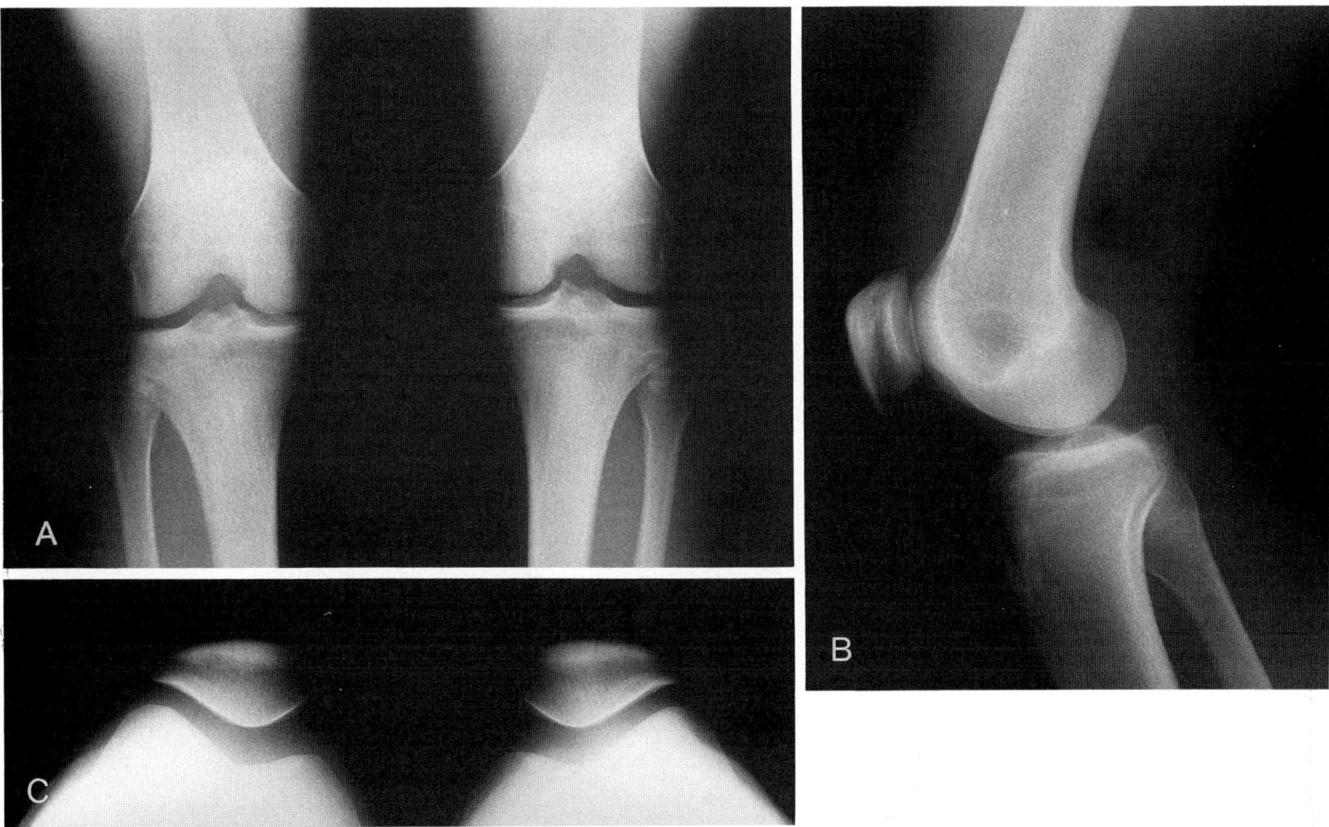

Figure 54.9. **A,** Standing AP radiograph. **B,** Standing lateral radiograph. **C,** Tangential view of the patella.

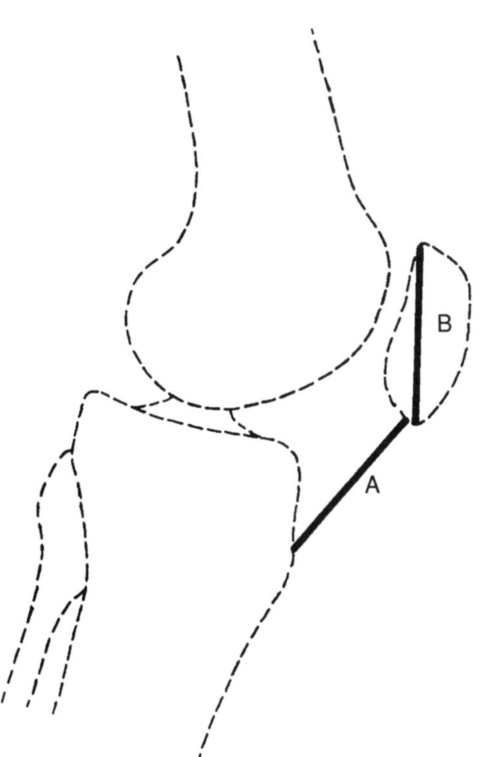

Figure 54.10. Insall and Salvati method of evaluating patella alta:baja by ratio of patellar tendon length (*A*) and greatest diagonal length of patella (*B*).

and 1.20 or greater represents patella alta. This is constant throughout the flexion range.

A second method, described by Blumensaat (22), measures patella alta from a lateral view with the knee flexed 30°. A line is drawn across the superior dome of the intercondylar notch. When this line is projected anteriorly, it should intersect the inferior pole of the patella. If the patella is above this line, it represents patella alta. This measurement is only applicable with the knee flexed 30° and may show variability based on the slope of the dome of the intercondylar notch.

On the AP view, if the tip of the patella is more than 20 mm above a line drawn across the distal margin of the femoral condyles, it is considered patella alta. AP views are also helpful in evaluating patellar fractures and bipartite patellae.

A tangential view is useful in evaluating the relationship of the patella to the trochlea. The most common methods of obtaining tangential views were described by Hughston (33), Merchant (34), and Laurin (35, 36). The techniques for obtaining these views are illustrated in Figure 54.11. The Hughston view is obtained with the knees flexed 55° and the patient prone. This position allows for assessment of lateral femoral condyle height and, therefore, bony restraint to lateral subluxation. This is, theoretically, the position in which the greatest lateral force on the patella is created and, therefore, is the most likely position to see lateral patellar subluxation (28, 33).

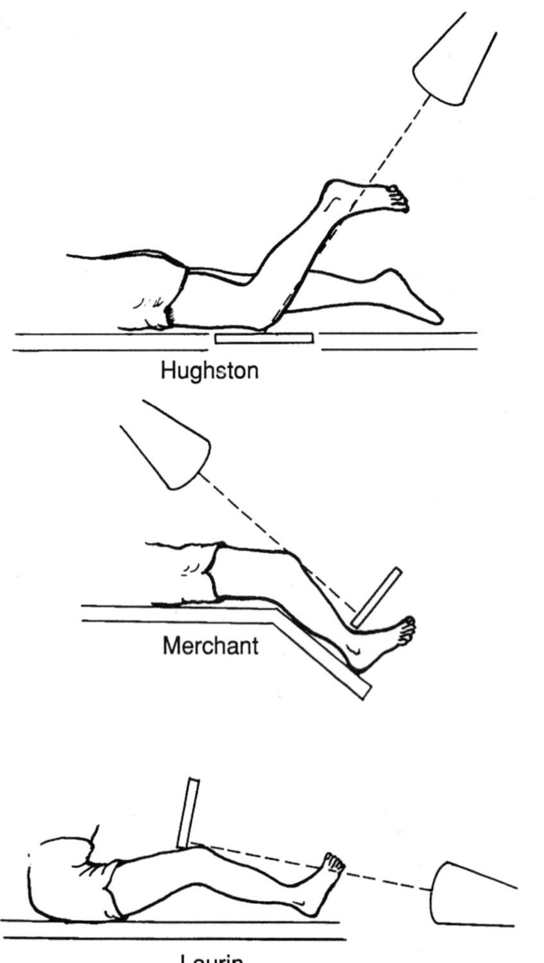

Figure 54.11. Hughston, Merchant, and Laurin tangential views of the patellofemoral articulation.

The Laurin view is taken with the knee flexed 20°. This view may be used to calculate the patellofemoral angle, which is useful in assessing patellar tilt. Patellofemoral angle is measured by drawing a line tangent to the femoral condyles and a second line along the lateral facet of the patella. The two lines should diverge laterally. Any deviation from this is considered abnormal and may reflect a tight lateral retinaculum and a tendency toward lateral subluxation or dislocation. A similar measurement may be made on the Merchant view.

Soft Tissue Injuries

Ruptures of the extensor mechanism are rare relative to the other types of knee injuries (37). Disruption may result from quadriceps tendon rupture, patellar fracture, tibial tubercle fracture, or patellar tendon rupture. Quadriceps and patellar tendon ruptures in the athlete likely represent the end result of repetitive microtrauma such as jumper's knee (38).

Bilateral tendon ruptures are unusual and are often associated with systemic disease or other underlying factors such as rheumatoid arthritis, systemic lupus erythematosus, chronic renal failure, diabetes mellitus, gout, hyperparathyroidism, polyarteritis nodosa, psoriatic arthritis, tuberculosis, acute rheumatic fever, chronic acidosis, Osgood-Schlatter's disease, and corticosteroid use (40, 41, 59).

Quadriceps Muscle Rupture

Ruptures of the quadriceps muscle are rare and occur in the midthigh, usually within the belly of the rectus femoris or vastus medialis muscle. This most commonly occurs with direct trauma to a maximally contracted muscle. Patients usually present with a history of a direct blow to the thigh and complain of pain and swelling in the middle third of the anterior thigh. A defect is often not palpable because of local hematoma formation.

Treatment of quadriceps muscle rupture is nonoperative. Only in the case of a large tear occurring in a high-performance athlete should operative repair be considered, and if so, it should be performed within 5 days of the injury. In general, immobilization of the knee for 2 to 3 weeks should allow for adequate scar formation to bridge the muscle gap. During this period, isometric exercises are performed to minimize quadriceps atrophy. Active flexion exercises are then begun, followed by straight-leg raising and progressive resistance exercises. Early motion is important to minimize stiffness and allow for organization of the scar tissue.

Quadriceps Tendon Rupture

Quadriceps tendon ruptures occur when the quadriceps contracts with the knee held in a slightly flexed position, more commonly in patients over 40 years old (39, 42). Ruptures may be confined to the tendon itself or may extend to the distal aponeurosis of the vastus muscles. The majority of the tears are incomplete and involve the rectus femoris tendon. The more extensive the tear, the more likely is the presence of a hematoma. There is mild to moderate tenderness to palpation and pain in the suprapatellar region. A defect may or may not be palpable, depending on the extent of the tear and the presence or absence of a hematoma. The patella may appear to lie more distally than the uninvolved side. Most strikingly, the patient will be unable to extend the knee against gravity or maintain the leg in extension. In the case of an incomplete rupture, the patient may be able to raise the leg from a supine position but not from a flexed position. With active quadriceps contraction, a defect may become palpable and the patella will not migrate proximally. Radiographs often reveal a patella baja or, occasionally, a bony avulsion fragment is seen off the superior pole of the patella. Calcification may be seen at the site of quadriceps or patellar tendon insertion, representing areas of previous microtrauma. Magnetic resonance imaging (MRI) is often helpful in distinguishing partial and complete tendon rupture.

Partial tendon ruptures may be treated nonoperatively by immobilizing the knee in full extension for 4 to 6 weeks. Complete tears require early surgical repair and may require augmentation with local tissue transfer, artificial material (Dacron weave), or allograft. Early repair or reconstruction provides good functional results, while late reconstruction may result in quadriceps weakness.

Patellar Tendon Rupture

Patellar tendon rupture occurs most commonly in patients less than 40 years old who have had a history of patellar tendinitis or jumper's knee; it results from a violent quadriceps muscle contraction against resistance in the extended knee. Physical examination reveals a defect in the patellar tendon and an inability to extend the knee. The patella may rest more proximally than the uninjured side and is seen to migrate proximally with active quadriceps contraction. Most commonly, the tendon ruptures off the inferior pole of the patella and may be accompanied by a bony fragment that is visible radiographically. X-rays will also reveal the associated patella alta. Ultrasound may be helpful in diagnosing a partial tear. Less frequently, the tendon is ruptured at its insertion on the tibial tubercle. This is usually associated with prior trauma, steroid injection, or Osgood-Schlatter's disease. The tendon is rarely ruptured in the midsubstance, except when associated with systemic disease. Patellar tendon rupture requires early surgical repair. If normal tendon length can be restored, functional results are excellent (39).

Acute Patellar Dislocation

Patellar dislocation most often results from external rotation of the tibia relative to the femur, producing a lateral patellar dislocation. It may also occur as the result of a direct lateral blow to the knee. The dislocation is usually reduced manually by the patient or as the knee is brought into extension before being seen by the physician. Physical examination is remarkable for a large hemarthrosis and tenderness along the medial retinaculum and patellofemoral and/or meniscopatellar ligament. Radiographs may reveal an osteochondral fragment off of either the medial facet of the patellar or the lateral femoral condylar edge of the trochlear groove.

If the patella is dislocated on examination, it is reduced by bringing the leg into extension and applying gentle pressure to the patella in a medial direction. If a significant osteochrondral fragment is present, it is repaired or excised. Avulsion of the medial soft tissue also requires surgical repair. Otherwise, the majority of primary dislocation may be treated nonoperatively with either an immobilizer, brace, or cylinder cast for 2 to 4 weeks. During this period, isometric quadriceps exercises should be performed. Many of these patients will have underlying malalignment problems that predispose them to redislocation. They require continued quadriceps strengthening and rehabilitation and, possibly, surgical intervention to correct an underlying condition (37, 43, 44).

Patellar Fracture

Patellar fractures occur in all age groups and result from either direct or indirect trauma. With the knee partially flexed, a strong quadriceps contraction may generate enough force to produce a transverse fracture of the patella. In addition, the location of the patella makes it susceptible to injury from a direct blow, such as a fall or dashboard injury. Fractures of the patella may be open (skin lacerated and bone exposed) or closed, transverse or comminuted, or displaced or nondisplaced. Fractures present with acute hemarthrosis, which is evident by inspection and palpation. The patient may or may not be able to perform a straight-leg raise or extend the knee, depending on the extent of the fracture and integrity of the surrounding retinaculum. AP and lateral radiographs will usually reveal a fracture. However, one must be careful to distinguish a bipartite patella from a fracture. A tangential view is helpful in determining any significant discontinuity of the fragments in the AP plane.

Treatment options vary from operative to nonoperative, with the goal of restoring continuity of the extensor mechanism. If the fracture is minimally displaced and the patient is able to perform a straight-leg raise or extend the knee (the extensor retinaculum is intact), then the fracture may be treated nonoperatively. Nonoperative treatment involves immobilization of the leg in full extension in a cylinder cast or brace for 4 to 6 weeks. During this time, the patient may ambulate with crutches and be partial weight bearing on the affected side. This is followed by an additional 4 to 6 weeks of protected weight bearing and range-of-motion exercises. Isometric quadriceps exercises should be performed to help prevent quadriceps muscle atrophy. Fractures that fail to meet the criteria for closed treatment and any open fracture should be treated surgically.

Ligamentous Injuries

Knee ligament injuries are common to athletics. The knee ligaments are composed of fibrous tissue, which attaches to adjacent bony structures. They are loaded in tension to provide both static and dynamic support to the knee. As noted previously, the knee rotates about three axes, thereby providing 6° of freedom. These motions are not limited to a single degree of freedom and as such are coupled. For example, anterior displacement of the tibia on the femur is coupled with internal rotation of the tibia. Similarly, posterior displacement is coupled with external rotation of the tibia. The ligamentous structures are intimately associated with coupling of motion and the inherent stability of the knee. It is, therefore, of utmost importance, to be able to perform an accurate examination of the ligamentous structures.

An understanding of the process of ligament healing is fundamental to the treatment of these problems. As research opens the doors to the understanding of ligament healing, the approach to the management of ligament healing continues to evolve. Warren (9) has stated that the ability of a ligament to heal depends on the blood supply, the approximation of the tissue, the stress placed across the ligament, and the timing of the stress.

The collateral ligaments receive a relatively rich blood

supply from the surrounding soft tissues. In contrast, the cruciate ligaments receive a more sparse vasculature from the synovial sheath and infrapatellar fat pad arising from branches of the middle and inferior geniculate arteries (45). Neither the collateral nor the cruciate ligaments receive significant vascular contributions from their bony attachment sites (45). The healing process is similar to that of other tissues. The initial fibrin clot formation stimulates an inflammatory response. Within the 1st week after injury, there is penetration of local vasculature and fibroblast proliferation. Collagen synthesis and degradation occur simultaneously, while overall collagen content increases. By 2 weeks, the fibroblasts become organized into a parallel network, with good tensile strength noted by 3 weeks. An essentially normal-appearing ligament is present by 8 weeks (45–47). In addition, although it was originally thought that early motion was detrimental to ligament healing, more recent data suggest that there is a beneficial effect of stress and strain on ligament healing. Animal models have shown that immobilization decreases the strength and energy-absorbing capacity of the ligament-bone junction (46, 47). In addition, it has been shown that medial collateral ligament injuries recover well without surgery or immobilization. It was suggested that the secondary restraints to valgus motion provided sufficient stability to allow for ligament healing, thus treatment protocols for ligament injuries continue to evolve. Surgical repair of medial collateral ligament injuries, rest, and immobilization are being deemphasized in favor of early controlled motion and functional rehabilitation.

Collateral Ligament

Medial and lateral collateral ligament injuries are referred to as sprains or strains. They may be further classified on the basis of comparison with the normal (unaffected) side. A grade 1 injury produces pain along the course of the ligament and may be accompanied by swelling. With varus of valgus stress testing, the joint line may open up to 5 mm more than the unaffected side. A grade 2 injury produces 5 to 10 mm of joint line opening relative to the unaffected side. The ligament may be stretched or partially torn; however, a firm end point is detectable with stress testing. A grade 3 injury produces more than 10 mm of opening relative to the unaffected side with no discernable end point. The ligament is completely torn and secondary capsular and ligamentous restrains are often disrupted. With any of these injuries, there also may be associated anterior cruciate ligament (ACL), posterior cruciate ligament (PCL), or meniscal pathology.

Medial Collateral Ligament

The primary restraint to valgus stress is the medial collateral ligament (MCL) with additional support afforded by the anterior cruciate ligament, posterior oblique ligament, and posteromedial capsule. Most commonly, the MCL is injured by a direct blow to the lateral side of the knee (valgus blow) with the foot planted. An isolated medial collateral ligament injury may produce localized swelling without a true knee effusion. Localization of tenderness to the medial epicondyle as opposed to the medial joint line helps to distinguish an MCL injury from a medial meniscal tear. However, a medial capsular strain or midsubstance MCL injury may produce joint line tenderness similar to a meniscal injury.

Clinical testing of medial laxity is performed with the patient in the supine position, allowing the thigh to rest on the examining table. The leg is supported over the edge of the table by the examiner's hand as depicted in Figure 54.12. A valgus or abduction stress test is then performed with the knee in 30° of flexion and in full extension, by placing valgus stress on the knee with gentle abduction of the tibia. At 30° of flexion, the cruciate ligaments and posterior capsule are relaxed, and testing is more specific for the medial collateral ligament. Laxity in full extension reflects a grade 3 injury with disruption of the MCL, posteromedial capsule, posterior oblique ligament, often the posterior cruciate ligament, and sometimes the anterior cruciate ligament.

Increasingly, isolated tears of the medial collateral ligament have been treated nonoperatively. Grade 3 MCL injuries that are associated with anterior or posterior cruciate ligament injuries or repairable meniscal injuries are occasionally treated surgically (48). Grade 1 injuries do not require bracing, while bracing of grade 2 injuries depends on the degree of stability, pain, and swelling and physician preference. Grade 3 injuries should be protected with a hinged brace. In grade 2 injuries requiring bracing and grade 3 injuries range of motion is limited to −10° to 75° of flexion for 4 weeks. Patients are allowed to bear weight as tolerated, using crutches as needed. In the early postinjury period, therapy includes patellar mobilization, active range of motion within pain-free limits for grade 1 and 2 injuries, and isometric quadriceps and hamstring exercises

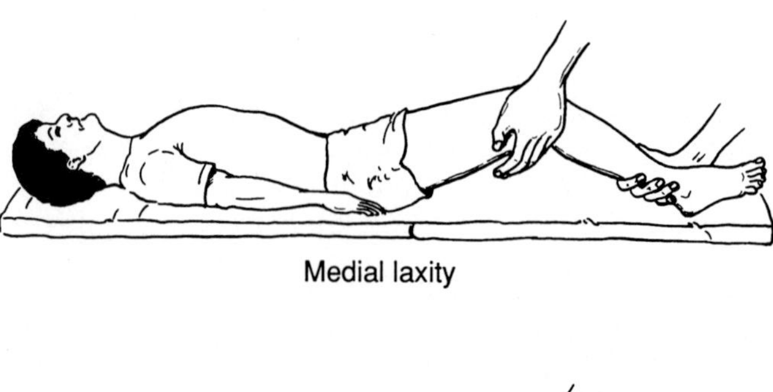

Figure 54.12. Testing for medial and lateral collateral ligament stability.

along with modalities such as whirlpool, electrical stimulation, and biofeedback. Once any bracing has been discontinued and a full range of motion has been achieved (3 to 6 weeks), the patient begins a flexibility and strengthening program. This includes leg presses, mini-squats, resisted knee flexion exercises, proprioceptive training, and swimming (no breast stroke). A functional, sport-specific training program is then introduced. Return to sport varies from 2 to 8 weeks, depending on the grade of injury and individual response. Patients are allowed to return to athletics when there are no signs of active inflammation, there is a full range of motion with normal flexibility, and peak torque and work values of the involved limb are within 85% of the uninvolved side, with a hamstring:quadriceps ratio of 65%.

Lateral Collateral Ligament

The lateral or fibular collateral ligament provides lateral restraint to varus stress, along with the arcuate ligament, posterolateral capsule, lateral capsular ligament, popliteus tendon, iliotibial band, and lateral head of the gastrocnemius (49). Most commonly, these structures are injured by a direct medial blow to the knee with the foot planted. Again, palpation of the lateral bony and ligamentous structures and lateral joint line is helpful in distinguishing the specific pathology. In addition, a joint effusion may or may not be present. Varus or adduction stress testing is performed in the same position as for valgus stress testing. With the examiner supporting the leg, a varus stress is produced as the tibia is adducted (see Fig. 54.12). With the knee in 30° of flexion, the posterior capsule and cruciate ligaments are relaxed, and the test is more specific for the lateral collateral ligament (LCL). Grading is as noted above. Laxity with the knee in full extension reflects additional injury to the posterolateral capsule, arcuate complex, and often the posterior cruciate ligament. This constitutes a grade 3 injury. In addition, with any LCL injury, it is important to evaluate the function of the common peroneal nerve. This nerve courses from posterior to anterior, emerging from behind the biceps tendon to pass around the fibular neck. The nerve divides distally into the superficial and deep peroneal nerves, providing motor function to the toe and foot dorsiflexors and foot everters as well as sensation to the anterior and lateral aspects of the lower leg and dorsum of the foot.

Treatment of an isolated lateral collateral ligament injury is nonoperative. The basic principles of rehabilitation are the same as those described for the medial collateral ligament. However, the majority of significant LCL injuries are accompanied by cruciate ligament injuries and are treated by surgical management of the associated injury.

Anterior Cruciate Ligament

The earliest description of the anterior cruciate ligament (ACL) dates back to Galen in A.D. 170. He described the anatomy of the "genu cruciate." Over the ensuing centuries the function and anatomy of the ligaments of the knee were further delineated. It was not, however, until 1850 that Stark recorded the first description of a rupture of the anterior cruciate ligament. Reports of injuries and attempted operative and nonoperative treatment of the ACL followed in the literature. In 1917, Hey-Groves (50) reported on an attempt to reconstruct the anterior cruciate ligament using a segment of fascia lata passed through a tibial tunnel. This formed the basis of current concepts of intraarticular reconstruction. Numerous others contributed to the expanding literature on ACL injuries and their management (51, 52). O'Donoghue's (53–57) work in the 1950s and 1960s further defined the concepts of ACL injuries and their surgical treatment. Since this landmark work, much has been accomplished in understanding the structure and function of the ACL. It is critical that one understand the role of the anterior cruciate ligament and its biomechanical function before addressing its injury and treatment.

Anatomy

Hey-Groves (16), in 1920, was the first to describe the anterior cruciate ligament's role as a stabilizer of the knee against anterior displacement of the tibia on the femur. Subsequently, Butler et al. (58) and others (59–65) have shown that the ACL acts as a primary restraint with the iliotibial band, medial collateral ligament, and lateral collateral ligament, with the medial and lateral capsules acting as secondary restraints. The secondary role of the ACL in the control of rotation and varus-valgus stability has also been elucidated. These roles are directly related to the anatomy and orientation of the ACL.

As Arnoczky (45) has clearly described, the femoral attachment of the anterior cruciate ligament is a semicircular region at the posterior aspect of the lateral femoral condyle within the intercondylar notch. The ACL then courses anteromedially through the notch beneath the transverse meniscal ligament to attach in a fossa slightly in front of and lateral to the anterior tibial spine (see Fig. 54.3).

The anterior cruciate ligament is composed of a series of fascicles that spiral laterally as the ligament courses from femur to tibia. The fascicles are divided into two major bundles: an anteromedial bundle and a posterolateral bundle. The anteromedial bundle or band is tight in flexion and relatively lax in extension. The posterolateral band is tightest in extension and relatively lax in flexion. The fascicles thus represent a continuum of fibers, some of which are taut throughout the entire range of knee motion.

Both cruciate ligaments derive the majority of their blood supply from surrounding synovial vessels originating primarily from the middle geniculate artery along with smaller contribution from terminal branches of the inferior geniculate arteries. In addition, branches of the tibial nerve course with the synovial and periligamentous vessels, providing mechanoreceptors and probably proprioceptive fibers to the ligament. Sensory nerve endings are limited within the ACL.

Biomechanics

The fundamental biomechanics and kinematics of knee motion have been described as a four-bar linkage system by Kapandji, Huson, and Menschik (4). Two rigid rods represent the anterior and posterior cruciate ligaments. The length of the rods is proportional to the lengths of the ACL and PCL. The rods are hinged at one end along a line that intersects a second line, representing the longitudinal axis of the femur at a 40° angle that represents the slope of the intercondylar roof. The free ends of the rods are attached to a coupler, representing the tibial plateau. As the coupler moves, a series of lines are produced that form tangents to a curve. The curve approximates the sagittal contour of the posterior half of the femoral condyles. The hinged bars, then, represent the positions of the cruciate ligaments as the knee is brought through a range of motion. The model also demonstrates the obligatory shifting of the bony contact points between femur and tibia as the knee changes position. Therefore, as the knee is flexed, the femur glides posteriorly on the tibial plateau so that the femoral shaft does not contact the posterior tibial plateau at terminal flexion. The ratio of rolling to gliding motion of the femoral condyle on the tibial plateau is 1:2 in early flexion and 1:4 in late flexion (4). It is important to understand these concepts when evaluating the function of the ACL and performing clinical diagnostic tests of ACL integrity.

History and Mechanism of Injury

The anterior cruciate ligament is most commonly injured by a twisting force accompanied by varus, valgus, or hyperextension stresses on a weight-bearing limb. ACL injuries are often accompanied by other structural injuries. In skiing, football, and soccer, the most frequent mechanism of injury occurs with valgus and external rotation forces producing damage to both the ACL and medial collateral ligaments. In basketball, the most common mechanism of injury involves hyperextension with internal rotation of the tibia, producing an ACL rupture as the player comes down from a rebound. Pure hyperextension may damage either the anterior or posterior cruciate ligament or both. The ACL also may be damaged by hyperflexion, but this is rare.

In approximately 40% of cases, the patient will describe a pop that is heard or felt. This is caused by the release of energy stored in the helicoid fibers of the anterior cruciate ligament and is the single factor in the history that most reliably indicates an ACL tear. The patient is usually unable to continue play and notes the gradual onset of an effusion over the ensuing 24 hr. A more rapid onset of effusion should clue the examiner in to the possibility of an osteochondral fracture. Also, there is minimal pain associated with a pure anterior cruciate ligament rupture. This is because of the relative paucity of pain fibers within the anterior cruciate ligament. More severe pain may occur if associated injuries are present or over time as swelling produces joint distention.

Various combinations of ligamentous injuries may result in different instability patterns. Anteromedial, anterolateral, posteromedial, posterolateral, varus, and valgus instability patterns may occur in different combinations, depending on the mechanism of injury and structural damage. The history is helpful in determining the specific instability pattern. For example, anterolateral rotatory instability secondary to ACL insufficiency produces a subluxation of the tibia on the femur as the knee approaches full extension (the pivot shift phenomenon). This results in the sensation of the knee suddenly giving out, which the patient will often describe.

Physical Examination

General inspection of the knee as described previously is the first step in assessment of any knee injury. It is often helpful to examine the unaffected knee first as a means of comparison as well as to relax the patient and allow him or her to gain confidence in the examiner's ability to perform the appropriate tests gently. Muscle resistance to ligamentous laxity testing not only makes testing difficult but also results in significant false-negative examinations.

Lachman Test. The Lachman test is the most sensitive test for ACL insufficiency and may be performed in the acute setting. The test is performed with the knee in 20° to 30° of knee flexion and the foot resting on the examination table. While the femur is held posteriorly with one hand, the tibia is gently drawn forward with the opposite hand (Fig. 54.13). The amount of tibial translation is compared with the unaffected knee and the degree of laxity is graded as previously described (grades 1 to 3). A false-negative test may occur if a bucket handle tear of the meniscus blocks anterior excursion of the tibia on the femur. If the limb is too large for adequate gripping, the test may be performed in the prone position. The leg is supported with the knee in 20° to 30° of flexion, and the tibia is gently drawn forward. In either case, the quality of the end point (firm or soft) should also be noted.

Anterior Drawer Test. The anterior drawer test is less sensitive than the Lachman test for ACL insufficiency. The test is performed with the patient lying supine, the hips flexed 45°, and the knee flexed between

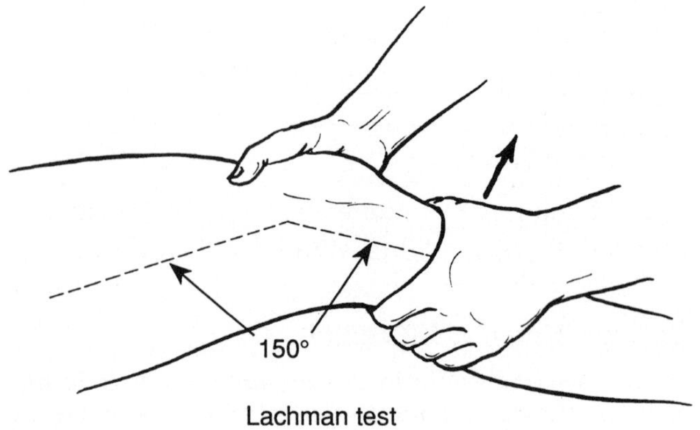

Figure 54.13. The Lachman test.

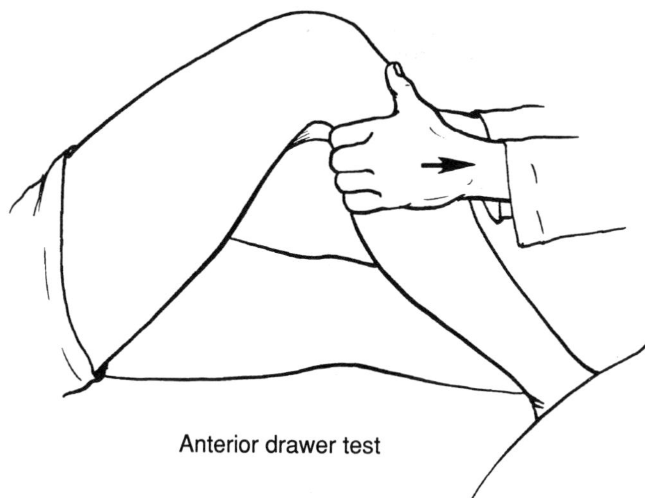

Figure 54.14. The anterior drawer test.

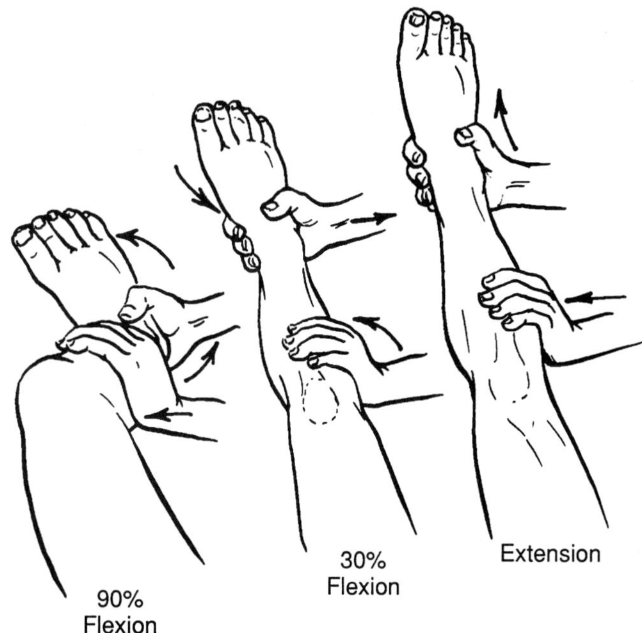

Figure 54.15. The pivot shift test. As the knee is brought into flexion, the iliotibial band reduces the tibia from its anteriorly subluxated position. Adapted from Insall JN. Examination of the knee. In: Insall JN, ed. Surgery of the knee. New York: Churchill Livingstone, 1984.

60° and 90°. With both thumbs placed on the joint line, the tibia is gently drawn forward, and excursion of the tibia is measured in comparison with the unaffected side (Fig. 54.14). Again, the quality of the end point should be noted. Grading is difficult and often depends on the examiner's level of experience. However, even in the chronic setting, anterior drawer testing under the best of circumstances still results in significant false-negative results.

Anterior drawer testing may be helpful in assessing the integrity of secondary restraints. When the test is performed with the foot in 15° of external rotation, increased excursion of the tibia reflects damage to some or all of the secondary medial restraints, which should be right in this position. Similarly, when the test is performed with the foot in 30° of internal rotation, the secondary lateral restraints should be tight. Increased excursion reflects damage to some or all of these structures.

Flexion-Rotation-Drawer Test. The flexion-rotation-drawer test is performed by providing an anterior tibial stress while the knee is flexed and extended (6, 65). As the knee is extended in an ACL-deficient knee, the tibia subluxates anteriorly and the lateral femoral condyle is observed to rotate externally as it falls off the convex slope of the lateral tibial plateau. Conversely, as the knee is flexed, the iliotibial band pulls the lateral tibial plateau posteriorly, the knee returns to its anatomic alignment, and the lateral femoral condyle is observed to rotate internally. Similar tests have been described by Hughston et al. (63) and Slocum et al. (66, 67), all of which are variations in testing for anterolateral rotatory instability.

In some cases of chronic ACL insufficiency and resulting anterolateral instability, a patient may be able to exhibit an active anterior drawer sign. With the patient either sitting up or lying down and the knee flexed 90° with the foot firmly planted, contraction of the gastrocnemius muscle may draw the tibia forward. In other patients, the same effect may be demonstrated as the patient flexes and extends the knee with a slight valgus stress applied, while the leg is partial weight bearing.

Pivot Shift. The pivot shift phenomenon describes the anterior subluxation of the lateral tibial plateau in extension in the ACL-deficient knee. With the knee in extension, the action of the quadriceps muscles and iliotibial band draws the tibia forward on the femur. As the knee is flexed, the axis of pull of the iliotibial band drops posteriorly and the tibia is pulled posteriorly, back to its normal anatomic position (Fig. 54.15). Numerous tests have been described to elicit this phenomenon (60–62, 68).

MacIntosh Test. The MacIntosh test was described in 1972 (60–62). With the knee extended and the foot internally rotated, a valgus stress is applied to the proximal tibia. The lateral tibial plateau is seen to subluxate anteriorly in the early phase of flexion. Then, as the knee reaches approximately 30° of flexion, the lateral tibial plateau reduces as a result of the action of the iliotibial band in flexion.

Losee Test. The Losee test is performed by grasping the foot of the affected leg with one hand. The thumb of the other hand is placed behind the fibular head, with the fingers resting on the patella. The knee is flexed approximately 40° and then slowly extended. As the knee is extended, the foot is internally rotated and the thumb pushes forward on the fibular head. As the knee reaches extension, the lateral tibial plateau is seen and felt to subluxate anteriorly (68, 69).

Instrumented Testing. Because clinical testing is subject to variability between examiners, attempts have been made to develop mechanical ligament testing devises. Three of the more commonly used devises are the KT-1000 arthrometer (Medmetric, San Diego, CA), the Genucom (Faro Medical Technologies, Inc., Montreal, Canada), and the Stryker Knee Laxity Tester

(Stryker Co., Kalamazoo, MI). By producing an anterior displacement force on the tibia with the femur stabilized, maximal tibial displacement may be quantified. Side-to-side measurement differences can be calculated between the injured and noninjured knees to evaluate the degree of instability.

Treatment of ACL Injuries

Over the past several years, the advances in knowledge regarding structure, function, and physiology of the ACL have allowed the treatment of ACL injuries to evolve. Numerous studies have suggested that progressive functional and anatomical deterioration of the knee results from chronic ACL deficiency. Further studies have gone on to elucidate the concepts of resulting meniscal damage, osteoarthritis, damage to secondary restraints, and overall decline of knee function (70–76). Still, numerous articles in the past have advocated conservative management of ACL injuries (77, 78), primarily because the results of such management did not differ significantly from operative management. More recent research, however, has led to improved understanding of ACL biomechanics, anatomy, and ligament healing and thus improved techniques for operative management and the recreation of a functional ligament.

Radiography. Plain radiographs will often reveal only a joint effusion. In some cases, a lateral capsular sign (Segond's sign) may be seen as a bony avulsion of the lateral capsular attachment to the tibia. In the chronic setting, "peaking" of the tibial spines may be evident. MRI scanning is often helpful in assessing both anterior and posterior cruciate ligament integrity as well as any associated pathology of the menisci or collateral ligaments (Fig. 54.16) (79–81).

Indications for Treatment. Treatment decisions must be individualized. The physician must consider the patient's physiologic age, activity level, ability and willingness to comply with a vigorous postoperative rehabilitation protocol, the additional anatomical considerations of associated collateral ligament injuries and meniscal injuries, and the patient's overall degree of generalized ligamentous laxity.

In general, a physiologically young person who remains active in sports that require cutting and deceleration and who does not wish to modify those activities is a candidate for surgical intervention. Surgery is further indicated in those patients with risk factors for recurrent instability or coexisting progression of intraarticular damage. This would include patients with associated grade 3 collateral ligament injuries, meniscal tears (particularly reparable tears), and generalized ligamentous laxity. Most authors agree that attempts to manage conservatively an ACL-deficient knee with associated grade 3 collateral ligament injury will result in functional instability of the knee. In addition, when a meniscal tear accompanies an acute ACL rupture, retear of the repaired meniscus or reinjury of the damaged meniscus is likely to occur if the ACL is not reconstructed. Rarely, repair of the meniscus may be performed in a chronically ACL-deficient knee without performing ACL reconstruction, if the knee is function-

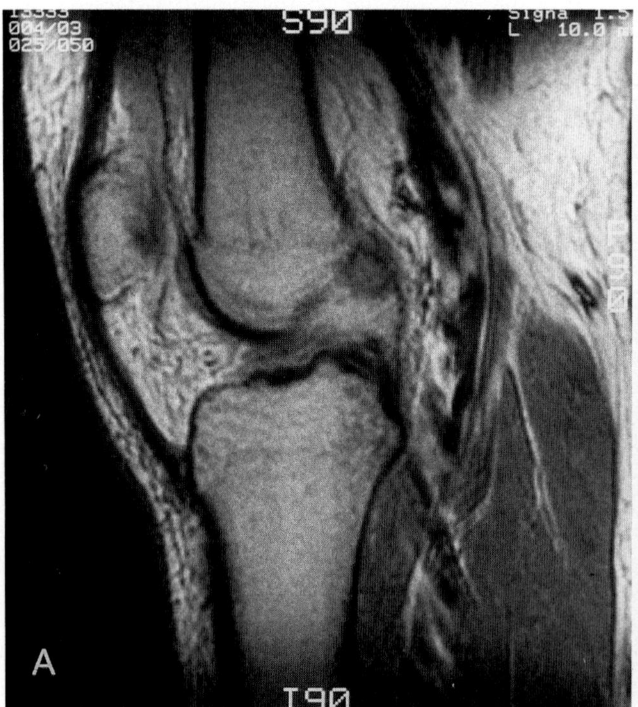

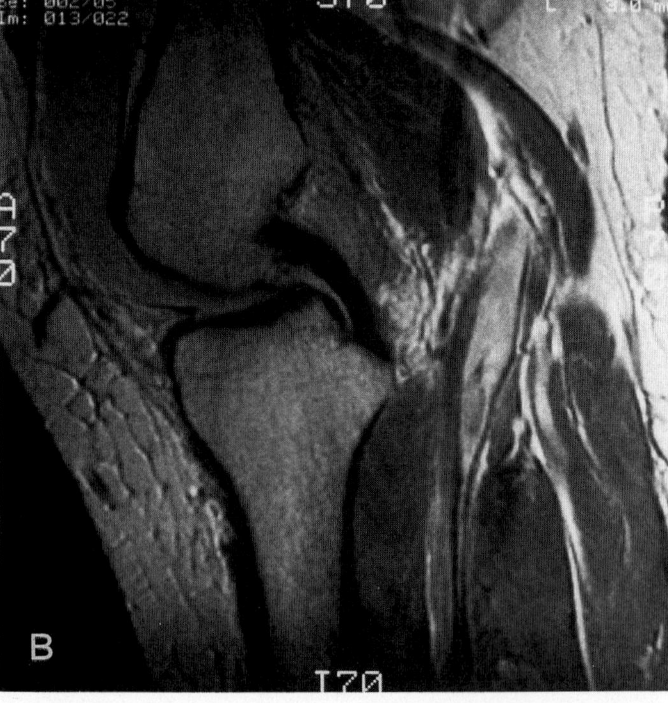

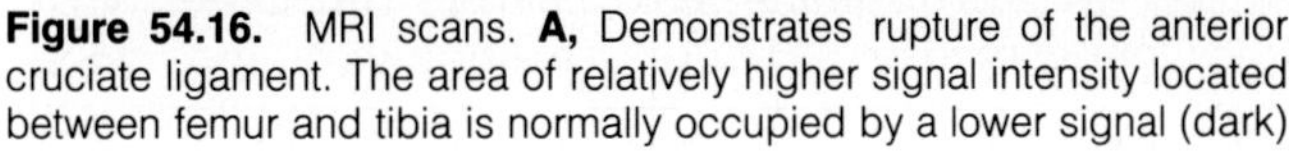

Figure 54.16. MRI scans. **A,** Demonstrates rupture of the anterior cruciate ligament. The area of relatively higher signal intensity located between femur and tibia is normally occupied by a lower signal (dark) band, representing the anterior cruciate ligament. **B,** Demonstrates the low signal band of an intact posterior cruciate ligament.

ally stable because of secondary restraints and the patient has a low-demand lifestyle.

Conservative treatment is warranted in the physiologically older athlete who has a less-demanding physical regimen (does not participate in cutting sports) or who is willing to modify his or her activity. This assumes that there is no associated grade 3 collateral ligament damage or meniscal damage.

Partial ACL Injury

Partial ACL ruptures occur in 10% to 28% of all ACL injuries (7, 78, 82). It is unclear whether the degree of fiber disruptuion can be correlated with the degree of instability and prognosis (82, 83), because it is difficult to assess the amount and effect of plastic deformation that likely occurs in the remaining ACL fibers. In these cases, one must assess the degree of instability through clinical testing as well as patient's history, symptomatology, and athletic demands. In some cases, examination under anesthesia and diagnostic arthroscopy may be necessary to evaluate the situation fully. Warner et al. (82) have suggested that a 25% tear of the ACL with a negative pivot shift may be treated conservately, whereas a 25% tear with a strongly positive pivot shift in an athletic individual should be treated with augmentation, using the semitendinosis and gracilis tendons.

Nonoperative Management

The ultimate goal of nonoperative care of an ACL injury is functional stability. The knee is treated symptomatically over the course of rehabilitation. A well-planned physical therapy regimen would include consideration of hamstring and quadriceps strengthening as dynamic knee stabilizers, patellofemoral biomechanics, proprioceptive training, and overall functional progression. The time needed to accomplish each step varies from patient to patient.

Early nonoperative and operative management of an ACL injury includes measures to reduce pain and swelling and restore full range of motion. Such measures are use of nonsteroidal antiinflammatory agents, ice, and physical therapy modalities. Crutches and a brace or knee immobilizer may be helpful in limiting discomfort but should be used for only a few days. Prolonged use promotes muscle atrophy and adhesion formation, resulting in a stiff knee. With the exception of associated collateral ligament injuries, braces or immobilizers are not necessary to protect the injured structures from daily activities involving full weight bearing. Other early rehabilitation goals include gait training, patellar mobilization, the initiation of neuromuscular activity, and patient education. Patients are counseled to avoid high-risk activities, at least until adequate strength and training have been accomplished.

Intermediate rehabilitation goals include range of motion, gait training, strengthening, and proprioceptive training. Once the effusion has dissipated and full range of motion has been attained, exercises such as swimming and bicycling are begun followed by light jogging (flat surface). The late phase of therapy should then include functional training of the athlete. The entire process may take 6 to 12 weeks before high-level activities can be resumed. This is reflected by muscle strength testing, which demonstrates quadriceps and hamstring strength within 90% of the unaffected side, along with completion of proprioceptive training and patient counseling. Bracing of the knee may provide a sense of reassurance to the athlete and prevent tibial translation at low levels of activity. However, there is no evidence to suggest that functional bracing can prevent tibial translation (pivot shifting) at higher demand levels. Therefore, bracing is not absolutely indicated.

It should be noted that nonoperative management does not mean that surgery is not indicated for associate pathology. In cases of meniscal injury or when a portion of the remaining ACL stump impinges in the joint, surgery may be necessary. Also, if nonoperative management is deemed unsuccessful by the patient and the physician because of recurrent episodes of instability, surgical reconstruction remains an option for treatment.

Operative Management

There are many accepted operative methods of treatment of an ACL-deficient knee. These include primary repair, repair with augmentation, reconstruction using autogenous graft tissue, reconstruction using a prosthetic ligament, reconstruction using both an autogenous graft and a prosthetic ligament, reconstruction with allograft tissue, and extraarticular reconstruction either alone or combined with other procedures. The results of primary repair alone are unpredictable (82, 84), but there have been reports of good results of primary ACL repair with extraarticular augmentation (82, 85). Primary repair is best performed when the ACL is avulsed proximally from its femoral attachment. This occurs uncommonly, and current recommendations are that repair should be performed in association with intraarticular or extraarticular augmentation, preferably intraarticular using the semitendinosis and gracilis tendons (82, 85).

Currently, the most common method of ACL reconstruction is autogenous graft reconstruction using the central one-third of the patellar tendon. Other structures that continue to be used include the hamstring tendons (gracilis and semitendinous) and iliotibial band. Noyes et al. (86, 87) documented the relative strengths of the various materials used for reconstruction. These data showed that with the exception of the bone-patellar–tendon-bone, all of the tissues were weaker than the normal ACL. In contrast, the bone-patellar–tendon-bone complex was 168% as strong as the normal ACL. In addition to its strength, the use of the bone-patellar—tendon-bone graft is preferable because of its availability and its immediate strong fixation to bone with interference screws as well as the bone plugs' rapid healing into the femoral and tibial bone tunnels in which they are fixed. The latter two of these allow for a more aggressive early rehabilitation program. These factors seem to outweigh the disadvantages, which include damage to the extensor mechanism, postoperative parapatellar pain, quadriceps weakness, and rare patella fracture and rupture of the patellar tendon. Thus reconstruction using the central third patellar tendon has become the operation of choice for most knee surgeons. Recent data have shown that more than 90% of patients are functionally stable, with excellent knee ligament rating scores (88, 89).

The hamstring tendons are somewhat easier to harvest. However, early fixation to bone is less secure than bone-patellar–tendon-bone, so early rehabilitation must be less aggressive. The hamstring tendons may be used for reconstruction of an ACL-deficient knee in which the secondary stabilizing ligaments and capsular structures are functioning. In cases in which autogenous graft reconstruction is selected and the secondary stabilizers are not functioning, the central third patellar tendon should be used.

The use of prosthetic devices and allograft material for intraarticular ACL reconstruction has significant appeal. The advantages include lower morbidity to the patient, because harvesting of autogenous tissues is avoided. In the case of prosthetic devices, there is immediate secure bony fixation, allowing for vigorous early rehabilitation. When used for augmentation, they provide immediate strength and load sharing during the revascularizing and remodeling phases of healing of the accompanying autogenous or allograft material. However, the current data on ligament augmentation devices have not shown them to be better than autogenous grafts alone (85, 90). Presently, there is limited use of prosthetic ligaments in the United States, but failure caused by fatigue, wear, and fretting has occurred at a high rate (85, 90).

Allograft reconstruction of the anterior cruciate ligament, using either the patellar tendon or the Achilles tendon, is gaining acceptance. Allograft reconstruction provides the benefits of autogenous graft reconstruction while eliminating the morbidity of graft harvesting. In addition, postoperative pain is diminished, cosmesis is improved as a smaller incision can be made, and operative tourniquet time is decreased. Of great concern is the transmission of viral disease. However, with current screening and sterilization techniques, the incidence of HIV transmission with allograft materal is 1:1,677,000 (91).

Allografts may be particularly useful in patients (*a*) over 40 years of age, (*b*) with preexisting patellofemoral chondrosis or extensor mechanism malalignment, (*c*) who require multiple ligament reconstruction (i.e., PCL and ACL), and (*d*) who require revision ACL reconstruction. Overall, results of allograft ACL reconstruction appear to be comparable with autograft reconstruction (92–94). In 33 patients followed at the University of Pittsburgh Center for Sports Medicine and Rehabilitation over a 44-month period, 73% of patients returned to their preoperative activity level, a figure comparable with most autograft studies.

Extraarticular reconstruction procedures (MacIntosh, Ellison, and Losee) are rarely used as isolated procedures for treatment of the ACL-deficient knee. Initially, it was felt that by extraarticular tenodesis of the posterolateral aspect of the knee, anterior translation of the tibia could be prevented. However, these tissues gradually stretch out with time and, therefore, eventually fail to provide stability. Such procedures may still be helpful in augmenting intraarticular repairs, particularly in the young athlete with open epiphyses, in whom the drilling of bone tunnels should be avoided.

Postoperative Rehabilitation

The postoperative rehabilitation process has evolved along with the changes in surgical techniques. As more is learned about biomechanics, and bone and soft tissue healing, these protocols will continue to change. However, protocols must be modified according to the type of repair or reconstruction performed, associated ligamentous and meniscal surgery, and the type of graft used. Rehabilitation has advanced from the long period of immobilization and nonweight bearing once recommended. Currently, the University of Pittsburgh Sports Medicine and Rehabilitation Center protocol for ACL reconstruction allows for immediate full passive extension and flexion. Early motion limits disuse atrophy, adhesion formation, and capsular contracture and promotes articular cartilage nutrition. Continuous passive motion is used during the 2-day hospital stay and often at home for the postoperative 1st week. The patient is allowed to weight bear as tolerated with the aid of crutches and the use of a brace locked in full extension. At 1 week postoperatively, the brace is unlocked; at 4 weeks, it is discontinued. Immediately postoperatively, straight-leg raises and quadriceps setting is begun. At 1 week, active range of motion is begun, along with patellar mobilization, hamstring sets, and active hip exercises. Within the 1st month, the patient begins isometric quadriceps exercises, partial squats, and leg presses. Between 4 and 8 weeks, the patient begins stationary bicycling and resistance exercises. During the 3rd month, resistance exercises are progressed along with balance and gait training. Once a full range of motion and normal gait pattern are reestablished, the patient may begin jogging on level surfaces. Strengthening and isokinetic training are advanced through the 4th month. Progression of the rehabilitation process must be individualized. Athletes may begin sports-specific rehabilitation as early as 4 months postsurgery, with the aim of a return to participation between 6 and 9 months postoperatively.

Posterior Cruciate Ligament and Posterolateral Corner

The primary function of the PCL is to act as a restraint to posterior tibial displacement. It also plays a role as a secondary stabilizer to varus and valgus stress and to external rotation. The origin of the PCl is a broad region, approximately 32 mm in anteroposterior diameter, along the lateral side of the medial femoral condyle, with the distal fibers approximately 3 mm proximal to the articular margin of the condyle (14, 95). The ligament averages 38 mm in length and 13 mm in width

(14, 84), and courses posteriorly and distally to a broad insertion site (approximately 13 mm) (14, 95) on the flat, posterior surface of the proximal tibia, approximately 1 cm below the tibial articular surface. The meniscofemoral ligaments (ligaments of Humphrey and Wrisberg) lie anterior and posterior to the PCL in about 70% of patients.

Posterior cruciate ligament injuries are less common than ACL injuries, but the true incidence is undetermined because until recently many have gone undetected. As more is learned about the anatomy and function of the posterior and posterolateral structures of the knee, the diagnosis has been made more frequently. A broad spectrum of disability may be caused by injuries to the PCL and posterolateral structures (arcuate complex, posterolateral capsule, biceps, and popliteus tendon) of the knee, ranging from no functional disability to severe disability. Isolated PCL injury results in posterior subluxation of the tibia on the femur, producing straight posterior instability. Injury to some or all of the posterolateral structures in addition to the PCL produces posterolateral rotatory instability, as the lateral tibial plateau subluxates posteriorly relative to the lateral femoral condyle. The intact posteromedial structures act as a pivot point. It should be noted that these injuries occur more commonly in conjunction with other knee ligament injuries, including ACL injury. PCL and posterolateral injuries account for about 8% of all knee ligament injuries (95).

Mechanism of Injury

The majority of PCL injuries occur in athletics and motor vehicle accidents, resulting from a direct blow to the flexed knee. In sports, this may occur when the flexed knee strikes the ground with the foot plantar flexed. This concentrates the force of the blow on the tibial tubercle, effectively creating a strong posterior drawer effect on the proximal tibia, thus rupturing the PCL. Similarly, vehicular trauma produces the same forces when the flexed knee strikes the dashboard, rupturing the PCL. Forced hyperflexion also may cause PCL rupture as the anterolateral fibers are stretched beyond their elastic limit.

Hyperextension injury has been shown to produce ACL and PCL rupture in combination, while a varus or valgus blow to the knee may produce a PCL rupture in association with collateral ligament injury. The posterolateral corner is most commonly injured by the "valgus side-swipe," which occurs when a blow is struck to the anteromedial aspect of the knee, producing hyperextension and a posterolaterally directed force (52, 63, 95, 96). Less commonly, posterolateral injury may occur with a severe external rotation force to the tibia.

History

As with other knee injuries, the history begins with a description of the mechanism of injury. In cases of chronic posterior or posterolateral instability, pain is a predominant feature (62, 95–97). The patient usually complains of posterolateral pain, and in more chronic cases patellofemoral symptoms may occur. Patients with chronic posterolateral instability will often complain of feelings of instability and that their knee gives way in extension or hyperextends. These patients will exhibit a varus and hyperextension deformity in the stance phase of gait (95, 97).

Physical Examination

These injuries have been commonly missed if a proper and thorough examination is not performed. The first key to examination is observation. Posterolateral ecchymosis and swelling, along with anterormedial ecchymosis, swelling and/or abrasion are suggestive of the mechanism of injury. Of note, it is important to remember that significant force is required to produce these injuries. Therefore, a thorough neurovascular examination should be part of the evaluation. One must always consider the possibility of a knee dislocation (see "Knee Dislocation," below). Also, assessment of peroneal nerve function is important because 10% to 30% of knees with lateral and posterolateral ligament damage have associated peroneal nerve injury (63, 95).

Posterior Drawer Test. The posterior drawer test is the most accurate way of assessing PCL competence. The test is performed in a similar fashion to the anterior drawer test, but with a posterior force directed on the tibia (Fig. 54.17). The examiner must assess the degree of posterior displacement and the quality of the end point (firm or soft). it is also helpful to palpate the medial joint line. Normally, there is a 1-cm step-off between the anterior medial tibial plateau and the medial femoral condyle. When the PCL is nonfunctional, the tibia sags posteriorly in the 90° flexed position and this step-off is eliminated.

External Rotation Recurvatum Test. The external rotation recurvatum test was described by Hughston et al. (63, 95, 97) and is performed with the patient in the supine position. The great toe is grasped, and the leg is elevated with the knee in full extension (Fig. 54.18). External rotation of the tibia and varus hypertension (recurvatum) of the knee reflect injury to the arcuate ligament complex, according to Hughston et al. However, it is now believed that pronounced hyperextension and external rotation are more likely produced by

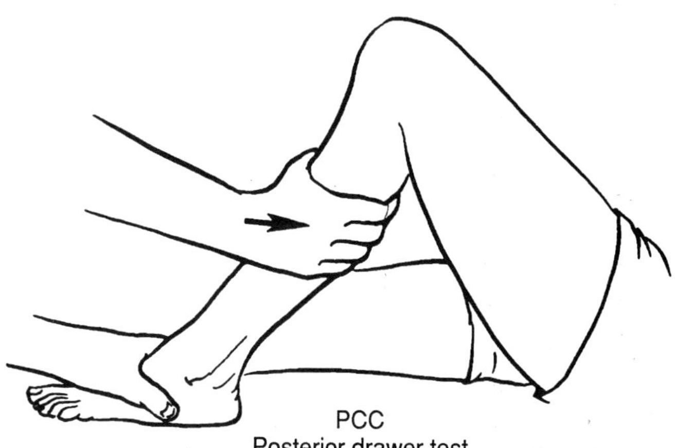

Figure 54.17. The posterior drawer test.

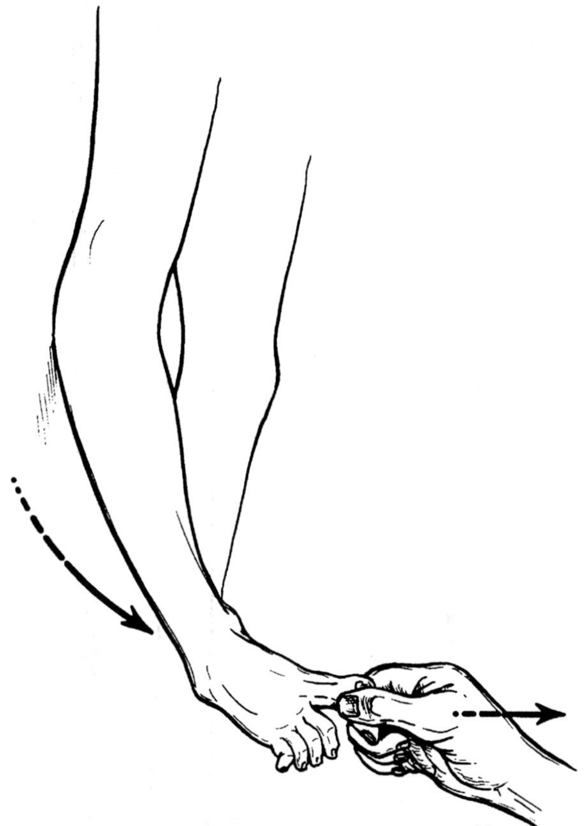

Figure 54.18. The external rotation recurvatum test.

arcuate complex injury accompanied by ACL and possibily PCL injury (95).

Quadriceps Active Drawer Test. Daniel et al. (98) described the quadriceps active drawer test as a means of assessing the resting position of the tibia in relationship to the femur. With the patient lying supine, the knee flexed 90°, and the foot firmly planted, the quadriceps muscle is actively contracted. In the PCL-deficient knee, the resting position of the tibia is posterior relative to the femur and to its normal resting position. When the quadriceps muscle is contracted in the PCL-deficient knee, the force vector is directed anteriorly, producing an anterior tibial translation that is visible to the examiner.

Tests for Posterolateral Instability. *Varus-Valgus Stress Testing.* Varus and valgus stress testing was described earlier; however, it should be noted that injury to the posterolateral structures may produce varus instability when tested in 30° of flexion and in full extension. It should be remembered, though, that most of these are combined LCL and posterolateral injuries, and that although PCL injury is not necessary to produce varus laxity in full extension, it is probably more commonly associated with these injuries than not (95).

Posterolateral Drawer Test. The posterolateral drawer test is performed in a similar manner to the posterior drawer test, but with the foot externally rotated 15°. As the tibia is pushed posteriorly the lateral tibial plateau moves posteriorly while the medial tibial plateau remains fixed. Evaluation of this test is somewhat subjective. Mild to moderate posterior displacement of the lateral tibial plateau is indicative of damage to the posterolateral structures, whereas marked posterior displacement is suggestive of combined injury, including PCL disruption.

Tibial External Rotation. Tibial external rotation evaluates the posterolateral structures by assessing external rotation of the tibia on the femur. The patient is either prone or supine and the feet are grasped so that the test may be performed on each knee for comparison. The test is performed at both 30° and 90° of knee flexion by maximally externally rotating the feet and comparing the relative amounts of external tibial rotation.

Reversed Pivot Shift. Jakob et al. (99) described the reversed pivot shift test, which is performed in a manner similar to the pivot shift test for ACL injury. As the knee is brought from 90° of flexion to full extension with a valgus stress applied and the foot is externally rotated, the lateral tibial plateau is observed to move from a posteriorly subluxed position to its reduced anatomical position. This is suggestive of a posterolateral injury but is not an absolute finding. The results of this test are most significant when there is asymmetry between the affected and the unaffected knee, as there may be false-positive tests in individuals with ligamentous laxity.

Instrumented testing of PCL laxity, such as the KT-1000 used for ACL testing, has been attempted, but currently no reproducible system has been perfected. This will likely be of benefit for quantification of laxity in the near future.

Radiographic Evaluation. Evidence of PCL or posterolateral ligament complex injury is sometimes seen on routine plain radiographs. The lateral radiograph commonly may show a posterior translation of the tibia relative to the femur or a bony avulsion at the tibial insertion site of the PCL. In cases of lateral and posterolateral injury, bony avulsions can be seen off of the fibular head or Gerdy's tubercle. In the case of chronic PCL insufficiency, radiographs may reveal evidence of medial compartment or patellofemoral arthritis. In addition, as with anterior cruciate ligament injury, magnetic resonance imaging can provide an excellent evaluation of PCL integrity.

Treatment

Isolated PCL Injury. In the case of isolated PCL injuries, most of these knees will regain normal or near normal function with nonoperative management and an appropriate physical therapy regimen. The majority of athletes are able to return fully to their sports. Even in cases of bony avulsion of the PCL, Cooper et al. (95) recommend surgery only in cases of combined injury or posterior translation of the tibia greater than 15 mm.

Indications for surgery include (*a*) combined ligamentous injuries, (*b*) chronic PCL instability with posterior tibial translation of more than 10 to 15 mm, (*c*) symptoms limiting daily activities despite conservative management, and (*d*) early degenerative changes (95, 100). Current surgical techniques involve primary repair, or the use of autogenous patellar tendon grafts, and occasionally patellar tendon or Achilles tendon allografts. The results of these procedures have become increasingly more successful. As with the ACL, PCL reconstruction may now be performed arthroscopically.

Posterolateral Instability. Posterolateral instability usually occurs in combination with PCL injury. These structures are best repaired in the acute setting (95, 96), repairing or reconstructing all involved components. In the chronic setting, surgical reconstruction is indicated in symptomatic cases in which there is a varus deformity of the knee and a lateral thrust during the stance phase of gait (95). In these cases, a valgus-producing high tibial osteotomy may be necessary to reduce the stress on ligamentous reconstruction.

Postoperative Rehabilitation

The general principles of postoperative rehabilitation of isloated PCL reconstruction requires no active hamstring work and protection against posterior tibial translation. In the early phase (1st week postoperation), the knee is braced in full extension and the patient is allowed to weight bear as tolerated. Quadriceps exercises in the form of quadriceps setting and straight-leg raising are begun. The brace is unlocked for ambulation only at 1 week postoperation, and with the patient in the prone position, active assisted knee flexion is begun. Hamstring and calf stretching are begun. At 4 weeks the brace is unlocked, and quadriceps exercises are progressed. Gradually, as a normal gait pattern returns, balance and proprioceptive training begin. Progress is individualized, according to function and symptoms. Patients generally return to full activitiy between 8 and 12 months.

Meniscal Injuries

The menisci function in both load transmission and stability of the knee. In 1948, Fairbank (101) described the radiographic appearance of knee joint changes after meniscectomy (Fig. 54.19). He demonstrated squaring of the contour of the femoral condyle, a medial ridge of the femoral condyle, and narrowing of the joint space. Since that time, several investigators have shown that removal of the menisci will result in increased contact stresses on the underlying cartilage and bone (102). This includes data that showed an increase in contact forces of greater than threefold with removal of 16% to 34% of the meniscus (93, 94, 103–105). Further studies have demonstrated the increased incidence of Fairbank's changes after meniscectomy in ACL-deficient knees (106–109). In addition, studies by Markolf (110) and Levy (111) have illustrated the stabilizing effect of the medial meniscus. It is, therefore, essential for the physician to be able to diagnose a meniscal injury, and for the orthopedic surgeon to assess the type and location of the tear to formulate an appropriate treatment plan.

Diagnosis

Characteristically, meniscal injuries result from a twisting injury with the foot planted. In the athletic population, a specific incident can usually be cited, although with degenerative meniscal tears in the older population this is often not the case. The inciting episode is accompanied by joint line pain and the onset of swelling over the next few hours. Symptoms may diminish over 1 to 2 weeks, but will usually recur when the patient resumes pivoting or cutting activities. Patients may complain of swelling, episodes of locking or catching in which the knee may not fully straighten, and joint line pain (112).

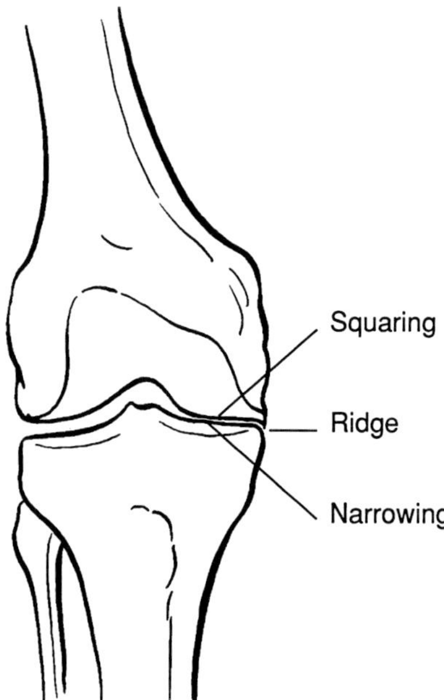

Figure 54.19. Fairbank's radiographic changes of the knee joint after meniscectomy.

Physical examination classically reveals an effusion, joint line tenderness, pain with squatting, and a positive McMurray test. The McMurray test is performed with the patient in the supine position. The knee is gently maximally flexed with one hand on the heel and the thumb of the other hand resting on the lateral joint line with the fingers across the medial joint line (Fig. 54.20). With a valgus stress to the knee and external rotation of the foot, the knee is extended. A palpable or audible click in the medial side is suggestive of a tear of the posterior horn of the medial meniscus. Similarly, extension of the knee with varus and external rotation tests for a lateral meniscal tear. It should also be noted that the so-called locked knee, which cannot reach full extension, may be caused by a "bucket handle" meniscal tear that has displaced centrally into the joint, blocking a full range of motion. Acute isolated meniscal injuries rarely produce changes on plain radiograph, whereas chronic meniscal pathology may produce the Fairbank's changes previously discussed. In light of recent advances with magnetic resonance imaging, arthrography is rarely performed. MRI imaging is useful in cases of questionable meniscal damage (Fig. 54.21).

Treatment

Arthroscopic meniscal surgery was introduced by the Japanese in the 1960s and was further refined by

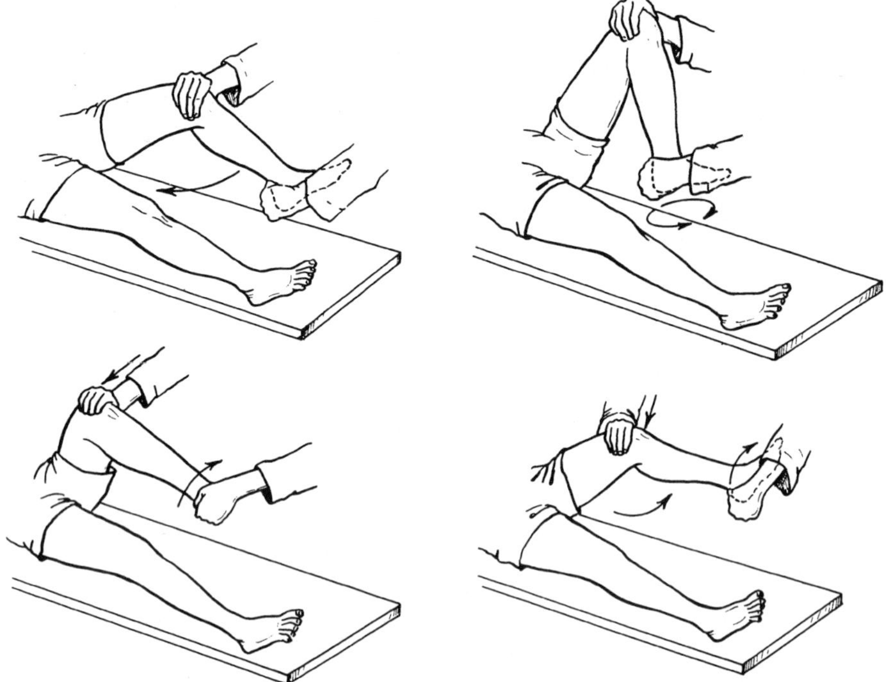

Figure 54.20. The McMurray test.

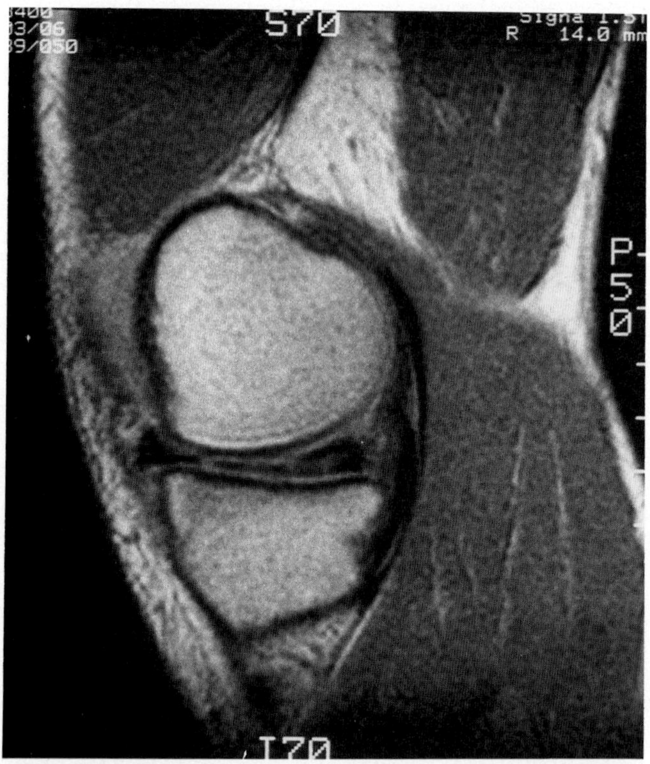

Figure 54.21. Increased signal intensity within the wedge-shaped meniscus indicative of a meniscal tear.

O'Connor in the 1970s. The advent of arthroscopic surgery drastically changed the treatment of meniscal tears. Meniscal tears may be resected or repair arthroscopically. There are four basic patterns of meniscal tears: (*a*) longitudinal; (*b*) horizontal; (*c*) oblique (flap); and (*d*) radial (Fig. 54.22). Complex tears involve a combination of these injuries. These distinctions are made at surgery and are important in the consideration of repair versus resection. Occasionally, however, meniscal tears may be managed nonoperatively.

Nonoperative Management

Nonoperatively managed tears represent approximately 5% of all meniscal injuries (104). Most commonly, these cases represent an incidental finding on physical examination or patients who complain of intermittent symptoms of pain, but no mechanical symptoms (locking, catching) and on physical examination have joint line tenderness but no effusion. McMurray testing may or may not be positive. Generally, these represent partial-thickness or small, full-thickness longitudinal tears that tend to be peripheral and, therefore, have blood supply to allow healing. These knees may be treated symptomatically with rest, ice, and nonsteroidal antiinflammatory agents. If symptoms persist for longer than 4 to 6 weeks or become debilitating, surgical intervention remains an option.

Operative Management

Arnoczky and Warren (113, 114, 115) have demonstrated the vascular anatomy of the meniscus. They showed that a perimeniscal capillary plexus, first described by Policard, supplied branches that pentrated the peripheral 10% to 30% of the menisci. The only exception is the posterolateral region of the lateral meniscus, immediately adjacent to the popliteal tendon, which is devoid of vasculature. Tears confined to the periph-

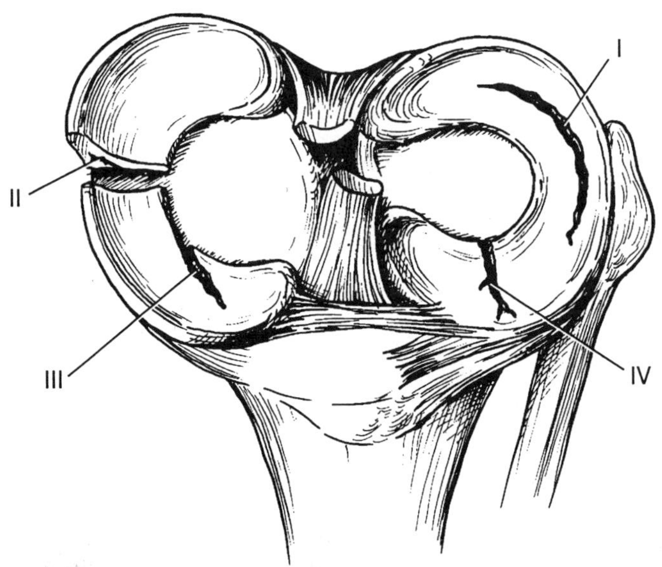

Figure 54.22. The four basic types of meniscal tear: *I*, longitudinal; *II*, horizontal; *III*, oblique; *IV*, radial. Adapted from Kalenak A, Hanks GA, et al. Arthroscopy of the knee. In: Evarts CM, ed. Surgery of the musculoskeletal system. New York: Churchill Livingstone, 1990:3349.

eral regions, therefore, are amenable to operative repair because of the potential for healing associated with vascularity, although the meniscus has been shown to heal by fibrous scar formation, not by regeneration (114, 115). Such tears are usually longitudinal in nature and may include the classic bucket handle tear. Other indications for repair include peripheral detachments through the coronary ligaments and selected peripheral, radial, and horizontal cleavage tears. Generally, tears within the peripheral 3 mm of the meniscus are amenable to repair, with a 90% to 95% success rate (116, 117). The region from 3 to 5 mm remains a gray zone in terms of repair, with data remaining somewhat controversial regarding success of healing within this zone; however, some authors have reported good results (116, 118, 119). Healing of menisci in regions greater than 5 or 6 mm from the periphery is unlikely, but some success has been reported, particularly in cases of repair accompanied by ACL reconstruction, for which results appear to be improved with all locations of meniscal tears.

There are two basic techniques for arthroscopic meniscal repair. The inside-out technique uses a cannula system to pass sutures in a horizontal mattress fashion across the tear and out through either a posteromedial or posterolateral incision (120). The outside-in method involves placement of needles percutaneously across the tear (116). Sutures are then passed through the needles and retrieved from the joint through one of the arthroscopic portals. A knot is tied in the end of the suture, which is then drawn back into the joint, pulling the ends of the tear into continuity. Fibrin clot may be used as an adjuvant to repair as a means of promoting healing (121). The advantages of arthroscopic meniscal repair include the ability to repair more central meniscal tears (2 to 6 mm) and posterolateral tears, which cannot be reached by open repair techniques. The risk of

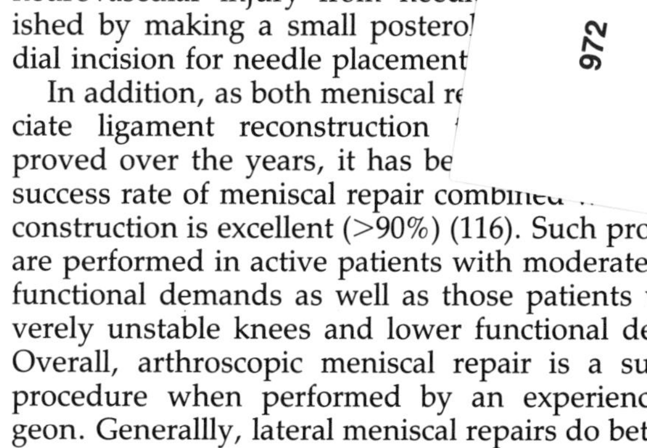

neurovascular injury from needl ished by making a small postero dial incision for needle placement

In addition, as both meniscal r ciate ligament reconstruction proved over the years, it has be success rate of meniscal repair combined construction is excellent (>90%) (116). Such procedures are performed in active patients with moderate to high functional demands as well as those patients with severely unstable knees and lower functional demands. Overall, arthroscopic meniscal repair is a successful procedure when performed by an experienced surgeon. Generallly, lateral meniscal repairs do better than medial, and increasing size of the tear correlates with an increasing failure rate (119, 122, 123).

Rehabilitation after Arthroscopic Meniscal Repair

The specific timing of the meniscal healing process remains unclear. However, it is widely accepted that it is necessary to protect the meniscal repair during the early healing phase, lasting for 4 to 6 weeks. The knee is protected from vigorous activity for 6 months to allow for maturation of the healing collagen. Thus the patient remains non–weight bearing or touch-down weight bearing for up to 6 weeks. If an anterior cruciate ligament repair has been performed simultaneously, the basic ACL rehabilitation protocol is then followed. In isolated meniscal repairs isometric quadriceps and hamstring exercises are begun immediately. Some surgeons prefer to avoid motion for up to 2 weeks, keeping the knee locked in a brace at 45° and then beginning limited motion (30° to 70°) until 6 weeks postoperatively. Others allow earlier full range of motion. Full weight bearing is allowed between 4 and 6 weeks, and a strengthening program is begun at 6 weeks. Once adequate strength is obtained along with a full range of motion without pain or effusion, the patient may begin jogging and half-speed running, cycling, and swimming. This occurs at about 3 months. By 6 months, the athlete is usually ready to return to full activities.

Open Meniscal Repair

Tears within the peripheral 1 to 2 mm of the anterior third of the menisci are amenable to open repair. Tears in the middle to posterior third require extensive exposure and, therefore, are better repaired arthroscopically. Open meniscal repair is typically performed on vertical longitudinal tears of 5 mm or more in length. Although these tears may also be repaired arthroscopically, some surgeons prefer the open technique, because it is felt that the repair bed may be better prepared, it is easier to place the vertically vented sutures, and there may be better anatomic orientation (122, 124). Postoperative rehabilitation is the same as for arthroscopic repair.

Arthroscopic Meniscectomy

Arthroscopic management of meniscal tears has replaced the historical open total meniscectomy. Arthro-

partial meniscectomy can be performed as an atient procedure, with minimal postoperative pain d morbidity and a rapid return to activities. This procedure is indicated in symptomatic patients who have a nonrepairable meniscal tear. At the time of surgery, only the torn portion of the meniscus is removed, leaving behind a stable capsular rim to help maintain joint stability. The remaining meniscal edge is smoothed and contoured to help prevent further meniscal injury. Overall, data on the long-term outcome of arthroscopic partial meniscectomy are unavailable. However, numerous authors have reported a high percentage of good to excellent results over a 5-year postoperative follow-up period (125).

Postoperative Rehabilitation

The patient is allowed to weight bear as tolerated and begin full range of motion along with isometric quadriceps exercises immediately postoperatively. These activities may be limited by pain and swelling, which can be treated with ice and pain medication. Ice is used throughout the rehabilitation process to diminish any effusion. After 1 week, isotonic and isokinetic exercises are begun, unless there is significant chondromalacia present, in which case these exercises are avoided for 4 to 6 weeks. Usually, the patient regains a full range of motion within the first 2 weeks, by which time cycling, walking, and swimming are begun. Once adequate strength is regained and there is no further pain and swelling, the patient may resume full activities. This is usually 6 to 8 weeks after surgery. Nonsteroidal antiinflammatory agents may be used for effusion or synovitis persisting for more than 2 to 3 weeks. Rarely is aspiration of an effusion indicated.

Discoid Lateral Meniscus

Occasionally, meniscal problems in children may be caused by a discoid lateral meniscus (2.4% to 4.2%) (126, 127). Discoid medial meniscus is less common. The clinical syndrome associated with discoid menisci was described by Kroiss in 1910 as a snapping or clicking. History is usually vague, as there is often no specific inciting episode. Patients may complain of pain, swelling, locking, snapping, or limited motion, although the lesions may be asymptomatic (128). Radiographs are helpful in ruling out other causes of the patient's symptoms. They are usually normal in the case of a discoid meniscus, although there has been some association with flattened or hypoplastic lateral femoral condyles, lateral joint space widening, hypoplasia of the lateral tibial spine, and elevation of the fibular head (126, 127, 129).

Asymptomatic or occasionally snapping discoid menisci require no treatment. However, the symptomatic or torn discoid meniscus poses a difficult surgical problem. Excision of the torn portion of discoid meniscus is technically challenging (130). Once this is achieved, it is important to be certain that a stable meniscal rim remains behind. This can be difficult in variants in which the meniscotibial ligament is congenitally absent. Postoperative management is the same as for routine partial meniscectomy.

Knee Dislocation

Dislocation of the knee is a potentially devastating injury that occurs as a result of major trauma. These injuries produce damage to multiple ligaments as well as to vascular structures in 30% to 50% of cases and nerve in up to 50% of cases (11, 131). As such, a knee dislocation is an orthopedic emergency. Obvious knee dislocations must be recognized and reduced quickly, and any knee with multiple ligament injuries including both cruciates should be suspected of being a spontaneously reduced dislocation.

Classification of knee dislocations is based on the direction of tibial displacement relative to the femur. Anterior and posterior dislocations are the most common types. Dislocations may also be medial, lateral, or rotatory. Rotatory dislocations are further classified as anteromedial, anterolateral, posteromedial, and posterolateral.

Another dislocation is caused by hyperextension resulting from a direct anterior blow to the knee. Most often this occurs in train and motor vehicle accidents, but it may also be produced by a football tackle when the helmet strikes the knee. Under such circumstances, the PCL and often the ACL are torn, and the popliteal artery may be stretched or torn.

Posterior dislocation results from a direct blow to the anterior, proximal tibia, driving it posteriorly. Again, both the ACL and PCL are disrupted. Also, the popliteal artery is stretched or torn as it is pushed posteriorly while tethered proximally at the adductor hiatus. The risk of vascular injury to the popliteal artery is highest with anterior and posterior dislocations.

Medial and lateral dislocations occur as a result of severe valgus or varus blows to the knee. These may produce both cruciate and collateral ligament damage, along with possible neurovascular injuries. Similarly, angular blows to the knee may produce rotatory instabilities, with motion hinged on the limited remaining intact structures.

Evaluation

Any knee with gross multiplanar instability should be considered as a frank or occult knee dislocation until proven otherwise. A thorough history of the injury, the amount of trauma involved, deformity, and spontaneous or manual reduction should be obtained in addition to performing a physical examination. The details of ligamentous examination of the knee were discussed above.

Any patient with a suspected knee dislocation is at risk for arterial injury and, therefore, should have an immediate arteriogram. In addition to complete rupture, arterial injuries may include initial tears or intraluminal thrombus formation. Therefore, signs and symptoms of arterial injury may not be present on the initial physical examination, despite an underlying problem. As a result, the foot may be pink, warm, have good capillary refill and a palpable pulse, despite arterial damage. Signs and symptoms may manifest hours to days after the injury.

In the case of an arteriogram revealing popliteal artery occlusion or tear, repair or grafting of the vessel should be completed within 6 to 8 hr of the injury to minimize the changes of ischemic damage to the limb and possible amputation.

Common peroneal nerve injuries occur in approximately 35% of cases (11, 131). These are most often associated with posterolateral dislocations. The injuries range from neurapraxia to complete disruption. Treatment of nerve injuries remains controversial. In general, if operative management of ligamentous injuries is pursued, the nerve may be examined at that time. If the nerve is completely disrupted, then repair or grafting may be undertaken at that time. Otherwise, observation and conservative management may be pursued.

Management

As already noted, initial management is directed toward the vascular status of the limb. A frankly dislocated knee should be immediately reduced. In an occult dislocation, physical examination is performed, and the examiner should quickly suspect a dislocation. In either case, an arteriogram is immediately obtained. Once the vascular assessment is completed, emergency repair or reconstruction of the vessel is performed, if necessary. Ligamentous reconstruction may be performed at the same operative sitting or within the ensuing 2 weeks. Operative techniques are the same as those described elsewhere in this chapter. Sisto and Warren (132) reported that postoperative knee stiffness was more of a problem than instability. However, with more recent advances in techniques of ligament reconstruction, allowing earlier motion and producing a lower incidence of stiff knee, this is less likely to be a problem (133), and the authors currently advocate operative stabilization. Nonoperative management involves bracing for 6 to 8 weeks, followed by physical therapy.

Postoperative treatment must be guided by the degree of associated arterial and neurologic injury and repair. Generally, an early range of motion should be established. Postoperative rehabilitation protocols may then be adapted for the specific complex of injuries sustained by each individual. Long-term prognosis for return of function depends primarily on the neurovascular status of the limb. If adequate arterial flow and neurologic function are reestablished, then the prognosis is good. Prognosis seems to be best for those limbs managed by surgical intervention. However, success with nonoperative management has been reported.

Tibial Plateau Fracture

Fractures of the tibial plateau are relatively rare in athletics. They result from severe varus or valgus forces combined with axial loading. Incidence, fracture pattern, and associated injuries largely depend on the age of the patient. It is generally believed that an intact, lateral collateral ligament acts as a hinge when a varus stress and axial load are applied. The medial femoral condyle is then driven into the medial tibial plateau, resulting in fracture. The same mechanism applies for the medial collateral ligament when valgus and axial forces are applied.

Signs and Symptoms

Patients present with pain and swelling of the knee. Examination should focus on the extent of swelling, tenderness, and ecchymosis. A hemarthrosis is usually present and may be aspirated. Fat droplets present in the aspirate are indicative of an intraarticular fracture. It should be noted that about 15% of tibial plateau fractures are associated with collateral ligament injuries, and 5% to 15% are associated with meniscal injuries (134). Neurovascular injuries and compartment syndromes are rare.

Radiographic Studies

Standard anteroposterior and lateral radiographs are often sufficient to reveal a fracture. If the fracture is not visualized on these views oblique, tangential, or tunnel views may be helpful. When no fracture line is seen, but there remains a high index of suspicion (fat droplets in aspirate), then a bone scan or MRI scan may be obtained. Once the radiographic diagnosis has been made it is helpful to delineate the amount of depression and displacement of the fracture. This may be done with AP and lateral tomograms or CT scans. Stress x-rays also may be helpful in assessment of instability.

Classification

Numerous classification systems exist for tibial plateau fractures. Probably the most commonly used system is the AO classification system. This includes four types: *(a)* wedge fracture; *(b)* depression fracture; *(c)* wedge and depression fracture; and *(d)* Y- and T-type split fractures. Young patients with strong bones most commonly sustain the wedge or split fracture.

Treatment

Treatment may be operative or nonoperative. The type of treatment is based on the amount of displacement or depression of the fracture, bone quality, age of the patient, and amount of associated instability. In general, a young patient with 6 mm or more of plateau depression or an unreducible displaced fragment is a candidate for surgical management. Depending on the type of fracture, this may involve closed reduction with percutaneous screw or pin fixation; arthroscopically aided reduction and bone grafting with pin or screw fixation; or open reduction and internal fixation with bone grafting, plate, and/or screw fixation.

Nonoperative management may be used for fractures with less than 6 mm of plateau depression, split fractures that can be reduced closed, stable knees (less than 5° to 10° of joint opening on varus or valgus stress testing), and older patients with poor bone quality. This involves the use of a cast, cast-brace, or brace with protected weight bearing for up to 12 weeks.

Tibial Spine and Intercondylar Eminence Fractures

Tibial spine and intercondylar eminence fractures are often seen as isolated injuries and are associated with knee instability. These fractures are most commonly caused by an athletic injury or motor vehicle accident. They result from violent hyperextension or hyperflexion, varus or valgus stress, or twisting injury. Hyperextension or hyperflexion usually causes an intercondylar eminence avulsion (with attached ACL), while twisting may produce a tibial fracture (135, 136).

Signs and Symptoms

The patient usually presents with complaints of pain and swelling. Often, the knee does not reach full extension. This is caused by a mechanical block as the intercondylar eminence is elevated into the intercondylar notch. The knee may also be unstable as a result of ACL or collateral ligament injury. Fracture is usually evident on standard anteroposterior and lateral views of the knee. However, CT scan or tomogram may be helpful in further evaluating the extent of the fracture and amount of displacement.

Treatment

An isolated tibial spine fracture can usually be reduced by placing the knee in full extension. In this case, it can be treated nonoperatively with a cast or brace in full extension for 4 to 6 weeks. However, if there is an associated ACL injury in a young, active patient, this may need to be addressed surgically (137).

Similarly, a minimally to moderately elevated intercondylar eminence fracture can usually be reduced by placing the knee in full extension. If this is the case, it may also be treated in full extension in a cast or brace for 4 to 6 weeks. However, if the fracture cannot be anatomically reduced by a closed method, operative intervention is indicated. This may be done arthroscopically, fixing the fragment with either a lag screw or suture placed around the fragment and tied over the anterior tibia.

REFERENCES

1. Seebacher JR, Inglis AE, Marshall JL, et al. The structure of the posterolateral aspect of the knee. J Bone Joint Surg 1982;64:536.
2. Warren LF, Marshall JL. The supportive structures and layers on the medial side of the knee. An anatomical analysis. J Bone Joint Surg 1979;61:56.
3. Allen WC, Hensdorf JR. Knee ligament reconstruction. In: Evarts CM, ed. Surgery of the musculoskeletal system. New York: Churchill Livingstone, 1990:3283.
4. Muller W. The knee: form, function, and ligament reconstruction. Berlin: Springer-Verlag, 1983.
5. Norwood LA, Cross MJ. Anterior cruciate ligament: functional anatomy of its bundles in rotatory instabilities. Am J Sports Med 1979;7:23.
6. Noyes FR, Grood ES, Butler DL, et al. Clinical biomechanics of the knee ligament restraints and functional stability. In: Funk J, ed. Symposium on the athlete's knee: surgical repair and reconstruction. St. Louis: CV Mosby, 1979:1–35.
7. Noyes, FR, Mooar PA, Matthews DS, Butler DL. The symptomatic anterior cruciate-deficient knee. I: The long-term functional disability in athletically active individuals. J Bone Joint Surg 1983;65A:154.
8. Reider B, Marshall JL. The anterior cruciate; guardian of the meniscus. Orthop Rev. 1979;7(5):83.
9. Warren RF. Acute ligament injuries. In: Insall JN, ed. Surgery of the knee. New York: Churchill Livingstone, 1984, pp. 261–294.
10. Arms SW, Pope MH, Johnson RJ, et al. The biomechanics of anterior cruciate ligament rehabilitation and reconstruction. Am J Sports Med 1984;12:8.
11. DeHaven KE. Acute ligament injuries and dislocations. In: Evarts CM, ed. Surgery of the musculoskeletal system. New York: Churchill Livingstone, 1990:3255.
12. Ellison AE. The pathogenesis and treatment of anterolateral rotary instability. Clin Orthop 1980;147:51.
13. Furman W, Marshall JL, Girgis FB. The anterior cruciate ligament. A functional analysis based on post mortem studies. J Bone Joint Surg 1976;58A:179.
14. Girgis FG, Marshall JL, Monajem AARS. The cruciate ligament of the knee joint. Anatomical, functional, and experimental analysis. Clin Orthop 1975;106:216.
15. Gollehon DL, Torzilli PA, Warren RF. The role of the posterolateral and cruciate ligaments in the stability of the human knee. J Bone Joint Surg 1987;69A:233.
16. Hey-Groves EW. The crucial ligaments of the knee joint: Their function, rupture and the operative treatment of the same. Br J Surg 1920;7:505.
17. Johnson RJ. Anatomy and biomechanics of the knee. In: Chapman MW, ed. Operative orthopaedics. Philadelphia: JB Lippincott, 1988:1617.
18. Kennedy JC, Weinberg HW, Wilson AS. The anatomy and function of the anterior cruciate ligament as determined by clinical and morphological studies. J Bone Joint Surg 1974;56A:223.
19. Collins HR. Screening of athletic knee injuries. Clin Sports Med 1985;4(2):217–230.
20. Jensen JE, Conn RB, Hazelrigg G, Hewett JE. Systematic evaluation of acute knee injuries. Clin Sports Med 1985;4(2):295–312.
21. Grana WA, Kriegshauser LA. Scientific basis of extensor mechanism disorders. Clin Sports Med 1985;4(2):247–258.
22. Insall JN. Disorders of the patella. In: Insall JN, ed. Surgery of the knee. New York: Churchill Livingstone, 1984, pp. 191–260.
23. Bassett FH III. Acute dislocation of the patella osteochondral fractures and injuries of the extensor mechanism of the knee. In: AAOS Instructional Course Lectures. Vol. 25. St. Louis: CV Mosby, 1976:40–49.
24. Ferguson AB, Brown TD, Fu FH, et al. Relief of patellofemoral contact stress by anterior displacement of the tibial tubercle. J Bone Joint Surg 1979;61A:159.
25. Albright JP. Musculotendinous problems about the knee. In: Evarts CM, ed. Surgery of the musculoskeletal system. New York: Churchill Livingstone, 1990:3499.
26. McBeath AA. The patellofemoral joint. In: Evarts CM, ed. Surgery of the musculoskeletal system. New York: Churchill Livingstone, 1990:3433.
27. Larson RL. Subluxation-dislocation of the patella. In: Kennedy JC, ed. The injured adolescent knee. Baltimore: Williams & Wilkins, 1979:161–204.
28. Carson WG Jr. Diagnosis of extensor mechanism disorders. Clin Sports Med 1985;4(2):231–246.
29. Carson WG Jr, James SL, Larson RL, et al. Patellofemoral disorders: physical and radiographic evaluation. I and II. Clin Orthop 1984;185:165.
30. Insall JN, Bullough PG, Burstein AH. Proximal "tube" realignment of the patella for chondromalacia patellae. Clin Orthop 1979;144:63.
31. Insall J, Goldberg V, Salvati E. Recurrent dislocation and the high-riding patella. Clin Orthop 1972;88:67.
32. Insall J, Salvati E. Patella position in the normal knee joint. Radiology 1971;101:101.
33. Hughston JC, Walsh WM. Proximal and distal reconstruction of the extensor mechanism for patellar subluxation. Clin Orthop 1979;144:36.
34. Merchant AC. Patellofemoral disorders: biomechanics, diagnosis,

and nonoperative treatment. In: McGinty JB, ed. Operative arthroscopy. New York: Raven Press. 1991, pp. 261–275.
35. Laurin CA, Dussault R, Levesque HP. The tangential x-ray investigation of the patellofemoral joint: x-ray technique, diagnostic criteria and their interpretation. Clin Orthop 1979;144:16.
36. Laurin CA, Levesque HP, Dussault R. The abnormal lateral patellofemoral angle: a diagnostic roentgenographic sign of recurrent patellar subluxation. J Bone Joint Surg 1978;60A:55.
37. Hawkins RJ, Bell RH, Anisette G. Acute patellar dislocations: the natural history. Am J Sports Med 1986;14:117.
38. Bassett F, Soucacos P, Carr W. Jumper's knees: patellar tendinitis and patellar tendon rupture. In: AAOS symposium on the athlete's knee. St. Louis: CV Mosby. 1978.
39. Kelly DW, Carter VS, Jobe FW, et al. Patellar and quadriceps tendon ruptures—jumper's knee. Am J Sports Med 1984;12:375.
40. Morgan J, McCarty D. Tendon ruptures in patients with systemic lupus erythematosus treated with cortical steroids. Arthrit Rheumat 1974;17:1033–1035.
41. Rao J, Siwek K. Bilateral spontaneous rupture of the patellar tendons. Orthop Rev 1978;7:51.
42. Scuderi C. Ruptures of the quadriceps tendon. Am J Surg 1958;95:626.
43. McManus F, Rang M, Heslin DJ. Acute dislocation of the patella in children: the natural history. Clin Orthop 1979;139:88.
44. Rorabeck CH, Bobechko WP. Acute dislocation of the patella with osteochondral fracture. J Bone Joint Surg 1976;58B:237.
45. Arnoczky SP. Basic science of anterior cruciate ligament repair and reconstruction. In Tullos HS (Ed). AAOS Instruc Course Lect 1991;40:201–212.
46. Woo SL-Y, Gomez MA, Sites TJ, et al. The biomechanical and morphological changes of the MCL following immobilization and remobilization. J Bone Joint Surg 1987;69A:1200.
47. Woo SL-Y, Gomez MA, Inoue M, et al. New experimental procedures to evaluate the biomechanical properties of healing canine medial collateral ligaments. J Orthop Res 1987;5:425.
48. Indelicato PA. Non-operative treatment of complete tears of the medial collateral ligament of the knee. J Bone Joint Surg 1983;65A:322.
49. Hughston JC, Andrews JR, Cross MJ, et al. Classification of knee ligament instabilities. Part II. The lateral compartment. J Bone Joint Surg 1976;58A:173.
50. Hey-Groves EW. Operation for the repair of crucial ligaments. Lancet 1917;2:674.
51. Palmer I. On the injuries to the ligaments of the knee joint. Acta Chir Scand 1938;81(suppl 53):3.
52. Bosworth DM, Bosworth BM. Use of fascia lata to stabilize the knee in cases of ruptured crucial ligaments. J Bone Joint Surg 1936;18A:178.
53. O'Donoghue DH. Surgical treatment of fresh injuries to the major ligaments of the knee. J Bone Joint Surg 1950;32A:721–738.
54. O'Donoghue DH. An analysis of the end results of surgical treatment of major injuries to the ligaments of the knee. J Bone Joint Surg 1955;37A:1.
55. O'Donoghue DH. A method for replacement of the anterior cruciate ligament of the knee. J Bone Joint Surg 1963;45A:905.
56. O'Donoghue DH. Reconstruction for medial instability of the knee. Technique and results in sixty cases. J Bone Joint Surg 1973;55A:941.
57. O'Donoghue DH, Frank GR, Jeter GL, et al. Repair and reconstruction of the anterior cruciate ligament in dogs. J Bone Joint Surg 1971;53A:710.
58. Butler DL, Noyes FR, Grood ES. Ligamentous restraints to anterior-posterior drawer in the human knee. J Bone Joint Surg 1980;62A:259.
59. Fetto JF, Marshall JL. Injury to the anterior cruciate ligament producing the pivot-shift sign. J Bone Joint Surg 1979;61A:710.
60. Galway R. Pivot-shift syndrome. J Bone Joint Surg 1972;54B:558.
61. Galway HR, Beaupre A, MacIntosh D. Pivot shift. A clinical sign of symptomatic anterior cruciate insufficiency. J Bone Joint Surg 1972;54B:763.
62. Galway HR, MacIntosh DL. The lateral pivot shift: symptom and sign of anterior cruciate ligament insufficiency. Clin Orthop 1980;147:45.
63. Hughston JC, Andrews JR, Cross MJ, et al. Classification of knee ligament instabilities. Part I. The medial compartment and cruciate ligaments. J Bone Joint Surg 1976;58A:159.
64. Kennedy JC, Fowler PJ. Medial and anterior instability of the knee. J Bone Joint Surg 1971;53A:1257.
65. Noyes FR, Grood ES, Butler DL, et al. Clinical laxity tests and functional stability of the knee: biomechanical concepts. Clin Orthop 1980;146:84.
66. Slocum DB, James SL, Larson RL, et al. Clinical test for anterolateral rotary instability of the knee. Clin Orthop 1976;118:63.
67. Slocum DB, Larson RL. Rotatory instability of the knee. Its pathogenesis and a clinical test to determine its presence. J Bone Joint Surg 1968;50A:211.
68. Losee RE. The pivot shift. In: Feagin JA, ed. The Crucial Ligaments. New York: Churchill Livingstone, 1988. pp. 301–316.
69. Losee RE, Johnson TR, Southwick WO. Anterior subluxation of the lateral tibial plateau. A diagnostic test and operative repair. J Bone Joint Surg 1978;60A:1015.
70. Arnold JA, Coker TP, Heaton LM, et al. Natural history of anterior cruciate tears. Am J Sports Med 1976;7(6):305.
71. Cabaud HE, Rodkey WG. Philosophy and rationale for the management of anterior cruciate injuries and the resultant deficiencies. Clin Sports Med 1985;4(2):313–324.
72. Feagin JA Jr. The syndrome of the torn anterior cruciate ligament. Orthop Clin North Am 1979;10:31.
73. Feagin JA, Curl WW. Isolated tear of the anterior cruciate ligament: 5 year follow up study. Am J Sports Med 1976;4:95.
74. Fetto JR, Marshall JL. The natural history and diagnosis of anterior cruciate ligament insufficiency. Clin Orthop 1980;147:29.
75. Funk FJ. Osteoarthritis of the knee following ligamentous injury. Clin Orthop 1983;172:154.
76. Holden DL, Jackson DW. Treatment selection in acute anterior cruciate ligament tears. Orthop Clin North Am 1985;16:99.
77. Kannus P, Jarvinen M. Conservatively treated tears of the anterior cruciate ligament. Long term results. J Bone Joint Surg 1987;69A:1007.
78. McDaniel WJ, Dameron TB. Untreated ruptures of the anterior cruciate ligament. A follow-up study. J Bone Joint Surg 1980;62A:696.
79. Bach BR, Warren RF. Radiographic indicators of anterior cruciate ligament injury. In: Feagin JA, ed. The crucial ligaments. New York: Churchill Livingstone, 1988; pp. 317–327.
80. Woods GW, Stanley RF, Tullos HS. Lateral capsular sign: x-ray clue to a significant knee instability. Am J Sport Med 1979;7:27.
81. Polly DW, Callaghan JJ. Magnetic resonance imaging of the cruciate ligaments. In: Feagin JA, ed. The Crucial Ligaments. New York: Churchill Livingstone, 1988,328–332.
82. Warner JJP, Warren RF, Cooper DE. Management of acute anterior cruciate ligament injury. In Tullos HS (ed.) AAOS Instruct Cours Lect 1991;40:219–232.
83. Noyes FR, DeLucas JL, Torrik PJ. Biomechanics of anterior cruciate ligament failure: an analysis of strain-rate sensitivity and mechanisms of failure in primates. J Bone Joint Surg 1979;56A:236.
84. Warren RF. Primary repair of the anterior cruciate ligament. Clin Orthop 1983;172:65.
85. Johnson RJ, Beynnon BD, et al. The treatment of injuries of the anterior cruciate ligament. J Bone Joint Surg 1992;74A:140.
86. Noyes FR, Butler DL, Paulos LE, Grood ES. Intraarticular cruciate reconstruction. I: Perspectives on graft strength, vascularization, and immediate motion after replacement. Clin Orthop 1983;172:71.
87. Butler DL, Noyes FR, Grood ES, et al. Mechanical properties of transplants for the anterior cruciate ligament. Trans Orthop Res Soc 1979;4:81.
88. O'Brien SJ, Warren RF, et al. Reconstruction of the chronically insufficient anterior cruciate ligament with the central third of the patellar ligament. J Bone Joint Surg 1991;73A:278.
89. Howe JG, Johnson RJ, et al. Anterior cruciate ligament reconstruction using quadriceps patellar tendon graft. Part I. Long-term follow up. Am J Sports Med 1992;19:447.
90. Woods GW. Synthetics in anterior cruciate ligament reconstruction: a review. Orthop Clin North Am 1985;16:227.
91. Czitrom AA, Axelrod T, Fernandes B. Antigen presenting cells

and bone allotransplantation. Clin Orthop 1985;197:27–31.
92. Shino K, Inoue M, Horibe S, et al. Reconstruction of the anterior cruciate ligament using allogeneic tendon. Long term follow-up. Am J Sports Med 1992;18:457.
93. Indelicato PA, Linton RC, Huegel M. The results of fresh-frozen patellar tendon allografts for chronic anterior cruciate ligament deficiency of the knee. Am J Sport Med 1992;20:118.
94. Noyes FR, Barber SD, Mangine RE. Bone-patellar ligament-bone and fascia lata allografts for reconstruction of the anterior cruciate ligament. J Bone Joint Surg 1990;72A:1125.
95. Cooper DE, Warren RF, Warner JJP. The posterior cruciate ligament and posterolateral structure of the knee: anatomy, function, and patterns of injury. In Tullo HS. (ed). AAOS Instruct Course Lect 1991;40:249–270.
96. Hughston JC, Barrett GR. Acute anteromedial rotatory instability. Long-term results of surgical repair. J Bone Joint Surg 1983;65A:145.
97. Hughston JC, Norwood LA. The posterolateral drawer test and external rotational recurvatum for posterolateral rotary instability of the knee. Clin Orthop 1980;147:82.
98. Insall JN. Examination of the knee. In: Insall JN, ed. Surgery of the knee. New York: Churchill Livingstone, 1984, pp. 55–72.
99. Jakob RP, Staubli HU, Deland JT. Grading the pivot shift. Objective tests with implications for treatment. J Bone Joint Surg 1987;69B:294.
100. Bergfeld JA, Parolia J. Non-operative treatment of isolated PCL injuries in the athlete. Am J Sports Med 1986;14(1):35.
101. Fairbank TJ. Knee joint changes after meniscectomy. J Bone Joint Surg 1948;30:B664.
102. Henning CE, Lynch MA. Current concepts of meniscal function and pathology. Clin Sports Med 4(2):259–266.
103. Seedhom BB, Hargreaves DJ. Transmission of the load in the knee joint with special reference to the role of the menisci. Part II. Experimental results, discussion, and conclusions. Eng Med 1979;8:220.
104. DeHaven KE. Rationale for meniscus repair or excision. Clin Sports Med 1985;4(2):267–274.
105. Radin EL, De LaMotte F, Maquet P. Role of the menisci in the distribution of stress in the knee. Clin Orthop 1984;185: 290.
106. Casscells SW. The torn or degenerated meniscus and its relationship to degeneration of the weight bearing areas of the femur and tibia. Clin Orthop 1978;132:196.
107. Casscells SW. The torn meniscus, the torn anterior cruciate ligament, and their relationship to degenerative joint disease. Arthroscopy 1985;1(1):28.
108. Cox JS, Nye CE, Schaefer WW, Woodstein IJ. The degenerative effects of partial and total resection of the medial meniscus in dog's knees. Clin Orthop 1975;109:178.
109. Dandy DJ, Jackson RW. The diagnosis of problems after meniscectomy pathology. Clin Orthop 1982;163:218.
110. Markolf KL, Bargar WL, Shoemaker SC, et al. The role of joint load in knee stability. J Bone Joint Surg (Am) 1981;63:570.
111. Levy IM, Torzilli PA, Warren RF. The effect of medial meniscectomy on anterior-posterior motion of the knee. J Bone Joint Surg (Am) 1982;64:883.
112. Daniel D, Daniels E, Aronson D. The diagnosis of meniscus pathology. Clin Orthop 1982;163:218.
113. Arnoczky SP, Warren RF. Microvasculature of the human meniscus. Am J Sports Med 1982;10:90.
114. Arnoczky SP, Warren RF. The microvasculature of the meniscus and its response to injury. An experimental study in the dog. Am J Sports Med 1983;11:131.
115. Arnoczky SP. The blood supply of the meniscus and its role in healing and repair. In: Finerman G, ed. AAOS symposium on sports medicine: the knee. St. Louis: CV Mosby, 1985:94–110.
116. Cannon WD. Arthroscopic meniscal repair. In: McGinty JB, ed. Operative arthroscopy. New York: Raven Press, 1991.
117. Rosenberg TD, Metcalf RW, Gurley WG. Arthroscopic meniscectomy. In: Bassett FH, ed. AAOS Instructional Course Lectures. Vol. 37. St. Louis: CV Mosby, 1988.
118. Henning CE. Arthroscopic repair of meniscus tears. Orthopedics 1983;6:1130.
119. Henning CE, Clark CE, Lynch MA, et al. Arthroscopic meniscus repair with a posterior incision. In: Bassett, FH III, ed. AAOS Instructional Course Lectures. Vol. 37. St. Louis: CV Mosby, 1988:209–221.
120. Warren RF. Arthroscopic meniscal repair. Arthroscopy 1985;1:170.
121. Arnoczky SP, McDevitt CA, Warren RF, et al. Meniscus repair using an exogenous fibrin clot—an experimental study in dogs. Orthop Trans 1986;10:327.
122. DeHaven KE. Meniscus repair—open vs. arthroscopic. Arthroscopy 1985;1:173.
123. Clancy WG Jr, Graf BK. Arthroscopic meniscal repair. Orthopaedics 1983;6:1125.
124. DeHaven KE. Open meniscus repair. In: McGinty JE, ed. Operative arthroscopy. New York: Raven Press, 1991, pp. 253–260.
125. Metcalf RW. Arthroscopic meniscal surgery. In: McGinty JB, ed. Operative arthroscopy. New York: Raven Press, 1991, pp. 203–236.
126. Kalenak A, Hanks GA, Sebastianelli WJ. Arthroscopy of the knee. In: Evarts CM, ed. Surgery of the musculoskeletal system. New York: Churchill Livingstone, 1990:3349.
127. Smillie IS. The congenital discoid meniscus. J Bone Joint Surg 1948;30B:671.
128. Dickhaut SC, DeLee JC. The discoid lateral-meniscus syndrome. J Bone Joint Surg 1982;64A:1068.
129. Fujikawa K, Iseki F, Mikura Y. Partial resection of the discoid meniscus in the child's knee. J Bone Joint Surg 1981;63B:391.
130. Ikeuchi H. Arthroscopic treatment of the discoid lateral meniscus. Clin Orthop 1982;167:19.
131. Larson RL. Dislocations and ligamentous injuries to the knee. In: Rockwood CA, Green DP, eds. Fractures. Philadelphia: JB Lippincott, 1975:1182.
132. Sisto DJ, Warren RF. Complete knee dislocation. A follow-up study of operative treatment. Clin Orthop Relat Res 1985;198:94–101.
133. Irrgang JJ, Harner CD, Fu RH, DiGiacmo R, Silbey MB. Loss of motion following ACL reconstruction: a second look. In preparation.
134. Bowes DN, Hohl M. Tibial condylar fractures. Evaluation of treatment and outcome. Clin Orthop 1982;171:104.
135. Meyers MH, McKeever FM. Fractures of the intercondylar eminence of the tibia. J Bone Joint Surg 1970;52A:1671.
136. Roberts JM, Lovell WW. Fractures of the intercondylar eminence of the tibia. J Bone Joint Surg 1970;52A:827.
137. Baxter MP, Wiley JJ. Fractures of the tibial spine in children. J Bone Joint Surg 1988;70B:228.

55 / ANKLE AND FOOT INJURIES

Jonathan S. Jaivin and Richard D. Ferkel

Biomechanics of the Ankle and Foot

Biomechanics, simply stated, is the application of mechanical laws to living structures. Understanding the biomechanics of the foot and ankle is critical to the study of foot and ankle injuries (1).

Gait is a complex process that involves all major body segments. The foot and ankle must be viewed as just one component of this system. Human gait is characteristically orthograde and bipedal with intraspecies variation (2). Ralston (3) notes that human gait evolved to take an individual from one point to another with minimal expenditure of energy. Energy is wasted with vertical displacement of an individual's center of gravity, a motion that serves no useful purpose. One need only try to walk a short distance with a limp to realize that any major aberration of normal gait will cause a major increase in energy expenditure. The key to understanding human gait lies in the realization that all body movements responsible for gait are interrelated and serve to minimize energy expenditure (4).

Gait is a cyclical process that is divided into two phases: the stance phase, in which one limb is in contact with the ground, and the swing phase, during which the same limb is propelled forward (2). For forward progression to occur, four requirements must be satisfied. The limb must be stable in stance, and step length must be adequate. The foot must be adequately prepositioned for ground contact and must clear the ground in swing.

The stance phase is divided into four periods (Fig. 55.1). Stance begins with initial contact, the point at which both limbs touch the floor. Initial contact evolves to loading response when body weight and momentum is accepted. Midstance is a period of single support at which time the contralateral limb and body advance over the stationary foot. Terminal stance begins at heel rise and ends with preswing, another period of double support. The swing phase is divided into three periods (see Fig. 55.1). Normally, the stance phase accounts for 60% of the gait cycle (2).

Running is not understood to the same degree as walking. One main difference between running and walking is that one limb is always in contact with the ground in walking. In running, the period of double support is replaced by an analogous period of double "float" when both feet are off the ground. The speed at which a person makes a transition between walking and running is predictable. Another difference between walking and running is the sharp increase in energy expenditure. The equation that energy is a function of mass multiplied by distance traveled does not hold true with the human machine. Running involves considerably more energy than walking (5).

The function of the foot may be divided into three general categories: accepting uneven terrain, providing a firm lever for pushoff, and absorbing shock. The ability to accept uneven terrain depends on the foot being pliable. The ability to change from pliable to rigid is accomplished by altering the position of the hind foot. In general, the hind foot is rigid in varus and pliable in valgus. Hind foot valgus or varus is largely a result of subtalar joint movement. The subtalar joint is formed by the undersurface of the talus and the dorsal surface of the calcaneus (Fig. 55.2). It consists of three closely approximated articulations or facets. The largest facet is the posterior facet. The anterior and middle facets differ from the posterior facet by virtue of the fact that the posterior facet is concave on the calcaneal surface and convex on the talar surface. This situation is opposite from the anterior and middle facets. The side-to-side motion of the subtalar joint can be likened to the rocking of a boat (2).

The axis of the subtalar joint is actually at a 45° axis from the ground and at a 16° angle from a longitudinal line drawn through the second metatarsal (see Fig. 55.2). This motion and the up-and-down motion of the foot at the tibiotalar joint combine to form a "universal joint."

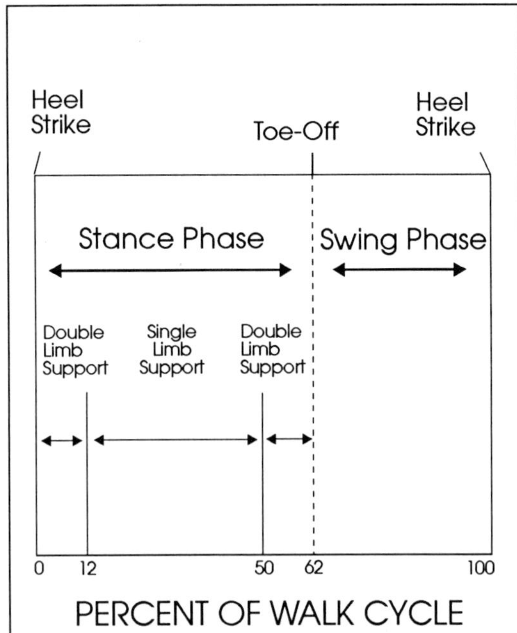

Figure 55.1. The gait cycle is divided into the stance phase and the swing phase. The stance phase occupies 62% of the gait cycle and is further divided into periods of single and double limb support.

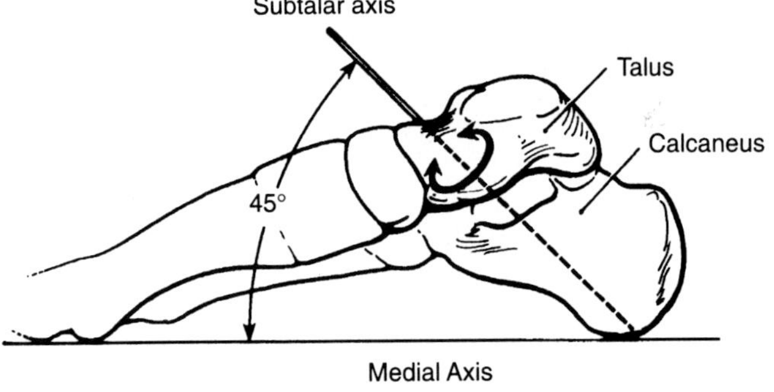

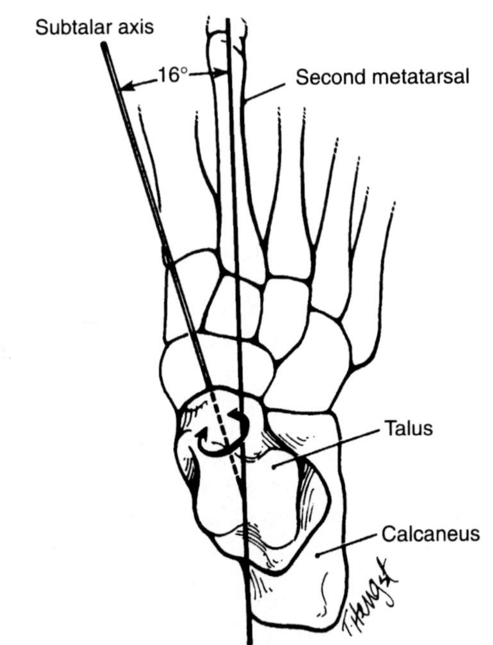

Figure 55.2. Motion about the subtalar joint occurs about an axis 45° from the floor and 16° medially from the central axis of the second metatarsal.

The foot is positioned by movements through both of these joints. When the hind foot is supinated, the geometry of the tibia and calcaneus is such that the bones are intimately joined together and the foot is stable. Hind foot pronation unlocks this relationship and a pliable foot is formed. In this way, the foot is controlled by the muscles of the leg to function in the gait cycle (2).

The athlete must strive to maximize performance by conserving energy. This is accomplished by eliminating movements or actions that do not serve a useful purpose. A seemingly insignificant foot injury may set up a pattern of compensatory movements that decrease an athlete's efficiency. Treatment of injuries in the athlete must be predicated on the fact that the foot/ankle unit is part of a larger and complex mechanism and the fact that altering motion at any body segment may have consequences distant to that site.

Epidemiology of Ankle and Foot Injuries

Every sport predisposes the athlete to a particular subset of foot and ankle injuries (6–9). Some sports are at high risk for injury. Knowledge of the types of injuries that occur in a given sport is important to prescribe safety gear and to recommend appropriate cross-training when an athlete is recovering from an injury. As one would expect, endurance athletes are prone to overuse injuries, whereas the collision sports have a higher incidence of strains, sprains, and fractures. A sprain may be defined as a ligamentous injury to a joint. A chronic sprain occurs because of persistent damage to the ligamentous support of a joint. A strain involves either overuse or stretching of muscles, tendons, and/or ligaments without significant tearing (10). A fracture is defined as a disruption of the integrity of bone. There are many types of fractures, two of which are germane to the subject of sports medicine. The first is secondary to direct or indirect forces applied across a bone, leading to fracture and soft tissue damage. The second type of fracture is a stress fracture. Subjecting normal bone to repeated stresses may lead to failure. The classic "march" fracture or stress fracture of a metatarsal provides an example of this mechanism. This injury is seen in athletes (or military recruits) who have increased the distance that they run, jog, or "march ." The stresses across the metatarsal are not unlike the stresses across a paper clip bent back and forth between one's fingers. No single bending motion is strong enough but the accumulated stresses will eventually break the metal clip.

Some sports are associated with unique problems caused by the use of special equipment or playing surfaces. For example, ice hockey is associated with a high percentage of lacerations, including lacerations of the tibial tendons and vessels because of ice skates (11). In contrast, most injuries associated with cross-country running are the result of overuse or training errors.

The Leg

Exertional Leg Pain

Running athletes are predisposed to exercise-related leg pain of many etiologies. A proper diagnosis is the first step in the treatment of this common complaint. Exertional leg pain may be divided into three general categories: medial tibial stress syndrome (shin splints), exertional compartment syndrome, and stress fracture.

The term *shin splints* is becoming outdated. The term *medial tibial stress syndrome* is preferred for leg pain and tenderness characteristically localized to the medial border of the distal one-third of the tibia without sensory, motor, vascular, or radiographic abnormalities. Three-phase radionuclide bone scanning reveals increased linear uptake along the posteromedial border of the tibia. This phenomenon is likely the result of periosteal inflammation along the posteromedial border of the tibia secondary to the soleus and/or the posterior tibial muscle (Fig. 55.3).

Pain is reproduced by resisted active plantarflexion and inversion of the foot or resisted active plantarflexion alone. There is palpation tenderness along the posteromedial border of the distal one-third of the tibia. Treatment consists of rest, cross-training, and emphasizing nonimpact activities. Nonsteroidal antiinflammatory drugs (NSAIDs) may be useful in some cases.

Exertional compartment syndromes are a form of chronic compartment syndromes and characteristically involve the anterior and lateral compartments and occasionally the superficial or deep posterior compartments of the leg (Fig. 55.4) (12). A compartment syndrome occurs in an athlete when the pressure within a fascial compartment increases enough to compromise

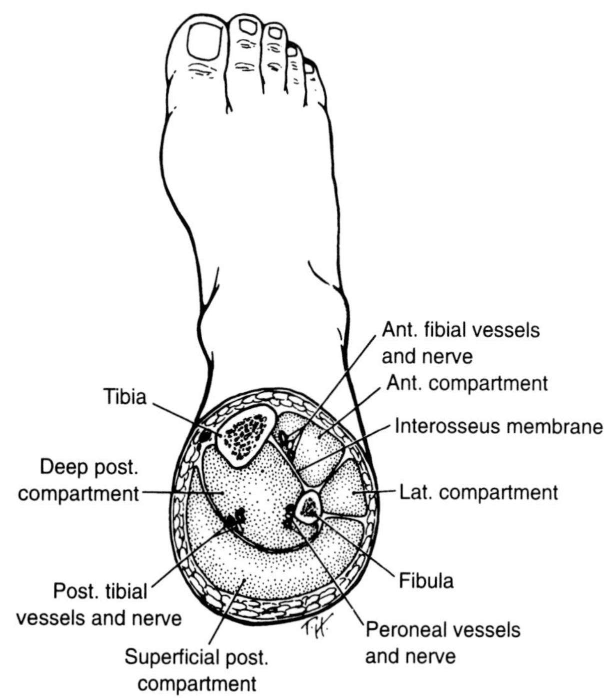

Figure 55.4. Compartments of the leg. There are four compartments of the leg divided by fascial compartments. The major nerves and vessels are consistently present in their respective compartments.

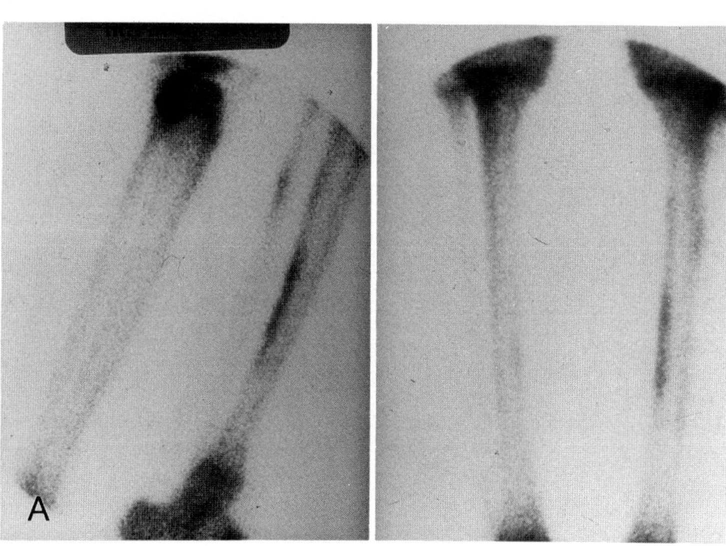

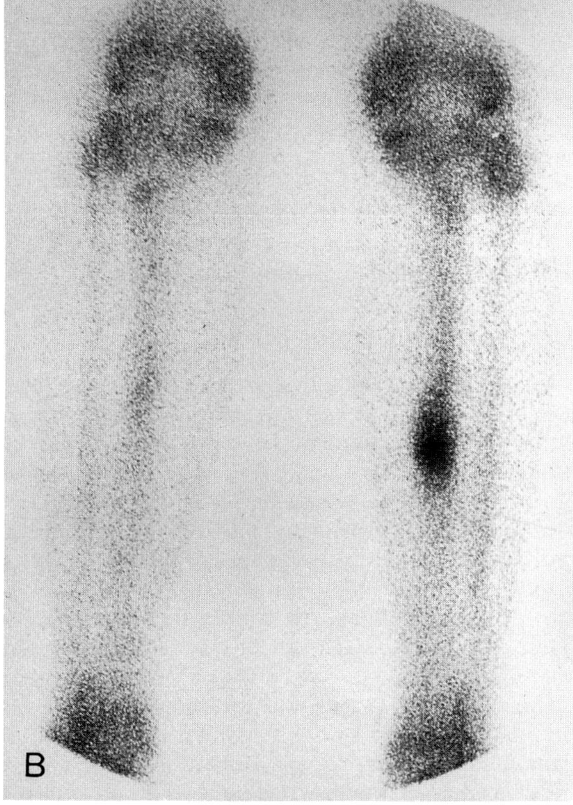

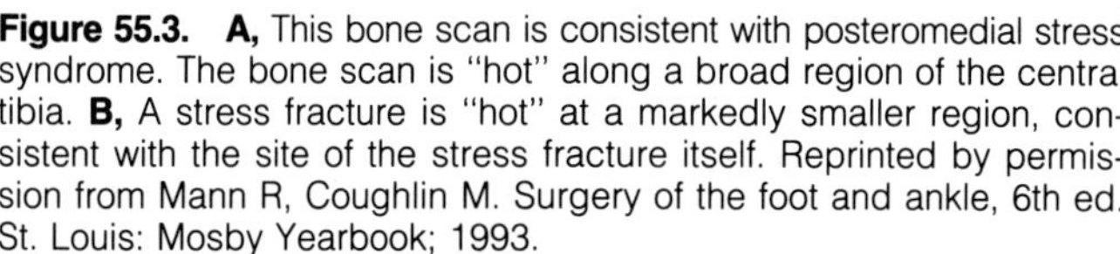

Figure 55.3. **A,** This bone scan is consistent with posteromedial stress syndrome. The bone scan is "hot" along a broad region of the central tibia. **B,** A stress fracture is "hot" at a markedly smaller region, consistent with the site of the stress fracture itself. Reprinted by permission from Mann R, Coughlin M. Surgery of the foot and ankle, 6th ed. St. Louis: Mosby Yearbook; 1993.

the neurovascular function within the space. Compartment pressure increases as muscle volume increases during exercise. Muscle volume may increase secondary to increased capillary permeability, anomalous venous or lymphatic return, or microhemorrhage. Patients will complain of bilateral (95% of the time) leg pain induced by activity, which is often consistently reproducible by the patient. This has led to the term "third lap syndrome." The discomfort may persist for hours after the activity and transient hypesthesia and/or weakness may result. A foot drop may occur. This is a markedly different presentation than an acute compartment syndrome. An acute compartment syndrome is a true surgical emergency and is a complication of trauma or postischemic edema. Treatment of the acute form is a decompressive fasciotomy to prevent myoneural necrosis (13–15).

Diagnosis of chronic compartment syndrome is confirmed with intracompartmental pressure measurements at rest, at peak activity, and at postactivity. Patients with chronic compartment syndrome usually will have a resting pressure greater than 15 mm Hg that may exceed 75 to 100 mm Hg during exercise and will remain elevated (>30 mm Hg) after exercise for 5 or more min. Treatment is fasciotomy of all involved compartments.

Tibial stress fractures are more common in women and may be either bilateral or unilateral. Physical findings, especially well-localized tenderness, edema, and erythema may be noticeable before radiographic changes. A bone scan may be positive anytime between 2 and 8 days after the onset of pain, whereas radiographs may take 2 to 3 weeks.

Treatment of stress fractures is rest and occasionally immobilization. Rarely, excision of the involved bone and bone grafting is necessary. After the stress fracture has resolved, the training regimen may need to be modified (training intensity, duration, and surfaces) to prevent recurrence. If the athlete has significant weakness or atrophy of the leg following treatment of the stress fracture, the authors believe a course of rehabilitation is necessary. But not all patients are placed in rehabilitation following stress fractures.

Medial Gastrocnemius Strain

A medial gastrocnemius strain, or "tennis leg," occurs when running or lifting, and an athlete will give a history of a sharp pain in the posterior calf. This injury has been called *coup de fouet* ("snap of the whip"). It was once thought that the pain was caused by the long plantaris tendon rupturing and recoiling through the medial gastrocnemius muscle. There has never been surgical or autopsy evidence supporting this conclusion. It is generally accepted that this injury represents a strain to the medial head of the gastrocnemius muscle (16).

The patient is typically a middle-aged male "weekend warrior." The entire proximal calf is tender and edematous. The medial gastrocnemius is generally more tender and walking may be quite difficult. With time, the foot may be ecchymotic secondary to pooling of the hematoma with gravity. The differential diagnosis includes rupture of the Achilles tendon and rupture of a Baker's cyst.

Treatment is symptomatic and depends on the severity of the injury. Mild tears can be treated with a lift, compression stocking, and ice. More moderate to severe tears may require a short leg cast for 2 to 3 weeks and then a cast boot for several weeks. In subsequent weeks, physiotherapy is necessary and a return to full activities can be expected in 6 to 12 weeks.

Achilles Tendon Rupture

Rupture of the Achilles tendon is a serious cause of leg pain and dysfunction in the athlete (17). The tendo Achilles is the only tendon crossing the ankle joint that is not encased in a synovial tendon sheath. There is a region of reduced blood supply to this tendon approximately 4 to 5 cm above its insertion into the calcaneus (17). The diagnosis of complete rupture of the tendo Achilles is made by a history of sudden posterior calf pain with exertion, a palpable gap in the tendon and a positive Thompson's test. The Thompson's test is performed by having the patient lie prone with the distal leg hanging off the edge of the table. The gastrocnemius-soleus muscle is compressed and the foot is observed. Rupture of the tendo Achilles results in lack of plantar flexion on the involved side (Fig. 55.5). Treat-

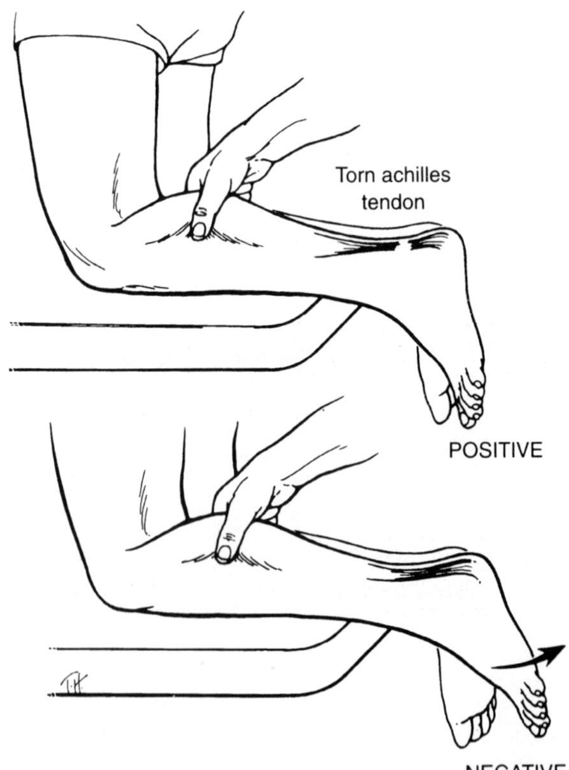

Figure 55.5. Thompson's test is a reliable clinical test to identify the presence of a complete tear in the Achilles tendon. When the Achilles tendon is torn, a positive test is elicited by squeezing the calf and seeing *no* plantar flexion of the foot. A negative test occurs when the calf is squeezed and plantar flexion occurs in the foot.

ment is either by open repair or equinus casting (18, 19). There is a slightly lower rate of rerupture and increased strength noted in those patients treated with surgery. Equinus casting remains an excellent treatment alternative in the elderly patient or those with low demands on this tendon. Before complete rupture, the Achilles tendon may become inflamed and interstitial degeneration may occur in the same region as the complete rupture. This problem is generally best treated with immobilization and antiinflammatory medication. Debridement of the involved tissues is an option for persistent cases.

The Ankle

Arthroscopy of the Ankle

Arthroscopic surgery of the ankle has led to further understanding of the etiology of ankle pain following sports injuries and has been instrumental in providing state-of-the-art treatment. Arthroscopy of the ankle allows direct visualization of all articular structures without the need for extensive surgical approach, arthrotomy, or malleolar osteotomy (20). Through direct inspection of the ankle, the articular and ligamentous surfaces can be assessed and intraoperative stress-testing maneuvers performed. A variety of surgical procedures may be accomplished by using arthroscopic techniques, including biopsy, debridement, synovectomy, and loose body removal. Postoperative advantages of the arthroscopic approach include decreased patient discomfort, decreased morbidity, faster rate of rehabilitation, and earlier return to daily and athletic activities.

The indications for arthroscopy of the ankle include unexplained pain, swelling, stiffness, instability, hemarthrosis, locking, and popping. The therapeutic indications for ankle arthroscopy include articular injury, soft tissue injury, bony impingement, arthrofibrosis, fracture, synovitis, loose bodies, osteophytes, osteochondral defects, and arthrodesis. The relative contraindications for ankle arthroscopy include moderate degenerative joint disease with restricted range of motion, significantly reduced joint space, severe edema, and tenuous vascular status; absolute contraindications include localized soft tissue infection and severe degenerative joint disease.

Arthroscopy can be performed supine, lateral decubitus, or with the knee flexed 90° over the table. Three anterior portals may be used for ankle arthroscopy, but only the anteromedial and anterolateral are recommended (Fig. 55.6). There are three posterior portals as well, but only the posterolateral is commonly used (Fig. 55.7) (21).

Both 4.0- and 2.7-mm arthroscopes are used for ankle arthroscopy (Fig. 55.8). In addition, small joint instrumentation is necessary to work in the small space between the tibia and talus. Visualization of the ankle can be significantly improved by the use of an ankle distractor to increase the space between the tibia and talus. Distraction methods applied to the ankle may be either invasive or noninvasive (Fig. 55.9). Noninvasive techniques include manual distraction, gravity distraction, or a soft tissue device hooked around the front and back of the foot. In cases in which the ankle is quite tight, an invasive distraction device may be necessary with a pin inserted in the tibia and the calcaneus (22).

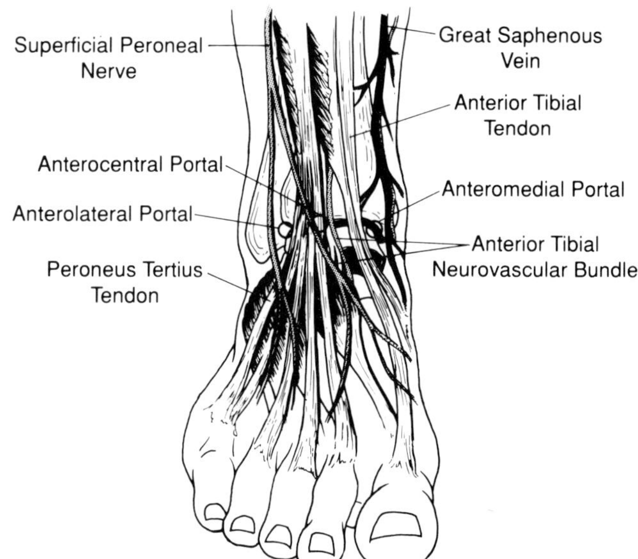

Figure 55.6. Anterior arthroscopic portals. The anteromedial and anterolateral are routinely used, and the anterocentral is rarely necessary. Reprinted by permission from Mann R, Coughlin M. Surgery of the foot and ankle. 6th ed. St. Louis: Mosby Yearbook, 1993.

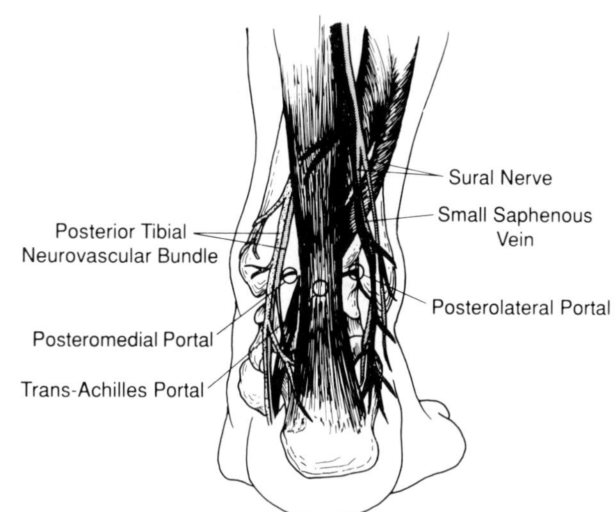

Figure 55.7. Posterior arthroscopic portals. The posterolateral portal is routinely used, and the posteromedial and trans-Achilles portals should be avoided. Reprinted by permission from Mann R, Coughlin M. Surgery of the foot and ankle. 6th ed. St. Louis: Mosby Yearbook, 1993.

Diagnosis and Treatment of Acute Sprains

One of the most common sports injuries encountered is the ankle sprain (23). The ankle joint is responsible for plantar flexion and dorsiflexion of the foot and is composed of the tibia, fibula, and talus. The tibia and fibula form a mortise or notch at their distal end for the body of the talus. This configuration is supported by three strong sets of ligaments (Fig. 55.10). The distal tibia and fibula are joined by the anterior and posterior inferior tibiofibular ligaments or syndesmotic ligaments. A strong medial deltoid ligament is composed of a deep and superficial portion. The deep portion consists of the anterior tibiotalar and posterior tibiotalar parts. The superficial portion consists of the tibionavicular, tibiocalcaneal, and posterior tibiotalar parts. The lateral ankle complex consists of four distinct ligaments: the anterior and posterior talofibular, the calcaneofibular, and the talocalcaneal ligaments.

A lateral ankle sprain is a twisting injury to the ankle, causing damage to the lateral ankle ligamentous complex. Inversion accounts for 85% of the ankle sprains that occur. The amount of force causing the injury is the main determinate of the degree of injury (24). The Standard Nomenclature of Athletic Injuries (25) defines a first-degree sprain as a mild injury, a second-degree sprain as a moderate injury, and a third-degree sprain as a severe injury. A severe injury would be a complete rupture of the supporting ligaments, tendons, and muscles (25).

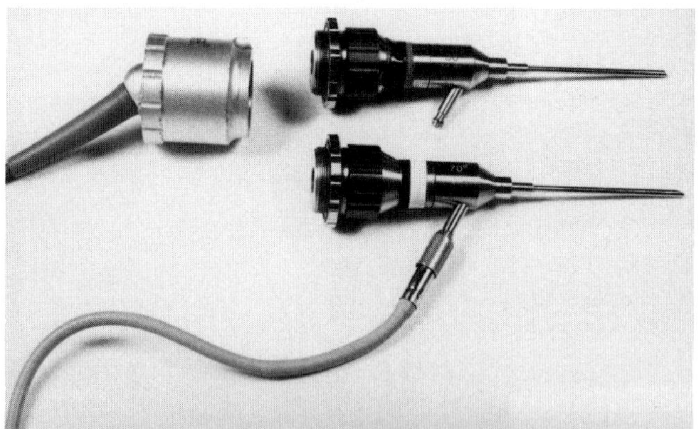

Figure 55.8. Typical video arthroscopes for the ankle. These arthroscopes are 2.7 mm in diameter, have an angulation at the tip of either 30° or 70°, and screw directly into the camera head.

The superficial location of the lateral ankle ligaments makes the proper diagnosis of an ankle sprain possible. This is particularly helpful to the team physician tending to an injured player on the playing field. Radiographic examination is often needed to complete the workup. Most postsprain ankle x-rays are normal, however, and the physical examination remains the keystone of diagnosis. An inversion injury is the injury responsible for a lateral ankle sprain. Clinical and cadaveric research has pointed to a predictable sequence of ligamentous damage occurring with inversion injuries to the ankle.

The body of the talus is widest anteriorly. Therefore, the ankle is most stable in dorsiflexion when the anterior aspect of the talus articulates with mortise (18). Most inversion ankle injuries occur in plantar flexion when the ankle is least stable. The first ligament injured is the anterior talofibular ligament. This ligament is actually a thickening in the anterior ankle capsule and blends imperceptibly into it. A torn anterior talofibular ligament is, therefore, a capsular injury. The next ligament injured is the calcaneofibular ligament. The anterior talofibular ligament need not necessarily be completely torn to allow damage to the calcaneofibular ligament. The calcaneofibular ligament is part of the medial wall of the peroneal tendon sheath. The calcaneofibular ligament may be injured without damage to the anterior talofibular ligament in the uncommon situation of inversion stress applied across a dorsiflexed ankle. The posterior talofibular ligament is rarely injured. An inversion injury may be likened to opening a book. The posterior talofibular ligament is located at the binding and, therefore, is not generally torn as the injury progresses (26).

Another popular classification scheme for ankle sprains was proposed by Leach (27). In this classification scheme, a first-degree sprain is defined as a partial or complete tear of the anterior talofibular ligament. A

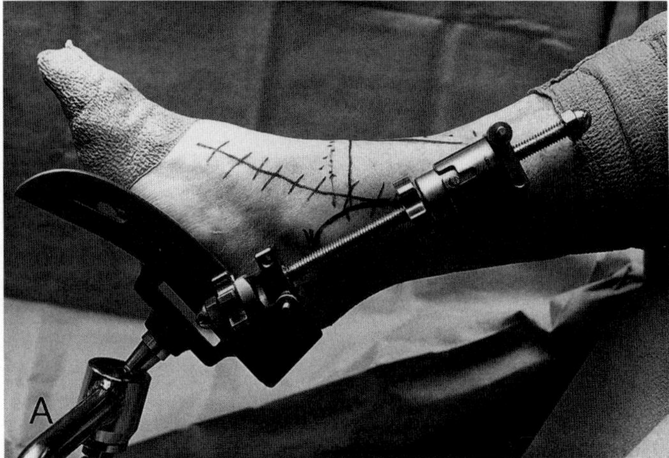

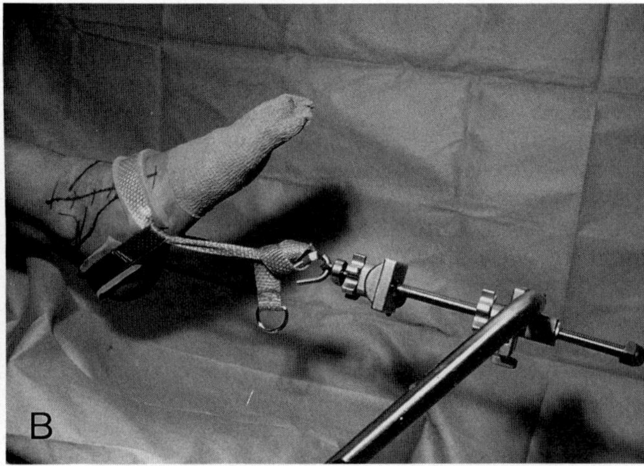

Figure 55.9. **A,** Invasive distraction on the lateral side of the ankle with the pin in the distal tibia and calcaneus. Note the strain gauge indicates the amount of force across the ankle. **B,** Noninvasive distraction. This type is most commonly used, and in the majority of cases, it will give adequate visualization.

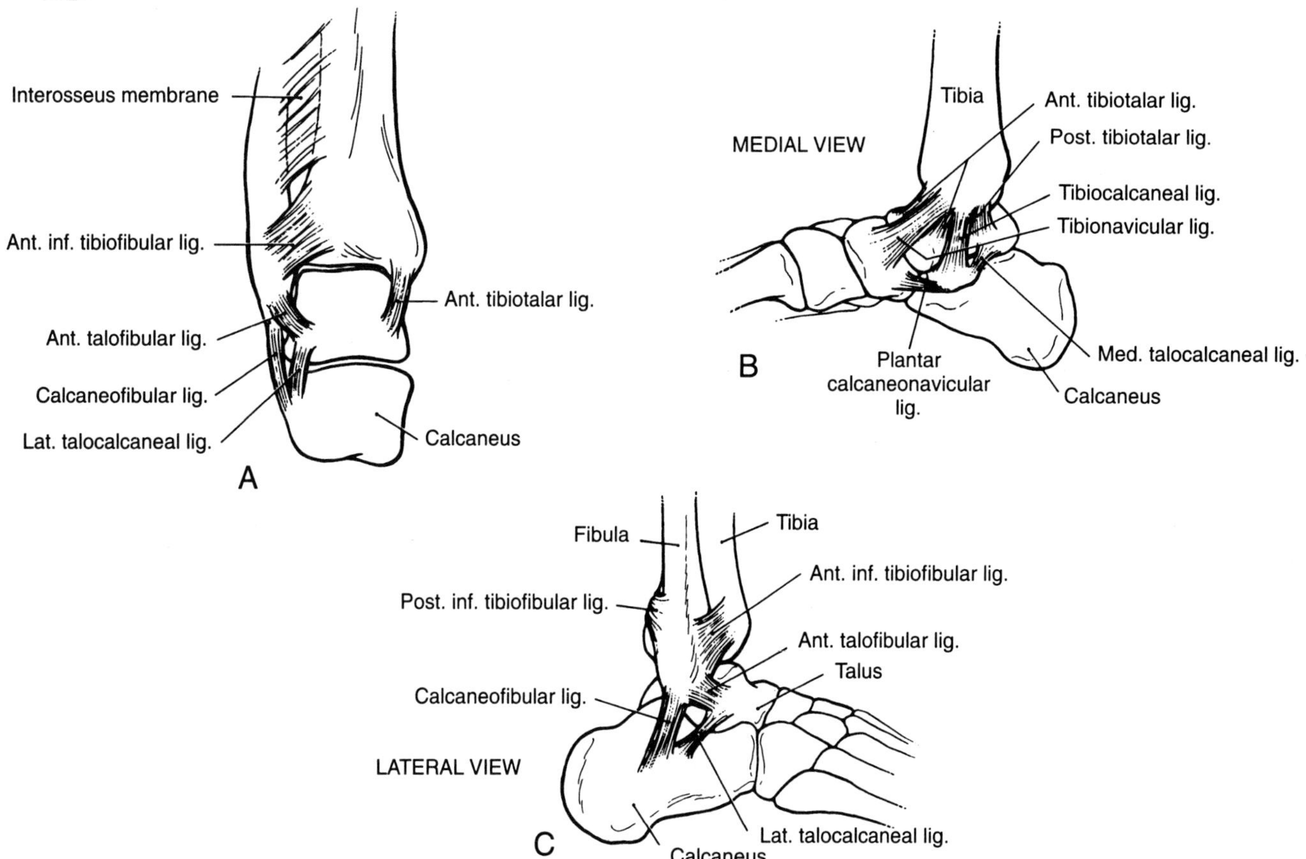

Figure 55.10. The ankle joint consists of the tibia, fibula, and talus and the supporting ligamentous structures. It is usually possible to identify which structures have been injured by careful palpation of the ankle joint because of the relative lack of subcutaneous fat and muscle.

second-degree sprain is characterized by injury to both the anterior talofibular and calcaneofibular ligaments. A third-degree sprain implies injury to all three lateral ligaments.

Unless the ankle is examined soon after injury, edema and hemorrhage may make determination of ligament tenderness difficult. This is particularly true in the case of the calcaneofibular ligament because of its position deep to the peroneal tendons. Similarly, the anterior talofibular ligament may produce significant regional tenderness to make the diagnosis of a syndesmotic sprain difficult. Serial examination may be needed to determine the prognosis of an ankle sprain for this reason.

Other classification schemes have been proposed that incorporate evaluation of anterior and lateral instability. These schemes use two simple clinical tests to determine the extent of ligamentous damage present. The first test is the anterior drawer test and is similar to the Lachman test used in the knee joint to evaluate the anterior cruciate ligament. In the ankle the test is performed by firmly grasping the heel with one hand and gently moving the foot forward while securing the tibia with the other hand. The test is done slowly with the patient relaxed. The foot is held in slight dorsiflexion and is always compared with the contralateral side (Fig. 55.11). The amount of individual difference is striking, and a "sloppy" feeling of instability on one side may

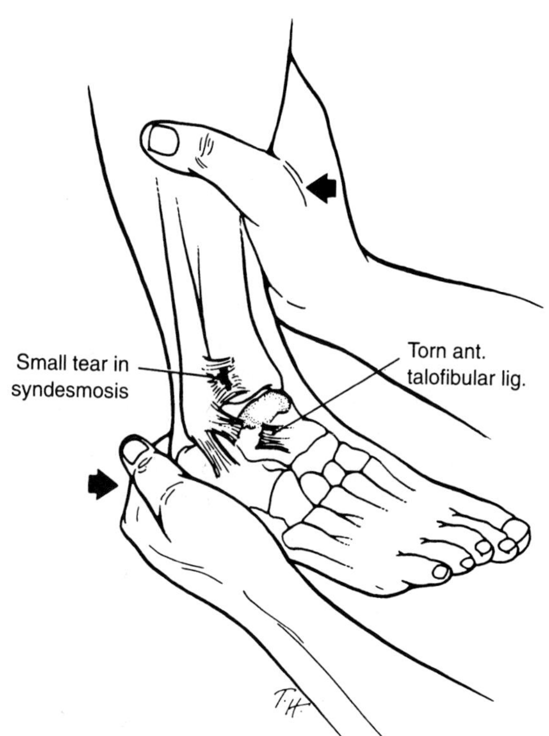

Figure 55.11. Anterior drawer test is performed by stabilizing the tibia and pulling the foot towards the examiner. A positive test identifies the presence of a torn anterior talofibular ligament.

be less meaningful if the examination of the opposite ankle is identical. As with ligamentous testing of the knee, a solid end point may be more meaningful than the presence of motion. The second test is lateral talar tilt. A feeling of instability with talar tilt testing may be confused with subtalar motion. This test is performed by gently applying a inversion stress across the tibiotalar (ankle) joint with the ankle in dorsiflexion (Fig. 55.12). Both tests may be documented radiographically (Fig. 55.13).

X-rays provide a quantified measurement of the degree of anterior drawer or inversion talar tilt by comparing the injured with the uninjured side. Stress x-rays can be done either manually or by using an instrument such as the Telos device. This device offers the advantages of reproducibility and decreased exposure of ionized radiation to the physician. Sauser et al. (28), using the Telos stress device, found a talar tilt of 10° or more to be associated with a lateral ligament injury in 99% of cases. Normal values for talar tilt have reported to range from 5° to 23° (29). Chrisman and Snook (30) noted when comparing both ankles that a difference of more than 10° was significant when measuring the anterior talofibular and calcaneofibular ligaments (see Fig. 55.13). The anterior drawer stress test specifically tests the integrity of the anterior talofibular ligament. Gould et al. (31) thought that an increase of 4 mm was indicative of instability in the anterior drawer test. However, Laurin et al (32) believed that an increase greater than 9 mm was abnormal. Overall, values of up to 5 mm of separation between the talus and distal tibia are considered to be normal, whereas values between 5 and 10 mm are probably abnormal, and values over 10 mm are grossly abnormal (Fig. 55.14). A working classification for ankle sprains can be developed by correlating the anatomic injury to the physical exam and to the radiologic stress test (33) (Table 55.1).

A medial ankle sprain results from an eversion injury (34). A patient with a moderate or severe lateral ankle sprain may also sprain the deltoid ligament with inversion stress. The medial ligamentous complex is collectively known as the deltoid ligament because of its triangular shape. The apex of the triangle is the insertion on the medial malleolus of the tibia. The deltoid

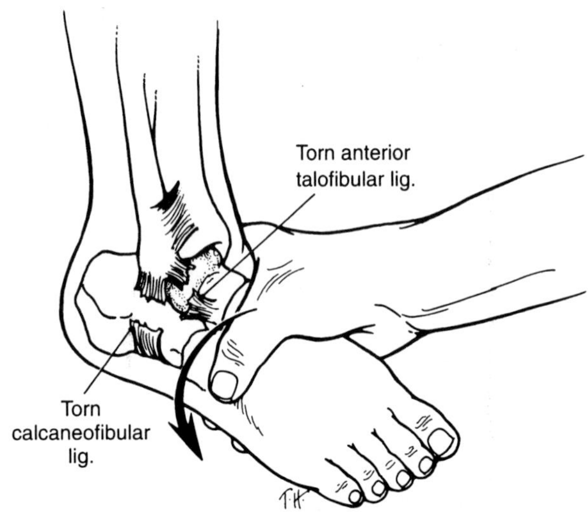

Figure 55.12. Talar tilt test is performed by inverting the foot and noting the amount of opening on the lateral side of the ankle. It is useful in determining the presence of a torn calcaneofibular ligament and, in some cases, a torn anterior talofibular ligament.

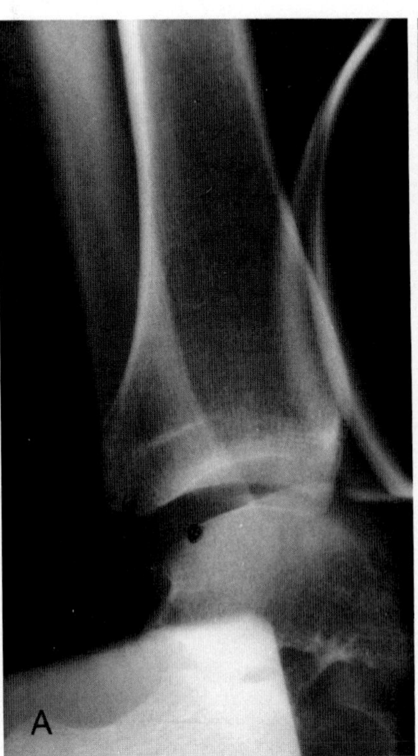

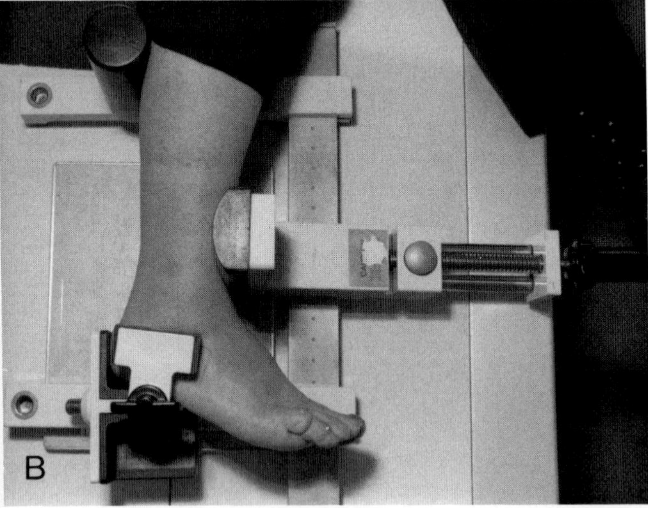

Figure 55.13. **A,** Anterior drawer stress x-ray using the Telos device. Note the talus comes forward in relation to the tibia, indicating a tear of the anterior talofibular ligament. **B,** The Telos device pulls the heel forward while stabilizing the distal tibia to perform an anterior drawer while an x-ray is taken.

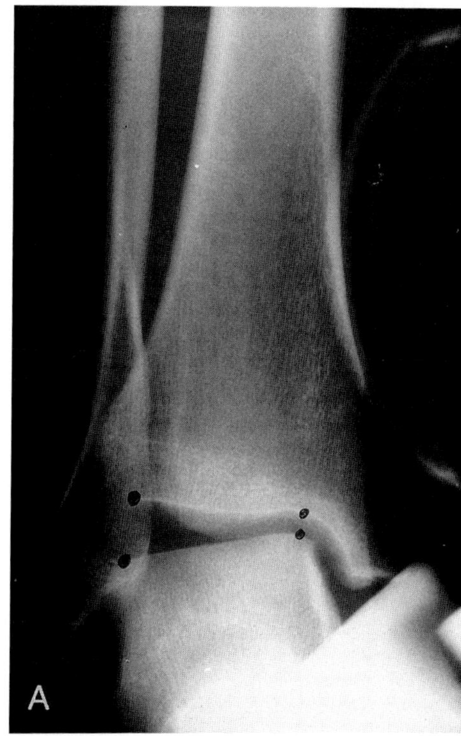

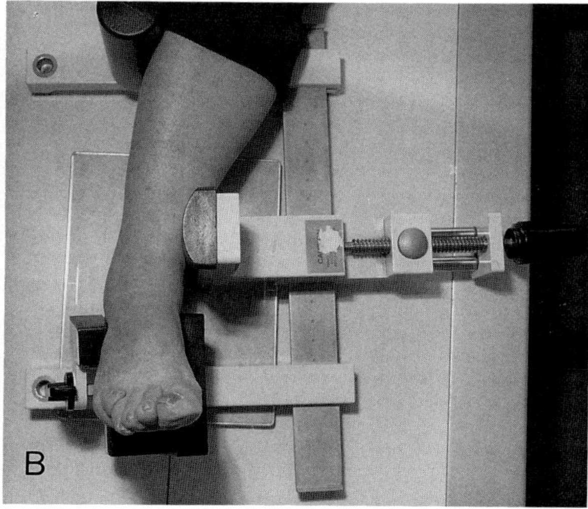

Figure 55.14. **A,** Inversion radiograph using the Telos device. Note the tilting of the talus in relation to the distal tibia. **B,** Inversion stress test using the Telos device.

Table 55.1.
Working Classification of Ankle Sprains

Grade	Anatomic Injury	Physical Examination (Drawer Sign)	X-Ray Findings
I	Partial tear; ATF or CF	Negative or 1+ drawer sign	Negative drawer sign; negative talar tilt
II	Torn ATF; intact CF	2+ drawer sign	Positive drawer sign; negative talar tilt
III	Torn ATF; torn CF	3+ drawer sign	Positive drawer sign; positive talar tilt

From Hamilton WG, Thompson FM, Snow SW. The modified Bröstrom procedure for lateral ankle instability. Foot Ankle 1993;14:1.

ligament has a superficial and deep portion. The superficial portion consists of three ligaments: the tibionavicular and the anterior and posterior tibiocalcaneal ligaments. The deep portion consists of the anterior and posterior tibiotalar ligaments. Medial instability resulting from a ligamentous eversion injury is distinctly uncommon. Commonly the medial malleolus will fracture prior to rupture of the deltoid ligament.

A syndesmotic or "high" ankle sprain may occur alone or in conjunction with a lateral ankle sprain. Syndesmotic sprains have been estimated to occur in as many as 10% of all ankle injuries and tend to be most commonly seen in collision sports such as ice hockey, football, and soccer. Syndesmotic sprains may involve any or all of the following structures: (*a*) anterior inferior tibiofibular ligament; (*b*) posterior inferior tibiofibular ligament, including its distal and deep component, the transverse ligament; and (*c*) interosseous membrane. Although not entirely clear, the mechanism of injury appears to be primarily an external rotation injury, although hyperdorsiflexion has been reported to lead to tears of the syndesmosis. Diagnosis is made by palpation directly over the syndesmosis more proximally along the interosseous membrane. The "squeeze test" is performed by compressing the fibula to the tibia above the midpoint of the calf; the test is considered positive when proximal compression produces distal pain in the area of the interosseous membrane and syndesmotic ligament (Fig. 55.15) (35). The external rotation stress test also is useful in diagnosing syndesmotic ankle sprains and is performed by applying external rotational stress to the foot and ankle with the knee held at 90° of flexion and the ankle in neutral position (36). A positive test produces pain over the anterior or posterior tibiofibular ligament(s) and over the interosseous membrane (Fig. 55.16). Radiographs help determine the degree of injury. Radiographic evidence of acute widening of the syndesmosis requires operative repair to restore the ankle mortise. Even in the absence of radiographic changes, athletes with this injury will miss significantly more games and practices than those athletes with lateral ankle sprains alone. Complete recovery may take 4 to 12 weeks.

One mistake that is easily prevented in the evaluation of ankle pain is to obtain a history and examine the patient *before* ordering x-rays. Often a patient will attribute pain in the lower extremity to an ankle sprain when the pathology may be in the foot. A preliminary exam may help localize the problem to the foot and ankle and occasionally the spine. Often a foot or ankle radiograph will mislead the examiner by the presence

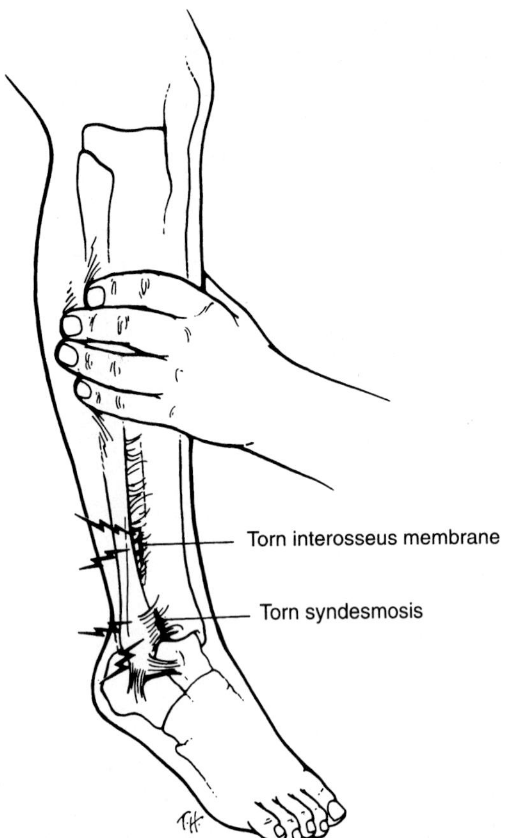

Figure 55.15. The squeeze test is used to detect tears of the syndesmosis. It is positive when squeezing the midcalf produces pain in the distal interosseous membrane and syndesmosis.

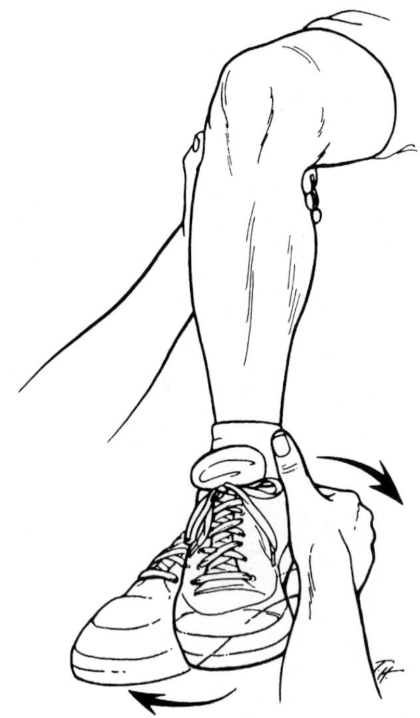

Figure 55.16. The external rotation test is used to detect tears of the syndesmosis and is performed by stabilizing the calf and externally rotating the foot.

of radiographic pathology unrelated to the patient's complaints.

The examination initially begins with observation of the patient. A person's ambulatory status is the first clue as to the severity of the injury. Edema and ecchymosis should be noted. Pulses should be palpated in both the dorsalis pedis and posterior tibial arteries and sensation tested. A quick guide to the presence of an acute compartment syndrome can be obtained by noting the firmness of the various compartments of the leg that are accessible to palpation; the posterior, anterior and lateral compartments. Passive flexion and extension of the toes is also helpful in this regard.

Palpation is then carried out in an unhurried manner taking care not to hurt the patient further with excessive force. The best starting point is the proximal fibula. If this is routinely done, a Maisonneuve fracture will not be missed. This fracture pattern is produced by external rotation of the talus separating the fibula from the tibia and tearing the syndesmotic ligament and interosseous membrane proximally to the level of a high fibular fracture (Fig. 55.17) (37). Tenderness at the proximal fibula may be indicative of a fracture. Often a patient will not relate lateral knee pain to an ankle injury. The consequences of missing the diagnosis is ankle arthritis secondary to altered weight bearing across the tibiotalar joint.

The examination proceeds with palpation of the lateral ligamentous complex, syndesmosis, sinus tarsi, and base of the fifth metatarsal. The medial ankle is systematically palpated beginning with the medial malleolus and the deltoid ligament. The insertion of the posterior tibial tendon is found just anterior to the talonavicular joint inferiorly. The metatarsal squeeze test is then performed by compressing the metatarsal heads together. The ankle, subtalar and metatarsophalangeal joints are evaluated and compared with the contralateral side.

A partial tear of the medial ligamentous complex may result in a small avulsion fracture from the medial malleolus. An avulsion fracture may be differentiated from a congenital ossicle by its ragged edges and a history of significant trauma. Generally, these lesions are asymptomatic, but occasionally pain may result from impingement of these fractures against the talus. Treatment would then consist of simple excision. This is accomplished through a small incision or by arthroscopic technique. An equivalent lesion may be seen laterally from the fibular attachment of the calcaneofibular ligament.

Considerable disability may result from a "simple" ankle sprain (38). Treatment of this injury consists of two phases. The first phase consists of addressing the acute injury. Rest, ice, compression, and elevation (RICE) make up an excellent treatment protocol for most acute ligamentous injuries. Immobilization is generally reserved for severe injuries and those with evidence of instability. The second phase consists of rehabilitation. Rehabilitation addresses the three problems associated with a subacute sprain: decreased range of motion; strength; and proprioception. A previous lateral ankle injury may predispose an athlete to a second injury.

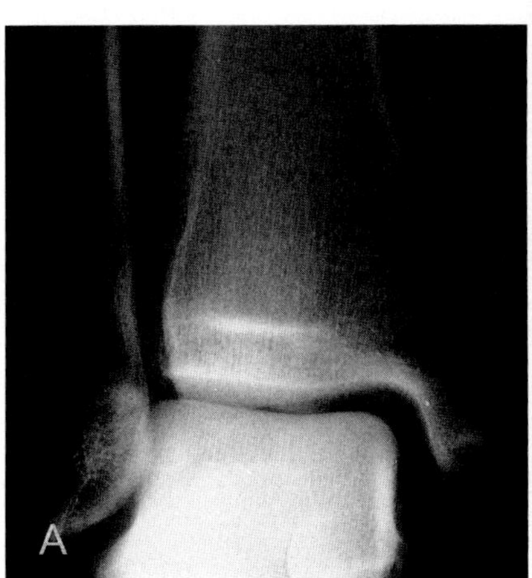

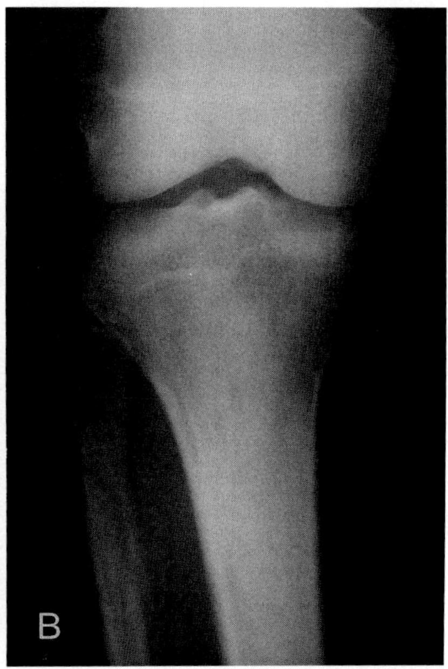

Figure 55.17. A, A Maisonneuve fracture consists of a proximal fibular fracture and a torn interosseous membrane and syndesmosis. A widened medial clear space with no obvious fracture laterally should alert the physician to x-ray the entire fibula. **B,** The same patient with the widened medial clear space and a fracture of the proximal fibula indicative of a Maisonneuve fracture.

Residual weakness of the ligaments after healing may occur so that less force is required to produce the same degree of damage. Strengthening the muscles across the ankle joint, especially the peroneal muscles, has been found to be an effective way to allow an athlete to return to a high level of function. Injuries to proprioceptive nerve fibers occur in conjunction with ankle sprains, and may give a feeling of instability in an otherwise stable joint. Proprioceptive training using a tilt board or similar device may be helpful in this regard. Elastic braces that offer no true mechanical support may function by providing tactile information to the brain regarding the relative position of the foot and ankle (39, 40).

Ankle taping in sports is a popular method of limiting the motion of the ankle and subtalar joints. It is used for both the treatment and prevention of injuries. Just how many injuries are prevented by ankle taping is controversial (41). The effectiveness of the taping depends on the quality of the taping job and how long the player has played with the tape in place. The effectiveness of tape decreases quickly with use and retaping may be needed. Although this seems like a trivial point, college and professional teams devote huge sums of money on the materials and the personnel needed to tape players. A lace-up canvas brace may offer the advantage of lower cost.

Many different types of ankle braces are available today for use in sports. These braces range in shape and form from tubular elastic supports or figure-eight straps to custom-molded orthotics that effectively limit subtalar motion. Intermediate designs include leather or synthetic lace-up designs with side compartments for placement of struts to limit motion. Prescribing the appropriate brace is a matter of determining the amount of support that the individual athlete requires to perform his or her chosen sport effectively. An off-the-shelf brace may be effective if sized correctly and of sufficient strength (Fig. 55.18).

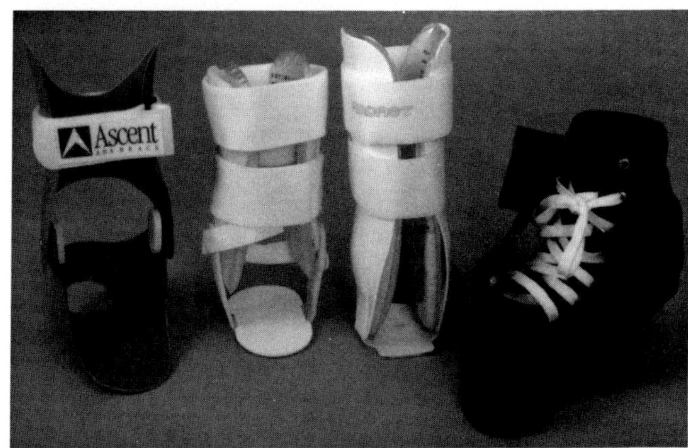

Figure 55.18. Functional ankle braces. The degree of injury and patient preference help determine the appropriate brace to use for each patient.

In the situation in which an athlete cannot return to sports secondary to persistent lateral ankle instability that is not well-controlled by bracing, or in the case in which activities of daily living are compromised by the presence of instability, reconstructive surgery of the lateral ankle may be considered (42). Although there are many different types of lateral ankle reconstruction procedures, athletes and ballet dancers often do quite well with the modified Bröstrom direct repair with imbrication (Fig. 55.19). This surgery consists of repairing and reinforcing the anterior talofibular ligament. The advantage of this procedure in an athlete is that no other musculotendinous units are sacrificed, patients generally have a reasonable range of motion following sur-

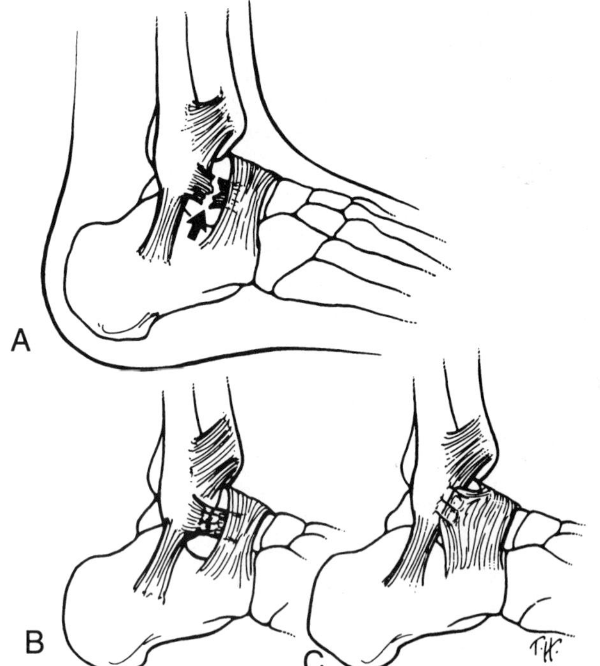

Figure 55.19. The modified Bröstrom procedure is one of many methods used to reconstruct the lateral ankle ligamentous complex after an injury. It is particularly useful in athletes and dancers.

gery, and are able to participate in their preinjury activities.

Chronic Sprain Pain

Differential Diagnosis

Ankle sprains are among the most common injuries in sports and at work. While many ankle sprains apparently recover well after conservative therapy, studies have shown that between 20% and 40% of patients may have residual problems. When evaluating an athlete with chronic ankle sprain pain, a number of etiologies must be considered in the differential diagnosis. This includes congenital abnormalities, soft tissue inflammation, trauma, nerve injury, tumor, and incomplete rehabilitation (43) (Table 55.2).

Although it is difficult to imagine that a midfoot sprain can be confused for an ankle sprain, this injury is a frequently "missed" injury. Diagnosis can be made by palpating the dorsum of the foot and gently stressing the tarsometatarsal joint, also known as the Lisfranc's joint. If the ligaments have been disrupted the foot may assume a valgus attitude.

Soft Tissue Impingement

Soft tissue impingement is the most common cause of chronic pain after an ankle sprain. This can occur along the syndesmosis anterior gutter, the interval between the tibia and fibula under the ankle, or posteriorly in the syndesmosis and posterior gutter (Fig. 55.20). Chronic lateral ankle pain is much more common than medial ankle pain after a sprain. Anterolateral impingement of the ankle is the most common type of soft tissue impingement that occurs (44). Typically, the patient complains of vague anterior pain, usually along the anterior and anterolateral aspect of the ankle, occasionally involving the syndesmosis and sinus tarsi. Pain is usually absent at rest and present with most

Table 55.2.
Differential Diagnosis of Chronic Sprain Pain

1. Congenital abnormalities
   - Tarsal coalition
   - Accessory navicular
   - Anomalous peroneal tendon and soleus muscle
2. Soft tissue inflammation
   - Anterolateral impingement
   - Posterolateral impingement
   - Syndesmotic impingement
   - Nonspecific synovitis
   - Inflammatory rheumatic synovitis
3. Trauma
   - Osteochondral and chondral lesions of the tibia and talus
   - Ligamentous injury
   - Tendon injury/subluxation
   - Avulsion fracture, stress fracture of physeal injury
   - Calcific ossicles
   - Degenerative joint disease
   - Subtalar dysfunction
4. Nerve injury
   - Entrapment
   - Neuropraxia
5. Tumor
   - Osteoid osteoma
   - Giant cell
   - Ganglion and cysts
   - Other benign and malignant tumors
6. Inadequate rehabilitation
   - Muscle atrophy
   - Loss of proprioception
   - Loss of motion and contracture
   - Arthrofibrosis of ankle and subtalar joint
   - RSD

Modified from Nachtigal MP, Grana WA. Hidden ankle injuries. Paper presented at the annual meeting of the Arthroscopy Association of North America, Orlando, FL, 1990.

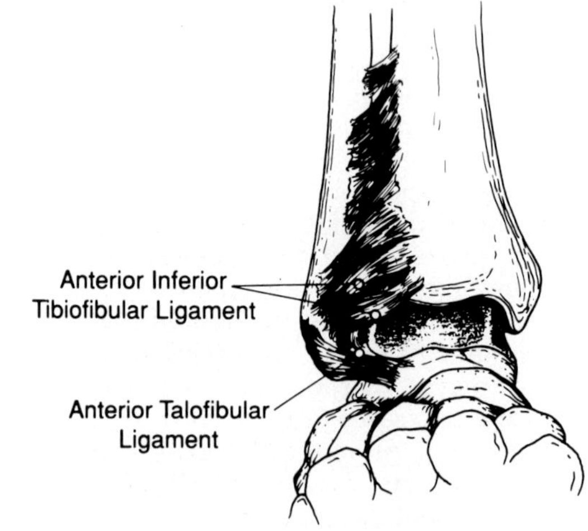

Figure 55.20. Anterior impingement sites. Anterior soft tissue impingement can occur along the anterior inferior tibiofibular ligament as well as the anterior talofibular ligament. Reprinted by permission from Mann R, Coughlin M. Surgery of the foot and ankle. 6th ed. St. Louis: Mosby Yearbook, 1993.

activities, limiting a patient's ability to participate in a given sport. Often the patient has seen several physicians and is frustrated by his or her lack of progress.

Physical exam may reveal tenderness along the syndesmosis anterior gutter, including the anterior talofibular ligament and calcaneofibular ligament, and many times the posterior subtalar joint and sinus tarsi are also involved. Radiologic evaluation may reveal calcification of heterotopic bone in the interosseous space, indicative of previous injury to the distal tibiofibular syndesmosis, or ossicles along the tip of the fibula and lateral dome, consistent with injuries to the anterior talofibular ligament. In many instances, the radiographs are normal, as are the bone scan and computed tomography scan. In some cases magnetic resonance imaging (MRI) may be helpful in indicating the abnormality in the lateral gutter, and occasionally a kinematic MRI is useful to show an impingement lesion. Stress radiographs in this group are usually negative.

Arthroscopy not only aids in the diagnosis of chronic sprain pain but is useful in its treatment (45). At surgery, patients may have synovitis and fibrosis of the lateral gutter and chondromalacia of the talus and fibula. In some patients, a thick band can be identified and excised. This lesion is an adhesion that develops along the lateral talomalleolar joint and may contain torn fibers of the capsule and ligament as well as chronic synovial tissue. Inflammatory tissue may be seen not only in the lateral gutter but also in the syndesmosis and articular space between the tibia and fibula (Fig. 55.21*A*). At surgery, debridement of the anterolateral gutter is done with removal of inflamed synovium, thickened adhesive bands, osteophytes, and loose bodies (Fig. 55.21*B*). Postoperatively, patients are weight bearing as tolerated with a compression bandage and crutches and usually start rehabilitation after 1 to 2 weeks. Sports are not resumed for 4 to 6 weeks. A sequence for the progression of chronic anterolateral ankle pain can be developed (Table 55.3).

Bassett et al. (46) found syndesmotic impingement occurring with a separate distal fascicle of the anterior inferior tibiofibular ligament. With tearing of the anterior talofibular ligament, laxity occurs and the talar dome extrudes in dorsiflexion, leading to impingement of the talus against the fascicle. Surgical treatment consists of either arthroscopic debridement of this ligament or, in some cases, resection of the intraarticular portion of the ligament. Postoperative treatment is similar to that described for anterolateral impingement problems.

Posterior impingement may also lead to ankle pain that usually occurs along the lateral side and involves the posterior inferior tibiofibular ligament, including the transverse tibiofibular ligament. This type is most commonly seen in ballet dancers and gymnasts whose activities require extreme plantar flexion (45).

Table 55.3.
Sequence of Lateral Ankle Pain

Inversion Sprain
↓
Torn Lateral Ligaments
↓
Repetitive Motion
↓
Inflamed Ligament Ends
↙ ↘
Synovitis Scar Tissue
↘ ↙
Hypertrophic Soft Tissue
↓
Impingement in Lateral Gutter
↓
Chronic Lateral Ankle Pain

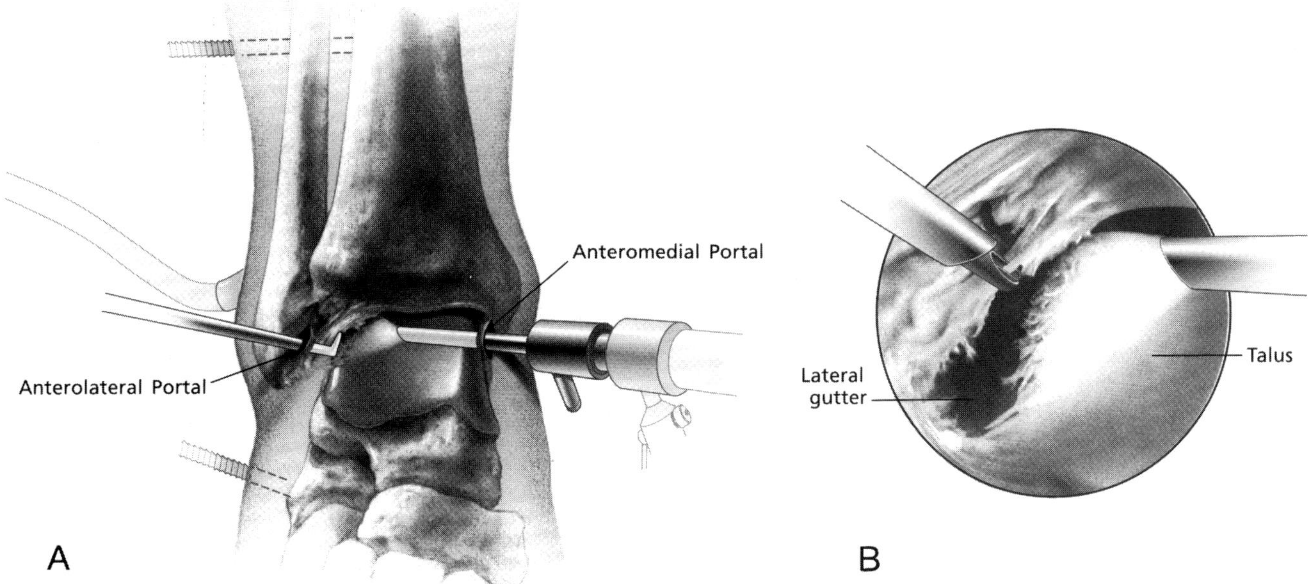

Figure 55.21. A, Soft tissue impingement of the lateral gutter and syndesmosis of the ankle. The arthroscope visualizes from the anteromedial portal and a probe is inserted through the anterolateral portal. **B,** The lateral gutter and syndesmosis are debrided by inserting a shaver through the anterolateral portal while visualizing through the anteromedial portal.

Posttraumatic lateral ankle pain may be caused by chronic subtalar synovitis, chondromalacia, or instability. Pain may be localized to the sinus tarsi, posterior subtalar joint, and the lateral gutter of the ankle. There are five ligaments securing the subtalar or talocalcaneal joint. The interosseous ligament is surrounded by the anterior, posterior, medial, and lateral talocalcaneal ligaments.

Examination consists of gently ranging the subtalar joint while holding the ankle joint stable. Pain elicited via this mechanism is likely indicative of a subtalar joint dysfunction. Injection of xylocaine into the sinus tarsi may also be helpful in securing this diagnosis. Initial therapy is conservative with antiinflammatories, physical therapy, and orthotics. If pain persists, arthroscopic evaluation of the subtalar and sinus tarsi areas is indicated. Occasionally, arthroscopic or open excision of the thickened fibrous and fatty tissue may be helpful in relieving persistent pain. An algorithm can be developed for the evaluation and treatment of chronic sprain pain (Table 55.4).

Peroneal Tendon Pathology

The peroneal tendons pass posterior to the lateral malleolus, running through a discreet tendon sheath. Stability is provided to the peroneal tendons by the superior and inferior peroneal retinaculae and the fibular groove. The peroneus brevis inserts in the base of the fifth metatarsal, a prominent bony landmark on the lateral side of the midportion of the foot. The peroneus longus runs deep to the peroneus brevis. It runs below the cuboid bone and the deep plantar layer of the foot and inserts on the base of the first metatarsal and medial cuneiform. The peroneus brevis, therefore, functions to evert the foot, while the peroneus longus contributes to eversion and also depresses the first metatarsal.

Injuries to the peroneal tendons may occur in conjunction with, or may be confused with, ankle sprains. Patients will usually give a history of a resisted inversion-type injury. The injury may result in a longitudinal tear in the peroneal tendons, especially the peroneus brevis (Fig. 55.22) (47). Tearing of the superior retinaculum sheath may cause anterior subluxation or dislocation of the peroneal tendons.

Acute injuries to the peroneal tendons results in swelling, tenderness, and ecchymosis in the groove on the posterior surface of the lateral malleolus, clinically resembling a lateral ankle sprain. In these patients, the greatest tenderness will be posterior to the lateral mal-

Table 55.4.
Chronic Ankle Pain

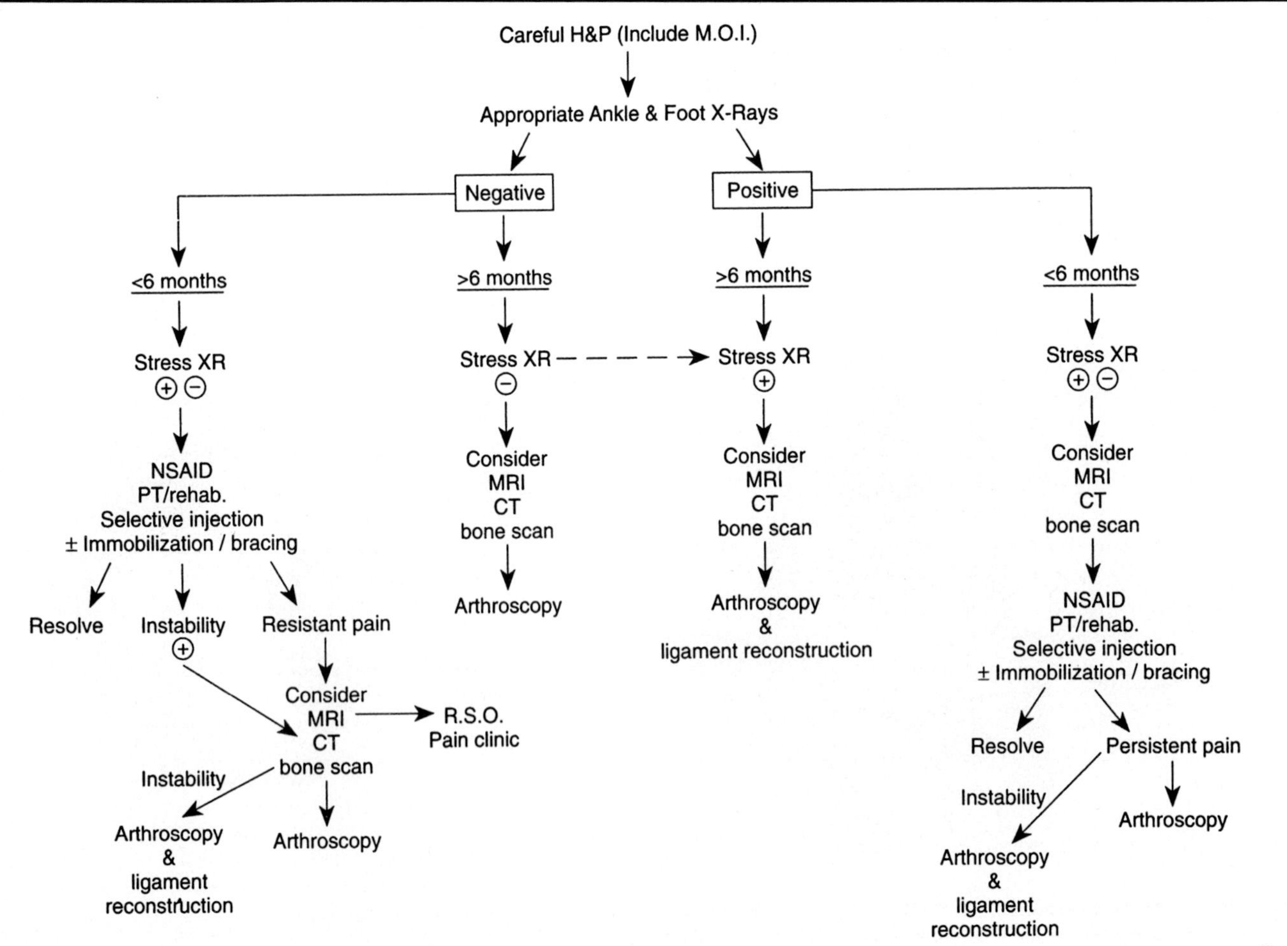

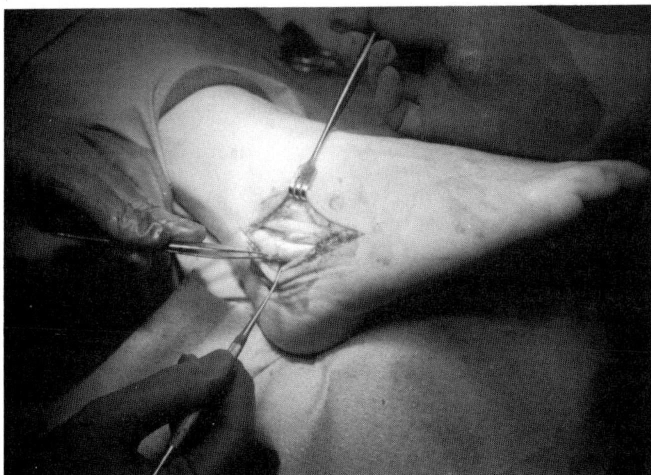

Figure 55.22. Longitudinal tear of the peroneal tendon. This often presents with evidence of thickening and pain over the tendon, and at surgery, a longitudinal split and thickening of the tendon can be seen.

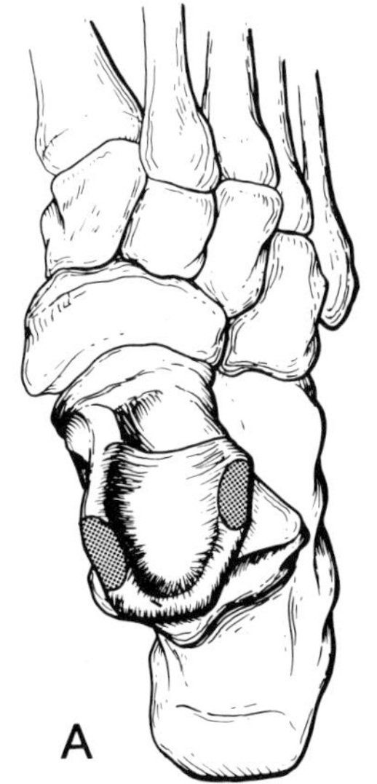

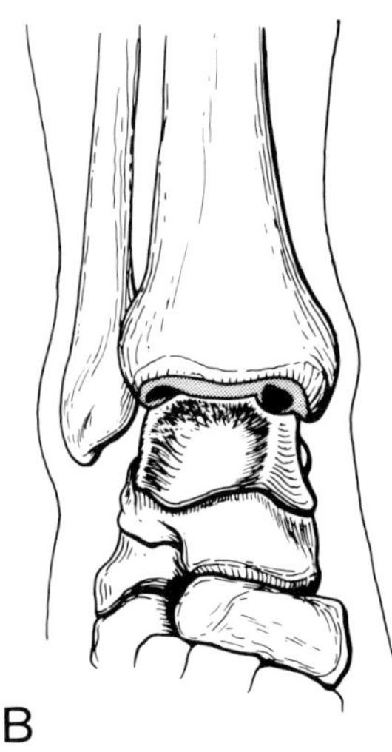

Figure 55.23. Osteochondral lesions of the talus. **A,** The location of the medial lesions tends to be more posterior, and the lateral lesions tend to be more anterior. **B,** The shape of the lateral lesions is usually shallow and wafer-like and frequently displaced; the medial lesions tend to be deeper, cup-shaped, and usually nondisplaced. Reprinted by permission from Mann R, Coughlin M. Surgery of the foot and ankle. 6th ed. St. Louis: Mosby Yearbook, 1993.

leolus in contrast to patients with classic ankle sprains in which the tenderness is greatest over the anterior talofibular ligament and anterolateral gutter. Usually routine radiographs are normal, but MRI may be helpful in diagnosing these problems.

If peroneal tendon injury is diagnosed acutely, immobilization in short leg cast with foot in slight equinus position may allow the injury to heal. Patients with chronic tenderness over the peroneal tendons or recurrent dislocations of these tendons should be treated operatively. There are numerous procedures to correct peroneal dislocation, including fibular grooving, reefing of the superior peroneal retinaculum, transferring the peroneal tendons under the calcaneofibular ligament, creation of an Achilles sling, and bone block procedures. Peroneal tears are usually longitudinal within the body of the peroneus brevis or longus and when present in isolation may be repaired primarily. Occasionally, these patients may present with peroneal tendon dislocation (48, 49).

Osteochondral Lesions of the Talus

Osteochondral lesions of the talus (OLT) are a common cause of pain following an inversion injury. Several different terms have been used to describe this lesion, including transchondral fracture, osteochondral fracture, osteochondritis dissecans, and talar dome fracture. Although the etiology of this problem remains controversial, many patients will give a history of a previous ankle sprain. Typically, such injury involves either the posteromedial or the anterolateral talar dome (Fig. 55.23). Lateral lesions are shallow and wafer shaped and are thought to result from impaction of the talus on the fibular by strong inversion of the dorsiflexed foot. Posteromedial lesions are deeper and cup shaped and may result from inversion, plantar flexion, and external rotation of the tibia on the talus. Osteochondral lesions must be considered in the differential diagnosis of the chronic ankle sprain, but a high index of suspicion is sometimes necessary to detect these problems. Patients will usually complain of a vague pain and are sometimes unable to localize their pain to a specific area. Physical exam also may be unremarkable or demonstrate some minor loss of motion and pain in a specific area. Standard AP, lateral, and mortise x-rays may occasionally be helpful in demonstrating the lesions. However, these lesions are frequently missed on conventional radiographs, and CT scanning in two planes has proven to be the best way to diagnose and accurately stage the lesion. Recently, the advent of MRI also has helped in the diagnosis of these problems. Osteochondral lesions occur bilaterally 10% of the time.

Table 55.5.
Computerized Tomographic Staging of Osteochondral Lesions of the Talus

Stage I	Cystic lesions with intact roof
Stage II	Lesion extends to articular surface
Stage III	Open lesion with nondisplaced fragment
Stage IV	Open lesion with displaced fragment

Several classification systems for these lesions have been devised, and the authors recently have developed a CT scan staging system that appears to correlate best to the pathology and subsequent results. These lesions are classified on a CT scan appearance at stage 1 through 4 (50) (Table 55.5).

Pritsch et al. (51) also developed an arthroscopic staging system to classify the cartilage quality overlying the lesion. They believed this system was a more useful indicator of the patient's prognosis. In this system, cartilage is considered to be grade I if it is intact, firm, and shiny; grade II is soft, spongy, and intact; in grade III, the cartilage is frayed.

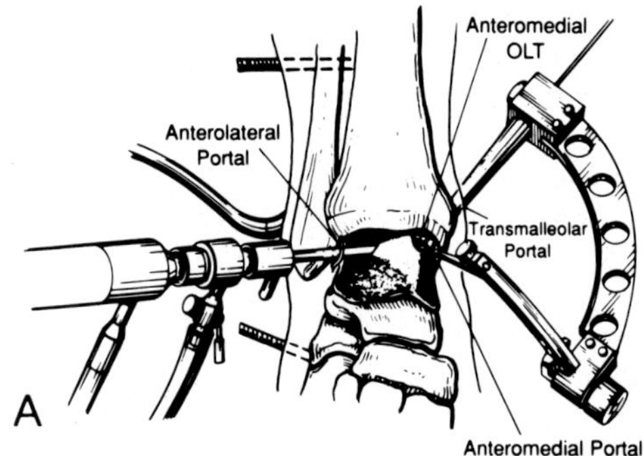

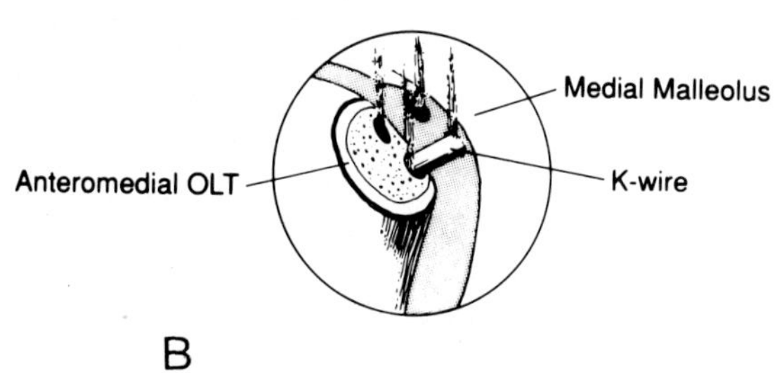

Figure 55.24. **A,** Transmalleolar drilling of an osteochondral lesion of the medial dome of the talus. Visualization is done through either the anterolateral portal or the posterolateral portal using a small joint drill guide. **B,** Drilling of the anteromedial osteochondral lesion of the talus to initiate new blood supply and cartilage healing. Reprinted by permission from Mann R, Coughlin M. Surgery of the foot and ankle. 6th ed. St. Louis: Mosby Yearbook, 1993.

Nonoperative treatment is followed for those with stage I or II lesions that can be adequately documented radiographically. Stage III lesions in young patients (≤18 years old) are to be treated initially conservatively, but if they do not respond, surgical treatment is indicated. In adults, all stage III and IV lesions that are symptomatic are treated surgically, and stage I and II lesions are treated surgically if they continued to be symptomatic despite all conservative treatment.

Currently, arthroscopy is the best way to assess and treat osteochondral lesions of the talus (51). Not only does it allow accurate diagnosis of the lesion, including whether it is loose or not, but it allows surgical treatment such as excision, debridement, and transmalleolar drilling (Fig. 55.24). Arthroscopic treatment also allows early range-of-motion and strengthening exercises, and in a large group of patients, 85% had good to excellent results (52).

Fractures

Excluding the high-energy fractures associated with falls and motor vehicle accidents, ankle fractures occurring in sports injuries are no different from fractures occurring in the general population (53). A complete discussion of this topic is beyond the scope of this chapter. There are several important principles of diagnosis and treatment that are useful to the nonorthopedic physician practicing sports medicine. These concepts will be emphasized here.

Fractures are classified in a variety of ways. An open or compound fracture is characterized by a wound exposing the fracture to the external environment. Most sports-related fractures are closed or simple. The radiographic appearance of the fracture is described as transverse, oblique, spiral, or comminuted. Another fracture classification scheme divides fractures into stable or unstable injuries. This classification is useful in that unstable fractures require stabilization for optimal treatment. A stable injury requires no reduction and is immobilized for comfort and to allow healing.

The fibula may be fractured below, at or above the joint line. This is the basis of the Danis-Weber classification scheme (Fig. 55.25). It is helpful to think of the soft tissue structures that are disrupted in conjunction with the fractures. The stability of the fracture pattern can then be determined.

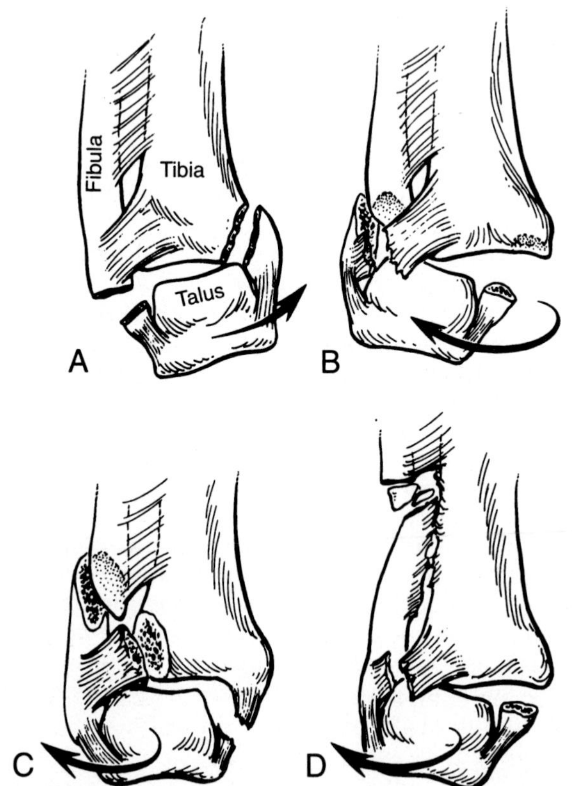

Figure 55.25. Danis-Weber classification of ankle fractures is based on the mechanism of injury.

The Foot

Running Footwear

Running footwear has blossomed into a multimillion-dollar business, and a wide variety of shoes are available to the athlete. With more choices available, there is understandably much confusion regarding the choice of one type of shoe over another. Although there are certain guidelines for the proper selection of footwear for a given sport, individual preference is a major factor in patient satisfaction. The selection of a shoe must take into consideration the sport, whether or not the shoe is for training or competition, the playing surface, and the ability of the shoe to accommodate the addition of orthotic and/or braces. An ideal athletic shoe would facilitate performance, protect from injury, and be economical. Runners and other athletes will usually find a specific brand and size of shoe (usually through trial and error) that they will be most comfortable in.

In general, running and jogging shoes should be self-fitting, lightweight, and aerated (Fig. 55.26). They should be contoured to provide some rocker effect. Shoe stability is a function of the last. A last is a model approximating the weight-bearing foot over which a shoe is made. This explains the differences in shoe sizes from manufacturer to manufacturer and why one brand of shoes may fit an individual better than a similarly sized shoe from another company. A straight-last shoe is the most rigid design and a curved or banana last is the most flexible. Most lasts are termed intermediate.

The midsole provides cushioning. A board last is designed to increase the support provided by the shoe. With this modification, the upper is glued to a firm board before being attached to the midsole. A slip last is very flexible by virtue of the fact that the upper is attached to the midsole without a stiffening board. A combination last has a board only in the rear of the shoe. A patient with pronation problems may benefit from the maximum stability provided by a straight-board last and a firm midsole. Similarly, a rigid cavus foot will benefit from a curved slip last with a soft midsole. When shoe instability is required, a firmer midsole may be needed.

The outsole is the interface between the shoe and playing surface. A stiff outsole tends to be heavier and more durable than a blown rubber outsole that is filled with air pockets. The outsole can be made from a combination of solid and blown rubber to provide increased durability at the heel while allowing greater flexibility in the forefoot. The treads are designed to aid in shock absorption and to provide traction. Individual preference and the playing surface play a large role in the selection of an appropriate tread pattern. Two common styles are the herringbone and waffle tread.

A beveled heel and outflared sole are modifications to provide maximum stability at heel contact. Plastic heel stabilizers act to reinforce the heel counter at the base.

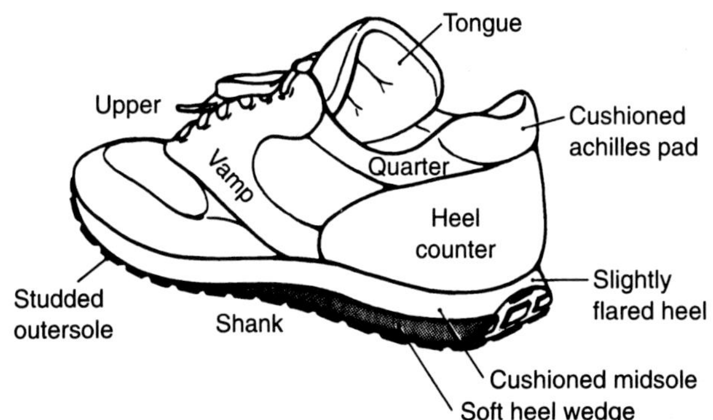

Figure 55.26. Running shoes differ by modifying different components of the same basic design.

Other modifications may be added to the shoe for specific problems. For example, pain secondary to posterior tibial tendinitis may be addressed by the addition of an arch support. A soft heel wedge may help the symptoms of Achilles tendinitis.

An orthotic must use sound principles based on the normal gait pattern. Orthotics are devices designed to maximize function in two ways. By correcting a biomechanical problem, an athlete need not waste energy compensating for a problem. Orthotics may also be used to reduce discomfort by changing the weight-bearing profile of the foot.

Orthotics may be classified as flexible, semirigid, and rigid (Fig. 55.27). A flexible orthotic acts mostly to cushion the foot and provides only minimal support. Semirigid orthotics balance the need for a device that will provide support yet accommodate for the changing shape of the foot in gait.

One of the most common indications for an orthotics prescription is to control subtalar pronation in a person with pes planus (flat feet). By reducing baseline pronation, the foot is able to assume a supinated position. Hind foot supination is necessary to form a rigid lever for stability at toe-off and heel strike. Fatigue is theoretically reduced by this mechanism. The high incidence of pes planus in the general population and the popularity of running sports create an environment of potential abuse of this technology. This is particularly true in the case of rigid orthotic. Rigid orthotics are generally manufactured of acrylic at great expense to the patient. Although they may be beneficial in some cases, they violate the principles of gait by not allowing the foot to move from a rigid lever to a flexible unit capable of accepting uneven ground and providing shock absorption. This may lead to neuroma formation, nerve impingement, heel pain syndrome, and stress fracture, especially with distance runners.

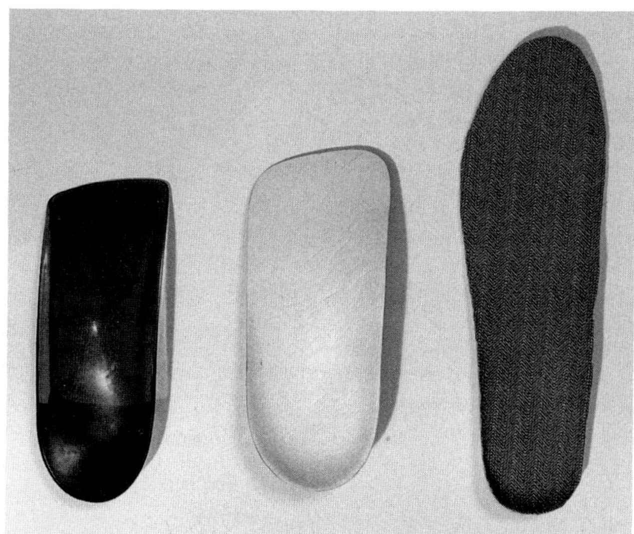

Figure 55.27. Foot orthotics. Rigid (*left*), semirigid (*middle*), and flexible (*right*) orthotics are shown.

Fractures

Recently there has been attention focused on a stress avulsion fracture of the tarsal navicular in athletes involved in sprinting and jumping. A small dorsal triangular fracture fragment is best seen in weight-bearing, lateral-view radiographs. Radionuclide scans and tomography are occasionally needed to confirm the diagnosis. Nonoperative treatment is recommended in all but the most symptomatic of cases.

The Jones fracture is a fracture of the base of the fifth metatarsal at the junction of the metaphysis and the diaphysis, and is named for Sir Robert Jones. Jones suffered this particular injury personally while dancing in the early part of this century. This fracture must be differentiated from the more common fracture of the base of the fifth metatarsal within the metaphyseal region. This second fracture pattern is a avulsion-type fracture from the peroneus brevis tendon insertion (Fig. 55.28). These latter fractures rarely displace and generally heal without complications. The Jones fracture may result from an acute injury or be a stress fracture. This injury has a high rate of nonunion, delayed union, and refracture. Treatment is controversial. It is clear that if cast immobilization is tried, the patient must be nonweight bearing. For earlier return to athletics, intramedullary screw fixation is a reasonable alternative. Nonunion is frequently seen, and bone grafting may be necessary to achieve union (54–57).

Tendinitis

Any tendon crossing the ankle joint to insert on the foot may be subject to tendinitis. Tendinitis is inflammation of a tendon and may be acute or chronic. Appropriate treatment depends on the accurate assessment of which tendon(s) is involved and to what degree.

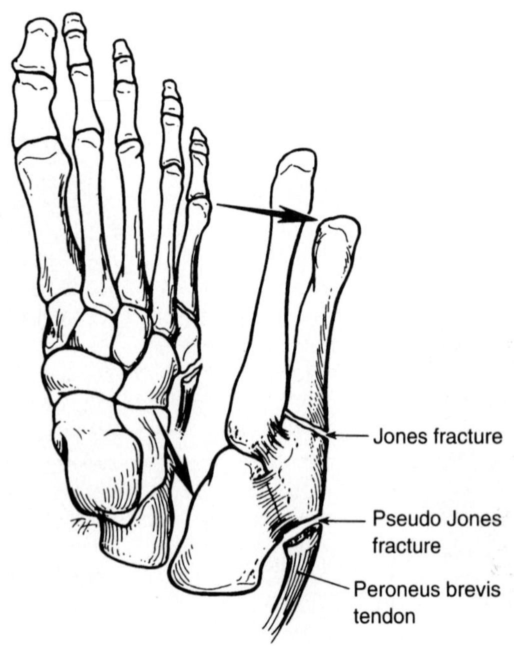

Figure 55.28. The Jones fracture and pseudo-Jones fracture differ with respect to both location and prognosis.

The treatment of tendinitis is initially immobilization, antiinflammatory medication is given, and gradual return to full function is achieved. Local measures such as icing the affected part after practice or games can be helpful for both treatment and pain relief. Stretching is an important part of both the rehabilitation and prevention of this problem.

The posterior tibial tendon may be inflamed at its insertion into the navicular or proximally as it winds around the medial malleolus. The athlete may have trouble standing on his or her toes or running because the posterior tibial tendon acts as both a strong plantar flexor and helps position the hind foot in pronation, the position of stability (Fig. 55.29).

The anterior tibial tendon is easily palpable anteriorly. Pain in this structure may be caused by a hyperplantar flexion injury of the foot as in football or soccer. Diagnosis is made by direct palpation of this tendon and by resisted dorsiflexion of the foot causing pain.

The flexor hallucis longus tendon may be inflamed as it passes between the medial and lateral posterior talar processes or as it winds around the medial malleolus. This problem is often seen in dancers and sprinters. Pain with resisted plantar flexion or a snapping sensation as the great toe is moved from a plantar flexed to a dorsiflexed position is the hallmark of diagnosis and in ballet dancers is called hallux saltans.

Plantar Heel Pain

The differential diagnosis of plantar heel pain includes both common and rare conditions (58). Diagnosis is often difficult, because there are many problems with similar presentations in a small anatomic region. Three primary tissues may be involved: nerve, bone, and connective tissue other than bone. Quite frequently, the source of pain is difficult to identify and is best called heel pain syndrome (HPS). The term *HPS* reconciles the fact that not all heel pain is true plantar fasciitis and implies inflammation of the entire plantar fascia. Most heel pain diagnosed as plantar fasciitis is actually best described as HPS, because true plantar fasciitis is rather uncommon. Heel pain syndrome is one

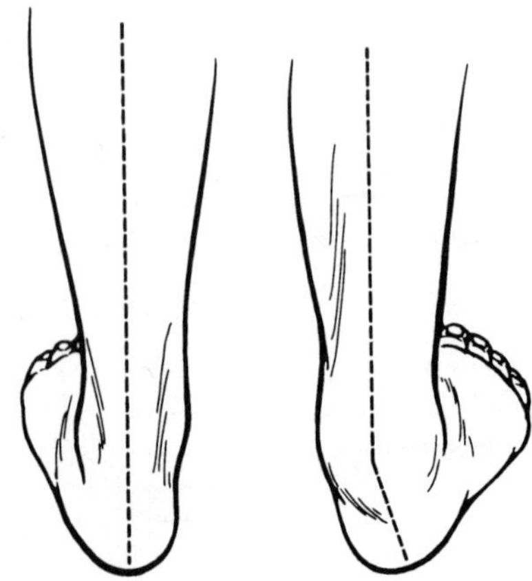

Figure 55.29. A tear of the posterior tibial tendon will cause a "too many toe sign" as seen from behind as well as increased valgus of the subtalar joint.

Table 55.6.
Differential Diagnosis of Focal Plantar Heel Pain

1. Nerve
   - Tarsal tunnel syndrome
   - Entrapment of the nerve to the abductor digiti quinti muscle
   - Medial calcaneal nerve neuroma
2. Bone
   - Medial calcaneal periostitis
   - Calcaneal stress fracture
   - Heel spur fracture
   - Tumor
3. Other connective tissues
   - Plantar fasciitis/rupture of the plantar fascia
   - Fat pad atrophy or inflammation
   - Heel pain syndrome

of the most common reasons for an athlete to visit a physician with a foot complaint. Unfortunately, the term *plantar fasciitis* is entrenched in the literature and is used interchangeably with HPS. Table 55.6 lists the focal causes for plantar heel pain by tissue type (59).

Plantar fasciitis may be unilateral or bilateral. When a patient presents with bilateral plantar fasciitis, the diagnosis of a systemic rheumatic disorder such as Reiter's syndrome must be entertained. Most commonly, a running athlete or patient who has either begun an exercise program, gained weight (including pregnancy), or increased the intensity of his or her training may be prone to this disorder. High-impact aerobics and occupations that require walking on hard surfaces may also lead to this painful disorder.

The plantar fascia is a strong band of collagen extending from the anterior aspect of the calcaneal tuberosity to the base of each proximal phalanx (Fig. 55.30). The distal attachment divides to allow the passage of the flexor tendons to the toes. Therefore, there are 10 distal attachments of the plantar fascia. The insertion of the plantar fascia distal to the metatarsophalangeal joints also gives rise to the windlass mechanism of the foot. The windlass mechanism elevates the longitudinal arch with toe dorsiflexion leading to greater foot stability.

A typical history for plantar fasciitis is stabbing heel pain with the first few steps in the morning after rising. The pain will gradually diminish during the day with walking. By the end of the day or in the early evening the heel will ache. The reason for the early morning pain is likely caused by the fact that the plantar fascia has not been stretched during the night and the first steps serve to release a contracture of this tissue.

Physical exam consists of palpation of the entire plantar fascia. The insertion of the fascia is more medial than lateral and is not generally beneath the calcaneus as much as along the anteromedial border. Occasionally, the pain may be distal to the insertion, especially when a history of discrete trauma to that area is elicited. Care must be taken to palpate a plantar fibroma or other mass in the fascia when the tender area is distal to the calcaneal insertion. Forceful sustained dorsiflexion of the toes and compression of the plantar

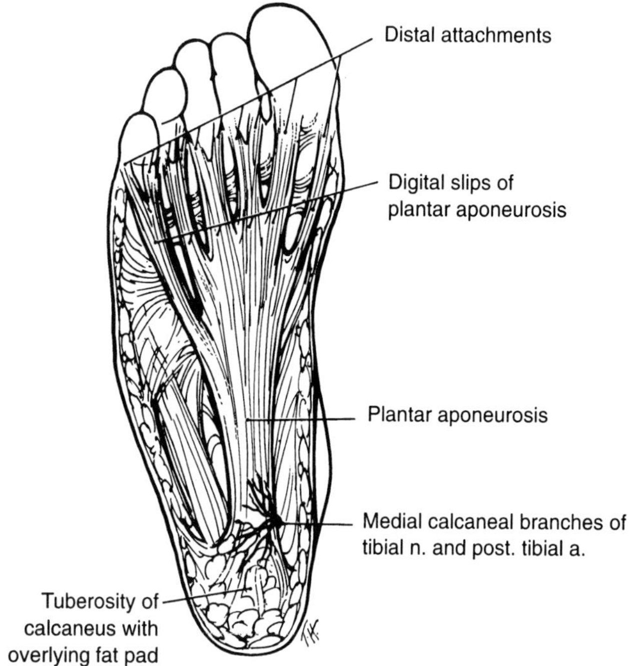

Figure 55.30. The plantar fascia attaches to the anteromedial calcaneal tuberosity and is usually the site of pain in runners with plantar fasciitis.

fascia in the midarch region inconsistently may cause pain at the insertion of the plantar fascia on the calcaneus.

Plantar fasciitis may be associated with a radiologic finding known as a heel spur. In actuality, the heel spur is a ridge of bone within the substance of the flexor digitorum brevis muscle, one of the intrinsic muscles of the foot. This bony ridge is seldom responsible for the heel pain. Rarely, the spur itself may fracture causing pain in this region. The spur is seen in a discreet percentage of feet without pain referable to the heel. The presence of a heel spur on a radiograph can never be considered synonymous with plantar fasciitis or HPS. The differential diagnosis of heel pain includes common and uncommon causes, and there is some controversy in the orthopedic literature as to the existence or importance of these various clinical entities.

Treatment consists of patient education and both pharmacologic and mechanical modalities. The natural history of this condition is such that resolution of the pain may take 1 or more years. The patient must be informed of the length of time that the condition may persist so that appropriate scheduling of athletic events, training, and cross-training may be done. It is helpful to develop an outline of the treatment hierarchy with the patient so that the inevitable frustration on the part of the patient (and physician!) is minimized. On the initial visit, a viscoelastic heel pad, NSAIDs, and appropriate patient information brochures may be recommended. The patient may be given a chance to try the heel pads in the office. Generally, heel pads are placed in both shoes. If the patient does not experience at least partial relief of the pain with heel pads, an off-the-shelf medial arch support is tried. Heel pads act to share the shock absorption function of the plantar fascia, whereas the medial arch support shares the function of the plantar fascia in maintaining the medial longitudinal arch of the foot. Use of night splints to increase flexibility of the gastrocnemius-soleus-Achilles tendon complex and the plantar fascia itself also are effective, especially to reduce morning stiffness and pain. Taping the arch is also effective in some situations. A prefabricated night splint that holds the ankle in 5° of dorsiflexion may be combined with a program of Achilles tendon stretching and conditioning.

Injection of a cortisone preparation with a local anesthetic into the insertion of the plantar fascia is another method of treatment and is best reserved for those patients who have failed an adequate trial of NSAIDs or who are unable to tolerate them (60). The injection is best performed medially to avoid leakage of cortisone into the heel pad. The skin can be sprayed with ethyl chloride before injection to decrease the pain from the needle or entry through the skin. Injection of the origin of the plantar fascia is then performed using 3 to 5 ml xylocaine and 1 ml corticosteroid (Fig. 55.31). The patient will usually experience good pain relief after injection, but it may take 7 to 10 days. The injection may be repeated if needed. In the authors' experience, a time interval of at least 6 weeks between injections and a limit of two to three injections total to each foot is a satisfactory protocol. Patients should be told that the heel may be quite tender for several days following the injection and that the pain relief following injection may be permanent or last days, weeks, or months. Rarely, rupture of the plantar fascia, usually with activity and after multiple cortisone injections, may occur (61). After the initial pain and edema has resolved, the patient will usually have little or no symptoms.

Surgery for plantar fasciitis is best reserved as a last resort for those patients with intractable pain for 1 or more years. Although there are many different operations described in the literature for the treatment of plantar fasciitis, the most commonly performed procedures are those intended to release the medial attachment of the plantar fascia from the anterior inferior aspect of the calcaneus. The release is performed through an oblique incision on the medial side of the foot that allows exploration of both the plantar fascia, abductor hallucis fascia, and plantar nerves. It also is unclear as to whether or not removing the heel spur is necessary or whether this only serves to perpetuate the myth that the symptoms of plantar fasciitis are secondary to the presence of the bony spur (62–64).

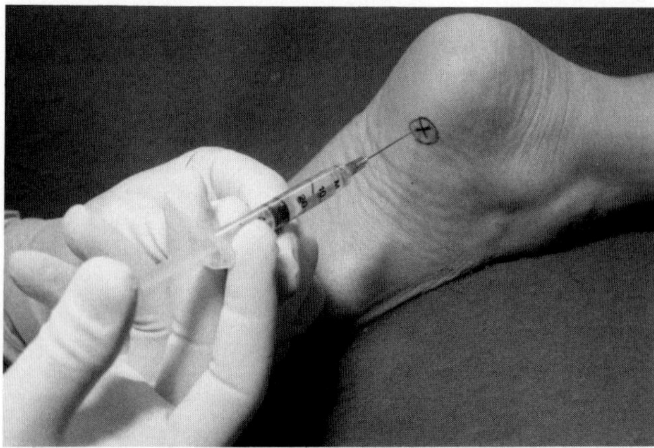

Figure 55.31. Injection of plantar fascia with cortisone. The patient in this picture was placed prone, and the injection was done along the medial calcaneal tuberosity at the site of maximum pain.

Posterior Heel Pain

Posterior heel pain may be caused by any one or more of the structures located in the retrotalar region. A careful history and physical exam combined with appropriate imaging studies will help secure the proper diagnosis.

The os trigonum is formed by the congenital nonunion of the lateral posterior talar process to the body of the talus. The flexor hallucis longus runs between the medial and lateral posterior talar processes. Impingement of the os trigonum on the posterior distal tibia may occur with extreme plantar flexion of the ankle as in ballet or soccer (Fig. 55.32). This problem has been termed the *talar compression syndrome* (65) and develops when the articular capsule is pinched between the tibia and the os trigonum, leading to soft tissue inflammation, thickening, and increased impingement-like symptoms. Posterior heel pain resulting from this injury is initially treated conservatively with rest, antiinflammatory medications, injections, and physical therapy. In some cases, the symptomatic os trigonum may be excised through a small incision behind the lateral malleolus or via subtalar arthroscopy.

Posterior heel pain may result from insertional Achilles tendinitis, an inflamed retrocalcaneal bursa, or a pump bump. A pump bump is a tender calcaneal exostosis and may be posteromedial, posterolateral, or di-

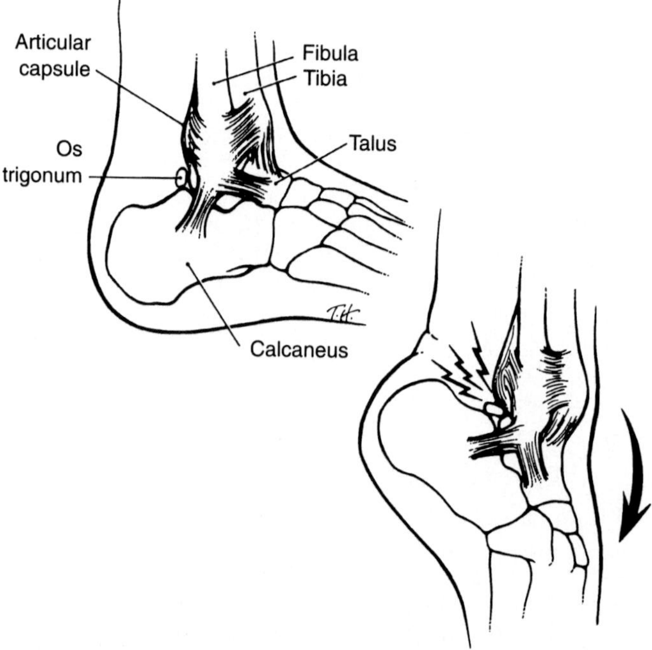

Figure 55.32. Talar compression is caused by forced plantar flexion of the ankle joint with the presence of an os trigonum or congenital nonunion of the lateral talar process.

rectly posterior. When the exostosis is posterior, it is commonly termed a Haglund's deformity (66–68).

Calcium deposits may form in the substance of the Achilles tendon following repetitive trauma and microhemorrhage. If excision of these deposits is elected, care must be taken not to disturb the surrounding normal fibers of the tendon.

Sesamoid Problems

The two sesamoids of the great toe lie within the tendon of the flexor hallucis brevis. They move anteriorly and posteriorly within medial and lateral grooves beneath the distal first metatarsal separated by a ridge or crista. Their primary function is to increase the mechanical advantage by increasing the lever arm of the flexor brevis in a similar manner to the patella of the knee joint. The ancient Hebrews believed that the medial sesamoid was indestructible and was the seat of individual resurrection. Although not indestructible, the sesamoids bear three times the weight of the body with the medial sesamoid taking the majority of the force. Unfortunately, these small but important bones and the investing structures are subject to a variety of acute and chronic injuries in the athletic individual. These problems may be quite debilitating and require prompt and accurate diagnosis for early return to sports. To confuse the issue, the sesamoid bones are formed from multiple ossification centers and nonunion of these centers leads to the radiographic appearance of bi-, tri- and quadripartite sesamoid bones (69, 70).

The most common sesamoid problem encountered in the athletic population is caused by repetitive stress from the sesamoid and is termed "sesamoiditis." This is a common problem in athletes from whom maximum dorsiflexion of the great toe is required. This population includes joggers, sprinters, figure skaters, ballet dancers, and basketball and football players. Sesamoiditis may be associated with direct pressure from a cleat in an athletic shoe. The problem is manifested by the insidious onset of pain and tenderness under the first metatarsal head in the region of the medial or lateral sesamoid. Treatment of sesamoiditis consists of changing the weight-bearing profile of the foot to decrease the load underneath the first metatarsal head. This is best accomplished through the use of orthotics. NSAIDs may be helpful. Some authors advocate the injection of corticosteroids into the tissue surrounding the affected sesamoid to decrease the inflammation but this must be done with extreme care as it may lead to permanent skin atrophy at the site of injection.

Sesamoiditis is a distinct entity from osteochondritis of the sesamoid in that osteochondritis will rarely respond to conservative treatment. Changes in the appearance of the sesamoid may not appear for 9 months to 1 year, however. With osteochondritis the sesamoid may undergo fragmentation, flattening, and enlargement, leading to a painful arthritis of the sesamoid-metatarsal articulation. The treatment of this problem is generally surgical excision of the affected sesamoid with careful attention to meticulous repair of the flexor tendon. A poor repair of the defect left from excision of the medial sesamoid may lead to hallux valgus, whereas an insufficient repair of the tendon after lateral sesamoid excision may lead to hallux varus.

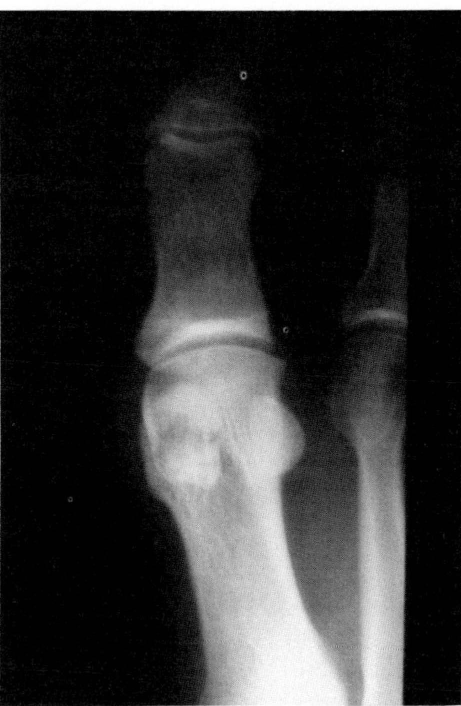

Figure 55.33. Fracture of the medial sesamoid. The edges of the fractured sesamoid are jagged, which is more suggestive of a fracture than of a bipartite sesamoid.

Neuritis of the medial plantar digital nerve is a rare posttraumatic injury that may masquerade as lateral sesamoiditis. The medial plantar digital nerve or Joplin's nerve passes plantar to the lateral sesamoid and passes dorsal to the flexor hallucis longus tendon. The diagnosis should be suspected when the pain beneath the lateral sesamoid is present with hypesthesia of the medial hallux. The treatment of the problem is initially to unload the lateral sesamoid although surgery is occasionally necessary with failure of conservative treatment.

Fractures of a sesamoid are generally the result of a fall from a height and are an uncommon sports injury (Fig. 55.33). Dorsal dislocation of the metatarsophalangeal joint with fracture of the sesamoids is more likely the result of high-energy trauma such as a motor vehicle accident. Rarely the intersesamoid ligament, a proportionately strong ligament between the medial and lateral sesamoids may rupture with a great toe dorsiflexion injury.

Accessory Navicular

The longitudinal arch of the foot serves to provide a shock absorber for the body with each step. Just as the outer side is the interface between the shoe and the ground, the foot is the interface between the body and the ground. By virtue of this fact, the foot must protect the other joints of the lower extremity by damping the energy imparted on the leg with each step.

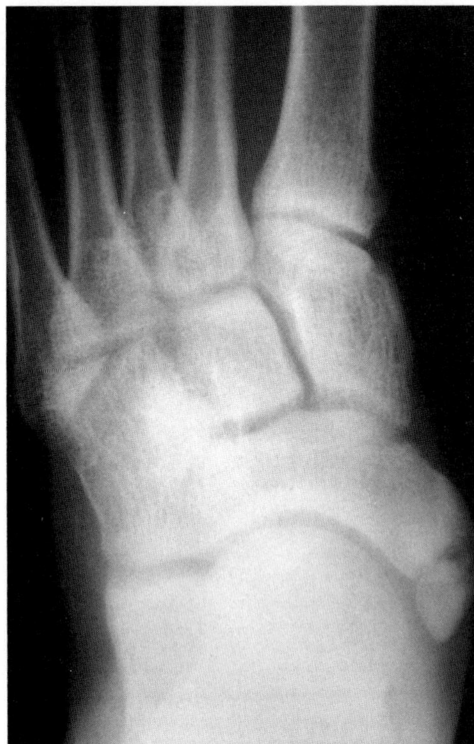

Figure 55.34. An accessory navicular appears as a separate bone on standard radiographs. It is actually connected to the main body of the navicular by a disc of cartilage.

The arch is supported by several intrinsic and extrinsic factors. The shape of the bones in the foot is such that a gentle arch is formed. Strong ligaments hold the bones of the foot together but allow motion to occur. The plantar fascia extends from the anterior aspect of the calcaneus inferiorly to the base of each proximal phalanx. The posterior tibial tendon winds behind the medial malleolus and inserts primarily on the plantar-medial surface of the navicular. The navicular is located at the apex of the longitudinal arch so that the posterior tibial tendon acts as a dynamic support of this configuration. A congenital nonunion of two centers of ossification may occur in the navicular with the smaller of the two halves in the medial position (Fig. 55.34). A portion of the posterior tibial tendon inserts on this medial piece and chronic stresses can cause a microfracture of the synchondrosis or cartilaginous connection between the two halves. This manifests itself as arch pain and weakness of the posterior tibial tendon function, as in posterior tibial tendinitis. Treatment is aimed at rest, immobilization, and reducing the associated inflammation. Excision of the accessory navicular is needed when conservative methods fail. After the accessory bone is excised, the tendon is reattached to the main body of the navicular (71).

Turf Toe

Turf toe refers to ligamentous injury of the first metatarsophalangeal joint and is a common injury to soccer and football. The term *turf toe* refers to the observation that the injury is more common on the artificial playing surfaces. The use of nonleather playing shoes has also been implicated. The mechanism of injury is typically a tackle in which the player's foot is planted on the nonyielding playing surface and the player or the opponent falls on the leg forcing the great toe into hyperdorsiflexion (Fig. 55.35). Ligamentous injury to the metatarsophalangeal joint may also occur by hyperplantar flexion and valgus forces. Sesamoid and midfoot injuries have the same mechanism of injury and must be considered in the differential diagnosis.

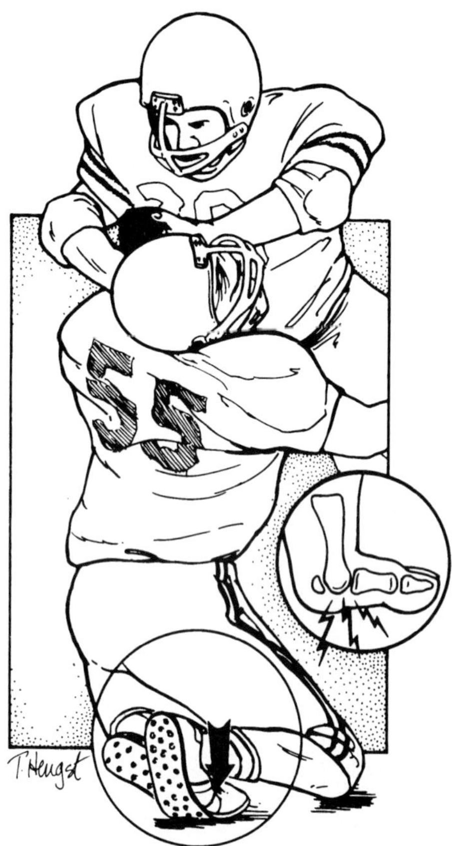

Figure 55.35. Turf toe occurs with hyperflexion of the metatarsophalangeal joint of the great toe and is commonly seen in football played on synthetic fields.

Treatment consists of local care (RICE), and return to competition may be facilitated by taping the great toe to limit motion or modifying shoe wear to reinforce the forefoot area. A 0.51-mm spring-steel insert is ideal for this purpose.

Miscellaneous Problems

Callous formation is a reaction by the skin to excessive pressure. It serves to protect against skin breakdown by increasing both the thickness and strength of the skin. Not only do callouses cause pain, but they usually are a sign that there is a problem with the distribution of pressure on the sole of the foot. When callouses form on the dorsum of the toes they are called corns. The moist environment between the toes may give rise to a soft corn when abnormal pressures are encountered in this area. Treatment is always aimed at reducing the pressure in the area of the callous. The weight-bearing profile of the foot must be considered and changes in footwear, orthotics, and surgery may be recommended.

Blisters result from shear forces over the skin. The skin over the blister should be kept intact if possible as it serves as a biologic dressing. If the skin does break, the loose skin should be gently debrided and the underlying tissue dressed and protected as appropriate.

The black toe of runners refers to the subungual hematoma that develops from repetitive shear forces over the great toenail in athletes whose feet rub on the top of their shoe distally with running or with the stop-and-start action in paddle or racquet sports. The great toenail is sometimes lost if the hematoma is large enough. Treatment here is aimed at finding the proper shoe wear to prevent this from occurring.

Rehabilitation of the Ankle and Foot

Although much has been written about the rehabilitation of joints such as the knee and the shoulder, little has been presented regarding the functional rehabilitation of the foot and ankle complex. The main goal of rehabilitation is to restore maximum functional potential. The goals remain the same postoperatively as compared to postacute injury.

Various rehabilitation modalities can be used to treat the foot and ankle. Numerous electrical stimulation devices that appear to provide some symptomatic relief to the patient are available on the market. Most rehabilitation programs use ice, heat, message, ultrasound (including phonophoresis and iontophoresis), and electrical stimulation. In addition, exercises—passive, active assisted, and/or active—are critical to the rehabilitation process.

The authors emphasize a team approach when rehabilitating a patient to maximum functional return. The team includes the patient, the physician, and the therapist. Although the physician gives primary input into the treatment protocol, the therapist contacts the patient on a much more frequent basis and can help indicate rehabilitation progress. The patient needs to be knowledgeable about what is occurring to encourage maximum effort during rehabilitation. The program can be divided into four general phases:

Phase 1. Acute postoperative and early rehabilitation.
Phase 2. Rehabilitation.
Phase 3. Functional return.
Phase 4. Specificity of sport or activity.

Phase 1 is defined as the acute or symptomatic phase and is immediately after surgery or postinjury. Rehabilitation goals are to decrease pain, edema, and inflammation and to increase pain-free range of motion and stimulate collagen alignment. In addition, restoration of flexibility and prevention of kinesthetic shutdown is important.

In Phase 2, the goals are to increase range of motion to full and diminish swelling as well as to increase strength. Progression should be made to weight-bearing exercises and improvement with kinesthetic and neuromuscular control.

Phase 3 continues strengthening and endurance from phase 2 as needed, and advances proprioceptive training in preparation for sports-specific drills, which will be used in phase 4, especially with multidirectional movements.

Phase 4 continues strengthening and endurance training while emphasizing more advanced proprioceptive training and return to the individual sport. The rate of progression from one phase to another varies among patients, depending on the type of surgery or injury, the patient, and the therapist's and physician's perceptions of progress.

Appropriate rehabilitation of the foot and ankle is absolutely necessary for the athlete to return to his or her sport at full performance without risk of reinjury (72).

REFERENCES

1. Mann RA. Biomechanical approach to the treatment of foot problems. Foot Ankle 1982;2:205–212.
2. Mann RA. Biomechanics of the foot and ankle. In: Mann RA, ed. Surgery of the foot. St. Louis: CV Mosby, 1986:1–30.
3. Ralston HJ. Energy-speed relation and optimal speed during level walking. Int Z Angew Physiol 1958;17:277.
4. Sammarco GJ. Biomechanics of the foot. In: Frankel VN, Nordin M, eds. Basic biomechanics of the musculoskeletal system. 2nd ed. Philadelphia: Lea & Febiger, 1989:163–181.
5. Czerniecki JM. Foot and ankle biomechanics in walking and running. Am J Phys Med Rehabil 1988;67:246–252.
6. Ferkel R, Mai L, Ullis K, Finerman G. An analysis of roller skating injuries. Am J Sports Med 1982;10:24–30.
7. Johansson C. Injuries in elite orienters. Am J Sports Med 1986;14:410–415.
8. Kiburz D, Jacobs R, Reckling F, Mason J. Bicycle accident and injuries among adult cyclists. Am J Sports Med 1986;14:416–419.
9. Clancy WG Jr. Lower extremity injuries in the jogger and distance runner. Phys Sportsmed 1974;2:47.
10. Nicholas JA. Ankle injuries in athletes. Orthop Clin North Am 1974;5:153–175.
11. Hovelius L, Palmgren H. Laceration of tibial tendons and vessels in ice hockey players: three case histories of a skate boot top injury. Am J Sports Med 1979;7:297.
12. Rarabeck CH. Exertional tibialis posterior compartment syndrome. Clin Orthop 1986;208:61–64.
13. Matsen FA III. A practical approach to compartmental syndromes: part I. Definition, therapy and pathogenesis. In: Evarts CM, ed. American Academy of Orthopaedic Surgeons Instructional Course Lectures. No. 32. St. Louis: CV Mosby, 1983:88–92.
14. Mubarak SJ. A practical approach to compartmental syndromes: part II. Diagnosis. In: Evarts CM, ed. American Academy of Orthopaedic Surgeons Instructional Course Lectures. No. 32. St. Louis: CV Mosby, 1983:92–102.
15. Rorabeck CH. A practical approach to compartmental syndromes: part III. Management. In: Evarts CM, ed. America Academy of Orthopaedic Surgeons Instructional Course Lectures. No. 32. St. Louis: CV Mosby, 1983:102–113.
16. Severanse HW, Bassett FH. Rupture of the plantaris—does it exist? J Bone Joint Surg 1982;64A:1387–1388.
17. Lagergren C, Lindholm A. Vascular distribution in the Achilles tendon: an angiographic and microangiographic study. Acta Chir Scand 1958–1959;116:491–495.
18. Inglis AE, Scott WN, Sculco TP, et al. Ruptures of the tendon Achilles: an objective assessment of surgical and non-surgical treatment. J Bone Joint Surg 1976;58A:990–993.
19. Nistor L. Surgical and non-surgical treatment of Achilles tendon rupture. J Bone Joint Surg 1981;63A:394–399.
20. Ferkel RD, Fischer, SP: Progress in ankle arthroscopy. Clin Orthop 1989;240:210–220.

21. Ferkel RD. Ankle arthroscopy. In: An illustrated guide to small joint arthroscopy. Andover, MA: Dyonics Inc., 1989:1–6.
22. Ferkel RD. Instrumentation. In: Ferkel RD. Arthroscopic surgery: the foot and ankle. Philadelphia: JB Lippincott, in press.
23. Leonard MH. A sprained ankle may be a more serious injury than a fracture. Am Surg 1954;20:660–663.
24. Singer KM, Jones DC. Soft tissue conditions of the ankle and foot. In: Nicholas JA, Hershmen EB, eds. The lower extremity and spine in sports medicine. St. Louis: CV Mosby, eds. The lower extremity and spine in sports medicine. St. Louis: CV Mosby, 1986;498–505.
25. Subcommittee on Classification of Sports Injuries, American Medical Association, Committee on the Medical Aspects of Sports. Standard nomenclature of athletic injuries. Chicago: American Medical Association, 1966.
26. Brostrom L. Sprained ankles: I. Anatomic lesions in recent sprains. Acta Chir Scand 1964;128:483–495.
27. Leach RE. Acute ankle sprains: vigorous treatment for best results. J Musculoskel Med 1983;1:68.
28. Sauser DD, Nelson RC, Laurine MH, et al. Acute injuries of the lateral ligaments of the ankle: comparison of stress radiography and arthrography. Radiology 1983;148:653.
29. Rubin G, Witten M. The talar tilt ankle and the fibular collateral ligaments: a method for the determination of talar tilt. J Bone Joint Surg 1960;42A:311.
30. Chrisman OD, Snook CA. A reconstruction of lateral ligament tears of the ankle: an experimental study and clinical evaluation of seven patients treated by a new modification of the Elmslie procedure. J Bone Joint Surg 1969;51A:904–912.
31. Gould N, Seligson D, Glassman J. Early and late repair of lateral ligaments of the ankle. Foot Ankle 1980;1:84.
32. Laurin CA, Ouellet R, St Jacques R. Talar and subtalar tilt: an experimental investigation. Can J Surg 1968;11:270.
33. Hamilton WG, Thompson FM, Snow SW. The modified Brostrom procedure for lateral ankle instability. Foot Ankle 1993;14;1–7.
34. Staples OS. Injuries to the medial ligaments of the ankle. J Bone Joint Surg 1960;42A:1287–1307.
35. Hopkinson WJ, St Pierre P, Ryan JB, Wheeler JH. Syndesmosis sprains of the ankle. Foot Ankle 1990;10:325–330.
36. Boytim MJ, Fischer DA, Neumann L. Syndesmotic ankle sprains. Am J Sports Med 1991;19:294–298.
37. Pankovich AM. Maisonneuve fracture of the fibula. J Bone Joint Surg 1976;58A:337–342.
38. Grana WA. Chronic pain persisting after ankle sprain. J Musculoskel Med 1990;7:35–49.
39. Smith RW, Reischl SF. Treatment of ankle sprains in young athletes. Am J Sports Med 1986;14:465–471.
40. Kay DE. The sprained ankle: current therapy. Foot Ankle 1985;6:22–28.
41. Rarick GL, Bigley G, Karst R, et al. The measurable support of the ankle joint by conventional methods of taping. J Bone Joint Surg 1962;44A:1183–1190.
42. Freeman MAR. Instability of the foot after injuries to the lateral ligament of the ankle. J Bone Joint Surg 1965;47B:669–677.
43. Nachtigal MP, Grana WA. Hidden ankle injuries. Paper presented at the annual meeting of the Arthroscopy Association of North America, Orlando, FL, 1990.
44. Ferkel RD, Karzel RP, Del Pizzo W, et al. Arthroscopic treatment of anterolateral impingement of the ankle. Am J Sports Med 1991;19:440–446.
45. Ferkel RD. Soft tissue pathology of the ankle. In: McGinty JB, ed. Operative arthroscopy. New York: Raven Press, 1991:713–725.
46. Bassett FH, Gates HS, Billys JB, et al. Talar impingement by the anteroinferior tibiofibular ligament. J Bone Joint Surg 1990;72A:55–59.
47. Woodward AH. Complications of lateral ankle sprain. In: Mann RA, Coughlin MJ, eds. Surgery of the foot and ankle. St. Louis: CV Mosby, 1992:196–206.
48. Gunn DR. Stenosing tenosynovitis of the common peroneal tendon sheath. Br Med J 1959:691–692.
49. Sobel M, Levy ME, Bohne WHO. Longitudinal attrition of the peroneus brevis tendon in the fibular groove: an anatomic study. Foot Ankle 1990;11:124–128.
50. Ferkel RD. Arthroscopy of the ankle and foot. In: Mann RA, Coughlin MJ, eds. Surgery of the foot and ankle. St. Louis: CV Mosby, 1992:1277–1310.
51. Pritsch M, Horoshovski H, Farine I. Arthroscopic treatment of osteochondral lesions of the talus. J Bone Joint Surg 1986;68A:862–865.
52. Ferkel RD, Sgaglione NA. Arthroscopic treatment of osteochondral lesions of the talus. Paper presented at the American Academy of Orthopaedic Surgeons annual meeting, San Francisco, 1993.
53. Zenker H, Nerlich M. Prognostic aspects in operated ankle fractures. Arch Orthop Trauma Surg 1982;100:237–241.
54. Kavanaugh JH, Brower TD, Mann RV. The Jones fracture revisited. J Bone Joint Surg 1978;60A:776–782.
55. Torg JS, Balduini FC, Zelko RR, Pavlov H, Peff TC, Das M. Fractures of the base of the fifth metatarsal distal to the tuberosity. J Bone Joint Surg 1984;66A:209–214.
56. Zogby RG, Baker BE. A review of nonoperative treatment of Jones' fracture. Am J Sports Med 1987;15:304–307.
57. DeLee JC, Evans JP, Julian J. Stress fracture of the fifth metatarsal. Am J Sports Med 1983;11:349–353.
58. Bordelon RL. Subcalcaneal pain: a method of evaluation and plan for treatment. Clin Orthop 1983;177:49–53.
59. Furey JG. Plantar fasciitis: the painful heel syndrome. J Bone Joint Surg 1975;57A:672–673.
60. Blockey NJ. The painful heel: a controlled trial of the value of hydrocortisone. Br Med J (Clin Res) 1956;1:1277–1278.
61. Leach R, Jones R, Silva T. Rupture of the plantar fascia in athletes. J Bone Joint Surg 1978;60A:537–539.
62. Leach RE, Seavey MS, Salter DK. Results of surgery in athletes with plantar fasciitis. Foot Ankle 1986;7:156–161.
63. Lutter LD. Surgical decisions in athletes' subcalcaneal pain. Am J Sports Med 1986;14:481–485.
64. Lester DK, Buchanan JR. Surgical treatment of plantar fasciitis. Clin Orthop 1984;186:202–204.
65. Brodsky AE, Khalil MA. Talar compression syndrome. Foot Ankle 1987;7:338–344.
66. Steffensen JCA, Evensen A. Bursitis retrocalcanea achilli. Acta Orthop Scand 1958;27:228–236.
67. Heneghan MA, Pavlov H. The Haglund painful heel syndrome. Clin Orthop 1984;1987:228–234.
68. Keck SW, Kelly PJ. Bursitis of the posterior part of the heel. J Bone Joint Surg 1965;47A:267–273.
69. Jahss MH. The sesamoids of the hallux. Clin Orthop 1981;157:88–97.
70. Yeventen EO. Sesamoid disorders and treatment—an update. Clin Orthop 1991;269:236–240.
71. Macnicol MF, Voutsinas S. Surgical treatment of the symptomatic accessory navicular. J Bone Joint Surg 1984;66B:218–226.
72. Ferkel RD, Reid M. Foot and ankle rehabilitation. In: Ferkel RD. Arthroscopic surgery: the foot and ankle. Philadelphia: JB Lippincott, in press.

SUGGESTED READINGS

Drez D Jr, Guhl JF, Gollehon DL. Ankle arthroscopy: technique and indications. Foot Ankle 1981;2:138–143.

Kvist M, Jozsa L, Jarvinen MJ, et al. Chronic Achilles paratenonitis in athletes: a histological and histochemical study. Pathology 1987;19:1–11.

Martin DF, Baker CL, Curl WW, et al. Operative ankle arthroscopy: long term follow-up. Am J Sports Med 1989;17:16–23.

McCarroll Jr, Schrader JW, Shelbourne KD, et al. Meniscoid lesions of the ankle in soccer players. Am J Sports Med 1987;15:255–257.

Orava S, Karpakka J, Hulkko A, Takala T. Stress avulsion fracture of the tarsal navicular. Am J Sports Med 1991;19:392–395.

Puddu G, Ippolito E, Postacchini F. A classification of Achilles tendon disease. Am J Sports Med 1976;4:145–150.

Quirk R. Talar compression syndrome in dancers. Foot Ankle 1982;3:65.

Stormont DM, Morrey BF, An K, et al. Stability of the loaded ankle: relation between articular restraint and primary and secondary static restraints. Am J Sports Med 1985;13:295–300.

Yates CK, Grana WA. A simple distraction technique for ankle arthroscopy. Arthroscopy 1988;4:103–105.

56 / ABDOMINAL INJURIES

Christine E. Haycock

Abdominal injuries to the athlete are not frequent, but they represent a significant number of deaths that are sports related. Because the majority of these injuries present as blunt trauma, they may not be recognized immediately on the playing field, hence the need for constant awareness of the potential danger they present by the team physician, trainer, and coach. Penetrating abdominal injuries occur in sports such as skiing, bicycle riding, and automobile racing and are usually obvious even to the untrained spectator, so that they normally receive immediate treatment.

The modern sports physician, trainer, and coach are generally well-aware of the possibility of abdominal injuries because of specialized sports medicine courses now available; but in many areas, because of financial difficulties, such well-trained individuals are not available, and the burden falls on a local family physician or on emergency medical personnel to treat the athlete. It is their responsibility to recognize what may be subtle signs of internal abdominal injury. Delay in recognition of such injuries can have fatal consequences (1).

Mechanisms of Injury

The abdomen can withstand the majority of blows received in the course of normal contact sports, because of the protection afforded by the bony pelvis below, the ribs above, and the musculoaponeuotic structures attached to them (Fig. 56.1). The degree to which the muscles and bones protect the internal abdominal structures depend on a number of factors. Among these are the force of the blow, the angle it strikes, how well-developed the muscles are, and whether penetration through the muscles occurs.

Most injuries are caused either by two athletes colliding (Fig. 56.2) or by a player being struck by a moving object (2). The velocity of the collision or the striking object is the most important factor, the second being the mass. This is based on the kinetic energy formula: $F=MV^2$. Obviously, if the collision is with a stationary object, the athlete will absorb the full force of the impact, and the injury may be greater than if the blow results from contact with another player.

The most commonly injured viscera is this type of trauma are the solid organs: the kidneys, spleen, liver, and pancreas. The spleen and kidneys represent the majority of such injuries, but the exact percentages vary by sport. The spleen is the most vulnerable, for example, in football, while boxers frequently suffer kidney injuries. These organs are relatively fragile and fixed in location, thus they are subject to acceleration or deceleration injuries, which can strip their capsules, disrupt their vascular supplies at the pedicles, tear off their peritoneal attachments, or fracture them.

Fortunately injury to the pancreas is rare because of its deep location. If such an injury does occur, it carries a high mortality rate. The mechanism in this type of injury with blunt trauma is a direct solar plexus blow that impinges the pancreas against the vertebrae, thus fracturing or crushing it (3). Such cases have been reported in children who crash their bicycles into objects and are thrown against the end of the handlebar (Fig. 56.3) (4). Hollow viscera injury is not common, because most of the gut is mobile and can role with the blow. The fixed areas such as the duodenum, the first part of the jejunum, and the cecum are more vulnerable. Rupture of the stomach, small and large intestines, and urinary bladder can occur with a sudden increase in intraabdominal pressure from a blow (5), a squeeze (6), or deceleration. There have been some unusual cases of ruptured stomachs reported caused by barometric pressure changes in scuba divers (7). A stomach full of food, or a distended urinary bladder are more injury prone, because they cannot absorb the force of a blow without bursting. Children tend to be more prone to intestinal injury than adults, because abdominal musculature is not strong enough to resist blows.

Hemorrhage is most likely to occur from damage to the vascular areas of the solid organs or from lacerations of the mesentary or mesocolon, but it is rarely

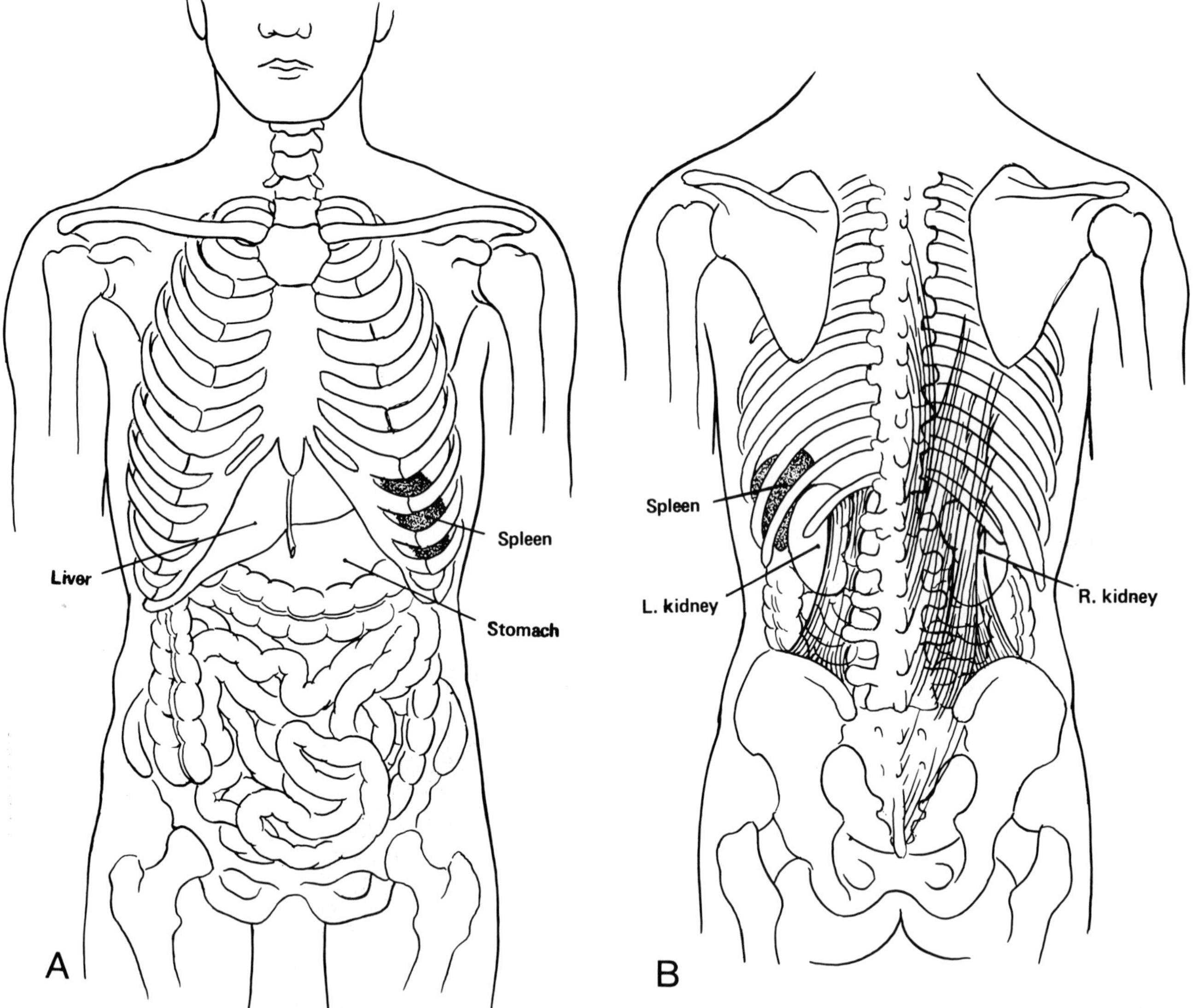

Figue 56.1. The solid abdominal viscera are fragile and easily injured but are well-protected by the musculoaponeurotic and skeletal components of the abdominal parietes. **A,** Anterior view. **B,** Posterior view.

from major vessel injuries in blunt trauma. In penetrating injuries, any structure can be damaged, including blood vessels as well as the urinary bladder and female reproductive organs, which are normally well-protected by the bony pelvis. Fractures of the ribs or pelvis may occur with or without injury to the adjacent organs, and conversely, they may not be injured by direct blows that damage internal structures impacted against them (Fig. 56.2).

Recognition of Injury

Penetrating wounds are obvious to the eye and do require immediate treatment but not always operative intervention. They may range from contusions and abrasions, to lacerations requiring closure, to intraabdominal wounds necessitating operative exploration (8, 9).

Blunt injuries are more difficult to diagnose and may escape initial detection. An astute observer who is trained to suspect possible serious injury should be present at the sports activity. What may seem to be a trivial blow to the abdomen in a collision, for example, can result in a fractured spleen or worse, depending on the way the injury occurred. Questions to ask include the following: Were the players concerned running? Was one stationary? Was a helmeted head involved? In addition, the athlete must be carefully questioned and examined at the time the injury occurs and then followed during (if he or she continues to participate) the game as well as afterward. If there is any question at all regarding the possibility of internal injury, the athlete must be taken immediately to a medical facility for further examination and testing. Failure to do so could result in an extremely serious situation or even death.

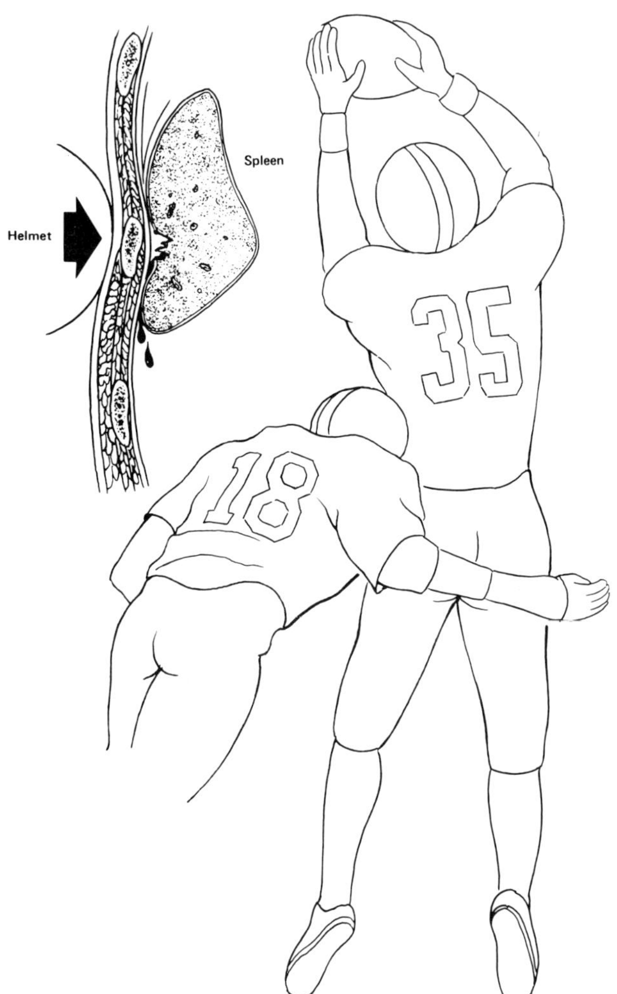

Figure 56.2. A direct blow may rupture a viscus without bony fracture. Hemorrhage may be slow and subtle or massive.

Initial Management

Management of the injured athlete begins on the playing field, whether that is a ski slope, a racetrack, or a stadium. In addition to, or perhaps in many cases instead of, a physician, a well-trained emergency medical squad is invaluable. The squad should have the responsibility of removing the injured athlete from the point of injury and transferring him or her to the proper medical facility. The emergency medical personnel are trained to administer CPR as required, ensure a proper airway, control external hemorrhage, and stabilize fractures.

The decision to remove the injured athlete from the playing field to a hospital should be based on observations made at the site, including state of consciousness, rapidity of pulse, pallor, difficulty breathing, inability to move or sense an extremity, obvious deformity indicating fracture or suspected fracture (especially of the cervical spine), or severe pain. Many professional teams have sophisticated equipment, including portable x-ray equipment in the trainer's room. But this is seldom available to the amateur athlete, so when in doubt, it is

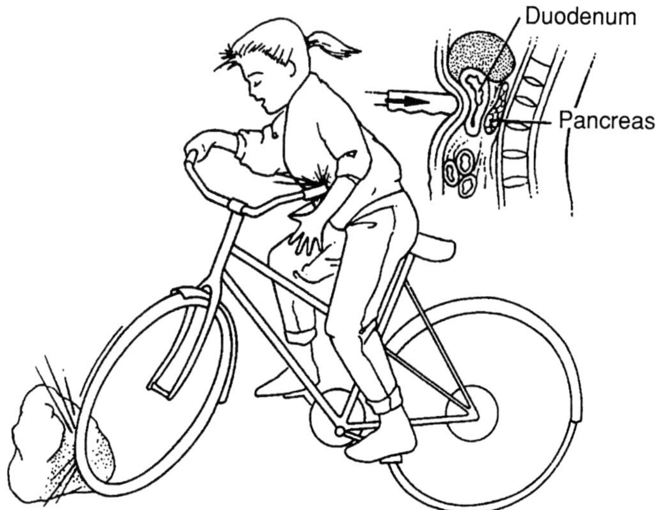

Figure 56.3. In bicycle handlebar trauma, force is applied to the abdominal and retroperitoneal structures, particularly the duodenum and pancreas, compressing them against the spinal column. Reprinted by permission from Valentine MW. Bicycle handlebar injuries in children. Emerg Med 1988;20:37.

best to err on the side of over caution and transport the athlete to the hospital. For example, it is not uncommon for the spleen to undergo a delayed rupture, hence the athlete who sustains a blow to the left upper abdomen or lower left rib cage is best transported if any of the above-mentioned signs are present (10–12).

Renal injuries might be suspected from a blow to the area followed by flank pain. One simple test at the site is to have the athlete void, and then look for blood in urine by sight and with a dip stick. If the first test is negative, wait 10 min and have the player void again, as a full bladder may preclude initial detection of blood. Hospital observation is indicated if positive. Recognition of injury to the duodenum or pancreas is not easily made in the early stages of the injury, so if a severe blow to the epigastrium is sustained followed by any persistent pain, hospitalization is advised. Just as with the spleen, delayed recognition of injury to the colon may also occur (13). Liver injuries may be suspected by blows to the right upper quadrant followed by immediate sharp pain that persists, but unless the liver is deeply lacerated, little bleeding may result, so no signs of shock may be manifest. If such signs are present, very rapid transport to a hospital is mandatory, as bleeding can be massive.

In the event of suspected intraabdominal injury as evidenced by signs of shock such as a rapid and thready pulse, low blood pressure, pallor, diaphoresis, abdominal pain with guarding, and faintness, the ambulance personnel should radio ahead to ensure the presence of a trained surgeon at the emergency department if it is not a trauma center (14).

Once at the hospital, a definitive examination is begun to assess vital signs further for indications of internal bleeding, blood is drawn for baseline blood studies (minimally complete blood count, blood chemistries, and blood typing and or cross-matching if bleeding appears obvious), and large-bore intravenous lines are placed as indicated with Ringer's lactate solution running.

If other injuries are present in addition to the suspected abdominal trauma, these must be dealt with appropriately as indicated. Special attention should be directed to suspected rib or pelvic fractures as these may be contributing to underlying abdominal injuries.

If the patient is able to communicate and time permits, a careful medical history should be obtained for allergies, previous abdominal surgery, and any medications the athlete may be taking for diseases such as diabetes. When splenic injury is suspected, special emphasis should be placed on the possibility that the athlete may have had mononucleosis within the past few years, as studies have found that as many as 44% of splenic injuries in sports are related to this disease (15, 16).

If examination suggests that intraabdominal hemorrhage exists, this may be confirmed quickly by peritoneal lavage or laparoscopy, which is now being used in the major trauma centers. The presence of gross blood would indicate immediate transfer of the patient to the operating room for exploratory laparotomy. If the lavage fluid return has a red blood count in excess of 100,000 mm^3 or a white cell count of over 500 mm^3, an intraabdominal injury should be suspected. A lower count is probably a negative finding. The test is considered about 95% accurate (17–19). If the patient is stable despite the positive test, or if the negative finding is doubted, then additional studies are indicated.

In most major trauma centers today, an immediate computerd tomography (CT) scan of such a patient would be the next step to determine the type and extent of injury of the nonurgent patient (20). Lacerations of the solid organs and retroperitoneal hemorrhage are readily visualized, and the extent of the injury can be determined as well as the presence of free blood in the abdomen (Fig. 56.4). If the injury appears minimal, especially for splenic lacerations in children, an observational approach may be taken to preserve this important organ. The use of contrast enhancement with the CT scan can ascertain vessel abnormalities and ruptured hollow organs and aid in diagnosing urinary extravasation.

If a CT scan is not available, ultrasound examination may be of some value in determining the need for laparotomy, but it is not as reliable (5). Flat or upright x-rays of the abdomen are of value only if they show free air under the diaphragm, indicating a possible ruptured viscus, or indicate an overall haziness, confirming a large quantity of blood. When kidney or urinary bladder injury is suspected, an intravenous pyelogram will provide valuable information. If the patient's condition permits, a chest x-ray is valuable to ascertain the status of the lungs and to determine if fractured ribs are present. Not infrequently free air in the abdomen under the diaphragm is better visualized by a chest film than an abdominal film. Although magnetic resonance imaging (MRI) can give good soft tissue views, it is not a practical tool for emergencies. The results of blood

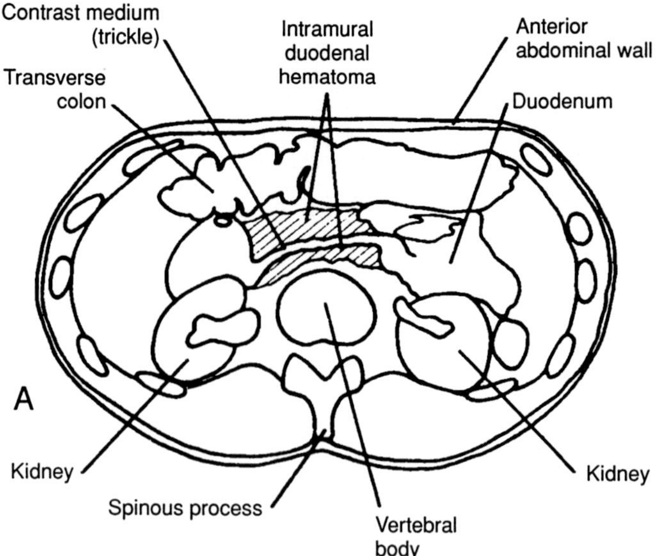

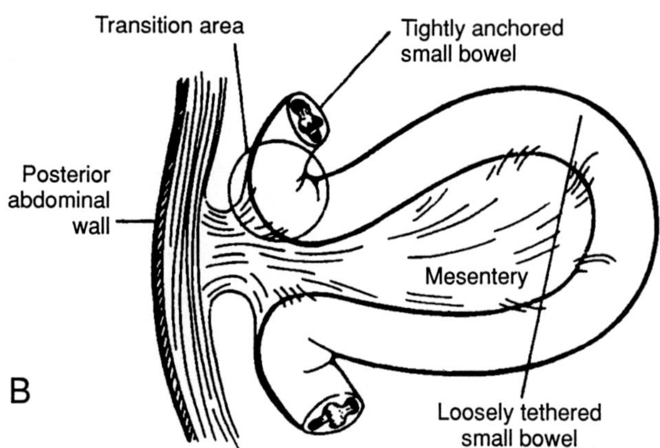

Figure 56.4. A, A cross-section, coronal plane, cephalad view of a CT scan of the abdomen showing an intramural duodenal hematoma, resulting from a football injury. **B,** The transition area of the duodenum between the tightly anchored and loosely tethered attachments of the small bowel to the mesentary. This transition area becomes stressed when an athlete is stopped suddenly, which can happen in football, cycling, or equestrian events. Reprinted by permission of MacGraw-Hill, Inc., from Henderson JM, Puffer JC. Abdominal pain in a football player. Phys Sportsmed 1989;17:48.

studies may be of diagnostic value for the patient who is not an immediate surgical candidate. A markedly elevated amylase that persists (21), a dropping hematocrit, or increasing liver enzymes during the observation period may indicate the need for eventual surgery. Other studies using peritoneal lavage fluid may also be helpful (22).

Because of the serious implications of a missed abdominal injury, it is best always to err on the side of over caution when dealing with blunt trauma to an athlete (1).

Penetrating trauma in sports occurs most often by equipment breaking (ski poles, pole vault poles or bars, bicycles, hockey sticks, and fencing foils), by falling (from horses and equipment), and by crashing (of vehicles) (4, 8). Management of these injuries differs from the blunt trauma patient only by the fact that the injury is usually obvious, only the depth of penetration is unknown. The majority of these cases will go directly to the operating room after stabilization for removal of the offending object (if it remains in place it should never be removed at the scene of the accident), debridement, and repair.

The majority of trauma cases with organ penetration will profit by the use of prophylactic antibiotics as will the blunt injury patients with fractured or ruptured organs. The choice of antibiotic used depends on the area of the injury and the surgeon.

The Abdominal Wall

Blows to the abdominal wall may not result in internal injury, but nevertheless can cause some uncomfortable if not serious injuries to the abdominal wall and groin structures. These may become painful and chronic soft tissue complaints such as adductor, psoas, or rectus femoris strains; tendinitis; and overuse syndromes. The pain is generally located in the groin or pubic areas and can be resistive to therapeutic modalities. For the athlete with groin pain that does not respond to physiotherapy, it is important to consider the possibility of hernia or nerve entrapment (12). Several studies reported of such individuals have shown an incidence as high as 49% of inguinal hernias, especially in male athletes. Both indirect and direct hernias have been present; the majority could be repaired, and the athlete returned to his or her sport (23–25).

Increased intraabdominal pressure may also result in an esophageal hiatus hernia. Weight lifters, obese wrestlers, and jumpers can develop this problem. The author has seen two such cases that were initially suspected of being either peptic ulcer disease or angina. The weight lifter had to be advised to discontinue his sport or tolerate the symptoms with medication as best he could. The wrestler was improved by weight loss. It has been shown that the use of a belt by weight lifters, while reducing the compressive forces on the spine, does increase intraabdominal pressure, and this may have been a factor contributing to the development of the hiatal hernia (6, 26).

The attachment of the rectus sheath to the suprapubic area can lead to an osteitis pubis when tears occur in that area. In the female athlete, especially runners, this is not an uncommon phenomena; however, it is important to rule out any underlying pelvic disorder that cause the persistence of pain (25).

Blows also may lead to hemorrhage in the abdominal muscles with resultant large hematomas, especially in the rectus sheath. A simple cross-table lateral x-ray or peritoneal lavage can usually rule out internal extension, and the majority of these lesions respond to conservative therapy. Occasionally, an expanding hematoma may require evacuation and ligation of the offending artery. One oddity reported was an omental mass secondary to a boxing blow that went on to calcify, causing pelvic pain sufficient to require operative removal (27).

Solid Organ Injury

Spleen

Solid organ injuries vary in frequency in different sports, but splenic rupture is the most common occurrence. Its anatomical location, just behind and slightly below the lower left ribs, combined with its size and fragile structure make it a vulnerable target, especially in contact sports. If the organ is enlarged as a result of a lymphoma or if the athlete has had mononucleosis (a common disease of young high school or college students), he or she is particularly vulnerable to splenic rupture (28). It is preferable for these individuals to avoid contact sports totally in the first instance, and to wait for at least 6 months after all symptoms have disappeared and blood studies are normal in the latter group. There has been some dispute about the length of time the athlete recovering from mononucleosis needs to avoid contact sports, but because no definitive study exists in this regard, the 6-month ban seems safest for the amateur athlete (and for the legal protection of the sports physician).

Splenic injury may range from a small subcapsular tear to total disruption of the organ (29). All such injuries will result in some degree of hemorrhage, which will manifest itself immediately if the injury is extensive or be delayed if it is initially contained within the splenic capsule. It is the latter case that may be the most dangerous, as treatment can be delayed owing to a missed diagnosis; this could have fatal results. Thus it is important that even the slightest suspicion of a splenic injury be aggressively investigated by peritoneal lavage as a rapid method when it seems obvious, and then followed through by a CT scan when the lavage is questionable or if suspicion remains high despite a negative lavage.

In the past, when severe injury resulted in evidence of shock caused by hypovolemia, the athlete was taken immediately to the operating room, a transfusion was given if blood loss was extreme, and the spleen was removed. Fortunately, in this modern era, that is no longer always the scenario. Because it is now known how important the spleen is to the immune system, especially in the young person, and that it plays a vital part in the body's defense against infection through its role in immunoglobin and opsonin production, every effort is made to preserve this organ. In fact, unless the injury directly involves the splenic pedicle, most spleens can be salvaged by use of coagulents such as microfibrillar collagen and topical thrombin combined with hemostatic suturing; the spleen may even be wrapped in mesh (Fig. 56.5).

The routine use of prophylactic antibiotics is advisable in any intraabdominal organ injury whether splenectomy is performed or not. Although the splenectomized patient is more prone to infection, there is always the immediate possibility in any intraabdominal trauma, hence at least 48-hr i.v. coverage is advised. The use of polyvalent pneumococcal vaccine (Pneumovax) after the recovery of the splenectomized patient is still advised as protection in later life against some se-

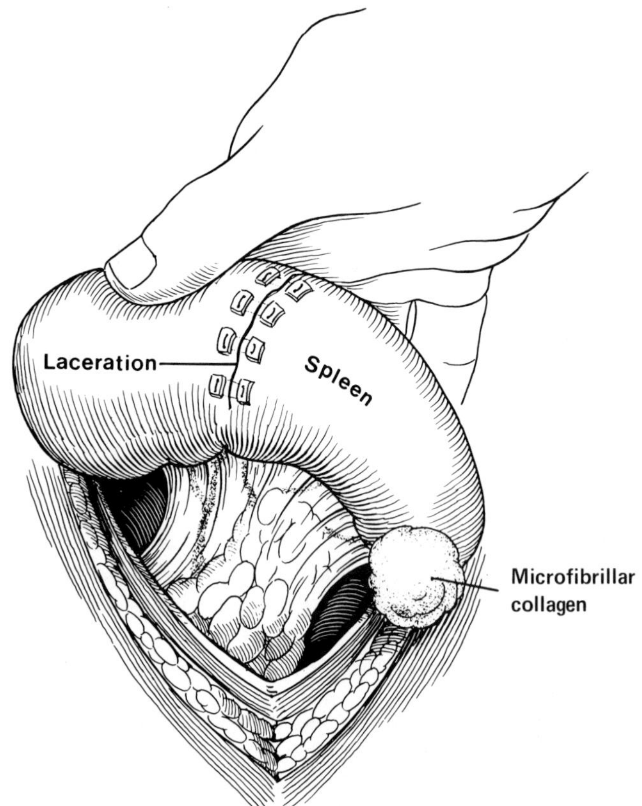

Figure 56.5. Fulminant sepsis is a rare but highly lethal late complication of splenectomy. Accordingly, splenic repair is attempted when feasible. Bleeding from larger vessels can be controlled with ligation or partial splenectomy, and bothersome oozing often is controlled with hemostatic agents such as microfibrillar collagen.

rotypes of pneumococci, and revaccination every 3 years is suggested. Because this athlete has impaired immune responses, any potential infective injury or procedure should be covered by appropriate antibiotics.

The potential of the AIDS virus being present in transfused blood, however remote, has made the routine use of transfusions less frequent. If the patient can be adequately sustained on electrolyte solutions such as Ringer's lactate, blood is administered only if blood loss is severe. The majority of athletes are generally in good physiologic condition when injured and can sustain considerable blood loss and maintain a hemodynamic balance with electrolyte solutions. The hemoglobin can then be restored by iron preparations in the postoperative course. However, this is an individual decision that must be made in each case.

Kidney

Almost as frequently injured as the spleen is the kidney, especially in sports such as soccer, horseback riding, skiing and boxing (1, 4, 11). American football players wear protective gear not used by their European counterparts that tends to reduce renal injury.

Symptomatically these patients usually present initially with relatively mild tenderness in the upper abdomen or flank and gross or microscopic hematuria. This then progresses to frank swelling and evidence of hypotension and increasing pain. This scenario generally leads to open exploration. Kidney salvage, if at all possible, is the aim of the surgeon.

In less obvious cases, CT scan is the choice for diagnosis when available, however an intravenous pylegram (IVP) may reveal the extent of the problem, especially if extravasation is present. Ultrasound imaging may also help, and angiography can be used, especially to define the extent of vascular disruption.

In many cases, renal injuries can be managed by conservative treatment, including bed rest, i.v. fluids, antibiotics, and careful observation. Most cases of microscopic hematuria merely indicate a mild contusion of the kidney. After a marathon run, the participants (it has been reported to have occurred in 18% in one study) may be found to have a transient hematuria as well as dysuria, a finding that, unless it recurs repeatedly, does not usually require investigation. In males it is felt to be caused by the impact of the base of the bladder and trigone against the prostate. Increased fluid intake to resolve any existing dehydration from the run, and a few days of rest from running are generally sufficient to resolve the problem (14). Ureter or urethral injuries are rare in sports, but the latter may occasionally be encountered in bicycling or straddle falls on bars in gymnastics.

Liver

Blunt trauma to the liver, despite its size, is not as frequent or serious in sports as experienced in high-speed vehicular accidents (1). About 50% of the injuries found are simply capsular tears or superficial parenchymal lacerations. The liver is a resilient organ and bleeding may be minimal and self-limited. If the injury is severe with massive bleeding caused by deep lacerations or rupture—as might occur in a fall from a horse, a collision of a skier with a tree, or to a auto race driver—immediate surgery is required. Such an injury may be fatal if the large vessels such as the vena cava, portal veins, or hepatic arteries are involved, but with recent advances in liver resection techniques, most liver trauma can be repaired by use of hemostatic agents, suturing, or resection of the severely fractured portion. Fortunately, the liver has excellent regenerative abilities so that survival with just a portion of the liver is possible.

The use of CT scanning can often determine the extent of the injury, and if the athlete is hemodynamically stable, no explorative surgery may be necessary. Occasionally, angiography can be employed as an adjunct to rule out active bleeding when doubt exists, but in such situations a paracentesis showing bright red blood is a better determinate. When the doubt cannot be resolved then surgical exploration is necessary.

It must be kept in mind that although bleeding may not be a problem, bile leakage can be. The onset of fever, nausea, and signs of peritoneal irritation that was not present initially but developed over a period of hours or days must arouse strong suspicion of bile peritonitis in the liver-injured athlete, whether exploratory surgery has been done or not. Even later, symptoms of jaundice and acholic stools may occur. It is very important during laparotomy when liver lacerations are found that careful examination of the duodenum by a Kocher maneuver is performed and that the entire extrahepatic biliary system is inspected.

The appearance of liver cysts with the use of anabolic steroids has given rise to some supposition that this might increase the vulnerability of the liver to injury. However, in general, liver cysts seen in the past of a congenital or disease origin have not led to increased trauma and are usually an incidental finding at surgery for some other reason, at least in the Western world. Hepatitis would put the athlete out of action during its acute phases and may result in cirrhosis or liver failure, but if the athlete is merely surface–antigen-antibody positive, there should be no problem after recovery.

Pancreas

Injuries to the pancreas are, fortunately, rare in sports, but failure to recognize the problem could have serious consequences. Signs and symptoms are often slow to appear, especially if other injuries are not present. A pseudocyst found even years later may have resulted from a forgotten blow to the abdomen. A high degree of suspicion must be aroused in the physician, especially when duodenal injury has occurred. Missed injury at exploration may lead to persistent fistulas that are difficult to resolve. Adequate drainage of suspected injury when none can be visualized is a wise course (30, 31).

Surgical treatment of a lacerated pancreas may require resection of the injured portion with implantation (Peaustow pancreaticojejunostomy with Roux-en-Y anastomosis) into the small bowel to allow drainage. Fortunately, minor lacerations that do not disrupt the pancreatic duct can be managed with suturing and adequate drainage, as can contusions.

Elevated amylase levels do not always occur, especially early because of transient secretory inhibition. Serial levels showing a rise with time are probably of help in questionable cases.

Hollow Viscera Injury

Small Bowel

Injury to the duodenum was mentioned in conjunction with liver and pancreatic injuries, but it may occur as an isolated injury. Unlike the ileum and most of the jejunum, the second and third parts of the duodenum are held in a fixed position, making them vulnerable to contusions caused by impaction against the vertebral column. A resulting hematoma in the duodenum may go unrecognized until vomiting, indicating a high obstruction, appears. If injury of the mesentary occurs adjacent to the wall of the bowel, some of the small vessels along the wall may be compromised, leading to necrosis and perforation several weeks after the injury and resultant peritonitis with serious consequences. Children, especially, should be carefully observed for such a possibility following injury.

For both pancreas and duodenum, CT scanning is essential for diagnosis as peritoneal lavage may be negative, and x-rays are of little value. Duodenal and occasional ileal or jejunal injuries usually occur when a narrow instrument such as a ski pole, a hockey stick, or a bike handle is the culprit. These injuries tend to be more prevalent in child athletes because of less-developed abdominal musculature (4).

Retroperitoneal hematomas have been reported after being seen by ultrasound or CT scan associated with duodenal and, occasionally, pancreatic injuries. If the patient is hemodynamically stable and exploration is deemed unnecessary, these hematomas normally resolve spontaneously. Even on exploration, it is usually best to leave them undisturbed unless they appear to be expanding.

Colon

Except for an occasional cecal injury, blunt trauma to the colon in athletes is a rarity. In addition to the gear worn in contact sports and rules prohibiting blows beneath the waist in sports such as boxing, the bony pelvis provides good protection not only to the colon but to the genitourinary structures as well.

Injury to the colon in blunt trauma may go unrecognized until signs of peritonitis develop, so if the athlete has sustained a lower abdominal injury in a high-speed motorcycle race, for example, a CT scan is essential, and laparotomy is done if a suspicious area is seen (11).

Diarrhea following a long-distance run is a common phenomena in marathoners, and occasionally this may be bloody. However, in the reported cases, extensive workups that include colonostomy and barium studies usually show nothing of importance. Occasionally, a colitis, a polyp, or in the older athlete a previously nonsymptomatic carcinoma has been found. It is probably wise always to work up the athlete who has bloody diarrhea, even though hemorrhoids or a rectal fissure is the usual finding.

The Surgical Wound

The first thing the athlete who sustains an abdominal injury wants to know is when he or she can return to participation in his or her chosen sport. If no surgical procedure is involved, all evidence of the internal injury must be absent and proven by follow-up studies. The return is determined by the type of sport involved. Obviously, return to a collision-type sport must follow a more conservative course than a noncollision type. This is a judgment call that must be made on an individual basis by the physician. For example, a football player sustaining a duodenal hematoma treated by observation should not return to football, but the same athlete could participate in basketball and baseball later in the year.

Wound healing depends on the overall status of the patient's health. Chronically ill patients heal poorly and wounds may disrupt. Fortunately, the athlete is generally in good physical condition, and the strength of the abdominal wall—which depends on basically three

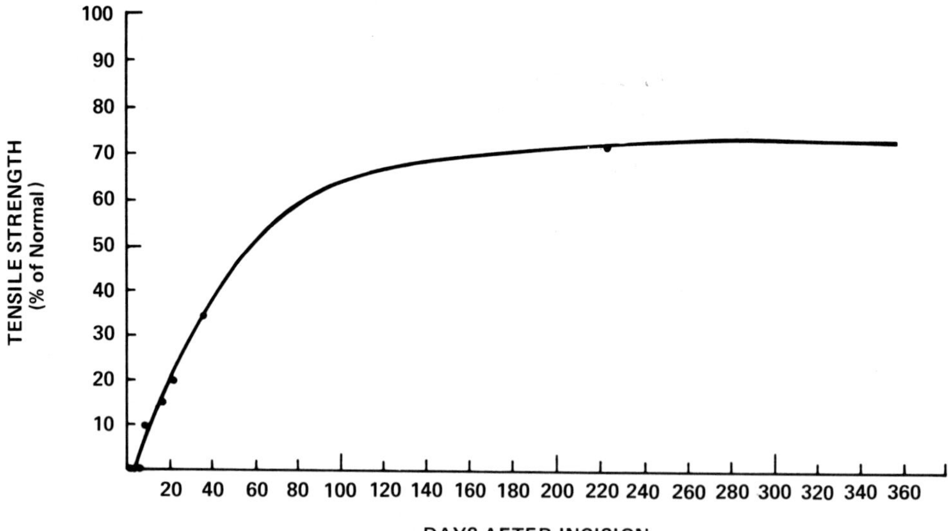

Figure 56.6. Tensil strength of healing wounds of the aponeurosis in relation to postoperative time. Modified from Douglas DM. The healing of aponeurotic incisions. Br J Surg 1952;40:79.

muscles (the internal and external oblique and the transverse abdominis) and their flat tendons (aponeuroses)—is above average. The skin and subcutaneous fascia along with some adipose tissues add a little support (28).

Midline abdominal incisions in uncomplicated cases require adequate time to heal, usually a minimum of 8 weeks for return to noncontact sports and 12 for contact sports. McBurney-type appendectomy incisions, because they split but do not cut the muscles, require less time away from sports participation. The healing wound can be disrupted by muscle contraction occurring at right angles to the aponeurotic incision in the midline or by abdominal distension and increased intraabdominal pressure. Coughing or straining can disrupt a poorly repaired incision or one in which healing is impaired by infection. If that has occurred, the athlete might be forced to remain inactive for an even longer period of time.

Hernia repairs, depending on the type and approach, may cause a loss of time of 2 to 6 weeks. With the advent of laparoscopic repairs, this time may decrease.

The tensile strength of healing wounds has been studied over the years and can be used as a guide in the decision to allow the athlete to return to participation (32, 33) (Fig. 56.6). Obvious complications such as wound infection, dehiscense, repeat explorations, or ventral hernias will greatly extend this elapsed time, and require individualized decisions.

The athlete with a midline incision can begin a supervised rehabilitation program in as little as 1 week. The program must ensure that no stress is placed on the abdominal wound during the first 3 weeks of healing, but the extremities can be exercised and conditioned.

The athlete is usually anxious to return to sport activity, but this desire must not be allowed to cause him or her to return too soon and cause further injury. The athlete, for the sake of his or her future, must not be allowed to make these decisions without professional guidance. The athlete should be carefully counseled as to the reasons why return to a sport requires adequate time or is delayed.

References

1. Haycock C. How I manage abdominal injuries. Phys Sportsmed 1986;14:86–99.
2. du Troit DF, Rademan F. Splenic rupture caused by a cricket ball. A case report. S Afr Med J 1987:796.
3. Speakman M. Gastric and pancreatic rupture due to a sports injury. Minn Med 1983;66:93–96.
4. Valentine MW. Bicycle handlebar injuries in children. Emerg Med 1988;20:37–42.
5. Foley LC. Ultrasound of epigastric injuries after blunt trauma. Am J Roentgenol 1979;132:593–598.
6. Harman EA, Rosenstein RM, Frykman, Nigro GA. Effects of a belt on intra-abdominal pressure during weight lifting. Med Sc Sports Exerc 1989;21:186–190.
7. Halpern P. Rupture of the stomach in a diving accident with attempted resuscitation. A case report. Br J Anesth 1986;58:1059–1061.
8. Carragher AM, Sulaiman SK, Panesar KJ. Scroto-abdominal impalement injury in a skateboard rider. J Emerg Med 1990;8:419–421.
9. Lanng C, Winther-Nielsen, Hougen HP. Intraperitoneal granulomatous foreign body reaction after accidental perforation of the abdominal wall. Case report. Acta Chir Scand 1988;154:683–684.
10. Mohanlal M. Anyone for tennis? Aust Fam Phys 1988;17:916.
11. Diamond DL. Sports-related abdominal trauma. Clin Sports Med 1989;21:91–99.
12. Balduini FC. Abdominal and groin injuries in tennis. Clin Sports Med 1988;7:349–357.
13. Lifschutz H, Kaufman CS. Delayed colon perforation in blunt abdominal trauma. Contem Surg 1983;22:93–100.
14. Kenney P. Abdominal pain in athletes. Clin Sports Med 1987;6:885–904.
15. Olsen WR, Polley TZ Jr. A second look at delayed splenic rupture. Arch Surg 1977;112:422–425.
16. Frelinger DP. The ruptured spleen in college athletes: a preliminary report. J Am Col Health Assoc 1978;26:217.

17. Root HD, Hauser CW, McKinley CR, LaFave JW, Mendoil RP Jr. Diagnostic peritoneal lavage. Surgery 1965;57:633–637.
18. Haycock CE, Machiedo G. The use of peritoneal lavage as a diagnostic tool in emergencies. J Am Col Emerg Phys 1974;3:397–400.
19. Olsen WR, Redeman HC, Hildreth DH. Quantitative peritoneal lavage in blunt abdominal trauma. Arch Surg 1972;104:536–539.
20. Olsen WR. The serum amylase in blunt abdominal trauma. J Trauma 1973;13:200–204.
21. Henderson JM, Puffer JC. Abdominal pain in a football player. Sportsmed 1989;17:47–52.
22. McAnena OJ, Marx JA, Moore EE. Contributions of peritoneal lavage enzyme determinations to the management of isolated hollow visceral abdominal injuries. Ann Emeg Med 1991;20–834–837.
23. Eckberg O, Persson NH, Abrahamsson PA, Westlin NE, Lilja B. Longstanding groin pain in athletes. A multidisciplinary approach. Sport Med 1988;6:56–61.
24. Zimmerman G. Groin pain in athletes. J Aust Fam Phys 1988;17:1046–1052.
25. Smedberg SG, Broome AE, Gullmo A. Roos H. Herniorraphy in athletes with groin pain. 1985;149:378–382.
26. Harmon EA, Rosenstein M, Frykman PN, Clagett ER, Kraemer WJ. Intra-abdominal and intra-thoracic pressures during lifting and jumping. Med Sci Sports Med 1988;20:195–201.
27. Doris PE, Johnston CC. Large calcified mass in a boxer. Am J Sports Med 1982;10:117–121.
28. Rutkow IM. Rupture of the spleen in infectious mononucleosis. A critical review. Arch Surg 1978;113:718–721.
29. Hughes JH. Unusual intra-abdominal bleeding [Letter to the Editor]. Ann Emerg Med 1980;132:647–648.
30. Majeski JA, Tyler G. Pancreatic trauma. Am Surg 1980;10:593–596.
31. Jordan LJ Jr. Pancreatic trauma. Contemp Surg 1985;26:11–17.
32. Van Winkle W Jr. The tensile strength of wounds and factors that influence it. Surg Gynecol Obstet 1969;129:819–823.
33. Mason ML, Allen HS. The rate of healing of tendons: An experimental study of tensile strength. Ann Surg 1941;113:424–427.

57 / CHEST INJURIES

Claire Chase and Stephen Z. Turney

Chest trauma is common in the United States, ranking third in incidence behind head and extremity injuries. The Major Trauma Outcome Study, reviewing nationwide data as of September 1987, reported a 30.6% incidence of chest injury in all types of trauma patients (1). A total of 10% were caused by a blunt mechanism. The chest wall was injured in 50% of these patients, pneumothorax or hemothorax was present in 45%, and pulmonary injury occurred in 26% of patients. Less common were cardiac (9%) and aortic/great vessel injuries (4%).

Although the most common cause of blunt chest trauma is the motor vehicle accident, many contact sports involve enough force to produce significant injury to the chest. The three most common mechanisms of injury to the thorax are acceleration/deceleration, compression, and high-speed impact. Acceleration/deceleration involves the delay in inertia of visceral organs compared with the skeletal inertia, resulting in injury to the viscera. This type of injury is typically seen in motor vehicle accidents, although any rapid change in velocity can be the cause. Compression injuries occur when the force applied to the chest exceeds the strength of the chest wall, as in falls or crush injury. High-speed impact entails injury produced by a projectile or blunt object impacting against a discrete area of a stationary body.

Chest Wall

The chest wall has two major functions: to protect and support the organs within it and to contribute to ventilatory efforts. To generate a greater negative intrathoracic pressure or inspiration, the thoracic cavity must expand. The intercostal muscles contract, causing an upward, outward movement of the chest wall. This, along with the descent of the diaphragm, is a principal factor in the maintenance of the ventilatory pump. Even relatively minor injuries such as rib fractures can cause a significant morbidity. The chest wall structures in their protective/supportive role can also absorb much of the energy directed to the thorax; fractures of these structures can provide a clue to the presence of massive forces and possible injury to internal viscera. These structures tend to be more compliant and flexible in the younger athlete, so that fracture may not occur, despite forces sufficient to damage seriously intrathoracic organs.

Rib Fractures

Rib fractures are the most common chest injuries and the most commonly fractured ribs are in the middle level, or the fourth through the seventh ribs. In the past, considerable efforts were made to diagnose each possible rib fracture radiographically. This resulted in a substantial expenditure of time and finance. With recent interest in cost containment, several studies have examined the efficacy of this practice (2–4).

The priorities of therapy are directed toward life-threatening intrathoracic injuries (e.g., pneumothorax, hemothorax, and pulmonary contusion) that can be detected on an anterior-posterior (AP) chest radiograph. The treatment for isolated rib fractures is analgesia alone. Therefore, special views to detect additional rib fractures are a waste of resources, as they will not change therapy.

There are notable exceptions to this rule: multiple rib fractures, especially in elderly patients or those with chronic lung disease, can cause serious difficulties in ventilation. These patients usually need to be admitted to the hospital for aggressive pulmonary care, even if the rib fractures are an isolated injury.

Another special circumstance that received considerable attention in recent years is fracture of the first rib. Because of the protected location and broad, thick dimensions of the first rib, it was assumed that a large amount of force is needed to fracture it. Thus the injury may serve as a "sentinel" to aortic rupture. Also, because of its close proximity to the lung and critical neurovascular structures, it was assumed that the ends of a fractured first rib have a greater likelihood to cause local serious damage (5). Routine angiography in all patients with first rib fracture (6) has given way to more selective use of contrast studies (7, 8). Current diagnostic protocols generally reserve arteriograms for the patient with documented upper extremity vascular or neurologic deficits, or other signs of aortic injury (discussed below).

Less well-documented in the literature but of comparable special concern are fractures of the lower ribs, especially on the left side. Because the energy needed to break the ribs overlying the spleen or liver could have been transmitted to the solid viscera, special care in the evaluation for intraabdominal injury is warranted in these patients.

Flail Chest

The term *flail chest* is used to describe the injury in which a segment of ribs has been isolated from the remainder of the chest wall secondary to multiple rib fractures. This segment is displaced outwardly during expiration (and inwardly during inspiration) in contrast to the rest of the thorax. Diagnosis is made on physical examination during respiration and may not be obvious initially. The understanding of the significance of the flail segment has changed over the past few decades. The typically serious respiratory difficulties encountered in patients with flail chest were at first hypothesized to be purely a result of futile pendulum-like exchange of air from one lung to another. Termed *pendelluft*, this theory fell into disfavor after such ventilatory movements could not be demonstrated in animal models (9). Currently, more importance is placed on the underlying pulmonary contusion to explain the respiratory manifestations of flail chest (10). However, factors related purely to ventilatory dysfunction such as retained secretions and atelectasis secondary to rib pain and splinting should not be discounted and need to be addressed in the care of the patient with flail chest. (Fig. 57.1).

Just as the knowledge of the pathophysiology of flail chest has undergone an evolution, so has the therapy of the injury. Mandatory prolonged mechanical ventilation for internal splinting, the standard of care for many years, has been gradually replaced by a protocol of selective endotracheal intubation, particularly in the younger, cooperative patient (11, 12). In this management plan, intubation is carried out only if the patient exhibits significant difficulties in oxygenation by arterial blood gas analysis or is in respiratory distress. Otherwise, therapy consists of aggressive pulmonary care and adequate analgesia. Major advancements have been made with the use of epidural narcotics or local anesthetics, providing pain relief while avoiding the respiratory depressive effects of systemic analgesia. This appears to be particularly true with epidural local anesthetics, such as bupivacaine (13).

Scapular Fractures

Another strong, well-protected bone of the thoracic cavity is the scapula. Because of the significant force required to damage it, fracture of the scapula (which is

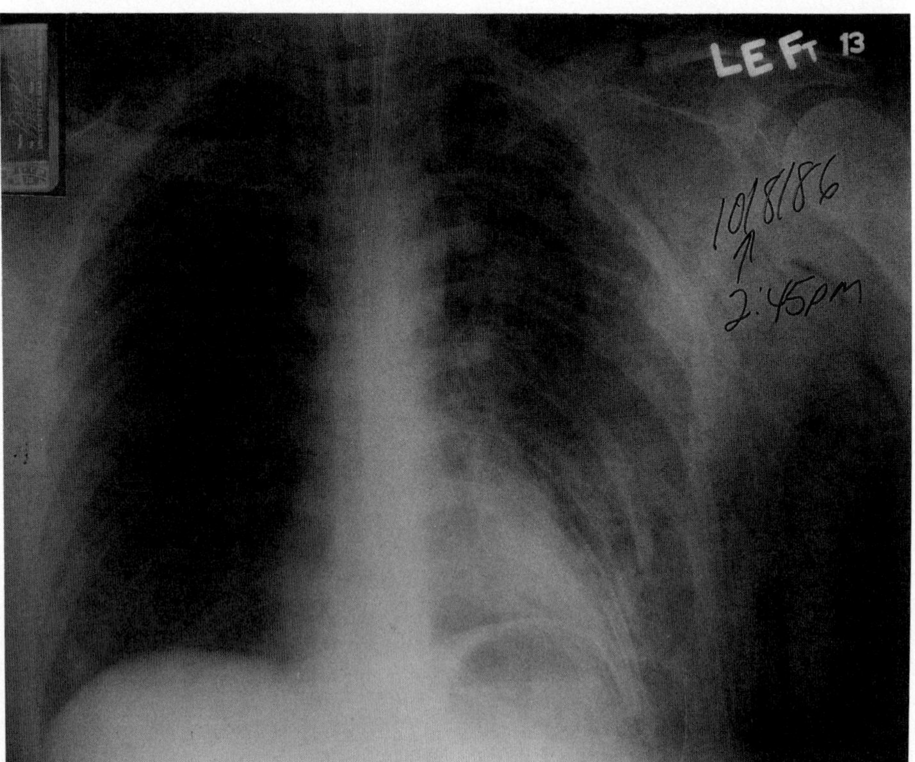

Figure 57.1. Chest film of a patient with left-sided flail chest. Multiple rib fractures and underlying lung contusion are evident. Reprinted by permission from Rodriguez A. Injuries of the chest wall, the lungs and the pleura. In: Turney SZ, Rodriguez A, Cowley RA, eds. Management of cardiothoracic trauma. Baltimore: Williams & Wilkins, 1991.

rare) has been cited as a marker for severe ipsilateral lung and chest wall injury. In one series of 56 patients with scapular fractures, 54% had pulmonary contusions; 12.5% had ipsilateral brachial plexus injuries; and 10.7% had ipsilateral subclavian, axillary, or brachial artery injury (14). Hospital admission is probably warranted, even in isolated scapular fracture, to evaluate for delayed pneumothorax or pulmonary injury. Because of the muscular encasement around the scapula, fractures usually heal without difficulty or permanent disability. However, severely comminuted neck and glenoid fractures occasionally require open reduction with internal fixation. An early program of range-of-motion exercises is essential in all patients with scapular fractures (15).

Sternal Fractures

The majority of sternal fractures occur secondary to motor vehicle accidents, usually related to impact on the steering wheel and possibly related to seat belt use. Much less commonly, the injury occurs after falls on direct blows to the chest. Once regarded as another sentinel injury suggesting possible myocardial contusion or aortic rupture, isolated sternal fracture was, in part, an indication for admission to a monitored unit and aortography. In recent studies, evidence is accumulating to show that there is no statistically significant increase in aortic rib or myocardial contusion in isolated sternal fracture (16, 17). As in the case of isolated first rib fracture, other findings of aortic rib must be present to lead to further diagnostic workup of that serious injury. Most sternal fractures are nondisplaced and require no therapy. The most common sites of fracture are at the junction of the body and manubrium and through the body. Occasionally, open reduction and internal fixation are required.

Costochondral Injuries

Separation of the costochondral or sternochondral articulations is quite common, even with relatively minor trauma to the chest. Pain, which can be severe, may be localized or radiating along the intercostal nerve distribution. Physical examination may reveal increased mobility or point tenderness over the involved articulation. Chest films are not usually helpful in the diagnosis because of the radiolucency of the costal cartilages. Initial management is conservative, with rest and application of local heat being the mainstays of treatment. If pain is persistent, instillation of local anesthetics or intercostal nerve block can be performed. In particularly severe cases, surgical resection of the involved cartilage may be necessary (13).

Clavicular Injuries

Clavicular fractures are common and can occur from either a direct blow to the clavicle or a lateral blow to the shoulders. Approximately 80% of these occur in the middle third of the bone. Most heal without difficulty with a "figure eight" dressing and immobilization. Occasionally, fractures with widely displaced fragments will require operative repair. Also, fragments of bone, especially in the distal third of the bone, may impinge on the subclavian vessels. Rare late side effects of callus formation include thoracic outlet obstruction with neurologic or vascular symptoms (18, 19).

Sternoclavicular dislocation is relatively unusual secondary to the strong ligamentous support of the joint. Anterior dislocation is much more common than posterior displacement. Either can occur from a lateral compression force applied to the shoulders. Posterior dislocation can occur from direct force and rarely results in injury to the underlying trachea and great vessels. The reduction can usually be performed with a closed technique and local anesthesia, although reduction of posterior dislocations may be performed more easily under general anesthesia.

Traumatic Asphyxia

A characteristic clinical syndrome of cyanotic discoloration of the neck and face with petechiae and subconjunctival hemorrhage can occur when a large force is applied to the chest. The cause of the cutaneous changes is thought to be reversal of blood flow through the valveless superior vena cava and jugular veins. Besides the constriction of the chest, an essential element in the pathophysiology of the syndrome appears to be closure of the glottis during full inspiration at the time of injury. Other than rare occurrence of prolonged coma secondary to anoxia, long-term neurologic sequelae do not appear to be significant (20). However, the underlying pulmonary and chest wall injury may be substantial (21). Recognition of the dramatic but benign cutaneous signs should alert the clinician that a careful evaluation for more serious associated injuries is necessary.

Pneumothorax

A pneumothorax results when the normally negative intrathoracic pressure is changed through the disruption of the pleura and air enters the pleural space. This can occur either with penetrating trauma with direct parenchymal injury and air leak or with blunt injuries. In the latter case, pneumothorax can result either from direct impact or from a fragment of fractured rib lacerating the lung.

Although the three types of pneumothorax (namely, tension, open, and simple) all require a tube thoracostomy, the initial approach varies somewhat. By far the most potentially lethal type is a tension pneumothorax, in which a flap valve mechanism allows the accumulation of inspired air in the pleural space without allowing its escape. This can eventually lead to mediastinal compression, hemodynamic compromise, and eventual death if not corrected. Prompt recognition of the physical signs of tension pneumothorax—absent or diminished breath sounds with possible shift of the trachea to the contralateral side, and especially if hypotension is present—should be followed by immediate decompression of the pneumothorax. If tube thoracostomy is not possible at that time, adequate initial treatment can be achieved even with placement of an intravenous catheter in the thorax. A general recommendation is insertion of a 14-gauge catheter into the second intercostal space in the midclavicular line. A rush of air can sometimes be evident, but not always. There is usually rapid improvement in vital signs if the pneumothorax was the major cause of the compromise. This is followed by placement of a tube thoracostomy as soon as it is feasible. Additional diagnostic evaluation may require bronchoscopy if there is persistent large air leak. This is rarely from major tracheobroncheal laceration or rupture.

An open pneumothorax occurs when there is a communication between the pleural cavity and the outside. If the opening is greater than two-thirds the diameter of the trachea, air will begin to flow preferentially through the chest wall defect rather than the trachea. To prevent ventilatory compromise, the wound should be covered and the covering secured on three sides with eventual placement of a chest tube at a site away from the wound. If a fully occlusive dressing is placed on the wound, a chest tube must be inserted promptly to avoid creation of a tension pneumothorax (Fig. 57.2).

A simple pneumothorax, unless it is small and reliable follow-up is possible, also requires a tube thoracostomy. However, this usually can be done with less urgency than in the previous two types of pneumothorax. The placement of chest tube for evacuation of air and/or fluid is now recommended in the fourth or fifth intercostal space in the anterior axillary line, posterior to the border of the pectoralis major muscle. Previous recommendations to use the second intercostal space in the midclavicular line has been abandoned, because of the need for dissection through the pectoralis major muscle and the lack of real benefit of using this position.

When there is a strong suggestion of the presence of a pneumothorax, such as when subcutaneous or mediastinal emphysema is present, but none can be detected on chest film, there are some instances in which insertions of a prophylactic chest tube is warranted. If the patient will not be followed reliably for a while, such as during transport to another facility and during an operative procedure, or if the patient will be maintained on positive pressure ventilation, the presence of the chest tube protects against the development of a tension pneumothorax.

Hemothorax

Hemothorax may result from injury to the great vessels, the bronchial circulation, the lung parenchyma, or the intercostal vessels. Accumulations greater than approximately 300 ml can be detected on chest x-ray. All pleural fluid collections in the acute trauma setting should be drained with a large-bore (at least 36 French) chest tube placed in the fifth intercostal space. This is usually the only treatment needed: bleeding resolves spontaneously, especially if the injury is the low pressure pulmonary vessels (22). However, if initial drainage is greater than 1500 ml, or continues at a rate of

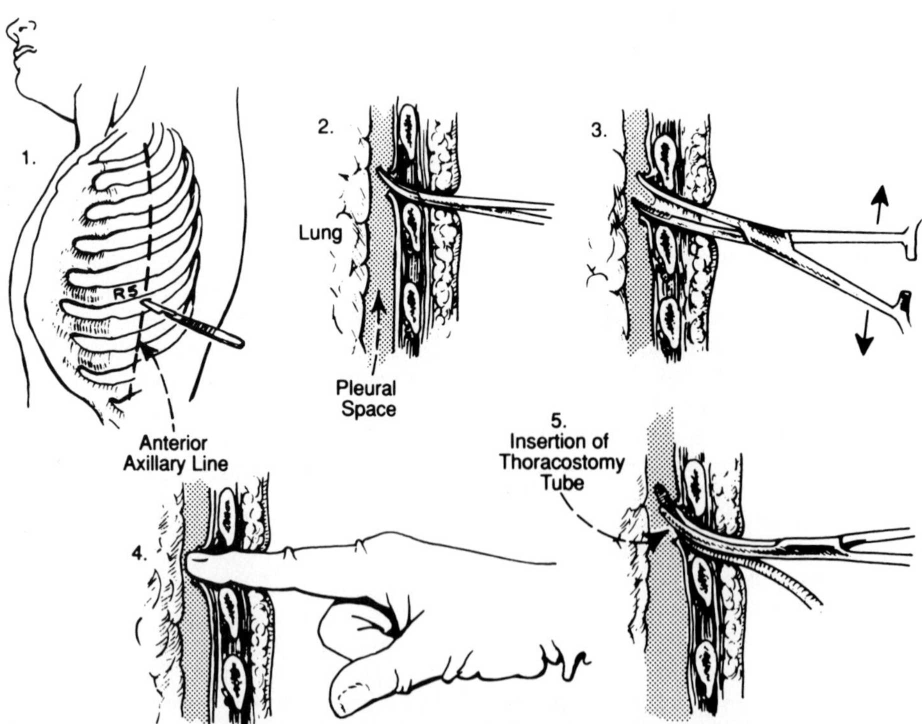

Figure 57.2. Schematic representation of technique for insertion of a chest tube. *1*, Proper location in the fifth intercostal space, anterior axillary line. *2*, Careful blunt dissection and penetration of the pleura with clamp. *3*, Spreading of intercostal tissues with clamp. *4*, Digital dilatation of tube tract and exploration of pleural cavity. *5*, Insertion of tube with clamp. Use of trocar is not recommended. Reprinted by permission from Baker JL. Management of thoracic trauma by the emergency physician. In: Turney SZ, Rodriguez A, Cowley RA, eds. Management of cardiothoracic trauma. Baltimore: Williams & Wilkins, 1991.

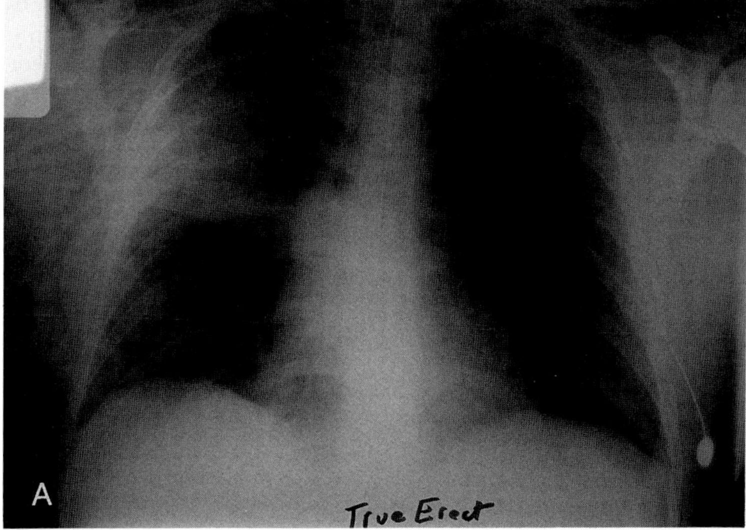

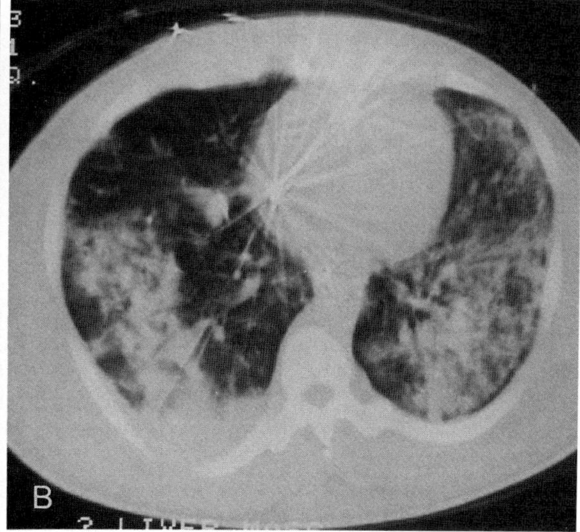

Figure 57.3. A, Chest film from patient with lung contusion. The contusion is seen as a fairly smooth density peripherally in the right upper lobe. **B,** CT of the chest from another patient with bilateral lung contusions. Mottled densities are present throughout both mid lung fields.

more than 300 ml/hr for 3 consecutive hours, then urgent thoracotomy is usually indicated (23).

Pulmonary Injuries

Blunt trauma to the thorax can result in injury to the lung parenchyma. With the increasing use of chest computed tomography (CT) in the evaluation of thoracic trauma, several distinct traumatic lung lesions have been described. Lung lacerations are being recognized more frequently with the use of chest CT (24). The injuries may be a result of shearing energy or a direct tear by a broken rib. These different causes may be clinically significant, because the lacerations secondary to pure blunt force may have more contused tissue present. This may result in more frequent problems with hypoxia and infection. Most lung lacerations can be managed simply with placement of the chest tube. Persistent air leak or bleeding may be an indication for thoracotomy.

Pulmonary hematoma results when the cavity formed by a laceration fills with blood. Radiographically, it can be distinguished from a contusion by the more distinct margins and greater density of a hematoma. Although hematomas take longer to resolve than contusions, they have a more benign clinical course with rarely any effect on pulmonary function evident.

Pulmonary contusion is classically diagnosed as a infiltrate developing within the setting of acute trauma (Fig. 57.3). The detection on plain chest film must be within approximately 6 hr of the injury, otherwise atelectasis or aspiration pneumonia may be the cause of the infiltrate. CT is more sensitive with immediate detection the rule (25). The lesion is of great clinical significance. Because of the architectural disruption of the alveoli and the adjacent microvasculature, the air space becomes filled with cells and fluid, causing shunting and subsequent hypoxia. There also is atelectasis in associated areas of the lung that are not directly injured.

Considerable controversy has surrounded the treatment of patients with pulmonary contusion. Because of the derangement in the permeability of the alveolar membrane, it was thought that fluid restriction along with colloid administration would prevent the severe sequelae of fluid overload (11). However, the current consensus is that euvolemia is the most appropriate goal and that judicious use of crystalloid is not deleterious in these patients. Efforts have been directed toward identifying a subset of patients in whom prompt intubation and mechanical ventilation are important. Several criteria have been established, the clearest of which are the following:

1. Hemodynamic instability.
2. Hypoxemia: the patient is unable to maintain a Pa_{O_2}:FI_{O_2} ratio greater than 350.
3. Hypoventilation: the patient is unable easily to maintain a vital capacity greater than 12 to 14 ml/kg or has sustained hypercarbia.

If nonmechanical ventilatory management is chosen, aggressive pulmonary therapy and adequate analgesia are mandatory.

Aortic Disruption

Blunt traumatic rupture of the thoracic aorta and its major branches is a life-threatening injury seen especially in high-speed motor vehicle accidents and falls. The hypothesized mechanism primarily involves deceleration (horizontal or vertical) or crushing chest injuries with some flexion of the spine. At least three factors appear to be present:

1. A relative fixation of one portion of the aorta compared with another, e.g., the aortic isthmus just distal to the origin of the left subclavian artery. Deceleration of the proximal and distal segments will occur at unequal rates, causing a shearing force.

2. Compressive and bending stress on the aorta over the vertebral column.
3. Intraluminal hypertension at the time of injury, causing a burst stress (26–28).

Autopsy studies have shown that most aortic ruptures occur at the isthmus, followed by the distal descending and the ascending aorta. Very few of the ascending aortic group survive long enough to present to a hospital (Fig. 57.4). The patients who do survive to be evaluated do so because of the containment of the hematoma within the fragile aortic adventitial tissue. As described in the original natural history of this lesion by Parmley et al. (29), if untreated, 25% of these survivors will have delayed rupture within 24 hr of presentation and an additional 5% will rupture each day for 2 weeks after initial presentation.

Diagnosis of aortic disruption often depends on the clinician's high index of suspicion based on mechanism of injury. All patients who have withstood sufficient deceleration or compressive forces to have possibly caused aortic rupture should be assumed to have injury until otherwise proven (Fig. 57.5). An upright chest film may demonstrate some of the many described radiologic signs suggestive of mediastinal hematoma. Among the most reliable are loss of the normal aortic knob contour, widening of the mediastinum greater than 8 cm, and shift of the trachea or nasogastric tube to the right. The diagnosis of aortic rupture is made definitively through aortography. Although there may be more of a role in the future for dynamic chest CT in this setting, at the current time, it is used as an ancillary study when the suspicion of the diagnosis is lower. If mediastinal hematoma is seen, it must be followed by aortogram (30). Prompt surgical repair is usually mandatory.

Myocardial Contusion

Blunt injury to the heart, whether secondary to steering column impact in a motor vehicle accident or a severe blow to the chest during contact sports, is common. The estimated incidence ranges from 10% to 38% in patients with chest trauma (31, 32). One of the great difficulties in clearly defining the incidence is the lack of a precise diagnostic test. Fortunately, most myocardial contusions do not cause severe clinical manifestations and heal without serious sequelae.

The histopathologic lesion is similar to that found with myocardial infarction, except that the contused tissue contains more areas of hemorrhage with more myonecrosis. Also, the boundary between normal and injured tissue is more clearly defined in contusions. The severity of injury can range from epicardial alone to full thickness (33).

The most common physical sign of myocardial contusion is sinus tachycardia, although any type of dysrhythmia is possible. Functional pump disturbance, i.e., cardiac failure, is uncommon except in the most severe cases of contusion. There are no distinctive symptoms of the injury other than nonspecific chest pain, which is not always present and may easily be a result of non-

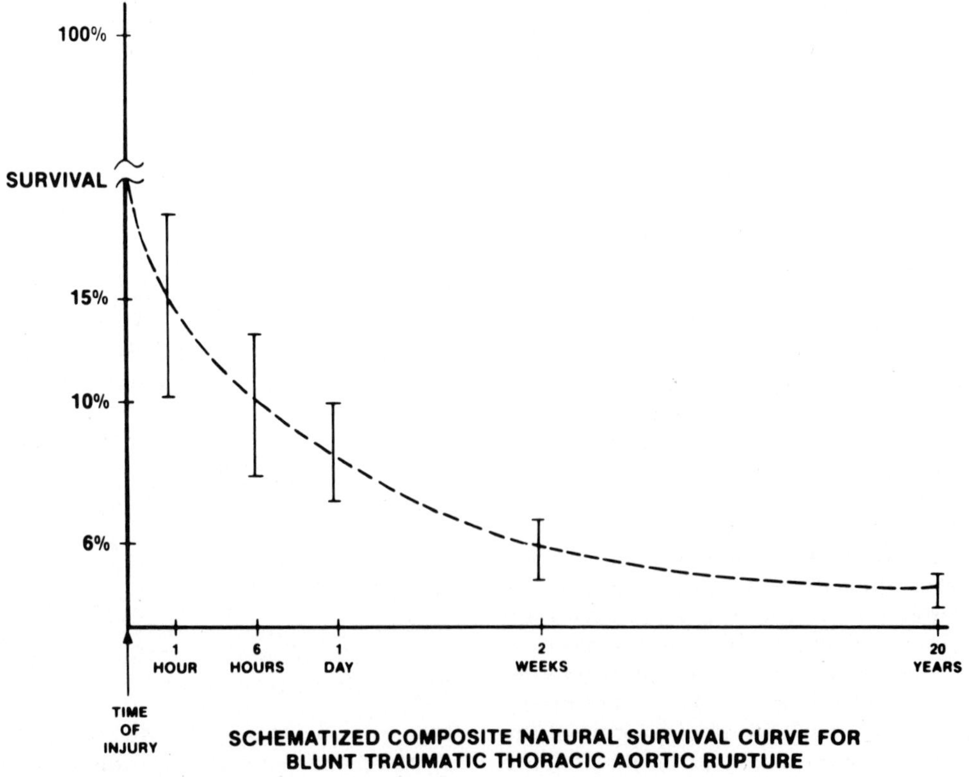

Figure 57.4. Hypothetical composite survival curve of *untreated* blunt traumatic aortic rupture. Reprinted by permission from Turney SZ, Rodriguez A. Injuries to the great thoracic vessels. In: Turney SZ, Rodriguez A, Cowley RA, eds. Management of cardiothoracic trauma. Baltimore: Williams & Wilkins, 1991.

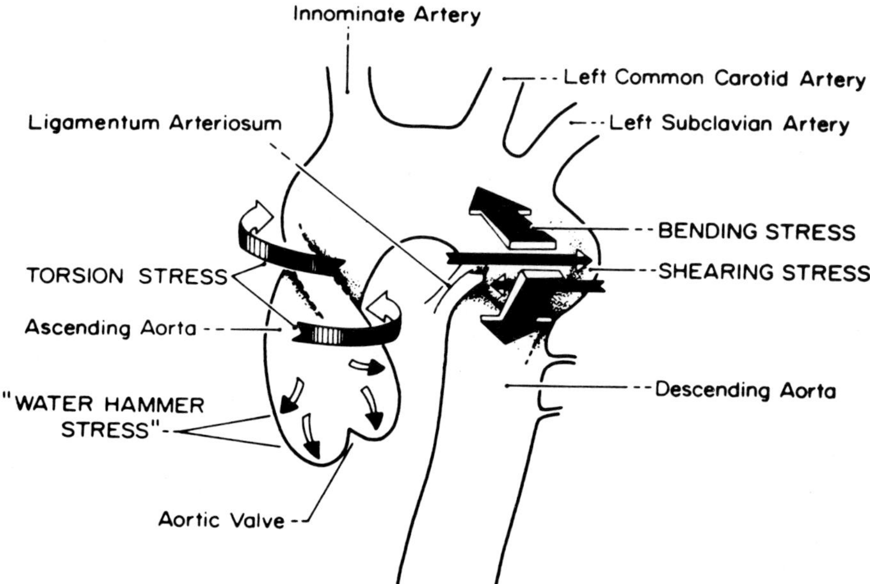

Figure 57.5. Possible forces acting on the aorta that result in blunt traumatic rupture. Reprinted by permission from Symbas PN. Cardiothoracic trauma. Philadelphia: WB Saunders, 1990.

cardiac thoracic injury. All of these factors result in myocardial contusion being a difficult diagnosis to establish on initial presentation of the patient.

A further complication in the evaluation of myocardial contusion is the lack of a clearly accepted diagnostic test. ECG is the easiest but is not sensitive or specific: Contusion may not be accompanied by dysrhythmia, and, conversely, rhythm disturbances may be the result of other causes. However, persistent ECG abnormalities are highly suggestive of contusion and the diagnosis should be pursued (26).

Creatine kinase MB band (CK MB) determinations have long been used to detect ischemically infarcted myocardium, and the application was extended to the diagnosis of contused tissue. There has been considerable controversy in the literature concerning the efficacy of the test, with varying reports of its specificity and sensitivity. However, CK MB serial determinations remain a screening test in patients suspected of having a myocardial contusion.

Once the diagnosis is probable, i.e., the ECG and/or CK MB determinations are positive, more focused evaluations are warranted. Again, the available tests have proven less than ideal. Radionuclide imaging with technetium-99 is less accurate than was previously hoped (34). Radionuclide angiography (MUGA scan) has also been proposed, with varying reported results (35, 36). Perhaps the most useful of the imaging evaluations is currently echocardiography, which can provide some indications of functional disturbance of wall motion and values as well as a measurement of any pericardial fluid present (37).

Because of the tendency toward dysrhythmias in injured cardiac tissue, once the diagnosis of contusion is established, cardiac monitoring should be instituted. No clear recommendations for the length of observation have been described, but it should certainly continue until no acute symptoms are present. Long-term sequelae such as ventricular aneurysms have been described but are rare.

Cardiac Rupture and Pericardial Tamponade

Severe blunt injury to the chest wall can result in disruption of a free cardiac wall or, less commonly, the intraventricular septum or valves. Most patients sustaining such an injury die quickly, particularly with free rupture into the pericardium with tamponade. However, 10%, to as many as 30% with lower pressure atrial ruptures, may survive long enough to be treated (38).

Free wall rupture will result in pericardial tamponade if the pericardium is intact, but massive hemothorax with hypovolemic shock may be the result if there is associated pericardial rupture. Pericardial tamponade, with its accompanying impaired cardiac filling and low output, has classically been diagnosed by the concurrence of shock, distended neck veins, and narrowed pulse pressure. Unfortunately, the classic physical signs may not be easy to appreciate in the setting of acute trauma. If the patient is relatively stable, the measurement of central venous pressure (CVP) may provide supporting evidence: An elevated CVP in the presence of low systemic blood pressure is presumptive evidence of cardiac tamponade. However, if shock is profound, CVP may not be elevated. Echocardiography will usually be conclusive diagnostically (39), but this requires specialized equipment and trained personnel.

The most direct method of diagnosis is an emergency subxyphoid retrosternal pericardiotomy performed in the operating room. Free blood in the pericardial cavity confirms the diagnosis. Preliminary pericardial aspiration of even 20 to 50 ml of blood, using a long subxyphoid needle, may improve hemodynamics temporarily, allowing time to prepare for surgery.

Iatrogenic Injuries Secondary to CPR

Cardiac arrest can occur during sports activity, whether seen in the increasing proportion of older people engaging in sports, in the small but definite subset of athletes who abuse arrhythogenic recreational drugs, or in persons with no known risk factors. With the prevalence of CPR training programs for the general population, closed cardiac massage is being started in the field by bystanders more frequently. Although these efforts are laudable, overzealous attempts at resuscitation (as well as mechanical cardiac resuscitation devices) can result in injury (40). Rib fractures, sternal fractures, aortic rupture, and right ventricular rapture have been reported especially with improper positioning of the hands on the sternum (they should be centrally located in the lower third of the sternum). The sports clinician should be aware of the possibility of these injuries occurring during CPR.

REFERENCES

1. LoCicero J, Mattox K. Epidemiology of chest trauma. Surg Clin North Am 1989;69:15–19.
2. Thompson BM. Rib radiographs for trauma: useful or wasteful? Ann Emerg Med 1986;15:261–265.
3. DeLuca SA, Rhea JT, O'Malley J. Radiographic evaluation of rib fractures. Am J Radiol 1982;138:91–92.
4. Danher J, Eyes BE, Kumar K. Are rib views after blunt trauma an unnecessary routine? Clin Res 1984;289:1271–1272.
5. Richardson JD, McElvein RB, Trinkle JK. First rib fracture: hallmark of severe trauma. Ann Surg 1975;181:251–254.
6. Strum JT, Strate RG, Nowlen A, et al. Blunt trauma of the subclavian artery. Surg Obstet Gynecol 1974;138:915–918.
7. Phillips EH, Rogers WF, Gaspar MR. First rib fractures: incidence of vascular injuries and indications for angiography. Surgery 1981;32:42–46.
8. Ablers JE, Rath RK, Glaser RS, et al. Severity of intrathoracic injuries associated wiht first rib fractures. Ann Thorac Surg 1982;33:614–618.
9. Maloney JV, Schmutzer KJ, Raschke E. Paradoxical respiration and "pendelluft." J Thorac Cardiovasc Surg 1961;41:291–296.
10. Richardson JD, Adams L, Flint LM. Selective management of flail chest and pulmonary contusion. Ann Surg 1992;196:481–487.
11. Trinkle JK, Richardson JD, Franz JL, et al. Management of flail chest without mechanical ventilation. Ann Thorac Surg 1975;19:355–363.
12. Shackford SR, Virgilio RW, Peters RM. Selective use of ventilator therapy in flail chest injury. J Thorac Cardiovasc Surg 1981;81:194–201.
13. Cicala RS, Voeller GR, Fox T, et al. Epidural analgesia in thoracic trauma: effects of lumbar morphine and thoracic bupivicaine on pulmonary function. Crit Care Med 1980;18:229–231.
14. Thompson DA, Flynn TC, Miller PW, et al. The significance of scapular fractures. J Trauma 1985;25:974–977.
15. McGinnis M, Dento J. Fractures of the scapula: a retrospective study of 40 fractured scapulae. J Trauma 1989;29:1488–1493.
16. Sturm JT. Does sternal fracture increase the risk of aortic rupture? Ann Thorac Surg 1989;48:697–698.
17. Wojcik JB. Sternal fractures—the natural history. Ann Emerg Med 1988;17:912–914.
18. Mulder DS, Greenwood FAH, Brooks CE. Post traumatic thoracic outlet syndrome. J Trauma 1973;113:706–715.
19. Rodriguez A. Injuries of the chest wall, the lungs and the pleura. In: Turney SZ, Rodriguez A, Cowley RA, eds. Management of cardiothoracic trauma. Baltimore: Williams & Wilkins, 1990:157–177.
20. Landercasper J, Cogbill T. Long-term followup after traumatic asphyxia. J Trauma 1985;25:838–841.
21. Newguist MJ, Sobel RM. Traumatic asphyxia: an indicator of significant pulmonary injury. Ann Emerg Med 1990;8:212–215.
22. Richardson JD. Indications for thoracotomy in thoracic trauma. Curr Surg 1985;42:361–364.
23. Beall AC, Crawford HW, De Bakey ME, Consideration in the management of acute traumatic hemothorax. J Thorac Cardiovasc Surg 1966;52:351–357.
24. Wagner RB, Crawford WO, Schimpf PP. Classification of parenchymal injuries of the lung. Radiology 1988;167:77–82.
25. Wagner RB, Jamieson PM. Pulmonary contusion: evaluation and classification by computed tomography. Surg Clin North Am 1989;69:31–40.
26. Symbas PN. Cardiothoracic trauma. 2nd ed. Philadelphia: WB Saunders, 1989.
27. Mattox KL. Injury to the thoracic great vessels. In: Moore EE, Mattox KL, Feliciano DV, eds. Trauma. East Norwalk, CT: Appleton & Lang, 1991:393–408.
28. Turney SZ, Rodriguez A. Injuries to the great thoracic vessels. In: Turney SZ, Rodriguez A, Cowley RA, eds. Management of cardiothoracic trauma. Baltimore: Williams & Wilkins. 1990:229–260.
29. Parmley LF, Mattingly TW, Mannion WC, et al. Non penetrating traumatic injury of the aorta circulation. 1957;17:1086–1101.
30. Mirvis SE. Imaging of thoracic trauma In: Turney SZ, Rodriguez A, Cowley RA, eds. Management of cardiothoracic trauma. Baltimore: Williams & Wilkins. 1990:27–93.
31. Jones JW, Hewitt RL, Drapanas T. Cardiac contusion: A capricious syndrome. Ann Surg 1975;181:567–574.
32. Watson JH, Bartholomae WM. Cardiac injury due to non penetrating chest trauma. Ann Int Med 1960;52:871–876.
33. Rodriguez A, Turney SZ. Blunt injuries of the heart and pericardium In: Turney SZ, Rodriguez A, Cowley RA, eds. Management of cardiothoracic trauma. Baltimore: Williams & Wilkins. 1990:261–284.
34. Rodriguez A, Shatney C. The value of technetrium 99 pyrophosphate scanning in the diagnosis of myocardial contusion. Am Surg 1982;48:472–474.
35. Torres-Mirabel P, Greenberg JC, Brown RS, et al. Spectrum of myocardial contusion. Am Surg 1982;48:383–389.
36. Rosenbaum RC, Johnston CC. Post traumatic cardiac dysfunction: assessment with radionuclide ventriculography. Radiology 1986;160:91–94.
37. King RM, Mucha P, Seward JB. Cardiac contusion: a new diagnostic approach utilizing 2 D echocardiography. J Trauma 1983;23:610.
38. Symbas PN. Cardiothoracic trauma. In: Wells SA, ed. Current problems in surgery. Vol. 28. St. Louis: Mosby Yearbook, 1991:770–771.
39. Mazurek B, Jehle D, Martin M. Emergency department echocardiography in the diagnosis and therapy of cardiac tamponade. J Emerg Med 1985;9:27–31.
40. Bodily K, Fischer RP. Aortic rupture and right ventricular rupture induced by closed chest cardiac massage. Minn Med 1979;52:225–227.

INDEX

Page numbers followed by "f" indicate figures; those followed by "t" indicate tables.

T